Trust Carol J. Buck and Elsevier
to take you through the levels of coding success

Step 4: Professional Resources

Step 3: Certify

Step 2: Practice

Step 1: Learn

With the resources you need for every level of coding success, Carol J. Buck and Elsevier are with you every step of your coding career. From beginning to advanced, from the classroom to the workplace, from application to certification, the Step Series products are your guides to greater opportunities and successful career advancement.

Keep climbing with the most trusted name in medical coding.

Author and Educator
Carol J. Buck, MS, CPC, CPC-H, CCS-P

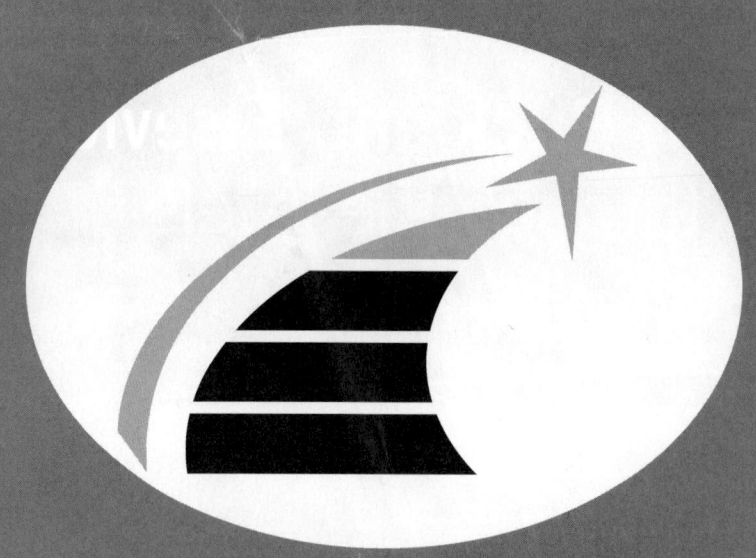

Step 4: Professional Resources

"Nothing is particularly hard if you divide it into small jobs."

— Henry Ford

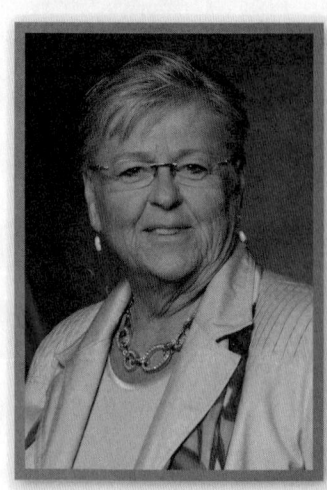

As you reach higher and more specialized levels of coding, I want to applaud you for taking this step in your career. You won't be disappointed. Specialized coders are like rare gems—***they are harder to find and greatly valued*** in the profession.

— Carol J. Buck, MS, CPC, CPC-H, CCS-P

Track your progress!

See the checklist in the back of this book to learn more about your steps toward coding success!

Standard Edition

2014
ICD-9-CM

FOR PHYSICIANS Volumes 1 & 2

INCLUDES NETTER'S ANATOMY ART

Standard Edition

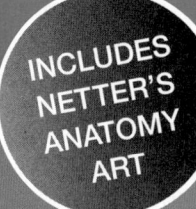
INCLUDES NETTER'S ANATOMY ART

2014
ICD-9-CM

FOR PHYSICIANS Volumes 1 & 2

Carol J. Buck
MS, CPC, CPC-H, CCS-P

Former Program Director
Medical Secretary Programs
Northwest Technical College
East Grand Forks, Minnesota

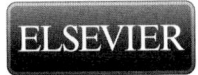

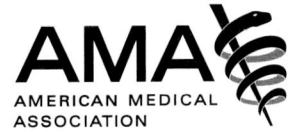
AMERICAN MEDICAL ASSOCIATION

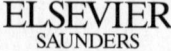

3251 Riverport Lane
St. Louis, Missouri 63043

2014 ICD-9-CM FOR PHYSICIANS, VOLUMES 1 & 2, STANDARD EDITION

ISBN: 978-0-323-18677-3

Copyright © 2014, 2013, 2012, 2011, 2010, 2009, 2008, 2007, 2006, 2005, 2004, 2003, 2002, 2001, 2000 by Saunders, an imprint of Elsevier Inc.

All rights reserved. No part of this publication may be reproduced or transmitted in any form or by any means, electronic or mechanical, including photocopying, recording, or any information storage and retrieval system, without permission in writing from the publisher. Details on how to seek permission, further information about the Publisher's permissions policies and our arrangements with organizations such as the Copyright Clearance Center and the Copyright Licensing Agency, can be found at our website: www.elsevier.com/permissions.

This book and the individual contributions contained in it are protected under copyright by the Publisher (other than as may be noted herein).

Notices

Knowledge and best practice in this field are constantly changing. As new research and experience broaden our understanding, changes in research methods, professional practices, or medical treatment may become necessary.

Practitioners and researchers must always rely on their own experience and knowledge in evaluating and using any information, methods, compounds, or experiments described herein. In using such information or methods they should be mindful of their own safety and the safety of others, including parties for whom they have a professional responsibility.

With respect to any drug or pharmaceutical products identified, readers are advised to check the most current information provided (i) on procedures featured or (ii) by the manufacturer of each product to be administered, to verify the recommended dose or formula, the method and duration of administration, and contraindications. It is the responsibility of practitioners, relying on their own experience and knowledge of their patients, to make diagnoses, to determine dosages and the best treatment for each individual patient, and to take all appropriate safety precautions.

To the fullest extent of the law, neither the Publisher nor the authors, contributors, or editors, assume any liability for any injury and/or damage to persons or property as a matter of products liability, negligence or otherwise, or from any use or operation of any methods, products, instructions, or ideas contained in the material herein.

Library of Congress Cataloging-in-Publication Data

Buck, Carol J., author.
  [ICD-9-CM for physicians volumes 1 & 2 (Standard edition)]
  2014 ICD-9-CM for physicians volumes 1 & 2 / Carol J. Buck. -- Standard edition.
     p. ; cm.
  ICD-9-CM for physicians
  Includes index.
  Preceded by 2013 ICD-9-CM for physicians volumes 1 & 2 / Carol J. Buck.
  Standard edition.
  ISBN 978-0-323-18677-3 (pbk. : alk. paper)
  I. Title. II. Title: ICD-9-CM for physicians.
  [DNLM: 1. International classification of diseases. 9th revision. Clinical modification. 2. International Classification of Diseases. 3. Forms and Records Control--methods. 4. Medical Records--classification. WB 15]
  RB115
  616.001'2--dc23

2013030582

Content Strategy Director: Jeanne R. Olson
Senior Content Development Specialist: Jenna Price
Publishing Services Manager: Pat Joiner
Design Direction: Amy Buxton

Printed in the United States of America

Last digit is the print number: 9 8 7 6 5 4 3 2 1

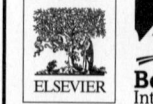 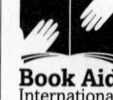

Working together to grow libraries in developing countries

www.elsevier.com • www.bookaid.org

Query Team:

Patricia Cordy Henricksen, MS, CHCA, CPC-I, CPC, CCP-P, ASC-PM
Auditing and Coding Educator
Soterion Medical Services
Lexington, Kentucky

Jacqueline Klitz Grass, MA, CPC
Coding and Reimbursement Specialist
Grand Forks, North Dakota

Kathleen Buchda, CPC, CPMA
Revenue Recognition
New Richmond, Wisconsin

Technical Collaborators:

Nancy Maguire, ACS, CRT, PCS, FCS, HCS-D, APC, AFC
Physician Consultant for Auditing and Education
Winchester, Virginia

Judith Neppel, RN, MS
Executive Director
Minnesota Rural Health Association
University of Minnesota, Crookston
Crookston, Minnesota

Elsevier/MC Strategies Revenue Cycle, Coding and Compliance Staff:

"Experts in providing e-learning on revenue cycle, coding and compliance."

Deborah Neville, RHIA, CCS-P
Director

Lynn-Marie D. Wozniak, MS, RHIT
Content Manager

Sandra L. Macica, MS, RHIA, CCS, ROCC
Product Specialist

Therese M. Jorwic, MPH, RHIA, CCS, CCS-P, FAHIMA
Product Specialist

CONTENTS

GUIDE TO USING THE 2014 ICD-9-CM FOR PHYSICIANS, VOLUMES 1 & 2, STANDARD EDITION x

SYMBOLS AND CONVENTIONS xii

Part I Introduction 1

ICD-9-CM BACKGROUND 1

COORDINATION AND MAINTENANCE COMMITTEE 1

CHARACTERISTICS OF ICD-9-CM 1
  The Disease Classification 2

ICD-9-CM OFFICIAL GUIDELINES FOR CODING AND REPORTING 2

Part II Alphabetic Index Volume 2 53

Section I Index to Diseases and Injuries 54
Section II Table of Drugs and Chemicals 490
Section III Index to External Causes of Injury (E Code) 613

Part III Diseases: Tabular List Volume 1 637

1. Infectious and Parasitic Diseases (001–139) 637
2. Neoplasms (140–239) 662
3. Endocrine, Nutritional and Metabolic Diseases, and Immunity Disorders (240–279) 685
4. Diseases of the Blood and Blood-Forming Organs (280–289) 697
5. Mental, Behavioral and Neurodevelopmental Disorders (290–319) 704
6. Diseases of the Nervous System and Sense Organs (320–389) 717
7. Diseases of the Circulatory System (390–459) 749
8. Diseases of the Respiratory System (460–519) 768
9. Diseases of the Digestive System (520–579) 779
10. Diseases of the Genitourinary System (580–629) 798
11. Complications of Pregnancy, Childbirth, and the Puerperium (630–679) 814
12. Diseases of the Skin and Subcutaneous Tissue (680–709) 828
13. Diseases of the Musculoskeletal System and Connective Tissue (710–739) 837
14. Congenital Anomalies (740–759) 850
15. Certain Conditions Originating in the Perinatal Period (760–779) 864
16. Symptoms, Signs, and Ill-Defined Conditions (780–799) 872
17. Injury and Poisoning (800–999) 885

Supplementary Classification of Factors Influencing Health Status and Contact with Health Services (V01–V91) 928

Supplementary Classification of External Causes of Injury and Poisoning (E000–E999) 956

Appendix A—Morphology of Neoplasms 995

Appendix B—Glossary of Mental Disorders (Deleted as of October 1, 2004) 1001

Appendix C—Classification of Drugs by American Hospital Formulary Services List Number and Their ICD-9-CM Equivalents 1002

Appendix D—Classification of Industrial Accidents According to Agency 1004

Appendix E—List of Three-Digit Categories 1006

Table A—Table of Bacterial Food Poisoning 1017

GUIDE TO USING THE 2014 ICD-9-CM FOR PHYSICIANS, VOLUMES 1 & 2, STANDARD EDITION

Medical coding has long been a part of the health care profession. Through the years medical coding systems have become more complex and extensive. Today, medical coding is an intricate and immense process that is present in every health care setting. The increased use of electronic submissions for health care services only increases the need for coders who understand the coding process.

2014 ICD-9-CM for Physicians, Volumes 1 & 2, Standard Edition was developed to help meet the needs of coding professionals at all levels by offering a comprehensive coding text at a reasonable price. This text combines the official coding guidelines and Volumes 1 and 2 of the ICD-9-CM in one book.

All material strictly adheres to the latest government versions available at the time of printing.

Updates from the FY2014 *Definitions of Medicare Code Edits* (MCE) will be posted to the companion website (www.codingupdates.com) when available.

ILLUSTRATIONS AND ITEMS

The ICD-9-CM, Volume 1, Tabular List contains illustrations, pictures, and items to assist you in understanding difficult terminology, diseases/conditions, or coding in a specific category. Items are always printed in ▌▌▌▌▌ ink so the added material is not mistaken for official notations or instructions. ▌▌▌▌▌ ink is used for other annotations in the text. Your ideas on what other descriptions or illustrations should be in future editions of this text are always appreciated.

Annotated

Throughout the volumes, revisions, additions, and deleted codes or words are indicated by the following symbols:

- ⬅ **Revised:** Revisions within the line or code from the previous edition are indicated by the arrow.

- ◀ **New:** Additions to the previous edition are indicated by the triangle.

- deleted **Deleted:** Deletions from the previous edition are struck through.

- ▌▌ **Omit code:** No code is to be assigned. The words "omit code" are highlighted in ▌▌ for easier reference.

ICD-9-CM, Volume 1, Tabular List Symbols

- ● **Use Additional Digit(s):** The colored dot cautions that the code requires additional digit(s) to ensure the greatest specificity.

- ▪ **Unspecified:** These have a square before the code because the code description states "classified elsewhere" or there is a "Code first" note that directs the assignment of another code before the code at this location is assigned.

- ● **Not first-listed DX:** The black dot before a code indicates that the code should not be reported as the first-listed (primary) diagnosis.

- OGCR **OGCR:** The *ICD-9-CM Official Guidelines for Coding and Reporting* symbol indicates the placement of a portion of a guideline as that guideline pertains to the code by which it is located. The complete OGCR are located in Part I.

- **Coding Clinic** identifies the year, quarter, and page number that presents information about an ICD-9-CM code in the American Hospital Association's *Coding Clinic for ICD-9-CM*.

- ▭ **Excludes:** Terms following the word "Excludes" are to be coded elsewhere and are highlighted in ▭ for easier reference.

Includes: This note appears immediately to further define or give examples of the content of codes and is highlighted in ▓▓▓▓ for easier reference.

Use additional: The words indicate an instructional note that another code may be needed and are highlighted in ▓▓▓▓ for easier reference.

Code first: The words indicate an instructional note that directs the coder to sequence the underlying condition before the manifestation. "Code first" is highlighted in ▓▓▓▓ for easier reference.

Omit code: No code is to be assigned. The words "omit code" are highlighted in ▓▓▓▓ for easier reference.

SYMBOLS AND CONVENTIONS

ICD-9-CM, Volumes 1 & 2
Symbols Used to Identify New, Revised, or Deleted Material

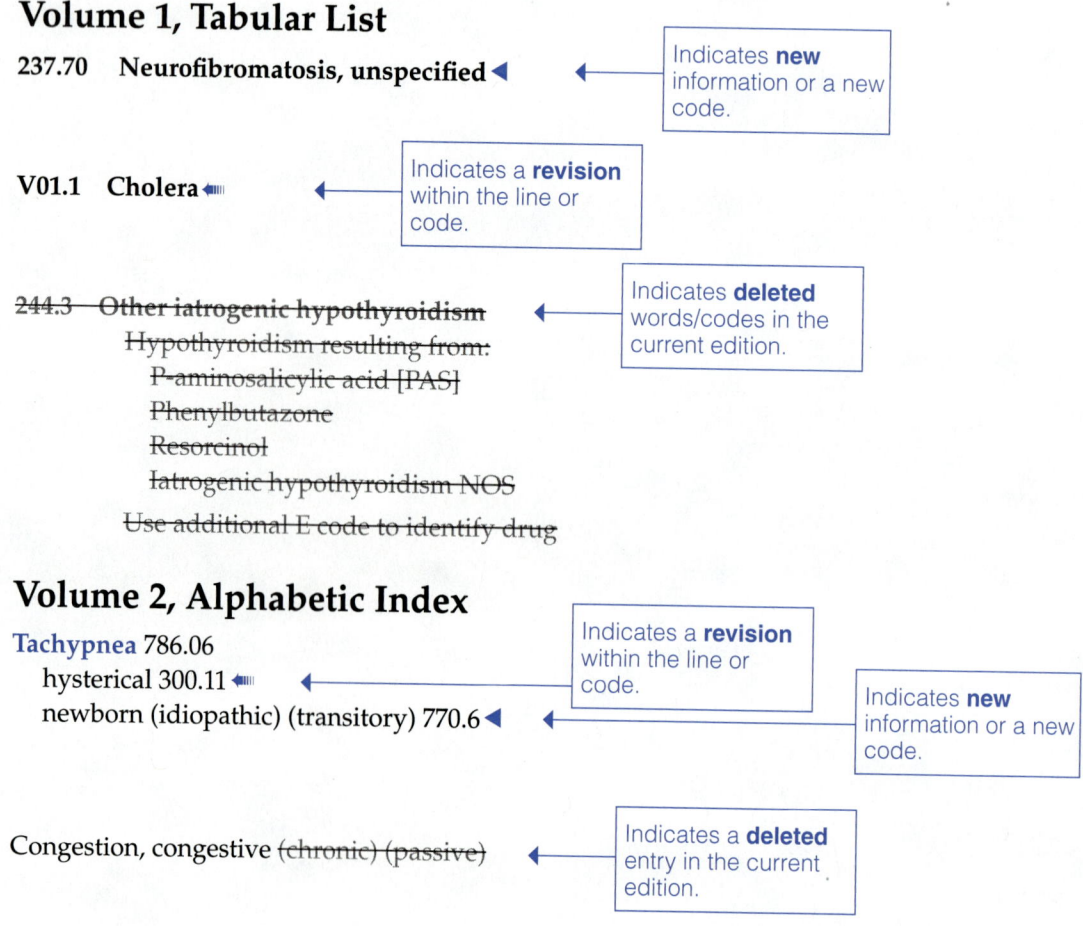

Codes or index entries are for purposes of illustration only and may not be current.

Symbols for Volume 1, Tabular List

Use Additional Digit(s): The colored dot cautions you that the code requires additional digit(s) to ensure the greatest specificity.

● 237.7 **Neurofibromatosis**
　　　　　von Recklinghausen's disease

■ 237.70 **Neurofibromatosis, unspecified**

Unspecified: These have a square before the code because the code description states "classified elsewhere" or there is a "Code first" note that directs the assignment of another code before the code at this location is assigned.

　007.4 **Cryptosporidiosis**
　　　　　Coding Clinic: 1997, Q4, P30-31

Indicates a Volume 1 reference in the American Hospital Association *Coding Clinic for ICD-9-CM*.

Codes with a black dot are not to be listed as the primary diagnosis.

● 284.2 *Myelophthisis*

Codes or index entries are for purposes of illustration only and may not be current.

Conventions for Volume 1, Tabular List
2. NEOPLASMS (140–239)

Notes define terms or give coding instructions.

→ **Notes**
1. Content
   This chapter contains the following broad groups:
   140–195   Malignant neoplasms, stated or presumed to be primary, of specified sites, except of lymphatic and hematopoietic tissue

510   Empyema
  Use additional code to identify infectious organism (041.0–041.9)

"Use additional" directs you to assign an additional code to give a more complete picture of the diagnosis.

Code first: The words indicate an instructional note that directs the coder to sequence the underlying condition (etiology) before the manifestation.

366.4   Cataract associated with other disorders
  366.41   Diabetic cataract
    Code first diabetes (249.5, 250.5)

A code with this note may be first listed (primary) if no causal condition is applicable or known.

428   Heart failure
  Code, if applicable, heart failure due to hypertension first (402.0–402.9, with fifth-digit 1 or 404.0–404.9 with fifth-digit 1 or 3)

Terms following the word "Excludes" are to be coded elsewhere. The term "Excludes" means "Do Not Code Here."

150.2   Abdominal esophagus
  Excludes   adenocarcinoma (151.0)
         cardio-esophageal junction (151.0)

The "Includes" note appears to further define, or give example of, the contents of the code.

087   Relapsing fever
  Includes   recurrent fever

Codes or index entries are for purposes of illustration only and may not be current.

474 Chronic disease of tonsils and adenoids

> "and" indicates a code that can be assigned if either of the conditions is present or if both of the conditions are present.

366.4 Cataract associated with other disorders

> "with" indicates a code that can be used only if both conditions are present.

> Identifies manifestations that are not sequenced as the first diagnosis.

● **420.0** *Acute pericarditis in disease classified elsewhere*

244.8 Other specified acquired hypothyroidism
Secondary hypothyroidism NEC

> "NEC" means Not Elsewhere Classifiable and is to be used only when the information at hand specifies a condition but there is no more specific code for that condition.

> **Bold** type is used for all codes and titles.

159.0 Intestinal tract, part unspecified
Intestine NOS

> "NOS" means Not Otherwise Specified and is the equivalent of "unspecified."

426.89 Other
Dissociation:
    atrioventricular [AV]

> Brackets are used to enclose synonyms, alternative wording, or explanatory phrases.

158.8 Specified parts of peritoneum
Cul-de-sac (of Douglas)
Mesentery

> Parentheses are used to enclose supplementary words that may be present or absent in the statement of a disease without affecting the code.

628.4 Of cervical or vaginal origin
Infertility associated with:
    anomaly of cervical mucus
    congenital structural anomaly

> A colon is used after an incomplete term that needs one or more of the modifiers that follow in order to make it assignable to a given category.

Codes or index entries are for purposes of illustration only and may not be current.

Conventions for Volume 2, Alphabetic Index

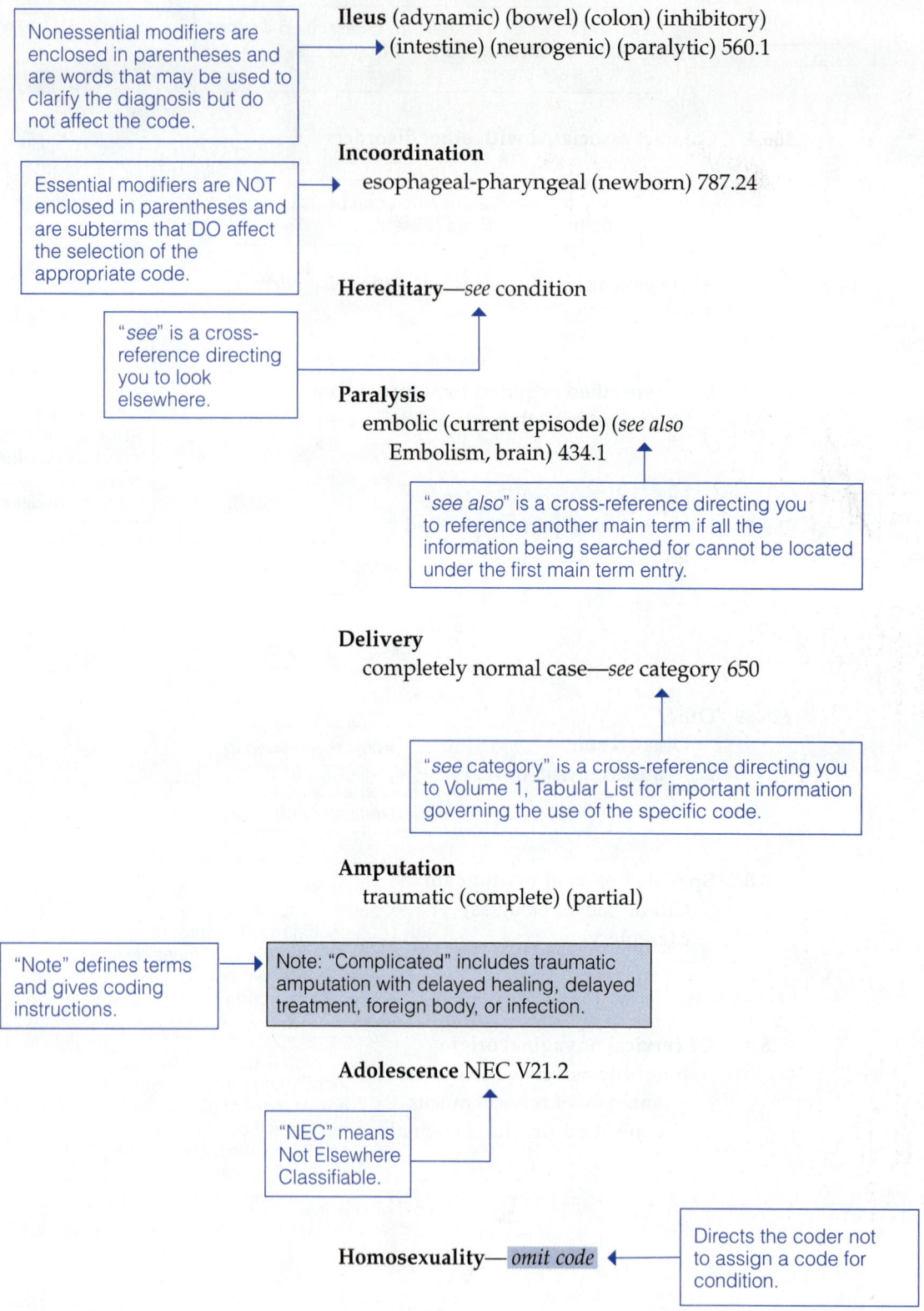

Codes or index entries are for purposes of illustration only and may not be current.

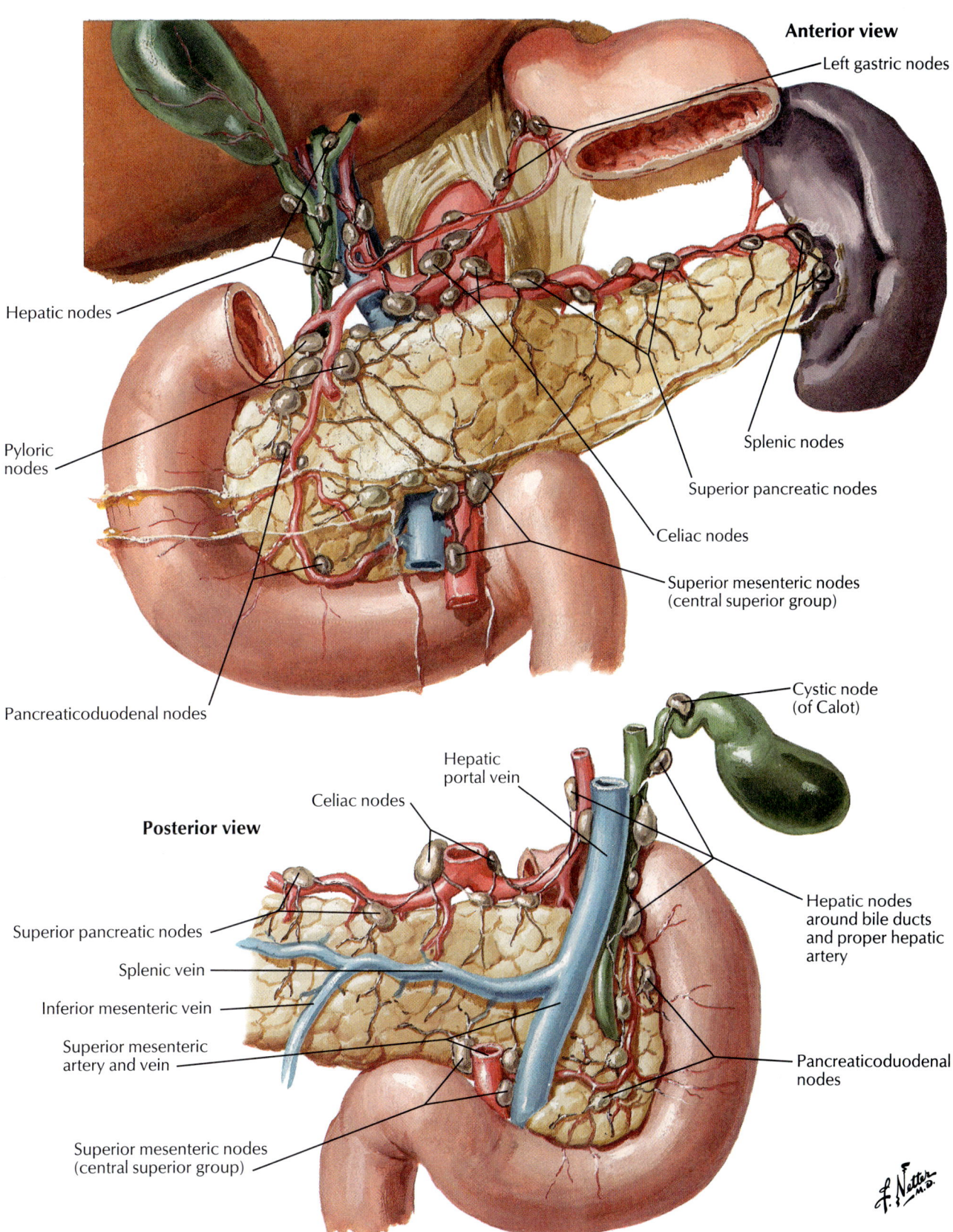

Plate 315 Lymph Vessels and Nodes of Pancreas. (Netter: Atlas of Human Anatomy, 4 ed, 2006, Saunders.)

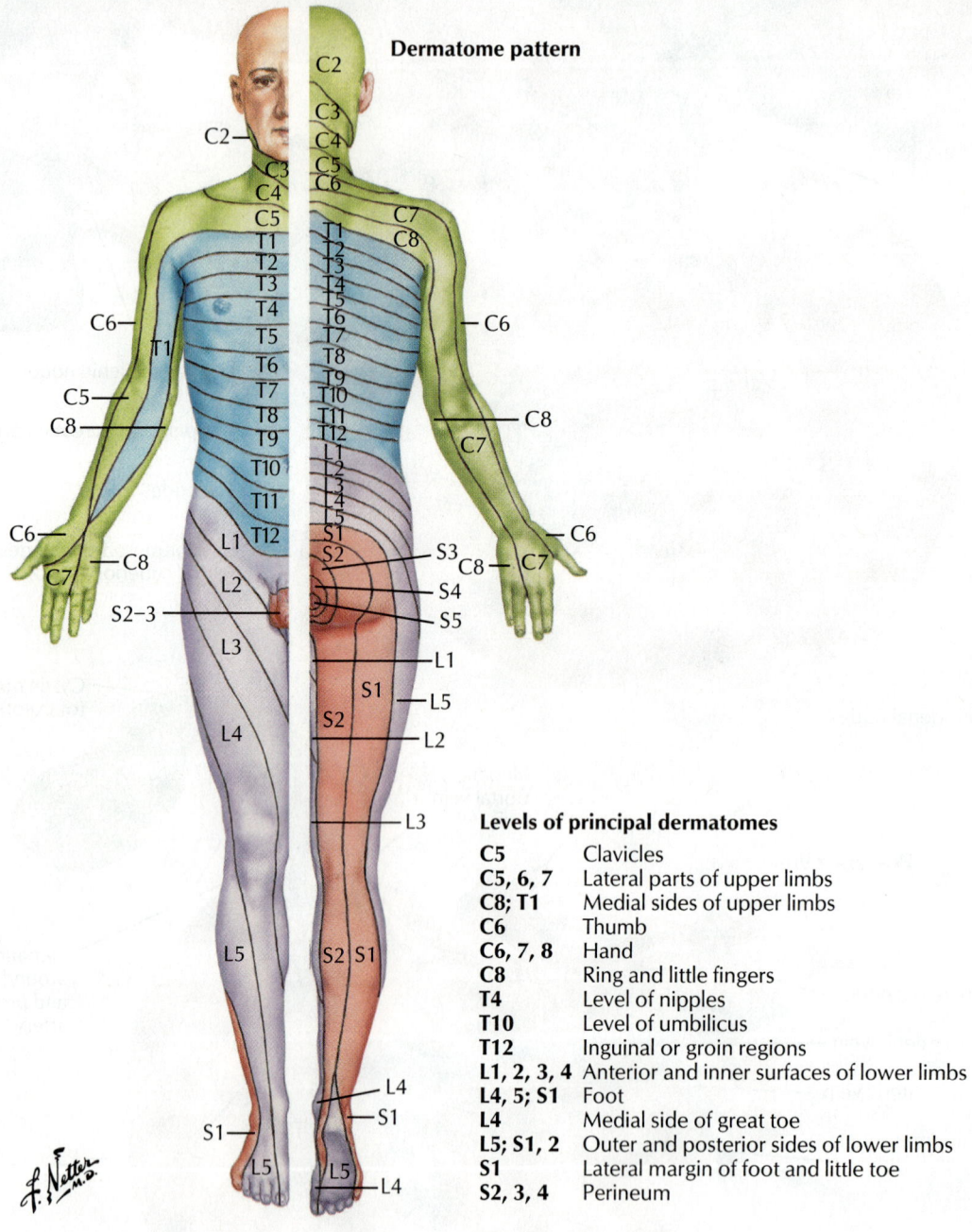

Plate 164 Dermatomes. (Netter: Atlas of Human Anatomy, 4 ed, 2006, Saunders.)

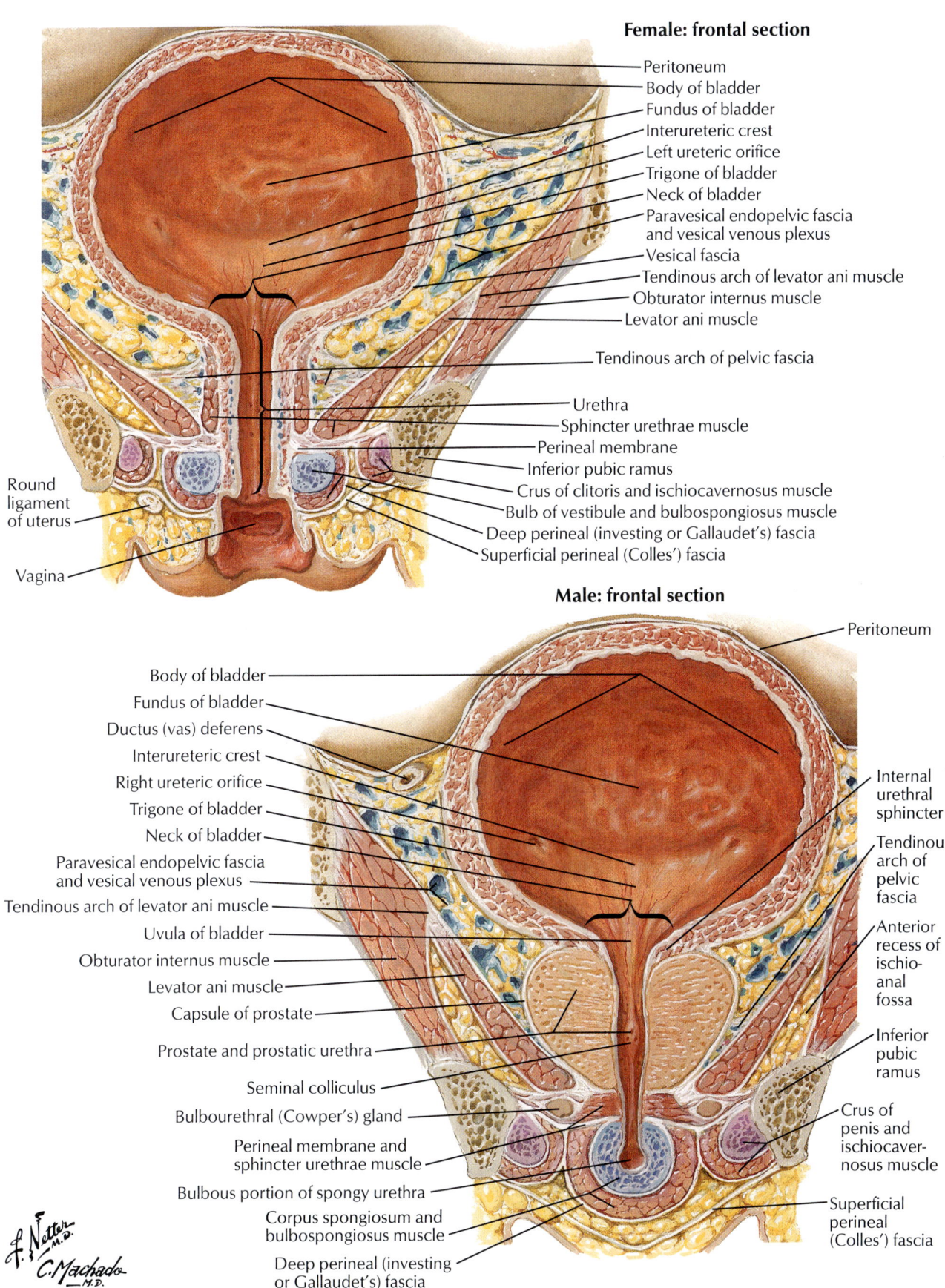

Plate 366 Urinary Bladder: Female and Male. (Netter: Atlas of Human Anatomy, 4 ed, 2006, Saunders.)

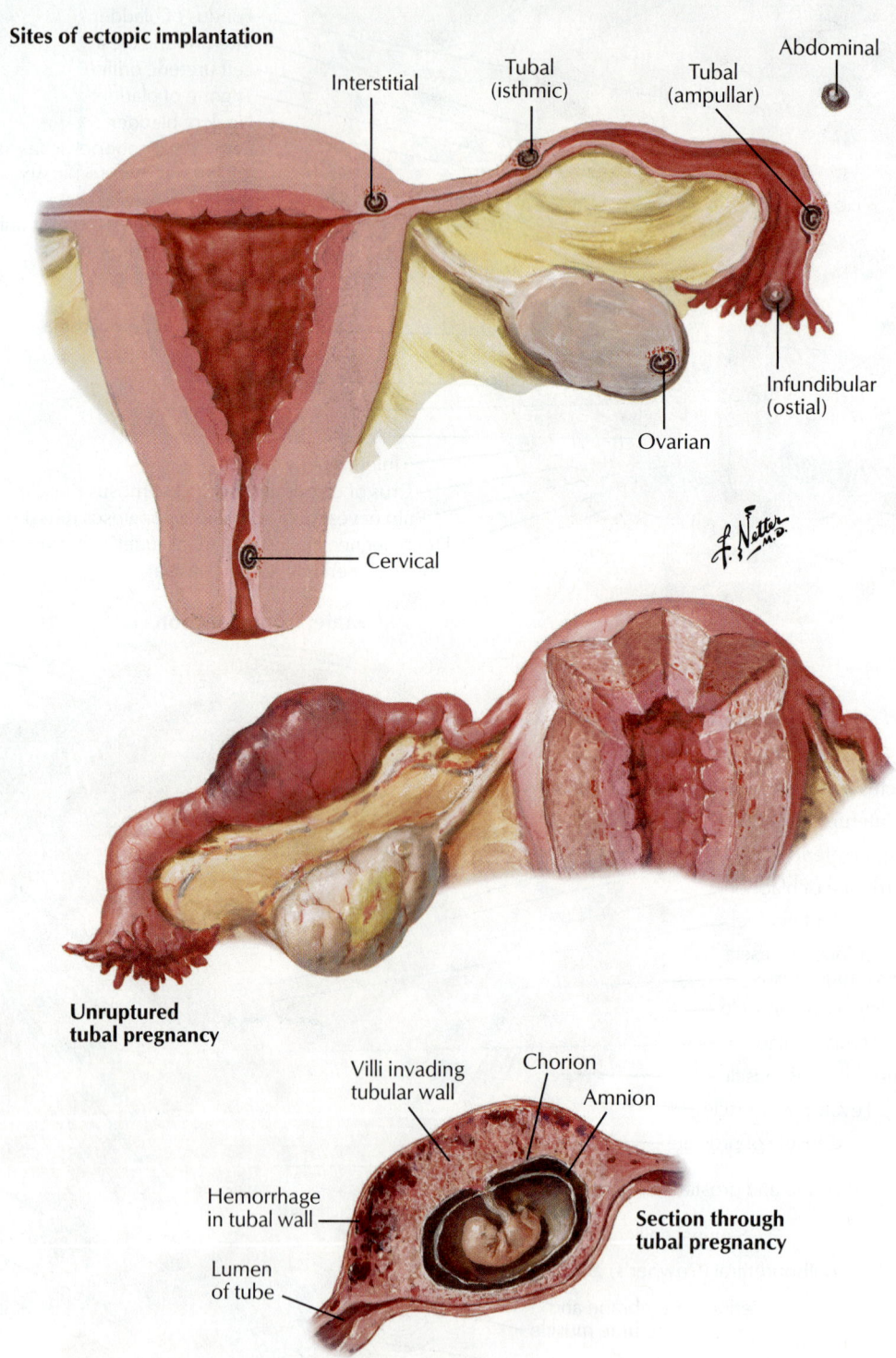

Plate 375　Ectopic Pregnancy. (Netter: Atlas of Human Anatomy, 4 ed, 2006, Saunders.)

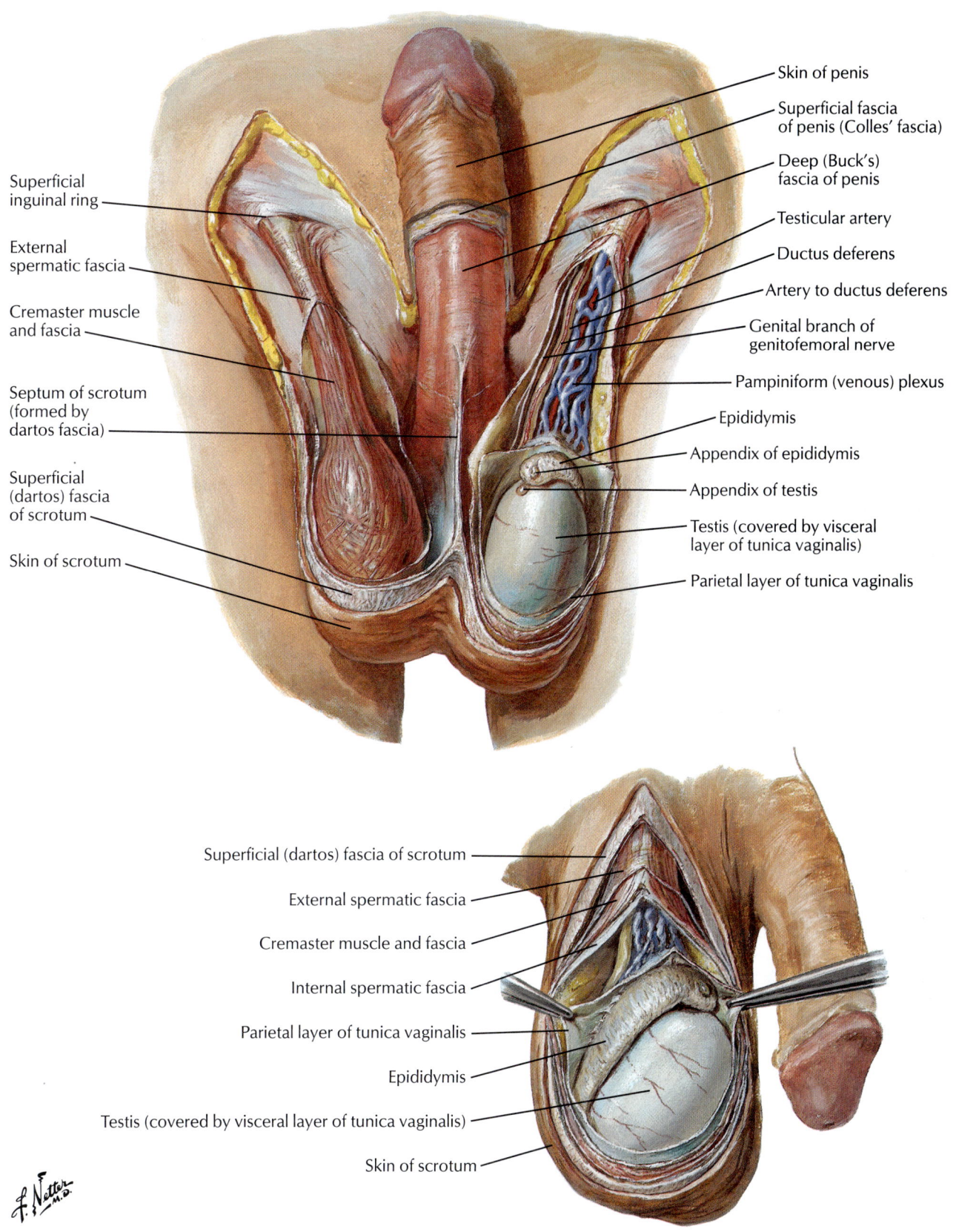

Plate 387 Scrotum and Contents. (Netter: Atlas of Human Anatomy, 4 ed, 2006, Saunders.)

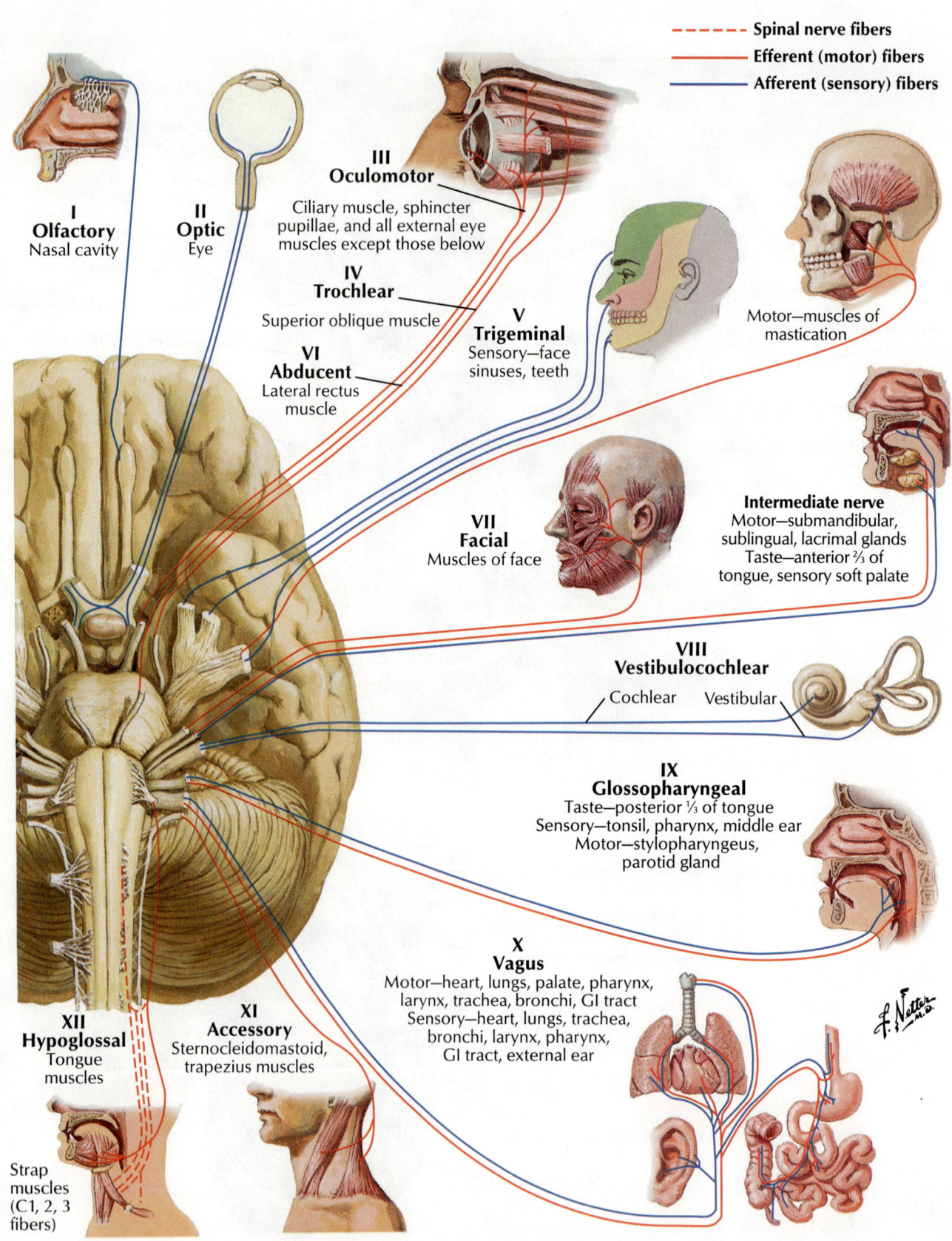

Plate 118 Cranial Nerves (Motor and Sensory Distribution): Schema. (Netter: Atlas of Human Anatomy, 4 ed, 2006, Saunders.)

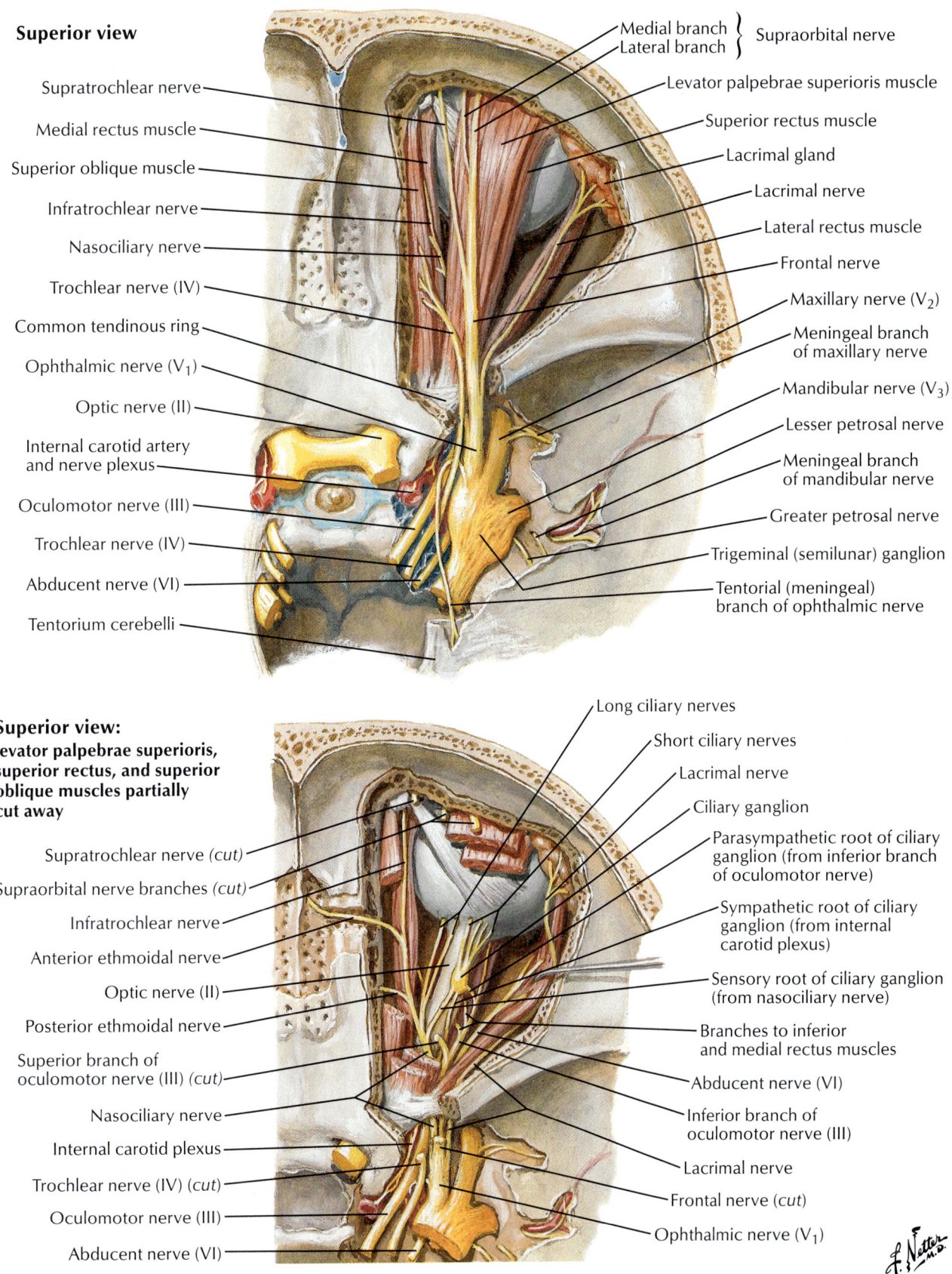

Plate 86 Nerves of Orbit. (Netter: Atlas of Human Anatomy, 4 ed, 2006, Saunders.)

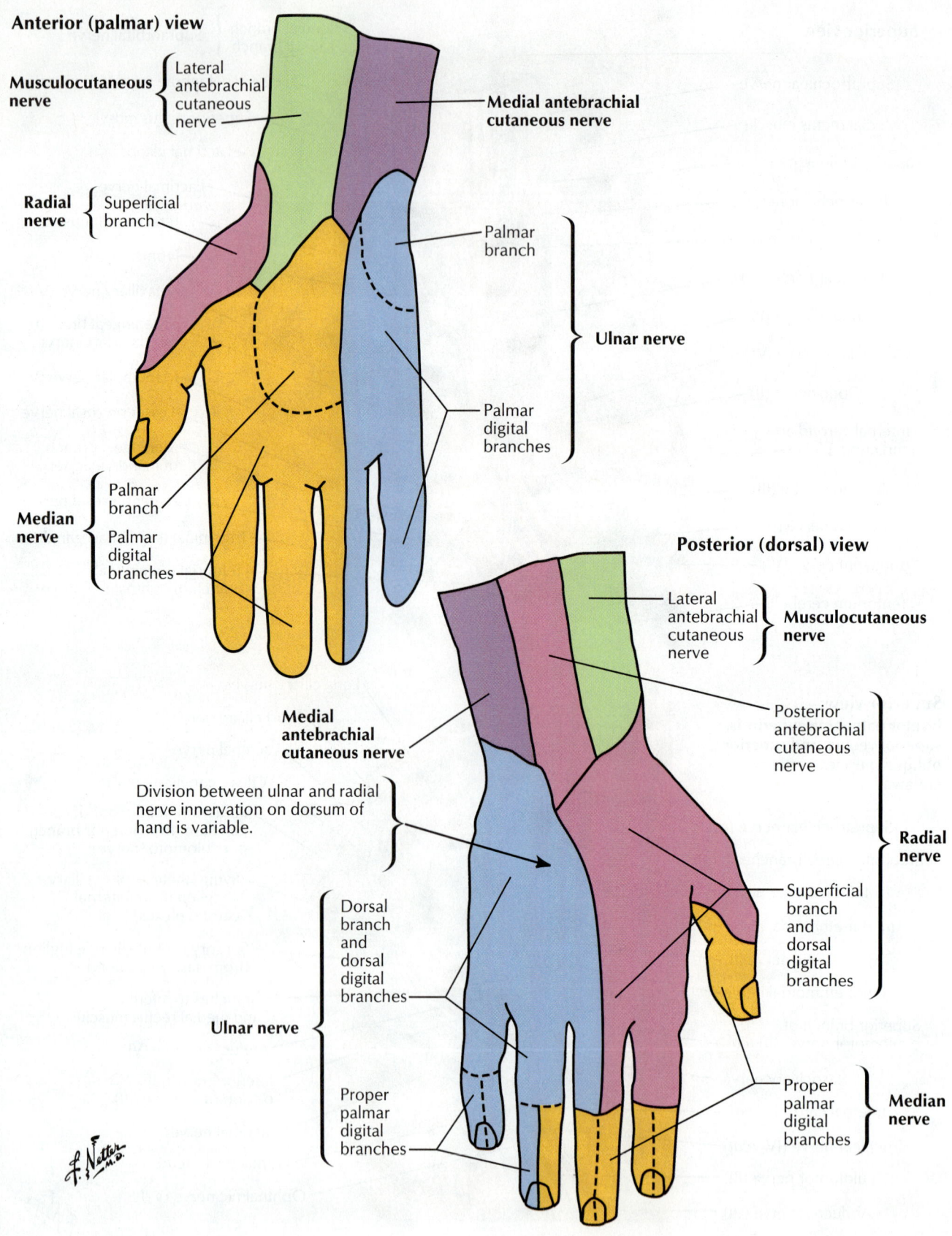

Plate 472 Cutaneous Innervation of Wrist and Hand. (Netter: Atlas of Human Anatomy, 4 ed, 2006, Saunders.)

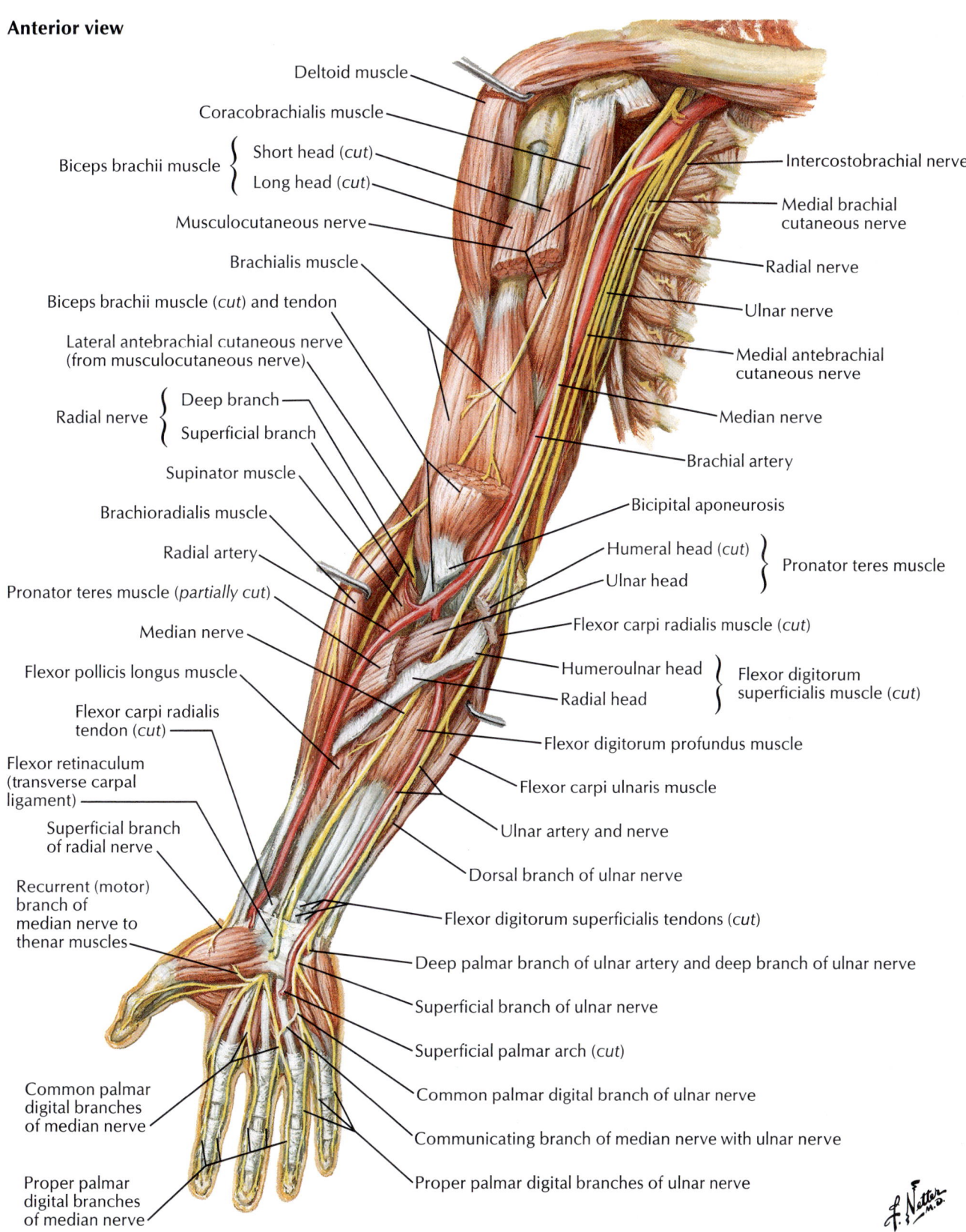

Plate 473 Arteries and Nerves of Upper Limb. (Netter: Atlas of Human Anatomy, 4 ed, 2006, Saunders.)

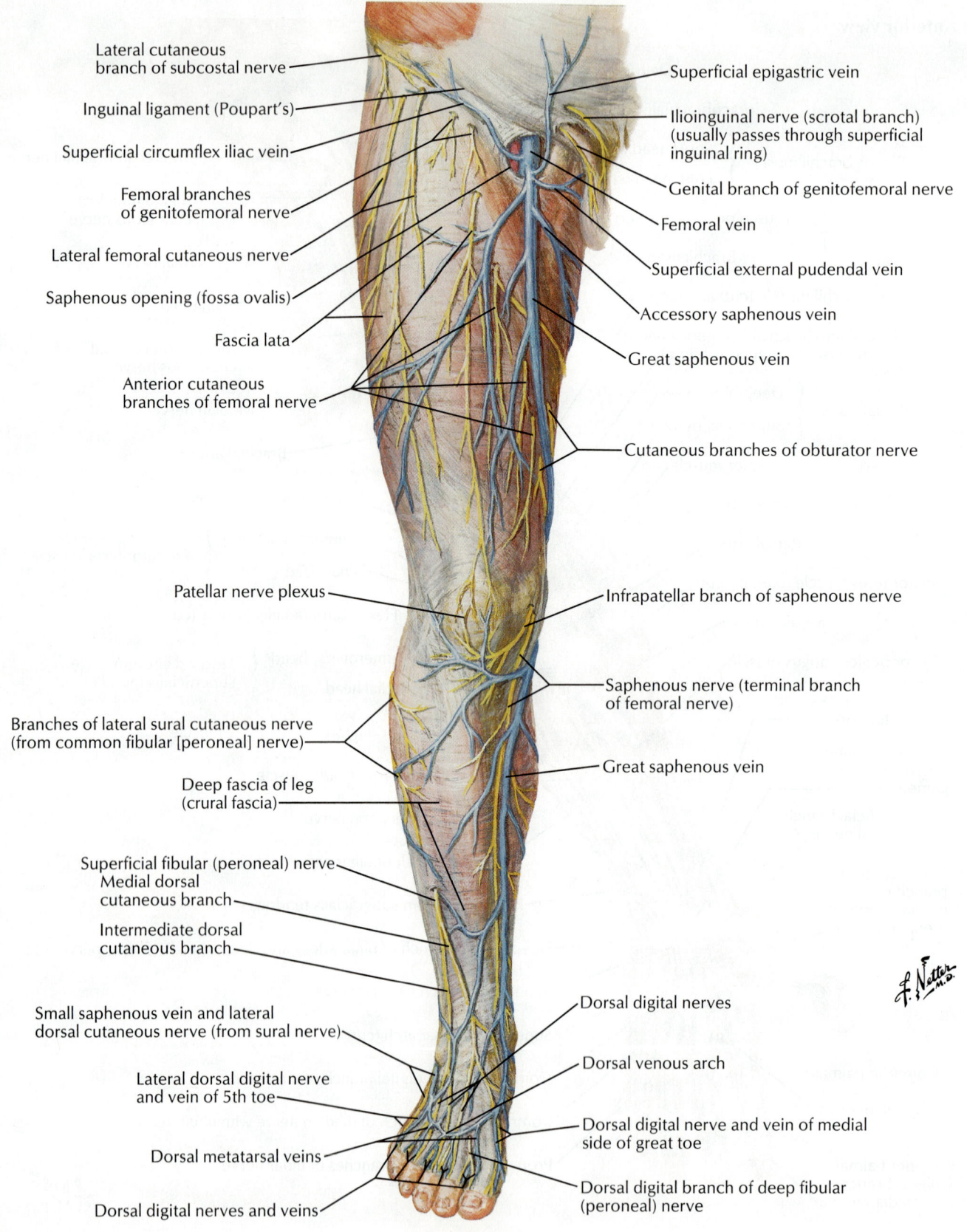

Plate 544 Superficial Nerves and Veins of Lower Limb: Anterior View. (Netter: Atlas of Human Anatomy, 4 ed, 2006, Saunders.)

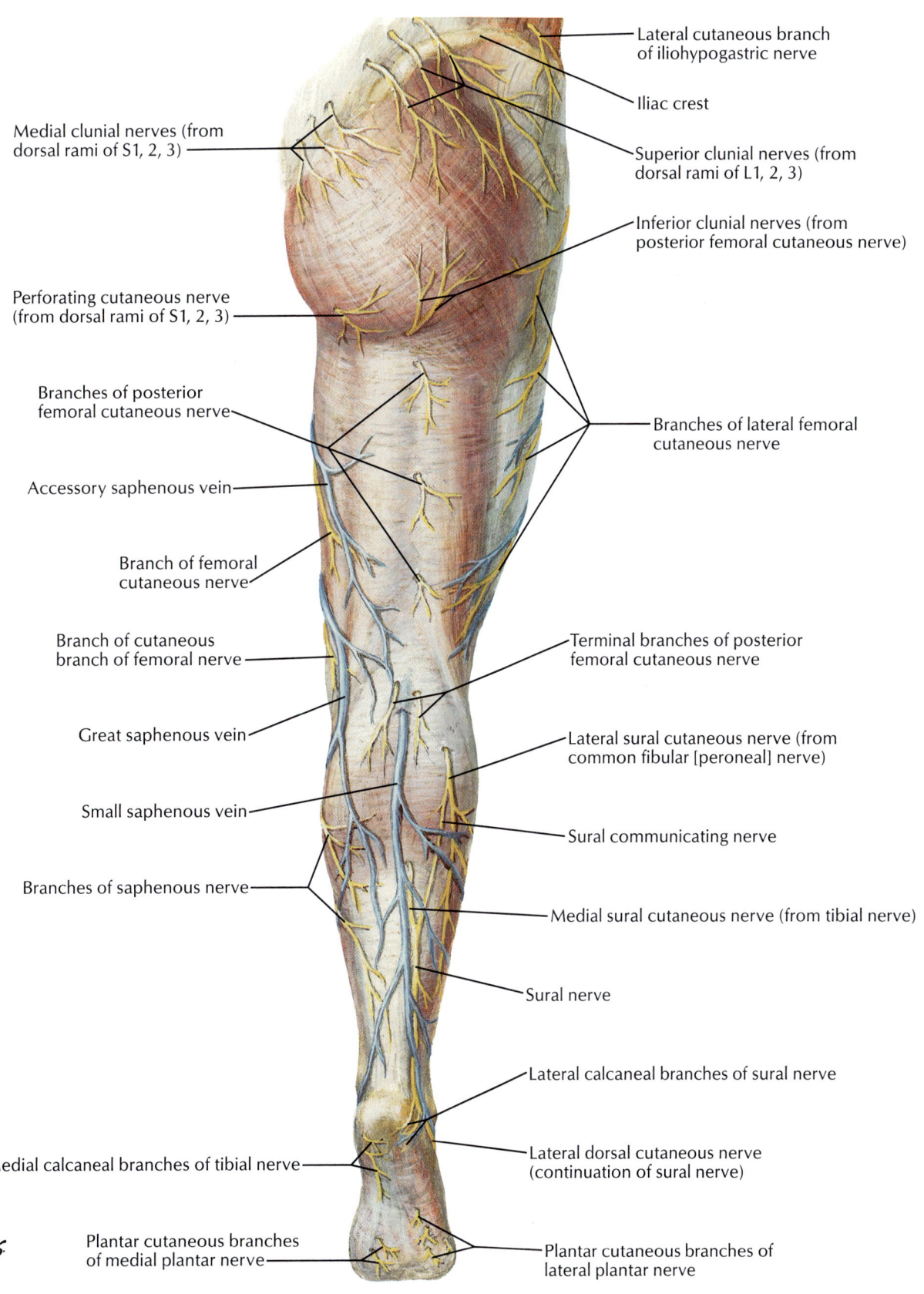

Plate 545 Superficial Nerves and Veins of Lower Limb: Posterior View. (Netter: Atlas of Human Anatomy, 4 ed, 2006, Saunders.)

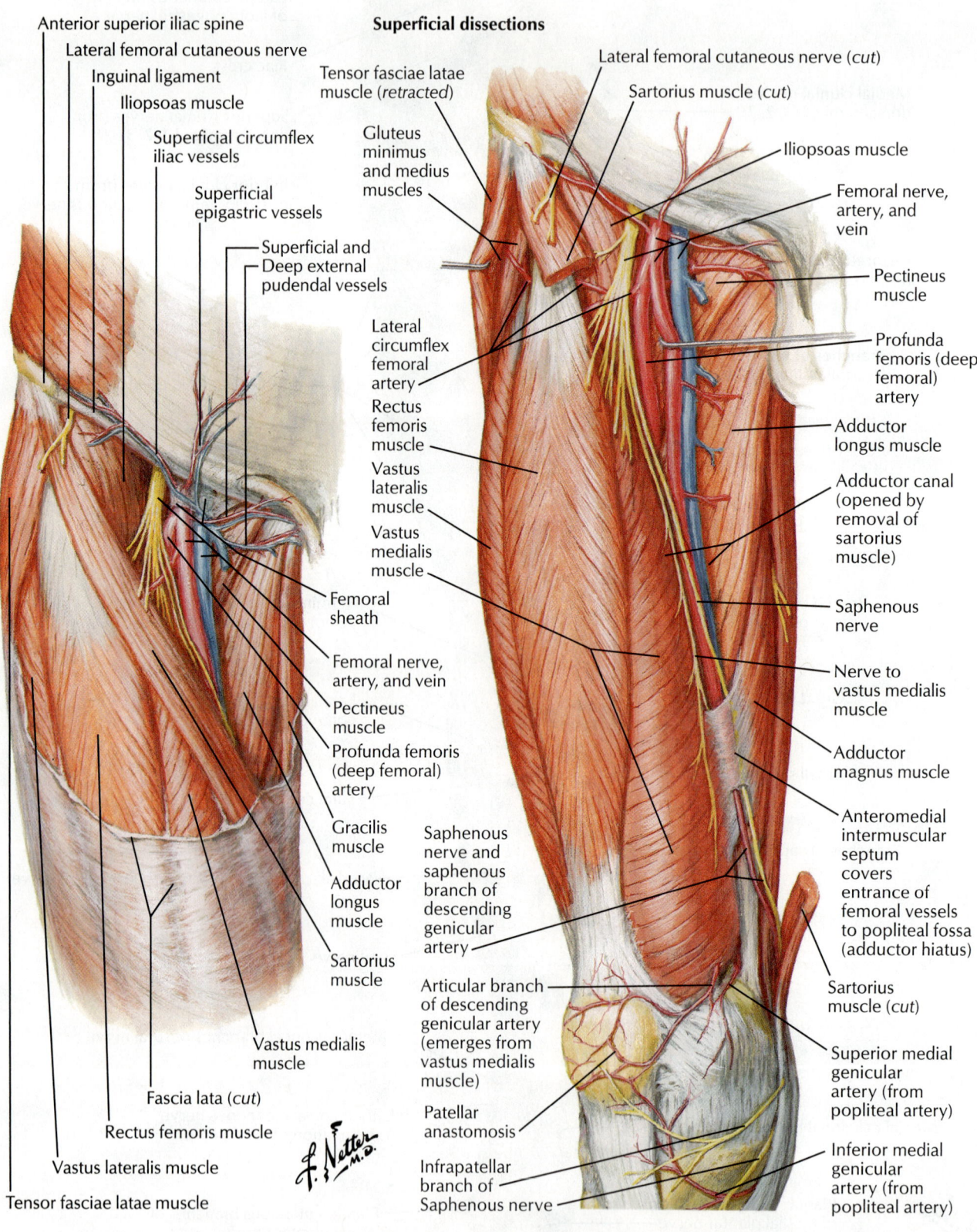

Plate 500 Arteries and Nerves of Thigh: Anterior View. (Netter: Atlas of Human Anatomy, 4 ed, 2006, Saunders.)

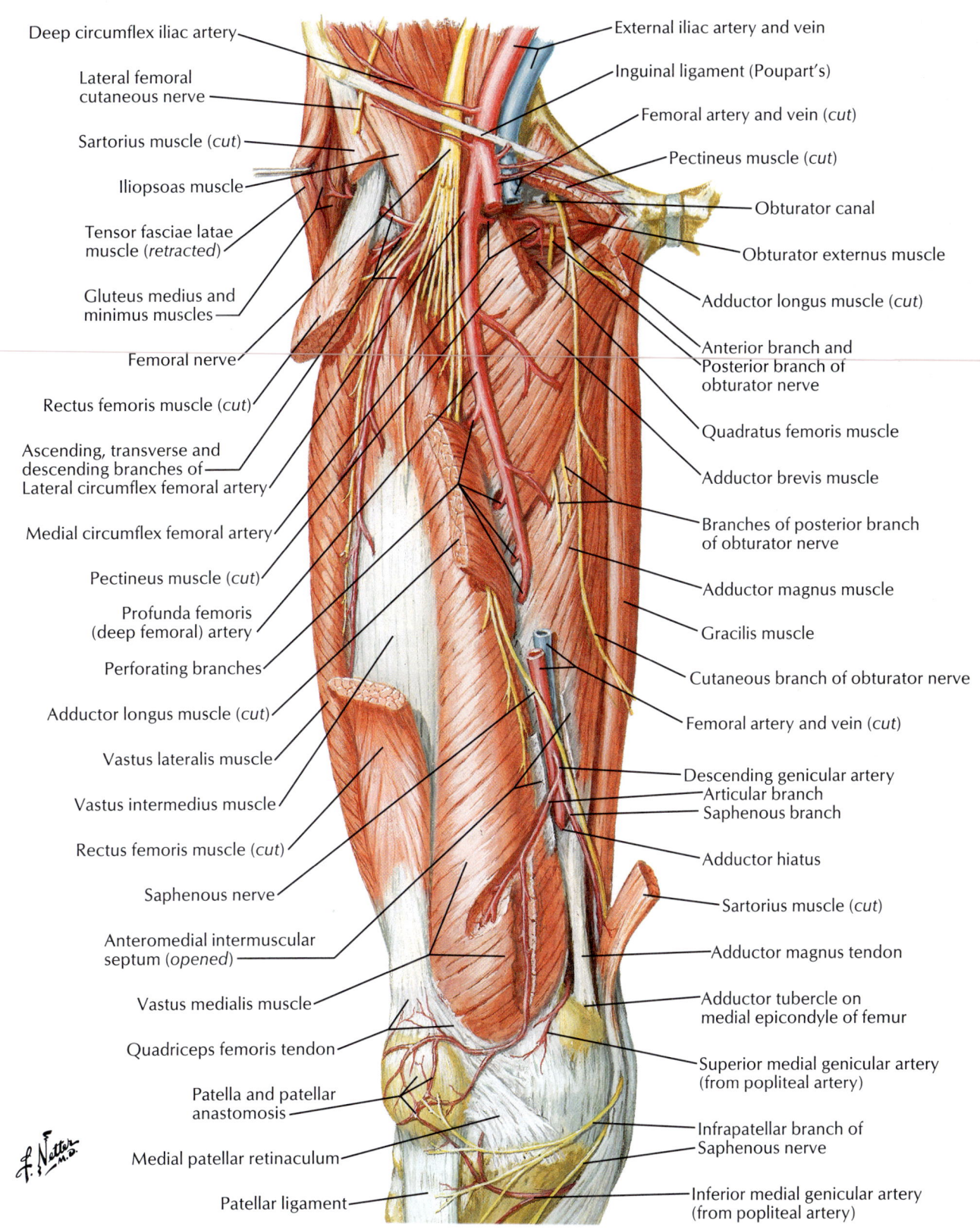

Plate 501 Arteries and Nerves of Thigh: Anterior View. (Netter: Atlas of Human Anatomy, 4 ed, 2006, Saunders.)

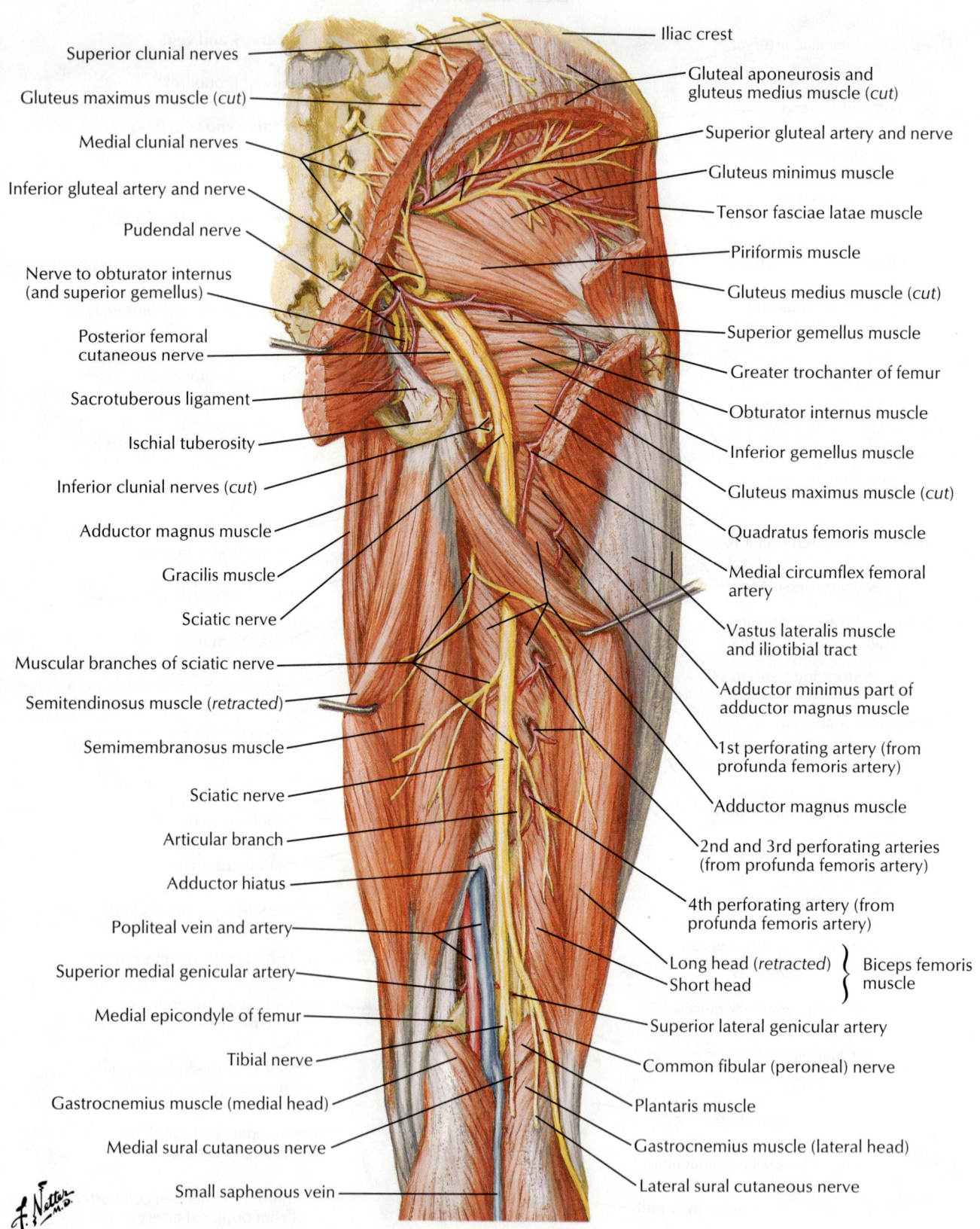

Plate 502 Arteries and Nerves of Thigh: Posterior View. (Netter: Atlas of Human Anatomy, 4 ed, 2006, Saunders.)

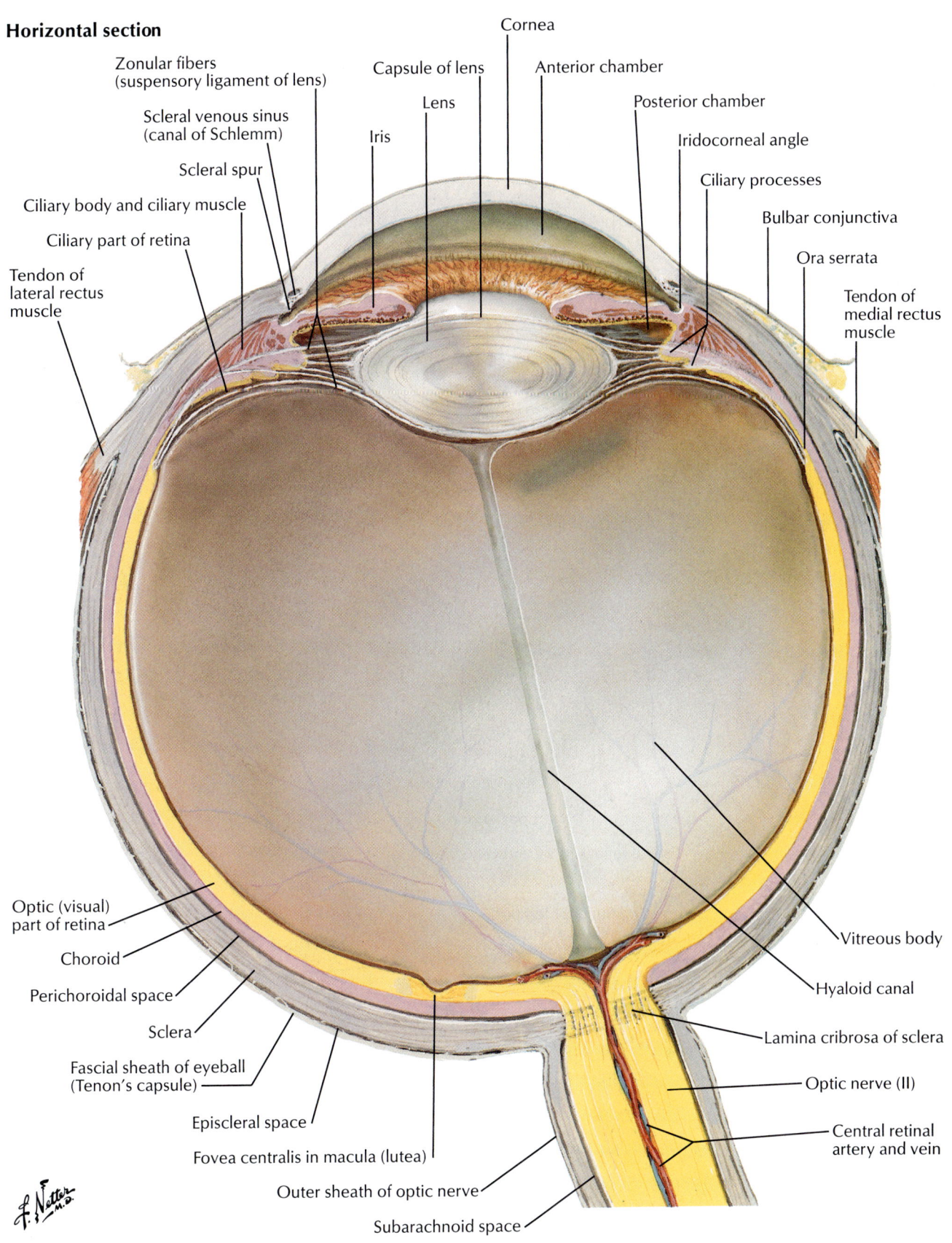

Plate 87 Eyeball. (Netter: Atlas of Human Anatomy, 4 ed, 2006, Saunders.)

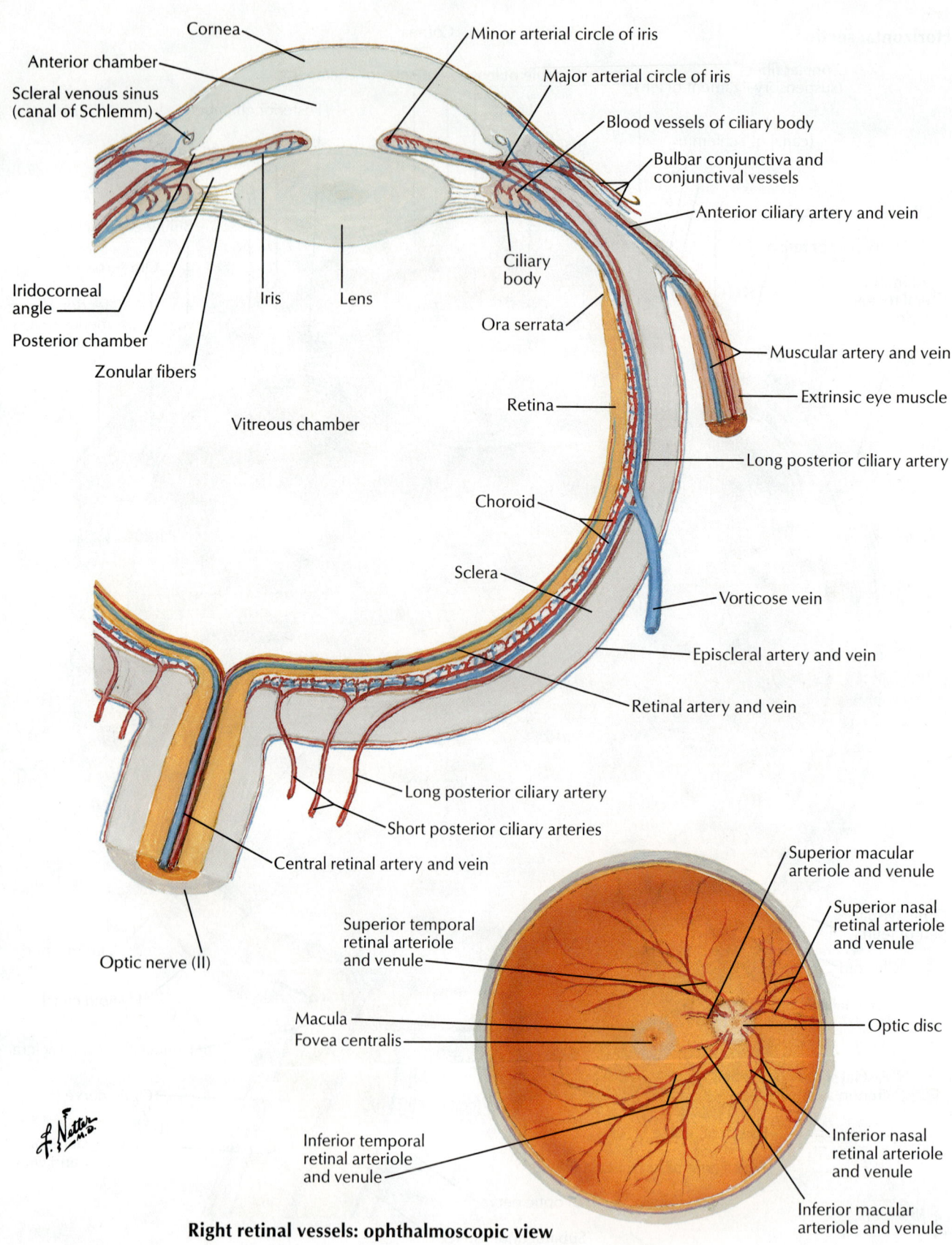

Plate 90 Intrinsic Arteries and Veins of Eye. (Netter: Atlas of Human Anatomy, 4 ed, 2006, Saunders.)

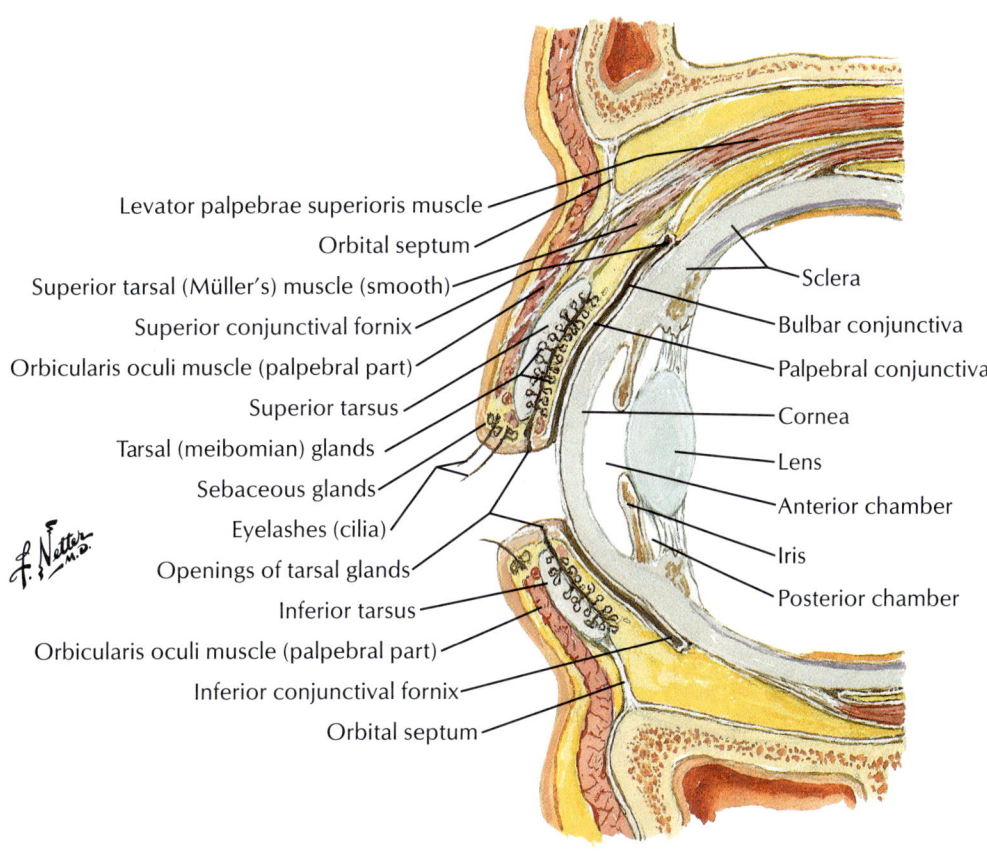

Plate 81, Middle Eyelid. (Netter: Atlas of Human Anatomy, 4 ed, 2006, Saunders.)

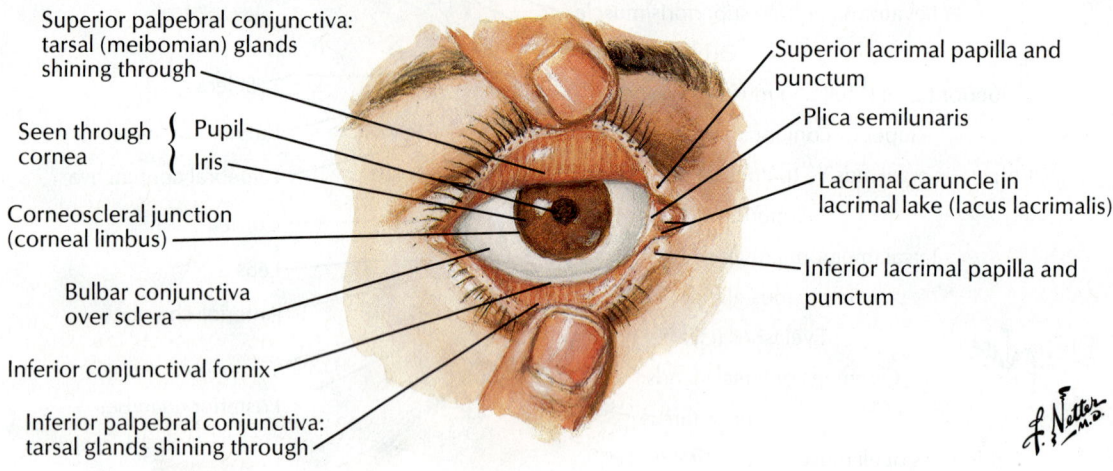

Plate 81, Upper Eyelid. (Netter: Atlas of Human Anatomy, 4 ed, 2006, Saunders.)

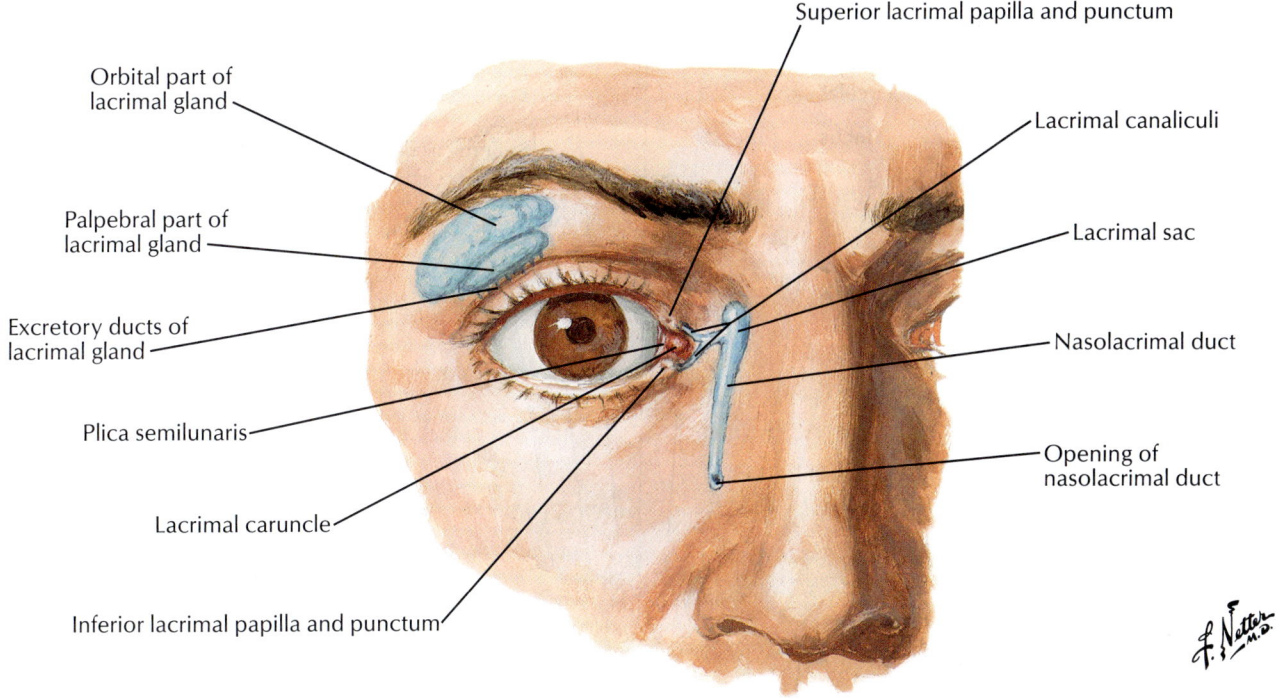
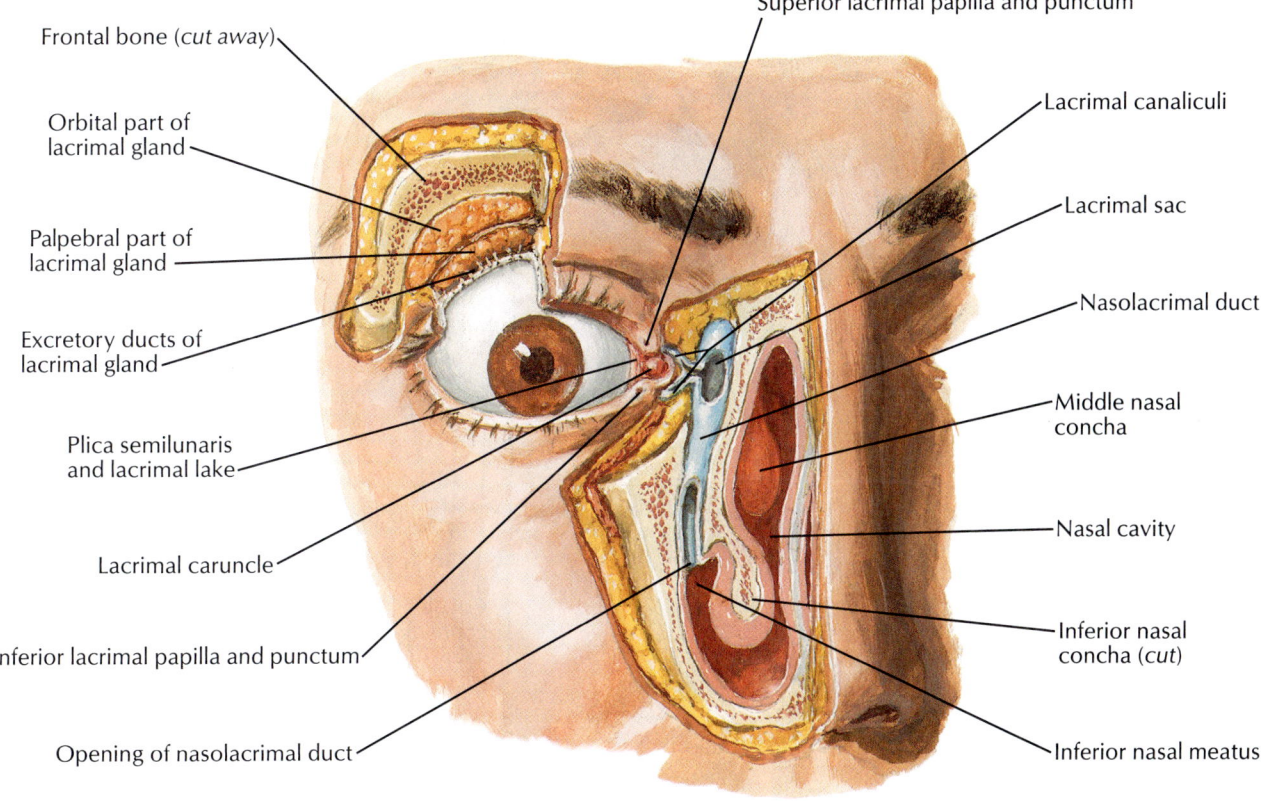

Plate 82 Lacrimal Apparatus. (Netter: Atlas of Human Anatomy, 4 ed, 2006, Saunders.)

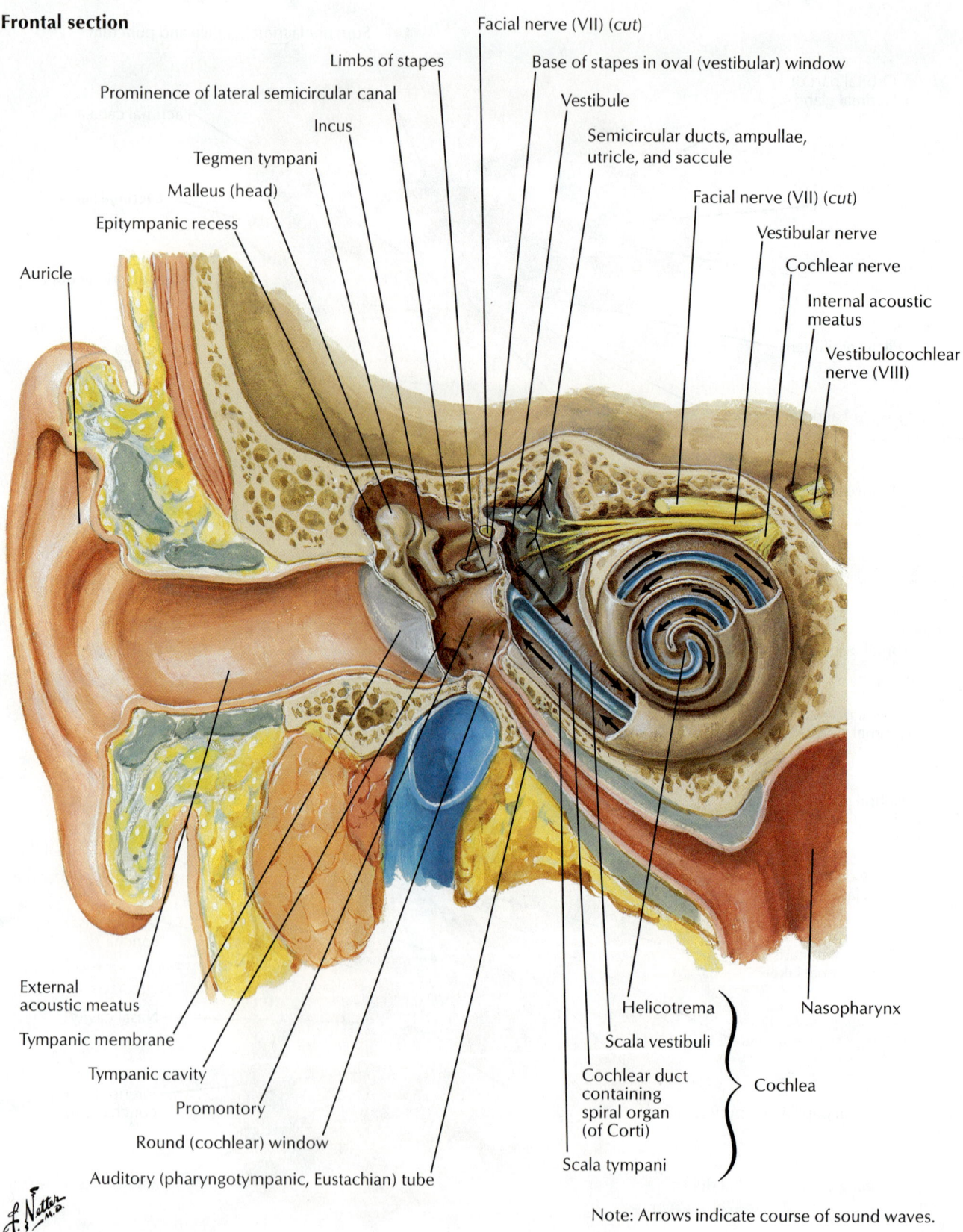

Plate 92 Pathway of Sound Reception. (Netter: Atlas of Human Anatomy, 4 ed, 2006, Saunders.)

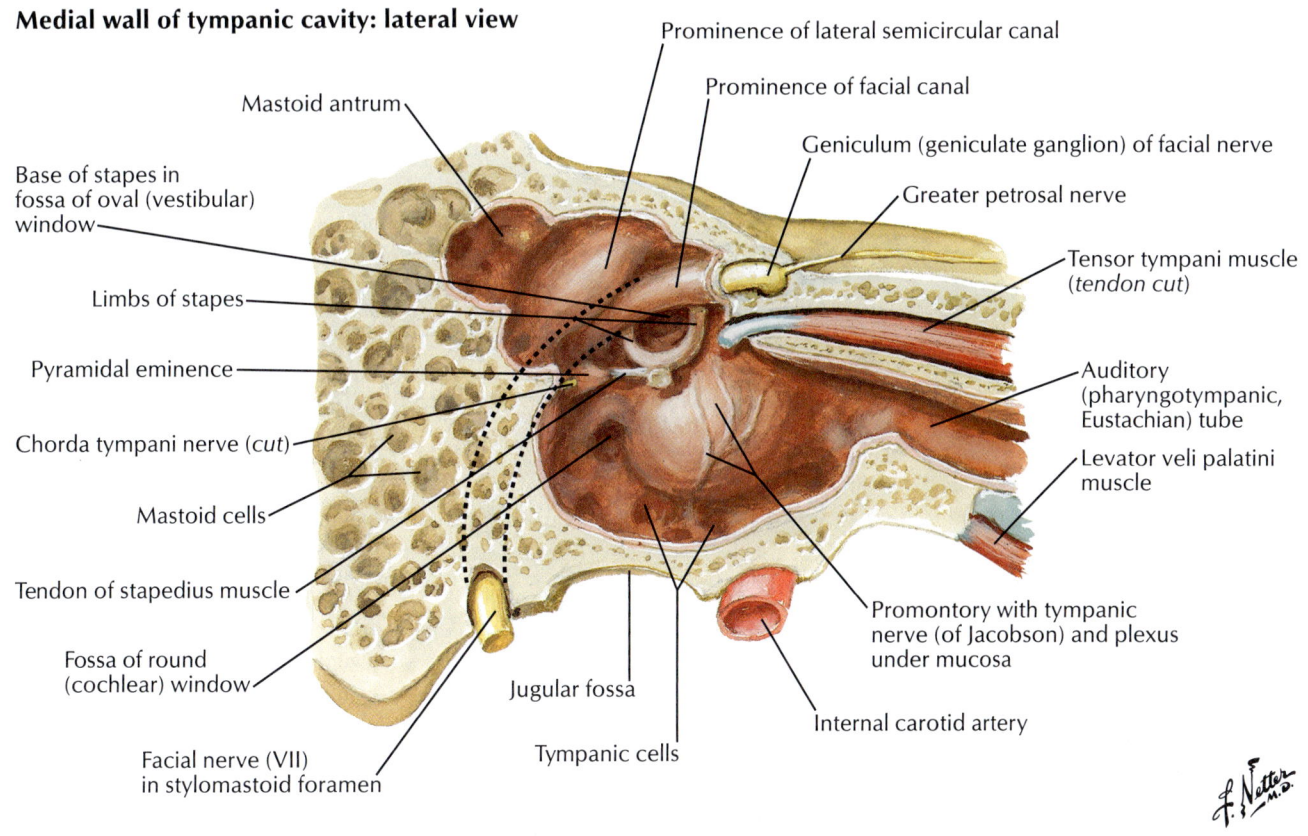

Plate 94 Tympanic Cavity. (Netter: Atlas of Human Anatomy, 4 ed, 2006, Saunders.)

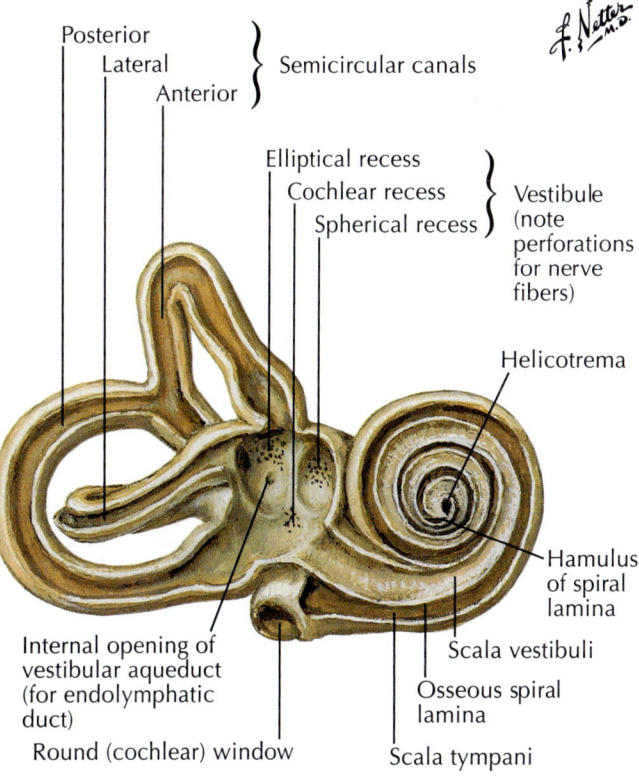

Plate 93 Tympanic Cavity. (Netter: Atlas of Human Anatomy, 4 ed, 2006, Saunders.)

Plate 95 Bony Membranous Labyrinth. (Netter: Atlas of Human Anatomy, 4 ed, 2006, Saunders.)

NAP-21

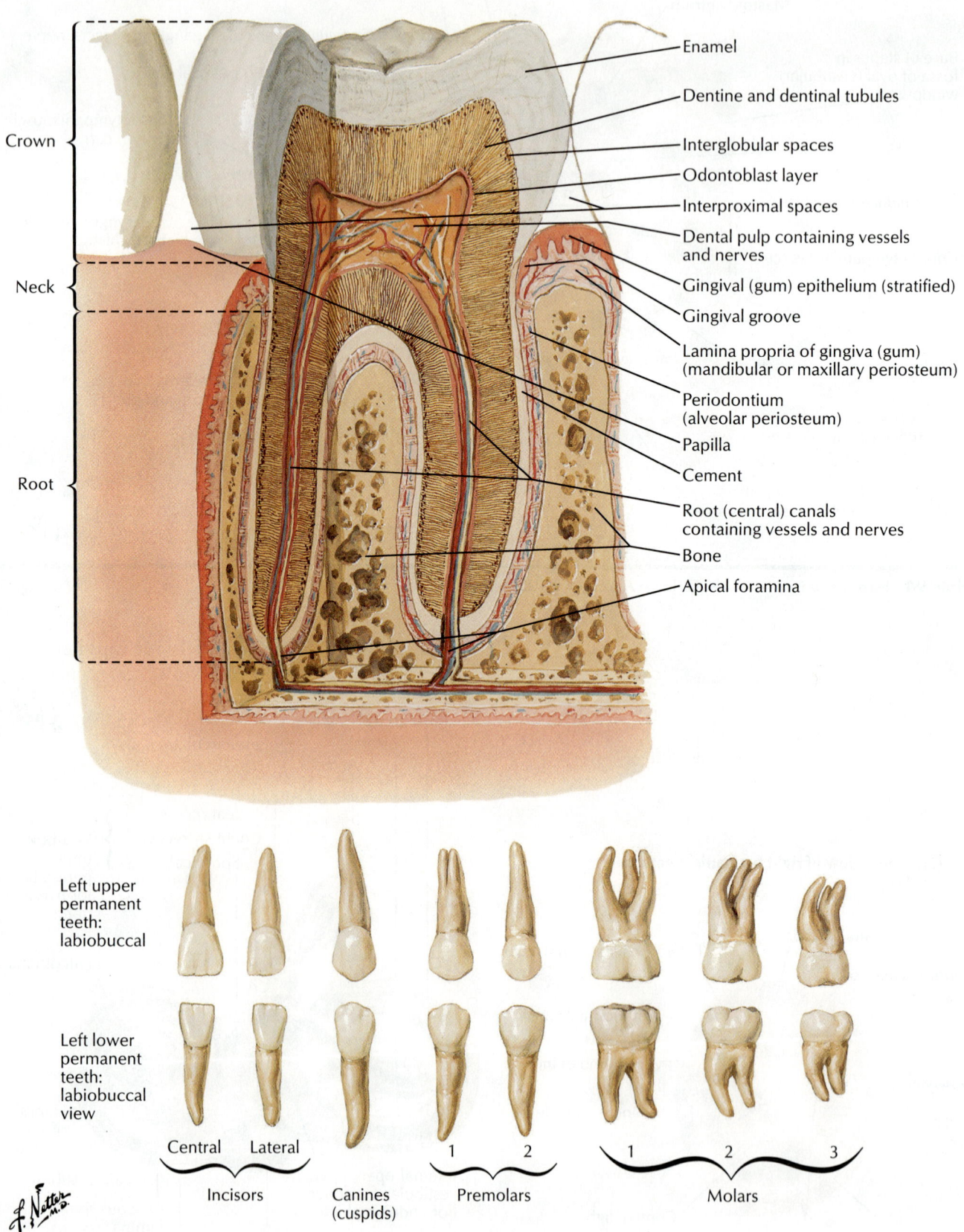

Plate 57 Teeth. (Netter: Atlas of Human Anatomy, 4 ed, 2006, Saunders.)

Tongue

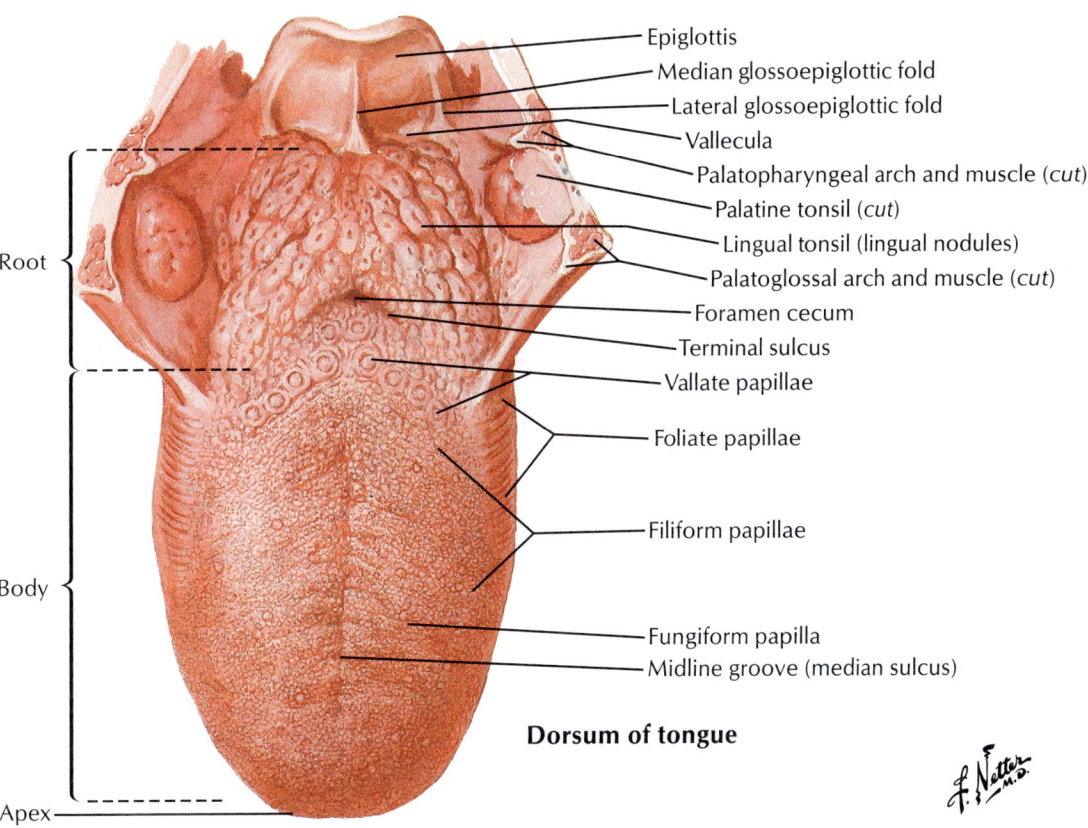

Plate 58 Tongue. (Netter: Atlas of Human Anatomy, 4 ed, 2006, Saunders.)

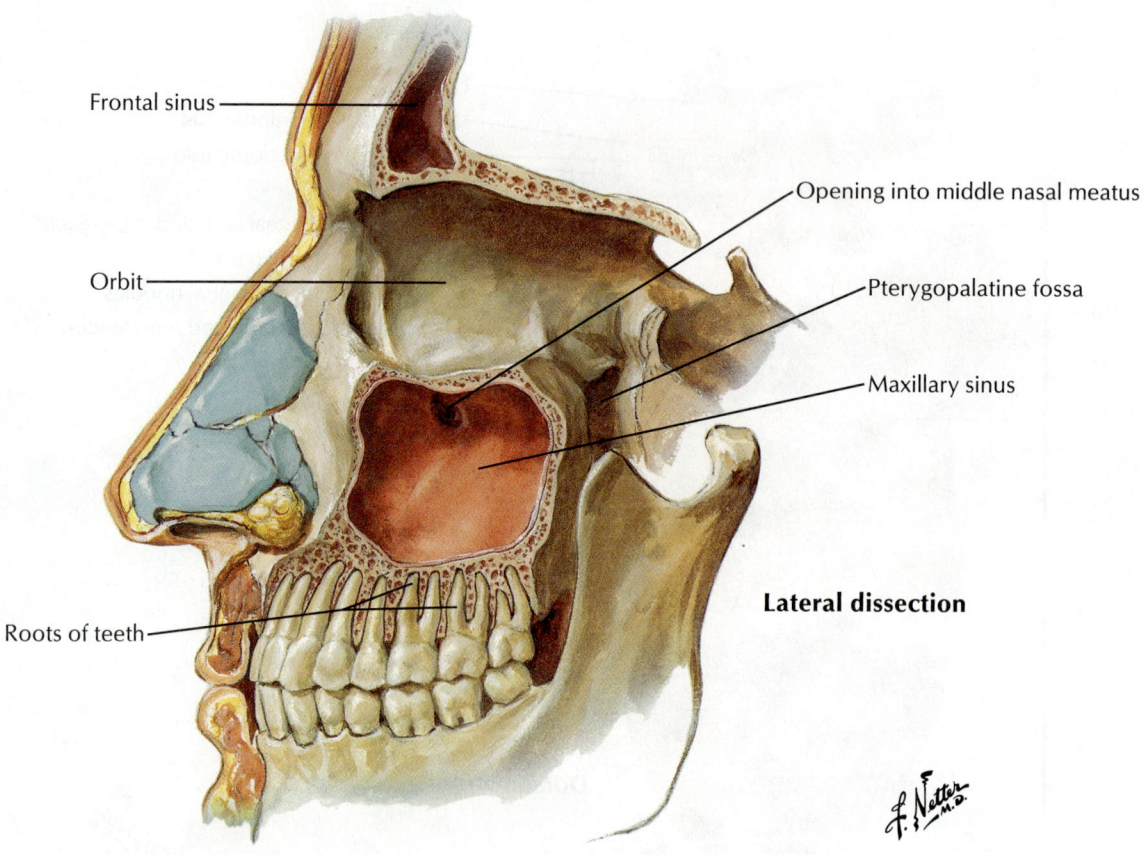

Plate 49 Paranasal Sinuses. (Netter: Atlas of Human Anatomy, 4 ed, 2006, Saunders.)

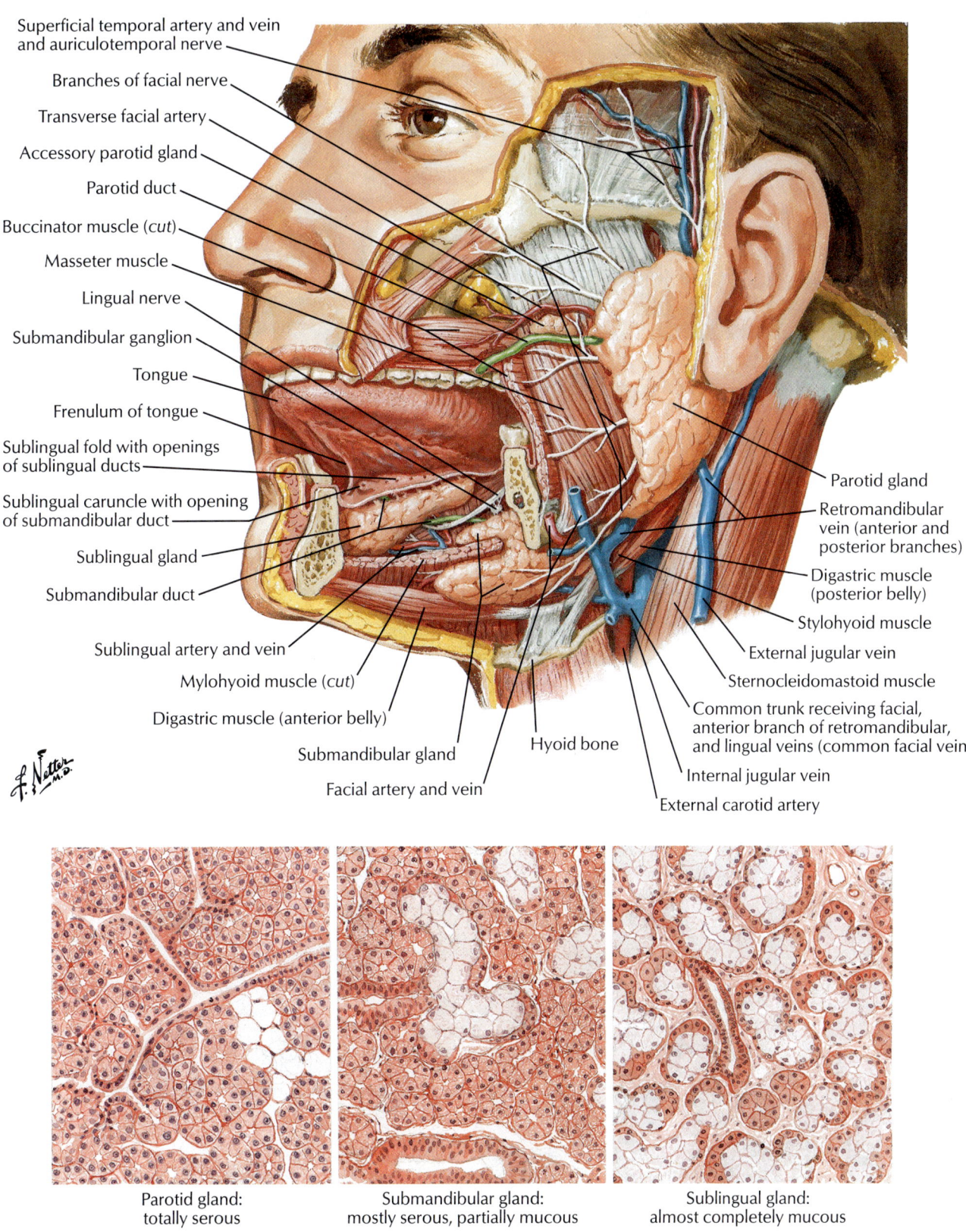

Plate 61 Salivary Glands. (Netter: Atlas of Human Anatomy, 4 ed, 2006, Saunders.)

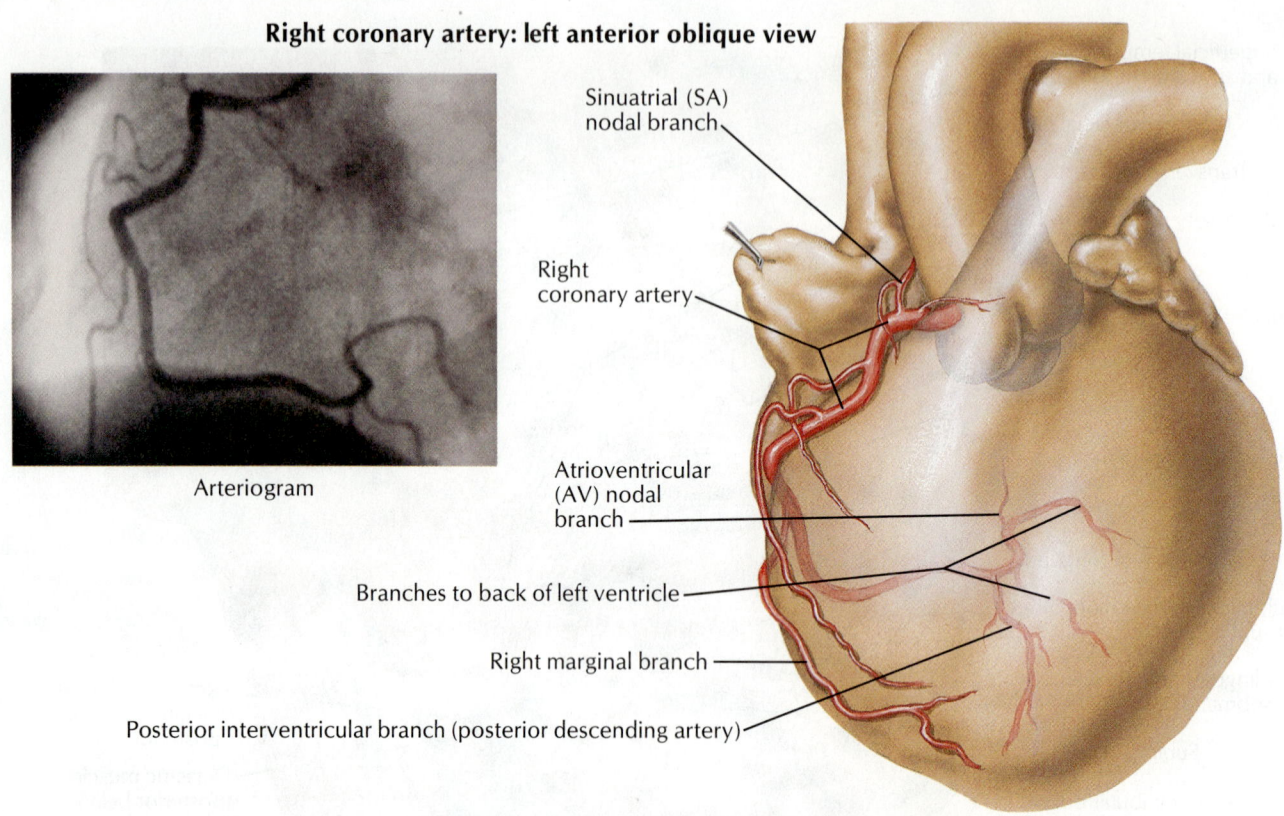

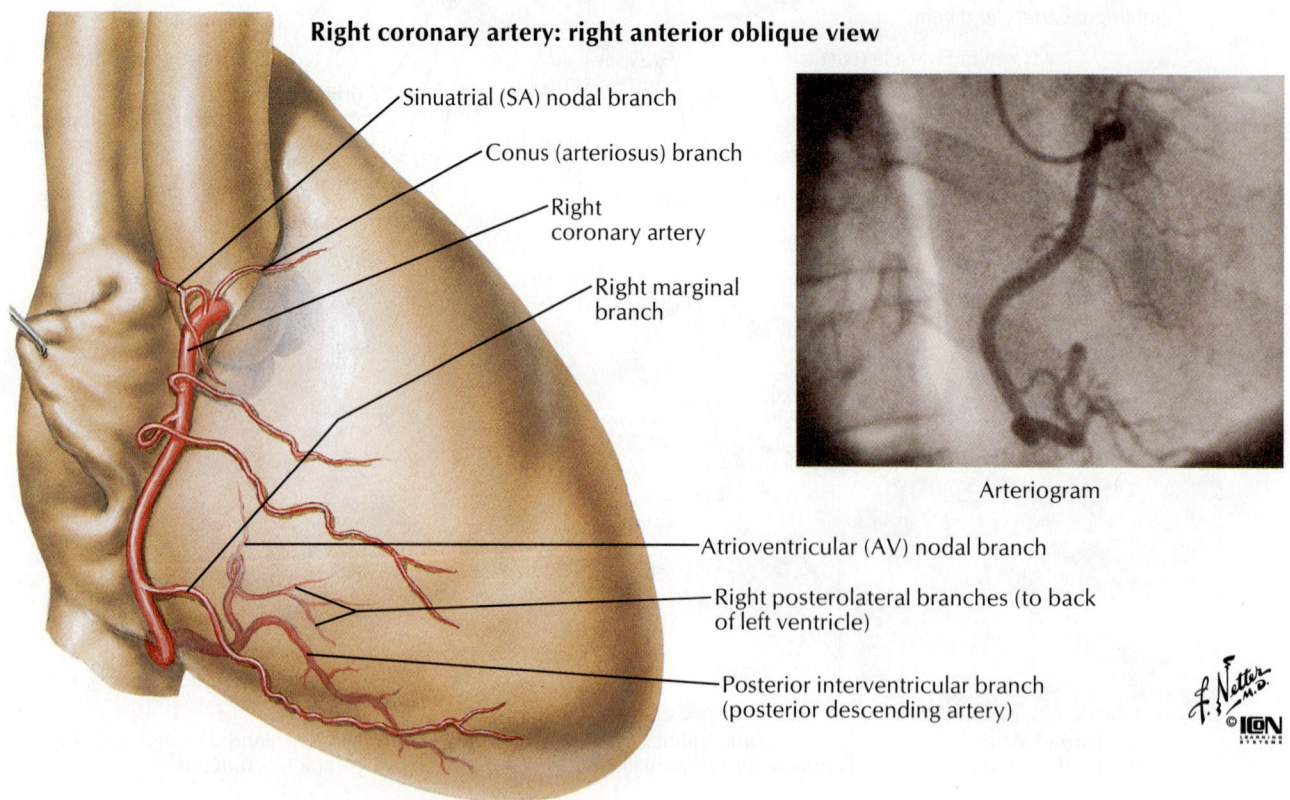

Plate 218 Coronary Arteries: Arteriographic Views. (Netter: Atlas of Human Anatomy, 4 ed, 2006, Saunders.)

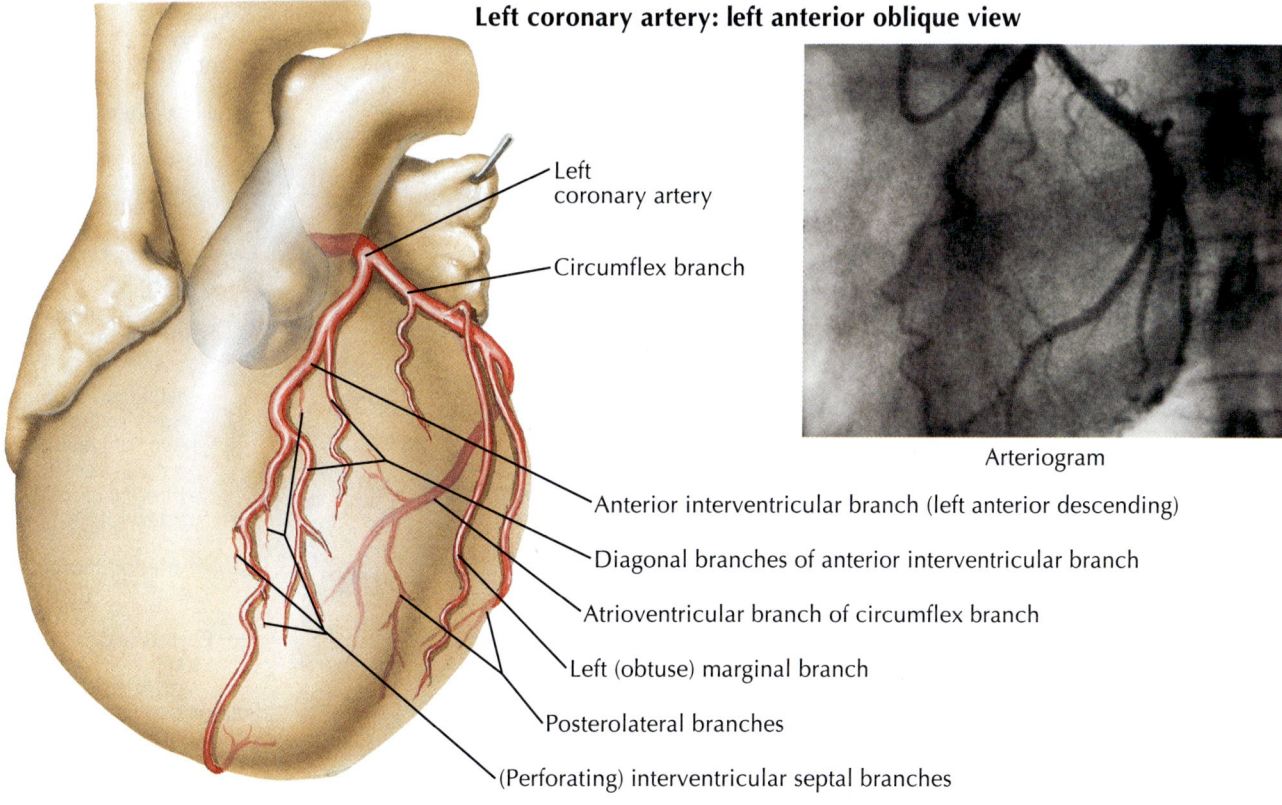
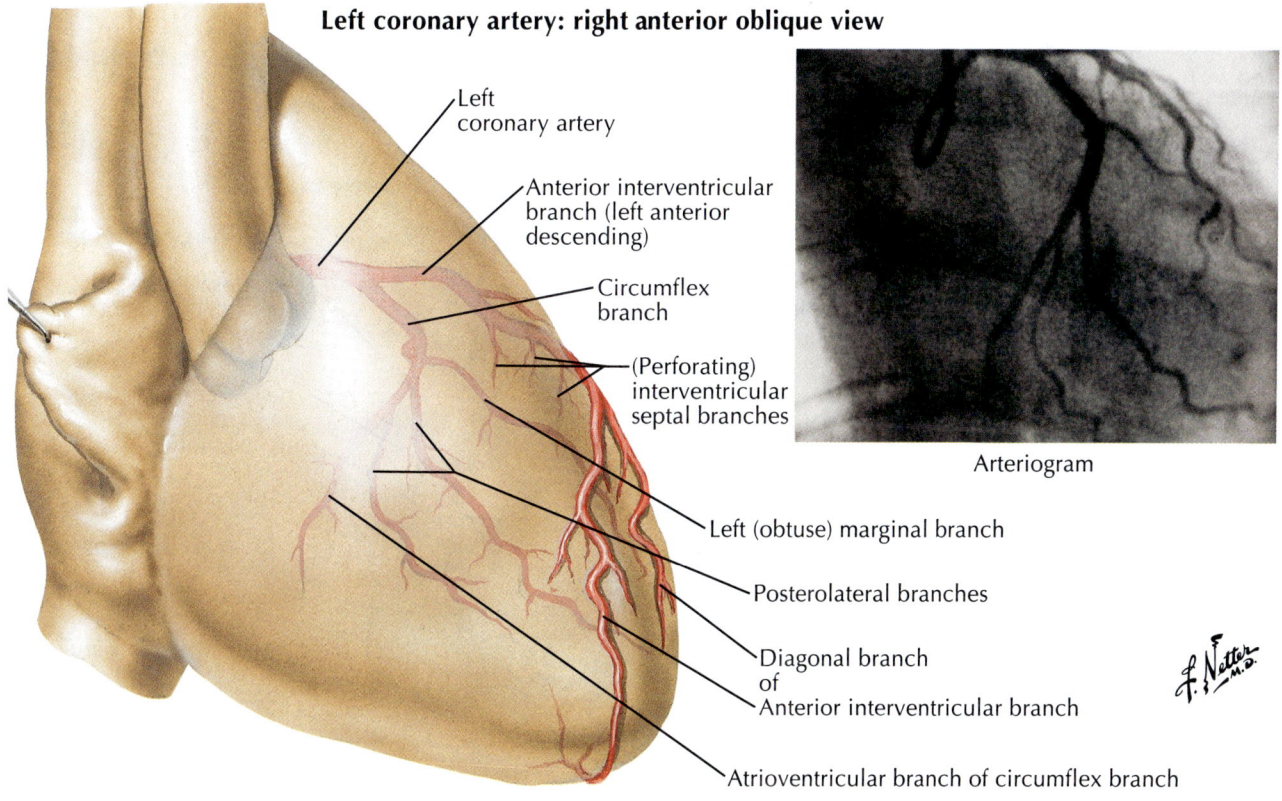

Plate 219 Coronary Arteries: Arteriographic Views. (Netter: Atlas of Human Anatomy, 4 ed, 2006, Saunders.)

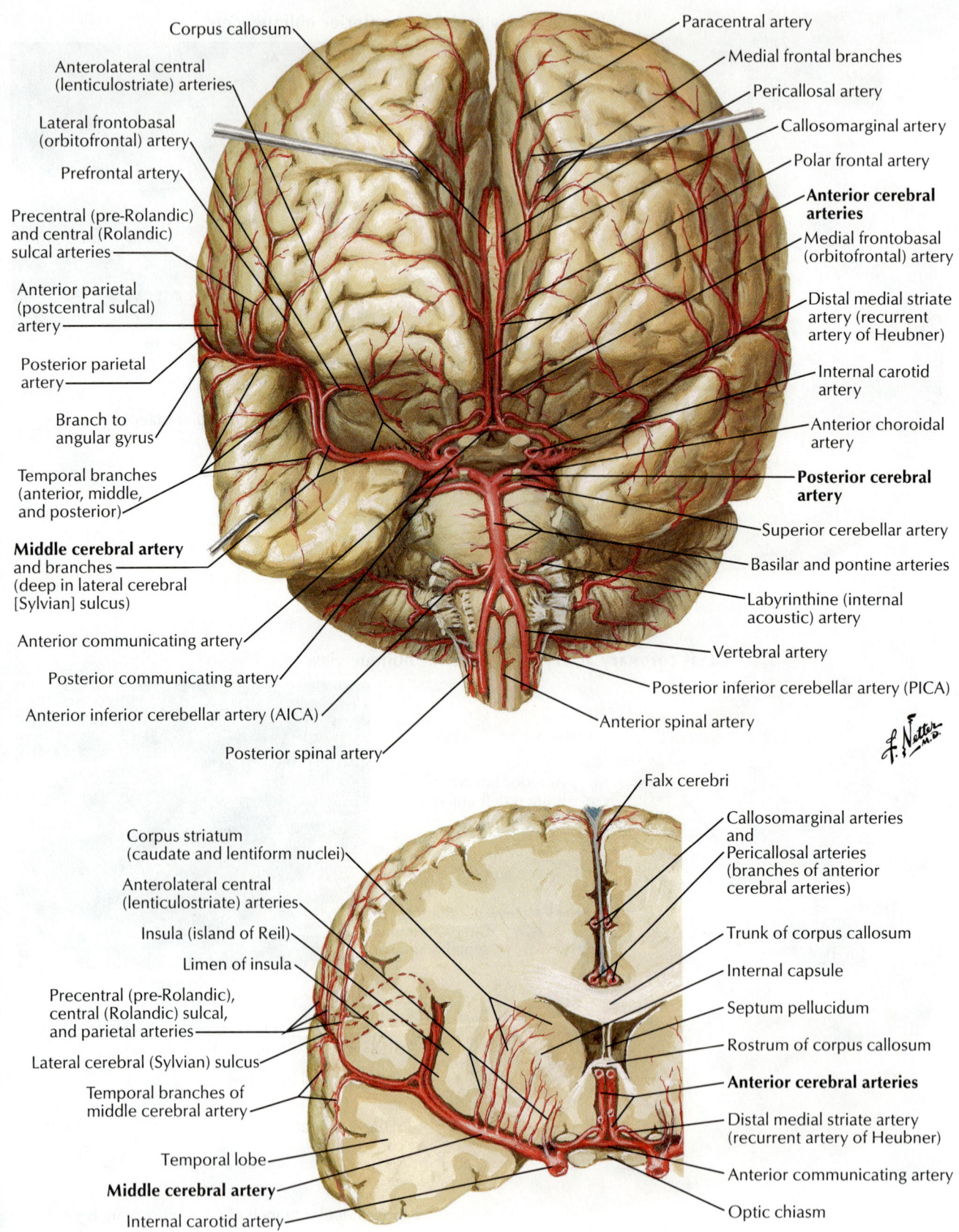

Plate 141 Arteries of Brain: Frontal View and Section. (Netter: Atlas of Human Anatomy, 4 ed, 2006, Saunders.)

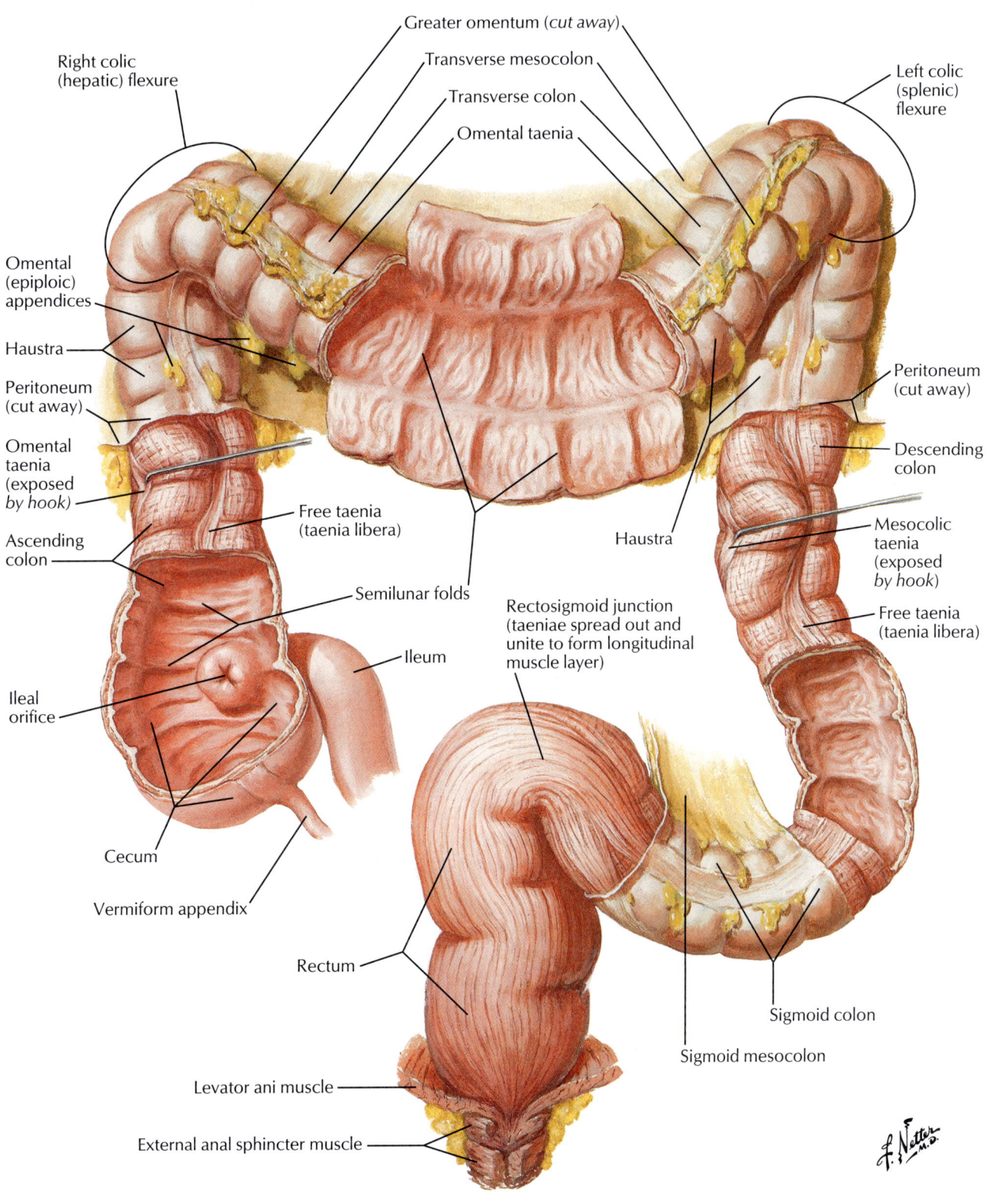

Plate 284 Mucosa and Musculature of Large Intestine. (Netter: Atlas of Human Anatomy, 4 ed, 2006, Saunders.)

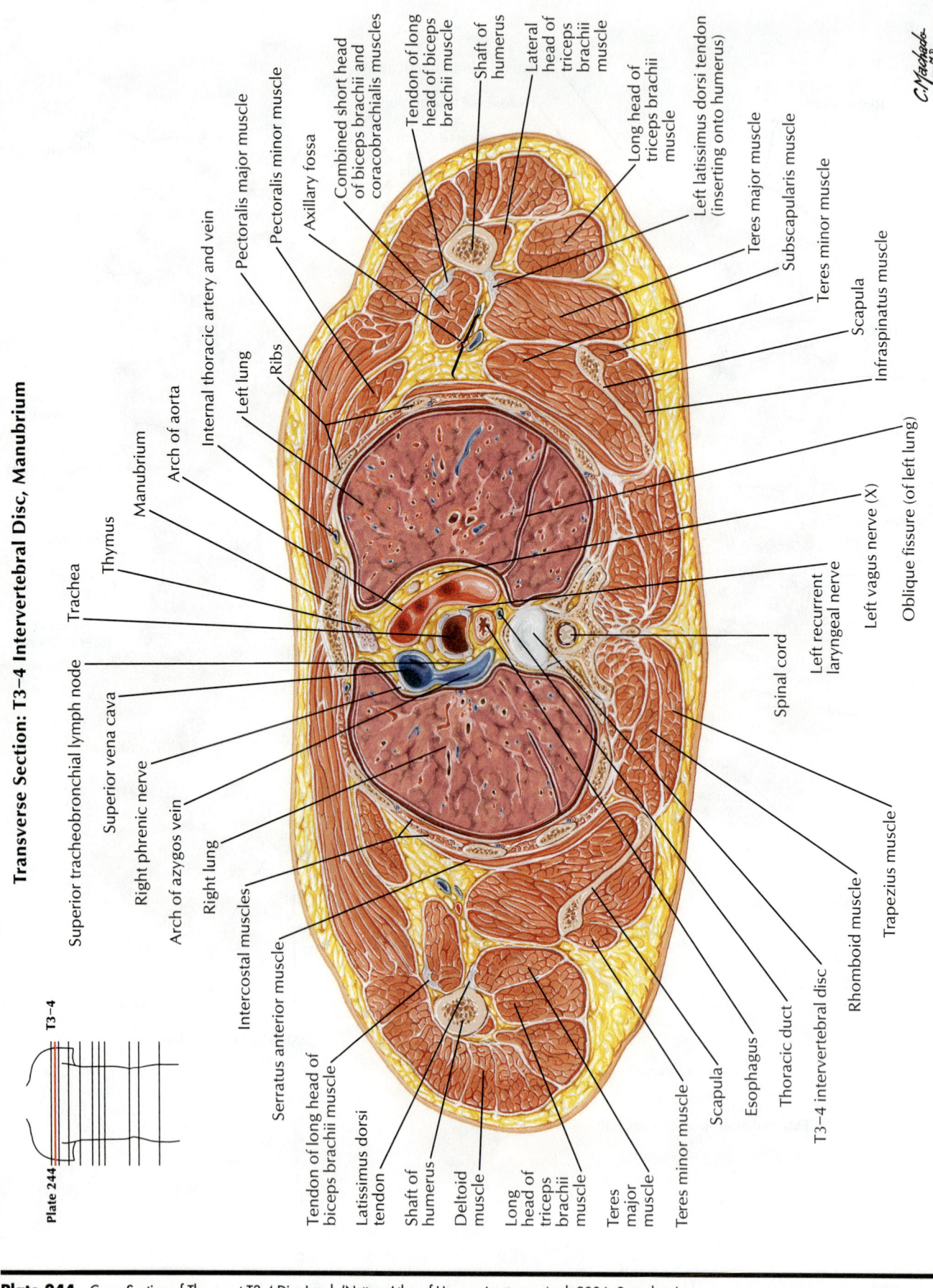

Plate 244 Cross Section of Thorax at T3-4 Disc Level. (Netter: Atlas of Human Anatomy, 4 ed, 2006, Saunders.)

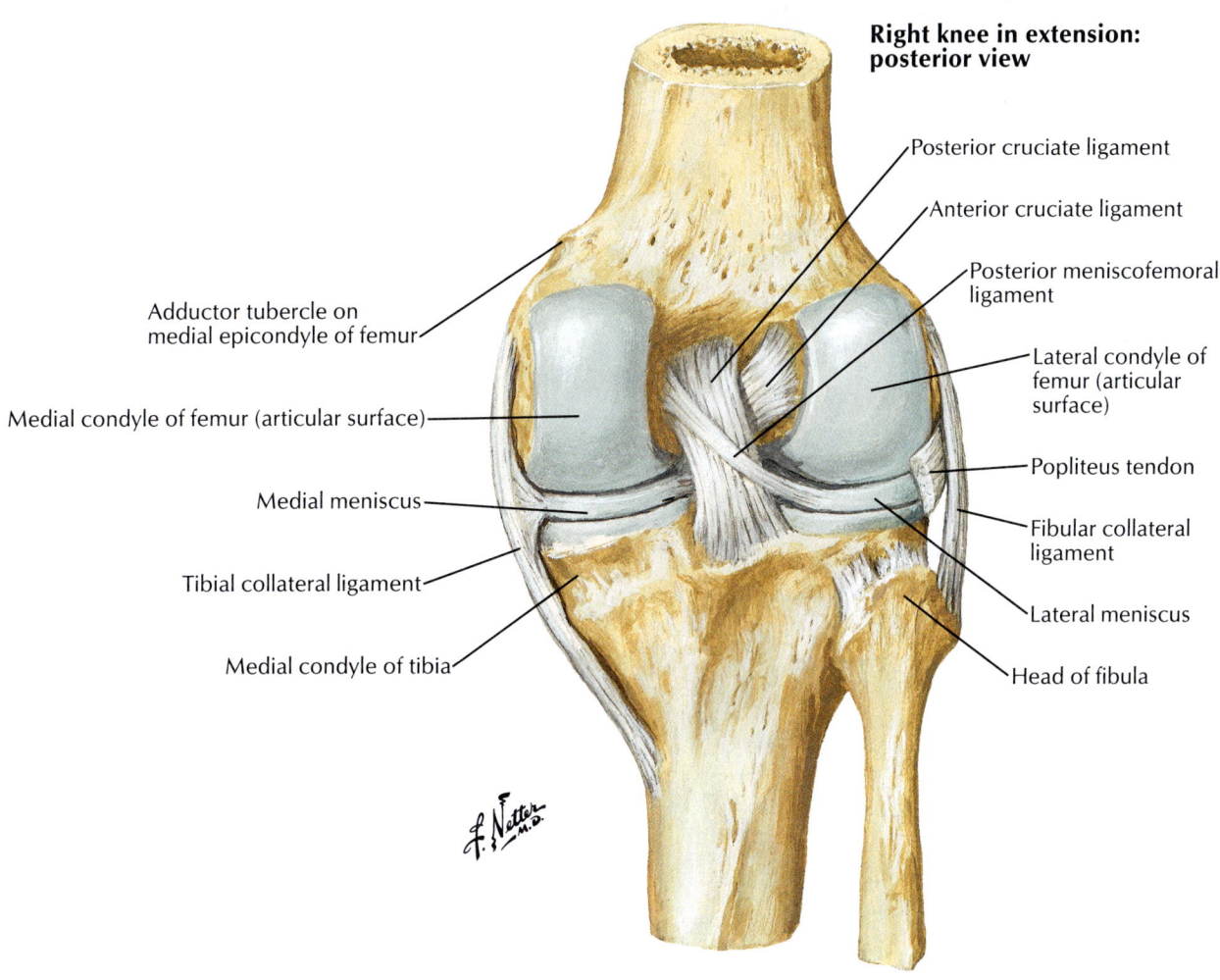

Plate 509 Knee: Cruciate and Collateral Ligaments. (Netter: Atlas of Human Anatomy, 4 ed, 2006, Saunders.)

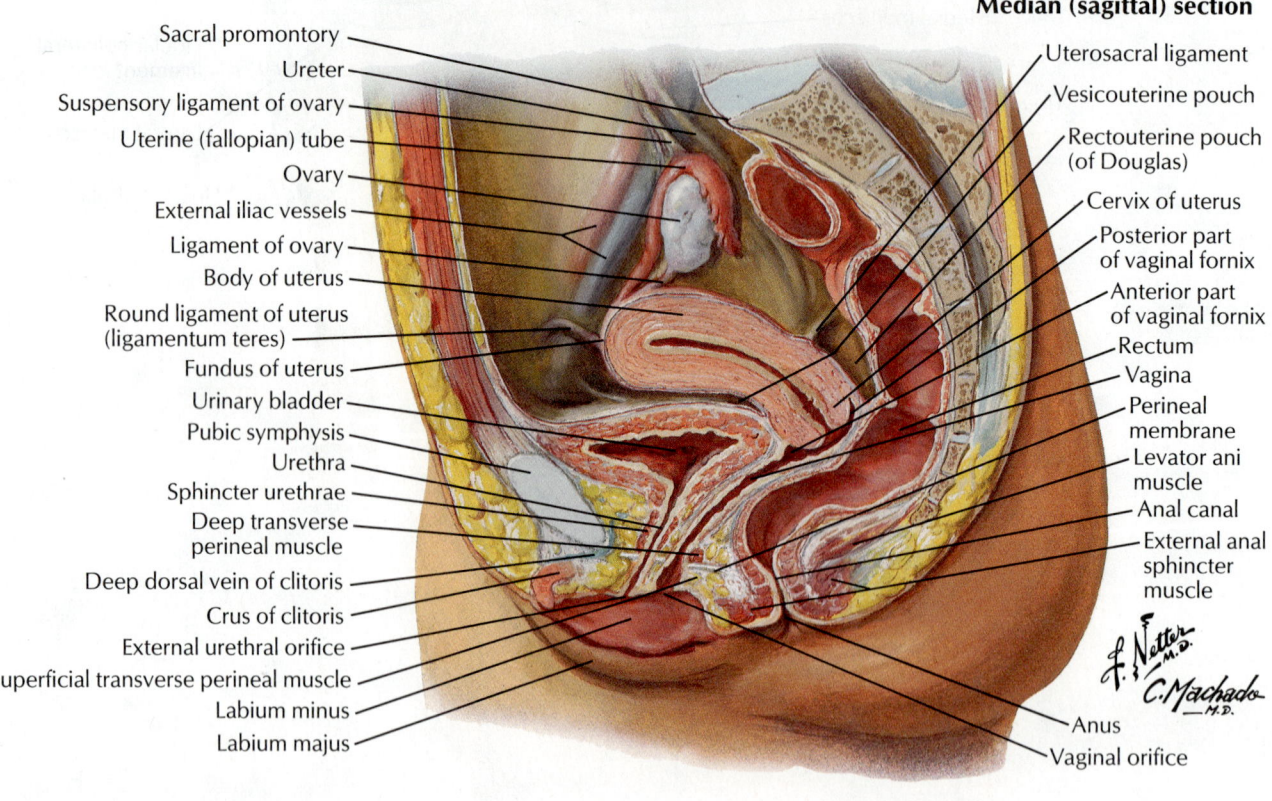

Plate 360   Pelvic Viscera and Perineum: Female. (Netter: Atlas of Human Anatomy, 4 ed, 2006, Saunders.)

PART 1

INTRODUCTION

ICD-9-CM BACKGROUND

The International Classification of Diseases, 9th Revision, Clinical Modification (ICD-9-CM) is based on the official version of the World Health Organization's 9th Revision, International Classification of Diseases (ICD-9). ICD-9 is designed for the classification of morbidity and mortality information for statistical purposes, and for the indexing of hospital records by disease and operations, for data storage and retrieval. The historical background of the International Classification of Diseases may be found in the Introduction to ICD-9 (Manual of the International Classification of Diseases, Injuries, and Causes of Death, World Health Organization, Geneva, Switzerland, 1977).

ICD-9-CM is a clinical modification of the World Health Organization's International Classification of Diseases, 9th Revision (ICD-9). The term "clinical" is used to emphasize the modification's intent: to serve as a useful tool in the area of classification of morbidity data for indexing of medical records, medical care review, and ambulatory and other medical care programs, as well as for basic health statistics. To describe the clinical picture of the patient, the codes must be more precise than those needed only for statistical groupings and trend analysis.

COORDINATION AND MAINTENANCE COMMITTEE

Annual modifications are made to the ICD-9-CM through the ICD-9-CM Coordination and Maintenance Committee (C&M). The Committee is made up of representatives from two Federal Government agencies, the National Center for Health Statistics and the Health Care Financing Administration. The Committee holds meetings twice a year which are open to the public. Modification proposals submitted to the Committee for consideration are presented at the meetings for public discussion. Those modification proposals which are approved are incorporated into the official government version of the ICD-9-CM and become effective for use October 1 of the year following their presentation. The C&M also prepares updates for use April 1 of each year. To date, no April 1 updates have been released.

CHARACTERISTICS OF ICD-9-CM

ICD-9-CM far exceeds its predecessors in the number of codes provided. The disease classification has been expanded to include health-related conditions and to provide greater specificity at the fifth-digit level of detail. These fifth digits are not optional; they are intended for use in recording the information substantiated in the clinical record.

Volume I of ICD-9-CM contains five appendices:

Appendix A	Morphology of Neoplasms
Appendix B	Glossary of Mental Disorders (Deleted in 2004)
Appendix C	Classification of Drugs by American Hospital Formulary Service List Number and Their ICD-9-CM Equivalents
Appendix D	Classification of Industrial Accidents According to Agency
Appendix E	List of Three-Digit Categories

These appendices are included as a reference to the user in order to provide further information about the patient's clinical picture, to further define a diagnostic statement, to aid in classifying new drugs, or to reference three-digit categories.

Volume 2 of ICD-9-CM contains many diagnostic terms which do not appear in Volume 1 since the index includes most diagnostic terms currently in use.

The Disease Classification

ICD-9-CM is totally compatible with its parent system, ICD-9, thus meeting the need for comparability of morbidity and mortality statistics at the international level. A few fourth-digit codes were created in existing three-digit rubrics only when the necessary detail could not be accommodated by the use of a fifth-digit subclassification. To ensure that each rubric of ICD-9-CM collapses back to its ICD-9 counterpart, the following specifications governed the ICD-9-CM disease classification:

Specifications for the Tabular List

1. Three-digit rubrics and their contents are unchanged from ICD-9.
2. The sequence of three-digit rubrics is unchanged from ICD-9.
3. Unsubdivided three-digit rubrics are subdivided where necessary to:
   a) Add clinical detail
   b) Isolate terms for clinical accuracy
4. The modification in ICD-9-CM is accomplished by the addition of a fifth digit to existing ICD-9 rubrics.
5. The optional dual classification in ICD-9 is modified.
   a) Duplicate rubrics are deleted:
      1) Four-digit manifestation categories duplicating etiology entries.
      2) Manifestation inclusion terms duplicating etiology entries.
   b) Manifestations of diseases are identified, to the extent possible, by creating five-digit codes in the etiology rubrics.
   c) When the manifestation of a disease cannot be included in the etiology rubrics, provision for its identification is made by retaining the ICD-9 rubrics used for classifying manifestations of disease.
6. The format of ICD-9-CM is revised from that used in ICD-9.
   a) American spelling of medical terms is used.
   b) Inclusion terms are indented beneath the titles of codes.
   c) Codes not to be used for principal tabulation of disease are printed with the notation, "Code first underlying disease."

Specifications for the Alphabetic Index

1. Format of the Alphabetic Index follows the format of ICD-9.
2. When two codes are required to indicate etiology and manifestation, the manifestation code appears in brackets, e.g., diabetic cataract 250.5X [366.41]. The etiology code is always sequenced first followed by the manifestation code.

The following guidelines were the most current at the time of publication. Check the website at http://codingupdates.com for the latest updates to the Guidelines.

ICD-9-CM OFFICIAL GUIDELINES FOR CODING AND REPORTING

Effective October 1, 2011
Narrative changes appear in bold text
Items underlined have been moved within the guidelines since October 1, 2010

The Centers for Medicare and Medicaid Services (CMS) and the National Center for Health Statistics (NCHS), two departments within the U.S. Federal Government's Department of Health and Human Services (DHHS) provide the following guidelines for coding and reporting using the International Classification of Diseases, 9th Revision, Clinical Modification (ICD-9-CM). These guidelines should be used as a companion document to the official version of the ICD-9-CM as published on CD-ROM by the U.S. Government Printing Office (GPO).

These guidelines have been approved by the four organizations that make up the Cooperating Parties for the ICD-9-CM: the American Hospital Association (AHA), the American Health Information Management Association (AHIMA), CMS, and NCHS. These guidelines are included on the official government version of the ICD-9-CM, and also appear in "Coding Clinic for ICD-9-CM" published by the AHA.

These guidelines are a set of rules that have been developed to accompany and complement the official conventions and instructions provided within the ICD-9-CM itself. The instructions and conventions of the classification take precedence over guidelines. These guidelines are based on the coding and sequencing instructions in Volumes I, II and III of ICD-9-CM, but provide additional instruction. Adherence to these guidelines when assigning ICD-9-CM diagnosis and procedure codes is required under the Health Insurance Portability and Accountability Act (HIPAA). The diagnosis codes (Volumes 1-2) have been adopted under HIPAA for all healthcare settings. Volume 3 procedure codes have been adopted for inpatient procedures reported by hospitals. A joint effort between the healthcare provider and the coder is essential to achieve complete and accurate documentation, code assignment, and reporting of diagnoses and procedures. These guidelines have been developed to assist both the healthcare provider and the coder in identifying those diagnoses and procedures that are to be reported. The importance of consistent, complete documentation in the medical record cannot be overemphasized. Without such documentation accurate coding cannot be achieved. The entire record should be reviewed to determine the specific reason for the encounter and the conditions treated.

The term encounter is used for all settings, including hospital admissions. In the context of these guidelines, the term provider is used throughout the guidelines to mean physician or any qualified health care practitioner who is legally accountable for establishing the patient's diagnosis. Only this set of guidelines, approved by the Cooperating Parties, is official.

The guidelines are organized into sections. Section I includes the structure and conventions of the classification and general guidelines that apply to the entire classification, and chapter-specific guidelines that correspond to the chapters as they are arranged in the classification. Section II includes guidelines for selection of principal diagnosis for non-outpatient settings. Section III includes guidelines for reporting additional diagnoses in non-outpatient settings. Section IV is for outpatient coding and reporting.

ICD-9-CM Official Guidelines for Coding and Reporting

Section I. Conventions, general coding guidelines and chapter specific guidelines

A. Conventions for the ICD-9-CM
1. Format:
2. Abbreviations
   a. Index abbreviations
   b. Tabular abbreviations
3. Punctuation
4. Includes and Excludes Notes and Inclusion terms
5. Other and Unspecified codes
   a. "Other" codes
   b. "Unspecified" codes
6. Etiology/manifestation convention ("code first", "use additional code" and "in diseases classified elsewhere" notes)
7. "And"
8. "With"
9. "See" and "See Also"

B. General Coding Guidelines
1. Use of Both Alphabetic Index and Tabular List
2. Locate each term in the Alphabetic Index
3. Level of Detail in Coding
4. Code or codes from 001.0 through V91.99
5. Selection of codes 001.0 through 999.9
6. Signs and symptoms
7. Conditions that are an integral part of a disease process
8. Conditions that are not an integral part of a disease process
9. Multiple coding for a single condition
10. Acute and Chronic Conditions
11. Combination Code
12. Late Effects
13. Impending or Threatened Condition
14. Reporting Same Diagnosis Code More than Once
15. Admissions/Encounters for Rehabilitation
16. Documentation for BMI and Pressure Ulcer Stages
17. Syndromes
18. **Documentation of Complications of care**

C. Chapter-Specific Coding Guidelines
1. Chapter 1: Infectious and Parasitic Diseases (001-139)
   a. Human Immunodeficiency Virus (HIV) Infections
   b. Septicemia, Systemic Inflammatory Response Syndrome (SIRS), Sepsis, Severe Sepsis, and Septic Shock
   c. Methicillin Resistant *Staphylococcus aureus* (MRSA) Conditions
2. Chapter 2: Neoplasms (140-239)
   a. Treatment directed at the malignancy
   b. Treatment of secondary site
   c. Coding and sequencing of complications
   d. Primary malignancy previously excised
   e. Admissions/Encounters involving chemotherapy, immunotherapy and radiation therapy
   f. Admission/encounter to determine extent of malignancy
   g. Symptoms, signs, and ill-defined conditions listed in Chapter 16 associated with neoplasms
   h. Admission/encounter for pain control/management
   i. Malignant neoplasm associated with transplanted organ
3. Chapter 3: Endocrine, Nutritional, and Metabolic Diseases and Immunity Disorders (240-279)
   a. Diabetes mellitus
4. Chapter 4: Diseases of Blood and Blood Forming Organs (280-289)
   a. Anemia of chronic disease
5. Chapter 5: Mental Disorders (290-319)
   Reserved for future guideline expansion
6. Chapter 6: Diseases of Nervous System and Sense Organs (320-389)
   a. Pain - Category 338
   b. Glaucoma
7. Chapter 7: Diseases of Circulatory System (390-459)
   a. Hypertension
   b. Cerebral infarction/stroke/cerebrovascular accident (CVA)
   c. Postoperative cerebrovascular accident
   d. Late Effects of Cerebrovascular Disease
   e. Acute myocardial infarction (AMI)
8. Chapter 8: Diseases of Respiratory System (460-519)
   a. Chronic Obstructive Pulmonary Disease [COPD] and Asthma
   b. Chronic Obstructive Pulmonary Disease [COPD] and Bronchitis
   c. Acute Respiratory Failure
   d. Influenza due to *certain* identified *viruses*

9. Chapter 9: Diseases of Digestive System (520-579)
   Reserved for future guideline expansion
10. Chapter 10: Diseases of Genitourinary System (580-629)
    a. Chronic kidney disease
11. Chapter 11: Complications of Pregnancy, Childbirth, and the Puerperium (630-679)
    a. General Rules for Obstetric Cases
    b. Selection of OB Principal or First-listed Diagnosis
    c. Fetal Conditions Affecting the Management of the Mother
    d. HIV Infection in Pregnancy, Childbirth and the Puerperium
    e. Current Conditions Complicating Pregnancy
    f. Diabetes mellitus in pregnancy
    g. Gestational diabetes
    h. Normal Delivery, Code 650
    i. The Postpartum and Peripartum Periods
    j. Code 677, Late effect of complication of pregnancy
    k. Abortions
12. Chapter 12: Diseases Skin and Subcutaneous Tissue (680-709)
    a. Pressure ulcer stage codes
13. Chapter 13: Diseases of Musculoskeletal and Connective Tissue (710-739)
    a. Coding of Pathologic Fractures
14. Chapter 14: Congenital Anomalies (740-759)
    a. Codes in categories 740-759, Congenital Anomalies
15. Chapter 15: Newborn (Perinatal) Guidelines (760-779)
    a. General Perinatal Rules
    b. Use of codes V30-V39
    c. Newborn transfers
    d. Use of category V29
    e. Use of other V codes on perinatal records
    f. Maternal Causes of Perinatal Morbidity
    g. Congenital Anomalies in Newborns
    h. Coding Additional Perinatal Diagnoses
    i. Prematurity and Fetal Growth Retardation
    j. Newborn sepsis
16. Chapter 16: Signs, Symptoms and Ill-Defined Conditions (780-799)
    Reserved for future guideline expansion
17. Chapter 17: Injury and Poisoning (800-999)
    a. Coding of Injuries
    b. Coding of Traumatic Fractures
    c. Coding of Burns
    d. Coding of Debridement of Wound, Infection, or Burn
    e. Adverse Effects, Poisoning and Toxic Effects
    f. Complications of care
    g. SIRS due to Non-infectious Process
18. Classification of Factors Influencing Health Status and Contact with Health Service (Supplemental V01-V91)
    a. Introduction
    b. V codes use in any healthcare setting
    c. V Codes indicate a reason for an encounter
    d. Categories of V Codes
    e. V Codes That May Only be Principal/ First-Listed Diagnosis
19. Supplemental Classification of External Causes of Injury and Poisoning (E-codes, E800-E999)
    a. General E Code Coding Guidelines
    b. Place of Occurrence Guideline
    c. Adverse Effects of Drugs, Medicinal and Biological Substances Guidelines
    d. Child and Adult Abuse Guideline
    e. Unknown or Suspected Intent Guideline
    f. Undetermined Cause
    g. Late Effects of External Cause Guidelines
    h. Misadventures and Complications of Care Guidelines
    i. Terrorism Guidelines
    j. Activity Code Guidelines
    k. External cause status

Section II. Selection of Principal Diagnosis

A. Codes for symptoms, signs, and ill-defined conditions
B. Two or more interrelated conditions, each potentially meeting the definition for principal diagnosis
C. Two or more diagnoses that equally meet the definition for principal diagnosis
D. Two or more comparative or contrasting conditions
E. A symptom(s) followed by contrasting/comparative diagnoses
F. Original treatment plan not carried out
G. Complications of surgery and other medical care
H. Uncertain Diagnosis
I. Admission from Observation Unit
   1. Admission Following Medical Observation
   2. Admission Following Post-Operative Observation
J. Admission from Outpatient Surgery

Section III. Reporting Additional Diagnoses

A. Previous conditions
B. Abnormal findings
C. Uncertain Diagnosis

Section IV. Diagnostic Coding and Reporting Guidelines for Outpatient Services

A. Selection of first-listed condition
  1. Outpatient Surgery
  2. Observation Stay
B. Codes from 001.0 through V91.99
C. Accurate reporting of ICD-9-CM diagnosis codes
D. Selection of codes 001.0 through 999.9
E. Codes that describe symptoms and signs
F. Encounters for circumstances other than a disease or injury
G. Level of Detail in Coding
  1. ICD-9-CM codes with 3, 4, or 5 digits
  2. Use of full number of digits required for a code
H. ICD-9-CM code for the diagnosis, condition, problem, or other reason for encounter/visit
I. Uncertain diagnosis
J. Chronic diseases
K. Code all documented conditions that coexist
L. Patients receiving diagnostic services only
M. Patients receiving therapeutic services only
N. Patients receiving preoperative evaluations only
O. Ambulatory surgery
P. Routine outpatient prenatal visits

Appendix I: Present on Admission Reporting Guidelines

Section I. Conventions, general coding guidelines and chapter specific guidelines

The conventions, general guidelines and chapter-specific guidelines are applicable to all health care settings unless otherwise indicated. The conventions and instructions of the classification take precedence over guidelines.

A. **Conventions for the ICD-9-CM**

  The conventions for the ICD-9-CM are the general rules for use of the classification independent of the guidelines. These conventions are incorporated within the index and tabular of the ICD-9-CM as instructional notes. The conventions are as follows:

  1. **Format:**
    The ICD-9-CM uses an indented format for ease in reference
  2. **Abbreviations**
    a. **Index abbreviations**
      NEC "Not elsewhere classifiable" This abbreviation in the index represents "other specified" when a specific code is not available for a condition the index directs the coder to the "other specified" code in the tabular.
    b. **Tabular abbreviations**
      NEC "Not elsewhere classifiable" This abbreviation in the tabular represents "other specified". When a specific code is not available for a condition the tabular includes an NEC entry under a code to identify the code as the "other specified" code. *(See Section I.A.5.a. "Other" codes)*.
      NOS "Not otherwise specified" This abbreviation is the equivalent of unspecified. *(See Section I.A.5.b., "Unspecified" codes)*
  3. **Punctuation**
    [ ] Brackets are used in the tabular list to enclose synonyms, alternative wording or explanatory phrases. Brackets are used in the index to identify manifestation codes. *(See Section I.A.6. "Etiology/manifestations")*
    ( ) Parentheses are used in both the index and tabular to enclose supplementary words that may be present or absent in the statement of a disease or procedure without affecting the code number to which it is assigned. The terms within the parentheses are referred to as nonessential modifiers.
    : Colons are used in the Tabular list after an incomplete term which needs one or more of the modifiers following the colon to make it assignable to a given category.
  4. **Includes and Excludes Notes and Inclusion terms**
    Includes: This note appears immediately under a three-digit code title to further define, or give examples of, the content of the category.
    Excludes: An excludes note under a code indicates that the terms excluded from the code are to be coded elsewhere. In some cases the codes for the excluded terms should not be used in conjunction with the code from which it is excluded. An example of this is a congenital condition excluded from an acquired form of the same condition. The congenital and acquired codes should not be used together. In other cases, the excluded terms may be used together with an excluded code. An example of this is when fractures of different bones are coded to different codes. Both codes may be used together if both types of fractures are present.
    Inclusion terms: List of terms is included under certain four and five digit codes. These terms are the conditions for which that code number is to be used. The terms may be synonyms of the code title, or, in the case of "other specified" codes, the terms are a list of the various conditions assigned to that code. The

inclusion terms are not necessarily exhaustive. Additional terms found only in the index may also be assigned to a code.

5. Other and Unspecified codes

a. "Other" codes

Codes titled "other" or "other specified" (usually a code with a 4th digit 8 or fifth-digit 9 for diagnosis codes) are for use when the information in the medical record provides detail for which a specific code does not exist. Index entries with NEC in the line designate "other" codes in the tabular. These index entries represent specific disease entities for which no specific code exists so the term is included within an "other" code.

b. "Unspecified" codes

Codes (usually a code with a 4th digit 9 or 5th digit 0 for diagnosis codes) titled "unspecified" are for use when the information in the medical record is insufficient to assign a more specific code.

6. Etiology/manifestation convention ("code first", "use additional code" and "in diseases classified elsewhere" notes)

Certain conditions have both an underlying etiology and multiple body system manifestations due to the underlying etiology. For such conditions, the ICD-9-CM has a coding convention that requires the underlying condition be sequenced first followed by the manifestation. Wherever such a combination exists, there is a "use additional code" note at the etiology code, and a "code first" note at the manifestation code. These instructional notes indicate the proper sequencing order of the codes, etiology followed by manifestation.

In most cases the manifestation codes will have in the code title, "in diseases classified elsewhere." Codes with this title are a component of the etiology/manifestation convention. The code title indicates that it is a manifestation code. "In diseases classified elsewhere" codes are never permitted to be used as first listed or principal diagnosis codes. They must be used in conjunction with an underlying condition code and they must be listed following the underlying condition.

There are manifestation codes that do not have "in diseases classified elsewhere" in the title. For such codes a "use additional code" note will still be present and the rules for sequencing apply.

In addition to the notes in the tabular, these conditions also have a specific index entry structure. In the index both conditions are listed together with the etiology code first followed by the manifestation codes in brackets. The code in brackets is always to be sequenced second.

The most commonly used etiology/manifestation combinations are the codes for Diabetes mellitus, category 250. For each code under category 250 there is a use additional code note for the manifestation that is specific for that particular diabetic manifestation. Should a patient have more than one manifestation of diabetes, more than one code from category 250 may be used with as many manifestation codes as are needed to fully describe the patient's complete diabetic condition. The category 250 diabetes codes should be sequenced first, followed by the manifestation codes.

"Code first" and "Use additional code" notes are also used as sequencing rules in the classification for certain codes that are not part of an etiology/manifestation combination.

See - Section I.B.9. "Multiple coding for a single condition".

7. "And"

The word "and" should be interpreted to mean either "and" or "or" when it appears in a title.

8. "With"

The word "with" should be interpreted to mean "associated with" or "due to" when it appears in a code title, the Alphabetic Index, or an instructional note in the Tabular List.

The word "with" in the alphabetic index is sequenced immediately following the main term, not in alphabetical order.

9. "See" and "See Also"

The "see" instruction following a main term in the index indicates that another term should be referenced. It is necessary to go to the main term referenced with the "see" note to locate the correct code.

A "see also" instruction following a main term in the index instructs that there is another main term that may also be referenced that may provide additional index entries that may be useful. It is not necessary to follow the "see also" note when the original main term provides the necessary code.

B. General Coding Guidelines

1. Use of Both Alphabetic Index and Tabular List

Use both the Alphabetic Index and the Tabular List when locating and assigning a code. Reliance on only the Alphabetic Index or the Tabular List leads to errors in code assignments and less specificity in code selection.

2. Locate each term in the Alphabetic Index

Locate each term in the Alphabetic Index and verify the code selected in the Tabular List. Read and be guided by instructional notations that appear in both the Alphabetic Index and the Tabular List.

3. Level of Detail in Coding

Diagnosis and procedure codes are to be used at their highest number of digits available.

ICD-9-CM diagnosis codes are composed of codes with 3, 4, or 5 digits. Codes with three digits are included in ICD-9-CM as the heading of a category of codes that may be further subdivided by the use of fourth and/or fifth digits, which provide greater detail.

A three-digit code is to be used only if it is not further subdivided. Where fourth-digit subcategories and/or fifth-digit subclassifications are provided, they must be assigned. A code is invalid if it has not been coded to the full number of digits required for that code. For example, Acute myocardial infarction, code 410, has fourth digits that describe the location of the infarction (e.g., 410.2, Of inferolateral wall), and fifth digits that identify the episode of care. It would be incorrect to report a code in category 410 without a fourth and fifth digit.

ICD-9-CM Volume 3 procedure codes are composed of codes with either 3 or 4 digits. Codes with two digits are included in ICD-9-CM as the heading of a category of codes that may be further subdivided by the use of third and/or fourth digits, which provide greater detail.

4. **Code or codes from 001.0 through V91.99**

   The appropriate code or codes from 001.0 through V91.99 must be used to identify diagnoses, symptoms, conditions, problems, complaints or other reason(s) for the encounter/visit.

5. **Selection of codes 001.0 through 999.9**

   The selection of codes 001.0 through 999.9 will frequently be used to describe the reason for the admission/encounter. These codes are from the section of ICD-9-CM for the classification of diseases and injuries (e.g., infectious and parasitic diseases; neoplasms; symptoms, signs, and ill-defined conditions, etc.).

6. **Signs and symptoms**

   Codes that describe symptoms and signs, as opposed to diagnoses, are acceptable for reporting purposes when a related definitive diagnosis has not been established (confirmed) by the provider. Chapter 16 of ICD-9-CM, Symptoms, Signs, and Ill-defined conditions (codes 780.0 - 799.9) contain many, but not all codes for symptoms.

7. **Conditions that are an integral part of a disease process**

   Signs and symptoms that are associated routinely with a disease process should not be assigned as additional codes, unless otherwise instructed by the classification.

8. **Conditions that are not an integral part of a disease process**

   Additional signs and symptoms that may not be associated routinely with a disease process should be coded when present.

9. **Multiple coding for a single condition**

   In addition to the etiology/manifestation convention that requires two codes to fully describe a single condition that affects multiple body systems, there are other single conditions that also require more than one code. "Use additional code" notes are found in the tabular at codes that are not part of an etiology/manifestation pair where a secondary code is useful to fully describe a condition. The sequencing rule is the same as the etiology/manifestation pair - , "use additional code" indicates that a secondary code should be added.

   For example, for infections that are not included in chapter 1, a secondary code from category 041, Bacterial infection in conditions classified elsewhere and of unspecified site, may be required to identify the bacterial organism causing the infection. A "use additional code" note will normally be found at the infectious disease code, indicating a need for the organism code to be added as a secondary code.

   "Code first" notes are also under certain codes that are not specifically manifestation codes but may be due to an underlying cause. When a "code first" note is present and an underlying condition is present the underlying condition should be sequenced first.

   "Code, if applicable, any causal condition first", notes indicate that this code may be assigned as a principal diagnosis when the causal condition is unknown or not applicable. If a causal condition is known, then the code for that condition should be sequenced as the principal or first-listed diagnosis.

   Multiple codes may be needed for late effects, complication codes and obstetric codes to more fully describe a condition. See the specific guidelines for these conditions for further instruction.

10. **Acute and Chronic Conditions**

    If the same condition is described as both acute (subacute) and chronic, and separate subentries exist in the Alphabetic Index at the same indentation level, code both and sequence the acute (subacute) code first.

11. **Combination Code**

    A combination code is a single code used to classify:
    Two diagnoses, or
    A diagnosis with an associated secondary process (manifestation)
    A diagnosis with an associated complication

    Combination codes are identified by referring to subterm entries in the Alphabetic Index and by reading the inclusion and exclusion notes in the Tabular List.

    Assign only the combination code when that code fully identifies the diagnostic conditions involved or when the Alphabetic Index so directs. Multiple coding should not be used when the classification provides a combination code that clearly identifies all of the elements documented in the diagnosis. When the combination code lacks necessary specificity in describing the manifestation or complication, an additional code should be used as a secondary code.

12. **Late Effects**

    A late effect is the residual effect (condition produced) after the acute phase of an illness or injury has terminated. There is no time limit on when a late effect code can be used. The residual may be apparent early, such as in cerebrovascular accident cases, or it may occur months or years later, such as that due to a previous injury. Coding of late effects generally requires two codes sequenced in the following order: The condition or nature of the late effect is sequenced first. The late effect code is sequenced second.

    Exceptions to the above guidelines are those instances where the late effect code has been expanded (at the fourth and fifth-digit levels) to include the manifestation(s) **or the classification instructs otherwise.** The code for the acute phase of an illness or injury that led to the late effect is never used with a code for the late effect.

13. **Impending or Threatened Condition**

    Code any condition described at the time of discharge as "impending" or "threatened" as follows:

    If it did occur, code as confirmed diagnosis.

    If it did not occur, reference the Alphabetic Index to determine if the condition has a subentry term for "impending" or "threatened" and also reference main term entries for "Impending" and for "Threatened."

    If the subterms are listed, assign the given code.

    If the subterms are not listed, code the existing underlying condition(s) and not the condition described as impending or threatened.

14. **Reporting Same Diagnosis Code More than Once**

    Each unique ICD-9-CM diagnosis code may be reported only once for an encounter. This applies to bilateral conditions or two different conditions classified to the same ICD-9-CM diagnosis code.

15. **Admissions/Encounters for Rehabilitation**

    When the purpose for the admission/encounter is rehabilitation, sequence the appropriate V code from category V57, Care involving use of rehabilitation procedures, as the principal/first-listed diagnosis. The code for the condition for which the service is being performed should be reported as an additional diagnosis.

    Only one code from category V57 is required. Code V57.89, Other specified rehabilitation procedures, should be assigned if more than one type of rehabilitation is performed during a single encounter. A procedure code should be reported to identify each type of rehabilitation therapy actually performed.

16. **Documentation for BMI and Pressure Ulcer Stages**

    For the Body Mass Index (BMI) and pressure ulcer stage codes, code assignment may be based on medical record documentation from clinicians who are not the patient's provider (i.e., physician or other qualified healthcare practitioner legally accountable for establishing the patient's diagnosis), since this information is typically documented by other clinicians involved in the care of the patient (e.g., a dietitian often documents the BMI and nurses often documents the pressure ulcer stages). However, the associated diagnosis (such as overweight, obesity, or pressure ulcer) must be documented by the patient's provider. If there is conflicting medical record documentation, either from the same clinician or different clinicians, the patient's attending provider should be queried for clarification.

    The BMI and pressure ulcer stage codes should only be reported as secondary diagnoses. As with all other secondary diagnosis codes, the BMI and pressure ulcer stage codes should only be assigned when they meet the definition of a reportable additional diagnosis (see Section III, Reporting Additional Diagnoses).

17. **Syndromes**

    Follow the Alphabetic Index guidance when coding syndromes. In the absence of index guidance, assign codes for the documented manifestations of the syndrome.

18. **Documentation of Complications of care**

    Code assignment is based on the provider's documentation of the relationship between the condition and the care or procedure. The guideline extends to any complications of care, regardless of the chapter the code is located in. It is important to note that not all conditions that occur during or following medical care or surgery are classified as complications. There must be a cause-and-effect relationship between the care provided and the condition, and an indication in the documentation that it is a complication. Query the provider for clarification, if the complication is not clearly documented.

C. **Chapter-Specific Coding Guidelines**

In addition to general coding guidelines, there are guidelines for specific diagnoses and/or conditions in the classification. Unless otherwise indicated, these guidelines apply to all health care settings. Please refer to Section II for guidelines on the selection of principal diagnosis.

1. **Chapter 1: Infectious and Parasitic Diseases (001-139)**

    a. **Human Immunodeficiency Virus (HIV) Infections**

    1) **Code only confirmed cases**

        Code only confirmed cases of HIV infection/illness. This is an exception to the hospital inpatient guideline Section II, H.

        In this context, "confirmation" does not require documentation of positive serology or culture for HIV; the provider's diagnostic statement that the patient is HIV positive, or has an HIV-related illness is sufficient.

2) **Selection and sequencing of HIV codes**

(a) **Patient admitted for HIV-related condition**

If a patient is admitted for an HIV-related condition, the principal diagnosis should be 042, followed by additional diagnosis codes for all reported HIV-related conditions.

(b) **Patient with HIV disease admitted for unrelated condition**

If a patient with HIV disease is admitted for an unrelated condition (such as a traumatic injury), the code for the unrelated condition (e.g., the nature of injury code) should be the principal diagnosis. Other diagnoses would be 042 followed by additional diagnosis codes for all reported HIV-related conditions.

(c) **Whether the patient is newly diagnosed**

Whether the patient is newly diagnosed or has had previous admissions/encounters for HIV conditions is irrelevant to the sequencing decision.

(d) **Asymptomatic human immunodeficiency virus**

V08 Asymptomatic human immunodeficiency virus [HIV] infection, is to be applied when the patient without any documentation of symptoms is listed as being "HIV positive," "known HIV," "HIV test positive," or similar terminology. Do not use this code if the term "AIDS" is used or if the patient is treated for any HIV-related illness or is described as having any condition(s) resulting from his/her HIV positive status; use 042 in these cases.

(e) **Patients with inconclusive HIV serology**

Patients with inconclusive HIV serology, but no definitive diagnosis or manifestations of the illness, may be assigned code 795.71, Inconclusive serologic test for Human Immunodeficiency Virus [HIV].

(f) **Previously diagnosed HIV-related illness**

Patients with any known prior diagnosis of an HIV-related illness should be coded to 042. Once a patient has developed an HIV-related illness, the patient should always be assigned code 042 on every subsequent admission/encounter. Patients previously diagnosed with any HIV illness (042) should never be assigned to 795.71 or V08.

(g) **HIV Infection in Pregnancy, Childbirth and the Puerperium**

During pregnancy, childbirth or the puerperium, a patient admitted (or presenting for a health care encounter) because of an HIV-related illness should receive a principal diagnosis code of 647.6X, Other specified infectious and parasitic diseases in the mother classifiable elsewhere, but complicating the pregnancy, childbirth or the puerperium, followed by 042 and the code(s) for the HIV-related illness(es). Codes from Chapter 15 always take sequencing priority.

Patients with asymptomatic HIV infection status admitted (or presenting for a health care encounter) during pregnancy, childbirth, or the puerperium should receive codes of 647.6X and V08.

(h) **Encounters for testing for HIV**

If a patient is being seen to determine his/her HIV status, use code V73.89, Screening for other specified viral disease. Use code V69.8, Other problems related to lifestyle, as a secondary code if an asymptomatic patient is in a known high risk group for HIV. Should a patient with signs or symptoms or illness, or a confirmed HIV related diagnosis be tested for HIV, code the signs and symptoms or the diagnosis. An additional counseling code V65.44 may be used if counseling is provided during the encounter for the test.

When a patient returns to be informed of his/her HIV test results use code V65.44, HIV counseling, if the results of the test are negative.

If the results are positive but the patient is asymptomatic use code V08, Asymptomatic HIV infection. If the results are positive and the patient is symptomatic use code 042, HIV infection, with codes for the HIV related symptoms or diagnosis. The HIV counseling code may also be used if counseling is provided for patients with positive test results.

b. **Septicemia, Systemic Inflammatory Response Syndrome (SIRS), Sepsis, Severe Sepsis, and Septic Shock**

1) **SIRS, Septicemia, and Sepsis**

    (a) The terms *septicemia* and *sepsis* are often used interchangeably by providers, however they are not considered synonymous terms. The following descriptions are provided for reference but do not preclude querying the provider for clarification about terms used in the documentation:

    (i) Septicemia generally refers to a systemic disease associated with the presence of pathological microorganisms or toxins in the blood, which can include bacteria, viruses, fungi or other organisms.

    (ii) Systemic inflammatory response syndrome (SIRS) generally refers to the systemic response to infection, trauma/burns, or other insult (such as cancer) with symptoms including fever, tachycardia, tachypnea, and leukocytosis.

    (iii) Sepsis generally refers to SIRS due to infection.

    (iv) Severe sepsis generally refers to sepsis with associated acute organ dysfunction.

    (b) **The Coding of SIRS, sepsis and severe sepsis**

    The coding of SIRS, sepsis and severe sepsis requires a minimum of 2 codes: a code for the underlying cause (such as infection or trauma) and a code from subcategory 995.9 Systemic inflammatory response syndrome (SIRS).

    (i) The code for the underlying cause (such as infection or trauma) must be sequenced before the code from subcategory 995.9 Systemic inflammatory response syndrome (SIRS).

    (ii) Sepsis and severe sepsis require a code for the systemic infection (038.xx, 112.5, etc.) and either code 995.91, Sepsis, or 995.92, Severe sepsis. If the causal organism is not documented, assign code 038.9, Unspecified septicemia.

    (iii) Severe sepsis requires additional code(s) for the associated acute organ dysfunction(s).

    (iv) If a patient has sepsis with multiple organ dysfunctions, follow the instructions for coding severe sepsis.

    (v) Either the term sepsis or SIRS must be documented to assign a code from subcategory 995.9.

    (vi) *See Section I.C.17.g), Injury and poisoning, for information regarding systemic inflammatory response syndrome (SIRS) due to trauma/burns and other non-infectious processes.*

    (c) Due to the complex nature of sepsis and severe sepsis, some cases may require querying the provider prior to assignment of the codes.

2) **Sequencing sepsis and severe sepsis**

    (a) **Sepsis and severe sepsis as principal diagnosis**

    If sepsis or severe sepsis is present on admission, and meets the definition of principal diagnosis, the systemic infection code (e.g., 038.xx, 112.5, etc) should be assigned as the principal diagnosis, followed by code 995.91, Sepsis, or 995.92, Severe sepsis, as required by the sequencing rules in the Tabular List. Codes from subcategory 995.9 can never be assigned as a principal diagnosis. A code should also be assigned for any localized infection, if present.

    If the sepsis or severe sepsis is due to a postprocedural infection, see Section I.C.1.b.10 for guidelines related to sepsis due to postprocedural infection.

    (b) **Sepsis and severe sepsis as secondary diagnoses**

    When sepsis or severe sepsis develops during the encounter (it was not present on admission), the systemic infection code and code 995.91 or 995.92 should be assigned as secondary diagnoses.

    (c) **Documentation unclear as to whether sepsis or severe sepsis is present on admission**

    Sepsis or severe sepsis may be present on admission but the diagnosis may not be confirmed until sometime after admission. If the documentation is not clear whether the sepsis or severe sepsis was present on admission, the provider should be queried.

3) **Sepsis/SIRS with Localized Infection**

    If the reason for admission is both sepsis, severe sepsis, or SIRS and a localized infection, such as pneumonia or cellulitis, a code for the systemic infection (038.xx,

112.5, etc) should be assigned first, then code 995.91 or 995.92, followed by the code for the localized infection. If the patient is admitted with a localized infection, such as pneumonia, and sepsis/SIRS doesn't develop until after admission, see guideline I.C.1.b.2.b).

If the localized infection is postprocedural, *see Section I.C.1.b.10 for guidelines related to sepsis due to postprocedural infection.*

Note: The term urosepsis is a nonspecific term. If that is the only term documented then only code 599.0 should be assigned based on the default for the term in the ICD-9-CM index, in addition to the code for the causal organism if known.

4) **Bacterial Sepsis and Septicemia**

   In most cases, it will be a code from category 038, Septicemia, that will be used in conjunction with a code from subcategory 995.9 such as the following:

   (a) **Streptococcal sepsis**

   If the documentation in the record states streptococcal sepsis, codes 038.0, Streptococcal septicemia, and code 995.91 should be used, in that sequence.

   (b) **Streptococcal septicemia**

   If the documentation states streptococcal septicemia, only code 038.0 should be assigned, however, the provider should be queried whether the patient has sepsis, an infection with SIRS.

5) **Acute organ dysfunction that is not clearly associated with the sepsis**

   If a patient has sepsis and an acute organ dysfunction, but the medical record documentation indicates that the acute organ dysfunction is related to a medical condition other than the sepsis, do not assign code 995.92, Severe sepsis. An acute organ dysfunction must be associated with the sepsis in order to assign the severe sepsis code. If the documentation is not clear as to whether an acute organ dysfunction is related to the sepsis or another medical condition, query the provider.

6) **Septic shock**

   (a) **Sequencing of septic shock and postprocedural septic shock**

   Septic shock generally refers to circulatory failure associated with severe sepsis, and, therefore, it represents a type of acute organ dysfunction.

   For cases of septic shock, the code for the systemic infection should be sequenced first, followed by codes 995.92, **Severe sepsis** and 785.52, **Septic shock or 998.02, Postoperative septic shock.** Any additional codes for other acute organ dysfunctions should also be assigned. As noted in the sequencing instructions in the Tabular List, the code for septic shock cannot be assigned as a principal diagnosis.

   (b) **Septic shock and postprocedural septic shock without documentation of severe sepsis**

   Since septic shock indicates the presence of severe sepsis, **c**ode 995.92, Severe sepsis, **can be** assigned with code 785.52, Septic shock, **or code 998.02 Postoperative shock, septic,** even if the term severe sepsis is not documented in the record.

7) **Sepsis and septic shock complicating abortion and pregnancy**

   Sepsis and septic shock complicating abortion, ectopic pregnancy, and molar pregnancy are classified to category codes in Chapter 11 (630-639).

   See section I.C.11.i.7 for information on the coding of puerperal sepsis.

8) **Negative or inconclusive blood cultures**

   Negative or inconclusive blood cultures do not preclude a diagnosis of septicemia or sepsis in patients with clinical evidence of the condition, however, the provider should be queried.

9) **Newborn sepsis**

   See Section I.C.15.j for information on the coding of newborn sepsis.

10) **Sepsis due to a Postprocedural Infection**

    (a) **Documentation of causal relationship**

    As with all postprocedural complications, code assignment is based on the provider's documentation of the relationship between the infection and the procedure.

    (b) **Sepsis due to postprocedural infection**

    In cases of postprocedural sepsis, the complication code, such as code 998.59, Other postoperative infection, or 674.3x, Other complications of obstetrical surgical wounds should be coded first followed by the appropriate sepsis codes (systemic infection code and either code 995.91 or 995.92). An additional code(s) for any acute organ dysfunction should also be assigned for cases of severe sepsis.

    See Section I.C.1.b.6 if the sepsis or severe sepsis results in postprocedural septic shock.

(c) **Postprocedural infection and postprocedural septic shock**

In cases where a postprocedural infection has occurred and has resulted in severe sepsis and postprocedural septic shock, the code for the precipitating complication such as code 998.59, Other postoperative infection, or 674.3x, Other complications of obstetrical surgical wounds should be coded first followed by the appropriate sepsis codes (systemic infection code and code 995.92). Code 998.02, Postoperative septic shock, should be assigned as an additional code. In cases of severe sepsis, an additional code(s) for any acute organ dysfunction should also be assigned.

11) **External cause of injury codes with SIRS**

Refer to Section I.C.19.a.7 for instruction on the use of external cause of injury codes with codes for SIRS resulting from trauma.

12) **Sepsis and Severe Sepsis Associated with Non-infectious Process**

In some cases, a non-infectious process, such as trauma, may lead to an infection which can result in sepsis or severe sepsis. If sepsis or severe sepsis is documented as associated with a non-infectious condition, such as a burn or serious injury, and this condition meets the definition for principal diagnosis, the code for the non-infectious condition should be sequenced first, followed by the code for the systemic infection and either code 995.91, Sepsis, or 995.92, Severe sepsis. Additional codes for any associated acute organ dysfunction(s) should also be assigned for cases of severe sepsis. If the sepsis or severe sepsis meets the definition of principal diagnosis, the systemic infection and sepsis codes should be sequenced before the non-infectious condition. When both the associated non-infectious condition and the sepsis or severe sepsis meet the definition of principal diagnosis, either may be assigned as principal diagnosis.

See Section I.C.1.b.2.a for guidelines pertaining to sepsis or severe sepsis as the principal diagnosis.

Only one code from subcategory 995.9 should be assigned. Therefore, when a non-infectious condition leads to an infection resulting in sepsis or severe sepsis, assign either code 995.91 or 995.92. Do not additionally assign code 995.93, Systemic inflammatory response syndrome due to non-infectious process without acute organ dysfunction, or 995.94, Systemic inflammatory response syndrome with acute organ dysfunction.

See Section I.C.17.g for information on the coding of SIRS due to trauma/burns or other non-infectious disease processes.

c. **Methicillin Resistant *Staphylococcus aureus* (MRSA) Conditions**

1) **Selection and sequencing of MRSA codes**

(a) **Combination codes for MRSA infection**

When a patient is diagnosed with an infection that is due to methicillin resistant *Staphylococcus aureus* (MRSA), and that infection has a combination code that includes the causal organism (e.g., septicemia, pneumonia) assign the appropriate code for the condition (e.g., code 038.12, Methicillin resistant Staphylococcus aureus septicemia or code 482.42, Methicillin resistant pneumonia due to Staphylococcus aureus). Do not assign code 041.12, Methicillin resistant Staphylococcus aureus, as an additional code because the code includes the type of infection and the MRSA organism. Do not assign a code from subcategory V09.0, Infection with microorganisms resistant to penicillins, as an additional diagnosis.

See Section C.1.b.1 for instructions on coding and sequencing of septicemia.

(b) **Other codes for MRSA infection**

When there is documentation of a current infection (e.g., wound infection, stitch abscess, urinary tract infection) due to MRSA, and that infection does not have a combination code that includes the causal organism, select the appropriate code to identify the condition along with code 041.12, Methicillin resistant Staphylococcus aureus, for the MRSA infection. Do not assign a code from subcategory V09.0, Infection with microorganisms resistant to penicillins.

(c) **Methicillin susceptible Staphylococcus aureus (MSSA) and MRSA colonization**

The condition or state of being colonized or carrying MSSA or MRSA is called colonization or carriage, while an individual person is described as being colonized or being a carrier. Colonization means that MSSA or MSRA is present on or in the body without necessarily causing illness. A positive MRSA colonization test might be documented by the provider as "MRSA screen positive" or "MRSA nasal swab positive".

Assign code V02.54, Carrier or suspected carrier, Methicillin resistant Staphylococcus aureus, for patients documented as having MRSA colonization. Assign code V02.53, Carrier or suspected carrier, Methicillin susceptible Staphylococcus aureus, for patient documented as having MSSA colonization. Colonization is not necessarily indicative of a disease process or as the cause of a specific condition the patient may have unless documented as such by the provider.

Code V02.59, Other specified bacterial diseases, should be assigned for other types of staphylococcal colonization (e.g., *S. epidermidis, S. saprophyticus*). Code V02.59 should not be assigned for colonization with any type of *Staphylococcus aureus* (MRSA, MSSA).

(d) **MRSA colonization and infection**

If a patient is documented as having both MRSA colonization and infection during a hospital admission, code V02.54, Carrier or suspected carrier, Methicillin resistant *Staphylococcus aureus*, and a code for the MRSA infection may both be assigned.

2. **Chapter 2: Neoplasms (140-239)**

<u>General guidelines</u>

Chapter 2 of the ICD-9-CM contains the codes for most benign and all malignant neoplasms. Certain benign neoplasms, such as prostatic adenomas, may be found in the specific body system chapters. To properly code a neoplasm it is necessary to determine from the record if the neoplasm is benign, in-situ, malignant, or of uncertain histologic behavior. If malignant, any secondary (metastatic) sites should also be determined.

The neoplasm table in the Alphabetic Index should be referenced first. However, if the histological term is documented, that term should be referenced first, rather than going immediately to the Neoplasm Table, in order to determine which column in the Neoplasm Table is appropriate. For example, if the documentation indicates "adenoma," refer to the term in the Alphabetic Index to review the entries under this term and the instructional note to "see also neoplasm, by site, benign." The table provides the proper code based on the type of neoplasm and the site. It is important to select the proper column in the table that corresponds to the type of neoplasm. The tabular should then be referenced to verify that the correct code has been selected from the table and that a more specific site code does not exist.

See Section I.C.18.d.4. for information regarding V codes for genetic susceptibility to cancer.

a. **Treatment directed at the malignancy**

If the treatment is directed at the malignancy, designate the malignancy as the principal diagnosis.

The only exception to this guideline is if a patient admission/encounter is solely for the administration of chemotherapy, immunotherapy or radiation therapy, assign the appropriate V58.x code as the first-listed or principal diagnosis, and the diagnosis or problem for which the service is being performed as a secondary diagnosis.

b. **Treatment of secondary site**

When a patient is admitted because of a primary neoplasm with metastasis and treatment is directed toward the secondary site only, the secondary neoplasm is designated as the principal diagnosis even though the primary malignancy is still present.

c. **Coding and sequencing of complications**

Coding and sequencing of complications associated with the malignancies or with the therapy thereof are subject to the following guidelines:

1) **Anemia associated with malignancy**

When admission/encounter is for management of an anemia associated with the malignancy, and the treatment is only for anemia, the appropriate anemia code (such as code 285.22, Anemia in neoplastic disease) is designated as the principal diagnosis and is followed by the appropriate code(s) for the malignancy.

Code 285.22 may also be used as a secondary code if the patient suffers from anemia and is being treated for the malignancy.

If anemia in neoplastic disease and anemia due to antineoplastic chemotherapy are both documented, **assign codes for both conditions**.

2) **Anemia associated with chemotherapy, immunotherapy and radiation therapy**

When the admission/encounter is for management of an anemia associated with chemotherapy, immunotherapy or radiotherapy and the only treatment is for the anemia, the anemia is sequenced first. The appropriate neoplasm code should be assigned as an additional code.

3) **Management of dehydration due to the malignancy**

When the admission/encounter is for management of dehydration due to the malignancy or the therapy, or a combination of both, and only the dehydration is being treated (intravenous rehydration), the dehydration is sequenced first, followed by the code(s) for the malignancy.

4) Treatment of a complication resulting from a surgical procedure

When the admission/encounter is for treatment of a complication resulting from a surgical procedure, designate the complication as the principal or first-listed diagnosis if treatment is directed at resolving the complication.

d. Primary malignancy previously excised

When a primary malignancy has been previously excised or eradicated from its site and there is no further treatment directed to that site and there is no evidence of any existing primary malignancy, a code from category V10, Personal history of malignant neoplasm, should be used to indicate the former site of the malignancy. Any mention of extension, invasion, or metastasis to another site is coded as a secondary malignant neoplasm to that site. The secondary site may be the principal or first-listed with the V10 code used as a secondary code.

e. Admissions/Encounters involving chemotherapy, immunotherapy and radiation therapy

1) Episode of care involves surgical removal of neoplasm

When an episode of care involves the surgical removal of a neoplasm, primary or secondary site, followed by adjunct chemotherapy or radiation treatment during the same episode of care, the neoplasm code should be assigned as principal or first-listed diagnosis, using codes in the 140-198 series or where appropriate in the 200-203 series.

2) Patient admission/encounter solely for administration of chemotherapy, immunotherapy and radiation therapy

If a patient admission/encounter is solely for the administration of chemotherapy, immunotherapy or radiation therapy assign code V58.0, Encounter for radiation therapy, or V58.11, Encounter for antineoplastic chemotherapy, or V58.12, Encounter for antineoplastic immunotherapy as the first-listed or principal diagnosis. If a patient receives more than one of these therapies during the same admission more than one of these codes may be assigned, in any sequence.

The malignancy for which the therapy is being administered should be assigned as a secondary diagnosis.

3) Patient admitted for radiotherapy/chemotherapy and immunotherapy and develops complications

When a patient is admitted for the purpose of radiotherapy, immunotherapy or chemotherapy and develops complications such as uncontrolled nausea and vomiting or dehydration, the principal or first-listed diagnosis is V58.0, Encounter for radiotherapy, or V58.11, Encounter for antineoplastic chemotherapy, or V58.12, Encounter for antineoplastic immunotherapy followed by any codes for the complications.

f. Admission/encounter to determine extent of malignancy

When the reason for admission/encounter is to determine the extent of the malignancy, or for a procedure such as paracentesis or thoracentesis, the primary malignancy or appropriate metastatic site is designated as the principal or first-listed diagnosis, even though chemotherapy or radiotherapy is administered.

g. Symptoms, signs, and ill-defined conditions listed in Chapter 16 associated with neoplasms

Symptoms, signs, and ill-defined conditions listed in Chapter 16 characteristic of, or associated with, an existing primary or secondary site malignancy cannot be used to replace the malignancy as principal or first-listed diagnosis, regardless of the number of admissions or encounters for treatment and care of the neoplasm.

h. Admission/encounter for pain control/management

See Section I.C.6.a.5 for information on coding admission/encounter for pain control/management.

i. Malignant neoplasm associated with transplanted organ

A malignant neoplasm of a transplanted organ should be coded as a transplant complication. Assign first the appropriate code from subcategory 996.8, Complications of transplanted organ, followed by code 199.2, Malignant neoplasm associated with transplanted organ. Use an additional code for the specific malignancy.

3. Chapter 3: Endocrine, Nutritional, and Metabolic Diseases and Immunity Disorders (240-279)

a. Diabetes mellitus

Codes under category 250, Diabetes mellitus, identify complications/manifestations associated with diabetes mellitus. A fifth-digit is required for all category 250 codes to identify the type of diabetes mellitus and whether the diabetes is controlled or uncontrolled.

See I.C.3.a.7 for secondary diabetes

1) Fifth-digits for category 250:

The following are the fifth-digits for the codes under category 250:

0   type II or unspecified type, not stated as uncontrolled

1   type I, [juvenile type], not stated as uncontrolled

2   type II or unspecified type, uncontrolled

3   type I, [juvenile type], uncontrolled

The age of a patient is not the sole determining factor, though most type I diabetics develop the condition before reaching puberty. For this reason type I diabetes mellitus is also referred to as juvenile diabetes.

2) **Type of diabetes mellitus not documented**

If the type of diabetes mellitus is not documented in the medical record the default is type II.

3) **Diabetes mellitus and the use of insulin**

All type I diabetics must use insulin to replace what their bodies do not produce. However, the use of insulin does not mean that a patient is a type I diabetic. Some patients with type II diabetes mellitus are unable to control their blood sugar through diet and oral medication alone and do require insulin. If the documentation in a medical record does not indicate the type of diabetes but does indicate that the patient uses insulin, the appropriate fifth-digit for type II must be used. For type II patients who routinely use insulin, code V58.67, Long-term (current) use of insulin, should also be assigned to indicate that the patient uses insulin. Code V58.67 should not be assigned if insulin is given temporarily to bring a type II patient's blood sugar under control during an encounter.

4) **Assigning and sequencing diabetes codes and associated conditions**

When assigning codes for diabetes and its associated conditions, the code(s) from category 250 must be sequenced before the codes for the associated conditions. The diabetes codes and the secondary codes that correspond to them are paired codes that follow the etiology/manifestation convention of the classification *(See Section I.A.6., Etiology/manifestation convention)*. Assign as many codes from category 250 as needed to identify all of the associated conditions that the patient has. The corresponding secondary codes are listed under each of the diabetes codes.

(a) **Diabetic retinopathy/diabetic macular edema**

Diabetic macular edema, code 362.07, is only present with diabetic retinopathy. Another code from subcategory 362.0, Diabetic retinopathy, must be used with code 362.07. Codes under subcategory 362.0 are diabetes manifestation codes, so they must be used following the appropriate diabetes code.

5) **Diabetes mellitus in pregnancy and gestational diabetes**

(a) For diabetes mellitus complicating pregnancy, see Section I.C.11.f., Diabetes mellitus in pregnancy.

(b) For gestational diabetes, see Section I.C.11, g., Gestational diabetes.

6) **Insulin pump malfunction**

(a) **Underdose of insulin due insulin pump failure**

An underdose of insulin due to an insulin pump failure should be assigned 996.57, Mechanical complication due to insulin pump, as the principal or first listed code, followed by the appropriate diabetes mellitus code based on documentation.

(b) **Overdose of insulin due to insulin pump failure**

The principal or first listed code for an encounter due to an insulin pump malfunction resulting in an overdose of insulin, should also be 996.57, Mechanical complication due to insulin pump, followed by code 962.3, Poisoning by insulins and antidiabetic agents, and the appropriate diabetes mellitus code based on documentation.

7) **Secondary Diabetes Mellitus**

Codes under category 249, Secondary diabetes mellitus, identify complications/manifestations associated with secondary diabetes mellitus. Secondary diabetes is always caused by another condition or event (e.g., cystic fibrosis, malignant neoplasm of pancreas, pancreatectomy, adverse effect of drug, or poisoning).

(a) **Fifth-digits for category 249:**

A fifth-digit is required for all category 249 codes to identify whether the diabetes is controlled or uncontrolled.

(b) **Secondary diabetes mellitus and the use of insulin**

For patients who routinely use insulin, code V58.67, Long-term (current) use of insulin, should also be assigned. Code V58.67 should not be assigned if insulin is given temporarily to bring a patient's blood sugar under control during an encounter.

(c) **Assigning and sequencing secondary diabetes codes and associated conditions**

When assigning codes for secondary diabetes and its associated conditions (e.g. renal manifestations), the code(s) from category 249 must be sequenced before the codes for the associated conditions. The secondary diabetes codes and the diabetic manifestation codes that correspond to them are paired codes that follow the etiology/manifestation convention of the classification. Assign as many codes from category 249 as needed to identify all of the associated conditions that the patient has. The corresponding codes for the associated conditions are listed under each of the secondary diabetes codes. For example, secondary diabetes with diabetic nephrosis is assigned to code 249.40, followed by 581.81.

(d) **Assigning and sequencing secondary diabetes codes and its causes**

The sequencing of the secondary diabetes codes in relationship to codes for the cause of the diabetes is based on the reason for the encounter, applicable ICD-9-CM sequencing conventions, and chapter-specific guidelines.

If a patient is seen for treatment of the secondary diabetes or one of its associated conditions, a code from category 249 is sequenced as the principal or first-listed diagnosis, with the cause of the secondary diabetes (e.g. cystic fibrosis) sequenced as an additional diagnosis.

If, however, the patient is seen for the treatment of the condition causing the secondary diabetes (e.g., malignant neoplasm of pancreas), the code for the cause of the secondary diabetes should be sequenced as the principal or first-listed diagnosis followed by a code from category 249.

(i) **Secondary diabetes mellitus due to pancreatectomy**

For postpancreatectomy diabetes mellitus (lack of insulin due to the surgical removal of all or part of the pancreas), assign code 251.3, Postsurgical hypoinsulinemia. Assign a code from subcategory 249, Secondary diabetes mellitus and a code from subcategory V88.1, Acquired absence of pancreas as additional codes. Code also any diabetic manifestations (e.g. diabetic nephrosis 581.81).

(ii) **Secondary diabetes due to drugs**

Secondary diabetes may be caused by an adverse effect of correctly administered medications, poisoning or late effect of poisoning.

See section I.C.17.e for coding of adverse effects and poisoning, and section I.C.19 for E code reporting.

4. **Chapter 4: Diseases of Blood and Blood Forming Organs (280-289)**

   a. **Anemia of chronic disease**

   Subcategory 285.2, Anemia in chronic illness, has codes for anemia in chronic kidney disease, code 285.21; anemia in neoplastic disease, code 285.22; and anemia in other chronic illness, code 285.29. These codes can be used as the principal/first listed code if the reason for the encounter is to treat the anemia. They may also be used as secondary codes if treatment of the anemia is a component of an encounter, but not the primary reason for the encounter. When using a code from subcategory 285 it is also necessary to use the code for the chronic condition causing the anemia.

   1) **Anemia in chronic kidney disease**

   When assigning code 285.21, Anemia in chronic kidney disease, it is also necessary to assign a code from category 585, Chronic kidney disease, to indicate the stage of chronic kidney disease.

   See I.C.10.a. Chronic kidney disease (CKD).

   2) **Anemia in neoplastic disease**

   When assigning code 285.22, Anemia in neoplastic disease, it is also necessary to assign the neoplasm code that is responsible for the anemia. Code 285.22 is for use for anemia that is due to the malignancy, not for anemia due to antineoplastic chemotherapy drugs. Assign **the appropriate code** for anemia due to antineoplastic chemotherapy.

   See I.C.2.c.1 Anemia associated with malignancy.

   See I.C.2.c.2 Anemia associated with chemotherapy, immunotherapy and radiation therapy.

   See I.C.17.e.1. Adverse effects.

5. **Chapter 5: Mental Disorders (290-319)**

   Reserved for future guideline expansion

6. **Chapter 6: Diseases of Nervous System and Sense Organs (320-389)**
   a. **Pain - Category 338**
      1) **General coding information**

         Codes in category 338 may be used in conjunction with codes from other categories and chapters to provide more detail about acute or chronic pain and neoplasm-related pain, unless otherwise indicated below.

         If the pain is not specified as acute or chronic, do not assign codes from category 338, except for post-thoracotomy pain, postoperative pain, neoplasm related pain, or central pain syndrome.

         A code from subcategories 338.1 and 338.2 should not be assigned if the underlying (definitive) diagnosis is known, unless the reason for the encounter is pain control/management and not management of the underlying condition.

         (a) **Category 338 Codes as Principal or First-Listed Diagnosis**

            Category 338 codes are acceptable as principal diagnosis or the first-listed code:

            - When pain control or pain management is the reason for the admission/encounter (e.g., a patient with displaced intervertebral disc, nerve impingement and severe back pain presents for injection of steroid into the spinal canal). The underlying cause of the pain should be reported as an additional diagnosis, if known.
            - When an admission or encounter is for a procedure aimed at treating the underlying condition (e.g., spinal fusion, kyphoplasty), a code for the underlying condition (e.g., vertebral fracture, spinal stenosis) should be assigned as the principal diagnosis. No code from category 338 should be assigned.
            - When a patient is admitted for the insertion of a neurostimulator for pain control, assign the appropriate pain code as the principal or first listed diagnosis. When an admission or encounter is for a procedure aimed at treating the underlying condition and a neurostimulator is inserted for pain control during the same admission/encounter, a code for the underlying condition should be assigned as the principal diagnosis and the appropriate pain code should be assigned as a secondary diagnosis.

         (b) **Use of Category 338 Codes in Conjunction with Site Specific Pain Codes**

            (i) **Assigning Category 338 Codes and Site-Specific Pain Codes**

               Codes from category 338 may be used in conjunction with codes that identify the site of pain (including codes from chapter 16) if the category 338 code provides additional information. For example, if the code describes the site of the pain, but does not fully describe whether the pain is acute or chronic, then both codes should be assigned.

            (ii) **Sequencing of Category 338 Codes with Site-Specific Pain Codes**

               The sequencing of category 338 codes with site-specific pain codes (including chapter 16 codes), is dependent on the circumstances of the encounter/admission as follows:

               - If the encounter is for pain control or pain management, assign the code from category 338 followed by the code identifying the specific site of pain (e.g., encounter for pain management for acute neck pain from trauma is assigned code 338.11, Acute pain due to trauma, followed by code 723.1, Cervicalgia, to identify the site of pain).
               - If the encounter is for any other reason except pain control or pain management, and a related definitive diagnosis has not been established (confirmed) by the provider, assign the code for the specific site of pain first, followed by the appropriate code from category 338.

      2) **Pain due to devices, implants and grafts**

         Pain associated with devices, implants or grafts left in a surgical site (for example painful hip prosthesis) is assigned to the appropriate code(s) found in Chapter 17, Injury and Poisoning. Use additional code(s) from category 338 to identify acute or chronic pain due to presence of the device, implant or graft (338.18-338.19 or 338.28-338.29).

3) Postoperative Pain

Post-thoracotomy pain and other postoperative pain are classified to subcategories 338.1 and 338.2, depending on whether the pain is acute or chronic. The default for post-thoracotomy and other postoperative pain not specified as acute or chronic is the code for the acute form.

Routine or expected postoperative pain immediately after surgery should not be coded.

(a) Postoperative pain not associated with specific postoperative complication

Postoperative pain not associated with a specific postoperative complication is assigned to the appropriate postoperative pain code in category 338.

(b) Postoperative pain associated with specific postoperative complication

Postoperative pain associated with a specific postoperative complication (such as painful wire sutures) is assigned to the appropriate code(s) found in Chapter 17, Injury and Poisoning. If appropriate, use additional code(s) from category 338 to identify acute or chronic pain (338.18 or 338.28). If pain control/management is the reason for the encounter, a code from category 338 should be assigned as the principal or first-listed diagnosis in accordance with *Section I.C.6.a.1.a above.*

(c) Postoperative pain as principal or first-listed diagnosis

Postoperative pain may be reported as the principal or first-listed diagnosis when the stated reason for the admission/encounter is documented as postoperative pain control/management.

(d) Postoperative pain as secondary diagnosis

Postoperative pain may be reported as a secondary diagnosis code when a patient presents for outpatient surgery and develops an unusual or inordinate amount of postoperative pain.

The provider's documentation should be used to guide the coding of postoperative pain, as well as *Section III. Reporting Additional Diagnoses* and *Section IV. Diagnostic Coding and Reporting in the Outpatient Setting.*

See Section II.I.2 for information on sequencing of diagnoses for patients admitted to hospital inpatient care following post-operative observation.

See Section II.J for information on sequencing of diagnoses for patients admitted to hospital inpatient care from outpatient surgery.

See Section IV.A.2 for information on sequencing of diagnoses for patients admitted for observation.

4) Chronic pain

Chronic pain is classified to subcategory 338.2. There is no time frame defining when pain becomes chronic pain. The provider's documentation should be used to guide use of these codes.

5) Neoplasm Related Pain

Code 338.3 is assigned to pain documented as being related, associated or due to cancer, primary or secondary malignancy, or tumor. This code is assigned regardless of whether the pain is acute or chronic.

This code may be assigned as the principal or first-listed code when the stated reason for the admission/encounter is documented as pain control/pain management. The underlying neoplasm should be reported as an additional diagnosis.

When the reason for the admission/encounter is management of the neoplasm and the pain associated with the neoplasm is also documented, code 338.3 may be assigned as an additional diagnosis.

See Section I.C.2 for instructions on the sequencing of neoplasms for all other stated reasons for the admission/encounter (except for pain control/pain management).

6) Chronic pain syndrome

This condition is different than the term "chronic pain," and therefore this code should only be used when the provider has specifically documented this condition.

b. Glaucoma

1) Glaucoma

For types of glaucoma classified to subcategories 365.1-365.6, an additional code should be assigned from subcategory 365.7, Glaucoma stage, to identify the glaucoma stage. Codes from 365.7, Glaucoma stage, may not be assigned as a principal or first-listed diagnosis.

2) Bilateral glaucoma with same stage

When a patient has bilateral glaucoma and both are documented as being the same type and stage, report only the code for the type of glaucoma and one code for the stage.

3) **Bilateral glaucoma stage with different stages**

When a patient has bilateral glaucoma and each eye is documented as having a different stage, assign one code for the type of glaucoma and one code for the highest glaucoma stage.

4) **Bilateral glaucoma with different types and different stages**

When a patient has bilateral glaucoma and each eye is documented as having a different type and a different stage, assign one code for each type of glaucoma and one code for the highest glaucoma stage.

5) **Patient admitted with glaucoma and stage evolves during the admission**

If a patient is admitted with glaucoma and the stage progresses during the admission, assign the code for highest stage documented.

6) **Indeterminate stage glaucoma**

Assignment of code 365.74, Indeterminate stage glaucoma, should be based on the clinical documentation. Code 365.74 is used for glaucomas whose stage cannot be clinically determined. This code should not be confused with code 365.70, Glaucoma stage, unspecified. Code 365.70 should be assigned when there is no documentation regarding the stage of the glaucoma.

7. **Chapter 7: Diseases of Circulatory System (390-459)**

   a. **Hypertension**

   Hypertension Table

   The Hypertension Table, found under the main term, "Hypertension", in the Alphabetic Index, contains a complete listing of all conditions due to or associated with hypertension and classifies them according to malignant, benign, and unspecified.

   1) **Hypertension, Essential, or NOS**

   Assign hypertension (arterial) (essential) (primary) (systemic) (NOS) to category code 401 with the appropriate fourth digit to indicate malignant (.0), benign (.1), or unspecified (.9). Do not use either .0 malignant or .1 benign unless medical record documentation supports such a designation.

   2) **Hypertension with Heart Disease**

   Heart conditions (425.8, 429.0-429.3, 429.8, 429.9) are assigned to a code from category 402 when a causal relationship is stated (due to hypertension) or implied (hypertensive). Use an additional code from category 428 to identify the type of heart failure in those patients with heart failure. More than one code from category 428 may be assigned if the patient has systolic or diastolic failure and congestive heart failure.

   The same heart conditions (425.8, 429.0-429.3, 429.8, 429.9) with hypertension, but without a stated causal relationship, are coded separately. Sequence according to the circumstances of the admission/encounter.

   3) **Hypertensive Chronic Kidney Disease**

   Assign codes from category 403, Hypertensive chronic kidney disease, when conditions classified to category 585 or code 587 are present with hypertension. Unlike hypertension with heart disease, ICD-9-CM presumes a cause-and-effect relationship and classifies chronic kidney disease (CKD) with hypertension as hypertensive chronic kidney disease.

   Fifth digits for category 403 should be assigned as follows:

   - 0 with CKD stage I through stage IV, or unspecified.
   - 1 with CKD stage V or end stage renal disease.

   The appropriate code from category 585, Chronic kidney disease, should be used as a secondary code with a code from category 403 to identify the stage of chronic kidney disease.

   See Section I.C.10.a for information on the coding of chronic kidney disease.

   4) **Hypertensive Heart and Chronic Kidney Disease**

   Assign codes from combination category 404, Hypertensive heart and chronic kidney disease, when both hypertensive kidney disease and hypertensive heart disease are stated in the diagnosis. Assume a relationship between the hypertension and the chronic kidney disease, whether or not the condition is so designated. Assign an additional code from category 428, to identify the type of heart failure. More than one code from category 428 may be assigned if the patient has systolic or diastolic failure and congestive heart failure.

   Fifth digits for category 404 should be assigned as follows:

   - 0 without heart failure and with chronic kidney disease (CKD) stage I through stage IV, or unspecified
   - 1 with heart failure and with CKD stage I through stage IV, or unspecified
   - 2 without heart failure and with CKD stage V or end stage renal disease
   - 3 with heart failure and with CKD stage V or end stage renal disease

The appropriate code from category 585, Chronic kidney disease, should be used as a secondary code with a code from category 404 to identify the stage of kidney disease.

See Section I.C.10.a for information on the coding of chronic kidney disease.

5) **Hypertensive Cerebrovascular Disease**

   First assign codes from 430-438, Cerebrovascular disease, then the appropriate hypertension code from categories 401-405.

6) **Hypertensive Retinopathy**

   Two codes are necessary to identify the condition. First assign the code from subcategory 362.11, Hypertensive retinopathy, then the appropriate code from categories 401-405 to indicate the type of hypertension.

7) **Hypertension, Secondary**

   Two codes are required: one to identify the underlying etiology and one from category 405 to identify the hypertension. Sequencing of codes is determined by the reason for admission/encounter.

8) **Hypertension, Transient**

   Assign code 796.2, Elevated blood pressure reading without diagnosis of hypertension, unless patient has an established diagnosis of hypertension. Assign code 642.3x for transient hypertension of pregnancy.

9) **Hypertension, Controlled**

   Assign appropriate code from categories 401-405. This diagnostic statement usually refers to an existing state of hypertension under control by therapy.

10) **Hypertension, Uncontrolled**

    Uncontrolled hypertension may refer to untreated hypertension or hypertension not responding to current therapeutic regimen. In either case, assign the appropriate code from categories 401-405 to designate the stage and type of hypertension. Code to the type of hypertension.

11) **Elevated Blood Pressure**

    For a statement of elevated blood pressure without further specificity, assign code 796.2, Elevated blood pressure reading without diagnosis of hypertension, rather than a code from category 401.

b. **Cerebral infarction/stroke/cerebrovascular accident (CVA)**

   The terms stroke and CVA are often used interchangeably to refer to a cerebral infarction. The terms stroke, CVA, and cerebral infarction NOS are all indexed to the default code 434.91, Cerebral artery occlusion, unspecified, with infarction.

   Additional code(s) should be assigned for any neurologic deficits associated with the acute CVA, regardless of whether or not the neurologic deficit resolves prior to discharge.

   See Section I.C.18.d.3 for information on coding status post administration of tPA in a different facility within the last 24 hours.

c. **Postoperative cerebrovascular accident**

   A cerebrovascular hemorrhage or infarction that occurs as a result of medical intervention is coded to 997.02, Iatrogenic cerebrovascular infarction or hemorrhage. Medical record documentation should clearly specify the cause-and-effect relationship between the medical intervention and the cerebrovascular accident in order to assign this code. A secondary code from the code range 430-432 or from a code from subcategories 433 or 434 with a fifth digit of "1" should also be used to identify the type of hemorrhage or infarct.

   This guideline conforms to the use additional code note instruction at category 997. Code 436, Acute, but ill-defined, cerebrovascular disease, should not be used as a secondary code with code 997.02.

d. **Late Effects of Cerebrovascular Disease**

   1) **Category 438, Late Effects of Cerebrovascular disease**

      Category 438 is used to indicate conditions classifiable to categories 430-437 as the causes of late effects (neurologic deficits), themselves classified elsewhere. These "late effects" include neurologic deficits that persist after initial onset of conditions classifiable to 430-437. The neurologic deficits caused by cerebrovascular disease may be present from the onset or may arise at any time after the onset of the condition classifiable to 430-437.

      Codes in category 438 are only for use for late effects of cerebrovascular disease, not for neurologic deficits associated with an acute CVA.

   2) **Codes from category 438 with codes from 430-437**

      Codes from category 438 may be assigned on a health care record with codes from 430-437, if the patient has a current cerebrovascular accident (CVA) and deficits from an old CVA.

   3) **Code V12.54**

      Assign code V12.54, Transient ischemic attack (TIA), and cerebral infarction without residual deficits (and not a code from category 438) as an additional code for history of cerebrovascular disease when no neurologic deficits are present.

e. **Acute myocardial infarction (AMI)**

  1) **ST elevation myocardial infarction (STEMI) and non ST elevation myocardial infarction (NSTEMI)**

     The ICD-9-CM codes for acute myocardial infarction (AMI) identify the site, such as anterolateral wall or true posterior wall. Subcategories 410.0-410.6 and 410.8 are used for ST elevation myocardial infarction (STEMI). Subcategory 410.7, Subendocardial infarction, is used for non ST elevation myocardial infarction (NSTEMI) and nontransmural MIs.

  2) **Acute myocardial infarction, unspecified**

     Subcategory 410.9 is the default for the unspecified term acute myocardial infarction. If only STEMI or transmural MI without the site is documented, query the provider as to the site, or assign a code from subcategory 410.9.

  3) **AMI documented as nontransmural or subendocardial but site provided**

     If an AMI is documented as nontransmural or subendocardial, but the site is provided, it is still coded as a subendocardial AMI. If NSTEMI evolves to STEMI, assign the STEMI code. If STEMI converts to NSTEMI due to thrombolytic therapy, it is still coded as STEMI.

     See Section I.C.18.d.3 for information on coding status post administration of tPA in a different facility within the last 24 hours.

8. **Chapter 8: Diseases of Respiratory System (460-519)**

   See I.C.17.f. for ventilator-associated pneumonia.

   a. **Chronic Obstructive Pulmonary Disease [COPD] and Asthma**

     1) **Conditions that comprise COPD and Asthma**

        The conditions that comprise COPD are obstructive chronic bronchitis, subcategory 491.2, and emphysema, category 492. All asthma codes are under category 493, Asthma. Code 496, Chronic airway obstruction, not elsewhere classified, is a nonspecific code that should only be used when the documentation in a medical record does not specify the type of COPD being treated.

     2) **Acute exacerbation of chronic obstructive bronchitis and asthma**

        The codes for chronic obstructive bronchitis and asthma distinguish between uncomplicated cases and those in acute exacerbation. An acute exacerbation is a worsening or a decompensation of a chronic condition. An acute exacerbation is not equivalent to an infection superimposed on a chronic condition, though an exacerbation may be triggered by an infection.

     3) **Overlapping nature of the conditions that comprise COPD and asthma**

        Due to the overlapping nature of the conditions that make up COPD and asthma, there are many variations in the way these conditions are documented. Code selection must be based on the terms as documented. When selecting the correct code for the documented type of COPD and asthma, it is essential to first review the index, and then verify the code in the tabular list. There are many instructional notes under the different COPD subcategories and codes. It is important that all such notes be reviewed to assure correct code assignment.

     4) **Acute exacerbation of asthma and status asthmaticus**

        An acute exacerbation of asthma is an increased severity of the asthma symptoms, such as wheezing and shortness of breath. Status asthmaticus refers to a patient's failure to respond to therapy administered during an asthmatic episode and is a life threatening complication that requires emergency care. If status asthmaticus is documented by the provider with any type of COPD or with acute bronchitis, the status asthmaticus should be sequenced first. It supersedes any type of COPD including that with acute exacerbation or acute bronchitis. It is inappropriate to assign an asthma code with 5th digit 2, with acute exacerbation, together with an asthma code with 5th digit 1, with status asthmatics. Only the 5th digit 1 should be assigned.

   b. **Chronic Obstructive Pulmonary Disease [COPD] and Bronchitis**

     1) **Acute bronchitis with COPD**

        Acute bronchitis, code 466.0, is due to an infectious organism. When acute bronchitis is documented with COPD, code 491.22, Obstructive chronic bronchitis with acute bronchitis, should be assigned. It is not necessary to also assign code 466.0. If a medical record documents acute bronchitis with COPD with acute exacerbation, only code 491.22 should be assigned. The acute bronchitis included in code 491.22 supersedes the acute exacerbation. If a medical record documents COPD with acute exacerbation without mention of acute bronchitis, only code 491.21 should be assigned.

c. **Acute Respiratory Failure**

1) **Acute respiratory failure as principal diagnosis**

   Acute respiratory failure, may be assigned as a principal diagnosis when it is the condition established after study to be chiefly responsible for occasioning the admission to the hospital, and the selection is supported by the Alphabetic Index and Tabular List. However, chapter-specific coding guidelines (such as obstetrics, poisoning, HIV, newborn) that provide sequencing direction take precedence.

2) **Acute respiratory failure as secondary diagnosis**

   Respiratory failure may be listed as a secondary diagnosis if it occurs after admission, or if it is present on admission, but does not meet the definition of principal diagnosis.

3) **Sequencing of acute respiratory failure and another acute condition**

   When a patient is admitted with respiratory failure and another acute condition, (e.g., myocardial infarction, cerebrovascular accident, aspiration pneumonia), the principal diagnosis will not be the same in every situation. This applies whether the other acute condition is a respiratory or nonrespiratory condition. Selection of the principal diagnosis will be dependent on the circumstances of admission. If both the respiratory failure and the other acute condition are equally responsible for occasioning the admission to the hospital, and there are no chapter-specific sequencing rules, the guideline regarding two or more diagnoses that equally meet the definition for principal diagnosis *(Section II, C.)* may be applied in these situations.

   If the documentation is not clear as to whether acute respiratory failure and another condition are equally responsible for occasioning the admission, query the provider for clarification.

d. **Influenza due to *certain* identified *viruses***

   Code only confirmed cases of avian influenza (codes 488.01-488.02, 488.09, Influenza due to indentified avian influenza virus), **2009** H1N1 influenza virus (codes 488.11-488.12, 488.19), **or novel influenza A (codes 488.81-488.82, 488.89, Influenza due to identified novel influenza A virus).** This is an exception to the hospital inpatient guideline Section II, H. (Uncertain Diagnosis).

   In this context, "confirmation" does not require documentation of positive laboratory testing specific for avian, **2009 H1N1** or novel influenza A virus. However, coding should be based on the provider's diagnostic statement that the patient has avian **influenza, 2009 H1N1 influenza,** or novel influenza **A.**

   If the provider records "suspected" or "possible" or "probable" avian, **2009 H1N1,** or novel influenza **A,** the appropriate influenza code from category 487**, Influenza** should be assigned. A code from category 488, Influenza due to certain identified avian influenza viruses, should not be assigned.

9. **Chapter 9: Diseases of Digestive System (520-579)**

   Reserved for future guideline expansion

10. **Chapter 10: Diseases of Genitourinary System (580-629)**

    a. **Chronic kidney disease**

    1) **Stages of chronic kidney disease (CKD)**

       The ICD-9-CM classifies CKD based on severity. The severity of CKD is designated by stages I-V. Stage II, code 585.2, equates to mild CKD; stage III, code 585.3, equates to moderate CKD; and stage IV, code 585.4, equates to severe CKD. Code 585.6, End stage renal disease (ESRD), is assigned when the provider has documented end-stage-renal disease (ESRD).

       If both a stage of CKD and ESRD are documented, assign code 585.6 only.

    2) **Chronic kidney disease and kidney transplant status**

       Patients who have undergone kidney transplant may still have some form of CKD, because the kidney transplant may not fully restore kidney function. Therefore, the presence of CKD alone does not constitute a transplant complication. Assign the appropriate 585 code for the patient's stage of CKD and code V42.0. If a transplant complication such as failure or rejection is documented, see section I.C.17.f.2.b for information on coding complications of a kidney transplant. If the documentation is unclear as to whether the patient has a complication of the transplant, query the provider.

    3) **Chronic kidney disease with other conditions**

       Patients with CKD may also suffer from other serious conditions, most commonly diabetes mellitus and hypertension. The sequencing of the CKD code in relationship to codes for other contributing conditions is based on the conventions in the tabular list.

       See I.C.3.a.4 for sequencing instructions for diabetes.

       See I.C.4.a.1 for anemia in CKD.

       See I.C.7.a.3 for hypertensive chronic kidney disease.

See I.C.17.f.2.b, Kidney transplant complications, for instructions on coding of documented rejection or failure.

11. **Chapter 11: Complications of Pregnancy, Childbirth, and the Puerperium (630-679)**
    a. **General Rules for Obstetric Cases**
       1) **Codes from chapter 11 and sequencing priority**

          Obstetric cases require codes from chapter 11, codes in the range 630-679, Complications of Pregnancy, Childbirth, and the Puerperium. Chapter 11 codes have sequencing priority over codes from other chapters. Additional codes from other chapters may be used in conjunction with chapter 11 codes to further specify conditions. Should the provider document that the pregnancy is incidental to the encounter, then code V22.2 should be used in place of any chapter 11 codes. It is the provider's responsibility to state that the condition being treated is not affecting the pregnancy.

       2) **Chapter 11 codes used only on the maternal record**

          Chapter 11 codes are to be used only on the maternal record, never on the record of the newborn.

       3) **Chapter 11 fifth-digits**

          Categories 640-649, 651-676 have required fifth-digits, which indicate whether the encounter is antepartum, postpartum and whether a delivery has also occurred.

       4) **Fifth-digits, appropriate for each code**

          The fifth-digits, which are appropriate for each code number, are listed in brackets under each code. The fifth-digits on each code should all be consistent with each other. That is, should a delivery occur all of the fifth-digits should indicate the delivery.

    b. **Selection of OB Principal or First-listed Diagnosis**
       1) **Routine outpatient prenatal visits**

          For routine outpatient prenatal visits when no complications are present codes V22.0, Supervision of normal first pregnancy, and V22.1, Supervision of other normal pregnancy, should be used as the first-listed diagnoses. These codes should not be used in conjunction with chapter 11 codes.

       2) **Prenatal outpatient visits for high-risk patients**

          For **routine** prenatal outpatient visits for patients with high-risk pregnancies, a code from category V23, Supervision of high-risk pregnancy, should be used as the first-listed diagnosis. Secondary chapter 11 codes may be used in conjunction with these codes if appropriate.

       3) **Episodes when no delivery occurs**

          In episodes when no delivery occurs, the principal diagnosis should correspond to the principal complication of the pregnancy, which necessitated the encounter. Should more than one complication exist, all of which are treated or monitored, any of the complications codes may be sequenced first.

       4) **When a delivery occurs**

          When a delivery occurs, the principal diagnosis should correspond to the main circumstances or complication of the delivery. In cases of cesarean delivery, the selection of the principal diagnosis should be the condition established after study that was responsible for the patient's admission. If the patient was admitted with a condition that resulted in the performance of a cesarean procedure, that condition should be selected as the principal diagnosis. If the reason for the admission/encounter was unrelated to the condition resulting in the cesarean delivery, the condition related to the reason for the admission/encounter should be selected as the principal diagnosis, even if a cesarean was performed.

       5) **Outcome of delivery**

          An outcome of delivery code, V27.0-V27.9, should be included on every maternal record when a delivery has occurred. These codes are not to be used on subsequent records or on the newborn record.

    c. **Fetal Conditions Affecting the Management of the Mother**
       1) **Codes from categories 655 and 656**

          Codes from categories 655, Known or suspected fetal abnormality affecting management of the mother, and 656, Other known or suspected fetal and placental problems affecting the management of the mother, are assigned only when the fetal condition is actually responsible for modifying the management of the mother, i.e., by requiring diagnostic studies, additional observation, special care, or termination of pregnancy. The fact that the fetal condition exists does not justify assigning a code from this series to the mother's record.

          See I.C.18.d. for suspected maternal and fetal conditions not found

       2) **In utero surgery**

          In cases when surgery is performed on the fetus, a diagnosis code from category 655, Known or suspected fetal abnormalities affecting management of the mother, should be assigned identifying the fetal condition. Procedure code 75.36, Correction of fetal defect, should be assigned on the hospital inpatient record.

No code from Chapter 15, the perinatal codes, should be used on the mother's record to identify fetal conditions. Surgery performed in utero on a fetus is still to be coded as an obstetric encounter.

d. HIV Infection in Pregnancy, Childbirth and the Puerperium

During pregnancy, childbirth or the puerperium, a patient admitted because of an HIV-related illness should receive a principal diagnosis of 647.6X, Other specified infectious and parasitic diseases in the mother classifiable elsewhere, but complicating the pregnancy, childbirth or the puerperium, followed by 042 and the code(s) for the HIV-related illness(es).

Patients with asymptomatic HIV infection status admitted during pregnancy, childbirth, or the puerperium should receive codes of 647.6X and V08.

e. Current Conditions Complicating Pregnancy

Assign a code from subcategory 648.x for patients that have current conditions when the condition affects the management of the pregnancy, childbirth, or the puerperium. Use additional secondary codes from other chapters to identify the conditions, as appropriate.

f. Diabetes mellitus in pregnancy

Diabetes mellitus is a significant complicating factor in pregnancy. Pregnant women who are diabetic should be assigned code 648.0x, Diabetes mellitus complicating pregnancy, and a secondary code from category 250, Diabetes mellitus, or category 249, Secondary diabetes to identify the type of diabetes.

Code V58.67, Long-term (current) use of insulin, should also be assigned if the diabetes mellitus is being treated with insulin.

g. Gestational diabetes

Gestational diabetes can occur during the second and third trimester of pregnancy in women who were not diabetic prior to pregnancy. Gestational diabetes can cause complications in the pregnancy similar to those of pre-existing diabetes mellitus. It also puts the woman at greater risk of developing diabetes after the pregnancy. Gestational diabetes is coded to 648.8x, Abnormal glucose tolerance. Codes 648.0x and 648.8x should never be used together on the same record.

Code V58.67, Long-term (current) use of insulin, should also be assigned if the gestational diabetes is being treated with insulin.

h. Normal Delivery, Code 650

1) **Normal delivery**

Code 650 is for use in cases when a woman is admitted for a full-term normal delivery and delivers a single, healthy infant without any complications antepartum, during the delivery, or postpartum during the delivery episode. Code 650 is always a principal diagnosis. It is not to be used if any other code from chapter 11 is needed to describe a current complication of the antenatal, delivery, or perinatal period. Additional codes from other chapters may be used with code 650 if they are not related to or are in any way complicating the pregnancy.

2) **Normal delivery with resolved antepartum complication**

Code 650 may be used if the patient had a complication at some point during her pregnancy, but the complication is not present at the time of the admission for delivery.

3) **V27.0, Single liveborn, outcome of delivery**

V27.0, Single liveborn, is the only outcome of delivery code appropriate for use with 650.

i. The Postpartum and Peripartum Periods

1) **Postpartum and peripartum periods**

The postpartum period begins immediately after delivery and continues for six weeks following delivery. The peripartum period is defined as the last month of pregnancy to five months postpartum.

2) **Postpartum complication**

A postpartum complication is any complication occurring within the six-week period.

3) **Pregnancy-related complications after 6 week period**

Chapter 11 codes may also be used to describe pregnancy-related complications after the six-week period should the provider document that a condition is pregnancy related.

4) **Postpartum complications occurring during the same admission as delivery**

Postpartum complications that occur during the same admission as the delivery are identified with a fifth digit of "2." Subsequent admissions/encounters for postpartum complications should be identified with a fifth digit of "4."

5) **Admission for routine postpartum care following delivery outside hospital**

When the mother delivers outside the hospital prior to admission and is admitted for routine postpartum care and no complications are noted, code V24.0, Postpartum care and examination immediately after delivery, should be assigned as the principal diagnosis.

6) **Admission following delivery outside hospital with postpartum conditions**

   A delivery diagnosis code should not be used for a woman who has delivered prior to admission to the hospital. Any postpartum conditions and/or postpartum procedures should be coded.

7) **Puerperal sepsis**

   Code 670.2x, Puerperal sepsis, should be assigned with a secondary code to identify the causal organism (e.g., for a bacterial infection, assign a code from category 041, Bacterial infections in conditions classified elsewhere and of unspecified site). A code from category 038, Septicemia, should not be used for puerperal sepsis. Do not assign code 995.91, Sepsis, as code 670.2x describes the sepsis. If applicable, use additional codes to identify severe sepsis (995.92) and any associated acute organ dysfunction.

j. **Code 677, Late effect of complication of pregnancy**

   1) **Code 677**

      Code 677, Late effect of complication of pregnancy, childbirth, and the puerperium is for use in those cases when an initial complication of a pregnancy develops a sequelae requiring care or treatment at a future date.

   2) **After the initial postpartum period**

      This code may be used at any time after the initial postpartum period.

   3) **Sequencing of Code 677**

      This code, like all late effect codes, is to be sequenced following the code describing the sequelae of the complication.

k. **Abortions**

   1) **Fifth-digits required for abortion categories**

      Fifth-digits are required for abortion categories 634-637. Fifth digit assignment is based on the status of the patient at the beginning (or start) of the encounter. Fifth-digit 1, incomplete, indicates that all of the products of conception have not been expelled from the uterus. Fifth-digit 2, complete, indicates that all products of conception have been expelled from the uterus.

   2) **Code from categories 640-649 and 651-659**

      A code from categories 640-649 and 651-659 may be used as additional codes with an abortion code to indicate the complication leading to the abortion.

      Fifth digit 3 is assigned with codes from these categories when used with an abortion code because the other fifth digits will not apply. Codes from the 660-669 series are not to be used for complications of abortion.

   3) **Code 639 for complications**

      Code 639 is to be used for all complications following abortion. Code 639 cannot be assigned with codes from categories 634-638.

   4) **Abortion with Liveborn Fetus**

      When an attempted termination of pregnancy results in a liveborn fetus assign code 644.21, Early onset of delivery, with an appropriate code from category V27, Outcome of Delivery. The procedure code for the attempted termination of pregnancy should also be assigned.

   5) **Retained Products of Conception following an abortion**

      Subsequent admissions for retained products of conception following a spontaneous or legally induced abortion are assigned the appropriate code from category 634, Spontaneous abortion, or 635 Legally induced abortion, with a fifth digit of "1" (incomplete). This advice is appropriate even when the patient was discharged previously with a discharge diagnosis of complete abortion.

12. **Chapter 12: Diseases Skin and Subcutaneous Tissue (680-709)**

    a. **Pressure ulcer stage codes**

       1) **Pressure ulcer stages**

          Two codes are needed to completely describe a pressure ulcer: A code from subcategory 707.0, Pressure ulcer, to identify the site of the pressure ulcer and a code from subcategory 707.2, Pressure ulcer stages.

          The codes in subcategory 707.2, Pressure ulcer stages, are to be used as an additional diagnosis with a code(s) from subcategory 707.0, Pressure Ulcer. Codes from 707.2, Pressure ulcer stages, may not be assigned as a principal or first-listed diagnosis. The pressure ulcer stage codes should only be used with pressure ulcers and not with other types of ulcers (e.g., stasis ulcer).

          The ICD-9-CM classifies pressure ulcer stages based on severity, which is designated by stages I-IV and unstageable.

       2) **Unstageable pressure ulcers**

          Assignment of code 707.25, Pressure ulcer, unstageable, should be based on the clinical documentation. Code 707.25 is used for pressure ulcers whose stage cannot be clinically determined (e.g., the ulcer is covered by eschar or has been treated with a skin or muscle graft) and pressure ulcers that are documented as deep tissue injury but not documented as due to trauma. This code should not be confused with code 707.20, Pressure ulcer, stage unspecified. Code 707.20 should be assigned when there is no documentation regarding the stage of the pressure ulcer.

3) **Documented pressure ulcer stage**

   Assignment of the pressure ulcer stage code should be guided by clinical documentation of the stage or documentation of the terms found in the index. For clinical terms describing the stage that are not found in the index, and there is no documentation of the stage, the provider should be queried.

4) **Bilateral pressure ulcers with same stage**

   When a patient has bilateral pressure ulcers (e.g., both buttocks) and both pressure ulcers are documented as being the same stage, only the code for the site and one code for the stage should be reported.

5) **Bilateral pressure ulcers with different stages**

   When a patient has bilateral pressure ulcers at the same site (e.g., both buttocks) and each pressure ulcer is documented as being at a different stage, assign one code for the site and the appropriate codes for the pressure ulcer stage.

6) **Multiple pressure ulcers of different sites and stages**

   When a patient has multiple pressure ulcers at different sites (e.g., buttock, heel, shoulder) and each pressure ulcer is documented as being at different stages (e.g., stage 3 and stage 4), assign the appropriate codes for each different site and a code for each different pressure ulcer stage.

7) **Patients admitted with pressure ulcers documented as healed**

   No code is assigned if the documentation states that the pressure ulcer is completely healed.

8) **Patients admitted with pressure ulcers documented as healing**

   Pressure ulcers described as healing should be assigned the appropriate pressure ulcer stage code based on the documentation in the medical record. If the documentation does not provide information about the stage of the healing pressure ulcer, assign code 707.20, Pressure ulcer stage, unspecified.

   If the documentation is unclear as to whether the patient has a current (new) pressure ulcer or if the patient is being treated for a healing pressure ulcer, query the provider.

9) **Patient admitted with pressure ulcer evolving into another stage during the admission**

   If a patient is admitted with a pressure ulcer at one stage and it progresses to a higher stage, assign the code for highest stage reported for that site.

13. **Chapter 13: Diseases of Musculoskeletal and Connective Tissue (710-739)**

   a. **Coding of Pathologic Fractures**

      1) **Acute Fractures vs. Aftercare**

         Pathologic fractures are reported using subcategory 733.1, when the fracture is newly diagnosed. Subcategory 733.1 may be used while the patient is receiving active treatment for the fracture. Examples of active treatment are: surgical treatment, emergency department encounter, evaluation and treatment by a new physician.

         Fractures are coded using the aftercare codes (subcategories V54.0, V54.2, V54.8 or V54.9) for encounters after the patient has completed active treatment of the fracture and is receiving routine care for the fracture during the healing or recovery phase. Examples of fracture aftercare are: cast change or removal, removal of external or internal fixation device, medication adjustment, and follow up visits following fracture treatment.

         Care for complications of surgical treatment for fracture repairs during the healing or recovery phase should be coded with the appropriate complication codes.

         Care of complications of fractures, such as malunion and nonunion, should be reported with the appropriate codes.

         See Section I.C.17.b for information on the coding of traumatic fractures.

14. **Chapter 14: Congenital Anomalies (740-759)**

   a. **Codes in categories 740-759, Congenital Anomalies**

      Assign an appropriate code(s) from categories 740-759, Congenital Anomalies, when an anomaly is documented. A congenital anomaly may be the principal/first listed diagnosis on a record or a secondary diagnosis.

      When a congenital anomaly does not have a unique code assignment, assign additional code(s) for any manifestations that may be present.

      When the code assignment specifically identifies the congenital anomaly, manifestations that are an inherent component of the anomaly should not be coded separately. Additional codes should be assigned for manifestations that are not an inherent component.

Codes from Chapter 14 may be used throughout the life of the patient. If a congenital anomaly has been corrected, a personal history code should be used to identify the history of the anomaly. Although present at birth, a congenital anomaly may not be identified until later in life. Whenever the condition is diagnosed by the physician, it is appropriate to assign a code from codes 740-759.

For the birth admission, the appropriate code from category V30, Liveborn infants, according to type of birth should be sequenced as the principal diagnosis, followed by any congenital anomaly codes, 740-759.

15. **Chapter 15: Newborn (Perinatal) Guidelines (760-779)**

   For coding and reporting purposes the perinatal period is defined as before birth through the 28th day following birth. The following guidelines are provided for reporting purposes. Hospitals may record other diagnoses as needed for internal data use.

   a. **General Perinatal Rules**

   1) **Chapter 15 Codes**

      They are never for use on the maternal record. Codes from Chapter 11, the obstetric chapter, are never permitted on the newborn record. Chapter 15 code may be used throughout the life of the patient if the condition is still present.

   2) **Sequencing of perinatal codes**

      Generally, codes from Chapter 15 should be sequenced as the principal/first-listed diagnosis on the newborn record, with the exception of the appropriate V30 code for the birth episode, followed by codes from any other chapter that provide additional detail. The "use additional code" note at the beginning of the chapter supports this guideline. If the index does not provide a specific code for a perinatal condition, assign code 779.89, Other specified conditions originating in the perinatal period, followed by the code from another chapter that specifies the condition. Codes for signs and symptoms may be assigned when a definitive diagnosis has not been established.

   3) **Birth process or community acquired conditions**

      If a newborn has a condition that may be either due to the birth process or community acquired and the documentation does not indicate which it is, the default is due to the birth process and the code from Chapter 15 should be used. If the condition is community-acquired, a code from Chapter 15 should not be assigned.

   4) **Code all clinically significant conditions**

      All clinically significant conditions noted on routine newborn examination should be coded. A condition is clinically significant if it requires:
      - clinical evaluation; or
      - therapeutic treatment; or
      - diagnostic procedures; or
      - extended length of hospital stay; or
      - increased nursing care and/or monitoring; or
      - has implications for future health care needs

      Note: The perinatal guidelines listed above are the same as the general coding guidelines for "additional diagnoses", except for the final point regarding implications for future health care needs. Codes should be assigned for conditions that have been specified by the provider as having implications for future health care needs. Codes from the perinatal chapter should not be assigned unless the provider has established a definitive diagnosis.

   b. **Use of codes V30-V39**

      When coding the birth of an infant, assign a code from categories V30-V39, according to the type of birth. A code from this series is assigned as a principal diagnosis, and assigned only once to a newborn at the time of birth.

   c. **Newborn transfers**

      If the newborn is transferred to another institution, the V30 series is not used at the receiving hospital.

   d. **Use of category V29**

   1) **Assigning a code from category V29**

      Assign a code from category V29, Observation and evaluation of newborns and infants for suspected conditions not found, to identify those instances when a healthy newborn is evaluated for a suspected condition that is determined after study not to be present. Do not use a code from category V29 when the patient has identified signs or symptoms of a suspected problem; in such cases, code the sign or symptom.

      A code from category V29 may also be assigned as a principal code for readmissions or encounters when the V30 code no longer applies. Codes from category V29 are for use only for healthy newborns and infants for which no condition after study is found to be present.

   2) **V29 code on a birth record**

      A V29 code is to be used as a secondary code after the V30, Outcome of delivery, code.

e. Use of other V codes on perinatal records

V codes other than V30 and V29 may be assigned on a perinatal or newborn record code. The codes may be used as a principal or first-listed diagnosis for specific types of encounters or for readmissions or encounters when the V30 code no longer applies.

See Section I.C.18 for information regarding the assignment of V codes.

f. Maternal Causes of Perinatal Morbidity

Codes from categories 760-763, Maternal causes of perinatal morbidity and mortality, are assigned only when the maternal condition has actually affected the fetus or newborn. The fact that the mother has an associated medical condition or experiences some complication of pregnancy, labor or delivery does not justify the routine assignment of codes from these categories to the newborn record.

g. Congenital Anomalies in Newborns

For the birth admission, the appropriate code from category V30, Liveborn infants according to type of birth, should be used, followed by any congenital anomaly codes, categories 740-759. Use additional secondary codes from other chapters to specify conditions associated with the anomaly, if applicable.

Also, see Section I.C.14 for information on the coding of congenital anomalies.

h. Coding Additional Perinatal Diagnoses

1) Assigning codes for conditions that require treatment

Assign codes for conditions that require treatment or further investigation, prolong the length of stay, or require resource utilization.

2) Codes for conditions specified as having implications for future health care needs

Assign codes for conditions that have been specified by the provider as having implications for future health care needs.

Note: This guideline should not be used for adult patients.

3) Codes for newborn conditions originating in the perinatal period

Assign a code for newborn conditions originating in the perinatal period (categories 760-779), as well as complications arising during the current episode of care classified in other chapters, only if the diagnoses have been documented by the responsible provider at the time of transfer or discharge as having affected the fetus or newborn.

i. Prematurity and Fetal Growth Retardation

Providers utilize different criteria in determining prematurity. A code for prematurity should not be assigned unless it is documented. The 5th digit assignment for codes from category 764 and subcategories 765.0 and 765.1 should be based on the recorded birth weight and estimated gestational age.

A code from subcategory 765.2, Weeks of gestation, should be assigned as an additional code with category 764 and codes from 765.0 and 765.1 to specify weeks of gestation as documented by the provider in the record.

j. Newborn sepsis

Code 771.81, Septicemia [sepsis] of newborn, should be assigned with a secondary code from category 041, Bacterial infections in conditions classified elsewhere and of unspecified site, to identify the organism. A code from category 038, Septicemia, should not be used on a newborn record. Do not assign code 995.91, Sepsis, as code 771.81 describes the sepsis. If applicable, use additional codes to identify severe sepsis (995.92) and any associated acute organ dysfunction.

16. Chapter 16: Signs, Symptoms and Ill-Defined Conditions (780-799)

Reserved for future guideline expansion

17. Chapter 17: Injury and Poisoning (800-999)

a. Coding of Injuries

When coding injuries, assign separate codes for each injury unless a combination code is provided, in which case the combination code is assigned. Multiple injury codes are provided in ICD-9-CM, but should not be assigned unless information for a more specific code is not available. These traumatic injury codes are not to be used for normal, healing surgical wounds or to identify complications of surgical wounds.

The code for the most serious injury, as determined by the provider and the focus of treatment, is sequenced first.

1) Superficial injuries

Superficial injuries such as abrasions or contusions are not coded when associated with more severe injuries of the same site.

2) Primary injury with damage to nerves/blood vessels

When a primary injury results in minor damage to peripheral nerves or blood vessels, the primary injury is sequenced first with additional code(s) from categories 950-957, Injury to nerves and spinal cord, and/or 900-904, Injury to blood vessels. When the primary injury is to the blood vessels or nerves, that injury should be sequenced first.

b. Coding of Traumatic Fractures

The principles of multiple coding of injuries should be followed in coding fractures. Fractures of specified sites are coded individually by site in accordance with both the provisions within categories 800-829 and the level of detail furnished by medical record content. Combination categories for multiple fractures are provided for use when there is insufficient detail in the medical record (such as trauma cases transferred to another hospital), when the reporting form limits the number of codes that can be used in reporting pertinent clinical data, or when there is insufficient specificity at the fourth-digit or fifth-digit level. More specific guidelines are as follows:

1) **Acute Fractures vs. Aftercare**

    Traumatic fractures are coded using the acute fracture codes (800-829) while the patient is receiving active treatment for the fracture. Examples of active treatment are: surgical treatment, emergency department encounter, and evaluation and treatment by a new physician.

    Fractures are coded using the aftercare codes (subcategories V54.0, V54.1, V54.8, or V54.9) for encounters after the patient has completed active treatment of the fracture and is receiving routine care for the fracture during the healing or recovery phase. Examples of fracture aftercare are: cast change or removal, removal of external or internal fixation device, medication adjustment, and follow up visits following fracture treatment.

    Care for complications of surgical treatment for fracture repairs during the healing or recovery phase should be coded with the appropriate complication codes.

    Care of complications of fractures, such as malunion and nonunion, should be reported with the appropriate codes.

    Pathologic fractures are not coded in the 800-829 range, but instead are assigned to subcategory 733.1. *See Section I.C.13.a for additional information.*

2) **Multiple fractures of same limb**

    Multiple fractures of same limb classifiable to the same three-digit or four-digit category are coded to that category.

3) **Multiple unilateral or bilateral fractures of same bone**

    Multiple unilateral or bilateral fractures of same bone(s) but classified to different fourth-digit subdivisions (bone part) within the same three-digit category are coded individually by site.

4) **Multiple fracture categories 819 and 828**

    Multiple fracture categories 819 and 828 classify bilateral fractures of both upper limbs (819) and both lower limbs (828), but without any detail at the fourth-digit level other than open and closed type of fractures.

5) **Multiple fractures sequencing**

    Multiple fractures are sequenced in accordance with the severity of the fracture. The provider should be asked to list the fracture diagnoses in the order of severity.

c. **Coding of Burns**

Current burns (940-948) are classified by depth, extent and by agent (E code). Burns are classified by depth as first degree (erythema), second degree (blistering), and third degree (full-thickness involvement).

1) **Sequencing of burn and related condition codes**

    Sequence first the code that reflects the highest degree of burn when more than one burn is present.

    a. When the reason for the admission or encounter is for treatment of external multiple burns, sequence first the code that reflects the burn of the highest degree.

    b. When a patient has both internal and external burns, the circumstances of admission govern the selection of the principal diagnosis or first-listed diagnosis.

    c. When a patient is admitted for burn injuries and other related conditions such as smoke inhalation and/or respiratory failure, the circumstances of admission govern the selection of the principal or first-listed diagnosis.

2) **Burns of the same local site**

    Classify burns of the same local site (three-digit category level, 940-947) but of different degrees to the subcategory identifying the highest degree recorded in the diagnosis.

3) **Non-healing burns**

    Non-healing burns are coded as acute burns.

    Necrosis of burned skin should be coded as a non-healed burn.

4) **Code 958.3, Posttraumatic wound infection**

    Assign code 958.3, Posttraumatic wound infection, not elsewhere classified, as an additional code for any documented infected burn site.

5) **Assign separate codes for each burn site**

    When coding burns, assign separate codes for each burn site. Category 946 Burns of Multiple specified sites, should only be used if the location of the burns are not documented. Category 949, Burn, unspecified, is extremely vague and should rarely be used.

6) Assign codes from category 948, Burns

Burns classified according to extent of body surface involved, when the site of the burn is not specified or when there is a need for additional data. It is advisable to use category 948 as additional coding when needed to provide data for evaluating burn mortality, such as that needed by burn units. It is also advisable to use category 948 as an additional code for reporting purposes when there is mention of a third-degree burn involving 20 percent or more of the body surface.

In assigning a code from category 948:

> Fourth-digit codes are used to identify the percentage of total body surface involved in a burn (all degree).
>
> Fifth-digits are assigned to identify the percentage of body surface involved in third-degree burn.
>
> Fifth-digit zero (0) is assigned when less than 10 percent or when no body surface is involved in a third-degree burn.
>
> Category 948 is based on the classic "rule of nines" in estimating body surface involved: head and neck are assigned nine percent, each arm nine percent, each leg 18 percent, the anterior trunk 18 percent, posterior trunk 18 percent, and genitalia one percent. Providers may change these percentage assignments where necessary to accommodate infants and children who have proportionately larger heads than adults and patients who have large buttocks, thighs, or abdomen that involve burns.

7) Encounters for treatment of late effects of burns

Encounters for the treatment of the late effects of burns (i.e., scars or joint contractures) should be coded to the residual condition (sequelae) followed by the appropriate late effect code (906.5-906.9). A late effect E code may also be used, if desired.

8) Sequelae with a late effect code and current burn

When appropriate, both a sequelae with a late effect code, and a current burn code may be assigned on the same record (when both a current burn and sequelae of an old burn exist).

d. Coding of Debridement of Wound, Infection, or Burn

Excisional debridement involves surgical removal or cutting away, as opposed to a mechanical (brushing, scrubbing, washing) debridement.

For coding purposes, excisional debridement is assigned to code 86.22.

Nonexcisional debridement is assigned to code 86.28.

e. Adverse Effects, Poisoning and Toxic Effects

The properties of certain drugs, medicinal and biological substances or combinations of such substances, may cause toxic reactions. The occurrence of drug toxicity is classified in ICD-9-CM as follows:

1) Adverse Effect

When the drug was correctly prescribed and properly administered, code the reaction plus the appropriate code from the E930-E949 series. Codes from the E930-E949 series must be used to identify the causative substance for an adverse effect of drug, medicinal and biological substances, correctly prescribed and properly administered. The effect, such as tachycardia, delirium, gastrointestinal hemorrhaging, vomiting, hypokalemia, hepatitis, renal failure, or respiratory failure, is coded and followed by the appropriate code from the E930-E949 series.

Adverse effects of therapeutic substances correctly prescribed and properly administered (toxicity, synergistic reaction, side effect, and idiosyncratic reaction) may be due to (1) differences among patients, such as age, sex, disease, and genetic factors, and (2) drug-related factors, such as type of drug, route of administration, duration of therapy, dosage, and bioavailability.

2) Poisoning

(a) Error was made in drug prescription

Errors made in drug prescription or in the administration of the drug by provider, nurse, patient, or other person, use the appropriate poisoning code from the 960-979 series.

(b) Overdose of a drug intentionally taken

If an overdose of a drug was intentionally taken or administered and resulted in drug toxicity, it would be coded as a poisoning (960-979 series).

(c) Nonprescribed drug taken with correctly prescribed and properly administered drug

If a nonprescribed drug or medicinal agent was taken in combination with a correctly prescribed and properly administered drug, any drug toxicity or other reaction resulting from the interaction of the two drugs would be classified as a poisoning.

   (d) **Interaction of drug(s) and alcohol**

   When a reaction results from the interaction of a drug(s) and alcohol, this would be classified as poisoning.

   (e) **Sequencing of poisoning**

   When coding a poisoning or reaction to the improper use of a medication (e.g., wrong dose, wrong substance, wrong route of administration) the poisoning code is sequenced first, followed by a code for the manifestation. If there is also a diagnosis of drug abuse or dependence to the substance, the abuse or dependence is coded as an additional code.

   See Section I.C.3.a.6.b. if poisoning is the result of insulin pump malfunctions and Section I.C.19 for general use of E-codes.

  3) **Toxic Effects**

   (a) **Toxic effect codes**

   When a harmful substance is ingested or comes in contact with a person, this is classified as a toxic effect. The toxic effect codes are in categories 980-989.

   (b) **Sequencing toxic effect codes**

   A toxic effect code should be sequenced first, followed by the code(s) that identify the result of the toxic effect.

   (c) **External cause codes for toxic effects**

   An external cause code from categories E860-E869 for accidental exposure, codes E950.6 or E950.7 for intentional self-harm, category E962 for assault, or categories E980-E982, for undetermined, should also be assigned to indicate intent.

f. **Complications of care**

 1) **General guidelines for complications of care**

   (a) **Documentation of complications of care**

   See Section I.B.18. for information on documentation of complications of care.

   (b) **Use additional code to identify nature of complication**

   An additional code identifying the complication should be assigned with codes in categories 996-999, Complications of Surgical and Medical Care NEC, when the additional code provides greater specificity as to the nature of the condition. If the complication code fully describes the condition, no additional code is necessary.

 2) **Transplant complications**

   (a) **Transplant complications other than kidney**

   Codes under subcategory 996.8, Complications of transplanted organ, are for use for both complications and rejection of transplanted organs. A transplant complication code is only assigned if the complication affects the function of the transplanted organ. Two codes are required to fully describe a transplant complication, the appropriate code from subcategory 996.8 and a secondary code that identifies the complication.

   Pre-existing conditions or conditions that develop after the transplant are not coded as complications unless they affect the function of the transplanted organs.

   See I.C.18.d.3) for transplant organ removal status

   See I.C.2.i for malignant neoplasm associated with transplanted organ.

   (b) **Kidney transplant complications**

   Patients who have undergone kidney transplant may still have some form of chronic kidney disease (CKD) because the kidney transplant may not fully restore kidney function. Code 996.81 should be assigned for documented complications of a kidney transplant, such as transplant failure or rejection or other transplant complication. Code 996.81 should not be assigned for post kidney transplant patients who have chronic kidney (CKD) unless a transplant complication such as transplant failure or rejection is documented. If the documentation is unclear as to whether the patient has a complication of the transplant, query the provider.

   Conditions that affect the function of the transplanted kidney, other than CKD, should be assigned code 996.81, Complications of transplanted organ, Kidney, and a secondary code that identifies the complication.

   For patients with CKD following a kidney transplant, but who do not have a complication such as failure or rejection, *see section I.C.10.a.2, Chronic kidney disease and kidney transplant status.*

3) Ventilator associated pneumonia

(a) Documentation of Ventilator associated Pneumonia

As with all procedural or postprocedural complications, code assignment is based on the provider's documentation of the relationship between the condition and the procedure.

Code 997.31, Ventilator associated pneumonia, should be assigned only when the provider has documented ventilator associated pneumonia (VAP). An additional code to identify the organism (e.g., Pseudomonas aeruginosa, code 041.7) should also be assigned. Do not assign an additional code from categories 480-484 to identify the type of pneumonia.

Code 997.31 should not be assigned for cases where the patient has pneumonia and is on a mechanical ventilator but the provider has not specifically stated that the pneumonia is ventilator-associated pneumonia.

If the documentation is unclear as to whether the patient has a pneumonia that is a complication attributable to the mechanical ventilator, query the provider.

(b) Patient admitted with pneumonia and develops VAP

A patient may be admitted with one type of pneumonia (e.g., code 481, Pneumococcal pneumonia) and subsequently develop VAP. In this instance, the principal diagnosis would be the appropriate code from categories 480-484 for the pneumonia diagnosed at the time of admission. Code 997.31, Ventilator associated pneumonia, would be assigned as an additional diagnosis when the provider has also documented the presence of ventilator associated pneumonia.

g. SIRS due to Non-infectious Process

The systemic inflammatory response syndrome (SIRS) can develop as a result of certain non-infectious disease processes, such as trauma, malignant neoplasm, or pancreatitis. When SIRS is documented with a noninfectious condition, and no subsequent infection is documented, the code for the underlying condition, such as an injury, should be assigned, followed by code 995.93, Systemic inflammatory response syndrome due to noninfectious process without acute organ dysfunction, or 995.94, Systemic inflammatory response syndrome due to non-infectious process with acute organ dysfunction. If an acute organ dysfunction is documented, the appropriate code(s) for the associated acute organ dysfunction(s) should be assigned in addition to code 995.94. If acute organ dysfunction is documented, but it cannot be determined if the acute organ dysfunction is associated with SIRS or due to another condition (e.g., directly due to the trauma), the provider should be queried.

When the non-infectious condition has led to an infection that results in SIRS, *see Section I.C.1.b.12 for the guideline for sepsis and severe sepsis associated with a non-infectious process.*

18. Classification of Factors Influencing Health Status and Contact with Health Service (Supplemental V01-*V91*)

Note: The chapter specific guidelines provide additional information about the use of V codes for specified encounters.

a. Introduction

ICD-9-CM provides codes to deal with encounters for circumstances other than a disease or injury. The Supplementary Classification of Factors Influencing Health Status and Contact with Health Services (V01.0 - V91.99) is provided to deal with occasions when circumstances other than a disease or injury (codes 001-999) are recorded as a diagnosis or problem.

There are four primary circumstances for the use of V codes:

1) A person who is not currently sick encounters the health services for some specific reason, such as to act as an organ donor, to receive prophylactic care, such as inoculations or health screenings, or to receive counseling on health related issues.

2) A person with a resolving disease or injury, or a chronic, long-term condition requiring continuous care, encounters the health care system for specific aftercare of that disease or injury (e.g., dialysis for renal disease; chemotherapy for malignancy; cast change). A diagnosis/symptom code should be used whenever a current, acute, diagnosis is being treated or a sign or symptom is being studied.

3) Circumstances or problems influence a person's health status but are not in themselves a current illness or injury.

4) Newborns, to indicate birth status

b. V codes use in any healthcare setting

V codes are for use in any healthcare setting. V codes may be used as either a first listed (principal diagnosis code in the inpatient setting) or secondary code, depending on the circumstances of the encounter. Certain V codes may only be used as first listed, others only as secondary codes.

See Section I.C.18.e, V Codes That May Only be Principal/First-Listed Diagnosis.

PART I / Introduction

c. **V Codes indicate a reason for an encounter**

They are not procedure codes. A corresponding procedure code must accompany a V code to describe the procedure performed.

d. **Categories of V Codes**

1) **Contact/Exposure**

    Category V01 indicates contact with or exposure to communicable diseases. These codes are for patients who do not show any sign or symptom of a disease but have been exposed to it by close personal contact with an infected individual or are in an area where a disease is epidemic. These codes may be used as a first listed code to explain an encounter for testing, or, more commonly, as a secondary code to identify a potential risk.

    Codes V15.84 – V15.86 describe contact with or (suspected) exposure to asbestos, potentially hazardous body fluids, and lead.

    Subcategories V87.0 – V87.3 describe contact with or (suspected) exposure to hazardous metals, aromatic compounds, other potentially hazardous chemicals, and other potentially hazardous substances.

2) **Inoculations and vaccinations**

    Categories V03-V06 are for encounters for inoculations and vaccinations. They indicate that a patient is being seen to receive a prophylactic inoculation against a disease. The injection itself must be represented by the appropriate procedure code. A code from V03-V06 may be used as a secondary code if the inoculation is given as a routine part of preventive health care, such as a well-baby visit.

3) **Status**

    Status codes indicate that a patient is a carrier of a disease, has the sequelae or residual of a past disease or condition, or has another factor influencing a person's health status. This includes such things as the presence of prosthetic or mechanical devices resulting from past treatment. A status code is informative, because the status may affect the course of treatment and its outcome. A status code is distinct from a history code. The history code indicates that the patient no longer has the condition.

    A status code should not be used with a diagnosis code from one of the body system chapters, if the diagnosis code includes the information provided by the status code. For example, code V42.1, Heart transplant status, should not be used with code 996.83, Complications of transplanted heart. The status code does not provide additional information. The complication code indicates that the patient is a heart transplant patient.

    The status V codes/categories are:

    V02   Carrier or suspected carrier of infectious diseases

            Carrier status indicates that a person harbors the specific organisms of a disease without manifest symptoms and is capable of transmitting the infection.

    V07.5X   Use of agents affecting estrogen receptors and estrogen level

            This code indicates when a patient is receiving a drug that affects estrogen receptors and estrogen levels for prevention of cancer.

    V08   Asymptomatic HIV infection status

            This code indicates that a patient has tested positive for HIV but has manifested no signs or symptoms of the disease.

    V09   Infection with drug-resistant microorganisms

            This category indicates that a patient has an infection that is resistant to drug treatment. Sequence the infection code first.

    V21   Constitutional states in development

    V22.2   Pregnant state, incidental

            This code is a secondary code only for use when the pregnancy is in no way complicating the reason for visit. Otherwise, a code from the obstetric chapter is required.

    V26.5x   Sterilization status

    V42   Organ or tissue replaced by transplant

    V43   Organ or tissue replaced by other means

    V44   Artificial opening status

    V45   Other postsurgical states

            Assign code V45.87, Transplant organ removal status, to indicate that a transplanted organ has been previously removed. This code should not be assigned for the encounter in which the transplanted organ is removed. The complication necessitating removal of the transplant organ should be assigned for that encounter.

See section I.C17.f.2. for information on the coding of organ transplant complications.

Assign code V45.88, Status post administration of tPA (rtPA) in a different facility within the last 24 hours prior to admission to the current facility, as a secondary diagnosis when a patient is received by transfer into a facility and documentation indicates they were administered tissue plasminogen activator (tPA) within the last 24 hours prior to admission to the current facility.

This guideline applies even if the patient is still receiving the tPA at the time they are received into the current facility.

The appropriate code for the condition for which the tPA was administered (such as cerebrovascular disease or myocardial infarction) should be assigned first.

Code V45.88 is only applicable to the receiving facility record and not to the transferring facility record.

V46	Other dependence on machines
V49.6	Upper limb amputation status
V49.7	Lower limb amputation status

Note: Categories V42-V46, and subcategories V49.6, V49.7 are for use only if there are no complications or malfunctions of the organ or tissue replaced, the amputation site or the equipment on which the patient is dependent.

V49.81	Asymptomatic postmenopausal status (age-related) (natural)
V49.82	Dental sealant status
V49.83	Awaiting organ transplant status
V49.86	Do not resuscitate status

This code may be used when it is documented by the provider that a patient is on do not resuscitate status at any time during the stay.

V49.87	Physical restraint status

This code may be used when it is documented by the provider that a patient has been put in restraints during the current encounter. Please note that this code should not be reported when it is documented by the provider that a patient is temporarily restrained during a procedure.

V58.6x	Long-term (current) drug use

Codes from this subcategory indicate a patient's continuous use of a prescribed drug (including such things as aspirin therapy) for the long-term treatment of a condition or for prophylactic use. It is not for use for patients who have addictions to drugs. This subcategory is not for use of medications for detoxification or maintenance programs to prevent withdrawal symptoms in patients with drug dependence (e.g., methadone maintenance for opiate dependence). Assign the appropriate code for the drug dependence instead.

Assign a code from subcategory V58.6, Long-term (current) drug use, if the patient is receiving a medication for an extended period as a prophylactic measure (such as for the prevention of deep vein thrombosis) or as treatment of a chronic condition (such as arthritis) or a disease requiring a lengthy course of treatment (such as cancer). Do not assign a code from subcategory V58.6 for medication being administered for a brief period of time to treat an acute illness or injury (such as a course of antibiotics to treat acute bronchitis).

V83	Genetic carrier status

Genetic carrier status indicates that a person carries a gene, associated with a particular disease, which may be passed to offspring who may develop that disease. The person does not have the disease and is not at risk of developing the disease.

V84	Genetic susceptibility status

Genetic susceptibility indicates that a person has a gene that increases the risk of that person developing the disease.

Codes from category V84, Genetic susceptibility to disease, should not be used as principal or first-listed codes. If the patient has the condition to which he/she is susceptible, and that condition is the reason for the encounter, the code for the current condition should be sequenced first. If the patient is being seen for follow-up after completed treatment for this condition, and the condition no longer exists, a follow-up code should be sequenced first, followed by the appropriate personal history and genetic susceptibility codes. If the purpose of the encounter is genetic counseling associated with procreative management, a code from subcategory V26.3, Genetic counseling and testing, should be assigned as the first-listed code, followed by a code from category V84. Additional codes should be assigned for any applicable family or personal history.

See Section I.C. 18.d.14 for information on prophylactic organ removal due to a genetic susceptibility.

V85 Body Mass Index (BMI)
V86 Estrogen receptor status
V88 Acquired absence of other organs and tissue
V90 Retained foreign body

4) History (of)

There are two types of history V codes, personal and family. Personal history codes explain a patient's past medical condition that no longer exists and is not receiving any treatment, but that has the potential for recurrence, and therefore may require continued monitoring. The exceptions to this general rule are category V14, Personal history of allergy to medicinal agents, and subcategory V15.0, Allergy, other than to medicinal agents. A person who has had an allergic episode to a substance or food in the past should always be considered allergic to the substance.

Family history codes are for use when a patient has a family member(s) who has had a particular disease that causes the patient to be at higher risk of also contracting the disease.

Personal history codes may be used in conjunction with follow-up codes and family history codes may be used in conjunction with screening codes to explain the need for a test or procedure. History codes are also acceptable on any medical record regardless of the reason for visit. A history of an illness, even if no longer present, is important information that may alter the type of treatment ordered.

The history V code categories are:

V10 Personal history of malignant neoplasm
V12 Personal history of certain other diseases
V13 Personal history of other diseases

Except: V13.4, Personal history of arthritis, and subcategory V13.6, Personal history of congenital (corrected) malformations. These conditions are life-long so are not true history codes.

V14 Personal history of allergy to medicinal agents
V15 Other personal history presenting hazards to health

Except: **Codes** V15.7, Personal history of contraception; **V15.84, Contact with and (suspected) exposure to asbestos; V15.85, Contact with and (suspected) exposure to potentially hazardous body fluids; V15.86, Contact with and (suspected) exposure to lead.**

V16 Family history of malignant neoplasm
V17 Family history of certain chronic disabling diseases
V18 Family history of certain other specific diseases
V19 Family history of other conditions
V87 Other specified personal exposures and history presenting hazards to health

Except: Subcategories V87.0, Contact with and (suspected) exposure to hazardous metals; V87.1, Contact with and (suspected) exposure to hazardous aromatic compounds; V87.2, Contact with and (suspected) exposure to other potentially hazardous chemicals; and V87.3, Contact with and (suspected) exposure to other potentially hazardous substances

5) Screening

Screening is the testing for disease or disease precursors in seemingly well individuals so that early detection and treatment can be provided for those who test positive for the disease. Screenings that are recommended for many subgroups in a population include: routine mammograms for women over 40, a fecal occult blood test for everyone over 50, an amniocentesis to rule out a fetal anomaly for pregnant women over 35, because the incidence of breast cancer and colon cancer in these subgroups is higher than in the general population, as is the incidence of Down's syndrome in older mothers.

The testing of a person to rule out or confirm a suspected diagnosis because the patient has some sign or symptom is a diagnostic examination, not a screening. In these cases, the sign or symptom is used to explain the reason for the test.

A screening code may be a first listed code if the reason for the visit is specifically the screening exam. It may also be used as an additional code if the screening is done during an office visit for other health problems. A screening code is not necessary if the screening is inherent to a routine examination, such as a pap smear done during a routine pelvic examination.

Should a condition be discovered during the screening then the code for the condition may be assigned as an additional diagnosis.

The V code indicates that a screening exam is planned. A procedure code is required to confirm that the screening was performed.

The screening V code categories:

V28 Antenatal screening

V73-V82 Special screening examinations

6) Observation

There are three observation V code categories. They are for use in very limited circumstances when a person is being observed for a suspected condition that is ruled out. The observation codes are not for use if an injury or illness or any signs or symptoms related to the suspected condition are present. In such cases the diagnosis/symptom code is used with the corresponding E code to identify any external cause.

The observation codes are to be used as principal diagnosis only. The only exception to this is when the principal diagnosis is required to be a code from the V30, Live born infant, category. Then the V29 observation code is sequenced after the V30 code. Additional codes may be used in addition to the observation code but only if they are unrelated to the suspected condition being observed.

Codes from subcategory V89.0, Suspected maternal and fetal conditions not found, may either be used as a first listed or as an additional code assignment depending on the case. They are for use in very limited circumstances on a maternal record when an encounter is for a suspected maternal or fetal condition that is ruled out during that encounter (for example, a maternal or fetal condition may be suspected due to an abnormal test result). These codes should not be used when the condition is confirmed. In those cases, the confirmed condition should be coded. In addition, these codes are not for use if an illness or any signs or symptoms related to the suspected condition or problem are present. In such cases the diagnosis/symptom code is used.

Additional codes may be used in addition to the code from subcategory V89.0, but only if they are unrelated to the suspected condition being evaluated.

Codes from subcategory V89.0 may not be used for encounters for antenatal screening of mother. *See Section I.C.18.d., Screening).*

For encounters for suspected fetal condition that are inconclusive following testing and evaluation, assign the appropriate code from category 655, 656, 657 or 658.

The observation V code categories:

V29 Observation and evaluation of newborns for suspected condition not found

For the birth encounter, a code from category V30 should be sequenced before the V29 code.

V71 Observation and evaluation for suspected condition not found

V89 Suspected maternal and fetal conditions not found

7) Aftercare

Aftercare visit codes cover situations when the initial treatment of a disease or injury has been performed and the patient requires continued care during the healing or recovery phase, or for the long-term consequences of the disease. The aftercare V code should not be used if treatment is directed at a current, acute disease or injury. The diagnosis code is to be used in these cases. Exceptions to this rule are codes V58.0, Radiotherapy, and codes from subcategory V58.1, Encounter for chemotherapy and immunotherapy for neoplastic conditions. These codes are to be first listed, followed by the diagnosis code when a patient's encounter is solely to receive radiation therapy or chemotherapy for the treatment of a neoplasm. Should a patient receive both chemotherapy and radiation therapy during the same encounter code V58.0 and V58.1 may be used together on a record with either one being sequenced first.

The aftercare codes are generally first listed to explain the specific reason for the encounter. An aftercare code may be used as an additional code when some type of aftercare is provided in addition to the reason for admission and no diagnosis code is applicable. An example of this would be the closure of a colostomy during an encounter for treatment of another condition.

Aftercare codes should be used in conjunction with any other aftercare codes or other diagnosis codes to provide better detail on the specifics of an aftercare encounter visit, unless otherwise directed by the classification. The sequencing of multiple aftercare codes is discretionary.

Certain aftercare V code categories need a secondary diagnosis code to describe the resolving condition or sequelae, for others, the condition is inherent in the code title.

Additional V code aftercare category terms include fitting and adjustment, and attention to artificial openings.

Status V codes may be used with aftercare V codes to indicate the nature of the aftercare. For example code V45.81, Aortocoronary bypass status, may be used with code V58.73, Aftercare following surgery of the circulatory system, NEC, to indicate the surgery for which the aftercare is being performed. Also, a transplant status code may be used following code V58.44, Aftercare following organ transplant, to identify the organ transplanted. A status code should not be used when the aftercare code indicates the type of status, such as using V55.0, Attention to tracheostomy with V44.0, Tracheostomy status.

See Section I.B.16 Admissions/Encounter for Rehabilitation

The aftercare V category/codes:

V51.0	Encounter for breast reconstruction following mastectomy
V52	Fitting and adjustment of prosthetic device and implant
V53	Fitting and adjustment of other device
V54	Other orthopedic aftercare
V55	Attention to artificial openings
V56	Encounter for dialysis and dialysis catheter care
V57	Care involving the use of rehabilitation procedures
V58.0	Radiotherapy
V58.11	Encounter for antineoplastic chemotherapy
V58.12	Encounter for antineoplastic immunotherapy
V58.3x	Attention to dressings and sutures
V58.41	Encounter for planned post-operative wound closure
V58.42	Aftercare, surgery, neoplasm
V58.43	Aftercare, surgery, trauma
V58.44	Aftercare involving organ transplant
V58.49	Other specified aftercare following surgery
V58.7x	Aftercare following surgery
V58.81	Fitting and adjustment of vascular catheter
V58.82	Fitting and adjustment of non-vascular catheter
V58.83	Monitoring therapeutic drug
V58.89	Other specified aftercare

8) **Follow-up**

The follow-up codes are used to explain continuing surveillance following completed treatment of a disease, condition, or injury. They imply that the condition has been fully treated and no longer exists. They should not be confused with aftercare codes that explain current treatment for a healing condition or its sequelae. Follow-up codes may be used in conjunction with history codes to provide the full picture of the healed condition and its treatment. The follow-up code is sequenced first, followed by the history code.

A follow-up code may be used to explain repeated visits. Should a condition be found to have recurred on the follow-up visit, then the diagnosis code should be used in place of the follow-up code.

The follow-up V code categories:

V24	Postpartum care and evaluation
V67	Follow-up examination

9) **Donor**

Category V59 is the donor codes. They are used for living individuals who are donating blood or other body tissue. These codes are only for individuals donating for others, not for self donations. They are not for use to identify cadaveric donations.

10) Counseling

Counseling V codes are used when a patient or family member receives assistance in the aftermath of an illness or injury, or when support is required in coping with family or social problems. They are not necessary for use in conjunction with a diagnosis code when the counseling component of care is considered integral to standard treatment.

The counseling V categories/codes:

V25.0	General counseling and advice for contraceptive management
V26.3	Genetic counseling
V26.4	General counseling and advice for procreative management
V61.X	Other family circumstances
V65.1	Person consulted on behalf of another person
V65.3	Dietary surveillance and counseling
V65.4	Other counseling, not elsewhere classified

11) Obstetrics and related conditions

See Section I.C.11., the Obstetrics guidelines for further instruction on the use of these codes.

V codes for pregnancy are for use in those circumstances when none of the problems or complications included in the codes from the Obstetrics chapter exist (a routine prenatal visit or postpartum care). Codes V22.0, Supervision of normal first pregnancy, and V22.1, Supervision of other normal pregnancy, are always first listed and are not to be used with any other code from the OB chapter.

The outcome of delivery, category V27, should be included on all maternal delivery records. It is always a secondary code.

V codes for family planning (contraceptive) or procreative management and counseling should be included on an obstetric record either during the pregnancy or the postpartum stage, if applicable.

Obstetrics and related conditions V code categories:

V22	Normal pregnancy
V23	Supervision of high-risk pregnancy
	Except: V23.2, Pregnancy with history of abortion. Code 646.3, Recurrent pregnancy loss, from the OB chapter is required to indicate a history of abortion during a pregnancy.
V24	Postpartum care and evaluation
V25	Encounter for contraceptive management
	Except V25.0x
	(See Section I.C.18.d.11, Counseling)
V26	Procreative management
	Except V26.5x, Sterilization status, V26.3 and V26.4
	(See Section I.C.18.d.11., Counseling)
V27	Outcome of delivery
V28	Antenatal screening
	(See Section I.C.18.d.6., Screening)
V91	Multiple gestation placenta status

12) Newborn, infant and child

See Section I.C.15, the Newborn guidelines for further instruction on the use of these codes.

Newborn V code categories:

V20	Health supervision of infant or child
V29	Observation and evaluation of newborns for suspected condition not found
	(See Section I.C.18.d.7, Observation)
V30-V39	Liveborn infant according to type of birth

13) Routine and administrative examinations

The V codes allow for the description of encounters for routine examinations, such as, a general check-up, or examinations for administrative purposes, such as a pre-employment physical. The codes are not to be used if the examination is for diagnosis of a suspected condition or for treatment purposes. In such cases the diagnosis code is used. During a routine exam, should a diagnosis or condition be discovered, it should be coded as an additional code. Pre-existing and chronic conditions and history codes may also be included as additional codes as long as the examination is for administrative purposes and not focused on any particular condition.

Pre-operative examination and pre-procedural laboratory examination V codes are for use only in those situations when a patient is being cleared for a procedure or surgery and no treatment is given.

The V codes categories/code for routine and administrative examinations:

V20.2	Routine infant or child health check
	Any injections given should have a corresponding procedure code.

V70	General medical examination		V58.5	Orthodontics
V72	Special investigations and examinations		V60	Housing, household, and economic circumstances

V70 General medical examination

V72 Special investigations and examinations

Codes V72.5 and V72.62 may be used if the reason for the patient encounter is for routine laboratory/radiology testing in the absence of any signs, symptoms, or associated diagnosis. If routine testing is performed during the same encounter as a test to evaluate a sign, symptom, or diagnosis, it is appropriate to assign both the V code and the code describing the reason for the non-routine test.

14) Miscellaneous V codes

The miscellaneous V codes capture a number of other health care encounters that do not fall into one of the other categories. Certain of these codes identify the reason for the encounter, others are for use as additional codes that provide useful information on circumstances that may affect a patient's care and treatment.

Prophylactic Organ Removal

For encounters specifically for prophylactic removal of breasts, ovaries, or another organ due to a genetic susceptibility to cancer or a family history of cancer, the principal or first listed code should be a code from subcategory V50.4, Prophylactic organ removal, followed by the appropriate genetic susceptibility code and the appropriate family history code.

If the patient has a malignancy of one site and is having prophylactic removal at another site to prevent either a new primary malignancy or metastatic disease, a code for the malignancy should also be assigned in addition to a code from subcategory V50.4. A V50.4 code should not be assigned if the patient is having organ removal for treatment of a malignancy, such as the removal of the testes for the treatment of prostate cancer.

Miscellaneous V code categories/codes:

V07 Need for isolation and other prophylactic or treatment measures

Except V07.5X, Use of agents affecting estrogen receptors and estrogen levels

V40.31 Wandering in diseases classified elsewhere

V50 Elective surgery for purposes other than remedying health states

V58.5 Orthodontics

V60 Housing, household, and economic circumstances

V62 Other psychosocial circumstances

V63 Unavailability of other medical facilities for care

V64 Persons encountering health services for specific procedures, not carried out

V66 Convalescence and Palliative Care

V68 Encounters for administrative purposes

V69 Problems related to lifestyle

V85 Body Mass Index

15) Nonspecific V codes

Certain V codes are so non-specific, or potentially redundant with other codes in the classification, that there can be little justification for their use in the inpatient setting. Their use in the outpatient setting should be limited to those instances when there is no further documentation to permit more precise coding. Otherwise, any sign or symptom or any other reason for visit that is captured in another code should be used.

Nonspecific V code categories/codes:

V11 Personal history of mental disorder

A code from the mental disorders chapter, with an in remission fifth-digit, should be used.

V13.4 Personal history of arthritis

V13.6 Personal history of congenital malformations

V15.7 Personal history of contraception

V23.2 Pregnancy with history of abortion

V40 Mental and behavioral problems

Exception:

V40.31 Wandering in diseases classified elsewhere

V41 Problems with special senses and other special functions

V47 Other problems with internal organs

V48 Problems with head, neck, and trunk

V49 Problems with limbs and other problems

Exceptions:

V49.6 Upper limb amputation status

V49.7	Lower limb amputation status	
V49.81	Asymptomatic postmenopausal status (age-related) (natural)	
V49.82	Dental sealant status	
V49.83	Awaiting organ transplant status	
V49.86	Do not resuscitate status	
V49.87	Physical restraints status	

V51.8	Other aftercare involving the use of plastic surgery
V58.2	Blood transfusion, without reported diagnosis
V58.9	Unspecified aftercare

See Section IV.K. and Section IV.L. of the Outpatient guidelines.

e. V Codes That May Only be Principal/First-Listed Diagnosis

The list of V codes/categories below may only be reported as the principal/first-listed diagnosis, except when there are multiple encounters on the same day and the medical records for the encounters are combined or when there is more than one V code that meets the definition of principal diagnosis (e.g., a patient is admitted to home healthcare for both aftercare and rehabilitation and they equally meet the definition of principal diagnosis). These codes should not be reported if they do not meet the definition of principal or first-listed diagnosis.

See Section II and Section IV.A for information on selection of principal and first-listed diagnosis.

See Section II.C for information on two or more diagnoses that equally meet the definition for principal diagnosis.

V20.X	Health supervision of infant or child
V22.0	Supervision of normal first pregnancy
V22.1	Supervision of other normal pregnancy
V24.X	Postpartum care and examination
V26.81	Encounter for assisted reproductive fertility procedure cycle
V26.82	Encounter for fertility preservation procedure
V30.X	Single liveborn
V31.X	Twin, mate liveborn
V32.X	Twin, mate stillborn
V33.X	Twin, unspecified
V34.X	Other multiple, mates all liveborn
V35.X	Other multiple, mates all stillborn
V36.X	Other multiple, mates live- and stillborn
V37.X	Other multiple, unspecified
V39.X	Unspecified
V46.12	Encounter for respirator dependence during power failure
V46.13	Encounter for weaning from respirator [ventilator]
V51.0	Encounter for breast reconstruction following mastectomy
V56.0	Extracorporeal dialysis
V57.X	Care involving use of rehabilitation procedures
V58.0	Radiotherapy
V58.11	Encounter for antineoplastic chemotherapy
V58.12	Encounter for antineoplastic immunotherapy
V59.X	Donors
V66.0	Convalescence and palliative care following surgery
V66.1	Convalescence and palliative care following radiotherapy
V66.2	Convalescence and palliative care following chemotherapy
V66.3	Convalescence and palliative care following psychotherapy and other treatment for mental disorder
V66.4	Convalescence and palliative care following treatment of fracture
V66.5	Convalescence and palliative care following other treatment
V66.6	Convalescence and palliative care following combined treatment
V66.9	Unspecified convalescence
V68.X	Encounters for administrative purposes
V70.0	Routine general medical examination at a health care facility
V70.1	General psychiatric examination, requested by the authority
V70.2	General psychiatric examination, other and unspecified
V70.3	Other medical examination for administrative purposes
V70.4	Examination for medicolegal reasons
V70.5	Health examination of defined subpopulations
V70.6	Health examination in population surveys
V70.8	Other specified general medical examinations
V70.9	Unspecified general medical examination

V71.X Observation and evaluation for suspected conditions not found

19. Supplemental Classification of External Causes of Injury and Poisoning (E-codes, E800-E999)

Introduction: These guidelines are provided for those who are currently collecting E codes in order that there will be standardization in the process. If your institution plans to begin collecting E codes, these guidelines are to be applied. The use of E codes is supplemental to the application of ICD-9-CM diagnosis codes.

External causes of injury and poisoning codes (categories E000 and E800-E999) are intended to provide data for injury research and evaluation of injury prevention strategies. Activity codes (categories E001-E030) are intended to be used to describe the activity of a person seeking care for injuries as well as other health conditions, when the injury or other health condition resulted from an activity or the activity contributed to a condition. E codes capture how the injury, poisoning, or adverse effect happened (cause), the intent (unintentional or accidental; or intentional, such as suicide or assault), the person's status (e.g. civilian, military), the associated activity and the place where the event occurred.

Some major categories of E codes include:

transport accidents

poisoning and adverse effects of drugs, medicinal substances and biologicals

accidental falls

accidents caused by fire and flames

accidents due to natural and environmental factors

late effects of accidents, assaults or self injury

assaults or purposely inflicted injury

suicide or self inflicted injury

These guidelines apply for the coding and collection of E codes from records in hospitals, outpatient clinics, emergency departments, other ambulatory care settings and provider offices, and nonacute care settings, except when other specific guidelines apply.

a. General E Code Coding Guidelines

1) **Used with any code in the range of 001-V91**

   An E code from categories E800-E999 may be used with any code in the range of 001-V91, which indicates an injury, poisoning, or adverse effect due to an external cause.

   An activity E code (categories E001-E030) may be used with any code in the range of 001-V91 that indicates an injury, or other health condition that resulted from an activity, or the activity contributed to a condition.

2) **Assign the appropriate E code for all initial treatments**

   Assign the appropriate E code for the initial encounter of an injury, poisoning, or adverse effect of drugs, not for subsequent treatment.

   External cause of injury codes (E-codes) may be assigned while the acute fracture codes are still applicable.

   See Section I.C.17.b.1 for coding of acute fractures.

3) **Use the full range of E codes**

   Use the full range of E codes (E800–E999) to completely describe the cause, the intent and the place of occurrence, if applicable, for all injuries, poisonings, and adverse effects of drugs.

   See a.1.), j.), and k.) in this section for information on the use of status and activity E codes.

4) **Assign as many E codes as necessary**

   Assign as many E codes as necessary to fully explain each cause.

5) **The selection of the appropriate E code**

   The selection of the appropriate E code is guided by the Index to External Causes, which is located after the alphabetical index to diseases and by Inclusion and Exclusion notes in the Tabular List.

6) **E code can never be a principal diagnosis**

   An E code can never be a principal (first listed) diagnosis.

7) **External cause code(s) with systemic inflammatory response syndrome (SIRS)**

   An external cause code is not appropriate with a code from subcategory 995.9, unless the patient also has another condition for which an E code would be appropriate (such as an injury, poisoning, or adverse effect of drugs.

8) **Multiple Cause E Code Coding Guidelines**

   More than one E-code is required to fully describe the external cause of an illness, injury or poisoning. The assignment of E-codes should be sequenced in the following priority:

   If two or more events cause separate injuries, an E code should be assigned for each cause. The first listed E code will be selected in the following order:

   E codes for child and adult abuse take priority over all other E codes.

   See Section I.C.19.e., Child and Adult abuse guidelines.

E codes for terrorism events take priority over all other E codes except child and adult abuse.

E codes for cataclysmic events take priority over all other E codes except child and adult abuse and terrorism.

E codes for transport accidents take priority over all other E codes except cataclysmic events, child and adult abuse and terrorism.

Activity and external cause status codes are assigned following all causal (intent) E codes.

The first-listed E code should correspond to the cause of the most serious diagnosis due to an assault, accident, or self-harm, following the order of hierarchy listed above.

9) **If the reporting format limits the number of E codes**

If the reporting format limits the number of E codes that can be used in reporting clinical data, report the code for the cause/intent most related to the principal diagnosis. If the format permits capture of additional E codes, the cause/intent, including medical misadventures, of the additional events should be reported rather than the codes for place, activity or external status.

b. **Place of Occurrence Guideline**

Use an additional code from category E849 to indicate the Place of Occurrence for injuries and poisonings. The Place of Occurrence describes the place where the event occurred and not the patient's activity at the time of the event.

Do not use E849.9 if the place of occurrence is not stated.

c. **Adverse Effects of Drugs, Medicinal and Biological Substances Guidelines**

1) **Do not code directly from the Table of Drugs**

Do not code directly from the Table of Drugs and Chemicals. Always refer back to the Tabular List.

2) **Use as many codes as necessary to describe**

Use as many codes as necessary to describe completely all drugs, medicinal or biological substances.

If the reporting format limits the number of E codes, and there are different fourth digit codes in the same three digit category, use the code for "Other specified" of that category of drugs, medicinal or biological substances. If there is no "Other specified" code in that category, use the appropriate "Unspecified" code in that category.

If the reporting format limits the number of E codes, and the codes are in different three digit categories, assign the appropriate E code for other multiple drugs and medicinal substances.

3) **If the same E code would describe the causative agent**

If the same E code would describe the causative agent for more than one adverse reaction, assign the code only once.

4) **If two or more drugs, medicinal or biological substances**

If two or more drugs, medicinal or biological substances are reported, code each individually unless the combination code is listed in the Table of Drugs and Chemicals. In that case, assign the E code for the combination.

5) **When a reaction results from the interaction of a drug(s)**

When a reaction results from the interaction of a drug(s) and alcohol, use poisoning codes and E codes for both.

6) **Codes from the E930-E949 series**

Codes from the E930-E949 series must be used to identify the causative substance for an adverse effect of drug, medicinal and biological substances, correctly prescribed and properly administered. The effect, such as tachycardia, delirium, gastrointestinal hemorrhaging, vomiting, hypokalemia, hepatitis, renal failure, or respiratory failure, is coded and followed by the appropriate code from the E930-E949 series.

d. **Child and Adult Abuse Guideline**

1) **Intentional injury**

When the cause of an injury or neglect is intentional child or adult abuse, the first listed E code should be assigned from categories E960-E968, Homicide and injury purposely inflicted by other persons, (except category E967). An E code from category E967, Child and adult battering and other maltreatment, should be added as an additional code to identify the perpetrator, if known.

2) **Accidental intent**

In cases of neglect when the intent is determined to be accidental E code E904.0, Abandonment or neglect of infant and helpless person, should be the first listed E code.

e. **Unknown or Suspected Intent Guideline**

1) **If the intent (accident, self-harm, assault) of the cause of an injury or poisoning is unknown**

If the intent (accident, self-harm, assault) of the cause of an injury or poisoning is unknown or unspecified, code the intent as undetermined E980-E989.

2) **If the intent (accident, self-harm, assault) of the cause of an injury or poisoning is questionable**

If the intent (accident, self-harm, assault) of the cause of an injury or poisoning is questionable, probable or suspected, code the intent as undetermined E980-E989.

f. **Undetermined Cause**

When the intent of an injury or poisoning is known, but the cause is unknown, use codes: E928.9, Unspecified accident, E958.9, Suicide and self-inflicted injury by unspecified means, and E968.9, Assault by unspecified means.

These E codes should rarely be used, as the documentation in the medical record, in both the inpatient outpatient and other settings, should normally provide sufficient detail to determine the cause of the injury.

g. **Late Effects of External Cause Guidelines**

1) **Late effect E codes**

Late effect E codes exist for injuries and poisonings but not for adverse effects of drugs, misadventures and surgical complications.

2) **Late effect E codes (E929, E959, E969, E977, E989, or E999.1)**

A late effect E code (E929, E959, E969, E977, E989, or E999.1) should be used with any report of a late effect or sequela resulting from a previous injury or poisoning (905-909).

3) **Late effect E code with a related current injury**

A late effect E code should never be used with a related current nature of injury code.

4) **Use of late effect E codes for subsequent visits**

Use a late effect E code for subsequent visits when a late effect of the initial injury or poisoning is being treated. There is no late effect E code for adverse effects of drugs.

Do not use a late effect E code for subsequent visits for follow-up care (e.g., to assess healing, to receive rehabilitative therapy) of the injury or poisoning when no late effect of the injury has been documented.

h. **Misadventures and Complications of Care Guidelines**

1) **Code range E870-E876**

Assign a code in the range of E870-E876 if misadventures are stated by the provider. When applying the E code guidelines pertaining to sequencing, these E codes are considered causal codes.

2) **Code range E878-E879**

Assign a code in the range of E878-E879 if the provider attributes an abnormal reaction or later complication to a surgical or medical procedure, but does not mention misadventure at the time of the procedure as the cause of the reaction.

i. **Terrorism Guidelines**

1) **Cause of injury identified by the Federal Government (FBI) as terrorism**

When the cause of an injury is identified by the Federal Government (FBI) as terrorism, the first-listed E-code should be a code from category E979, Terrorism. The definition of terrorism employed by the FBI is found at the inclusion note at E979. The terrorism E-code is the only E-code that should be assigned. Additional E codes from the assault categories should not be assigned.

2) **Cause of an injury is suspected to be the result of terrorism**

When the cause of an injury is suspected to be the result of terrorism a code from category E979 should not be assigned. Assign a code in the range of E codes based circumstances on the documentation of intent and mechanism.

3) **Code E979.9, Terrorism, secondary effects**

Assign code E979.9, Terrorism, secondary effects, for conditions occurring subsequent to the terrorist event. This code should not be assigned for conditions that are due to the initial terrorist act.

4) **Statistical tabulation of terrorism codes**

For statistical purposes these codes will be tabulated within the category for assault, expanding the current category from E960-E969 to include E979 and E999.1.

j. **Activity Code Guidelines**

Assign a code from category E001-E030 to describe the activity that caused or contributed to the injury or other health condition.

Unlike other E codes, activity E codes may be assigned to indicate a health condition (not just injuries) resulted from an activity, or the activity contributed to the condition.

The activity codes are not applicable to poisonings, adverse effects, misadventures or late effects.

Do not assign E030, Unspecified activity, if the activity is not stated.

k. **External cause status**

A code from category E000, External cause status, should be assigned whenever any other E code is assigned for an encounter, including an Activity

E code, except for the events noted below. Assign a code from category E000, External cause status, to indicate the work status of the person at the time the event occurred. The status code indicates whether the event occurred during military activity, whether a non-military person was at work, whether an individual including a student or volunteer was involved in a non-work activity at the time of the causal event.

A code from E000, External cause status, should be assigned, when applicable, with other external cause codes, such as transport accidents and falls. The external cause status codes are not applicable to poisonings, adverse effects, misadventures or late effects.

Do not assign a code from category E000 if no other E codes (cause, activity) are applicable for the encounter.

Do not assign code E000.9, Unspecified external cause status, if the status is not stated.

Section II. Selection of Principal Diagnosis

The circumstances of inpatient admission always govern the selection of principal diagnosis. The principal diagnosis is defined in the Uniform Hospital Discharge Data Set (UHDDS) as "that condition established after study to be chiefly responsible for occasioning the admission of the patient to the hospital for care."

The UHDDS definitions are used by hospitals to report inpatient data elements in a standardized manner. These data elements and their definitions can be found in the July 31, 1985, Federal Register (Vol. 50, No, 147), pp. 31038-40.

Since that time the application of the UHDDS definitions has been expanded to include all non-outpatient settings (acute care, short term, long term care and psychiatric hospitals; home health agencies; rehab facilities; nursing homes, etc).

In determining principal diagnosis the coding conventions in the ICD-9-CM, Volumes I and II take precedence over these official coding guidelines.

(See Section I.A., Conventions for the ICD-9-CM)

The importance of consistent, complete documentation in the medical record cannot be overemphasized. Without such documentation the application of all coding guidelines is a difficult, if not impossible, task.

A. **Codes for symptoms, signs, and ill-defined conditions**

   Codes for symptoms, signs, and ill-defined conditions from Chapter 16 are not to be used as principal diagnosis when a related definitive diagnosis has been established.

B. **Two or more interrelated conditions, each potentially meeting the definition for principal diagnosis.**

   When there are two or more interrelated conditions (such as diseases in the same ICD-9-CM chapter or manifestations characteristically associated with a certain disease) potentially meeting the definition of principal diagnosis, either condition may be sequenced first, unless the circumstances of the admission, the therapy provided, the Tabular List, or the Alphabetic Index indicate otherwise.

C. **Two or more diagnoses that equally meet the definition for principal diagnosis**

   In the unusual instance when two or more diagnoses equally meet the criteria for principal diagnosis as determined by the circumstances of admission, diagnostic workup and/or therapy provided, and the Alphabetic Index, Tabular List, or another coding guidelines does not provide sequencing direction, any one of the diagnoses may be sequenced first.

D. **Two or more comparative or contrasting conditions.**

   In those rare instances when two or more contrasting or comparative diagnoses are documented as "either/or" (or similar terminology), they are coded as if the diagnoses were confirmed and the diagnoses are sequenced according to the circumstances of the admission. If no further determination can be made as to which diagnosis should be principal, either diagnosis may be sequenced first.

E. **A symptom(s) followed by contrasting/comparative diagnoses**

   When a symptom(s) is followed by contrasting/comparative diagnoses, the symptom code is sequenced first. All the contrasting/comparative diagnoses should be coded as additional diagnoses.

F. **Original treatment plan not carried out**

   Sequence as the principal diagnosis the condition, which after study occasioned the admission to the hospital, even though treatment may not have been carried out due to unforeseen circumstances.

G. **Complications of surgery and other medical care**

   When the admission is for treatment of a complication resulting from surgery or other medical care, the complication code is sequenced as the principal diagnosis. If the complication is classified to the 996-999 series and the code lacks the necessary specificity in describing the complication, an additional code for the specific complication should be assigned.

H. **Uncertain Diagnosis**

   If the diagnosis documented at the time of discharge is qualified as "probable", "suspected", "likely", "questionable", "possible", or "still to be ruled out", or other similar terms indicating uncertainty, code the condition as if it existed or was established. The bases for these guidelines are the diagnostic workup, arrangements for further workup or observation, and initial therapeutic approach that correspond most closely with the established diagnosis.

   Note: This guideline is applicable only to inpatient admissions to short-term, acute, long-term care and psychiatric hospitals.

I. **Admission from Observation Unit**

   1. **Admission Following Medical Observation**

      When a patient is admitted to an observation unit for a medical condition, which either worsens or does not improve, and is subsequently admitted as an inpatient of the same hospital for this same medical condition, the principal diagnosis would be the medical condition which led to the hospital admission.

   2. **Admission Following Post-Operative Observation**

      When a patient is admitted to an observation unit to monitor a condition (or complication) that develops following outpatient surgery, and then is subsequently admitted as an inpatient of the same hospital, hospitals should apply the Uniform Hospital Discharge Data Set (UHDDS) definition of principal diagnosis as "that condition established after study to be chiefly responsible for occasioning the admission of the patient to the hospital for care."

J. **Admission from Outpatient Surgery**

   When a patient receives surgery in the hospital's outpatient surgery department and is subsequently admitted for continuing inpatient care at the same hospital, the following guidelines should be followed in selecting the principal diagnosis for the inpatient admission:

   - If the reason for the inpatient admission is a complication, assign the complication as the principal diagnosis.
   - If no complication, or other condition, is documented as the reason for the inpatient admission, assign the reason for the outpatient surgery as the principal diagnosis.
   - If the reason for the inpatient admission is another condition unrelated to the surgery, assign the unrelated condition as the principal diagnosis.

Section III. Reporting Additional Diagnoses

GENERAL RULES FOR OTHER (ADDITIONAL) DIAGNOSES

For reporting purposes the definition for "other diagnoses" is interpreted as additional conditions that affect patient care in terms of requiring:

   clinical evaluation; or
   therapeutic treatment; or
   diagnostic procedures; or
   extended length of hospital stay; or
   increased nursing care and/or monitoring.

The UHDDS item #11-b defines Other Diagnoses as "all conditions that coexist at the time of admission, that develop subsequently, or that affect the treatment received and/or the length of stay. Diagnoses that relate to an earlier episode which have no bearing on the current hospital stay are to be excluded." UHDDS definitions apply to inpatients in acute care, short-term, long term care and psychiatric hospital setting. The UHDDS definitions are used by acute care short-term hospitals to report inpatient data elements in a standardized manner. These data elements and their definitions can be found in the July 31, 1985, Federal Register (Vol. 50, No, 147), pp. 31038-40.

Since that time the application of the UHDDS definitions has been expanded to include all non-outpatient settings (acute care, short term, long term care and psychiatric hospitals; home health agencies; rehab facilities; nursing homes, etc).

The following guidelines are to be applied in designating "other diagnoses" when neither the Alphabetic Index nor the Tabular List in ICD-9-CM provide direction. The listing of the diagnoses in the patient record is the responsibility of the attending provider.

A. **Previous conditions**

   If the provider has included a diagnosis in the final diagnostic statement, such as the discharge summary or the face sheet, it should ordinarily be coded. Some providers include in the diagnostic statement resolved conditions or diagnoses and status-post procedures from previous admission that have no bearing on the current stay. Such conditions are not to be reported and are coded only if required by hospital policy.

   However, history codes (V10-V19) may be used as secondary codes if the historical condition or family history has an impact on current care or influences treatment.

B. **Abnormal findings**

   Abnormal findings (laboratory, x-ray, pathologic, and other diagnostic results) are not coded and reported unless the provider indicates their clinical significance. If the findings are outside the normal range and the attending provider has ordered other tests to evaluate the condition or prescribed treatment, it is appropriate to ask the provider whether the abnormal finding should be added.

   Please note: This differs from the coding practices in the outpatient setting for coding encounters for diagnostic tests that have been interpreted by a provider.

C. **Uncertain Diagnosis**

   If the diagnosis documented at the time of discharge is qualified as "probable", "suspected", "likely", "questionable", "possible", or "still to be ruled out" or other similar terms indicating uncertainty, code the condition as if it existed or was established. The bases for these guidelines are the diagnostic workup, arrangements for further workup or observation, and initial therapeutic approach that correspond most closely with the established diagnosis.

   Note: This guideline is applicable only to inpatient admissions to short-term, acute, long-term care and psychiatric hospitals.

Section IV. Diagnostic Coding and Reporting Guidelines for Outpatient Services

These coding guidelines for outpatient diagnoses have been approved for use by hospitals/providers in coding and reporting hospital-based outpatient services and provider-based office visits.

Information about the use of certain abbreviations, punctuation, symbols, and other conventions used in the ICD-9-CM Tabular List (code numbers and titles), can be found in Section IA of these guidelines, under "Conventions Used in the Tabular List." Information about the correct sequence to use in finding a code is also described in Section I.

The terms encounter and visit are often used interchangeably in describing outpatient service contacts and, therefore, appear together in these guidelines without distinguishing one from the other.

Though the conventions and general guidelines apply to all settings, coding guidelines for outpatient and provider reporting of diagnoses will vary in a number of instances from those for inpatient diagnoses, recognizing that:

The Uniform Hospital Discharge Data Set (UHDDS) definition of principal diagnosis applies only to inpatients in acute, short-term, long-term care and psychiatric hospitals.

Coding guidelines for inconclusive diagnoses (probable, suspected, rule out, etc.) were developed for inpatient reporting and do not apply to outpatients.

A. Selection of first-listed condition

In the outpatient setting, the term first-listed diagnosis is used in lieu of principal diagnosis.

In determining the first-listed diagnosis the coding conventions of ICD-9-CM, as well as the general and disease specific guidelines take precedence over the outpatient guidelines.

Diagnoses often are not established at the time of the initial encounter/visit. It may take two or more visits before the diagnosis is confirmed.

The most critical rule involves beginning the search for the correct code assignment through the Alphabetic Index. Never begin searching initially in the Tabular List as this will lead to coding errors.

1. Outpatient Surgery

When a patient presents for outpatient surgery, code the reason for the surgery as the first-listed diagnosis (reason for the encounter), even if the surgery is not performed due to a contraindication.

2. Observation Stay

When a patient is admitted for observation for a medical condition, assign a code for the medical condition as the first-listed diagnosis.

When a patient presents for outpatient surgery and develops complications requiring admission to observation, code the reason for the surgery as the first reported diagnosis (reason for the encounter), followed by codes for the complications as secondary diagnoses.

B. Codes from 001.0 through V91.99

The appropriate code or codes from 001.0 through V91.99 must be used to identify diagnoses, symptoms, conditions, problems, complaints, or other reason(s) for the encounter/visit.

C. Accurate reporting of ICD-9-CM diagnosis codes

For accurate reporting of ICD-9-CM diagnosis codes, the documentation should describe the patient's condition, using terminology which includes specific diagnoses as well as symptoms, problems, or reasons for the encounter. There are ICD-9-CM codes to describe all of these.

D. Selection of codes 001.0 through 999.9

The selection of codes 001.0 through 999.9 will frequently be used to describe the reason for the encounter. These codes are from the section of ICD-9-CM for the classification of diseases and injuries (e.g. infectious and parasitic diseases; neoplasms; symptoms, signs, and ill-defined conditions, etc.).

E. Codes that describe symptoms and signs

Codes that describe symptoms and signs, as opposed to diagnoses, are acceptable for reporting purposes when a diagnosis has not been established (confirmed) by the provider. Chapter 16 of ICD-9-CM, Symptoms, Signs, and Ill-defined conditions (codes 780.0 - 799.9) contain many, but not all codes for symptoms.

F. Encounters for circumstances other than a disease or injury

ICD-9-CM provides codes to deal with encounters for circumstances other than a disease or injury. The Supplementary Classification of factors Influencing Health Status and Contact with Health Services (V01.0- V91.99) is provided to deal with occasions when circumstances other than a disease or injury are recorded as diagnosis or problems. *See Section I.C.18 for information on V-codes.*

G. Level of Detail in Coding

1. ICD-9-CM codes with 3, 4, or 5 digits

ICD-9-CM is composed of codes with either 3, 4, or 5 digits. Codes with three digits are included in ICD-9-CM as the heading of a category of codes that may be further subdivided by the use of fourth and/or fifth digits, which provide greater specificity.

2. Use of full number of digits required for a code

A three-digit code is to be used only if it is not further subdivided. Where fourth-digit subcategories and/or fifth-digit subclassifications are provided, they must be assigned. A code is invalid if it has not been coded to the full number of digits required for that code.

See also discussion under Section I.b.3., General Coding Guidelines, Level of Detail in Coding.

H. ICD-9-CM code for the diagnosis, condition, problem, or other reason for encounter/visit

List first the ICD-9-CM code for the diagnosis, condition, problem, or other reason for encounter/visit shown in the medical record to be chiefly responsible for the services provided. List additional codes that describe any coexisting conditions. In some cases the first-listed diagnosis may be a symptom when a diagnosis has not been established (confirmed) by the physician.

I. Uncertain diagnosis

Do not code diagnoses documented as "probable", "suspected," "questionable," "rule out," or "working diagnosis" or other similar terms indicating uncertainty. Rather, code the condition(s) to the highest degree of certainty for that encounter/visit, such as symptoms, signs, abnormal test results, or other reason for the visit.

Please note: This differs from the coding practices used by short-term, acute care, long-term care and psychiatric hospitals.

J. Chronic diseases

Chronic diseases treated on an ongoing basis may be coded and reported as many times as the patient receives treatment and care for the condition(s)

K. Code all documented conditions that coexist

Code all documented conditions that coexist at the time of the encounter/visit, and require or affect patient care treatment or management. Do not code conditions that were previously treated and no longer exist. However, history codes (V10-V19) may be used as secondary codes if the historical condition or family history has an impact on current care or influences treatment.

L. Patients receiving diagnostic services only

For patients receiving diagnostic services only during an encounter/visit, sequence first the diagnosis, condition, problem, or other reason for encounter/visit shown in the medical record to be chiefly responsible for the outpatient services provided during the encounter/visit. Codes for other diagnoses (e.g., chronic conditions) may be sequenced as additional diagnoses.

For encounters for routine laboratory/radiology testing in the absence of any signs, symptoms, or associated diagnosis, assign V72.5 and/or a code from subcategory V72.6. If routine testing is performed during the same encounter as a test to evaluate a sign, symptom, or diagnosis, it is appropriate to assign both the V code and the code describing the reason for the non-routine test.

For outpatient encounters for diagnostic tests that have been interpreted by a physician, and the final report is available at the time of coding, code any confirmed or definitive diagnosis(es) documented in the interpretation. Do not code related signs and symptoms as additional diagnoses.

Please note: This differs from the coding practice in the hospital inpatient setting regarding abnormal findings on test results.

M. Patients receiving therapeutic services only

For patients receiving therapeutic services only during an encounter/visit, sequence first the diagnosis, condition, problem, or other reason for encounter/visit shown in the medical record to be chiefly responsible for the outpatient services provided during the encounter/visit. Codes for other diagnoses (e.g., chronic conditions) may be sequenced as additional diagnoses.

The only exception to this rule is that when the primary reason for the admission/encounter is chemotherapy, radiation therapy, or rehabilitation, the appropriate V code for the service is listed first, and the diagnosis or problem for which the service is being performed listed second.

N. Patients receiving preoperative evaluations only

For patients receiving preoperative evaluations only, sequence first a code from category V72.8, Other specified examinations, to describe the pre-op consultations. Assign a code for the condition to describe the reason for the surgery as an additional diagnosis. Code also any findings related to the pre-op evaluation.

O. Ambulatory surgery

For ambulatory surgery, code the diagnosis for which the surgery was performed. If the postoperative diagnosis is known to be different from the preoperative diagnosis at the time the diagnosis is confirmed, select the postoperative diagnosis for coding, since it is the most definitive.

P. Routine outpatient prenatal visits

For routine outpatient prenatal visits when no complications are present, codes V22.0, Supervision of normal first pregnancy, or V22.1, Supervision of other normal pregnancy, should be used as the principal diagnosis. These codes should not be used in conjunction with chapter 11 codes.

Appendix I Present on Admission Reporting Guidelines

Introduction

These guidelines are to be used as a supplement to the *ICD-9-CM Official Guidelines for Coding and Reporting* to facilitate the assignment of the Present on Admission (POA) indicator for each diagnosis and external cause of injury code reported on claim forms (UB-04 and 837 Institutional).

These guidelines are not intended to replace any guidelines in the main body of the *ICD-9-CM Official Guidelines for Coding and Reporting.* The POA guidelines are not intended to provide guidance on when a condition should be coded, but rather, how to apply the POA indicator to the final set of diagnosis codes that have been assigned in accordance with Sections I, II, and III of the official coding guidelines. Subsequent to the assignment of the ICD-9-CM codes, the POA indicator should then be assigned to those conditions that have been coded.

As stated in the Introduction to the ICD-9-CM Official Guidelines for Coding and Reporting, a joint effort between the healthcare provider and the coder is essential to achieve complete and accurate documentation, code assignment, and reporting of diagnoses and procedures. The importance of consistent, complete documentation in the medical record cannot be overemphasized. Medical record documentation from any provider involved in the care and treatment of the patient may be used to support the determination of whether a condition was present on admission or not. In the context of the official coding guidelines, the term "provider" means a physician or any qualified healthcare practitioner who is legally accountable for establishing the patient's diagnosis.

These guidelines are not a substitute for the provider's clinical judgment as to the determination of whether a condition was/was not present on admission. The provider should be queried regarding issues related to the linking of signs/symptoms, timing of test results, and the timing of findings.

General Reporting Requirements

All claims involving inpatient admissions to general acute care hospitals or other facilities that are subject to a law or regulation mandating collection of present on admission information.

Present on admission is defined as present at the time the order for inpatient admission occurs — conditions that develop during an outpatient encounter, including emergency department, observation, or outpatient surgery, are considered as present on admission.

POA indicator is assigned to principal and secondary diagnoses (as defined in Section II of the Official Guidelines for Coding and Reporting) and the external cause of injury codes.

Issues related to inconsistent, missing, conflicting or unclear documentation must still be resolved by the provider.

If a condition would not be coded and reported based on UHDDS definitions and current official coding guidelines, then the POA indicator would not be reported.

Reporting Options

Y - Yes
N - No
U - Unknown
W – Clinically undetermined
Unreported/Not used (or "1" for Medicare usage) – (Exempt from POA reporting)

Reporting Definitions

Y = present at the time of inpatient admission
N = not present at the time of inpatient admission
U = documentation is insufficient to determine if condition is present on admission
W = provider is unable to clinically determine whether condition was present on admission or not

Timeframe for POA Identification and Documentation

There is no required timeframe as to when a provider (per the definition of "provider" used in these guidelines) must identify or document a condition to be present on admission. In some clinical situations, it may not be possible for a provider to make a definitive diagnosis (or a condition may not be recognized or reported by the patient) for a period of time after admission. In some cases it may be several days before the provider arrives at a definitive diagnosis. This does not mean that the condition was not present on admission. Determination of whether the condition was present on admission or not will be based on the applicable POA guideline as identified in this document, or on the provider's best clinical judgment.

If at the time of code assignment the documentation is unclear as to whether a condition was present on admission or not, it is appropriate to query the provider for clarification.

Assigning the POA Indicator

Condition is on the "Exempt from Reporting" list

Leave the "present on admission" field blank if the condition is on the list of ICD-9-CM codes for which this field is not applicable. This is the only circumstance in which the field may be left blank.

POA Explicitly Documented

Assign Y for any condition the provider explicitly documents as being present on admission.

Assign N for any condition the provider explicitly documents as not present at the time of admission.

Conditions diagnosed prior to inpatient admission

Assign "Y" for conditions that were diagnosed prior to admission (example: hypertension, diabetes mellitus, asthma).

Conditions diagnosed during the admission but clearly present before admission

Assign "Y" for conditions diagnosed during the admission that were clearly present but not diagnosed until after admission occurred.

Diagnoses subsequently confirmed after admission are considered present on admission if at the time of admission they are documented as suspected, possible, rule out, differential diagnosis, or constitute an underlying cause of a symptom that is present at the time of admission.

Condition develops during outpatient encounter prior to inpatient admission

Assign Y for any condition that develops during an outpatient encounter prior to a written order for inpatient admission.

Documentation does not indicate whether condition was present on admission

Assign "U" when the medical record documentation is unclear as to whether the condition was present on admission. "U" should not be routinely assigned and used only in very limited circumstances. Coders are encouraged to query the providers when the documentation is unclear.

Documentation states that it cannot be determined whether the condition was or was not present on admission

Assign "W" when the medical record documentation indicates that it cannot be clinically determined whether or not the condition was present on admission.

Chronic condition with acute exacerbation during the admission

If the code is a combination code that identifies both the chronic condition and the acute exacerbation, see POA guidelines pertaining to combination codes.

If the combination code only identifies the chronic condition and not the acute exacerbation (e.g., acute exacerbation of chronic leukemia), assign "Y."

Conditions documented as possible, probable, suspected, or rule out at the time of discharge

If the final diagnosis contains a possible, probable, suspected, or rule out diagnosis, and this diagnosis was based on signs, symptoms, or clinical findings suspected at the time of inpatient admission, assign "Y."

If the final diagnosis contains a possible, probable, suspected, or rule out diagnosis, and this diagnosis was based on signs, symptoms or clinical findings that were not present on admission, assign "N".

Conditions documented as impending or threatened at the time of discharge

If the final diagnosis contains an impending or threatened diagnosis, and this diagnosis is based on symptoms or clinical findings that were present on admission, assign "Y".

If the final diagnosis contains an impending or threatened diagnosis, and this diagnosis is based on symptoms or clinical findings that were not present on admission, assign "N".

Acute and Chronic Conditions

Assign "Y" for acute conditions that are present at time of admission and N for acute conditions that are not present at time of admission.

Assign "Y" for chronic conditions, even though the condition may not be diagnosed until after admission.

If a single code identifies both an acute and chronic condition, see the POA guidelines for combination codes.

Combination Codes

Assign "N" if any part of the combination code was not present on admission (e.g., obstructive chronic bronchitis with acute exacerbation and the exacerbation was not present on admission; gastric ulcer that does not start bleeding until after admission; asthma patient develops status asthmaticus after admission)

Assign "Y" if all parts of the combination code were present on admission (e.g., patient with diabetic nephropathy is admitted with uncontrolled diabetes)

If the final diagnosis includes comparative or contrasting diagnoses, and both were present, or suspected, at the time of admission, assign "Y".

For infection codes that include the causal organism, assign "Y" if the infection (or signs of the infection) was present on admission, even though the culture results may not be known until after admission (e.g., patient is admitted with pneumonia and the provider documents pseudomonas as the causal organism a few days later).

Same Diagnosis Code for Two or More Conditions

When the same ICD-9-CM diagnosis code applies to two or more conditions during the same encounter (e.g. bilateral condition, or two separate conditions classified to the same ICD-9-CM diagnosis code):

Assign "Y" if all conditions represented by the single ICD-9-CM code were present on admission (e.g. bilateral fracture of the same bone, same site, and both fractures were present on admission)

Assign "N" if any of the conditions represented by the single ICD-9-CM code was not present on admission (e.g. dehydration with hyponatremia is assigned to code 276.1, but only one of these conditions was present on admission).

Obstetrical conditions

Whether or not the patient delivers during the current hospitalization does not affect assignment of the POA indicator. The determining factor for POA assignment is whether the pregnancy complication or obstetrical condition described by the code was present at the time of admission or not.

If the pregnancy complication or obstetrical condition was present on admission (e.g., patient admitted in preterm labor), assign "Y".

If the pregnancy complication or obstetrical condition was not present on admission (e.g., 2nd degree laceration during delivery, postpartum hemorrhage that occurred during current hospitalization, fetal distress develops after admission), assign "N".

If the obstetrical code includes more than one diagnosis and any of the diagnoses identified by the code were not present on admission assign "N".

(e.g., Code 642.7, Pre-eclampsia or eclampsia superimposed on pre-existing hypertension).

If the obstetrical code includes information that is not a diagnosis, do not consider that information in the POA determination.

(e.g. Code 652.1x, Breech or other malpresentation successfully converted to cephalic presentation should be reported as present on admission if the fetus was breech on admission but was converted to cephalic presentation after admission (since the conversion to cephalic presentation does not represent a diagnosis, the fact that the conversion occurred after admission has no bearing on the POA determination).

Perinatal conditions

Newborns are not considered to be admitted until after birth. Therefore, any condition present at birth or that developed in utero is considered present at admission and should be assigned "Y". This includes conditions that occur during delivery (e.g., injury during delivery, meconium aspiration, exposure to streptococcus B in the vaginal canal).

Congenital conditions and anomalies

Assign "Y" for congenital conditions and anomalies, **except for categories 740-759, Congenital anomalies, which are on the exempt list.** Congenital conditions are always considered present on admission.

External cause of injury codes

Assign "Y" for any E code representing an external cause of injury or poisoning that occurred prior to inpatient admission (e.g., patient fell out of bed at home, patient fell out of bed in emergency room prior to admission)

Assign "N" for any E code representing an external cause of injury or poisoning that occurred during inpatient hospitalization (e.g., patient fell out of hospital bed during hospital stay, patient experienced an adverse reaction to a medication administered after inpatient admission)

Categories and Codes Exempt from Diagnosis Present on Admission Requirement

Effective Date: October 1, 2008

Note: "Diagnosis present on admission" for these code categories are exempt because they represent circumstances regarding the healthcare encounter or factors influencing health status that do not represent a current disease or injury or are always present on admission.

Categories or subcategories listed are inclusive of all codes within those categories or subcategories, unless otherwise indicated. In order to streamline the POA exempt list and make it easier to read, where all of the codes in a code range are POA exempt, only the code range is shown, rather than listing each of the individual codes in the range.

137-139, Late effects of infectious and parasitic diseases

268.1, Rickets, late effect

326, Late effects of intracranial abscess or pyogenic infection

412, Old myocardial infarction

438, Late effects of cerebrovascular disease

650, Normal delivery

660.7, Failed forceps or vacuum extractor, unspecified

677, Late effect of complication of pregnancy, childbirth, and the puerperium

740-759, Congenital anomalies

905-909, Late effects of injuries, poisonings, toxic effects, and other external causes

V02, Carrier or suspected carrier of infectious diseases

V03, Need for prophylactic vaccination and inoculation against bacterial diseases

V04, Need for prophylactic vaccination and inoculation against certain viral diseases

V05, Need for other prophylactic vaccination and inoculation against single diseases

V06, Need for prophylactic vaccination and inoculation against combinations of diseases

V07, Need for isolation and other prophylactic or treatment measures

V10, Personal history of malignant neoplasm

V11, Personal history of mental disorder

V12, Personal history of certain other diseases

V13, Personal history of other diseases

V14, Personal history of allergy to medicinal agents

V15, Other personal history presenting hazards to health

V16, Family history of malignant neoplasm

V17, Family history of certain chronic disabling diseases

V18, Family history of certain other specific conditions

V19, Family history of other conditions

V20, Health supervision of infant or child

V21, Constitutional states in development

V22, Normal pregnancy

V23, Supervision of high-risk pregnancy

V24, Postpartum care and examination

V25, Encounter for contraceptive management

V26, Procreative management

V27, Outcome of delivery

V28, Antenatal screening

V29, Observation and evaluation of newborns for suspected condition not found

V30-V39, Liveborn infants according to type of birth

V42, Organ or tissue replaced by transplant

V43, Organ or tissue replaced by other means

V44, Artificial opening status

V45, Other postprocedural states

V46, Other dependence on machines and devices

V49.60-V49.77, Upper and lower limb amputation status

V49.81-V49.85, Other specified conditions influencing health status

V50, Elective surgery for purposes other than remedying health states

V51, Aftercare involving the use of plastic surgery

PART I / Introduction

V52, Fitting and adjustment of prosthetic device and implant

V53, Fitting and adjustment of other device

V54, Other orthopedic aftercare

V55, Attention to artificial openings

V56, Encounter for dialysis and dialysis catheter care

V57, Care involving use of rehabilitation procedures

V58, Encounter for other and unspecified procedures and aftercare

V59, Donors

V60, Housing, household, and economic circumstances

V61, Other family circumstances

V62, Other psychosocial circumstances

V64, Persons encountering health services for specific procedures, not carried out

V65, Other persons seeking consultation

V66, Convalescence and palliative care

V67, Follow-up examination

V68, Encounters for administrative purposes

V69, Problems related to lifestyle

V70, General medical examination

V71, Observation and evaluation for suspected condition not found

V72, Special investigations and examinations

V73, Special screening examination for viral and chlamydial diseases

V74, Special screening examination for bacterial and spirochetal diseases

V75, Special screening examination for other infectious diseases

V76, Special screening for malignant neoplasms

V77, Special screening for endocrine, nutritional, metabolic, and immunity disorders

V78, Special screening for disorders of blood and blood-forming organs

V79, Special screening for mental disorders and developmental handicaps

V80, Special screening for neurological, eye, and ear diseases

V81, Special screening for cardiovascular, respiratory, and genitourinary diseases

V82, Special screening for other conditions

V83, Genetic carrier status

V84, Genetic susceptibility to disease

V85, Body Mass Index

V86, Estrogen receptor status

V87.32, Contact with and (suspected) exposure to algae bloom

V87.4, Personal history of drug therapy

V88, Acquired absence of other organs and tissue

V89, Suspected maternal and fetal conditions not found

V90, Retained foreign body

V91, Multiple gestation placenta status

E000, External cause status

E001-E030, Activity

E800-E807, Railway accidents

E810-E819, Motor vehicle traffic accidents

E820-E825, Motor vehicle nontraffic accidents

E826-E829, Other road vehicle accidents

E830-E838, Water transport accidents

E840-E845, Air and space transport accidents

E846-E848, Vehicle accidents not elsewhere classifiable

E849, Place of occurrence (Except E849.7)

E883.1, Accidental fall into well

E883.2, Accidental fall into storm drain or manhole

E884.0, Fall from playground equipment

E884.1, Fall from cliff

E885.0, Fall from (nonmotorized) scooter

E885.1, Fall from roller skates

E885.2, Fall from skateboard

E885.3, Fall from skis

E885.4, Fall from snowboard

E886.0, Fall on same level from collision, pushing, or shoving, by or with other person, In sports

E890.0-E890.9, Conflagration in private dwelling

E893.0, Accident caused by ignition of clothing, from controlled fire in private dwelling

E893.2, Accident caused by ignition of clothing, from controlled fire not in building or structure

E894, Ignition of highly inflammable material

E895, Accident caused by controlled fire in private dwelling

E897, Accident caused by controlled fire not in building or structure

E917.0, Striking against or struck accidentally by objects or persons, in sports without subsequent fall

E917.1, Striking against or struck accidentally by objects or persons, caused by a crowd, by collective fear or panic without subsequent fall

E917.2, Striking against or struck accidentally by objects or persons, in running water without subsequent fall

E917.5, Striking against or struck accidentally by objects or persons, object in sports with subsequent fall

E917.6, Striking against or struck accidentally by objects or persons, caused by a crowd, by collective fear or panic with subsequent fall

E919, Accident caused by machinery (Except E919.2)

E921, Accident caused by explosion of pressure vessel

E922, Accident caused by firearm and air gun missile

E926.2, Visible and ultraviolet light sources

E928.0-E928.8, Other and unspecified environmental and accidental causes

E929.0-E929.9, Late effects of accidental injury

E959, Late effects of self-inflicted injury

E970-E978, Legal intervention

E979, Terrorism

E981, Poisoning by gases in domestic use, undetermined whether accidentally or purposely inflicted

E982, Poisoning by other gases, undetermined whether accidentally or purposely inflicted

E985, Injury by firearms, air guns and explosives, undetermined whether accidentally or purposely inflicted

E987.0, Falling from high place, undetermined whether accidentally or purposely inflicted, residential premises

E987.2, Falling from high place, undetermined whether accidentally or purposely inflicted, natural sites

E989, Late effects of injury, undetermined whether accidentally or purposely inflicted

E990-E999, Injury resulting from operations of war

POA Examples

The POA examples have been removed from the guidelines.

PART II

ALPHABETIC INDEX VOLUME 2

SECTION I INDEX TO DISEASES AND INJURIES

A

AAT (alpha-1 antitrypsin) deficiency 273.4
AAV (disease) (illness) (infection) - *see* Human immunodeficiency virus (disease) (illness) (infection)
Abactio - *see* Abortion, induced
Abactus venter - *see* Abortion, induced
Abarognosis 781.99
Abasia (-astasia) 307.9
   atactica 781.3
   choreic 781.3
   hysterical 300.11
   paroxysmal trepidant 781.3
   spastic 781.3
   trembling 781.3
   trepidans 781.3
Abderhalden-Kaufmann-Lignac syndrome (cystinosis) 270.0
Abdomen, abdominal - *see also* condition
   accordion 306.4
   acute 789.0
   angina 557.1
   burst 868.00
   convulsive equivalent (*see also* Epilepsy) 345.5
   heart 746.87
   muscle deficiency syndrome 756.79
   obstipum 756.79
Abdominalgia 789.0
   periodic 277.31
Abduction contracture, hip or other joint - *see* Contraction, joint
Abercrombie's syndrome (amyloid degeneration) 277.39
Aberrant (congenital) - *see also* Malposition, congenital
   adrenal gland 759.1
   blood vessel NEC 747.60
      arteriovenous NEC 747.60
      cerebrovascular 747.81
      gastrointestinal 747.61
      lower limb 747.64
      renal 747.62
      spinal 747.82
      upper limb 747.63
   breast 757.6
   endocrine gland NEC 759.2
   gastrointestinal vessel (peripheral) 747.61
   hepatic duct 751.69
   lower limb vessel (peripheral) 747.64
   pancreas 751.7
   parathyroid gland 759.2
   peripheral vascular vessel NEC 747.60
   pituitary gland (pharyngeal) 759.2
   renal blood vessel 747.62
   sebaceous glands, mucous membrane, mouth 750.26
   spinal vessel 747.82
   spleen 759.0
   testis (descent) 752.51
   thymus gland 759.2
   thyroid gland 759.2
   upper limb vessel (peripheral) 747.63
Aberratio
   lactis 757.6
   testis 752.51
Aberration - *see also* Anomaly
   chromosome - *see* Anomaly, chromosome(s)
   distantial 368.9
   mental (*see also* Disorder, mental, nonpsychotic) 300.9
Abetalipoproteinemia 272.5
Abionarce 780.79
Abiotrophy 799.89
Ablatio
   placentae - *see* Placenta, ablatio
   retinae (*see also* Detachment, retina) 361.9

Ablation
   pituitary (gland) (with hypofunction) 253.7
   placenta - *see* Placenta, ablatio
   uterus 621.8
Ablepharia, ablepharon, ablephary 743.62
Ablepsia - *see* Blindness
Ablepsy - *see* Blindness
Ablutomania 300.3
Abnormal, abnormality, abnormalities - *see also* Anomaly
   acid-base balance 276.4
      fetus or newborn - *see* Distress, fetal
   adaptation curve, dark 368.63
   alveolar ridge 525.9
   amnion 658.9
      affecting fetus or newborn 762.9
   anatomical relationship NEC 759.9
   apertures, congenital, diaphragm 756.6
   auditory perception NEC 388.40
   autosomes NEC 758.5
      13 758.1
      18 758.2
      21 or 22 758.0
      D_1 758.1
      E_3 758.2
      G 758.0
   ballistocardiogram 794.39
   basal metabolic rate (BMR) 794.7
   biosynthesis, testicular androgen 257.2
   blood level (of)
      cobalt 790.6
      copper 790.6
      iron 790.6
      lead 790.6
      lithium 790.6
      magnesium 790.6
      mineral 790.6
      zinc 790.6
   blood pressure
      elevated (without diagnosis of hypertension) 796.2
      low (*see also* Hypotension) 458.9
         reading (incidental) (isolated) (nonspecific) 796.3
   blood sugar 790.29
   bowel sounds 787.5
   breathing behavior - *see* Respiration
   caloric test 794.19
   cervix (acquired) NEC 622.9
      congenital 752.40
      in pregnancy or childbirth 654.6
         causing obstructed labor 660.2
            affecting fetus or newborn 763.1
   chemistry, blood NEC 790.6
   chest sounds 786.7
   chorion 658.9
      affecting fetus or newborn 762.9
   chromosomal NEC 758.89
      analysis, nonspecific result 795.2
      autosomes (*see also* Abnormal, autosomes NEC) 758.5
      fetal, (suspected) affecting management of pregnancy 655.1
      sex 758.81
   clinical findings NEC 796.4
   communication - *see* Fistula
   configuration of pupils 379.49
   coronary
      artery 746.85
      vein 746.9
   cortisol-binding globulin 255.8
   course, Eustachian tube 744.24
   creatinine clearance 794.4
   dentofacial NEC 524.9
      functional 524.50
      specified type NEC 524.89
   development, developmental NEC 759.9
      bone 756.9
      central nervous system 742.9
   direction, teeth 524.30

Abnormal, abnormality, abnormalities
   (*Continued*)
   dynia (*see also* Defect, coagulation) 286.9
   Ebstein 746.2
   echocardiogram 793.2
   echoencephalogram 794.01
   echogram NEC - *see* Findings, abnormal, structure
   electrocardiogram (ECG) (EKG) 794.31
   electroencephalogram (EEG) 794.02
   electromyogram (EMG) 794.17
      ocular 794.14
   electro-oculogram (EOG) 794.12
   electroretinogram (ERG) 794.11
   erythrocytes 289.9
      congenital, with perinatal jaundice 282.9 [774.0]
   eustachian valve 746.9
   excitability under minor stress 301.9
   fat distribution 782.9
   feces 787.7
   fetal heart rate - *see* Distress, fetal
   fetus NEC
      affecting management of pregnancy - *see* Pregnancy, management affected by, fetal
      causing disproportion 653.7
         affecting fetus or newborn 763.1
         causing obstructed labor 660.1
            affecting fetus or newborn 763.1
   findings without manifest disease - *see* Findings, abnormal
   fluid
      amniotic 792.3
      cerebrospinal 792.0
      peritoneal 792.9
      pleural 792.9
      synovial 792.9
      vaginal 792.9
   forces of labor NEC 661.9
      affecting fetus or newborn 763.7
   form, teeth 520.2
   function studies
      auditory 794.15
      bladder 794.9
      brain 794.00
      cardiovascular 794.30
      endocrine NEC 794.6
      kidney 794.4
      liver 794.8
      nervous system
         central 794.00
         peripheral 794.19
      oculomotor 794.14
      pancreas 794.9
      placenta 794.9
      pulmonary 794.2
      retina 794.11
      special senses 794.19
      spleen 794.9
      thyroid 794.5
      vestibular 794.16
   gait 781.2
      hysterical 300.11
   gastrin secretion 251.5
   globulin
      cortisol-binding 255.8
      thyroid-binding 246.8
   glucagon secretion 251.4
   glucose 790.29
      in pregnancy, childbirth, or puerperium 648.8
      fetus or newborn 775.0
      non-fasting 790.29
   gravitational (G) forces or states 994.9
   hair NEC 704.2
   hard tissue formation in pulp 522.3
   head movement 781.0

Abnormal, abnormality, abnormalities
(Continued)
- heart
  - rate
    - fetus, affecting liveborn infant
      - before the onset of labor 763.81
      - during labor 763.82
      - unspecified as to time of onset 763.83
    - intrauterine
      - before the onset of labor 763.81
      - during labor 763.82
      - unspecified as to time of onset 763.83
    - newborn
      - before the onset of labor 763.81
      - during labor 763.82
      - unspecified as to time of onset 763.83
  - shadow 793.2
  - sounds NEC 785.3
- hemoglobin (see also Disease, hemoglobin) 282.7
  - trait - see Trait, hemoglobin, abnormal
- hemorrhage, uterus - see Hemorrhage, uterus
- histology NEC 795.4
- increase in
  - appetite 783.6
  - development 783.9
- involuntary movement 781.0
- jaw closure 524.51
- karyotype 795.2
- knee jerk 796.1
- labor NEC 661.9 ●
  - affecting fetus or newborn 763.7
- laboratory findings - see Findings, abnormal
- length, organ or site, congenital - see Distortion
- liver function test 790.6
- loss of height 781.91
- loss of weight 783.21
- lung shadow 793.19
- mammogram 793.80
  - calcification 793.89
  - calculus 793.89
  - microcalcification 793.81
- Mantoux test 795.51
- membranes (fetal)
  - affecting fetus or newborn 762.9
  - complicating pregnancy 658.8 ●
- menstruation - see Menstruation
- metabolism (see also condition) 783.9
- movement 781.0
  - disorder NEC 333.90
    - sleep related, unspecified 780.58
    - specified NEC 333.99
  - head 781.0
  - involuntary 781.0
  - specified type NEC 333.99
- muscle contraction, localized 728.85
- myoglobin (Aberdeen) (Annapolis) 289.9
- narrowness, eyelid 743.62
- optokinetic response 379.57
- organs or tissues of pelvis NEC
  - in pregnancy or childbirth 654.9 ●
    - affecting fetus or newborn 763.89
    - causing obstructed labor 660.2 ●
      - affecting fetus or newborn 763.1
- origin - see Malposition, congenital
- palmar creases 757.2
- Papanicolaou (smear)
  - anus 796.70
    - with
      - atypical squamous cells
        - cannot exclude high grade squamous intraepithelial lesion (ASC-H) 796.72
        - of undetermined significance (ASC-US) 796.71
      - cytologic evidence of malignancy 796.76

Abnormal, abnormality, abnormalities
(Continued)
- Papanicolaou (Continued)
  - anus (Continued)
    - with (Continued)
      - high grade squamous intraepithelial lesion (HGSIL) 796.74
      - low grade squamous intraepithelial lesion (LGSIL) 796.73
      - glandular 796.70
      - specified finding NEC 796.79
  - cervix 795.00
    - with
      - atypical squamous cells
        - cannot exclude high grade squamous intraepithelial lesion (ASC-H) 795.02
        - of undetermined significance (ASC-US) 795.01
      - cytologic evidence of malignancy 795.06
      - high grade squamous intraepithelial lesion (HGSIL) 795.04
      - low grade squamous intraepithelial lesion (LGSIL) 795.03
      - nonspecific finding NEC 795.09
    - other site 796.9
  - vagina 795.10
    - with
      - atypical squamous cells
        - cannot exclude high grade squamous intraepithelial lesion (ASC-H) 795.12
        - of undetermined significance (ASC-US) 795.11
      - cytologic evidence of malignancy 795.16
      - high grade squamous intraepithelial lesion (HGSIL) 795.14
      - low grade squamous intraepithelial lesion (LGSIL) 795.13
      - glandular 795.10
      - specified finding NEC 795.19
- parturition
  - affecting fetus or newborn 763.9
  - mother - see Delivery, complicated
- pelvis (bony) - see Deformity, pelvis
- percussion, chest 786.7
- periods (grossly) (see also Menstruation) 626.9
- phonocardiogram 794.39
- placenta - see Placenta, abnormal
- plantar reflex 796.1
- plasma protein - see Deficiency, plasma, protein
- pleural folds 748.8
- position - see also Malposition
  - gravid uterus 654.4 ●
    - causing obstructed labor 660.2 ●
      - affecting fetus or newborn 763.1
- posture NEC 781.92
- presentation (fetus) - see Presentation, fetus, abnormal
- product of conception NEC 631.8
- puberty - see Puberty
- pulmonary
  - artery 747.39
  - function, newborn 770.89
  - test results 794.2
  - ventilation, newborn 770.89
    - hyperventilation 786.01
- pulsations in neck 785.1
- pupil reflexes 379.40
- quality of milk 676.8 ●
- radiological examination 793.99
  - abdomen NEC 793.6
  - biliary tract 793.3

Abnormal, abnormality, abnormalities
(Continued)
- radiological examination (Continued)
  - breast 793.89
    - mammogram NOS 793.80
    - mammographic
      - calcification 793.89
      - calculus 793.89
      - microcalcification 793.81
  - gastrointestinal tract 793.4
  - genitourinary organs 793.5
  - head 793.0
  - image test inconclusive due to excess body fat 793.91
  - intrathoracic organ NEC 793.2
  - lung (field) 793.19
  - musculoskeletal system 793.7
  - retroperitoneum 793.6
  - skin and subcutaneous tissue 793.99
  - skull 793.0
- red blood cells 790.09
  - morphology 790.09
  - volume 790.09
- reflex NEC 796.1
- renal function test 794.4
- respiration signs - see Respiration
- response to nerve stimulation 794.10
- retinal correspondence 368.34
- rhythm, heart - see also Arrhythmia
  - fetus - see Distress, fetal
- saliva 792.4
- scan
  - brain 794.09
  - kidney 794.4
  - liver 794.8
  - lung 794.2
  - thyroid 794.5
- secretion
  - gastrin 251.5
  - glucagon 251.4
- semen 792.2
- serum level (of)
  - acid phosphatase 790.5
  - alkaline phosphatase 790.5
  - amylase 790.5
  - enzymes NEC 790.5
  - lipase 790.5
- shape
  - cornea 743.41
  - gallbladder 751.69
  - gravid uterus 654.4 ●
    - affecting fetus or newborn 763.89
    - causing obstructed labor 660.2 ●
      - affecting fetus or newborn 763.1
  - head (see also Anomaly, skull) 756.0
  - organ or site, congenital NEC - see Distortion
- sinus venosus 747.40
- size
  - fetus, complicating delivery 653.5 ●
    - causing obstructed labor 660.1 ●
  - gallbladder 751.69
  - head (see also Anomaly, skull) 756.0
  - organ or site, congenital NEC - see Distortion
  - teeth 520.2
- skin and appendages, congenital NEC 757.9
- soft parts of pelvis - see Abnormal, organs or tissues of pelvis
- spermatozoa 792.2
- sputum (amount) (color) (excessive) (odor) (purulent) 786.4
- stool NEC 787.7
  - bloody 578.1
    - occult 792.1
  - bulky 787.7
  - color (dark) (light) 792.1
  - content (fat) (mucus) (pus) 792.1
  - occult blood 792.1
- synchondrosis 756.9

SECTION I INDEX TO DISEASES AND INJURIES / Abnormal, abnormality, abnormalities

Abnormal, abnormality, abnormalities *(Continued)*
- test results without manifest disease - *see* Findings, abnormal
- thebesian valve 746.9
- thermography - *see* Findings, abnormal, structure
- threshold, cones or rods (eye) 368.63
- thyroid-binding globulin 246.8
- thyroid product 246.8
- toxicology (findings) NEC 796.0
- tracheal cartilage (congenital) 748.3
- transport protein 273.8
- ultrasound results - *see* Findings, abnormal, structure
- umbilical cord
  - affecting fetus or newborn 762.6
  - complicating delivery 663.9●
  - specified NEC 663.8●
- union
  - cricoid cartilage and thyroid cartilage 748.3
  - larynx and trachea 748.3
  - thyroid cartilage and hyoid bone 748.3
- urination NEC 788.69
  - psychogenic 306.53
  - stream
    - intermittent 788.61
    - slowing 788.62
    - splitting 788.61
    - weak 788.62
  - urgency 788.63
- urine (constituents) NEC 791.9
- uterine hemorrhage (*see also* Hemorrhage, uterus) 626.9
  - climacteric 627.0
  - postmenopausal 627.1
- vagina (acquired) (congenital)
  - in pregnancy or childbirth 654.7●
    - affecting fetus or newborn 763.89
    - causing obstructed labor 660.2●
      - affecting fetus or newborn 763.1
- vascular sounds 785.9
- vectorcardiogram 794.39
- visually evoked potential (VEP) 794.13
- vulva (acquired) (congenital)
  - in pregnancy or childbirth 654.8●
    - affecting fetus or newborn 763.89
    - causing obstructed labor 660.2●
      - affecting fetus or newborn 763.1
- weight
  - gain 783.1
    - of pregnancy 646.1●
      - with hypertension - *see* Toxemia, of pregnancy
  - loss 783.21
- x-ray examination - *see* Abnormal, radiological examination

Abnormally formed uterus - *see* Anomaly, uterus

Abnormity (any organ or part) - *see* Anomaly

ABO
- hemolytic disease 773.1
- incompatibility (due to transfusion of blood or blood products)
  - with hemolytic transfusion reaction (HTR) (not specified as acute or delayed) 999.61
    - 24 hours or more after transfusion 999.63
    - acute 999.62
    - delayed 999.63
    - less than 24 hours after transfusion 999.62
    - unspecified time after transfusion 999.61
  - reaction 999.60
    - specified NEC 999.69

Abocclusion 524.20

Abolition, language 784.69

Aborter, habitual or recurrent NEC
- without current pregnancy 629.81
- current abortion (*see also* Abortion, spontaneous) 634.9●
  - affecting fetus or newborn 761.8
- observation in current pregnancy 646.3●

Abortion (complete) (incomplete) (inevitable) (with retained products of conception) 637.9●

> Note: Use the following fifth-digit subclassification with categories 634-637:
> 0 unspecified
> 1 incomplete
> 2 complete

- with
  - complication(s) (any) following previous abortion - *see* category 639
  - damage to pelvic organ (laceration) (rupture) (tear) 637.2●
  - embolism (air) (amniotic fluid) (blood clot) (pulmonary) (pyemic) (septic) (soap) 637.6●
  - genital tract and pelvic infection 637.0●
  - hemorrhage, delayed or excessive 637.1●
  - metabolic disorder 637.4●
  - renal failure (acute) 637.3●
  - sepsis (genital tract) (pelvic organ) 637.0●
    - urinary tract 637.7●
  - shock (postoperative) (septic) 637.5●
  - specified complication NEC 637.7●
  - toxemia 637.3●
  - unspecified complication(s) 637.8●
  - urinary tract infection 637.7●
- accidental - *see* Abortion, spontaneous
- artificial - *see* Abortion, induced
- attempted (failed) - *see* Abortion, failed
- criminal - *see* Abortion, illegal
- early - *see* Abortion, spontaneous
- elective - *see* Abortion, legal
- failed (legal) 638.9
  - with
    - damage to pelvic organ (laceration) (rupture) (tear) 638.2
    - embolism (air) (amniotic fluid) (blood clot) (pulmonary) (pyemic) (septic) (soap) 638.6
    - genital tract and pelvic infection 638.0
    - hemorrhage, delayed or excessive 638.1
    - metabolic disorder 638.4
    - renal failure (acute) 638.3
    - sepsis (genital tract) (pelvic organ) 638.0
      - urinary tract 638.7
    - shock (postoperative) (septic) 638.5
    - specified complication NEC 638.7
    - toxemia 638.3
    - unspecified complication(s) 638.8
    - urinary tract infection 638.7
- fetal indication - *see* Abortion, legal
- fetus 779.6
- following threatened abortion - *see* Abortion, by type
- habitual or recurrent (care during pregnancy) 646.3●
  - with current abortion (*see also* Abortion, spontaneous) 634.9●
    - affecting fetus or newborn 761.8
  - without current pregnancy 629.81
- homicidal - *see* Abortion, illegal
- illegal 636.9●
  - with
    - damage to pelvic organ (laceration) (rupture) (tear) 636.2●
    - embolism (air) (amniotic fluid) (blood clot) (pulmonary) (pyemic) (septic) (soap) 636.6●
    - genital tract and pelvic infection 636.0●

Abortion *(Continued)*
- illegal *(Continued)*
  - with *(Continued)*
    - hemorrhage, delayed or excessive 636.1●
    - metabolic disorder 636.4●
    - renal failure 636.3●
    - sepsis (genital tract) (pelvic organ) 636.0●
      - urinary tract 636.7●
    - shock (postoperative) (septic) 636.5●
    - specified complication NEC 636.7●
    - toxemia 636.3●
    - unspecified complication(s) 636.8●
    - urinary tract infection 636.7●
  - fetus 779.6
- induced 637.9●
  - illegal - *see* Abortion, illegal
  - legal indications - *see* Abortion, legal
  - medical indications - *see* Abortion, legal
  - therapeutic - *see* Abortion, legal
- late - *see* Abortion, spontaneous
- legal (legal indication) (medical indication) (under medical supervision) 635.9●
  - with
    - damage to pelvic organ (laceration) (rupture) (tear) 635.2●
    - embolism (air) (amniotic fluid) (blood clot) (pulmonary) (pyemic) (septic) (soap) 635.6●
    - genital tract and pelvic infection 635.0●
    - hemorrhage, delayed or excessive 635.1●
    - metabolic disorder 635.4●
    - renal failure (acute) 635.3●
    - sepsis (genital tract) (pelvic organ) 635.0●
      - urinary tract 635.7●
    - shock (postoperative) (septic) 635.5●
    - specified complication NEC 635.7●
    - toxemia 635.3●
    - unspecified complication(s) 635.8●
    - urinary tract infection 635.7●
  - fetus 779.6
- medical indication - *see* Abortion, legal
- mental hygiene problem - *see* Abortion, legal
- missed 632
- operative - *see* Abortion, legal
- psychiatric indication - *see* Abortion, legal
- recurrent - *see* Abortion, spontaneous
- self-induced - *see* Abortion, illegal
- septic - *see* Abortion, by type, with sepsis
- spontaneous 634.9●
  - with
    - damage to pelvic organ (laceration) (rupture) (tear) 634.2●
    - embolism (air) (amniotic fluid) (blood clot) (pulmonary) (pyemic) (septic) (soap) 634.6●
    - genital tract and pelvic infection 634.0●
    - hemorrhage, delayed or excessive 634.1●
    - metabolic disorder 634.4●
    - renal failure 634.3●
    - sepsis (genital tract) (pelvic organ) 634.0●
      - urinary tract 634.7●
    - shock (postoperative) (septic) 634.5●
    - specified complication NEC 634.7●
    - toxemia 634.3●
    - unspecified complication(s) 634.8●
    - urinary tract infection 634.7●
  - fetus 761.8
  - threatened 640.0●
    - affecting fetus or newborn 762.1
- surgical - *see* Abortion, legal
- therapeutic - *see* Abortion, legal
- threatened 640.0●
  - affecting fetus or newborn 762.1

SECTION I INDEX TO DISEASES AND INJURIES / Abscess

Abortion (Continued)
  tubal - see Pregnancy, tubal
  voluntary - see Abortion, legal
Abortus fever 023.9
Aboulomania 301.6
Abrachia 755.20
Abrachiatism 755.20
Abrachiocephalia 759.89
Abrachiocephalus 759.89
Abrami's disease (acquired hemolytic jaundice) 283.9
Abramov-Fiedler myocarditis (acute isolated myocarditis) 422.91
Abrasion - see also Injury, superficial, by site
  cornea 918.1
  dental 521.20
    extending into
      dentine 521.22
      pulp 521.23
    generalized 521.25
    limited to enamel 521.21
    localized 521.24
  teeth, tooth (dentifrice) (habitual) (hard tissues) (occupational) (ritual) (traditional) (wedge defect) (see also Abrasion, dental) 521.20
Abrikossov's tumor (M9580/0) - see also Neoplasm, connective tissue, benign
  malignant (M9580/3) - see Neoplasm, connective tissue, malignant
Abrism 988.8
Abruption, placenta - see Placenta, abruptio
Abruptio placentae - see Placenta, abruptio
Abscess (acute) (chronic) (infectional) (lymphangitic) (metastatic) (multiple) (pyogenic) (septic) (with lymphangitis) (see also Cellulitis) 682.9
  abdomen, abdominal
    cavity 567.22
    wall 682.2
  abdominopelvic 567.22
  accessory sinus (chronic) (see also Sinusitis) 473.9
  adrenal (capsule) (gland) 255.8
  alveolar 522.5
    with sinus 522.7
  amebic 006.3
    bladder 006.8
    brain (with liver or lung abscess) 006.5
    liver (without mention of brain or lung abscess) 006.3
      with
        brain abscess (and lung abscess) 006.5
        lung abscess 006.4
    lung (with liver abscess) 006.4
      with brain abscess 006.5
    seminal vesicle 006.8
    specified site NEC 006.8
    spleen 006.8
  anaerobic 040.0
  ankle 682.6
  anorectal 566
  antecubital space 682.3
  antrum (chronic) (Highmore) (see also Sinusitis, maxillary) 473.0
  anus 566
  apical (tooth) 522.5
    with sinus (alveolar) 522.7
  appendix 540.1
  areola (acute) (chronic) (nonpuerperal) 611.0
    puerperal, postpartum 675.1●
  arm (any part, above wrist) 682.3
  artery (wall) 447.2
  atheromatous 447.2
  auditory canal (external) 380.10
  auricle (ear) (staphylococcal) (streptococcal) 380.10
  axilla, axillary (region) 682.3
    lymph gland or node 683
  back (any part) 682.2

Abscess (Continued)
  Bartholin's gland 616.3
    with
      abortion - see Abortion, by type, with sepsis
      ectopic pregnancy (see also categories 633.0-633.9) 639.0
      molar pregnancy (see also categories 630-632) 639.0
    complicating pregnancy or puerperium 646.6●
    following
      abortion 639.0
      ectopic or molar pregnancy 639.0
  bartholinian 616.3
  Bezold's 383.01
  bile, biliary, duct or tract (see also Cholecystitis) 576.8
  bilharziasis 120.1
  bladder (wall) 595.89
    amebic 006.8
  bone (subperiosteal) (see also Osteomyelitis) 730.0●
    accessory sinus (chronic) (see also Sinusitis) 473.9
    acute 730.0●
    chronic or old 730.1●
    jaw (lower) (upper) 526.4
    mastoid - see Mastoiditis, acute
    petrous (see also Petrositis) 383.20
    spinal (tuberculous) (see also Tuberculosis) 015.0● [730.88]
    nontuberculous 730.08
  bowel 569.5
  brain (any part) 324.0
    amebic (with liver or lung abscess) 006.5
    cystic 324.0
    late effect - see category 326
    otogenic 324.0
    tuberculous (see also Tuberculosis) 013.3●
  breast (acute) (chronic) (nonpuerperal) 611.0
    newborn 771.5
    puerperal, postpartum 675.1●
    tuberculous (see also Tuberculosis) 017.9●
  broad ligament (chronic) (see also Disease, pelvis, inflammatory) 614.4
    acute 614.3
  Brodie's (chronic) (localized) (see also Osteomyelitis) 730.1●
  bronchus 519.19
  buccal cavity 528.3
  bulbourethral gland 597.0
  bursa 727.89
    pharyngeal 478.29
  buttock 682.5
  canaliculus, breast 611.0
  canthus 372.20
  cartilage 733.99
  cecum 569.5
    with appendicitis 540.1
  cerebellum, cerebellar 324.0
    late effect - see category 326
  cerebral (embolic) 324.0
    late effect - see category 326
  cervical (neck region) 682.1
    lymph gland or node 683
    stump (see also Cervicitis) 616.0
  cervix (stump) (uteri) (see also Cervicitis) 616.0
  cheek, external 682.0
    inner 528.3
  chest 510.9
    with fistula 510.0
    wall 682.2
  chin 682.0
  choroid 363.00
  ciliary body 364.3
  circumtonsillar 475
  cold (tuberculous) - see also Tuberculosis, abscess
    articular - see Tuberculosis, joint

Abscess (Continued)
  colon (wall) 569.5
  colostomy or enterostomy 569.61
  conjunctiva 372.00
  connective tissue NEC 682.9
  cornea 370.55
    with ulcer 370.00
  corpus
    cavernosum 607.2
    luteum (see also Salpingo-oophoritis) 614.2
  Cowper's gland 597.0
  cranium 324.0
  cul-de-sac (Douglas') (posterior) (see also Disease, pelvis, inflammatory) 614.4
    acute 614.3
  dental 522.5
    with sinus (alveolar) 522.7
  dentoalveolar 522.5
    with sinus (alveolar) 522.7
  diaphragm, diaphragmatic 567.22
  digit NEC 681.9
  Douglas' cul-de-sac or pouch (see also Disease, pelvis, inflammatory) 614.4
    acute 614.3
  Dubois' 090.5
  ductless gland 259.8
  ear
    acute 382.00
    external 380.10
    inner 386.30
    middle - see Otitis media
  elbow 682.3
  endamebic - see Abscess, amebic
  entamebic - see Abscess, amebic
  enterostomy 569.61
  epididymis 604.0
  epidural 324.9
    brain 324.0
    late effect - see category 326
    spinal cord 324.1
  epiglottis 478.79
  epiploon, epiploic 567.22
  erysipelatous (see also Erysipelas) 035
  esophagostomy 530.86
  esophagus 530.19
  ethmoid (bone) (chronic) (sinus) (see also Sinusitis, ethmoidal) 473.2
  external auditory canal 380.10
  extradural 324.9
    brain 324.0
    late effect - see category 326
    spinal cord 324.1
  extraperitoneal - see Abscess, peritoneum
  eye 360.00
  eyelid 373.13
  face (any part, except eye) 682.0
  fallopian tube (see also Salpingo-oophoritis) 614.2
  fascia 728.89
  fauces 478.29
  fecal 569.5
  femoral (region) 682.6
  filaria, filarial (see also Infestation, filarial) 125.9
  finger (any) (intrathecal) (periosteal) (subcutaneous) (subcuticular) 681.00
  fistulous NEC 682.9
  flank 682.2
  foot (except toe) 682.7
  forearm 682.3
  forehead 682.0
  frontal (sinus) (chronic) (see also Sinusitis, frontal) 473.1
  gallbladder (see also Cholecystitis, acute) 575.0
  gastric 535.0●

Abscess (Continued)
genital organ or tract NEC
  female 616.9
    with
      abortion - see Abortion, by type, with sepsis
      ectopic pregnancy (see also categories 633.0-633.9) 639.0
      molar pregnancy (see also categories 630-632) 639.0
      following
        abortion 639.0
        ectopic or molar pregnancy 639.0
      puerperal, postpartum, childbirth 670.8●
  male 608.4
genitourinary system, tuberculous (see also Tuberculosis) 016.9●
gingival 523.30
gland, glandular (lymph) (acute) NEC 683
glottis 478.79
gluteal (region) 682.5
gonorrheal NEC (see also Gonococcus) 098.0
groin 682.2
gum 523.30
hand (except finger or thumb) 682.4
head (except face) 682.8
heart 429.89
heel 682.7
helminthic (see also Infestation, by specific parasite) 128.9
hepatic 572.0
  amebic (see also Abscess, liver, amebic) 006.3
  duct 576.8
hip 682.6
  tuberculous (active) (see also Tuberculosis) 015.1●
ileocecal 540.1
ileostomy (bud) 569.61
iliac (region) 682.2
  fossa 540.1
iliopsoas 567.31
  tuberculous (see also Tuberculosis) 015.0● [730.88]
infraclavicular (fossa) 682.3
inguinal (region) 682.2
  lymph gland or node 683
intersphincteric (anus) 566
intestine, intestinal 569.5
  rectal 566
intra-abdominal (see also Abscess, peritoneum) 567.22
  postoperative 998.59
intracranial 324.0
  late effect - see category 326
intramammary - see Abscess, breast
intramastoid (see also Mastoiditis, acute) 383.00
intraorbital 376.01
intraperitoneal 567.22
intraspinal 324.1
  late effect - see category 326
intratonsillar 475
iris 364.3
ischiorectal 566
jaw (bone) (lower) (upper) 526.4
  skin 682.0
joint (see also Arthritis, pyogenic) 711.0●
  vertebral (tuberculous) (see also Tuberculosis) 015.0● [730.88]
  nontuberculous 724.8
kidney 590.2
  with
    abortion - see Abortion, by type, with urinary tract infection
    calculus 592.0
    ectopic pregnancy (see also categories 633.0-633.9) 639.8
    molar pregnancy (see also categories 630-632) 639.8

Abscess (Continued)
kidney (Continued)
  with (Continued)
    complicating pregnancy or puerperium 646.6●
    affecting fetus or newborn 760.1
  following
    abortion 639.8
    ectopic or molar pregnancy 639.8
knee 682.6
  joint 711.06
  tuberculous (active) (see also Tuberculosis) 015.2●
labium (majus) (minus) 616.4
  complicating pregnancy, childbirth, or puerperium 646.6●
lacrimal (passages) (sac) (see also Dacryocystitis) 375.30
  caruncle 375.30
  gland (see also Dacryoadenitis) 375.00
lacunar 597.0
larynx 478.79
lateral (alveolar) 522.5
  with sinus 522.7
leg, except foot 682.6
lens 360.00
lid 373.13
lingual 529.0
  tonsil 475
lip 528.5
Littre's gland 597.0
liver 572.0
  amebic 006.3
    with
      brain abscess (and lung abscess) 006.5
      lung abscess 006.4
    due to Entamoeba histolytica 006.3
  dysenteric (see also Abscess, liver, amebic) 006.3
  pyogenic 572.0
  tropical (see also Abscess, liver, amebic) 006.3
loin (region) 682.2
lumbar (tuberculous) (see also Tuberculosis) 015.0● [730.88]
  nontuberculous 682.2
lung (miliary) (putrid) 513.0
  amebic (with liver abscess) 006.4
    with brain abscess 006.5
lymph, lymphatic, gland or node (acute) 683
  any site, except mesenteric 683
  mesentery 289.2
lymphangitic, acute - see Cellulitis
malar 526.4
mammary gland - see Abscess, breast
marginal (anus) 566
mastoid (process) (see also Mastoiditis, acute) 383.00
  subperiosteal 383.01
maxilla, maxillary 526.4
  molar (tooth) 522.5
    with sinus 522.7
  premolar 522.5
  sinus (chronic) (see also Sinusitis, maxillary) 473.0
mediastinum 513.1
meibomian gland 373.12
meninges (see also Meningitis) 320.9
mesentery, mesenteric 567.22
mesosalpinx (see also Salpingo-oophoritis) 614.2
milk 675.1●
Monro's (psoriasis) 696.1
mons pubis 682.2
mouth (floor) 528.3
multiple sites NEC 682.9
mural 682.2
muscle 728.89
  psoas 567.31
myocardium 422.92

Abscess (Continued)
nabothian (follicle) (see also Cervicitis) 616.0
nail (chronic) (with lymphangitis) 681.9
  finger 681.02
  toe 681.11
nasal (fossa) (septum) 478.19
  sinus (chronic) (see also Sinusitis) 473.9
nasopharyngeal 478.29
nates 682.5
navel 682.2
  newborn NEC 771.4
neck (region) 682.1
  lymph gland or node 683
nephritic (see also Abscess, kidney) 590.2
nipple 611.0
  puerperal, postpartum 675.0●
nose (septum) 478.19
  external 682.0
omentum 567.22
operative wound 998.59
orbit, orbital 376.01
ossifluent - see Abscess, bone
ovary, ovarian (corpus luteum) (see also Salpingo-oophoritis) 614.2
oviduct (see also Salpingo-oophoritis) 614.2
palate (soft) 528.3
  hard 526.4
palmar (space) 682.4
pancreas (duct) 577.0
paradontal 523.30
parafrenal 607.2
parametric, parametrium (chronic) (see also Disease, pelvis, inflammatory) 614.4
  acute 614.3
paranephric 590.2
parapancreatic 577.0
parapharyngeal 478.22
pararectal 566
parasinus (see also Sinusitis) 473.9
parauterine (see also Disease, pelvis, inflammatory) 614.4
  acute 614.3
paravaginal (see also Vaginitis) 616.10
parietal region 682.8
parodontal 523.30
parotid (duct) (gland) 527.3
  region 528.3
parumbilical 682.2
  newborn 771.4
pectoral (region) 682.2
pelvirectal 567.22
pelvis, pelvic
  female (chronic) (see also Disease, pelvis, inflammatory) 614.4
    acute 614.3
  male, peritoneal (cellular tissue) - see Abscess, peritoneum
  tuberculous (see also Tuberculosis) 016.9●
penis 607.2
  gonococcal (acute) 098.0
  chronic or duration of 2 months or over 098.2
perianal 566
periapical 522.5
  with sinus (alveolar) 522.7
periappendiceal 540.1
pericardial 420.99
pericecal 540.1
pericemental 523.30
pericholecystic (see also Cholecystitis, acute) 575.0
pericoronal 523.30
peridental 523.30
perigastric 535.0●
perimetric (see also Disease, pelvis, inflammatory) 614.4
  acute 614.3
perinephric, perinephritic (see also Abscess, kidney) 590.2

Abscess (Continued)
  perineum, perineal (superficial) 682.2
    deep (with urethral involvement) 597.0
    urethra 597.0
  periodontal (parietal) 523.31
    apical 522.5
  periosteum, periosteal (see also Periostitis) 730.3●
    with osteomyelitis (see also Osteomyelitis) 730.2●
      acute or subacute 730.0●
      chronic or old 730.1●
  peripleuritic 510.9
    with fistula 510.0
  periproctic 566
  periprostatic 601.2
  perirectal (staphylococcal) 566
  perirenal (tissue) (see also Abscess, kidney) 590.2
  perisinuous (nose) (see also Sinusitis) 473.9
  peritoneum, peritoneal (perforated) (ruptured) 567.22
    with
      abortion - see Abortion, by type, with sepsis
      appendicitis 540.1
      ectopic pregnancy (see also categories 633.0-633.9) 639.0
      molar pregnancy (see also categories 630-632) 639.0
    following
      abortion 639.0
      ectopic or molar pregnancy 639.0
    pelvic, female (see also Disease, pelvis, inflammatory) 614.4
      acute 614.3
    postoperative 998.59
    puerperal, postpartum, childbirth 670.8●
    tuberculous (see also Tuberculosis) 014.0●
  peritonsillar 475
  perityphlic 540.1
  periureteral 593.89
  periurethral 597.0
    gonococcal (acute) 098.0
      chronic or duration of 2 months or over 098.2
  periuterine (see also Disease, pelvis, inflammatory) 614.4
    acute 614.3
  perivesical 595.89
  pernicious NEC 682.9
  petrous bone - see Petrositis
  phagedenic NEC 682.9
    chancroid 099.0
  pharynx, pharyngeal (lateral) 478.29
  phlegmonous NEC 682.9
  pilonidal 685.0
  pituitary (gland) 253.8
  pleura 510.9
    with fistula 510.0
  popliteal 682.6
  postanal 566
  postcecal 540.1
  postlaryngeal 478.79
  postnasal 478.19
  postpharyngeal 478.24
  posttonsillar 475
  posttyphoid 002.0
  Pott's (see also Tuberculosis) 015.0● [730.88]
  pouch of Douglas (chronic) (see also Disease, pelvis, inflammatory) 614.4
  premammary - see Abscess, breast
  prepatellar 682.6
  prostate (see also Prostatitis) 601.2
    gonococcal (acute) 098.12
      chronic or duration of 2 months or over 098.32
  psoas 567.31
    tuberculous (see also Tuberculosis) 015.0● [730.88]
  pterygopalatine fossa 682.8

Abscess (Continued)
  pubis 682.2
  puerperal - see Puerperal, abscess, by site
  pulmonary - see Abscess, lung
  pulp, pulpal (dental) 522.0
    finger 681.01
    toe 681.10
  pyemic - see Septicemia
  pyloric valve 535.0●
  rectovaginal septum 569.5
  rectovesical 595.89
  rectum 566
  regional NEC 682.9
  renal (see also Abscess, kidney) 590.2
  retina 363.00
  retrobulbar 376.01
  retrocecal 567.22
  retrolaryngeal 478.79
  retromammary - see Abscess, breast
  retroperineal 682.2
  retroperitoneal 567.38
    postprocedural 998.59
  retropharyngeal 478.24
    tuberculous (see also Tuberculosis) 012.8●
  retrorectal 566
  retrouterine (see also Disease, pelvis, inflammatory) 614.4
    acute 614.3
  retrovesical 595.89
  root, tooth 522.5
    with sinus (alveolar) 522.7
  round ligament (see also Disease, pelvis, inflammatory) 614.4
    acute 614.3
  rupture (spontaneous) NEC 682.9
  sacrum (tuberculous) (see also Tuberculosis) 015.0● [730.88]
    nontuberculous 730.08
  salivary duct or gland 527.3
  scalp (any part) 682.8
  scapular 730.01
  sclera 379.09
  scrofulous (see also Tuberculosis) 017.2●
  scrotum 608.4
  seminal vesicle 608.0
    amebic 006.8
  septal, dental 522.5
    with sinus (alveolar) 522.7
  septum (nasal) 478.19
  serous (see also Periostitis) 730.3●
  shoulder 682.3
  side 682.2
  sigmoid 569.5
  sinus (accessory) (chronic) (nasal) (see also Sinusitis) 473.9
    intracranial venous (any) 324.0
      late effect - see category 326
  Skene's duct or gland 597.0
  skin NEC 682.9
    tuberculous (primary) (see also Tuberculosis) 017.0●
  sloughing NEC 682.9
  specified site NEC 682.8
    amebic 006.8
  spermatic cord 608.4
  sphenoidal (sinus) (see also Sinusitis, sphenoidal) 473.3
  spinal
    cord (any part) (staphylococcal) 324.1
      tuberculous (see also Tuberculosis) 013.5●
    epidural 324.1
  spine (column) (tuberculous) (see also Tuberculosis) 015.0● [730.88]
    nontuberculous 730.08
  spleen 289.59
    amebic 006.8
  staphylococcal NEC 682.9
  stitch 998.59
  stomach (wall) 535.0●

Abscess (Continued)
  strumous (tuberculous) (see also Tuberculosis) 017.2●
  subarachnoid 324.9
    brain 324.0
    cerebral 324.0
    late effect - see category 326
    spinal cord 324.1
  subareolar - see also Abscess, breast
    puerperal, postpartum 675.1●
  subcecal 540.1
  subcutaneous NEC 682.9
  subdiaphragmatic 567.22
  subdorsal 682.2
  subdural 324.9
    brain 324.0
    late effect - see category 326
    spinal cord 324.1
  subgaleal 682.8
  subhepatic 567.22
  sublingual 528.3
    gland 527.3
  submammary - see Abscess, breast
  submandibular (region) (space) (triangle) 682.0
    gland 527.3
  submaxillary (region) 682.0
    gland 527.3
  submental (pyogenic) 682.0
    gland 527.3
  subpectoral 682.2
  subperiosteal - see Abscess, bone
  subperitoneal 567.22
  subphrenic - see also Abscess, peritoneum 567.22
    postoperative 998.59
  subscapular 682.2
  subungual 681.9
  suburethral 597.0
  sudoriparous 705.89
  suppurative NEC 682.9
  supraclavicular (fossa) 682.3
  suprahepatic 567.22
  suprapelvic (see also Disease, pelvis, inflammatory) 614.4
    acute 614.3
  suprapubic 682.2
  suprarenal (capsule) (gland) 255.8
  sweat gland 705.89
  syphilitic 095.8
  teeth, tooth (root) 522.5
    with sinus (alveolar) 522.7
    supporting structures NEC 523.30
  temple 682.0
  temporal region 682.0
  temporosphenoidal 324.0
    late effect - see category 326
  tendon (sheath) 727.89
  testicle - see Orchitis
  thecal 728.89
  thigh (acquired) 682.6
  thorax 510.9
    with fistula 510.0
  throat 478.29
  thumb (intrathecal) (periosteal) (subcutaneous) (subcuticular) 681.00
  thymus (gland) 254.1
  thyroid (gland) 245.0
  toe (any) (intrathecal) (periosteal) (subcutaneous) (subcuticular) 681.10
  tongue (staphylococcal) 529.0
  tonsil(s) (lingual) 475
  tonsillopharyngeal 475
  tooth, teeth (root) 522.5
    with sinus (alveolar) 522.7
    supporting structure NEC 523.30
  trachea 478.9
  trunk 682.2
  tubal (see also Salpingo-oophoritis) 614.2
  tuberculous - see Tuberculosis, abscess

Abscess (Continued)
- tubo-ovarian (see also Salpingo-oophoritis) 614.2
- tunica vaginalis 608.4
- umbilicus NEC 682.2
  - newborn 771.4
- upper arm 682.3
- upper respiratory 478.9
- urachus 682.2
- urethra (gland) 597.0
- urinary 597.0
- uterus, uterine (wall) (see also Endometritis) 615.9
  - ligament (see also Disease, pelvis, inflammatory) 614.4
    - acute 614.3
  - neck (see also Cervicitis) 616.0
- uvula 528.3
- vagina (wall) (see also Vaginitis) 616.10
- vaginorectal (see also Vaginitis) 616.10
- vas deferens 608.4
- vermiform appendix 540.1
- vertebra (column) (tuberculous) (see also Tuberculosis) 015.0● [730.88]
  - nontuberculous 730.0●
- vesical 595.89
- vesicouterine pouch (see also Disease, pelvis, inflammatory) 614.4
- vitreous (humor) (pneumococcal) 360.04
- vocal cord 478.5
- von Bezold's 383.01
- vulva 616.4
  - complicating pregnancy, childbirth, or puerperium 646.6●
- vulvovaginal gland (see also Vaginitis) 616.3
- web-space 682.4
- wrist 682.4

Absence (organ or part) (complete or partial)
- acoustic nerve 742.8
- adrenal (gland) (congenital) 759.1
  - acquired V45.79
- albumin (blood) 273.8
- alimentary tract (complete) (congenital) (partial) 751.8
  - lower 751.5
  - upper 750.8
- alpha-fucosidase 271.8
- alveolar process (acquired) 525.8
  - congenital 750.26
- anus, anal (canal) (congenital) 751.2
- aorta (congenital) 747.22
- aortic valve (congenital) 746.89
- appendix, congenital 751.2
- arm (acquired) V49.60
  - above elbow V49.66
  - below elbow V49.65
  - congenital (see also Deformity, reduction, upper limb) 755.20
    - lower - see Absence, forearm, congenital
    - upper (complete) (partial) (with absence of distal elements, incomplete) 755.24
      - with
        - complete absence of distal elements 755.21
        - forearm (incomplete) 755.23
- artery (congenital) (peripheral) NEC (see also Anomaly, peripheral vascular system) 747.60
  - brain 747.81
  - cerebral 747.81
  - coronary 746.85
  - pulmonary 747.31
  - umbilical 747.5
- atrial septum 745.69
- auditory canal (congenital) (external) 744.01
- auricle (ear) (with stenosis or atresia of auditory canal), congenital 744.01
- bile, biliary duct (common) or passage (congenital) 751.61

Absence (Continued)
- bladder (acquired) V45.74
  - congenital 753.8
- bone (congenital) NEC 756.9
  - marrow 284.9
    - acquired (secondary) 284.89
    - congenital 284.09
    - hereditary 284.09
    - idiopathic 284.9
  - skull 756.0
- bowel sounds 787.5
- brain 740.0
  - specified part 742.2
- breast(s) (acquired) V45.71
  - congenital 757.6
- broad ligament (congenital) 752.19
- bronchus (congenital) 748.3
- calvarium, calvaria (skull) 756.0
- canaliculus lacrimalis, congenital 743.65
- carpal(s) (congenital) (complete) (partial) (with absence of distal elements, incomplete) (see also Deformity, reduction, upper limb) 755.28
  - with complete absence of distal elements 755.21
- cartilage 756.9
- caudal spine 756.13
- cecum (acquired) (postoperative) (posttraumatic) V45.72
  - congenital 751.2
- cementum 520.4
- cerebellum (congenital) (vermis) 742.2
- cervix (acquired) (uteri) V88.01
  - with remaining uterus V88.03
  - and uterus V88.01
  - congenital 752.43
- chin, congenital 744.89
- cilia (congenital) 743.63
  - acquired 374.89
- circulatory system, part NEC 747.89
- clavicle 755.51
- clitoris (congenital) 752.49
- coccyx, congenital 756.13
- cold sense (see also Disturbance, sensation) 782.0
- colon (acquired) (postoperative) V45.72
  - congenital 751.2
- congenital
  - lumen - see Atresia
  - organ or site NEC - see Agenesis
  - septum - see Imperfect, closure
- corpus callosum (congenital) 742.2
- cricoid cartilage 748.3
- diaphragm (congenital) (with hernia) 756.6
  - with obstruction 756.6
- digestive organ(s) or tract, congenital (complete) (partial) 751.8
  - acquired V45.79
  - lower 751.5
  - upper 750.8
- ductus arteriosus 747.89
- duodenum (acquired) (postoperative) V45.72
  - congenital 751.1
- ear, congenital 744.09
  - acquired V45.79
  - auricle 744.01
  - external 744.01
  - inner 744.05
  - lobe, lobule 744.21
  - middle, except ossicles 744.03
    - ossicles 744.04
  - ossicles 744.04
- ejaculatory duct (congenital) 752.89
- endocrine gland NEC (congenital) 759.2
- epididymis (congenital) 752.89
  - acquired V45.77
- epiglottis, congenital 748.3
- epileptic (atonic) (typical) (see also Epilepsy) 345.0●
- erythrocyte 284.9

Absence (Continued)
- erythropoiesis 284.9
  - congenital 284.01
- esophagus (congenital) 750.3
- eustachian tube (congenital) 744.24
- extremity (acquired)
  - congenital (see also Deformity, reduction) 755.4
  - lower V49.70
  - upper V49.60
- extrinsic muscle, eye 743.69
- eye (acquired) V45.78
  - adnexa (congenital) 743.69
  - congenital 743.00
  - muscle (congenital) 743.69
- eyelid (fold), congenital 743.62
  - acquired 374.89
- face
  - bones NEC 756.0
  - specified part NEC 744.89
- fallopian tube(s) (acquired) V45.77
  - congenital 752.19
- femur, congenital (complete) (partial) (with absence of distal elements, incomplete) (see also Deformity, reduction, lower limb) 755.34
  - with
    - complete absence of distal elements 755.31
    - tibia and fibula (incomplete) 755.33
- fibrin 790.92
- fibrinogen (congenital) 286.3
  - acquired 286.6
- fibula, congenital (complete) (partial) (with absence of distal elements, incomplete) (see also Deformity, reduction, lower limb) 755.37
  - with
    - complete absence of distal elements 755.31
    - tibia 755.35
      - with
        - complete absence of distal elements 755.31
        - femur (incomplete) 755.33
          - with complete absence of distal elements 755.31
- finger (acquired) V49.62
  - congenital (complete) (partial) (see also Deformity, reduction, upper limb) 755.29
    - meaning all fingers (complete) (partial) 755.21
    - transverse 755.21
- fissures of lungs (congenital) 748.5
- foot (acquired) V49.73
  - congenital (complete) 755.31
- forearm (acquired) V49.65
  - congenital (complete) (partial) (with absence of distal elements, incomplete) (see also Deformity, reduction, upper limb) 755.25
    - with
      - complete absence of distal elements (hand and fingers) 755.21
      - humerus (incomplete) 755.23
- fovea centralis 743.55
- fucosidase 271.8
- gallbladder (acquired) V45.79
  - congenital 751.69
- gamma globulin (blood) 279.00
- genital organs
  - acquired V45.77
  - congenital
    - female 752.89
      - external 752.49
      - internal NEC 752.89
    - male 752.89
      - penis 752.69
- genitourinary organs, congenital NEC 752.89
- glottis 748.3

Absence *(Continued)*
  gonadal, congenital NEC 758.6
  hair (congenital) 757.4
    acquired - *see* Alopecia
  hand (acquired) V49.63
    congenital (complete) (*see also* Deformity, reduction, upper limb) 755.21
  heart (congenital) 759.89
    acquired - *see* Status, organ replacement
  heat sense (*see also* Disturbance, sensation) 782.0
  humerus, congenital (complete) (partial) (with absence of distal elements, incomplete) (*see also* Deformity, reduction, upper limb) 755.24
    with
      complete absence of distal elements 755.21
      radius and ulna (incomplete) 755.23
  hymen (congenital) 752.49
  ileum (acquired) (postoperative) (posttraumatic) V45.72
    congenital 751.1
  immunoglobulin, isolated NEC 279.03
    IgA 279.01
    IgG 279.03
    IgM 279.02
  incus (acquired) 385.24
    congenital 744.04
  internal ear (congenital) 744.05
  intestine (acquired) (small) V45.72
    congenital 751.1
      large 751.2
    large V45.72
      congenital 751.2
  iris (congenital) 743.45
  jaw - *see* Absence, mandible
  jejunum (acquired) V45.72
    congenital 751.1
  joint (acquired) (following prior explantation of joint prosthesis) (with or without presence of antibiotic-impregnated cement spacer) NEC V88.29
    congenital NEC 755.8
    hip V88.21
    knee V88.22
  kidney(s) (acquired) V45.73
    congenital 753.0
  labium (congenital) (majus) (minus) 752.49
  labyrinth, membranous 744.05
  lacrimal apparatus (congenital) 743.65
  larynx (congenital) 748.3
  leg (acquired) V49.70
    above knee V49.76
    below knee V49.75
    congenital (partial) (unilateral) (*see also* Deformity, reduction, lower limb) 755.31
      lower (complete) (partial) (with absence of distal elements, incomplete) 755.35
        with
          complete absence of distal elements (foot and toes) 755.31
        thigh (incomplete) 755.33
          with complete absence of distal elements 755.31
      upper - *see* Absence, femur
  lens (congenital) 743.35
    acquired 379.31
  ligament, broad (congenital) 752.19
  limb (acquired)
    congenital (complete) (partial) (*see also* Deformity, reduction) 755.4
      lower 755.30
        complete 755.31
        incomplete 755.32
        longitudinal - *see* Deficiency, lower limb, longitudinal
        transverse 755.31

Absence *(Continued)*
  limb *(Continued)*
    congenital *(Continued)*
      upper 755.20
        complete 755.21
        incomplete 755.22
        longitudinal - *see* Deficiency, upper limb, longitudinal
        transverse 755.21
    lower NEC V49.70
    upper NEC V49.60
  lip 750.26
  liver (congenital) (lobe) 751.69
  lumbar (congenital) (vertebra) 756.13
    isthmus 756.11
    pars articularis 756.11
  lumen - *see* Atresia
  lung (bilateral) (congenital) (fissure) (lobe) (unilateral) 748.5
    acquired (any part) V45.76
  mandible (congenital) 524.09
  maxilla (congenital) 524.09
  menstruation 626.0
  metacarpal(s), congenital (complete) (partial) (with absence of distal elements, incomplete) (*see also* Deformity, reduction, upper limb) 755.28
    with all fingers, complete 755.21
  metatarsal(s), congenital (complete) (partial) (with absence of distal elements, incomplete) (*see also* Deformity, reduction, lower limb) 755.38
    with complete absence of distal elements 755.31
  muscle (congenital) (pectoral) 756.81
    ocular 743.69
  musculoskeletal system (congenital) NEC 756.9
  nail(s) (congenital) 757.5
  neck, part 744.89
  nerve 742.8
  nervous system, part NEC 742.8
  neutrophil 288.00
  nipple (congenital) 757.6
    acquired V45.71
  nose (congenital) 748.1
    acquired 738.0
  nuclear 742.8
  ocular muscle (congenital) 743.69
  organ
    of Corti (congenital) 744.05
    or site
      acquired V45.79
      congenital NEC 759.89
  osseous meatus (ear) 744.03
  ovary (acquired) V45.77
    congenital 752.0
  oviduct (acquired) V45.77
    congenital 752.19
  pancreas (congenital) 751.7
    acquired (postoperative) (posttraumatic) V88.11
      partial V88.12
      total V88.11
  parathyroid gland (congenital) 759.2
  parotid gland(s) (congenital) 750.21
  patella, congenital 755.64
  pelvic girdle (congenital) 755.69
  penis (congenital) 752.69
    acquired V45.77
  pericardium (congenital) 746.89
  perineal body (congenital) 756.81
  phalange(s), congenital 755.4
    lower limb (complete) (intercalary) (partial) (terminal) (*see also* Deformity, reduction, lower limb) 755.39
      meaning all toes (complete) (partial) 755.31
      transverse 755.31

Absence *(Continued)*
  phalange(s) *(Continued)*
    upper limb (complete) (intercalary) (partial) (terminal) (*see also* Deformity, reduction, upper limb) 755.29
      meaning all digits (complete) (partial) 755.21
      transverse 755.21
  pituitary gland (congenital) 759.2
  postoperative - *see* Absence, by site, acquired
  prostate (congenital) 752.89
    acquired V45.77
  pulmonary
    artery 747.31
    trunk 747.31
    valve (congenital) 746.01
    vein 747.49
  punctum lacrimale (congenital) 743.65
  radius, congenital (complete) (partial) (with absence of distal elements, incomplete) 755.26
    with
      complete absence of distal elements 755.21
      ulna 755.25
        with
          complete absence of distal elements 755.21
          humerus (incomplete) 755.23
  ray, congenital 755.4
    lower limb (complete) (partial) (*see also* Deformity, reduction, lower limb) 755.38
      meaning all rays 755.31
      transverse 755.31
    upper limb (complete) (partial) (*see also* Deformity, reduction, upper limb) 755.28
      meaning all rays 755.21
      transverse 755.21
  rectum (congenital) 751.2
    acquired V45.79
  red cell 284.9
    acquired (secondary) 284.81
    congenital 284.01
    hereditary 284.01
    idiopathic 284.9
  respiratory organ (congenital) NEC 748.9
  rib (acquired) 738.3
    congenital 756.3
  roof of orbit (congenital) 742.0
  round ligament (congenital) 752.89
  sacrum, congenital 756.13
  salivary gland(s) (congenital) 750.21
  scapula 755.59
  scrotum, congenital 752.89
  seminal tract or duct (congenital) 752.89
    acquired V45.77
  septum (congenital) - *see also* Imperfect, closure, septum
    atrial 745.69
      and ventricular 745.7
    between aorta and pulmonary artery 745.0
    ventricular 745.3
      and atrial 745.7
  sex chromosomes 758.81
  shoulder girdle, congenital (complete) (partial) 755.59
  skin (congenital) 757.39
  skull bone 756.0
    with
      anencephalus 740.0
      encephalocele 742.0
      hydrocephalus 742.3
        with spina bifida (*see also* Spina bifida) 741.0●
      microcephalus 742.1
  spermatic cord (congenital) 752.89
  spinal cord 742.59

SECTION 1 INDEX TO DISEASES AND INJURIES / Absence

Absence (Continued)
  spine, congenital 756.13
  spleen (congenital) 759.0
    acquired V45.79
  sternum, congenital 756.3
  stomach (acquired) (partial) (postoperative) V45.75
    with postgastric surgery syndrome 564.2
    congenital 750.7
  submaxillary gland(s) (congenital) 750.21
  superior vena cava (congenital) 747.49
  tarsal(s), congenital (complete) (partial) (with absence of distal elements, incomplete) (see also Deformity, reduction, lower limb) 755.38
  teeth, tooth (congenital) 520.0
    with abnormal spacing 524.30
    acquired 525.10
      with malocclusion 524.30
      due to
        caries 525.13
        extraction 525.10
        periodontal disease 525.12
        trauma 525.11
  tendon (congenital) 756.81
  testis (congenital) 752.89
    acquired V45.77
  thigh (acquired) 736.89
  thumb (acquired) V49.61
    congenital 755.29
  thymus gland (congenital) 759.2
  thyroid (gland) (surgical) 246.8
    with hypothyroidism 244.0
    cartilage, congenital 748.3
    congenital 243
  tibia, congenital (complete) (partial) (with absence of distal elements, incomplete) (see also Deformity, reduction, lower limb) 755.36
    with
      complete absence of distal elements 755.31
      fibula 755.35
        with
          complete absence of distal elements 755.31
          femur (incomplete) 755.33
            with complete absence of distal elements 755.31
  toe (acquired) V49.72
    congenital (complete) (partial) 755.39
      meaning all toes 755.31
      transverse 755.31
    great V49.71
  tongue (congenital) 750.11
  tooth, teeth (congenital) 520.0
    with abnormal spacing 524.30
    acquired 525.10
      with malocclusion 524.30
      due to
        caries 525.13
        extraction 525.10
        periodontal disease 525.12
        trauma 525.11
  trachea (cartilage) (congenital) (rings) 748.3
  transverse aortic arch (congenital) 747.21
  tricuspid valve 746.1
  ulna, congenital (complete) (partial) (with absence of distal elements, incomplete) (see also Deformity, reduction, upper limb) 755.27
    with
      complete absence of distal elements 755.21
      radius 755.25
        with
          complete absence of distal elements 755.21
          humerus (incomplete) 755.23
  umbilical artery (congenital) 747.5

Absence (Continued)
  ureter (congenital) 753.4
    acquired V45.74
  urethra, congenital 753.8
    acquired V45.74
  urinary system, part NEC, congenital 753.8
    acquired V45.74
  uterus (acquired) V88.01
    with remaining cervical stump V88.02
    and cervix V88.01
    congenital 752.31
  uvula (congenital) 750.26
  vagina, congenital 752.45
    acquired V45.77
  vas deferens (congenital) 752.89
    acquired V45.77
  vein (congenital) (peripheral) NEC (see also Anomaly, peripheral vascular system) 747.60
    brain 747.81
    great 747.49
    portal 747.49
    pulmonary 747.49
  vena cava (congenital) (inferior) (superior) 747.49
  ventral horn cell 742.59
  ventricular septum 745.3
  vermis of cerebellum 742.2
  vertebra, congenital 756.13
  vulva, congenital 752.49

Absentia epileptica (see also Epilepsy) 345.0●
Absinthemia (see also Dependence) 304.6●
Absinthism (see also Dependence) 304.6●
Absorbent system disease 459.89
Absorption
  alcohol, through placenta or breast milk 760.71
  antibiotics, through placenta or breast milk 760.74
  anticonvulsants, through placenta or breast milk 760.77
  antifungals, through placenta or breast milk 760.74
  anti-infective, through placenta or breast milk 760.74
  antimetabolics, through placenta or breast milk 760.78
  chemical NEC 989.9
    specified chemical or substance - see Table of Drugs and Chemicals
    through placenta or breast milk (fetus or newborn) 760.70
      alcohol 760.71
      anticonvulsants 760.77
      antifungals 760.74
      anti-infective agents 760.74
      antimetabolics 760.78
      cocaine 760.75
      "crack" 760.75
      diethylstilbestrol [DES] 760.76
      hallucinogenic agents 760.73
      medicinal agents NEC 760.79
      narcotics 760.72
      obstetric anesthetic or analgesic drug 763.5
      specified agent NEC 760.79
      suspected, affecting management of pregnancy 655.5●
  cocaine, through placenta or breast milk 760.75
  drug NEC (see also Reaction, drug)
    through placenta or breast milk (fetus or newborn) 760.70
      alcohol 760.71
      anticonvulsants 760.77
      antifungals 760.74
      anti-infective agents 760.74
      antimetabolics 760.78
      cocaine 760.75
      "crack" 760.75
      diethylstilbestrol (DES) 760.76

Absorption (Continued)
  drug NEC (Continued)
    through placenta or breast milk (Continued)
      hallucinogenic agents 760.73
      medicinal agents NEC 760.79
      narcotics 760.72
      obstetric anesthetic or analgesic drug 763.5
      specified agent NEC 760.79
      suspected, affecting management of pregnancy 655.5●
  fat, disturbance 579.8
  hallucinogenic agents, through placenta or breast milk 760.73
  immune sera, through placenta or breast milk 760.79
  lactose defect 271.3
  medicinal agents NEC, through placenta or breast milk 760.79
  narcotics, through placenta or breast milk 760.72
  noxious substance - see Absorption, chemical
  protein, disturbance 579.8
  pus or septic, general - see Septicemia
  quinine, through placenta or breast milk 760.74
  toxic substance - see Absorption, chemical
  uremic - see Uremia

Abstinence symptoms or syndrome
  alcohol 291.81
  drug 292.0
  neonatal 779.5

Abt-Letterer-Siwe syndrome (acute histiocytosis X) (M9722/3) 202.5●
Abulia 799.89
Abulomania 301.6
Abuse
  adult 995.80
    emotional 995.82
    multiple forms 995.85
    neglect (nutritional) 995.84
    physical 995.81
    psychological 995.82
    sexual 995.83
  alcohol (see also Alcoholism) 305.0●
    dependent 303.9●
    nondependent 305.0●
  child 995.50
    counseling
      perpetrator
        non-parent V62.83
        parent V61.22
      victim V61.21
    emotional 995.51
    multiple forms 995.59
    neglect (nutritional) 995.52
    physical 995.54
      shaken infant syndrome 995.55
    psychological 995.51
    sexual 995.53
  drugs, nondependent 305.9●

> Note: Use the following fifth-digit subclassification with the following codes: 305.0, 305.2-305.9:
>
> 0   unspecified
> 1   continuous
> 2   episodic
> 3   in remission

    amphetamine type 305.7●
    antidepressants 305.8●
    anxiolytic 305.4●
    barbiturates 305.4●
    caffeine 305.9●
    cannabis 305.2●
    cocaine type 305.6●
    hallucinogens 305.3●
    hashish 305.2●
    hypnotic 305.4●

Abuse (Continued)
  drugs, nondependent (Continued)
    inhalant 305.9●
    LSD 305.3●
    marijuana 305.2●
    mixed 305.9●
    morphine type 305.5●
    opioid type 305.5●
    phencyclidine (PCP) 305.9●
    sedative 305.4●
    specified NEC 305.9●
    tranquilizers 305.4●
  spouse 995.80
  tobacco 305.1
Acalcerosis 275.40
Acalcicosis 275.40
Acalculia 784.69
  developmental 315.1
Acanthocheilonemiasis 125.4
Acanthocytosis 272.5
Acanthokeratodermia 701.1
Acantholysis 701.8
  bullosa 757.39
Acanthoma (benign) (M8070/0) - see also
    Neoplasm, by site, benign
  malignant (M8070/3) - see Neoplasm, by site,
    malignant
Acanthosis (acquired) (nigricans) 701.2
  adult 701.2
  benign (congenital) 757.39
  congenital 757.39
  glycogenic
    esophagus 530.89
  juvenile 701.2
  tongue 529.8
Acanthrocytosis 272.5
Acapnia 276.3
Acarbia 276.2
Acardia 759.89
Acardiacus amorphus 759.89
Acardiotrophia 429.1
Acardius 759.89
Acariasis 133.9
  sarcoptic 133.0
Acaridiasis 133.9
Acarinosis 133.9
Acariosis 133.9
Acarodermatitis 133.9
  urticarioides 133.9
Acarophobia 300.29
Acatalasemia 277.89
Acatalasia 277.89
Acatamathesia 784.69
Acataphasia 784.59
Acathisia 781.0
  due to drugs 333.99
Acceleration, accelerated
  atrioventricular conduction 426.7
  idioventricular rhythm 427.89
Accessory (congenital)
  adrenal gland 759.1
  anus 751.5
  appendix 751.5
  atrioventricular conduction 426.7
  auditory ossicles 744.04
  auricle (ear) 744.1
  autosome(s) NEC 758.5
    21 or 22 758.0
  biliary duct or passage 751.69
  bladder 753.8
  blood vessels (peripheral) (congenital) NEC
    (see also Anomaly, peripheral vascular
    system) 747.60
      cerebral 747.81
      coronary 746.85
  bone NEC 756.9
    foot 755.67
  breast tissue, axilla 757.6
  carpal bones 755.56
  cecum 751.5
  cervix 752.44

Accessory (Continued)
  chromosome(s) NEC 758.5
    13-15 758.1
    16-18 758.2
    21 or 22 758.0
    autosome(s) NEC 758.5
    D_1 758.1
    E_3 758.2
    G 758.0
    sex 758.81
  coronary artery 746.85
  cusp(s), heart valve NEC 746.89
    pulmonary 746.09
  cystic duct 751.69
  digits 755.00
  ear (auricle) (lobe) 744.1
  endocrine gland NEC 759.2
  external os 752.44
  eyelid 743.62
  eye muscle 743.69
  face bone(s) 756.0
  fallopian tube (fimbria) (ostium) 752.19
  fingers 755.01
  foreskin 605
  frontonasal process 756.0
  gallbladder 751.69
  genital organ(s)
    female 752.89
      external 752.49
      internal NEC 752.89
    male NEC 752.89
      penis 752.69
  genitourinary organs NEC 752.89
  heart 746.89
    valve NEC 746.89
      pulmonary 746.09
  hepatic ducts 751.69
  hymen 752.49
  intestine (large) (small) 751.5
  kidney 753.3
  lacrimal canal 743.65
  leaflet, heart valve NEC 746.89
    pulmonary 746.09
  ligament, broad 752.19
  liver (duct) 751.69
  lobule (ear) 744.1
  lung (lobe) 748.69
  muscle 756.82
  navicular of carpus 755.56
  nervous system, part NEC 742.8
  nipple 757.6
  nose 748.1
  organ or site NEC - see Anomaly, specified
    type NEC
  ovary 752.0
  oviduct 752.19
  pancreas 751.7
  parathyroid gland 759.2
  parotid gland (and duct) 750.22
  pituitary gland 759.2
  placental lobe - see Placenta, abnormal
  preauricular appendage 744.1
  prepuce 605
  renal arteries (multiple) 747.62
  rib 756.3
    cervical 756.2
  roots (teeth) 520.2
  salivary gland 750.22
  sesamoids 755.8
  sinus - see Condition
  skin tags 757.39
  spleen 759.0
  sternum 756.3
  submaxillary gland 750.22
  tarsal bones 755.67
  teeth, tooth 520.1
    causing crowding 524.31
  tendon 756.89
  thumb 755.01
  thymus gland 759.2
  thyroid gland 759.2

Accessory (Continued)
  toes 755.02
  tongue 750.13
  tragus 744.1
  ureter 753.4
  urethra 753.8
  urinary organ or tract NEC 753.8
  uterus 752.2
  vagina 752.49
  valve, heart NEC 746.89
    pulmonary 746.09
  vertebra 756.19
  vocal cords 748.3
  vulva 752.49
Accident, accidental - see also condition
  birth NEC 767.9
  cardiovascular (see also Disease,
    cardiovascular) 429.2
  cerebral (see also Disease, cerebrovascular,
    acute) 434.91
  cerebrovascular (current) (CVA) (see also
    Disease, cerebrovascular, acute)
    434.91
    aborted 434.91
    embolic 434.11
    healed or old V12.54
    hemorrhagic - see Hemorrhage, brain
    impending 435.9
    ischemic 434.91
    late effect - see Late effect(s) (of)
      cerebrovascular disease
    postoperative 997.02
    thrombotic 434.01
  coronary (see also Infarct, myocardium)
    410.9●
  craniovascular (see also Disease,
    cerebrovascular, acute) 436
  during pregnancy, to mother, affecting fetus
    or newborn 760.5
  heart, cardiac (see also Infarct, myocardium)
    410.9●
  intrauterine 779.89
  vascular - see Disease, cerebrovascular, acute
Accommodation
  disorder of 367.51
    drug-induced 367.89
    toxic 367.89
  insufficiency of 367.4
  paralysis of 367.51
    hysterical 300.11
  spasm of 367.53
Accouchement - see Delivery
Accreta placenta (without hemorrhage) 667.0●
  with hemorrhage 666.0●
Accretio cordis (nonrheumatic) 423.1
Accretions on teeth 523.6
Accumulation secretion, prostate 602.8
Acephalia, acephalism, acephaly 740.0
Acephalic 740.0
Acephalobrachia 759.89
Acephalocardia 759.89
Acephalocardius 759.89
Acephalochiria 759.89
Acephalochirus 759.89
Acephalogaster 759.89
Acephalostomus 759.89
Acephalothorax 759.89
Acephalus 740.0
Acetonemia 790.6
  diabetic 250.1●
    due to secondary diabetes 249.1●
Acetonglycosuria 982.8
Acetonuria 791.6
Achalasia 530.0
  cardia 530.0
  digestive organs congenital NEC 751.8
  esophagus 530.0
  pelvirectal 751.3
  psychogenic 306.4
  pylorus 750.5
  sphincteral NEC 564.89

Achard-Thiers syndrome (adrenogenital) 255.2
Ache(s) - see Pain
Acheilia 750.26
Acheiria 755.21
Achillobursitis 726.71
Achillodynia 726.71
Achlorhydria, achlorhydric 536.0
 anemia 280.9
 diarrhea 536.0
 neurogenic 536.0
 postvagotomy 564.2
 psychogenic 306.4
 secondary to vagotomy 564.2
Achloroblepsia 368.52
Achloropsia 368.52
Acholia 575.8
Acholuric jaundice (familial) (splenomegalic) (see also Spherocytosis) 282.0
 acquired 283.9
Achondroplasia 756.4
Achrestic anemia 281.8
Achroacytosis, lacrimal gland 375.00
 tuberculous (see also Tuberculosis) 017.3
Achroma, cutis 709.00
Achromate (congenital) 368.54
Achromatopia 368.54
Achromatopsia (congenital) 368.54
Achromia
 congenital 270.2
 parasitica 111.0
 unguium 703.8
Achylia
 gastrica 536.8
  neurogenic 536.3
  psychogenic 306.4
 pancreatica 577.1
Achylosis 536.8
Acid
 burn - see also Burn, by site
  from swallowing acid - see Burn, internal organs
 deficiency
  amide nicotinic 265.2
  amino 270.9
  ascorbic 267
  folic 266.2
  nicotinic (amide) 265.2
  pantothenic 266.2
 intoxication 276.2
 peptic disease 536.8
 stomach 536.8
  psychogenic 306.4
Acidemia 276.2
 arginosuccinic 270.6
 fetal
  affecting management of pregnancy 656.3
  before onset of labor, in liveborn infant 768.2
  during labor and delivery, in liveborn infant 768.3
  intrauterine 656.3
  unspecified as to time of onset, in liveborn infant 768.4
 newborn 775.81
 pipecolic 270.7
Acidity, gastric (high) (low) 536.8
 psychogenic 306.4
Acidocytopenia 288.59
Acidocytosis 288.3
Acidopenia 288.59
Acidosis 276.2
 diabetic 250.1
  due to secondary diabetes 249.1
 fetal, affecting management of pregnancy 656.8
 fetal, affecting newborn 775.81
 kidney tubular 588.89
 lactic 276.2

Acidosis (Continued)
 metabolic NEC 276.2
  with respiratory acidosis 276.4
  of newborn 775.81
  late, of newborn 775.7
 newborn 775.81
 renal
  hyperchloremic 588.89
  tubular (distal) (proximal) 588.89
 respiratory 276.2
  complicated by
   metabolic acidosis 276.4
    of newborn 775.81
   metabolic alkalosis 276.4
Aciduria 791.9
 arginosuccinic 270.6
 beta-aminoisobutyric (BAIB) 277.2
 glutaric
  type I 270.7
  type II (type IIA, IIB, IIC) 277.85
  type III 277.86
 glycolic 271.8
 methylmalonic 270.3
  with glycinemia 270.7
 organic 270.9
 orotic (congenital) (hereditary) (pyrimidine deficiency) 281.4
Acladiosis 111.8
 skin 111.8
Aclasis
 diaphyseal 756.4
 tarsoepiphyseal 756.59
Acleistocardia 745.5
Aclusion 524.4
Acmesthesia 782.0
Acne (pustular) (vulgaris) 706.1
 agminata (see also Tuberculosis) 017.0
 artificialis 706.1
 atrophica 706.0
 cachecticorum (Hebra) 706.1
 conglobata 706.1
 conjunctiva 706.1
 cystic 706.1
 decalvans 704.09
 erythematosa 695.3
 eyelid 706.1
 frontalis 706.0
 indurata 706.1
 keloid 706.1
 lupoid 706.0
 necrotic, necrotica 706.0
  miliaris 704.8
 neonatal 706.1
 nodular 706.1
 occupational 706.1
 papulosa 706.1
 rodens 706.0
 rosacea 695.3
 scorbutica 267
 scrofulosorum (Bazin) (see also Tuberculosis) 017.0
 summer 692.72
 tropical 706.1
 varioliformis 706.0
Acneiform drug eruptions 692.3
Acnitis (primary) (see also Tuberculosis) 017.0
Acomia 704.00
Acontractile bladder 344.61
Aconuresis (see also Incontinence) 788.30
Acosta's disease 993.2
Acousma 780.1
Acoustic - see condition
Acousticophobia 300.29
Acquired - see condition
Acquired immune deficiency syndrome - see Human immunodeficiency virus (disease) (illness) (infection)
Acquired immunodeficiency syndrome - see Human immunodeficiency virus (disease) (illness) (infection)
Acragnosis 781.99

Acrania 740.0
Acroagnosis 781.99
Acroangiodermatitis 448.9
Acroasphyxia, chronic 443.89
Acrobrachycephaly 756.0
Acrobystiolith 608.89
Acrobystitis 607.2
Acrocephalopolysyndactyly 755.55
Acrocephalosyndactyly 755.55
Acrocephaly 756.0
Acrochondrohyperplasia 759.82
Acrocyanosis 443.89
 newborn 770.83
  meaning transient blue hands and feet - omit code
Acrodermatitis 686.8
 atrophicans (chronica) 701.8
 continua (Hallopeau) 696.1
 enteropathica 686.8
 Hallopeau's 696.1
 perstans 696.1
 pustulosa continua 696.1
 recalcitrant pustular 696.1
Acrodynia 985.0
Acrodysplasia 755.55
Acrohyperhidrosis (see also Hyperhidrosis) 780.8
Acrokeratosis verruciformis 757.39
Acromastitis 611.0
Acromegaly, acromegalia (skin) 253.0
Acromelalgia 443.82
Acromicria, acromikria 756.59
Acronyx 703.0
Acropachy, thyroid (see also Thyrotoxicosis) 242.9
Acropachyderma 757.39
Acroparesthesia 443.89
 simple (Schultz's type) 443.89
 vasomotor (Nothnagel's type) 443.89
Acropathy thyroid (see also Thyrotoxicosis) 242.9
Acrophobia 300.29
Acroposthitis 607.2
Acroscleriasis (see also Scleroderma) 710.1
Acroscleroderma (see also Scleroderma) 710.1
Acrosclerosis (see also Scleroderma) 710.1
Acrosphacelus 785.4
Acrosphenosyndactylia 755.55
Acrospiroma, eccrine (M8402/0) - see Neoplasm, skin, benign
Acrostealgia 732.9
Acrosyndactyly (see also Syndactylism) 755.10
Acrotrophodynia 991.4
Actinic - see also condition
 cheilitis (due to sun) 692.72
  chronic NEC 692.74
  due to radiation, except from sun 692.82
 conjunctivitis 370.24
 dermatitis (due to sun) (see also Dermatitis, actinic) 692.70
 due to
  roentgen rays or radioactive substance 692.82
  ultraviolet radiation, except from sun 692.82
  sun NEC 692.70
 elastosis solare 692.74
 granuloma 692.73
 keratitis 370.24
 ophthalmia 370.24
 reticuloid 692.73
Actinobacillosis, general 027.8
Actinobacillus
 lignieresii 027.8
 mallei 024
 muris 026.1
Actinocutitis NEC (see also Dermatitis, actinic) 692.70
Actinodermatitis NEC (see also Dermatitis, actinic) 692.70

Actinomyces
    israelii (infection) - *see* Actinomycosis
    muris-ratti (infection) 026.1
Actinomycosis, actinomycotic 039.9
    with
        pneumonia 039.1
    abdominal 039.2
    cervicofacial 039.3
    cutaneous 039.0
    pulmonary 039.1
    specified site NEC 039.8
    thoracic 039.1
Actinoneuritis 357.89
Action, heart
    disorder 427.9
        postoperative 997.1
    irregular 427.9
        postoperative 997.1
        psychogenic 306.2
Active - *see* condition
Activity decrease, functional 780.99
Acute - *see also* condition
    abdomen NEC 789.0 ●
    gallbladder (*see also* Cholecystitis, acute) 575.0
Acyanoblepsia 368.53
Acyanopsia 368.53
Acystia 753.8
Acystinervia - *see* Neurogenic, bladder
Acystineuria - *see* Neurogenic, bladder
Adactylia, adactyly (congenital) 755.4
    lower limb (complete) (intercalary) (partial) (terminal) (*see also* Deformity, reduction, lower limb) 755.39
        meaning all digits (complete) (partial) 755.31
        transverse (complete) (partial) 755.31
    upper limb (complete) (intercalary) (partial) (terminal) (*see also* Deformity, reduction, upper limb) 755.29
        meaning all digits (complete) (partial) 755.21
        transverse (complete) (partial) 755.21
Adair-Dighton syndrome (brittle bones and blue sclera, deafness) 756.51
Adamantinoblastoma (M9310/0) - *see* Ameloblastoma
Adamantinoma (M9310/0) - *see* Ameloblastoma
Adamantoblastoma (M9310/0) - *see* Ameloblastoma
Adams-Stokes (-Morgagni) disease or syndrome (syncope with heart block) 426.9
Adaptation reaction (*see also* Reaction, adjustment) 309.9
Addiction - *see* Dependence
    absinthe 304.6 ●
    alcoholic (ethyl) (methyl) (wood) 303.9 ●
        complicating pregnancy, childbirth, or puerperium 648.4 ●
            affecting fetus or newborn 760.71
        suspected damage to fetus affecting management of pregnancy 655.4 ●
    drug (*see also* Dependence) 304.9 ●
    ethyl alcohol 303.9 ●
    heroin 304.0 ●
    hospital 301.51
    methyl alcohol 303.9 ●
    methylated spirit 303.9 ●
    morphine (-like substances) 304.0 ●
    nicotine 305.1
    opium 304.0 ●
    tobacco 305.1
    wine 303.9 ●
Addison's
    anemia (pernicious) 281.0
    disease (bronze) (primary adrenal insufficiency) 255.41
        tuberculous (*see also* Tuberculosis) 017.6 ●
    keloid (morphea) 701.0

Addison's (*Continued*)
    melanoderma (adrenal cortical hypofunction) 255.41
Addison-Biermer anemia (pernicious) 281.0
Addison-Gull disease - *see* Xanthoma
Addisonian crisis or melanosis (acute adrenocortical insufficiency) 255.41
Additional - *see also* Accessory
    chromosome(s) 758.5
        13-15 758.1
        16-18 758.2
        21 758.0
        autosome(s) NEC 758.5
        sex 758.81
Adduction contracture, hip or other joint - *see* Contraction, joint
ADEM (acute disseminated encephalomy-elitis) (postinfectious) 136.9 [323.61]
    infectious 136.9 [323.61]
    noninfectious 323.81
Adenasthenia gastrica 536.0
Aden fever 061
Adenitis (*see also* Lymphadenitis) 289.3
    acute, unspecified site 683
        epidemic infectious 075
    axillary 289.3
        acute 683
        chronic or subacute 289.1
    Bartholin's gland 616.89
    bulbourethral gland (*see also* Urethritis) 597.89
    cervical 289.3
        acute 683
        chronic or subacute 289.1
    chancroid (Ducrey's bacillus) 099.0
    chronic (any lymph node, except mesenteric) 289.1
        mesenteric 289.2
    Cowper's gland (*see also* Urethritis) 597.89
    epidemic, acute 075
    gangrenous 683
    gonorrheal NEC 098.89
    groin 289.3
        acute 683
        chronic or subacute 289.1
    infectious 075
    inguinal (region) 289.3
        acute 683
        chronic or subacute 289.1
    lymph gland or node, except mesenteric 289.3
        acute 683
        chronic or subacute 289.1
        mesenteric (acute) (chronic) (nonspecific) (subacute) 289.2
    mesenteric (acute) (chronic) (nonspecific) (subacute) 289.2
        due to Pasteurella multocida (P. septica) 027.2
    parotid gland (suppurative) 527.2
    phlegmonous 683
    salivary duct or gland (any) (recurring) (suppurative) 527.2
    scrofulous (*see also* Tuberculosis) 017.2 ●
    septic 289.3
    Skene's duct or gland (*see also* Urethritis) 597.89
    strumous, tuberculous (*see also* Tuberculosis) 017.2 ●
    subacute, unspecified site 289.1
    sublingual gland (suppurative) 527.2
    submandibular gland (suppurative) 527.2
    submaxillary gland (suppurative) 527.2
    suppurative 683
    tuberculous - *see* Tuberculosis, lymph gland
    urethral gland (*see also* Urethritis) 597.89
    venereal NEC 099.8
    Wharton's duct (suppurative) 527.2

Adenoacanthoma (M8570/3) - *see* Neoplasm, by site, malignant
Adenoameloblastoma (M9300/0) 213.1
    upper jaw (bone) 213.0
Adenocarcinoma (M8140/3) - *see also* Neoplasm, by site, malignant

> Note: The list of adjectival modifiers below is not exhaustive. A description of adenocarcinoma that does not appear in this list should be coded in the same manner as carcinoma with that description. Thus, "mixed acidophil-basophil adenocarcinoma," should be coded in the same manner as "mixed acidophil-basophil carcinoma," which appears in the list under "Carcinoma."
>
> Except where otherwise indicated, the morphological varieties of adenocarcinoma in the list below should be coded by site as for "Neoplasm, malignant."

    with
        apocrine metaplasia (M8573/3)
        cartilaginous (and osseous) metaplasia (M8571/3)
        osseous (and cartilaginous) metaplasia (M8571/3)
        spindle cell metaplasia (M8572/3)
        squamous metaplasia (M8570/3)
    acidophil (M8280/3)
        specified site - *see* Neoplasm, by site, malignant
        unspecified site 194.3
    acinar (M8550/3)
    acinic cell (M8550/3)
    adrenal cortical (M8370/3) 194.0
    alveolar (M8251/3)
        and
            epidermoid carcinoma, mixed (M8560/3)
            squamous cell carcinoma, mixed (M8560/3)
    apocrine (M8401/3)
        breast - *see* Neoplasm, breast, malignant
        specified site NEC - *see* Neoplasm, skin, malignant
        unspecified site 173.99
    basophil (M8300/3)
        specified site - *see* Neoplasm, by site, malignant
        unspecified site 194.3
    bile duct type (M8160/3)
        liver 155.1
        specified site NEC - *see* Neoplasm, by site, malignant
        unspecified site 155.1
    bronchiolar (M8250/3) - *see* Neoplasm, lung, malignant
    ceruminous (M8420/3) 173.29
    chromophobe (M8270/3)
        specified site - *see* Neoplasm, by site, malignant
        unspecified site 194.3
    clear cell (mesonephroid type) (M8310/3)
    colloid (M8480/3)
    cylindroid type (M8200/3)
    diffuse type (M8145/3)
        specified site - *see* Neoplasm, by site, malignant
        unspecified site 151.9
    duct (infiltrating) (M8500/3)
        with Paget's disease (M8541/3) - *see* Neoplasm, breast, malignant
        specified site - *see* Neoplasm, by site, malignant
        unspecified site 174.9
    embryonal (M9070/3)
    endometrioid (M8380/3) - *see* Neoplasm, by site, malignant

SECTION 1 INDEX TO DISEASES AND INJURIES / Adenocarcinoma

Adenocarcinoma (Continued)
  eosinophil (M8280/3)
    specified site - see Neoplasm, by site, malignant
    unspecified site 194.3
  follicular (M8330/3)
    and papillary (M8340/3) 193
      moderately differentiated type (M8332/3) 193
    pure follicle type (M8331/3) 193
    specified site - see Neoplasm, by site, malignant
    trabecular type (M8332/3) 193
    unspecified type 193
    well differentiated type (M8331/3) 193
  gelatinous (M8480/3)
  granular cell (M8320/3)
  Hürthle cell (M8290/3) 193
  in
    adenomatous
      polyp (M8210/3)
      polyposis coli (M8220/3) 153.9
    polypoid adenoma (M8210/3)
    tubular adenoma (M8210/3)
    villous adenoma (M8261/3)
  infiltrating duct (M8500/3)
    with Paget's disease (M8541/3) - see Neoplasm, breast, malignant
    specified site - see Neoplasm, by site, malignant
    unspecified site 174.9
  inflammatory (M8530/3)
    specified site - see Neoplasm, by site, malignant
    unspecified site 174.9
  in situ (M8140/2) - see Neoplasm, by site, in situ
  intestinal type (M8144/3)
    specified site - see Neoplasm, by site, malignant
    unspecified site 151.9
  intraductal (noninfiltrating) (M8500/2)
    papillary (M8503/2)
      specified site - see Neoplasm, by site, in situ
      unspecified site 233.0
    specified site - see Neoplasm, by site, in situ
    unspecified site 233.0
  islet cell (M8150/3)
    and exocrine, mixed (M8154/3)
      specified site - see Neoplasm, by site, malignant
      unspecified site 157.9
    pancreas 157.4
    specified site NEC - see Neoplasm, by site, malignant
    unspecified site 157.4
  lobular (M8520/3)
    specified site - see Neoplasm, by site, malignant
    unspecified site 174.9
  medullary (M8510/3)
  mesonephric (M9110/3)
  mixed cell (M8323/3)
  mucinous (M8480/3)
  mucin-producing (M8481/3)
  mucoid (M8480/3) - see also Neoplasm, by site, malignant
    cell (M8300/3)
      specified site - see Neoplasm, by site, malignant
      unspecified site 194.3
  nonencapsulated sclerosing (M8350/3) 193
  oncocytic (M8290/3)
  oxyphilic (M8290/3)
  papillary (M8260/3)
    and follicular (M8340/3) 193
    intraductal (noninfiltrating) (M8503/2)
      specified site - see Neoplasm, by site, in situ
      unspecified site 233.0

Adenocarcinoma (Continued)
  papillary (Continued)
    serous (M8460/3)
      specified site - see Neoplasm, by site, malignant
      unspecified site 183.0
    papillocystic (M8450/3)
      specified site - see Neoplasm, by site, malignant
      unspecified site 183.0
    pseudomucinous (M8470/3)
      specified site - see Neoplasm, by site, malignant
      unspecified site 183.0
    renal cell (M8312/3) 189.0
    sebaceous (M8410/3)
    serous (M8441/3) - see also Neoplasm, by site, malignant
      papillary
        specified site - see Neoplasm, by site, malignant
        unspecified site 183.0
    signet ring cell (M8490/3)
    superficial spreading (M8143/3)
    sweat gland (M8400/3) - see Neoplasm, skin, malignant
    trabecular (M8190/3)
    tubular (M8211/3)
    villous (M8262/3)
    water-clear cell (M8322/3) 194.1
Adenofibroma (M9013/0)
  clear cell (M8313/0) - see Neoplasm, by site, benign
  endometrioid (M8381/0) 220
    borderline malignancy (M8381/1) 236.2
    malignant (M8381/3) 183.0
  mucinous (M9015/0)
    specified site - see Neoplasm, by site, benign
    unspecified site 220
  prostate 600.20
    with
      other lower urinary tract symptoms (LUTS) 600.21
      urinary
        obstruction 600.21
        retention 600.21
  serous (M9014/0)
    specified site - see Neoplasm, by site, benign
    unspecified site 220
  specified site - see Neoplasm, by site, benign
  unspecified site 220
Adenofibrosis
  breast 610.2
  endometrioid 617.0
Adenoiditis 474.01
  acute 463
  chronic 474.01
    with chronic tonsillitis 474.02
Adenoids (congenital) (of nasal fossa) 474.9
  hypertrophy 474.12
  vegetations 474.2
Adenolipomatosis (symmetrical) 272.8
Adenolymphoma (M8561/0)
  specified site - see Neoplasm, by site, benign
  unspecified 210.2
Adenoma (sessile) (M8140/0) - see also Neoplasm, by site, benign

> Note: Except where otherwise indicated, the morphological varieties of adenoma in the list below should be coded by site as for "Neoplasm, benign."

  acidophil (M8280/0)
    specified site - see Neoplasm, by site, benign
    unspecified site 227.3
  acinar (cell) (M8550/0)
  acinic cell (M8550/0)

Adenoma (Continued)
  adrenal (cortex) (cortical) (functioning) (M8370/0) 227.0
    clear cell type (M8373/0) 227.0
    compact cell type (M8371/0) 227.0
    glomerulosa cell type (M8374/0) 227.0
    heavily pigmented variant (M8372/0) 227.0
    mixed cell type (M8375/0) 227.0
  alpha cell (M8152/0)
    pancreas 211.7
    specified site NEC - see Neoplasm, by site, benign
    unspecified site 211.7
  alveolar (M8251/0)
  apocrine (M8401/0)
    breast 217
    specified site NEC - see Neoplasm, skin, benign
    unspecified site 216.9
  basal cell (M8147/0)
  basophil (M8300/0)
    specified site - see Neoplasm, by site, benign
    unspecified site 227.3
  beta cell (M8151/0)
    pancreas 211.7
    specified site NEC - see Neoplasm, by site, benign
    unspecified site 211.7
  bile duct (M8160/0) 211.5
  black (M8372/0) 227.0
  bronchial (M8140/1) 235.7
    carcinoid type (M8240/3) - see Neoplasm, lung, malignant
    cylindroid type (M8200/3) - see Neoplasm, lung, malignant
  ceruminous (M8420/0) 216.2
  chief cell (M8321/0) 227.1
  chromophobe (M8270/0)
    specified site - see Neoplasm, by site, benign
    unspecified site 227.3
  clear cell (M8310/0)
  colloid (M8334/0)
    specified site - see Neoplasm, by site, benign
    unspecified site 226
  cylindroid type, bronchus (M8200/3) - see Neoplasm, lung, malignant
  duct (M8503/0)
  embryonal (M8191/0)
  endocrine, multiple (M8360/1)
    single specified site - see Neoplasm, by site, uncertain behavior
    two or more specified sites 237.4
    unspecified site 237.4
  endometrioid (M8380/0) - see also Neoplasm, by site, benign
    borderline malignancy (M8380/1) - see Neoplasm, by site, uncertain behavior
  eosinophil (M8280/0)
    specified site - see Neoplasm, by site, benign
    unspecified site 227.3
  fetal (M8333/0)
    specified site - see Neoplasm, by site, benign
    unspecified site 226
  follicular (M8330/0)
    specified site - see Neoplasm, by site, benign
    unspecified site 226
  hepatocellular (M8170/0) 211.5
  Hürthle cell (M8290/0) 226
  intracystic papillary (M8504/0)
  islet cell (functioning) (M8150/0)
    pancreas 211.7
    specified site NEC - see Neoplasm, by site, benign
    unspecified site 211.7

Adenoma (Continued)
 liver cell (M8170/0) 211.5
 macrofollicular (M8334/0)
  specified site NEC - see Neoplasm, by site, benign
  unspecified site 226
 malignant, malignum (M8140/3) - see Neoplasm, by site, malignant
 mesonephric (M9110/0)
 microfollicular (M8333/0)
  specified site - see Neoplasm, by site, benign
  unspecified site 226
 mixed cell (M8323/0)
 monomorphic (M8146/0)
 mucinous (M8480/0)
 mucoid cell (M8300/0)
  specified site - see Neoplasm, by site, benign
  unspecified site 227.3
 multiple endocrine (M8360/1)
  single specified site - see Neoplasm, by site, uncertain behavior
  two or more specified sites 237.4
  unspecified site 237.4
 nipple (M8506/0) 217
 oncocytic (M8290/0)
 oxyphilic (M8290/0)
 papillary (M8260/0) - see also Neoplasm, by site, benign
  intracystic (M8504/0)
 papillotubular (M8263/0)
 Pick's tubular (M8640/0)
  specified site - see Neoplasm, by site, benign
  unspecified site
   female 220
   male 222.0
 pleomorphic (M8940/0)
 polypoid (M8210/0)
 prostate (benign) 600.20
  with
   other lower urinary tract symptoms (LUTS) 600.21
   urinary
    obstruction 600.21
    retention 600.21
 rete cell 222.0
 sebaceous, sebaceum (gland) (senile) (M8410/0) - see also Neoplasm, skin, benign
  disseminata 759.5
 Sertoli cell (M8640/0)
  specified site - see Neoplasm, by site, benign
  unspecified site
   female 220
   male 222.0
 skin appendage (M8390/0) - see Neoplasm, skin, benign
 sudoriferous gland (M8400/0) - see Neoplasm, skin, benign
 sweat gland or duct (M8400/0) - see Neoplasm, skin, benign
 testicular (M8640/0)
  specified site - see Neoplasm, by site, benign
  unspecified site
   female 220
   male 222.0
 thyroid 226
 trabecular (M8190/0)
 tubular (M8211/0) - see also Neoplasm, by site, benign
  papillary (M8460/3)
  Pick's (M8640/0)
   specified site - see Neoplasm, by site, benign
   unspecified site
    female 220
    male 222.0

Adenoma (Continued)
 tubulovillous (M8263/0)
 villoglandular (M8263/0)
 villous (M8261/1) - see Neoplasm, by site, uncertain behavior
 water-clear cell (M8322/0) 227.1
 wolffian duct (M9110/0)
Adenomatosis (M8220/0)
 endocrine (multiple) (M8360/1)
  single specified site - see Neoplasm, by site, uncertain behavior
  two or more specified sites 237.4
  unspecified site 237.4
 erosive of nipple (M8506/0) 217
 pluriendocrine - see Adenomatosis, endocrine
 pulmonary (M8250/1) 235.7
  malignant (M8250/3) - see Neoplasm, lung, malignant
 specified site - see Neoplasm, by site, benign
 unspecified site 211.3
Adenomatous
 cyst, thyroid (gland) - see Goiter, nodular
 goiter (nontoxic) (see also Goiter, nodular) 241.9
  toxic or with hyperthyroidism 242.3●
Adenomyoma (M8932/0) - see also Neoplasm, by site, benign
 prostate 600.20
  with
   other lower urinary tract symptoms (LUTS) 600.21
   urinary
    obstruction 600.21
    retention 600.21
Adenomyometritis 617.0
Adenomyosis (uterus) (internal) 617.0
Adenopathy (lymph gland) 785.6
 inguinal 785.6
 mediastinal 785.6
 mesentery 785.6
 syphilitic (secondary) 091.4
 tracheobronchial 785.6
  tuberculous (see also Tuberculosis) 012.1●
   primary, progressive 010.8●
 tuberculous (see also Tuberculosis, lymph gland) 017.2●
  tracheobronchial 012.1●
   primary, progressive 010.8●
Adenopharyngitis 462
Adenophlegmon 683
Adenosalpingitis 614.1
Adenosarcoma (M8960/3) 189.0
Adenosclerosis 289.3
Adenosis
 breast (sclerosing) 610.2
 vagina, congenital 752.49
Adentia (complete) (partial) (see also Absence, teeth) 520.0
Adherent
 labium (minus) 624.4
 pericardium (nonrheumatic) 423.1
  rheumatic 393
 placenta 667.0●
  with hemorrhage 666.0●
 prepuce 605
 scar (skin) NEC 709.2
 tendon in scar 709.2
Adhesion(s), adhesive (postinfectional) (postoperative)
 abdominal (wall) (see also Adhesions, peritoneum) 568.0
 amnion to fetus 658.8●
  affecting fetus or newborn 762.8
 appendix 543.9
 arachnoiditis - see Meningitis
 auditory tube (Eustachian) 381.89
 bands - see also Adhesions, peritoneum
  cervix 622.3
  uterus 621.5
 bile duct (any) 576.8

Adhesion(s) (Continued)
 bladder (sphincter) 596.89
 bowel (see also Adhesions, peritoneum) 568.0
 cardiac 423.1
  rheumatic 398.99
 cecum (see also Adhesions, peritoneum) 568.0
 cervicovaginal 622.3
  congenital 752.49
  postpartal 674.8●
   old 622.3
 cervix 622.3
 clitoris 624.4
 colon (see also Adhesions, peritoneum) 568.0
 common duct 576.8
 congenital - see also Anomaly, specified type NEC
  fingers (see also Syndactylism, fingers) 755.11
  labium (majus) (minus) 752.49
  omental, anomalous 751.4
  ovary 752.0
  peritoneal 751.4
  toes (see also Syndactylism, toes) 755.13
  tongue (to gum or roof of mouth) 750.12
 conjunctiva (acquired) (localized) 372.62
  congenital 743.63
  extensive 372.63
 cornea - see Opacity, cornea
 cystic duct 575.8
 diaphragm (see also Adhesions, peritoneum) 568.0
 due to foreign body - see Foreign body
 duodenum (see also Adhesions, peritoneum) 568.0
  with obstruction 537.3
 ear, middle - see Adhesions, middle ear
 epididymis 608.89
 epidural - see Adhesions, meninges
 epiglottis 478.79
 Eustachian tube 381.89
 eyelid 374.46
  postoperative 997.99
  surgically created V45.69
 gallbladder (see also Disease, gallbladder) 575.8
 globe 360.89
 heart 423.1
  rheumatic 398.99
 ileocecal (coil) (see also Adhesions, peritoneum) 568.0
 ileum (see also Adhesions, peritoneum) 568.0
 intestine (postoperative) (see also Adhesions, peritoneum) 568.0
  with obstruction 560.81
   with hernia - see also Hernia, by site, with obstruction
    gangrenous - see Hernia, by site, with gangrene
 intra-abdominal (see also Adhesions, peritoneum) 568.0
 iris 364.70
  to corneal graft 996.79
 joint (see also Ankylosis) 718.5●
 kidney 593.89
 labium (majus) (minus), congenital 752.49
 liver 572.8
 lung 511.0
 mediastinum 519.3
 meninges 349.2
  cerebral (any) 349.2
   congenital 742.4
  congenital 742.8
  spinal (any) 349.2
   congenital 742.59
  tuberculous (cerebral) (spinal) (see also Tuberculosis, meninges) 013.0●
 mesenteric (see also Adhesions, peritoneum) 568.0

SECTION 1 INDEX TO DISEASES AND INJURIES / Adhesion(s)

Adhesion(s) (Continued)
- middle ear (fibrous) 385.10
  - drum head 385.19
    - to
      - incus 385.11
      - promontorium 385.13
      - stapes 385.12
    - specified NEC 385.19
- nasal (septum) (to turbinates) 478.19
- nerve NEC 355.9
  - spinal 355.9
    - root 724.9
      - cervical NEC 723.4
      - lumbar NEC 724.4
      - lumbosacral 724.4
      - thoracic 724.4
- ocular muscle 378.60
- omentum (see also Adhesions, peritoneum) 568.0
- organ or site, congenital NEC - see Anomaly, specified type NEC
- ovary 614.6
  - congenital (to cecum, kidney, or omentum) 752.0
- parauterine 614.6
- parovarian 614.6
- pelvic (peritoneal)
  - female (postoperative) (postinfection) 614.6
  - male (postoperative) (postinfection) (see also Adhesions, peritoneum) 568.0
  - postpartal (old) 614.6
  - tuberculous (see also Tuberculosis) 016.9●
- penis to scrotum (congenital) 752.69
- periappendiceal (see also Adhesions, peritoneum) 568.0
- pericardium (nonrheumatic) 423.1
  - rheumatic 393
  - tuberculous (see also Tuberculosis) 017.9● [420.0]
- pericholecystic 575.8
- perigastric (see also Adhesions, peritoneum) 568.0
- periovarian 614.6
- periprostatic 602.8
- perirectal (see also Adhesions, peritoneum) 568.0
- perirenal 593.89
- peritoneum, peritoneal (fibrous) (postoperative) 568.0
  - with obstruction (intestinal) 560.81
    - with hernia - see also Hernia, by site, with obstruction
      - gangrenous - see Hernia, by site, with gangrene
  - duodenum 537.3
  - congenital 751.4
  - female (postoperative) (postinfective) 614.6
  - pelvic, female 614.6
  - pelvic, male 568.0
  - postpartal, pelvic 614.6
  - to uterus 614.6
- peritubal 614.6
- periureteral 593.89
- periuterine 621.5
- perivesical 596.89
- perivesicular (seminal vesicle) 608.89
- pleura, pleuritic 511.0
  - tuberculous (see also Tuberculosis, pleura) 012.0●
- pleuropericardial 511.0
- postoperative (gastrointestinal tract) (see also Adhesions, peritoneum)
  - eyelid 997.99
    - surgically created V45.69
  - pelvic, female 614.9
  - pelvic, male 568.0
  - urethra 598.2

Adhesion(s) (Continued)
- postpartal, old 624.4
- preputial, prepuce 605
- pulmonary 511.0
- pylorus (see also Adhesions, peritoneum) 568.0
- Rosenmüller's fossa 478.29
- sciatic nerve 355.0
- seminal vesicle 608.89
- shoulder (joint) 726.0
- sigmoid flexure (see also Adhesions, peritoneum) 568.0
- spermatic cord (acquired) 608.89
  - congenital 752.89
- spinal canal 349.2
  - nerve 355.9
    - root 724.9
      - cervical NEC 723.4
      - lumbar NEC 724.4
      - lumbosacral 724.4
      - thoracic 724.4
- stomach (see also Adhesions, peritoneum) 568.0
- subscapular 726.2
- tendonitis 726.90
  - shoulder 726.0
- testicle 608.89
- tongue (congenital) (to gum or roof of mouth) 750.12
  - acquired 529.8
- trachea 519.19
- tubo-ovarian 614.6
- tunica vaginalis 608.89
- ureter 593.89
- uterus 621.5
  - to abdominal wall 614.6
    - in pregnancy or childbirth 654.4●
      - affecting fetus or newborn 763.89
- vagina (chronic) (postoperative) (postradiation) 623.2
- vaginitis (congenital) 752.49
- vesical 596.89
- vitreomacular adhesion 379.27
- vitreous 379.29

Adie (-Holmes) syndrome (tonic pupillary reaction) 379.46
Adiponecrosis neonatorum 778.1
Adiposa dolorosa 272.8
Adiposalgia 272.8
Adiposis
- cerebralis 253.8
- dolorosa 272.8
- tuberosa simplex 272.8

Adiposity 278.02
- heart (see also Degeneration, myocardial) 429.1
- localized 278.1

Adiposogenital dystrophy 253.8
Adjustment
- prosthesis or other device - see Fitting of
- reaction - see Reaction, adjustment

Administration, prophylactic
- antibiotics, long-term V58.62
  - short-term use - omit code
- antitoxin, any V07.2
- antivenin V07.2
- chemotherapeutic agent NEC V07.39
- chemotherapy NEC V07.39
- diphtheria antitoxin V07.2
- fluoride V07.31
- gamma globulin V07.2
- immune sera (gamma globulin) V07.2
- passive immunization agent V07.2
- RhoGAM V07.2

Admission (encounter)
- as organ donor - see Donor
- by mistake V68.9
- for
  - adequacy testing (for)
    - hemodialysis V56.31
    - peritoneal dialysis V56.32

Admission (Continued)
- for (Continued)
  - adjustment (of)
    - artificial
      - arm (complete) (partial) V52.0
      - eye V52.2
      - leg (complete) (partial) V52.1
    - brain neuropacemaker V53.02
    - breast
      - implant V52.4
        - exchange (different material) (different size) V52.4
      - prosthesis V52.4
    - cardiac device V53.39
      - defibrillator, automatic implantable (with synchronous cardiac pacemaker) V53.32
      - pacemaker V53.31
        - carotid sinus V53.39
    - catheter
      - non-vascular V58.82
      - vascular V58.81
    - cerebral ventricle (communicating) shunt V53.01
    - colostomy belt V55.3
    - contact lenses V53.1
    - cystostomy device V53.6
    - dental prosthesis V52.3
    - device, unspecified type V53.90
      - abdominal V53.59
      - cardiac V53.39
        - defibrillator, automatic implantable (with synchronous cardiac pacemaker) V53.32
        - pacemaker V53.31
          - carotid sinus V53.39
      - cerebral ventricle (communicating) shunt V53.01
      - gastrointestinal NEC V53.59
      - insulin pump V53.91
      - intestinal V53.50
      - nervous system V53.09
      - orthodontic V53.4
      - other device V53.99
      - prosthetic V52.9
        - breast V52.4
        - dental V52.3
        - eye V52.2
        - specified type NEC V52.8
      - special senses V53.09
      - substitution
        - auditory V53.09
        - nervous system V53.09
        - visual V53.09
      - urinary V53.6
    - dialysis catheter
      - extracorporeal V56.1
      - peritoneal V56.2
    - diaphragm (contraceptive) V25.02
    - gastric lap band V53.51
    - gastrointestinal appliance and device NEC V53.59
    - growth rod V54.02
    - hearing aid V53.2
    - ileostomy device V55.2
    - intestinal appliance and device V53.50
    - neuropacemaker (brain) (peripheral nerve) (spinal cord) V53.02
    - orthodontic device V53.4
    - orthopedic (device) V53.7
      - brace V53.7
      - cast V53.7
      - shoes V53.7
    - pacemaker
      - brain V53.02
      - cardiac V53.31
      - carotid sinus V53.39
      - peripheral nerve V53.02
      - spinal cord V53.02

SECTION I INDEX TO DISEASES AND INJURIES / Admission

Admission (Continued)
　for (Continued)
　　adjustment (of) (Continued)
　　　prosthesis V52.9
　　　　arm (complete) (partial) V52.0
　　　　breast V52.4
　　　　dental V52.3
　　　　eye V52.2
　　　　leg (complete) (partial) V52.1
　　　　specified type NEC V52.8
　　　spectacles V53.1
　　　wheelchair V53.8
　　adoption referral or proceedings V68.89
　　aftercare (see also Aftercare) V58.9
　　　cardiac pacemaker V53.31
　　　chemotherapy (oral) (intravenous) V58.11
　　　dialysis
　　　　extracorporeal (renal) V56.0
　　　　peritoneal V56.8
　　　　renal V56.0
　　　fracture (see also Aftercare, fracture) V54.9
　　　medical NEC V58.89
　　　organ transplant V58.44
　　　orthopedic V54.9
　　　　following explantation of joint prosthesis (for joint prosthesis insertion) (staged procedure) V54.82
　　　　specified care NEC V54.89
　　　pacemaker device
　　　　brain V53.02
　　　　cardiac V53.31
　　　　carotid sinus V53.39
　　　　nervous system V53.02
　　　　spinal cord V53.02
　　　postoperative NEC V58.49
　　　　wound closure, planned V58.41
　　　postpartum
　　　　immediately after delivery V24.0
　　　　routine follow-up V24.2
　　　postradiation V58.0
　　　radiation therapy V58.0
　　　removal of
　　　　non-vascular catheter V58.82
　　　　vascular catheter V58.81
　　　specified NEC V58.89
　　　surgical NEC V58.49
　　　　wound closure, planned V58.41
　　antineoplastic
　　　chemotherapy (oral) (intravenous) V58.11
　　　immunotherapy V58.12
　　artificial insemination V26.1
　　assisted reproductive fertility procedure cycle V26.81
　　attention to artificial opening (of) V55.9
　　　artificial vagina V55.7
　　　colostomy V55.3
　　　cystostomy V55.5
　　　enterostomy V55.4
　　　gastrostomy V55.1
　　　ileostomy V55.2
　　　jejunostomy V55.4
　　　nephrostomy V55.6
　　　specified site NEC V55.8
　　　　intestinal tract V55.4
　　　　urinary tract V55.6
　　　tracheostomy V55.0
　　　ureterostomy V55.6
　　　urethrostomy V55.6
　　battery replacement
　　　cardiac pacemaker V53.31
　　blood typing V72.86
　　　Rh typing V72.86
　　boarding V65.0

Admission (Continued)
　for (Continued)
　　breast
　　　augmentation or reduction V50.1
　　　implant exchange (different material) (different size) V52.4
　　　reconstruction following mastectomy V51.0
　　　removal
　　　　prophylactic V50.41
　　　　tissue expander without synchronous insertion of permanent implant V52.4
　　change of
　　　cardiac pacemaker (battery) 53.31
　　　carotid sinus pacemaker V53.39
　　　catheter in artificial opening - see Attention to, artificial, opening
　　　drains V58.49
　　　dressing
　　　　wound V58.30
　　　　　nonsurgical V58.30
　　　　　surgical V58.31
　　　fixation device
　　　　external V54.89
　　　　internal V54.01
　　　Kirschner wire V54.89
　　　neuropacemaker device (brain) (peripheral nerve) (spinal cord) V53.02
　　　nonsurgical wound dressing V58.30
　　　pacemaker device
　　　　brain V53.02
　　　　cardiac V53.31
　　　　carotid sinus V53.39
　　　　nervous system V53.02
　　　plaster cast V54.89
　　　splint, external V54.89
　　　Steinmann pin V54.89
　　　surgical wound dressing V58.31
　　　traction device V54.89
　　　wound packing V58.30
　　　　nonsurgical V58.30
　　　　surgical V58.31
　　checkup only V70.0
　　chemotherapy, (oral) (intravenous)
　　　antineoplastic V58.11
　　circumcision, ritual or routine (in absence of medical indication) V50.2
　　clinical research investigation (control) (normal comparison) (participant) V70.7
　　closure of artificial opening - see Attention to, artificial, opening
　　contraceptive
　　　counseling V25.09
　　　　emergency V25.03
　　　　postcoital V25.03
　　　management V25.9
　　　　specified type NEC V25.8
　　convalescence following V66.9
　　　chemotherapy V66.2
　　　psychotherapy V66.3
　　　radiotherapy V66.1
　　　surgery V66.0
　　　treatment (for) V66.5
　　　　combined V66.6
　　　　fracture V66.4
　　　　mental disorder NEC V66.3
　　　　specified condition NEC V66.5
　　cosmetic surgery NEC V50.1
　　　breast reconstruction following mastectomy V51.0
　　　following healed injury or operation V51.8
　　counseling (see also Counseling) V65.40
　　　without complaint or sickness V65.49
　　　contraceptive management V25.09
　　　　emergency V25.03
　　　　postcoital V25.03
　　　dietary V65.3

Admission (Continued)
　for (Continued)
　　counseling (Continued)
　　　exercise V65.41
　　　fertility preservation (prior to cancer therapy) (prior to surgical removal of gonads) V26.42
　　　for
　　　　nonattending third party V65.19
　　　　pediatric
　　　　　pre-adoption visit for adoptive parent(s) V65.11
　　　　　pre-birth visit for expectant parent(s) V65.11
　　　　victim of abuse
　　　　　child V61.21
　　　　　partner or spouse V61.11
　　　genetic V26.33
　　　gonorrhea V65.45
　　　HIV V65.44
　　　human immunodeficiency virus V65.44
　　　injury prevention V65.43
　　　insulin pump training V65.46
　　　natural family planning
　　　　procreative V26.41
　　　　to avoid pregnancy V25.04
　　　procreative management V26.49
　　　　using natural family planning V26.41
　　　sexually transmitted disease NEC V65.45
　　　　HIV V65.44
　　　specified reason NEC V65.49
　　　substance use and abuse V65.42
　　　syphilis V65.45
　　　victim of abuse
　　　　child V61.21
　　　　partner or spouse V61.11
　　desensitization to allergens V07.1
　　dialysis V56.0
　　　catheter
　　　　fitting and adjustment
　　　　　extracorporeal V56.1
　　　　　peritoneal V56.2
　　　　removal or replacement
　　　　　extracorporeal V56.1
　　　　　peritoneal V56.2
　　　extracorporeal (renal) V56.0
　　　peritoneal V56.8
　　　renal V56.0
　　dietary surveillance and counseling V65.3
　　drug monitoring, therapeutic V58.83
　　ear piercing V50.3
　　elective surgery
　　　breast
　　　　augmentation or reduction V50.1
　　　　reconstruction following mastectomy V51.0
　　　　removal, prophylactic V50.41
　　　circumcision, ritual or routine (in absence of medical indication) V50.2
　　　cosmetic NEC V50.1
　　　　breast reconstruction following mastectomy V51.0
　　　　following healed injury or operation V51.8
　　　ear piercing V50.3
　　　face-lift V50.1
　　　hair transplant V50.0
　　　plastic
　　　　breast reconstruction following mastectomy V51.0
　　　　cosmetic NEC V50.1
　　　　following healed injury or operation V51.8
　　　prophylactic organ removal V50.49
　　　　breast V50.41
　　　　ovary V50.42
　　　repair of scarred tissue (following healed injury or operation) V51.8
　　　specified type NEC V50.8

SECTION 1 INDEX TO DISEASES AND INJURIES / Admission

Admission (Continued)
  for (Continued)
    end-of-life care V66.7
    examination (see also Examination)
      V70.9
      administrative purpose NEC V70.3
      adoption V70.3
      allergy V72.7
      antibody response V72.61
      at health care facility V70.0
      athletic team V70.3
      camp V70.3
      cardiovascular, preoperative V72.81
      clinical research investigation (control)
        (participant) V70.7
      dental V72.2
      developmental testing (child) (infant)
        V20.2
      donor (potential) V70.8
      driver's license V70.3
      ear V72.19
      employment V70.5
      eye V72.0
      follow-up (routine) - see Examination,
        follow-up
      for admission to
        old age home V70.3
        school V70.3
      general V70.9
        specified reason NEC V70.8
      gynecological V72.31
      health supervision
        child (over 28 days old) V20.2
        infant (over 28 days old) V20.2
        newborn
          8 to 28 days old V20.32
          under 8 days old V20.31
      hearing V72.19
        following failed hearing screening
          V72.11
      immigration V70.3
      infant
        8 to 28 days old V20.32
        over 28 days old, routine V20.2
        under 8 days old V20.31
      insurance certification V70.3
      laboratory V72.60
        ordered as part of a routine
          general medical examination
          V72.62
        pre-operative V72.63
        pre-procedural V72.63
        specified NEC V72.69
      marriage license V70.3
      medical (general) (see also Examination,
        medical) V70.9
      medicolegal reasons V70.4
      naturalization V70.3
      pelvic (annual) (periodic) V72.31
      postpartum checkup V24.2
      pregnancy (possible) (unconfirmed)
        V72.40
        negative result V72.41
        positive result V72.42
      preoperative V72.84
        cardiovascular V72.81
        respiratory V72.82
        specified NEC V72.83
      preprocedural V72.84
        cardiovascular V72.81
        general physical V72.83
        respiratory V72.82
        specified NEC V72.83
      prior to chemotherapy V72.83
      prison V70.3
      psychiatric (general) V70.2
        requested by authority V70.1
      radiological NEC V72.5
      respiratory, preoperative V72.82
      school V70.3
      screening - see Screening

Admission (Continued)
  for (Continued)
    examination (Continued)
      skin hypersensitivity V72.7
      specified type NEC V72.85
      sport competition V70.3
      vision V72.0
      well baby and child care V20.2
    exercise therapy V57.1
    face-lift, cosmetic reason V50.1
    fertility preservation (prior to cancer
      therapy) (prior to surgical removal
      of gonads) V26.82
    fitting (of)
      artificial
        arm (complete) (partial) V52.0
        eye V52.2
        leg (complete) (partial) V52.1
      biliary drainage tube V58.82
      brain neuropacemaker V53.02
      breast V52.4
        implant V52.4
        prosthesis V52.4
      cardiac pacemaker V53.31
      catheter
        non-vascular V58.82
        vascular V58.81
      cerebral ventricle (communicating)
        shunt V53.01
      chest tube V58.82
      colostomy belt V55.2
      contact lenses V53.1
      cystostomy device V53.6
      dental prosthesis V52.3
      device, unspecified type V53.90
        abdominal V53.59
        cerebral ventricle (communicating)
          shunt V53.01
        gastrointestinal NEC V53.59
        insulin pump V53.91
        intestinal V53.50
        intrauterine contraceptive
          insertion V25.11
          removal V25.12
            and reinsertion V25.13
          replacement V25.13
        nervous system V53.09
        orthodontic V53.4
        other device V53.99
        prosthetic V52.9
          breast V52.4
          dental V52.3
          eye V52.2
        special senses V53.09
        substitution
          auditory V53.09
          nervous system V53.09
          visual V53.09
      diaphragm (contraceptive) V25.02
      fistula (sinus tract) drainage tube
        V58.82
      gastric lap band V53.51
      gastrointestinal appliance and device
        NEC V53.59
      growth rod V54.02
      hearing aid V53.2
      ileostomy device V55.2
      intestinal appliance and device
        V53.50
      intrauterine contraceptive device
        insertion V25.11
        removal V25.12
          and reinsertion V25.13
        replacement V25.13
      neuropacemaker (brain) (peripheral
        nerve) (spinal cord) V53.02
      orthodontic device V53.4
      orthopedic (device) V53.7
        brace V53.7
        cast V53.7
        shoes V53.7

Admission (Continued)
  for (Continued)
    fitting (of) (Continued)
      pacemaker
        brain V53.02
        cardiac V53.31
        carotid sinus V53.39
        spinal cord V53.02
      pleural drainage tube V58.82
      portacath V58.81
      prosthesis V52.9
        arm (complete) (partial) V52.0
        breast V52.4
        dental V52.3
        eye V52.2
        leg (complete) (partial) V52.1
        specified type NEC V52.8
      spectacles V53.1
      wheelchair V53.8
    follow-up examination (routine)
      (following) V67.9
      cancer chemotherapy V67.2
      chemotherapy V67.2
      high-risk medication NEC V67.51
      injury NEC V67.59
      psychiatric V67.3
      psychotherapy V67.3
      radiotherapy V67.1
      specified surgery NEC V67.09
      surgery V67.00
        vaginal pap smear V67.01
      treatment (for) V67.9
        combined V67.6
        fracture V67.4
        involving high-risk medication
          NEC V67.51
        mental disorder V67.3
        specified NEC V67.59
    hair transplant, for cosmetic reason
      V50.0
    health advice, education, or instruction
      V65.4
    hearing conservation and treatment
      V72.12
    hormone replacement therapy
      (postmenopausal) V07.4
    hospice care V66.7
    immunizations (childhood) appropriate
      for age V20.2
    immunotherapy, antineoplastic V58.12
    insertion (of)
      intrauterine contraceptive device
        V25.11
      subdermal implantable contraceptive
        V25.5
    insulin pump titration V53.91
    insulin pump training V65.46
    intrauterine device
      insertion V25.11
      management V25.42
      removal V25.12
        and reinsertion V25.13
      replacement V25.13
    investigation to determine further
      disposition V63.8
    in vitro fertilization cycle V26.81
    isolation V07.0
    issue of
      disability examination certificate
        V68.01
      medical certificate NEC V68.09
      repeat prescription NEC V68.1
        contraceptive device NEC V25.49
    kidney dialysis V56.0
    lengthening of growth rod V54.02
    mental health evaluation V70.2
      requested by authority V70.1
    natural family planning counseling and
      advice
      procreative V26.41
      to avoid pregnancy V25.04

SECTION 1 INDEX TO DISEASES AND INJURIES / Admission

Admission (Continued)
  for (Continued)
    nonmedical reason NEC V68.89
    nursing care evaluation V63.8
    observation (without need for further
        medical care) (see also Observation)
        V71.9
      accident V71.4
      alleged rape or seduction V71.5
      criminal assault V71.6
      following accident V71.4
        at work V71.3
      foreign body ingestion V71.89
      growth and development variations,
        childhood V21.0
      inflicted injury NEC V71.6
      ingestion of deleterious agent or
        foreign body V71.89
      injury V71.6
      malignant neoplasm V71.1
      mental disorder V71.09
      newborn - see Observation, suspected,
        condition, newborn
      rape V71.5
      specified NEC V71.89
        disorder V71.9
          abuse V71.81
          accident V71.4
            at work V71.3
          benign neoplasm V71.89
          cardiovascular V71.7
          exposure
            anthrax V71.82
            biological agent NEC
              V71.83
            SARS V71.83
          heart V71.7
          inflicted injury NEC V71.6
          malignant neoplasm V71.1
          mental NEC V71.09
          neglect V71.81
          specified condition NEC
            V71.89
          tuberculosis V71.2
      maternal and fetal problem not
        found
          amniotic cavity and membrane
            V89.01
          cervical shortening V89.05
          fetal anomaly V89.03
          fetal growth V89.04
          oligohydramnios V89.01
          other specified NEC V89.09
          placenta V89.02
          polyhydramnios V89.01
      tuberculosis V71.2
    occupational therapy V57.21
    organ transplant, donor - see Donor
    ovary, ovarian removal, prophylactic
      V50.42
    palliative care V66.7
    Papanicolaou smear
      cervix V76.2
        for suspected malignant neoplasm
          V76.2
        no disease found V71.1
        routine, as part of gynecological
          examination V72.31
        to confirm findings of recent
          normal smear following
            initial abnormal smear
            V72.32
      vaginal V76.47
        following hysterectomy for
          malignant condition V67.01
    passage of sounds or bougie in artificial
      opening - see Attention to, artificial,
      opening
    paternity testing V70.4
    peritoneal dialysis V56.32
    physical therapy NEC V57.1

Admission (Continued)
  for (Continued)
    plastic surgery
      breast reconstruction following
        mastectomy V51.0
      cosmetic NEC V50.1
      following healed injury or operation
        V51.8
    postmenopausal hormone replacement
      therapy V07.4
    postpartum observation
      immediately after delivery V24.0
      routine follow-up V24.2
    poststerilization (for restoration) V26.0
    procreative management V26.9
      assisted reproductive fertility
        procedure cycle V26.81
      in vitro fertilization cycle V26.81
      specified type NEC V26.89
    prophylactic
      administration of
        antibiotics, long-term V58.62
          short-term use - omit code
        antitoxin, any V07.2
        antivenin V07.2
        chemotherapeutic agent NEC
          V07.39
        chemotherapy NEC V07.39
        diphtheria antitoxin V07.2
        fluoride V07.31
        gamma globulin V07.2
        immune sera (gamma globulin)
          V07.2
        RhoGAM V07.2
        tetanus antitoxin V07.2
      breathing exercises V57.0
      chemotherapy NEC V07.39
        fluoride V07.31
      measure V07.9
        specified type NEC V07.8
      organ removal V50.49
        breast V50.41
        ovary V50.42
    psychiatric examination (general)
      V70.2
      requested by authority V70.1
    radiation management V58.0
    radiotherapy V58.0
    reconstruction following mastectomy
      V51.0
    reforming of artificial opening - see
      Attention to, artificial, opening
    rehabilitation V57.9
      multiple types V57.89
      occupational V57.21
      orthoptic V57.4
      orthotic V57.81
      physical NEC V57.1
      specified type NEC V57.89
      speech (-language) V57.3
      vocational V57.22
    removal of
      breast tissue expander without
        synchronous insertion of
        permanent implant V52.4
      cardiac pacemaker V53.31
      cast (plaster) V54.89
      catheter from artificial opening - see
        Attention to, artificial, opening
      cerebral ventricle (communicating)
        shunt V53.01
      cystostomy catheter V55.5
      device
        cerebral ventricle (communicating)
          shunt V53.01
        fixation
          external V54.89
          internal V54.01
        intrauterine contraceptive V25.12
        traction, external V54.89
      drains V58.49

Admission (Continued)
  for (Continued)
    removal of (Continued)
      dressing
        wound V58.30
          nonsurgical V58.30
          surgical V58.31
      fixation device
        external V54.89
        internal V54.01
      intrauterine contraceptive device
        V25.12
      Kirschner wire V54.89
      neuropacemaker (brain) (peripheral
        nerve) (spinal cord) V53.02
      nonsurgical wound dressing V58.30
      orthopedic fixation device
        external V54.89
        internal V54.01
      pacemaker device
        brain V53.02
        cardiac V53.31
        carotid sinus V53.39
        nervous system V53.02
      plaster cast V54.89
      plate (fracture) V54.01
      rod V54.01
      screw (fracture) V54.01
      splint, traction V54.89
      staples V58.32
      Steinmann pin V54.89
      subdermal implantable contraceptive
        V25.43
      surgical wound dressing V58.31
      sutures V58.32
      traction device, external V54.89
      ureteral stent V53.6
      wound packing V58.30
        nonsurgical V58.30
        surgical V58.31
    repair of scarred tissue (following healed
      injury or operation) V51.8
    replacement of intrauterine contraceptive
      device V25.13
    reprogramming of cardiac pacemaker
      V53.31
    respirator [ventilator] dependence
      during
        mechanical failure V46.14
        power failure V46.12
      for weaning V46.13
    restoration of organ continuity
      (poststerilization) (tuboplasty)
      (vasoplasty) V26.0
    Rh typing V72.86
    routine infant and child vision and
      hearing testing V20.2
    sensitivity test - see also Test, skin
      allergy NEC V72.7
      bacterial disease NEC V74.9
      Dick V74.8
      Kveim V82.89
      Mantoux V74.1
      mycotic infection NEC V75.4
      parasitic disease NEC V75.8
      Schick V74.3
      Schultz-Charlton V74.8
    social service (agency) referral or
      evaluation V63.8
    speech (-language) therapy V57.3
    sterilization V25.2
    suspected disorder (ruled out) (without
      need for further care) - see
      Observation
    terminal care V66.7
    tests only - see Test
    therapeutic drug monitoring V58.83
    therapy
      blood transfusion, without reported
        diagnosis V58.2
      breathing exercises V57.0

SECTION I INDEX TO DISEASES AND INJURIES / Admission

Admission (Continued)
  for (Continued)
    therapy (Continued)
      chemotherapy, antineoplastic V58.11
        prophylactic NEC V07.39
          fluoride V07.31
      dialysis (intermittent) (treatment)
        extracorporeal V56.0
        peritoneal V56.8
        renal V56.0
        specified type NEC V56.8
      exercise (remedial) NEC V57.1
        breathing V57.0
      immunotherapy, antineoplastic V58.12
      long-term (current) (prophylactic)
        drug use NEC V58.69
          antibiotics V58.62
            short-term use - *omit code*
          anticoagulants V58.61
          anti-inflammatories, non-steroidal (NSAID) V58.64
          antiplatelets V58.63
          antithrombotics V58.63
          aspirin V58.66
          bisphosphonates V58.68
          high-risk medications NEC V58.69
          insulin V58.67
          methadone for pain control V58.69
          opiate analgesic V58.69
          steroids V58.65
      occupational V57.21
      orthoptic V57.4
      physical NEC V57.1
      radiation V58.0
      speech (-language) V57.3
      vocational V57.22
    toilet or cleaning
      of artificial opening - *see* Attention to, artificial, opening
      of non-vascular catheter V58.82
      of vascular catheter V58.81
    treatment
      measure V07.9
        specified type NEC V07.8
    tubal ligation V25.2
    tuboplasty for previous sterilization V26.0
    ultrasound, routine fetal V28.3
    vaccination, prophylactic (against)
      arthropod-borne virus, viral NEC V05.1
        disease NEC V05.1
        encephalitis V05.0
      Bacille Calmette Guérin (BCG) V03.2
      BCG V03.2
      chickenpox V05.4
      cholera alone V03.0
        with typhoid-paratyphoid (cholera + TAB) V06.0
      common cold V04.7
      dengue V05.1
      diphtheria alone V03.5
      diphtheria-tetanus-pertussis (DTP) (DTaP) V06.1
        with
          poliomyelitis (DTP polio) V06.3
          typhoid-paratyphoid (DTP + TAB) V06.2
      diphtheria-tetanus [Td] [DT] without pertussis V06.5
      disease (single) NEC V05.9
        bacterial NEC V03.9
          specified type NEC V03.89
        combinations NEC V06.9
          specified type NEC V06.8
        specified type NEC V05.8
        viral NEC V04.89
      encephalitis, viral, arthropod-borne V05.0
      Hemophilus influenzae, type B [Hib] V03.81
      hepatitis, viral V05.3

Admission (Continued)
  for (Continued)
    vaccination, prophylactic (Continued)
      human papillomavirus (HPV) V04.89
      immune sera (gamma globulin) V07.2
      influenza V04.81
        with
          Streptococcus pneumoniae [pneumococcus] V06.6
      Leishmaniasis V05.2
      measles alone V04.2
      measles-mumps-rubella (MMR) V06.4
      mumps alone V04.6
        with measles and rubella (MMR) V06.4
      not done because of contraindication V64.09
      pertussis alone V03.6
      plague V03.3
      pneumonia V03.82
      poliomyelitis V04.0
        with diphtheria-tetanus-pertussis (DTP polio) V06.3
      rabies V04.5
      respiratory syncytial virus (RSV) V04.82
      rubella alone V04.3
        with measles and mumps (MMR) V06.4
      smallpox V04.1
      specified type NEC V05.8
      Streptococcus pneumoniae [pneumococcus] V03.82
        with
          influenza V06.6
      tetanus toxoid alone V03.7
        with diphtheria [Td] [DT] V06.5
        and pertussis (DTP) (DTaP) V06.1
      tuberculosis (BCG) V03.2
      tularemia V03.4
      typhoid alone V03.1
        with diphtheria-tetanus-pertussis (TAB + DTP) V06.2
      typhoid-paratyphoid alone (TAB) V03.1
      typhus V05.8
      varicella (chicken pox) V05.4
      viral encephalitis, arthropod-borne V05.0
      viral hepatitis V05.3
      yellow fever V04.4
    vasectomy V25.2
    vasoplasty for previous sterilization V26.0
    vision examination V72.0
    vocational therapy V57.22
    waiting period for admission to other facility V63.2
      undergoing social agency investigation V63.8
    well baby and child care V20.2
    x-ray of chest
      for suspected tuberculosis V71.2
      routine V72.5

Adnexitis (suppurative) (*see also* Salpingo-oophoritis) 614.2
Adolescence NEC V21.2
Adoption
  agency referral V68.89
  examination V70.3
  held for V68.89
Adrenal gland - *see* condition
Adrenalism 255.9
  tuberculous (*see also* Tuberculosis) 017.6●
Adrenalitis, adrenitis 255.8
  meningococcal hemorrhagic 036.3
Adrenarche, precocious 259.1
Adrenocortical syndrome 255.2
Adrenogenital syndrome (acquired) (congenital) 255.2
  iatrogenic, fetus or newborn 760.79

Adrenoleukodystrophy 277.86
  neonatal 277.86
  x-linked 277.86
Adrenomyeloneuropathy 277.86
Adventitious bursa - *see* Bursitis
Adynamia (episodica) (hereditary) (periodic) 359.3
Adynamic
  ileus or intestine (*see also* Ileus) 560.1
  ureter 753.22
Aeration lung, imperfect, newborn 770.5
Aerobullosis 993.3
Aerocele - *see* Embolism, air
Aerodermectasia
  subcutaneous (traumatic) 958.7
    surgical 998.81
  surgical 998.81
Aerodontalgia 993.2
Aeroembolism 993.3
Aerogenes capsulatus infection (*see also* Gangrene, gas) 040.0
Aero-otitis media 993.0
Aerophagy, aerophagia 306.4
  psychogenic 306.4
Aerosinusitis 993.1
Aerotitis 993.0
Affection, affections - *see also* Disease
  sacroiliac (joint), old 724.6
  shoulder region NEC 726.2
Afibrinogenemia 286.3
  acquired 286.6
  congenital 286.3
  postpartum 666.3●
African
  sleeping sickness 086.5
  tick fever 087.1
  trypanosomiasis 086.5
    Gambian 086.3
    Rhodesian 086.4
Aftercare V58.9
  amputation stump V54.89
  artificial openings - *see* Attention to, artificial, opening
  blood transfusion without reported diagnosis V58.2
  breathing exercise V57.0
  cardiac device V53.39
    defibrillator, automatic implantable (with synchronous cardiac pacemaker) V53.32
    pacemaker V53.31
      carotid sinus V53.39
  carotid sinus pacemaker V53.39
  cerebral ventricle (communicating) shunt V53.01
  chemotherapy (oral) (intravenous) session (adjunctive) (maintenance) V58.11
  defibrillator, automatic implantable cardiac (with synchronous cardiac pacemaker) V53.32
  exercise (remedial) (therapeutic) V57.1
    breathing V57.0
  extracorporeal dialysis (intermittent) (treatment) V56.0
  following surgery NEC V58.49
    for
      injury V58.43
      neoplasm V58.42
      organ transplant V58.44
      trauma V58.43
    joint
      explantation of prosthesis (staged procedure) V54.82
      replacement V54.81
    of
      circulatory system V58.73
      digestive system V58.75
      genital organs V58.76
      genitourinary system V58.76
      musculoskeletal system V58.78
      nervous system V58.72

SECTION I INDEX TO DISEASES AND INJURIES / Agenesis

Aftercare *(Continued)*
- following surgery NEC *(Continued)*
  - of *(Continued)*
    - oral cavity V58.75
    - respiratory system V58.74
    - sense organs V58.71
    - skin V58.77
    - subcutaneous tissue V58.77
    - teeth V58.75
    - urinary system V58.76
  - spinal - *see* Aftercare, following surgery, of, specified body system
  - wound closure, planned V58.41
- fracture V54.9
  - healing V54.89
    - pathologic
      - ankle V54.29
      - arm V54.20
        - lower V54.22
        - upper V54.21
      - finger V54.29
      - foot V54.29
      - hand V54.29
      - hip V54.23
      - leg V54.24
        - lower V54.26
        - upper V54.25
      - pelvis V54.29
      - specified site NEC V54.29
      - toe(s) V54.29
      - vertebrae V54.27
      - wrist V54.29
    - traumatic
      - ankle V54.19
      - arm V54.10
        - lower V54.12
        - upper V54.11
      - finger V54.19
      - foot V54.19
      - hand V54.19
      - hip V54.13
      - leg V54.14
        - lower V54.16
        - upper V54.15
      - pelvis V54.19
      - specified site NEC V54.19
      - toe(s) V54.19
      - vertebrae V54.17
      - wrist V54.19
  - removal of
    - external fixation device V54.89
    - internal fixation device V54.01
  - specified care NEC V54.89
- gait training V57.1
  - for use of artificial limb(s) V57.81
- internal fixation device V54.09
- involving
  - dialysis (intermittent) (treatment)
    - extracorporeal V56.0
    - peritoneal V56.8
    - renal V56.0
  - gait training V57.1
    - for use of artificial limb(s) V57.81
  - growth rod
    - adjustment V54.02
    - lengthening V54.02
  - internal fixation device V54.09
  - orthoptic training V57.4
  - orthotic training V57.81
  - radiotherapy session V58.0
  - removal of
    - drains V58.49
    - dressings
      - wound V58.30
        - nonsurgical V58.30
        - surgical V58.31
    - fixation device
      - external V54.89
      - internal V54.01
    - fracture plate V54.01
    - nonsurgical wound dressing V58.30

Aftercare *(Continued)*
- involving *(Continued)*
  - removal of *(Continued)*
    - pins V54.01
    - plaster cast V54.89
    - rods V54.01
    - screws V54.01
    - staples V58.32
    - surgical wound dressings V58.31
    - sutures V58.32
    - traction device, external V54.89
    - wound packing V58.30
      - nonsurgical V58.30
      - surgical V58.31
  - neuropacemaker (brain) (peripheral nerve) (spinal cord) V53.02
  - occupational therapy V57.21
  - orthodontic V58.5
  - orthopedic V54.9
    - change of external fixation or traction device V54.89
    - following joint
      - explantation of prosthesis (staged procedure) V54.82
      - replacement V54.81
    - internal fixation device V54.09
    - removal of fixation device
      - external V54.89
      - internal V54.01
    - specified care NEC V54.89
  - orthoptic training V57.4
  - orthotic training V57.81
  - pacemaker
    - brain V53.02
    - cardiac V53.31
    - carotid sinus V53.39
    - peripheral nerve V53.02
    - spinal cord V53.02
  - peritoneal dialysis (intermittent) (treatment) V56.8
  - physical therapy NEC V57.1
    - breathing exercises V57.0
  - radiotherapy session V58.0
  - rehabilitation procedure V57.9
    - breathing exercises V57.0
    - multiple types V57.89
    - occupational V57.21
    - orthoptic V57.4
    - orthotic V57.81
    - physical therapy NEC V57.1
    - remedial exercises V57.1
    - specified type NEC V57.89
    - speech (-language) V57.3
    - therapeutic exercises V57.1
    - vocational V57.22
  - renal dialysis (intermittent) (treatment) V56.0
  - specified type NEC V58.89
    - removal of non-vascular cathether V58.82
    - removal of vascular catheter V58.81
  - speech (-language) therapy V57.3
  - stump, amputation V54.89
  - vocational rehabilitation V57.22
After-cataract 366.50
- obscuring vision 366.53
- specified type, not obscuring vision 366.52
Agalactia 676.4●
Agammaglobulinemia 279.00
- with lymphopenia 279.2
- acquired (primary) (secondary) 279.06
- Bruton's X-linked 279.04
- infantile sex-linked (Bruton's) (congenital) 279.04
- Swiss-type 279.2
Aganglionosis (bowel) (colon) 751.3
Age (old) *(see also* Senile) 797
Agenesis - *see also* Absence, by site, congenital
- acoustic nerve 742.8
- adrenal (gland) 759.1

Agenesis *(Continued)*
- alimentary tract (complete) (partial) NEC 751.8
  - lower 751.2
  - upper 750.8
- anus, anal (canal) 751.2
- aorta 747.22
- appendix 751.2
- arm (complete) (partial) (*see also* Deformity, reduction, upper limb) 755.20
- artery (peripheral) NEC (*see also* Anomaly, peripheral vascular system) 747.60
  - brain 747.81
  - coronary 746.85
  - pulmonary 747.31
  - umbilical 747.5
- auditory (canal) (external) 744.01
- auricle (ear) 744.01
- bile, biliary duct or passage 751.61
- bone NEC 756.9
- brain 740.0
  - specified part 742.2
- breast 757.6
- bronchus 748.3
- canaliculus lacrimalis 743.65
- carpus NEC (*see also* Deformity, reduction, upper limb) 755.28
- cartilage 756.9
- cecum 751.2
- cerebellum 742.2
- cervix 752.43
- chin 744.89
- cilia 743.63
- circulatory system, part NEC 747.89
- clavicle 755.51
- clitoris 752.49
- coccyx 756.13
- colon 751.2
- corpus callosum 742.2
- cricoid cartilage 748.3
- diaphragm (with hernia) 756.6
- digestive organ(s) or tract (complete) (partial) NEC 751.8
  - lower 751.2
  - upper 750.8
- ductus arteriosus 747.89
- duodenum 751.1
- ear NEC 744.09
  - auricle 744.01
  - lobe 744.21
- ejaculatory duct 752.89
- endocrine (gland) NEC 759.2
- epiglottis 748.3
- esophagus 750.3
- Eustachian tube 744.24
- extrinsic muscle, eye 743.69
- eye 743.00
  - adnexa 743.69
- eyelid (fold) 743.62
- face
  - bones NEC 756.0
  - specified part NEC 744.89
- fallopian tube 752.19
- femur NEC (*see also* Absence, femur, congenital) 755.34
- fibula NEC (*see also* Absence, fibula, congenital) 755.37
- finger NEC (*see also* Absence, finger, congenital) 755.29
- foot (complete) (*see also* Deformity, reduction, lower limb) 755.31
- gallbladder 751.69
- gastric 750.8
- genitalia, genital (organ)
  - female 752.89
    - external 752.49
    - internal NEC 752.89
  - male 752.89
    - penis 752.69
- glottis 748.3
- gonadal 758.6

◀ New ◀ Revised ~~deleted~~ Deleted ● Use Additional Digit(s) Omit code

73

SECTION 1 INDEX TO DISEASES AND INJURIES / Agenesis

Agenesis (Continued)
  hair 757.4
  hand (complete) (see also Deformity,
      reduction, upper limb) 755.21
  heart 746.89
    valve NEC 746.89
      aortic 746.89
      mitral 746.89
      pulmonary 746.01
  hepatic 751.69
  humerus NEC (see also Absence, humerus,
      congenital) 755.24
  hymen 752.49
  ileum 751.1
  incus 744.04
  intestine (small) 751.1
    large 751.2
  iris (dilator fibers) 743.45
  jaw 524.09
  jejunum 751.1
  kidney(s) (partial) (unilateral) 753.0
  labium (majus) (minus) 752.49
  labyrinth, membranous 744.05
  lacrimal apparatus (congenital) 743.65
  larynx 748.3
  leg NEC (see also Deformity, reduction, lower
      limb) 755.30
  lens 743.35
  limb (complete) (partial) (see also Deformity,
      reduction) 755.4
    lower NEC 755.30
    upper 755.20
  lip 750.26
  liver 751.69
  lung (bilateral) (fissures) (lobe) (unilateral)
      748.5
  mandible 524.09
  maxilla 524.09
  metacarpus NEC 755.28
  metatarsus NEC 755.38
  muscle (any) 756.81
  musculoskeletal system NEC 756.9
  nail(s) 757.5
  neck, part 744.89
  nerve 742.8
  nervous system, part NEC 742.8
  nipple 757.6
  nose 748.1
  nuclear 742.8
  organ
    of Corti 744.05
    or site not listed - see Anomaly, specified
      type NEC
  osseous meatus (ear) 744.03
  ovary 752.0
  oviduct 752.19
  pancreas 751.7
  parathyroid (gland) 759.2
  patella 755.64
  pelvic girdle (complete) (partial) 755.69
  penis 752.69
  pericardium 746.89
  perineal body 756.81
  pituitary (gland) 759.2
  prostate 752.89
  pulmonary
    artery 747.31
    trunk 747.31
    vein 747.49
  punctum lacrimale 743.65
  radioulnar NEC (see also Absence, forearm,
      congenital) 755.25
  radius NEC (see also Absence, radius,
      congenital) 755.26
  rectum 751.2
  renal 753.0
  respiratory organ NEC 748.9
  rib 756.3
  roof of orbit 742.0
  round ligament 752.89
  sacrum 756.13

Agenesis (Continued)
  salivary gland 750.21
  scapula 755.59
  scrotum 752.89
  seminal duct or tract 752.89
  septum
    atrial 745.69
    between aorta and pulmonary artery 745.0
    ventricular 745.3
  shoulder girdle (complete) (partial) 755.59
  skull (bone) 756.0
    with
      anencephalus 740.0
      encephalocele 742.0
      hydrocephalus 742.3
        with spina bifida (see also Spina
          bifida) 741.0●
      microcephalus 742.1
  spermatic cord 752.89
  spinal cord 742.59
  spine 756.13
    lumbar 756.13
      isthmus 756.11
      pars articularis 756.11
  spleen 759.0
  sternum 756.3
  stomach 750.7
  tarsus NEC 755.38
  tendon 756.81
  testicular 752.89
  testis 752.89
  thymus (gland) 759.2
  thyroid (gland) 243
    cartilage 748.3
  tibia NEC (see also Absence, tibia, congenital)
      755.36
  tibiofibular NEC 755.35
  toe (complete) (partial) (see also Absence, toe,
      congenital) 755.39
  tongue 750.11
  trachea (cartilage) 748.3
  ulna NEC (see also Absence, ulna, congenital)
      755.27
  ureter 753.4
  urethra 753.8
  urinary tract NEC 753.8
  uterus 752.31
  uvula 750.26
  vagina (total) (partial) 752.45
  vas deferens 752.89
  vein(s) (peripheral) NEC (see also Anomaly,
      peripheral vascular system) 747.60
    brain 747.81
    great 747.49
    portal 747.49
    pulmonary 747.49
    vena cava (inferior) (superior) 747.49
  vermis of cerebellum 742.2
  vertebra 756.13
    lumbar 756.13
      isthmus 756.11
      pars articularis 756.11
  vulva 752.49
Ageusia (see also Disturbance, sensation) 781.1
Aggressiveness 301.3
Aggressive outburst (see also Disturbance,
      conduct) 312.0●
  in children or adolescents 313.9
Aging skin 701.8
Agitated - see condition
Agitation 307.9
  catatonic (see also Schizophrenia) 295.2●
Aglossia (congenital) 750.11
Aglycogenosis 271.0
Agnail (finger) (with lymphangitis) 681.02
Agnosia (body image) (tactile) 784.69
  verbal 784.69
    auditory 784.69
      secondary to organic lesion 784.69
    developmental 315.8
    secondary to organic lesion 784.69

Agnosia (Continued)
  visual 368.16
    object 368.16
Agoraphobia 300.22
  with panic disorder 300.21
Agrammatism 784.69
Agranulocytopenia (see also Agranulocytosis)
    288.09
Agranulocytosis (see also Neutropenia) 288.09
  chronic 288.09
  cyclical 288.02
  due to infection 288.04
  genetic 288.01
  infantile 288.01
  periodic 288.02
  pernicious 288.09
Agraphia (absolute) 784.69
  with alexia 784.61
  developmental 315.39
Agrypnia (see also Insomnia) 780.52
Ague (see also Malaria) 084.6
  brass-founders' 985.8
  dumb 084.6
  tertian 084.1
Agyria 742.2
AHTR (acute hemolytic transfusion reaction) -
    see Complications, transfusion
Ahumada-del Castillo syndrome
    (nonpuerperal galactorrhea and
    amenorrhea) 253.1
AIDS 042
AIDS-associated retrovirus (disease) (illness)
    042
  infection - see Human immunodeficiency
    virus, infection
AIDS-associated virus (disease) (illness) 042
  infection - see Human immunodeficiency
    virus, infection
AIDS-like disease (illness) (syndrome) 042
AIDS-related complex 042
AIDS-related conditions 042
AIDS-related virus (disease) (illness) 042
  infection - see Human immunodeficiency
    virus, infection
AIDS virus (disease) (illness) 042
  infection - see Human immunodeficiency
    virus, infection
Ailment, heart - see Disease, heart
Ailurophobia 300.29
AIN I (anal intraepithelial neoplasia I)
    (histologically confirmed) 569.44
AIN II (anal intraepithelial neoplasia II)
    (histologically confirmed) 569.44
AIN III (anal intraepithelial neoplasia III) 230.6
  anal canal 230.5
Ainhum (disease) 136.0
AIPHI (acute idiopathic pulmonary hemorrhage
    in infants (over 28 days old)) 786.31
Air
  anterior mediastinum 518.1
  compressed, disease 993.3
  embolism (any site) (artery) (cerebral) 958.0
    with
      abortion - see Abortion, by type, with
        embolism
      ectopic pregnancy (see also categories
        633.0-633.9) 639.6
      molar pregnancy (see also categories
        630-632) 639.6
    due to implanted device - see
      Complications, due to (presence of)
      any device, implant, or graft
      classified to 996.0-996.5 NEC
    following
      abortion 639.6
      ectopic or molar pregnancy 639.6
      infusion, perfusion, or transfusion
        999.1
    in pregnancy, childbirth, or puerperium
      673.0●
    traumatic 958.0

SECTION I INDEX TO DISEASES AND INJURIES / Allergy, allergic

Air *(Continued)*
  hunger 786.09
    psychogenic 306.1
  leak (lung) (pulmonary) (thorax) 512.84
    iatrogenic 512.1
    persistent 512.84
    postoperative 512.2
  rarefied, effects of - *see* Effect, adverse, high altitude
  sickness 994.6
Airplane sickness 994.6
Akathisia, acathisia 781.0
  due to drugs 333.99
  neuroleptic-induced acute 333.99
Akinesia algera 352.6
Akiyami 100.89
Akureyri disease (epidemic neuromyasthenia) 049.8
Alacrima (congenital) 743.65
Alactasia (hereditary) 271.3
Alagille syndrome 759.89
Alalia 784.3
  developmental 315.31
    receptive-expressive 315.32
  secondary to organic lesion 784.3
Alaninemia 270.8
Alastrim 050.1
Albarrán's disease (colibacilluria) 791.9
Albers-Schönberg's disease (marble bones) 756.52
Albert's disease 726.71
Albinism, albino (choroid) (cutaneous) (eye) (generalized) (isolated) (ocular) (oculocutaneous) (partial) 270.2
Albinismus 270.2
Albright (-Martin) (-Bantam) disease (pseudohypoparathyroidism) 275.49
Albright (-McCune) (-Sternberg) syndrome (osteitis fibrosa disseminata) 756.59
Albuminous - *see* Condition
Albuminuria, albuminuric (acute) (chronic) (subacute) 791.0
  Bence-Jones 791.0
  cardiac 785.9
  complicating pregnancy, childbirth, or puerperium 646.2●
    with hypertension - *see* Toxemia, of pregnancy
    affecting fetus or newborn 760.1
  cyclic 593.6
  gestational 646.2●
  gravidarum 646.2●
    with hypertension - *see* Toxemia, of pregnancy
    affecting fetus or newborn 760.1
  heart 785.9
  idiopathic 593.6
  orthostatic 593.6
  postural 593.6
  pre-eclamptic (mild) 642.4●
    affecting fetus or newborn 760.0
    severe 642.5●
      affecting fetus or newborn 760.0
  recurrent physiologic 593.6
  scarlatinal 034.1
Albumosuria 791.0
  Bence-Jones 791.0
  myelopathic (M9730/3) 203.0●
Alcaptonuria 270.2
Alcohol, alcoholic
  abstinence 291.81
  acute intoxication 305.0●
    with dependence 303.0●
  addiction (*see also* Alcoholism) 303.9●
    maternal
      with suspected fetal damage affecting management of pregnancy 655.4●
      affecting fetus or newborn 760.71
  amnestic disorder, persisting 291.1
  anxiety 291.89

Alcohol, alcoholic *(Continued)*
  brain syndrome, chronic 291.2
  cardiopathy 425.5
  chronic (*see also* Alcoholism) 303.9●
  cirrhosis (liver) 571.2
  delirium 291.0
    acute 291.0
    chronic 291.1
    tremens 291.0
    withdrawal 291.0
  dementia NEC 291.2
  deterioration 291.2
  drunkenness (simple) 305.0●
  hallucinosis (acute) 291.3
  induced
    circadian rhythm sleep disorder 291.82
    hypersomnia 291.82
    insomnia 291.82
    mental disorder 291.9
      anxiety 291.89
      mood 291.89
      sexual 291.89
      sleep 291.82
      specified type 291.89
    parasomnia 291.82
    persisting
      amnestic disorder 291.1
      dementia 291.2
    psychotic disorder
      with
        delusions 291.5
        hallucinations 291.3
    sleep disorder 291.82
  insanity 291.9
  intoxication (acute) 305.0●
    with dependence 303.0●
    pathological 291.4
  jealousy 291.5
  Korsakoff's, Korsakov's, Korsakow's 291.1
  liver NEC 571.3
    acute 571.1
    chronic 571.2
  mania (acute) (chronic) 291.9
  mood 291.89
  paranoia 291.5
  paranoid (type) psychosis 291.5
  pellagra 265.2
  poisoning, accidental (acute) NEC 980.9
    specified type of alcohol - *see* Table of Drugs and Chemicals
  psychosis (*see also* Psychosis, alcoholic) 291.9
    Korsakoff's, Korsakov's, Korsakow's 291.1
    polyneuritic 291.1
    with
      delusions 291.5
      hallucinations 291.3
  related disorder 291.9
  withdrawal symptoms, syndrome NEC 291.81
    delirium 291.0
    hallucinosis 291.3
Alcoholism 303.9●

Note: Use the following fifth-digit subclassification with category 303:
  0 unspecified
  1 continuous
  2 episodic
  3 in remission

  with psychosis (*see also* Psychosis, alcoholic) 291.9
  acute 303.0●
  chronic 303.9●
    with psychosis 291.9
  complicating pregnancy, childbirth, or puerperium 648.4●
    affecting fetus or newborn 760.71
  history V11.3
  Korsakoff's, Korsakov's, Korsakow's 291.1

Alcoholism *(Continued)*
  suspected damage to fetus affecting management of pregnancy 655.4●
Alder's anomaly or syndrome (leukocyte granulation anomaly) 288.2
Alder-Reilly anomaly (leukocyte granulation) 288.2
Aldosteronism (primary) 255.10
  congenital 255.10
  familial type I 255.11
  glucocorticoid-remediable 255.11
  secondary 255.14
Aldosteronoma (M8370/1) 237.2
Aldrich (-Wiskott) syndrome (eczema-thrombocytopenia) 279.12
Aleppo boil 085.1
Aleukemic - *see* condition
Aleukia
  congenital 288.09
  hemorrhagica 284.9
    acquired (secondary) 284.89
    congenital 284.09
    idiopathic 284.9
  splenica 289.4
Alexia (congenital) (developmental) 315.01
  secondary to organic lesion 784.61
Algoneurodystrophy 733.7
Algophobia 300.29
Alibert's disease (mycosis fungoides) (M9700/3) 202.1●
Alibert-Bazin disease (M9700/3) 202.1●
Alice in Wonderland syndrome 293.89
Alienation, mental (*see also* Psychosis) 298.9
Alkalemia 276.3
Alkalosis 276.3
  metabolic 276.3
    with respiratory acidosis 276.4
  respiratory 276.3
Alkaptonuria 270.2
Allen-Masters syndrome 620.6
Allergic bronchopulmonary aspergillosis 518.6
Allergy, allergic (reaction) 995.3
  air-borne substance (*see also* Fever, hay) 477.9
    specified allergen NEC 477.8
  alveolitis (extrinsic) 495.9
    due to
      Aspergillus clavatus 495.4
      cryptostroma corticale 495.6
      organisms (fungal, thermophilic actinomycete, other) growing in ventilation (air conditioning systems) 495.7
    specified type NEC 495.8
  anaphylactic reaction or shock 995.0
    due to food - *see* Anaphylactic reaction or shock, due to, food
  angioedema 995.1
  angioneurotic edema 995.1
  animal (cat) (dog) (epidermal) 477.8
    dander 477.2
    hair 477.2
  arthritis (*see also* Arthritis, allergic) 716.2●
  asthma - *see* Asthma
  bee sting (anaphylactic shock) 989.5
  biological - *see* Allergy, drug
  bronchial asthma - *see* Asthma
  conjunctivitis (eczematous) 372.14
  dander, animal (cat) (dog) 477.2
  dandruff 477.8
  dermatitis (venenata) - *see* Dermatitis
  diathesis V15.09
  drug, medicinal substance, and biological (any) (correct medicinal substance properly administered) (external) (internal) 995.27
    wrong substance given or taken NEC 977.9
      specified drug or substance - *see* Table of Drugs and Chemicals
  dust (house) (stock) 477.8
  eczema - *see* Eczema

◀ New   ⬅ Revised   ~~deleted~~ Deleted   ● Use Additional Digit(s)   Omit code   75

Allergy, allergic *(Continued)*
- endophthalmitis 360.19
- epidermal (animal) 477.8
- existing dental restorative material 525.66
- feathers 477.8
- food (any) (ingested) 693.1
  - atopic 691.8
  - in contact with skin 692.5
- gastritis 535.4
- gastroenteritis 558.3
- gastrointestinal 558.3
- grain 477.0
- grass (pollen) 477.0
  - asthma (see also Asthma) 493.0
  - hay fever 477.0
- hair, animal (cat) (dog) 477.2
- hay fever (grass) (pollen) (ragweed) (tree) (see also Fever, hay) 477.9
- history (of) V15.09
  - to
    - arachnid bite V15.06
    - eggs V15.03
    - food additives V15.05
    - insect bite V15.06
    - latex V15.07
    - milk products V15.02
    - nuts V15.05
      - peanuts V15.01
    - radiographic dye V15.08
    - seafood V15.04
    - specified food NEC V15.05
    - spider bite V15.06
- horse serum - see Allergy, serum
- inhalant 477.9
  - dust 477.8
  - pollen 477.0
  - specified allergen other than pollen 477.8
- kapok 477.8
- medicine - see Allergy, drug
- migraine 339.00
- milk protein 558.3
- pannus 370.62
- pneumonia 518.3
- pollen (any) (hay fever) 477.0
  - asthma (see also Asthma) 493.0
- primrose 477.0
- primula 477.0
- purpura 287.0
- ragweed (pollen) (Senecio jacobae) 477.0
  - asthma (see also Asthma) 493.0
  - hay fever 477.0
- respiratory (see also Allergy, inhalant) 477.9
  - due to
    - drug - see Allergy, drug
    - food - see Allergy, food
- rhinitis (see also Fever, hay) 477.9
  - due to food 477.1
- rose 477.0
- Senecio jacobae 477.0
- serum (prophylactic) (therapeutic) 999.59
  - anaphylactic reaction or shock 999.49
- shock (anaphylactic) (due to adverse effect of correct medicinal substance properly administered) 995.0
  - food - see Anaphylactic reaction or shock, due to, food
  - from
    - administration of blood and blood products 999.41
    - immunization 999.42
    - serum NEC 999.49
- sinusitis (see also Fever, hay) 477.9
- skin reaction 692.9
  - specified substance - see Dermatitis, due to
- tree (any) (hay fever) (pollen) 477.0
  - asthma (see also Asthma) 493.0
- upper respiratory (see also Fever, hay) 477.9
- urethritis 597.89
- urticaria 708.0
- vaccine - see Allergy, serum

Allescheriosis 117.6
Alligator skin disease (ichthyosis congenita) 757.1
- acquired 701.1

Allocheiria, allochiria (see also Disturbance, sensation) 782.0
Almeida's disease (Brazilian blastomycosis) 116.1
Alopecia (atrophicans) (pregnancy) (premature) (senile) 704.00
- adnata 757.4
- areata 704.01
- celsi 704.01
- cicatrisata 704.09
- circumscripta 704.01
- congenital, congenitalis 757.4
- disseminata 704.01
- effluvium (telogen) 704.02
- febrile 704.09
- generalisata 704.09
- hereditaria 704.09
- marginalis 704.01
- mucinosa 704.09
- postinfectional 704.09
- seborrheica 704.09
- specific 091.82
- syphilitic (secondary) 091.82
- telogen effluvium 704.02
- totalis 704.09
- toxica 704.09
- universalis 704.09
- x-ray 704.09

Alpers' disease 330.8
Alpha-lipoproteinemia 272.4
Alpha thalassemia 282.43
Alphos 696.1
Alpine sickness 993.2
Alport's syndrome (hereditary hematuria-nephropathy-deafness) 759.89
ALPS (autoimmune lymphoproliferative syndrome) 279.41
ALTE (apparent life threatening event) in newborn and infant 799.82
Alteration (of), altered
- awareness 780.09
  - transient 780.02
- consciousness 780.09
  - persistent vegetative state 780.03
  - transient 780.02
- mental status 780.97
  - amnesia (retrograde) 780.93
  - memory loss 780.93

Alternaria (infection) 118
Alternating - see condition
Altitude, high (effects) - see Effect, adverse, high altitude
Aluminosis (of lung) 503
Alvarez syndrome (transient cerebral ischemia) 435.9
Alveolar capillary block syndrome 516.64
Alveolitis
- allergic (extrinsic) 495.9
  - due to organisms (fungal, thermophilic actinomycete, other) growing in ventilation (air conditioning systems) 495.7
  - specified type NEC 495.8
- due to
  - Aspergillus clavatus 495.4
  - Cryptostroma corticale 495.6
- fibrosing (chronic) (cryptogenic) (lung) 516.31
  - idiopathic 516.30
  - rheumatoid 714.81
- jaw 526.5
- sicca dolorosa 526.5

Alveolus, alveolar - see condition
Alymphocytosis (pure) 279.2
Alymphoplasia, thymic 279.2

Alzheimer's
- dementia (senile)
  - with behavioral disturbance 331.0 [294.11]
  - without behavioral disturbance 331.0 [294.10]
- disease or sclerosis 331.0
  - with dementia - see Alzheimer's, dementia

Amastia (see also Absence, breast) 611.89
Amaurosis (acquired) (congenital) (see also Blindness) 369.00
- fugax 362.34
- hysterical 300.11
- Leber's (congenital) 362.76
- tobacco 377.34
- uremic - see Uremia

Amaurotic familial idiocy (infantile) (juvenile) (late) 330.1
Ambisexual 752.7
Amblyopia (acquired) (congenital) (partial) 368.00
- color 368.59
  - acquired 368.55
- deprivation 368.02
- ex anopsia 368.00
- hysterical 300.11
- nocturnal 368.60
  - vitamin A deficiency 264.5
- refractive 368.03
- strabismic 368.01
- suppression 368.01
- tobacco 377.34
- toxic NEC 377.34
- uremic - see Uremia

Ameba, amebic (histolytica) - see also Amebiasis
- abscess 006.3
  - bladder 006.8
  - brain (with liver and lung abscess) 006.5
  - liver 006.3
    - with
      - brain abscess (and lung abscess) 006.5
      - lung abscess 006.4
  - lung (with liver abscess) 006.4
    - with brain abscess 006.5
  - seminal vesicle 006.8
  - spleen 006.8
- carrier (suspected of) V02.2
- meningoencephalitis
  - due to Naegleria (gruberi) 136.29
  - primary 136.29

Amebiasis NEC 006.9
- with
  - brain abscess (with liver or lung abscess) 006.5
  - liver abscess (without mention of brain or lung abscess) 006.3
  - lung abscess (with liver abscess) 006.4
    - with brain abscess 006.5
- acute 006.0
- bladder 006.8
- chronic 006.1
- cutaneous 006.6
- cutis 006.6
- due to organism other than Entamoeba histolytica 007.8
- hepatic (see also Abscess, liver, amebic) 006.3
- nondysenteric 006.2
- seminal vesicle 006.8
- specified
  - organism NEC 007.8
  - site NEC 006.8

Ameboma 006.8
Amelia 755.4
- lower limb 755.31
- upper limb 755.21

SECTION I INDEX TO DISEASES AND INJURIES / Anarthritic rheumatoid disease

Ameloblastoma (M9310/0) 213.1
    jaw (bone) (lower) 213.1
        upper 213.0
    long bones (M9261/3) - see Neoplasm, bone, malignant
    malignant (M9310/3) 170.1
        jaw (bone) (lower) 170.1
            upper 170.0
    mandible 213.1
    tibial (M9261/3) 170.7
Amelogenesis imperfecta 520.5
    nonhereditaria (segmentalis) 520.4
Amenorrhea (primary) (secondary) 626.0
    due to ovarian dysfunction 256.8
    hyperhormonal 256.8
Amentia (see also Disability, intellectual) 319
    Meynert's (nonalcoholic) 294.0
        alcoholic 291.1
    nevoid 759.6
American
    leishmaniasis 085.5
    mountain tick fever 066.1
    trypanosomiasis - see Trypanosomiasis, American
Ametropia (see also Disorder, accommodation) 367.9
Amianthosis 501
Amimia 784.69
Amino acid
    deficiency 270.9
        anemia 281.4
    metabolic disorder (see also Disorder, amino acid) 270.9
Aminoaciduria 270.9
    imidazole 270.5
Amnesia (retrograde) 780.93
    auditory 784.69
        developmental 315.31
        secondary to organic lesion 784.69
    dissociative 300.12
    hysterical or dissociative type 300.12
    psychogenic 300.12
    transient global 437.7
Amnestic (confabulatory) syndrome 294.0
    alcohol-induced persisting 291.1
    drug-induced persisting 292.83
    posttraumatic 294.0
Amniocentesis screening (for) V28.2
    alphafetoprotein level, raised V28.1
    chromosomal anomalies V28.0
Amnion, amniotic - see also condition
    nodosum 658.8 ●
Amnionitis (complicating pregnancy) 658.4 ●
    affecting fetus or newborn 762.7
Amoral trends 301.7
Amotio retinae (see also Detachment, retina) 361.9
Ampulla
    lower esophagus 530.89
    phrenic 530.89
Amputation
    any part of fetus, to facilitate delivery 763.89
    cervix (supravaginal) (uteri) 622.8
        in pregnancy or childbirth 654.6 ●
            affecting fetus or newborn 763.89
    clitoris - see Wound, open, clitoris
    congenital
        lower limb 755.31
        upper limb 755.21
    neuroma (traumatic) - see also Injury, nerve, by site
    surgical complication (late) 997.61
    penis - see Amputation, traumatic, penis
    status (without complication) - see Absence, by site, acquired
    stump (surgical) (posttraumatic)
        abnormal, painful, or with complication (late) 997.60
        healed or old NEC - see also Absence, by site, acquired
            lower V49.70
            upper V49.60

Amputation (Continued)
    traumatic (complete) (partial)

> Note: "Complicated" includes traumatic amputation with delayed healing, delayed treatment, foreign body, or infection.

        arm 887.4
            at or above elbow 887.2
                complicated 887.3
            below elbow 887.0
                complicated 887.1
            both (bilateral) (any level(s)) 887.6
                complicated 887.7
            complicated 887.5
        finger(s) (one or both hands) 886.0
            with thumb(s) 885.0
                complicated 885.1
            complicated 886.1
        foot (except toe(s) only) 896.0
            and other leg 897.6
                complicated 897.7
            both (bilateral) 896.2
                complicated 896.3
            complicated 896.1
        toe(s) only (one or both feet) 895.0
            complicated 895.1
        genital organ(s) (external) NEC 878.8
            complicated 878.9
        hand (except finger(s) only) 887.0
            and other arm 887.6
                complicated 887.7
            both (bilateral) 887.6
                complicated 887.7
            complicated 887.1
            finger(s) (one or both hands) 886.0
                with thumb(s) 885.0
                      complicated 885.1
                complicated 886.1
            thumb(s) (with fingers of either hand) 885.0
                complicated 885.1
        head 874.9
        late effect - see Late, effects (of), amputation
        leg 897.4
            and other foot 897.6
                complicated 897.7
            at or above knee 897.2
                complicated 897.3
            below knee 897.0
                complicated 897.1
            both (bilateral) 897.6
                complicated 897.7
            complicated 897.5
        lower limb(s) except toe(s) - see Amputation, traumatic, leg
        nose - see Wound, open, nose
        penis 878.0
            complicated 878.1
        sites other than limbs - see Wound, open, by site
        thumb(s) (with finger(s) of either hand) 885.0
            complicated 885.1
        toe(s) (one or both feet) 895.0
            complicated 895.1
        upper limb(s) - see Amputation, traumatic, arm
Amputee (bilateral) (old) - see also Absence, by site, acquired V49.70
Amusia 784.69
    developmental 315.39
    secondary to organic lesion 784.69
Amyelencephalus 740.0
Amyelia 742.59
Amygdalitis - see Tonsillitis
Amygdalolith 474.8
Amyloid disease or degeneration 277.30
    heart 277.39 [425.7]

Amyloidosis (familial) (general) (generalized) (genetic) (primary) 277.30
    with lung involvement 277.39 [517.8]
    cardiac, hereditary 277.39
    heart 277.39 [425.7]
    nephropathic 277.39 [583.81]
    neuropathic (Portuguese) (Swiss) 277.39 [357.4]
    pulmonary 277.39 [517.8]
    secondary 277.39
    systemic, inherited 277.39
Amylopectinosis (brancher enzyme deficiency) 271.0
Amylophagia 307.52
Amyoplasia, congenita 756.89
Amyotonia 728.2
    congenita 358.8
Amyotrophia, amyotrophy, amyotrophic 728.2
    congenita 756.89
    diabetic 250.6 ● [353.5]
        due to secondary diabetes 249.6 ● [353.5]
    lateral sclerosis (syndrome) 335.20
    neuralgic 353.5
    sclerosis (lateral) 335.20
    spinal progressive 335.21
Anacidity, gastric 536.0
    psychogenic 306.4
Anaerosis of newborn 770.88
Analbuminemia 273.8
Analgesia (see also Anesthesia) 782.0
Analphalipoproteinemia 272.5
Anaphylactic reaction or shock (correct substance properly administered) 995.0
    due to
        administration of blood and blood products 999.41
        chemical - see Table of Drugs and Chemicals
        correct medicinal substance properly administered 995.0
        drug or medicinal substance
            correct substance properly administered 995.0
            overdose or wrong substance given or taken 977.9
            specified drug - see Table of Drugs and Chemicals
        following sting(s) 989.5
        food 995.60
            additives 995.66
            crustaceans 995.62
            eggs 995.68
            fish 995.65
            fruits 995.63
            milk products 995.67
            nuts (tree) 995.64
            peanuts 995.61
            seeds 995.64
            specified NEC 995.69
            tree nuts 995.64
            vegetables 995.63
        immunization 999.42
        overdose or wrong substance given or taken 977.9
            specified drug - see Table of Drugs and Chemicals
        serum NEC 999.49
    following sting(s) 989.5
    purpura 287.0
    serum NEC 999.49
Anaphylactoid reaction or shock - see Anaphylactic reaction or shock
Anaphylaxis - see Anaphylactic reaction or shock
Anaplasia, cervix 622.10
Anaplasmosis, human 082.49
Anarthria 784.51
Anarthritic rheumatoid disease 446.5

SECTION I INDEX TO DISEASES AND INJURIES / Anasarca

Anasarca 782.3
   cardiac (see also Failure, heart) 428.0
   fetus or newborn 778.0
   lung 514
   nutritional 262
   pulmonary 514
   renal (see also Nephrosis) 581.9
Anaspadias 752.62
Anastomosis
   aneurysmal - see Aneurysm
   arteriovenous, congenital NEC (see also
      Anomaly, arteriovenous) 747.60
      ruptured, of brain (see also Hemorrhage,
         subarachnoid) 430
      intestinal 569.89
         complicated NEC 997.49
            involving urinary tract 997.5
      retinal and choroidal vessels 743.58
         acquired 362.17
Anatomical narrow angle (glaucoma)
   365.02
Ancylostoma (infection) (infestation)
   126.9
   americanus 126.1
   braziliense 126.2
   caninum 126.8
   ceylanicum 126.3
   duodenale 126.0
   Necator americanus 126.1
Ancylostomiasis (intestinal) 126.9
   ancylostoma
      americanus 126.1
      caninum 126.8
      ceylanicum 126.3
      duodenale 126.0
   braziliense 126.2
   Necator americanus 126.1
Anders' disease or syndrome (adiposis
   tuberosa simplex) 272.8
Andersen's glycogen storage disease
   271.0
Anderson's disease 272.7
Andes disease 993.2
Andrews' disease (bacterid) 686.8
Androblastoma (M8630/1)
   benign (M8630/0)
      specified site - see Neoplasm, by site,
         benign
      unspecified site
         female 220
         male 222.0
   malignant (M8630/3)
      specified site - see Neoplasm, by site,
         malignant
      unspecified site
         female 183.0
         male 186.9
   specified site - see Neoplasm, by site,
      uncertain behavior
   tubular (M8640/0)
      with lipid storage (M8641/0)
         specified site - see Neoplasm, by site,
            benign
         unspecified site
            female 220
            male 222.0
      specified site - see Neoplasm, by site,
         benign
      unspecified site
         female 220
         male 222.0
   unspecified site
      female 236.2
      male 236.4
Android pelvis 755.69
   with disproportion (fetopelvic) 653.3●
      affecting fetus or newborn 763.1
      causing obstructed labor 660.1●
         affecting fetus or newborn 763.1
Anectasis, pulmonary (newborn or fetus)
   770.5

Anemia 285.9
   with
      disorder of
         anaerobic glycolysis 282.3
         pentose phosphate pathway 282.2
      koilonychia 280.9
   6-phosphogluconic dehydrogenase
      deficiency 282.2
   achlorhydric 280.9
   achrestic 281.8
   Addison's (pernicious) 281.0
   Addison-Biermer (pernicious) 281.0
   agranulocytic 288.09
   amino acid deficiency 281.4
   antineoplastic chemotherapy induced 285.3
   aplastic 284.9
      acquired (secondary) 284.89
      congenital 284.01
      constitutional 284.01
      due to
         antineoplastic chemotherapy 284.89
         chronic systemic disease 284.89
         drugs 284.89
         infection 284.89
         radiation 284.89
      idiopathic 284.9
      myxedema 244.9
      of or complicating pregnancy 648.2●
      red cell (acquired) (adult) (with
         thymoma) 284.81
         congenital 284.01
         pure 284.01
      specified type NEC 284.89
      toxic (paralytic) 284.89
   aregenerative 284.9
      congenital 284.01
   asiderotic 280.9
   atypical (primary) 285.9
   autohemolysis of Selwyn and Dacie (type I)
      282.2
   autoimmune hemolytic 283.0
   Baghdad Spring 282.2
   Balantidium coli 007.0
   Biermer's (pernicious) 281.0
   blood loss (chronic) 280.0
      acute 285.1
   bothriocephalus 123.4
   brickmakers' (see also Ancylostomiasis) 126.9
   cerebral 437.8
   childhood 282.9
   chlorotic 280.9
   chronic 285.9
      blood loss 280.0
      hemolytic 282.9
         idiopathic 283.9
      simple 281.9
   chronica congenita aregenerativa 284.01
   combined system disease NEC 281.0 [336.2]
      due to dietary deficiency 281.1 [336.2]
   complicating pregnancy or childbirth 648.2●
   congenital (following fetal blood loss) 776.5
      aplastic 284.01
      due to isoimmunization NEC 773.2
      Heinz-body 282.7
      hereditary hemolytic NEC 282.9
      nonspherocytic
         type I 282.2
         type II 282.3
      pernicious 281.0
      spherocytic (see also Spherocytosis) 282.0
   Cooley's (erythroblastic) 282.44
   crescent - see Disease, sickle-cell
   cytogenic 281.0
   Dacie's (nonspherocytic)
      type I 282.2
      type II 282.3
   Davidson's (refractory) 284.9
   deficiency 281.9
      2, 3 diphosphoglycurate mutase 282.3
      2, 3 PG 282.3
      6-PGD 282.2

Anemia (Continued)
   deficiency (Continued)
      6-phosphogluronic dehydrogenase 282.2
      amino acid 281.4
      combined B_{12} and folate 281.3
      enzyme, drug-induced (hemolytic) 282.2
      erythrocytic glutathione 282.2
      folate 281.2
         dietary 281.2
         drug-induced 281.2
      folic acid 281.2
         dietary 281.2
         drug-induced 281.2
      G-6-PD 282.2
      GGS-R 282.2
      glucose-6-phosphate dehydrogenase
         (G-6-PD) 282.2
      glucose-phosphate isomerase 282.3
      glutathione peroxidase 282.2
      glutathione reductase 282.2
      glyceraldehyde phosphate
         dehydrogenase 282.3
      GPI 282.3
      G SH 282.2
      hexokinase 282.3
      iron (Fe) 280.9
         specified NEC 280.8
      nutritional 281.9
         with
            poor iron absorption 280.9
            specified deficiency NEC 281.8
         due to inadequate dietary iron intake
            280.1
         specified type NEC 281.8
      of or complicating pregnancy 648.2●
      pentose phosphate pathway 282.2
      PFK 282.3
      phosphofructo-aldolase 282.3
      phosphofructokinase 282.3
      phosphoglycerate kinase 282.3
      PK 282.3
      protein 281.4
      pyruvate kinase (PK) 282.3
      TPI 282.3
      triosephosphate isomerase 282.3
      vitamin B_{12} NEC 281.1
         dietary 281.1
         pernicious 281.0
   Diamond-Blackfan (congenital hypoplastic)
      284.01
   dibothriocephalus 123.4
   dimorphic 281.9
   diphasic 281.8
   diphtheritic 032.89
   Diphyllobothrium 123.4
   drepanocytic (see also Disease, sickle-cell)
      282.60
   due to
      antineoplastic chemotherapy 285.3
      blood loss (chronic) 280.0
         acute 285.1
      chemotherapy, antineoplastic 285.3
      defect of Embden-Meyerhof pathway
         glycolysis 282.3
      disorder of glutathione metabolism 282.2
      drug - see Anemia, by type (see also Table
         of Drugs and Chemicals)
         chemotherapy, antineoplastic 285.3
      fetal blood loss 776.5
      fish tapeworm (D. latum) infestation
         123.4
      glutathione metabolism disorder 282.2
      hemorrhage (chronic) 280.0
         acute 285.1
      hexose monophosphate (HMP) shunt
         deficiency 282.2
      impaired absorption 280.9
      loss of blood (chronic) 280.0
         acute 285.1
      myxedema 244.9
      Necator americanus 126.1

Anemia (Continued)
due to (Continued)
prematurity 776.6
selective vitamin B$_{12}$ malabsorption with proteinuria 281.1
Dyke-Young type (secondary) (symptomatic) 283.9
dyserythropoietic (congenital) (types I, II, III) 285.8
dyshemopoietic (congenital) 285.8
Egypt (see also Ancylostomiasis) 126.9
elliptocytosis (see also Elliptocytosis) 282.1
enzyme deficiency, drug-induced 282.2
epidemic (see also Ancylostomiasis) 126.9
EPO resistant 285.21
erythroblastic
familial 282.44
fetus or newborn (see also Disease, hemolytic) 773.2
late 773.5
erythrocytic glutathione deficiency 282.2
erythropoietin-resistant (EPO resistant anemia) 285.21
essential 285.9
Faber's (achlorhydric anemia) 280.9
factitious (self-induced bloodletting) 280.0
familial erythroblastic (microcytic) 282.44
Fanconi's (congenital pancytopenia) 284.09
favism 282.2
fetal 678.0 ●
following blood loss, affecting newborn 776.5
fetus or newborn
due to
ABO
antibodies 773.1
incompatibility, maternal/fetal 773.1
isoimmunization 773.1
Rh
antibodies 773.0
incompatibility, maternal/fetal 773.0
isoimmunization 773.0
following fetal blood loss 776.5
fish tapeworm (D. latum) infestation 123.4
folate (folic acid) deficiency 281.2
dietary 281.2
drug-induced 281.2
folate malabsorption, congenital 281.2
folic acid deficiency 281.2
dietary 281.2
drug-induced 281.2
G-6-PD 282.2
general 285.9
glucose-6-phosphate dehydrogenase deficiency 282.2
glutathione-reductase deficiency 282.2
goat's milk 281.2
granulocytic 288.09
Heinz-body, congenital 282.7
hemoglobin deficiency 285.9
hemolytic 283.9
acquired 283.9
with hemoglobinuria NEC 283.2
autoimmune (cold type) (idiopathic) (primary) (secondary) (symptomatic) (warm type) 283.0
due to
cold reactive antibodies 283.0
drug exposure 283.0
warm reactive antibodies 283.0
fragmentation 283.19
idiopathic (chronic) 283.9
infectious 283.19
autoimmune 283.0
non-autoimmune 283.10
toxic 283.19
traumatic cardiac 283.19

Anemia (Continued)
hemolytic (Continued)
acute 283.9
due to enzyme deficiency NEC 282.3
fetus or newborn (see also Disease, hemolytic) 773.2
late 773.5
Lederer's (acquired infectious hemolytic anemia) 283.19
autoimmune (acquired) 283.0
chronic 282.9
idiopathic 283.9
cold type (secondary) (symptomatic) 283.0
congenital (spherocytic) (see also Spherocytosis) 282.0
nonspherocytic - see Anemia, hemolytic, nonspherocytic, congenital
drug-induced 283.0
enzyme deficiency 282.2
due to
cardiac conditions 283.19
drugs 283.0
enzyme deficiency NEC 282.3
drug-induced 282.2
presence of shunt or other internal prosthetic device 283.19
thrombotic thrombocytopenic purpura 446.6
elliptocytotic (see also Elliptocytosis) 282.1
familial 282.9
hereditary 282.9
due to enzyme deficiency NEC 282.3
specified NEC 282.8
idiopathic (chronic) 283.9
infectious (acquired) 283.19
mechanical 283.19
microangiopathic 283.19
nonautoimmune 283.10
nonspherocytic
congenital or hereditary NEC 282.3
glucose-6-phosphate dehydrogenase deficiency 282.2
pyruvate kinase (PK) deficiency 282.3
type I 282.2
type II 282.3
type I 282.2
type II 282.3
of or complicating pregnancy 648.2 ●
resulting from presence of shunt or other internal prosthetic device 283.19
secondary 283.19
autoimmune 283.0
sickle-cell - see Disease, sickle-cell
Stransky-Regala type (Hb-E) (see also Disease, hemoglobin) 282.7
symptomatic 283.19
autoimmune 283.0
toxic (acquired) 283.19
uremic (adult) (child) 283.11
warm type (secondary) (symptomatic) 283.0
hemorrhagic (chronic) 280.0
acute 285.1
HEMPAS 285.8
hereditary erythroblast multinuclearity-positive acidified serum test 285.8
Herrick's (hemoglobin S disease) 282.61
hexokinase deficiency 282.3
high A$_2$ 282.46
hookworm (see also Ancylostomiasis) 126.9
hypochromic (idiopathic) (microcytic) (normoblastic) 280.9
with iron loading 285.0
due to blood loss (chronic) 280.0
acute 285.1
familial sex linked 285.0
pyridoxine-responsive 285.0

Anemia (Continued)
hypoplasia, red blood cells 284.81
congenital or familial 284.01
hypoplastic (idiopathic) 284.9
congenital 284.01
familial 284.01
of childhood 284.09
idiopathic 285.9
hemolytic, chronic 283.9
in (due to) (with)
chronic illness NEC 285.29
chronic kidney disease 285.21
end-stage renal disease 285.21
neoplastic disease 285.22
infantile 285.9
infective, infectional 285.9
intertropical (see also Ancylostomiasis) 126.9
iron (Fe) deficiency 280.9
due to blood loss (chronic) 280.0
acute 285.1
of or complicating pregnancy 648.2 ●
specified NEC 280.8
Jaksch's (pseudoleukemia infantum) 285.8
Joseph-Diamond-Blackfan (congenital hypoplastic) 284.01
labyrinth 386.50
Lederer's (acquired infectious hemolytic anemia) 283.19
leptocytosis (hereditary) 282.40
leukoerythroblastic 284.2
macrocytic 281.9
nutritional 281.2
of or complicating pregnancy 648.2 ●
tropical 281.2
malabsorption (familial), selective B$_{12}$ with proteinuria 281.1
malarial (see also Malaria) 084.6
malignant (progressive) 281.0
malnutrition 281.9
marsh (see also Malaria) 084.6
Mediterranean 282.40
with hemoglobinopathy 282.49
megaloblastic 281.9
combined B$_{12}$ and folate deficiency 281.3
nutritional (of infancy) 281.2
of infancy 281.2
of or complicating pregnancy 648.2 ●
refractory 281.3
specified NEC 281.3
megalocytic 281.9
microangiopathic hemolytic 283.19
microcytic (hypochromic) 280.9
due to blood loss (chronic) 280.0
acute 285.1
familial 282.49
hypochromic 280.9
microdrepanocytosis 282.41
miners' (see also Ancylostomiasis) 126.9
myelopathic 285.8
myelophthisic (normocytic) 284.2
newborn (see also Disease, hemolytic) 773.2
due to isoimmunization (see also Disease, hemolytic) 773.2
late, due to isoimmunization 773.5
posthemorrhagic 776.5
nonregenerative 284.9
nonspherocytic hemolytic - see Anemia, hemolytic, nonspherocytic
normocytic (infectional) (not due to blood loss) 285.9
due to blood loss (chronic) 280.0
acute 285.1
myelophthisic 284.2
nutritional (deficiency) 281.9
with
poor iron absorption 280.9
specified deficiency NEC 281.8
due to inadequate dietary iron intake 280.1
megaloblastic (of infancy) 281.2
of childhood 282.9

SECTION I INDEX TO DISEASES AND INJURIES / Anemia

Anemia (Continued)
  of chronic
    disease NEC 285.29
    illness NEC 285.29
  of or complicating pregnancy 648.2●
    affecting fetus or newborn 760.8
  of prematurity 776.6
  orotic aciduric (congenital) (hereditary) 281.4
  osteosclerotic 289.89
  ovalocytosis (hereditary) (see also
    Elliptocytosis) 282.1
  paludal (see also Malaria) 084.6
  pentose phosphate pathway deficiency 282.2
  pernicious (combined system disease)
    (congenital) (dorsolateral spinal
    degeneration) (juvenile) (myelopathy)
    (neuropathy) (posterior sclerosis)
    (primary) (progressive) (spleen) 281.0
    of or complicating pregnancy 648.2●
  pleochromic 285.9
    of sprue 281.8
  portal 285.8
  posthemorrhagic (chronic) 280.0
    acute 285.1
    newborn 776.5
  postoperative
    due to (acute) blood loss 285.1
      chronic blood loss 280.0
    other 285.9
  postpartum 648.2●
  pressure 285.9
  primary 285.9
  profound 285.9
  progressive 285.9
    malignant 281.0
    pernicious 281.0
  protein-deficiency 281.4
  pseudoleukemica infantum 285.8
  puerperal 648.2●
  pure red cell 284.81
    congenital 284.01
  pyridoxine-responsive (hypochromic)
    285.0
  pyruvate kinase (PK) deficiency 282.3
  refractoria sideroblastica 238.72
  refractory (primary) 238.72
    with
      excess
        blasts-1 (RAEB-1) 238.72
        blasts-2 (RAEB-2) 238.73
      hemochromatosis 238.72
      ringed sideroblasts (RARS) 238.72
    due to
      drug 285.0
      myelodysplastic syndrome 238.72
      toxin 285.0
    hereditary 285.0
    idiopathic 238.72
    megaloblastic 281.3
    sideroblastic 238.72
      hereditary 285.0
    sideropenic 280.9
  Rietti-Greppi-Micheli (thalassemia minor)
    282.46
  scorbutic 281.8
  secondary (to) 285.9
    blood loss (chronic) 280.0
      acute 285.1
    hemorrhage 280.0
      acute 285.1
    inadequate dietary iron intake 280.1
  semiplastic 284.9
  septic 285.9
  sickle-cell (see also Disease, sickle-cell)
    282.60
  sideroachrestic 285.0
  sideroblastic (acquired) (any type)
    (congenital) (drug-induced) (due to
    disease) (hereditary) (primary)
    (secondary) (sex-linked hypochromic)
    (vitamin B_6 responsive) 285.0

Anemia (Continued)
  sideroblastic (Continued)
    refractory 238.72
      congenital 285.0
      drug-induced 285.0
      hereditary 285.0
      sex-linked hypochromic 285.0
      vitamin B_6-responsive 285.0
  sideropenic 280.9
    due to blood loss (chronic) 280.0
      acute 285.1
  simple chronic 281.9
  specified type NEC 285.8
  spherocytic (hereditary) (see also
    Spherocytosis) 282.0
  splenic 285.8
    familial (Gaucher's) 272.7
  splenomegalic 285.8
  stomatocytosis 282.8
  syphilitic 095.8
  target cell (oval) 285.8
    with thalassemia - see Thalassemia
  thalassemia 282.40
  thrombocytopenic (see also
    Thrombocytopenia) 287.5
  toxic 284.89
  triosephosphate isomerase deficiency 282.3
  tropical, macrocytic 281.2
  tuberculous (see also Tuberculosis) 017.9●
  Vegan's 281.1
  vitamin
    B_6-responsive 285.0
    B_{12} deficiency (dietary) 281.1
      pernicious 281.0
  von Jaksch's (pseudoleukemia infantum) 285.8
  Witts' (achlorhydric anemia) 280.9
  Zuelzer (-Ogden) (nutritional megaloblastic
    anemia) 281.2

Anencephalus, anencephaly 740.0
  fetal, affecting management of pregnancy
    655.0●
Anergasia (see also Psychosis, organic) 294.9
  senile 290.0
Anesthesia, anesthetic 782.0
  complication or reaction NEC 995.22
    due to
      correct substance properly
        administered 995.22
      overdose or wrong substance given
        968.4
        specified anesthetic - see Table of
          Drugs and Chemicals
  cornea 371.81
  death from
    correct substance properly administered
      995.4
    during delivery 668.9●
    overdose or wrong substance given 968.4
      specified anesthetic - see Table of Drugs
        and Chemicals
  eye 371.81
  functional 300.11
  hyperesthetic, thalamic 338.0
  hysterical 300.11
  local skin lesion 782.0
  olfactory 781.1
  sexual (psychogenic) 302.72
  shock
    due to
      correct substance properly
        administered 995.4
      overdose or wrong substance given
        968.4
        specified anesthetic - see Table of
          Drugs and Chemicals
  skin 782.0
  tactile 782.0
  testicular 608.9
  thermal 782.0
Anetoderma (maculosum) 701.3
Aneuploidy NEC 758.5

Aneurin deficiency 265.1
Aneurysm (anastomotic) (artery) (cirsoid)
  (diffuse) (false) (fusiform) (multiple)
  (ruptured) (saccular) (varicose) 442.9
  abdominal (aorta) 441.4
    ruptured 441.3
    syphilitic 093.0
  aorta, aortic (nonsyphilitic) 441.9
    abdominal 441.4
      dissecting 441.02
      ruptured 441.3
      syphilitic 093.0
    arch 441.2
      ruptured 441.1
    arteriosclerotic NEC 441.9
      ruptured 441.5
    ascending 441.2
      ruptured 441.1
    congenital 747.29
    descending 441.9
      abdominal 441.4
        ruptured 441.3
      ruptured 441.5
      thoracic 441.2
        ruptured 441.1
    dissecting 441.00
      abdominal 441.02
      thoracic 441.01
      thoracoabdominal 441.03
    due to coarctation (aorta) 747.10
    ruptured 441.5
    sinus, right 747.29
    syphilitic 093.0
    thoracoabdominal 441.7
      ruptured 441.6
    thorax, thoracic (arch) (nonsyphilitic)
      441.2
      dissecting 441.01
      ruptured 441.1
      syphilitic 093.0
    transverse 441.2
      ruptured 441.1
    valve (heart) (see also Endocarditis, aortic)
      424.1
  arteriosclerotic NEC 442.9
    cerebral 437.3
      ruptured (see also Hemorrhage,
        subarachnoid) 430
  arteriovenous (congenital) (peripheral) NEC
    (see also Anomaly, arteriovenous)
    747.60
    acquired NEC 447.0
      brain 437.3
        ruptured (see also Hemorrhage,
          subarachnoid) 430
      coronary 414.11
      pulmonary 417.0
    brain (cerebral) 747.81
      ruptured (see also Hemorrhage,
        subarachnoid) 430
    coronary 746.85
    pulmonary 747.32
    retina 743.58
    specified site NEC 747.89
      acquired 447.0
    traumatic (see also Injury, blood vessel, by
      site) 904.9
  basal - see Aneurysm, brain
  berry (congenital) (ruptured) (see also
    Hemorrhage, subarachnoid) 430
    nonruptured 437.3
  brain 437.3
    arteriosclerotic 437.3
      ruptured (see also Hemorrhage,
        subarachnoid) 430
    arteriovenous 747.81
      acquired 437.3
        ruptured (see also Hemorrhage,
          subarachnoid) 430
      ruptured (see also Hemorrhage,
        subarachnoid) 430

Aneurysm (Continued)
  brain (Continued)
    berry (congenital) (ruptured) (see also Hemorrhage, subarachnoid) 430
      nonruptured 437.3
    congenital 747.81
      ruptured (see also Hemorrhage, subarachnoid) 430
    meninges 437.3
      ruptured (see also Hemorrhage, subarachnoid) 430
    miliary (congenital) (ruptured) (see also Hemorrhage, subarachnoid) 430
    mycotic 421.0
      ruptured (see also Hemorrhage, subarachnoid) 430
    nonruptured 437.3
    ruptured (see also Hemorrhage, subarachnoid) 430
    syphilitic 094.87
    syphilitic (hemorrhage) 094.87
    traumatic - see Injury, intracranial
  cardiac (false) (see also Aneurysm, heart) 414.10
  carotid artery (common) (external) 442.81
    internal (intracranial portion) 437.3
      extracranial portion 442.81
      ruptured into brain (see also Hemorrhage, subarachnoid) 430
    syphilitic 093.89
      intracranial 094.87
  cavernous sinus (see also Aneurysm, brain) 437.3
    arteriovenous 747.81
      ruptured (see also Hemorrhage, subarachnoid) 430
    congenital 747.81
      ruptured (see also Hemorrhage, subarachnoid) 430
  celiac 442.84
  central nervous system, syphilitic 094.89
  cerebral - see Aneurysm, brain
  chest - see Aneurysm, thorax
  circle of Willis (see also Aneurysm, brain) 437.3
    congenital 747.81
      ruptured (see also Hemorrhage, subarachnoid) 430
    ruptured (see also Hemorrhage, subarachnoid) 430
  common iliac artery 442.2
  congenital (peripheral) NEC 747.60
    brain 747.81
      ruptured (see also Hemorrhage, subarachnoid) 430
    cerebral - see Aneurysm, brain, congenital
    coronary 746.85
    gastrointestinal 747.61
    lower limb 747.64
    pulmonary 747.32
    renal 747.62
    retina 743.58
    specified site NEC 747.89
    spinal 747.82
    upper limb 747.63
  conjunctiva 372.74
  conus arteriosus (see also Aneurysm, heart) 414.10
  coronary (arteriosclerotic) (artery) (vein) (see also Aneurysm, heart) 414.11
    arteriovenous 746.85
    congenital 746.85
    syphilitic 093.89
  cylindrical 441.9
    ruptured 441.5
    syphilitic 093.9
  dissecting 442.9
    aorta 441.00
      abdominal 441.02
      thoracic 441.01
      thoracoabdominal 441.03
    syphilitic 093.9

Aneurysm (Continued)
  ductus arteriosus 747.0
  embolic - see Embolism, artery
  endocardial, infective (any valve) 421.0
  femoral 442.3
  gastroduodenal 442.84
  gastroepiploic 442.84
  heart (chronic or with a stated duration of over 8 weeks) (infectional) (wall) 414.10
    acute or with a stated duration of 8 weeks or less (see also Infarct, myocardium) 410.9●
    congenital 746.89
    valve - see Endocarditis
  hepatic 442.84
  iliac (common) 442.2
  infective (any valve) 421.0
  innominate (nonsyphilitic) 442.89
    syphilitic 093.89
  interauricular septum (see also Aneurysm, heart) 414.10
  interventricular septum (see also Aneurysm, heart) 414.10
  intracranial - see Aneurysm, brain
  intrathoracic (nonsyphilitic) 441.2
    ruptured 441.1
    syphilitic 093.0
  jugular vein (acute) 453.89
    chronic 453.76
  lower extremity 442.3
  lung (pulmonary artery) 417.1
  malignant 093.9
  mediastinal (nonsyphilitic) 442.89
    syphilitic 093.89
  miliary (congenital) (ruptured) (see also Hemorrhage, subarachnoid) 430
  mitral (heart) (valve) 424.0
  mural (arteriovenous) (heart) (see also Aneurysm, heart) 414.10
  mycotic, any site 421.0
    without endocarditis - see Aneurysm, by site
    ruptured, brain (see also Hemorrhage, subarachnoid) 430
  myocardium (see also Aneurysm, heart) 414.10
  neck 442.81
  pancreaticoduodenal 442.84
  patent ductus arteriosus 747.0
  peripheral NEC 442.89
    congenital NEC (see also Aneurysm, congenital) 747.60
  popliteal 442.3
  pulmonary 417.1
    arteriovenous 747.32
      acquired 417.0
    syphilitic 093.89
    valve (heart) (see also Endocarditis, pulmonary) 424.3
  racemose 442.9
    congenital (peripheral) NEC 747.60
  radial 442.0
  Rasmussen's (see also Tuberculosis) 011.2●
  renal 442.1
  retinal (acquired) 362.17
    congenital 743.58
    diabetic 250.5● [362.01]
      due to secondary diabetes 249.5● [362.01]
  sinus, aortic (of Valsalva) 747.29
  specified site NEC 442.89
  spinal (cord) 442.89
    congenital 747.82
    syphilitic (hemorrhage) 094.89
  spleen, splenic 442.83
  subclavian 442.82
    syphilitic 093.89
  superior mesenteric 442.84

Aneurysm (Continued)
  syphilitic 093.9
    aorta 093.0
    central nervous system 094.89
    congenital 090.5
    spine, spinal 094.89
  thoracoabdominal 441.7
    ruptured 441.6
  thorax, thoracic (arch) (nonsyphilitic) 441.2
    dissecting 441.01
    ruptured 441.1
    syphilitic 093.0
  traumatic (complication) (early) - see Injury, blood vessel, by site
  tricuspid (heart) (valve) - see Endocarditis, tricuspid
  ulnar 442.0
  upper extremity 442.0
  valve, valvular - see Endocarditis
  venous 456.8
    congenital NEC (see also Aneurysm, congenital) 747.60
  ventricle (arteriovenous) (see also Aneurysm, heart) 414.10
  visceral artery NEC 442.84
Angiectasis 459.89
Angiectopia 459.9
Angiitis 447.6
  allergic granulomatous 446.4
  hypersensitivity 446.20
    Goodpasture's syndrome 446.21
    specified NEC 446.29
  necrotizing 446.0
  Wegener's (necrotizing respiratory granulomatosis) 446.4
Angina (attack) (cardiac) (chest) (effort) (heart) (pectoris) (syndrome) (vasomotor) 413.9
  abdominal 557.1
  accelerated 411.1
  agranulocytic 288.03
  aphthous 074.0
  catarrhal 462
  crescendo 411.1
  croupous 464.4
  cruris 443.9
    due to atherosclerosis NEC (see also Arteriosclerosis, extremities) 440.20
  decubitus 413.0
  diphtheritic (membranous) 032.0
  equivalent 413.9
  erysipelatous 034.0
  erythematous 462
  exudative, chronic 476.0
  faucium 478.29
  gangrenous 462
    diphtheritic 032.0
  infectious 462
  initial 411.1
  intestinal 557.1
  ludovici 528.3
  Ludwig's 528.3
  malignant 462
    diphtheritic 032.0
  membranous 464.4
    diphtheritic 032.0
  mesenteric 557.1
  monocytic 075
  nocturnal 413.0
  phlegmonous 475
    diphtheritic 032.0
  preinfarctional 411.1
  Prinzmetal's 413.1
  progressive 411.1
  pseudomembranous 101
  psychogenic 306.2
  pultaceous, diphtheritic 032.0
  scarlatinal 034.1
  septic 034.0
  simple 462
  stable NEC 413.9
  staphylococcal 462

SECTION 1 INDEX TO DISEASES AND INJURIES / Angina

Angina (Continued)
  streptococcal 034.0
  stridulous, diphtheritic 032.3
  syphilitic 093.9
    congenital 090.5
  tonsil 475
  trachealis 464.4
  unstable 411.1
  variant 413.1
  Vincent's 101
Angioblastoma (M9161/1) - see Neoplasm, connective tissue, uncertain behavior
Angiocholecystitis (see also Cholecystitis, acute) 575.0
Angiocholitis (see also Cholecystitis, acute) 576.1
Angiodysgensis spinalis 336.1
Angiodysplasia (intestinalis) (intestine) 569.84
  with hemorrhage 569.85
  duodenum 537.82
    with hemorrhage 537.83
  stomach 537.82
    with hemorrhage 537.83
Angioedema (allergic) (any site) (with urticaria) 995.1
  hereditary 277.6
Angioendothelioma (M9130/1) - see also Neoplasm, by site, uncertain behavior
  benign (M9130/0) (see also Hemangioma, by site) 228.00
  bone (M9260/3) - see Neoplasm, bone, malignant
  Ewing's (M9260/3) - see Neoplasm, bone, malignant
  nervous system (M9130/0) 228.09
Angiofibroma (M9160/0) - see also Neoplasm, by site, benign
  juvenile (M9160/0) 210.7
    specified site - see Neoplasm, by site, benign
    unspecified site 210.7
Angiohemophilia (A) (B) 286.4
Angioid streaks (choroid) (retina) 363.43
Angiokeratoma (M9141/0) - see also Neoplasm, skin, benign
  corporis diffusum 272.7
Angiokeratosis
  diffuse 272.7
Angioleiomyoma (M8894/0) - see Neoplasm, connective tissue, benign
Angioleucitis 683
Angiolipoma (M8861/0) (see also Lipoma, by site) 214.9
  infiltrating (M8861/1) - see Neoplasm, connective tissue, uncertain behavior
Angioma (M9120/0) (see also Hemangioma, by site) 228.00
  capillary 448.1
  hemorrhagicum hereditaria 448.0
  malignant (M9120/3) - see Neoplasm, connective tissue, malignant
  pigmentosum et atrophicum 757.33
  placenta - see Placenta, abnormal
  plexiform (M9131/0) - see Hemangioma, by site
  senile 448.1
  serpiginosum 709.1
  spider 448.1
  stellate 448.1
Angiomatosis 757.32
  bacillary 083.8
  corporis diffusum universale 272.7
  cutaneocerebral 759.6
  encephalocutanea 759.6
  encephalofacial 759.6
  encephalotrigeminal 759.6
  hemorrhagic familial 448.0
  hereditary familial 448.0
  heredofamilial 448.0
  meningo-oculofacial 759.6
  multiple sites 228.09

Angiomatosis (Continued)
  neuro-oculocutaneous 759.6
  retina (Hippel's disease) 759.6
  retinocerebellosa 759.6
  retinocerebral 759.6
  systemic 228.09
Angiomyolipoma (M8860/0)
  specified site - see Neoplasm, connective tissue, benign
  unspecified site 223.0
Angiomyoliposarcoma (M8860/3) - see Neoplasm, connective tissue, malignant
Angiomyoma (M8894/0) - see Neoplasm, connective tissue, benign
Angiomyosarcoma (M8894/3) - see Neoplasm, connective tissue, malignant
Angioneurosis 306.2
Angioneurotic edema (allergic) (any site) (with urticaria) 995.1
  hereditary 277.6
Angiopathia, angiopathy 459.9
  diabetic (peripheral) 250.7 ● [443.81]
    due to secondary diabetes 249.7 ● [443.81]
  peripheral 443.9
    diabetic 250.7 ● [443.81]
      due to secondary diabetes 249.7 ● [443.81]
    specified type NEC 443.89
  retinae syphilitica 093.89
  retinalis (juvenilis) 362.18
    background 362.10
    diabetic 250.5 ● [362.01]
      due to secondary diabetes 249.5 ● [362.01]
    proliferative 362.29
    tuberculous (see also Tuberculosis) 017.3 ● [362.18]
Angiosarcoma (M9120/3) - see Neoplasm, connective tissue, malignant
Angiosclerosis - see Arteriosclerosis
Angioscotoma, enlarged 368.42
Angiospasm 443.9
  brachial plexus 353.0
  cerebral 435.9
  cervical plexus 353.2
  nerve
    arm 354.9
      axillary 353.0
      median 354.1
      ulnar 354.2
    autonomic (see also Neuropathy, peripheral, autonomic) 337.9
    axillary 353.0
    leg 355.8
      plantar 355.6
    lower extremity - see Angiospasm, nerve, leg
    median 354.1
    peripheral NEC 355.9
    spinal NEC 355.9
    sympathetic (see also Neuropathy, peripheral, autonomic) 337.9
    ulnar 354.2
    upper extremity - see Angiospasm, nerve, arm
  peripheral NEC 443.9
  traumatic 443.9
    foot 443.9
    leg 443.9
  vessel 443.9
Angiospastic disease or edema 443.9
Angle's
  class I 524.21
  class II 524.22
  class III 524.23
Anguillulosis 127.2
Angulation
  cecum (see also Obstruction, intestine) 560.9
  coccyx (acquired) 738.6
    congenital 756.19

Angulation (Continued)
  femur (acquired) 736.39
    congenital 755.69
  intestine (large) (small) (see also Obstruction, intestine) 560.9
  sacrum (acquired) 738.5
    congenital 756.19
  sigmoid (flexure) (see also Obstruction, intestine) 560.9
  spine (see also Curvature, spine) 737.9
  tibia (acquired) 736.89
    congenital 755.69
  ureter 593.3
  wrist (acquired) 736.09
    congenital 755.59
Angulus infectiosus 686.8
Anhedonia 780.99
Anhidrosis (lid) (neurogenic) (thermogenic) 705.0
Anhydration 276.51
  with
    hypernatremia 276.0
    hyponatremia 276.1
Anhydremia 276.52
  with
    hypernatremia 276.0
    hyponatremia 276.1
Anidrosis 705.0
Aniridia (congenital) 743.45
Anisakiasis (infection) (infestation) 127.1
Anisakis larva infestation 127.1
Aniseikonia 367.32
Anisocoria (pupil) 379.41
  congenital 743.46
Anisocytosis 790.09
Anisometropia (congenital) 367.31
Ankle - see condition
Ankyloblepharon (acquired) (eyelid) 374.46
  filiforme (adnatum) (congenital) 743.62
  total 743.62
Ankylodactly (see also Syndactylism) 755.10
Ankyloglossia 750.0
Ankylosis (fibrous) (osseous) 718.50
  ankle 718.57
  any joint, produced by surgical fusion V45.4
  cricoarytenoid (cartilage) (joint) (larynx) 478.79
  dental 521.6
  ear ossicle NEC 385.22
    malleus 385.21
  elbow 718.52
  finger 718.54
  hip 718.55
  incostapedial joint (infectional) 385.22
  joint, produced by surgical fusion NEC V45.4
  knee 718.56
  lumbosacral (joint) 724.6
  malleus 385.21
  multiple sites 718.59
  postoperative (status) V45.4
  sacroiliac (joint) 724.6
  shoulder 718.51
  specified site NEC 718.58
  spine NEC 724.9
  surgical V45.4
  teeth, tooth (hard tissues) 521.6
  temporomandibular joint 524.61
  wrist 718.53
Ankylostoma - see Ancylostoma
Ankylostomiasis (intestinal) - see Ancylostomiasis
Ankylurethria (see also Stricture, urethra) 598.9
Annular - see also condition
  detachment, cervix 622.8
  organ or site, congenital NEC - see Distortion
  pancreas (congenital) 751.7

Anodontia (complete) (partial) (vera) 520.0
  with abnormal spacing 524.30
  acquired 525.10
    causing malocclusion 524.30
    due to
      caries 525.13
      extraction 525.10
      periodontal disease 525.12
      trauma 525.11
Anomaly, anomalous (congenital) (unspecified type) 759.9
  abdomen 759.9
  abdominal wall 756.70
  acoustic nerve 742.9
  adrenal (gland) 759.1
  Alder (-Reilly) (leukocyte granulation) 288.2
  alimentary tract 751.9
    lower 751.5
    specified type NEC 751.8
    upper (any part, except tongue) 750.9
      tongue 750.10
        specified type NEC 750.19
  alveolar 524.70
    ridge (process) 525.8
    specified NEC 524.79
  ankle (joint) 755.69
  anus, anal (canal) 751.5
  aorta, aortic 747.20
    arch 747.21
    coarctation (postductal) (preductal) 747.10
    cusp or valve NEC 746.9
    septum 745.0
    specified type NEC 747.29
  aorticopulmonary septum 745.0
  apertures, diaphragm 756.6
  appendix 751.5
  aqueduct of Sylvius 742.3
    with spina bifida (see also Spina bifida) 741.0●
  arm 755.50
    reduction (see also Deformity, reduction, upper limb) 755.20
  arteriovenous (congenital) (peripheral) NEC 747.60
    brain 747.81
    cerebral 747.81
    coronary 746.85
    gastrointestinal 747.61
      acquired - see Angiodysplasia
    lower limb 747.64
    renal 747.62
    specified site NEC 747.69
    spinal 747.82
    upper limb 747.63
  artery (see also Anomaly, peripheral vascular system) NEC 747.60
    brain 747.81
    cerebral 747.81
    coronary 746.85
    eye 743.9
    pulmonary 747.39
    renal 747.62
    retina 743.9
    umbilical 747.5
  arytenoepiglottic folds 748.3
  atrial
    bands 746.9
    folds 746.9
    septa 745.5
  atrioventricular
    canal 745.69
    common 745.69
    conduction 426.7
    excitation 426.7
    septum 745.4
  atrium - see Anomaly, atrial
  auditory canal 744.3
    specified type NEC 744.29
      with hearing impairment 744.02

Anomaly, anomalous (Continued)
  auricle
    ear 744.3
      causing impairment of hearing 744.02
    heart 746.9
      septum 745.5
  autosomes, autosomal NEC 758.5
  Axenfeld's 743.44
  back 759.9
  band
    atrial 746.9
    heart 746.9
    ventricular 746.9
  Bartholin's duct 750.9
  biliary duct or passage 751.60
    atresia 751.61
  bladder (neck) (sphincter) (trigone) 753.9
    specified type NEC 753.8
  blood vessel 747.9
    artery - see Anomaly, artery
    peripheral vascular - see Anomaly, peripheral vascular system
    vein - see Anomaly, vein
  bone NEC 756.9
    ankle 755.69
    arm 755.50
    chest 756.3
    cranium 756.0
    face 756.0
    finger 755.50
    foot 755.67
    forearm 755.50
    frontal 756.0
    head 756.0
    hip 755.63
    leg 755.60
    lumbosacral 756.10
    nose 748.1
    pelvic girdle 755.60
    rachitic 756.4
    rib 756.3
    shoulder girdle 755.50
    skull 756.0
      with
        anencephalus 740.0
        encephalocele 742.0
        hydrocephalus 742.3
          with spina bifida (see also Spina bifida) 741.0●
        microcephalus 742.1
    toe 755.66
  brain 742.9
    multiple 742.4
    reduction 742.2
    specified type NEC 742.4
    vessel 747.81
  branchial cleft NEC 744.49
    cyst 744.42
    fistula 744.41
    persistent 744.41
    sinus (external) (internal) 744.41
  breast 757.6
  broad ligament 752.10
    specified type NEC 752.19
  bronchus 748.3
  bulbar septum 745.0
  bulbus cordis 745.9
    persistent (in left ventricle) 745.8
  bursa 756.9
  canal of Nuck 752.9
  canthus 743.9
  capillary NEC (see also Anomaly, peripheral vascular system) 747.60
  cardiac 746.9
    septal closure 745.9
      acquired 429.71
    valve NEC 746.9
      pulmonary 746.00
      specified type NEC 746.89

Anomaly, anomalous (Continued)
  cardiovascular system 746.9
    complicating pregnancy, childbirth, or puerperium 648.5●
  carpus 755.50
  cartilage, trachea 748.3
  cartilaginous 756.9
  caruncle, lacrimal, lachrymal 743.9
  cascade stomach 750.7
  cauda equina 742.59
  cecum 751.5
  cerebral - see also Anomaly, brain vessels 747.81
  cerebrovascular system 747.81
  cervix (uterus) 752.40
    with doubling of vagina and uterus 752.2
    in pregnancy or childbirth 654.6●
      affecting fetus or newborn 763.89
    causing obstructed labor 660.2●
      affecting fetus or newborn 763.1
  Chédiak-Higashi (-Steinbrinck) (congenital gigantism of peroxidase granules) 288.2
  cheek 744.9
  chest (wall) 756.3
  chin 744.9
    specified type NEC 744.89
  chordae tendineae 746.9
  choroid 743.9
    plexus 742.9
  chromosomes, chromosomal 758.9
    13 (13-15) 758.1
    18 (16-18) 758.2
    21 or 22 758.0
    autosomes NEC (see also Abnormal, autosomes) 758.5
    deletion 758.39
    Christchurch 758.39
    D_1 758.1
    E_3 758.2
    G 758.0
    mitochondrial 758.9
    mosaics 758.89
    sex 758.81
      complement, XO 758.6
      complement, XXX 758.81
      complement, XXY 758.7
      complement, XYY 758.81
      gonadal dysgenesis 758.6
      Klinefelter's 758.7
      Turner's 758.6
    trisomy 21 758.0
  cilia 743.9
  circulatory system 747.9
    specified type NEC 747.89
  clavicle 755.51
  clitoris 752.40
  coccyx 756.10
  colon 751.5
  common duct 751.60
  communication
    coronary artery 746.85
    left ventricle with right atrium 745.4
  concha (ear) 744.3
  connection
    renal vessels with kidney 747.62
    total pulmonary venous 747.41
  connective tissue 756.9
    specified type NEC 756.89
  cornea 743.9
    shape 743.41
    size 743.41
    specified type NEC 743.49
  coronary
    artery 746.85
    vein 746.89
  cranium - see Anomaly, skull
  cricoid cartilage 748.3
  cushion, endocardial 745.60
    specified type NEC 745.69
  cystic duct 751.60

SECTION 1 INDEX TO DISEASES AND INJURIES / Anomaly, anomalous

Anomaly, anomalous (Continued)
- dental arch 524.20
  - specified NEC 524.29
- dental arch relationship 524.20
  - angle's class I 524.21
  - angle's class II 524.22
  - angle's class III 524.23
  - articulation
    - anterior 524.27
    - posterior 524.27
    - reverse 524.27
  - disto-occlusion 524.22
    - division I 524.22
    - division II 524.22
  - excessive horizontal overlap 524.26
  - interarch distance (excessive) (inadequate) 524.28
  - mesio-occlusion 524.23
  - neutro-occlusion 524.21
  - open
    - anterior occlusal relationship 524.24
    - posterior occlusal relationship 524.25
  - specified NEC 524.29
- dentition 520.6
- dentofacial NEC 524.9
  - functional 524.50
  - specified type NEC 524.89
- dermatoglyphic 757.2
- Descemet's membrane 743.9
  - specified type NEC 743.49
- development
  - cervix 752.40
  - vagina 752.40
  - vulva 752.40
- diaphragm, diaphragmatic (apertures) NEC 756.6
- digestive organ(s) or system 751.9
  - lower 751.5
  - specified type NEC 751.8
  - upper 750.9
- distribution, coronary artery 746.85
- ductus
  - arteriosus 747.0
  - Botalli 747.0
- duodenum 751.5
- dura 742.9
  - brain 742.4
  - spinal cord 742.59
- ear 744.3
  - causing impairment of hearing 744.00
    - specified type NEC 744.09
  - external 744.3
    - causing impairment of hearing 744.02
    - specified type NEC 744.29
  - inner (causing impairment of hearing) 744.05
  - middle, except ossicles (causing impairment of hearing) 744.03
    - ossicles 744.04
  - ossicles 744.04
  - prominent auricle 744.29
  - specified type NEC 744.29
  - with hearing impairment 744.09
- Ebstein's (heart) 746.2
  - tricuspid valve 746.2
- ectodermal 757.9
- Eisenmenger's (ventricular septal defect) 745.4
- ejaculatory duct 752.9
  - specified type NEC 752.89
- elbow (joint) 755.50
- endocardial cushion 745.60
  - specified type NEC 745.69
- endocrine gland NEC 759.2
- epididymis 752.9
- epiglottis 748.3
- esophagus 750.9
  - specified type NEC 750.4
- Eustachian tube 744.3
  - specified type NEC 744.24

Anomaly, anomalous (Continued)
- eye (any part) 743.9
  - adnexa 743.9
    - specified type NEC 743.69
  - anophthalmos 743.00
  - anterior
    - chamber and related structures 743.9
      - angle 743.9
        - specified type NEC 743.44
      - specified type NEC 743.44
    - segment 743.9
      - combined 743.48
      - multiple 743.48
      - specified type NEC 743.49
  - cataract (see also Cataract) 743.30
  - glaucoma (see also Buphthalmia) 743.20
  - lid 743.9
    - specified type NEC 743.63
  - microphthalmos (see also Microphthalmos) 743.10
  - posterior segment 743.9
    - specified type NEC 743.59
    - vascular 743.58
    - vitreous 743.9
      - specified type NEC 743.51
  - ptosis (eyelid) 743.61
  - retina 743.9
    - specified type NEC 743.59
  - sclera 743.9
    - specified type NEC 743.47
  - specified type NEC 743.8
- eyebrow 744.89
- eyelid 743.9
  - specified type NEC 743.63
- face (any part) 744.9
  - bone(s) 756.0
  - specified type NEC 744.89
- fallopian tube 752.10
  - specified type NEC 752.19
- fascia 756.9
  - specified type NEC 756.89
- femur 755.60
- fibula 755.60
- finger 755.50
  - supernumerary 755.01
  - webbed (see also Syndactylism, fingers) 755.11
- fixation, intestine 751.4
- flexion (joint) 755.9
  - hip or thigh (see also Dislocation, hip, congenital) 754.30
- folds, heart 746.9
- foot 755.67
- foramen
  - Botalli 745.5
  - ovale 745.5
- forearm 755.50
- forehead (see also Anomaly, skull) 756.0
- form, teeth 520.2
- fovea centralis 743.9
- frontal bone (see also Anomaly, skull) 756.0
- gallbladder 751.60
- Gartner's duct 752.41
- gastrointestinal tract 751.9
  - specified type NEC 751.8
  - vessel 747.61
- genitalia, genital organ(s) or system
  - female 752.9
    - external 752.40
      - specified type NEC 752.49
    - internal NEC 752.9
  - male (external and internal) 752.9
    - epispadias 752.62
    - hidden penis 752.65
    - hydrocele, congenital 778.6
    - hypospadias 752.61
    - micropenis 752.64
    - testis, undescended 752.51
      - retractile 752.52
    - specified type NEC 752.89
- genitourinary NEC 752.9

Anomaly, anomalous (Continued)
- Gerbode 745.4
- globe (eye) 743.9
- glottis 748.3
- granulation or granulocyte, genetic 288.2
  - constitutional 288.2
  - leukocyte 288.2
- gum 750.9
- gyri 742.9
- hair 757.9
  - specified type NEC 757.4
- hand 755.50
- hard tissue formation in pulp 522.3
- head (see also Anomaly, skull) 756.0
- heart 746.9
  - auricle 746.9
  - bands 746.9
  - fibroelastosis cordis 425.3
  - folds 746.9
  - malposition 746.87
  - maternal, affecting fetus or newborn 760.3
  - obstructive NEC 746.84
  - patent ductus arteriosus (Botalli) 747.0
  - septum 745.9
    - acquired 429.71
    - aortic 745.0
    - aorticopulmonary 745.0
    - atrial 745.5
    - auricular 745.5
    - between aorta and pulmonary artery 745.0
    - endocardial cushion type 745.60
      - specified type NEC 745.69
    - interatrial 745.5
    - interventricular 745.4
      - with pulmonary stenosis or atresia, dextraposition of aorta, and hypertrophy of right ventricle 745.2
      - acquired 429.71
    - specified type NEC 745.8
    - ventricular 745.4
      - with pulmonary stenosis or atresia, dextraposition of aorta, and hypertrophy of right ventricle 745.2
      - acquired 429.71
  - specified type NEC 746.89
  - tetralogy of Fallot 745.2
  - valve NEC 746.9
    - aortic 746.9
      - atresia 746.89
      - bicuspid valve 746.4
      - insufficiency 746.4
      - specified type NEC 746.89
      - stenosis 746.3
        - subaortic 746.81
        - supravalvular 747.22
    - mitral 746.9
      - atresia 746.89
      - insufficiency 746.6
      - specified type NEC 746.89
      - stenosis 746.5
    - pulmonary 746.00
      - atresia 746.01
      - insufficiency 746.09
      - stenosis 746.02
        - infundibular 746.83
        - subvalvular 746.83
    - tricuspid 746.9
      - atresia 746.1
      - stenosis 746.1
  - ventricle 746.9
- heel 755.67
- Hegglin's 288.2
- hemianencephaly 740.0
- hemicephaly 740.0
- hemicrania 740.0

SECTION I INDEX TO DISEASES AND INJURIES / Anomaly, anomalous

Anomaly, anomalous (Continued)
  hepatic duct 751.60
  hip (joint) 755.63
  hourglass
    bladder 753.8
    gallbladder 751.69
    stomach 750.7
  humerus 755.50
  hymen 752.40
  hypersegmentation of neutrophils, hereditary 288.2
  hypophyseal 759.2
  ileocecal (coil) (valve) 751.5
  ileum (intestine) 751.5
  ilium 755.60
  integument 757.9
    specified type NEC 757.8
  interarch distance (excessive) (inadequate) 524.28
  intervertebral cartilage or disc 756.10
  intestine (large) (small) 751.5
    fixational type 751.4
  iris 743.9
    specified type NEC 743.46
  ischium 755.60
  jaw NEC 524.9
    closure 524.51
    size (major) NEC 524.00
    specified type NEC 524.89
  jaw-cranial base relationship 524.10
    specified NEC 524.19
  jejunum 751.5
  joint 755.9
    hip
      dislocation (see also Dislocation, hip, congenital) 754.30
      predislocation (see also Subluxation, congenital, hip) 754.32
      preluxation (see also Subluxation, congenital, hip) 754.32
      subluxation (see also Subluxation, congenital, hip) 754.32
    lumbosacral 756.10
      spondylolisthesis 756.12
      spondylosis 756.11
    multiple arthrogryposis 754.89
    sacroiliac 755.69
  Jordan's 288.2
  kidney(s) (calyx) (pelvis) 753.9
    vessel 747.62
  Klippel-Feil (brevicollis) 756.16
  knee (joint) 755.64
  labium (majus) (minus) 752.40
  labyrinth, membranous (causing impairment of hearing) 744.05
  lacrimal
    apparatus, duct or passage 743.9
      specified type NEC 743.65
    gland 743.9
      specified type NEC 743.64
  Langdon Down (mongolism) 758.0
  larynx, laryngeal (muscle) 748.3
    web, webbed 748.2
  leg (lower) (upper) 755.60
    reduction NEC (see also Deformity, reduction, lower limb) 755.30
  lens 743.9
    shape 743.36
    specified type NEC 743.39
  leukocytes, genetic 288.2
    granulation (constitutional) 288.2
  lid (fold) 743.9
  ligament 756.9
    broad 752.10
    round 752.9
  limb, except reduction deformity 755.8
    lower 755.60
      reduction deformity (see also Deformity, reduction, lower limb) 755.30
      specified type NEC 755.69

Anomaly, anomalous (Continued)
  limb (Continued)
    upper 755.50
      reduction deformity (see also Deformity, reduction, upper limb) 755.20
      specified type NEC 755.59
  lip 750.9
    harelip (see also Cleft, lip) 749.10
    specified type NEC 750.26
  liver (duct) 751.60
    atresia 751.69
  lower extremity 755.60
    vessel 747.64
  lumbosacral (joint) (region) 756.10
  lung (fissure) (lobe) NEC 748.60
    agenesis 748.5
    specified type NEC 748.69
  lymphatic system 759.9
  Madelung's (radius) 755.54
  mandible 524.9
    size NEC 524.00
  maxilla 524.90
    size NEC 524.00
  May (-Hegglin) 288.2
  meatus urinarius 753.9
    specified type NEC 753.8
  meningeal bands or folds, constriction of 742.8
  meninges 742.9
    brain 742.4
    spinal 742.59
  meningocele (see also Spina bifida) 741.9●
    acquired 349.2
  mesentery 751.9
  metacarpus 755.50
  metatarsus 755.67
  middle ear, except ossicles (causing impairment of hearing) 744.03
    ossicles 744.04
  mitral (leaflets) (valve) 746.9
    atresia 746.89
    insufficiency 746.6
    specified type NEC 746.89
    stenosis 746.5
  mouth 750.9
    specified type NEC 750.26
  multiple NEC 759.7
    specified type NEC 759.89
  muscle 756.9
    eye 743.9
      specified type NEC 743.69
    specified type NEC 756.89
  musculoskeletal system, except limbs 756.9
    specified type NEC 756.9
  nail 757.9
    specified type NEC 757.5
  narrowness, eyelid 743.62
  nasal sinus or septum 748.1
  neck (any part) 744.9
    specified type NEC 744.89
  nerve 742.9
    acoustic 742.9
      specified type NEC 742.8
    optic 742.9
      specified type NEC 742.8
    specified type NEC 742.8
  nervous system NEC 742.9
    brain 742.9
      specified type NEC 742.4
    specified type NEC 742.8
  neurological 742.9
  nipple 757.6
  nonteratogenic NEC 754.89
  nose, nasal (bone) (cartilage) (septum) (sinus) 748.1
  ocular muscle 743.9
  omphalomesenteric duct 751.0
  opening, pulmonary veins 747.49

Anomaly, anomalous (Continued)
  optic
    disc 743.9
      specified type NEC 743.57
    nerve 742.9
  opticociliary vessels 743.9
  orbit (eye) 743.9
    specified type NEC 743.66
  organ
    of Corti (causing impairment of hearing) 744.05
    or site 759.9
      specified type NEC 759.89
  origin
    both great arteries from same ventricle 745.11
    coronary artery 746.85
    innominate artery 747.69
    left coronary artery from pulmonary artery 746.85
    pulmonary artery 747.39
    renal vessels 747.62
    subclavian artery (left) (right) 747.21
  osseous meatus (ear) 744.03
  ovary 752.0
  oviduct 752.10
  palate (hard) (soft) 750.9
    cleft (see also Cleft, palate) 749.00
  pancreas (duct) 751.7
  papillary muscles 746.9
  parathyroid gland 759.2
  paraurethral ducts 753.9
  parotid (gland) 750.9
  patella 755.64
  Pelger-Huët (hereditary hyposegmentation) 288.2
  pelvic girdle 755.60
    specified type NEC 755.69
  pelvis (bony) 755.60
    complicating delivery 653.0●
    rachitic 268.1
      fetal 756.4
  penis (glans) 752.69
  pericardium 746.89
  peripheral vascular system NEC 747.60
    gastrointestinal 747.61
    lower limb 747.64
    renal 747.62
    specified site NEC 747.69
    spinal 747.82
    upper limb 747.63
  Peter's 743.44
  pharynx 750.9
    branchial cleft 744.41
    specified type NEC 750.29
  Pierre Robin 756.0
  pigmentation 709.00
    congenital 757.33
    specified NEC 709.09
  pituitary (gland) 759.2
  pleural folds 748.8
  portal vein 747.40
  position tooth, teeth 524.30
    crowding 524.31
    displacement 524.30
      horizontal 524.33
      vertical 524.34
    distance
      interocclusal
        excessive 524.37
        insufficient 524.36
    excessive spacing 524.32
    rotation 524.35
    specified NEC 524.39
  preauricular sinus 744.46
  prepuce 752.9
  prostate 752.9
  pulmonary 748.60
    artery 747.39
    circulation 747.39

SECTION 1 INDEX TO DISEASES AND INJURIES / Anomaly, anomalous

Anomaly, anomalous (Continued)
- pulmonary (Continued)
  - specified type NEC 748.69
  - valve 746.00
    - atresia 746.01
    - insufficiency 746.09
    - specified type NEC 746.09
    - stenosis 746.02
      - infundibular 746.83
      - subvalvular 746.83
  - vein 747.40
  - venous
    - connection 747.49
      - partial 747.42
      - total 747.41
    - return 747.49
      - partial 747.42
      - total (TAPVR) (complete) (subdiaphragmatic) (supradiaphragmatic) 747.41
- pupil 743.9
- pylorus 750.9
  - hypertrophy 750.5
  - stenosis 750.5
- rachitic, fetal 756.4
- radius 755.50
- rectovaginal (septum) 752.40
- rectum 751.5
- refraction 367.9
- renal 753.9
  - vessel 747.62
- respiratory system 748.9
  - specified type NEC 748.8
- rib 756.3
  - cervical 756.2
- Rieger's 743.44
- rings, trachea 748.3
- rotation - see also Malrotation
  - hip or thigh (see also Subluxation, congenital, hip) 754.32
- round ligament 752.9
- sacroiliac (joint) 755.69
- sacrum 756.10
- saddle
  - back 754.2
  - nose 754.0
    - syphilitic 090.5
- salivary gland or duct 750.9
  - specified type NEC 750.26
- scapula 755.50
- sclera 743.9
  - specified type NEC 743.47
- scrotum 752.9
- sebaceous gland 757.9
- seminal duct or tract 752.9
- sense organs 742.9
  - specified type NEC 742.8
- septum
  - heart - see Anomaly, heart, septum
  - nasal 748.1
- sex chromosomes NEC (see also Anomaly, chromosomes) 758.81
- shoulder (girdle) (joint) 755.50
  - specified type NEC 755.59
- sigmoid (flexure) 751.5
- sinus of Valsalva 747.29
- site NEC 759.9
- skeleton generalized NEC 756.50
- skin (appendage) 757.9
  - specified type NEC 757.39
- skull (bone) 756.0
  - with
    - anencephalus 740.0
    - encephalocele 742.0
    - hydrocephalus 742.3
      - with spina bifida (see also Spina bifida) 741.0●
    - microcephalus 742.1

Anomaly, anomalous (Continued)
- specified type NEC
  - adrenal (gland) 759.1
  - alimentary tract (complete) (partial) 751.8
    - lower 751.5
    - upper 750.8
  - ankle 755.69
  - anus, anal (canal) 751.5
  - aorta, aortic 747.29
    - arch 747.21
  - appendix 751.5
  - arm 755.59
  - artery (peripheral) NEC (see also Anomaly, peripheral vascular system) 747.60
    - brain 747.81
    - coronary 746.85
    - eye 743.58
    - pulmonary 747.39
    - retinal 743.58
    - umbilical 747.5
  - auditory canal 744.29
    - causing impairment of hearing 744.02
  - bile duct or passage 751.69
  - bladder 753.8
    - neck 753.8
  - bone(s) 756.9
    - arm 755.59
    - face 756.0
    - leg 755.69
    - pelvic girdle 755.69
    - shoulder girdle 755.59
    - skull 756.0
      - with
        - anencephalus 740.0
        - encephalocele 742.0
        - hydrocephalus 742.3
          - with spina bifida (see also Spina bifida) 741.0●
        - microcephalus 742.1
  - brain 742.4
  - breast 757.6
  - broad ligament 752.19
  - bronchus 748.3
  - canal of Nuck 752.89
  - cardiac septal closure 745.8
  - carpus 755.59
  - cartilaginous 756.9
  - cecum 751.5
  - cervix 752.49
  - chest (wall) 756.3
  - chin 744.89
  - ciliary body 743.46
  - circulatory system 747.89
  - clavicle 755.51
  - clitoris 752.49
  - coccyx 756.19
  - colon 751.5
  - common duct 751.69
  - connective tissue 756.89
  - cricoid cartilage 748.3
  - cystic duct 751.69
  - diaphragm 756.6
  - digestive organ(s) or tract 751.8
    - lower 751.5
    - upper 750.8
  - duodenum 751.5
  - ear 744.29
    - auricle 744.29
      - causing impairment of hearing 744.02
    - causing impairment of hearing 744.09
    - inner (causing impairment of hearing) 744.05
    - middle, except ossicles 744.03
      - ossicles 744.04
  - ejaculatory duct 752.89
  - endocrine 759.2
  - epiglottis 748.3
  - esophagus 750.4
  - eustachian tube 744.24

Anomaly, anomalous (Continued)
- specified type NEC (Continued)
  - eye 743.8
    - lid 743.63
    - muscle 743.69
  - face 744.89
    - bone(s) 756.0
  - fallopian tube 752.19
  - fascia 756.89
  - femur 755.69
  - fibula 755.69
  - finger 755.59
  - foot 755.67
  - fovea centralis 743.55
  - gallbladder 751.69
  - Gartner's duct 752.89
  - gastrointestinal tract 751.8
  - genitalia, genital organ(s)
    - female 752.89
      - external 752.49
      - internal NEC 752.89
    - male 752.89
      - penis 752.69
      - scrotal transposition 752.81
  - genitourinary tract NEC 752.89
  - glottis 748.3
  - hair 757.4
  - hand 755.59
  - heart 746.89
    - valve NEC 746.89
      - pulmonary 746.09
  - hepatic duct 751.69
  - hydatid of Morgagni 752.89
  - hymen 752.49
  - integument 757.8
  - intestine (large) (small) 751.5
    - fixational type 751.4
  - iris 743.46
  - jejunum 751.5
  - joint 755.8
  - kidney 753.3
  - knee 755.64
  - labium (majus) (minus) 752.49
  - labyrinth, membranous 744.05
  - larynx 748.3
  - leg 755.69
  - lens 743.39
  - limb, except reduction deformity 755.8
    - lower 755.69
      - reduction deformity (see also Deformity, reduction, lower limb) 755.30
    - upper 755.59
      - reduction deformity (see also Deformity, reduction, upper limb) 755.20
  - lip 750.26
  - liver 751.69
  - lung (fissure) (lobe) 748.69
  - meatus urinarius 753.8
  - metacarpus 755.59
  - mouth 750.26
  - Müllerian
    - cervix 752.49
    - uterus 752.39
    - vagina 752.49
  - muscle 756.89
    - eye 743.69
  - musculoskeletal system, except limbs 756.9
  - nail 757.5
  - neck 744.89
  - nerve 742.8
    - acoustic 742.8
    - optic 742.8
  - nervous system 742.8
  - nipple 757.6
  - nose 748.1
  - organ NEC 759.89
    - of Corti 744.05
  - osseous meatus (ear) 744.03

SECTION I INDEX TO DISEASES AND INJURIES / Anosognosia

Anomaly, anomalous *(Continued)*
　　specified type NEC *(Continued)*
　　　ovary 752.0
　　　oviduct 752.19
　　　pancreas 751.7
　　　parathyroid 759.2
　　　patella 755.64
　　　pelvic girdle 755.69
　　　penis 752.69
　　　pericardium 746.89
　　　peripheral vascular system NEC *(see also* Anomaly, peripheral vascular system) 747.60
　　　pharynx 750.29
　　　pituitary 759.2
　　　prostate 752.89
　　　radius 755.59
　　　rectum 751.5
　　　respiratory system 748.8
　　　rib 756.3
　　　round ligament 752.89
　　　sacrum 756.19
　　　salivary duct or gland 750.26
　　　scapula 755.59
　　　sclera 743.47
　　　scrotum 752.89
　　　　transposition 752.81
　　　seminal duct or tract 752.89
　　　shoulder girdle 755.59
　　　site NEC 759.89
　　　skin 757.39
　　　skull (bone(s)) 756.0
　　　　with
　　　　　anencephalus 740.0
　　　　　encephalocele 742.0
　　　　　hydrocephalus 742.3
　　　　　　with spina bifida *(see also* Spina bifida) 741.0●
　　　　　microcephalus 742.1
　　　specified organ or site NEC 759.89
　　　spermatic cord 752.89
　　　spinal cord 742.59
　　　spine 756.19
　　　spleen 759.0
　　　sternum 756.3
　　　stomach 750.7
　　　tarsus 755.67
　　　tendon 756.89
　　　testis 752.89
　　　thorax (wall) 756.3
　　　thymus 759.2
　　　thyroid (gland) 759.2
　　　　cartilage 748.3
　　　tibia 755.69
　　　toe 755.66
　　　tongue 750.19
　　　trachea (cartilage) 748.3
　　　ulna 755.59
　　　urachus 753.7
　　　ureter 753.4
　　　　obstructive 753.29
　　　urethra 753.8
　　　　obstructive 753.6
　　　urinary tract 753.8
　　　uterus (Müllerian) 752.39
　　　uvula 750.26
　　　vagina 752.49
　　　vascular NEC *(see also* Anomaly, peripheral vascular system) 747.60
　　　　brain 747.81
　　　vas deferens 752.89
　　　vein(s) (peripheral) NEC *(see also* Anomaly, peripheral vascular system) 747.60
　　　　brain 747.81
　　　　great 747.49
　　　　portal 747.49
　　　　pulmonary 747.49
　　　vena cava (inferior) (superior) 747.49
　　　vertebra 756.19
　　　vulva 752.49

Anomaly, anomalous *(Continued)*
　　spermatic cord 752.9
　　spine, spinal 756.10
　　　column 756.10
　　　cord 742.9
　　　　meningocele *(see also* Spina bifida) 741.9●
　　　　specified type NEC 742.59
　　　　spina bifida *(see also* Spina bifida) 741.9●
　　　　vessel 747.82
　　　meninges 742.59
　　　nerve root 742.9
　　spleen 759.0
　　Sprengel's 755.52
　　sternum 756.3
　　stomach 750.9
　　　specified type NEC 750.7
　　submaxillary gland 750.9
　　superior vena cava 747.40
　　talipes - *see* Talipes
　　tarsus 755.67
　　　with complete absence of distal elements 755.31
　　teeth, tooth NEC 520.9
　　　position 524.30
　　　　crowding 524.31
　　　　displacement 524.30
　　　　　horizontal 524.33
　　　　　vertical 524.34
　　　　distance
　　　　　interocclusal
　　　　　　excessive 524.37
　　　　　　insufficient 524.36
　　　　excessive spacing 524.32
　　　　rotation 524.35
　　　　specified NEC 524.39
　　　spacing 524.30
　　tendon 756.9
　　　specified type NEC 756.89
　　termination
　　　coronary artery 746.85
　　testis 752.9
　　thebesian valve 746.9
　　thigh 755.60
　　　flexion *(see also* Subluxation, congenital, hip) 754.32
　　thorax (wall) 756.3
　　throat 750.9
　　thumb 755.50
　　　supernumerary 755.01
　　thymus gland 759.2
　　thyroid (gland) 759.2
　　　cartilage 748.3
　　tibia 755.60
　　　saber 090.5
　　toe 755.66
　　　supernumerary 755.02
　　　webbed *(see also* Syndactylism, toes) 755.13
　　tongue 750.10
　　　specified type NEC 750.19
　　trachea, tracheal 748.3
　　　cartilage 748.3
　　　rings 748.3
　　tragus 744.3
　　transverse aortic arch 747.21
　　trichromata 368.59
　　trichromatopsia 368.59
　　tricuspid (leaflet) (valve) 746.9
　　　atresia 746.1
　　　Ebstein's 746.2
　　　specified type NEC 746.89
　　　stenosis 746.1
　　trunk 759.9
　　Uhl's (hypoplasia of myocardium, right ventricle) 746.84
　　ulna 755.50
　　umbilicus 759.9
　　　artery 747.5
　　union, trachea with larynx 748.3

Anomaly, anomalous *(Continued)*
　　unspecified site 759.9
　　upper extremity 755.50
　　　vessel 747.63
　　urachus 753.7
　　　specified type NEC 753.7
　　ureter 753.9
　　　obstructive 753.20
　　　specified type NEC 753.4
　　　　obstructive 753.29
　　urethra (valve) 753.9
　　　obstructive 753.6
　　　specified type NEC 753.8
　　urinary tract or system (any part, except urachus) 753.9
　　　specified type NEC 753.8
　　　urachus 753.7
　　uterus 752.39
　　　with only one functioning horn 752.33
　　　in pregnancy or childbirth 654.0●
　　　　affecting fetus or newborn 763.89
　　　　causing obstructed labor 660.2●
　　　　　affecting fetus or newborn 763.1
　　uvula 750.9
　　vagina 752.40
　　valleculae 748.3
　　valve (heart) NEC 746.9
　　　formation, ureter 753.29
　　　pulmonary 746.00
　　　specified type NEC 746.89
　　vascular NEC *(see also* Anomaly, peripheral vascular system) 747.60
　　　ring 747.21
　　vas deferens 752.9
　　vein(s) (peripheral) NEC *(see also* Anomaly, peripheral vascular system) 747.60
　　　brain 747.81
　　　cerebral 747.81
　　　coronary 746.89
　　　great 747.40
　　　　specified type NEC 747.49
　　　portal 747.40
　　　pulmonary 747.40
　　　retina 743.9
　　vena cava (inferior) (superior) 747.40
　　venous - *see* Anomaly, vein
　　venous return (pulmonary) 747.49
　　　partial 747.42
　　　total 747.41
　　ventricle, ventricular (heart) 746.9
　　　bands 746.9
　　　folds 746.9
　　　septa 745.4
　　vertebra 756.10
　　vesicourethral orifice 753.9
　　vessels NEC *(see also* Anomaly, peripheral vascular system) 747.60
　　　optic papilla 743.9
　　vitelline duct 751.0
　　vitreous humor 743.9
　　　specified type NEC 743.51
　　vulva 752.40
　　wrist (joint) 755.50

Anomia 784.69
Anonychia 757.5
　　acquired 703.8
Anophthalmos, anophthalmus (clinical) (congenital) (globe) 743.00
　　acquired V45.78
Anopsia (altitudinal) (quadrant) 368.46
Anorchia 752.89
Anorchism, anorchidism 752.89
Anorexia 783.0
　　hysterical 300.11
　　nervosa 307.1
Anosmia *(see also* Disturbance, sensation) 781.1
　　hysterical 300.11
　　postinfectional 478.9
　　psychogenic 306.7
　　traumatic 951.8
Anosognosia 780.99

Anosphrasia 781.1
Anosteoplasia 756.50
Anotia 744.09
Anovulatory cycle 628.0
Anoxemia 799.02
   newborn 770.88
Anoxia 799.02
   altitude 993.2
   cerebral 348.1
      with
         abortion - see Abortion, by type, with specified complication NEC
         ectopic pregnancy (see also categories 633.0-633.9) 639.8
         molar pregnancy (see also categories 630-632) 639.8
      complicating
         delivery (cesarean) (instrumental) 669.4●
         ectopic or molar pregnancy 639.8
         obstetric anesthesia or sedation 668.2●
      during or resulting from a procedure 997.01
      following
         abortion 639.8
         ectopic or molar pregnancy 639.8
      newborn (see also Distress, fetal, liveborn infant) 770.88
   due to drowning 994.1
   fetal, affecting newborn 770.88
   heart - see Insufficiency, coronary
   high altitude 993.2
   intrauterine
      fetal death (before onset of labor) 768.0
      during labor 768.1
   liveborn infant - see Distress, fetal, liveborn infant
   myocardial - see Insufficiency, coronary
   newborn 768.9
      mild or moderate 768.6
      severe 768.5
   pathological 799.02
Anteflexion - see Anteversion
Antenatal
   care, normal pregnancy V22.1
      first V22.0
   sampling
      chorionic villus V28.89
   screening of mother (for) V28.9
      based on amniocentesis NEC V28.2
         chromosomal anomalies V28.0
         raised alphafetoprotein levels V28.1
      chromosomal anomalies V28.0
      fetal growth retardation using ultrasonics V28.4
      genomic V28.89
      isoimmunization V28.5
      malformations using ultrasonics V28.3
      proteomic V28.89
      raised alphafetoprotein levels in amniotic fluid V28.1
      risk
         pre-term labor V28.82
      specified condition NEC V28.89
      Streptococcus B V28.6
   survey
      fetal anatomic V28.81
   testing
      nuchal translucency V28.89
Antepartum - see condition
Anterior - see also condition
   spinal artery compression syndrome 721.1
Antero-occlusion 524.24
Anteversion
   cervix - see Anteversion, uterus
   femur (neck), congenital 755.63

Anteversion (Continued)
   uterus, uterine (cervix) (postinfectional) (postpartal, old) 621.6
      congenital 752.39
      in pregnancy or childbirth 654.4●
         affecting fetus or newborn 763.89
         causing obstructed labor 660.2●
            affecting fetus or newborn 763.1
Anthracosilicosis (occupational) 500
Anthracosis (lung) (occupational) 500
   lingua 529.3
Anthrax 022.9
   with pneumonia 022.1 [484.5]
   colitis 022.2
   cutaneous 022.0
   gastrointestinal 022.2
   intestinal 022.2
   pulmonary 022.1
   respiratory 022.1
   septicemia 022.3
   specified manifestation NEC 022.8
Anthropoid pelvis 755.69
   with disproportion (fetopelvic) 653.2●
      affecting fetus or newborn 763.1
      causing obstructed labor 660.1●
         affecting fetus or newborn 763.1
Anthropophobia 300.29
Antibioma, breast 611.0
Antibodies
   maternal (blood group) (see also Incompatibility) 656.2●
   anti-D, cord blood 656.1●
      fetus or newborn 773.0
Antibody
   anticardiolipin 795.79
      with
         hemorrhagic disorder 286.53
         hypercoagulable state 289.81
   antiphosphatidylglycerol 795.79
      with
         hemorrhagic disorder 286.53
         hypercoagulable state 289.81
   antiphosphatidylinositol 795.79
      with
         hemorrhagic disorder 286.53
         hypercoagulable state 289.81
   antiphosphatidylserine 795.79
      with
         hemorrhagic disorder 286.53
         hypercoagulable state 289.81
   antiphospholipid 795.79
      with
         hemorrhagic disorder 286.53
         hypercoagulable state 289.81
   deficiency syndrome
      agammaglobulinemic 279.00
      congenital 279.04
      hypogammaglobulinemic 279.00
Anticoagulant
   intrinsic, circulating, causing hemorrhagic disorder (see also Circulating, anticoagulants) 286.59
   lupus (LAC) 795.79
      with
         hemorrhagic disorder 286.53
         hypercoagulable state 289.81
Antimongolism syndrome 758.39
Antimonial cholera 985.4
Antisocial personality 301.7
Antithrombinemia (see also Circulating anticoagulants) 286.59
Antithromboplastinemia (see also Circulating anticoagulants) 286.59
Antithromboplastinogenemia (see also Circulating anticoagulants) 286.59
Antitoxin complication or reaction - see Complications, vaccination
Anton (-Babinski) syndrome (hemiasomatognosia) 307.9

Antritis (chronic) 473.0
   maxilla 473.0
      acute 461.0
   stomach 535.4●
Antrum, antral - see condition
Anuria 788.5
   with
      abortion - see Abortion, by type, with renal failure
      ectopic pregnancy (see also categories 633.0-633.9) 639.3
      molar pregnancy (see also categories 630-632) 639.3
   calculus (impacted) (recurrent) 592.9
      kidney 592.0
      ureter 592.1
   congenital 753.3
   due to a procedure 997.5
   following
      abortion 639.3
      ectopic or molar pregnancy 639.3
   newborn 753.3
   postrenal 593.4
   puerperal, postpartum, childbirth 669.3●
   specified as due to a procedure 997.5
   sulfonamide
      correct substance properly administered 788.5
      overdose or wrong substance given or taken 961.0
   traumatic (following crushing) 958.5
Anus, anal - see also condition
   high risk human papillomavirus (HPV) DNA test positive 796.75
   low risk human papillomavirus (HPV) DNA test positive 796.79
Anusitis 569.49
Anxiety (neurosis) (reaction) (state) 300.00
   alcohol-induced 291.89
   depression 300.4
   drug-induced 292.89
   due to or associated with physical condition 293.84
   generalized 300.02
   hysteria 300.20
   in
      acute stress reaction 308.0
      transient adjustment reaction 309.24
   panic type 300.01
   separation, abnormal 309.21
   syndrome (organic) (transient) 293.84
Aorta, aortic - see condition
Aortectasia (see also Ectasia, aortic) 447.70
   with aneurysm 441.9
Aortitis (nonsyphilitic) 447.6
   arteriosclerotic 440.0
   calcific 447.6
   Döhle-Heller 093.1
   luetic 093.1
   rheumatic (see also Endocarditis, acute, rheumatic) 391.1
   rheumatoid - see Arthritis, rheumatoid
   specific 093.1
   syphilitic 093.1
      congenital 090.5
Apathetic 799.25
   thyroid storm (see also Thyrotoxicosis) 242.9●
Apathy 799.25
Apepsia 536.8
   achlorhydric 536.0
   psychogenic 306.4
Aperistalsis, esophagus 530.0
Apert's syndrome (acrocephalosyndactyly) 755.55
Apert-Gallais syndrome (adrenogenital) 255.2
Apertognathia 524.20
Aphagia 787.20
   psychogenic 307.1
Aphakia (acquired) (bilateral) (postoperative) (unilateral) 379.31
   congenital 743.35

SECTION 1 INDEX TO DISEASES AND INJURIES / Appetite

Aphalangia (congenital) 755.4
   lower limb (complete) (intercalary) (partial) (terminal) 755.39
      meaning all digits (complete) (partial) 755.31
      transverse 755.31
   upper limb (complete) (intercalary) (partial) (terminal) 755.29
      meaning all digits (complete) (partial) 755.21
      transverse 755.21
Aphasia (amnestic) (ataxic) (auditory) (Broca's) (choreatic) (classic) (expressive) (global) (ideational) (ideokinetic) (ideomotor) (jargon) (motor) (nominal) (receptive) (semantic) (sensory) (syntactic) (verbal) (visual) (Wernicke's) 784.3
   developmental 315.31
   syphilis, tertiary 094.89
   uremic - see Uremia
Aphemia 784.3
   uremic - see Uremia
Aphonia 784.41
   clericorum 784.49
   hysterical 300.11
   organic 784.41
   psychogenic 306.1
Aphthae, aphthous - see also condition
   Bednar's 528.2
   cachectic 529.0
   epizootic 078.4
   fever 078.4
   oral 528.2
   stomatitis 528.2
   thrush 112.0
   ulcer (oral) (recurrent) 528.2
      genital organ(s) NEC
         female 616.50
         male 608.89
      larynx 478.79
Apical - see condition
Apical ballooning syndrome 429.83
Aplasia - see also Agenesis
   alveolar process (acquired) 525.8
      congenital 750.26
   aorta (congenital) 747.22
   aortic valve (congenital) 746.89
   axialis extracorticalis (congenital) 330.0
   bone marrow (myeloid) 284.9
      acquired (secondary) 284.89
      congenital 284.01
      idiopathic 284.9
   brain 740.0
      specified part 742.2
   breast 757.6
   bronchus 748.3
   cementum 520.4
   cerebellar 742.2
   congenital (pure) red cell 284.01
   corpus callosum 742.2
   erythrocyte 284.81
      congenital 284.01
   extracortical axial 330.0
   eye (congenital) 743.00
   fovea centralis (congenital) 743.55
   germinal (cell) 606.0
   iris 743.45
   labyrinth, membranous 744.05
   limb (congenital) 755.4
      lower NEC 755.30
      upper NEC 755.20
   lung (bilateral) (congenital) (unilateral) 748.5
   nervous system NEC 742.8
   nuclear 742.8
   ovary 752.0
   Pelizaeus-Merzbacher 330.0
   prostate (congenital) 752.89
   red cell (with thymoma) 284.81
      acquired (secondary) 284.81
         due to drugs 284.81
      adult 284.81

Aplasia (Continued)
   red cell (Continued)
      congenital 284.01
      hereditary 284.01
      of infants 284.01
      primary 284.01
      pure 284.01
         due to drugs 284.81
   round ligament (congenital) 752.89
   salivary gland 750.21
   skin (congenital) 757.39
   spinal cord 742.59
   spleen 759.0
   testis (congenital) 752.89
   thymic, with immunodeficiency 279.2
   thyroid 243
   uterus 752.39
   ventral horn cell 742.59
Apleuria 756.3
Apnea, apneic (spells) 786.03
   newborn, neonatorum 770.81
      essential 770.81
      obstructive 770.82
      primary 770.81
      sleep 770.81
      specified NEC 770.82
   psychogenic 306.1
   sleep 780.57
      with
         hypersomnia, unspecified 780.53
         hyposomnia, unspecified 780.51
         insomnia, unspecified 780.51
         sleep disturbance 780.57
      central, in conditions classified elsewhere 327.27
      obstructive (adult) (pediatric) 327.23
      organic 327.20
         other 327.29
      primary central 327.21
Apneumatosis newborn 770.4
Apodia 755.31
Apophysitis (bone) (see also Osteochondrosis) 732.9
   calcaneus 732.5
   juvenile 732.6
Apoplectiform convulsions (see also Disease, cerebrovascular, acute) 436
Apoplexia, apoplexy, apoplectic (see also Disease, cerebrovascular, acute) 436
   abdominal 569.89
   adrenal 036.3
   attack 436
   basilar (see also Disease, cerebrovascular, acute) 436
   brain (see also Disease, cerebrovascular, acute) 436
   bulbar (see also Disease, cerebrovascular, acute) 436
   capillary (see also Disease, cerebrovascular, acute) 436
   cardiac (see also Infarct, myocardium) 410.9●
   cerebral (see also Disease, cerebrovascular, acute) 436
   chorea (see also Disease, cerebrovascular, acute) 436
   congestive (see also Disease, cerebrovascular, acute) 436
      newborn 767.4
   embolic (see also Embolism, brain) 434.1●
   fetus 767.0
   fit (see also Disease, cerebrovascular, acute) 436
   healed or old V12.54
   heart (auricle) (ventricle) (see also Infarct, myocardium) 410.9●
   heat 992.0
   hemiplegia (see also Disease, cerebrovascular, acute) 436

Apoplexia, apoplexy, apoplectic (Continued)
   hemorrhagic (stroke) (see also Hemorrhage, brain) 432.9
   ingravescent (see also Disease, cerebrovascular, acute) 436
   late effect - see Late effect(s) (of) cerebrovascular disease
   lung - see Embolism, pulmonary
   meninges, hemorrhagic (see also Hemorrhage, subarachnoid) 430
   neonatorum 767.0
   newborn 767.0
   pancreatitis 577.0
   placenta 641.2●
   progressive (see also Disease, cerebrovascular, acute) 436
   pulmonary (artery) (vein) - see Embolism, pulmonary
   sanguineous (see also Disease, cerebrovascular, acute) 436
   seizure (see also Disease, cerebrovascular, acute) 436
   serous (see also Disease, cerebrovascular, acute) 436
   spleen 289.59
   stroke (see also Disease, cerebrovascular, acute) 436
   thrombotic (see also Thrombosis, brain) 434.0●
   uremic - see Uremia
   uteroplacental 641.2●
Appendage
   fallopian tube (cyst of Morgagni) 752.11
   intestine (epiploic) 751.5
   preauricular 744.1
   testicular (organ of Morgagni) 752.89
Appendicitis 541
   with
      perforation, peritonitis (generalized), or rupture 540.0
         with peritoneal abscess 540.1
      peritoneal abscess 540.1
   acute (catarrhal) (fulminating) (gangrenous) (inflammatory) (obstructive) (retrocecal) (suppurative) 540.9
      with
         perforation, peritonitis, or rupture 540.0
            with peritoneal abscess 540.1
         peritoneal abscess 540.1
   amebic 006.8
   chronic (recurrent) 542
   exacerbation - see Appendicitis, acute
   fulminating - see Appendicitis, acute
   gangrenous - see Appendicitis, acute
   healed (obliterative) 542
   interval 542
   neurogenic 542
   obstructive 542
   pneumococcal 541
   recurrent 542
   relapsing 542
   retrocecal 541
   subacute (adhesive) 542
   subsiding 542
   suppurative - see Appendicitis, acute
   tuberculous (see also Tuberculosis) 014.8●
Appendiclausis 543.9
Appendicolithiasis 543.9
Appendicopathia oxyurica 127.4
Appendix, appendicular - see also condition
   Morgagni (male) 752.89
      fallopian tube 752.11
Appetite
   depraved 307.52
   excessive 783.6
      psychogenic 307.51
   lack or loss (see also Anorexia) 783.0
      nonorganic origin 307.59
   perverted 307.52
      hysterical 300.11

Apprehension, apprehensiveness (abnormal) (state) 300.00
  specified type NEC 300.09
Approximal wear 521.10
Apraxia (classic) (ideational) (ideokinetic) (ideomotor) (motor) 784.69
  oculomotor, congenital 379.51
  verbal 784.69
Aptyalism 527.5
Aqueous misdirection 365.83
Arabicum elephantiasis (see also Infestation, filarial) 125.9
Arachnidism 989.5
Arachnitis - see Meningitis
Arachnodactyly 759.82
Arachnoidism 989.5
Arachnoiditis (acute) (adhesive) (basic) (brain) (cerebrospinal) (chiasmal) (chronic) (spinal) (see also Meningitis) 322.9
  meningococcal (chronic) 036.0
  syphilitic 094.2
  tuberculous (see also Tuberculosis, meninges) 013.0●
Araneism 989.5
Arboencephalitis, Australian 062.4
Arborization block (heart) 426.6
Arbor virus, arbovirus (infection) NEC 066.9
ARC 042
Arches - see condition
Arcuate uterus 752.36
Arcuatus uterus 752.36
Arcus (cornea)
  juvenilis 743.43
    interfering with vision 743.42
  senilis 371.41
Arc-welders' lung 503
Arc-welders' syndrome (photokeratitis) 370.24
Areflexia 796.1
Areola - see condition
Argentaffinoma (M8241/1) - see also Neoplasm, by site, uncertain behavior
  benign (M8241/0) - see Neoplasm, by site, benign
  malignant (M8241/3) - see Neoplasm, by site, malignant
  syndrome 259.2
Argentinian hemorrhagic fever 078.7
Arginosuccinicaciduria 270.6
Argonz-Del Castillo syndrome (nonpuerperal galactorrhea and amenorrhea) 253.1
Argyll-Robertson phenomenon, pupil, or syndrome (syphilitic) 094.89
  atypical 379.45
  nonluetic 379.45
  nonsyphilitic 379.45
  reversed 379.45
Argyria, argyriasis NEC 985.8
  conjunctiva 372.55
  cornea 371.16
  from drug or medicinal agent
    correct substance properly administered 709.09
    overdose or wrong substance given or taken 961.2
Arhinencephaly 742.2
Arias-Stella phenomenon 621.30
Ariboflavinosis 266.0
Arizona enteritis 008.1
Arm - see condition
Armenian disease 277.31
Arnold-Chiari obstruction or syndrome (see also Spina bifida) 741.0●
  type I 348.4
  type II (see also Spina bifida) 741.0●
  type III 742.0
  type IV 742.2
Arousals
  confusional 327.41

Arrest, arrested
  active phase of labor 661.1●
    affecting fetus or newborn 763.7
  any plane in pelvis
    complicating delivery 660.1●
      affecting fetus or newborn 763.1
  bone marrow (see also Anemia, aplastic) 284.9
  cardiac 427.5
    with
      abortion - see Abortion, by type, with specified complication NEC
      ectopic pregnancy (see also categories 633.0-633.9) 639.8
      molar pregnancy (see also categories 630-632) 639.8
    complicating
      anesthesia
        correct substance properly administered 427.5
        obstetric 668.1●
        overdose or wrong substance given 968.4
          specified anesthetic - see Table of Drugs and Chemicals
      delivery (cesarean) (instrumental) 669.4●
      ectopic or molar pregnancy 639.8
      surgery (nontherapeutic) (therapeutic) 997.1
    fetus or newborn 779.85
    following
      abortion 639.8
      ectopic or molar pregnancy 639.8
    personal history, successfully rescuscitated V12.53
    postoperative (immediate) 997.1
      long-term effect of cardiac surgery 429.4
  cardiorespiratory (see also Arrest, cardiac) 427.5
  deep transverse 660.3●
    affecting fetus or newborn 763.1
  development or growth
    bone 733.91
    child 783.40
    fetus 764.9●
      affecting management of pregnancy 656.5●
    tracheal rings 748.3
  epiphyseal 733.91
  granulopoiesis 288.09
  heart - see Arrest, cardiac
  respiratory 799.1
    newborn 770.87
  sinus 426.6
  transverse (deep) 660.3●
    affecting fetus or newborn 763.1
Arrhenoblastoma (M8630/1)
  benign (M8630/0)
    specified site - see Neoplasm, by site, benign
    unspecified site
      female 220
      male 222.0
  malignant (M8630/3)
    specified site - see Neoplasm, by site, malignant
    unspecified site
      female 183.0
      male 186.9
  specified site - see Neoplasm, by site, uncertain behavior
  unspecified site
    female 236.2
    male 236.4
Arrhinencephaly 742.2
  due to
    trisomy 13 (13-15) 758.1
    trisomy 18 (16-18) 758.2

Arrhythmia (auricle) (cardiac) (cordis) (gallop rhythm) (juvenile) (nodal) (reflex) (sinus) (supraventricular) (transitory) (ventricle) 427.9
  bigeminal rhythm 427.89
  block 426.9
  bradycardia 427.89
  contractions, premature 427.60
  coronary sinus 427.89
  ectopic 427.89
  extrasystolic 427.60
  postoperative 997.1
  psychogenic 306.2
  vagal 780.2
Arrillaga-Ayerza syndrome (pulmonary artery sclerosis with pulmonary hypertension) 416.0
Arsenical
  dermatitis 692.4
  keratosis 692.4
  pigmentation 985.1
    from drug or medicinal agent
      correct substance properly administered 709.09
      overdose or wrong substance given or taken 961.1
Arsenism 985.1
  from drug or medicinal agent
    correct substance properly administered 692.4
    overdose or wrong substance given or taken 961.1
Arterial - see condition
Arteriectasis 447.8
Arteriofibrosis - see Arteriosclerosis
Arteriolar sclerosis - see Arteriosclerosis
Arteriolith - see Arteriosclerosis
Arteriolitis 447.6
  necrotizing, kidney 447.5
  renal - see Hypertension, kidney
Arteriolosclerosis - see Arteriosclerosis
Arterionephrosclerosis (see also Hypertension, kidney) 403.90
Arteriopathy 447.9
Arteriosclerosis, arteriosclerotic (artery) (deformans) (diffuse) (disease) (endarteritis) (general) (obliterans) (obliterative) (occlusive) (senile) (with calcification) 440.9
  with
    gangrene 440.24
    psychosis (see also Psychosis, arteriosclerotic) 290.40
    ulceration 440.23
  aorta 440.0
  arteries of extremities - see Arteriosclerosis, extremities
  basilar (artery) (see also Occlusion, artery, basilar) 433.0●
  brain 437.0
  bypass graft
    coronary artery 414.05
      autologous artery (gastroepiploic) (internal mammary) 414.04
      autologous vein 414.02
      nonautologous biological 414.03
      of transplanted heart 414.07
    extremity 440.30
      autologous vein 440.31
      nonautologous biological 440.32
  cardiac - see Arteriosclerosis, coronary
  cardiopathy - see Arteriosclerosis, coronary
  cardiorenal (see also Hypertension, cardiorenal) 404.90
  cardiovascular (see also Disease, cardiovascular) 429.2
  carotid (artery) (common) (internal) (see also Occlusion, artery, carotid) 433.1●
  central nervous system 437.0

SECTION I INDEX TO DISEASES AND INJURIES / Arthritis, arthritic

Arteriosclerosis, arteriosclerotic *(Continued)*
  cerebral 437.0
    late effect - *see* Late effect(s) (of)
        cerebrovascular disease
  cerebrospinal 437.0
  cerebrovascular 437.0
  coronary (artery) 414.00
    due to
        calcified coronary lesion (severely)
            414.4
        graft - *see* Arteriosclerosis, bypass graft
            native artery 414.01
            of transplanted heart 414.06
        lipid rich plaque 414.3
  extremities (native artery) NEC 440.20
    bypass graft 440.30
        autologous vein 440.31
        nonautologous biological 440.32
    claudication (intermittent) 440.21
        and
            gangrene 440.24
            rest pain 440.22
                and
                    gangrene 440.24
                    ulceration 440.23
                        and gangrene 440.24
            ulceration 440.23
                and gangrene 440.24
    gangrene 440.24
    rest pain 440.22
        and
            gangrene 440.24
            ulceration 440.23
                and gangrene 440.24
    specified site NEC 440.29
    ulceration 440.23
        and gangrene 440.24
  heart (disease) - *see also* Arteriosclerosis,
      coronary
    valve 424.99
        aortic 424.1
        mitral 424.0
        pulmonary 424.3
        tricuspid 424.2
  iliac 440.8
  kidney (*see also* Hypertension, kidney) 403.90
  labyrinth, labyrinthine 388.00
  medial NEC (*see also* Arteriosclerosis,
      extremities) 440.20
  mesentery (artery) 557.1
  Mönckeberg's (*see also* Arteriosclerosis,
      extremities) 440.20
  myocarditis 429.0
  nephrosclerosis (*see also* Hypertension,
      kidney) 403.90
  peripheral (of extremities) - *see*
      Arteriosclerosis, extremities
  precerebral 433.9●
      specified artery NEC 433.8●
  pulmonary (idiopathic) 416.0
  renal (*see also* Hypertension, kidney) 403.90
      arterioles (*see also* Hypertension, kidney)
          403.90
      artery 440.1
  retinal (vascular) 440.8 [362.13]
  specified artery NEC 440.8
      with gangrene 440.8 [785.4]
  spinal (cord) 437.0
  vertebral (artery) (*see also* Occlusion, artery,
      vertebral) 433.2●

Arteriospasm 443.9
Arteriovenous - *see* condition
Arteritis 447.6
  allergic (*see also* Angiitis, hypersensitivity)
      446.20
  aorta (nonsyphilitic) 447.6
      syphilitic 093.1
  aortic arch 446.7
  brachiocephalica 446.7
  brain 437.4
      syphilitic 094.89

Arteritis *(Continued)*
  branchial 446.7
  cerebral 437.4
    late effect - *see* Late effect(s) (of)
        cerebrovascular disease
    syphilitic 094.89
  coronary (artery) - *see also* Arteriosclerosis,
      coronary
      rheumatic 391.9
          chronic 398.99
      syphilitic 093.89
  cranial (left) (right) 446.5
  deformans - *see* Arteriosclerosis
  giant cell 446.5
  necrosing or necrotizing 446.0
  nodosa 446.0
  obliterans - *see also* Arteriosclerosis
      subclaviocarotica 446.7
  pulmonary 417.8
  retina 362.18
  rheumatic - *see* Fever, rheumatic
  senile - *see* Arteriosclerosis
  suppurative 447.2
  syphilitic (general) 093.89
      brain 094.89
      coronary 093.89
      spinal 094.89
  temporal 446.5
  young female, syndrome 446.7
Artery, arterial - *see* condition
Arthralgia (*see also* Pain, joint) 719.4●
  allergic (*see also* Pain, joint) 719.4●
  in caisson disease 993.3
  psychogenic 307.89
  rubella 056.71
  Salmonella 003.23
  temporomandibular joint 524.62
Arthritis, arthritic (acute) (chronic) (subacute)
    716.9●
  meaning Osteoarthritis - *see* Osteoarthrosis

> Note: Use the following fifth-digit
> subclassification with categories 711-712,
> 715-716:
>
> 0   site unspecified
> 1   shoulder region
> 2   upper arm
> 3   forearm
> 4   hand
> 5   pelvic region and thigh
> 6   lower leg
> 7   ankle and foot
> 8   other specified sites
> 9   multiple sites

  allergic 716.2●
  ankylosing (crippling) (spine) 720.0 [713.2]
      sites other than spine 716.9●
  atrophic 714.0
      spine 720.9
  back (*see also* Arthritis, spine) 721.90
  Bechterew's (ankylosing spondylitis) 720.0
  blennorrhagic 098.50 [711.6]●
  cervical, cervicodorsal (*see also* Spondylosis,
      cervical) 721.0
  Charcôt's 094.0 [713.5]
      diabetic 250.6● [713.5]
          due to secondary diabetes 249.6●
              [713.5]
      syringomyelic 336.0 [713.5]
      tabetic 094.0 [713.5]
  chylous (*see also* Filariasis) 125.9 [711.7]●
  climacteric NEC 716.3●
  coccyx 721.8
  cricoarytenoid 478.79
  crystal (-induced) - *see* Arthritis, due to
      crystals
  deformans (*see also* Osteoarthrosis)
      715.9●
      spine 721.90
          with myelopathy 721.91

Arthritis, arthritic *(Continued)*
  degenerative (*see also* Osteoarthrosis) 715.9●
      idiopathic 715.09
      polyarticular 715.09
      spine 721.90
          with myelopathy 721.91
  dermatoarthritis, lipoid 272.8 [713.0]
  due to or associated with
      acromegaly 253.0 [713.0]
      actinomycosis 039.8 [711.4]●
      amyloidosis 277.39 [713.7]
      bacterial disease NEC 040.89 [711.4]●
      Behçet's syndrome 136.1 [711.2]●
      blastomycosis 116.0 [711.6]●
      brucellosis (*see also* Brucellosis) 023.9
          [711.4]●
      caisson disease 993.3
      coccidioidomycosis 114.3 [711.6]●
      coliform (Escherichia coli) 711.0●
      colitis, ulcerative (*see also* Colitis,
          ulcerative) 556.9 [713.1]
      cowpox 051.01 [711.5]●
      crystals (*see also* Gout)
          dicalcium phosphate 275.49 [712.1]●
          pyrophosphate 275.49 [712.2]●
          specified NEC 275.49 [712.8]●
      dermatoarthritis, lipoid 272.8 [713.0]
      dermatological disorder NEC 709.9
          [713.3]
      diabetes 250.6● [713.5]
          due to secondary diabetes 249.6●
              [713.5]
      diphtheria 032.89 [711.4]●
      dracontiasis 125.7 [711.7]●
      dysentery 009.0 [711.3]●
      endocrine disorder NEC 259.9 [713.0]
      enteritis NEC 009.1 [711.3]●
          infectious (*see also* Enteritis, infectious)
              009.0 [711.3]●
          specified organism NEC 008.8
              [711.3]●
          regional (*see also* Enteritis, regional)
              555.9 [713.1]
          specified organism NEC 008.8 [711.3]●
      epiphyseal slip, nontraumatic (old)
          716.8●
      erysipelas 035 [711.4]●
      erythema
          epidemic 026.1
          multiforme 695.10 [713.3]
          nodosum 695.2 [713.3]
      Escherichia coli 711.0●
      filariasis NEC 125.9 [711.7]●
      gastrointestinal condition NEC 569.9
          [713.1]
      glanders 024 [711.4]●
      Gonococcus 098.50
      gout 274.00
      H. influenzae 711.0●
      helminthiasis NEC 128.9 [711.7]●
      hematological disorder NEC 289.9 [713.2]
      hemochromatosis 275.03 [713.0]
      hemoglobinopathy NEC (*see also* Disease,
          hemoglobin) 282.7 [713.2]
      hemophilia (*see also* Hemophilia) 286.0
          [713.2]
      Hemophilus influenzae (H. influenzae)
          711.0●
      Henoch (-Schönlein) purpura 287.0 [713.6]
      histoplasmosis NEC (*see also*
          Histoplasmosis) 115.99 [711.6]●
      human parvovirus 079.83 [711.5]●
      hyperparathyroidism 252.00 [713.0]
      hypersensitivity reaction NEC 995.3
          [713.6]
      hypogammaglobulinemia (*see also*
          Hypogammaglobulinemia) 279.00
          [713.0]
      hypothyroidism NEC 244.9 [713.0]
      infection (*see also* Arthritis, infectious)
          711.9●

SECTION I INDEX TO DISEASES AND INJURIES / Arthritis, arthritic

Arthritis, arthritic (Continued)
  due to or associated with (Continued)
    infectious disease NEC 136.9 [711.8]●
    leprosy (see also Leprosy) 030.9 [711.4]●
    leukemia NEC (M9800/3) 208.9● [713.2]
    lipoid dermatoarthritis 272.8 [713.0]
    Lyme disease 088.81 [711.8]●
    Mediterranean fever, familial 277.31 [713.7]
    meningococcal infection 036.82
    metabolic disorder NEC 277.9 [713.0]
    multiple myelomatosis (M9730/3) 203.0● [713.2]
    mumps 072.79 [711.5]●
    mycobacteria 031.8 [711.4]●
    mycosis NEC 117.9 [711.6]●
    neurological disorder NEC 349.9 [713.5]
    ochronosis 270.2 [713.0]
    O'Nyong Nyong 066.3 [711.5]●
    parasitic disease NEC 136.9 [711.8]●
    paratyphoid fever (see also Fever, paratyphoid) 002.9 [711.3]●
    parvovirus B19 079.83 [711.5]●
    Pneumococcus 711.0●
    poliomyelitis (see also Poliomyelitis) 045.9● [711.5]●
    Pseudomonas 711.0●
    psoriasis 696.0
    pyogenic organism (E. coli) (H. influenzae) (Pseudomonas) (Streptococcus) 711.0●
    rat-bite fever 026.1 [711.4]●
    regional enteritis (see also Enteritis, regional) 555.9 [713.1]
    Reiter's disease 099.3 [711.1]●
    respiratory disorder NEC 519.9 [713.4]
    reticulosis, malignant (M9720/3) 202.3● [713.2]
    rubella 056.71
    salmonellosis 003.23
    sarcoidosis 135 [713.7]
    serum sickness 999.59 [713.6]
    Staphylococcus 711.0●
    Streptococcus 711.0●
    syphilis (see also Syphilis) 094.0 [711.4]●
    syringomyelia 336.0 [713.5]
    thalassemia (see also Thalassemia) 282.40 [713.2]
    tuberculosis (see also Tuberculosis, arthritis) 015.9● [711.4]●
    typhoid fever 002.0 [711.3]●
    ulcerative colitis (see also Colitis, ulcerative) 556.9 [713.1]
    urethritis
      nongonococcal (see also Urethritis, nongonococcal) 099.40 [711.1]●
      nonspecific (see also Urethritis, nongonococcal) 099.40 [711.1]●
      Reiter's 099.3 [711.1]●
    viral disease NEC 079.99 [711.5]●
  erythema epidemic 026.1
  gonococcal 098.50
  gouty 274.00
    acute 274.01
  hypertrophic (see also Osteoarthrosis) 715.9●
    spine 721.90
      with myelopathy 721.91
  idiopathic, blennorrheal 099.3
  in caisson disease 993.3 [713.8]
  infectious or infective (acute) (chronic) (subacute) NEC 711.9●
    nonpyogenic 711.9●
    spine 720.9
  inflammatory NEC 714.9
  juvenile rheumatoid (chronic) (polyarticular) 714.30
    acute 714.31
    monoarticular 714.33
    pauciarticular 714.32
  lumbar (see also Spondylosis, lumbar) 721.3
  meningococcal 036.82

Arthritis, arthritic (Continued)
  menopausal NEC 716.3●
  migratory - see Fever, rheumatic
  neuropathic (Charcôt's) 094.0 [713.5]
    diabetic 250.6● [713.5]
      due to secondary diabetes 249.6● [713.5]
    nonsyphilitic NEC 349.9 [713.5]
    syringomyelic 336.0 [713.5]
    tabetic 094.0 [713.5]
  nodosa (see also Osteoarthrosis) 715.9●
    spine 721.90
      with myelopathy 721.91
  nonpyogenic NEC 716.9●
    spine 721.90
      with myelopathy 721.91
  ochronotic 270.2 [713.0]
  palindromic (see also Rheumatism, palindromic) 719.3●
  pneumococcal 711.0●
  postdysenteric 009.0 [711.3]●
  postrheumatic, chronic (Jaccoud's) 714.4
  primary progressive 714.0
    spine 720.9
  proliferative 714.0
    spine 720.0
  psoriatic 696.0
  purulent 711.0●
  pyogenic or pyemic 711.0●
  reactive 099.3
  rheumatic 714.0
    acute or subacute - see Fever, rheumatic
    chronic 714.0
    spine 720.9
  rheumatoid (nodular) 714.0
    with
      splenoadenomegaly and leukopenia 714.1
      visceral or systemic involvement 714.2
    aortitis 714.89
    carditis 714.2
    heart disease 714.2
    juvenile (chronic) (polyarticular) 714.30
      acute 714.31
      monoarticular 714.33
      pauciarticular 714.32
    spine 720.0
  rubella 056.71
  sacral, sacroiliac, sacrococcygeal (see also Spondylosis, sacral) 721.3
  scorbutic 267
  senile or senescent (see also Osteoarthrosis) 715.9●
    spine 721.90
      with myelopathy 721.91
  septic 711.0●
  serum (nontherapeutic) (therapeutic) 999.59 [713.6]
  specified form NEC 716.8●
  spine 721.90
    with myelopathy 721.91
    atrophic 720.9
    degenerative 721.90
      with myelopathy 721.91
    hypertrophic (with deformity) 721.90
      with myelopathy 721.91
    infectious or infective NEC 720.9
    Marie-Strümpell 720.0
    nonpyogenic 721.90
      with myelopathy 721.91
    pyogenic 720.9
    rheumatoid 720.0
    traumatic (old) 721.7
    tuberculous (see also Tuberculosis) 015.0● [720.81]
  staphylococcal 711.0●
  streptococcal 711.0●
  suppurative 711.0●
  syphilitic 094.0 [713.5]
    congenital 090.49 [713.5]
  syphilitica deformans (Charcôt) 094.0 [713.5]

Arthritis, arthritic (Continued)
  temporomandibular joint 524.69
  thoracic (see also Spondylosis, thoracic) 721.2
  toxic of menopause 716.3●
  transient 716.4●
  traumatic (chronic) (old) (post) 716.1●
    current injury - see nature of injury
  tuberculous (see also Tuberculosis, arthritis) 015.9● [711.4]●
  urethritica 099.3 [711.1]●
  urica, uratic 274.00
  venereal 099.3 [711.1]●
  vertebral (see also Arthritis, spine) 721.90
  villous 716.8●
  von Bechterew's 720.0
Arthrocele (see also Effusion, joint) 719.0●
Arthrochondritis - see Arthritis
Arthrodesis status V45.4
Arthrodynia (see also Pain, joint) 719.4●
  psychogenic 307.89
Arthrodysplasia 755.9
Arthrofibrosis, joint (see also Ankylosis) 718.5●
Arthrogryposis 728.3
  multiplex, congenita 754.89
Arthrokatadysis 715.35
Arthrolithiasis 274.00
Arthro-onychodysplasia 756.89
Arthro-osteo-onychodysplasia 756.89
Arthropathy (see also Arthritis) 716.9●

> Note: Use the following fifth-digit subclassification with categories 711-712, 716:
>
> 0 site unspecified
> 1 shoulder region
> 2 upper arm
> 3 forearm
> 4 hand
> 5 pelvic region and thigh
> 6 lower leg
> 7 ankle and foot
> 8 other specified sites
> 9 multiple sites

  Behçet's 136.1 [711.2]●
  Charcôt's 094.0 [713.5]
    diabetic 250.6● [713.5]
      due to secondary diabetes 249.6● [713.5]
    syringomyelic 336.0 [713.5]
    tabetic 094.0 [713.5]
  crystal (-induced) - see Arthritis, due to crystals
  gouty 274.00
    acute 274.01
    chronic (without mention of tophus (tophi)) 274.02
      with tophus (tophi) 274.03
  neurogenic, neuropathic (Charcôt's) (tabetic) 094.0 [713.5]
    diabetic 250.6● [713.5]
      due to secondary diabetes 249.6● [713.5]
    nonsyphilitic NEC 349.9 [713.5]
    syringomyelic 336.0 [713.5]
  postdysenteric NEC 009.0 [711.3]●
  postrheumatic, chronic (Jaccoud's) 714.4
  psoriatic 696.0
  pulmonary 731.2
  specified NEC 716.8●
  syringomyelia 336.0 [713.5]
  tabes dorsalis 094.0 [713.5]
  tabetic 094.0 [713.5]
  transient 716.4●
  traumatic 716.1●
  uric acid 274.00
Arthrophyte (see also Loose, body, joint) 718.1●
Arthrophytis 719.80
  ankle 719.87
  elbow 719.82
  foot 719.87
  hand 719.84

SECTION I INDEX TO DISEASES AND INJURIES / Aspiration

Arthrophytis *(Continued)*
    hip 719.85
    knee 719.86
    multiple sites 719.89
    pelvic region 719.85
    shoulder (region) 719.81
    specified site NEC 719.88
    wrist 719.83
Arthropyosis *(see also* Arthritis, pyogenic) 711.0●
Arthroscopic surgical procedure converted to open procedure V64.43
Arthrosis (deformans) (degenerative) *(see also* Osteoarthrosis) 715.9●
    Charcôt's 094.0 [713.5]
    polyarticular 715.09
    spine *(see also* Spondylosis) 721.90
Arthus phenomenon 995.21
    due to
        correct substance properly administered 995.21
        overdose or wrong substance given or taken 977.9
            specified drug - *see* Table of Drugs and Chemicals
        serum 999.59
Articular - *see also* condition
    disc disorder (reducing or non-reducing) 524.63
    spondylolisthesis 756.12
Articulation
    anterior 524.27
    posterior 524.27
    reverse 524.27
Artificial
    device (prosthetic) - *see* Fitting, device
    insemination V26.1
    menopause (states) (symptoms) (syndrome) 627.4
    opening status (functioning) (without complication) V44.9
        anus (colostomy) V44.3
        colostomy V44.3
        cystostomy V44.50
            appendico-vesicostomy V44.52
            cutaneous-vesicostomy V44.51
            specified type NEC V44.59
        enterostomy V44.4
        gastrostomy V44.1
        ileostomy V44.2
        intestinal tract NEC V44.4
        jejunostomy V44.4
        nephrostomy V44.6
        specified site NEC V44.8
        tracheostomy V44.0
        ureterostomy V44.6
        urethrostomy V44.6
        urinary tract NEC V44.6
        vagina V44.7
        vagina status V44.7
    ARV (disease) (illness) (infection) - *see* Human immunodeficiency virus (disease) (illness) (infection)
Arytenoid - *see* condition
Asbestosis (occupational) 501
Asboe-Hansen's disease (incontinentia pigmenti) 757.33
Ascariasis (intestinal) (lung) 127.0
Ascaridiasis 127.0
Ascaridosis 127.0
Ascaris 127.0
    lumbricoides (infestation) 127.0
    pneumonia 127.0
Ascending - *see* condition
Aschoff's bodies *(see also* Myocarditis, rheumatic) 398.0
Ascites 789.59
    abdominal NEC 789.59
    cancerous (M8000/6) 789.51
    cardiac 428.0
    chylous (nonfilarial) 457.8
        filarial *(see also* Infestation, filarial) 125.9

Ascites *(Continued)*
    congenital 778.0
    due to S. japonicum 120.2
    fetal, causing fetopelvic disproportion 653.7●
    heart 428.0
    joint *(see also* Effusion, joint) 719.0●
    malignant (M8000/6) 789.51
    pseudochylous 789.59
    syphilitic 095.2
    tuberculous *(see also* Tuberculosis) 014.0●
Ascorbic acid (vitamin C) deficiency (scurvy) 267
ASC-H (atypical squamous cells cannot exclude high grade squamous intraepithelial lesion)
    anus 796.72
    cervix 795.02
    vagina 795.12
ASC-US (atypical squamous cells of undetermined significance)
    anus 796.71
    cervix 795.01
    vagina 795.11
ASCVD (arteriosclerotic cardiovascular disease) 429.2
Aseptic - *see* condition
Asherman's syndrome 621.5
Asialia 527.7
Asiatic cholera *(see also* Cholera) 001.9
Asocial personality or trends 301.7
Asomatognosia 781.8
Aspergillosis 117.3
    with pneumonia 117.3 [484.6]
    allergic bronchopulmonary 518.6
    nonsyphilitic NEC 117.3
Aspergillus (flavus) (fumigatus) (infection) (terreus) 117.3
Aspermatogenesis 606.0
Aspermia (testis) 606.0
Asphyxia, asphyxiation (by) 799.01
    antenatal - *see* Distress, fetal
    bedclothes 994.7
    birth *(see also* Asphyxia, newborn) 768.9
    bunny bag 994.7
    carbon monoxide 986
    caul *(see also* Asphyxia, newborn) 768.9
    cave-in 994.7
        crushing - *see* Injury, internal, intrathoracic organs
    constriction 994.7
    crushing - *see* Injury, internal, intrathoracic organs
    drowning 994.1
    fetal, affecting newborn 768.9
    food or foreign body (in larynx) 933.1
        bronchioles 934.8
        bronchus (main) 934.1
        lung 934.8
        nasopharynx 933.0
        nose, nasal passages 932
        pharynx 933.0
        respiratory tract 934.9
            specified part NEC 934.8
        throat 933.0
        trachea 934.0
    gas, fumes, or vapor NEC 987.9
        specified - *see* Table of Drugs and Chemicals
    gravitational changes 994.7
    hanging 994.7
    inhalation - *see* Inhalation
    intrauterine
        fetal death (before onset of labor) 768.0
            during labor 768.1
        liveborn infant - *see* Distress, fetal, liveborn infant
    local 443.0
    mechanical 994.7
        during birth *(see also* Distress, fetal) 768.9

Asphyxia, asphyxiation *(Continued)*
    mucus 933.1
        bronchus (main) 934.1
        larynx 933.1
        lung 934.8
        nasal passages 932
        newborn 770.18
        pharynx 933.0
        respiratory tract 934.9
            specified part NEC 934.8
        throat 933.0
        trachea 934.0
        vaginal (fetus or newborn) 770.18
    newborn 768.9
        with neurologic involvement 768.5
        blue 768.6
        livida 768.6
        mild or moderate 768.6
        pallida 768.5
        severe 768.5
        white 768.5
    pathological 799.01
    plastic bag 994.7
    postnatal *(see also* Asphyxia, newborn) 768.9
        mechanical 994.7
    pressure 994.7
    reticularis 782.61
    strangulation 994.7
    submersion 994.1
    traumatic NEC - *see* Injury, internal, intrathoracic organs
    vomiting, vomitus - *see* Asphyxia, food or foreign body
Aspiration
    acid pulmonary (syndrome) 997.39
        obstetric 668.0●
    amniotic fluid 770.13
        with respiratory symptoms 770.14
    bronchitis 507.0
    clear amniotic fluid 770.13
        with
            pneumonia 770.14
            pneumonitis 770.14
            respiratory symptoms 770.14
    contents of birth canal 770.17
        with respiratory symptoms 770.18
    fetal 770.10
        blood 770.15
            with
                pneumonia 770.16
                pneumonitis 770.16
        pneumonitis 770.18
    food, foreign body, or gasoline (with asphyxiation) - *see* Asphyxia, food or foreign body
    meconium 770.11
        with
            pneumonia 770.12
            pneumonitis 770.12
            respiratory symptoms 770.12
        below vocal cords 770.11
            with respiratory symptoms 770.12
    mucus 933.1
        into
            bronchus (main) 934.1
            lung 934.8
            respiratory tract 934.9
                specified part NEC 934.8
            trachea 934.0
        newborn 770.17
        vaginal (fetus or newborn) 770.17
    newborn 770.10
        with respiratory symptoms 770.18
        blood 770.15
            with
                pneumonia 770.16
                pneumonitis 770.16
                respiratory symptoms 770.16
    pneumonia 507.0
        fetus or newborn 770.18
            meconium 770.12

Aspiration (Continued)
  pneumonitis 507.0
    fetus or newborn 770.18
      meconium 770.12
    obstetric 668.0●
  postnatal stomach contents 770.85
    with
      pneumonia 770.86
      pneumonitis 770.86
      respiratory symptoms 770.86
  syndrome of newborn (massive) 770.18
    meconium 770.12
  vernix caseosa 770.17
Asplenia 759.0
  with mesocardia 746.87
Assam fever 085.0
Assimilation, pelvis
  with disproportion 653.2●
    affecting fetus or newborn 763.1
    causing obstructed labor 660.1●
      affecting fetus or newborn 763.1
Assmann's focus (see also Tuberculosis) 011.0●
Astasia (-abasia) 307.9
  hysterical 300.11
Asteatosis 706.8
  cutis 706.8
Astereognosis 780.99
Asterixis 781.3
  in liver disease 572.8
Asteroid hyalitis 379.22
Asthenia, asthenic 780.79
  cardiac (see also Failure, heart) 428.9
    psychogenic 306.2
  cardiovascular (see also Failure, heart) 428.9
    psychogenic 306.2
  heart (see also Failure, heart) 428.9
    psychogenic 306.2
  hysterical 300.11
  myocardial (see also Failure, heart) 428.9
    psychogenic 306.2
  nervous 300.5
  neurocirculatory 306.2
  neurotic 300.5
  psychogenic 300.5
  psychoneurotic 300.5
  psychophysiologic 300.5
  reaction, psychoneurotic 300.5
  senile 797
  Stiller's 780.79
  tropical anhidrotic 705.1
Asthenopia 368.13
  accommodative 367.4
  hysterical (muscular) 300.11
  psychogenic 306.7
Asthenospermia 792.2
Asthma, asthmatic (bronchial) (catarrh) (spasmodic) 493.9●

> Note: The following fifth digit subclassification is for use with codes 493.0-493.2, 493.9:
>
> 0 unspecified
> 1 with status asthmaticus
> 2 with (acute) exacerbation

  with
    chronic obstructive pulmonary disease (COPD) 493.2●
    hay fever 493.0●
    rhinitis, allergic 493.0●
  allergic 493.9●
    stated cause (external allergen) 493.0●
  atopic 493.0●
  cardiac (see also Failure, ventricular, left) 428.1
  cardiobronchial (see also Failure, ventricular, left) 428.1
  cardiorenal (see also Hypertension, cardiorenal) 404.90
  childhood 493.0●
  Colliers' 500

Asthma, asthmatic (Continued)
  cough variant 493.82
  croup 493.9●
  detergent 507.8
  due to
    detergent 507.8
    inhalation of fumes 506.3
    internal immunological process 493.0●
  endogenous (intrinsic) 493.1●
  eosinophilic 518.3
  exercise induced bronchospasm 493.81
  exogenous (cosmetics) (dander or dust) (drugs) (dust) (feathers) (food) (hay) (platinum) (pollen) 493.0●
  extrinsic 493.0●
  grinders' 502
  hay 493.0●
  heart (see also Failure, ventricular, left) 428.1
  IgE 493.0●
  infective 493.1●
  intrinsic 493.1●
  Kopp's 254.8
  late-onset 493.1●
  meat-wrappers' 506.9
  Millar's (laryngismus stridulus) 478.75
  millstone makers' 502
  miners' 500
  Monday morning 504
  New Orleans (epidemic) 493.0●
  platinum 493.0●
  pneumoconiotic (occupational) NEC 505
  potters' 502
  psychogenic 316 [493.9]●
  pulmonary eosinophilic 518.3
  red cedar 495.8
  Rostan's (see also Failure, ventricular, left) 428.1
  sandblasters' 502
  sequoiosis 495.8
  stonemasons' 502
  thymic 254.8
  tuberculous (see also Tuberculosis, pulmonary) 011.9●
  Wichmann's (laryngismus stridulus) 478.75
  wood 495.8
Astigmatism (compound) (congenital) 367.20
  irregular 367.22
  regular 367.21
Astroblastoma (M9430/3)
  nose 748.1
  specified site - see Neoplasm, by site, malignant
  unspecified site 191.9
Astrocytoma (cystic) (M9400/3)
  anaplastic type (M9401/3)
    specified site - see Neoplasm, by site, malignant
    unspecified site 191.9
  fibrillary (M9420/3)
    specified site - see Neoplasm, by site, malignant
    unspecified site 191.9
  fibrous (M9420/3)
    specified site - see Neoplasm, by site, malignant
    unspecified site 191.9
  gemistocytic (M9411/3)
    specified site - see Neoplasm, by site, malignant
    unspecified site 191.9
  juvenile (M9421/3)
    specified site - see Neoplasm, by site, malignant
    unspecified site 191.9
  nose 748.1
  pilocytic (M9421/3)
    specified site - see Neoplasm, by site, malignant
    unspecified site 191.9

Astrocytoma (Continued)
  piloid (M9421/3)
    specified site - see Neoplasm, by site, malignant
    unspecified site 191.9
  protoplasmic (M9410/3)
    specified site - see Neoplasm, by site, malignant
    unspecified site 191.9
  specified site - see Neoplasm, by site, malignant
  subependymal (M9383/1) 237.5
    giant cell (M9384/1) 237.5
  unspecified site 191.9
Astroglioma (M9400/3)
  nose 748.1
  specified site - see Neoplasm, by site, malignant
  unspecified site 191.9
Asymbolia 784.60
Asymmetrical breathing 786.09
Asymmetry - see also Distortion
  breast, between native and reconstructed 612.1
  chest 786.9
  face 754.0
  jaw NEC 524.12
    maxillary 524.11
  pelvis with disproportion 653.0●
    affecting fetus or newborn 763.1
    causing obstructed labor 660.1●
      affecting fetus or newborn 763.1
Asynergia 781.3
Asynergy 781.3
  ventricular 429.89
Asystole (heart) (see also Arrest, cardiac) 427.5
At risk for falling V15.88
Ataxia, ataxy, ataxic 781.3
  acute 781.3
  brain 331.89
  cerebellar 334.3
    hereditary (Marie's) 334.2
    in
      alcoholism 303.9● [334.4]
      myxedema (see also Myxedema) 244.9 [334.4]
      neoplastic disease NEC 239.9 [334.4]
  cerebral 331.89
  family, familial 334.2
    cerebral (Marie's) 334.2
    spinal (Friedreich's) 334.0
  Friedreich's (heredofamilial) (spinal) 334.0
  frontal lobe 781.3
  gait 781.2
    hysterical 300.11
  general 781.3
  hereditary NEC 334.2
    cerebellar 334.2
    spastic 334.1
    spinal 334.0
  heredofamilial (Marie's) 334.2
  hysterical 300.11
  locomotor (progressive) 094.0
    diabetic 250.6● [337.1]
      due to secondary diabetes 249.6● [337.1]
  Marie's (cerebellar) (heredofamilial) 334.2
  nonorganic origin 307.9
  partial 094.0
  postchickenpox 052.7
  progressive locomotor 094.0
  psychogenic 307.9
  Sanger-Brown's 334.2
  spastic 094.0
    hereditary 334.1
    syphilitic 094.0
  spinal
    hereditary 334.0
    progressive locomotor 094.0
  telangiectasia 334.8

Ataxia-telangiectasia 334.8
Atelectasis (absorption collapse) (complete)
    (compression) (massive) (partial)
    (postinfective) (pressure collapse)
    (pulmonary) (relaxation) 518.0
  newborn (congenital) (partial) 770.5
    primary 770.4
  primary 770.4
  tuberculous (see also Tuberculosis,
    pulmonary) 011.9●
Ateleiosis, ateliosis 253.3
Atelia - see Distortion
Ateliosis 253.3
Atelocardia 746.9
Atelomyelia 742.59
Athelia 757.6
Atheroembolism
  extremity
    lower 445.02
    upper 445.01
  kidney 445.81
  specified site NEC 445.89
Atheroma, atheromatous (see also
    Arteriosclerosis) 440.9
  aorta, aortic 440.0
    valve (see also Endocarditis, aortic) 424.1
  artery - see Arteriosclerosis
  basilar (artery) (see also Occlusion, artery,
    basilar) 433.0●
  carotid (artery) (common) (internal) (see also
    Occlusion, artery, carotid) 433.1●
  cerebral (arteries) 437.0
  coronary (artery) - see Arteriosclerosis,
    coronary
  degeneration - see Arteriosclerosis
  heart, cardiac - see Arteriosclerosis, coronary
  mitral (valve) 424.0
  myocardium, myocardial - see
    Arteriosclerosis, coronary
  pulmonary valve (heart) (see also
    Endocarditis, pulmonary) 424.3
  skin 706.2
  tricuspid (heart) (valve) 424.2
  valve, valvular - see Endocarditis
  vertebral (artery) (see also Occlusion, artery,
    vertebral) 433.2●
Atheromatosis - see also Arteriosclerosis
  arterial, congenital 272.8
Atherosclerosis - see Arteriosclerosis
Athetosis (acquired) 781.0
  bilateral 333.79
  congenital (bilateral) 333.6
  double 333.71
  unilateral 781.0
Athlete's
  foot 110.4
  heart 429.3
Athletic team examination V70.3
Athrepsia 261
Athyrea (acquired) (see also Hypothyroidism)
    244.9
  congenital 243
Athyreosis (congenital) 243
  acquired - see Hypothyroidism
Athyroidism (acquired) (see also
    Hypothyroidism) 244.9
  congenital 243
Atmospheric pyrexia 992.0
Atonia, atony, atonic
  abdominal wall 728.2
  bladder (sphincter) 596.4
    neurogenic NEC 596.54
      with cauda equina syndrome 344.61
  capillary 448.9
  cecum 564.89
    psychogenic 306.4
  colon 564.89
    psychogenic 306.4
  congenital 779.89
  dyspepsia 536.3
    psychogenic 306.4

Atonia, atony, atonic (Continued)
  intestine 564.89
    psychogenic 306.4
  stomach 536.3
    neurotic or psychogenic 306.4
    psychogenic 306.4
  uterus 661.2●
    with hemorrhage (postpartum) 666.1●
      affecting fetus or newborn 763.7
    without hemorrhage
      intrapartum 661.2●
      postpartum 669.8●
  vesical 596.4
Atopy NEC V15.09
Atransferrinemia, congenital 273.8
Atresia, atretic (congenital) 759.89
  alimentary organ or tract NEC 751.8
    lower 751.2
    upper 750.8
  ani, anus, anal (canal) 751.2
  aorta 747.22
    with hypoplasia of ascending aorta and
      defective development of left
      ventricle (with mitral valve atresia)
      746.7
    arch 747.11
    ring 747.21
  aortic (orifice) (valve) 746.89
    arch 747.11
  aqueduct of Sylvius 742.3
    with spina bifida (see also Spina bifida)
      741.0●
  artery NEC (see also Atresia, blood vessel)
    747.60
    cerebral 747.81
    coronary 746.85
    eye 743.58
    pulmonary 747.31
    umbilical 747.5
  auditory canal (external) 744.02
  bile, biliary duct (common) or passage
    751.61
    acquired (see also Obstruction, biliary)
      576.2
  bladder (neck) 753.6
  blood vessel (peripheral) NEC 747.60
    cerebral 747.81
    gastrointestinal 747.61
    lower limb 747.64
    pulmonary artery 747.31
    renal 747.62
    spinal 747.82
    upper limb 747.63
  bronchus 748.3
  canal, ear 744.02
  cardiac
    valve 746.89
      aortic 746.89
      mitral 746.89
      pulmonary 746.01
      tricuspid 746.1
  cecum 751.2
  cervix (acquired) 622.4
    congenital 752.43
    in pregnancy or childbirth 654.6●
      affecting fetus or newborn 763.89
      causing obstructed labor 660.2●
        affecting fetus or newborn 763.1
  choana 748.0
  colon 751.2
  cystic duct 751.61
    acquired 575.8
      with obstruction (see also Obstruction,
        gallbladder) 575.2
  digestive organs NEC 751.8
  duodenum 751.1
  ear canal 744.02
  ejaculatory duct 752.89
  epiglottis 748.3
  esophagus 750.3
  Eustachian tube 744.24

Atresia, atretic (Continued)
  fallopian tube (acquired) 628.2
    congenital 752.19
  follicular cyst 620.0
  foramen of
    Luschka 742.3
      with spina bifida (see also Spina bifida)
        741.0●
    Magendie 742.3
      with spina bifida (see also Spina bifida)
        741.0●
  gallbladder 751.69
  genital organ
    external
      female 752.49
      male NEC 752.89
        penis 752.69
    internal
      female 752.89
      male 752.89
  glottis 748.3
  gullet 750.3
  heart
    valve NEC 746.89
      aortic 746.89
      mitral 746.89
      pulmonary 746.01
      tricuspid 746.1
  hymen 752.42
    acquired 623.3
    postinfective 623.3
  ileum 751.1
  intestine (small) 751.1
    large 751.2
  iris, filtration angle (see also Buphthalmia)
    743.20
  jejunum 751.1
  kidney 753.3
  lacrimal, apparatus 743.65
    acquired - see Stenosis, lacrimal
  larynx 748.3
  ligament, broad 752.19
  lung 748.5
  meatus urinarius 753.6
  mitral valve 746.89
    with atresia or hypoplasia of aortic orifice
      or valve, with hypoplasia of
      ascending aorta and defective
      development of left ventricle
      746.7
  nares (anterior) (posterior) 748.0
  nasolacrimal duct 743.65
  nasopharynx 748.8
  nose, nostril 748.0
    acquired 738.0
  organ or site NEC - see Anomaly, specified
    type NEC
  osseous meatus (ear) 744.03
  oviduct (acquired) 628.2
    congenital 752.19
  parotid duct 750.23
    acquired 527.8
  pulmonary (artery) 747.31
    valve 746.01
    vein 747.49
  pulmonic 746.01
  pupil 743.46
  rectum 751.2
  salivary duct or gland 750.23
    acquired 527.8
  sublingual duct 750.23
    acquired 527.8
  submaxillary duct or gland 750.23
    acquired 527.8
  trachea 748.3
  tricuspid valve 746.1
  ureter 753.29
  ureteropelvic junction 753.21
  ureterovesical orifice 753.22
  urethra (valvular) 753.6
  urinary tract NEC 753.29

Atresia, atretic *(Continued)*
  uterus 752.31
    acquired 621.8
  vagina (acquired) 623.2
    congenital (total) (partial) 752.45
    postgonococcal (old) 098.2
    postinfectional 623.2
    senile 623.2
  vascular NEC *(see also* Atresia, blood vessel) 747.60
    cerebral 747.81
  vas deferens 752.89
  vein NEC *(see also* Atresia, blood vessel) 747.60
    cardiac 746.89
    great 747.49
    portal 747.49
    pulmonary 747.49
  vena cava (inferior) (superior) 747.49
  vesicourethral orifice 753.6
  vulva 752.49
    acquired 624.8
Atrichia, atrichosis 704.00
  congenital (universal) 757.4
Atrioventricularis commune 745.69
Atrophia - *see also* Atrophy
  alba 709.09
  cutis 701.8
    idiopathica progressiva 701.8
    senilis 701.8
  dermatological, diffuse (idiopathic) 701.8
  flava hepatis (acuta) (subacuta) *(see also* Necrosis, liver) 570
  gyrata of choroid and retina (central) 363.54
    generalized 363.57
  senilis 797
    dermatological 701.8
  unguium 703.8
    congenita 757.5
Atrophoderma, atrophodermia 701.9
  diffusum (idiopathic) 701.8
  maculatum 701.3
    et striatum 701.3
      due to syphilis 095.8
    syphilitic 091.3
  neuriticum 701.8
  pigmentosum 757.33
  reticulatum symmetricum faciei 701.8
  senile 701.8
  symmetrical 701.8
  vermiculata 701.8
Atrophy, atrophic
  adrenal (autoimmune) (capsule) (cortex) (gland) 255.41
    with hypofunction 255.41
  alveolar process or ridge (edentulous) 525.20
    mandible 525.20
      minimal 525.21
      moderate 525.22
      severe 525.23
    maxilla 525.20
      minimal 525.24
      moderate 525.25
      severe 525.26
  appendix 543.9
  Aran-Duchenne muscular 335.21
  arm 728.2
  arteriosclerotic - *see* Arteriosclerosis
  arthritis 714.0
    spine 720.9
  bile duct (any) 576.8
  bladder 596.89
  blanche (of Milian) 701.3
  bone (senile) 733.99
    due to
      disuse 733.7
      infection 733.99
        tabes dorsalis (neurogenic) 094.0
    posttraumatic 733.99

Atrophy, atrophic *(Continued)*
  brain (cortex) (progressive) 331.9
    with dementia 290.10
    Alzheimer's 331.0
      with dementia - *see* Alzheimer's, dementia
    circumscribed (Pick's) 331.11
      with dementia
        with behavioral disturbance 331.11 [294.11]
        without behavioral disturbance 331.11 [294.10]
    congenital 742.4
    hereditary 331.9
    senile 331.2
  breast 611.4
    puerperal, postpartum 676.3●
  buccal cavity 528.9
  cardiac (brown) (senile) *(see also* Degeneration, myocardial) 429.1
  cartilage (infectional) (joint) 733.99
  cast, plaster of Paris 728.2
  cerebellar - *see* Atrophy, brain
  cerebral - *see* Atrophy, brain
  cervix (endometrium) (mucosa) (myometrium) (senile) (uteri) 622.8
    menopausal 627.8
  Charcôt-Marie-Tooth 356.1
  choroid 363.40
    diffuse secondary 363.42
    hereditary *(see also* Dystrophy, choroid) 363.50
      gyrate
        central 363.54
        diffuse 363.57
        generalized 363.57
    senile 363.41
  ciliary body 364.57
  colloid, degenerative 701.3
  conjunctiva (senile) 372.89
  corpus cavernosum 607.89
  cortical *(see also* Atrophy, brain) 331.9
  Cruveilhier's 335.21
  cystic duct 576.8
  dacryosialadenopathy 710.2
  degenerative
    colloid 701.3
    senile 701.3
  Déjérine-Thomas 333.0
  diffuse idiopathic, dermatological 701.8
  disuse
    bone 733.7
    muscle 728.2
    pelvic muscles and anal sphincter 618.83
  Duchenne-Aran 335.21
  ear 388.9
  edentulous alveolar ridge 525.20
    mandible 525.20
      minimal 525.21
      moderate 525.22
      severe 525.23
    maxilla 525.20
      minimal 525.24
      moderate 525.25
      severe 525.26
  emphysema, lung 492.8
  endometrium (senile) 621.8
    cervix 622.8
  enteric 569.89
  epididymis 608.3
  eyeball, cause unknown 360.41
  eyelid (senile) 374.50
  facial (skin) 701.9
  facioscapulohumeral (Landouzy-Déjérine) 359.1
  fallopian tube (senile), acquired 620.3
  fatty, thymus (gland) 254.8
  gallbladder 575.8
  gastric 537.89
  gastritis (chronic) 535.1●
  gastrointestinal 569.89

Atrophy, atrophic *(Continued)*
  genital organ, male 608.89
  glandular 289.3
  globe (phthisis bulbi) 360.41
  gum *(see also* Recession, gingival) 523.20
  hair 704.2
  heart (brown) (senile) *(see also* Degeneration, myocardial) 429.1
  hemifacial 754.0
    Romberg 349.89
  hydronephrosis 591
  infantile 261
    paralysis, acute *(see also* Poliomyelitis, with paralysis) 045.1●
  intestine 569.89
  iris (generalized) (postinfectional) (sector shaped) 364.59
    essential 364.51
    progressive 364.51
    sphincter 364.54
  kidney (senile) *(see also* Sclerosis, renal) 587
    with hypertension *(see also* Hypertension, kidney) 403.90
    congenital 753.0
    hydronephrotic 591
    infantile 753.0
  lacrimal apparatus (primary) 375.13
    secondary 375.14
  Landouzy-Déjérine 359.1
  laryngitis, infection 476.0
  larynx 478.79
  Leber's optic 377.16
  lip 528.5
  liver (acute) (subacute) *(see also* Necrosis, liver) 570
    chronic (yellow) 571.8
    yellow (congenital) 570
      with
        abortion - *see* Abortion, by type, with specified complication NEC
        ectopic pregnancy *(see also* categories 633.0-633.9) 639.8
        molar pregnancy *(see also* categories 630-632) 639.8
      chronic 571.8
      complicating pregnancy 646.7●
      following
        abortion 639.8
        ectopic or molar pregnancy 639.8
      from injection, inoculation or transfusion (onset within 8 months after administration) - *see* Hepatitis, viral
      healed 571.5
      obstetric 646.7●
      postabortal 639.8
      postimmunization - *see* Hepatitis, viral
      posttransfusion - *see* Hepatitis, viral
      puerperal, postpartum 674.8●
  lung (senile) 518.89
    congenital 748.69
  macular (dermatological) 701.3
    syphilitic, skin 091.3
      striated 095.8
  muscle, muscular 728.2
    disuse 728.2
    Duchenne-Aran 335.21
    extremity (lower) (upper) 728.2
    familial spinal 335.11
    general 728.2
    idiopathic 728.2
    infantile spinal 335.0
    myelopathic (progressive) 335.10
    myotonic 359.21
    neuritic 356.1
    neuropathic (peroneal) (progressive) 356.1
    peroneal 356.1
    primary (idiopathic) 728.2

Atrophy, atrophic (Continued)
    muscle, muscular (Continued)
        progressive (familial) (hereditary) (pure) 335.21
            adult (spinal) 335.19
            infantile (spinal) 335.0
            juvenile (spinal) 335.11
            spinal 335.10
                adult 335.19
                hereditary or familial 335.11
                infantile 335.0
        pseudohypertrophic 359.1
        spinal (progressive) 335.10
            adult 335.19
            Aran-Duchenne 335.21
            familial 335.11
            hereditary 335.11
            infantile 335.0
            juvenile 335.11
        syphilitic 095.6
    myocardium (see also Degeneration, myocardial) 429.1
    myometrium (senile) 621.8
        cervix 622.8
    myotatic 728.2
    myotonia 359.21
    nail 703.8
        congenital 757.5
    nasopharynx 472.2
    nerve - see also Disorder, nerve
        abducens 378.54
        accessory 352.4
        acoustic or auditory 388.5
        cranial 352.9
            first (olfactory) 352.0
            second (optic) (see also Atrophy, optic nerve) 377.10
            third (oculomotor) (partial) 378.51
                total 378.52
            fourth (trochlear) 378.53
            fifth (trigeminal) 350.8
            sixth (abducens) 378.54
            seventh (facial) 351.8
            eighth (auditory) 388.5
            ninth (glossopharyngeal) 352.2
            tenth (pneumogastric) (vagus) 352.3
            eleventh (accessory) 352.4
            twelfth (hypoglossal) 352.5
        facial 351.8
        glossopharyngeal 352.2
        hypoglossal 352.5
        oculomotor (partial) 378.51
            total 378.52
        olfactory 352.0
        peripheral 355.9
        pneumogastric 352.3
        trigeminal 350.8
        trochlear 378.53
        vagus (pneumogastric) 352.3
    nervous system, congenital 742.8
    neuritic (see also Disorder, nerve) 355.9
    neurogenic NEC 355.9
        bone
            tabetic 094.0
    nutritional 261
    old age 797
    olivopontocerebellar 333.0
    optic nerve (ascending) (descending) (infectional) (nonfamilial) (papillomacular bundle) (postretinal) (secondary NEC) (simple) 377.10
        associated with retinal dystrophy 377.13
        dominant hereditary 377.16
        glaucomatous 377.14
        hereditary (dominant) (Leber's) 377.16
        Leber's (hereditary) 377.16
        partial 377.15
        postinflammatory 377.12
        primary 377.11

Atrophy, atrophic (Continued)
    optic nerve (Continued)
        syphilitic 094.84
            congenital 090.49
            tabes dorsalis 094.0
    orbit 376.45
    ovary (senile), acquired 620.3
    oviduct (senile), acquired 620.3
    palsy, diffuse 335.20
    pancreas (duct) (senile) 577.8
    papillary muscle 429.81
    paralysis 355.9
    parotid gland 527.0
    patches skin 701.3
        senile 701.8
    penis 607.89
    pharyngitis 472.1
    pharynx 478.29
    pluriglandular 258.8
    polyarthritis 714.0
    prostate 602.2
    pseudohypertrophic 359.1
    renal (see also Sclerosis, renal) 587
    reticulata 701.8
    retina (see also Degeneration, retina) 362.60
        hereditary (see also Dystrophy, retina) 362.70
    rhinitis 472.0
    salivary duct or gland 527.0
    scar NEC 709.2
    sclerosis, lobar (of brain) 331.0
        with dementia
            with behavioral disturbance 331.0 [294.11]
            without behavioral disturbance 331.0 [294.10]
    scrotum 608.89
    seminal vesicle 608.89
    senile 797
        degenerative, of skin 701.3
    skin (patches) (senile) 701.8
    spermatic cord 608.89
    spinal (cord) 336.8
        acute 336.8
        muscular (chronic) 335.10
            adult 335.19
            familial 335.11
            juvenile 335.10
        paralysis 335.10
            acute (see also Poliomyelitis, with paralysis) 045.1
    spine (column) 733.99
    spleen (senile) 289.59
    spots (skin) 701.3
        senile 701.8
    stomach 537.89
    striate and macular 701.3
        syphilitic 095.8
    subcutaneous 701.9
        due to injection 999.9
    sublingual gland 527.0
    submaxillary gland 527.0
    Sudeck's 733.7
    suprarenal (autoimmune) (capsule) (gland) 255.41
        with hypofunction 255.41
    tarso-orbital fascia, congenital 743.66
    testis 608.3
    thenar, partial 354.0
    throat 478.29
    thymus (fat) 254.8
    thyroid (gland) 246.8
        with
            cretinism 243
            myxedema 244.9
        congenital 243
    tongue (senile) 529.8
        papillae 529.4
        smooth 529.4
    trachea 519.19
    tunica vaginalis 608.89

Atrophy, atrophic (Continued)
    turbinate 733.99
    tympanic membrane (nonflaccid) 384.82
        flaccid 384.81
    ulcer (see also Ulcer, skin) 707.9
    upper respiratory tract 478.9
    uterus, uterine (acquired) (senile) 621.8
        cervix 622.8
        due to radiation (intended effect) 621.8
    vagina (senile) 627.3
    vascular 459.89
    vas deferens 608.89
    vertebra (senile) 733.99
    vulva (primary) (senile) 624.1
    Werdnig-Hoffmann 335.0
    yellow (acute) (congenital) (liver) (subacute) (see also Necrosis, liver) 570
        chronic 571.8
        resulting from administration of blood, plasma, serum, or other biological substance (within 8 months of administration) - see Hepatitis, viral

Attack
    akinetic (see also Epilepsy) 345.0 ●
    angina - see Angina
    apoplectic (see also Disease, cerebrovascular, acute) 436
    benign shuddering 333.93
    bilious - see Vomiting
    cataleptic 300.11
    cerebral (see also Disease, cerebrovascular, acute) 436
    coronary (see also Infarct, myocardium) 410.9 ●
    cyanotic, newborn 770.83
    epileptic (see also Epilepsy) 345.9 ●
    epileptiform 780.39
    heart (see also Infarct, myocardium) 410.9 ●
    hemiplegia (see also Disease, cerebrovascular, acute) 436
    hysterical 300.11
    jacksonian (see also Epilepsy) 345.5 ●
    myocardium, myocardial (see also Infarct, myocardium) 410.9 ●
    myoclonic (see also Epilepsy) 345.1 ●
    panic 300.01
    paralysis (see also Disease, cerebrovascular, acute) 436
    paroxysmal 780.39
    psychomotor (see also Epilepsy) 345.4 ●
    salaam (see also Epilepsy) 345.6 ●
    schizophreniform (see also Schizophrenia) 295.4 ●
    sensory and motor 780.39
    syncope 780.2
    toxic, cerebral 780.39
    transient ischemic (TIA) 435.9
    unconsciousness 780.2
        hysterical 300.11
    vasomotor 780.2
    vasovagal (idiopathic) (paroxysmal) 780.2

Attention to
    artificial
        opening (of) V55.9
            digestive tract NEC V55.4
            specified site NEC V55.8
            urinary tract NEC V55.6
        vagina V55.7
    colostomy V55.3
    cystostomy V55.5
    dressing
        wound V58.30
            nonsurgical V58.30
            surgical V58.31
    gastrostomy V55.1
    ileostomy V55.2
    jejunostomy V55.4
    nephrostomy V55.6
    surgical dressings V58.31
    sutures V58.32
    tracheostomy V55.0

SECTION I INDEX TO DISEASES AND INJURIES / Attention to

Attention to (Continued)
  ureterostomy V55.6
  urethrostomy V55.6
Attrition
  gum (see also Recession, gingival) 523.20
  teeth (hard tissues) 521.10
    excessive 521.10
      extending into
        dentine 521.12
        pulp 521.13
      generalized 521.15
      limited to enamel 521.11
      localized 521.14
Atypical - see also condition
  cells
    endocervical 795.00
    endometrial 795.00
    glandular
      anus 796.70
      cervical 795.00
      vaginal 795.10
  distribution, vessel (congenital) (peripheral) NEC 747.60
  endometrium 621.9
  kidney 593.89
Atypism, cervix 622.10
Audible tinnitus (see also Tinnitus) 388.30
Auditory - see condition
Audry's syndrome (acropachyderma) 757.39
Aujeszky's disease 078.89
Aura
  jacksonian (see also Epilepsy) 345.5
  persistent migraine 346.5
    with cerebral infarction 346.6
    without cerebral infarction 346.5
Aurantiasis, cutis 278.3
Auricle, auricular - see condition
Auriculotemporal syndrome 350.8
Australian
  Q fever 083.0
  X disease 062.4
Autism, autistic (child) (infantile) 299.0
Autodigestion 799.89
Autoerythrocyte sensitization 287.2
Autographism 708.3
Autoimmune
  cold sensitivity 283.0
  disease NEC 279.49
  hemolytic anemia 283.0
  inhibitors to clotting factors 286.52
  lymphoproliferative syndrome (ALPS) 279.41
  thyroiditis 245.2
Autoinfection, septic - see Septicemia
Autointoxication 799.89
Automatism 348.89
  with temporal sclerosis 348.81
  epileptic (see also Epilepsy) 345.4

Automatism (Continued)
  paroxysmal, idiopathic (see also Epilepsy) 345.4
Autonomic, autonomous
  bladder 596.54
    neurogenic 596.54
      with cauda equina 344.61
  dysreflexia 337.3
  faciocephalalgia (see also Neuropathy, peripheral, autonomic) 337.9
  hysterical seizure 300.11
  imbalance (see also Neuropathy, peripheral, autonomic 337.9
Autophony 388.40
Autosensitivity, erythrocyte 287.2
Autotopagnosia 780.99
Autotoxemia 799.89
Autumn - see condition
Avellis' syndrome 344.89
Aversion
  oral 783.3
    newborn 779.31
    nonorganic origin 307.59
Aviators
  disease or sickness (see also Effect, adverse, high altitude) 993.2
  ear 993.0
  effort syndrome 306.2
Avitaminosis (multiple NEC) (see also Deficiency, vitamin) 269.2
  A 264.9
  B 266.9
    with
      beriberi 265.0
      pellagra 265.2
  B_1 265.1
  B_2 266.0
  B_6 266.1
  B_{12} 266.2
  C (with scurvy) 267
  D 268.9
    with
      osteomalacia 268.2
      rickets 268.0
  E 269.1
  G 266.0
  H 269.1
  K 269.0
  multiple 269.2
  nicotinic acid 265.2
  P 269.1
Avulsion (traumatic) 879.8
  blood vessel - see Injury, blood vessel, by site
  cartilage - see also Dislocation, by site
    knee, current (see also Tear, meniscus) 836.2
    symphyseal (inner), complicating delivery 665.6

Avulsion (Continued)
  complicated 879.9
  diaphragm - see Injury, internal, diaphragm
  ear - see Wound, open, ear
  epiphysis of bone - see Fracture, by site
  external site other than limb - see Wound, open, by site
  eye 871.3
  fingernail - see Wound, open, finger
  fracture - see Fracture, by site
  genital organs, external - see Wound, open, genital organs
  head (intracranial) NEC - see also Injury, intracranial, with open intracranial wound
    complete 874.9
    external site NEC 873.8
      complicated 873.9
  internal organ or site - see Injury, internal, by site
  joint - see also Dislocation, by site
    capsule - see Sprain, by site
  ligament - see Sprain, by site
  limb - see also Amputation, traumatic, by site
    skin and subcutaneous tissue - see Wound, open, by site
  muscle - see Sprain, by site
  nerve (root) - see Injury, nerve, by site
  scalp - see Wound, open, scalp
  skin and subcutaneous tissue - see Wound, open, by site
  symphyseal cartilage (inner), complicating delivery 665.6
  tendon - see also Sprain, by site
    with open wound - see Wound, open, by site
  toenail - see Wound, open, toe(s)
  tooth 873.63
    complicated 873.73
Awaiting organ transplant status V49.83
Awareness of heart beat 785.1
Axe grinders' disease 502
Axenfeld's anomaly or syndrome 743.44
Axilla, axillary - see also condition
  breast 757.6
Axonotmesis - see Injury, nerve, by site
Ayala's disease 756.89
Ayerza's disease or syndrome (pulmonary artery sclerosis with pulmonary hypertension) 416.0
Azoospermia 606.0
Azorean disease (of the nervous system) 334.8
Azotemia 790.6
  meaning uremia (see also Uremia) 586
Aztec ear 744.29
Azygos lobe, lung (fissure) 748.69

B

Baader's syndrome (erythema multiforme exudativum) 695.19
Baastrup's syndrome 721.5
Babesiasis 088.82
Babesiosis 088.82
Babington's disease (familial hemorrhagic telangiectasia) 448.0
Babinski's syndrome (cardiovascular syphilis) 093.89
Babinski-Fröhlich syndrome (adiposogenital dystrophy) 253.8
Babinski-Nageotte syndrome 344.89
Bacillary - see condition
Bacilluria 791.9
    asymptomatic, in pregnancy or puerperium 646.5●
    tuberculous (see also Tuberculosis) 016.9●
Bacillus - see also Infection, bacillus
    abortus infection 023.1
    anthracis infection 022.9
    coli
        infection 041.49
            generalized 038.42
            intestinal 008.00
        pyemia 038.42
        septicemia 038.42
    Flexner's 004.1
    fusiformis infestation 101
    mallei infection 024
    Shiga's 004.0
    suipestifer infection (see also Infection, Salmonella) 003.9
Back - see condition
Backache (postural) 724.5
    psychogenic 307.89
    sacroiliac 724.6
Backflow (pyelovenous) (see also Disease, renal) 593.9
Backknee (see also Genu, recurvatum) 736.5
Bacteremia 790.7
    newborn 771.83
Bacteria
    in blood (see also Bacteremia) 790.7
    in urine (see also Bacteriuria) 791.9
Bacterial - see condition
Bactericholia (see also Cholecystitis, acute) 575.0
Bacterid, bacteride (Andrews' pustular) 686.8
Bacteriuria, bacteruria 791.9
    with
        urinary tract infection 599.0
    asymptomatic 791.9
        in pregnancy or puerperium 646.5●
            affecting fetus or newborn 760.1
Bad
    breath 784.99
    heart - see Disease, heart
    trip (see also Abuse, drugs, nondependent) 305.3●
Baehr-Schiffrin disease (thrombotic thrombocytopenic purpura) 446.6
Baelz's disease (cheilitis glandularis apostematosa) 528.5
Baerensprung's disease (eczema marginatum) 110.3
Bagassosis (occupational) 495.1
Baghdad boil 085.1
Bagratuni's syndrome (temporal arteritis) 446.5
Baker's
    cyst (knee) 727.51
        tuberculous (see also Tuberculosis) 015.2●
    itch 692.89
Bakwin-Krida syndrome (craniometa-physeal dysplasia) 756.89
Balanitis (circinata) (gangraenosa) (infectious) (vulgaris) 607.1
    amebic 006.8
    candidal 112.2
    chlamydial 099.53
    due to Ducrey's bacillus 099.0

Balanitis (Continued)
    erosiva circinata et gangraenosa 607.1
    gangrenous 607.1
    gonococcal (acute) 098.0
        chronic or duration of 2 months or over 098.2
    nongonococcal 607.1
    phagedenic 607.1
    venereal NEC 099.8
    xerotica obliterans 607.81
Balanoposthitis 607.1
    chlamydial 099.53
    gonococcal (acute) 098.0
        chronic or duration of 2 months or over 098.2
    ulcerative NEC 099.8
Balanorrhagia - see Balanitis
Balantidiasis 007.0
Balantidiosis 007.0
Balbuties, balbutio (see also Disorder, fluency) 315.35
Bald
    patches on scalp 704.00
    tongue 529.4
Baldness (see also Alopecia) 704.00
Balfour's disease (chloroma) 205.3●
Balint's syndrome (psychic paralysis of visual fixation) 368.16
Balkan grippe 083.0
Ball
    food 938
    hair 938
Ballantyne (-Runge) syndrome (postmaturity) 766.22
Balloon disease (see also Effect, adverse, high altitude) 993.2
Ballooning posterior leaflet syndrome 424.0
Baló's disease or concentric sclerosis 341.1
Bamberger's disease (hypertrophic pulmonary osteoarthropathy) 731.2
Bamberger-Marie disease (hypertrophic pulmonary osteoarthropathy) 731.2
Bamboo spine 720.0
Bancroft's filariasis 125.0
Band(s)
    adhesive (see also Adhesions, peritoneum) 568.0
    amniotic 658.8●
        affecting fetus or newborn 762.8
    anomalous or congenital - see also Anomaly, specified type NEC
        atrial 746.9
        heart 746.9
        intestine 751.4
        omentum 751.4
        ventricular 746.9
    cervix 622.3
    gallbladder (congenital) 751.69
    intestinal (adhesive) (see also Adhesions, peritoneum) 568.0
        congenital 751.4
        obstructive (see also Obstruction, intestine) 560.81
    periappendiceal (congenital) 751.4
    peritoneal (adhesive) (see also Adhesions, peritoneum) 568.0
        with intestinal obstruction 560.81
        congenital 751.4
    uterus 621.5
    vagina 623.2
Bandemia (without diagnosis of specific infection) 288.66
Bandl's ring (contraction)
    complicating delivery 661.4●
        affecting fetus or newborn 763.7
Bang's disease (Brucella abortus) 023.1
Bangkok hemorrhagic fever 065.4
Bannister's disease 995.1
Bantam-Albright-Martin disease (pseudohypoparathyroidism) 275.49

Banti's disease or syndrome (with cirrhosis) (with portal hypertension) - see Cirrhosis, liver
Bar
    calcaneocuboid 755.67
    calcaneonavicular 755.67
    cubonavicular 755.67
    prostate 600.90
        with
            other lower urinary tract symptoms (LUTS) 600.91
            urinary
                obstruction 600.91
                retention 600.91
    talocalcaneal 755.67
Baragnosis 780.99
Barasheh, barashek 266.2
Barcoo disease or rot (see also Ulcer, skin) 707.9
Bard-Pic syndrome (carcinoma, head of pancreas) 157.0
Bärensprung's disease (eczema marginatum) 110.3
Baritosis 503
Barium lung disease 503
Barlow's syndrome (meaning mitral valve prolapse) 424.0
Barlow (-Möller) disease or syndrome (meaning infantile scurvy) 267
Barodontalgia 993.2
Baron Münchausen syndrome 301.51
Barosinusitis 993.1
Barotitis 993.0
Barotrauma 993.2
    odontalgia 993.2
    otitic 993.0
    sinus 993.1
Barraquer's disease or syndrome (progressive lipodystrophy) 272.6
Barré-Guillain syndrome 357.0
Barré-Liéou syndrome (posterior cervical sympathetic) 723.2
Barrel chest 738.3
Barrett's esophagus 530.85
Barrett's syndrome or ulcer (chronic peptic ulcer of esophagus) 530.85
Bársony-Polgár syndrome (corkscrew esophagus) 530.5
Bársony-Teschendorf syndrome (corkscrew esophagus) 530.5
Barth syndrome 759.89
Bartholin's
    adenitis (see also Bartholinitis) 616.89
    gland - see condition
Bartholinitis (suppurating) 616.89
    gonococcal (acute) 098.0
        chronic or duration of 2 months or over 098.2
Bartonellosis 088.0
Bartter's syndrome (secondary hyperaldosteronism with juxtaglomerular hyperplasia) 255.13
Basal - see condition
Basan's (hidrotic) ectodermal dysplasia 757.31
Baseball finger 842.13
Basedow's disease or syndrome (exophthalmic goiter) 242.0●
Basic - see condition
Basilar - see condition
Bason's (hidrotic) ectodermal dysplasia 757.31
Basopenia 288.59
Basophilia 288.65
Basophilism (corticoadrenal) (Cushing's) (pituitary) (thymic) 255.0
Bassen-Kornzweig syndrome (abetalipoproteinemia) 272.5
Bat ear 744.29
Bateman's
    disease 078.0
    purpura (senile) 287.2
Bathing cramp 994.1
Bathophobia 300.23

SECTION 1 INDEX TO DISEASES AND INJURIES / Batten's disease, retina

Batten's disease, retina 330.1 [362.71]
Batten-Mayou disease 330.1 [362.71]
Batten-Steinert syndrome 359.21
Battered
    adult (syndrome) 995.81
    baby or child (syndrome) 995.54
    spouse (syndrome) 995.81
Battey mycobacterium infection 031.0
Battledore placenta - see Placenta, abnormal
Battle exhaustion (see also Reaction, stress, acute) 308.9
Baumgarten-Cruveilhier (cirrhosis) disease, or syndrome 571.5
Bauxite
    fibrosis (of lung) 503
    workers' disease 503
Bayle's disease (dementia paralytica) 094.1
Bazin's disease (primary) (see also Tuberculosis) 017.1●
Beach ear 380.12
Beaded hair (congenital) 757.4
Beals syndrome 759.82
Beard's disease (neurasthenia) 300.5
Bearn-Kunkel (-Slater) syndrome (lupoid hepatitis) 571.49
Beat
    elbow 727.2
    hand 727.2
    knee 727.2
Beats
    ectopic 427.60
    escaped, heart 427.60
        postoperative 997.1
    premature (nodal) 427.60
        atrial 427.61
        auricular 427.61
        postoperative 997.1
        specified type NEC 427.69
        supraventricular 427.61
        ventricular 427.69
Beau's
    disease or syndrome (see also Degeneration, myocardial) 429.1
    lines (transverse furrows on fingernails) 703.8
Bechterew's disease (ankylosing spondylitis) 720.0
Bechterew-Strümpell-Marie syndrome (ankylosing spondylitis) 720.0
Beck's syndrome (anterior spinal artery occlusion) 433.8●
Becker's
    disease
        idiopathic mural endomyocardial disease 425.2
        myotonia congenita, recessive form 359.22
    dystrophy 359.22
Beckwith (-Wiedemann) syndrome 759.89
Bedbugs bite(s) - see Injury, superficial, by site
Bedclothes, asphyxiation or suffocation by 994.7
Bed confinement status V49.84
Bednar's aphthae 528.2
Bedsore (see also Ulcer, pressure) 707.00
    with gangrene 707.00 [785.4]
Bedwetting (see also Enuresis) 788.36
Beer-drinkers' heart (disease) 425.5
Bee sting (with allergic or anaphylactic shock) 989.5
Begbie's disease (exophthalmic goiter) 242.0●
Behavior disorder, disturbance - see also
    Disturbance, conduct
    antisocial, without manifest psychiatric disorder
        adolescent V71.02
        adult V71.01
        child V71.02
    dyssocial, without manifest psychiatric disorder
        adolescent V71.02
        adult V71.01
        child V71.02
    high-risk- see problem

Behçet's syndrome 136.1
Behr's disease 362.50
Beigel's disease or morbus (white piedra) 111.2
Bejel 104.0
Bekhterev's disease (ankylosing spondylitis) 720.0
Bekhterev-Strümpell-Marie syndrome (ankylosing spondylitis) 720.0
Belching (see also Eructation) 787.3
Bell's
    disease (see also Psychosis, affective) 296.0●
    mania (see also Psychosis, affective) 296.0●
    palsy, paralysis 351.0
        infant 767.5
        newborn 767.5
        syphilitic 094.89
    spasm 351.0
Bence-Jones albuminuria, albuminosuria, or proteinuria 791.0
Bends 993.3
Benedikt's syndrome (paralysis) 344.89
Benign - see also condition
    cellular changes, cervix 795.09
    prostate
        hyperplasia 600.20
            with
                other lower urinary tract symptoms (LUTS) 600.21
                urinary
                      obstruction 600.21
                      retention 600.21
        neoplasm 222.2
Bennett's
    disease (leukemia) 208.9●
    fracture (closed) 815.01
        open 815.11
Benson's disease 379.22
Bent
    back (hysterical) 300.11
    nose 738.0
        congenital 754.0
Bereavement V62.82
    as adjustment reaction 309.0
Berger's paresthesia (lower limb) 782.0
Bergeron's disease (hysteroepilepsy) 300.11
Beriberi (acute) (atrophic) (chronic) (dry) (subacute) (wet) 265.0
    with polyneuropathy 265.0 [357.4]
    heart (disease) 265.0 [425.7]
    leprosy 030.1
    neuritis 265.0 [357.4]
Berlin's disease or edema (traumatic) 921.3
Berloque dermatitis 692.72
Bernard-Horner syndrome (see also Neuropathy, peripheral, autonomic) 337.9
Bernard-Sergent syndrome (acute adrenocortical insufficiency) 255.41
Bernard-Soulier disease or thrombopathy 287.1
Bernhardt's disease or paresthesia 355.1
Bernhardt-Roth disease or syndrome (parasthesia) 355.1
Bernheim's syndrome (see also Failure, heart) 428.0
Bertielliasis 123.8
Bertolotti's syndrome (sacralization of fifth lumbar vertebra) 756.15
Berylliosis (acute) (chronic) (lung) (occupational) 503
Besnier's
    lupus pernio 135
    prurigo (atopic dermatitis) (infantile eczema) 691.8
Besnier-Boeck disease or sarcoid 135
Besnier-Boeck-Schaumann disease (sarcoidosis) 135
Best's disease 362.76
Bestiality 302.1
Beta-adrenergic hyperdynamic circulatory state 429.82
Beta-aminoisobutyric aciduria 277.2

Beta-mercaptolactate-cysteine disulfiduria 270.0
Beta thalassemia (mixed) 282.44
    major 282.44
    minor 282.46
Beurmann's disease (sporotrichosis) 117.1
Bezoar 938
    intestine 936
    stomach 935.2
Bezold's abscess (see also Mastoiditis) 383.01
Bianchi's syndrome (aphasia-apraxia-alexia) 784.69
Bicornuate or bicornis uterus (complete) (partial) 752.34
    in pregnancy or childbirth 654.0●
        with obstructed labor 660.2●
            affecting fetus or newborn 763.1
        affecting fetus or newborn 763.89
Bicuspid aortic valve 746.4
Biedl-Bardet syndrome 759.89
Bielschowsky's disease 330.1
Bielschowsky-Jansky
    amaurotic familial idiocy 330.1
    disease 330.1
Biemond's syndrome (obesity, polydactyly, and intellectual disabilities) 759.89
Biermer's anemia or disease (pernicious anemia) 281.0
Biett's disease 695.4
Bifid (congenital) - see also Imperfect, closure
    apex, heart 746.89
    clitoris 752.49
    epiglottis 748.3
    kidney 753.3
    nose 748.1
    patella 755.64
    scrotum 752.89
    toe 755.66
    tongue 750.13
    ureter 753.4
    uterus 752.34
    uvula 749.02
        with cleft lip (see also Cleft, palate, with cleft lip) 749.20
Biforis uterus (suprasimplex) 752.34
Bifurcation (congenital) - see also Imperfect, closure
    gallbladder 751.69
    kidney pelvis 753.3
    renal pelvis 753.3
    rib 756.3
    tongue 750.13
    trachea 748.3
    ureter 753.4
    urethra 753.8
    uvula 749.02
        with cleft lip (see also Cleft, palate, with cleft lip) 749.20
    vertebra 756.19
Bigeminal pulse 427.89
Bigeminy 427.89
Big spleen syndrome 289.4
Bilateral - see condition
Bile duct - see condition
Bile pigments in urine 791.4
Bilharziasis (see also Schistosomiasis) 120.9
    chyluria 120.0
    cutaneous 120.3
    galacturia 120.0
    hematochyluria 120.0
    intestinal 120.1
    lipemia 120.9
    lipuria 120.0
    Oriental 120.2
    piarhemia 120.9
    pulmonary 120.2
    tropical hematuria 120.0
    vesical 120.0
Biliary - see condition
Bilious (attack) - see also Vomiting
    fever, hemoglobinuric 084.8

Bilirubinuria 791.4
Biliuria 791.4
Billroth's disease
    meningocele (see also Spina bifida) 741.9
Bilobate placenta - see Placenta, abnormal
Bilocular
    heart 745.7
    stomach 536.8
Bing-Horton syndrome (histamine cephalgia) 339.00
Binswanger's disease or dementia 290.12
Biörck (-Thorson) syndrome (malignant carcinoid) 259.2
Biparta, bipartite - see also Imperfect, closure
    carpal scaphoid 755.59
    patella 755.64
    placenta - see Placenta, abnormal
    vagina 752.49
Bird
    face 756.0
    fanciers' lung or disease 495.2
    flu (see also Influenza, avian) 488.02
Bird's disease (oxaluria) 271.8
Birth
    abnormal fetus or newborn 763.9
    accident, fetus or newborn - see Birth, injury
    complications in mother - see Delivery, complicated
    compression during NEC 767.9
    defect - see Anomaly
    delayed, fetus 763.9
    difficult NEC, affecting fetus or newborn 763.9
    dry, affecting fetus or newborn 761.1
    forced, NEC, affecting fetus or newborn 763.89
    forceps, affecting fetus or newborn 763.2
    hematoma of sternomastoid 767.8
    immature 765.1
        extremely 765.0
    inattention, after or at 995.52
    induced, affecting fetus or newborn 763.89
    infant - see Newborn
    injury NEC 767.9
        adrenal gland 767.8
        basal ganglia 767.0
        brachial plexus (paralysis) 767.6
        brain (compression) (pressure) 767.0
        cerebellum 767.0
        cerebral hemorrhage 767.0
        conjunctiva 767.8
        eye 767.8
        fracture
            bone, any except clavicle or spine 767.3
            clavicle 767.2
            femur 767.3
            humerus 767.3
            long bone 767.3
            radius and ulna 767.3
            skeleton NEC 767.3
            skull 767.3
            spine 767.4
            tibia and fibula 767.3
        hematoma 767.8
            liver (subcapsular) 767.8
            mastoid 767.8
            skull 767.19
            sternomastoid 767.8
            testes 767.8
            vulva 767.8
        intracranial (edema) 767.0
        laceration
            brain 767.0
            by scalpel 767.8
            peripheral nerve 767.7
        liver 767.8
        meninges
            brain 767.0
            spinal cord 767.4
        nerves (cranial, peripheral) 767.7
            brachial plexus 767.6
            facial 767.5

Birth (Continued)
    injury NEC (Continued)
        paralysis 767.7
            brachial plexus 767.6
            Erb (-Duchenne) 767.6
            facial nerve 767.5
            Klumpke (-Déjérine) 767.6
            radial nerve 767.6
            spinal (cord) (hemorrhage) (laceration) (rupture) 767.4
        rupture
            intracranial 767.0
            liver 767.8
            spinal cord 767.4
            spleen 767.8
            viscera 767.8
        scalp 767.19
        scalpel wound 767.8
        skeleton NEC 767.3
        specified NEC 767.8
        spinal cord 767.4
        spleen 767.8
        subdural hemorrhage 767.0
        tentorial, tear 767.0
        testes 767.8
        vulva 767.8
    instrumental, NEC, affecting fetus or newborn 763.2
    lack of care, after or at 995.52
    multiple
        affected by maternal complications of pregnancy 761.5
        healthy liveborn - see Newborn, multiple
    neglect, after or at 995.52
    newborn - see Newborn
    palsy or paralysis NEC 767.7
    precipitate, fetus or newborn 763.6
    premature (infant) 765.1
    prolonged, affecting fetus or newborn 763.9
    retarded, fetus or newborn 763.9
    shock, newborn 779.89
    strangulation or suffocation
        due to aspiration of clear amniotic fluid 770.13
            with respiratory symptoms 770.14
        mechanical 767.8
    trauma NEC 767.9
    triplet
        affected by maternal complications of pregnancy 761.5
        healthy liveborn - see Newborn, multiple
    twin
        affected by maternal complications of pregnancy 761.5
        healthy liveborn - see Newborn, twin
    ventouse, affecting fetus or newborn 763.3
Birthmark 757.32
Birt-Hogg-Dube syndrome 759.89
Bisalbuminemia 273.8
Biskra button 085.1
Bite(s)
    with intact skin surface - see Contusion
    animal - see Wound, open, by site
        intact skin surface - see Contusion
    bedbug - see Injury, superficial, by site
    centipede 989.5
    chigger 133.8
    fire ant 989.5
    flea - see Injury, superficial, by site
    human (open wound) - see also Wound, open, by site
        intact skin surface - see Contusion
    insect
        nonvenomous - see Injury, superficial, by site
        venomous 989.5
    mad dog (death from) 071
    open
        anterior 524.24
        posterior 524.25
    poisonous 989.5

Bite(s) (Continued)
    red bug 133.8
    reptile 989.5
        nonvenomous - see Wound, open, by site
    snake 989.5
        nonvenomous - see Wound, open, by site
    spider (venomous) 989.5
        nonvenomous - see Injury, superficial, by site
    venomous 989.5
Biting
    cheek or lip 528.9
    nail 307.9
Black
    death 020.9
    eye NEC 921.0
    hairy tongue 529.3
    heel 924.20
    lung disease 500
    palm 923.20
Blackfan-Diamond anemia or syndrome (congenital hypoplastic anemia) 284.01
Blackhead 706.1
Blackout 780.2
Blackwater fever 084.8
Bladder - see condition
Blast
    blindness 921.3
    concussion - see Blast, injury
    injury 869.0
        with open wound into cavity 869.1
        abdomen or thorax - see Injury, internal, by site
        brain (see also Concussion, brain) 850.9
            with skull fracture - see Fracture, skull
        ear (acoustic nerve trauma) 951.5
            with perforation, tympanic membrane - see Wound, open, ear, drum
        lung (see also Injury, internal, lung) 861.20
        otitic (explosive) 388.11
Blastomycosis, blastomycotic (chronic) (cutaneous) (disseminated) (lung) (pulmonary) (systemic) 116.0
    Brazilian 116.1
    European 117.5
    keloidal 116.2
    North American 116.0
    primary pulmonary 116.0
    South American 116.1
Bleb(s) 709.8
    emphysematous (bullous) (diffuse) (lung) (ruptured) (solitary) 492.0
    filtering, eye (postglaucoma) (status) V45.69
        with complication 997.99
        postcataract extraction (complication) 997.99
    lung (ruptured) 492.0
        congenital 770.5
    subpleural (emphysematous) 492.0
Bleeder (familial) (hereditary) (see also Defect, coagulation) 286.9
    nonfamilial 286.9
Bleeding (see also Hemorrhage) 459.0
    anal 569.3
    anovulatory 628.0
    atonic, following delivery 666.1
    capillary 448.9
    due to subinvolution 621.1
        puerperal 666.2
    ear 388.69
    excessive, associated with menopausal onset 627.0
    familial (see also Defect, coagulation) 286.9
    following intercourse 626.7
    gastrointestinal 578.9
    gums 523.8
    hemorrhoids - see Hemorrhoids, bleeding
    intermenstrual
        irregular 626.6
        regular 626.5

SECTION I INDEX TO DISEASES AND INJURIES / Bleeding

Bleeding (Continued)
  intraoperative 998.11
  irregular NEC 626.4
  menopausal 627.0
  mouth 528.9
  nipple 611.79
  nose 784.7
  ovulation 626.5
  postclimacteric 627.1
  postcoital 626.7
  postmenopausal 627.1
    following induced menopause 627.4
  postoperative 998.11
  preclimacteric 627.0
  puberty 626.3
    excessive, with onset of menstrual periods 626.3
  rectum, rectal 569.3
  tendencies (see also Defect, coagulation) 286.9
  throat 784.8
  umbilical stump 772.3
  umbilicus 789.9
  unrelated to menstrual cycle 626.6
  uterus, uterine 626.9
    climacteric 627.0
    dysfunctional 626.8
    functional 626.8
    unrelated to menstrual cycle 626.6
  vagina, vaginal 623.8
    functional 626.8
  vicarious 625.8

Blennorrhagia, blennorrhagic - see Blennorrhea

Blennorrhea (acute) 098.0
  adultorum 098.40
  alveolaris 523.40
  chronic or duration of 2 months or over 098.2
  gonococcal (neonatorum) 098.40
  inclusion (neonatal) (newborn) 771.6
  neonatorum 098.40

Blepharelosis (see also Entropion) 374.00

Blepharitis (eyelid) 373.00
  angularis 373.01
  ciliaris 373.00
    with ulcer 373.01
  marginal 373.00
    with ulcer 373.01
  scrofulous (see also Tuberculosis) 017.3 ● [373.00]
  squamous 373.02
  ulcerative 373.01

Blepharochalasis 374.34
  congenital 743.62

Blepharoclonus 333.81

Blepharoconjunctivitis (see also Conjunctivitis) 372.20
  angular 372.21
  contact 372.22

Blepharophimosis (eyelid) 374.46
  congenital 743.62

Blepharoplegia 374.89

Blepharoptosis 374.30
  congenital 743.61

Blepharopyorrhea 098.49

Blepharospasm 333.81
  due to drugs 333.85

Blessig's cyst 362.62

Blighted ovum 631.8

Blind
  bronchus (congenital) 748.3
  eye - see also Blindness
    hypertensive 360.42
    hypotensive 360.41
  loop syndrome (postoperative) 579.2
  sac, fallopian tube (congenital) 752.19
  spot, enlarged 368.42
  tract or tube (congenital) NEC - see Atresia

Blindness (acquired) (congenital) (both eyes) 369.00
  with deafness V49.85
  blast 921.3
    with nerve injury - see Injury, nerve, optic

Blindness (Continued)
  Bright's - see Uremia
  color (congenital) 368.59
    acquired 368.55
    blue 368.53
    green 368.52
    red 368.51
    total 368.54
  concussion 950.9
  cortical 377.75
  day 368.10
    acquired 368.10
    congenital 368.10
    hereditary 368.10
    specified type NEC 368.10
  due to
    injury NEC 950.9
    refractive error - see Error, refractive
  eclipse (total) 363.31
  emotional 300.11
  face 368.16
  hysterical 300.11
  legal (both eyes) (USA definition) 369.4
    with impairment of better (less impaired) eye
      near-total 369.02
        with
          lesser eye impairment 369.02
            near-total 369.04
            total 369.03
      profound 369.05
        with
          lesser eye impairment 369.05
            near-total 369.07
            profound 369.08
            total 369.06
      severe 369.21
        with
          lesser eye impairment 369.21
            blind 369.11
            near-total 369.13
            profound 369.14
            severe 369.22
            total 369.12
      total
        with lesser eye impairment
          total 369.01
  mind 784.69
  moderate
    both eyes 369.25
      with impairment of lesser eye (specified as)
        blind, not further specified 369.15
        low vision, not further specified 369.23
        near-total 369.17
        profound 369.18
        severe 369.24
        total 369.16
    one eye 369.74
      with vision of other eye (specified as)
        near-normal 369.75
        normal 369.76
  near-total
    both eyes 369.04
      with impairment of lesser eye (specified as)
        blind, not further specified 369.02
        total 369.03
    one eye 369.64
      with vision of other eye (specified as)
        near-normal 369.65
        normal 369.66
  night 368.60
    acquired 368.62
    congenital (Japanese) 368.61
    hereditary 368.61
    specified type NEC 368.69
    vitamin A deficiency 264.5
  nocturnal - see Blindness, night

Blindness (Continued)
  one eye 369.60
    with low vision of other eye 369.10
  profound
    both eyes 369.08
      with impairment of lesser eye (specified as)
        blind, not further specified 369.05
        near-total 369.07
        total 369.06
    one eye 369.67
      with vision of other eye (specified as)
        near-normal 369.68
        normal 369.69
  psychic 784.69
  severe
    both eyes 369.22
      with impairment of lesser eye (specified as)
        blind, not further specified 369.11
        low vision, not further specified 369.21
        near-total 369.13
        profound 369.14
        total 369.12
    one eye 369.71
      with vision of other eye (specified as)
        near-normal 369.72
        normal 369.73
  snow 370.24
  sun 363.31
  temporary 368.12
  total
    both eyes 369.01
    one eye 369.61
      with vision of other eye (specified as)
        near-normal 369.62
        normal 369.63
  transient 368.12
  traumatic NEC 950.9
  word (developmental) 315.01
    acquired 784.61
    secondary to organic lesion 784.61

Blister - see also Injury, superficial, by site
  beetle dermatitis 692.89
  due to burn - see Burn, by site, second degree
  fever 054.9
  fracture - *omit code*
  multiple, skin, nontraumatic 709.8

Bloating 787.3

Bloch-Siemens syndrome (incontinentia pigmenti) 757.33

Bloch-Stauffer dyshormonal dermatosis 757.33

Bloch-Sulzberger disease or syndrome (incontinentia pigmenti) (melanoblastosis) 757.33

Block
  alveolar capillary 516.8
  arborization (heart) 426.6
  arrhythmic 426.9
  atrioventricular (AV) (incomplete) (partial) 426.10
    with
      2:1 atrioventricular response block 426.13
      atrioventricular dissociation 426.0
    first degree (incomplete) 426.11
    second degree (Mobitz type I) 426.13
      Mobitz (type II) 426.12
    third degree 426.0
    complete 426.0
      congenital 746.86
    congenital 746.86
    Mobitz (incomplete)
      type I (Wenckebach's) 426.13
      type II 426.12
    partial 426.13

Block (Continued)
    auriculoventricular (see also Block, atrioventricular) 426.10
        complete 426.0
            congenital 746.86
        congenital 746.86
    bifascicular (cardiac) 426.53
    bundle branch (complete) (false) (incomplete) 426.50
        bilateral 426.53
        left (complete) (main stem) 426.3
            with right bundle branch block 426.53
            anterior fascicular 426.2
                with
                    posterior fascicular block 426.3
                    right bundle branch block 426.52
            hemiblock 426.2
            incomplete 426.2
                with right bundle branch block 426.53
            posterior fascicular 426.2
                with
                    anterior fascicular block 426.3
                    right bundle branch block 426.51
        right 426.4
            with
                left bundle branch block (incomplete) (main stem) 426.53
                left fascicular block 426.53
                    anterior 426.52
                    posterior 426.51
        Wilson's type 426.4
    cardiac 426.9
    conduction 426.9
        complete 426.0
    Eustachian tube (see also Obstruction, Eustachian tube) 381.60
    fascicular (left anterior) (left posterior) 426.2
    foramen Magendie (acquired) 331.3
        congenital 742.3
            with spina bifida (see also Spina bifida) 741.0●
    heart 426.9
        first degree (atrioventricular) 426.11
        second degree (atrioventricular) 426.13
        third degree (atrioventricular) 426.0
        bundle branch (complete) (false) (incomplete) 426.50
            bilateral 426.53
            left (see also Block, bundle branch, left) 426.3
            right (see also Block, bundle branch, right) 426.4
        complete (atrioventricular) 426.0
        congenital 746.86
        incomplete 426.13
        intra-atrial 426.6
        intraventricular NEC 426.6
        sinoatrial 426.6
        specified type NEC 426.6
    hepatic vein 453.0
    intraventricular (diffuse) (myofibrillar) 426.6
        bundle branch (complete) (false) (incomplete) 426.50
            bilateral 426.53
            left (see also Block, bundle branch, left) 426.3
            right (see also Block, bundle branch, right) 426.4
    kidney (see also Disease, renal) 593.9
        postcystoscopic 997.5
    myocardial (see also Block, heart) 426.9
    nodal 426.10
    optic nerve 377.49
    organ or site (congenital) NEC - see Atresia
    parietal 426.6
    peri-infarction 426.6
    portal (vein) 452
    sinoatrial 426.6
    sinoauricular 426.6
    spinal cord 336.9

Block (Continued)
    trifascicular 426.54
    tubal 628.2
    vein NEC 453.9
Blocq's disease or syndrome (astasia-abasia) 307.9
Blood
    constituents, abnormal NEC 790.6
    disease 289.9
        specified NEC 289.89
    donor V59.01
        other blood components V59.09
        stem cells V59.02
        whole blood V59.01
    dyscrasia 289.9
        with
            abortion - see Abortion, by type, with hemorrhage, delayed or excessive
            ectopic pregnancy (see also categories 633.0–633.9) 639.1
            molar pregnancy (see also categories 630–632) 639.1
        following
            abortion 639.1
            ectopic or molar pregnancy 639.1
        newborn NEC 776.9
        puerperal, postpartum 666.3●
    flukes NEC (see also Infestation, Schistosoma) 120.9
    in
        feces (see also Melena) 578.1
            occult 792.1
        urine (see also Hematuria) 599.70
    mole 631.8
    occult 792.1
    poisoning (see also Septicemia) 038.9
    pressure
        decreased, due to shock following injury 958.4
        fluctuating 796.4
        high (see also Hypertension) 401.9
            borderline 796.2
            incidental reading (isolated) (nonspecific), without diagnosis of hypertension 796.2
        low (see also Hypotension) 458.9
            incidental reading (isolated) (nonspecific), without diagnosis of hypotension 796.3
    spitting (see also Hemoptysis) 786.30
    staining cornea 371.12
    transfusion
        without reported diagnosis V58.2
        donor V59.01
            stem cells V59.02
        reaction or complication - see Complications, transfusion
    tumor - see Hematoma
    vessel rupture - see Hemorrhage
    vomiting (see also Hematemesis) 578.0
Blood-forming organ disease 289.9
Bloodgood's disease 610.1
Bloodshot eye 379.93
Bloom (-Machacek) (-Torre) syndrome 757.39
Blotch, palpebral 372.55
Blount's disease (tibia vara) 732.4
Blount-Barber syndrome (tibia vara) 732.4
Blue
    baby 746.9
    bloater 491.20
        with
            acute bronchitis 491.22
            exacerbation (acute) 491.21
    diaper syndrome 270.0
    disease 746.9
    dome cyst 610.0
    drum syndrome 381.02
    sclera 743.47
        with fragility of bone and deafness 756.51
    toe syndrome 445.02

Blueness (see also Cyanosis) 782.5
Blurring, visual 368.8
Blushing (abnormal) (excessive) 782.62
BMI (body mass index)
    adult
        25.0–25.9 V85.21
        26.0–26.9 V85.22
        27.0–27.9 V85.23
        28.0–28.9 V85.24
        29.0–29.9 V85.25
        30.0–30.9 V85.30
        31.0–31.9 V85.31
        32.0–32.9 V85.32
        33.0–33.9 V85.33
        34.0–34.9 V85.34
        35.0–35.9 V85.35
        36.0–36.9 V85.36
        37.0–37.9 V85.37
        38.0–38.9 V85.38
        39.0–39.9 V85.39
        40.0-44.9 V85.41
        45.0-49.9 V85.42
        50.0-59.9 V85.43
        60.0-69.9 V85.44
        70 and over V85.45
        between 19–24 V85.1
        less than 19 V85.0
    pediatric
        5th percentile to less than 85th percentile for age V85.52
        85th percentile to less than 95th percentile for age V85.53
        greater than or equal to 95th percentile for age V85.54
        less than 5th percentile for age V85.51
Boarder, hospital V65.0
    infant V65.0
Bockhart's impetigo (superficial folliculitis) 704.8
Bodechtel-Guttmann disease (subacute sclerosing panencephalitis) 046.2
Boder-Sedgwick syndrome (ataxia-telangiectasia) 334.8
Body, bodies
    Aschoff (see also Myocarditis, rheumatic) 398.0
    asteroid, vitreous 379.22
    choroid, colloid (degenerative) 362.57
        hereditary 362.77
    cytoid (retina) 362.82
    drusen (retina) (see also Drusen) 362.57
        optic disc 377.21
    fibrin, pleura 511.0
    foreign - see Foreign body
    Hassall-Henle 371.41
    loose
        joint (see also Loose, body, joint) 718.1●
            knee 717.6
        knee 717.6
        sheath, tendon 727.82
    Mallory's 034.1
    mass index (BMI)
        adult
            25.0–25.9 V85.21
            26.0–26.9 V85.22
            27.0–27.9 V85.23
            28.0–28.9 V85.24
            29.0–29.9 V85.25
            30.0–30.9 V85.30
            31.0–31.9 V85.31
            32.0–32.9 V85.32
            33.0–33.9 V85.33
            34.0–34.9 V85.34
            35.0–35.9 V85.35
            36.0–36.9 V85.36
            37.0–37.9 V85.37
            38.0–38.9 V85.38
            39.0–39.9 V85.39
            40.0-44.9 V85.41
            45.0-49.9 V85.42
            50.0-59.9 V85.43

Body, bodies (Continued)
   mass index (BMI) (Continued)
      adult (Continued)
         60.0-69.9 V85.44
         70 and over V85.45
         between 19–24 V85.1
         less than 19 V85.0
      pediatric
         5th percentile to less than 85th percentile for age V85.52
         85th percentile to less than 95th percentile for age V85.53
         greater than or equal to 95th percentile for age V85.54
         less than 5th percentile for age V85.51
   Mooser 081.0
   Negri 071
   rice (joint) (see also Loose, body, joint) 718.1●
      knee 717.6
   rocking 307.3
Boeck's
   disease (sarcoidosis) 135
   lupoid (miliary) 135
   sarcoid 135
Boerhaave's syndrome (spontaneous esophageal rupture) 530.4
Boggy
   cervix 622.8
   uterus 621.8
Boil (see also Carbuncle) 680.9
   abdominal wall 680.2
   Aleppo 085.1
   ankle 680.6
   anus 680.5
   arm (any part, above wrist) 680.3
   auditory canal, external 680.0
   axilla 680.3
   back (any part) 680.2
   Baghdad 085.1
   breast 680.2
   buttock 680.5
   chest wall 680.2
   corpus cavernosum 607.2
   Delhi 085.1
   ear (any part) 680.0
   eyelid 373.13
   face (any part, except eye) 680.0
   finger (any) 680.4
   flank 680.2
   foot (any part) 680.7
   forearm 680.3
   Gafsa 085.1
   genital organ, male 608.4
   gluteal (region) 680.5
   groin 680.2
   hand (any part) 680.4
   head (any part, except face) 680.8
   heel 680.7
   hip 680.6
   knee 680.6
   labia 616.4
   lacrimal (see also Dacryocystitis) 375.30
      gland (see also Dacryoadenitis) 375.00
      passages (duct) (sac) (see also Dacryocystitis) 375.30
   leg, any part, except foot 680.6
   multiple sites 680.9
   natal 085.1
   neck 680.1
   nose (external) (septum) 680.0
   orbit, orbital 376.01
   partes posteriores 680.5
   pectoral region 680.2
   penis 607.2
   perineum 680.2
   pinna 680.0
   scalp (any part) 680.8
   scrotum 608.4
   seminal vesicle 608.0
   shoulder 680.3
   skin NEC 680.9

Boil (Continued)
   specified site NEC 680.8
   spermatic cord 608.4
   temple (region) 680.0
   testis 608.4
   thigh 680.6
   thumb 680.4
   toe (any) 680.7
   tropical 085.1
   trunk 680.2
   tunica vaginalis 608.4
   umbilicus 680.2
   upper arm 680.3
   vas deferens 608.4
   vulva 616.4
   wrist 680.4
Bold hives (see also Urticaria) 708.9
Bolivian hemorrhagic fever 078.7
Bombé, iris 364.74
Bomford-Rhoads anemia (refractory) 238.72
Bone - see condition
Bonnevie-Ullrich syndrome 758.6
Bonnier's syndrome 386.19
Bonvale Dam fever 780.79
Bony block of joint 718.80
   ankle 718.87
   elbow 718.82
   foot 718.87
   hand 718.84
   hip 718.85
   knee 718.86
   multiple sites 718.89
   pelvic region 718.85
   shoulder (region) 718.81
   specified site NEC 718.88
   wrist 718.83
BOOP (bronchiolitis obliterans organized pneumonia) 516.8
Borderline
   diabetes mellitus 790.29
   hypertension 796.2
   intellectual functioning V62.89
   osteopenia 733.90
   pelvis 653.1●
      with obstruction during labor 660.1●
         affecting fetus or newborn 763.1
   psychosis (see also Schizophrenia) 295.5●
      of childhood (see also Psychosis, childhood) 299.8●
   schizophrenia (see also Schizophrenia) 295.5●
Borna disease 062.9
Bornholm disease (epidemic pleurodynia) 074.1
Borrelia vincentii (mouth) (pharynx) (tonsils) 101
Bostock's catarrh (see also Fever, hay) 477.9
Boston exanthem 048
Botalli, ductus (patent) (persistent) 747.0
Bothriocephalus latus infestation 123.4
Botulism 005.1
   food poisoning 005.1
   infant 040.41
   non-foodborne 040.42
   wound 040.42
Bouba (see also Yaws) 102.9
Bouffée délirante 298.3
Bouillaud's disease or syndrome (rheumatic heart disease) 391.9
Bourneville's disease (tuberous sclerosis) 759.5
Boutonneuse fever 082.1
Boutonniere
   deformity (finger) 736.21
   hand (intrinsic) 736.21
Bouveret (-Hoffmann) disease or syndrome (paroxysmal tachycardia) 427.2
Bovine heart - see Hypertrophy, cardiac
Bowel - see condition
Bowen's
   dermatosis (precancerous) (M8081/2) - see Neoplasm, skin, in situ
   disease (M8081/2) - see Neoplasm, skin, in situ

Bowen's (Continued)
   epithelioma (M8081/2) - see Neoplasm, skin, in situ
   type
      epidermoid carcinoma in situ (M8081/2) - see Neoplasm, skin, in situ
      intraepidermal squamous cell carcinoma (M8081/2) - see Neoplasm, skin, in situ
Bowing
   femur 736.89
      congenital 754.42
   fibula 736.89
      congenital 754.43
   forearm 736.09
      away from midline (cubitus valgus) 736.01
      toward midline (cubitus varus) 736.02
   leg(s), long bones, congenital 754.44
   radius 736.09
      away from midline (cubitus valgus) 736.01
      toward midline (cubitus varus) 736.02
   tibia 736.89
      congenital 754.43
Bowleg(s) 736.42
   congenital 754.44
   rachitic 268.1
Boyd's dysentery 004.2
Brachial - see condition
Brachman-de Lange syndrome (Amsterdam dwarf, intellectual disabilities, and brachycephaly) 759.89
Brachycardia 427.89
Brachycephaly 756.0
Brachymorphism and ectopia lentis 759.89
Bradley's disease (epidemic vomiting) 078.82
Bradycardia 427.89
   chronic (sinus) 427.81
   newborn 779.81
   nodal 427.89
   postoperative 997.1
   reflex 337.09
   sinoatrial 427.89
      with paroxysmal tachyarrhythmia or tachycardia 427.81
      chronic 427.81
   sinus 427.89
      with paroxysmal tachyarrhythmia or tachycardia 427.81
      chronic 427.81
      persistent 427.81
      severe 427.81
   tachycardia syndrome 427.81
   vagal 427.89
Bradykinesia 781.0
Bradypnea 786.09
Brailsford's disease 732.3
   radial head 732.3
   tarsal scaphoid 732.5
Brailsford-Morquio disease or syndrome (mucopolysaccharidosis IV) 277.5
Brain - see also condition
   death 348.82
   syndrome (acute) (chronic) (nonpsychotic) (organic) (with neurotic reaction) (with behavioral reaction) (see also Syndrome, brain) 310.9
      with
         presenile brain disease 290.10
         psychosis, psychotic reaction (see also Psychosis, organic) 294.9
      congenital (see also Disability, intellectual) 319
Branched-chain amino-acid disease 270.3
Branchial - see condition
Brandt's syndrome (acrodermatitis enteropathica) 686.8
Brash (water) 787.1
Brass-founders' ague 985.8

Bravais-Jacksonian epilepsy (see also Epilepsy) 345.5 •
Braxton Hicks contractions 644.1 •
Braziers' disease 985.8
Brazilian
 blastomycosis 116.1
 leishmaniasis 085.5
BRBPR (bright red blood per rectum) 569.3
Break
 cardiorenal - see Hypertension, cardiorenal
 retina (see also Defect, retina) 361.30
Breakbone fever 061
Breakdown
 device, implant, or graft - see Complications, mechanical
 nervous (see also Disorder, mental, nonpsychotic) 300.9
 perineum 674.2 •
Breast - see also condition
 buds 259.1
  in newborn 779.89
 dense 793.82
 nodule 793.89
Breast feeding difficulties 676.8 •
Breath
 foul 784.99
 holder, child 312.81
 holding spells 786.9
 shortness 786.05
Breathing
 asymmetrical 786.09
 bronchial 786.09
 exercises V57.0
 labored 786.09
 mouth 784.99
  causing malocclusion 524.59
 periodic 786.09
  high altitude 327.22
 tic 307.20
Breathlessness 786.09
Breda's disease (see also Yaws) 102.9
Breech
 delivery, affecting fetus or newborn 763.0
 extraction, affecting fetus or newborn 763.0
 presentation (buttocks) (complete) (frank) 652.2 •
  with successful version 652.1 •
  before labor, affecting fetus or newborn 761.7
  during labor, affecting fetus or newborn 763.0
Breisky's disease (kraurosis vulvae) 624.09
Brennemann's syndrome (acute mesenteric lymphadenitis) 289.2
Brenner's
 tumor (benign) (M9000/0) 220
  borderline malignancy (M9000/1) 236.2
  malignant (M9000/3) 183.0
  proliferating (M9000/1) 236.2
Bretonneau's disease (diphtheritic malignant angina) 032.0
Breus' mole 631.8
Brevicollis 756.16
Bricklayers' itch 692.89
Brickmakers' anemia 126.9
Bridge
 myocardial 746.85
Bright red blood per rectum (BRBPR) 569.3
Bright's
 blindness - see Uremia
 disease (see also Nephritis) 583.9
  arteriosclerotic (see also Hypertension, kidney) 403.90
Brill's disease (recrudescent typhus) 081.1
 flea-borne 081.0
 louse-borne 081.1
Brill-Symmers disease (follicular lymphoma) (M9690/3) 202.0 •
Brill-Zinsser disease (recrudescent typhus) 081.1

Brinton's disease (linitis plastica) (M8142/3) 151.9
Brion-Kayser disease (see also Fever, paratyphoid) 002.9
Briquet's disorder or syndrome 300.81
Brissaud's
 infantilism (infantile myxedema) 244.9
 motor-verbal tic 307.23
Brissaud-Meige syndrome (infantile myxedema) 244.9
Brittle
 bones (congenital) 756.51
 nails 703.8
  congenital 757.5
Broad - see also condition
 beta disease 272.2
 ligament laceration syndrome 620.6
Brock's syndrome (atelectasis due to enlarged lymph nodes) 518.0
Brocq's disease 691.8
 atopic (diffuse) neurodermatitis 691.8
 lichen simplex chronicus 698.3
 parakeratosis psoriasiformis 696.2
 parapsoriasis 696.2
Brocq-Duhring disease (dermatitis herpetiformis) 694.0
Brodie's
 abscess (localized) (chronic) (see also Osteomyelitis) 730.1 •
 disease (joint) (see also Osteomyelitis) 730.1 •
Broken
 arches 734
  congenital 755.67
 back - see Fracture, vertebra, by site
 bone - see Fracture, by site
 compensation - see Disease, heart
 heart syndrome 429.83
 implant or internal device - see listing under Complications, mechanical
 neck - see Fracture, vertebra, cervical
 nose 802.0
  open 802.1
 tooth, teeth 873.63
  complicated 873.73
Bromhidrosis 705.89
Bromidism, bromism
 acute 967.3
  correct substance properly administered 349.82
  overdose or wrong substance given or taken 967.3
 chronic (see also Dependence) 304.1 •
Bromidrosiphobia 300.23
Bromidrosis 705.89
Bronchi, bronchial - see condition
Bronchiectasis (cylindrical) (diffuse) (fusiform) (localized) (moniliform) (postinfectious) (recurrent) (saccular) 494.0
 with acute exacerbation 494.1
 congenital 748.61
 tuberculosis (see also Tuberculosis) 011.5 •
Bronchiolectasis - see Bronchiectasis
Bronchiolitis (acute) (infectious) (subacute) 466.19
 with
  bronchospasm or obstruction 466.19
  influenza, flu, or grippe (see also Influenza) 487.1
 catarrhal (acute) (subacute) 466.19
 chemical 506.0
  chronic 506.4
 chronic (obliterative) 491.8
 due to external agent - see Bronchitis, acute, due to
 fibrosa obliterans 491.8
 influenzal (see also Influenza) 487.1
 obliterans 491.8
  with organizing pneumonia (BOOP) 516.8
  status post lung transplant 996.84

Bronchiolitis (Continued)
 obliterative (chronic) (diffuse) (subacute) 491.8
 due to fumes or vapors 506.4
 respiratory syncytial virus 466.11
 vesicular - see Pneumonia, broncho-
Bronchitis (diffuse) (hypostatic) (infectious) (inflammatory) (simple) 490
 with
  emphysema - see Emphysema
  influenza, flu, or grippe (see also Influenza) 487.1
  obstruction airway, chronic 491.20
   with
    acute bronchitis 491.22
    exacerbation (acute) 491.21
  tracheitis 490
   acute or subacute 466.0
    with bronchospasm or obstruction 466.0
   chronic 491.8
 acute or subacute 466.0
  with
   bronchiectasis 494.1
   bronchospasm 466.0
   obstruction 466.0
   tracheitis 466.0
  chemical (due to fumes or vapors) 506.0
  due to
   fumes or vapors 506.0
   radiation 508.8
 allergic (acute) (see also Asthma) 493.9 •
 arachidic 934.1
 aspiration 507.0
  due to fumes or vapors 506.0
 asthmatic (acute) 493.90
  with
   acute exacerbation 493.92
   status asthmaticus 493.91
  chronic 493.2 •
 capillary 466.19
  with bronchospasm or obstruction 466.19
  chronic 491.8
 caseous (see also Tuberculosis) 011.3 •
 Castellani's 104.8
 catarrhal 490
  acute - see Bronchitis, acute
  chronic 491.0
 chemical (acute) (subacute) 506.0
  chronic 506.4
  due to fumes or vapors (acute) (subacute) 506.0
   chronic 506.4
 chronic 491.9
  with
   tracheitis (chronic) 491.8
  asthmatic 493.2 •
  catarrhal 491.0
  chemical (due to fumes and vapors) 506.4
  due to
   fumes or vapors (chemical) (inhalation) 506.4
   radiation 508.8
   tobacco smoking 491.0
  mucopurulent 491.1
  obstructive 491.20
   with
    acute bronchitis 491.22
    exacerbation (acute) 491.21
  purulent 491.1
  simple 491.0
  specified type NEC 491.8
 croupous 466.0
  with bronchospasm or obstruction 466.0
  due to fumes or vapors 506.0
 emphysematous 491.20
  with
   acute bronchitis 491.22
   exacerbation (acute) 491.21
 exudative 466.0
 fetid (chronic) (recurrent) 491.1

Bronchitis (Continued)
   fibrinous, acute or subacute 466.0
      with bronchospasm or obstruction 466.0
   grippal (see also Influenza) 487.1
   influenzal (see also Influenza) 487.1
   membranous, acute or subacute 466.0
      with bronchospasm or obstruction 466.0
   moulders' 502
   mucopurulent (chronic) (recurrent) 491.1
      acute or subacute 466.0
   obliterans 491.8
   obstructive (chronic) 491.20
      with
         acute bronchitis 491.22
         exacerbation (acute) 491.21
   pituitous 491.1
   plastic (inflammatory) 466.0
   pneumococcal, acute or subacute 466.0
      with bronchospasm or obstruction 466.0
   pseudomembranous 466.0
   purulent (chronic) (recurrent) 491.1
      acute or subacute 466.0
         with bronchospasm or obstruction 466.0
   putrid 491.1
   scrofulous (see also Tuberculosis) 011.3●
   senile 491.9
   septic, acute or subacute 466.0
      with bronchospasm or obstruction 466.0
   smokers' 491.0
   spirochetal 104.8
   suffocative, acute or subacute 466.0
   summer (see also Asthma) 493.9●
   suppurative (chronic) 491.1
      acute or subacute 466.0
   tuberculous (see also Tuberculosis) 011.3●
   ulcerative 491.8
      Vincent's 101
   Vincent's 101
   viral, acute or subacute 466.0
Bronchoalveolitis 485
Bronchoaspergillosis 117.3
Bronchocele
   meaning
      dilatation of bronchus 519.19
      goiter 240.9
Bronchogenic carcinoma 162.9
Bronchohemisporosis 117.9
Broncholithiasis 518.89
   tuberculous (see also Tuberculosis) 011.3●
Bronchomalacia 748.3
Bronchomoniliasis 112.89
Bronchomycosis 112.89
Bronchonocardiosis 039.1
Bronchopleuropneumonia - see Pneumonia, broncho-
Bronchopneumonia - see Pneumonia, broncho-
Bronchopneumonitis - see Pneumonia, broncho-
Bronchopulmonary - see condition
Bronchopulmonitis - see Pneumonia, broncho-
Bronchorrhagia 786.30
   newborn 770.3
   tuberculous (see also Tuberculosis) 011.3●
Bronchorrhea (chronic) (purulent) 491.0
   acute 466.0
Bronchospasm 519.11
   with
      asthma - see Asthma
      bronchiolitis, acute 466.19
         due to respiratory syncytial virus 466.11
      bronchitis - see Bronchitis
      chronic obstructive pulmonary disease (COPD) 496
      emphysema - see Emphysema
         due to external agent - see Condition, respiratory, acute, due to
   acute 519.11
   exercise induced 493.81

Bronchospirochetosis 104.8
Bronchostenosis 519.19
Bronchus - see condition
Bronze, bronzed
   diabetes 275.01
   disease (Addison's) (skin) 255.41
      tuberculous (see also Tuberculosis) 017.6●
Brooke's disease or tumor (M8100/0) - see Neoplasm, skin, benign
Brown's tendon sheath syndrome 378.61
Brown enamel of teeth (hereditary) 520.5
Brown-Séquard's paralysis (syndrome) 344.89
Brow presentation complicating delivery 652.4●
Brucella, brucellosis (infection) 023.9
   abortus 023.1
   canis 023.3
   dermatitis, skin 023.9
   melitensis 023.0
   mixed 023.8
   suis 023.2
Bruck's disease 733.99
Bruck-de Lange disease or syndrome (Amsterdam dwarf, intellectual disabilities, and brachycephaly) 759.89
Brugada syndrome 746.89
Brug's filariasis 125.1
Brugsch's syndrome (acropachyderma) 757.39
Bruhl's disease (splenic anemia with fever) 285.8
Bruise (skin surface intact) - see also Contusion
   with
      fracture - see Fracture, by site
      open wound - see Wound, open, by site
      internal organ (abdomen, chest, or pelvis) - see Injury, internal, by site
   umbilical cord 663.6●
      affecting fetus or newborn 762.6
Bruit 785.9
   arterial (abdominal) (carotid) 785.9
   supraclavicular 785.9
Brushburn - see Injury, superficial, by site
Bruton's X-linked agammaglobulinemia 279.04
Bruxism 306.8
   sleep related 327.53
Bubbly lung syndrome 770.7
Bubo 289.3
   blennorrhagic 098.89
   chancroidal 099.0
   climatic 099.1
   due to Hemophilus ducreyi 099.0
   gonococcal 098.89
   indolent NEC 099.8
   inguinal NEC 099.8
      chancroidal 099.0
      climatic 099.1
      due to H. ducreyi 099.0
   scrofulous (see also Tuberculosis) 017.2●
   soft chancre 099.0
   suppurating 683
   syphilitic 091.0
      congenital 090.0
   tropical 099.1
   venereal NEC 099.8
   virulent 099.0
Bubonic plague 020.0
Bubonocele - see Hernia, inguinal
Buccal - see condition
Buchanan's disease (juvenile osteochondrosis of iliac crest) 732.1
Buchem's syndrome (hyperostosis corticalis) 733.3
Buchman's disease (osteochondrosis, juvenile) 732.1
Bucket handle fracture (semilunar cartilage) (see also Tear, meniscus) 836.2
Budd-Chiari syndrome (hepatic vein thrombosis) 453.0
Budgerigar-fanciers' disease or lung 495.2
Büdinger-Ludloff-Läwen disease 717.89

Buds
   breast 259.1
   in newborn 779.89
Buerger's disease (thromboangiitis obliterans) 443.1
Bulbar - see condition
Bulbus cordis 745.9
   persistent (in left ventricle) 745.8
Bulging fontanels (congenital) 756.0
Bulimia 783.6
   nervosa 307.51
   nonorganic origin 307.51
Bulky uterus 621.2
Bulla(e) 709.8
   lung (emphysematous) (solitary) 492.0
Bullet wound - see also Wound, open, by site
   fracture - see Fracture, by site, open
   internal organ (abdomen, chest, or pelvis) - see Injury, internal, by site, with open wound
   intracranial - see Laceration, brain, with open wound
Bullis fever 082.8
Bullying (see also Disturbance, conduct) 312.0●
Bundle
   branch block (complete) (false) (incomplete) 426.50
      bilateral 426.53
      left (see also Block, bundle branch, left) 426.3
         hemiblock 426.2
      right (see also Block, bundle branch, right) 426.4
   of His - see condition
   of Kent syndrome (anomalous atrioventricular excitation) 426.7
Bungpagga 040.81
Bunion 727.1
Bunionette 727.1
Bunyamwera fever 066.3
Buphthalmia, buphthalmos (congenital) 743.20
   associated with
      keratoglobus, congenital 743.22
      megalocornea 743.22
      ocular anomalies NEC 743.22
   isolated 743.21
   simple 743.21
Bürger-Grütz disease or syndrome (essential familial hyperlipemia) 272.3
Buried roots 525.3
Burke's syndrome 577.8
Burkitt's
   tumor (M9750/3) 200.2●
   type malignant, lymphoma, lymphoblastic, or undifferentiated (M9750/3) 200.2●
Burn (acid) (cathode ray) (caustic) (chemical) (electric heating appliance) (electricity) (fire) (flame) (hot liquid or object) (irradiation) (lime) (radiation) (steam) (thermal) (x-ray) 949.0

> Note: Use the following fifth-digit subclassification with category 948 to indicate the percent of body surface with third degree burn:
>
> 0   less than 10 percent or unspecified
> 1   10–19 percent
> 2   20–29 percent
> 3   30–39 percent
> 4   40–49 percent
> 5   50–59 percent
> 6   60–69 percent
> 7   70–79 percent
> 8   80–89 percent
> 9   90 percent or more of body surface

   with
      blisters - see Burn, by site, second degree
      erythema - see Burn, by site, first degree

SECTION I INDEX TO DISEASES AND INJURIES / Burn

Burn *(Continued)*
   with *(Continued)*
      skin loss (epidermal) - *see also* Burn, by site, second degree
      full thickness - *see also* Burn, by site, third degree
        with necrosis of underlying tissues - *see* Burn, by site, third degree, deep
   first degree - *see* Burn, by site, first degree
   second degree - *see* Burn, by site, second degree
   third degree - *see also* Burn, by site, third degree
      deep - *see* Burn, by site, third degree, deep
   abdomen, abdominal (muscle) (wall) 942.03
      with
        trunk - *see* Burn, trunk, multiple sites
      first degree 942.13
      second degree 942.23
      third degree 942.33
        deep 942.43
          with loss of body part 942.53
   ankle 945.03
      with
        lower limb(s) - *see* Burn, leg, multiple sites
      first degree 945.13
      second degree 945.23
      third degree 945.33
        deep 945.43
          with loss of body part 945.53
   anus - *see* Burn, trunk, specified site NEC
   arm(s) 943.00
      first degree 943.10
      second degree 943.20
      third degree 943.30
        deep 943.40
          with loss of body part 943.50
      lower - *see* Burn, forearm(s)
      multiple sites, except hand(s) or wrist(s) 943.09
        first degree 943.19
        second degree 943.29
        third degree 943.39
          deep 943.49
            with loss of body part 943.59
      upper 943.03
        first degree 943.13
        second degree 943.23
        third degree 943.33
          deep 943.43
            with loss of body part 943.53
   auditory canal (external) - *see* Burn, ear
   auricle (ear) - *see* Burn, ear
   axilla 943.04
      with
        upper limb(s), except hand(s) or wrist(s) - *see* Burn, arm(s), multiple sites
      first degree 943.14
      second degree 943.24
      third degree 943.34
        deep 943.44
          with loss of body part 943.54
   back 942.04
      with
        trunk - *see* Burn, trunk, multiple sites
      first degree 942.14
      second degree 942.24
      third degree 942.34
        deep 942.44
          with loss of body part 942.54
   biceps
      brachii - *see* Burn, arm(s), upper
      femoris - *see* Burn, thigh
   breast(s) 942.01
      with
        trunk - *see* Burn, trunk, multiple sites
      first degree 942.11
      second degree 942.21

Burn *(Continued)*
   breast(s) *(Continued)*
      third degree 942.31
        deep 942.41
          with loss of body part 942.51
   brow - *see* Burn, forehead
   buttock(s) - *see* Burn, back
   canthus (eye) 940.1
      chemical 940.0
   cervix (uteri) 947.4
   cheek (cutaneous) 941.07
      with
        face or head - *see* Burn, head, multiple sites
      first degree 941.17
      second degree 941.27
      third degree 941.37
        deep 941.47
          with loss of body part 941.57
   chest wall (anterior) 942.02
      with
        trunk - *see* Burn, trunk, multiple sites
      first degree 942.12
      second degree 942.22
      third degree 942.32
        deep 942.42
          with loss of body part 942.52
   chin 941.04
      with
        face or head - *see* Burn, head, multiple sites
      first degree 941.14
      second degree 941.24
      third degree 941.34
        deep 941.44
          with loss of body part 941.54
   clitoris - *see* Burn, genitourinary organs, external
   colon 947.3
   conjunctiva (and cornea) 940.4
      chemical
        acid 940.3
        alkaline 940.2
   cornea (and conjunctiva) 940.4
      chemical
        acid 940.3
        alkaline 940.2
   costal region - *see* Burn, chest wall
   due to ingested chemical agent - *see* Burn, internal organs
   ear (auricle) (canal) (drum) (external) 941.01
      with
        face or head - *see* Burn, head, multiple sites
      first degree 941.11
      second degree 941.21
      third degree 941.31
        deep 941.41
          with loss of a body part 941.51
   elbow 943.02
      with
        hand(s) and wrist(s) - *see* Burn, multiple specified sites
        upper limb(s), except hand(s) or wrist(s) - *see also* Burn, arm(s), multiple sites
      first degree 943.12
      second degree 943.22
      third degree 943.32
        deep 943.42
          with loss of body part 943.52
   electricity, electric current - *see* Burn, by site
   entire body - *see* Burn, multiple, specified sites
   epididymis - *see* Burn, genitourinary organs, external
   epigastric region - *see* Burn, abdomen
   epiglottis 947.1
   esophagus 947.2

Burn *(Continued)*
   extent (percent of body surface)
      less than 10 percent 948.0 ●
      10–19 percent 948.1 ●
      20–29 percent 948.2 ●
      30–39 percent 948.3 ●
      40–49 percent 948.4 ●
      50–59 percent 948.5 ●
      60–69 percent 948.6 ●
      70–79 percent 948.7 ●
      80–89 percent 948.8 ●
      90 percent or more 948.9 ●
   extremity
      lower - *see* Burn, leg
      upper - *see* Burn, arm(s)
   eye(s) (and adnexa) (only) 940.9
      with
        face, head, or neck 941.02
        first degree 941.12
        second degree 941.22
        third degree 941.32
          deep 941.42
            with loss of body part 941.52
        other sites (classifiable to more than one category in 940–945) - *see* Burn, multiple, specified sites
        resulting rupture and destruction of eyeball 940.5
      specified part - *see* Burn, by site
   eyeball - *see also* Burn, eye
      with resulting rupture and destruction of eyeball 940.5
   eyelid(s) 940.1
      chemical 940.0
   face - *see* Burn, head
   finger (nail) (subungual) 944.01
      with
        hand(s) - *see* Burn, hand(s), multiple sites
        other sites - *see* Burn, multiple, specified sites
        thumb 944.04
          first degree 944.14
          second degree 944.24
          third degree 944.34
            deep 944.44
              with loss of body part 944.54
      first degree 944.11
      second degree 944.21
      third degree 944.31
        deep 944.41
          with loss of body part 944.51
      multiple (digits) 944.03
        with thumb - *see* Burn, finger, with thumb
        first degree 944.13
        second degree 944.23
        third degree 944.33
          deep 944.43
            with loss of body part 944.53
   flank - *see* Burn, abdomen
   foot 945.02
      with
        lower limb(s) - *see* Burn, leg, multiple sites
      first degree 945.12
      second degree 945.22
      third degree 945.32
        deep 945.42
          with loss of body part 945.52
   forearm(s) 943.01
      with
        upper limb(s), except hand(s) or wrist(s) - *see* Burn, arm(s), multiple sites
      first degree 943.11
      second degree 943.21
      third degree 943.31
        deep 943.41
          with loss of body part 943.51

SECTION 1 INDEX TO DISEASES AND INJURIES / Burn

Burn (Continued)
   forehead 941.07
     with
       face or head - see Burn, head, multiple sites
     first degree 941.17
     second degree 941.27
     third degree 945.37
       deep 941.47
         with loss of body part 941.57
   fourth degree - see Burn, by site, third degree, deep
   friction - see Injury, superficial, by site
   from swallowing caustic or corrosive substance NEC - see Burn, internal organs
   full thickness - see Burn, by site, third degree
   gastrointestinal tract 947.3
   genitourinary organs
     external 942.05
       with
         trunk - see Burn, trunk, multiple sites
       first degree 942.15
       second degree 942.25
       third degree 942.35
         deep 942.45
           with loss of body part 942.55
     internal 947.8
   globe (eye) - see Burn, eyeball
   groin - see Burn, abdomen
   gum 947.0
   hand(s) (phalanges) (and wrist) 944.00
     first degree 944.10
     second degree 944.20
     third degree 944.30
       deep 944.40
         with loss of body part 944.50
     back (dorsal surface) 944.06
       first degree 944.16
       second degree 944.26
       third degree 944.36
         deep 944.46
           with loss of body part 944.56
     multiple sites 944.08
       first degree 944.18
       second degree 944.28
       third degree 944.38
         deep 944.48
           with loss of body part 944.58
   head (and face) 941.00
     eye(s) only 940.9
       specified part - see Burn, by site
     first degree 941.10
     second degree 941.20
     third degree 941.30
       deep 941.40
         with loss of body part 941.50
     multiple sites 941.09
       with eyes - see Burn, eyes, with face, head, or neck
       first degree 941.19
       second degree 941.29
       third degree 941.39
         deep 941.49
           with loss of body part 941.59
   heel - see Burn, foot
   hip - see Burn, trunk, specified site NEC
   iliac region - see Burn, trunk, specified site NEC
   infected 958.3
   inhalation (see also Burn, internal organs) 947.9
   internal organs 947.9
     from caustic or corrosive substance (swallowing) NEC 947.9
     specified NEC (see also Burn, by site) 947.8
   interscapular region - see Burn, back

Burn (Continued)
   intestine (large) (small) 947.3
   iris - see Burn, eyeball
   knee 945.05
     with
       lower limb(s) - see Burn, leg, multiple sites
     first degree 945.15
     second degree 945.25
     third degree 945.35
       deep 945.45
         with loss of body part 945.55
   labium (majus) (minus) - see Burn, genitourinary organs, external
   lacrimal apparatus, duct, gland, or sac 940.1
     chemical 940.0
   larynx 947.1
   late effect - see Late, effects (of), burn
   leg 945.00
     first degree 945.10
     second degree 945.20
     third degree 945.30
       deep 945.40
         with loss of body part 945.50
     lower 945.04
       with other part(s) of lower limb(s) - see Burn, leg, multiple sites
       first degree 945.14
       second degree 945.24
       third degree 945.34
         deep 945.44
           with loss of body part 945.54
     multiple sites 945.09
       first degree 945.19
       second degree 945.29
       third degree 945.39
         deep 945.49
           with loss of body part 945.59
     upper - see Burn, thigh
   lightning - see Burn, by site
   limb(s)
     lower (including foot or toe(s)) - see Burn, leg
     upper (except wrist and hand) - see Burn, arm(s)
   lip(s) 941.03
     with
       face or head - see Burn, head, multiple sites
     first degree 941.13
     second degree 941.23
     third degree 941.33
       deep 941.43
         with loss of body part 941.53
   lumbar region - see Burn, back
   lung 947.1
   malar region - see Burn, cheek
   mastoid region - see Burn, scalp
   membrane, tympanic - see Burn, ear
   midthoracic region - see Burn, chest wall
   mouth 947.0
   multiple (see also Burn, unspecified) 949.0
     specified sites classifiable to more than one category in 940–945 946.0
       first degree 946.1
       second degree 946.2
       third degree 946.3
         deep 946.4
           with loss of body part 946.5
   muscle, abdominal - see Burn, abdomen
   nasal (septum) - see Burn, nose
   neck 941.08
     with
       face or head - see Burn, head, multiple sites
     first degree 941.18
     second degree 941.28
     third degree 941.38
       deep 941.48
         with loss of body part 941.58

Burn (Continued)
   nose (septum) 941.05
     with
       face or head - see Burn, head, multiple sites
     first degree 941.15
     second degree 941.25
     third degree 941.35
       deep 941.45
         with loss of body part 941.55
   occipital region - see Burn, scalp
   orbit region 940.1
     chemical 940.0
   oronasopharynx 947.0
   palate 947.0
   palm(s) 944.05
     with
       hand(s) and wrist(s) - see Burn, hand(s), multiple sites
     first degree 944.15
     second degree 944.25
     third degree 944.35
       deep 944.45
         with loss of a body part 944.55
   parietal region - see Burn, scalp
   penis - see Burn, genitourinary organs, external
   perineum - see Burn, genitourinary organs, external
   periocular area 940.1
     chemical 940.0
   pharynx 947.0
   pleura 947.1
   popliteal space - see Burn, knee
   prepuce - see Burn, genitourinary organs, external
   pubic region - see Burn, genitourinary organs, external
   pudenda - see Burn, genitourinary organs, external
   rectum 947.3
   sac, lacrimal 940.1
     chemical 940.0
   sacral region - see Burn, back
   salivary (ducts) (glands) 947.0
   scalp 941.06
     with
       face or neck - see Burn, head, multiple sites
     first degree 941.16
     second degree 941.26
     third degree 941.36
       deep 941.46
         with loss of body part 941.56
   scapular region 943.06
     with
       upper limb(s), except hand(s) or wrist(s) - see Burn, arm(s), multiple sites
     first degree 943.16
     second degree 943.26
     third degree 943.36
       deep 943.46
         with loss of body part 943.56
   sclera - see Burn, eyeball
   scrotum - see Burn, genitourinary organs, external
   septum, nasal - see Burn, nose
   shoulder(s) 943.05
     with
       hand(s) and wrist(s) - see Burn, multiple, specified sites
       upper limb(s), except hand(s) or wrist(s) - see Burn, arm(s), multiple sites
     first degree 943.15
     second degree 943.25
     third degree 943.35
       deep 943.45
         with loss of body part 943.55
   skin NEC (see also Burn, unspecified) 949.0

Burn *(Continued)*
  skull - *see* Burn, head
  small intestine 947.3
  sternal region - *see* Burn, chest wall
  stomach 947.3
  subconjunctival - *see* Burn, conjunctiva
  subcutaneous - *see* Burn, by site, third degree
  submaxillary region - *see* Burn, head
  submental region - *see* Burn, chin
  sun - *see* Sunburn
  supraclavicular fossa - *see* Burn, neck
  supraorbital - *see* Burn, forehead
  temple - *see* Burn, scalp
  temporal region - *see* Burn, scalp
  testicle - *see* Burn, genitourinary organs, external
  testis - *see* Burn, genitourinary organs, external
  thigh 945.06
    with
      lower limb(s) - *see* Burn, leg, multiple sites
      first degree 945.16
      second degree 945.26
      third degree 945.36
        deep 945.46
          with loss of body part 945.56
  thorax (external) - *see* Burn, chest wall
  throat 947.0
  thumb(s) (nail) (subungual) 944.02
    with
      finger(s) - *see* Burn, finger, with other sites, thumb
      hand(s) and wrist(s) - *see* Burn, hand(s), multiple sites
      first degree 944.12
      second degree 944.22
      third degree 944.32
        deep 944.42
          with loss of body part 944.52
  toe (nail) (subungual) 945.01
    with
      lower limb(s) - *see* Burn, leg, multiple sites
      first degree 945.11
      second degree 945.21
      third degree 945.31
        deep 945.41
          with loss of body part 945.51
  tongue 947.0
  tonsil 947.0
  trachea 947.1
  trunk 942.00
    first degree 942.10
    second degree 942.20
    third degree 942.30
      deep 942.40
        with loss of body part 942.50
    multiple sites 942.09
      first degree 942.19
      second degree 942.29
      third degree 942.39
        deep 942.49
          with loss of body part 942.59

Burn *(Continued)*
  trunk *(Continued)*
    specified site NEC 942.09
      first degree 942.19
      second degree 942.29
      third degree 942.39
        deep 942.49
          with loss of body part 942.59
  tunica vaginalis - *see* Burn, genitourinary organs, external
  tympanic membrane - *see* Burn, ear
  tympanum - *see* Burn, ear
  ultraviolet 692.82
  unspecified site (multiple) 949.0
    with extent of body surface involved specified
      less than 10 percent 948.0 ●
      10–19 percent 948.1 ●
      20–29 percent 948.2 ●
      30–39 percent 948.3 ●
      40–49 percent 948.4 ●
      50–59 percent 948.5 ●
      60–69 percent 948.6 ●
      70–79 percent 948.7 ●
      80–89 percent 948.8 ●
      90 percent or more 948.9 ●
    first degree 949.1
    second degree 949.2
    third degree 949.3
      deep 949.4
        with loss of body part 949.5
  uterus 947.4
  uvula 947.0
  vagina 947.4
  vulva - *see* Burn, genitourinary organs, external
  wrist(s) 944.07
    with
      hand(s) - *see* Burn, hand(s), multiple sites
      first degree 944.17
      second degree 944.27
      third degree 944.37
        deep 944.47
          with loss of body part 944.57
Burnett's syndrome (milk-alkali) 275.42
Burnier's syndrome (hypophyseal dwarfism) 253.3
Burning
  feet syndrome 266.2
  sensation (*see also* Disturbance, sensation) 782.0
  tongue 529.6
Burns' disease (osteochondrosis, lower ulna) 732.3
Bursa - *see also* condition
  pharynx 478.29
Bursitis NEC 727.3
  Achilles tendon 726.71
  adhesive 726.90
    shoulder 726.0

Bursitis NEC *(Continued)*
  ankle 726.79
  buttock 726.5
  calcaneal 726.79
  collateral ligament
    fibular 726.63
    tibial 726.62
  Duplay's 726.2
  elbow 726.33
  finger 726.8
  foot 726.79
  gonococcal 098.52
  hand 726.4
  hip 726.5
  infrapatellar 726.69
  ischiogluteal 726.5
  knee 726.60
  occupational NEC 727.2
  olecranon 726.33
  pes anserinus 726.61
  pharyngeal 478.29
  popliteal 727.51
  prepatellar 726.65
  radiohumeral 727.3
  scapulohumeral 726.19
    adhesive 726.0
  shoulder 726.10
    adhesive 726.0
  subacromial 726.19
    adhesive 726.0
  subcoracoid 726.19
  subdeltoid 726.19
    adhesive 726.0
  subpatellar 726.69
  syphilitic 095.7
  Thornwaldt's, Tornwaldt's (pharyngeal) 478.29
  toe 726.79
  trochanteric area 726.5
  wrist 726.4
Burst stitches or sutures (complication of surgery) (external) (*see also* Dehiscence) 998.32
  internal 998.31
Buruli ulcer 031.1
Bury's disease (erythema elevatum diutinum) 695.89
Buschke's disease or scleredema (adultorum) 710.1
Busquet's disease (osteoperiostitis) (*see also* Osteomyelitis) 730.1 ●
Busse-Buschke disease (cryptococcosis) 117.5
Buttock - *see* condition
Button
  Biskra 085.1
  Delhi 085.1
  oriental 085.1
Buttonhole hand (intrinsic) 736.21
Bwamba fever (encephalitis) 066.3
Byssinosis (occupational) 504
Bywaters' syndrome 958.5

C

Cacergasia 300.9
Cachexia 799.4
    cancerous - see also Neoplasm, by site,
            malignant 799.4
    cardiac - see Disease, heart
    dehydration 276.51
        with
            hypernatremia 276.0
            hyponatremia 276.1
    due to malnutrition 799.4
    exophthalmic 242.0●
    heart - see Disease, heart
    hypophyseal 253.2
    hypopituitary 253.2
    lead 984.9
        specified type of lead - see Table of Drugs
            and Chemicals
    malaria 084.9
    malignant see also Neoplasm, by site,
            malignant 799.4
    marsh 084.9
    nervous 300.5
    old age 797
    pachydermic - see Hypothyroidism
    paludal 084.9
    pituitary (postpartum) 253.2
    renal (see also Disease, renal) 593.9
    saturnine 984.9
        specified type of lead - see Table of Drugs
            and Chemicals
    senile 797
    Simmonds' (pituitary cachexia) 253.2
    splenica 289.59
    strumipriva (see also Hypothyroidism) 244.9
    tuberculous NEC (see also Tuberculosis)
            011.9●
Café au lait spots 709.09
Caffey's disease or syndrome (infantile cortical
        hyperostosis) 756.59
Caisson disease 993.3
Caked breast (puerperal, postpartum) 676.2●
Cake kidney 753.3
Calabar swelling 125.2
Calcaneal spur 726.73
Calcaneoapophysitis 732.5
Calcaneonavicular bar 755.67
Calcareous - see condition
Calcicosis (occupational) 502
Calciferol (vitamin D) deficiency 268.9
    with
        osteomalacia 268.2
        rickets (see also Rickets) 268.0
Calcification
    adrenal (capsule) (gland) 255.41
        tuberculous (see also Tuberculosis) 017.6●
    aorta 440.0
    artery (annular) - see Arteriosclerosis
    auricle (ear) 380.89
    bladder 596.89
        due to S. hematobium 120.0
    brain (cortex) - see Calcification, cerebral
    bronchus 519.19
    bursa 727.82
    cardiac (see also Degeneration, myocardial)
            429.1
    cartilage (postinfectional) 733.99
    cerebral (cortex) 348.89
        artery 437.0
    cervix (uteri) 622.8
    choroid plexus 349.2
    conjunctiva 372.54
    corpora cavernosa (penis) 607.89
    cortex (brain) - see Calcification, cerebral
    dental pulp (nodular) 522.2
    dentinal papilla 520.4
    disc, intervertebral 722.90
        cervical, cervicothoracic 722.91
        lumbar, lumbosacral 722.93
        thoracic, thoracolumbar 722.92

Calcification (Continued)
    fallopian tube 620.8
    falx cerebri - see Calcification, cerebral
    fascia 728.89
    gallbladder 575.8
    general 275.40
    heart (see also Degeneration, myocardial)
            429.1
        valve - see Endocarditis
    intervertebral cartilage or disc
            (postinfectional) 722.90
        cervical, cervicothoracic 722.91
        lumbar, lumbosacral 722.93
        thoracic, thoracolumbar 722.92
    intracranial - see Calcification, cerebral
    intraspinal ligament 728.89
    joint 719.80
        ankle 719.87
        elbow 719.82
        foot 719.87
        hand 719.84
        hip 719.85
        knee 719.86
        multiple sites 719.89
        pelvic region 719.85
        shoulder (region) 719.81
        specified site NEC 719.88
        wrist 719.83
    kidney 593.89
        tuberculous (see also Tuberculosis)
            016.0●
    larynx (senile) 478.79
    lens 366.8
    ligament 728.89
        intraspinal 728.89
        knee (medial collateral) 717.89
    lung 518.89
        active 518.89
        postinfectional 518.89
        tuberculous (see also Tuberculosis,
            pulmonary) 011.9●
    lymph gland or node (postinfectional)
            289.3
        tuberculous (see also Tuberculosis, lymph
            gland) 017.2●
    mammographic 793.89
    massive (paraplegic) 728.10
    medial (see also Arteriosclerosis, extremities)
            440.20
    meninges (cerebral) 349.2
    metastatic 275.40
    Mönckeberg's - see Arteriosclerosis
    muscle 728.10
        heterotopic, postoperative 728.13
    myocardium, myocardial (see also
            Degeneration, myocardial) 429.1
    ovary 620.8
    pancreas 577.8
    penis 607.89
    periarticular 728.89
    pericardium (see also Pericarditis) 423.8
    pineal gland 259.8
    pleura 511.0
        postinfectional 518.89
        tuberculous (see also Tuberculosis, pleura)
            012.0●
    pulp (dental) (nodular) 522.2
    renal 593.89
    Rider's bone 733.99
    sclera 379.16
    semilunar cartilage 717.89
    spleen 289.59
    subcutaneous 709.3
    suprarenal (capsule) (gland) 255.41
    tendon (sheath) 727.82
        with bursitis, synovitis or tenosynovitis
            727.82
    trachea 519.19
    ureter 593.89
    uterus 621.8
    vitreous 379.29

Calcified - see also Calcification
    hematoma NEC 959.9
Calcinosis (generalized) (interstitial) (tumoral)
        (universalis) 275.49
    circumscripta 709.3
    cutis 709.3
    intervertebralis 275.49 [722.90]
    Raynaud's phenomenon
        sclerodactylytelangiectasis (CRST)
        710.1
Calciphylaxis (see also Calcification, by site)
        275.49
Calcium
    blood
        high (see also Hypercalcemia) 275.42
        low (see also Hypocalcemia) 275.41
    deposits - see also Calcification, by site
        in bursa 727.82
        in tendon (sheath) 727.82
            with bursitis, synovitis or
                tenosynovitis 727.82
    salts or soaps in vitreous 379.22
Calciuria 791.9
Calculi - see Calculus
Calculosis, intrahepatic - see
    Choledocholithiasis
Calculus, calculi, calculous 592.9
    ampulla of Vater - see Choledocholithiasis
    anuria (impacted) (recurrent) 592.0
    appendix 543.9
    bile duct (any) - see Choledocholithiasis
    biliary - see Cholelithiasis
    bilirubin, multiple - see Cholelithiasis
    bladder (encysted) (impacted) (urinary)
            594.1
        diverticulum 594.0
    bronchus 518.89
    calyx (kidney) (renal) 592.0
        congenital 753.3
    cholesterol (pure) (solitary) - see
        Cholelithiasis
    common duct (bile) - see Choledocholithiasis
    conjunctiva 372.54
    cystic 594.1
        duct - see Cholelithiasis
    dental 523.6
        subgingival 523.6
        supragingival 523.6
    epididymis 608.89
    gallbladder - see also Cholelithiasis
        congenital 751.69
    hepatic (duct) - see Choledocholithiasis
    intestine (impaction) (obstruction) 560.39
    kidney (impacted) (multiple) (pelvis)
            (recurrent) (staghorn) 592.0
        congenital 753.3
    lacrimal (passages) 375.57
    liver (impacted) - see Choledocholithiasis
    lung 518.89
    mammographic 793.89
    nephritic (impacted) (recurrent) 592.0
    nose 478.19
    pancreas (duct) 577.8
    parotid gland 527.5
    pelvis, encysted 592.0
    prostate 602.0
    pulmonary 518.89
    renal (impacted) (recurrent) 592.0
        congenital 753.3
    salivary (duct) (gland) 527.5
    seminal vesicle 608.89
    staghorn 592.0
    Stensen's duct 527.5
    sublingual duct or gland 527.5
        congenital 750.26
    submaxillary duct, gland, or region 527.5
    suburethral 594.8
    tonsil 474.8
    tooth, teeth 523.6
    tunica vaginalis 608.89
    ureter (impacted) (recurrent) 592.1

SECTION 1 INDEX TO DISEASES AND INJURIES / Carcinoma

Calculus, calculi, calculous (Continued)
 urethra (impacted) 594.2
 urinary (duct) (impacted) (passage) (tract) 592.9
  lower tract NEC 594.9
   specified site 594.8
 vagina 623.8
 vesical (impacted) 594.1
 Wharton's duct 527.5
Caliectasis 593.89
California
 disease 114.0
 encephalitis 062.5
Caligo cornea 371.03
Callositas, callosity (infected) 700
Callus (infected) 700
 bone 726.91
 excessive, following fracture - *see also* Late, effect (of), fracture
Calvé (-Perthes) disease (osteochondrosis, femoral capital) 732.1
Calvities (*see also* Alopecia) 704.00
Cameroon fever (*see also* Malaria) 084.6
Camptocormia 300.11
Camptodactyly (congenital) 755.59
Camurati-Engelmann disease (diaphyseal sclerosis) 756.59
Canal - *see* condition
Canaliculitis (lacrimal) (acute) 375.31
 Actinomyces 039.8
 chronic 375.41
Canavan's disease 330.0
Cancer (M8000/3) - *see also* Neoplasm, by site, malignant

> Note: The term "cancer" when modified by an adjective or adjectival phrase indicating a morphological type should be coded in the same manner as "carcinoma" with that adjective or phrase. Thus, "squamous-cell cancer" should be coded in the same manner as "squamous-cell carcinoma," which appears in the list under "Carcinoma."

 bile duct type (M8160/3), liver 155.1
 hepatocellular (M8170/3) 155.0
Cancerous (M8000/3) - *see* Neoplasm, by site, malignant
Cancerphobia 300.29
Cancrum oris 528.1
Candidiasis, candidal 112.9
 with pneumonia 112.4
 balanitis 112.2
 congenital 771.7
 disseminated 112.5
 endocarditis 112.81
 esophagus 112.84
 intertrigo 112.3
 intestine 112.85
 lung 112.4
 meningitis 112.83
 mouth 112.0
 nails 112.3
 neonatal 771.7
 onychia 112.3
 otitis externa 112.82
 otomycosis 112.82
 paronychia 112.3
 perionyxis 112.3
 pneumonia 112.4
 pneumonitis 112.4
 skin 112.3
 specified site NEC 112.89
 systemic 112.5
 urogenital site NEC 112.2
 vagina 112.1
 vulva 112.1
 vulvovaginitis 112.1
Candidiosis - *see* Candidiasis
Candiru infection or infestation 136.8

Canities (premature) 704.3
 congenital 757.4
Canker (mouth) (sore) 528.2
 rash 034.1
Cannabinosis 504
Canton fever 081.9
Cap
 cradle 690.11
Capillariasis 127.5
Capillary - *see* condition
Caplan's syndrome 714.81
Caplan-Colinet syndrome 714.81
Capsule - *see* condition
Capsulitis (joint) 726.90
 adhesive (shoulder) 726.0
 hip 726.5
 knee 726.60
 labyrinthine 387.8
 thyroid 245.9
 wrist 726.4
Caput
 crepitus 756.0
 medusae 456.8
 succedaneum 767.19
Carapata disease 087.1
Carate - *see* Pinta
Carbohydrate-deficient glycoprotein syndrome (CDGS) 271.8
Carboxyhemoglobinemia 986
Carbuncle 680.9
 abdominal wall 680.2
 ankle 680.6
 anus 680.5
 arm (any part, above wrist) 680.3
 auditory canal, external 680.0
 axilla 680.3
 back (any part) 680.2
 breast 680.2
 buttock 680.5
 chest wall 680.2
 corpus cavernosum 607.2
 ear (any part) (external) 680.0
 eyelid 373.13
 face (any part, except eye) 680.0
 finger (any) 680.4
 flank 680.2
 foot (any part) 680.7
 forearm 680.3
 genital organ (male) 608.4
 gluteal (region) 680.5
 groin 680.2
 hand (any part) 680.4
 head (any part, except face) 680.8
 heel 680.7
 hip 680.6
 kidney (*see also* Abscess, kidney) 590.2
 knee 680.6
 labia 616.4
 lacrimal
  gland (*see also* Dacryoadenitis) 375.00
  passages (duct) (sac) (*see also* Dacryocystitis) 375.30
 leg, any part except foot 680.6
 lower extremity, any part except foot 680.6
 malignant 022.0
 multiple sites 680.9
 neck 680.1
 nose (external) (septum) 680.0
 orbit, orbital 376.01
 partes posteriores 680.5
 pectoral region 680.2
 penis 607.2
 perineum 680.2
 pinna 680.0
 scalp (any part) 680.8
 scrotum 608.4
 seminal vesicle 608.0
 shoulder 680.3
 skin NEC 680.9
 specified site NEC 680.8
 spermatic cord 608.4

Carbuncle (Continued)
 temple (region) 680.0
 testis 608.4
 thigh 680.6
 thumb 680.4
 toe (any) 680.7
 trunk 680.2
 tunica vaginalis 608.4
 umbilicus 680.2
 upper arm 680.3
 urethra 597.0
 vas deferens 608.4
 vulva 616.4
 wrist 680.4
Carbunculus (*see also* Carbuncle) 680.9
Carcinoid (tumor) (M8240/1) - *see* Tumor, carcinoid
Carcinoidosis 259.2
Carcinoma (M8010/3) - *see also* Neoplasm, by site, malignant

> Note: Except where otherwise indicated, the morphological varieties of carcinoma in the list below should be coded by site as for "Neoplasm, malignant."

 with
  apocrine metaplasia (M8573/3)
  cartilaginous (and osseous) metaplasia (M8571/3)
  osseous (and cartilaginous) metaplasia (M8571/3)
  productive fibrosis (M8141/3)
  spindle cell metaplasia (M8572/3)
  squamous metaplasia (M8570/3)
 acidophil (M8280/3)
  specified site - *see* Neoplasm, by site, malignant
  unspecified site 194.3
 acidophil-basophil, mixed (M8281/3)
  specified site - *see* Neoplasm, by site, malignant
  unspecified site 194.3
 acinar (cell) (M8550/3)
 acinic cell (M8550/3)
 adenocystic (M8200/3)
 adenoid
  cystic (M8200/3)
  squamous cell (M8075/3)
 adenosquamous (M8560/3)
 adnexal (skin) (M8390/3) - *see* Neoplasm, skin, malignant
 adrenal cortical (M8370/3) 194.0
 alveolar (M8251/3)
  cell (M8250/3) - *see* Neoplasm, lung, malignant
 anaplastic type (M8021/3)
 apocrine (M8401/3)
  breast - *see* Neoplasm, breast, malignant
  specified site NEC - *see* Neoplasm, skin, malignant
  unspecified site 173.99
 basal cell (pigmented) (M8090/3) - *see also* Neoplasm, skin, malignant 173.91
  fibro-epithelial type (M8093/3) - *see* Neoplasm, skin, malignant
  morphea type (M8092/3) - *see* Neoplasm, skin, malignant
  multicentric (M8091/3) - *see* Neoplasm, skin, malignant
 basaloid (M8123/3)
 basal-squamous cell, mixed (M8094/3) - *see* Neoplasm, skin, malignant
 basophil (M8300/3)
  specified site - *see* Neoplasm, by site, malignant
  unspecified site 194.3
 basophil-acidophil, mixed (M8281/3)
  specified site - *see* Neoplasm, by site, malignant
  unspecified site 194.3

Carcinoma (Continued)
  basosquamous (M8094/3) - see Neoplasm, skin, malignant
  bile duct type (M8160/3)
    and hepatocellular, mixed (M8180/3) 155.0
    liver 155.1
    specified site NEC - see Neoplasm, by site, malignant
    unspecified site 155.1
  branchial or branchiogenic 146.8
  bronchial or bronchogenic - see Neoplasm, lung, malignant
  bronchiolar (terminal) (M8250/3) - see Neoplasm, lung, malignant
  bronchiolo-alveolar (M8250/3) - see Neoplasm, lung, malignant
  bronchogenic (epidermoid) 162.9
  C cell (M8510/3)
    specified site - see Neoplasm, by site, malignant
    unspecified site 193
  ceruminous (M8420/3) 173.29
  chorionic (M9100/3)
    specified site - see Neoplasm, by site, malignant
    unspecified site
      female 181
      male 186.9
  chromophobe (M8270/3)
    specified site - see Neoplasm, by site, malignant
    unspecified site 194.3
  clear cell (mesonephroid type) (M8310/3)
  cloacogenic (M8124/3)
    specified site - see Neoplasm, by site, malignant
    unspecified site 154.8
  colloid (M8480/3)
  cribriform (M8201/3)
  cylindroid type (M8200/3)
  diffuse type (M8145/3)
    specified site - see Neoplasm, by site, malignant
    unspecified site 151.9
  duct (cell) (M8500/3)
    with Paget's disease (M8541/3) - see Neoplasm, breast, malignant
    infiltrating (M8500/3)
      specified site - see Neoplasm, by site, malignant
      unspecified site 174.9
  ductal (M8500/3)
  ductular, infiltrating (M8521/3)
  embryonal (M9070/3)
    and teratoma, mixed (M9081/3)
    combined with choriocarcinoma (M9101/3) - see Neoplasm, by site, malignant
    infantile type (M9071/3)
    liver 155.0
    polyembryonal type (M9072/3)
  endometrioid (M8380/3)
  eosinophil (M8280/3)
    specified site - see Neoplasm, by site, malignant
    unspecified site 194.3
  epidermoid (M8070/3) - see also Carcinoma, squamous cell
    and adenocarcinoma, mixed (M8560/3)
    in situ, Bowen's type (M8081/2) - see Neoplasm, skin, in situ
    intradermal - see Neoplasm, skin, in situ
  fibroepithelial type basal cell (M8093/3) - see Neoplasm, skin, malignant
  follicular (M8330/3)
    and papillary (mixed) (M8340/3) 193
    moderately differentiated type (M8332/3) 193
    pure follicle type (M8331/3) 193

Carcinoma (Continued)
  follicular (Continued)
    specified site - see Neoplasm, by site, malignant
    trabecular type (M8332/3) 193
    unspecified site 193
    well differentiated type (M8331/3) 193
  gelatinous (M8480/3)
  giant cell (M8031/3)
    and spindle cell (M8030/3)
  granular cell (M8320/3)
  granulosa cell (M8620/3) 183.0
  hepatic cell (M8170/3) 155.0
  hepatocellular (M8170/3) 155.0
    and bile duct, mixed (M8180/3) 155.0
  hepatocholangiolitic (M8180/3) 155.0
  Hürthle cell (thyroid) 193
  hypernephroid (M8311/3)
  in
    adenomatous
      polyp (M8210/3)
      polyposis coli (M8220/3) 153.9
    pleomorphic adenoma (M8940/3)
    polypoid adenoma (M8210/3)
    situ (M8010/3) - see Carcinoma, in situ
    tubular adenoma (M8210/3)
    villous adenoma (M8261/3)
  infiltrating duct (M8500/3)
    with Paget's disease (M8541/3) - see Neoplasm, breast, malignant
    specified site - see Neoplasm, by site, malignant
    unspecified site 174.9
  inflammatory (M8530/3)
    specified site - see Neoplasm, by site, malignant
    unspecified site 174.9
  in situ (M8010/2) - see also Neoplasm, by site, in situ
    epidermoid (M8070/2) - see also Neoplasm, by site, in situ
      with questionable stromal invasion (M8076/2)
        specified site - see Neoplasm, by site, in situ
        unspecified site 233.1
      Bowen's type (M8081/2) - see Neoplasm, skin, in situ
    intraductal (M8500/2)
      specified site - see Neoplasm, by site, in situ
      unspecified site 233.0
    lobular (M8520/2)
      specified site - see Neoplasm, by site, in situ
      unspecified site 233.0
    papillary (M8050/2) - see Neoplasm, by site, in situ
    squamous cell (M8070/2) - see also Neoplasm, by site, in situ
      with questionable stromal invasion (M8076/2)
        specified site - see Neoplasm, by site, in situ
        unspecified site 233.1
    transitional cell (M8120/2) - see Neoplasm, by site, in situ
  intestinal type (M8144/3)
    specified site - see Neoplasm, by site, malignant
    unspecified site 151.9
  intraductal (noninfiltrating) (M8500/2)
    papillary (M8503/2)
      specified site - see Neoplasm, by site, in situ
      unspecified site 233.0
    specified site - see Neoplasm, by site, in situ
    unspecified site 233.0

Carcinoma (Continued)
  intraepidermal (M8070/2) - see also Neoplasm, skin, in situ
    squamous cell, Bowen's type (M8081/2) - see Neoplasm, skin, in situ
  intraepithelial (M8010/2) - see also Neoplasm, by site, in situ
    squamous cell (M8072/2) - see Neoplasm, by site, in situ
  intraosseous (M9270/3) 170.1
    upper jaw (bone) 170.0
  islet cell (M8150/3)
    and exocrine, mixed (M8154/3)
      specified site - see Neoplasm, by site, malignant
      unspecified site 157.9
    pancreas 157.4
    specified site NEC - see Neoplasm, by site, malignant
    unspecified site 157.4
  juvenile, breast (M8502/3) - see Neoplasm, breast, malignant
  Kulchitsky's cell (carcinoid tumor of intestine) 259.2
  large cell (M8012/3)
    squamous cell, non-keratinizing type (M8072/3)
  Leydig cell (testis) (M8650/3)
    specified site - see Neoplasm, by site, malignant
    unspecified site 186.9
      female 183.0
      male 186.9
  liver cell (M8170/3) 155.0
  lobular (infiltrating) (M8520/3)
    noninfiltrating (M8520/3)
      specified site - see Neoplasm, by site, in situ
      unspecified site 233.0
    specified site - see Neoplasm, by site, malignant
    unspecified site 174.9
  lymphoepithelial (M8082/3)
  medullary (M8510/3)
    with
      amyloid stroma (M8511/3)
        specified site - see Neoplasm, by site, malignant
        unspecified site 193
      lymphoid stroma (M8512/3)
        specified site - see Neoplasm, by site, malignant
        unspecified site 174.9
  Merkel cell 209.36
    buttock 209.36
    ear 209.31
    eyelid, including canthus 209.31
    face 209.31
    genitals 209.36
    lip 209.31
    lower limb 209.34
    neck 209.32
    nodal presentation 209.75
    scalp 209.32
    secondary (any site) 209.75
    specified site NEC 209.36
    trunk 209.35
    unknown primary site 209.75
    upper limb 209.33
    visceral metastatic presentation 209.75
  mesometanephric (M9110/3)
  mesonephric (M9110/3)
  metastatic (M8010/6) - see Metastasis, cancer
  metatypical (M8095/3) - see Neoplasm, skin, malignant
  morphea type basal cell (M8092/3) - see Neoplasm, skin, malignant
  mucinous (M8480/3)
  mucin-producing (M8481/3)
  mucin-secreting (M8481/3)
  mucoepidermoid (M8430/3)

SECTION I INDEX TO DISEASES AND INJURIES / Cardiomyopathy

Carcinoma (Continued)
  mucoid (M8480/3)
    cell (M8300/3)
      specified site - see Neoplasm, by site, malignant
      unspecified site 194.3
  mucous (M8480/3)
  neuroendocrine
    high grade (M8240/3) 209.30
    malignant poorly differentiated (M8240/3) 209.30
  nonencapsulated sclerosing (M8350/3) 193
  noninfiltrating
    intracystic (M8504/2) - see Neoplasm, by site, in situ
    intraductal (M8500/2)
      papillary (M8503/2)
        specified site - see Neoplasm, by site, in situ
        unspecified site 233.0
      specified site - see Neoplasm, by site, in situ
      unspecified site 233.0
    lobular (M8520/2)
      specified site - see Neoplasm, by site, in situ
      unspecified site 233.0
  oat cell (M8042/3)
    specified site - see Neoplasm, by site, malignant
    unspecified site 162.9
  odontogenic (M9270/3) 170.1
    upper jaw (bone) 170.0
  onocytic (M8290/3)
  oxyphilic (M8290/3)
  papillary (M8050/3)
    and follicular (mixed) (M8340/3) 193
    epidermoid (M8052/3)
    intraductal (noninfiltrating) (M8503/2)
      specified site - see Neoplasm, by site, in situ
      unspecified site 233.0
    serous (M8460/3)
      specified site - see Neoplasm, by site, malignant
      surface (M8461/3)
        specified site - see Neoplasm, by site, malignant
        unspecified site 183.0
      unspecified site 183.0
    squamous cell (M8052/3)
    transitional cell (M8130/3)
  papillocystic (M8450/3)
    specified site - see Neoplasm, by site, malignant
    unspecified site 183.0
  parafollicular cell (M8510/3)
    specified site - see Neoplasm, by site, malignant
    unspecified site 193
  pleomorphic (M8022/3)
  polygonal cell (M8034/3)
  prickle cell (M8070/3)
  pseudoglandular, squamous cell (M8075/3)
  pseudomucinous (M8470/3)
    specified site - see Neoplasm, by site, malignant
    unspecified site 183.0
  pseudosarcomatous (M8033/3)
  regaud type (M8082/3) - see Neoplasm, nasopharynx, malignant
  renal cell (M8312/3) 189.0
  reserve cell (M8041/3)
  round cell (M8041/3)
  Schmincke (M8082/3) - see Neoplasm, nasopharynx, malignant
  Schneiderian (M8121/3)
    specified site - see Neoplasm, by site, malignant
    unspecified site 160.0

Carcinoma (Continued)
  scirrhous (M8141/3)
  sebaceous (M8410/3) - see Neoplasm, skin, malignant
  secondary (M8010/6) - see Neoplasm, by site, malignant, secondary
  secretory, breast (M8502/3) - see Neoplasm, breast, malignant
  serous (M8441/3)
    papillary (M8460/3)
      specified site - see Neoplasm, by site, malignant
      unspecified site 183.0
    surface, papillary (M8461/3)
      specified site - see Neoplasm, by site, malignant
      unspecified site 183.0
  Sertoli cell (M8640/3)
    specified site - see Neoplasm, by site, malignant
    unspecified site 186.9
  signet ring cell (M8490/3)
    metastatic (M8490/6) - see Neoplasm, by site, secondary
  simplex (M8231/3)
  skin appendage (M8390/3) - see Neoplasm, skin, malignant
  small cell (M8041/3)
    fusiform cell type (M8043/3)
    squamous cell, nonkeratinizing type (M8073/3)
  solid (M8230/3)
    with amyloid stroma (M8511/3)
      specified site - see Neoplasm, by site, malignant
      unspecified site 193
  spheroidal cell (M8035/3)
  spindle cell (M8032/3)
    and giant cell (M8030/3)
  spinous cell (M8070/3)
  squamous (cell) (M8070/3)
    adenoid type (M8075/3)
    and adenocarcinoma, mixed (M8560/3)
    intraepidermal, Bowen's type - see Neoplasm, skin, in situ
    keratinizing type (large cell) (M8071/3)
    large cell, nonkeratinizing type (M8072/3)
    microinvasive (M8076/3)
      specified site - see Neoplasm, by site, malignant
      unspecified site 180.9
    nonkeratinizing type (M8072/3)
    papillary (M8052/3)
    pseudoglandular (M8075/3)
    skin (see also Neoplasm, skin, malignant) 173.92
    small cell, nonkeratinizing type (M8073/3)
    spindle cell type (M8074/3)
    verrucous (M8051/3)
  superficial spreading (M8143/3)
  sweat gland (M8400/3) - see Neoplasm, skin, malignant
  theca cell (M8600/3) 183.0
  thymic (M8580/3) 164.0
  trabecular (M8190/3)
  transitional (cell) (M8120/3)
    papillary (M8130/3)
    spindle cell type (M8122/3)
  tubular (M8211/3)
  undifferentiated type (M8020/3)
  urothelial (M8120/3)
  ventriculi 151.9
  verrucous (epidermoid) (squamous cell) (M8051/3)
  villous (M8262/3)
  water-clear cell (M8322/3) 194.1
  wolffian duct (M9110/3)

Carcinomaphobia 300.29
Carcinomatosis
  peritonei (M8010/6) 197.6
  specified site NEC (M8010/3) - see Neoplasm, by site, malignant
  unspecified site (M8010/6) 199.0
Carcinosarcoma (M8980/3) - see also Neoplasm, by site, malignant
  embryonal type (M8981/3) - see Neoplasm, by site, malignant
Cardia, cardial - see condition
Cardiac - see also condition
  death - see Disease, heart
  device
    defibrillator, automatic implantable (with synchronous cardiac pacemaker) V45.02
    in situ NEC V45.00
    pacemaker
      cardiac
        fitting or adjustment V53.31
        in situ V45.01
      carotid sinus
        fitting or adjustment V53.39
        in situ V45.09
  pacemaker - see Cardiac, device, pacemaker
  tamponade 423.3
Cardialgia (see also Pain, precordial) 786.51
Cardiectasis - see Hypertrophy, cardiac
Cardiochalasia 530.81
Cardiomalacia (see also Degeneration, myocardial) 429.1
Cardiomegalia glycogenica diffusa 271.0
Cardiomegaly (see also Hypertrophy, cardiac) 429.3
  congenital 746.89
  glycogen 271.0
  hypertensive (see also Hypertension, heart) 402.90
  idiopathic 425.4
Cardiomyoliposis (see also Degeneration, myocardial) 429.1
Cardiomyopathy (congestive) (constrictive) (familial) (infiltrative) (obstructive) (restrictive) (sporadic) 425.4
  alcoholic 425.5
  amyloid 277.39 [425.7]
  beriberi 265.0 [425.7]
  cobalt-beer 425.5
  congenital 425.3
  due to
    amyloidosis 277.39 [425.7]
    beriberi 265.0 [425.7]
    cardiac glycogenosis 271.0 [425.7]
    Chagas' disease 086.0
    Friedreich's ataxia 334.0 [425.8]
    hypertension - see Hypertension, with, heart involvement
    mucopolysaccharidosis 277.5 [425.7]
    myotonia atrophica 359.21 [425.8]
    progressive muscular dystrophy 359.1 [425.8]
    sarcoidosis 135 [425.8]
  glycogen storage 271.0 [425.7]
  hypertensive - see Hypertension, with, heart involvement
  hypertrophic 425.18
    nonobstructive 425.18
    obstructive 425.11
      congenital 746.84
  idiopathic (concentric) 425.4
  in
    Chagas' disease 086.0
    sarcoidosis 135 [425.8]
  ischemic 414.8
  metabolic NEC 277.9 [425.7]
    amyloid 277.39 [425.7]
    thyrotoxic (see also Thyrotoxicosis) 242.9● [425.7]
    thyrotoxicosis (see also Thyrotoxicosis) 242.9● [425.7]

Cardiomyopathy (Continued)
  newborn 425.4
    congenital 425.3
  nutritional 269.9 [425.7]
    beriberi 265.0 [425.7]
  obscure of Africa 425.2
  peripartum 674.5●
  postpartum 674.5●
  primary 425.4
  secondary 425.9
  stress induced 429.83
  takotsubo 429.83
  thyrotoxic (see also Thyrotoxicosis) 242.9●
    [425.7]
  toxic NEC 425.9
  tuberculous (see also Tuberculosis) 017.9●
    [425.8]
Cardionephritis - see Hypertension, cardiorenal
Cardionephropathy - see Hypertension, cardiorenal
Cardionephrosis - see Hypertension, cardiorenal
Cardioneurosis 306.2
Cardiopathia nigra 416.0
Cardiopathy (see also Disease, heart) 429.9
  hypertensive (see also Hypertension, heart) 402.90
  idiopathic 425.4
  mucopolysaccharidosis 277.5 [425.7]
Cardiopericarditis (see also Pericarditis) 423.9
Cardiophobia 300.29
Cardioptosis 746.87
Cardiorenal - see condition
Cardiorrhexis (see also Infarct, myocardium) 410.9●
Cardiosclerosis - see Arteriosclerosis, coronary
Cardiosis - see Disease, heart
Cardiospasm (esophagus) (reflex) (stomach) 530.0
  congenital 750.7
Cardiostenosis - see Disease, heart
Cardiosymphysis 423.1
Cardiothyrotoxicosis - see Hyperthyroidism
Cardiovascular - see condition
Carditis (acute) (bacterial) (chronic) (subacute) 429.89
  Coxsackie 074.20
  hypertensive (see also Hypertension, heart) 402.90
  meningococcal 036.40
  rheumatic - see Disease, heart, rheumatic
  rheumatoid 714.2
Care (of)
  child (routine) V20.1
  convalescent following V66.9
    chemotherapy V66.2
    medical NEC V66.5
    psychotherapy V66.3
    radiotherapy V66.1
    surgery V66.0
    surgical NEC V66.0
    treatment (for) V66.5
      combined V66.6
      fracture V66.4
      mental disorder NEC V66.3
      specified type NEC V66.5
  end-of-life V66.7
  family member (handicapped) (sick)
    creating problem for family V61.49
    provided away from home for holiday relief V60.5
    unavailable, due to
      absence (person rendering care) (sufferer) V60.4
      inability (any reason) of person rendering care V60.4
    holiday relief V60.5
  hospice V66.7
  lack of (at or after birth) (infant) (child) 995.52
    adult 995.84

Care (Continued)
  lactation of mother V24.1
  palliative V66.7
  postpartum
    immediately after delivery V24.0
    routine follow-up V24.2
  prenatal V22.1
    first pregnancy V22.0
    high-risk pregnancy V23.9
      inconclusive fetal viability V23.87
      specified problem NEC V23.89
  terminal V66.7
  unavailable, due to
    absence of person rendering care V60.4
    inability (any reason) of person rendering care V60.4
  well baby V20.1
Caries (bone) (see also Tuberculosis, bone) 015.9● [730.8]●
  arrested 521.04
  cementum 521.03
  cerebrospinal (tuberculous) 015.0● [730.88]
  dental (acute) (chronic) (incipient) (infected) 521.00
    with pulp exposure 521.03
    extending to
      dentine 521.02
      pulp 521.03
    other specified NEC 521.09
    pit and fissure 521.06
    primary
      pit and fissure origin 521.06
      root surface 521.08
      smooth surface origin 521.07
    root surface 521.08
    smooth surface 521.07
  dentin (acute) (chronic) 521.02
  enamel (acute) (chronic) (incipient) 521.01
  external meatus 380.89
  hip (see also Tuberculosis) 015.1● [730.85]
  initial 521.01
  knee 015.2● [730.86]
  labyrinth 386.8
  limb NEC 015.7● [730.88]
  mastoid (chronic) (process) 383.1
  middle ear 385.89
  nose 015.7● [730.88]
  orbit 015.7● [730.88]
  ossicle 385.24
  petrous bone 383.20
  sacrum (tuberculous) 015.0● [730.88]
  spine, spinal (column) (tuberculous) 015.0● [730.88]
  syphilitic 095.5
    congenital 090.0 [730.8]●
  teeth (internal) 521.00
    initial 521.01
  vertebra (column) (tuberculous) 015.0● [730.88]
Carini's syndrome (ichthyosis congenita) 757.1
Carious teeth 521.00
Carneous mole 631.8
Carnosinemia 270.5
Carotid body or sinus syndrome 337.01
Carotidynia 337.01
Carotinemia (dietary) 278.3
Carotinosis (cutis) (skin) 278.3
Carpal tunnel syndrome 354.0
Carpenter's syndrome 759.89
Carpopedal spasm (see also Tetany) 781.7
Carpoptosis 736.05
Carrier (suspected) of
  amebiasis V02.2
  bacterial disease (meningococcal, staphylococcal) NEC V02.59
  cholera V02.0
  cystic fibrosis gene V83.81
  defective gene V83.89
  diphtheria V02.4
  dysentery (bacillary) V02.3
    amebic V02.2

Carrier (Continued)
  Endamoeba histolytica V02.2
  gastrointestinal pathogens NEC V02.3
  genetic defect V83.89
  gonorrhea V02.7
  group B streptococcus V02.51
  HAA (hepatitis Australian-antigen) V02.61
  hemophilia A (asymptomatic) V83.01
    symptomatic V83.02
  hepatitis V02.60
    Australian-antigen (HAA) V02.61
    B V02.61
    C V02.62
    specified type NEC V02.69
    serum V02.61
    viral V02.60
  infective organism NEC V02.9
  malaria V02.9
  paratyphoid V02.3
  Salmonella V02.3
    typhosa V02.1
  serum hepatitis V02.61
  Shigella V02.3
  Staphylococcus NEC V02.59
    methicillin
      resistant Staphylococcus aureus V02.54
      susceptible Staphylococcus aureus V02.53
  Streptococcus NEC V02.52
    group B V02.51
  typhoid V02.1
  venereal disease NEC V02.8
Carrión's disease (Bartonellosis) 088.0
Car sickness 994.6
Carter's
  relapsing fever (Asiatic) 087.0
Cartilage - see condition
Caruncle (inflamed)
  abscess, lacrimal (see also Dacryocystitis) 375.30
  conjunctiva 372.00
    acute 372.00
  eyelid 373.00
  labium (majus) (minus) 616.89
  lacrimal 375.30
  urethra (benign) 599.3
  vagina (wall) 616.89
Cascade stomach 537.6
Caseation lymphatic gland (see also Tuberculosis) 017.2●
Caseous
  bronchitis - see Tuberculosis, pulmonary
  meningitis 013.0●
  pneumonia - see Tuberculosis, pulmonary
Cassidy (-Scholte) syndrome (malignant carcinoid) 259.2
Castellani's bronchitis 104.8
Castleman's tumor or lymphoma (mediastinal lymph node hyperplasia) 785.6
Castration, traumatic 878.2
  complicated 878.3
Casts in urine 791.7
Cat's ear 744.29
Catalepsy 300.11
  catatonic (acute) (see also Schizophrenia) 295.2●
  hysterical 300.11
  schizophrenic (see also Schizophrenia) 295.2●
Cataphasia (see also Disorder, fluency) 315.35
Cataplexy (idiopathic) see also Narcolepsy
Cataract (anterior cortical) (anterior polar) (black) (capsular) (central) (cortical) (hypermature) (immature) (incipient) (mature) 366.9
  anterior
    and posterior axial embryonal 743.33
    pyramidal 743.31
    subcapsular polar
      infantile, juvenile, or presenile 366.01
      senile 366.13

Cataract (Continued)
　associated with
　　calcinosis 275.40 [366.42]
　　craniofacial dysostosis 756.0 [366.44]
　　galactosemia 271.1 [366.44]
　　hypoparathyroidism 252.1 [366.42]
　　myotonic disorders 359.21 [366.43]
　　neovascularization 366.33
　blue dot 743.39
　cerulean 743.39
　complicated NEC 366.30
　congenital 743.30
　　capsular or subcapsular 743.31
　　cortical 743.32
　　nuclear 743.33
　　specified type NEC 743.39
　　total or subtotal 743.34
　　zonular 743.32
　coronary (congenital) 743.39
　　acquired 366.12
　cupuliform 366.14
　diabetic 250.5● [366.41]
　　due to secondary diabetes 249.5● [366.41]
　drug-induced 366.45
　due to
　　chalcosis 360.24 [366.34]
　　chronic choroiditis (see also Choroiditis) 363.20 [366.32]
　　degenerative myopia 360.21 [366.34]
　　glaucoma (see also Glaucoma) 365.9 [366.31]
　　infection, intraocular NEC 366.32
　　inflammatory ocular disorder NEC 366.32
　　iridocyclitis, chronic 364.10 [366.33]
　　pigmentary retinal dystrophy 362.74 [366.34]
　　radiation 366.46
　electric 366.46
　glassblowers' 366.46
　heat ray 366.46
　heterochromic 366.33
　in eye disease NEC 366.30
　infantile (see also Cataract, juvenile) 366.00
　intumescent 366.12
　irradiational 366.46
　juvenile 366.00
　　anterior subcapsular polar 366.01
　　combined forms 366.09
　　cortical 366.03
　　lamellar 366.03
　　nuclear 366.04
　　posterior subcapsular polar 366.02
　　specified NEC 366.09
　　zonular 366.03
　lamellar 743.32
　　infantile juvenile, or presenile 366.03
　morgagnian 366.18
　myotonic 359.21 [366.43]
　myxedema 244.9 [366.44]
　　nuclear 366.16
　posterior, polar (capsular) 743.31
　　infantile, juvenile, or presenile 366.02
　　senile 366.14
　presenile (see also Cataract, juvenile) 366.00
　punctate
　　acquired 366.12
　　congenital 743.39
　secondary (membrane) 366.50
　　obscuring vision 366.53
　　specified type, not obscuring vision 366.52
　senile 366.10
　　anterior subcapsular polar 366.13
　　combined forms 366.19
　　cortical 366.15
　　hypermature 366.18
　　immature 366.12
　　incipient 366.12
　　mature 366.17
　　nuclear 366.16
　　posterior subcapsular polar 366.14
　　specified NEC 366.19
　　total or subtotal 366.17

Cataract (Continued)
　snowflake 250.5● [366.41]
　　due to secondary diabetes 249.5● [366.41]
　specified NEC 366.8
　subtotal (senile) 366.17
　　congenital 743.34
　sunflower 360.24 [366.34]
　tetanic NEC 252.1 [366.42]
　total (mature) (senile) 366.17
　　congenital 743.34
　　localized 366.21
　　traumatic 366.22
　toxic 366.45
　traumatic 366.20
　　partially resolved 366.23
　　total 366.22
　zonular (perinuclear) 743.32
　　infantile, juvenile, or presenile 366.03
Cataracta 366.10
　brunescens 366.16
　cerulea 743.39
　complicata 366.30
　congenita 743.30
　coralliformis 743.39
　coronaria (congenital) 743.39
　　acquired 366.12
　diabetic 250.5● [366.41]
　　due to secondary diabetes 249.5● [366.41]
　floriformis 360.24 [366.34]
　membranacea
　　accreta 366.50
　　congenita 743.39
　nigra 366.16
Catarrh, catarrhal (inflammation) (see also condition) 460
　acute 460
　asthma, asthmatic (see also Asthma) 493.9●
　Bostock's (see also Fever, hay) 477.9
　bowel - see Enteritis
　bronchial 490
　　acute 466.0
　　chronic 491.0
　　subacute 466.0
　cervix, cervical (canal) (uteri) - see Cervicitis
　chest (see also Bronchitis) 490
　chronic 472.0
　congestion 472.0
　conjunctivitis 372.03
　due to syphilis 095.9
　　congenital 090.0
　enteric - see Enteritis
　epidemic (see also Influenza) 487.1
　Eustachian 381.50
　eye (acute) (vernal) 372.03
　fauces (see also Pharyngitis) 462
　febrile 460
　fibrinous acute 466.0
　gastroenteric - see Enteritis
　gastrointestinal - see Enteritis
　gingivitis 523.00
　hay (see also Fever, hay) 477.9
　infectious 460
　intestinal - see Enteritis
　larynx (see also Laryngitis, chronic) 476.0
　liver 070.1
　　with hepatic coma 070.0
　lung (see also Bronchitis) 490
　　acute 466.0
　　chronic 491.0
　middle ear (chronic) - see Otitis media, chronic
　mouth 528.00
　nasal (chronic) (see also Rhinitis) 472.0
　　acute 460
　nasobronchial 472.2
　nasopharyngeal (chronic) 472.2
　　acute 460
　nose - see Catarrh, nasal
　ophthalmia 372.03
　pneumococcal, acute 466.0

Catarrh, catarrhal (Continued)
　pulmonary (see also Bronchitis) 490
　　acute 466.0
　　chronic 491.0
　spring (eye) 372.13
　suffocating (see also Asthma) 493.9●
　summer (hay) (see also Fever, hay) 477.9
　throat 472.1
　tracheitis 464.10
　　with obstruction 464.11
　tubotympanal 381.4
　　acute (see also Otitis media, acute, nonsuppurative) 381.00
　　chronic 381.10
　vasomotor (see also Fever, hay) 477.9
　vesical (bladder) - see Cystitis
Catarrhus aestivus (see also Fever, hay) 477.9
Catastrophe, cerebral (see also Disease, cerebrovascular, acute) 436
Catatonia, catatonic (acute) 781.99
　with
　　affective psychosis - see Psychosis, affective
　agitation 295.2●
　dementia (praecox) 295.2●
　due to or associated with physical condition 293.89
　excitation 295.2●
　excited type 295.2●
　in conditions classified elsewhere 293.89
　schizophrenia 295.2●
　stupor 295.2●
Cat-scratch - see also Injury, superficial
　disease or fever 078.3
Cauda equina - see also condition
　syndrome 344.60
Cauliflower ear 738.7
Caul over face 768.9
Causalgia 355.9
　lower limb 355.71
　upper limb 354.4
Cause
　external, general effects NEC 994.9
　not stated 799.9
　unknown 799.9
Caustic burn - see also Burn, by site
　from swallowing caustic or corrosive substance - see Burn, internal organs
Cavare's disease (familial periodic paralysis) 359.3
Cave-in, injury
　crushing (severe) (see also Crush, by site) 869.1
　suffocation 994.7
Cavernitis (penis) 607.2
　lymph vessel - see Lymphangioma
Cavernositis 607.2
Cavernous - see condition
Cavitation of lung (see also Tuberculosis) 011.2●
　nontuberculous 518.89
　primary, progressive 010.8●
Cavity
　lung - see Cavitation of lung
　optic papilla 743.57
　pulmonary - see Cavitation of lung
　teeth 521.00
　vitreous (humor) 379.21
Cavovarus foot, congenital 754.59
Cavus foot (congenital) 754.71
　acquired 736.73
Cazenave's
　disease (pemphigus) NEC 694.4
　lupus (erythematosus) 695.4
CDGS (carbohydrate-deficient glycoprotein syndrome) 271.8
Cecitis - see Appendicitis
Cecocele - see Hernia
Cecum - see condition
Celiac
　artery compression syndrome 447.4
　disease 579.0
　infantilism 579.0

 New　　　Revised　　~~deleted~~ Deleted　　● Use Additional Digit(s)　　　Omit code

SECTION I INDEX TO DISEASES AND INJURIES / Cell, cellular

Cell, cellular - *see also* condition
- anterior chamber (eye) (positive aqueous ray) 364.04

Cellulitis (diffuse) (with lymphangitis) (*see also* Abscess) 682.9
- abdominal wall 682.2
- anaerobic (*see also* Gas gangrene) 040.0
- ankle 682.6
- anus 566
- areola 611.0
- arm (any part, above wrist) 682.3
- auditory canal (external) 380.10
- axilla 682.3
- back (any part) 682.2
- breast 611.0
  - postpartum 675.1●
- broad ligament (*see also* Disease, pelvis, inflammatory) 614.4
  - acute 614.3
- buttock 682.5
- cervical (neck region) 682.1
- cervix (uteri) (*see also* Cervicitis) 616.0
- cheek, external 682.0
  - internal 528.3
- chest wall 682.2
- chronic NEC 682.9
- colostomy 569.61
- corpus cavernosum 607.2
- digit 681.9
- Douglas' cul-de-sac or pouch (chronic) (*see also* Disease, pelvis, inflammatory) 614.4
  - acute 614.3
- drainage site (following operation) 998.59
- ear, external 380.10
- enterostomy 569.61
- erysipelar (*see also* Erysipelas) 035
- esophagostomy 530.86
- eyelid 373.13
- face (any part, except eye) 682.0
- finger (intrathecal) (periosteal) (subcutaneous) (subcuticular) 681.00
- flank 682.2
- foot (except toe) 682.7
- forearm 682.3
- gangrenous (*see also* Gangrene) 785.4
- genital organ NEC
  - female - *see* Abscess, genital organ, female
  - male 608.4
- glottis 478.71
- gluteal (region) 682.5
- gonococcal NEC 098.0
- groin 682.2
- hand (except finger or thumb) 682.4
- head (except face) NEC 682.8
- heel 682.7
- hip 682.6
- jaw (region) 682.0
- knee 682.6
- labium (majus) (minus) (*see also* Vulvitis) 616.10
- larynx 478.71
- leg, except foot 682.6
- lip 528.5
- mammary gland 611.0
- mouth (floor) 528.3
- multiple sites NEC 682.9
- nasopharynx 478.21
- navel 682.2
  - newborn NEC 771.4
- neck (region) 682.1
- nipple 611.0
- nose 478.19
  - external 682.0
- orbit, orbital 376.01
- palate (soft) 528.3
- pectoral (region) 682.2
- pelvis, pelvic
  - with
    - abortion - *see* Abortion, by type, with sepsis

Cellulitis (Continued)
- pelvis, pelvic (Continued)
  - with (Continued)
    - ectopic pregnancy (*see also* categories 633.0–633.9) 639.0
    - molar pregnancy (*see also* categories 630–632) 639.0
  - female (*see also* Disease, pelvis, inflammatory) 614.4
    - acute 614.3
  - following
    - abortion 639.0
    - ectopic or molar pregnancy 639.0
  - male 567.21
  - puerperal, postpartum, childbirth 670.8●
- penis 607.2
- perineal, perineum 682.2
- perirectal 566
- peritonsillar 475
- periurethral 597.0
- periuterine (*see also* Disease, pelvis, inflammatory) 614.4
  - acute 614.3
- pharynx 478.21
- phlegmonous NEC 682.9
- rectum 566
- retromammary 611.0
- retroperitoneal (*see also* Peritonitis) 567.38
- round ligament (*see also* Disease, pelvis, inflammatory) 614.4
  - acute 614.3
- scalp (any part) 682.8
  - dissecting 704.8
- scrotum 608.4
- seminal vesicle 608.0
- septic NEC 682.9
- shoulder 682.3
- specified sites NEC 682.8
- spermatic cord 608.4
- submandibular (region) (space) (triangle) 682.0
  - gland 527.3
- submaxillary 528.3
  - gland 527.3
- submental (pyogenic) 682.0
  - gland 527.3
- suppurative NEC 682.9
- testis 608.4
- thigh 682.6
- thumb (intrathecal) (periosteal) (subcutaneous) (subcuticular) 681.00
- toe (intrathecal) (periosteal) (subcutaneous) (subcuticular) 681.10
- tonsil 475
- trunk 682.2
- tuberculous (primary) (*see also* Tuberculosis) 017.0●
- tunica vaginalis 608.4
- umbilical 682.2
  - newborn NEC 771.4
- vaccinal 999.39
- vagina - *see* Vaginitis
- vas deferens 608.4
- vocal cords 478.5
- vulva (*see also* Vulvitis) 616.10
- wrist 682.4

Cementoblastoma, benign (M9273/0) 213.1
- upper jaw (bone) 213.0

Cementoma (M9273/0) 213.1
- gigantiform (M9275/0) 213.1
  - upper jaw (bone) 213.0
- upper jaw (bone) 213.0

Cementoperiostitis 523.40
- acute 523.33
- apical 523.40

Cephalgia, cephalagia (*see also* Headache) 784.0
- histamine 339.00
- nonorganic origin 307.81
- other trigeminal autonomic (TACS) 339.09
- psychogenic 307.81
- tension 307.81

Cephalhematocele, cephalematocele
- due to birth injury 767.19
- fetus or newborn 767.19
- traumatic (*see also* Contusion, head) 920

Cephalhematoma, cephalematoma (calcified)
- due to birth injury 767.19
- fetus or newborn 767.19
- traumatic (*see also* Contusion, head) 920

Cephalic - *see* condition
Cephalitis - *see* Encephalitis
Cephalocele 742.0
Cephaloma - *see* Neoplasm, by site, malignant
Cephalomenia 625.8
Cephalopelvic - *see* condition
Cercomoniasis 007.3
Cerebellitis - *see* Encephalitis
Cerebellum (cerebellar) - *see* condition
Cerebral - *see* condition
Cerebritis - *see* Encephalitis
Cerebrohepatorenal syndrome 759.89
Cerebromacular degeneration 330.1
Cerebromalacia (*see also* Softening, brain) 348.89
- due to cerebrovascular accident 438.89

Cerebrosidosis 272.7
Cerebrospasticity - *see* Palsy, cerebral
Cerebrospinal - *see* condition
Cerebrum - *see* condition
Ceroid storage disease 272.7
Cerumen (accumulation) (impacted) 380.4
Cervical - *see also* condition
- auricle 744.43
- high risk human papillomavirus (HPV) DNA test positive 795.05
- intraepithelial glandular neoplasia 233.1
- low risk human papillomavirus (HPV) DNA test positive 795.09
- rib 756.2
- shortening - *see* Short, cervical

Cervicalgia 723.1
Cervicitis (acute) (chronic) (nonvenereal) (subacute) (with erosion or ectropion) 616.0
- with
  - abortion - *see* Abortion, by type, with sepsis
  - ectopic pregnancy (*see also* categories 633.0-633.9) 639.0
  - molar pregnancy (*see also* categories 630-632) 639.0
  - ulceration 616.0
- chlamydial 099.53
- complicating pregnancy or puerperium 646.6●
  - affecting fetus or newborn 760.8
- following
  - abortion 639.0
  - ectopic or molar pregnancy 639.0
- gonococcal (acute) 098.15
  - chronic or duration of 2 months or more 098.35
- senile (atrophic) 616.0
- syphilitic 095.8
- trichomonal 131.09
- tuberculous (*see also* Tuberculosis) 016.7●

Cervicoaural fistula 744.49
Cervicocolpitis (emphysematosa) (*see also* Cervicitis) 616.0
Cervix - *see* condition
Cesarean delivery, operation or section NEC 669.7●
- affecting fetus or newborn 763.4
- (planned) occurring after 37 completed weeks of gestation but before 39 completed weeks gestation due to (spontaneous) onset of labor 649.8●
- post mortem, affecting fetus or newborn 761.6
- previous, affecting management of pregnancy 654.2●

Céstan's syndrome 344.89
Céstan-Chenais paralysis 344.89

Céstan-Raymond syndrome 433.8●
Cestode infestation NEC 123.9
    specified type NEC 123.8
Cestodiasis 123.9
CGF (congenital generalized fibromatosis) 759.89
Chabert's disease 022.9
Chacaleh 266.2
Chafing 709.8
Chagas' disease (see also Trypanosomiasis, American) 086.2
    with heart involvement 086.0
Chagres fever 084.0
Chalasia (cardiac sphincter) 530.81
Chalazion 373.2
Chalazoderma 757.39
Chalcosis 360.24
    cornea 371.15
    crystalline lens 360.24 [366.34]
    retina 360.24
Chalicosis (occupational) (pulmonum) 502
Chancre (any genital site) (hard) (indurated) (infecting) (primary) (recurrent) 091.0
    congenital 090.0
    conjunctiva 091.2
    Ducrey's 099.0
    extragenital 091.2
    eyelid 091.2
    Hunterian 091.0
    lip (syphilis) 091.2
    mixed 099.8
    nipple 091.2
    Nisbet's 099.0
    of
        carate 103.0
        pinta 103.0
        yaws 102.0
    palate, soft 091.2
    phagedenic 099.0
    Ricord's 091.0
    Rollet's (syphilitic) 091.0
    seronegative 091.0
    seropositive 091.0
    simple 099.0
    soft 099.0
        bubo 099.0
    urethra 091.0
    yaws 102.0
Chancriform syndrome 114.1
Chancroid 099.0
    anus 099.0
    penis (Ducrey's bacillus) 099.0
    perineum 099.0
    rectum 099.0
    scrotum 099.0
    urethra 099.0
    vulva 099.0
Chandipura fever 066.8
Chandler's disease (osteochondritis dissecans, hip) 732.7
Change(s) (of) - see also Removal of
    arteriosclerotic - see Arteriosclerosis
    battery
        cardiac pacemaker V53.31
    bone 733.90
        diabetic 250.8● [731.8]
            due to secondary diabetes 249.8● [731.8]
        in disease, unknown cause 733.90
    bowel habits 787.99
    cardiorenal (vascular) (see also Hypertension, cardiorenal) 404.90
    cardiovascular - see Disease, cardiovascular
    circulatory 459.9
    cognitive or personality change of other type, nonpsychotic 310.1
    color, teeth, tooth
        during formation 520.8
        extrinsic 523.6
        intrinsic posteruptive 521.7
    contraceptive device V25.42

Change(s) (Continued)
    cornea, corneal
        degenerative NEC 371.40
        membrane NEC 371.30
        senile 371.41
    coronary (see also Ischemia, heart) 414.9
    degenerative
        chamber angle (anterior) (iris) 364.56
        ciliary body 364.57
        spine or vertebra (see also Spondylosis) 721.90
    dental pulp, regressive 522.2
    drains V58.49
    dressing
        wound V58.30
            nonsurgical V58.30
            surgical V58.31
    fixation device V54.89
        external V54.89
        internal V54.01
    heart - see also Disease, heart
    hip joint 718.95
    hyperplastic larynx 478.79
    hypertrophic
        nasal sinus (see also Sinusitis) 473.9
        turbinate, nasal 478.0
        upper respiratory tract 478.9
    inflammatory - see Inflammation
    joint (see also Derangement, joint) 718.90
        sacroiliac 724.6
    Kirschner wire V54.89
    knee 717.9
    macular, congenital 743.55
    malignant (M----/3) - see also Neoplasm, by site, malignant

    Note: For malignant change occurring in a neoplasm, use the appropriate M code with behavior digit/3 e.g., malignant change in uterine fibroid-M8890/3. For malignant change occurring in a nonneoplastic condition (e.g., gastric ulcer) use the M code M8000/3.

    mental (status) NEC 780.97
        due to or associated with physical condition - see Syndrome, brain
    myocardium, myocardial - see Degeneration, myocardial
    of life (see also Menopause) 627.2
    pacemaker battery (cardiac) V53.31
    peripheral nerve 355.9
    personality (nonpsychotic) NEC 310.1
    plaster cast V54.89
    refractive, transient 367.81
    regressive, dental pulp 522.2
    retina 362.9
        myopic (degenerative) (malignant) 360.21
        vascular appearance 362.13
    sacroiliac joint 724.6
    scleral 379.19
        degenerative 379.16
    senile (see also Senility) 797
    sensory (see also Disturbance, sensation) 782.0
    skin texture 782.8
    spinal cord 336.9
    splint, external V54.89
    subdermal implantable contraceptive V25.5
    suture V58.32
    traction device V54.89
    trophic 355.9
        arm NEC 354.9
        leg NEC 355.8
        lower extremity NEC 355.8
        upper extremity NEC 354.9
    vascular 459.9
    vasomotor 443.9
    voice 784.49
        psychogenic 306.1

Change(s) (Continued)
    wound packing V58.30
        nonsurgical V58.30
        surgical V58.31
Changing sleep-work schedule, affecting sleep 327.36
Changuinola fever 066.0
Chapping skin 709.8
Character
    depressive 301.12
Charcôt's
    arthropathy 094.0 [713.5]
    cirrhosis - see Cirrhosis, biliary
    disease 094.0
        spinal cord 094.0
    fever (biliary) (hepatic) (intermittent) - see Choledocholithiasis
    joint (disease) 094.0 [713.5]
        diabetic 250.6● [713.5]
            due to secondary diabetes 249.6● [713.5]
        syringomyelic 336.0 [713.5]
    syndrome (intermittent claudication) 443.9
        due to atherosclerosis 440.21
Charcôt-Marie-Tooth disease, paralysis, or syndrome 356.1
CHARGE association (syndrome) 759.89
Charleyhorse (quadriceps) 843.8
    muscle, except quadriceps - see Sprain, by site
Charlouis' disease (see also Yaws) 102.9
Chauffeur's fracture - see Fracture, ulna, lower end
Cheadle (-Möller) (-Barlow) disease or syndrome (infantile scurvy) 267
Checking (of)
    contraceptive device (intrauterine) V25.42
    device
        fixation V54.89
            external V54.89
            internal V54.09
        traction V54.89
    Kirschner wire V54.89
    plaster cast V54.89
    splint, external V54.89
Checkup
    following treatment - see Examination
    health V70.0
    infant (over 28 days old) (not sick) V20.2
    newborn, routine
        8 to 28 days old V20.32
        over 28 days old, routine V20.2
        under 8 days old V20.31
        weight V20.32
    pregnancy (normal) V22.1
        first V22.0
        high-risk pregnancy V23.9
            inconclusive fetal viability V23.87
            specified problem NEC V23.89
Chédiak-Higashi (-Steinbrinck) anomaly, disease, or syndrome (congenital gigantism of peroxidase granules) 288.2
Cheek - see also condition
    biting 528.9
Cheese itch 133.8
Cheese washers' lung 495.8
Cheilitis 528.5
    actinic (due to sun) 692.72
        chronic NEC 692.74
            due to radiation, except from sun 692.82
        due to radiation, except from sun 692.82
    acute 528.5
    angular 528.5
    catarrhal 528.5
    chronic 528.5
    exfoliative 528.5
    gangrenous 528.5
    glandularis apostematosa 528.5
    granulomatosa 351.8
    infectional 528.5

Cheilitis (Continued)
  membranous 528.5
  Miescher's 351.8
  suppurative 528.5
  ulcerative 528.5
  vesicular 528.5
Cheilodynia 528.5
Cheilopalatoschisis (see also Cleft, palate, with cleft lip) 749.20
Cheilophagia 528.9
Cheiloschisis (see also Cleft, lip) 749.10
Cheilosis 528.5
  with pellagra 265.2
  angular 528.5
  due to
    dietary deficiency 266.0
    vitamin deficiency 266.0
Cheiromegaly 729.89
Cheiropompholyx 705.81
Cheloid (see also Keloid) 701.4
Chemical burn - see also Burn, by site
  from swallowing chemical - see Burn, internal organs
Chemodectoma (M8693/1) - see Paraganglioma, nonchromaffin
Chemoprophylaxis NEC V07.39
Chemosis, conjunctiva 372.73
Chemotherapy
  convalescence V66.2
  encounter (for) (oral) (intravenous) V58.11
  maintenance (oral) (intravenous) V58.11
  prophylactic NEC V07.39
    fluoride V07.31
Cherubism 526.89
Chest - see condition
Cheyne-Stokes respiration (periodic) 786.04
Chiari's
  disease or syndrome (hepatic vein thrombosis) 453.0
  malformation
    type I 348.4
    type II (see also Spina bifida) 741.0●
    type III 742.0
    type IV 742.2
  network 746.89
Chiari-Frommel syndrome 676.6●
Chicago disease (North American blastomycosis) 116.0
Chickenpox (see also Varicella) 052.9
  exposure to V01.71
  vaccination and inoculation (prophylactic) V05.4
Chiclero ulcer 085.4
Chiggers 133.8
Chignon 111.2
  fetus or newborn (from vacuum extraction) 767.19
Chigoe disease 134.1
Chikungunya fever 066.3
Chilaiditi's syndrome (subphrenic displacement, colon) 751.4
Chilblains 991.5
  lupus 991.5
Child
  behavior causing concern V61.20
    adopted child V61.24
    biological child V61.23
    foster child V61.25
Childbed fever 670.8●
Childbirth - see also Delivery
  puerperal complications - see Puerperal
Childhood, period of rapid growth V21.0
Chill(s) 780.64
  with fever 780.60
  without fever 780.64
  congestive 780.99
    in malarial regions 084.6
  septic - see Septicemia
  urethral 599.84

Chilomastigiasis 007.8
Chin - see condition
Chinese dysentery 004.9
Chiropractic dislocation (see also Lesion, nonallopathic, by site) 739.9
Chitral fever 066.0
Chlamydia, chlamydial - see condition
Chloasma 709.09
  cachecticorum 709.09
  eyelid 374.52
    congenital 757.33
    hyperthyroid 242.0●
  gravidarum 646.8●
  idiopathic 709.09
  skin 709.09
  symptomatic 709.09
Chloroma (M9930/3) 205.3●
Chlorosis 280.9
  Egyptian (see also Ancylostomiasis) 126.9
  miners' (see also Ancylostomiasis) 126.9
Chlorotic anemia 280.9
Chocolate cyst (ovary) 617.1
Choked
  disk or disc - see Papilledema
  on food, phlegm, or vomitus NEC (see also Asphyxia, food) 933.1
  phlegm 933.1
  while vomiting NEC (see also Asphyxia, food) 933.1
Chokes (resulting from bends) 993.3
Choking sensation 784.99
Cholangiectasis (see also Disease, gallbladder) 575.8
Cholangiocarcinoma (M8160/3)
  and hepatocellular carcinoma, combined (M8180/3) 155.0
  liver 155.1
  specified site NEC - see Neoplasm, by site, malignant
  unspecified site 155.1
Cholangiohepatitis 575.8
  due to fluke infestation 121.1
Cholangiohepatoma (M8180/3) 155.0
Cholangiolitis (acute) (chronic) (extrahepatic) (gangrenous) 576.1
  intrahepatic 575.8
  paratyphoidal (see also Fever, paratyphoid) 002.9
  typhoidal 002.0
Cholangioma (M8160/0) 211.5
  malignant - see Cholangiocarcinoma
Cholangitis (acute) (ascending) (catarrhal) (chronic) (infective) (malignant) (primary) (recurrent) (sclerosing) (secondary) (stenosing) (suppurative) 576.1
  chronic nonsuppurative destructive 571.6
  nonsuppurative destructive (chronic) 571.6
Cholecystdocholithiasis - see Choledocholithiasis
Cholecystitis 575.10
  with
    calculus, stones in
      bile duct (common) (hepatic) - see Choledocholithiasis
      gallbladder - see Cholelithiasis
  acute 575.0
  acute and chronic 575.12
  chronic 575.11
  emphysematous (acute) (see also Cholecystitis, acute) 575.0
  gangrenous (see also Cholecystitis, acute) 575.0
  paratyphoidal, current (see also Fever, paratyphoid) 002.9
  suppurative (see also Cholecystitis, acute) 575.0
  typhoidal 002.0
Choledochitis (suppurative) 576.1
Choledocholith - see Choledocholithiasis

Choledocholithiasis 574.5●

> Note: Use the following fifth-digit subclassification with category 574:
> 0 without mention of obstruction
> 1 with obstruction

  with
    cholecystitis 574.4●
      acute 574.3●
      chronic 574.4●
    cholelithiasis 574.9●
      with
        cholecystitis 574.7●
          acute 574.6●
            and chronic 574.8●
          chronic 574.7●
Cholelithiasis (impacted) (multiple) 574.2●

> Note: Use the following fifth-digit subclassification with category 574:
> 0 without mention of obstruction
> 1 with obstruction

  with
    cholecystitis 574.1●
      acute 574.0●
      chronic 574.1●
    choledocholithiasis 574.9●
      with
        cholecystitis 574.7●
          acute 574.6●
            and chronic 574.8●
          chronic cholecystitis 574.7●
Cholemia (see also Jaundice) 782.4
  familial 277.4
  Gilbert's (familial nonhemolytic) 277.4
Cholemic gallstone - see Cholelithiasis
Choleperitoneum, choleperitonitis (see also Disease, gallbladder) 567.81
Cholera (algid) (Asiatic) (asphyctic) (epidemic) (gravis) (Indian) (malignant) (morbus) (pestilential) (spasmodic) 001.9
  antimonial 985.4
  carrier (suspected) of V02.0
  classical 001.0
  contact V01.0
  due to
    Vibrio
      cholerae (Inaba, Ogawa, Hikojima serotypes) 001.0
      el Tor 001.1
  el Tor 001.1
  exposure to V01.0
  vaccination, prophylactic (against) V03.0
Cholerine (see also Cholera) 001.9
Cholestasis 576.8
  due to total parenteral nutrition (TPN) 573.8
Cholesteatoma (ear) 385.30
  attic (primary) 385.31
  diffuse 385.35
  external ear (canal) 380.21
  marginal (middle ear) 385.32
    with involvement of mastoid cavity 385.33
  secondary (with middle ear involvement) 385.33
  mastoid cavity 385.30
  middle ear (secondary) 385.32
    with involvement of mastoid cavity 385.33
  postmastoidectomy cavity (recurrent) 383.32
  primary 385.31
  recurrent, postmastoidectomy cavity 383.32
  secondary (middle ear) 385.32
    with involvement of mastoid cavity 385.33
Cholesteatosis (middle ear) (see also Cholesteatoma) 385.30
  diffuse 385.35
Cholesteremia 272.0

Cholesterin
  granuloma, middle ear 385.82
  in vitreous 379.22
Cholesterol
  deposit
    retina 362.82
    vitreous 379.22
  elevated (high) 272.0
    with elevated (high) triglycerides 272.2
  imbibition of gallbladder (see also Disease, gallbladder) 575.6
Cholesterolemia 272.0
  essential 272.0
  familial 272.0
  hereditary 272.0
Cholesterosis, cholesterolosis (gallbladder) 575.6
  with
    cholecystitis - see Cholecystitis
    cholelithiasis - see Cholelithiasis
  middle ear (see also Cholesteatoma) 385.30
Cholocolic fistula (see also Fistula, gallbladder) 575.5
Choluria 791.4
Chondritis (purulent) 733.99
  auricle 380.03
  costal 733.6
    Tietze's 733.6
  patella, posttraumatic 717.7
  pinna 380.03
  posttraumatica patellae 717.7
  tuberculous (active) (see also Tuberculosis) 015.9 ●
    intervertebral 015.0 ● [730.88]
Chondroangiopathia calcarea seu punctate 756.59
Chondroblastoma (M9230/0) - see also
  Neoplasm, bone, benign
  malignant (M9230/3) - see Neoplasm, bone, malignant
Chondrocalcinosis (articular) (crystal deposition) (dihydrate) (see also Arthritis, due to, crystals) 275.49 [712.3] ●
  due to
    calcium pyrophosphate 275.49 [712.2] ●
    dicalcium phosphate crystals 275.49 [712.1] ●
    pyrophosphate crystals 275.49 [712.2] ●
Chondrodermatitis nodularis helicis 380.00
Chondrodysplasia 756.4
  angiomatose 756.4
  calcificans congenita 756.59
  epiphysialis punctata 756.59
  hereditary deforming 756.4
  rhizomelic punctata 277.86
Chondrodystrophia (fetalis) 756.4
  calcarea 756.4
  calcificans congenita 756.59
  fetalis hypoplastica 756.59
  hypoplastica calcinosa 756.59
  punctata 756.59
  tarda 277.5
Chondrodystrophy (familial) (hypoplastic) 756.4
  myotonic (congenital) 359.23
Chondroectodermal dysplasia 756.55
Chondrolysis 733.99
Chondroma (M9220/0) - see also Neoplasm, cartilage, benign
  juxtacortical (M9221/0) - see Neoplasm, bone, benign
  periosteal (M9221/0) - see Neoplasm, bone, benign
Chondromalacia 733.92
  epiglottis (congenital) 748.3
  generalized 733.92
  knee 717.7
  larynx (congenital) 748.3
  localized, except patella 733.92
  patella, patellae 717.7
  systemic 733.92

Chondromalacia (Continued)
  tibial plateau 733.92
  trachea (congenital) 748.3
Chondromatosis (M9220/1) - see Neoplasm, cartilage, uncertain behavior
Chondromyxosarcoma (M9220/3) - see Neoplasm, cartilage, malignant
Chondro-osteodysplasia (Morquio-Brailsford type) 277.5
Chondro-osteodystrophy 277.5
Chondro-osteoma (M9210/0) - see Neoplasm, bone, benign
Chondropathia tuberosa 733.6
Chondrosarcoma (M9220/3) - see also
  Neoplasm, cartilage, malignant
  juxtacortical (M9221/3) - see Neoplasm, bone, malignant
  mesenchymal (M9240/3) - see Neoplasm, connective tissue, malignant
Chordae tendineae rupture (chronic) 429.5
Chordee (nonvenereal) 607.89
  congenital 752.63
  gonococcal 098.2
Chorditis (fibrinous) (nodosa) (tuberosa) 478.5
Chordoma (M9370/3) - see Neoplasm, by site, malignant
Chorea (gravis) (minor) (spasmodic) 333.5
  with
    heart involvement - see Chorea with rheumatic heart disease
    rheumatic heart disease (chronic, inactive, or quiescent) (conditions classifiable to 393–398) - see- rheumatic heart condition involved,
      active or acute (conditions classifiable to 391) 392.0
  acute - see Chorea, Sydenham's
  apoplectic (see also Disease, cerebrovascular, acute) 436
  chronic 333.4
  electric 049.8
  gravidarum - see Eclampsia, pregnancy
  habit 307.22
  hereditary 333.4
  Huntington's 333.4
  posthemiplegic 344.89
  pregnancy - see Eclampsia, pregnancy
  progressive 333.4
    chronic 333.4
    hereditary 333.4
  rheumatic (chronic) 392.9
    with heart disease or involvement - see Chorea, with rheumatic heart disease
  senile 333.5
  Sydenham's 392.9
    with heart involvement - see Chorea, with rheumatic heart disease
    nonrheumatic 333.5
  variabilis 307.23
Choreoathetosis (paroxysmal) 333.5
Chorioadenoma (destruens) (M9100/1) 236.1
Chorioamnionitis 658.4 ●
  affecting fetus or newborn 762.7
Chorioangioma (M9120/0) 219.8
Choriocarcinoma (M9100/3)
  combined with
    embryonal carcinoma (M9101/3) - see Neoplasm, by site, malignant
    teratoma (M9101/3) - see Neoplasm, by site, malignant
  specified site - see Neoplasm, by site, malignant
  unspecified site
    female 181
    male 186.9
Chorioencephalitis, lymphocytic (acute) (serous) 049.0
Chorioepithelioma (M9100/3) - see Choriocarcinoma

Choriomeningitis (acute) (benign) (lymphocytic) (serous) 049.0
Chorionepithelioma (M9100/3) - see Choriocarcinoma
Chorionitis (see also Scleroderma) 710.1
Chorioretinitis 363.20
  disseminated 363.10
    generalized 363.13
    in
      neurosyphilis 094.83
      secondary syphilis 091.51
    peripheral 363.12
    posterior pole 363.11
    tuberculous (see also Tuberculosis) 017.3 ● [363.13]
  due to
    histoplasmosis (see also Histoplasmosis) 115.92
    toxoplasmosis (acquired) 130.2
      congenital (active) 771.2
  focal 363.00
    juxtapapillary 363.01
    peripheral 363.04
    posterior pole NEC 363.03
  juxtapapillaris, juxtapapillary 363.01
  progressive myopia (degeneration) 360.21
  syphilitic (secondary) 091.51
    congenital (early) 090.0 [363.13]
    late 090.5 [363.13]
    late 095.8 [363.13]
  tuberculous (see also Tuberculosis) 017.3 ● [363.13]
Choristoma - see Neoplasm, by site, benign
Choroid - see condition
Choroideremia, choroidermia (initial stage) (late stage) (partial or total atrophy) 363.55
Choroiditis (see also Chorioretinitis) 363.20
  leprous 030.9 [363.13]
  senile guttate 363.41
  sympathetic 360.11
  syphilitic (secondary) 091.51
    congenital (early) 090.0 [363.13]
    late 090.5 [363.13]
    late 095.8 [363.13]
  Tay's 363.41
  tuberculous (see also Tuberculosis) 017.3 ● [363.13]
Choroidopathy NEC 363.9
  degenerative (see also Degeneration, choroid) 363.40
  hereditary (see also Dystrophy, choroid) 363.50
  specified type NEC 363.8
Choroidoretinitis - see Chorioretinitis
Choroidosis, central serous 362.41
Choroidretinopathy, serous 362.41
Christian's syndrome (chronic histiocytosis X) 277.89
Christian-Weber disease (nodular nonsuppurative panniculitis) 729.30
Christmas disease 286.1
Chromaffinoma (M8700/0) - see also Neoplasm, by site, benign
  malignant (M8700/3) - see Neoplasm, by site, malignant
Chromatopsia 368.59
Chromhidrosis, chromidrosis 705.89
Chromoblastomycosis 117.2
Chromomycosis 117.2
Chromophytosis 111.0
Chromotrichomycosis 111.8
Chronic - see condition
Churg-Strauss syndrome 446.4
Chyle cyst, mesentery 457.8
Chylocele (nonfilarial) 457.8
  filarial (see also Infestation, filarial) 125.9
  tunica vaginalis (nonfilarial) 608.84
    filarial (see also Infestation, filarial) 125.9
Chylomicronemia (fasting) (with hyperprebetalipoproteinemia) 272.3

SECTION I INDEX TO DISEASES AND INJURIES / Chylopericardium

Chylopericardium (acute) 420.90
Chylothorax (nonfilarial) 457.8
   filarial (*see also* Infestation, filarial) 125.9
Chylous
   ascites 457.8
   cyst of peritoneum 457.8
   hydrocele 603.9
   hydrothorax (nonfilarial) 457.8
      filarial (*see also* Infestation, filarial) 125.9
Chyluria 791.1
   bilharziasis 120.0
   due to
      Brugia (malayi) 125.1
      Wuchereria (bancrofti) 125.0
         malayi 125.1
   filarial (*see also* Infestation, filarial) 125.9
   filariasis (*see also* Infestation, filarial) 125.9
   nonfilarial 791.1
Cicatricial (deformity) - *see* Cicatrix
Cicatrix (adherent) (contracted) (painful)
      (vicious) 709.2
   adenoid 474.8
   alveolar process 525.8
   anus 569.49
   auricle 380.89
   bile duct (*see also* Disease, biliary) 576.8
   bladder 596.89
   bone 733.99
   brain 348.89
   cervix (postoperative) (postpartal) 622.3
      in pregnancy or childbirth 654.6●
         causing obstructed labor 660.2●
   chorioretinal 363.30
      disseminated 363.35
      macular 363.32
      peripheral 363.34
      posterior pole NEC 363.33
   choroid - *see* Cicatrix, chorioretinal
   common duct (*see also* Disease, biliary) 576.8
   congenital 757.39
   conjunctiva 372.64
   cornea 371.00
      tuberculous (*see also* Tuberculosis) 017.3●
         [371.05]
   duodenum (bulb) 537.3
   esophagus 530.3
   eyelid 374.46
      with
         ectropion - *see* Ectropion
         entropion - *see* Entropion
   hypopharynx 478.29
   knee, semilunar cartilage 717.5
   lacrimal
      canaliculi 375.53
      duct
         acquired 375.56
            neonatal 375.55
      punctum 375.52
      sac 375.54
   larynx 478.79
   limbus (cystoid) 372.64
   lung 518.89
   macular 363.32
      disseminated 363.35
      peripheral 363.34
   middle ear 385.89
   mouth 528.9
   muscle 728.89
   nasolacrimal duct
      acquired 375.56
      neonatal 375.55
   nasopharynx 478.29
   palate (soft) 528.9
   penis 607.89
   prostate 602.8
   rectum 569.49
   retina 363.30
      disseminated 363.35
      macular 363.32
      peripheral 363.34
      posterior pole NEC 363.33

Cicatrix (*Continued*)
   semilunar cartilage - *see* Derangement,
      meniscus
   seminal vesicle 608.89
   skin 709.2
      infected 686.8
      postinfectional 709.2
      tuberculous (*see also* Tuberculosis)
         017.0●
      specified site NEC 709.2
   throat 478.29
   tongue 529.8
   tonsil (and adenoid) 474.8
   trachea 478.9
   tuberculous NEC (*see also* Tuberculosis)
      011.9●
   ureter 593.89
   urethra 599.84
   uterus 621.8
   vagina 623.4
      in pregnancy or childbirth
         654.7●
            causing obstructed labor
               660.2●
   vocal cord 478.5
   wrist, constricting (annular) 709.2
CIDP (chronic inflammatory demyelinating
      polyneuropathy) 357.81
CIN I (cervical intraepithelial neoplasia I)
   622.11
CIN II (cervical intraepithelial neoplasia II)
   622.12
CIN III (cervical intraepithelial neoplasia III)
   233.1
Cinchonism
   correct substance properly administered
      386.9
   overdose or wrong substance given or taken
      961.4
Circine herpes 110.5
Circle of Willis - *see* condition
Circular - *see also* condition
   hymen 752.49
Circulating anticoagulants, antibodies, or
      inhibitors (*see also* Anticoagulants)
      286.59
   extrinsic 287.8
   following childbirth 666.3●
   intrinsic, causing hemorrhagic disorder
      286.59
      with
         acquired hemophilia 286.52
         antiphospholipid antibody
            286.53
   postpartum 666.3●
Circulation
   collateral (venous), any site 459.89
   defective 459.9
      congenital 747.9
      lower extremity 459.89
   embryonic 747.9
   failure 799.89
      fetus or newborn 779.89
      peripheral 785.59
   fetal, persistent 747.83
   heart, incomplete 747.9
Circulatory system - *see* condition
Circulus senilis 371.41
Circumcision
   in absence of medical indication
      V50.2
   ritual V50.2
   routine V50.2
Circumscribed - *see* condition
Circumvallata placenta - *see* Placenta,
      abnormal
Cirrhosis, cirrhotic 571.5
   with alcoholism 571.2
   alcoholic (liver) 571.2
   atrophic (of liver) - *see* Cirrhosis, portal
   Baumgarten-Cruveilhier 571.5

Cirrhosis, cirrhotic (*Continued*)
   biliary (cholangiolitic) (cholangitic)
      (cholestatic) (extrahepatic)
      (hypertrophic) (intrahepatic)
      (nonobstructive) (obstructive)
      (pericholangiolitic) (posthepatic)
      (primary) (secondary) (xanthomatous)
      571.6
      due to
         clonorchiasis 121.1
         flukes 121.3
   brain 331.9
   capsular - *see* Cirrhosis, portal
   cardiac 571.5
      alcoholic 571.2
   central (liver) - *see* Cirrhosis, liver
   Charcôt's 571.6
   cholangiolitic - *see* Cirrhosis, biliary
   cholangitic - *see* Cirrhosis, biliary
   cholestatic - *see* Cirrhosis, biliary
   clitoris (hypertrophic) 624.2
   coarsely nodular 571.5
   congestive (liver) - *see* Cirrhosis, cardiac
   Cruveilhier-Baumgarten 571.5
   cryptogenic (of liver) 571.5
      alcoholic 571.2
   dietary (*see also* Cirrhosis, portal) 571.5
   due to
      bronzed diabetes 275.01
      congestive hepatomegaly - *see* Cirrhosis,
         cardiac
      cystic fibrosis 277.00
      hemochromatosis (*see also*
         Hemochromatosis) 275.03
      hepatolenticular degeneration 275.1
      passive congestion (chronic) - *see*
         Cirrhosis, cardiac
      Wilson's disease 275.1
      xanthomatosis 272.2
   extrahepatic (obstructive) - *see* Cirrhosis,
      biliary
   fatty 571.8
      alcoholic 571.0
   florid 571.2
   Glisson's - *see* Cirrhosis, portal
   Hanot's (hypertrophic) - *see* Cirrhosis,
      biliary
   hepatic - *see* Cirrhosis, liver
   hepatolienal - *see* Cirrhosis, liver
   hobnail - *see* Cirrhosis, portal
   hypertrophic - *see also* Cirrhosis, liver
      biliary - *see* Cirrhosis, biliary
      Hanot's - *see* Cirrhosis, biliary
   infectious NEC - *see* Cirrhosis, portal
   insular - *see* Cirrhosis, portal
   intrahepatic (obstructive) (primary)
      (secondary) - *see* Cirrhosis, biliary
   juvenile (*see also* Cirrhosis, portal) 571.5
   kidney (*see also* Sclerosis, renal) 587
   Laennec's (of liver) 571.2
      nonalcoholic 571.5
   liver (chronic) (hepatolienal) (hypertrophic)
      (nodular) (splenomegalic) (unilobar)
      571.5
      with alcoholism 571.2
      alcoholic 571.2
      congenital (due to failure of obliteration
         of umbilical vein) 777.8
      cryptogenic 571.5
         alcoholic 571.2
      fatty 571.8
         alcoholic 571.0
      macronodular 571.5
         alcoholic 571.2
      micronodular 571.5
         alcoholic 571.2
      nodular, diffuse 571.5
         alcoholic 571.2
      pigmentary 275.01
      portal 571.5
         alcoholic 571.2

Cirrhosis, cirrhotic *(Continued)*
 liver *(Continued)*
  postnecrotic 571.5
   alcoholic 571.2
   syphilitic 095.3
  lung (chronic) *(see also* Fibrosis, lung) 515
  macronodular (of liver) 571.5
   alcoholic 571.2
  malarial 084.9
  metabolic NEC 571.5
  micronodular (of liver) 571.5
   alcoholic 571.2
  monolobular - *see* Cirrhosis, portal
  multilobular - *see* Cirrhosis, portal
  nephritis *(see also* Sclerosis, renal) 587
  nodular - *see* Cirrhosis, liver
  nutritional (fatty) 571.5
  obstructive (biliary) (extrahepatic)
    (intrahepatic) - *see* Cirrhosis, biliary
  ovarian 620.8
  paludal 084.9
  pancreas (duct) 577.8
  pericholangiolitic - *see* Cirrhosis, biliary
  periportal - *see* Cirrhosis, portal
  pigment, pigmentary (of liver) 275.01
  portal (of liver) 571.5
   alcoholic 571.2
  posthepatitic *(see also* Cirrhosis, postnecrotic) 571.5
  postnecrotic (of liver) 571.5
   alcoholic 571.2
  primary (intrahepatic) - *see* Cirrhosis, biliary
  pulmonary *(see also* Fibrosis, lung) 515
  renal *(see also* Sclerosis, renal) 587
  septal *(see also* Cirrhosis, postnecrotic) 571.5
  spleen 289.51
  splenomegalic (of liver) - *see* Cirrhosis, liver
  stasis (liver) - *see* Cirrhosis, liver
  stomach 535.4●
  Todd's *(see also* Cirrhosis, biliary) 571.6
  toxic (nodular) - *see* Cirrhosis, postnecrotic
  trabecular - *see* Cirrhosis, postnecrotic
  unilobar - *see* Cirrhosis, liver
  vascular (of liver) - *see* Cirrhosis, liver
  xanthomatous (biliary) *(see also* Cirrhosis, biliary) 571.6
   due to xanthomatosis (familial) (metabolic) (primary) 272.2
Cistern, subarachnoid 793.0
Citrullinemia 270.6
Citrullinuria 270.6
Ciuffini-Pancoast tumor (M8010/3) (carcinoma, pulmonary apex) 162.3
Civatte's disease or poikiloderma 709.09
CJD (Creutzfeldt-Jakob disease) 046.19
 variant (vCJD) 046.11
CLABSI (central line-associated bloodstream infection) 999.32
Clam diggers' itch 120.3
Clap - *see* Gonorrhea
Clark's paralysis 343.9
Clarke-Hadfield syndrome (pancreatic infantilism) 577.8
Clastothrix 704.2
Claude's syndrome 352.6
Claude Bernard-Horner syndrome *(see also* Neuropathy, peripheral, autonomic) 337.9
Claudication, intermittent 443.9
 cerebral (artery) *(see also* Ischemia, cerebral, transient) 435.9
 due to atherosclerosis 440.21
 spinal cord (arteriosclerotic) 435.1
  syphilitic 094.89
 spinalis 435.1
 venous (axillary) 453.89
Claudicatio venosa intermittens 453.89
Claustrophobia 300.29
Clavus (infected) 700
Clawfoot (congenital) 754.71
 acquired 736.74

Clawhand (acquired) 736.06
 congenital 755.59
Clawtoe (congenital) 754.71
 acquired 735.5
Clay eating 307.52
Clay shovelers' fracture - *see* Fracture, vertebra, cervical
Cleansing of artificial opening *(see also* Attention to artificial opening) V55.9
Cleft (congenital) - *see also* Imperfect, closure
 alveolar process 525.8
 branchial (persistent) 744.41
  cyst 744.42
 clitoris 752.49
 cricoid cartilage, posterior 748.3
 facial *(see also* Cleft, lip) 749.10
 lip 749.10
  with cleft palate 749.20
   bilateral (lip and palate) 749.24
    with unilateral lip or palate 749.25
    complete 749.23
    incomplete 749.24
   unilateral (lip and palate) 749.22
    with bilateral lip or palate 749.25
    complete 749.21
    incomplete 749.22
  bilateral 749.14
   with cleft palate, unilateral 749.25
   complete 749.13
   incomplete 749.14
  unilateral 749.12
   with cleft palate, bilateral 749.25
   complete 749.11
   incomplete 749.12
 nose 748.1
 palate 749.00
  with cleft lip 749.20
   bilateral (lip and palate) 749.24
    with unilateral lip or palate 749.25
    complete 749.23
    incomplete 749.24
   unilateral (lip and palate) 749.22
    with bilateral lip or palate 749.25
    complete 749.21
    incomplete 749.22
  bilateral 749.04
   with cleft lip, unilateral 749.25
   complete 749.03
   incomplete 749.04
  unilateral 749.02
   with cleft lip, bilateral 749.25
   complete 749.01
   incomplete 749.02
 penis 752.69
 posterior, cricoid cartilage 748.3
 scrotum 752.89
 sternum (congenital) 756.3
 thyroid cartilage (congenital) 748.3
 tongue 750.13
 uvula 749.02
  with cleft lip *(see also* Cleft, lip, with cleft palate) 749.20
 water 366.12
Cleft hand (congenital) 755.58
Cleidocranial dysostosis 755.59
Cleidotomy, fetal 763.89
Cleptomania 312.32
Clérambault's syndrome 297.8
 erotomania 302.89
Clergyman's sore throat 784.49
Click, clicking
 systolic syndrome 785.2
Clifford's syndrome (postmaturity) 766.22
Climacteric *(see also* Menopause) 627.2
 arthritis NEC *(see also* Arthritis, climacteric) 716.3●
 depression *(see also* Psychosis, affective) 296.2●
 disease 627.2
  recurrent episode 296.3●
  single episode 296.2●

Climacteric *(Continued)*
 female (symptoms) 627.2
 male (symptoms) (syndrome) 608.89
 melancholia *(see also* Psychosis, affective) 296.2●
  recurrent episode 296.3●
  single episode 296.2●
 paranoid state 297.2
 paraphrenia 297.2
 polyarthritis NEC 716.39
  male 608.89
 symptoms (female) 627.2
Clinical research investigation (control) (participant) V70.7
Clinodactyly 755.59
Clitoris - *see* condition
Cloaca, persistent 751.5
Clonorchiasis 121.1
Clonorchiosis 121.1
Clonorchis infection, liver 121.1
Clonus 781.0
Closed bite 524.20
Closed surgical procedure converted to open procedure
 arthroscopic V64.43
 laparoscopic V64.41
 thoracoscopic V64.42
Closure
 artificial opening *(see also* Attention to artificial opening) V55.9
 congenital, nose 748.0
 cranial sutures, premature 756.0
 defective or imperfect NEC - *see* Imperfect, closure
 fistula, delayed - *see* Fistula
 fontanelle, delayed 756.0
 foramen ovale, imperfect 745.5
 hymen 623.3
 interauricular septum, defective 745.5
 interventricular septum, defective 745.4
 lacrimal duct 375.56
  congenital 743.65
  neonatal 375.55
 nose (congenital) 748.0
  acquired 738.0
 primary angle without glaucoma damage 365.06
 vagina 623.2
 valve - *see* Endocarditis
 vulva 624.8
Clot (blood)
 artery (obstruction) (occlusion) *(see also* Embolism) 444.9
 atrial appendage 429.89
 bladder 596.7
 brain (extradural or intradural) *(see also* Thrombosis, brain) 434.0●
  late effect - *see* Late effect(s) (of) cerebrovascular disease
 circulation 444.9
 heart *(see also* Infarct, myocardium) 410.9●
  without myocardial infarction 429.89
 vein *(see also* Thrombosis) 453.9
Clotting defect NEC *(see also* Defect, coagulation) 286.9
Clouded state 780.09
 epileptic *(see also* Epilepsy) 345.9●
 paroxysmal (idiopathic) *(see also* Epilepsy) 345.9●
Clouding
 corneal graft 996.51
Cloudy
 antrum, antra 473.0
 dialysis effluent 792.5
Clouston's (hidrotic) ectodermal dysplasia 757.31
Clubbing of fingers 781.5
Clubfinger 736.29
 acquired 736.29
 congenital 754.89

Clubfoot (congenital) 754.70
    acquired 736.71
    equinovarus 754.51
    paralytic 736.71
Club hand (congenital) 754.89
    acquired 736.07
Clubnail (acquired) 703.8
    congenital 757.5
Clump kidney 753.3
Clumsiness 781.3
    syndrome 315.4
Cluttering (see also Disorder, fluency) 315.35
Clutton's joints 090.5
Coagulation, intravascular (diffuse) (disseminated) (see also Fibrinolysis) 286.6
    newborn 776.2
Coagulopathy (see also Defect, coagulation) 286.9
    consumption 286.6
    intravascular (disseminated) NEC 286.6
        newborn 776.2
Coalition
    calcaneoscaphoid 755.67
    calcaneus 755.67
    tarsal 755.67
Coal miners'
    elbow 727.2
    lung 500
Coal workers' lung or pneumoconiosis 500
Coarctation
    aorta (postductal) (preductal) 747.10
    pulmonary artery 747.31
Coated tongue 529.3
Coats' disease 362.12
Cocainism (see also Dependence) 304.2●
Coccidioidal granuloma 114.3
Coccidioidomycosis 114.9
    with pneumonia 114.0
    cutaneous (primary) 114.1
    disseminated 114.3
    extrapulmonary (primary) 114.1
    lung 114.5
        acute 114.0
        chronic 114.4
        primary 114.0
    meninges 114.2
    primary (pulmonary) 114.0
        acute 114.0
    prostate 114.3
    pulmonary 114.5
        acute 114.0
        chronic 114.4
        primary 114.0
    specified site NEC 114.3
Coccidioidosis 114.9
    lung 114.5
        acute 114.0
        chronic 114.4
        primary 114.0
    meninges 114.2
Coccidiosis (colitis) (diarrhea) (dysentery) 007.2
Cocciuria 791.9
Coccus in urine 791.9
Coccydynia 724.79
Coccygodynia 724.79
Coccyx - see condition
Cochin-China
    diarrhea 579.1
        anguilluliasis 127.2
    ulcer 085.1
Cock's peculiar tumor 706.2
Cockayne's disease or syndrome (microcephaly and dwarfism) 759.89
Cockayne-Weber syndrome (epidermolysis bullosa) 757.39
Cocked-up toe 735.2
Codman's tumor (benign chondroblastoma) (M9230/0) - see Neoplasm, bone, benign
Coenurosis 123.8
Coffee workers' lung 495.8

Cogan's syndrome 370.52
    congenital oculomotor apraxia 379.51
    nonsyphilitic interstitial keratitis 370.52
Coiling, umbilical cord - see Complications, umbilical cord
Coitus, painful (female) 625.0
    male 608.89
    psychogenic 302.76
Cold 460
    with influenza, flu, or grippe (see also Influenza) 487.1
    abscess - see also Tuberculosis, abscess
        articular - see Tuberculosis, joint
    agglutinin
        disease (chronic) or syndrome 283.0
        hemoglobinuria 283.0
            paroxysmal (cold) (nocturnal) 283.2
    allergic (see also Fever, hay) 477.9
    bronchus or chest - see Bronchitis
        with grippe or influenza (see also Influenza) 487.1
    common (head) 460
        vaccination, prophylactic (against) V04.7
    deep 464.10
    effects of 991.9
        specified effect NEC 991.8
    excessive 991.9
        specified effect NEC 991.8
    exhaustion from 991.8
    exposure to 991.9
        specified effect NEC 991.8
    grippy (see also Influenza) 487.1
    head 460
    injury syndrome (newborn) 778.2
    intolerance 780.99
    on lung - see Bronchitis
    rose 477.0
    sensitivity, autoimmune 283.0
    virus 460
Coldsore (see also Herpes, simplex) 054.9
Colibacillosis 041.49
    generalized 038.42
Colibacilluria 791.9
Colic (recurrent) 789.7
    abdomen 789.7
        psychogenic 307.89
    appendicular 543.9
    appendix 543.9
    bile duct - see Choledocholithiasis
    biliary - see Cholelithiasis
    bilious - see Cholelithiasis
    common duct - see Choledocholithiasis
    Devonshire NEC 984.9
        specified type of lead - see Table of Drugs and Chemicals
    flatulent 787.3
    gallbladder or gallstone - see Cholelithiasis
    gastric 536.8
    hepatic (duct) - see Choledocholithiasis
    hysterical 300.11
    in
        adult 789.0
        child over 12 months old 789.0
        infant 789.7
    infantile 789.7
    intestinal 789.7
    kidney 788.0
    lead NEC 984.9
        specified type of lead - see Table of Drugs and Chemicals
    liver (duct) - see Choledocholithiasis
    mucous 564.9
        psychogenic 316 [564.9]
    nephritic 788.0
    Painter's NEC 984.9
    pancreas 577.8
    psychogenic 306.4
    renal 788.0
    saturnine NEC 984.9
        specified type of lead - see Table of Drugs and Chemicals

Colic (Continued)
    spasmodic 789.7
    ureter 788.0
    urethral 599.84
        due to calculus 594.2
    uterus 625.8
        menstrual 625.3
    vermicular 543.9
    virus 460
    worm NEC 128.9
Colicystitis (see also Cystitis) 595.9
Colitis (acute) (catarrhal) (croupous) (cystica superficialis) (exudative) (hemorrhagic) (noninfectious) (phlegmonous) (presumed noninfectious) 558.9
    adaptive 564.9
    allergic 558.3
    amebic (see also Amebiasis) 006.9
        nondysenteric 006.2
    anthrax 022.2
    bacillary (see also Infection, Shigella) 004.9
    balantidial 007.0
    chronic 558.9
        ulcerative (see also Colitis, ulcerative) 556.9
    coccidial 007.2
    dietetic 558.9
    due to radiation 558.1
    eosinophilic 558.42
    functional 558.9
    gangrenous 009.0
    giardial 007.1
    granulomatous 555.1
    gravis (see also Colitis, ulcerative) 556.9
    infectious (see also Enteritis, due to, specific organism) 009.0
        presumed 009.1
    ischemic 557.9
        acute 557.0
        chronic 557.1
        due to mesenteric artery insufficiency 557.1
    membranous 564.9
        psychogenic 316 [564.9]
    mucous 564.9
        psychogenic 316 [564.9]
    necrotic 009.0
    polyposa (see also Colitis, ulcerative) 556.9
    protozoal NEC 007.9
    pseudomembranous 008.45
    pseudomucinous 564.9
    regional 555.1
    segmental 555.1
    septic (see also Enteritis, due to, specific organism) 009.0
    spastic 564.9
        psychogenic 316 [564.9]
    Staphylococcus 008.41
        food 005.0
    thromboulcerative 557.0
    toxic 558.2
    transmural 555.1
    trichomonal 007.3
    tuberculous (ulcerative) 014.8●
    ulcerative (chronic) (idiopathic) (nonspecific) 556.9
        entero- 556.0
        fulminant 557.0
        ileo- 556.1
        left-sided 556.5
        procto- 556.2
        proctosigmoid 556.3
        psychogenic 316 [556]
        specified NEC 556.8
        universal 556.6
Collagen disease NEC 710.9
    nonvascular 710.9
    vascular (allergic) (see also Angiitis, hypersensitivity) 446.20
Collagenosis (see also Collagen disease) 710.9
    cardiovascular 425.4
    mediastinal 519.3

Collapse 780.2
adrenal 255.8
cardiorenal (see also Hypertension, cardiorenal) 404.90
cardiorespiratory 785.51
  fetus or newborn 779.85
cardiovascular (see also Disease, heart) 785.51
  fetus or newborn 779.85
circulatory (peripheral) 785.59
  with
    abortion - see Abortion, by type, with shock
    ectopic pregnancy (see also categories 633.0–633.9) 639.5
    molar pregnancy (see also categories 630–632) 639.5
  during or after labor and delivery 669.1●
  fetus or newborn 779.85
  following
    abortion 639.5
    ectopic or molar pregnancy 639.5
  during or after labor and delivery 669.1●
  fetus or newborn 779.89
  during or resulting from a surgical procedure 998.00
external ear canal 380.50
  secondary to
    inflammation 380.53
    surgery 380.52
    trauma 380.51
general 780.2
heart - see Disease, heart
heat 992.1
hysterical 300.11
labyrinth, membranous (congenital) 744.05
lung (massive) (see also Atelectasis) 518.0
  pressure, during labor 668.0●
myocardial - see Disease, heart
nervous (see also Disorder, mental, nonpsychotic) 300.9
neurocirculatory 306.2
nose 738.0
postoperative (cardiovascular) 998.09
pulmonary (see also Atelectasis) 518.0
  fetus or newborn 770.5
    partial 770.5
    primary 770.4
thorax 512.89
  iatrogenic 512.1
  postoperative 512.1
trachea 519.19
valvular - see Endocarditis
vascular (peripheral) 785.59
  with
    abortion - see Abortion, by type, with shock
    ectopic pregnancy (see also categories 633.0–633.9) 639.5
    molar pregnancy (see also categories 630–632) 639.5
  cerebral (see also Disease, cerebrovascular, acute) 436
  during or after labor and delivery 669.1●
  fetus or newborn 779.89
  following
    abortion 639.5
    ectopic or molar pregnancy 639.5
vasomotor 785.59
vertebra 733.13
Collateral - see also condition
circulation (venous) 459.89
dilation, veins 459.89
Colles' fracture (closed) (reversed) (separation) 813.41
open 813.51
Collet's syndrome 352.6
Collet-Sicard syndrome 352.6
Colliculitis urethralis (see also Urethritis) 597.89

Colliers'
asthma 500
lung 500
phthisis (see also Tuberculosis) 011.4●
Collodion baby (ichthyosis congenita) 757.1
Colloid milium 709.3
Coloboma NEC 743.49
choroid 743.59
fundus 743.52
iris 743.46
lens 743.36
lids 743.62
optic disc (congenital) 743.57
  acquired 377.23
retina 743.56
sclera 743.47
Coloenteritis - see Enteritis
Colon - see condition
Colonization
MRSA (methicillin resistant Staphylococcus aureus) V02.54
MSSA (methicillin susceptible Staphylococcus aureus) V02.53
Coloptosis 569.89
Color
amblyopia NEC 368.59
  acquired 368.55
blindness NEC (congenital) 368.59
  acquired 368.55
Colostomy
attention to V55.3
fitting or adjustment V55.3
malfunctioning 569.62
status V44.3
Colpitis (see also Vaginitis) 616.10
Colpocele 618.6
Colpocystitis (see also Vaginitis) 616.10
Colporrhexis 665.4●
Colpospasm 625.1
Column, spinal, vertebral - see condition
Coma 780.01
apoplectic (see also Disease, cerebrovascular, acute) 436
diabetic (with ketoacidosis) 250.3●
  due to secondary diabetes 249.3●
  hyperosmolar 250.2●
    due to secondary diabetes 249.2●
eclamptic (see also Eclampsia) 780.39
epileptic 345.3
hepatic 572.2
hyperglycemic 250.2●
  due to secondary diabetes 249.2●
hyperosmolar (diabetic) (nonketotic) 250.2●
  due to secondary diabetes 249.2●
hypoglycemic 251.0
  diabetic 250.3●
    due to secondary diabetes 249.3●
  insulin 250.3●
    due to secondary diabetes 249.3●
    hyperosmolar 250.2●
      due to secondary diabetes 249.2●
  nondiabetic 251.0
  organic hyperinsulinism 251.0
Kussmaul's (diabetic) 250.3●
  due to secondary diabetes 249.3●
liver 572.2
newborn 779.2
prediabetic 250.2●
  due to secondary diabetes 249.2●
uremic - see Uremia
Combat fatigue (see also Reaction, stress, acute) 308.9
Combined - see condition
Comedo 706.1
Comedocarcinoma (M8501/3) - see also Neoplasm, breast, malignant
noninfiltrating (M8501/2)
  specified site - see Neoplasm, by site, in situ
  unspecified site 233.0
Comedomastitis 610.4

Comedones 706.1
lanugo 757.4
Comma bacillus, carrier (suspected) of V02.3
Comminuted fracture - see Fracture, by site
Common
aortopulmonary trunk 745.0
atrioventricular canal (defect) 745.69
atrium 745.69
cold (head) 460
  vaccination, prophylactic (against) V04.7
truncus (arteriosus) 745.0
ventricle 745.3
Commotio (current)
cerebri (see also Concussion, brain) 850.9
  with skull fracture - see Fracture, skull, by site
retinae 921.3
spinalis - see Injury, spinal, by site
Commotion (current)
brain (without skull fracture) (see also Concussion, brain) 850.9
  with skull fracture - see Fracture, skull, by site
spinal cord - see Injury, spinal, by site
Communication
abnormal - see also Fistula
  between
    base of aorta and pulmonary artery 745.0
    left ventricle and right atrium 745.4
    pericardial sac and pleural sac 748.8
    pulmonary artery and pulmonary vein 747.39
  congenital, between uterus and anterior abdominal wall 752.39
    bladder 752.39
    intestine 752.39
    rectum 752.39
  left ventricular-right atrial 745.4
  pulmonary artery-pulmonary vein 747.39
Compartment syndrome - see Syndrome, compartment
Compensation
broken - see Failure, heart
failure - see Failure, heart
neurosis, psychoneurosis 300.11
Complaint - see also Disease
bowel, functional 564.9
  psychogenic 306.4
intestine, functional 564.9
  psychogenic 306.4
kidney (see also Disease, renal) 593.9
liver 573.9
miners' 500
Complete - see condition
Complex
cardiorenal (see also Hypertension, cardiorenal) 404.90
castration 300.9
Costen's 524.60
ego-dystonic homosexuality 302.0
Eisenmenger's (ventricular septal defect) 745.4
homosexual, ego-dystonic 302.0
hypersexual 302.89
inferiority 301.9
jumped process
  spine - see Dislocation, vertebra
primary, tuberculosis (see also Tuberculosis) 010.0●
regional pain syndrome 355.9
  type I 337.20
    lower limb 337.22
    specified site NEC 337.29
    upper limb 337.21
  type II
    lower limb 355.71
    upper limb 354.4
Taussig-Bing (transposition, aorta and overriding pulmonary artery) 745.11

SECTION I INDEX TO DISEASES AND INJURIES / Complications

Complications
- abortion NEC - *see* categories 634–639
- accidental puncture or laceration during a procedure 998.2
- amniocentesis, fetal 679.1●
- amputation stump (late) (surgical) 997.60
  - traumatic - *see* Amputation, traumatic
- anastomosis (and bypass) - *see also* Complications, due to (presence of) any device, implant, or graft classified to 996.0–996.5 NEC
  - hemorrhage NEC 998.11
  - intestinal (internal) NEC 997.49
    - involving urinary tract 997.5
  - mechanical - *see* Complications, mechanical, graft
  - urinary tract (involving intestinal tract) 997.5
- anesthesia, anesthetic NEC (*see also* Anesthesia, complication) 995.22
  - in labor and delivery 668.9●
    - affecting fetus or newborn 763.5
    - cardiac 668.1●
    - central nervous system 668.2●
    - pulmonary 668.0●
    - specified type NEC 668.8●
- aortocoronary (bypass) graft 996.03
  - atherosclerosis - *see* Arteriosclerosis, coronary
  - embolism 996.72
  - occlusion NEC 996.72
  - thrombus 996.72
- arthroplasty (*see also* Complications, prosthetic joint) 996.49
- artificial opening
  - cecostomy 569.60
  - colostomy 569.60
  - cystostomy 596.83
    - infection 596.81
    - mechanical 596.82
    - specified complication NEC 596.83
  - enterostomy 569.60
  - esophagostomy 530.87
    - infection 530.86
    - mechanical 530.87
  - gastrostomy 536.40
  - ileostomy 569.60
  - jejunostomy 569.60
  - nephrostomy 997.5
  - tracheostomy 519.00
  - ureterostomy 997.5
  - urethrostomy 997.5
- bariatric surgery
  - gastric band procedure 539.09
    - infection 539.01
  - specified procedure NEC 539.89
    - infection 539.81
- bile duct implant (prosthetic) NEC 996.79
  - infection or inflammation 996.69
  - mechanical 996.59
- bleeding (intraoperative) (postoperative) 998.11
- blood vessel graft 996.1
  - aortocoronary 996.03
    - atherosclerosis - *see* Arteriosclerosis, coronary
    - embolism 996.72
    - occlusion NEC 996.72
    - thrombus 996.72
  - atherosclerosis - *see* Arteriosclerosis, extremities
  - embolism 996.74
  - occlusion NEC 996.74
  - thrombus 996.74
- bone growth stimulator NEC 996.78
  - infection or inflammation 996.67
- bone marrow transplant 996.85
- breast implant (prosthetic) NEC 996.79
  - infection or inflammation 996.69
  - mechanical 996.54

Complications (*Continued*)
- bypass - *see also* Complications, anastomosis
  - aortocoronary 996.03
    - atherosclerosis - *see* Arteriosclerosis, coronary
    - embolism 996.72
    - occlusion NEC 996.72
    - thrombus 996.72
  - carotid artery 996.1
    - atherosclerosis - *see* Arteriosclerosis, coronary
    - embolism 996.74
    - occlusion NEC 996.74
    - thrombus 996.74
- cardiac (*see also* Disease, heart) 429.9
  - device, implant, or graft NEC 996.72
    - infection or inflammation 996.61
    - long-term effect 429.4
    - mechanical (*see also* Complications, mechanical, by type) 996.00
      - valve prosthesis 996.71
        - infection or inflammation 996.61
  - postoperative NEC 997.1
    - long-term effect 429.4
- cardiorenal (*see also* Hypertension, cardiorenal) 404.90
- carotid artery bypass graft 996.1
  - atherosclerosis - *see* Arteriosclerosis, coronary
  - embolism 996.74
  - occlusion NEC 996.74
  - thrombus 996.74
- cataract fragments in eye 998.82
- catheter device NEC - *see also* Complications, due to (presence of) any device, implant, or graft classified to 996.0–996.5 NEC
  - mechanical - *see* Complications, mechanical, catheter
- cecostomy 569.60
- cesarean section wound 674.3●
- chemotherapy (antineoplastic) 995.29
- chin implant (prosthetic) NEC 996.79
  - infection or inflammation 996.69
  - mechanical 996.59
- colostomy (enterostomy) 569.60
  - specified type NEC 569.69
- contraceptive device, intrauterine NEC 996.76
  - infection 996.65
  - inflammation 996.65
  - mechanical 996.32
- cord (umbilical) - *see* Complications, umbilical cord
- cornea
  - due to
    - contact lens 371.82
- coronary (artery) bypass (graft) NEC 996.03
  - atherosclerosis - *see* Arteriosclerosis, coronary
  - embolism 996.72
  - infection or inflammation 996.61
  - mechanical 996.03
  - occlusion NEC 996.72
  - specified type NEC 996.72
  - thrombus 996.72
- cystostomy 596.83
  - infection 596.81
  - mechanical 596.82
  - specified complication NEC 596.83
- delivery 669.9●
  - procedure (instrumental) (manual) (surgical) 669.4●
  - specified type NEC 669.8●

Complications (*Continued*)
- dialysis (hemodialysis) (peritoneal) (renal) NEC 999.9
- catheter NEC - *see also* Complications, due to (presence of) any device, implant, or graft classified to 996.0–996.5 NEC
  - infection or inflammation 996.62
    - peritoneal 996.68
  - mechanical 996.1
    - peritoneal 996.56
- drug NEC 995.29
- due to (presence of) any device, implant, or graft classified to 996.0–996.5 NEC
  - with infection or inflammation - *see* Complications, infection or inflammation, due to (presence of) any device, implant, or graft classified to 996.0–996.5 NEC
  - arterial NEC 996.74
    - coronary NEC 996.03
      - atherosclerosis - *see* Arteriosclerosis, coronary
      - embolism 996.72
      - occlusion NEC 996.72
      - specified type NEC 996.72
      - thrombus 996.72
    - renal dialysis 996.73
  - arteriovenous fistula or shunt NEC 996.74
  - bone growth stimulator 996.78
  - breast NEC 996.79
  - cardiac NEC 996.72
    - defibrillator 996.72
    - pacemaker 996.72
    - valve prosthesis 996.71
  - catheter NEC 996.79
    - spinal 996.75
    - urinary, indwelling 996.76
    - vascular NEC 996.74
      - renal dialysis 996.73
    - ventricular shunt 996.75
  - coronary (artery) bypass (graft) NEC 996.03
    - atherosclerosis - *see* Arteriosclerosis, coronary
    - embolism 996.72
    - occlusion NEC 996.72
    - thrombus 996.72
  - electrodes
    - brain 996.75
    - heart 996.72
  - esophagostomy 530.87
  - gastrointestinal NEC 996.79
  - genitourinary NEC 996.76
  - heart valve prosthesis NEC 996.71
  - infusion pump 996.74
  - insulin pump 996.57
  - internal
    - joint prosthesis 996.77
    - orthopedic NEC 996.78
    - specified type NEC 996.79
  - intrauterine contraceptive device NEC 996.76
  - joint prosthesis, internal NEC 996.77
  - mechanical - *see* Complications, mechanical
  - nervous system NEC 996.75
  - ocular lens NEC 996.79
  - orbital NEC 996.79
  - orthopedic NEC 996.78
    - joint, internal 996.77
  - renal dialysis 996.73
  - specified type NEC 996.79
  - urinary catheter, indwelling 996.76
  - vascular NEC 996.74
  - ventricular shunt 996.75
- during dialysis NEC 999.9
- ectopic or molar pregnancy NEC 639.9
- electroshock therapy NEC 999.9
- enterostomy 569.60
  - specified type NEC 569.69

124 ◀ New ◀║║ Revised ~~deleted~~ Deleted ● Use Additional Digit(s) ▓ Omit code

SECTION 1 INDEX TO DISEASES AND INJURIES / Complications

Complications (Continued)
  esophagostomy 530.87
    infection 530.86
    mechanical 530.87
  external (fixation) device with internal component(s) NEC 996.78
    infection or inflammation 996.67
    mechanical 996.49
  extracorporeal circulation NEC 999.9
  eye implant (prosthetic) NEC 996.79
    infection or inflammation 996.69
    mechanical
      ocular lens 996.53
      orbital globe 996.59
  fetal, from amniocentesis 679.1●
  gastrointestinal, postoperative NEC (see also Complications, surgical procedures) 997.49
  gastrostomy 536.40
    specified type NEC 536.49
  genitourinary device, implant or graft NEC 996.76
    erosion of implanted vaginal mesh 629.31
    exposure of implanted vaginal mesh 629.32
    infection or inflammation 996.65
      urinary catheter, indwelling 996.64
    mechanical (see also Complications, mechanical, by type) 996.30
      specified NEC 996.39
  graft (bypass) (patch) - see also Complications, due to (presence of) any device, implant, or graft classified to 996.0–996.5 NEC
    bone marrow 996.85
    corneal NEC 996.79
      infection or inflammation 996.69
      rejection or reaction 996.51
      retroprosthetic membrane 996.51
    mechanical - see Complications, mechanical, graft
    organ (immune or nonimmune cause) (partial) (total) 996.80
      bone marrow 996.85
      heart 996.83
      intestines 996.87
      kidney 996.81
      liver 996.82
      lung 996.84
      pancreas 996.86
      specified NEC 996.89
    skin NEC 996.79
      infection or inflammation 996.69
      rejection 996.52
        artificial 996.55
        decellularized allodermis 996.55
  heart - see also Disease, heart transplant (immune or nonimmune cause) 996.83
  hematoma (intraoperative) (postoperative) 998.12
  hemorrhage (intraoperative) (postoperative) 998.11
  hyperalimentation therapy NEC 999.9
  immunization (procedure) - see Complications, vaccination
  implant - see also Complications, due to (presence of) any device, implant, or graft classified to 996.0–996.5 NEC
    dental placement, hemorrhagic 525.71
    mechanical, - see Complications, mechanical, implant
  infection and inflammation
    due to (presence of) any device, implant or graft classified to 996.0–996.5 NEC 996.60
      arterial NEC 996.62
        coronary 996.61
        renal dialysis 996.62
      arteriovenous fistula or shunt 996.62
      artificial heart 996.61
      bone growth stimulator 996.67

Complications (Continued)
  infection and inflammation (Continued)
    due to (Continued)
      breast 996.69
      cardiac 996.61
      catheter NEC 996.69
        central venous 999.31
          bloodstream 999.32
          localized 999.33
        Hickman 999.31
          bloodstream 999.32
          localized 999.33
        peripherally inserted central (PICC) 999.31
          bloodstream 999.32
          localized 999.33
        peritoneal 996.68
        portacath (port-a-cath) 999.31
          bloodstream 999.32
          localized 999.33
        spinal 996.63
        triple lumen 999.31
          bloodstream 999.32
          localized 999.33
        umbilical venous 999.31
          bloodstream 999.32
          localized 999.33
        urinary, indwelling 996.64
        vascular (arterial) (dialysis) (peripheral venous) NEC 996.62
        ventricular shunt 996.63
      central venous catheter 999.31
        bloodstream 999.32
        localized 999.33
      coronary artery bypass 996.61
      electrodes
        brain 996.63
        heart 996.61
      gastrointestinal NEC 996.69
      genitourinary NEC 996.65
        indwelling urinary catheter 996.64
      heart assist device 996.61
      heart valve 996.61
      Hickman catheter 999.31
        bloodstream 999.32
        localized 999.33
      infusion pump 996.62
      insulin pump 996.69
      intrauterine contraceptive device 996.65
      joint prosthesis, internal 996.66
      ocular lens 996.69
      orbital (implant) 996.69
      orthopedic NEC 996.67
        joint, internal 996.66
      peripherally inserted central catheter (PICC) 999.31
        bloodstream 999.32
        localized 999.33
      portacath (port-a-cath) 999.31
        bloodstream 999.32
        localized 999.33
      specified type NEC 996.69
      triple lumen catheter 999.31
        bloodstream 999.32
        localized 999.33
      umbilical venous catheter 999.31
        bloodstream 999.32
        localized 999.33
      urinary catheter, indwelling 996.64
      ventricular shunt 996.63
  infusion (procedure) 999.88
    blood - see Complications, transfusion
    infection NEC 999.39
    sepsis NEC 999.39
  inhalation therapy NEC 999.9
  injection (procedure) 999.9
    drug reaction (see also Reaction, drug) 995.27
    infection NEC 999.39

Complications (Continued)
  injection (Continued)
    sepsis NEC 999.39
    serum (prophylactic) (therapeutic) - see Complications, vaccination
    vaccine (any) - see Complications, vaccination
  inoculation (any) - see Complications, vaccination
  insulin pump 996.57
  internal device (catheter) (electronic) (fixation) (prosthetic) - see also Complications, due to (presence of) any device, implant, or graft classified to 996.0–996.5 NEC
    mechanical - see Complications, mechanical
  intestinal pouch, specified NEC 569.79
  intestinal transplant (immune or nonimmune cause) 996.87
  intraoperative bleeding or hemorrhage 998.11
  intrauterine contraceptive device (see also Complications, contraceptive device) 996.76
    with fetal damage affecting management of pregnancy 655.8●
    infection or inflammation 996.65
  in utero procedure
    fetal 679.1●
    maternal 679.0●
  jejunostomy 569.60
  kidney transplant (immune or nonimmune cause) 996.81
  labor 669.9●
    specified condition NEC 669.8●
  liver transplant (immune or nonimmune cause) 996.82
  lumbar puncture 349.0
  mechanical
    anastomosis - see Complications, mechanical, graft
    artificial heart 996.09
    bypass - see Complications, mechanical, graft
    catheter NEC 996.59
      cardiac 996.09
      cystostomy 596.82
      dialysis (hemodialysis) 996.1
        peritoneal 996.56
      during a procedure 998.2
      urethral, indwelling 996.31
    colostomy 569.62
    device NEC 996.59
      balloon (counterpulsation), intra-aortic 996.1
      cardiac 996.00
        automatic implantable defibrillator 996.04
        long-term effect 429.4
        specified NEC 996.09
      contraceptive, intrauterine 996.32
      counterpulsation, intra-aortic 996.1
      fixation, external, with internal components 996.49
      fixation, internal (nail, rod, plate) 996.40
      genitourinary 996.30
        specified NEC 996.39
      insulin pump 996.57
      nervous system 996.2
      orthopedic, internal 996.40
        prosthetic joint (see also Complications, mechanical, device, orthopedic, prosthetic, joint) 996.47
      prosthetic NEC 996.59
        joint 996.47
          articular bearing surface wear 996.46
          aseptic loosening 996.41

SECTION I INDEX TO DISEASES AND INJURIES / Complications

Complications *(Continued)*
  mechanical *(Continued)*
    device NEC *(Continued)*
      prosthetic NEC *(Continued)*
        joint *(Continued)*
          breakage 996.43
          dislocation 996.42
          failure 996.47
          fracture 996.43
            around prosthetic 996.44
            peri-prosthetic 996.44
          instability 996.42
          loosening 996.41
          peri-prosthetic osteolysis 996.45
          subluxation 996.42
          wear 996.46
      umbrella, vena cava 996.1
      vascular 996.1
    dorsal column stimulator 996.2
    electrode NEC 996.59
      brain 996.2
      cardiac 996.01
      spinal column 996.2
    enterostomy 569.62
    esophagostomy 530.87
    fistula, arteriovenous, surgically created 996.1
    gastrostomy 536.42
    graft NEC 996.52
      aortic (bifurcation) 996.1
      aortocoronary bypass 996.03
      blood vessel NEC 996.1
      bone 996.49
      cardiac 996.00
      carotid artery bypass 996.1
      cartilage 996.49
      corneal 996.51
      coronary bypass 996.03
      decellularized allodermis 996.55
      genitourinary 996.30
        specified NEC 996.39
      muscle 996.49
      nervous system 996.2
      organ (immune or nonimmune cause) 996.80
        heart 996.83
        intestines 996.87
        kidney 996.81
        liver 996.82
        lung 996.84
        pancreas 996.86
        specified NEC 996.89
      orthopedic, internal 996.49
      peripheral nerve 996.2
      prosthetic NEC 996.59
      skin 996.52
        artificial 996.55
      specified NEC 996.59
      tendon 996.49
      tissue NEC 996.52
      tooth 996.59
      ureter, without mention of resection 996.39
      vascular 996.1
    heart valve prosthesis 996.02
      long-term effect 429.4
    implant NEC 996.59
      cardiac 996.00
        automatic implantable defibrillator 996.04
        long-term effect 429.4
        specified NEC 996.09
      electrode NEC 996.59
        brain 996.2
        cardiac 996.01
        spinal column 996.2
      genitourinary 996.30
      nervous system 996.2
      orthopedic, internal 996.49

Complications *(Continued)*
  mechanical *(Continued)*
    implant NEC *(Continued)*
      prosthetic NEC 996.59
        in
          bile duct 996.59
          breast 996.54
          chin 996.59
          eye
            ocular lens 996.53
            orbital globe 996.59
        vascular 996.1
    insulin pump 996.57
    nonabsorbable surgical material 996.59
    pacemaker NEC 996.59
      brain 996.2
      cardiac 996.01
      nerve (phrenic) 996.2
    patch - *see* Complications, mechanical, graft
    prosthesis NEC 996.59
      bile duct 996.59
      breast 996.54
      chin 996.59
      ocular lens 996.53
      reconstruction, vas deferens 996.39
    reimplant NEC 996.59
      extremity (*see also* Complications, reattached, extremity) 996.90
      organ (*see also* Complications, transplant, organ, by site) 996.80
    repair - *see* Complications, mechanical, graft
    respirator [ventilator] V46.14
    shunt NEC 996.59
      arteriovenous, surgically created 996.1
      ventricular (communicating) 996.2
    stent NEC 996.59
    tracheostomy 519.02
    vas deferens reconstruction 996.39
    ventilator [respirator] V46.14
  medical care NEC 999.9
    cardiac NEC 997.1
    gastrointestinal NEC 997.49
    nervous system NEC 997.00
    peripheral vascular NEC 997.2
    respiratory NEC 997.39
    urinary NEC 997.5
    vascular
      mesenteric artery 997.71
      other vessels 997.79
      peripheral vessels 997.2
      renal artery 997.72
  nephrostomy 997.5
  nervous system
    device, implant, or graft NEC 349.1
      mechanical 996.2
    postoperative NEC 997.00
  obstetric 669.9 ●
    procedure (instrumental) (manual) (surgical) 669.4 ●
    specified NEC 669.8 ●
    surgical wound 674.3 ●
  ocular lens implant NEC 996.79
    infection or inflammation 996.69
    mechanical 996.53
  organ transplant - *see* Complications, transplant, organ, by site
  orthopedic device, implant, or graft
    internal (fixation) (nail) (plate) (rod) NEC 996.78
      infection or inflammation 996.67
      joint prosthesis 996.77
        infection or inflammation 996.66
      mechanical 996.40
  pacemaker (cardiac) 996.72
    infection or inflammation 996.61
    mechanical 996.01
  pancreas transplant (immune or nonimmune cause) 996.86
  perfusion NEC 999.9

Complications *(Continued)*
  perineal repair (obstetrical) 674.3 ●
    disruption 674.2 ●
  pessary (uterus) (vagina) - *see* Complications, contraceptive device
  phototherapy 990
  postcystoscopic 997.5
  postmastoidectomy NEC 383.30
  postoperative - *see* Complications, surgical procedures
  pregnancy NEC 646.9 ●
    affecting fetus or newborn 761.9
  prosthetic device, internal - *see also* Complications, due to (presence of) any device, implant or graft classified to 996.0–996.5 NEC
    mechanical NEC (*see also* Complications, mechanical) 996.59
  puerperium NEC (*see also* Puerperal) 674.9 ●
  puncture, spinal 349.0
  pyelogram 997.5
  radiation 990
  radiotherapy 990
  reattached
    body part, except extremity 996.99
    extremity (infection) (rejection) 996.90
      arm(s) 996.94
      digit(s) (hand) 996.93
        foot 996.95
      finger(s) 996.93
      foot 996.95
      forearm 996.91
      hand 996.92
      leg 996.96
      lower NEC 996.96
      toe(s) 996.95
      upper NEC 996.94
  reimplant NEC - *see also* Complications, due to (presence of) any device, implant, or graft classified to 996.0–996.5 NEC
    bone marrow 996.85
    extremity (*see also* Complications, reattached, extremity) 996.90
      due to infection 996.90
    mechanical - *see* Complications, mechanical, reimplant
    organ (immune or nonimmune cause) (partial) (total) (*see also* Complications, transplant, organ, by site) 996.80
  renal allograft 996.81
  renal dialysis - *see* Complications, dialysis
  respirator [ventilator], mechanical V46.14
  respiratory 519.9
    device, implant or graft NEC 996.79
      infection or inflammation 996.69
      mechanical 996.59
    distress syndrome, adult, following trauma and surgery 518.52
    insufficiency, acute, postoperative 518.52
    postoperative NEC 997.39
    therapy NEC 999.9
  sedation during labor and delivery 668.9 ●
    affecting fetus or newborn 763.5
    cardiac 668.1 ●
    central nervous system 668.2 ●
    pulmonary 668.0 ●
    specified type NEC 668.8 ●
  seroma (intraoperative) (postoperative) (noninfected) 998.13
    infected 998.51
  shunt - *see also* Complications, due to (presence of) any device, implant, or graft classified to 996.0–996.5 NEC
    mechanical - *see* Complications, mechanical, shunt

Complications (Continued)
- specified body system NEC
  - device, implant, or graft - see
    - Complications, due to (presence of) any device, implant, or graft classified to 996.0–996.5 NEC
  - postoperative NEC 997.99
- spinal puncture or tap 349.0
- stoma, external
  - gastrointestinal tract
    - colostomy 569.60
    - enterostomy 569.60
    - esophagostomy 530.87
      - infection 530.86
      - mechanical 530.87
    - gastrostomy 536.40
  - urinary tract 596.83
- stomach banding 539.09
- stomach stapling 539.89
- surgical procedures 998.9
  - accidental puncture or laceration 998.2
  - amputation stump (late) 997.60
  - anastomosis - see Complications, anastomosis
  - burst stitches or sutures (external) (see also Dehiscence) 998.32
    - internal 998.31
  - cardiac 997.1
    - long-term effect following cardiac surgery 429.4
  - catheter device - see Complications, catheter device
  - cataract fragments in eye 998.82
  - cecostomy malfunction 569.62
  - colostomy malfunction 569.62
  - cystostomy malfunction 596.82
    - infection 596.81
    - mechanical 596.82
    - specified complication NEC 596.83
  - dehiscence (of incision) (external) (see also Dehiscence) 998.32
    - internal 998.31
  - dialysis NEC (see also Complications, dialysis) 999.9
  - disruption (see also Dehiscence)
    - anastomosis (internal) - see Complications, mechanical, graft
    - internal suture (line) 998.31
    - wound (external) 998.32
      - internal 998.31
  - dumping syndrome (postgastrectomy) 564.2
  - elephantiasis or lymphedema 997.99
    - postmastectomy 457.0
  - emphysema (surgical) 998.81
  - enterostomy malfunction 569.62
  - esophagostomy malfunction 530.87
  - evisceration 998.32
  - fistula (persistent postoperative) 998.6
  - foreign body inadvertently left in wound (sponge) (suture) (swab) 998.4
  - from nonabsorbable surgical material (Dacron) (mesh) (permanent suture) (reinforcing) (Teflon) - see Complications due to (presence of) any device, implant, or graft classified to 996.0–996.5 NEC
  - gastrointestinal NEC 997.49
  - gastrostomy malfunction 536.42
  - hematoma 998.12
  - hemorrhage 998.11
  - ileostomy malfunction 569.62
  - internal prosthetic device NEC (see also Complications, internal device) 996.70
    - hemolytic anemia 283.19
    - infection or inflammation 996.60
    - malfunction - see Complications, mechanical

Complications (Continued)
- surgical procedures (Continued)
  - internal prosthetic device NEC (Continued)
    - mechanical complication - see Complications, mechanical
    - thrombus 996.70
  - jejunostomy malfunction 569.62
  - nervous system NEC 997.00
  - obstruction, internal anastomosis - see Complications, mechanical, graft
  - other body system NEC 997.99
  - peripheral vascular NEC 997.2
  - postcardiotomy syndrome 429.4
  - postcholecystectomy syndrome 576.0
  - postcommissurotomy syndrome 429.4
  - postgastrectomy dumping syndrome 564.2
  - postmastectomy lymphedema syndrome 457.0
  - postmastoidectomy 383.30
    - cholesteatoma, recurrent 383.32
    - cyst, mucosal 383.31
    - granulation 383.33
    - inflammation, chronic 383.33
  - postvagotomy syndrome 564.2
  - postvalvulotomy syndrome 429.4
  - reattached extremity (infection) (rejection) (see also Complications, reattached, extremity) 996.90
  - respiratory NEC 997.39
  - seroma 998.13
  - shock (endotoxic) (septic) 998.02
    - hypovolemic 998.09
  - shunt, prosthetic (thrombus) - see also Complications, due to (presence of) any device, implant, or graft classified to 996.0–996.5 NEC
    - hemolytic anemia 283.19
  - specified complication NEC 998.89
  - stitch abscess 998.59
  - transplant - see Complications, graft
  - ureterostomy malfunction 997.5
  - urethrostomy malfunction 997.5
  - urinary NEC 997.5
  - vascular
    - mesenteric artery 997.71
    - other vessels 997.79
    - peripheral vessels 997.2
    - renal artery 997.72
  - wound infection 998.59
- therapeutic misadventure NEC 999.9
  - surgical treatment 998.9
- tracheostomy 519.00
- transfusion (blood) (lymphocytes) (plasma) 999.80
  - acute lung injury (TRALI) 518.7
  - atrophy, liver, yellow, subacute (within 8 months of administration) - see Hepatitis, viral
  - bone marrow 996.85
  - embolism
    - air 999.1
    - thrombus 999.2
  - febrile nonhemolytic reaction (FNHTR) 780.66
  - hemolysis NEC 999.89
    - bone marrow 996.85
  - hemolytic reaction, incompatibility unspecified 999.83
    - acute 999.84
    - delayed 999.85
  - hepatitis (serum) (type B) (within 8 months after administration) - see Hepatitis, viral
  - incompatibility reaction
    - ABO 999.60
      - with hemolytic transfusion reaction (HTR) (not specified as acute or delayed) 999.61
        - acute 999.62
        - delayed 999.63
      - specified type NEC 999.69

Complications (Continued)
- transfusion (Continued)
  - incompatibility reaction (Continued)
    - minor blood group 999.89
    - non-ABO (minor antigens) (Duffy) (Kell) (Kidd) (Lewis) (M) (N) (P) (S) 999.75
      - with hemolytic transfusion reaction (HTR) (not specified as acute or delayed) 999.76
        - acute 999.77
        - delayed 999.78
      - specified type NEC 999.79
    - Rh antigen (C) (c) (D) (E) (e) (factor) 999.70
      - with hemolytic transfusion reaction (HTR) (not specified as acute or delayed) 999.71
        - acute 999.72
        - delayed 999.73
      - specified type NEC 999.74
  - infection 999.39
    - acute 999.34
  - jaundice (serum) (within 8 months after administration) - see Hepatitis, viral
  - sepsis 999.39
  - shock or reaction NEC 999.89
    - bone marrow 996.85
  - specified reaction NEC 999.89
  - subacute yellow atrophy of liver (within 8 months after administration) - see Hepatitis, viral
  - thromboembolism 999.2
- transplant NEC - see also Complications, due to (presence of) any device, implant, or graft classified to 996.0–996.5 NEC
  - bone marrow 996.85
  - organ (immune or nonimmune cause) (partial) (total) 996.80
    - bone marrow 996.85
    - heart 996.83
    - intestines 996.87
    - kidney 996.81
    - liver 996.82
    - lung 996.84
    - pancreas 996.86
    - specified NEC 996.89
  - stem cell(s) 996.88
    - from
      - peripheral blood 996.88
      - umbilical cord 996.88
- trauma NEC (early) 958.8
- ultrasound therapy NEC 999.9
- umbilical cord
  - affecting fetus or newborn 762.6
  - complicating delivery 663.9●
    - affecting fetus or newborn 762.6
  - specified type NEC 663.8●
- urethral catheter NEC 996.76
  - infection or inflammation 996.64
  - mechanical 996.31
- urinary, postoperative NEC 997.5
- vaccination 999.9
  - anaphylaxis NEC 999.42
  - cellulitis 999.39
  - encephalitis or encephalomyelitis 323.51
  - hepatitis (serum) (type B) (within 8 months after administration) - see Hepatitis, viral
  - infection (general) (local) NEC 999.39
  - jaundice (serum) (within 8 months after administration) - see Hepatitis, viral
  - meningitis 997.09 [321.8]
  - myelitis 323.52
  - protein sickness 999.52
  - reaction (allergic) 999.52
    - serum 999.52
  - sepsis 999.39
  - serum intoxication, sickness, rash, or other serum reaction NEC 999.52
  - shock (allergic) (anaphylactic) 999.49

SECTION 1 INDEX TO DISEASES AND INJURIES / Complications

Complications (Continued)
  vaccination (Continued)
    subacute yellow atrophy of liver (within 8 months after administration) - see Hepatitis, viral
    vaccinia (generalized) 999.0
      localized 999.39
  vascular
    device, implant, or graft NEC 996.74
      infection or inflammation 996.62
      mechanical NEC 996.1
        cardiac (see also Complications, mechanical, by type) 996.00
    following infusion, perfusion, or transfusion 999.2
    postoperative NEC 997.2
      mesenteric artery 997.71
      other vessels 997.79
      peripheral vessels 997.2
      renal artery 997.72
  ventilation therapy NEC 999.9
  ventilator [respirator], mechanical V46.14

Compound presentation, complicating delivery 652.8 ●
  causing obstructed labor 660.0 ●

Compressed air disease 993.3

Compression
  with injury - see specific injury
  arm NEC 354.9
  artery 447.1
    celiac, syndrome 447.4
  brachial plexus 353.0
  brain (stem) 348.4
    due to
      contusion, brain - see Contusion, brain
      injury NEC - see also Hemorrhage, brain, traumatic
        birth - see Birth, injury, brain
      laceration, brain - see Laceration, brain
    osteopathic 739.0
  bronchus 519.19
  by cicatrix - see Cicatrix
  cardiac 423.9
  cauda equina 344.60
    with neurogenic bladder 344.61
  celiac (artery) (axis) 447.4
  cerebral - see Compression, brain
  cervical plexus 353.2
  cord (umbilical) - see Compression, umbilical cord
  cranial nerve 352.9
    second 377.49
    third (partial) 378.51
      total 378.52
    fourth 378.53
    fifth 350.8
    sixth 378.54
    seventh 351.8
  divers' squeeze 993.3
  duodenum (external) (see also Obstruction, duodenum) 537.3
  during birth 767.9
  esophagus 530.3
    congenital, external 750.3
  Eustachian tube 381.63
  facies (congenital) 754.0
  fracture - see Fracture, by site
  heart - see Disease, heart
  intestine (see also Obstruction, intestine) 560.9
    with hernia - see Hernia, by site, with obstruction
  laryngeal nerve, recurrent 478.79
  leg NEC 355.8
  lower extremity NEC 355.8
  lumbosacral plexus 353.1
  lung 518.89
  lymphatic vessel 457.1
  medulla - see Compression, brain

Compression (Continued)
  nerve NEC - see also Disorder, nerve
    arm NEC 354.9
    autonomic nervous system (see also Neuropathy, peripheral, autonomic) 337.9
    axillary 353.0
    cranial NEC 352.9
    due to displacement of intervertebral disc 722.2
      with myelopathy 722.70
      cervical 722.0
        with myelopathy 722.71
      lumbar, lumbosacral 722.10
        with myelopathy 722.73
      thoracic, thoracolumbar 722.11
        with myelopathy 722.72
    iliohypogastric 355.79
    ilioinguinal 355.79
    leg NEC 355.8
    lower extremity NEC 355.8
    median (in carpal tunnel) 354.0
    obturator 355.79
    optic 377.49
    plantar 355.6
    posterior tibial (in tarsal tunnel) 355.5
    root (by scar tissue) NEC 724.9
      cervical NEC 723.4
      lumbar NEC 724.4
      lumbosacral 724.4
      thoracic 724.4
    saphenous 355.79
    sciatic (acute) 355.0
    sympathetic 337.9
    traumatic - see Injury, nerve
    ulnar 354.2
    upper extremity NEC 354.9
  peripheral - see Compression, nerve
  spinal (cord) (old or nontraumatic) 336.9
    by displacement of intervertebral disc - see Displacement, intervertebral disc
    nerve
      root NEC 724.9
        postoperative 722.80
          cervical region 722.81
          lumbar region 722.83
          thoracic region 722.82
        traumatic - see Injury, nerve, spinal
      traumatic - see Injury, nerve, spinal
    spondylogenic 721.91
      cervical 721.1
      lumbar, lumbosacral 721.42
      thoracic 721.41
    traumatic - see also Injury, spinal, by site
      with fracture, vertebra - see Fracture, vertebra, by site, with spinal cord injury
  spondylogenic - see Compression, spinal cord, spondylogenic
  subcostal nerve (syndrome) 354.8
  sympathetic nerve NEC 337.9
  syndrome 958.5
  thorax 512.89
    iatrogenic 512.1
    postoperative 512.1
  trachea 519.19
    congenital 748.3
  ulnar nerve (by scar tissue) 354.2
  umbilical cord
    affecting fetus or newborn 762.5
      cord prolapsed 762.4
    complicating delivery 663.2 ●
      cord around neck 663.1 ●
      cord prolapsed 663.0 ●
  upper extremity NEC 354.9
  ureter 593.3
  urethra - see Stricture, urethra
  vein 459.2
  vena cava (inferior) (superior) 459.2
  vertebral NEC - see Compression, spinal (cord)

Compulsion, compulsive
  eating 307.51
  neurosis (obsessive) 300.3
  personality 301.4
  states (mixed) 300.3
  swearing 300.3
    in Gilles de la Tourette's syndrome 307.23
  tics and spasms 307.22
  water drinking NEC (syndrome) 307.9

Concato's disease (pericardial polyserositis) 423.2
  peritoneal 568.82
  pleural - see Pleurisy

Concavity, chest wall 738.3

Concealed
  hemorrhage NEC 459.0
  penis 752.65

Concentric fading 368.12

Concern (normal) about sick person in family V61.49

Concrescence (teeth) 520.2

Concretio cordis 423.1
  rheumatic 393

Concretion - see also Calculus
  appendicular 543.9
  canaliculus 375.57
  clitoris 624.8
  conjunctiva 372.54
  eyelid 374.56
  intestine (impaction) (obstruction) 560.39
  lacrimal (passages) 375.57
  prepuce (male) 605
    female (clitoris) 624.8
  salivary gland (any) 527.5
  seminal vesicle 608.89
  stomach 537.89
  tonsil 474.8

Concussion (current) 850.9
  with
    loss of consciousness 850.5
      brief (less than one hour)
        30 minutes or less 850.11
        31–59 minutes 850.12
      moderate (1–24 hours) 850.2
      prolonged (more than 24 hours) (with complete recovery) (with return to pre-existing conscious level) 850.3
        without return to pre-existing conscious level 850.4
    mental confusion or disorientation (without loss of consciousness) 850.0
      with loss of consciousness - see Concussion, with, loss of consciousness
  without loss of consciousness 850.0
  blast (air) (hydraulic) (immersion) (underwater) 869.0
    with open wound into cavity 869.1
    abdomen or thorax - see Injury, internal, by site
    brain - see Concussion, brain
    ear (acoustic nerve trauma) 951.5
      with perforation, tympanic membrane - see Wound, open, ear drum
    thorax - see Injury, internal, intrathoracic organs NEC
  brain or cerebral (without skull fracture) 850.9
    with
      loss of consciousness 850.5
        brief (less than one hour)
          30 minutes or less 850.11
          31–59 minutes 850.12
        moderate (1–24 hours) 850.2

SECTION I INDEX TO DISEASES AND INJURIES / Conjunctivitis

Compression *(Continued)*
  brain or cerebral *(Continued)*
    with *(Continued)*
      loss of consciousness *(Continued)*
        prolonged (more than 24 hours)
          (with complete recovery)
          (with return to pre-existing
            conscious level) 850.3
          without return to pre-existing
            conscious level 850.4
        mental confusion or disorientation
          (without loss of consciousness)
            850.0
        with loss of consciousness - *see*
          Concussion, brain, with, loss
          of consciousness
      skull fracture - *see* Fracture, skull, by site
    without loss of consciousness 850.0
  cauda equina 952.4
  cerebral - *see* Concussion, brain
  conus medullaris (spine) 952.4
  hydraulic - *see* Concussion, blast
  internal organs - *see* Injury, internal, by site
  labyrinth - *see* Injury, intracranial
  ocular 921.3
  osseous labyrinth - *see* Injury, intracranial
  spinal (cord) - *see also* Injury, spinal, by site
    due to
      broken
        back - *see* Fracture, vertebra, by site,
          with spinal cord injury
        neck - *see* Fracture, vertebra,
          cervical, with spinal cord
          injury
      fracture, fracture dislocation, or
        compression fracture of spine or
        vertebra - *see* Fracture, vertebra,
        by site, with spinal cord injury
  syndrome 310.2
  underwater blast - *see* Concussion, blast
Condition - *see also* Disease
  fetal hematologic 678.0 ●
  psychiatric 298.9
  respiratory NEC 519.9
    acute or subacute NEC 519.9
      due to
        external agent 508.9
          specified type NEC 508.8
        fumes or vapors (chemical)
          (inhalation) 506.3
        radiation 508.0
    chronic NEC 519.9
      due to
        external agent 508.9
          specified type NEC 508.8
        fumes or vapors (chemical)
          (inhalation) 506.4
        radiation 508.1
      due to
        external agent 508.9
          specified type NEC 508.8
        fumes or vapors (chemical) inhalation
          506.9
        smoke inhalation 508.2
Conduct disturbance *(see also* Disturbance,
    conduct) 312.9
  adjustment reaction 309.3
  hyperkinetic 314.2
Condyloma NEC 078.11
  acuminatum 078.11
  gonorrheal 098.0
  latum 091.3
  syphilitic 091.3
    congenital 090.0
  venereal, syphilitic 091.3
Confinement - *see* Delivery
Conflagration - *see also* Burn, by site
  asphyxia (by inhalation of gases, fumes, or
    vapors) 987.9
      specified agent - *see* Table of Drugs and
        Chemicals

Conflict
  family V61.9
    specified circumstance NEC V61.8
  interpersonal NEC V62.81
  marital V61.10
    involving
      divorce V61.03
      estrangement V61.09
  parent (guardian)-child V61.20
    adopted child V61.24
    biological child V61.23
    foster child V61.25
  partner V61.10
Confluent - *see* condition
Confusion, confused (mental) (state) *(see also*
    State, confusional) 298.9
  acute 293.0
  epileptic 293.0
  postoperative 293.9
  psychogenic 298.2
  reactive (from emotional stress,
    psychological trauma) 298.2
  subacute 293.1
Confusional arousals 327.41
Congelation 991.9
Congenital - *see also* condition
  aortic septum 747.29
  generalized fibromatosis (CGF) 759.89
  intrinsic factor deficiency 281.0
  malformation - *see* Anomaly
Congestion, congestive
  asphyxia, newborn 768.9
  bladder 596.89
  bowel 569.89
  brain *(see also* Disease, cerebrovascular NEC)
    437.8
    malarial 084.9
  breast 611.79
  bronchi 519.19
  bronchial tube 519.19
  catarrhal 472.0
  cerebral - *see* Congestion, brain
  cerebrospinal - *see* Congestion, brain
  chest 786.9
  chill 780.99
    malarial *(see also* Malaria) 084.6
  circulatory NEC 459.9
  conjunctiva 372.71
  due to disturbance of circulation 459.9
  duodenum 537.3
  enteritis - *see* Enteritis
  eye 372.71
  fibrosis syndrome (pelvic) 625.5
  gastroenteritis - *see* Enteritis
  general 799.89
  glottis 476.0
  heart *(see also* Failure, heart) 428.0
  hepatic 573.0
  hypostatic (lung) 514
  intestine 569.89
  intracranial - *see* Congestion, brain
  kidney 593.89
  labyrinth 386.50
  larynx 476.0
  liver 573.0
  lung 786.9
    active or acute *(see also* Pneumonia) 486
      congenital 770.0
    chronic 514
    hypostatic 514
    idiopathic, acute 518.52
    passive 514
  malaria, malarial (brain) (fever) *(see also*
    Malaria) 084.6
  medulla - *see* Congestion, brain
  nasal 478.19
  nose 478.19
  orbit, orbital 376.33
    inflammatory (chronic) 376.10
      acute 376.00
  ovary 620.8

Congestion, congestive *(Continued)*
  pancreas 577.8
  pelvic, female 625.5
  pleural 511.0
  prostate (active) 602.1
  pulmonary - *see* Congestion, lung
  renal 593.89
  retina 362.89
  seminal vesicle 608.89
  spinal cord 336.1
  spleen 289.51
    chronic 289.51
  stomach 537.89
  trachea 464.11
  urethra 599.84
  uterus 625.5
    with subinvolution 621.1
  viscera 799.89
Congestive - *see* Congestion
Conical
  cervix 622.6
  cornea 371.60
  teeth 520.2
Conjoined twins 759.4
  causing disproportion (fetopelvic) 678.1 ●
  fetal 678.1 ●
Conjugal maladjustment V61.10
  involving
    divorce V61.03
    estrangement V61.09
Conjunctiva - *see* condition
Conjunctivitis (exposure) (infectious)
    (nondiphtheritic) (pneumococcal)
    (pustular) (staphylococcal) (streptococcal)
    NEC 372.30
  actinic 370.24
  acute 372.00
    atopic 372.05
    chemical 372.06
    contagious 372.03
    follicular 372.02
    hemorrhagic (viral) 077.4
    toxic 372.06
  adenoviral (acute) 077.3
  allergic (chronic) 372.14
    with hay fever 372.05
  anaphylactic 372.05
  angular 372.03
  Apollo (viral) 077.4
  atopic 372.05
  blennorrhagic (neonatorum) 098.40
  catarrhal 372.03
  chemical 372.06
    allergic 372.05
    meaning corrosion - *see* Burn, conjunctiva
  chlamydial 077.98
    due to
      Chlamydia trachomatis - *see* Trachoma
    paratrachoma 077.0
  chronic 372.10
    allergic 372.14
    follicular 372.12
    simple 372.11
    specified type NEC 372.14
    vernal 372.13
  diphtheritic 032.81
  due to
    dust 372.05
    enterovirus type 70 077.4
    erythema multiforme 695.1 [372.33]
    filariasis *(see also* Filariasis) 125.9 [372.15]
    mucocutaneous
      disease NEC 372.33
      leishmaniasis 085.5 [372.15]
    Reiter's disease 099.3 [372.33]
    syphilis 095.8 [372.10]
    toxoplasmosis (acquired) 130.1
      congenital (active) 771.2
    trachoma - *see* Trachoma
  dust 372.05
  eczematous 370.31

 New   Revised   ~~deleted~~ Deleted   ● Use Additional Digit(s)   Omit code

SECTION I INDEX TO DISEASES AND INJURIES / Conjunctivitis

Conjunctivitis (Continued)
   epidemic 077.1
      hemorrhagic 077.4
   follicular (acute) 372.02
      adenoviral (acute) 077.3
         chronic 372.12
   glare 370.24
   gonococcal (neonatorum) 098.40
   granular (trachomatous) 076.1
      late effect 139.1
   hemorrhagic (acute) (epidemic) 077.4
   herpetic (simplex) 054.43
      zoster 053.21
   inclusion 077.0
   infantile 771.6
   influenzal 372.03
   Koch-Weeks 372.03
   light 372.05
   medicamentosa 372.05
   membranous 372.04
   meningococcic 036.89
   Morax-Axenfeld 372.02
   mucopurulent NEC 372.03
   neonatal 771.6
      gonococcal 098.40
   Newcastle's 077.8
   nodosa 360.14
   of Beal 077.3
   parasitic 372.15
      filariasis (see also Filariasis) 125.9 [372.15]
      mucocutaneous leishmaniasis 085.5 [372.15]
   Parinaud's 372.02
   petrificans 372.39
   phlyctenular 370.31
   pseudomembranous 372.04
      diphtheritic 032.81
   purulent 372.03
   Reiter's 099.3 [372.33]
   rosacea 695.3 [372.31]
   serous 372.01
      viral 077.99
   simple chronic 372.11
   specified NEC 372.39
   sunlamp 372.04
   swimming pool 077.0
   toxic 372.06
   trachomatous (follicular) 076.1
      acute 076.0
      late effect 139.1
   traumatic NEC 372.39
   tuberculous (see also Tuberculosis) 017.3● [370.31]
   tularemic 021.3
   tularensis 021.3
   vernal 372.13
      limbar 372.13 [370.32]
   viral 077.99
      acute hemorrhagic 077.4
      specified NEC 077.8
Conjunctivochalasis 372.81
Conjunctoblepharitis - see Conjunctivitis
Conn (-Louis) syndrome (primary aldosteronism) 255.12
Connective tissue - see condition
Conradi (-Hünermann) syndrome or disease (chondrodysplasia calcificans congenita) 756.59
Consanguinity V19.7
Consecutive - see condition
Consolidated lung (base) - see Pneumonia, lobar
Constipation 564.00
   atonic 564.09
   drug induced
      correct substance properly administered 564.09
      overdose or wrong substance given or taken 977.9
         specified drug - see Table of Drugs and Chemicals

Constipation (Continued)
   neurogenic 564.09
   other specified NEC 564.09
   outlet dysfunction 564.02
   psychogenic 306.4
   simple 564.00
   slow transit 564.01
   spastic 564.09
Constitutional - see also condition
   arterial hypotension (see also Hypotension) 458.9
   obesity 278.00
      morbid 278.01
   psychopathic state 301.9
   short stature in childhood 783.43
   state, developmental V21.9
      specified development NEC V21.8
   substandard 301.6
Constitutionally substandard 301.6
Constriction
   anomalous, meningeal bands or folds 742.8
   aortic arch (congenital) 747.10
   asphyxiation or suffocation by 994.7
   bronchus 519.19
   canal, ear (see also Stricture, ear canal, acquired) 380.50
   duodenum 537.3
   gallbladder (see also Obstruction, gallbladder) 575.2
      congenital 751.69
   intestine (see also Obstruction, intestine) 560.9
   larynx 478.74
      congenital 748.3
   meningeal bands or folds, anomalous 742.8
   organ or site, congenital NEC - see Atresia
   prepuce (congenital) 605
   pylorus 537.0
      adult hypertrophic 537.0
      congenital or infantile 750.5
      newborn 750.5
   ring (uterus) 661.4●
      affecting fetus or newborn 763.7
   spastic - see also Spasm
      ureter 593.3
      urethra - see Stricture, urethra
   stomach 537.89
   ureter 593.3
   urethra - see Stricture, urethra
   visual field (functional) (peripheral) 368.45
Constrictive - see condition
Consultation V65.9
   medical - see also Counseling, medical
   specified reason NEC V65.8
   without complaint or sickness V65.9
      feared complaint unfounded V65.5
      specified reason NEC V65.8
Consumption - see Tuberculosis
Contact - see also Exposure (suspected)
   with
      AIDS virus V01.79
      anthrax V01.81
      asbestos V15.84
      cholera V01.0
      communicable disease V01.9
         specified type NEC V01.89
         viral NEC V01.79
      Escherichia coli (E. coli) V01.83
      German measles V01.4
      gonorrhea V01.6
      HIV V01.79
      human immunodeficiency virus V01.79
      lead V15.86
      meningococcus V01.84
      parasitic disease NEC V01.89
      poliomyelitis V01.2
      potentially hazardous body fluids V15.85
      rabies V01.5
      rubella V01.4
      SARS-associated coronavirus V01.82
      smallpox V01.3
      syphilis V01.6

Contact (Continued)
   with (Continued)
      tuberculosis V01.1
      varicella V01.71
      venereal disease V01.6
      viral disease NEC V01.79
   dermatitis - see Dermatitis
Contamination, food (see also Poisoning, food) 005.9
Contraception, contraceptive
   advice NEC V25.09
      family planning V25.09
      fitting of diaphragm V25.02
      prescribing or use of
         oral contraceptive agent V25.01
         specified agent NEC V25.02
   counseling NEC V25.09
      emergency V25.03
      family planning V25.09
      fitting of diaphragm V25.02
      prescribing or use of
         oral contraceptive agent V25.01
            emergency V25.03
            postcoital V25.03
         specified agent NEC V25.02
   device (in situ) V45.59
      causing menorrhagia 996.76
      checking V25.42
      complications 996.32
      insertion V25.11
      intrauterine V45.51
      reinsertion V25.13
      removal V25.12
         and reinsertion V25.13
      replacement V25.13
      subdermal V45.52
   fitting of diaphragm V25.02
   insertion
      intrauterine contraceptive device V25.11
      subdermal implantable V25.5
   maintenance V25.40
      examination V25.40
         intrauterine device V25.42
         oral contraceptive V25.41
         specified method NEC V25.49
         subdermal implantable V25.43
      intrauterine device V25.42
      oral contraceptive V25.41
      specified method NEC V25.49
      subdermal implantable V25.43
   management NEC V25.49
   prescription
      oral contraceptive agent V25.01
         emergency V25.03
         postcoital V25.03
         repeat V25.41
      specified agent NEC V25.02
         repeat V25.49
   sterilization V25.2
   surveillance V25.40
      intrauterine device V25.42
      oral contraceptive agent V25.41
      specified method NEC V25.49
      subdermal implantable V25.43
Contraction, contracture, contracted
   Achilles tendon (see also Short, tendon, Achilles) 727.81
   anus 564.89
   axilla 729.90
   bile duct (see also Disease, biliary) 576.8
   bladder 596.89
      neck or sphincter 596.0
   bowel (see also Obstruction, intestine) 560.9
   Braxton Hicks 644.1●
   breast implant, capsular 611.83
   bronchus 519.19
   burn (old) - see Cicatrix
   capsular, of breast implant 611.83
   cecum (see also Obstruction, intestine) 560.9
   cervix (see also Stricture, cervix) 622.4
      congenital 752.49

SECTION 1 INDEX TO DISEASES AND INJURIES / Contusion

Contraction, contracture, contracted
(Continued)
cicatricial - see Cicatrix
colon (see also Obstruction, intestine) 560.9
conjunctiva, trachomatous, active 076.1
   late effect 139.1
Dupuytren's 728.6
eyelid 374.41
eye socket (after enucleation) 372.64
face 729.90
fascia (lata) (postural) 728.89
   Dupuytren's 728.6
   palmar 728.6
   plantar 728.71
finger NEC 736.29
   congenital 755.59
   joint (see also Contraction, joint) 718.44
flaccid, paralytic
   joint (see also Contraction, joint) 718.4●
   muscle 728.85
      ocular 378.50
gallbladder (see also Obstruction, gallbladder) 575.2
hamstring 728.89
   tendon 727.81
heart valve - see Endocarditis
Hicks' 644.1●
hip (see also Contraction, joint) 718.4●
hourglass
   bladder 596.89
      congenital 753.8
   gallbladder (see also Obstruction, gallbladder) 575.2
      congenital 751.69
   stomach 536.8
      congenital 750.7
      psychogenic 306.4
   uterus 661.4●
      affecting fetus or newborn 763.7
hysterical 300.11
infantile (see also Epilepsy) 345.6●
internal os (see also Stricture, cervix) 622.4
intestine (see also Obstruction, intestine) 560.9
joint (abduction) (acquired) (adduction) (flexion) (rotation) 718.40
   ankle 718.47
   congenital NEC 755.8
      generalized or multiple 754.89
         lower limb joints 754.89
      hip (see also Subluxation, congenital, hip) 754.32
      lower limb (including pelvic girdle) not involving hip 754.89
      upper limb (including shoulder girdle) 755.59
   elbow 718.42
   foot 718.47
   hand 718.44
   hip 718.45
   hysterical 300.11
   knee 718.46
   multiple sites 718.49
   pelvic region 718.45
   shoulder (region) 718.41
   specified site NEC 718.48
   wrist 718.43
kidney (granular) (secondary) (see also Sclerosis, renal) 587
   congenital 753.3
   hydronephritic 591
   pyelonephritic (see also Pyelitis, chronic) 590.00
   tuberculous (see also Tuberculosis) 016.0●
ligament 728.89
   congenital 756.89
liver - see Cirrhosis, liver
muscle (postinfectional) (postural) NEC 728.85
   congenital 756.89
      sternocleidomastoid 754.1
   extraocular 378.60

Contraction, contracture, contracted
(Continued)
muscle NEC (Continued)
   eye (extrinsic) (see also Strabismus) 378.9
      paralytic (see also Strabismus, paralytic) 378.50
   flaccid 728.85
   hysterical 300.11
   ischemic (Volkmann's) 958.6
   paralytic 728.85
   posttraumatic 958.6
   psychogenic 306.0
      specified as conversion reaction 300.11
myotonic 728.85
neck (see also Torticollis) 723.5
   congenital 754.1
   psychogenic 306.0
ocular muscle (see also Strabismus) 378.9
   paralytic (see also Strabismus, paralytic) 378.50
organ or site, congenital NEC - see Atresia
outlet (pelvis) - see Contraction, pelvis
palmar fascia 728.6
paralytic
   joint (see also Contraction, joint) 718.4●
   muscle 728.85
      ocular (see also Strabismus, paralytic) 378.50
pelvis (acquired) (general) 738.6
   affecting fetus or newborn 763.1
   complicating delivery 653.1●
      causing obstructed labor 660.1●
   generally contracted 653.1●
      causing obstructed labor 660.1●
   inlet 653.2●
      causing obstructed labor 660.1●
   midpelvic 653.8●
      causing obstructed labor 660.1●
   midplane 653.8●
      causing obstructed labor 660.1●
   outlet 653.3●
      causing obstructed labor 660.1●
plantar fascia 728.71
premature
   atrial 427.61
   auricular 427.61
   auriculoventricular 427.61
   heart (junctional) (nodal) 427.60
   supraventricular 427.61
   ventricular 427.69
prostate 602.8
pylorus (see also Pylorospasm) 537.81
rectosigmoid (see also Obstruction, intestine) 560.9
rectum, rectal (sphincter) 564.89
   psychogenic 306.4
ring (Bandl's) 661.4●
   affecting fetus or newborn 763.7
scar - see Cicatrix
sigmoid (see also Obstruction, intestine) 560.9
socket, eye 372.64
spine (see also Curvature, spine) 737.9
stomach 536.8
   hourglass 536.8
      congenital 750.7
      psychogenic 306.4
   psychogenic 306.4
tendon (sheath) (see also Short, tendon) 727.81
toe 735.9
ureterovesical orifice (postinfectional) 593.3
urethra 599.84
uterus 621.8
   abnormal 661.9●
      affecting fetus or newborn 763.7
   clonic, hourglass or tetanic 661.4●
      affecting fetus or newborn 763.7
   dyscoordinate 661.4●
      affecting fetus or newborn 763.7
   hourglass 661.4●
      affecting fetus or newborn 763.7

Contraction, contracture, contracted
(Continued)
uterus (Continued)
   hypotonic NEC 661.2●
      affecting fetus or newborn 763.7
   incoordinate 661.4●
      affecting fetus or newborn 763.7
   inefficient or poor 661.2●
      affecting fetus or newborn 763.7
   irregular 661.2●
      affecting fetus or newborn 763.7
   tetanic 661.4●
      affecting fetus or newborn 763.7
vagina (outlet) 623.2
vesical 596.89
   neck or urethral orifice 596.0
visual field, generalized 368.45
Volkmann's (ischemic) 958.6

Contusion (skin surface intact) 924.9
with
   crush injury - see Crush
   dislocation - see Dislocation, by site
   fracture - see Fracture, by site
   internal injury - see also Injury, internal, by site
      heart - see Contusion, cardiac
      kidney - see Contusion, kidney
      liver - see Contusion, liver
      lung - see Contusion, lung
      spleen - see Contusion, spleen
   intracranial injury - see Injury, intracranial
   nerve injury - see Injury, nerve
   open wound - see Wound, open, by site
abdomen, abdominal (muscle) (wall) 922.2
   organ(s) NEC 868.00
adnexa, eye NEC 921.9
ankle 924.21
   with other parts of foot 924.20
arm 923.9
   lower (with elbow) 923.10
   upper 923.03
      with shoulder or axillary region 923.09
auditory canal (external) (meatus) (and other part(s) of neck, scalp, or face, except eye) 920
auricle, ear (and other part(s) of neck, scalp, or face except eye) 920
axilla 923.02
   with shoulder or upper arm 923.09
back 922.31
bone NEC 924.9
brain (cerebral) (membrane) (with hemorrhage) 851.8●

Note: Use the following fifth-digit subclassification with categories 851–854:

0 unspecified state of consciousness
1 with no loss of consciousness
2 with brief [less than one hour] loss of consciousness
3 with moderate [1-24 hours] loss of consciousness
4 with prolonged [more than 24 hours] loss of consciousness and return to pre-existing conscious level
5 with prolonged [more than 24 hours] loss of consciousness, without return to pre-existing conscious level

Use fifth-digit 5 to designate when a patient is unconscious and dies before regaining consciousness, regardless of the duration of the loss of consciousness

6 with loss of consciousness of unspecified duration
9 with concussion, unspecified

with
   open intracranial wound 851.9●
   skull fracture - see Fracture, skull, by site

131

SECTION I INDEX TO DISEASES AND INJURIES / Contusion

Contusion (Continued)
  brain (Continued)
    cerebellum 851.4●
      with open intracranial wound 851.5●
    cortex 851.0●
      with open intracranial wound 851.1●
    occipital lobe 851.4●
      with open intracranial wound 851.5●
    stem 851.4●
      with open intracranial wound 851.5●
  breast 922.0
  brow (and other part(s) of neck, scalp, or face, except eye) 920
  buttock 922.32
  canthus 921.1
  cardiac 861.01
    with open wound into thorax 861.11
  cauda equina (spine) 952.4
  cerebellum - *see* Contusion, brain, cerebellum
  cerebral - *see* Contusion, brain
  cheek(s) (and other part(s) of neck, scalp, or face, except eye) 920
  chest (wall) 922.1
  chin (and other part(s) of neck, scalp, or face, except eye) 920
  clitoris 922.4
  conjunctiva 921.1
  conus medullaris (spine) 952.4
  cornea 921.3
  corpus cavernosum 922.4
  cortex (brain) (cerebral) - *see* Contusion, brain, cortex
  costal region 922.1
  ear (and other part(s) of neck, scalp, or face except eye) 920
  elbow 923.11
    with forearm 923.10
  epididymis 922.4
  epigastric region 922.2
  eye NEC 921.9
  eyeball 921.3
  eyelid(s) (and periocular area) 921.1
  face (and neck, or scalp, any part, except eye) 920
  femoral triangle 922.2
  fetus or newborn 772.6
  finger(s) (nail) (subungual) 923.3
  flank 922.2
  foot (with ankle) (excluding toe(s)) 924.20
  forearm (and elbow) 923.10
  forehead (and other part(s) of neck, scalp, or face, except eye) 920
  genital organs, external 922.4
  globe (eye) 921.3
  groin 922.2
  gum(s) (and other part(s) of neck, scalp, or face, except eye) 920
  hand(s) (except fingers alone) 923.20
  head (any part, except eye) (and face) (and neck) 920
  heart - *see* Contusion, cardiac
  heel 924.20
  hip 924.01
    with thigh 924.00
  iliac region 922.2
  inguinal region 922.2
  internal organs (abdomen, chest, or pelvis) NEC - *see* Injury, internal, by site
  interscapular region 922.33
  iris (eye) 921.3
  kidney 866.01
    with open wound into cavity 866.11
  knee 924.11
    with lower leg 924.10
  labium (majus) (minus) 922.4
  lacrimal apparatus, gland, or sac 921.1
  larynx (and other part(s) of neck, scalp, or face, except eye) 920
  late effect - *see* Late, effects (of), contusion
  leg 924.5
    lower (with knee) 924.10

Contusion (Continued)
  lens 921.3
  lingual (and other part(s) of neck, scalp, or face, except eye) 920
  lip(s) (and other part(s) of neck, scalp, or face, except eye) 920
  liver 864.01
    with
      laceration - *see* Laceration, liver
      open wound into cavity 864.11
  lower extremity 924.5
    multiple sites 924.4
  lumbar region 922.31
  lung 861.21
    with open wound into thorax 861.31
  malar region (and other part(s) of neck, scalp, or face, except eye) 920
  mandibular joint (and other part(s) of neck, scalp, or face, except eye) 920
  mastoid region (and other part(s) of neck, scalp, or face, except eye) 920
  membrane, brain - *see* Contusion, brain
  midthoracic region 922.1
  mouth (and other part(s) of neck, scalp, or face, except eye) 920
  multiple sites (not classifiable to same three-digit category) 924.8
    lower limb 924.4
    trunk 922.8
    upper limb 923.8
  muscle NEC 924.9
  myocardium - *see* Contusion, cardiac
  nasal (septum) (and other part(s) of neck, scalp, or face, except eye) 920
  neck (and scalp, or face, any part, except eye) 920
  nerve - *see* Injury, nerve, by site
  nose (and other part(s) of neck, scalp, or face, except eye) 920
  occipital region (scalp) (and neck or face, except eye) 920
    lobe - *see* Contusion, brain, occipital lobe
  orbit (region) (tissues) 921.2
  palate (soft) (and other part(s) of neck, scalp, or face, except eye) 920
  parietal region (scalp) (and neck, or face, except eye) 920
    lobe - *see* Contusion, brain
  penis 922.4
  pericardium - *see* Contusion, cardiac
  perineum 922.4
  periocular area 921.1
  pharynx (and other part(s) of neck, scalp, or face, except eye) 920
  popliteal space (*see also* Contusion, knee) 924.11
  prepuce 922.4
  pubic region 922.4
  pudenda 922.4
  pulmonary - *see* Contusion, lung
  quadriceps femoralis 924.00
  rib cage 922.1
  sacral region 922.32
  salivary ducts or glands (and other part(s) of neck, scalp, or face, except eye) 920
  scalp (and neck, or face, any part, except eye) 920
  scapular region 923.01
    with shoulder or upper arm 923.09
  sclera (eye) 921.3
  scrotum 922.4
  shoulder 923.00
    with upper arm or axillar regions 923.09
  skin NEC 924.9
  skull 920
  spermatic cord 922.4
  spinal cord - *see also* Injury, spinal, by site
    cauda equina 952.4
    conus medullaris 952.4
  spleen 865.01
    with open wound into cavity 865.11

Contusion (Continued)
  sternal region 922.1
  stomach - *see* Injury, internal, stomach
  subconjunctival 921.1
  subcutaneous NEC 924.9
  submaxillary region (and other part(s) of neck, scalp, or face, except eye) 920
  submental region (and other part(s) of neck, scalp, or face, except eye) 920
  subperiosteal NEC 924.9
  supraclavicular fossa (and other part(s) of neck, scalp, or face, except eye) 920
  supraorbital (and other part(s) of neck, scalp, or face, except eye) 920
  temple (region) (and other part(s) of neck, scalp, or face, except eye) 920
  testis 922.4
  thigh (and hip) 924.00
  thorax 922.1
    organ - *see* Injury, internal, intrathoracic
  throat (and other part(s) of neck, scalp, or face, except eye) 920
  thumb(s) (nail) (subungual) 923.3
  toe(s) (nail) (subungual) 924.3
  tongue (and other part(s) of neck, scalp, or face, except eye) 920
  trunk 922.9
    multiple sites 922.8
    specified site - *see* Contusion, by site
  tunica vaginalis 922.4
  tympanum (membrane) (and other part(s) of neck, scalp, or face, except eye) 920
  upper extremity 923.9
    multiple sites 923.8
  uvula (and other part(s) of neck, scalp, or face, except eye) 920
  vagina 922.4
  vocal cord(s) (and other part(s) of neck, scalp, or face, except eye) 920
  vulva 922.4
  wrist 923.21
    with hand(s), except finger(s) alone 923.20

Conus (any type) (congenital) 743.57
  acquired 371.60
  medullaris syndrome 336.8

Convalescence (following) V66.9
  chemotherapy V66.2
  medical NEC V66.5
  psychotherapy V66.3
  radiotherapy V66.1
  surgery NEC V66.0
  treatment (for) NEC V66.5
    combined V66.6
    fracture V66.4
    mental disorder NEC V66.3
    specified disorder NEC V66.5

Conversion
  closed surgical procedure to open procedure
    arthroscopic V64.43
    laparoscopic V64.41
    thoracoscopic V64.42
  hysteria, hysterical, any type 300.11
  neurosis, any 300.11
  reaction, any 300.11

Converter, tuberculosis (test reaction) 795.51

Convulsions (idiopathic) 780.39
  apoplectiform (*see also* Disease, cerebrovascular, acute) 436
  brain 780.39
  cerebral 780.39
  cerebrospinal 780.39
  due to trauma NEC - *see* Injury, intracranial
  eclamptic (*see also* Eclampsia) 780.39
  epileptic (*see also* Epilepsy) 345.9●
  epileptiform (*see also* Seizure, epileptiform) 780.39
  epileptoid (*see also* Seizure, epileptiform) 780.39

Convulsions (Continued)
  ether
    anesthetic
      correct substance properly administered 780.39
      overdose or wrong substance given 968.2
    other specified type - see Table of Drugs and Chemicals
  febrile (simple) 780.31
    complex 780.32
  generalized 780.39
  hysterical 300.11
  infantile 780.39
    epilepsy - see Epilepsy
  internal 780.39
  jacksonian (see also Epilepsy) 345.5 ●
  myoclonic 333.2
  newborn 779.0
  paretic 094.1
  pregnancy (nephritic) (uremic) - see Eclampsia, pregnancy
  psychomotor (see also Epilepsy) 345.4 ●
  puerperal, postpartum - see Eclampsia, pregnancy
  recurrent 780.39
    epileptic - see Epilepsy
  reflex 781.0
  repetitive 780.39
    epileptic - see Epilepsy
  salaam (see also Epilepsy) 345.6 ●
  scarlatinal 034.1
  spasmodic 780.39
  tetanus, tetanic (see also Tetanus) 037
  thymic 254.8
  uncinate 780.39
  uremic 586
Convulsive - see also Convulsions
  disorder or state 780.39
    epileptic - see Epilepsy
  equivalent, abdominal (see also Epilepsy) 345.5 ●
Cooke-Apert-Gallais syndrome (adrenogenital) 255.2
Cooley's anemia (erythroblastic) 282.44
Coolie itch 126.9
Cooper's
  disease 610.1
  hernia - see Hernia, Cooper's
Coordination disturbance 781.3
Copper wire arteries, retina 362.13
Copra itch 133.8
Coprolith 560.39
Coprophilia 302.89
Coproporphyria, hereditary 277.1
Coprostasis 560.32
  with hernia - see also Hernia, by site, with obstruction
    gangrenous - see Hernia, by site, with gangrene
Cor
  biloculare 745.7
  bovinum - see Hypertrophy, cardiac
  bovis - see also Hypertrophy, cardiac
  pulmonale (chronic) 416.9
    acute 415.0
  triatriatum, triatrium 746.82
  triloculare 745.8
    biatriatum 745.3
    biventriculare 745.69
Corbus' disease 607.1
Cord - see also condition
  around neck (tightly) (with compression)
    affecting fetus or newborn 762.5
    complicating delivery 663.1 ●
      without compression 663.3 ●
        affecting fetus or newborn 762.6
  bladder NEC 344.61
    tabetic 094.0

Cord (Continued)
  prolapse
    affecting fetus or newborn 762.4
    complicating delivery 663.0 ●
Cord's angiopathy (see also Tuberculosis) 017.3 ● [362.18]
Cordis ectopia 746.87
Corditis (spermatic) 608.4
Corectopia 743.46
Cori type glycogen storage disease - see Disease, glycogen storage
Cork-handlers' disease or lung 495.3
Corkscrew esophagus 530.5
Corlett's pyosis (impetigo) 684
Corn (infected) 700
Cornea - see also condition
  donor V59.5
  guttata (dystrophy) 371.57
  plana 743.41
Cornelia de Lange's syndrome (Amsterdam dwarf, intellectual disabilities, and brachycephaly) 759.89
Cornual gestation or pregnancy - see Pregnancy, cornual
Cornu cutaneum 702.8
Coronary (artery) - see also condition
  arising from aorta or pulmonary trunk 746.85
Corpora - see also condition
  amylacea (prostate) 602.8
  cavernosa - see condition
Corpulence (see also Obesity)
Corpus - see condition
Corrigan's disease - see Insufficiency, aortic
Corrosive burn - see Burn, by site
Corsican fever (see also Malaria) 084.6
Cortical - see also condition
  blindness 377.75
  necrosis, kidney (bilateral) 583.6
Corticoadrenal - see condition
Corticosexual syndrome 255.2
Coryza (acute) 460
  with grippe or influenza (see also Influenza) 487.1
  syphilitic 095.8
    congenital (chronic) 090.0
Costen's syndrome or complex 524.60
Costiveness (see also Constipation) 564.00
Costochondritis 733.6
Cotard's syndrome (paranoia) 297.1
Cot death 798.0
Cotia virus 059.8
Cotungo's disease 724.3
Cough 786.2
  with hemorrhage (see also Hemoptysis) 786.39
  affected 786.2
  bronchial 786.2
    with grippe or influenza (see also Influenza) 487.1
  chronic 786.2
  epidemic 786.2
  functional 306.1
  hemorrhagic 786.39
  hysterical 300.11
  laryngeal, spasmodic 786.2
  nervous 786.2
  psychogenic 306.1
  smokers' 491.0
  tea tasters' 112.89
Counseling NEC V65.40
  without complaint or sickness V65.49
  abuse victim NEC V62.89
    child V61.21
    partner V61.11
    spouse V61.11
  child abuse, maltreatment, or neglect V61.21

Counseling NEC (Continued)
  contraceptive NEC V25.09
    device (intrauterine) V25.02
    maintenance V25.40
      intrauterine contraceptive device V25.42
      oral contraceptive (pill) V25.41
      specified type NEC V25.49
      subdermal implantable V25.43
    management NEC V25.9
    oral contraceptive (pill) V25.01
      emergency V25.03
      postcoital V25.03
    prescription NEC V25.02
      oral contraceptive (pill) V25.01
        emergency V25.03
        postcoital V25.03
      repeat prescription V25.41
    repeat prescription V25.40
    subdermal implantable V25.43
    surveillance NEC V25.40
  dietary V65.3
  exercise V65.41
  expectant parent(s)
    pediatric pre-adoption visit V65.11
    pediatric pre-birth visit V65.11
  explanation of
    investigation finding NEC V65.49
    medication NEC V65.49
  family planning V25.09
    natural
      procreative V26.41
      to avoid pregnancy V25.04
  for nonattending third party V65.19
  genetic V26.33
  gonorrhea V65.45
  health (advice) (education) (instruction) NEC V65.49
  HIV V65.44
  human immunodeficiency virus V65.44
  injury prevention V65.43
  insulin pump training V65.46
  marital V61.10
  medical (for) V65.9
    boarding school resident V60.6
    condition not demonstrated V65.5
    feared complaint and no disease found V65.5
    institutional resident V60.6
    on behalf of another V65.19
    person living alone V60.3
  natural family planning
    procreative V26.41
    to avoid pregnancy V25.04
  parent (guardian)-child conflict V61.20
    adopted child V61.24
    biological child V61.23
    foster child V61.25
    specified problem NEC V61.29
  partner abuse
    perpetrator V61.12
    victim V61.11
  pediatric
    pre-adoption visit for adoptive parent(s) V65.11
    pre-birth visit for expectant parents V65.11
  perpetrator of
    child abuse V62.83
      parental V61.22
    partner abuse V61.12
    spouse abuse V61.12
  procreative V65.49
  sex NEC V65.49
    transmitted disease NEC V65.45
    HIV V65.44
  specified reason NEC V65.49
  spousal abuse
    perpetrator V61.12
    victim V61.11
  substance use and abuse V65.42
  syphilis V65.45

SECTION I INDEX TO DISEASES AND INJURIES / Counseling NEC

Counseling NEC (Continued)
  victim (of)
    abuse NEC V62.89
    child abuse V61.21
    partner abuse V61.11
    spousal abuse V61.11
Coupled rhythm 427.89
Couvelaire uterus (complicating delivery) - *see* Placenta, separation
Cowper's gland - *see* condition
Cowperitis (*see also* Urethritis) 597.89
  gonorrheal (acute) 098.0
    chronic or duration of 2 months or over 098.2
Cowpox (abortive) 051.01
  due to vaccination 999.0
  eyelid 051.01 [373.5]
    postvaccination 999.0 [373.5]
Coxa
  plana 732.1
  valga (acquired) 736.31
    congenital 755.61
    late effect of rickets 268.1
  vara (acquired) 736.32
    congenital 755.62
    late effect of rickets 268.1
Coxae malum senilis 715.25
Coxalgia (nontuberculous) 719.45
  tuberculous (*see also* Tuberculosis) 015.1● [730.85]
Coxalgic pelvis 736.30
Coxitis 716.65
Coxsackie (infection) (virus) 079.2
  central nervous system NEC 048
  endocarditis 074.22
  enteritis 008.67
  meningitis (aseptic) 047.0
  myocarditis 074.23
  pericarditis 074.21
  pharyngitis 074.0
  pleurodynia 074.1
  specific disease NEC 074.8
Crabs, meaning pubic lice 132.2
Crack baby 760.75
Cracked
  nipple 611.2
    puerperal, postpartum 676.1●
  tooth 521.81
Cradle cap 690.11
Craft neurosis 300.89
Craigiasis 007.8
Cramp(s) 729.82
  abdominal 789.0●
  bathing 994.1
  colic 789.7
    infantile 789.7
    psychogenic 306.4
  due to immersion 994.1
  extremity (lower) (upper) NEC 729.82
  fireman 992.2
  heat 992.2
  hysterical 300.11
  immersion 994.1
  intestinal 789.0●
    psychogenic 306.4
  linotypist's 300.89
    organic 333.84
  muscle (extremity) (general) 729.82
    due to immersion 994.1
    hysterical 300.11
  occupational (hand) 300.89
    organic 333.84
  psychogenic 307.89
  salt depletion 276.1
  sleep related leg 327.52
  stoker 992.2
  stomach 789.0●
  telegraphers' 300.89
    organic 333.84
  typists' 300.89
    organic 333.84

Cramp(s) (Continued)
  uterus 625.8
    menstrual 625.3
  writers' 333.84
    organic 333.84
    psychogenic 300.89
Cranial - *see* condition
Cranioclasis, fetal 763.89
Craniocleidodysostosis 755.59
Craniofenestria (skull) 756.0
Craniolacunia (skull) 756.0
Craniopagus 759.4
Craniopathy, metabolic 733.3
Craniopharyngeal - *see* condition
Craniopharyngioma (M9350/1) 237.0
Craniorachischisis (totalis) 740.1
Cranioschisis 756.0
Craniostenosis 756.0
Craniosynostosis 756.0
Craniotabes (cause unknown) 733.3
  rachitic 268.1
  syphilitic 090.5
Craniotomy, fetal 763.89
Cranium - *see* condition
Craw-craw 125.3
CRBSI (catheter-related bloodstream infection) 999.31
Creaking joint 719.60
  ankle 719.67
  elbow 719.62
  foot 719.67
  hand 719.64
  hip 719.65
  knee 719.66
  multiple sites 719.69
  pelvic region 719.65
  shoulder (region) 719.61
  specified site NEC 719.68
  wrist 719.63
Creeping
  eruption 126.9
  palsy 335.21
  paralysis 335.21
Crenated tongue 529.8
Creotoxism 005.9
Crepitus
  caput 756.0
  joint 719.60
    ankle 719.67
    elbow 719.62
    foot 719.67
    hand 719.64
    hip 719.65
    knee 719.66
    multiple sites 719.69
    pelvic region 719.65
    shoulder (region) 719.61
    specified site NEC 719.68
    wrist 719.63
Crescent or conus choroid, congenital 743.57
Cretin, cretinism (athyrotic) (congenital) (endemic) (metabolic) (nongoitrous) (sporadic) 243
  goitrous (sporadic) 246.1
  pelvis (dwarf type) (male type) 243
    with disproportion (fetopelvic) 653.1●
      affecting fetus or newborn 763.1
    causing obstructed labor 660.1●
      affecting fetus or newborn 763.1
  pituitary 253.3
Cretinoid degeneration 243
Creutzfeldt-Jakob disease (CJD) (syndrome) 046.19
  with dementia
    with behavioral disturbance 046.19 [294.11]
    without behavioral disturbance 046.19 [294.10]
  familial 046.19
  iatrogenic 046.19
  specified NEC 046.19

Creutzfeldt-Jakob disease (Continued)
  sporadic 046.19
  variant (vCJD) 046.11
    with dementia
      with behavioral disturbance 046.11 [294.11]
      without behavioral disturbance 046.11 [294.10]
Crib death 798.0
Cribriform hymen 752.49
Cri-du-chat syndrome 758.31
Crigler-Najjar disease or syndrome (congenital hyperbilirubinemia) 277.4
Crimean hemorrhagic fever 065.0
Criminalism 301.7
Crisis
  abdomen 789.0●
  addisonian (acute adrenocortical insufficiency) 255.41
  adrenal (cortical) 255.41
  asthmatic - *see* Asthma
  brain, cerebral (*see also* Disease, cerebrovascular, acute) 436
  celiac 579.0
  Dietl's 593.4
  emotional NEC 309.29
    acute reaction to stress 308.0
    adjustment reaction 309.9
    specific to childhood or adolescence 313.9
  gastric (tabetic) 094.0
  glaucomatocyclitic 364.22
  heart (*see also* Failure, heart) 428.9
  hypertensive - *see* Hypertension
  nitritoid
    correct substance properly administered 458.29
    overdose or wrong substance given or taken 961.1
  oculogyric 378.87
    psychogenic 306.7
  Pel's 094.0
  psychosexual identity 302.6
  rectum 094.0
  renal 593.81
  sickle cell 282.62
  stomach (tabetic) 094.0
  tabetic 094.0
  thyroid (*see also* Thyrotoxicosis) 242.9●
  thyrotoxic (*see also* Thyrotoxicosis) 242.9●
  vascular - *see* Disease, cerebrovascular, acute
Crocq's disease (acrocyanosis) 443.89
Crohn's disease (*see also* Enteritis, regional) 555.9
Cronkhite-Canada syndrome 211.3
Crooked septum, nasal 470
Cross
  birth (of fetus) complicating delivery 652.3●
    with successful version 652.1●
    causing obstructed labor 660.0●
  bite, anterior or posterior 524.27
  eye (*see also* Esotropia) 378.00
Crossed ectopia of kidney 753.3
Crossfoot 754.50
Croup, croupous (acute) (angina) (catarrhal) (infective) (inflammatory) (laryngeal) (membranous) (nondiphtheritic) (pseudomembranous) 464.4
  asthmatic (*see also* Asthma) 493.9●
  bronchial 466.0
  diphtheritic (membranous) 032.3
  false 478.75
  spasmodic 478.75
    diphtheritic 032.3
  stridulous 478.75
    diphtheritic 032.3
Crouzon's disease (craniofacial dysostosis) 756.0
Crowding, teeth 524.31
CRST syndrome (cutaneous systemic sclerosis) 710.1
Cruchet's disease (encephalitis lethargica) 049.8

Cruelty in children (see also Disturbance, conduct) 312.9
Crural ulcer (see also Ulcer, lower extremity) 707.10
Crush, crushed, crushing (injury) 929.9
　abdomen 926.19
　　internal - see Injury, internal, abdomen
　ankle 928.21
　　with other parts of foot 928.20
　arm 927.9
　　lower (and elbow) 927.10
　　upper 927.03
　　　with shoulder or axillary region 927.09
　axilla 927.02
　　with shoulder or upper arm 927.09
　back 926.11
　breast 926.19
　buttock 926.12
　cheek 925.1
　chest - see Injury, internal, chest
　ear 925.1
　elbow 927.11
　　with forearm 927.10
　face 925.1
　finger(s) 927.3
　　with hand(s) 927.20
　　　and wrist(s) 927.21
　flank 926.19
　foot, excluding toe(s) alone (with ankle) 928.20
　forearm (and elbow) 927.10
　genitalia, external (female) (male) 926.0
　　internal - see Injury, internal, genital organ NEC
　hand, except finger(s) alone (and wrist) 927.20
　head - see Fracture, skull, by site
　heel 928.20
　hip 928.01
　　with thigh 928.00
　internal organ (abdomen, chest, or pelvis) - see Injury, internal, by site
　knee 928.11
　　with leg, lower 928.10
　labium (majus) (minus) 926.0
　larynx 925.2
　late effect - see Late, effects (of), crushing
　leg 928.9
　　lower 928.10
　　　and knee 928.11
　　upper 928.00
　limb
　　lower 928.9
　　　multiple sites 928.8
　　upper 927.9
　　　multiple sites 927.8
　multiple sites NEC 929.0
　neck 925.2
　nerve - see Injury, nerve, by site
　nose 802.0
　　open 802.1
　penis 926.0
　pharynx 925.2
　scalp 925.1
　scapular region 927.01
　　with shoulder or upper arm 927.09
　scrotum 926.0
　shoulder 927.00
　　with upper arm or axillary region 927.09
　skull or cranium - see Fracture, skull, by site
　spinal cord - see Injury, spinal, by site
　syndrome (complication of trauma) 958.5
　testis 926.0
　thigh (with hip) 928.00
　throat 925.2
　thumb(s) (and fingers) 927.3
　toe(s) 928.3
　　with foot 928.20
　　　and ankle 928.21
　tonsil 925.2

Crush, crushed, crushing (Continued)
　trunk 926.9
　　chest - see Injury, internal, intrathoracic organs NEC
　　internal organ - see Injury, internal, by site
　　multiple sites 926.8
　　specified site NEC 926.19
　vulva 926.0
　wrist 927.21
　　with hand(s), except fingers alone 927.20
Crusta lactea 690.11
Crusts 782.8
Crutch paralysis 953.4
Cruveilhier's disease 335.21
Cruveilhier-Baumgarten cirrhosis, disease, or syndrome 571.5
Cruz-Chagas disease (see also Trypanosomiasis) 086.2
Crying
　constant, continuous
　　adolescent 780.95
　　adult 780.95
　　baby 780.92
　　child 780.95
　　infant 780.92
　　newborn 780.92
　excessive
　　adolescent 780.95
　　adult 780.95
　　baby 780.92
　　child 780.95
　　infant 780.92
　　newborn 780.92
Cryofibrinogenemia 273.2
Cryoglobulinemia (mixed) 273.2
Crypt (anal) (rectal) 569.49
Cryptitis (anal) (rectal) 569.49
Cryptococcosis (European) (pulmonary) (systemic) 117.5
Cryptococcus 117.5
　epidermicus 117.5
　neoformans, infection by 117.5
Cryptopapillitis (anus) 569.49
Cryptophthalmos (eyelid) 743.06
Cryptorchid, cryptorchism, cryptorchidism 752.51
Cryptosporidiosis 007.4
　hepatobiliary 136.8
　respiratory 136.8
Cryptotia 744.29
Crystallopathy
　calcium pyrophosphate (see also Arthritis) 275.49 [712.2] ●
　dicalcium phosphate (see also Arthritis) 275.49 [712.1] ●
　gouty 274.00
　pyrophosphate NEC (see also Arthritis) 275.49 [712.2] ●
　uric acid 274.00
Crystalluria 791.9
Csillag's disease (lichen sclerosus et atrophicus) 701.0
Cuban itch 050.1
Cubitus
　valgus (acquired) 736.01
　　congenital 755.59
　　late effect of rickets 268.1
　varus (acquired) 736.02
　　congenital 755.59
　　late effect of rickets 268.1
Cultural deprivation V62.4
Cupping of optic disc 377.14
Curling's ulcer - see Ulcer, duodenum
Curling esophagus 530.5
Curschmann (-Batten) (-Steinert) disease or syndrome 359.21
Curvature
　organ or site, congenital NEC - see Distortion
　penis (lateral) 752.69
　Pott's (spinal) (see also Tuberculosis) 015.0 ● [737.43]

Curvature (Continued)
　radius, idiopathic, progressive (congenital) 755.54
　spine (acquired) (angular) (idiopathic) (incorrect) (postural) 737.9
　　congenital 754.2
　　due to or associated with
　　　Charcôt-Marie-Tooth disease 356.1 [737.40]
　　　mucopolysaccharidosis 277.5 [737.40]
　　　neurofibromatosis 237.71 [737.40]
　　　osteitis
　　　　deformans 731.0 [737.40]
　　　　fibrosa cystica 252.01 [737.40]
　　　osteoporosis (see also Osteoporosis) 733.00 [737.40]
　　　poliomyelitis (see also Poliomyelitis) 138 [737.40]
　　　tuberculosis (Pott's curvature) (see also Tuberculosis) 015.0 ● [737.43]
　　kyphoscoliotic (see also Kyphoscoliosis) 737.30
　　kyphotic (see also Kyphosis) 737.10
　　late effect of rickets 268.1 [737.40]
　　Pott's 015.0 ● [737.40]
　　scoliotic (see also Scoliosis) 737.30
　　specified NEC 737.8
　　tuberculous 015.0 ● [737.40]
Cushing's
　basophilism, disease, or syndrome (iatrogenic) (idiopathic) (pituitary basophilism) (pituitary dependent) 255.0
　ulcer - see Ulcer, peptic
Cushingoid due to steroid therapy
　correct substance properly administered 255.0
　overdose or wrong substance given or taken 962.0
Cut (external) - see Wound, open, by site
Cutaneous - see also condition
　hemorrhage 782.7
　horn (cheek) (eyelid) (mouth) 702.8
　larva migrans 126.9
Cutis - see also condition
　hyperelastic 756.83
　　acquired 701.8
　laxa 756.83
　　senilis 701.8
　marmorata 782.61
　osteosis 709.3
　pendula 756.83
　　acquired 701.8
　rhomboidalis nuchae 701.8
　verticis gyrata 757.39
　　acquired 701.8
Cyanopathy, newborn 770.83
Cyanosis 782.5
　autotoxic 289.7
　common atrioventricular canal 745.69
　congenital 770.83
　conjunctiva 372.71
　due to
　　endocardial cushion defect 745.60
　　nonclosure, foramen botalli 745.5
　　patent foramen botalli 745.5
　　persistent foramen ovale 745.5
　enterogenous 289.7
　fetus or newborn 770.83
　ostium primum defect 745.61
　paroxysmal digital 443.0
　retina, retinal 362.10
Cycle
　anovulatory 628.0
　menstrual, irregular 626.4
Cyclencephaly 759.89
Cyclical vomiting 536.2
　associated with migraine 346.2 ●
　psychogenic 306.4
Cyclitic membrane 364.74

SECTION I INDEX TO DISEASES AND INJURIES / Cyclitis

Cyclitis (see also Iridocyclitis) 364.3
   acute 364.00
      primary 364.01
      recurrent 364.02
   chronic 364.10
      in
         sarcoidosis 135 [364.11]
         tuberculosis (see also Tuberculosis)
            017.3● [364.11]
   Fuchs' heterochromic 364.21
   granulomatous 364.10
   lens induced 364.23
   nongranulomatous 364.00
   posterior 363.21
   primary 364.01
   recurrent 364.02
   secondary (noninfectious) 364.04
      infectious 364.03
   subacute 364.00
      primary 364.01
      recurrent 364.02
Cyclokeratitis - see Keratitis
Cyclophoria 378.44
Cyclopia, cyclops 759.89
Cycloplegia 367.51
Cyclospasm 367.53
Cyclosporiasis 007.5
Cyclothymia 301.13
Cyclothymic personality 301.13
Cyclotropia 378.33
Cyesis - see Pregnancy
Cylindroma (M8200/3) - see also Neoplasm, by site, malignant
   eccrine dermal (M8200/0) - see Neoplasm, skin, benign
   skin (M8200/0) - see Neoplasm, skin, benign
Cylindruria 791.7
Cyllosoma 759.89
Cynanche
   diphtheritic 032.3
   tonsillaris 475
Cynorexia 783.6
Cyphosis - see Kyphosis
Cyprus fever (see also Brucellosis) 023.9
Cyriax's syndrome (slipping rib) 733.99
Cyst (mucus) (retention) (serous) (simple)

> Note: In general, cysts are not neoplastic and are classified to the appropriate category for disease of the specified anatomical site. This generalization does not apply to certain types of cysts which are neoplastic in nature, for example, dermoid, nor does it apply to cysts of certain structures, for example, branchial cleft, which are classified as developmental anomalies.
>
> The following listing includes some of the most frequently reported sites of cysts as well as qualifiers which indicate the type of cyst. The latter qualifiers usually are not repeated under the anatomical sites. Since the code assignment for a given site may vary depending upon the type of cyst, the coder should refer to the listings under the specified type of cyst before consideration is given to the site.

   accessory, fallopian tube 752.11
   adenoid (infected) 474.8
   adrenal gland 255.8
      congenital 759.1
   air, lung 518.89
   allantoic 753.7
   alveolar process (jaw bone) 526.2
   amnion, amniotic 658.8●
   anterior chamber (eye) 364.60
      exudative 364.62
      implantation (surgical) (traumatic) 364.61
      parasitic 360.13
   anterior nasopalatine 526.1
   antrum 478.19

Cyst (Continued)
   anus 569.49
   apical (periodontal) (tooth) 522.8
   appendix 543.9
   arachnoid, brain 348.0
   arytenoid 478.79
   auricle 706.2
   Baker's (knee) 727.51
      tuberculous (see also Tuberculosis) 015.2●
   Bartholin's gland or duct 616.2
   bile duct (see also Disease, biliary) 576.8
   bladder (multiple) (trigone) 596.89
   Blessig's 362.62
   blood, endocardial (see also Endocarditis) 424.90
   blue dome 610.0
   bone (local) 733.20
      aneurysmal 733.22
      jaw 526.2
         developmental (odontogenic) 526.0
         fissural 526.1
         latent 526.89
      solitary 733.21
      unicameral 733.21
   brain 348.0
      congenital 742.4
      hydatid (see also Echinococcus) 122.9
      third ventricle (colloid) 742.4
   branchial (cleft) 744.42
   branchiogenic 744.42
   breast (benign) (blue dome) (pedunculated) (solitary) (traumatic) 610.0
      involution 610.4
      sebaceous 610.8
   broad ligament (benign) 620.8
      embryonic 752.11
   bronchogenic (mediastinal) (sequestration) 518.89
      congenital 748.4
   buccal 528.4
   bulbourethral gland (Cowper's) 599.89
   bursa, bursal 727.49
      pharyngeal 478.26
   calcifying odontogenic (M9301/0) 213.1
      upper jaw (bone) 213.0
   canal of Nuck (acquired) (serous) 629.1
      congenital 752.41
   canthus 372.75
   carcinomatous (M8010/3) - see Neoplasm, by site, malignant
   cartilage (joint) - see Derangement, joint
   cauda equina 336.8
   cavum septi pellucidi NEC 348.0
   celomic (pericardium) 746.89
   cerebellopontine (angle) - see Cyst, brain
   cerebellum - see Cyst, brain
   cerebral - see Cyst, brain
   cervical lateral 744.42
   cervix 622.8
      embryonal 752.41
      nabothian (gland) 616.0
   chamber, anterior (eye) 364.60
      exudative 364.62
      implantation (surgical) (traumatic) 364.61
      parasitic 360.13
   chiasmal, optic NEC (see also Lesion, chiasmal) 377.54
   chocolate (ovary) 617.1
   choledochal (congenital) 751.69
      acquired 576.8
   choledochus 751.69
   chorion 658.8●
   choroid plexus 348.0
   chyle, mesentery 457.8
   ciliary body 364.60
      exudative 364.64
      implantation 364.61
      primary 364.63
   clitoris 624.8
   coccyx (see also Cyst, bone) 733.20

Cyst (Continued)
   colloid
      third ventricle (brain) 742.4
      thyroid gland - see Goiter
   colon 569.89
   common (bile) duct (see also Disease, biliary) 576.8
   congenital NEC 759.89
      adrenal glands 759.1
      epiglottis 748.3
      esophagus 750.4
      fallopian tube 752.11
      kidney 753.10
         multiple 753.19
         single 753.11
      larynx 748.3
      liver 751.62
      lung 748.4
      mediastinum 748.8
      ovary 752.0
      oviduct 752.11
      pancreas 751.7
      periurethral (tissue) 753.8
      prepuce NEC 752.69
         penis 752.69
      sublingual 750.26
      submaxillary gland 750.26
      thymus (gland) 759.2
      tongue 750.19
      ureterovesical orifice 753.4
      vulva 752.41
   conjunctiva 372.75
   cornea 371.23
   corpora quadrigemina 348.0
   corpus
      albicans (ovary) 620.2
      luteum (ruptured) 620.1
   Cowper's gland (benign) (infected) 599.89
   cranial meninges 348.0
   craniobuccal pouch 253.8
   craniopharyngeal pouch 253.8
   cystic duct (see also Disease, gallbladder) 575.8
   Cysticercus (any site) 123.1
   Dandy-Walker 742.3
      with spina bifida (see also Spina bifida) 741.0●
   dental 522.8
      developmental 526.0
      eruption 526.0
      lateral periodontal 526.0
      primordial (keratocyst) 526.0
      root 522.8
   dentigerous 526.0
      mandible 526.0
      maxilla 526.0
   dermoid (M9084/0) - see also Neoplasm, by site, benign
      with malignant transformation (M9084/3) 183.0
      implantation
         external area or site (skin) NEC 709.8
         iris 364.61
         skin 709.8
         vagina 623.8
         vulva 624.8
      mouth 528.4
      oral soft tissue 528.4
      sacrococcygeal 685.1
         with abscess 685.0
   developmental of ovary, ovarian 752.0
   dura (cerebral) 348.0
      spinal 349.2
   ear (external) 706.2
   echinococcal (see also Echinococcus) 122.9
   embryonal
      cervix uteri 752.41
      genitalia, female external 752.41
      uterus 752.39
      vagina 752.41

Cyst *(Continued)*
- endometrial 621.8
  - ectopic 617.9
- endometrium (uterus) 621.8
  - ectopic - *see* Endometriosis
- enteric 751.5
- enterogenous 751.5
- epidermal (inclusion) (*see also* Cyst, skin) 706.2
- epidermoid (inclusion) (*see also* Cyst, skin) 706.2
  - mouth 528.4
  - not of skin - *see* Cyst, by site
  - oral soft tissue 528.4
- epididymis 608.89
- epiglottis 478.79
- epiphysis cerebri 259.8
- epithelial (inclusion) (*see also* Cyst, skin) 706.2
- epoophoron 752.11
- eruption 526.0
- esophagus 530.89
- ethmoid sinus 478.19
- eye (retention) 379.8
  - congenital 743.03
  - posterior segment, congenital 743.54
- eyebrow 706.2
- eyelid (sebaceous) 374.84
  - infected 373.13
  - sweat glands or ducts 374.84
- falciform ligament (inflammatory) 573.8
- fallopian tube 620.8
  - congenital 752.11
- female genital organs NEC 629.89
- fimbrial (congenital) 752.11
- fissural (oral region) 526.1
- follicle (atretic) (graafian) (ovarian) 620.0
  - nabothian (gland) 616.0
- follicular (atretic) (ovarian) 620.0
  - dentigerous 526.0
- frontal sinus 478.19
- gallbladder or duct 575.8
- ganglion 727.43
- Gartner's duct 752.41
- gas, of mesentery 568.89
- gingiva 523.8
- gland of moll 374.84
- globulomaxillary 526.1
- graafian follicle 620.0
- granulosal lutein 620.2
- hemangiomatous (M9121/0) (*see also* Hemangioma) 228.00
- hydatid (*see also* Echinococcus) 122.9
  - fallopian tube (Morgagni) 752.11
  - liver NEC 122.8
  - lung NEC 122.9
  - Morgagni 752.89
    - fallopian tube 752.11
  - specified site NEC 122.9
- hymen 623.8
  - embryonal 752.41
- hypopharynx 478.26
- hypophysis, hypophyseal (duct) (recurrent) 253.8
  - cerebri 253.8
- implantation (dermoid)
  - anterior chamber (eye) 364.61
  - external area or site (skin) NEC 709.8
  - iris 364.61
  - vagina 623.8
  - vulva 624.8
- incisor, incisive canal 526.1
- inclusion (epidermal) (epithelial) (epidermoid) (mucous) (squamous) (*see also* Cyst, skin) 706.2
  - not of skin - *see* Neoplasm, by site, benign
- intestine (large) (small) 569.89
- intracranial - *see* Cyst, brain
- intraligamentous 728.89
  - knee 717.89
- intrasellar 253.8

Cyst *(Continued)*
- iris (idiopathic) 364.60
  - exudative 364.62
  - implantation (surgical) (traumatic) 364.61
  - miotic pupillary 364.55
  - parasitic 360.13
- Iwanoff's 362.62
- jaw (bone) (aneurysmal) (extravasation) (hemorrhagic) (traumatic) 526.2
  - developmental (odontogenic) 526.0
  - fissural 526.1
- keratin 706.2
- kidney (congenital) 753.10
  - acquired 593.2
  - calyceal (*see also* Hydronephrosis) 591
  - multiple 753.19
  - pyelogenic (*see also* Hydronephrosis) 591
  - simple 593.2
  - single 753.11
  - solitary (not congenital) 593.2
- labium (majus) (minus) 624.8
  - sebaceous 624.8
- lacrimal
  - apparatus 375.43
  - gland or sac 375.12
- larynx 478.79
- lens 379.39
  - congenital 743.39
- lip (gland) 528.5
- liver 573.8
  - congenital 751.62
  - hydatid (*see also* Echinococcus) 122.8
    - granulosis 122.0
    - multilocularis 122.5
- lung 518.89
  - congenital 748.4
  - giant bullous 492.0
- lutein 620.1
- lymphangiomatous (M9173/0) 228.1
- lymphoepithelial
  - mouth 528.4
  - oral soft tissue 528.4
- macula 362.54
- malignant (M8000/3) - *see* Neoplasm, by site, malignant
- mammary gland (sweat gland) (*see also* Cyst, breast) 610.0
- mandible 526.2
  - dentigerous 526.0
  - radicular 522.8
- maxilla 526.2
  - dentigerous 526.0
  - radicular 522.8
- median
  - anterior maxillary 526.1
  - palatal 526.1
- mediastinum (congenital) 748.8
- meibomian (gland) (retention) 373.2
  - infected 373.12
- membrane, brain 348.0
- meninges (cerebral) 348.0
  - spinal 349.2
- meniscus knee 717.5
- mesentery, mesenteric (gas) 568.89
  - chyle 457.8
  - gas 568.89
- mesonephric duct 752.89
- mesothelial
  - peritoneum 568.89
  - pleura (peritoneal) 568.89
- milk 611.5
- miotic pupillary (iris) 364.55
- Morgagni (hydatid) 752.89
  - fallopian tube 752.11
- mouth 528.4
- Müllerian duct 752.89
  - appendix testis 608.89
  - cervix (embryonal) 752.41
  - fallopian tube 752.11
  - prostatic utricle 599.89
  - vagina (embryonal) 752.41

Cyst *(Continued)*
- multilocular (ovary) (M8000/1) 239.5
- myometrium 621.8
- nabothian (follicle) (ruptured) 616.0
- nasal sinus 478.19
- nasoalveolar 528.4
- nasolabial 528.4
- nasopalatine (duct) 526.1
  - anterior 526.1
- nasopharynx 478.26
- neoplastic (M8000/1) - *see also* Neoplasm, by site, unspecified nature
  - benign (M8000/0) - *see* Neoplasm, by site, benign
  - uterus 621.8
- nervous system - *see* Cyst, brain
- neuroenteric 742.59
- neuroepithelial ventricle 348.0
- nipple 610.0
- nose 478.19
  - skin of 706.2
- odontogenic, developmental 526.0
- omentum (lesser) 568.89
  - congenital 751.8
- oral soft tissue (dermoid) (epidermoid) (lymphoepithelial) 528.4
- ora serrata 361.19
- orbit 376.81
- ovary, ovarian (twisted) 620.2
  - adherent 620.2
  - chocolate 617.1
  - corpus
    - albicans 620.2
    - luteum 620.1
  - dermoid (M9084/0) 220
  - developmental 752.0
  - due to failure of involution NEC 620.2
  - endometrial 617.1
  - follicular (atretic) (graafian) (hemorrhagic) 620.0
  - hemorrhagic 620.2
  - in pregnancy or childbirth 654.4
    - affecting fetus or newborn 763.89
    - causing obstructed labor 660.2
      - affecting fetus or newborn 763.1
  - multilocular (M8000/1) 239.5
  - pseudomucinous (M8470/0) 220
  - retention 620.2
  - serous 620.2
  - theca lutein 620.2
  - tuberculous (*see also* Tuberculosis) 016.6
  - unspecified 620.2
- oviduct 620.8
- palatal papilla (jaw) 526.1
- palate 526.1
  - fissural 526.1
  - median (fissural) 526.1
- palatine, of papilla 526.1
- pancreas, pancreatic 577.2
  - congenital 751.7
  - false 577.2
  - hemorrhagic 577.2
  - true 577.2
- paralabral
  - hip 718.85
  - shoulder 840.7
- paramesonephric duct - *see* Cyst, Müllerian duct
- paranephric 593.2
- paraovarian 752.11
- paraphysis, cerebri 742.4
- parasitic NEC 136.9
- parathyroid (gland) 252.8
- paratubal (fallopian) 620.8
- paraurethral duct 599.5
- paroophoron 752.11
- parotid gland 527.6
  - mucous extravasation or retention 527.6
- parovarian 752.11

SECTION I INDEX TO DISEASES AND INJURIES / Cyst

Cyst *(Continued)*
- pars planus 364.60
  - exudative 364.64
  - primary 364.63
- pelvis, female
  - in pregnancy or childbirth 654.4●
    - affecting fetus or newborn 763.89
    - causing obstructed labor 660.2●
      - affecting fetus or newborn 763.1
- penis (sebaceous) 607.89
- periapical 522.8
- pericardial (congenital) 746.89
  - acquired (secondary) 423.8
- pericoronal 526.0
- perineural (Tarlov's) 355.9
- periodontal 522.8
  - lateral 526.0
- peripancreatic 577.2
- peripelvic (lymphatic) 593.2
- peritoneum 568.89
  - chylous 457.8
- pharynx (wall) 478.26
- pilar 704.41
- pilonidal (infected) (rectum) 685.1
  - with abscess 685.0
  - malignant (M9084/3) 173.59
- pituitary (duct) (gland) 253.8
- placenta (amniotic) - *see* Placenta, abnormal
- pleura 519.8
- popliteal 727.51
- porencephalic 742.4
  - acquired 348.0
- postanal (infected) 685.1
  - with abscess 685.0
- posterior segment of eye, congenital 743.54
- postmastoidectomy cavity 383.31
- preauricular 744.47
- prepuce 607.89
  - congenital 752.69
- primordial (jaw) 526.0
- prostate 600.3
- pseudomucinous (ovary) (M8470/0) 220
- pudenda (sweat glands) 624.8
- pupillary, miotic 364.55
  - sebaceous 624.8
- radicular (residual) 522.8
- radiculodental 522.8
- ranular 527.6
- Rathke's pouch 253.8
- rectum (epithelium) (mucous) 569.49
- renal - *see* Cyst, kidney
- residual (radicular) 522.8
- retention (ovary) 620.2
- retina 361.19
  - macular 362.54
  - parasitic 360.13
  - primary 361.13
  - secondary 361.14
- retroperitoneal 568.89
- sacrococcygeal (dermoid) 685.1
  - with abscess 685.0
- salivary gland or duct 527.6
  - mucous extravasation or retention 527.6
- Sampson's 617.1
- sclera 379.19
- scrotum (sebaceous) 706.2
  - sweat glands 706.2
- sebaceous (duct) (gland) 706.2
  - breast 610.8
  - eyelid 374.84
  - genital organ NEC
    - female 629.89
    - male 608.89
  - scrotum 706.2
- semilunar cartilage (knee) (multiple) 717.5
- seminal vesicle 608.89
- serous (ovary) 620.2
- sinus (antral) (ethmoidal) (frontal) (maxillary) (nasal) (sphenoidal) 478.19
- Skene's gland 599.89

Cyst *(Continued)*
- skin (epidermal) (epidermoid, inclusion) (epithelial) (inclusion) (retention) (sebaceous) 706.2
  - breast 610.8
  - eyelid 374.84
  - genital organ NEC
    - female 629.89
    - male 608.89
  - neoplastic 216.3
  - scrotum 706.2
  - sweat gland or duct 705.89
- solitary
  - bone 733.21
  - kidney 593.2
- spermatic cord 608.89
- sphenoid sinus 478.19
- spinal meninges 349.2
- spine (*see also* Cyst, bone) 733.20
- spleen NEC 289.59
  - congenital 759.0
  - hydatid (*see also* Echinococcus) 122.9
- spring water (pericardium) 746.89
- subarachnoid 348.0
  - intrasellar 793.0
- subdural (cerebral) 348.0
  - spinal cord 349.2
- sublingual gland 527.6
  - mucous extravasation or retention 527.6
- submaxillary gland 527.6
  - mucous extravasation or retention 527.6
- suburethral 599.89
- suprarenal gland 255.8
- suprasellar - *see* Cyst, brain
- sweat gland or duct 705.89
- sympathetic nervous system 337.9
- synovial 727.40
  - popliteal space 727.51
- Tarlov's 355.9
- tarsal 373.2
- tendon (sheath) 727.42
- testis 608.89
- theca-lutein (ovary) 620.2
- Thornwaldt's, Tornwaldt's 478.26
- thymus (gland) 254.8
- thyroglossal (duct) (infected) (persistent) 759.2
- thyroid (gland) 246.2
  - adenomatous - *see* Goiter, nodular
  - colloid (*see also* Goiter) 240.9
- thyrolingual duct (infected) (persistent) 759.2
- tongue (mucous) 529.8
- tonsil 474.8
- tooth (dental root) 522.8
- trichilemmal (proliferating) 704.42
- tubo-ovarian 620.8
  - inflammatory 614.1
- tunica vaginalis 608.89
- turbinate (nose) (*see also* Cyst, bone) 733.20
- Tyson's gland (benign) (infected) 607.89
- umbilicus 759.89
- urachus 753.7
- ureter 593.89
- ureterovesical orifice 593.89
  - congenital 753.4
- urethra 599.84
- urethral gland (Cowper's) 599.89
- uterine
  - ligament 620.8
    - embryonic 752.11
  - tube 620.8
- uterus (body) (corpus) (recurrent) 621.8
  - embryonal 752.39
- utricle (ear) 386.8
  - prostatic 599.89
- utriculus masculinus 599.89
- vagina, vaginal (squamous cell) (wall) 623.8
  - embryonal 752.41
  - implantation 623.8
  - inclusion 623.8
- vallecula, vallecular 478.79

Cyst *(Continued)*
- ventricle, neuroepithelial 348.0
- verumontanum 599.89
- vesical (orifice) 596.89
- vitreous humor 379.29
- vulva (sweat glands) 624.8
  - congenital 752.41
  - implantation 624.8
  - inclusion 624.8
  - sebaceous gland 624.8
- vulvovaginal gland 624.8
- wolffian 752.89

Cystadenocarcinoma (M8440/3) - *see also* Neoplasm, by site, malignant
- bile duct type (M8161/3) 155.1
- endometrioid (M8380/3) - *see* Neoplasm, by site, malignant
- mucinous (M8470/3)
  - papillary (M8471/3)
    - specified site - *see* Neoplasm, by site, malignant
    - unspecified site 183.0
  - specified site - *see* Neoplasm, by site, malignant
  - unspecified site 183.0
- papillary (M8450/3)
  - mucinous (M8471/3)
    - specified site - *see* Neoplasm, by site, malignant
    - unspecified site 183.0
  - pseudomucinous (M8471/3)
    - specified site - *see* Neoplasm, by site, malignant
    - unspecified site 183.0
  - serous (M8460/3)
    - specified site - *see* Neoplasm, by site, malignant
    - unspecified site 183.0
  - specified site - *see* Neoplasm, by site, malignant
  - unspecified site 183.0
- pseudomucinous (M8470/3)
  - papillary (M8471/3)
    - specified site - *see* Neoplasm, by site, malignant
    - unspecified site 183.0
  - specified site - *see* Neoplasm, by site, malignant
  - unspecified site 183.0
- serous (M8441/3)
  - papillary (M8460/3)
    - specified site - *see* Neoplasm, by site, malignant
    - unspecified site 183.0
  - specified site - *see* Neoplasm, by site, malignant
  - unspecified site 183.0

Cystadenofibroma (M9013/0)
- clear cell (M8313/0) - *see* Neoplasm, by site, benign
- endometrioid (M8381/0) 220
  - borderline malignancy (M8381/1) 236.2
  - malignant (M8381/3) 183.0
- mucinous (M9015/0)
  - specified site - *see* Neoplasm, by site, benign
  - unspecified site 220
- serous (M9014/0)
  - specified site - *see* Neoplasm, by site, benign
  - unspecified site 220
- specified site - *see* Neoplasm, by site, benign
- unspecified site 220

Cystadenoma (M8440/0) - *see also* Neoplasm, by site, benign
- bile duct (M8161/0) 211.5
- endometrioid (M8380/0) - *see also* Neoplasm, by site, benign
  - borderline malignancy (M8380/1) - *see* Neoplasm, by site, uncertain behavior

Cystadenoma (Continued)
- malignant (M8440/3) - see Neoplasm, by site, malignant
- mucinous (M8470/0)
  - borderline malignancy (M8470/1)
    - specified site - see Neoplasm, uncertain behavior
    - unspecified site 236.2
  - papillary (M8471/0)
    - borderline malignancy (M8471/1)
      - specified site - see Neoplasm, by site, uncertain behavior
      - unspecified site 236.2
    - specified site - see Neoplasm, by site, benign
    - unspecified site 220
  - specified site - see Neoplasm, by site, benign
  - unspecified site 220
- papillary (M8450/0)
  - borderline malignancy (M8450/1)
    - specified site - see Neoplasm, by site, uncertain behavior
    - unspecified site 236.2
  - lymphomatosum (M8561/0) 210.2
  - mucinous (M8471/0)
    - borderline malignancy (M8471/1)
      - specified site - see Neoplasm, by site, uncertain behavior
      - unspecified site 236.2
    - specified site - see Neoplasm, by site, benign
    - unspecified site 220
  - pseudomucinous (M8471/0)
    - borderline malignancy (M8471/1)
      - specified site - see Neoplasm, by site uncertain behavior
      - unspecified site 236.2
    - specified site - see Neoplasm, by site, benign
    - unspecified site 220
  - serous (M8460/0)
    - borderline malignancy (M8460/1)
      - specified site - see Neoplasm, by site, uncertain behavior
      - unspecified site 236.2
    - specified site - see Neoplasm, by site, benign
    - unspecified site 220
  - specified site - see Neoplasm, by site, benign
  - unspecified site 220
- pseudomucinous (M8470/0)
  - borderline malignancy (M8470/1)
    - specified site - see Neoplasm, by site uncertain behavior
    - unspecified site 236.2
  - papillary (M8471/0)
    - borderline malignancy (M8471/1)
      - specified site - see Neoplasm, by site uncertain behavior
      - unspecified site 236.2
    - specified site - see Neoplasm, by site, benign
    - unspecified site 220
  - specified site - see Neoplasm, by site, benign
  - unspecified site 220
- serous (M8441/0)
  - borderline malignancy (M8441/1)
    - specified site - see Neoplasm, by site, uncertain behavior
    - unspecified site 236.2
  - papillary (M8460/0)
    - borderline malignancy (M8460/1)
      - specified site - see Neoplasm, by site, uncertain behavior
      - unspecified site 236.2
    - specified site - see Neoplasm, by site, benign
    - unspecified site 220

Cystadenoma (Continued)
- serous (Continued)
  - specified site - see Neoplasm, by site, benign
  - unspecified site 220
- thyroid 226

Cystathioninemia 270.4
Cystathioninuria 270.4
Cystic - see also condition
- breast, chronic 610.1
- corpora lutea 620.1
- degeneration, congenital
  - brain 742.4
  - kidney (see also Cystic, disease, kidney) 753.10
- disease
  - breast, chronic 610.1
  - kidney, congenital 753.10
    - medullary 753.16
    - multiple 753.19
    - polycystic - see Polycystic, kidney
    - single 753.11
    - specified NEC 753.19
  - liver, congenital 751.62
  - lung 518.89
    - congenital 748.4
  - pancreas, congenital 751.7
  - semilunar cartilage 717.5
- duct - see condition
- eyeball, congenital 743.03
- fibrosis (pancreas) 277.00
  - with
    - manifestations
      - gastrointestinal 277.03
      - pulmonary 277.02
      - specified NEC 277.09
    - meconium ileus 277.01
    - pulmonary exacerbation 277.02
- hygroma (M9173/0) 228.1
- kidney, congenital 753.10
  - medullary 753.16
  - multiple 753.19
  - polycystic - see Polycystic, kidney
  - single 753.11
  - specified NEC 753.19
- liver, congenital 751.62
- lung 518.89
  - congenital 748.4
- mass - see Cyst
- mastitis, chronic 610.1
- ovary 620.2
- pancreas, congenital 751.7

Cysticerciasis 123.1
Cysticercosis (mammary) (subretinal) 123.1
Cysticercus 123.1
- cellulosae infestation 123.1

Cystinosis (malignant) 270.0
Cystinuria 270.0
Cystitis (bacillary) (colli) (diffuse) (exudative) (hemorrhagic) (purulent) (recurrent) (septic) (suppurative) (ulcerative) 595.9
- with
  - abortion - see Abortion, by type, with urinary tract infection
  - ectopic pregnancy (see also categories 633.0–633.9) 639.8
  - fibrosis 595.1
  - leukoplakia 595.1
  - malakoplakia 595.1
  - metaplasia 595.1
  - molar pregnancy (see also categories 630–632) 639.8
- actinomycotic 039.8 [595.4]
- acute 595.0
  - of trigone 595.3
- allergic 595.89
- amebic 006.8 [595.4]
- bilharzial 120.9 [595.4]
- blennorrhagic (acute) 098.11
  - chronic or duration of 2 months or more 098.31

Cystitis (Continued)
- bullous 595.89
- calculous 594.1
- chlamydial 099.53
- chronic 595.2
  - interstitial 595.1
  - of trigone 595.3
- complicating pregnancy, childbirth, or puerperium 646.6●
  - affecting fetus or newborn 760.1
- cystic(a) 595.81
- diphtheritic 032.84
- echinococcal
  - glanulosus 122.3 [595.4]
  - multilocularis 122.6 [595.4]
- emphysematous 595.89
- encysted 595.81
- follicular 595.3
- following
  - abortion 639.8
  - ectopic or molar pregnancy 639.8
- gangrenous 595.89
- glandularis 595.89
- gonococcal (acute) 098.11
  - chronic or duration of 2 months or more 098.31
- incrusted 595.89
- interstitial 595.1
- irradiation 595.82
- irritation 595.89
- malignant 595.89
- monilial 112.2
- of trigone 595.3
- panmural 595.1
- polyposa 595.89
- prostatic 601.3
- radiation 595.82
- Reiter's (abacterial) 099.3
- specified NEC 595.89
- subacute 595.2
- submucous 595.1
- syphilitic 095.8
- trichomoniasis 131.09
- tuberculous (see also Tuberculosis) 016.1●
- ulcerative 595.1

Cystocele
- female (without uterine prolapse) 618.01
  - with uterine prolapse 618.4
    - complete 618.3
    - incomplete 618.2
  - lateral 618.02
  - midline 618.01
  - paravaginal 618.02
- in pregnancy or childbirth 654.4●
  - affecting fetus or newborn 763.89
  - causing obstructed labor 660.2●
    - affecting fetus or newborn 763.1
- male 596.89

Cystoid
- cicatrix limbus 372.64
- degeneration macula 362.53

Cystolithiasis 594.1
Cystoma (M8440/0) - see also Neoplasm, by site, benign
- endometrial, ovary 617.1
- mucinous (M8470/0)
  - specified site - see Neoplasm, by site, benign
  - unspecified site 220
- serous (M8441/0)
  - specified site - see Neoplasm, by site, benign
  - unspecified site 220
- simple (ovary) 620.2

Cystoplegia 596.53
Cystoptosis 596.89
Cystopyelitis (see also Pyelitis) 590.80
Cystorrhagia 596.89

Cystosarcoma phyllodes (M9020/1) 238.3
　benign (M9020/0) 217
　malignant (M9020/3) - see Neoplasm, breast, malignant
Cystostomy status V44.50
　with complication 596.83
　　infection 596.81
　　mechanical 596.82
　　specified complication NEC 596.83
　appendico-vesicostomy V44.52

Cystostomy status (Continued)
　cutaneous-vesicostomy V44.51
　specified type NEC V44.59
Cystourethritis (see also Urethritis) 597.89
Cystourethrocele (see also Cystocele)
　female (without uterine prolapse) 618.09
　　with uterine prolapse 618.4
　　　complete 618.3
　　　incomplete 618.2
　male 596.89

Cytomegalic inclusion disease 078.5
　congenital 771.1
Cytomycosis, reticuloendothelial (see also Histoplasmosis, American) 115.00
Cytopenia 289.9
　refractory
　　with
　　　multilineage dysplasia (RCMD) 238.72
　　　　and ringed sideroblasts (RCMD-RS) 238.72

D

Daae (-Finsen) **disease** (epidemic pleurodynia) 074.1
Dabney's grip 074.1
Da Costa's syndrome (neurocirculatory asthenia) 306.2
Dacryoadenitis, dacryadenitis 375.00
    acute 375.01
    chronic 375.02
Dacryocystitis 375.30
    acute 375.32
    chronic 375.42
    neonatal 771.6
    phlegmonous 375.33
    syphilitic 095.8
        congenital 090.0
    trachomatous, active 076.1
        late effect 139.1
    tuberculous (see also Tuberculosis) 017.3●
Dacryocystoblenorrhea 375.42
Dacryocystocele 375.43
Dacryolith, dacryolithiasis 375.57
Dacryoma 375.43
Dacryopericystitis (acute) (subacute) 375.32
    chronic 375.42
Dacryops 375.11
Dacryosialadenopathy, atrophic 710.2
Dacryostenosis 375.56
    congenital 743.65
Dactylitis
    bone (see also Osteomyelitis) 730.2●
    sickle-cell 282.62
        Hb-C 282.64
        Hb-SS 282.62
        specified NEC 282.69
    syphilitic 095.5
    tuberculous (see also Tuberculosis) 015.5●
Dactylolysis spontanea 136.0
Dactylosymphysis (see also Syndactylism) 755.10
Damage
    arteriosclerotic - see Arteriosclerosis
    brain 348.9
        anoxic, hypoxic 348.1
            during or resulting from a procedure 997.01
            ischemic, in newborn 768.70
                mild 768.71
                moderate 768.72
                severe 768.73
        child NEC 343.9
        due to birth injury 767.0
        minimal (child) (see also Hyperkinesia) 314.9
        newborn 767.0
    cardiac - see also Disease, heart
    cardiorenal (vascular) (see also Hypertension, cardiorenal) 404.90
    central nervous system - see Damage, brain
    cerebral NEC - see Damage, brain
    coccyx, complicating delivery 665.6●
    coronary (see also Ischemia, heart) 414.9
    eye, birth injury 767.8
    heart - see also Disease, heart
        valve - see Endocarditis
    hypothalamus NEC 348.9
    liver 571.9
        alcoholic 571.3
    medication 995.20
    myocardium (see also Degeneration, myocardial) 429.1
    pelvic
        joint or ligament, during delivery 665.6●
        organ NEC
            with
                abortion - see Abortion, by type, with damage to pelvic organs
                ectopic pregnancy (see also categories 633.0–633.9) 639.2
                molar pregnancy (see also categories 630–632) 639.2

Damage (Continued)
    pelvic (Continued)
        organ NEC (Continued)
            during delivery 665.5●
            following
                abortion 639.2
                ectopic or molar pregnancy 639.2
    renal (see also Disease, renal) 593.9
    skin, solar 692.79
        acute 692.72
        chronic 692.74
    subendocardium, subendocardial (see also Degeneration, myocardial) 429.1
    vascular 459.9
Dameshek's syndrome (erythroblastic anemia) 282.49
Dana-Putnam syndrome (subacute combined sclerosis with pernicious anemia) 281.0 [336.2]
Danbolt (-Closs) **syndrome** (acrodermatitis enteropathica) 686.8
Dandruff 690.18
Dandy fever 061
Dandy-Walker deformity or syndrome (atresia, foramen of Magendie) 742.3
    with spina bifida (see also Spina bifida) 741.0●
Dangle foot 736.79
Danielssen's disease (anesthetic leprosy) 030.1
Danlos' syndrome 756.83
Darier's disease (congenital) (keratosis follicularis) 757.39
    due to vitamin A deficiency 264.8
    meaning erythema annulare centrifugum 695.0
Darier-Roussy sarcoid 135
Dark area on retina 239.81
Darling's
    disease (see also Histoplasmosis, American) 115.00
    histoplasmosis (see also Histoplasmosis, American) 115.00
Dartre 054.9
Darwin's tubercle 744.29
Davidson's anemia (refractory) 284.9
Davies' disease 425.0
Davies-Colley syndrome (slipping rib) 733.99
Dawson's encephalitis 046.2
Day blindness (see also Blindness, day) 368.60
Dead
    fetus
        retained (in utero) 656.4●
            early pregnancy (death before 22 completed weeks' gestation) 632
            late (death after 22 completed weeks' gestation) 656.4●
        syndrome 641.3●
    labyrinth 386.50
    ovum, retained 631.8
Deaf and dumb NEC 389.7
Deaf mutism (acquired) (congenital) NEC 389.7
    endemic 243
    hysterical 300.11
    syphilitic, congenital 090.0
Deafness (acquired) (complete) (congenital) (hereditary) (middle ear) (partial) 389.9
    with
        blindness V49.85
        blue sclera and fragility of bone 756.51
    auditory fatigue 389.9
    aviation 993.0
        nerve injury 951.5
    boilermakers' 951.5
    central 389.14
        with conductive hearing loss 389.20
            bilateral 389.22
            unilateral 389.21
    conductive (air) 389.00
        with sensorineural hearing loss 389.20
            bilateral 389.22
            unilateral 389.21
        bilateral 389.06

Deafness (Continued)
    conductive (Continued)
        combined types 389.08
        external ear 389.01
        inner ear 389.04
        middle ear 389.03
        multiple types 389.08
        tympanic membrane 389.02
        unilateral 389.05
    emotional (complete) 300.11
    functional (complete) 300.11
    high frequency 389.8
    hysterical (complete) 300.11
    injury 951.5
    low frequency 389.8
    mental 784.69
    mixed conductive and sensorineural 389.20
        bilateral 389.22
        unilateral 389.21
    nerve
        with conductive hearing loss 389.20
            bilateral 389.22
            unilateral 389.21
        bilateral 389.12
        unilateral 389.13
    neural
        with conductive hearing loss 389.20
            bilateral 389.22
            unilateral 389.21
        bilateral 389.12
        unilateral 389.13
    noise-induced 388.12
        nerve injury 951.5
    nonspeaking 389.7
    perceptive 389.10
        with conductive hearing loss 389.20
            bilateral 389.22
            unilateral 389.21
        central 389.14
        neural
            bilateral 389.12
            unilateral 389.13
        sensorineural 389.10
            asymmetrical 389.16
            bilateral 389.18
            unilateral 389.15
        sensory
            bilateral 389.11
            unilateral 389.17
    psychogenic (complete) 306.7
    sensorineural (see also Deafness, perceptive) 389.10
        asymmetrical 389.16
        bilateral 389.18
        unilateral 389.15
    sensory
        with conductive hearing loss 389.20
            bilateral 389.22
            unilateral 389.21
        bilateral 389.11
        unilateral 389.17
    specified type NEC 389.8
    sudden NEC 388.2
    syphilitic 094.89
    transient ischemic 388.02
    transmission - see Deafness, conductive
    traumatic 951.5
    word (secondary to organic lesion) 784.69
        developmental 315.31
Death
    after delivery (cause not stated) (sudden) 674.9●
    anesthetic
        due to
            correct substance properly administered 995.4
            overdose or wrong substance given 968.4
                specified anesthetic - see Table of Drugs and Chemicals
        during delivery 668.9●

Death (Continued)
   brain 348.82
   cardiac (sudden) (SCD) - *code to* underlying condition
      family history of V17.41
      personal history of, successfully resuscitated V12.53
   cause unknown 798.2
   cot (infant) 798.0
   crib (infant) 798.0
   fetus, fetal (cause not stated) (intrauterine) 779.9
      early, with retention (before 22 completed weeks' gestation) 632
      from asphyxia or anoxia (before labor) 768.0
         during labor 768.1
      late, affecting management of pregnancy (after 22 completed weeks' gestation) 656.4●
   from pregnancy NEC 646.9●
   instantaneous 798.1
   intrauterine (*see also* Death, fetus) 779.9
      complicating pregnancy 656.4●
   maternal, affecting fetus or newborn 761.6
   neonatal NEC 779.9
   sudden (cause unknown) 798.1
      cardiac (SCD)
         family history of V17.41
         personal history of, successfully resuscitated V12.53
      during delivery 669.9●
      under anesthesia NEC 668.9●
      infant, syndrome (SIDS) 798.0
      puerperal, during puerperium 674.9●
   unattended (cause unknown) 798.9
   under anesthesia NEC
      due to
         correct substance properly administered 995.4
         overdose or wrong substance given 968.4
            specified anesthetic - *see* Table of Drugs and Chemicals
      during delivery 668.9●
   violent 798.1
de Beurmann-Gougerot disease (sporotrichosis) 117.1
Debility (general) (infantile) (postinfectional) 799.3
   with nutritional difficulty 269.9
   congenital or neonatal NEC 779.9
   nervous 300.5
   old age 797
   senile 797
Débove's disease (splenomegaly) 789.2
Decalcification
   bone (*see also* Osteoporosis) 733.00
   teeth 521.89
Decapitation 874.9
   fetal (to facilitate delivery) 763.89
Decapsulation, kidney 593.89
Decay
   dental 521.00
   senile 797
   tooth, teeth 521.00
Decensus, uterus - *see* Prolapse, uterus
Deciduitis (acute)
   with
      abortion - *see* Abortion, by type, with sepsis
      ectopic pregnancy (*see also* categories 633.0–633.9) 639.0
      molar pregnancy (*see also* categories 630–632) 639.0
   affecting fetus or newborn 760.8
   following
      abortion 639.0
      ectopic or molar pregnancy 639.0
   in pregnancy 646.6●
   puerperal, postpartum 670.1●

Deciduoma malignum (M9100/3) 181
Deciduous tooth (retained) 520.6
Decline (general) (*see also* Debility) 799.3
Decompensation
   cardiac (acute) (chronic) (*see also* Disease, heart) 429.9
      failure - *see* Failure, heart
   cardiorenal (*see also* Hypertension, cardiorenal) 404.90
   cardiovascular (*see also* Disease, cardiovascular) 429.2
   heart (*see also* Disease, heart) 429.9
      failure - *see* Failure, heart
   hepatic 572.2
   myocardial (acute) (chronic) (*see also* Disease, heart) 429.9
      failure - *see* Failure, heart
   respiratory 519.9
Decompression sickness 993.3
Decrease, decreased
   blood
      platelets (*see also* Thrombocytopenia) 287.5
      pressure 796.3
         due to shock following
            injury 958.4
            operation 998.00
      white cell count 288.50
         specified NEC 288.59
   cardiac reserve - *see* Disease, heart
   estrogen 256.39
      postablative 256.2
   fetal movements 655.7●
   fragility of erythrocytes 289.89
   function
      adrenal (cortex) 255.41
         medulla 255.5
      ovary in hypopituitarism 253.4
      parenchyma of pancreas 577.8
      pituitary (gland) (lobe) (anterior) 253.2
         posterior (lobe) 253.8
   functional activity 780.99
   glucose 790.29
   haptoglobin (serum) NEC 273.8
   leukocytes 288.50
   libido 799.81
   lymphocytes 288.51
   platelets (*see also* Thrombocytopenia) 287.5
   pulse pressure 785.9
   respiration due to shock following injury 958.4
   sexual desire 799.81
   tear secretion NEC 375.15
   tolerance
      fat 579.8
      salt and water 276.9
   vision NEC 369.9
   white blood cell count 288.50
Decubital gangrene (*see also* Ulcer, pressure) 707.00 [785.4]
Decubiti (*see also* Ulcer, pressure) 707.00
Decubitus (ulcer) (*see also* Ulcer, pressure) 707.00
   with gangrene 707.00 [785.4]
   ankle 707.06
   back
      lower 707.03
      upper 707.02
   buttock 707.05
   coccyx 707.03
   elbow 707.01
   head 707.09
   heel 707.07
   hip 707.04
   other site 707.09
   sacrum 707.03
   shoulder blades 707.02
Deepening acetabulum 718.85
Defect, defective 759.9
   3-beta-hydroxysteroid dehydrogenase 255.2
   11-hydroxylase 255.2

Defect, defective (Continued)
   21-hydroxylase 255.2
   abdominal wall, congenital 756.70
   aorticopulmonary septum 745.0
   aortic septal 745.0
   atrial septal (ostium secundum type) 745.5
      acquired 429.71
      ostium primum type 745.61
      sinus venosus 745.8
   atrioventricular
      canal 745.69
      septum 745.4
         acquired 429.71
   atrium secundum 745.5
      acquired 429.71
   auricular septal 745.5
      acquired 429.71
   bilirubin excretion 277.4
   biosynthesis, testicular androgen 257.2
   bridge 525.60
   bulbar septum 745.0
   butanol-insoluble iodide 246.1
   chromosome - *see* Anomaly, chromosome
   circulation (acquired) 459.9
      congenital 747.9
      newborn 747.9
   clotting NEC (*see also* Defect, coagulation) 286.9
   coagulation (factor) (*see also* Deficiency, coagulation factor) 286.9
      with
         abortion - *see* Abortion, by type, with hemorrhage
         ectopic pregnancy (*see also* categories 634–638) 639.1
         molar pregnancy (*see also* categories 630–632) 639.1
      acquired (any) 286.7
      antepartum or intrapartum 641.3●
         affecting fetus or newborn 762.1
      causing hemorrhage of pregnancy or delivery 641.3●
      complicating pregnancy, childbirth, or puerperium 649.3●
      due to
         liver disease 286.7
         vitamin K deficiency 286.7
      newborn, transient 776.3
      postpartum 666.3●
      specified type NEC 286.9
   conduction (heart) 426.9
      bone (*see also* Deafness, conductive) 389.00
   congenital, organ or site NEC - *see also* Anomaly
      circulation 747.9
      Descemet's membrane 743.9
         specified type NEC 743.49
      diaphragm 756.6
      ectodermal 757.9
      esophagus 750.9
      pulmonic cusps - *see* Anomaly, heart valve
      respiratory system 748.9
         specified type NEC 748.8
   crown 525.60
   cushion endocardial 745.60
   dental restoration 525.60
   dentin (hereditary) 520.5
   Descemet's membrane (congenital) 743.9
      acquired 371.30
      specific type NEC 743.49
   deutan 368.52
   developmental - *see also* Anomaly, by site
      cauda equina 742.59
      left ventricle 746.9
         with atresia or hypoplasia of aortic orifice or valve, with hypoplasia of ascending aorta 746.7
         in hypoplastic left heart syndrome 746.7
      testis 752.9
      vessel 747.9

Defect, defective (Continued)
  diaphragm
    with elevation, eventration, or hernia - see Hernia, diaphragm
    congenital 756.6
      with elevation, eventration, or hernia 756.6
        gross (with elevation, eventration, or hernia) 756.6
  ectodermal, congenital 757.9
  Eisenmenger's (ventricular septal defect) 745.4
  endocardial cushion 745.60
    specified type NEC 745.69
  esophagus, congenital 750.9
  extensor retinaculum 728.9
  fibrin polymerization (see also Defect, coagulation) 286.3
  filling
    biliary tract 793.3
    bladder 793.5
    dental 525.60
    gallbladder 793.3
    kidney 793.5
    stomach 793.4
    ureter 793.5
  fossa ovalis 745.5
  gene, carrier (suspected) of V83.89
  Gerbode 745.4
  glaucomatous, without elevated tension 365.89
  Hageman (factor) (see also Defect, coagulation) 286.3
  hearing (see also Deafness) 389.9
  high grade 317
  homogentisic acid 270.2
  interatrial septal 745.5
    acquired 429.71
  interauricular septal 745.5
    acquired 429.71
  interventricular septal 745.4
    with pulmonary stenosis or atresia, dextraposition of aorta, and hypertrophy of right ventricle 745.2
    acquired 429.71
    in tetralogy of Fallot 745.2
  iodide trapping 246.1
  iodotyrosine dehalogenase 246.1
  kynureninase 270.2
  learning, specific 315.2
  major osseous 731.3
  mental (see also Disability, intellectual) 319
  osseous, major 731.3
  osteochondral NEC 738.8
  ostium
    primum 745.61
    secundum 745.5
  pericardium 746.89
  peroxidase-binding 246.1
  placental blood supply - see Placenta, insufficiency
  platelet (qualitative) 287.1
    constitutional 286.4
  postural, spine 737.9
  protan 368.51
  pulmonic cusps, congenital 746.00
  renal pelvis 753.9
    obstructive 753.29
    specified type NEC 753.3
  respiratory system, congenital 748.9
    specified type NEC 748.8
  retina, retinal 361.30
    with detachment (see also Detachment, retina, with retinal defect) 361.00
      multiple 361.33
        with detachment 361.02
      nerve fiber bundle 362.85
      single 361.30
        with detachment 361.01

Defect, defective (Continued)
  septal (closure) (heart) NEC 745.9
    acquired 429.71
    atrial 745.5
    specified type NEC 745.8
  speech NEC 784.59
    developmental 315.39
    late effect of cerebrovascular disease - see Late effect(s) (of) cerebrovascular disease, speech and language deficit
    secondary to organic lesion 784.59
    Taussig-Bing (transposition, aorta and overriding pulmonary artery) 745.11
  teeth, wedge 521.20
  thyroid hormone synthesis 246.1
  tritan 368.53
  ureter 753.9
    obstructive 753.29
  vascular (acquired) (local) 459.9
    congenital (peripheral) NEC 747.60
      gastrointestinal 747.61
      lower limb 747.64
      renal 747.62
      specified NEC 747.69
      spinal 747.82
      upper limb 747.63
  ventricular septal 745.4
    with pulmonary stenosis or atresia, dextraposition of aorta, and hypertrophy of right ventricle 745.2
    acquired 429.71
    atrioventricular canal type 745.69
    between infundibulum and anterior portion 745.4
    in tetralogy of Fallot 745.2
    isolated anterior 745.4
  vision NEC 369.9
  visual field 368.40
    arcuate 368.43
    heteronymous, bilateral 368.47
    homonymous, bilateral 368.46
    localized NEC 368.44
    nasal step 368.44
    peripheral 368.44
    sector 368.43
  voice and resonance 784.40
  wedge, teeth (abrasion) 521.20
Defeminization syndrome 255.2
Deferentitis 608.4
  gonorrheal (acute) 098.14
    chronic or duration of 2 months or over 098.34
Defibrination syndrome (see also Fibrinolysis) 286.6
Deficiency, deficient
  3-beta-hydroxysteroid dehydrogenase 255.2
  6-phosphogluconic dehydrogenase (anemia) 282.2
  11-beta-hydroxylase 255.2
  17-alpha-hydroxylase 255.2
  18-hydroxysteroid dehydrogenase 255.2
  20-alpha-hydroxylase 255.2
  21-hydroxylase 255.2
  AAT (alpha-1 antitrypsin) 273.4
  abdominal muscle syndrome 756.79
  accelerator globulin (Ac G) (blood) (see also Defect, coagulation) 286.3
  AC globulin (congenital) (see also Defect, coagulation) 286.3
    acquired 286.7
  activating factor (blood) (see also Defect, coagulation) 286.3
  adenohypophyseal 253.2
  adenosine deaminase 277.2
  aldolase (hereditary) 271.2
  alpha-1-antitrypsin 273.4
  alpha-1-trypsin inhibitor 273.4
  alpha-fucosidase 271.8
  alpha-lipoprotein 272.5
  alpha-mannosidase 271.8

Deficiency, deficient (Continued)
  amino acid 270.9
  anemia - see Anemia, deficiency
  aneurin 265.1
    with beriberi 265.0
  antibody NEC 279.00
  antidiuretic hormone 253.5
  antihemophilic
    factor (A) 286.0
    B 286.1
    C 286.2
    globulin (AHG) NEC 286.0
  antithrombin III 289.81
  antitrypsin 273.4
  argininosuccinate synthetase or lyase 270.6
  ascorbic acid (with scurvy) 267
  autoprothrombin
    I (see also Defect, coagulation) 286.3
    II 286.1
    C (see also Defect, coagulation) 286.3
  bile salt 579.8
  biotin 266.2
  biotinidase 277.6
  bradykinase-1 277.6
  brancher enzyme (amylopectinosis) 271.0
  calciferol 268.9
    with
      osteomalacia 268.2
      rickets (see also Rickets) 268.0
  calcium 275.40
    dietary 269.3
  calorie, severe 261
  carbamyl phosphate synthetase 270.6
  cardiac (see also Insufficiency, myocardial) 428.0
  carnitine 277.81
    due to
      hemodialysis 277.83
      inborn errors of metabolism 277.82
      valproic acid therapy 277.83
    iatrogenic 277.83
    palmitoyltransferase (CPT1, CPT2) 277.85
    palmityl transferase (CPT1, CPT2) 277.85
    primary 277.81
    secondary 277.84
  carotene 264.9
  Carr factor (see also Defect, coagulation) 286.9
  central nervous system 349.9
  ceruloplasmin 275.1
  cevitamic acid (with scurvy) 267
  choline 266.2
  Christmas factor 286.1
  chromium 269.3
  citrin 269.1
  clotting (blood) (see also Defect, coagulation) 286.9
  coagulation factor NEC 286.9
    with
      abortion - see Abortion, by type, with hemorrhage
      ectopic pregnancy (see also categories 634–638) 639.1
      molar pregnancy (see also categories 630–632) 639.1
    acquired (any) 286.7
    antepartum or intrapartum 641.3 ●
      affecting fetus or newborn 762.1
    complicating pregnancy, childbirth, or puerperium 649.3 ●
    due to
      liver disease 286.7
      vitamin K deficiency 286.7
    newborn, transient 776.3
    postpartum 666.3 ●
    specified type NEC 286.3
  color vision (congenital) 368.59
    acquired 368.55
  combined glucocorticoid and mineralocorticoid 255.41
  combined, two or more coagulation factors (see also Defect, coagulation) 286.9

SECTION I INDEX TO DISEASES AND INJURIES / Deficiency, deficient

Deficiency, deficient (Continued)
- complement factor NEC 279.8
- contact factor (see also Defect, coagulation) 286.3
- copper NEC 275.1
- corticoadrenal 255.41
- craniofacial axis 756.0
- cyanocobalamin (vitamin B_{12}) 266.2
- debrancher enzyme (limit dextrinosis) 271.0
- desmolase 255.2
- diet 269.9
- dihydrofolate reductase 281.2
- dihydropteridine reductase 270.1
- dihydropyrimidine dehydrogenase (DPD) 277.6
- disaccharidase (intestinal) 271.3
- disease NEC 269.9
- ear(s) V48.8
- edema 262
- endocrine 259.9
- enzymes, circulating NEC (see also Deficiency, by specific enzyme) 277.6
- ergosterol 268.9
  - with
    - osteomalacia 268.2
    - rickets (see also Rickets) 268.0
- erythrocytic glutathione (anemia) 282.2
- eyelid(s) V48.8
- factor (see also Defect, coagulation) 286.9
  - I (congenital) (fibrinogen) 286.3
    - antepartum or intrapartum 641.3●
      - affecting fetus or newborn 762.1
    - newborn, transient 776.3
    - postpartum 666.3●
  - II (congenital) (prothrombin) 286.3
  - V (congenital) (labile) 286.3
  - VII (congenital) (stable) 286.3
  - VIII (congenital) (functional) 286.0
    - with
      - functional defect 286.0
      - vascular defect 286.4
  - IX (Christmas) (congenital) (functional) 286.1
  - X (congenital) (Stuart-Prower) 286.3
  - XI (congenital) (plasma thromboplastin antecedent) 286.2
  - XII (congenital) (Hageman) 286.3
  - XIII (congenital) (fibrin stabilizing) 286.3
  - Hageman 286.3
  - multiple (congenital) 286.9
    - acquired 286.7
- fibrinase (see also Defect, coagulation) 286.3
- fibrinogen (congenital) (see also Defect, coagulation) 286.3
  - acquired 286.6
- fibrin-stabilizing factor (congenital) (see also Defect, coagulation) 286.3
  - acquired 286.7
- finger - see Absence, finger
- fletcher factor (see also Defect, coagulation) 286.9
- fluorine 269.3
- folate, anemia 281.2
- folic acid (vitamin B_C) 266.2
  - anemia 281.3
- follicle-stimulating hormone (FSH) 253.4
- fructokinase 271.2
- fructose-1, 6-diphosphate 271.2
- fructose-1-phosphate aldolase 271.2
- FSH (follicle-stimulating hormone) 253.4
- fucosidase 271.8
- galactokinase 271.1
- galactose-1-phosphate uridyl transferase 271.1
- gamma globulin in blood 279.00
- glass factor (see also Defect, coagulation) 286.3
- glucocorticoid 255.41
- glucose-6-phosphatase 271.0
- glucose-6-phosphate dehydrogenase anemia 282.2

Deficiency, deficient (Continued)
- glucuronyl transferase 277.4
- glutathione-reductase (anemia) 282.2
- glycogen synthetase 271.0
- growth hormone 253.3
- Hageman factor (congenital) (see also Defect, coagulation) 286.3
- head V48.0
- hemoglobin (see also Anemia) 285.9
- hepatophosphorylase 271.0
- hexose monophosphate (HMP) shunt 282.2
- HGH (human growth hormone) 253.3
- HG-PRT 277.2
- homogentisic acid oxidase 270.2
- hormone - see also Deficiency, by specific hormone
  - anterior pituitary (isolated) (partial) NEC 253.4
    - growth (human) 253.3
  - follicle-stimulating 253.4
  - growth (human) (isolated) 253.3
  - human growth 253.3
  - interstitial cell-stimulating 253.4
  - luteinizing 253.4
  - melanocyte-stimulating 253.4
  - testicular 257.2
- human growth hormone 253.3
- humoral 279.00
  - with
    - hyper-IgM 279.05
      - autosomal recessive 279.05
      - X-linked 279.05
    - increased IgM 279.05
  - congenital hypogammaglobulinemia 279.04
  - non-sex-linked 279.06
  - selective immunoglobulin NEC 279.03
    - IgA 279.01
    - IgG 279.03
    - IgM 279.02
      - increased 279.05
  - specified NEC 279.09
- hydroxylase 255.2
- hypoxanthine-guanine phosphoribosyltransferase (HG-PRT) 277.2
- ICSH (interstitial cell-stimulating hormone) 253.4
- immunity NEC 279.3
  - cell-mediated 279.10
    - with
      - hyperimmunoglobulinemia 279.2
      - thrombocytopenia and eczema 279.12
    - specified NEC 279.19
  - combined (severe) 279.2
    - syndrome 279.2
  - common variable 279.06
  - humoral NEC 279.00
  - IgA (secretory) 279.01
  - IgG 279.03
  - IgM 279.02
- immunoglobulin, selective NEC 279.03
  - IgA 279.01
  - IgG 279.03
  - IgM 279.02
- inositol (B complex) 266.2
- interferon 279.49
- internal organ V47.0
- interstitial cell-stimulating hormone (ICSH) 253.4
- intrinsic factor (Castle's) (congenital) 281.0
- intrinsic (urethral) sphincter (ISD) 599.82
- invertase 271.3
- iodine 269.3
- iron, anemia 280.9
- labile factor (congenital) (see also Defect, coagulation) 286.3
  - acquired 286.7
- lacrimal fluid (acquired) 375.15
  - congenital 743.64

Deficiency, deficient (Continued)
- lactase 271.3
- Laki-Lorand factor (see also Defect, coagulation) 286.3
- lecithin-cholesterol acyltranferase 272.5
- LH (luteinizing hormone) 253.4
- limb V49.0
  - lower V49.0
    - congenital (see also Deficiency, lower limb, congenital) 755.30
  - upper V49.0
    - congenital (see also Deficiency, upper limb, congenital) 755.20
- lipocaic 577.8
- lipoid (high-density) 272.5
- lipoprotein (familial) (high-density) 272.5
- liver phosphorylase 271.0
- long chain 3-hydroxyacyl CoA dehydrogenase (LCHAD) 277.85
- long chain/very long chain acyl CoA dehydrogenase (LCAD, VLCAD) 277.85
- lower limb V49.0
  - congenital 755.30
    - with complete absence of distal elements 755.31
    - longitudinal (complete) (partial) (with distal deficiencies, incomplete) 755.32
      - with complete absence of distal elements 755.31
      - combined femoral, tibial, fibular (incomplete) 755.33
      - femoral 755.34
      - fibular 755.37
      - metatarsal(s) 755.38
      - phalange(s) 755.39
        - meaning all digits 755.31
      - tarsal(s) 755.38
      - tibia 755.36
      - tibiofibular 755.35
    - transverse 755.31
- luteinizing hormone (LH) 253.4
- lysosomal alpha-1, 4 glucosidase 271.0
- magnesium 275.2
- mannosidase 271.8
- medium chain acyl CoA dehydrogenase (MCAD) 277.85
- melanocyte-stimulating hormone (MSH) 253.4
- menadione (vitamin K) 269.0
  - newborn 776.0
- mental (familial) (hereditary) (see also Disability, intellectual) 319
- methylenetetrahydrofolate reductase (MTHFR) 270.4
- mineral NEC 269.3
- mineralocorticoid 255.42
- molybdenum 269.3
- moral 301.7
- multiple, syndrome 260
- myocardial (see also Insufficiency, myocardial) 428.0
- myophosphorylase 271.0
- NADH (DPNH)-methemoglobin-reductase (congenital) 289.7
- NADH diaphorase or reductase (congenital) 289.7
- neck V48.1
- niacin (amide) (-tryptophan) 265.2
- nicotinamide 265.2
- nicotinic acid (amide) 265.2
- nose V48.8
- number of teeth (see also Anodontia) 520.0
- nutrition, nutritional 269.9
  - specified NEC 269.8
- ornithine transcarbamylase 270.6
- ovarian 256.39
- oxygen (see also Anoxia) 799.02
- pantothenic acid 266.2
- parathyroid (gland) 252.1

SECTION 1 INDEX TO DISEASES AND INJURIES / **Deformity**

Deficiency, deficient (Continued)
  phenylalanine hydroxylase 270.1
  phosphoenolpyruvate carboxykinase 271.8
  phosphofructokinase 271.2
  phosphoglucomutase 271.0
  phosphohexosisomerase 271.0
  phosphomannomutase 271.8
  phosphomannose isomerase 271.8
  phosphomannosyl mutase 271.8
  phosphorylase kinase, liver 271.0
  pituitary (anterior) 253.2
    posterior 253.5
  placenta - see Placenta, insufficiency
  plasma
    cell 279.00
    protein (paraproteinemia)
        (pyroglobulinemia) 273.8
      gamma globulin 279.00
    thromboplastin
      antecedent (PTA) 286.2
      component (PTC) 286.1
  platelet NEC 287.1
    constitutional 286.4
  polyglandular 258.9
  potassium (K) 276.8
  proaccelerin (congenital) (see also Defect,
      congenital) 286.3
    acquired 286.7
  proconvertin factor (congenital) (see also
      Defect, coagulation) 286.3
    acquired 286.7
  prolactin 253.4
  protein 260
    anemia 281.4
    C 289.81
    plasma - see Deficiency, plasma, protein
    S 289.81
  prothrombin (congenital) (see also Defect,
      coagulation) 286.3
    acquired 286.7
  Prower factor (see also Defect, coagulation)
      286.3
  PRT 277.2
  pseudocholinesterase 289.89
  psychobiological 301.6
  PTA 286.2
  PTC 286.1
  purine nucleoside phosphorylase 277.2
  pyracin (alpha) (beta) 266.1
  pyridoxal 266.1
  pyridoxamine 266.1
  pyridoxine (derivatives) 266.1
  pyruvate carboxylase 271.8
  pyruvate dehydrogenase 271.8
  pyruvate kinase (PK) 282.3
  riboflavin (vitamin B_2) 266.0
  saccadic eye movements 379.57
  salivation 527.7
  salt 276.1
  secretion
    ovary 256.39
    salivary gland (any) 527.7
    urine 788.5
  selenium 269.3
  serum
    antitrypsin, familial 273.4
    protein (congenital) 273.8
  short chain acyl CoA dehydrogenase (SCAD)
      277.85
  short stature homeobox gene (SHOX)
      with
    dyschondrosteosis 756.89
      short stature (idiopathic) 783.43
      Turner's syndrome 758.6
  smooth pursuit movements (eye) 379.58
  sodium (Na) 276.1
  SPCA (see also Defect, coagulation) 286.3
  specified NEC 269.8
  stable factor (congenital) (see also Defect,
      coagulation) 286.3
    acquired 286.7

Deficiency, deficient (Continued)
  Stuart (-Prower) factor (see also Defect,
      coagulation) 286.3
  sucrase 271.3
  sucrase-isomaltase 271.3
  sulfite oxidase 270.0
  syndrome, multiple 260
  thiamine, thiaminic (chloride) 265.1
  thrombokinase (see also Defect, coagulation)
      286.3
    newborn 776.0
  thrombopoieten 287.39
  thymolymphatic 279.2
  thyroid (gland) 244.9
  tocopherol 269.1
  toe - see Absence, toe
  tooth bud (see also Anodontia) 520.0
  trunk V48.1
  UDPG-glycogen transferase 271.0
  upper limb V49.0
    congenital 755.20
      with complete absence of distal
          elements 755.21
      longitudinal (complete) (partial) (with
          distal deficiencies, incomplete)
          755.22
        carpal(s) 755.28
        combined humeral, radial, ulnar
            (incomplete) 755.23
        humeral 755.24
        metacarpal(s) 755.28
        phalange(s) 755.29
          meaning all digits 755.21
        radial 755.26
        radioulnar 755.25
        ulnar 755.27
      transverse (complete) (partial) 755.21
  vascular 459.9
  vasopressin 253.5
  viosterol (see also Deficiency, calciferol) 268.9
  vitamin (multiple) NEC 269.2
    A 264.9
      with
        Bitôt's spot 264.1
        corneal 264.2
          with corneal ulceration 264.3
        keratomalacia 264.4
        keratosis, follicular 264.8
        night blindness 264.5
        scar of cornea, xerophthalmic 264.6
        specified manifestation NEC 264.8
          ocular 264.7
      xeroderma 264.8
      xerophthalmia 264.7
      xerosis
        conjunctival 264.0
          with Bitôt's spot 264.1
        corneal 264.2
          with corneal ulceration 264.3
    B (complex) NEC 266.9
      with
        beriberi 265.0
        pellagra 265.2
      specified type NEC 266.2
    B_1 NEC 265.1
      beriberi 265.0
    B_2 266.0
    B_6 266.1
    B_{12} 266.2
    B_C (folic acid) 266.2
    C (ascorbic acid) (with scurvy) 267
    D (calciferol) (ergosterol) 268.9
      with
        osteomalacia 268.2
        rickets (see also Rickets) 268.0
    E 269.1
    folic acid 266.2
    G 266.0
    H 266.2
    K 269.0
      of newborn 776.0

Deficiency, deficient (Continued)
  vitamin NEC (Continued)
    nicotinic acid 265.2
    P 269.1
    PP 265.2
    specified NEC 269.1
    zinc 269.3
Deficient - see also Deficiency
  blink reflex 374.45
  craniofacial axis 756.0
  number of teeth (see also Anodontia) 520.0
  secretion of urine 788.5
Deficit
  attention 799.51
  cognitive communication 799.52
  concentration 799.51
  executive function 799.55
  frontal lobe 799.55
  neurologic NEC 781.99
    due to
      cerebrovascular lesion (see also
          Disease, cerebrovascular, acute)
          436
      late effect - see Late effect(s) (of)
          cerebrovascular disease
      transient ischemic attack 435.9
    ischemic
      reversible (RIND) 434.91
        history of (personal) V12.54
      prolonged (PRIND) 434.91
        history of (personal) V12.54
  oxygen 799.02
  psychomotor 799.54
  visuospatial 799.53
Deflection
  radius 736.09
  septum (acquired) (nasal) (nose) 470
  spine - see Curvature, spine
  turbinate (nose) 470
Defluvium
  capillorum (see also Alopecia) 704.00
  ciliorum 374.55
  unguium 703.8
Deformity 738.9
  abdomen, congenital 759.9
  abdominal wall
    acquired 738.8
    congenital 756.70
    muscle deficiency syndrome 756.79
  acquired (unspecified site) 738.9
    specified site NEC 738.8
  adrenal gland (congenital) 759.1
  alimentary tract, congenital 751.9
    lower 751.5
    specified type NEC 751.8
    upper (any part, except tongue) 750.9
      specified type NEC 750.8
      tongue 750.10
        specified type NEC 750.19
  ankle (joint) (acquired) 736.70
    abduction 718.47
    congenital 755.69
    contraction 718.47
    specified NEC 736.79
  anus (congenital) 751.5
    acquired 569.49
  aorta (congenital) 747.20
    acquired 447.8
    arch 747.21
      acquired 447.8
      coarctation 747.10
    aortic
      arch 747.21
        acquired 447.8
      cusp or valve (congenital) 746.9
        acquired (see also Endocarditis, aortic)
            424.1
      ring 747.21
  appendix 751.5
  arm (acquired) 736.89
    congenital 755.50

145

SECTION I INDEX TO DISEASES AND INJURIES / Deformity

Deformity (Continued)
- arteriovenous (congenital) (peripheral) NEC 747.60
  - gastrointestinal 747.61
  - lower limb 747.64
  - renal 747.62
  - specified NEC 747.69
  - spinal 747.82
  - upper limb 747.63
- artery (congenital) (peripheral) NEC (*see also* Deformity, vascular) 747.60
  - acquired 447.8
  - cerebral 747.81
  - coronary (congenital) 746.85
    - acquired (*see also* Ischemia, heart) 414.9
  - retinal 743.9
  - umbilical 747.5
- atrial septal (congenital) (heart) 745.5
- auditory canal (congenital) (external) (*see also* Deformity, ear) 744.3
  - acquired 380.50
- auricle
  - ear (congenital) (*see also* Deformity, ear) 744.3
    - acquired 380.32
  - heart (congenital) 746.9
- back (acquired) - *see* Deformity, spine
- Bartholin's duct (congenital) 750.9
- bile duct (congenital) 751.60
  - acquired 576.8
    - with calculus, choledocholithiasis, or stones - *see* Choledocholithiasis
- biliary duct or passage (congenital) 751.60
  - acquired 576.8
    - with calculus, choledocholithiasis, or stones - *see* Choledocholithiasis
- bladder (neck) (sphincter) (trigone) (acquired) 596.89
  - congenital 753.9
- bone (acquired) NEC 738.9
  - congenital 756.9
  - turbinate 738.0
- boutonniere (finger) 736.21
- brain (congenital) 742.9
  - acquired 348.89
  - multiple 742.4
  - reduction 742.2
  - vessel (congenital) 747.81
- breast (acquired) 611.89
  - congenital 757.6
  - reconstructed 612.0
- bronchus (congenital) 748.3
  - acquired 519.19
- bursa, congenital 756.9
- canal of Nuck 752.9
- canthus (congenital) 743.9
  - acquired 374.89
- capillary (acquired) 448.9
  - congenital NEC (*see also* Deformity, vascular) 747.60
- cardiac - *see* Deformity, heart
- cardiovascular system (congenital) 746.9
- caruncle, lacrimal (congenital) 743.9
  - acquired 375.69
- cascade, stomach 537.6
- cecum (congenital) 751.5
  - acquired 569.89
- cerebral (congenital) 742.9
  - acquired 348.89
- cervix (acquired) (uterus) 622.8
  - congenital 752.40
- cheek (acquired) 738.19
  - congenital 744.9
- chest (wall) (acquired) 738.3
  - congenital 754.89
  - late effect of rickets 268.1
- chin (acquired) 738.19
  - congenital 744.9

Deformity (Continued)
- choroid (congenital) 743.9
  - acquired 363.8
  - plexus (congenital) 742.9
    - acquired 349.2
- cicatricial - *see* Cicatrix
- cilia (congenital) 743.9
  - acquired 374.89
- circulatory system (congenital) 747.9
- clavicle (acquired) 738.8
  - congenital 755.51
- clitoris (congenital) 752.40
  - acquired 624.8
- clubfoot - *see* Clubfoot
- coccyx (acquired) 738.6
  - congenital 756.10
- colon (congenital) 751.5
  - acquired 569.89
- concha (ear) (congenital) (*see also* Deformity, ear) 744.3
  - acquired 380.32
- congenital, organ or site not listed (*see also* Anomaly) 759.9
- cornea (congenital) 743.9
  - acquired 371.70
- coronary artery (congenital) 746.85
  - acquired (*see also* Ischemia, heart) 414.9
- cranium (acquired) 738.19
  - congenital (*see also* Deformity, skull, congenital) 756.0
- cricoid cartilage (congenital) 748.3
  - acquired 478.79
- cystic duct (congenital) 751.60
  - acquired 575.8
- Dandy-Walker 742.3
  - with spina bifida (*see also* Spina bifida) 741.0 ●
- diaphragm (congenital) 756.6
  - acquired 738.8
- digestive organ(s) or system (congenital) NEC 751.9
  - specified type NEC 751.8
- ductus arteriosus 747.0
- duodenal bulb 537.89
- duodenum (congenital) 751.5
  - acquired 537.89
- dura (congenital) 742.9
  - brain 742.4
    - acquired 349.2
  - spinal 742.59
    - acquired 349.2
- ear (congenital) 744.3
  - acquired 380.32
  - auricle 744.3
    - causing impairment of hearing 744.02
  - causing impairment of hearing 744.00
  - external 744.3
    - causing impairment of hearing 744.02
  - internal 744.05
  - lobule 744.3
  - middle 744.03
    - ossicles 744.04
  - ossicles 744.04
- ectodermal (congenital) NEC 757.9
  - specified type NEC 757.8
- ejaculatory duct (congenital) 752.9
  - acquired 608.89
- elbow (joint) (acquired) 736.00
  - congenital 755.50
  - contraction 718.42
- endocrine gland NEC 759.2
- epididymis (congenital) 752.9
  - acquired 608.89
  - torsion 608.24
- epiglottis (congenital) 748.3
  - acquired 478.79
- esophagus (congenital) 750.9
  - acquired 530.89
- Eustachian tube (congenital) NEC 744.3
  - specified type NEC 744.24

Deformity (Continued)
- extremity (acquired) 736.9
  - congenital, except reduction deformity 755.9
    - lower 755.60
    - upper 755.50
  - reduction - *see* Deformity, reduction
- eye (congenital) 743.9
  - acquired 379.8
  - muscle 743.9
- eyebrow (congenital) 744.89
- eyelid (congenital) 743.9
  - acquired 374.89
  - specified type NEC 743.62
- face (acquired) 738.19
  - congenital (any part) 744.9
    - due to intrauterine malposition and pressure 754.0
- fallopian tube (congenital) 752.10
  - acquired 620.8
- femur (acquired) 736.89
  - congenital 755.60
- fetal
  - with fetopelvic disproportion 653.7 ●
    - affecting fetus or newborn 763.1
  - causing obstructed labor 660.1 ●
    - affecting fetus or newborn 763.1
  - known or suspected, affecting management of pregnancy 655.9 ●
- finger (acquired) 736.20
  - boutonniere type 736.21
  - congenital 755.50
  - flexion contracture 718.44
  - swan neck 736.22
- flexion (joint) (acquired) 736.9
  - congenital NEC 755.9
  - hip or thigh (acquired) 736.39
    - congenital (*see also* Subluxation, congenital, hip) 754.32
- foot (acquired) 736.70
  - cavovarus 736.75
    - congenital 754.59
  - congenital NEC 754.70
    - specified type NEC 754.79
  - valgus (acquired) 736.79
    - congenital 754.60
      - specified type NEC 754.69
  - varus (acquired) 736.79
    - congenital 754.50
      - specified type NEC 754.59
- forearm (acquired) 736.00
  - congenital 755.50
- forehead (acquired) 738.19
  - congenital (*see also* Deformity, skull, congenital) 756.0
- frontal bone (acquired) 738.19
  - congenital (*see also* Deformity, skull, congenital) 756.0
- gallbladder (congenital) 751.60
  - acquired 575.8
- gastrointestinal tract (congenital) NEC 751.9
  - acquired 569.89
  - specified type NEC 751.8
- genitalia, genital organ(s) or system NEC
  - congenital 752.9
  - female (congenital) 752.9
    - acquired 629.89
    - external 752.40
    - internal 752.9
  - male (congenital) 752.9
    - acquired 608.89
- globe (eye) (congenital) 743.9
  - acquired 360.89
- gum (congenital) 750.9
  - acquired 523.9
- gunstock 736.02
- hand (acquired) 736.00
  - claw 736.06
  - congenital 755.50
  - minus (and plus) (intrinsic) 736.09
  - pill roller (intrinsic) 736.09

Deformity (Continued)
  hand (Continued)
    plus (and minus) (intrinsic) 736.09
    swan neck (intrinsic) 736.09
  head (acquired) 738.10
    congenital (see also Deformity, skull, congenital) 756.0
    specified NEC 738.19
  heart (congenital) 746.9
    auricle (congenital) 746.9
    septum 745.9
      auricular 745.5
      specified type NEC 745.8
      ventricular 745.4
    valve (congenital) NEC 746.9
      acquired - see Endocarditis
      pulmonary (congenital) 746.00
      specified type NEC 746.89
    ventricle (congenital) 746.9
  heel (acquired) 736.76
    congenital 755.67
  hepatic duct (congenital) 751.60
    acquired 576.8
      with calculus, choledocholithiasis, or stones - see Choledocholithiasis
  hip (joint) (acquired) 736.30
    congenital NEC 755.63
    flexion 718.45
      congenital (see also Subluxation, congenital, hip) 754.32
  hourglass - see Contraction, hourglass
  humerus (acquired) 736.89
    congenital 755.50
  hymen (congenital) 752.40
  hypophyseal (congenital) 759.2
  ileocecal (coil) (valve) (congenital) 751.5
    acquired 569.89
  ileum (intestine) (congenital) 751.5
    acquired 569.89
  ilium (acquired) 738.6
    congenital 755.60
  integument (congenital) 757.9
  intervertebral cartilage or disc (acquired) - see also Displacement, intervertebral disc
    congenital 756.10
  intestine (large) (small) (congenital) 751.5
    acquired 569.89
  iris (acquired) 364.75
    congenital 743.9
    prolapse 364.89
  ischium (acquired) 738.6
    congenital 755.60
  jaw (acquired) (congenital) NEC 524.9
    due to intrauterine malposition and pressure 754.0
  joint (acquired) NEC 738.8
    congenital 755.9
    contraction (abduction) (adduction) (extension) (flexion) - see Contraction, joint
  kidney(s) (calyx) (pelvis) (congenital) 753.9
    acquired 593.89
    vessel 747.62
      acquired 459.9
  Klippel-Feil (brevicollis) 756.16
  knee (acquired) NEC 736.6
    congenital 755.64
  labium (majus) (minus) (congenital) 752.40
    acquired 624.8
  lacrimal apparatus or duct (congenital) 743.9
    acquired 375.69
  larynx (muscle) (congenital) 748.3
    acquired 478.79
    web (glottic) (subglottic) 748.2
  leg (lower) (upper) (acquired) NEC 736.89
    congenital 755.60
      reduction - see Deformity, reduction, lower limb
  lens (congenital) 743.9
    acquired 379.39

Deformity (Continued)
  lid (fold) (congenital) 743.9
    acquired 374.89
  ligament (acquired) 728.9
    congenital 756.9
  limb (acquired) 736.9
    congenital, except reduction deformity 755.9
      lower 755.60
        reduction (see also Deformity, reduction, lower limb) 755.30
      upper 755.50
        reduction (see also Deformity, reduction, lower limb) 755.20
    specified NEC 736.89
  lip (congenital) NEC 750.9
    acquired 528.5
    specified type NEC 750.26
  liver (congenital) 751.60
    acquired 573.8
    duct (congenital) 751.60
      acquired 576.8
        with calculus, choledocholithiasis, or stones - see Choledocholithiasis
  lower extremity - see Deformity, leg
  lumbosacral (joint) (region) (congenital) 756.10
    acquired 738.5
  lung (congenital) 748.60
    acquired 518.89
    specified type NEC 748.69
  lymphatic system, congenital 759.9
  Madelung's (radius) 755.54
  maxilla (acquired) (congenital) 524.9
  meninges or membrane (congenital) 742.9
    brain 742.4
      acquired 349.2
    spinal (cord) 742.59
      acquired 349.2
  mesentery (congenital) 751.9
    acquired 568.89
  metacarpus (acquired) 736.00
    congenital 755.50
  metatarsus (acquired) 736.70
    congenital 754.70
  middle ear, except ossicles (congenital) 744.03
    ossicles 744.04
  mitral (leaflets) (valve) (congenital) 746.9
    acquired - see Endocarditis, mitral
    Ebstein's 746.89
    parachute 746.5
    specified type NEC 746.89
    stenosis, congenital 746.5
  mouth (acquired) 528.9
    congenital NEC 750.9
      specified type NEC 750.26
  multiple, congenital NEC 759.7
    specified type NEC 759.89
  muscle (acquired) 728.9
    congenital 756.9
      specified type NEC 756.89
      sternocleidomastoid (due to intrauterine malposition and pressure) 754.1
  musculoskeletal system, congenital NEC 756.9
    specified type NEC 756.9
  nail (acquired) 703.9
    congenital 757.9
  nasal - see Deformity, nose
  neck (acquired) NEC 738.2
    congenital (any part) 744.9
      sternocleidomastoid 754.1
  nervous system (congenital) 742.9
  nipple (congenital) 757.6
    acquired 611.89

Deformity (Continued)
  nose, nasal (cartilage) (acquired) 738.0
    bone (turbinate) 738.0
    congenital 748.1
      bent 754.0
      squashed 754.0
    saddle 738.0
      syphilitic 090.5
    septum 470
      congenital 748.1
    sinus (wall) (congenital) 748.1
      acquired 738.0
    syphilitic (congenital) 090.5
      late 095.8
  ocular muscle (congenital) 743.9
    acquired 378.60
  opticociliary vessels (congenital) 743.9
  orbit (congenital) (eye) 743.9
    acquired NEC 376.40
      associated with craniofacial deformities 376.44
      due to
        bone disease 376.43
        surgery 376.47
        trauma 376.47
  organ of Corti (congenital) 744.05
  ovary (congenital) 752.0
    acquired 620.8
  oviduct (congenital) 752.10
    acquired 620.8
  palate (congenital) 750.9
    acquired 526.89
    cleft (congenital) (see also Cleft, palate) 749.00
    hard, acquired 526.89
    soft, acquired 528.9
  pancreas (congenital) 751.7
    acquired 577.8
  parachute, mitral valve 746.5
  parathyroid (gland) 759.2
  parotid (gland) (congenital) 750.9
    acquired 527.8
  patella (acquired) 736.6
    congenital 755.64
  pelvis, pelvic (acquired) (bony) 738.6
    with disproportion (fetopelvic) 653.0●
      affecting fetus or newborn 763.1
      causing obstructed labor 660.1●
        affecting fetus or newborn 763.1
    congenital 755.60
    rachitic (late effect) 268.1
  penis (glans) (congenital) 752.9
    acquired 607.89
  pericardium (congenital) 746.9
    acquired - see Pericarditis
  pharynx (congenital) 750.9
    acquired 478.29
  Pierre Robin (congenital) 756.0
  pinna (acquired) 380.32
    congenital 744.3
  pituitary (congenital) 759.2
  pleural folds (congenital) 748.8
  portal vein (congenital) 747.40
  posture - see Curvature, spine
  prepuce (congenital) 752.9
    acquired 607.89
  prostate (congenital) 752.9
    acquired 602.8
  pulmonary valve - see Endocarditis, pulmonary
  pupil (congenital) 743.9
    acquired 364.75
  pylorus (congenital) 750.9
    acquired 537.89
  rachitic (acquired), healed or old 268.1
  radius (acquired) 736.00
    congenital 755.50
    reduction - see Deformity, reduction, upper limb
  rectovaginal septum (congenital) 752.40
    acquired 623.8

Deformity (Continued)
- rectum (congenital) 751.5
  - acquired 569.49
- reduction (extremity) (limb) 755.4
  - brain 742.2
  - lower limb 755.30
    - with complete absence of distal elements 755.31
    - longitudinal (complete) (partial) (with distal deficiencies, incomplete) 755.32
      - with complete absence of distal elements 755.31
      - combined femoral, tibial, fibular (incomplete) 755.33
      - femoral 755.34
      - fibular 755.37
      - metatarsal(s) 755.38
      - phalange(s) 755.39
        - meaning all digits 755.31
      - tarsal(s) 755.38
      - tibia 755.36
      - tibiofibular 755.35
    - transverse 755.31
  - upper limb 755.20
    - with complete absence of distal elements 755.21
    - longitudinal (complete) (partial) (with distal deficiencies, incomplete) 755.22
      - with complete absence of distal elements 755.21
      - carpal(s) 755.28
      - combined humeral, radial, ulnar (incomplete) 755.23
      - humeral 755.24
      - metacarpal(s) 755.28
      - phalange(s) 755.29
        - meaning all digits 755.21
      - radial 755.26
      - radioulnar 755.25
      - ulnar 755.27
    - transverse (complete) (partial) 755.21
- renal - see Deformity, kidney
- respiratory system (congenital) 748.9
  - specified type NEC 748.8
- rib (acquired) 738.3
  - congenital 756.3
    - cervical 756.2
- rotation (joint) (acquired) 736.9
  - congenital 755.9
  - hip or thigh 736.39
    - congenital (see also Subluxation, congenital, hip) 754.32
- sacroiliac joint (congenital) 755.69
  - acquired 738.5
- sacrum (acquired) 738.5
  - congenital 756.10
- saddle
  - back 737.8
  - nose 738.0
    - syphilitic 090.5
- salivary gland or duct (congenital) 750.9
  - acquired 527.8
- scapula (acquired) 736.89
  - congenital 755.50
- scrotum (congenital) 752.9
  - acquired 608.89
- sebaceous gland, acquired 706.8
- seminal tract or duct (congenital) 752.9
  - acquired 608.89
- septum (nasal) (acquired) 470
  - congenital 748.1
- shoulder (joint) (acquired) 736.89
  - congenital 755.50
    - specified type NEC 755.59
  - contraction 718.41
- sigmoid (flexure) (congenital) 751.5
  - acquired 569.89
- sinus of Valsalva 747.29

Deformity (Continued)
- skin (congenital) 757.9
  - acquired NEC 709.8
- skull (acquired) 738.19
  - congenital 756.0
    - with
      - anencephalus 740.0
      - encephalocele 742.0
      - hydrocephalus 742.3
        - with spina bifida (see also Spina bifida) 741.0●
      - microcephalus 742.1
    - due to intrauterine malposition and pressure 754.0
- soft parts, organs or tissues (of pelvis)
  - in pregnancy or childbirth NEC 654.9●
    - affecting fetus or newborn 763.89
    - causing obstructed labor 660.2●
      - affecting fetus or newborn 763.1
- spermatic cord (congenital) 752.9
  - acquired 608.89
    - torsion 608.22
      - extravaginal 608.21
      - intravaginal 608.22
- spinal
  - column - see Deformity, spine
  - cord (congenital) 742.9
    - acquired 336.8
    - vessel (congenital) 747.82
  - nerve root (congenital) 742.9
    - acquired 724.9
- spine (acquired) NEC 738.5
  - congenital 756.10
    - due to intrauterine malposition and pressure 754.2
  - kyphoscoliotic (see also Kyphoscoliosis) 737.30
  - kyphotic (see also Kyphosis) 737.10
  - lordotic (see also Lordosis) 737.20
  - rachitic 268.1
  - scoliotic (see also Scoliosis) 737.30
- spleen
  - acquired 289.59
  - congenital 759.0
- Sprengel's (congenital) 755.52
- sternum (acquired) 738.3
  - congenital 756.3
- stomach (congenital) 750.9
  - acquired 537.89
- submaxillary gland (congenital) 750.9
  - acquired 527.8
- swan neck (acquired)
  - finger 736.22
  - hand 736.09
- talipes - see Talipes
- teeth, tooth NEC 520.9
- testis (congenital) 752.9
  - acquired 608.89
    - torsion 608.20
- thigh (acquired) 736.89
  - congenital 755.60
- thorax (acquired) (wall) 738.3
  - congenital 754.89
  - late effect of rickets 268.1
- thumb (acquired) 736.20
  - congenital 755.50
- thymus (tissue) (congenital) 759.2
- thyroid (gland) (congenital) 759.2
  - cartilage 748.3
    - acquired 478.79
- tibia (acquired) 736.89
  - congenital 755.60
  - saber 090.5
- toe (acquired) 735.9
  - congenital 755.66
  - specified NEC 735.8
- tongue (congenital) 750.10
  - acquired 529.8
- tooth, teeth NEC 520.9
- trachea (rings) (congenital) 748.3
  - acquired 519.19

Deformity (Continued)
- transverse aortic arch (congenital) 747.21
- tricuspid (leaflets) (valve) (congenital) 746.9
  - acquired - see Endocarditis, tricuspid
  - atresia or stenosis 746.1
  - specified type NEC 746.89
- trunk (acquired) 738.3
  - congenital 759.9
- ulna (acquired) 736.00
  - congenital 755.50
- upper extremity - see Deformity, arm
- urachus (congenital) 753.7
- ureter (opening) (congenital) 753.9
  - acquired 593.89
- urethra (valve) (congenital) 753.9
  - acquired 599.84
- urinary tract or system (congenital) 753.9
  - urachus 753.7
- uterus (congenital) 752.39
  - acquired 621.8
- uvula (congenital) 750.9
  - acquired 528.9
- vagina (congenital) 752.40
  - acquired 623.8
- valve, valvular (heart) (congenital) 746.9
  - acquired - see Endocarditis
  - pulmonary 746.00
  - specified type NEC 746.89
- vascular (congenital) (peripheral) NEC 747.60
  - acquired 459.9
  - gastrointestinal 747.61
  - lower limb 747.64
  - renal 747.62
  - specified site NEC 747.69
  - spinal 747.82
  - upper limb 747.63
- vas deferens (congenital) 752.9
  - acquired 608.89
- vein (congenital) NEC (see also Deformity, vascular) 747.60
  - brain 747.81
  - coronary 746.9
  - great 747.40
- vena cava (inferior) (superior) (congenital) 747.40
- vertebra - see Deformity, spine
- vesicourethral orifice (acquired) 596.89
  - congenital NEC 753.9
    - specified type NEC 753.8
- vessels of optic papilla (congenital) 743.9
- visual field (contraction) 368.45
- vitreous humor (congenital) 743.9
  - acquired 379.29
- vulva (congenital) 752.40
  - acquired 624.8
- wrist (joint) (acquired) 736.00
  - congenital 755.50
  - contraction 718.43
  - valgus 736.03
    - congenital 755.59
  - varus 736.04
    - congenital 755.59

Degeneration, degenerative
- adrenal (capsule) (gland) 255.8
  - with hypofunction 255.41
  - fatty 255.8
  - hyaline 255.8
  - infectional 255.8
  - lardaceous 277.39
- amyloid (any site) (general) 277.39
- anterior cornua, spinal cord 336.8
- anterior labral 840.8
- aorta, aortic 440.0
  - fatty 447.8
  - valve (heart) (see also Endocarditis, aortic) 424.1
- arteriovascular - see Arteriosclerosis

Degeneration, degenerative (Continued)
    artery, arterial (atheromatous) (calcareous) -
        see also Arteriosclerosis
        amyloid 277.39
        lardaceous 277.39
        medial NEC (*see also* Arteriosclerosis,
            extremities) 440.20
    articular cartilage NEC (*see also* Disorder,
        cartilage, articular) 718.0●
        elbow 718.02
        knee 717.5
        patella 717.7
        shoulder 718.01
        spine (*see also* Spondylosis) 721.90
    atheromatous - *see* Arteriosclerosis
    bacony (any site) 277.39
    basal nuclei or ganglia NEC 333.0
    bone 733.90
    brachial plexus 353.0
    brain (cortical) (progressive) 331.9
        arteriosclerotic 437.0
        childhood 330.9
            specified type NEC 330.8
        congenital 742.4
        cystic 348.0
            congenital 742.4
        familial NEC 331.89
        grey matter 330.8
        heredofamilial NEC 331.89
        in
            alcoholism 303.9● [331.7]
            beriberi 265.0 [331.7]
            cerebrovascular disease 437.9 [331.7]
            congenital hydrocephalus 742.3 [331.7]
                with spina bifida (*see also* Spina
                    bifida) 741.0● [331.7]
            Babry's disease 272.7 [330.2]
            Gaucher's disease 272.7 [330.2]
            Hunter's disease or syndrome 277.5
                [330.3]
            lipidosis
                cerebral 330.1
                generalized 272.7 [330.2]
            mucopolysaccharidosis 277.5 [330.3]
            myxedema (*see also* Myxedema) 244.9
                [331.7]
            neoplastic disease NEC (M8000/1)
                239.9 [331.7]
            Niemann-Pick disease 272.7 [330.2]
            sphingolipidosis 272.7 [330.2]
            vitamin B_{12} deficiency 266.2 [331.7]
        motor centers 331.89
        senile 331.2
        specified type NEC 331.89
    breast - *see* Disease, breast
    Bruch's membrane 363.40
    bundle of His 426.50
        left 426.3
        right 426.4
    calcareous NEC 275.49
    capillaries 448.9
        amyloid 277.39
        fatty 448.9
        lardaceous 277.39
    cardiac (brown) (calcareous) (fatty) (fibrous)
        (hyaline) (mural) (muscular)
        (pigmentary) (senile) (with
        arteriosclerosis) (*see also* Degeneration,
        myocardial) 429.1
        valve, valvular - *see* Endocarditis
    cardiorenal (*see also* Hypertension,
        cardiorenal) 404.90
    cardiovascular (*see also* Disease,
        cardiovascular) 429.2
        renal (*see also* Hypertension, cardiorenal)
            404.90
    cartilage (joint) - *see* Derangement, joint
    cerebellar NEC 334.9
        primary (hereditary) (sporadic) 334.2
    cerebral - *see* Degeneration, brain
    cerebromacular 330.1

Degeneration, degenerative (Continued)
    cerebrovascular 437.1
        due to hypertension 437.2
        late effect - *see* Late effect(s) (of)
            cerebrovascular disease
    cervical plexus 353.2
    cervix 622.8
        due to radiation (intended effect) 622.8
            adverse effect or misadventure 622.8
    changes, spine or vertebra (*see also*
        Spondylosis) 721.90
    chitinous 277.39
    chorioretinal 363.40
        congenital 743.53
        hereditary 363.50
    choroid (colloid) (drusen) 363.40
        hereditary 363.50
        senile 363.41
            diffuse secondary 363.42
    cochlear 386.8
    collateral ligament (knee) (medial) 717.82
        lateral 717.81
    combined (spinal cord) (subacute) 266.2
        [336.2]
        with anemia (pernicious) 281.0 [336.2]
            due to dietary deficiency 281.1 [336.2]
        due to vitamin B_{12} deficiency anemia
            (dietary) 281.1 [336.2]
    conjunctiva 372.50
        amyloid 277.39 [372.50]
    cornea 371.40
        calcerous 371.44
        familial (hereditary) (*see also* Dystrophy,
            cornea) 371.50
            macular 371.55
            reticular 371.54
        hyaline (of old scars) 371.41
        marginal (Terrien's) 371.48
        mosaic (shagreen) 371.41
        nodular 371.46
        peripheral 371.48
        senile 371.41
    cortical (cerebellar) (parenchymatous) 334.2
        alcoholic 303.9● [334.4]
        diffuse, due to arteriopathy 437.0
    corticobasal 331.6
    corticostriatal-spinal 334.8
    cretinoid 243
    cruciate ligament (knee) (posterior) 717.84
        anterior 717.83
    cutis 709.3
        amyloid 277.39
    dental pulp 522.2
    disc disease - *see* Degeneration, intervertebral
        disc
    dorsolateral (spinal cord) - *see* Degeneration,
        combined
    endocardial 424.90
    extrapyramidal NEC 333.90
    eye NEC 360.40
        macular (*see also* Degeneration, macula)
            362.50
            congenital 362.75
            hereditary 362.76
    fatty (diffuse) (general) 272.8
        liver 571.8
            alcoholic 571.0
        localized site - *see* Degeneration, by site,
            fatty
        placenta - *see* Placenta, abnormal
    globe (eye) NEC 360.40
        macular - *see* Degeneration, macula
    grey matter 330.8
    heart (brown) (calcareous) (fatty) (fibrous)
        (hyaline) (mural) (muscular)
        (pigmentary) (senile) (with
        arteriosclerosis) (*see also* Degeneration,
        myocardial) 429.1
        amyloid 277.39 [425.7]
        atheromatous - *see* Arteriosclerosis,
            coronary

Degeneration, degenerative (Continued)
    heart (Continued)
        gouty 274.82
        hypertensive (*see also* Hypertension,
            heart) 402.90
        ischemic 414.9
        valve, valvular - *see* Endocarditis
    hepatolenticular (Wilson's) 275.1
    hepatorenal 572.4
    heredofamilial
        brain NEC 331.89
        spinal cord NEC 336.8
    hyaline (diffuse) (generalized) 728.9
        localized - *see also* Degeneration, by site
            cornea 371.41
            keratitis 371.41
    hypertensive vascular - *see* Hypertension
    infrapatellar fat pad 729.31
    internal semilunar cartilage 717.3
    intervertebral disc 722.6
        with myelopathy 722.70
        cervical, cervicothoracic 722.4
            with myelopathy 722.71
        lumbar, lumbosacral 722.52
            with myelopathy 722.73
        thoracic, thoracolumbar 722.51
            with myelopathy 722.72
    intestine 569.89
        amyloid 277.39
        lardaceous 277.39
    iris (generalized) (*see also* Atrophy, iris)
        364.59
        pigmentary 364.53
        pupillary margin 364.54
    ischemic - *see* Ischemia
    joint disease (*see also* Osteoarthrosis) 715.9●
        multiple sites 715.09
        spine (*see also* Spondylosis) 721.90
    kidney (*see also* Sclerosis, renal) 587
        amyloid 277.39 [583.81]
        cyst, cystic (multiple) (solitary) 593.2
            congenital (*see also* Cystic, disease,
                kidney) 753.10
        fatty 593.89
        fibrocystic (congenital) 753.19
        lardaceous 277.39 [583.81]
        polycystic (congenital) 753.12
            adult type (APKD) 753.13
            autosomal dominant 753.13
            autosomal recessive 753.14
            childhood type (CPKD) 753.14
            infantile type 753.14
        waxy 277.39 [583.81]
    Kuhnt-Junius (retina) 362.52
    labyrinth, osseous 386.8
    lacrimal passages, cystic 375.12
    lardaceous (any site) 277.39
    lateral column (posterior), spinal cord (*see
        also* Degeneration, combined) 266.2
        [336.2]
    lattice 362.63
    lens 366.9
        infantile, juvenile, or presenile 366.00
        senile 366.10
    lenticular (familial) (progressive) (Wilson's)
        (with cirrhosis of liver) 275.1
        striate artery 437.0
    lethal ball, prosthetic heart valve 996.02
    ligament
        collateral (knee) (medial) 717.82
            lateral 717.81
        cruciate (knee) (posterior) 717.84
            anterior 717.83
    liver (diffuse) 572.8
        amyloid 277.39
        congenital (cystic) 751.62
        cystic 572.8
            congenital 751.62
        fatty 571.8
            alcoholic 571.0
        hypertrophic 572.8

Degeneration, degenerative (Continued)
   liver (Continued)
      lardaceous 277.39
      parenchymatous, acute or subacute (see also Necrosis, liver) 570
      pigmentary 572.8
      toxic (acute) 573.8
      waxy 277.39
   lung 518.89
   lymph gland 289.3
      hyaline 289.3
      lardaceous 277.39
   macula (acquired) (senile) 362.50
      atrophic 362.51
      Best's 362.76
      congenital 362.75
      cystic 362.54
      cystoid 362.53
      disciform 362.52
      dry 362.51
      exudative 362.52
      familial pseudoinflammatory 362.77
      hereditary 362.76
      hole 362.54
      juvenile (Stargardt's) 362.75
      nonexudative 362.51
      pseudohole 362.54
      wet 362.52
   medullary - see Degeneration, brain
   membranous labyrinth, congenital (causing impairment of hearing) 744.05
   meniscus - see Derangement, joint
   microcystoid 362.62
   mitral - see Insufficiency, mitral
   Mönckeberg's (see also Arteriosclerosis, extremities) 440.20
   moral 301.7
   motor centers, senile 331.2
   mural (see also Degeneration, myocardial) 429.1
      heart, cardiac (see also Degeneration, myocardial) 429.1
      myocardium, myocardial (see also Degeneration, myocardial) 429.1
   muscle 728.9
      fatty 728.9
      fibrous 728.9
      heart (see also Degeneration, myocardial) 429.1
      hyaline 728.9
   muscular progressive 728.2
   myelin, central nervous system NEC 341.9
   myocardium, myocardial (brown) (calcareous) (fatty) (fibrous) (hyaline) (mural) (muscular) (pigmentary) (senile) (with arteriosclerosis) 429.1
      with rheumatic fever (conditions classifiable to 390) 398.0
        active, acute, or subacute 391.2
          with chorea 392.0
        inactive or quiescent (with chorea) 398.0
      amyloid 277.39 [425.7]
      congenital 746.89
      fetus or newborn 779.89
      gouty 274.82
      hypertensive (see also Hypertension, heart) 402.90
      ischemic 414.8
      rheumatic (see also Degeneration, myocardium, with rheumatic fever) 398.0
      syphilitic 093.82
   nasal sinus (mucosa) (see also Sinusitis) 473.9
      frontal 473.1
      maxillary 473.0
   nerve - see Disorder, nerve

Degeneration, degenerative (Continued)
   nervous system 349.89
      amyloid 277.39 [357.4]
      autonomic (see also Neuropathy, peripheral, autonomic) 337.9
      fatty 349.89
      peripheral autonomic NEC (see also Neuropathy, peripheral, autonomic) 337.9
   nipple 611.9
   nose 478.19
   oculoacousticocerebral, congenital (progressive) 743.8
   olivopontocerebellar (familial) (hereditary) 333.0
   osseous labyrinth 386.8
   ovary 620.8
      cystic 620.2
      microcystic 620.2
   pallidal, pigmentary (progressive) 333.0
   pancreas 577.8
      tuberculous (see also Tuberculosis) 017.9●
   papillary muscle 429.81
   paving stone 362.61
   penis 607.89
   peritoneum 568.89
   pigmentary (diffuse) (general)
      localized - see Degeneration, by site
      pallidal (progressive) 333.0
      secondary 362.65
   pineal gland 259.8
   pituitary (gland) 253.8
   placenta (fatty) (fibrinoid) (fibroid) - see Placenta, abnormal
   popliteal fat pad 729.31
   posterolateral (spinal cord) (see also Degeneration, combined) 266.2 [336.2]
   pulmonary valve (heart) (see also Endocarditis, pulmonary) 424.3
   pulp (tooth) 522.2
   pupillary margin 364.54
   renal (see also Sclerosis, renal) 587
      fibrocystic 753.19
      polycystic 753.12
        adult type (APKD) 753.13
        autosomal dominant 753.13
        autosomal recessive 753.14
        childhood type (CPKD) 753.14
        infantile type 753.14
   reticuloendothelial system 289.89
   retina (peripheral) 362.60
      with retinal defect (see also Detachment, retina, with retinal defect) 361.00
      cystic (senile) 362.50
      cystoid 362.53
      hereditary (see also Dystrophy, retina) 362.70
        cerebroretinal 362.71
        congenital 362.75
        juvenile (Stargardt's) 362.75
        macula 362.76
      Kuhnt-Junius 362.52
      lattice 362.63
      macular (see also Degeneration, macula) 362.50
      microcystoid 362.62
      palisade 362.63
      paving stone 362.61
      pigmentary (primary) 362.74
        secondary 362.65
      posterior pole (see also Degeneration, macula) 362.50
      secondary 362.66
      senile 362.60
        cystic 362.53
        reticular 362.64
   saccule, congenital (causing impairment of hearing) 744.05
   sacculocochlear 386.8

Degeneration, degenerative (Continued)
   senile 797
      brain 331.2
      cardiac, heart, or myocardium (see also Degeneration, myocardial) 429.1
      motor centers 331.2
      reticule 362.64
      retina, cystic 362.50
      vascular - see Arteriosclerosis
   silicone rubber poppet (prosthetic valve) 996.02
   sinus (cystic) (see also Sinusitis) 473.9
      polypoid 471.1
   skin 709.3
      amyloid 277.39
      colloid 709.3
   spinal (cord) 336.8
      amyloid 277.39
      column 733.90
      combined (subacute) (see also Degeneration, combined) 266.2 [336.2]
        with anemia (pernicious) 281.0 [336.2]
      dorsolateral (see also Degeneration, combined) 266.2 [336.2]
      familial NEC 336.8
      fatty 336.8
      funicular (see also Degeneration, combined) 266.2 [336.2]
      heredofamilial NEC 336.8
      posterolateral (see also Degeneration, combined) 266.2 [336.2]
      subacute combined - see Degeneration, combined
      tuberculous (see also Tuberculosis) 013.8●
   spine 733.90
   spleen 289.59
      amyloid 277.39
      lardaceous 277.39
   stomach 537.89
      lardaceous 277.39
   strionigral 333.0
   sudoriparous (cystic) 705.89
   suprarenal (capsule) (gland) 255.8
      with hypofunction 255.41
   sweat gland 705.89
   synovial membrane (pulpy) 727.9
   tapetoretinal 362.74
      adult or presenile form 362.50
   testis (postinfectional) 608.89
   thymus (gland) 254.8
      fatty 254.8
      lardaceous 277.39
   thyroid (gland) 246.8
   tricuspid (heart) (valve) - see Endocarditis, tricuspid
   tuberculous NEC (see also Tuberculosis) 011.9●
   turbinate 733.90
   uterus 621.8
      cystic 621.8
   vascular (senile) - see also Arteriosclerosis
      hypertensive - see Hypertension
   vitreoretinal (primary) 362.73
      secondary 362.66
   vitreous humor (with infiltration) 379.21
   wallerian NEC - see Disorder, nerve
   waxy (any site) 277.39
   Wilson's hepatolenticular 275.1

Deglutition
   paralysis 784.99
      hysterical 300.11
   pneumonia 507.0

Degos' disease or syndrome 447.8

Degradation disorder, branched-chain amino-acid 270.3

Dehiscence
   anastomosis - see Complications, anastomosis
   cesarean wound 674.1●

Dehiscence (Continued)
    closure of
        cornea 998.32
        fascia, superficial or muscular 998.31
        internal organ 998.31
        mucosa 998.32
        muscle or muscle flap 998.31
        ribs or rib cage 998.31
        skin 998.32
        skull or craniotomy 998.31
        sternum or sternotomy 998.31
        subcutaneous tissue 998.32
        tendon or ligament 998.31
        traumatic laceration (external) (internal) 998.33
    episiotomy 674.2●
    operation wound 998.32
        deep 998.31
        external 998.32
        internal 998.31
        superficial 998.32
    perineal wound (postpartum) 674.2●
    postoperative 998.32
        abdomen 998.32
            internal 998.31
        internal 998.31
    traumatic injury wound repair 998.33
    uterine wound 674.1●
Dehydration (cachexia) 276.51
    with
        hypernatremia 276.0
        hyponatremia 276.1
    newborn 775.5
Deiters' nucleus syndrome 386.19
Déjérine's disease 356.0
Déjérine-Klumpke paralysis 767.6
Déjérine-Roussy syndrome 338.0
Déjérine-Sottas disease or neuropathy (hypertrophic) 356.0
Déjérine-Thomas atrophy or syndrome 333.0
de Lange's syndrome (Amsterdam dwarf, intellectual disabilities, and brachycephaly) 759.89
Delay, delayed
    adaptation, cones or rods 368.63
    any plane in pelvis
        affecting fetus or newborn 763.1
        complicating delivery 660.1●
    birth or delivery NEC 662.1●
        affecting fetus or newborn 763.9
        second twin, triplet, or multiple mate 662.3●
    closure - see also Fistula
        cranial suture 756.0
        fontanel 756.0
    coagulation NEC 790.92
    conduction (cardiac) (ventricular) 426.9
    delivery NEC 662.1●
        second twin, triplet, etc. 662.3●
            affecting fetus or newborn 763.89
    development
        in childhood 783.40
            physiological 783.40
        intellectual NEC 315.9
        learning NEC 315.2
        reading 315.00
        sexual 259.0
        speech 315.39
            and language due to hearing loss 315.34
            associated with hyperkinesis 314.1
        spelling 315.09
    gastric emptying 536.8
    menarche 256.39
        due to pituitary hypofunction 253.4
    menstruation (cause unknown) 626.8
    milestone in childhood 783.42
    motility - see Hypomotility
    passage of meconium (newborn) 777.1
    primary respiration 768.9
    puberty 259.0

Delay, delayed (Continued)
    separation of umbilical cord 779.83
    sexual maturation, female 259.0
    vaccination V64.00
Del Castillo's syndrome (germinal aplasia) 606.0
Deleage's disease 359.89
Deletion syndrome
    5p 758.31
    22q11.2 758.32
    autosomal NEC 758.39
    constitutional 5q deletion 758.39
Delhi (boil) (button) (sore) 085.1
Delinquency (juvenile) 312.9
    group (see also Disturbance, conduct) 312.2●
    neurotic 312.4
Delirium, delirious 780.09
    acute 780.09
        due to conditions classified elsewhere 293.0
    alcoholic 291.0
        acute 291.0
        chronic 291.1
    alcoholicum 291.0
    chronic (see also Psychosis) 293.89
        due to or associated with physical condition - see Psychosis, organic
    drug-induced 292.81
    due to conditions classified elsewhere 293.0
    eclamptic (see also Eclampsia) 780.39
    exhaustion (see also Reaction, stress, acute) 308.9
    hysterical 300.11
    in
        presenile dementia 290.11
        senile dementia 290.3
    induced by drug 292.81
    manic, maniacal (acute) (see also Psychosis, affective) 296.0●
        recurrent episode 296.1●
        single episode 296.0●
    puerperal 293.9
    senile 290.3
    subacute (psychotic) 293.1
    thyroid (see also Thyrotoxicosis) 242.9●
    traumatic - see also Injury, intracranial
        with
            lesion, spinal cord - see Injury, spinal, by site
            shock, spinal - see Injury, spinal, by site
    tremens (impending) 291.0
    uremic - see Uremia
    withdrawal
        alcoholic (acute) 291.0
            chronic 291.1
        drug 292.0
Delivery

> Note: Use the following fifth-digit subclassification with categories 640–649, 651–676:
>
> 0   unspecified as to episode of care
> 1   delivered, with or without mention of antepartum condition
> 2   delivered, with mention of postpartum complication
> 3   antepartum condition or complication
> 4   postpartum condition or complication

    breech (assisted) (buttocks) (complete) (frank) (spontaneous) 652.2●
        affecting fetus or newborn 763.0
        extraction NEC 669.6●
    cesarean (for) 669.7●
        abnormal
            cervix 654.6●
            pelvic organs of tissues 654.9●
            pelvis (bony) (major) NEC 653.0●

Delivery (Continued)
    cesarean (Continued)
        abnormal (Continued)
            (planned) occurring after 37 completed weeks of gestation but before 39 completed weeks gestation due to (spontaneous) onset of labor 649.8●
            presentation or position 652.9●
                in multiple gestation 652.6●
            size, fetus 653.5●
            soft parts (of pelvis) 654.9●
            uterus, congenital 654.0●
            vagina 654.7●
            vulva 654.8●
        abruptio placentae 641.2●
        acromion presentation 652.8●
        affecting fetus or newborn 763.4
        anteversion, cervix or uterus 654.4●
        atony, uterus 661.2●
            with hemorrhage 666.1●
        bicornis or bicornuate uterus 654.0●
        breech presentation (buttocks) (complete) (frank) 652.2●
        brow presentation 652.4●
        cephalopelvic disproportion (normally formed fetus) 653.4●
        chin presentation 652.4●
        cicatrix of cervix 654.6●
        contracted pelvis (general) 653.1●
            inlet 653.2●
            outlet 653.3●
        cord presentation or prolapse 663.0●
        cystocele 654.4●
        deformity (acquired) (congenital)
            pelvic organs or tissues NEC 654.9●
            pelvis (bony) NEC 653.0●
        displacement, uterus NEC 654.4●
        disproportion NEC 653.9●
        distress
            fetal 656.8●
            maternal 669.0●
        eclampsia 642.6●
        face presentation 652.4●
        failed
            forceps 660.7●
            trial of labor NEC 660.6●
            vacuum extraction 660.7●
            ventouse 660.7●
        fetal deformity 653.7●
        fetal-maternal hemorrhage 656.0●
        fetus, fetal
            distress 656.8●
            prematurity 656.8●
        fibroid (tumor) (uterus) 654.1●
        footling 652.8●
            with successful version 652.1●
        hemorrhage (antepartum) (intrapartum) NEC 641.9●
        hydrocephalic fetus 653.6●
        incarceration of uterus 654.3●
        incoordinate uterine action 661.4●
        inertia, uterus 661.2●
            primary 661.0●
            secondary 661.1●
        lateroversion, uterus or cervix 654.4●
        mal lie 652.9●
        malposition
            fetus 652.9●
                in multiple gestation 652.6●
            pelvic organs or tissues NEC 654.9●
            uterus NEC or cervix 654.4●
        malpresentation NEC 652.9●
            in multiple gestation 652.6●
        maternal
            diabetes mellitus (conditions classifiable to 249 and 250) 648.0●
            heart disease NEC 648.6●
        meconium in liquor 656.8●
            staining only 792.3

SECTION 1 INDEX TO DISEASES AND INJURIES / Delivery

Delivery (Continued)
- cesarean (Continued)
  - oblique presentation 652.3
  - oversize fetus 653.5
  - pelvic tumor NEC 654.9
  - placental insufficiency 656.5
  - placenta previa 641.0
    - with hemorrhage 641.1
  - poor dilation, cervix 661.0
  - pre-eclampsia 642.4
    - severe 642.5
  - previous
    - cesarean delivery, section 654.2
    - surgery (to)
      - cervix 654.6
      - gynecological NEC 654.9
      - rectum 654.8
      - uterus NEC 654.9
        - previous cesarean delivery, section 654.2
      - vagina 654.7
  - prolapse
    - arm or hand 652.7
    - uterus 654.4
  - prolonged labor 662.1
  - rectocele 654.4
  - retroversion, uterus or cervix 654.3
  - rigid
    - cervix 654.6
    - pelvic floor 654.4
    - perineum 654.8
    - vagina 654.7
    - vulva 654.8
  - sacculation, pregnant uterus 654.4
  - scar(s)
    - cervix 654.6
    - cesarean delivery, section 654.2
    - uterus NEC 654.9
      - due to previous cesarean delivery, section 654.2
  - Shirodkar suture in situ 654.5
  - shoulder presentation 652.8
  - stenosis or stricture, cervix 654.6
  - transverse presentation or lie 652.3
  - tumor, pelvic organs or tissues NEC 654.4
  - umbilical cord presentation or prolapse 663.0
- completely normal case - see category 650
- complicated (by) NEC 669.9
  - abdominal tumor, fetal 653.7
    - causing obstructed labor 660.1
  - abnormal, abnormality of
    - cervix 654.6
      - causing obstructed labor 660.2
    - forces of labor 661.9
    - formation of uterus 654.0
    - pelvic organs or tissues 654.9
      - causing obstructed labor 660.2
    - pelvis (bony) (major) NEC 653.0
      - causing obstructed labor 660.1
    - presentation or position NEC 652.9
      - causing obstructed labor 660.0
    - size, fetus 653.5
      - causing obstructed labor 660.1
    - soft parts (of pelvis) 654.9
      - causing obstructed labor 660.2
    - uterine contractions NEC 661.9
    - uterus (formation) 654.0
      - causing obstructed labor 660.2
    - vagina 654.7
      - causing obstructed labor 660.2
  - abnormally formed uterus (any type) (congenital) 654.0
    - causing obstructed labor 660.2
  - acromion presentation 652.8
    - causing obstructed labor 660.0
  - adherent placenta 667.0
    - with hemorrhage 666.0
  - adhesions, uterus (to abdominal wall) 654.4

Delivery (Continued)
- complicated NEC (Continued)
  - advanced maternal age NEC 659.6
    - multigravida 659.6
    - primigravida 659.5
  - air embolism 673.0
  - amnionitis 658.4
  - amniotic fluid embolism 673.1
  - anesthetic death 668.9
  - annular detachment, cervix 665.3
  - antepartum hemorrhage - see Delivery, complicated, hemorrhage
  - anteversion, cervix or uterus 654.4
    - causing obstructed labor 660.2
  - apoplexy 674.0
    - placenta 641.2
  - arrested active phase 661.1
  - asymmetrical pelvis bone 653.0
    - causing obstructed labor 660.1
  - atony, uterus with hemorrhage (hypotonic) (inertia) 666.1
    - hypertonic 661.4
  - Bandl's ring 661.4
  - Battledore placenta - see Placenta, abnormal
  - bicornis or bicornuate uterus 654.0
    - causing obstructed labor 660.2
  - birth injury to mother NEC 665.9
  - bleeding (see also Delivery, complicated, hemorrhage) 641.9
  - breech presentation (assisted) (buttocks) (complete) (frank) (spontaneous) 652.2
    - with successful version 652.1
  - brow presentation 652.4
  - cephalopelvic disproportion (normally formed fetus) 653.4
    - causing obstructed labor 660.1
  - cerebral hemorrhage 674.0
  - cervical dystocia 661.2
  - chin presentation 652.4
    - causing obstructed labor 660.0
  - cicatrix
    - cervix 654.6
      - causing obstructed labor 660.2
    - vagina 654.7
      - causing obstructed labor 660.2
  - coagulation defect 649.3
  - colporrhexis 665.4
    - with perineal laceration 664.0
  - compound presentation 652.8
    - causing obstructed labor 660.0
  - compression of cord (umbilical) 663.2
    - around neck 663.1
    - cord prolapsed 663.0
  - contraction, contracted pelvis 653.1
    - causing obstructed labor 660.1
    - general 653.1
      - causing obstructed labor 660.1
    - inlet 653.2
      - causing obstructed labor 660.1
    - midpelvic 653.8
      - causing obstructed labor 660.1
    - midplane 653.8
      - causing obstructed labor 660.1
    - outlet 653.3
      - causing obstructed labor 660.1
  - contraction ring 661.4
  - cord (umbilical) 663.9
    - around neck, tightly or with compression 663.1
      - without compression 663.3
    - bruising 663.6
    - complication NEC 663.9
      - specified type NEC 663.8
    - compression NEC 663.2
    - entanglement NEC 663.3
      - with compression 663.2
    - forelying 663.0
    - hematoma 663.6
    - marginal attachment 663.8

Delivery (Continued)
- complicated NEC (Continued)
  - cord (Continued)
    - presentation 663.0
    - prolapse (complete) (occult) (partial) 663.0
    - short 663.4
    - specified complication NEC 663.8
    - thrombosis (vessels) 663.6
    - vascular lesion 663.6
    - velamentous insertion 663.8
  - Couvelaire uterus 641.2
  - cretin pelvis (dwarf type) (male type) 653.1
    - causing obstructed labor 660.1
  - crossbirth 652.3
    - with successful version 652.1
    - causing obstructed labor 660.0
  - cyst (Gartner's duct) 654.7
  - cystocele 654.4
    - causing obstructed labor 660.2
  - death of fetus (near term) 656.4
    - early (before 22 completed weeks' gestation) 632
  - deformity (acquired) (congenital)
    - fetus 653.7
      - causing obstructed labor 660.1
    - pelvic organs or tissues NEC 654.9
      - causing obstructed labor 660.2
    - pelvis (bony) NEC 653.0
      - causing obstructed labor 660.1
  - delay, delayed
    - delivery in multiple pregnancy 662.3
      - due to locked mates 660.5
    - following rupture of membranes (spontaneous) 658.2
      - artificial 658.3
  - depressed fetal heart tones 659.7
  - diastasis recti 665.8
  - dilatation
    - bladder 654.4
      - causing obstructed labor 660.2
    - cervix, incomplete, poor or slow 661.0
  - diseased placenta 656.7
  - displacement uterus NEC 654.4
    - causing obstructed labor 660.2
  - disproportion NEC 653.9
    - causing obstructed labor 660.1
  - disruptio uteri - see Delivery, complicated, rupture, uterus
  - distress
    - fetal 656.8
    - maternal 669.0
  - double uterus (congenital) 654.0
    - causing obstructed labor 660.2
  - dropsy amnion 657
  - dysfunction, uterus 661.9
    - hypertonic 661.4
    - hypotonic 661.2
      - primary 661.0
      - secondary 661.1
    - incoordinate 661.4
  - dystocia
    - cervical 661.2
    - fetal - see Delivery, complicated, abnormal, presentation
    - maternal - see Delivery, complicated, prolonged labor
    - pelvic - see Delivery, complicated, contraction pelvis
    - positional 652.8
    - shoulder girdle 660.4
  - eclampsia 642.6
  - ectopic kidney 654.4
    - causing obstructed labor 660.2
  - edema, cervix 654.6
    - causing obstructed labor 660.2
  - effusion, amniotic fluid 658.1
  - elderly multigravida 659.6
  - elderly primigravida 659.5

Delivery *(Continued)*
  complicated NEC *(Continued)*
    embolism (pulmonary) 673.2●
      air 673.0●
      amniotic fluid 673.1●
      blood-clot 673.2●
      cerebral 674.0●
      fat 673.8●
      pyemic 673.3●
      septic 673.3●
    entanglement, umbilical cord 663.3●
      with compression 663.2●
      around neck (with compression) 663.1●
    eversion, cervix or uterus 665.2●
    excessive
      fetal growth 653.5●
        causing obstructed labor 660.1●
      size of fetus 653.5●
        causing obstructed labor 660.1●
    face presentation 652.4●
      causing obstructed labor 660.0●
      to pubes 660.3●
    failure, fetal head to enter pelvic brim 652.5●
      causing obstructed labor 660.0●
    female genital mutilation 660.8●
    fetal
      acid-base balance 656.8●
      death (near term) NEC 656.4●
        early (before 22 completed weeks' gestation) 632
      deformity 653.7●
        causing obstructed labor 660.1●
      distress 656.8●
      heart rate or rhythm 659.7●
      reduction of multiple fetuses reduced to single fetus 651.7●
    fetopelvic disproportion 653.4●
      causing obstructed labor 660.1●
    fever during labor 659.2●
    fibroid (tumor) (uterus) 654.1●
      causing obstructed labor 660.2●
    fibromyomata 654.1●
      causing obstructed labor 660.2●
    forelying umbilical cord 663.0●
    fracture of coccyx 665.6●
    hematoma 664.5●
      broad ligament 665.7●
      ischial spine 665.7●
      pelvic 665.7●
      perineum 664.5●
      soft tissues 665.7●
      subdural 674.0●
      umbilical cord 663.6●
      vagina 665.7●
      vulva or perineum 664.5●
    hemorrhage (uterine) (antepartum) (intrapartum) (pregnancy) 641.9●
      accidental 641.2●
      associated with
        afibrinogenemia 641.3●
        coagulation defect 641.3●
          hyperfibrinolysis 641.3●
          hypofibrinogenemia 641.3●
      cerebral 674.0●
      due to
        low-lying placenta 641.1●
        placenta previa 641.1●
        premature separation of placenta (normally implanted) 641.2●
        retained placenta 666.0●
        trauma 641.8●
        uterine leiomyoma 641.8●
      marginal sinus rupture 641.2●
      placenta NEC 641.9●
      postpartum (atonic) (immediate) (within 24 hours) 666.1●
        with retained or trapped placenta 666.0●
        delayed 666.2●

Delivery *(Continued)*
  complicated NEC *(Continued)*
    hemorrhage *(Continued)*
      postpartum *(Continued)*
        secondary 666.2●
        third stage 666.0●
    hourglass contraction, uterus 661.4●
    hydramnios 657●
    hydrocephalic fetus 653.6●
      causing obstructed labor 660.1●
    hydrops fetalis 653.7●
      causing obstructed labor 660.1●
    hypertension - *see* Hypertension, complicating pregnancy
    hypertonic uterine dysfunction 661.4●
    hypotonic uterine dysfunction 661.2●
    impacted shoulders 660.4●
    incarceration, uterus 654.3●
      causing obstructed labor 660.2●
    incomplete dilation (cervix) 661.0●
    incoordinate uterus 661.4●
    indication NEC 659.9●
      specified type NEC 659.8●
    inertia, uterus 661.2●
      hypertonic 661.4●
      hypotonic 661.2●
      primary 661.0●
      secondary 661.1●
    infantile
      genitalia 654.4●
        causing obstructed labor 660.2●
      uterus (os) 654.4●
        causing obstructed labor 660.2●
    injury (to mother) NEC 665.9●
    intrauterine fetal death (near term) NEC 656.4●
      early (before 22 completed weeks' gestation) 632
    inversion, uterus 665.2●
    kidney, ectopic 654.4●
      causing obstructed labor 660.2●
    knot (true), umbilical cord 663.2●
    labor
      onset (spontaneous) after 37 completed weeks of gestation but before 39 completed weeks gestation with delivery by (planned) cesarean section 649.8●
      premature (before 37 completed weeks gestation) 644.2●
    laceration 664.9●
      anus (sphincter) (healed) (old) 654.7●
        with mucosa 664.3●
        not associated with third-degree perineal laceration 664.6●
      bladder (urinary) 665.5●
      bowel 665.5●
      central 664.4●
      cervix (uteri) 665.3●
      fourchette 664.0●
      hymen 664.0●
      labia (majora) (minora) 664.0●
      pelvic
        floor 664.1●
        organ NEC 665.5●
      perineum, perineal 664.4●
        first degree 664.0●
        second degree 664.1●
        third degree 664.2●
        fourth degree 664.3●
        central 664.4●
        extensive NEC 664.4●
        muscles 664.1●
        skin 664.0●
        slight 664.0●
      peritoneum (pelvic) 665.5●
      periurethral tissue 664.8●

Delivery *(Continued)*
  complicated NEC *(Continued)*
    laceration *(Continued)*
      rectovaginal (septum) (without perineal laceration) 665.4●
        with perineum 664.2●
          with anal or rectal mucosa 664.3●
      skin (perineum) 664.0●
      specified site or type NEC 664.8●
      sphincter ani (healed) (old) 654.8●
        with mucosa 664.3●
        not associated with third-degree perineal laceration 664.6●
      urethra 665.5●
      uterus 665.1●
        before labor 665.0●
      vagina, vaginal (deep) (high) (sulcus) (wall) (without perineal laceration) 665.4●
        with perineum 664.0●
        muscles, with perineum 664.1●
      vulva 664.0●
    lateroversion, uterus or cervix 654.4●
      causing obstructed labor 660.2●
    locked mates 660.5●
    low implantation of placenta - *see* Delivery, complicated, placenta, previa
    mal lie 652.9●
    malposition
      fetus NEC 652.9●
        causing obstructed labor 660.0●
      pelvic organs or tissues NEC 654.9●
        causing obstructed labor 660.2●
      placenta 641.1●
        without hemorrhage 641.0●
      uterus NEC or cervix 654.4●
        causing obstructed labor 660.2●
    malpresentation 652.9●
      causing obstructed labor 660.0●
    marginal sinus (bleeding) (rupture) 641.2●
    maternal hypotension syndrome 669.2●
    meconium in liquor 656.8●
    membranes, retained - *see* Delivery, complicated, placenta, retained
    mentum presentation 652.4●
      causing obstructed labor 660.0●
    metrorrhagia (myopathia) - *see* Delivery, complicated, hemorrhage
    metrorrhexis - *see* Delivery, complicated, rupture, uterus
    multiparity (grand) 659.4●
    myelomeningocele, fetus 653.7●
      causing obstructed labor 660.1●
    Nägele's pelvis 653.0●
      causing obstructed labor 660.1●
    nonengagement, fetal head 652.5●
      causing obstructed labor 660.0●
    oblique presentation 652.3●
      causing obstructed labor 660.0●
    obstetric
      shock 669.1●
      trauma NEC 665.9●
    obstructed labor 660.9●
      due to
        abnormality of pelvic organs or tissues (conditions classifiable to 654.0–654.9) 660.2●
        deep transverse arrest 660.3●
        impacted shoulders 660.4●
        locked twins 660.5●
        malposition and malpresentation of fetus (conditions classifiable to 652.0–652.9) 660.0●
        persistent occipitoposterior 660.3●
        shoulder dystocia 660.4●
    occult prolapse of umbilical cord 663.0●
    oversize fetus 653.5●
      causing obstructed labor 660.1●

SECTION I INDEX TO DISEASES AND INJURIES / Delivery

Delivery *(Continued)*
   complicated NEC *(Continued)*
      pathological retraction ring, uterus 661.4
      pelvic
         arrest (deep) (high) (of fetal head)
            (transverse) 660.3
         deformity (bone) - *see also* Deformity,
            pelvis, with disproportion
            soft tissue 654.9
               causing obstructed labor 660.2
         tumor NEC 654.9
            causing obstructed labor 660.2
      penetration, pregnant uterus by
         instrument 665.1
      perforation - *see* Delivery, complicated,
         laceration
      persistent
         hymen 654.8
            causing obstructed labor 660.2
         occipitoposterior 660.3
      placenta, placental
         ablatio 641.2
         abnormality 656.7
            with hemorrhage 641.2
         abruptio 641.2
         accreta 667.0
            with hemorrhage 666.0
         adherent (without hemorrhage) 667.0
            with hemorrhage 666.0
         apoplexy 641.2
         Battledore - *see* Placenta, abnormal
         detachment (premature) 641.2
         disease 656.7
         hemorrhage NEC 641.9
         increta (without hemorrhage) 667.0
            with hemorrhage 666.0
         low (implantation) 641.1
            without hemorrhage 641.0
         malformation 656.7
            with hemorrhage 641.2
         malposition 641.1
            without hemorrhage 641.0
         marginal sinus rupture 641.2
         percreta 667.0
            with hemorrhage 666.0
         premature separation 641.2
         previa (central) (lateral) (marginal)
            (partial) 641.1
            without hemorrhage 641.0
         retained (with hemorrhage) 666.0
            without hemorrhage 667.0
         rupture of marginal sinus 641.2
         separation (premature) 641.2
         trapped 666.0
            without hemorrhage 667.0
         vicious insertion 641.1
      polyhydramnios 657
      polyp, cervix 654.6
         causing obstructed labor 660.2
      precipitate labor 661.3
      premature
         labor (before 37 completed weeks'
            gestation) 644.2
         rupture, membranes 658.1
            delayed delivery following 658.2
      presenting umbilical cord 663.0
      previous
         cesarean delivery, section 654.2
         surgery
            cervix 654.6
               causing obstructed labor 660.2
            gynecological NEC 654.9
               causing obstructed labor 660.2
            perineum 654.8
            rectum 654.8
            uterus NEC 654.9
               due to previous cesarean
                  delivery, section 654.2
            vagina 654.7
               causing obstructed labor 660.2
            vulva 654.8

Delivery *(Continued)*
   complicated NEC *(Continued)*
      primary uterine inertia 661.0
      primipara, elderly or old 659.5
      prolapse
         arm or hand 652.7
            causing obstructed labor 660.0
         cord (umbilical) 663.0
         fetal extremity 652.8
         foot or leg 652.8
            causing obstructed labor 660.0
         umbilical cord (complete) (occult)
            (partial) 663.0
         uterus 654.4
            causing obstructed labor 660.2
      prolonged labor 662.1
         first stage 662.0
         second stage 662.2
         active phase 661.2
         due to
            cervical dystocia 661.2
            contraction ring 661.4
            tetanic uterus 661.4
            uterine inertia 661.2
               primary 661.0
               secondary 661.1
         latent phase 661.0
      pyrexia during labor 659.2
      rachitic pelvis 653.2
         causing obstructed labor 660.1
      rectocele 654.4
         causing obstructed labor 660.2
      retained membranes or portions of
         placenta 666.2
         without hemorrhage 667.1
      retarded (prolonged) birth 662.1
      retention secundines (with hemorrhage)
         666.2
         without hemorrhage 667.1
      retroversion, uterus or cervix 654.3
         causing obstructed labor 660.2
      rigid
         cervix 654.6
            causing obstructed labor 660.2
         pelvic floor 654.4
            causing obstructed labor 660.2
         perineum or vulva 654.8
            causing obstructed labor 660.2
         vagina 654.7
            causing obstructed labor 660.2
      Robert's pelvis 653.0
         causing obstructed labor 660.1
      rupture - *see also* Delivery, complicated,
         laceration
         bladder (urinary) 665.5
         cervix 665.3
         marginal sinus 641.2
         membranes, premature 658.1
         pelvic organ NEC 665.5
         perineum (without mention of other
            laceration) - *see* Delivery,
            complicated, laceration,
            perineum
         peritoneum (pelvic) 665.5
         urethra 665.5
         uterus (during labor) 665.1
            before labor 665.0
      sacculation, pregnant uterus 654.4
      sacral teratomas, fetal 653.7
         causing obstructed labor 660.1
      scar(s)
         cervix 654.6
            causing obstructed labor 660.2
         cesarean delivery, section 654.2
            causing obstructed labor 660.2
         perineum 654.8
            causing obstructed labor 660.2
         uterus NEC 654.9
            causing obstructed labor 660.2
            due to previous cesarean delivery,
               section 654.2

Delivery *(Continued)*
   complicated NEC *(Continued)*
      scar(s) *(Continued)*
         vagina 654.7
            causing obstructed labor 660.2
         vulva 654.8
            causing obstructed labor 660.2
      scoliotic pelvis 653.0
         causing obstructed labor 660.1
      secondary uterine inertia 661.1
      secundines, retained - *see* Delivery,
         complicated, placenta, retained
      separation
         placenta (premature) 641.2
         pubic bone 665.6
         symphysis pubis 665.6
      septate vagina 654.7
         causing obstructed labor 660.2
      shock (birth) (obstetric) (puerperal)
         669.1
      short cord syndrome 663.4
      shoulder
         girdle dystocia 660.4
         presentation 652.8
            causing obstructed labor 660.0
      Siamese twins 678.1
      slow slope active phase 661.2
      spasm
         cervix 661.4
         uterus 661.4
      spondylolisthesis, pelvis 653.3
         causing obstructed labor 660.1
      spondylolysis (lumbosacral) 653.3
         causing obstructed labor 660.1
      spondylosis 653.0
         causing obstructed labor 660.1
      stenosis or stricture
         cervix 654.6
            causing obstructed labor 660.2
         vagina 654.7
            causing obstructed labor 660.2
      sudden death, unknown cause 669.9
      tear (pelvic organ) (*see also* Delivery,
         complicated, laceration) 664.9
         anal sphincter (healed) (old) 654.8
            not associated with third-degree
               perineal laceration 664.6
      teratomas, sacral, fetal 653.7
         causing obstructed labor 660.1
      tetanic uterus 661.4
      tipping pelvis 653.0
         causing obstructed labor 660.1
      transverse
         arrest (deep) 660.3
         presentation or lie 652.3
            with successful version 652.1
            causing obstructed labor 660.0
      trauma (obstetrical) NEC 665.9
         periurethral 664.8
      tumor
         abdominal, fetal 653.7
            causing obstructed labor 660.1
         pelvic organs or tissues NEC 654.9
            causing obstructed labor 660.2
      umbilical cord (*see also* Delivery,
         complicated, cord) 663.9
         around neck tightly, or with
            compression 663.1
         entanglement NEC 663.3
            with compression 663.2
         prolapse (complete) (occult) (partial)
            663.0
      unstable lie 652.0
         causing obstructed labor 660.0
      uterine
         inertia (*see also* Delivery, complicated,
            inertia, uterus) 661.2
         spasm 661.4
      vasa previa 663.5
      velamentous insertion of cord 663.8
      young maternal age 659.8

Delivery *(Continued)*
  delayed NEC 662.1●
    following rupture of membranes
      (spontaneous) 658.2●
        artificial 658.3●
    second twin, triplet, etc. 662.3●
  difficult NEC 669.9●
    previous, affecting management of
      pregnancy or childbirth V23.49
    specified type NEC 669.8●
  early onset (spontaneous) 644.2●
  footling 652.8●
    with successful version 652.1●
  forceps NEC 669.5●
    affecting fetus or newborn 763.2
  missed (at or near term) 656.4●
  multiple gestation NEC 651.9●
    with fetal loss and retention of one or
      more fetus(es) 651.6●
    following (elective) fetal reduction 651.7●
    specified type NEC 651.8●
      with fetal loss and retention of one or
        more fetus(es) 651.6●
      following (elective) fetal reduction
        651.7●
  nonviable infant 656.4●
  normal - *see* category 650
  precipitate 661.3●
    affecting fetus or newborn 763.6
  premature NEC (before 37 completed weeks'
    gestation) 644.2●
    previous, affecting management of
      pregnancy V23.41
  quadruplet NEC 651.2●
    with fetal loss and retention of one or
      more fetus(es) 651.5●
    following (elective) fetal reduction
      651.7●
  quintuplet NEC 651.8●
    with fetal loss and retention of one or
      more fetus(es) 651.6●
    following (elective) fetal reduction
      651.7●
  sextuplet NEC 651.8●
    with fetal loss and retention of one or
      more fetus(es) 651.6●
    following (elective) fetal reduction
      651.7●
  specified complication NEC 669.8●
  stillbirth (near term) NEC 656.4●
    early (before 22 completed weeks'
      gestation) 632
  term pregnancy (live birth) NEC - *see*
    category 650
    stillbirth NEC 656.4●
  threatened premature 644.2●
  triplets NEC 651.1●
    with fetal loss and retention of one or
      more fetus(es) 651.4●
    delayed delivery (one or more mates)
      662.3●
    following (elective) fetal reduction
      651.7●
    locked mates 660.5●
  twins NEC 651.0●
    with fetal loss and retention of one fetus
      651.3●
    delayed delivery (one or more mates)
      662.3●
    following (elective) fetal reduction 651.7●
    locked mates 660.5●
  uncomplicated - *see* category 650
  vacuum extractor NEC 669.5●
    affecting fetus or newborn 763.3
  ventouse NEC 669.5●
    affecting fetus or newborn 763.3
Dellen, cornea 371.41
Delusions (paranoid) 297.9
  grandiose 297.1
  parasitosis 300.29
  systematized 297.1

Dementia 294.20
  with behavioral disturbance (aggressive)
    (combative) (violent) 294.21
  alcohol-induced persisting (*see also*
    Psychosis, alcoholic) 291.2
  Alzheimer's - *see* Alzheimer's, dementia
  arteriosclerotic (simple type)
    (uncomplicated) 290.40
    with
      acute confusional state 290.41
      delirium 290.41
      delusions 290.42
      depressed mood 290.43
    depressed type 290.43
    paranoid type 290.42
  Binswanger's 290.12
  catatonic (acute) (*see also* Schizophrenia)
    295.2
  congenital (*see also* Disability, intellectual)
    319
  degenerative 290.9
    presenile-onset - *see* Dementia, presenile
    senile-onset - *see* Dementia, senile
  developmental (*see also* Schizophrenia) 295.9●
  dialysis 294.8
    transient 293.9
  drug-induced persisting (*see also* Psychosis,
    drug) 292.82
  due to or associated with condition(s)
    classified elsewhere
    Alzheimer's
      with behavioral disturbance 331.0
        [294.11]
      without behavioral disturbance 331.0
        [294.10]
    cerebral lipidoses
      with behavioral disturbance 330.1
        [294.11]
      without behavioral disturbance 330.1
        [294.10]
    epilepsy
      with behavioral disturbance 345.9●
        [294.11]
      without behavioral disturbance 345.9●
        [294.10]
    hepatolenticular degeneration
      with behavioral disturbance 275.1
        [294.11]
      without behavioral disturbance 275.1
        [294.10]
    HIV
      with behavioral disturbance 042
        [294.11]
      without behavioral disturbance 042
        [294.10]
    Huntington's chorea
      with behavioral disturbance 333.4
        [294.11]
      without behavioral disturbance 333.4
        [294.10]
    Jakob-Creutzfeldt disease (CJD)
      with behavioral disturbance 046.19
        [294.11]
      without behavioral disturbance 046.19
        [294.10]
      variant (vCJD) 046.11
        with dementia
          with behavioral disturbance
            046.11 [294.11]
          without behavioral disturbance
            046.11 [294.10]
    Lewy bodies
      with behavioral disturbance 331.82
        [294.11]
      without behavioral disturbance 331.82
        [294.10]
    multiple sclerosis
      with behavioral disturbance 340
        [294.11]
      without behavioral disturbance 340
        [294.10]

Dementia *(Continued)*
  due to or associated with condition(s)
    classified elsewhere *(Continued)*
    neurosyphilis
      with behavioral disturbance 094.9
        [294.11]
      without behavioral disturbance 094.9
        [294.10]
    Parkinsonism
      with behavioral disturbance 331.82
        [294.11]
      without behavioral disturbance 331.82
        [294.10]
    Parkinson's disease
      with behavioral disturbance 332.0
        [294.11]
      without behavioral disturbance 332.0
        [294.10]
    Pelizaeus-Merzbacher disease
      with behavioral disturbance 333.0
        [294.11]
      without behavioral disturbance 333.0
        [294.10]
    Pick's disease
      with behavioral disturbance 331.11
        [294.11]
      without behavioral disturbance 331.11
        [294.10]
    polyarteritis nodosa
      with behavioral disturbance 446.0
        [294.11]
      without behavioral disturbance 446.0
        [294.10]
    syphilis
      with behavioral disturbance 094.1
        [294.11]
      without behavioral disturbance 094.1
        [294.10]
    Wilson's disease
      with behavioral disturbance 275.1
        [294.11]
      without behavioral disturbance 275.1
        [294.10]
  frontal 331.19
    with behavioral disturbance 331.19
      [294.11]
    without behavioral disturbance 331.19
      [294.10]
  frontotemporal 331.19
    with behavioral disturbance 331.19
      [294.11]
    without behavioral disturbance 331.19
      [294.10]
  hebephrenic (acute) 295.1●
  Heller's (infantile psychosis) (*see also*
    Psychosis, childhood) 299.1●
  idiopathic 290.9
    presenile-onset - *see* Dementia, presenile
    senile-onset - *see* Dementia, senile
  in
    arteriosclerotic brain disease 290.40
    senility 290.0
  induced by drug 292.82
  infantile, infantilia (*see also* Psychosis,
    childhood) 299.0●
  Lewy body 331.82
    with behavioral disturbance 331.82
      [294.11]
    without behavioral disturbance 331.82
      [294.10]
  multi-infarct (cerebrovascular) (*see also*
    Dementia, arteriosclerotic) 290.40
  old age 290.0
  paralytica, paralytic 094.1
    juvenilis 090.40
    syphilitic 094.1
      congenital 090.40
    tabetic form 094.1
  paranoid (*see also* Schizophrenia) 295.3●
  paraphrenic (*see also* Schizophrenia) 295.3●
  paretic 094.1

SECTION I INDEX TO DISEASES AND INJURIES / Dementia

Dementia (Continued)
- praecox (see also Schizophrenia) 295.9
- presenile 290.10
  - with
    - acute confusional state 290.11
    - delirium 290.11
    - delusional features 290.12
    - depressive features 290.13
  - depressed type 290.13
  - paranoid type 290.12
  - simple type 290.10
  - uncomplicated 290.10
- primary (acute) (see also Schizophrenia) 295.0
- progressive, syphilitic 094.1
- puerperal - see Psychosis, puerperal
- schizophrenic (see also Schizophrenia) 295.9
- senile 290.0
  - with
    - acute confusional state 290.3
    - delirium 290.3
    - delusional features 290.20
    - depressive features 290.21
  - depressed type 290.21
  - exhaustion 290.0
  - paranoid type 290.20
- simple type (acute) (see also Schizophrenia) 295.0
- simplex (acute) (see also Schizophrenia) 295.0
- syphilitic 094.1
- uremic - see Uremia
- vascular 290.40
  - with
    - delirium 290.41
    - delusions 290.42
    - depressed mood 290.43

Demerol dependence (see also Dependence) 304.0

Demineralization, ankle (see also Osteoporosis) 733.00

Demodex folliculorum (infestation) 133.8

Demoralization 799.25

de Morgan's spots (senile angiomas) 448.1

Demyelinating
- polyneuritis, chronic inflammatory 357.81

Demyelination, demyelinization
- central nervous system 341.9
  - specified NEC 341.8
- corpus callosum (central) 341.8
- global 340

Dengue (fever) 061
- sandfly 061
- vaccination, prophylactic (against) V05.1
- virus hemorrhagic fever 065.4

Dens
- evaginatus 520.2
- in dente 520.2
- invaginatus 520.2

Dense
- breast(s) 793.82

Density
- increased, bone (disseminated) (generalized) (spotted) 733.99
- lung (nodular) 518.89

Dental - see also condition
- examination only V72.2

Dentia praecox 520.6

Denticles (in pulp) 522.2

Dentigerous cyst 526.0

Dentin
- irregular (in pulp) 522.3
- opalescent 520.5
- secondary (in pulp) 522.3
- sensitive 521.89

Dentinogenesis imperfecta 520.5

Dentinoma (M9271/0) 213.1
- upper jaw (bone) 213.0

Dentition 520.7
- abnormal 520.6
- anomaly 520.6

Dentition (Continued)
- delayed 520.6
- difficult 520.7
- disorder of 520.6
- precocious 520.6
- retarded 520.6

Denture sore (mouth) 528.9

Dependence

> Note: Use the following fifth-digit subclassification with category 304:
> 0 unspecified
> 1 continuous
> 2 episodic
> 3 in remission

- with
  - withdrawal symptoms
    - alcohol 291.81
    - drug 292.0
- 14-hydroxy-dihydromorphinone 304.0
- absinthe 304.6
- acemorphan 304.0
- acetanilid(e) 304.6
- acetophenetidin 304.6
- acetorphine 304.0
- acetyldihydrocodeine 304.0
- acetyldihydrocodeinone 304.0
- Adalin 304.1
- Afghanistan black 304.3
- agrypnal 304.1
- alcohol, alcoholic (ethyl) (methyl) (wood) 303.9
  - maternal, with suspected fetal damage affecting management of pregnancy 655.4
- allobarbitone 304.1
- allonal 304.1
- allylisopropylacetylurea 304.1
- alphaprodine (hydrochloride) 304.0
- Alurate 304.1
- Alvodine 304.0
- amethocaine 304.6
- amidone 304.0
- amidopyrine 304.6
- aminopyrine 304.6
- amobarbital 304.1
- amphetamine(s) (type) (drugs classifiable to 969.72) 304.4
- amylene hydrate 304.6
- amylobarbitone 304.1
- amylocaine 304.6
- Amytal (sodium) 304.1
- analgesic (drug) NEC 304.6
  - synthetic with morphine-like effect 304.0
- anesthetic (agent) (drug) (gas) (general) (local) NEC 304.6
- Angel dust 304.6
- anileridine 304.0
- antipyrine 304.6
- anxiolytic 304.1
- aprobarbital 304.1
- aprobarbitone 304.1
- atropine 304.6
- Avertin (bromide) 304.6
- barbenyl 304.1
- barbital(s) 304.1
- barbitone 304.1
- barbiturate(s) (compounds) (drugs classifiable to 967.0) 304.1
- barbituric acid (and compounds) 304.1
- benzedrine 304.4
- benzylmorphine 304.0
- Beta-chlor 304.1
- bhang 304.3
- blue velvet 304.0
- Brevital 304.1
- bromal (hydrate) 304.1
- bromide(s) NEC 304.1
- bromine compounds NEC 304.1

Dependence (Continued)
- bromisovalum 304.1
- bromoform 304.1
- Bromo-seltzer 304.1
- bromural 304.1
- butabarbital (sodium) 304.1
- butabarpal 304.1
- butallylonal 304.1
- butethal 304.1
- buthalitone (sodium) 304.1
- Butisol 304.1
- butobarbitone 304.1
- butyl chloral (hydrate) 304.1
- caffeine 304.4
- cannabis (indica) (sativa) (resin) (derivatives) (type) 304.3
- carbamazepine 304.6
- Carbrital 304.1
- carbromal 304.1
- carisoprodol 304.6
- Catha (edulis) 304.4
- chloral (betaine) (hydrate) 304.1
- chloralamide 304.1
- chloralformamide 304.1
- chloralose 304.1
- chlordiazepoxide 304.1
- Chloretone 304.1
- chlorobutanol 304.1
- chlorodyne 304.1
- chloroform 304.6
- Cliradon 304.0
- coca (leaf) and derivatives 304.2
- cocaine 304.2
  - hydrochloride 304.2
  - salt (any) 304.2
- codeine 304.0
- combination of drugs (excluding morphine or opioid type drug) NEC 304.8
  - morphine or opioid type drug with any other drug 304.7
- croton-chloral 304.1
- cyclobarbital 304.1
- cyclobarbitone 304.1
- dagga 304.3
- Delvinal 304.1
- Demerol 304.0
- desocodeine 304.0
- desomorphine 304.0
- desoxyephedrine 304.4
- DET 304.5
- dexamphetamine 304.4
- dexedrine 304.4
- dextromethorphan 304.0
- dextromoramide 304.0
- dextronorpseudoephedrine 304.4
- dextrorphan 304.0
- diacetylmorphine 304.0
- Dial 304.1
- diallylbarbituric acid 304.1
- diamorphine 304.0
- diazepam 304.1
- dibucaine 304.6
- dichloroethane 304.6
- diethyl barbituric acid 304.1
- diethylsulfone-diethylmethane 304.1
- difencloxazine 304.0
- dihydrocodeine 304.0
- dihydrocodeinone 304.0
- dihydrohydroxycodeinone 304.0
- dihydroisocodeine 304.0
- dihydromorphine 304.0
- dihydromorphinone 304.0
- dihydroxcodeinone 304.0
- Dilaudid 304.0
- dimenhydrinate 304.6
- dimethylmeperidine 304.0
- dimethyltriptamine 304.5
- Dionin 304.0
- diphenoxylate 304.6
- dipipanone 304.0
- d-lysergic acid diethylamide 304.5

Dependence (Continued)
DMT 304.5
Dolophine 304.0
DOM 304.2
doriden 304.1
dormiral 304.1
Dormison 304.1
Dromoran 304.0
drug NEC 304.9
    analgesic NEC 304.6
    combination (excluding morphine or opioid type drug) NEC 304.8
    morphine or opioid type drug with any other drug 304.7
    complicating pregnancy, childbirth, or puerperium 648.3
        affecting fetus or newborn 779.5
    hallucinogenic 304.5
    hypnotic NEC 304.1
    narcotic NEC 304.9
    psychostimulant NEC 304.4
    sedative 304.1
    soporific NEC 304.1
    specified type NEC 304.6
    suspected damage to fetus affecting management of pregnancy 655.5
    synthetic, with morphine-like effect 304.0
    tranquilizing 304.1
duboisine 304.6
ectylurea 304.1
Endocaine 304.6
Equanil 304.1
Eskabarb 304.1
ethchlorvynol 304.1
ether (ethyl) (liquid) (vapor) (vinyl) 304.6
ethidene 304.6
ethinamate 304.1
ethoheptazine 304.6
ethyl
    alcohol 303.9
    bromide 304.6
    carbamate 304.6
    chloride 304.6
    morphine 304.0
ethylene (gas) 304.6
    dichloride 304.6
ethylidene chloride 304.6
etilfen 304.1
etorphine 304.0
etoval 304.1
eucodal 304.0
euneryl 304.1
Evipal 304.1
Evipan 304.1
fentanyl 304.0
ganja 304.3
gardenal 304.1
gardenpanyl 304.1
gelsemine 304.6
Gelsemium 304.6
Gemonil 304.1
glucochloral 304.1
glue (airplane) (sniffing) 304.6
glutethimide 304.1
hallucinogenics 304.5
hashish 304.3
headache powder NEC 304.6
Heavenly Blue 304.5
hedonal 304.1
hemp 304.3
heptabarbital 304.1
Heptalgin 304.0
heptobarbitone 304.1
heroin 304.0
    salt (any) 304.0
hexethal (sodium) 304.1
hexobarbital 304.1
Hycodan 304.0
hydrocodone 304.0
hydromorphinol 304.0

Dependence (Continued)
hydromorphinone 304.0
hydromorphone 304.0
hydroxycodeine 304.0
hypnotic NEC 304.1
Indian hemp 304.3
inhalant 304.6
intranarcon 304.1
Kemithal 304.1
ketobemidone 304.0
khat 304.4
kif 304.3
Lactuca (virosa) extract 304.1
lactucarium 304.1
laudanum 304.0
Lebanese red 304.3
Leritine 304.0
lettuce opium 304.1
Levanil 304.1
Levo-Dromoran 304.0
levo-iso-methadone 304.0
levorphanol 304.0
Librium 304.1
Lomotil 304.6
Lotusate 304.1
LSD (-25) (and derivatives) 304.5
Luminal 304.1
lysergic acid 304.5
    amide 304.5
maconha 304.3
magic mushroom 304.5
marihuana 304.3
MDA (methylene dioxyamphetamine) 304.4
Mebaral 304.1
Medinal 304.1
Medomin 304.1
megahallucinogenics 304.5
meperidine 304.0
mephobarbital 304.1
meprobamate 304.1
mescaline 304.5
methadone 304.0
methamphetamine(s) 304.4
methaqualone 304.1
metharbital 304.1
methitural 304.1
methobarbitone 304.1
methohexital 304.1
methopholine 304.6
methyl
    alcohol 303.9
    bromide 304.6
    morphine 304.0
    sulfonal 304.1
methylated spirit 303.9
methylbutinol 304.6
methyldihydromorphinone 304.0
methylene
    chloride 304.6
    dichloride 304.6
    dioxyamphetamine (MDA) 304.4
methylparafynol 304.1
methylphenidate 304.4
methyprylone 304.1
metopon 304.0
Miltown 304.1
morning glory seeds 304.5
morphinan(s) 304.0
morphine (sulfate) (sulfite) (type) (drugs classifiable to 965.00–965.09) 304.0
morphine or opioid type drug (drugs classifiable to 965.00–965.09) with any other drug 304.7
morphinol(s) 304.0
morphinon 304.0
morpholinylethylmorphine 304.0
mylomide 304.1
myristicin 304.5
narcotic (drug) NEC 304.9
nealbarbital 304.1

Dependence (Continued)
nealbarbitone 304.1
Nembutal 304.1
Neonal 304.1
Neraval 304.1
Neravan 304.1
neurobarb 304.1
nicotine 305.1
Nisentil 304.0
nitrous oxide 304.6
Noctec 304.1
Noludar 304.1
nonbarbiturate sedatives and tranquilizers with similar effect 304.1
noptil 304.1
normorphine 304.0
noscapine 304.0
Novocaine 304.6
Numorphan 304.0
nunol 304.1
Nupercaine 304.6
Oblivon 304.1
on
    aspirator V46.0
    hemodialysis V45.11
    hyperbaric chamber V46.8
    iron lung V46.11
    machine (enabling) V46.9
        specified type NEC V46.8
    peritoneal dialysis V45.11
    Possum (patient-operated-selector-mechanism) V46.8
    renal dialysis machine V45.11
    respirator [ventilator] V46.11
        encounter
            during
                power failure V46.12
                mechanical failure V46.14
            for weaning V46.13
    supplemental oxygen V46.2
    wheelchair V46.3
opiate 304.0
opioids 304.0
opioid type drug 304.0
    with any other drug 304.7
opium (alkaloids) (derivatives) (tincture) 304.0
ortal 304.1
oxazepam 304.1
oxycodone 304.0
oxymorphone 304.0
Palfium 304.0
Panadol 304.6
pantopium 304.0
pantopon 304.0
papaverine 304.0
paracetamol 304.6
paracodin 304.0
paraldehyde 304.1
paregoric 304.0
Parzone 304.0
PCP (phencyclidine) 304.6
Pearly Gates 304.5
pentazocine 304.0
pentobarbital 304.1
pentobarbitone (sodium) 304.1
Pentothal 304.1
Percaine 304.6
Percodan 304.0
Perichlor 304.1
Pernocton 304.1
Pernoston 304.1
peronine 304.0
pethidine (hydrochloride) 304.0
petrichloral 304.1
peyote 304.5
Phanodorn 304.1
phenacetin 304.6
phenadoxone 304.0
phenaglycodol 304.1
phenazocine 304.0

SECTION I INDEX TO DISEASES AND INJURIES / Dependence

Dependence (Continued)
  phencyclidine 304.6
  phenmetrazine 304.4
  phenobal 304.1
  phenobarbital 304.1
  phenobarbitone 304.1
  phenomorphan 304.0
  phenonyl 304.1
  phenoperidine 304.0
  pholcodine 304.0
  piminodine 304.0
  Pipadone 304.0
  Pitkin's solution 304.6
  Placidyl 304.1
  polysubstance 304.8
  Pontocaine 304.6
  pot 304.3
  potassium bromide 304.1
  Preludin 304.4
  Prinadol 304.0
  probarbital 304.1
  procaine 304.6
  propanal 304.1
  propoxyphene 304.6
  psilocibin 304.5
  psilocin 304.5
  psilocybin 304.5
  psilocyline 304.5
  psilocyn 304.5
  psychedelic agents 304.5
  psychostimulant NEC 304.4
  psychotomimetic agents 304.5
  pyrahexyl 304.3
  Pyramidon 304.6
  quinalbarbitone 304.1
  racemoramide 304.0
  racemorphan 304.0
  Rela 304.6
  scopolamine 304.6
  secobarbital 304.1
  seconal 304.1
  sedative NEC 304.1
    nonbarbiturate with barbiturate effect 304.1
  Sedormid 304.1
  sernyl 304.1
  sodium bromide 304.1
  Soma 304.6
  Somnal 304.1
  Somnos 304.1
  Soneryl 304.1
  soporific (drug) NEC 304.1
  specified drug NEC 304.6
  speed 304.4
  spinocaine 304.6
  stovaine 304.6
  STP 304.5
  stramonium 304.6
  Sulfonal 304.1
  sulfonethylmethane 304.1
  sulfonmethane 304.1
  Surital 304.1
  synthetic drug with morphine-like effect 304.0
  talbutal 304.1
  tetracaine 304.6
  tetrahydrocannabinol 304.3
  tetronal 304.1
  THC 304.3
  thebacon 304.0
  thebaine 304.0
  thiamil 304.1
  thiamylal 304.1
  thiopental 304.1
  tobacco 305.1
  toluene, toluol 304.6
  tranquilizer NEC 304.1
    nonbarbiturate with barbiturate effect 304.1
  tribromacetaldehyde 304.6
  tribromethanol 304.6

Dependence (Continued)
  tribromomethane 304.6
  trichloroethanol 304.6
  trichoroethyl phosphate 304.1
  triclofos 304.1
  Trional 304.1
  Tuinal 304.1
  Turkish green 304.3
  urethan(e) 304.6
  Valium 304.1
  Valmid 304.1
  veganin 304.0
  veramon 304.1
  Veronal 304.1
  versidyne 304.6
  vinbarbital 304.1
  vinbarbitone 304.1
  vinyl bitone 304.1
  vitamin B_6 266.1
  wine 303.9
  Zactane 304.6
Dependency
  passive 301.6
  reactions 301.6
Depersonalization (episode, in neurotic state) (neurotic) (syndrome) 300.6
Depletion
  carbohydrates 271.9
  complement factor 279.8
  extracellular fluid 276.52
  plasma 276.52
  potassium 276.8
    nephropathy 588.89
  salt or sodium 276.1
    causing heat exhaustion or prostration 992.4
    nephropathy 593.9
  volume 276.50
    extracellular fluid 276.52
    plasma 276.52
Deployment (military)
  personal history of V62.22
  returned from V62.22
  status V62.21
Deposit
  argentous, cornea 371.16
  bone, in Boeck's sarcoid 135
  calcareous, calcium - see Calcification
  cholesterol
    retina 362.82
    skin 709.3
    vitreous (humor) 379.22
  conjunctival 372.56
  cornea, corneal NEC 371.10
    argentous 371.16
    in
      cystinosis 270.0 [371.15]
      mucopolysaccharidosis 277.5 [371.15]
  crystalline, vitreous (humor) 379.22
  hemosiderin, in old scars of cornea 371.11
  metallic, in lens 366.45
  skin 709.3
  teeth, tooth (betel) (black) (green) (materia alba) (orange) (soft) (tobacco) 523.6
  urate, in kidney (see also Disease, renal) 593.9
Depraved appetite 307.52
Depression 311
  acute (see also Psychosis, affective) 296.2
    recurrent episode 296.3
    single episode 296.2
  agitated (see also Psychosis, affective) 296.2
    recurrent episode 296.3
    single episode 296.2
  anaclitic 309.21
  anxiety 300.4
  arches 734
    congenital 754.61
  autogenous (see also Psychosis, affective) 296.2
    recurrent episode 296.3
    single episode 296.2

Depression (Continued)
  basal metabolic rate (BMR) 794.7
  bone marrow 289.9
  central nervous system 799.1
    newborn 779.2
  cerebral 331.9
    newborn 779.2
  cerebrovascular 437.8
    newborn 779.2
  chest wall 738.3
  endogenous (see also Psychosis, affective) 296.2
    recurrent episode 296.3
    single episode 296.2
  functional activity 780.99
  hysterical 300.11
  involutional, climacteric, or menopausal (see also Psychosis, affective) 296.2
    recurrent episode 296.3
    single episode 296.2
  major 296.2
    recurrent episode 296.3
    single episode 296.2
  manic (see also Psychosis, affective) 296.80
  medullary 348.89
    newborn 779.2
  mental 300.4
  metatarsal heads - see Depression, arches
  metatarsus - see Depression, arches
  monopolar (see also Psychosis, affective) 296.2
    recurrent episode 296.3
    single episode 296.2
  nervous 300.4
  neurotic 300.4
  nose 738.0
  postpartum 648.4
  psychogenic 300.4
    reactive 298.0
  psychoneurotic 300.4
  psychotic (see also Psychosis, affective) 296.2
    reactive 298.0
    recurrent episode 296.3
    single episode 296.2
  reactive 300.4
    neurotic 300.4
    psychogenic 298.0
    psychoneurotic 300.4
    psychotic 298.0
  recurrent 296.3
  respiratory center 348.89
    newborn 770.89
  scapula 736.89
  senile 290.21
  situational (acute) (brief) 309.0
    prolonged 309.1
  skull 754.0
  sternum 738.3
  visual field 368.40
Depressive reaction - see also Reaction, depressive
  acute (transient) 309.0
    with anxiety 309.28
  prolonged 309.1
  situational (acute) 309.0
    prolonged 309.1
Deprivation
  cultural V62.4
  emotional V62.89
    affecting
      adult 995.82
      infant or child 995.51
  food 994.2
    specific substance NEC 269.8
  protein (familial) (kwashiorkor) 260
  sleep V69.4
  social V62.4
    affecting
      adult 995.82
      infant or child 995.51

Deprivation (Continued)
  symptoms, syndrome
    alcohol 291.81
    drug 292.0
  vitamins (see also Deficiency, vitamin) 269.2
  water 994.3
de Quervain's
  disease (tendon sheath) 727.04
  syndrome 259.51
  thyroiditis (subacute granulomatous thyroiditis) 245.1
Derangement
  ankle (internal) 718.97
    current injury (see also Dislocation, ankle) 837.0
    recurrent 718.37
  cartilage (articular) NEC (see also Disorder, cartilage, articular) 718.0●
    knee 717.9
      recurrent 718.36
    recurrent 718.3●
  collateral ligament (knee) (medial) (tibial) 717.82
    current injury 844.1
      lateral (fibular) 844.0
    lateral (fibular) 717.81
      current injury 844.0
  cruciate ligament (knee) (posterior) 717.84
    anterior 717.83
      current injury 844.2
    current injury 844.2
  elbow (internal) 718.92
    current injury (see also Dislocation, elbow) 832.00
    recurrent 718.32
  gastrointestinal 536.9
  heart - see Disease, heart
  hip (joint) (internal) (old) 718.95
    current injury (see also Dislocation, hip) 835.00
    recurrent 718.35
  intervertebral disc - see Displacement, intervertebral disc
  joint (internal) 718.90
    ankle 718.97
    current injury - see also Dislocation, by site
      knee (venom, meniscus or cartilage (see also Tear, meniscus) 836.2
    elbow 718.92
    foot 718.97
    hand 718.94
    hip 718.95
    knee 717.9
    multiple sites 718.99
    pelvic region 718.95
    recurrent 718.30
      ankle 718.37
      elbow 718.32
      foot 718.37
      hand 718.34
      hip 718.35
      knee 718.36
      multiple sites 718.39
      pelvic region 718.35
      shoulder (region) 718.31
      specified site NEC 718.38
      temporomandibular (old) 524.69
      wrist 718.33
    shoulder (region) 718.91
    specified site NEC 718.98
    spine NEC 724.9
    temporomandibular 524.69
    wrist 718.93
  knee (cartilage) (internal) 717.9
    current injury (see also Tear, meniscus) 836.2
    ligament 717.89
      capsular 717.85
        collateral - see Derangement, collateral ligament

Derangement (Continued)
  knee (Continued)
    ligament (Continued)
      cruciate - see Derangement, cruciate ligament
      specified NEC 717.85
    recurrent 718.36
  low back NEC 724.9
  meniscus NEC (knee) 717.5
    current injury (see also Tear, meniscus) 836.2
    lateral 717.40
      anterior horn 717.42
      posterior horn 717.43
      specified NEC 717.49
    medial 717.3
      anterior horn 717.1
      posterior horn 717.2
    recurrent 718.3●
    site other than knee - see Disorder, cartilage, articular
  mental (see also Psychosis) 298.9
  rotator cuff (recurrent) (tear) 726.10
    current 840.4
  sacroiliac (old) 724.6
    current - see Dislocation, sacroiliac
  semilunar cartilage (knee) 717.5
    current injury 836.2
      lateral 836.1
      medial 836.0
    recurrent 718.3●
  shoulder (internal) 718.91
    current injury (see also Dislocation, shoulder) 831.00
    recurrent 718.31
  spine (recurrent) NEC 724.9
    current - see Dislocation, spine
  temporomandibular (internal) (joint) (old) 524.69
    current - see Dislocation, jaw
Dercum's disease or syndrome (adiposis dolorosa) 272.8
Derealization (neurotic) 300.6
Dermal - see condition
Dermaphytid - see Dermatophytosis
Dermatergosis - see Dermatitis
Dermatitis (allergic) (contact) (occupational) (venenata) 692.9
  ab igne 692.82
  acneiform 692.9
  actinic (due to sun) 692.70
    acute 692.72
    chronic NEC 692.74
    other than from sun NEC 692.82
  ambustionis
    due to
      burn or scald - see Burn, by site
      sunburn (see also Sunburn) 692.71
  amebic 006.6
  ammonia 691.0
  anaphylactoid NEC 692.9
  arsenical 692.4
  artefacta 698.4
    psychogenic 316 [698.4]
  asthmatic 691.8
  atopic (allergic) (intrinsic) 691.8
    psychogenic 316 [691.8]
  atrophicans 701.8
    diffusa 701.8
    maculosa 701.3
  autoimmune progesterone 279.49
  berlock, berloque 692.72
  blastomycetic 116.0
  blister beetle 692.89
  Brucella NEC 023.9
  bullosa 694.9
    striata pratensis 692.6
  bullous 694.9
    mucosynechial, atrophic 694.60
      with ocular involvement 694.61
    seasonal 694.8

Dermatitis (Continued)
  calorica
    due to
      burn or scald - see Burn, by site
      cold 692.89
      sunburn (see also Sunburn) 692.71
  caterpillar 692.89
  cercarial 120.3
  combustionis
    due to
      burn or scald - see Burn, by site
      sunburn (see also Sunburn) 692.71
  congelationis 991.5
  contusiformis 695.2
  diabetic 250.8●
  diaper 691.0
  diphtheritica 032.85
  due to
    acetone 692.2
    acids 692.4
    adhesive plaster 692.4
    alcohol (skin contact) (substances classifiable to 980.0–980.9) 692.4
      taken internally 693.8
    alkalis 692.4
    allergy NEC 692.9
    ammonia (household) (liquid) 692.4
    animal
      dander (cat) (dog) 692.84
      hair (cat) (dog) 692.84
    arnica 692.3
    arsenic 692.4
      taken internally 693.8
    blister beetle 692.89
    cantharides 692.3
    carbon disulphide 692.2
    caterpillar 692.89
    caustics 692.4
    cereal (ingested) 693.1
      contact with skin 692.5
    chemical(s) NEC 692.4
      internal 693.8
      irritant NEC 692.4
      taken internally 693.8
    chlorocompounds 692.2
    coffee (ingested) 693.1
      contact with skin 692.5
    cold weather 692.89
    cosmetics 692.81
    cyclohexanes 692.2
    dander, animal (cat) (dog) 692.84
    deodorant 692.81
    detergents 692.0
    dichromate 692.4
    drugs and medicinals (correct substance properly administered) (internal use) 693.0
      external (in contact with skin) 692.3
        wrong substance given or taken 976.9
          specified substance - see Table of Drugs and Chemicals
      wrong substance given or taken 977.9
        specified substance - see Table of Drugs and Chemicals
    dyes 692.89
      hair 692.89
    epidermophytosis - see Dermatophytosis
    esters 692.2
    external irritant NEC 692.9
      specified agent NEC 692.89
    eye shadow 692.81
    fish (ingested) 693.1
      contact with skin 692.5
    flour (ingested) 693.1
      contact with skin 692.5
    food (ingested) 693.1
      in contact with skin 692.5
    fruit (ingested) 693.1
      contact with skin 692.5
    fungicides 692.3

SECTION I INDEX TO DISEASES AND INJURIES / Dermatitis

Dermatitis (Continued)
  due to (Continued)
    furs 692.84
    glycols 692.2
    greases NEC 692.1
    hair, animal (cat) (dog) 692.84
    hair dyes 692.89
    hot
      objects and materials - see Burn, by site
      weather or places 692.89
    hydrocarbons 692.2
    infrared rays, except from sun 692.82
      solar NEC (see also Dermatitis, due to, sun) 692.70
    ingested substance 693.9
      drugs and medicinals (see also Dermatitis, due to, drugs and medicinals) 693.0
      food 693.1
      specified substance NEC 693.8
    ingestion or injection of
      chemical 693.8
      drug (correct substance properly administered) 693.0
        wrong substance given or taken 977.9
          specified substance - see Table of Drugs and Chemicals
    insecticides 692.4
    internal agent 693.9
      drugs and medicinals (see also Dermatitis, due to, drugs and medicinals) 693.0
      food (ingested) 693.1
        in contact with skin 692.5
      specified agent NEC 693.8
    iodine 692.3
    iodoform 692.3
    irradiation 692.82
    jewelry 692.83
    keratolytics 692.3
    ketones 692.2
    lacquer tree (Rhus verniciflua) 692.6
    light (sun) NEC (see also Dermatitis, due to, sun) 692.70
      other 692.82
    low temperature 692.89
    mascara 692.81
    meat (ingested) 693.1
      contact with skin 692.5
    mercury, mercurials 692.3
    metals 692.83
    milk (ingested) 693.1
      contact with skin 692.5
    Neomycin 692.3
    nylon 692.4
    oils NEC 692.1
    paint solvent 692.2
    pediculocides 692.3
    petroleum products (substances classifiable to 981) 692.4
    phenol 692.3
    photosensitiveness, photosensitivity (sun) 692.72
      other light 692.82
    plants NEC 692.6
    plasters, medicated (any) 692.3
    plastic 692.4
    poison
      ivy (Rhus toxicodendron) 692.6
      oak (Rhus diversiloba) 692.6
      plant or vine 692.6
      sumac (Rhus venenata) 692.6
      vine (Rhus radicans) 692.6
    preservatives 692.89
    primrose (primula) 692.6
    primula 692.6
    radiation 692.82
      sun NEC (see also Dermatitis, due to, sun) 692.70
      tanning bed 692.82

Dermatitis (Continued)
  due to (Continued)
    radioactive substance 692.82
    radium 692.82
    ragweed (Senecio jacobae) 692.6
    Rhus (diversiloba) (radicans) (toxicodendron) (venenata) (verniciflua) 692.6
    rubber 692.4
    scabicides 692.3
    Senecio jacobae 692.6
    solar radiation - see Dermatitis, due to, sun
    solvents (any) (substances classifiable to 982.0–982.8) 692.2
      chlorocompound group 692.2
      cyclohexane group 692.2
      ester group 692.2
      glycol group 692.2
      hydrocarbon group 692.2
      ketone group 692.2
      paint 692.2
    specified agent NEC 692.89
    sun 692.70
      acute 692.72
      chronic NEC 692.74
      specified NEC 692.79
      sunburn (see also Sunburn) 692.71
    sunshine NEC (see also Dermatitis, due to, sun) 692.70
    tanning bed 692.82
    tetrachlorethylene 692.2
    toluene 692.2
    topical medications 692.3
    turpentine 692.2
    ultraviolet rays, except from sun 692.82
      sun NEC (see also Dermatitis, due to, sun) 692.70
    vaccine or vaccination (correct substance properly administered) 693.0
      wrong substance given or taken
        bacterial vaccine 978.8
          specified - see Table of Drugs and Chemicals
        other vaccines NEC 979.9
          specified - see Table of Drugs and Chemicals
    varicose veins (see also Varicose, vein, inflamed or infected) 454.1
    x-rays 692.82
  dyshydrotic 705.81
  dysmenorrheica 625.8
  eczematoid NEC 692.9
    infectious 690.8
  eczematous NEC 692.9
  epidemica 695.89
  erysipelatosa 695.81
  escharotica - see Burn, by site
  exfoliativa, exfoliative 695.89
    generalized 695.89
    infantum 695.81
    neonatorum 695.81
  eyelid 373.31
    allergic 373.32
    contact 373.32
    eczematous 373.31
    herpes (zoster) 053.20
      simplex 054.41
    infective 373.5
      due to
        actinomycosis 039.3 [373.5]
        herpes
          simplex 054.41
          zoster 053.20
        impetigo 684 [373.5]
        leprosy (see also Leprosy) 030.0 [373.4]
        lupus vulgaris (tuberculous) (see also Tuberculosis) 017.0 ● [373.4]

Dermatitis (Continued)
  eyelid (Continued)
    infective (Continued)
      due to (Continued)
        mycotic dermatitis (see also Dermatomycosis) 111.9 [373.5]
          vaccinia 051.02 [373.5]
            postvaccination 999.0 [373.5]
          yaws (see also Yaws) 102.9 [373.4]
  facta, factitia 698.4
    psychogenic 316 [698.4]
  ficta 698.4
    psychogenic 316 [698.4]
  flexural 691.8
  follicularis 704.8
  friction 709.8
  fungus 111.9
    specified type NEC 111.8
  gangrenosa, gangrenous (infantum) (see also Gangrene) 785.4
  gestationis 646.8 ●
  gonococcal 098.89
  gouty 274.89
  harvest mite 133.8
  heat 692.89
  herpetiformis (bullous) (erythematous) (pustular) (vesicular) 694.0
    juvenile 694.2
    senile 694.5
  hiemalis 692.89
  hypostatic, hypostatica 454.1
    with ulcer 454.2
  impetiginous 684
  infantile (acute) (chronic) (intertriginous) (intrinsic) (seborrheic) 690.12
  infectiosa eczematoides 690.8
  infectious (staphylococcal) (streptococcal) 686.9
    eczematoid 690.8
  infective eczematoid 690.8
  Jacquet's (diaper dermatitis) 691.0
  leptus 133.8
  lichenified NEC 692.9
  lichenoid, chronic 701.0
  lichenoides purpurica pigmentosa 709.1
  meadow 692.6
  medicamentosa (correct substance properly administered) (internal use) (see also Dermatitis, due to, drugs or medicinals) 693.0
    due to contact with skin 692.3
  mite 133.8
  multiformis 694.0
    juvenile 694.2
    senile 694.5
  napkin 691.0
  neuro 698.3
  neurotica 694.0
  nummular NEC 692.9
  osteatosis, osteatotic 706.8
  papillaris capillitii 706.1
  pellagrous 265.2
  perioral 695.3
  perstans 696.1
  photosensitivity (sun) 692.72
    other light 692.82
  pigmented purpuric lichenoid 709.1
  polymorpha dolorosa 694.0
  primary irritant 692.9
  pruriginosa 694.0
  pruritic NEC 692.9
  psoriasiform nodularis 696.2
  psychogenic 316
  purulent 686.00
  pustular contagious 051.2
  pyococcal 686.00
  pyocyaneus 686.09
  pyogenica 686.00
  radiation 692.82
  repens 696.1
  Ritter's (exfoliativa) 695.81

Dermatitis *(Continued)*
  Schamberg's (progressive pigmentary dermatosis) 709.09
  schistosome 120.3
  seasonal bullous 694.8
  seborrheic 690.10
    infantile 690.12
  sensitization NEC 692.9
  septic *(see also* Septicemia) 686.00
    gonococcal 098.89
  solar, solare NEC *(see also* Dermatitis, due to, sun) 692.70
  stasis 454.1
    due to
      postphlebitic syndrome 459.12
        with ulcer 459.13
      varicose veins - *see* Varicose
    ulcerated or with ulcer (varicose) 454.2
  sunburn *(see also* Sunburn) 692.71
  suppurative 686.00
  traumatic NEC 709.8
  trophoneurotica 694.0
  ultraviolet, except from sun 692.82
    due to sun NEC *(see also* Dermatitis, due to, sun) 692.70
  varicose 454.1
    with ulcer 454.2
  vegetans 686.8
  verrucosa 117.2
  xerotic 706.8
Dermatoarthritis, lipoid 272.8 [713.0]
Dermatochalasia, dermatochalasis 374.87
Dermatofibroma (lenticulare) (M8832/0) - *see also* Neoplasm, skin, benign
  protuberans (M8832/1) - *see* Neoplasm, skin, uncertain behavior
Dermatofibrosarcoma (protuberans) (M8832/3) - *see* Neoplasm, skin, malignant
Dermatographia 708.3
Dermatolysis (congenital) (exfoliativa) 757.39
  acquired 701.8
  eyelids 374.34
  palpebrarum 374.34
  senile 701.8
Dermatomegaly NEC 701.8
Dermatomucomyositis 710.3
Dermatomycosis 111.9
  furfuracea 111.0
  specified type NEC 111.8
Dermatomyositis (acute) (chronic) 710.3
Dermatoneuritis of children 985.0
Dermatophiliasis 134.1
Dermatophytide - *see* Dermatophytosis
Dermatophytosis (Epidermophyton) (infection) (microsporum) (tinea) (Trichophyton) 110.9
  beard 110.0
  body 110.5
  deep seated 110.6
  fingernails 110.1
  foot 110.4
  groin 110.3
  hand 110.2
  nail 110.1
  perianal (area) 110.3
  scalp 110.0
  scrotal 110.8
  specified site NEC 110.8
  toenails 110.1
  vulva 110.8
Dermatopolyneuritis 985.0
Dermatorrhexis 756.83
  acquired 701.8
Dermatosclerosis *(see also* Scleroderma) 710.1
  localized 701.0
Dermatosis 709.9
  Andrews' 686.8
  atopic 691.8
  Bowen's (M8081/2) - *see* Neoplasm, skin, in situ

Dermatosis *(Continued)*
  bullous 694.9
    specified type NEC 694.8
  erythematosquamous 690.8
  exfoliativa 695.89
  factitial 698.4
  gonococcal 098.89
  herpetiformis 694.0
    juvenile 694.2
    senile 694.5
  hysterical 300.11
  linear IgA 694.8
  menstrual NEC 709.8
  neutrophilic, acute febrile 695.89
  occupational *(see also* Dermatitis) 692.9
  papulosa nigra 709.8
  pigmentary NEC 709.00
    progressive 709.09
    Schamberg's 709.09
    Siemens-Bloch 757.33
  progressive pigmentary 709.09
  psychogenic 316
  pustular subcorneal 694.1
  Schamberg's (progressive pigmentary) 709.09
  senile NEC 709.3
  specified NEC 702.8
  Unna's (seborrheic dermatitis) 690.10
Dermographia 708.3
Dermographism 708.3
Dermoid (cyst) (M9084/0) - *see also* Neoplasm, by site, benign
  with malignant transformation (M9084/3) 183.0
Dermopathy
  infiltrative, with thyrotoxicosis 242.0 ●
  nephrogenic fibrosing 701.8
  senile NEC 709.3
Dermophytosis - *see* Dermatophytosis
Descemet's membrane - *see* condition
Descemetocele 371.72
Descending - *see* condition
Descensus uteri (complete) (incomplete) (partial) (without vaginal wall prolapse) 618.1
  with mention of vaginal wall prolapse - *see* Prolapse, uterovaginal
Desensitization to allergens V07.1
Desert
  rheumatism 114.0
  sore *(see also* Ulcer, skin) 707.9
Desertion (child) (newborn) 995.52
  adult 995.84
Desmoid (extra-abdominal) (tumor) (M8821/1) - *see also* Neoplasm, connective tissue, uncertain behavior
  abdominal (M8822/1) - *see* Neoplasm, connective tissue, uncertain behavior
Despondency 300.4
Desquamative dermatitis NEC 695.89
Destruction
  articular facet *(see also* Derangement, joint) 718.9 ●
    vertebra 724.9
  bone 733.90
    syphilitic 095.5
  joint *(see also* Derangement, joint) 718.9 ●
    sacroiliac 724.6
  kidney 593.89
  live fetus to facilitate birth NEC 763.89
  ossicles (ear) 385.24
  rectal sphincter 569.49
  septum (nasal) 478.19
  tuberculous NEC *(see also* Tuberculosis) 011.9 ●
  tympanic membrane 384.82
  tympanum 385.89
  vertebral disc - *see* Degeneration, intervertebral disc
Destructiveness *(see also* Disturbance, conduct) 312.9
  adjustment reaction 309.3

Detachment
  cartilage - *see also* Sprain, by site
    knee - *see* Tear, meniscus
  cervix, annular 622.8
    complicating delivery 665.3 ●
  choroid (old) (postinfectional) (simple) (spontaneous) 363.70
    hemorrhagic 363.72
    serous 363.71
  knee, medial meniscus (old) 717.3
    current injury 836.0
  ligament - *see* Sprain, by site
  placenta (premature) - *see* Placenta, separation
  retina (recent) 361.9
    with retinal defect (rhegmatogenous) 361.00
      giant tear 361.03
      multiple 361.02
      partial
        with
          giant tear 361.03
          multiple defects 361.02
          retinal dialysis (juvenile) 361.04
          single defect 361.01
      retinal dialysis (juvenile) 361.04
      single 361.01
      subtotal 361.05
      total 361.05
    delimited (old) (partial) 361.06
    old
      delimited 361.06
      partial 361.06
      total or subtotal 361.07
    pigment epithelium (RPE) (serous) 362.42
      exudative 362.42
      hemorrhagic 362.43
    rhegmatogenous *(see also* Detachment, retina, with retinal defect) 361.00
    serous (without retinal defect) 361.2
    specified type NEC 361.89
    traction (with vitreoretinal organization) 361.81
  vitreous humor 379.21
Detergent asthma 507.8
Deterioration
  epileptic
    with behavioral disturbance 345.9 ● [294.11]
    without behavioral disturbance 345.9 ● [294.10]
  heart, cardiac *(see also* Degeneration, myocardial) 429.1
  mental *(see also* Psychosis) 298.9
  myocardium, myocardial *(see also* Degeneration, myocardial) 429.1
  senile (simple) 797
  transplanted organ - *see* Complications, transplant, organ, by site
de Toni-Fanconi syndrome (cystinosis) 270.0
Deuteranomaly 368.52
Deuteranopia (anomalous trichromat) (complete) (incomplete) 368.52
Deutschländer's disease - *see* Fracture, foot
Development
  abnormal, bone 756.9
  arrested 783.40
    bone 733.91
    child 783.40
    due to malnutrition (protein-calorie) 263.2
    fetus or newborn 764.9 ●
    tracheal rings (congenital) 748.3
  defective, congenital - *see also* Anomaly
    cauda equina 742.59
    left ventricle 746.9
      with atresia or hypoplasia of aortic orifice or valve with hypoplasia of ascending aorta 746.7
      in hypoplastic left heart syndrome 746.7

SECTION I INDEX TO DISEASES AND INJURIES / Development

Development (Continued)
  delayed (see also Delay, development) 783.40
    arithmetical skills 315.1
    language (skills) 315.31
      and speech due to hearing loss 315.34
      expressive 315.31
      mixed receptive-expressive 315.32
    learning skill, specified NEC 315.2
    mixed skills 315.5
    motor coordination 315.4
    reading 315.00
    specified
      learning skill NEC 315.2
      type NEC, except learning 315.8
    speech 315.39
      and language due to hearing loss 315.34
      associated with hyperkinesia 314.1
      phonological 315.39
    spelling 315.09
    written expression 315.2
  imperfect, congenital - see also Anomaly
    heart 746.9
    lungs 748.60
  improper (fetus or newborn) 764.9●
  incomplete (fetus or newborn) 764.9●
    affecting management of pregnancy 656.5●
    bronchial tree 748.3
    organ or site not listed - see Hypoplasia
    respiratory system 748.9
  sexual, precocious NEC 259.1
  tardy, mental (see also Disability, intellectual) 319

Developmental - see condition
Devergie's disease (pityriasis rubra pilaris) 696.4
Deviation
  conjugate (eye) 378.87
    palsy 378.81
    spasm, spastic 378.82
  esophagus 530.89
  eye, skew 378.87
  mandible, opening and closing 524.53
  midline (jaw) (teeth) 524.29
    specified site NEC - see Malposition
  occlusal plane 524.76
  organ or site, congenital NEC - see Malposition, congenital
  septum (acquired) (nasal) 470
    congenital 754.0
  sexual 302.9
    bestiality 302.1
    coprophilia 302.89
    ego-dystonic
      homosexuality 302.0
      lesbianism 302.0
    erotomania 302.89
      Clérambault's 297.8
    exhibitionism (sexual) 302.4
    fetishism 302.81
      transvestic 302.3
    frotteurism 302.89
    homosexuality, ego-dystonic 302.0
      pedophilic 302.2
    lesbianism, ego-dystonic 302.0
    masochism 302.83
    narcissism 302.89
    necrophilia 302.89
    nymphomania 302.89
    pederosis 302.2
    pedophilia 302.2
    sadism 302.84
    sadomasochism 302.84
    satyriasis 302.89
    specified type NEC 302.89
    transvestic fetishism 302.3
    transvestism 302.3
    voyeurism 302.82
    zoophilia (erotica) 302.1

Deviation (Continued)
  teeth, midline 524.29
  trachea 519.19
  ureter (congenital) 753.4
Devic's disease 341.0
Device
  cerebral ventricle (communicating) in situ V45.2
  contraceptive - see Contraceptive, device
  drainage, cerebrospinal fluid V45.2
Devil's
  grip 074.1
  pinches (purpura simplex) 287.2
Devitalized tooth 522.9
Devonshire colic 984.9
  specified type of lead - see Table of Drugs and Chemicals
Dextraposition, aorta 747.21
  with ventricular septal defect, pulmonary stenosis or atresia, and hypertrophy of right ventricle 745.2
  in tetralogy of Fallot 745.2
Dextratransposition, aorta 745.11
Dextrinosis, limit (debrancher enzyme deficiency) 271.0
Dextrocardia (corrected) (false) (isolated) (secondary) (true) 746.87
  with
    complete transposition of viscera 759.3
    situs inversus 759.3
Dextroversion, kidney (left) 753.3
Dhobie itch 110.3
DHTR (delayed hemolytic transfusion reaction) - see Complications, transfusion
Diabetes, diabetic (brittle) (congenital) (familial) (mellitus) (severe) (slight) (without complication) 250.0●

> Note: Use the following fifth-digit subclassification with category 250:
>
> 0   type II or unspecified type, not stated as uncontrolled
>
> Fifth-digit 0 is for use for type II patients, even if the patient requires insulin
>
> 1   type I [juvenile type], not stated as uncontrolled
>
> 2   type II or unspecified type, uncontrolled
>
> Fifth-digit 2 is for use for type II patients, even if the patient requires insulin
>
> 3   type I [juvenile type], uncontrolled

  with
    coma (with ketoacidosis) 250.3●
      due to secondary diabetes 249.3●
    hyperosmolar (nonketotic) 250.2●
      due to secondary diabetes 249.2●
    complication NEC 250.9●
      due to secondary diabetes 249.9●
      specified NEC 250.8●
        due to secondary diabetes 249.8●
    gangrene 250.7● [785.4]
      due to secondary diabetes 249.7● [785.4]
    hyperglycemia - code to Diabetes, by type, with 5th digit for not stated as uncontrolled
    hyperosmolarity 250.2●
      due to secondary diabetes 249.2●
    ketosis, ketoacidosis 250.1●
      due to secondary diabetes 249.1●
    loss of protective sensation (LOPS) - see Diabetes, neuropathy
    osteomyelitis 250.8● [731.8]
      due to secondary diabetes 249.8● [731.8]
    specified manifestations NEC 250.8●
      due to secondary diabetes 249.8●

Diabetes, diabetic (Continued)
  acetonemia 250.1●
    due to secondary diabetes 249.1●
  acidosis 250.1●
    due to secondary diabetes 249.1●
  amyotrophy 250.6● [353.5]
    due to secondary diabetes 249.6● [353.5]
  angiopathy, peripheral 250.7● [443.81]
    due to secondary diabetes 249.7● [443.81]
  asymptomatic 790.29
  autonomic neuropathy (peripheral) 250.6● [337.1]
    due to secondary diabetes 249.6● [337.1]
  bone change 250.8● [731.8]
    due to secondary diabetes 249.8● [731.8]
  borderline 790.29
  bronze, bronzed 275.01
  cataract 250.5● [366.41]
    due to secondary diabetes 249.5● [366.41]
  chemical induced - see Diabetes, secondary
  complicating pregnancy, childbirth, or puerperium 648.0●
  coma (with ketoacidosis) 250.3●
    due to secondary diabetes 249.3●
    hyperglycemic 250.3●
      due to secondary diabetes 249.3●
    hyperosmolar (nonketotic) 250.2●
      due to secondary diabetes 249.2●
    hypoglycemic 250.3●
      due to secondary diabetes 249.3●
    insulin 250.3●
      due to secondary diabetes 249.3●
  complicating pregnancy, childbirth, or puerperium (maternal) (conditions classifiable to 249 and 250) 648.0●
    affecting fetus or newborn 775.0
  complication NEC 250.9●
    due to secondary diabetes 249.9●
    specified NEC 250.8●
      due to secondary diabetes 249.8●
  dorsal sclerosis 250.6● [340]
    due to secondary diabetes 249.6● [340]
  drug-induced - see also Diabetes, secondary
    overdose or wrong substance given or taken - see Table of Drugs and Chemicals
  due to
    cystic fibrosis - see Diabetes, secondary
    infection - see Diabetes, secondary
  dwarfism-obesity syndrome 258.1
  gangrene 250.7● [785.4]
    due to secondary diabetes 249.7● [785.4]
  gastroparesis 250.6● [536.3]
    due to secondary diabetes 249.6● [536.3]
  gestational 648.8●
    complicating pregnancy, childbirth, or puerperium 648.8●
  glaucoma 250.5● [365.44]
    due to secondary diabetes 249.5● [365.44]
  glomerulosclerosis (intercapillary) 250.4● [581.81]
    due to secondary diabetes 249.4● [581.81]
  glycogenosis, secondary 250.8● [259.8]
    due to secondary diabetes 249.8● [259.8]
  hemochromatosis (see also Hemochromatosis) 275.03
  hyperosmolar coma 250.2●
    due to secondary diabetes 249.2●
  hyperosmolarity 250.2●
    due to secondary diabetes 249.2●
  hypertension-nephrosis syndrome 250.4● [581.81]
    due to secondary diabetes 249.4● [581.81]
  hypoglycemia 250.8●
    due to secondary diabetes 249.8●
  hypoglycemic shock 250.8●
    due to secondary diabetes 249.8●
  inadequately controlled - code to Diabetes, by type, with 5th digit for not stated as uncontrolled

Diabetes, diabetic (Continued)
- insipidus 253.5
  - nephrogenic 588.1
  - pituitary 253.5
  - vasopression-resistant 588.1
- intercapillary glomerulosclerosis 250.4● [581.81]
  - due to secondary diabetes 249.4● [581.81]
- iritis 250.5● [364.42]
  - due to secondary diabetes 249.5● [364.42]
- ketosis, ketoacidosis 250.1●
  - due to secondary diabetes 249.1●
- Kimmelstiel (-Wilson) disease or syndrome (intercapillary glomerulosclerosis) 250.4● [581.81]
  - due to secondary diabetes 249.4● [581.81]
- Lancereaux's (diabetes mellitus with marked emaciation) 250.8● [261]
  - due to secondary diabetes 249.8● [261]
- latent (chemical) - *see* Diabetes, secondary
- complicating pregnancy, childbirth, or puerperium 648.0●
- lipoidosis 250.8● [272.7]
  - due to secondary diabetes 249.8● [272.7]
- macular edema 250.5● [362.07]
  - due to secondary diabetes 249.5● [362.07]
- maternal
  - with manifest disease in the infant 775.1
  - affecting fetus or newborn 775.0
- microaneurysms, retinal 250.5● [362.01]
  - due to secondary diabetes 249.5● [362.01]
- mononeuropathy 250.6● [355.9]
  - due to secondary diabetes 249.6● [355.9]
- neonatal, transient 775.1
- nephropathy 250.4● [583.81]
  - due to secondary diabetes 249.4● [583.81]
- nephrosis (syndrome) 250.4● [581.81]
  - due to secondary diabetes 249.4● [583.81]
- neuralgia 250.6● [357.2]
  - due to secondary diabetes 249.6● [357.2]
- neuritis 250.6● [357.2]
  - due to secondary diabetes 249.6● [357.2]
- neurogenic arthropathy 250.6● [713.5]
  - due to secondary diabetes 249.6● [713.5]
- neuropathy 250.6● [357.2]
  - autonomic (peripheral) 250.6● [337.1]
    - due to secondary diabetes 249.6 [337.1]
  - due to secondary diabetes 249.6● [357.2]
- nonclinical 790.29
- osteomyelitis 250.8● [731.8]
  - due to secondary diabetes 249.8● [731.8]
- out of control - *code to* Diabetes, by type, with 5th digit for uncontrolled
- peripheral autonomic neuropathy 250.6● [337.1]
  - due to secondary diabetes 249.6● [337.1]
- phosphate 275.3
- polyneuropathy 250.6● [357.2]
  - due to secondary diabetes 249.6● [357.2]
- poorly controlled - *code to* Diabetes, by type, with 5th digit for not stated as uncontrolled
- renal (true) 271.4
- retinal
  - edema 250.5● [362.07]
    - due to secondary diabetes 249.5● [362.07]
  - hemorrhage 250.5● [362.01]
    - due to secondary diabetes 249.5● [362.01]
  - microaneurysms 250.5● [362.01]
    - due to secondary diabetes 249.5● [362.01]
  - retinitis 250.5● [362.01]
    - due to secondary diabetes 249.5● [362.01]
  - retinopathy 250.5● [362.01]
    - due to secondary diabetes 249.5● [362.01]
    - background 250.5● [362.01]
      - due to secondary diabetes 249.5● [362.01]

Diabetes, diabetic (Continued)
- retinopathy (Continued)
  - nonproliferative 250.5● [362.03]
    - due to secondary diabetes 249.5● [362.03]
    - mild 250.5● [362.04]
      - due to secondary diabetes 249.5● [362.04]
    - moderate 250.5● [362.05]
      - due to secondary diabetes 249.5● [362.05]
    - severe 250.5● [362.06]
      - due to secondary diabetes 249.5● [362.06]
  - proliferative 250.5● [362.02]
    - due to secondary diabetes 249.5● [362.02]
- secondary (chemical-induced) (due to chronic condition) (due to infection) (drug-induced) 249.0●
  - with
    - coma (with ketoacidosis) 249.3●
      - hyperosmolar (nonketotic) 249.2●
    - complication NEC 249.9●
      - specified NEC 249.8●
    - gangrene 249.7● [785.4]
    - hyperosmolarity 249.2●
    - ketosis, ketoacidosis 249.1●
    - osteomyelitis 249.8● [731.8]
    - specified manifestations NEC 249.8●
  - acetonemia 249.1●
  - acidosis 249.1●
  - amyotrophy 249.6● [353.5]
  - angiopathy, peripheral 249.7● [443.81]
  - autonomic neuropathy (peripheral) 249.6● [337.1]
  - bone change 249.8● [731.8]
  - cataract 249.5● [366.41]
  - coma (with ketoacidosis) 249.3●
    - hyperglycemic 249.3●
    - hyperosmolar (nonketotic) 249.2●
    - hypoglycemic 249.3●
    - insulin 249.3●
  - complicating pregnancy, childbirth, or puerperium (maternal) 648.0●
    - affecting fetus or newborn 775.0
  - complication NEC 249.9●
    - specified NEC 249.8●
  - dorsal sclerosis 249.6● [340]
  - due to overdose or wrong substance given or taken - *see* Table of Drugs and Chemicals
  - gangrene 249.7● [785.4]
  - gastroparesis 249.6● [536.3]
  - glaucoma 249.5● [365.44]
  - glomerulosclerosis (intercapillary) 249.4● [581.81]
  - glycogenosis, secondary 249.8● [259.8]
  - hyperosmolar coma 249.2●
  - hyperosmolarity 249.2●
  - hypertension-nephrosis syndrome 249.4● [581.81]
  - hypoglycemia 249.8●
  - hypoglycemic shock 249.8●
  - intercapillary glomerulosclerosis 249.4● [581.81]
  - iritis 249.5● [364.42]
  - ketosis, ketoacidosis 249.1●
  - Kimmelstiel (-Wilson) disease or syndrome (intercapillary glomerulosclerosis) 249.4● [581.81]
  - Lancereaux's (diabetes mellitus with marked emaciation) 249.8● [261]
  - lipoidosis 249.8● [272.7]
  - macular edema 249.5● [362.07]
  - maternal
    - with manifest disease in the infant 775.1
    - affecting fetus or newborn 775.0
  - microaneurysms, retinal 249.5● [362.01]
  - mononeuropathy 249.6● [355.9]

Diabetes, diabetic (Continued)
- secondary (Continued)
  - nephropathy 249.4● [583.81]
  - nephrosis (syndrome) 249.4● [581.81]
  - neuralgia 249.6● [357.2]
  - neuritis 249.6● [357.2]
  - neurogenic arthropathy 249.6● [713.5]
  - neuropathy 249.6● [357.2]
    - autonomic (peripheral) 249.6 [337.1]
  - osteomyelitis 249.8● [731.8]
  - peripheral autonomic neuropathy 249.6● [337.1]
  - polyneuropathy 249.6● [357.2]
  - retinal
    - edema 249.5● [362.07]
    - hemorrhage 249.5● [362.01]
    - microaneurysms 249.5● [362.01]
  - retinitis 249.5● [362.01]
  - retinopathy 249.5● [362.01]
    - background 249.5● [362.01]
    - nonproliferative 249.5● [362.03]
      - mild 249.5● [362.04]
      - moderate 249.5● [362.05]
      - severe 249.5● [362.06]
    - proliferative 249.5● [362.02]
  - ulcer (skin) 249.8● [707.9]
    - lower extremity 249.8● [707.10]
      - ankle 249.8● [707.13]
      - calf 249.8● [707.12]
      - foot 249.8● [707.15]
      - heel 249.8● [707.14]
      - knee 249.8● [707.19]
      - specified site NEC 249.8● [707.19]
      - thigh 249.8● [707.11]
      - toes 249.8● [707.15]
    - specified site NEC 249.8● [707.8]
  - xanthoma 249.8● [272.2]
- steroid induced - *see also* Diabetes, secondary
  - overdose or wrong substance given or taken 962.0
- stress 790.29
- subclinical 790.29
- subliminal 790.29
- sugar 250.0●
- ulcer (skin) 250.8● [707.9]
  - due to secondary diabetes 249.8● [707.9]
  - lower extremity 250.8● [707.10]
    - due to secondary diabetes 249.8● [707.10]
    - ankle 250.8● [707.13]
      - due to secondary diabetes 249.8● [707.13]
    - calf 250.8● [707.12]
      - due to secondary diabetes 249.8● [707.12]
    - foot 250.8● [707.15]
      - due to secondary diabetes 249.8● [707.15]
    - heel 250.8● [707.14]
      - due to secondary diabetes 249.8● [707.14]
    - knee 250.8● [707.19]
      - due to secondary diabetes 249.8● [707.19]
    - specified site NEC 250.8● [707.19]
      - due to secondary diabetes 249.8● [707.19]
    - thigh 250.8● [707.11]
      - due to secondary diabetes 249.8● [707.11]
    - toes 250.8● [707.15]
      - due to secondary diabetes 249.8● [707.15]
  - specified site NEC 250.8● [707.8]
    - due to secondary diabetes 249.8● [707.8]
- xanthoma 250.8● [272.2]
  - due to secondary diabetes 249.8● [272.2]

Diacyclothrombopathia 287.1
Diagnosis deferred 799.9

Dialysis (intermittent) (treatment)
- anterior retinal (juvenile) (with detachment) 361.04
- extracorporeal V56.0
- hemodialysis V56.0
  - status only V45.11
- peritoneal V56.8
  - status only V45.11
- renal V56.0
  - status only V45.11
- specified type NEC V56.8

Diamond-Blackfan anemia or syndrome (congenital hypoplastic anemia) 284.01

Diamond-Gardener syndrome (autoerythrocyte sensitization) 287.2

Diaper rash 691.0

Diaphoresis (excessive) NEC (see also Hyperhidrosis) 780.8

Diaphragm - see condition

Diaphragmalgia 786.52

Diaphragmitis 519.4

Diaphyseal aclasis 756.4

Diaphysitis 733.99

Diarrhea, diarrheal (acute) (autumn) (bilious) (bloody) (catarrhal) (choleraic) (chronic) (gravis) (green) (infantile) (lienteric) (noninfectious) (presumed noninfectious) (putrefactive) (secondary) (sporadic) (summer) (symptomatic) (thermic) 787.91
- achlorhydric 536.0
- allergic 558.3
- amebic (see also Amebiasis) 006.9
  - with abscess - see Abscess, amebic
  - acute 006.0
  - chronic 006.1
  - nondysenteric 006.2
- bacillary - see Dysentery, bacillary
- bacterial NEC 008.5
- balantidial 007.0
- bile salt-induced 579.8
- cachectic NEC 787.91
- chilomastix 007.8
- choleriformis 001.1
- coccidial 007.2
- Cochin-China 579.1
  - anguilluliasis 127.2
  - psilosis 579.1
- Dientamoeba 007.8
- dietetic 787.91
- due to
  - achylia gastrica 536.8
  - Aerobacter aerogenes 008.2
  - Bacillus coli - see Enteritis, E. coli
  - bacteria NEC 008.5
  - bile salts 579.8
  - Capillaria
    - hepatica 128.8
    - philippinensis 127.5
  - Clostridium perfringens (C) (F) 008.46
  - Enterobacter aerogenes 008.2
  - enterococci 008.49
  - Escherichia coli - see Enteritis, E. coli
  - Giardia lamblia 007.1
  - Heterophyes heterophyes 121.6
  - irritating foods 787.91
  - Metagonimus yokogawai 121.5
  - Necator americanus 126.1
  - Paracolobactrum arizonae 008.1
  - Paracolon bacillus NEC 008.47
    - Arizona 008.1
  - Proteus (bacillus) (mirabilis) (Morganii) 008.3
  - Pseudomonas aeruginosa 008.42
  - S. japonicum 120.2
  - specified organism NEC 008.8
    - bacterial 008.49
    - viral NEC 008.69
  - Staphylococcus 008.41
  - Streptococcus 008.49
    - anaerobic 008.46
  - Strongyloides stercoralis 127.2

Diarrhea, diarrheal (Continued)
- due to (Continued)
  - Trichuris trichiuria 127.3
  - virus NEC (see also Enteritis, viral) 008.69
- dysenteric 009.2
  - due to specified organism NEC 008.8
- dyspeptic 787.91
- endemic 009.3
  - due to specified organism NEC 008.8
- epidemic 009.2
  - due to specified organism NEC 008.8
- fermentative 787.91
- flagellate 007.9
- Flexner's (ulcerative) 004.1
- functional 564.5
  - following gastrointestinal surgery 564.4
  - psychogenic 306.4
- giardial 007.1
- Giardia lamblia 007.1
- hill 579.1
- hyperperistalsis (nervous) 306.4
- infectious 009.2
  - due to specified organism NEC 008.8
  - presumed 009.3
- inflammatory 787.91
  - due to specified organism NEC 008.8
- malarial (see also Malaria) 084.6
- mite 133.8
- mycotic 117.9
- nervous 306.4
- neurogenic 564.5
- parenteral NEC 009.2
- postgastrectomy 564.4
- postvagotomy 564.4
- prostaglandin induced 579.8
- protozoal NEC 007.9
- psychogenic 306.4
- septic 009.2
  - due to specified organism NEC 008.8
- specified organism NEC 008.8
  - bacterial 008.49
  - viral NEC 008.69
- Staphylococcus 008.41
- Streptococcus 008.49
  - anaerobic 008.46
- toxic 558.2
- travelers' 009.2
  - due to specified organism NEC 008.8
- trichomonal 007.3
- tropical 579.1
- tuberculous 014.8 ●
- ulcerative (chronic) (see also Colitis, ulcerative) 556.9
- viral (see also Enteritis, viral) 008.8
- zymotic NEC 009.2

Diastasis
- cranial bones 733.99
  - congenital 756.0
- joint (traumatic) - see Dislocation, by site
- muscle 728.84
  - congenital 756.89
- recti (abdomen) 728.84
  - complicating delivery 665.8 ●
  - congenital 756.79

Diastema, teeth, tooth 524.30

Diastematomyelia 742.51

Diataxia, cerebral, infantile 343.0

Diathesis
- allergic V15.09
- bleeding (familial) 287.9
- cystine (familial) 270.0
- gouty 274.9
- hemorrhagic (familial) 287.9
  - newborn NEC 776.0
- oxalic 271.8
- scrofulous (see also Tuberculosis) 017.2 ●
- spasmophilic (see also Tetany) 781.7
- ulcer 536.9
- uric acid 274.9

Diaz's disease or osteochondrosis 732.5

Dibothriocephaliasis 123.4
- larval 123.5

Dibothriocephalus (infection) (infestation) (latus) 123.4
- larval 123.5

Dicephalus 759.4

Dichotomy, teeth 520.2

Dichromat, dichromata (congenital) 368.59

Dichromatopsia (congenital) 368.59

Dichuchwa 104.0

Dicroceliasis 121.8

Didelphys, didelphic (see also Double uterus) 752.2

Didymitis (see also Epididymitis) 604.90

Died - see also Death
- without
  - medical attention (cause unknown) 798.9
  - sign of disease 798.2

Dientamoeba diarrhea 007.8

Dietary
- inadequacy or deficiency 269.9
- surveillance and counseling V65.3

Dietl's crisis 593.4

Dieulafoy lesion (hemorrhagic)
- of
  - duodenum 537.84
  - esophagus 530.82
  - intestine 569.86
  - stomach 537.84

Difficult
- birth, affecting fetus or newborn 763.9
- delivery NEC 669.9 ●

Difficulty
- feeding 783.3
  - adult 783.3
  - breast 676.8 ●
  - child 783.3
  - elderly 783.3
  - infant 783.3
  - newborn 779.31
  - nonorganic (infant) NEC 307.59
- mechanical, gastroduodenal stoma 537.89
- reading 315.00
- specific, spelling 315.09
- swallowing (see also Dysphagia) 787.20
- walking 719.7

Diffuse - see condition

Diffused ganglion 727.42

Di George's syndrome (thymic hypoplasia) 279.11

Digestive - see condition

Di Guglielmo's disease or syndrome (M9841/3) 207.0 ●

Dihydropyrimidine dehydrogenase disease (DPD) 277.6

Diktyoma (M9051/3) - see Neoplasm, by site, malignant

Dilaceration, tooth 520.4

Dilatation
- anus 564.89
  - venule - see Hemorrhoids
- aorta (focal) (general) (see also Ectasia, aortic) 447.70
  - with aneurysm 441.9
  - congenital 747.29
  - infectional 093.0
  - ruptured 441.5
  - syphilitic 093.0
- appendix (cystic) 543.9
- artery 447.8
- bile duct (common) (congenital) 751.69
  - acquired 576.8
- bladder (sphincter) 596.89
  - congenital 753.8
  - in pregnancy or childbirth 654.4 ●
    - causing obstructed labor 660.2 ●
      - affecting fetus or newborn 763.1
- blood vessel 459.89
- bronchus, bronchi 494.0
  - with acute exacerbation 494.1
- calyx (due to obstruction) 593.89

Dilatation (Continued)
  capillaries 448.9
  cardiac (acute) (chronic) (see also
      Hypertrophy, cardiac) 429.3
    congenital 746.89
      valve NEC 746.89
        pulmonary 746.09
    hypertensive (see also Hypertension,
        heart) 402.90
  cavum septi pellucidi 742.4
  cecum 564.89
    psychogenic 306.4
  cervix (uteri) - see also Incompetency, cervix
    incomplete, poor, slow
      affecting fetus or newborn 763.7
      complicating delivery 661.0 ●
        affecting fetus or newborn 763.7
  colon 564.7
    congenital 751.3
    due to mechanical obstruction 560.89
    psychogenic 306.4
  common bile duct (congenital) 751.69
    acquired 576.8
      with calculus, choledocholithiasis, or
          stones - see Choledocholithiasis
  cystic duct 751.69
    acquired (any bile duct) 575.8
  duct, mammary 610.4
  duodenum 564.89
  esophagus 530.89
    congenital 750.4
    due to
      achalasia 530.0
      cardiospasm 530.0
  Eustachian tube, congenital 744.24
  fontanel 756.0
  gallbladder 575.8
    congenital 751.69
  gastric 536.8
    acute 536.1
    psychogenic 306.4
  heart (acute) (chronic) (see also Hypertrophy,
      cardiac) 429.3
    congenital 746.89
    hypertensive (see also Hypertension,
        heart) 402.90
    valve - see also Endocarditis
      congenital 746.89
  ileum 564.89
    psychogenic 306.4
  inguinal rings - see Hernia, inguinal
  jejunum 564.89
    psychogenic 306.4
  kidney (calyx) (collecting structures) (cystic)
      (parenchyma) (pelvis) 593.89
  lacrimal passages 375.69
  lymphatic vessel 457.1
  mammary duct 610.4
  Meckel's diverticulum (congenital) 751.0
  meningeal vessels, congenital 742.8
  myocardium (acute) (chronic) (see also
      Hypertrophy, cardiac) 429.3
  organ or site, congenital NEC - see Distortion
  pancreatic duct 577.8
  pelvis, kidney 593.89
  pericardium - see Pericarditis
  pharynx 478.29
  prostate 602.8
  pulmonary
    artery (idiopathic) 417.8
      congenital 747.39
    valve, congenital 746.09
  pupil 379.43
  rectum 564.89
  renal 593.89
  saccule vestibularis, congenital 744.05
  salivary gland (duct) 527.8
  sphincter ani 564.89
  stomach 536.8
    acute 536.1
    psychogenic 306.4

Dilatation (Continued)
  submaxillary duct 527.8
  trachea, congenital 748.3
  ureter (idiopathic) 593.89
    congenital 753.20
    due to obstruction 593.5
  urethra (acquired) 599.84
  vasomotor 443.9
  vein 459.89
  ventricular, ventricle (acute) (chronic)
      (see also Hypertrophy, cardiac)
      429.3
    cerebral, congenital 742.4
    hypertensive (see also Hypertension,
        heart) 402.90
  venule 459.89
    anus - see Hemorrhoids
  vesical orifice 596.89
Dilated, dilation - see Dilatation
Diminished
  hearing (acuity) (see also Deafness)
      389.9
  pulse pressure 785.9
  vision NEC 369.9
  vital capacity 794.2
Diminuta taenia 123.6
Diminution, sense or sensation (cold) (heat)
    (tactile) (vibratory) (see also Disturbance,
    sensation) 782.0
Dimitri-Sturge-Weber disease
    (encephalocutaneous angiomatosis)
    759.6
Dimple
  parasacral 685.1
    with abscess 685.0
  pilonidal 685.1
    with abscess 685.0
  postanal 685.1
    with abscess 685.0
Dioctophyma renale (infection) (infestation)
    128.8
Dipetalonemiasis 125.4
Diphallus 752.69
Diphtheria, diphtheritic (gangrenous)
    (hemorrhagic) 032.9
  carrier (suspected) of V02.4
  cutaneous 032.85
  cystitis 032.84
  faucial 032.0
  infection of wound 032.85
  inoculation (anti) (not sick) V03.5
  laryngeal 032.3
  myocarditis 032.82
  nasal anterior 032.2
  nasopharyngeal 032.1
  neurological complication 032.89
  peritonitis 032.83
  specified site NEC 032.89
Diphyllobothriasis (intestine) 123.4
  larval 123.5
Diplacusis 388.41
Diplegia (upper limbs) 344.2
  brain or cerebral 437.8
  congenital 343.0
  facial 351.0
    congenital 352.6
  infantile or congenital (cerebral) (spastic)
      (spinal) 343.0
  lower limbs 344.1
  syphilitic, congenital 090.49
Diplococcus, diplococcal - see condition
Diplomyelia 742.59
Diplopia 368.2
  refractive 368.15
Dipsomania (see also Alcoholism) 303.9 ●
  with psychosis (see also Psychosis, alcoholic)
      291.9
Dipylidiasis 123.8
  intestine 123.8
Direction, teeth, abnormal 524.30
Dirt-eating child 307.52

Disability, disabilities
  heart - see Disease, heart
  intellectual 319
    borderline V62.89
    mild, IQ 50-70 317
    moderate, IQ 35-49 318.0
    profound, IQ under 20 318.2
    severe, IQ 20-34 318.1
  learning NEC 315.2
  special spelling 315.09
Disarticulation (see also Derangement, joint)
    718.9 ●
  meaning
    amputation
      status - see Absence, by site
      traumatic - see Amputation, traumatic
    dislocation, traumatic or congenital - see
        Dislocation
Disaster, cerebrovascular (see also Disease,
    cerebrovascular, acute) 436
Discharge
  anal NEC 787.99
  breast (female) (male) 611.79
  conjunctiva 372.89
  continued locomotor idiopathic (see also
      Epilepsy) 345.5 ●
  diencephalic autonomic idiopathic (see also
      Epilepsy) 345.5 ●
  ear 388.60
    blood 388.69
    cerebrospinal fluid 388.61
  excessive urine 788.42
  eye 379.93
  nasal 478.19
  nipple 611.79
  patterned motor idiopathic (see also Epilepsy)
      345.5 ●
  penile 788.7
  postnasal - see Sinusitis
  sinus, from mediastinum 510.0
  umbilicus 789.9
  urethral 788.7
    bloody 599.84
  vaginal 623.5
Discitis 722.90
  cervical, cervicothoracic 722.91
  lumbar, lumbosacral 722.93
  thoracic, thoracolumbar 722.92
Discogenic syndrome - see Displacement,
    intervertebral disc
Discoid
  kidney 753.3
  meniscus, congenital 717.5
  semilunar cartilage 717.5
Discoloration
  mouth 528.9
  nails 703.8
  teeth 521.7
    due to
      drugs 521.7
      metals (copper) (silver) 521.7
      pulpal bleeding 521.7
    during formation 520.8
    extrinsic 523.6
    intrinsic posteruptive 521.7
Discomfort
  chest 786.59
  visual 368.13
Discomycosis - see Actinomycosis
Discontinuity, ossicles, ossicular chain
    385.23
Discrepancy
  centric occlusion
    maximum intercuspation 524.55
    of teeth 524.55
  leg length (acquired) 736.81
    congenital 755.30
  uterine size-date 649.6 ●
Discrimination
  political V62.4
  racial V62.4

◀ New   ◀▬▬ Revised   d̶e̶l̶e̶t̶e̶d̶ Deleted   Use Additional Digit(s)   Omit code

SECTION 1 INDEX TO DISEASES AND INJURIES / Discrimination

Discrimination (Continued)
   religious V62.4
   sex V62.4
Disease, diseased - see also Syndrome
   Abrami's (acquired hemolytic jaundice) 283.9
   absorbent system 459.89
   accumulation - see Thesaurismosis
   acid-peptic 536.8
   Acosta's 993.2
   Adams-Stokes (-Morgagni) (syncope with heart block) 426.9
   Addison's (bronze) (primary adrenal insufficiency) 255.41
      anemia (pernicious) 281.0
      tuberculous (see also Tuberculosis) 017.6●
   Addison-Gull - see Xanthoma
   adenoids (and tonsils) (chronic) 474.9
   adrenal (gland) (capsule) (cortex) 255.9
      hyperfunction 255.3
      hypofunction 255.41
      specified type NEC 255.8
   ainhum (dactylolysis spontanea) 136.0
   akamushi (scrub typhus) 081.2
   Akureyri (epidemic neuromyasthenia) 049.8
   Albarrán's (colibacilluria) 791.9
   Albers-Schönberg's (marble bones) 756.52
   Albert's 726.71
   Albright (-Martin) (-Bantam) 275.49
   Alibert's (mycosis fungoides) (M9700/3) 202.1●
   Alibert-Bazin (M9700/3) 202.1●
   alimentary canal 569.9
   alligator skin (ichthyosis congenita) 757.1
      acquired 701.1
   Almeida's (Brazilian blastomycosis) 116.1
   Alpers' 330.8
   alpine 993.2
   altitude 993.2
   alveoli, teeth 525.9
   Alzheimer's - see Alzheimer's
   amyloid (any site) 277.30
   anarthritic rheumatoid 446.5
   Anders' (adiposis tuberosa simplex) 272.8
   Andersen's (glycogenosis IV) 271.0
   Anderson's (angiokeratoma corporis diffusum) 272.7
   Andes 993.2
   Andrews' (bacterid) 686.8
   angiopastic, angiospasmodic 443.9
      cerebral 435.9
         with transient neurologic deficit 435.9
      vein 459.89
   anterior
      chamber 364.9
      horn cell 335.9
      specified type NEC 335.8
   antral (chronic) 473.0
      acute 461.0
   anus NEC 569.49
   aorta (nonsyphilitic) 447.9
      syphilitic NEC 093.89
   aortic (heart) (valve) (see also Endocarditis, aortic) 424.1
   apollo 077.4
   aponeurosis 726.90
   appendix 543.9
   aqueous (chamber) 364.9
   arc-welders' lung 503
   Armenian 277.31
   Arnold-Chiari (see also Spina bifida) 741.0●
   arterial 447.9
      occlusive (see also Occlusion, by site) 444.22
         with embolus or thrombus - see Occlusion, by site
         due to stricture or stenosis 447.1
      specified type NEC 447.8
   arteriocardiorenal (see also Hypertension, cardiorenal) 404.90

Disease, diseased (Continued)
   arteriolar (generalized) (obliterative) 447.90
      specified type NEC 447.8
   arteriorenal - see Hypertension, kidney
   arteriosclerotic - see also Arteriosclerosis
      cardiovascular 429.2
      coronary - see Arteriosclerosis, coronary
      heart - see Arteriosclerosis, coronary
      vascular - see Arteriosclerosis
   artery 447.9
      cerebral 437.9
      coronary - see Arteriosclerosis, coronary
      specified type NEC 447.8
   arthropod-borne NEC 088.9
      specified type NEC 088.89
   Asboe-Hansen's (incontinentia pigmenti) 757.33
   atticoantral, chronic (with posterior or superior marginal perforation of ear drum) 382.2
   auditory canal, ear 380.9
   Aujeszky's 078.89
   auricle, ear NEC 380.30
   Australian X 062.4
   autoimmune NEC 279.49
      hemolytic (cold type) (warm type) 283.0
      parathyroid 252.1
      thyroid 245.2
   aviators' (see also Effect, adverse, high altitude) 993.2
   ax(e)-grinders' 502
   Ayala's 756.89
   Ayerza's (pulmonary artery sclerosis with pulmonary hypertension) 416.0
   Azorean (of the nervous system) 334.8
   Babington's (familial hemorrhagic telangiectasia) 448.0
   back bone NEC 733.90
   bacterial NEC 040.89
      zoonotic NEC 027.9
      specified type NEC 027.8
   Baehr-Schiffrin (thrombotic thrombocytopenic purpura) 446.6
   Baelz's (cheilitis glandularis apostematosa) 528.5
   Baerensprung's (eczema marginatum) 110.3
   Balfour's (chloroma) 205.3●
   balloon (see also Effect, adverse, high altitude) 993.2
   Baló's 341.1
   Bamberger (-Marie) (hypertrophic pulmonary osteoarthropathy) 731.2
   Bang's (Brucella abortus) 023.1
   Bannister's 995.1
   Banti's (with cirrhosis) (with portal hypertension) - see Cirrhosis, liver
   Barcoo (see also Ulcer, skin) 707.9
   barium lung 503
   Barlow (-Möller) (infantile scurvy) 267
   barometer makers' 985.0
   Barraquer (-Simons) (progressive lipodystrophy) 272.6
   basal ganglia 333.90
      degenerative NEC 333.0
      specified NEC 333.89
   Basedow's (exophthalmic goiter) 242.0●
   basement membrane NEC 583.89
      with
         pulmonary hemorrhage (Goodpasture's syndrome) 446.21 [583.81]
   Bateman's 078.0
      purpura (senile) 287.2
   Batten's 330.1 [362.71]
   Batten-Mayou (retina) 330.1 [362.71]
   Batten-Steinert 359.21
   Battey 031.0
   Baumgarten-Cruveilhier (cirrhosis of liver) 571.5
   bauxite-workers' 503
   Bayle's (dementia paralytica) 094.1

Disease, diseased (Continued)
   Bazin's (primary) (see also Tuberculosis) 017.1●
   Beard's (neurasthenia) 300.5
   Beau's (see also Degeneration, myocardial) 429.1
   Bechterew's (ankylosing spondylitis) 720.0
   Becker's
      idiopathic mural endomyocardial disease 425.2
      myotonia congenita, recessive form 359.22
   Begbie's (exophthalmic goiter) 242.0●
   Behr's 362.50
   Beigel's (white piedra) 111.2
   Bekhterev's (ankylosing spondylitis) 720.0
   Bell's (see also Psychosis, affective) 296.0●
   Bennett's (leukemia) 208.9●
   Benson's 379.22
   Bergeron's (hysteroepilepsy) 300.11
   Berlin's 921.3
   Bernard-Soulier (thrombopathy) 287.1
   Bernhardt (-Roth) 355.1
   beryllium 503
   Besnier-Boeck (-Schaumann) (sarcoidosis) 135
   Best's 362.76
   Beurmann's (sporotrichosis) 117.1
   Bielschowsky (-Jansky) 330.1
   Biermer's (pernicious anemia) 281.0
   Biett's (discoid lupus erythematosus) 695.4
   bile duct (see also Disease, biliary) 576.9
   biliary (duct) (tract) 576.9
      with calculus, choledocholithiasis, or stones - see Choledocholithiasis
   Billroth's (meningocele) (see also Spina bifida) 741.9●
   Binswanger's 290.12
   Bird's (oxaluria) 271.8
   bird fanciers' 495.2
   black lung 500
   bladder 596.9
      specified NEC 596.89
   bleeder's 286.0
   Bloch-Sulzberger (incontinentia pigmenti) 757.33
   Blocq's (astasia-abasia) 307.9
   blood (-forming organs) 289.9
      specified NEC 289.89
      vessel 459.9
   Bloodgood's 610.1
   Blount's (tibia vara) 732.4
   blue 746.9
   Bodechtel-Guttmann (subacute sclerosing panencephalitis) 046.2
   Boeck's (sarcoidosis) 135
   bone 733.90
      fibrocystic NEC 733.29
         jaw 526.2
      marrow 289.9
      Paget's (osteitis deformans) 731.0
      specified type NEC 733.99
      von Recklinghausen's (osteitis fibrosa cystica) 252.01
   Bonfils' - see Disease, Hodgkin's
   Borna 062.9
   Bornholm (epidemic pleurodynia) 074.1
   Bostock's (see also Fever, hay) 477.9
   Bouchard's (myopathic dilatation of the stomach) 536.1
   Bouillaud's (rheumatic heart disease) 391.9
   Bourneville (-Brissaud) (tuberous sclerosis) 759.5
   Bouveret (-Hoffmann) (paroxysmal tachycardia) 427.2
   bowel 569.9
      functional 564.9
      psychogenic 306.4
   Bowen's (M8081/2) - see Neoplasm, skin, in situ
   Bozzolo's (multiple myeloma) (M9730/3) 203.0●

Disease, diseased (Continued)
    Bradley's (epidemic vomiting) 078.82
    Brailsford's 732.3
        radius, head 732.3
        tarsal, scaphoid 732.5
    Brailsford-Morquio (mucopolysaccharidosis IV) 277.5
    brain 348.9
        Alzheimer's 331.0
            with dementia - see Alzheimer's, dementia
        arterial, artery 437.9
        arteriosclerotic 437.0
        congenital 742.9
        degenerative - see Degeneration, brain
        inflammatory - see also Encephalitis
            late effect - see category 326
        organic 348.9
            arteriosclerotic 437.0
        parasitic NEC 123.9
        Pick's 331.11
            with dementia
                with behavioral disturbance 331.11 [294.11]
                without behavioral disturbance 331.11 [294.10]
        senile 331.2
    braziers' 985.8
    breast 611.9
        cystic (chronic) 610.1
        fibrocystic 610.1
        inflammatory 611.0
        Paget's (M8540/3) 174.0
        puerperal, postpartum NEC 676.3 ●
        specified NEC 611.89
    Breda's (see also Yaws) 102.9
    Breisky's (kraurosis vulvae) 624.09
    Bretonneau's (diphtheritic malignant angina) 032.0
    Bright's (see also Nephritis) 583.9
        arteriosclerotic (see also Hypertension, kidney) 403.90
    Brill's (recrudescent typhus) 081.1
        flea-borne 081.0
        louse-borne 081.1
    Brill-Symmers (follicular lymphoma) (M9690/3) 202.0 ●
    Brill-Zinsser (recrudescent typhus) 081.1
    Brinton's (leather bottle stomach) (M8142/3) 151.9
    Brion-Kayser (see also Fever, paratyphoid) 002.9
    broad
        beta 272.2
        ligament, noninflammatory 620.9
            specified NEC 620.8
    Brocq's 691.8
        meaning
            atopic (diffuse) neurodermatitis 691.8
            dermatitis herpetiformis 694.0
            lichen simplex chronicus 698.3
            parapsoriasis 696.2
            prurigo 698.2
    Brocq-Duhring (dermatitis herpetiformis) 694.0
    Brodie's (joint) (see also Osteomyelitis) 730.1 ●
    bronchi 519.19
    bronchopulmonary 519.19
    bronze (Addison's) 255.41
        tuberculous (see also Tuberculosis) 017.6 ●
    Brown-Séquard 344.89
    Bruck's 733.99
    Bruck-de Lange (Amsterdam dwarf, intellectual disabilities, and brachycephaly) 759.89
    Bruhl's (splenic anemia with fever) 285.8
    Bruton's (X-linked agammaglobulinemia) 279.04
    buccal cavity 528.9
    Buchanan's (juvenile osteochondrosis, iliac crest) 732.1

Disease, diseased (Continued)
    Buchman's (osteochondrosis juvenile) 732.1
    Budgerigar-Fanciers' 495.2
    Budinger-Ludloff-Läwen 717.89
    Büerger's (thromboangiitis obliterans) 443.1
    Burger-Grütz (essential familial hyperlipemia) 272.3
    Burns' (lower ulna) 732.3
    bursa 727.9
    Bury's (erythema elevatum diutinum) 695.89
    Buschke's 710.1
    Busquet's (see also Osteomyelitis) 730.1 ●
    Busse-Buschke (cryptococcosis) 117.5
    C_2 (see also Alcoholism) 303.9 ●
    Caffey's (infantile cortical hyperostosis) 756.59
    caisson 993.3
    calculus 592.9
    California 114.0
    Calvé (-Perthes) (osteochondrosis, femoral capital) 732.1
    Camurati-Engelmann (diaphyseal sclerosis) 756.59
    Canavan's 330.0
    capillaries 448.9
    Carapata 087.1
    cardiac - see Disease, heart
    cardiopulmonary, chronic 416.9
    cardiorenal (arteriosclerotic) (hepatic) (hypertensive) (vascular) (see also Hypertension, cardiorenal) 404.90
    cardiovascular (arteriosclerotic) 429.2
        congenital 746.9
        hypertensive (see also Hypertension, heart) 402.90
            benign 402.10
            malignant 402.00
        renal (see also Hypertension, cardiorenal) 404.90
        syphilitic (asymptomatic) 093.9
    carotid gland 259.8
    Carrión's (Bartonellosis) 088.0
    cartilage NEC 733.90
        specified NEC 733.99
    Castellani's 104.8
    cat-scratch 078.3
    Cavare's (familial periodic paralysis) 359.3
    Cazenave's (pemphigus) 694.4
    cecum 569.9
    celiac (adult) 579.0
        infantile 579.0
    cellular tissue NEC 709.9
    central core 359.0
    cerebellar, cerebellum - see Disease, brain
    cerebral (see also Disease, brain) 348.9
        arterial, artery 437.9
        degenerative - see Degeneration, brain
    cerebrospinal 349.9
    cerebrovascular NEC 437.9
        acute 436
            embolic - see Embolism, brain
            late effect - see Late effect(s) (of) cerebrovascular disease
            puerperal, postpartum, childbirth 674.0 ●
            thrombotic - see Thrombosis, brain
        arteriosclerotic 437.0
        embolic - see Embolism, brain
        ischemic, generalized NEC 437.1
        late effect - see Late effect(s) (of) cerebrovascular disease
        occlusive 437.1
        puerperal, postpartum, childbirth 674.0 ●
        specified type NEC 437.8
        thrombotic - see Thrombosis, brain
    ceroid storage 272.7
    cervix (uteri)
        inflammatory 616.0
        noninflammatory 622.9
            specified NEC 622.8
    Chabert's 022.9

Disease, diseased (Continued)
    Chagas' (see also Trypanosomiasis, American) 086.2
    Chandler's (osteochondritis dissecans, hip) 732.7
    Charcôt's (joint) 094.0 [713.5]
        spinal cord 094.0
    Charcôt-Marie-Tooth 356.1
    Charlouis' (see also Yaws) 102.9
    Cheadle (-Möller) (-Barlow) (infantile scurvy) 267
    Chédiak-Steinbrinck (-Higashi) (congenital gigantism of peroxidase granules) 288.2
    cheek, inner 528.9
    chest 519.9
    Chiari's (hepatic vein thrombosis) 453.0
    Chicago (North American blastomycosis) 116.0
    chignon (white piedra) 111.2
    chigoe, chigo (jigger) 134.1
    childhood granulomatous 288.1
    Chinese liver fluke 121.1
    chlamydial NEC 078.88
    cholecystic (see also Disease, gallbladder) 575.9
    choroid 363.9
        degenerative (see also Degeneration, choroid) 363.40
        hereditary (see also Dystrophy, choroid) 363.50
        specified type NEC 363.8
    Christian's (chronic histiocytosis X) 277.89
    Christian-Weber (nodular nonsuppurative panniculitis) 729.30
    Christmas 286.1
    ciliary body 364.9
        specified NEC 364.89
    circulatory (system) NEC 459.9
        chronic, maternal, affecting fetus or newborn 760.3
        specified NEC 459.89
        syphilitic 093.9
            congenital 090.5
    Civatte's (poikiloderma) 709.09
    climacteric 627.2
        male 608.89
    coagulation factor deficiency (congenital) (see also Defect, coagulation) 286.9
    Coats' 362.12
    coccidioidal pulmonary 114.5
        acute 114.0
        chronic 114.4
        primary 114.0
        residual 114.4
    Cockayne's (microcephaly and dwarfism) 759.89
    Cogan's 370.52
    cold
        agglutinin 283.0
            or hemoglobinuria 283.0
                paroxysmal (cold) (nocturnal) 283.2
        hemagglutinin (chronic) 283.0
    collagen NEC 710.9
        nonvascular 710.9
        specified NEC 710.8
        vascular (allergic) (see also Angiitis, hypersensitivity) 446.20
    colon 569.9
        functional 564.9
            congenital 751.3
        ischemic 557.0
    combined system (of spinal cord) 266.2 [336.2]
        with anemia (pernicious) 281.0 [336.2]
    compressed air 993.3
    Concato's (pericardial polyserositis) 423.2
        peritoneal 568.82
        pleural - see Pleurisy
    congenital NEC 799.89

SECTION 1 INDEX TO DISEASES AND INJURIES / Disease, diseased

Disease, diseased (Continued)
   conjunctiva 372.9
      chlamydial 077.98
         specified NEC 077.8
      specified type NEC 372.89
      viral 077.99
         specified NEC 077.8
   connective tissue, diffuse (see also Disease, collagen) 710.9
   Conor and Bruch's (boutonneuse fever) 082.1
   Conradi (-Hünermann) 756.59
   Cooley's (erythroblastic anemia) 282.44
   Cooper's 610.1
   Corbus' 607.1
   cork-handlers' 495.3
   cornea (see also Keratopathy) 371.9
   coronary (see also Ischemia, heart) 414.9
      congenital 746.85
      ostial, syphilitic 093.20
         aortic 093.22
         mitral 093.21
         pulmonary 093.24
         tricuspid 093.23
   Corrigan's - see Insufficiency, aortic
   Cotugno's 724.3
   Coxsackie (virus) NEC 074.8
   cranial nerve NEC 352.9
   Creutzfeldt-Jakob (CJD) 046.19
      with dementia
         with behavioral disturbance 046.19 [294.11]
         without behavioral disturbance 046.19 [294.10]
      familial 046.19
      iatrogenic 046.19
      specified NEC 046.19
      sporadic 046.19
      variant (vCJD) 046.11
         with dementia
            with behavioral disturbance 046.11 [294.11]
            without behavioral disturbance 046.11 [294.10]
   Crigler-Najjar (congenital hyperbilirubinemia) 277.4
   Crocq's (acrocyanosis) 443.89
   Crohn's (intestine) (see also Enteritis, regional) 555.9
   Crouzon's (craniofacial dysostosis) 756.0
   Cruchet's (encephalitis lethargica) 049.8
   Cruveilhier's 335.21
   Cruz-Chagas (see also Trypanosomiasis, American) 086.2
   crystal deposition (see also Arthritis, due to, crystals) 712.9●
   Csillag's (lichen sclerosus et atrophicus) 701.0
   Curschmann's 359.21
   Cushing's (pituitary basophilism) 255.0
   cystic
      breast (chronic) 610.1
      kidney, congenital (see also Cystic, disease, kidney) 753.10
      liver, congenital 751.62
      lung 518.89
         congenital 748.4
      pancreas 577.2
         congenital 751.7
      renal, congenital (see also Cystic, disease, kidney) 753.10
      semilunar cartilage 717.5
   cysticercus 123.1
   cystine storage (with renal sclerosis) 270.0
   cytomegalic inclusion (generalized) 078.5
      with
         pneumonia 078.5 [484.1]
      congenital 771.1
   Daae (-Finsen) (epidemic pleurodynia) 074.1
   dancing 297.8
   Danielssen's (anesthetic leprosy) 030.1

Disease, diseased (Continued)
   Darier's (congenital) (keratosis follicularis) 757.39
      erythema annulare centrifugum 695.0
      vitamin A deficiency 264.8
   Darling's (histoplasmosis) (see also Histoplasmosis, American) 115.00
   Davies' 425.0
   de Beurmann-Gougerot (sporotrichosis) 117.1
   Débove's (splenomegaly) 789.2
   deer fly (see also Tularemia) 021.9
   deficiency 269.9
   degenerative - see also Degeneration
      disc - see Degeneration, intervertebral disc
   Degos' 447.8
   Déjérine (-Sottas) 356.0
   Déleage's 359.89
   demyelinating, demyelinizating (brain stem) (central nervous system) 341.9
      multiple sclerosis 340
      specified NEC 341.8
   de Quervain's (tendon sheath) 727.04
      thyroid (subacute granulomatous thyroiditis) 245.1
   Dercum's (adiposis dolorosa) 272.8
   Deutschländer's - see Fracture, foot
   Devergie's (pityriasis rubra pilaris) 696.4
   Devic's 341.0
   diaphorase deficiency 289.7
   diaphragm 519.4
   diarrheal, infectious 009.2
   diatomaceous earth 502
   Diaz' (osteochondrosis astragalus) 732.5
   digestive system 569.9
   Di Guglielmo's (erythemic myelosis) (M9841/3) 207.0●
   Dimitri-Sturge-Weber (encephalocutaneous angiomatosis) 759.6
   disc, degenerative - see Degeneration, intervertebral disc
   discogenic (see also Disease, intervertebral disc) 722.90
   diverticular - see Diverticula
   Down's (mongolism) 758.0
   Dubini's (electric chorea) 049.8
   Dubois' (thymus gland) 090.5
   Duchenne's 094.0
      locomotor ataxia 094.0
      muscular dystrophy 359.1
      paralysis 335.22
      pseudohypertrophy, muscles 359.1
   Duchenne-Griesinger 359.1
   ductless glands 259.9
   Duhring's (dermatitis herpetiformis) 694.0
   Dukes (-Filatov) 057.8
   duodenum NEC 537.9
      specified NEC 537.89
   Duplay's 726.2
   Dupré's (meningism) 781.6
   Dupuytren's (muscle contracture) 728.6
   Durand-Nicolas-Favre (climatic bubo) 099.1
   Duroziez's (congenital mitral stenosis) 746.5
   Dutton's (trypanosomiasis) 086.9
   Eales' 362.18
   ear (chronic) (inner) NEC 388.9
      middle 385.9
         adhesive (see also Adhesions, middle ear) 385.10
         specified NEC 385.89
   Eberth's (typhoid fever) 002.0
   Ebstein's
      heart 746.2
      meaning diabetes 250.4● [581.81]
         due to secondary diabetes 249.4● [581.81]
   Echinococcus (see also Echinococcus) 122.9
   ECHO virus NEC 078.89
   Economo's (encephalitis lethargica) 049.8
   Eddowes' (brittle bones and blue sclera) 756.51

Disease, diseased (Continued)
   Edsall's 992.2
   Eichstedt's (pityriasis versicolor) 111.0
   Ellis-van Creveld (chondroectodermal dysplasia) 756.55
   endocardium - see Endocarditis
   endocrine glands or system NEC 259.9
      specified NEC 259.8
   endomyocardial, idiopathic mural 425.2
   Engel-von Recklinghausen (osteitis fibrosa cystica) 252.01
   Engelmann's (diaphyseal sclerosis) 756.59
   English (rickets) 268.0
   Engman's (infectious eczematoid dermatitis) 690.8
   enteroviral, enterovirus NEC 078.89
      central nervous system NEC 048
   epidemic NEC 136.9
   epididymis 608.9
   epigastric, functional 536.9
      psychogenic 306.4
   Erb (-Landouzy) 359.1
   Erb-Goldflam 358.00
   Erdheim-Chester (ECD) 277.89
   Erichsen's (railway spine) 300.16
   esophagus 530.9
      functional 530.5
      psychogenic 306.4
   Eulenburg's (congenital paramyotonia) 359.29
   Eustachian tube 381.9
   Evans' (thrombocytopenic purpura) 287.32
   external auditory canal 380.9
   extrapyramidal NEC 333.90
   eye 379.90
      anterior chamber 364.9
      inflammatory NEC 364.3
      muscle 378.9
   eyeball 360.9
   eyelid 374.9
   eyeworm of Africa 125.2
   Fabry's (angiokeratoma corporis diffusum) 272.7
   facial nerve (seventh) 351.9
      newborn 767.5
   Fahr-Volhard (malignant nephrosclerosis) 403.00
   fallopian tube, noninflammatory 620.9
      specified NEC 620.8
   familial periodic 277.31
      paralysis 359.3
   Fanconi's (congenital pancytopenia) 284.09
   Farber's (disseminated lipogranulomatosis) 272.8
   fascia 728.9
      inflammatory 728.9
   Fauchard's (periodontitis) 523.40
   Favre-Durand-Nicolas (climatic bubo) 099.1
   Favre-Racouchot (elastoidosis cutanea nodularis) 701.8
   Fede's 529.0
   Feer's 985.0
   Felix's (juvenile osteochondrosis, hip) 732.1
   Fenwick's (gastric atrophy) 537.89
   Fernels' (aortic aneurysm) 441.9
   fibrocaseous, of lung (see also Tuberculosis, pulmonary) 011.9●
   fibrocystic - see also Fibrocystic, disease
      newborn 277.01
   Fiedler's (leptospiral jaundice) 100.0
   fifth 057.0
   Filatoff's (infectious mononucleosis) 075
   Filatov's (infectious mononucleosis) 075
   file-cutters' 984.9
      specified type of lead - see Table of Drugs and Chemicals
   filterable virus NEC 078.89
   fish skin 757.1
      acquired 701.1
   Flajani (-Basedow) (exophthalmic goiter) 242.0●

SECTION I INDEX TO DISEASES AND INJURIES / Disease, diseased

Disease, diseased (Continued)
Flatau-Schilder 341.1
flax-dressers' 504
Fleischner's 732.3
flint 502
fluke - see Infestation, fluke
Følling's (phenylketonuria) 270.1
foot and mouth 078.4
foot process 581.3
Forbes' (glycogenosis III) 271.0
Fordyce's (ectopic sebaceous glands) (mouth) 750.26
Fordyce-Fox (apocrine miliaria) 705.82
Fothergill's
    meaning scarlatina anginosa 034.1
    neuralgia (see also Neuralgia, trigeminal) 350.1
Fournier's 608.83
    female 616.89
fourth 057.8
Fox (-Fordyce) (apocrine miliaria) 705.82
Francis' (see also Tularemia) 021.9
Franklin's (heavy chain) 273.2
Frei's (climatic bubo) 099.1
Freiberg's (flattening metatarsal) 732.5
Friedländer's (endarteritis obliterans) - see Arteriosclerosis
Friedreich's
    combined systemic or ataxia 334.0
    facial hemihypertrophy 756.0
    myoclonia 333.2
Fröhlich's (adiposogenital dystrophy) 253.8
Frommel's 676.6 ●
frontal sinus (chronic) 473.1
    acute 461.1
Fuller's earth 502
fungus, fungous NEC 117.9
Gaisböck's (polycythemia hypertonica) 289.0
gallbladder 575.9
    congenital 751.60
Gamna's (siderotic splenomegaly) 289.51
Gamstorp's (adynamia episodica hereditaria) 359.3
Gandy-Nanta (siderotic splenomegaly) 289.51
Gannister (occupational) 502
Garré's (see also Osteomyelitis) 730.1 ●
gastric (see also Disease, stomach) 537.9
gastroesophageal reflux (GERD) 530.81
gastrointestinal (tract) 569.9
    amyloid 277.39
    functional 536.9
        psychogenic 306.4
Gaucher's (adult) (cerebroside lipidosis) (infantile) 272.7
Gayet's (superior hemorrhagic polioencephalitis) 265.1
Gee (-Herter) (-Heubner) (-Thaysen) (nontropical sprue) 579.0
generalized neoplastic (M8000/6) 199.0
genital organs NEC
    female 629.9
        specified NEC 629.89
    male 608.9
Gerhardt's (erythromelalgia) 443.82
Gerlier's (epidemic vertigo) 078.81
Gibert's (pityriasis rosea) 696.3
Gibney's (perispondylitis) 720.9
Gierke's (glycogenosis I) 271.0
Gilbert's (familial nonhemolytic jaundice) 277.4
Gilchrist's (North American blastomycosis) 116.0
Gilford (-Hutchinson) (progeria) 259.8
Gilles de la Tourette's (motor-verbal tic) 307.23
Giovannini's 117.9
gland (lymph) 289.9
Glanzmann's (hereditary hemorrhagic thrombasthenia) 287.1
glassblowers' 527.1

Disease, diseased (Continued)
Glénard's (enteroptosis) 569.89
Glisson's (see also Rickets) 268.0
glomerular
    membranous, idiopathic 581.1
    minimal change 581.3
glycogen storage (Andersen's) (Cori types 1-7) (Forbes') (McArdle-Schmid-Pearson) (Pompe's) (types I-VII) 271.0
    cardiac 271.0 [425.7]
    generalized 271.0
    glucose-6-phosphatase deficiency 271.0
    heart 271.0 [425.7]
    hepatorenal 271.0
    liver and kidneys 271.0
    myocardium 271.0 [425.7]
    von Gierke's (glycogenosis I) 271.0
Goldflam-Erb 358.00
Goldscheider's (epidermolysis bullosa) 757.39
Goldstein's (familial hemorrhagic telangiectasia) 448.0
gonococcal NEC 098.0
Goodall's (epidemic vomiting) 078.82
Gordon's (exudative enteropathy) 579.8
Gougerot's (trisymptomatic) 709.1
Gougerot-Carteaud (confluent reticulate papillomatosis) 701.8
Gougerot-Hailey-Hailey (benign familial chronic pemphigus) 757.39
graft-versus-host 279.50
    acute 279.51
    on chronic 279.53
    chronic 279.52
grain-handlers' 495.8
Grancher's (splenopneumonia) - see Pneumonia
granulomatous (childhood) (chronic) 288.1
graphite lung 503
Graves' (exophthalmic goiter) 242.0 ●
Greenfield's 330.0
green monkey 078.89
Griesinger's (see also Ancylostomiasis) 126.9
grinders' 502
Grisel's 723.5
Gruby's (tinea tonsurans) 110.0
Guertin's (electric chorea) 049.8
Guillain-Barré 357.0
Guinon's (motor-verbal tic) 307.23
Gull's (thyroid atrophy with myxedema) 244.8
Gull and Sutton's - see Hypertension, kidney
gum NEC 523.9
Günther's (congenital erythropoietic porphyria) 277.1
gynecological 629.9
    specified NEC 629.89
H 270.0
Haas' 732.3
Habermann's (acute parapsoriasis varioliformis) 696.2
Haff 985.1
Hageman (congenital factor XII deficiency) (see also Defect, congenital) 286.3
Haglund's (osteochondrosis os tibiale externum) 732.5
Hagner's (hypertrophic pulmonary osteoarthropathy) 731.2
Hailey-Hailey (benign familial chronic pemphigus) 757.39
hair (follicles) NEC 704.9
    specified type NEC 704.8
Hallervorden-Spatz 333.0
Hallopeau's (lichen sclerosus et atrophicus) 701.0
Hamman's (spontaneous mediastinal emphysema) 518.1
hand, foot, and mouth 074.3
Hand-Schüller-Christian (chronic histiocytosis X) 277.89
Hanot's - see Cirrhosis, biliary

Disease, diseased (Continued)
Hansen's (leprosy) 030.9
    benign form 030.1
    malignant form 030.0
Harada's 363.22
Harley's (intermittent hemoglobinuria) 283.2
Hart's (pellagra-cerebellar ataxia-renal aminoaciduria) 270.0
Hartnup (pellagra-cerebellar ataxia-renal aminoaciduria) 270.0
Hashimoto's (struma lymphomatosa) 245.2
Hb - see Disease, hemoglobin
heart (organic) 429.9
    with
        acute pulmonary edema (see also Failure, ventricular, left) 428.1
        hypertensive 402.91
            with renal failure 404.92
            benign 402.11
                with renal failure 404.12
            malignant 402.01
                with renal failure 404.02
        kidney disease - see Hypertension, cardiorenal
        rheumatic fever (conditions classifiable to 390)
            active 391.9
                with chorea 392.0
            inactive or quiescent (with chorea) 398.90
    amyloid 277.39 [425.7]
    aortic (valve) (see also Endocarditis, aortic) 424.1
    arteriosclerotic or sclerotic (minimal) (senile) - see Arteriosclerosis, coronary
    artery, arterial - see Arteriosclerosis, coronary
    atherosclerotic - see Arteriosclerosis, coronary
    beer drinkers' 425.5
    beriberi 265.0 [425.7]
    black 416.0
    congenital NEC 746.9
        cyanotic 746.9
        maternal, affecting fetus or newborn 760.3
        specified type NEC 746.89
    congestive (see also Failure, heart) 428.0
    coronary 414.9
    cryptogenic 429.9
    due to
        amyloidosis 277.39 [425.7]
        beriberi 265.0 [425.7]
        cardiac glycogenosis 271.0 [425.7]
        Friedreich's ataxia 334.0 [425.8]
        gout 274.82
        mucopolysaccharidosis 277.5 [425.7]
        myotonia atrophica 359.21 [425.8]
        progressive muscular dystrophy 359.1 [425.8]
        sarcoidosis 135 [425.8]
    fetal 746.9
        inflammatory 746.89
    fibroid (see also Myocarditis) 429.0
    functional 427.9
        postoperative 997.1
        psychogenic 306.2
    glycogen storage 271.0 [425.7]
    gonococcal NEC 098.85
    gouty 274.82
    hypertensive (see also Hypertension, heart) 402.90
        benign 402.10
        malignant 402.00
    hyperthyroid (see also Hyperthyroidism) 242.9 ● [425.7]
    incompletely diagnosed - see Disease, heart

SECTION I INDEX TO DISEASES AND INJURIES / Disease, diseased

Disease, diseased (Continued)
  heart (Continued)
    ischemic (chronic) (see also Ischemia, heart) 414.9
      acute (see also Infarct, myocardium) 410.9●
        without myocardial infarction 411.89
          with coronary (artery) occlusion 411.81
        asymptomatic 412
        diagnosed on ECG or other special investigation but currently presenting no symptoms 412
    kyphoscoliotic 416.1
    mitral (see also Endocarditis, mitral) 394.9
    muscular (see also Degeneration, myocardial) 429.1
    postpartum 674.8●
    psychogenic (functional) 306.2
    pulmonary (chronic) 416.9
      acute 415.0
      specified NEC 416.8
    rheumatic (chronic) (inactive) (old) (quiescent) (with chorea) 398.90
      active or acute 391.9
        with chorea (active) (rheumatic) (Sydenham's) 392.0
        specified type NEC 391.8
      maternal, affecting fetus or newborn 760.3
    rheumatoid - see Arthritis, rheumatoid
    sclerotic - see Arteriosclerosis, coronary
    senile (see also Myocarditis) 429.0
    specified type NEC 429.89
    syphilitic 093.89
      aortic 093.1
        aneurysm 093.0
      asymptomatic 093.89
      congenital 090.5
    thyroid (gland) (see also Hyperthyroidism) 242.9● [425.7]
    thyrotoxic (see also Thyrotoxicosis) 242.9● [425.7]
    tuberculous (see also Tuberculosis) 017.9● [425.8]
    valve, valvular (obstructive) (regurgitant) - see Endocarditis
      congenital NEC (see also Anomaly, heart, valve) 746.9
        pulmonary 746.00
        specified type NEC 746.89
    vascular - see Disease, cardiovascular
  heavy-chain (gamma G) 273.2
  Heberden's 715.04
  Hebra's
    dermatitis exfoliativa 695.89
    erythema multiforme exudativum 695.19
    pityriasis
      maculata et circinata 696.3
      rubra 695.89
      pilaris 696.4
    prurigo 698.2
  Heerfordt's (uveoparotitis) 135
  Heidenhain's 290.10
    with dementia 290.10
  Heilmeyer-Schöner (M9842/3) 207.1●
  Heine-Medin (see also Poliomyelitis) 045.9●
  Heller's (see also Psychosis, childhood) 299.1●
  Heller-Döhle (syphilitic aortitis) 093.1
  hematopoietic organs 289.9
  hemoglobin (Hb) 282.7
    with thalassemia 282.49
    abnormal (mixed) NEC 282.7
      with thalassemia 282.49
    AS genotype 282.5
    Bart's 282.43

Disease, diseased (Continued)
  hemoglobin (Hb) (Continued)
    C (Hb-C) 282.7
      with other abnormal hemoglobin NEC 282.7
      elliptocytosis 282.7
      Hb-S (without crisis) 282.63
        with
          crisis 282.64
          vaso-occlusive pain 282.64
      sickle-cell (without crisis) 282.63
        with
          crisis 282.64
          vaso-occlusive pain 282.64
      thalassemia 282.49
    constant spring 282.7
    D (Hb-D) 282.7
      with other abnormal hemoglobin NEC 282.7
      Hb-S (without crisis) 282.68
        with crisis 282.69
      sickle-cell (without crisis) 282.68
        with crisis 282.69
      thalassemia 282.49
    E (Hb-E) 282.7
      with other abnormal hemoglobin NEC 282.7
      Hb-S (without crisis) 282.68
        with crisis 282.69
      sickle-cell (without crisis) 282.68
        with crisis 282.69
      thalassemia 282.47
    elliptocytosis 282.7
    F (Hb-F) 282.7
    G (Hb-G) 282.7
    H (Hb-H) 282.43
    hereditary persistence, fetal (HPFH) ("Swiss variety") 282.7
    high fetal gene 282.7
    I thalassemia 282.49
    M 289.7
    S - see also Disease, sickle-cell, Hb-S
      thalassemia (without crisis) 282.41
        with
          crisis 282.42
          vaso-occlusive pain 282.42
    spherocytosis 282.7
    unstable, hemolytic 282.7
    Zurich (Hb-Zurich) 282.7
  hemolytic (fetus) (newborn) 773.2
    autoimmune (cold type) (warm type) 283.0
    due to or with
      incompatibility
        ABO (blood group) 773.1
        blood (group) (Duffy) (Kell) (Kidd) (Lewis) (M) (S) NEC 773.2
        Rh (blood group) (factor) 773.0
          Rh negative mother 773.0
    unstable hemoglobin 282.7
  hemorrhagic 287.9
    newborn 776.0
  Henoch (-Schönlein) (purpura nervosa) 287.0
  hepatic - see Disease, liver
  hepatolenticular 275.1
  heredodegenerative NEC
    brain 331.89
    spinal cord 336.8
  Hers' (glycogenosis VI) 271.0
  Herter (-Gee) (-Heubner) (nontropical sprue) 579.0
  Herxheimer's (diffuse idiopathic cutaneous atrophy) 701.8
  Heubner's 094.89
  Heubner-Herter (nontropical sprue) 579.0
  high fetal gene or hemoglobin thalassemia (see also Thalassemia) 282.40
  Hildenbrand's (typhus) 081.9

Disease, diseased (Continued)
  hip (joint) NEC 719.95
    congenital 755.63
    suppurative 711.05
    tuberculous (see also Tuberculosis) 015.1● [730.85]
  Hippel's (retinocerebral angiomatosis) 759.6
  Hirschfeld's (acute diabetes mellitus) (see also Diabetes) 250.0●
    due to secondary diabetes 249.0●
  Hirschsprung's (congenital megacolon) 751.3
  His (-Werner) (trench fever) 083.1
  HIV 042
  Hodgkin's (M9650/3) 201.9●

> Note: Use the following fifth-digit subclassification with category 201:
> 0 unspecified site
> 1 lymph nodes of head, face, and neck
> 2 intrathoracic lymph nodes
> 3 intra-abdominal lymph nodes
> 4 lymph nodes of axilla and upper limb
> 5 lymph nodes of inguinal region and lower limb
> 6 intrapelvic lymph nodes
> 7 spleen
> 8 lymph nodes of multiple sites

  lymphocytic
    depletion (M9653/3) 201.7●
      diffuse fibrosis (M9654/3) 201.7●
      reticular type (M9655/3) 201.7●
    predominance (M9651/3) 201.4●
  lymphocytic-histiocytic predominance (M9651/3) 201.4●
  mixed cellularity (M9652/3) 201.6●
  nodular sclerosis (M9656/3) 201.5●
    cellular phase (M9657/3) 201.5●
  Hodgson's 441.9
    ruptured 441.5
  Hoffa (-Kastert) (liposynovitis prepatellaris) 272.8
  Holla (see also Spherocytosis) 282.0
  homozygous-Hb-S 282.61
  hoof and mouth 078.4
  hookworm (see also Ancylostomiasis) 126.9
  Horton's (temporal arteritis) 446.5
  host-versus-graft (immune or nonimmune cause) 279.50
  HPFH (hereditary persistence of fetal hemoglobin) ("Swiss variety") 282.7
  Huchard's (continued arterial hypertension) 401.9
  Huguier's (uterine fibroma) 218.9
  human immunodeficiency (virus) 042
  hunger 251.1
  Hunt's
    dyssynergia cerebellaris myoclonica 334.2
    herpetic geniculate ganglionitis 053.11
  Huntington's 333.4
  Huppert's (multiple myeloma) (M9730/3) 203.0●
  Hurler's (mucopolysaccharidosis I) 277.5
  Hutchinson's, meaning
    angioma serpiginosum 709.1
    cheiropompholyx 705.81
    prurigo estivalis 692.72
  Hutchinson-Boeck (sarcoidosis) 135
  Hutchinson-Gilford (progeria) 259.8
  hyaline (diffuse) (generalized) 728.9
    membrane (lung) (newborn) 769
  hydatid (see also Echinococcus) 122.9
  Hyde's (prurigo nodularis) 698.3
  hyperkinetic (see also Hyperkinesia) 314.9
    heart 429.82
  hypertensive (see also Hypertension) 401.9
  hypophysis 253.9
    hyperfunction 253.1
    hypofunction 253.2
  Iceland (epidemic neuromyasthenia) 049.8
  I cell 272.7

SECTION I INDEX TO DISEASES AND INJURIES / Disease, diseased

Disease, diseased (Continued)
  ill-defined 799.89
  immunologic NEC 279.9
  immunoproliferative 203.8 ●
  inclusion 078.5
    salivary gland 078.5
  infancy, early NEC 779.9
  infective NEC 136.9
  inguinal gland 289.9
  internal semilunar cartilage, cystic 717.5
  intervertebral disc 722.90
    with myelopathy 722.70
    cervical, cervicothoracic 722.91
      with myelopathy 722.71
    lumbar, lumbosacral 722.93
      with myelopathy 722.73
    thoracic, thoracolumbar 722.92
      with myelopathy 722.72
  intestine 569.9
    functional 564.9
      congenital 751.3
      psychogenic 306.4
    lardaceous 277.39
    organic 569.9
    protozoal NEC 007.9
  iris 364.9
    specified NEC 364.89
  iron
    metabolism (see also Hemochromatosis) 275.09
    storage (see also Hemochromatosis) 275.03
  Isambert's (see also Tuberculosis, larynx) 012.3 ●
  Iselin's (osteochondrosis, fifth metatarsal) 732.5
  island (scrub typhus) 081.2
  itai-itai 985.5
  Jadassohn's (maculopapular erythroderma) 696.2
  Jadassohn-Pellizari's (anetoderma) 701.3
  Jakob-Creutzfeldt (CJD) 046.19
    with dementia
      with behavioral disturbance 046.19 [294.11]
      without behavioral disturbance 046.19 [294.10]
    familial 046.19
    iatrogenic 046.19
    specified NEC 046.19
    sporadic 046.19
    variant (vCJD) 046.11
      with dementia
        with behavioral disturbance 046.11 [294.11]
        without behavioral disturbance 046.11 [294.10]
  Jaksch (-Luzet) (pseudoleukemia infantum) 285.8
  Janet's 300.89
  Jansky-Bielschowsky 330.1
  jaw NEC 526.9
    fibrocystic 526.2
  Jensen's 363.05
  Jeune's (asphyxiating thoracic dystrophy) 756.4
  Jigger 134.1
  Johnson-Stevens (erythema multiforme exudativum) 695.13
  joint NEC 719.9 ●
    ankle 719.97
    Charcôt 094.0 [713.5]
    degenerative (see also Osteoarthrosis) 715.9 ●
      multiple 715.09
      spine (see also Spondylosis) 721.90
    elbow 719.92
    foot 719.97
    hand 719.94
    hip 719.95

Disease, diseased (Continued)
  joint NEC (Continued)
    hypertrophic (chronic) (degenerative) (see also Osteoarthrosis) 715.9 ●
      spine (see also Spondylosis) 721.90
    knee 719.96
    Luschka 721.90
    multiple sites 719.99
    pelvic region 719.95
    sacroiliac 724.6
    shoulder (region) 719.91
    specified site NEC 719.98
    spine NEC 724.9
      pseudarthrosis following fusion 733.82
      sacroiliac 724.6
    wrist 719.93
  Jourdain's (acute gingivitis) 523.00
  Jüngling's (sarcoidosis) 135
  Kahler (-Bozzolo) (multiple myeloma) (M9730/3) 203.0 ●
  Kalischer's 759.6
  Kaposi's 757.33
    lichen ruber 697.8
      acuminatus 696.4
      moniliformis 697.8
    xeroderma pigmentosum 757.33
  Kaschin-Beck (endemic polyarthritis) 716.00
    ankle 716.07
    arm 716.02
      lower (and wrist) 716.03
      upper (and elbow) 716.02
    foot (and ankle) 716.07
    forearm (and wrist) 716.03
    hand 716.04
    leg 716.06
      lower 716.06
      upper 716.05
    multiple sites 716.09
    pelvic region (hip) (thigh) 716.05
    shoulder region 716.01
    specified site NEC 716.08
  Katayama 120.2
  Kawasaki 446.1
  Kedani (scrub typhus) 081.2
  kidney (functional) (pelvis) (see also Disease, renal) 593.9
    chronic 585.9
      requiring chronic dialysis 585.6
      stage
        I 585.1
        II (mild) 585.2
        III (moderate) 585.3
        IV (severe) 585.4
        V 585.5
    cystic (congenital) 753.10
      multiple 753.19
      single 753.11
      specified NEC 753.19
    fibrocystic (congenital) 753.19
    in gout 274.10
    polycystic (congenital) 753.12
      adult type (APKD) 753.13
      autosomal dominant 753.13
      autosomal recessive 753.14
      childhood type (CPKD) 753.14
      infantile type 753.14
  Kienböck's (carpal lunate) (wrist) 732.3
  Kimmelstiel (-Wilson) (intercapillary glomerulosclerosis) 250.4 ● [581.81]
    due to secondary diabetes 249.4 ● [581.81]
  Kinnier Wilson's (hepatolenticular degeneration) 275.1
  kissing 075
  Kleb's (see also Nephritis) 583.9
  Klinger's 446.4
  Klippel's 723.8
  Klippel-Feil (brevicollis) 756.16
  Knight's 911.1
  Köbner's (epidermolysis bullosa) 757.39
  Koenig-Wichmann (pemphigus) 694.4

Disease, diseased (Continued)
  Köhler's
    first (osteoarthrosis juvenilis) 732.5
    second (Freiberg's infraction, metatarsal head) 732.5
    patellar 732.4
    tarsal navicular (bone) (osteoarthrosis juvenilis) 732.5
  Köhler-Freiberg (infraction, metatarsal head) 732.5
  Köhler-Mouchet (osteoarthrosis juvenilis) 732.5
  Köhler-Pellegrini-Stieda (calcification, knee joint) 726.62
  Kok 759.89
  König's (osteochondritis dissecans) 732.7
  Korsakoff's (nonalcoholic) 294.0
    alcoholic 291.1
  Kostmann's (infantile genetic agranulocytosis) 288.01
  Krabbe's 330.0
  Kraepelin-Morel (see also Schizophrenia) 295.9 ●
  Kraft-Weber-Dimitri 759.6
  Kufs' 330.1
  Kugelberg-Welander 335.11
  Kuhnt-Junius 362.52
  Kümmell's (-Verneuil) (spondylitis) 721.7
  Kundrat's (lymphosarcoma) 200.1 ●
  kuru 046.0
  Kussmaul (-Meier) (polyarteritis nodosa) 446.0
  Kyasanur Forest 065.2
  Kyrle's (hyperkeratosis follicularis in cutem penetrans) 701.1
  labia
    inflammatory 616.10
    noninflammatory 624.9
      specified NEC 624.8
  labyrinth, ear 386.8
  lacrimal system (apparatus) (passages) 375.9
    gland 375.00
    specified NEC 375.89
  Lafora's 333.2
  Lagleyze-von Hippel (retinocerebral angiomatosis) 759.6
  Lancereaux-Mathieu (leptospiral jaundice) 100.0
  Landry's 357.0
  Lane's 569.89
  lardaceous (any site) 277.39
  Larrey-Weil (leptospiral jaundice) 100.0
  Larsen (-Johansson) (juvenile osteopathia patellae) 732.4
  larynx 478.70
  Lasègue's (persecution mania) 297.9
  Leber's 377.16
  Lederer's (acquired infectious hemolytic anemia) 283.19
  Legg's (capital femoral osteochondrosis) 732.1
  Legg-Calvé-Perthes (capital femoral osteochondrosis) 732.1
  Legg-Calvé-Waldenström (femoral capital osteochondrosis) 732.1
  Legg-Perthes (femoral capital osteochondosis) 732.1
  Legionnaires' 482.84
  Leigh's 330.8
  Leiner's (exfoliative dermatitis) 695.89
  Leloir's (lupus erythematosus) 695.4
  Lenegre's 426.0
  lens (eye) 379.39
  Leriche's (osteoporosis, posttraumatic) 733.7
  Letterer-Siwe (acute histiocytosis X) (M9722/3) 202.5 ●
  Lev's (acquired complete heart block) 426.0
  Lewandowski's (see also Tuberculosis) 017.0 ●
  Lewandowski-Lutz (epidermodysplasia verruciformis) 078.19

◀ New   ◀▮▮▮ Revised   ~~deleted~~ Deleted   ● Use Additional Digit(s)   ▮ Omit code

Disease, diseased (Continued)
 Lewy body 331.82
  with dementia
   with behavioral disturbance 331.82
    [294.11]
   without behavioral disturbance 331.82
    [294.10]
 Leyden's (periodic vomiting) 536.2
 Libman-Sacks (verrucous endocarditis) 710.0
  [424.91]
 Lichtheim's (subacute combined sclerosis
   with pernicious anemia) 281.0
   [336.2]
 ligament 728.9
 light chain 203.0●
 Lightwood's (renal tubular acidosis)
   588.89
 Lignac's (cystinosis) 270.0
 Lindau's (retinocerebral angiomatosis)
   759.6
 Lindau-von Hippel (angiomatosis
   retinocerebellosa) 759.6
 lip NEC 528.5
 lipidosis 272.7
 lipoid storage NEC 272.7
 Lipschütz's 616.50
 Little's - *see* Palsy, cerebral
 liver 573.9
  alcoholic 571.3
   acute 571.1
   chronic 571.3
  chronic 571.9
   alcoholic 571.3
  cystic, congenital 751.62
  drug-induced 573.3
  due to
   chemicals 573.3
    fluorinated agents 573.3
    hypersensitivity drugs 573.3
    isoniazids 573.3
  end stage NEC 572.8
   due to hepatitis - *see* Hepatitis
  fibrocystic (congenital) 751.62
  glycogen storage 271.0
  organic 573.9
  polycystic (congenital) 751.62
 Lobo's (keloid blastomycosis) 116.2
 Lobstein's (brittle bones and blue sclera)
   756.51
 locomotor system 334.9
 Lorain's (pituitary dwarfism) 253.3
 Lou Gehrig's 335.20
 Lucas-Championnière (fibrinous bronchitis)
   466.0
 Ludwig's (submaxillary cellulitis)
   528.3
 luetic - *see* Syphilis
 lumbosacral region 724.6
 lung NEC 518.89
  black 500
  congenital 748.60
  cystic 518.89
   congenital 748.4
  fibroid (chronic) (*see also* Fibrosis, lung)
    515
  fluke 121.2
   oriental 121.2
  in
   amyloidosis 277.39 [517.8]
   polymyositis 710.4 [517.8]
   sarcoidosis 135 [517.8]
   Sjögren's syndrome 710.2 [517.8]
   syphilis 095.1
   systemic lupus erythematosus 710.0
    [517.8]
   systemic sclerosis 710.1 [517.2]
  interstitial (chronic) 515
   acute 136.3
   respiratory bronchiolitis
    516.34
  nonspecific, chronic 496

Disease, diseased (Continued)
 lung NEC (Continued)
  obstructive (chronic) (COPD) 496
   with
    acute
     bronchitis 491.22
     exacerbation NEC 491.21
    alveolitis, allergic (*see also* Alveolitis,
      allergic) 495.9
    asthma (chronic) (obstructive)
      493.2●
    bronchiectasis 494.0
     with acute exacerbation 494.1
    bronchitis (chronic) 491.20
     with
      acute bronchitis 491.22
      exacerbation (acute) 491.21
     decompensated 491.21
      with exacerbation 491.21
    emphysema NEC 492.8
   diffuse (with fibrosis) 496
   of childhood, specified NEC 516.69
   polycystic 518.89
    asthma (chronic) (obstructive) 493.2●
    congenital 748.4
   purulent (cavitary) 513.0
   restrictive 518.89
   rheumatoid 714.81
    diffuse interstitial 714.81
   specified NEC 518.89
 Lutembacher's (atrial septal defect with
   mitral stenosis) 745.5
 Lutz-Miescher (elastosis perforans
   serpiginosa) 701.1
 Lutz-Splendore-de Almeida (Brazilian
   blastomycosis) 116.1
 Lyell's (toxic epidermal necrolysis) 695.15
  due to drug
   correct substance properly
    administered 695.15
   overdose or wrong substance given or
    taken 977.9
   specific drug - *see* Table of Drugs
    and Chemicals
 Lyme 088.81
 lymphatic (gland) (system) 289.9
  channel (noninfective) 457.9
  vessel (noninfective) 457.9
   specified NEC 457.8
 lymphoproliferative (chronic) (M9970/1)
   238.79
  X linked 759.89
 Machado-Joseph 334.8
 Madelung's (lipomatosis) 272.8
 Madura (actinomycotic) 039.9
  mycotic 117.4
 Magitot's 526.4
 Majocchi's (purpura annularis
   telangiectodes) 709.1
 malarial (*see also* Malaria) 084.6
 Malassez's (cystic) 608.89
 Malibu 919.8
  infected 919.9
 malignant (M8000/3) - *see also* Neoplasm, by
   site, malignant
  previous, affecting management of
    pregnancy V23.89
 Manson's 120.1
 maple bark 495.6
 maple syrup (urine) 270.3
 Marburg (virus) 078.89
 Marchiafava (-Bignami) 341.8
 Marfan's 090.49
  congenital syphilis 090.49
  meaning Marfan's syndrome 759.82
 Marie-Bamberger (hypertrophic pulmonary
   osteoarthropathy) (secondary) 731.2
  primary or idiopathic (acropachyderma)
    757.39
  pulmonary (hypertrophic
    osteoarthropathy) 731.2

Disease, diseased (Continued)
 Marie-Strümpell (ankylosing spondylitis)
   720.0
 Marion's (bladder neck obstruction) 596.0
 Marsh's (exophthalmic goiter) 242.0●
 Martin's 715.27
 mast cell 757.33
  systemic (M9741/3) 202.6●
 mastoid (*see also* Mastoiditis) 383.9
  process 385.9
 maternal, unrelated to pregnancy NEC,
   affecting fetus or newborn 760.9
 Mathieu's (leptospiral jaundice) 100.0
 Mauclaire's 732.3
 Mauriac's (erythema nodosum syphiliticum)
   091.3
 Maxcy's 081.0
 McArdle (-Schmid-Pearson) (glycogenosis V)
   271.0
 mediastinum NEC 519.3
 Medin's (*see also* Poliomyelitis) 045.9●
 Mediterranean 282.40
  with hemoglobinopathy 282.49
 medullary center (idiopathic) (respiratory)
   348.89
 Meige's (chronic hereditary edema) 757.0
 Meleda 757.39
 Ménétrier's (hypertrophic gastritis) 535.2●
 Ménière's (active) 386.00
  cochlear 386.02
  cochleovestibular 386.01
  inactive 386.04
  in remission 386.04
  vestibular 386.03
 meningeal - *see* Meningitis
 mental (*see also* Psychosis) 298.9
 Merzbacher-Pelizaeus 330.0
 mesenchymal 710.9
 mesenteric embolic 557.0
 metabolic NEC 277.9
 metal polishers' 502
 metastatic - *see* Metastasis
 Mibelli's 757.39
 microdrepanocytic 282.41
 microvascular - *code to* condition
 microvillus
  atrophy 751.5
  inclusion (MVD) 751.5
 Miescher's 709.3
 Mikulicz's (dryness of mouth, absent or
   decreased lacrimation) 527.1
 Milkman (-Looser) (osteomalacia with
   pseudofractures) 268.2
 Miller's (osteomalacia) 268.2
 Mills' 335.29
 Milroy's (chronic hereditary edema) 757.0
 Minamata 985.0
 Minor's 336.1
 Minot's (hemorrhagic disease, newborn)
   776.0
 Minot-von Willebrand-Jürgens
   (angiohemophilia) 286.4
 Mitchell's (erythromelalgia) 443.82
 mitral - *see* Endocarditis, mitral
 Mljet (mal de Meleda) 757.39
 Möbius', Moebius' 346.2●
 Möeller's 267
 Möller (-Barlow) (infantile scurvy) 267
 Mönckeberg's (*see also* Arteriosclerosis,
   extremities) 440.20
 Mondor's (thrombophlebitis of breast) 451.89
 Monge's 993.2
 Morel-Kraepelin (*see also* Schizophrenia)
   295.9●
 Morgagni's (syndrome) (hyperostosis
   frontalis interna) 733.3
 Morgagni-Adams-Stokes (syncope with
   heart block) 426.9
 Morquio (-Brailsford) (-Ullrich)
   (mucopolysaccharidosis IV) 277.5
 Morton's (with metatarsalgia) 355.6

SECTION I INDEX TO DISEASES AND INJURIES / Disease, diseased

Disease, diseased (Continued)
- Morvan's 336.0
- motor neuron (bulbar) (mixed type) 335.20
- Mouchet's (juvenile osteochondrosis, foot) 732.5
- mouth 528.9
- Moyamoya 437.5
- Mucha's (acute parapsoriasis varioliformis) 696.2
- mu-chain 273.2
- mucolipidosis (I) (II) (III) 272.7
- Münchmeyer's (exostosis luxurians) 728.11
- Murri's (intermittent hemoglobinuria) 283.2
- muscle 359.9
    - inflammatory 728.9
    - ocular 378.9
- musculoskeletal system 729.90
- mushroom workers' 495.5
- Myà's (congenital dilation, colon) 751.3
- mycotic 117.9
- myeloproliferative (chronic) (M9960/1) 238.79
- myocardium, myocardial (see also Degeneration, myocardial) 429.1
    - hypertensive (see also Hypertension, heart) 402.90
    - primary (idiopathic) 425.4
- myoneural 358.9
- Naegeli's 287.1
- nail 703.9
    - specified type NEC 703.8
- Nairobi sheep 066.1
- nasal 478.19
    - cavity NEC 478.19
    - sinus (chronic) - see Sinusitis
- navel (newborn) NEC 779.89
    - delayed separation of umbilical cord 779.83
- nemaline body 359.0
- neoplastic, generalized (M8000/6) 199.0
- nerve - see Disorder, nerve
- nervous system (central) 349.9
    - autonomic, peripheral (see also Neuropathy, peripheral, autonomic) 337.9
    - congenital 742.9
    - inflammatory - see Encephalitis
    - parasympathetic (see also Neuropathy, peripheral, autonomic) 337.9
    - peripheral NEC 355.9
    - prion NEC 046.79
    - specified NEC 349.89
    - sympathetic (see also Neuropathy, peripheral, autonomic) 337.9
    - vegetative (see also Neuropathy, peripheral, autonomic) 337.9
- Nettleship's (urticaria pigmentosa) 757.33
- Neumann's (pemphigus vegetans) 694.4
- neurologic (central) NEC (see also Disease, nervous system) 349.9
    - peripheral NEC 355.9
- neuromuscular system NEC 358.9
- Newcastle 077.8
- Nicolas (-Durand) -Favre (climatic bubo) 099.1
- Niemann-Pick (lipid histiocytosis) 272.7
- nipple 611.9
    - Paget's (M8540/3) 174.0
- Nishimoto (-Takeuchi) 437.5
- nonarthropod-borne NEC 078.89
    - central nervous system NEC 049.9
    - enterovirus NEC 078.89
- nonautoimmune hemolytic NEC 283.10
- Nonne-Milroy-Meige (chronic hereditary edema) 757.0
- Norrie's (congenital progressive oculoacousticocerebral degeneration) 743.8
- nose 478.19
- nucleus pulposus - see Disease, intervertebral disc

Disease, diseased (Continued)
- nutritional 269.9
    - maternal, affecting fetus or newborn 760.4
- oasthouse, urine 270.2
- obliterative vascular 447.1
- Odelberg's (juvenile osteochondrosis) 732.1
- Oguchi's (retina) 368.61
- Ohara's (see also Tularemia) 021.9
- Ollier's (chondrodysplasia) 756.4
- Opitz's (congestive splenomegaly) 289.51
- Oppenheim's 358.8
- Oppenheim-Urbach (necrobiosis lipoidica diabeticorum) 250.8● [709.3]
    - due to secondary diabetes 249.8● [709.3]
- optic nerve NEC 377.49
- orbit 376.9
    - specified NEC 376.89
- Oriental liver fluke 121.1
- Oriental lung fluke 121.2
- Ormond's 593.4
- Osgood's tibia (tubercle) 732.4
- Osgood-Schlatter 732.4
- Osler (-Vaquez) (polycythemia vera) (M9950/1) 238.4
- Osler-Rendu (familial hemorrhagic telangiectasia) 448.0
- osteofibrocystic 252.01
- Otto's 715.35
- outer ear 380.9
- ovary (noninflammatory) NEC 620.9
    - cystic 620.2
    - polycystic 256.4
    - specified NEC 620.8
- Owren's (congenital) (see also Defect, coagulation) 286.3
- Paas' 756.59
- Paget's (osteitis deformans) 731.0
    - with infiltrating duct carcinoma of the breast (M8541/3) - see Neoplasm, breast, malignant
    - bone 731.0
        - osteosarcoma in (M9184/3) - see Neoplasm, bone, malignant
    - breast (M8540/3) 174.0
    - extramammary (M8542/3) - see also Neoplasm, skin, malignant
        - anus 154.3
        - skin 173.59
    - malignant (M8540/3)
        - breast 174.0
        - specified site NEC (M8542/3) - see Neoplasm, skin, malignant
        - unspecified site 174.0
    - mammary (M8540/3) 174.0
    - nipple (M8540/3) 174.0
- palate (soft) 528.9
- Paltauf-Sternberg 201.9●
- pancreas 577.9
    - cystic 577.2
        - congenital 751.7
    - fibrocystic 277.00
- Panner's 732.3
    - capitellum humeri 732.3
    - head of humerus 732.3
    - tarsal navicular (bone) (osteochondrosis) 732.5
- panvalvular - see Endocarditis, mitral
- parametrium 629.9
- parasitic NEC 136.9
    - cerebral NEC 123.9
    - intestinal NEC 129
    - mouth 112.0
    - skin NEC 134.9
    - specified type - see Infestation
    - tongue 112.0
- parathyroid (gland) 252.9
    - specified NEC 252.8
- Parkinson's 332.0
- parodontal 523.9
- Parrot's (syphilitic osteochondritis) 090.0
- Parry's (exophthalmic goiter) 242.0●

Disease, diseased (Continued)
- Parson's (exophthalmic goiter) 242.0●
- Pavy's 593.6
- Paxton's (white piedra) 111.2
- Payr's (splenic flexure syndrome) 569.89
- pearl-workers' (chronic osteomyelitis) (see also Osteomyelitis) 730.1●
- Pel-Ebstein - see Disease, Hodgkin's
- Pelizaeus-Merzbacher 330.0
    - with dementia
        - with behavioral disturbance 330.0 [294.11]
        - without behavioral disturbance 330.0 [294.10]
- Pellegrini-Stieda (calcification, knee joint) 726.62
- pelvis, pelvic
    - female NEC 629.9
        - specified NEC 629.89
    - gonococcal (acute) 098.19
        - chronic or duration of 2 months or over 098.39
    - infection (see also Disease, pelvis, inflammatory) 614.9
    - inflammatory (female) (PID) 614.9
        - with
            - abortion - see Abortion, by type, with sepsis
            - ectopic pregnancy (see also categories 633.0–633.9) 639.0
            - molar pregnancy (see also categories 630–632) 639.0
        - acute 614.3
        - chronic 614.4
        - complicating pregnancy 646.6●
            - affecting fetus or newborn 760.8
        - following
            - abortion 639.0
            - ectopic or molar pregnancy 639.0
        - peritonitis (acute) 614.5
            - chronic NEC 614.7
        - puerperal, postpartum, childbirth 670.8●
        - specified NEC 614.8
    - organ, female NEC 629.9
        - specified NEC 629.89
    - peritoneum, female NEC 629.9
        - specified NEC 629.89
- penis 607.9
    - inflammatory 607.2
- peptic NEC 536.9
    - acid 536.8
- periapical tissues NEC 522.9
- pericardium 423.9
    - specified type NEC 423.8
- perineum
    - female
        - inflammatory 616.9
            - specified NEC 616.89
        - noninflammatory 624.9
            - specified NEC 624.8
    - male (inflammatory) 682.2
- periodic (familial) (Reimann's) NEC 277.31
    - paralysis 359.3
- periodontal NEC 523.9
    - specified NEC 523.8
- periosteum 733.90
- peripheral
    - arterial 443.9
    - autonomic nervous system (see also Neuropathy, autonomic) 337.9
    - nerve NEC (see also Neuropathy) 356.9
        - multiple - see Polyneuropathy
    - vascular 443.9
        - specified type NEC 443.89
- peritoneum 568.9
    - pelvic, female 629.9
        - specified NEC 629.89
- Perrin-Ferraton (snapping hip) 719.65

SECTION 1 INDEX TO DISEASES AND INJURIES / Disease, diseased

Disease, diseased (Continued)
- persistent mucosal (middle ear) (with posterior or superior marginal perforation of ear drum) 382.2
- Perthes' (capital femoral osteochondrosis) 732.1
- Petit's (see also Hernia, lumbar) 553.8
- Peutz-Jeghers 759.6
- Peyronie's 607.85
- Pfeiffer's (infectious mononucleosis) 075
- pharynx 478.20
- Phocas' 610.1
- photochromogenic (acid-fast bacilli)
  - (pulmonary) 031.0
  - nonpulmonary 031.9
- Pick's
  - brain 331.11
    - with dementia
      - with behavioral disturbance 331.11 [294.11]
      - without behavioral disturbance 331.11 [294.10]
  - cerebral atrophy 331.11
    - with dementia
      - with behavioral disturbance 331.11 [294.11]
      - without behavioral disturbance 331.11 [294.10]
  - lipid histiocytosis 272.7
  - liver (pericardial pseudocirrhosis of liver) 423.2
  - pericardium (pericardial pseudocirrhosis of liver) 423.2
  - polyserositis (pericardial pseudocirrhosis of liver) 423.2
- Pierson's (osteochondrosis) 732.1
- pigeon fanciers' or breeders' 495.2
- pineal gland 259.8
- pink 985.0
- Pinkus' (lichen nitidus) 697.1
- pinworm 127.4
- pituitary (gland) 253.9
  - hyperfunction 253.1
  - hypofunction 253.2
- pituitary snuff-takers' 495.8
- placenta
  - affecting fetus or newborn 762.2
  - complicating pregnancy or childbirth 656.7●
- pleura (cavity) (see also Pleurisy) 511.0
- Plummer's (toxic nodular goiter) 242.3●
- pneumatic
  - drill 994.9
  - hammer 994.9
- policeman's 729.2
- Pollitzer's (hidradenitis suppurativa) 705.83
- polycystic (congenital) 759.89
  - kidney or renal 753.12
    - adult type (APKD) 753.13
    - autosomal dominant 753.13
    - autosomal recessive 753.14
    - childhood type (CPKD) 753.14
    - infantile type 753.14
  - liver or hepatic 751.62
  - lung or pulmonary 518.89
    - congenital 748.4
  - ovary, ovaries 256.4
  - spleen 759.0
- polyethylene 996.45
- Pompe's (glycogenosis II) 271.0
- Poncet's (tuberculous rheumatism) (see also Tuberculosis) 015.9●
- Posada-Wernicke 114.9
- Potain's (pulmonary edema) 514
- Pott's (see also Tuberculosis) 015.0● [730.88]
  - osteomyelitis 015.0● [730.88]
  - paraplegia 015.0● [730.88]
  - spinal curvature 015.0● [737.43]
  - spondylitis 015.0● [720.81]
- Potter's 753.0
- Poulet's 714.2

Disease, diseased (Continued)
- pregnancy NEC (see also Pregnancy) 646.9●
- Preiser's (osteoporosis) 733.09
- Pringle's (tuberous sclerosis) 759.5
- Profichet's 729.90
- prostate 602.9
  - specified type NEC 602.8
- protozoal NEC 136.8
  - intestine, intestinal NEC 007.9
- pseudo-Hurler's (mucolipidosis III) 272.7
- psychiatric (see also Psychosis) 298.9
- psychotic (see also Psychosis) 298.9
- Puente's (simple glandular cheilitis) 528.5
- puerperal NEC (see also Puerperal) 674.9●
- pulmonary - see also Disease, lung
  - amyloid 277.39 [517.8]
  - artery 417.9
  - circulation, circulatory 417.9
    - specified NEC 417.8
  - diffuse obstructive (chronic) 496
    - with
      - acute bronchitis 491.22
      - asthma (chronic) (obstructive) 493.2●
      - exacerbation NEC (acute) 491.21
  - heart (chronic) 416.9
    - specified NEC 416.8
  - hypertensive (vascular) 416.0
    - cardiovascular 416.0
  - obstructive diffuse (chronic) 496
    - with
      - acute bronchitis 491.22
      - asthma (chronic) (obstructive) 493.2●
      - bronchitis (chronic) 491.20
        - with
          - exacerbation (acute) 491.21
        - acute 491.22
      - exacerbation NEC (acute) 491.21
    - decompensated 491.21
      - with exacerbation 491.21
  - valve (see also Endocarditis, pulmonary) 424.3
- pulp (dental) NEC 522.9
- pulseless 446.7
- Putnam's (subacute combined sclerosis with pernicious anemia) 281.0 [336.2]
- Pyle (-Cohn) (craniometaphyseal dysplasia) 756.89
- pyramidal tract 333.90
- Quervain's
  - tendon sheath 727.04
  - thyroid (subacute granulomatous thyroiditis) 245.1
- Quincke's - see Edema, angioneurotic
- Quinquaud (acne decalvans) 704.09
- rag sorters' 022.1
- Raynaud's (paroxysmal digital cyanosis) 443.0
- reactive airway - see Asthma
- Recklinghausen's (M9540/1) 237.71
  - bone (osteitis fibrosa cystica) 252.01
- Recklinghausen-Applebaum (hemochromatosis) (see also Hemochromatosis) 275.03
- Reclus' (cystic) 610.1
- rectum NEC 569.49
- Refsum's (heredopathia atactica polyneuritiformis) 356.3
- Reichmann's (gastrosuccorrhea) 536.8
- Reimann's (periodic) 277.31
- Reiter's 099.3
- renal (functional) (pelvis) (see also Disease, kidney) 593.9
  - with
    - edema (see also Nephrosis) 581.9
    - exudative nephritis 583.89
    - lesion of interstitial nephritis 583.89
    - stated generalized cause - see Nephritis
  - acute 593.9

Disease, diseased (Continued)
- renal (Continued)
  - basement membrane NEC 583.89
    - with
      - pulmonary hemorrhage (Goodpasture's syndrome) 446.21 [583.81]
  - chronic (see also Disease, kidney, chronic) 585.9
  - complicating pregnancy or puerperium NEC 646.2●
    - with hypertension - see Toxemia, of pregnancy
    - affecting fetus or newborn 760.1
  - cystic, congenital (see also Cystic, disease, kidney) 753.10
  - diabetic 250.4● [583.81]
    - due to secondary diabetes 249.4● [581.81]
  - due to
    - amyloidosis 277.39 [583.81]
    - diabetes mellitus 250.4● [583.81]
      - due to secondary diabetes 249.4● [581.81]
    - systemic lupus erythematosis 710.0 [583.81]
  - end-stage 585.6
  - exudative 583.89
  - fibrocystic (congenital) 753.19
  - gonococcal 098.19 [583.81]
  - gouty 274.10
  - hypertensive (see also Hypertension, kidney) 403.90
  - immune complex NEC 583.89
  - interstitial (diffuse) (focal) 583.89
  - lupus 710.0 [583.81]
  - maternal, affecting fetus or newborn 760.1
    - hypertensive 760.0
  - phosphate-losing (tubular) 588.0
  - polycystic (congenital) 753.12
    - adult type (APKD) 753.13
    - autosomal dominant 753.13
    - autosomal recessive 753.14
    - childhood type (CPKD) 753.14
    - infantile type 753.14
  - specified lesion or cause NEC (see also Glomerulonephritis) 583.89
  - subacute 581.9
  - syphilitic 095.4
  - tuberculous (see also Tuberculosis) 016.0● [583.81]
  - tubular (see also Nephrosis, tubular) 584.5
- Rendu-Osler-Weber (familial hemorrhagic telangiectasia) 448.0
- renovascular (arteriosclerotic) (see also Hypertension, kidney) 403.90
- respiratory (tract) 519.9
  - acute or subacute (upper) NEC 465.9
    - due to fumes or vapors 506.3
    - multiple sites NEC 465.8
    - noninfectious 478.9
    - streptococcal 034.0
  - chronic 519.9
    - arising in the perinatal period 770.7
    - due to fumes or vapors 506.4
  - due to
    - aspiration of liquids or solids 508.9
    - external agents NEC 508.9
      - specified NEC 508.8
    - fumes or vapors 506.9
      - acute or subacute NEC 506.3
      - chronic 506.4
  - fetus or newborn NEC 770.9
  - obstructive 496
  - smoke inhalation 508.2
  - specified type NEC 519.8
  - upper (acute) (infectious) NEC 465.9
    - multiple sites NEC 465.8
    - noninfectious NEC 478.9
    - streptococcal 034.0

Disease, diseased (Continued)
  retina, retinal NEC 362.9
    Batten's or Batten-Mayou 330.1 *[362.71]*
    degeneration 362.89
    vascular lesion 362.17
  rheumatic (*see also* Arthritis) 716.8 ●
    heart - *see* Disease, heart, rheumatic
  rheumatoid (heart) - *see* Arthritis, rheumatoid
  rickettsial NEC 083.9
    specified type NEC 083.8
  Riedel's (ligneous thyroiditis) 245.3
  Riga (-Fede) (cachectic aphthae) 529.0
  Riggs' (compound periodontitis) 523.40
  Ritter's 695.81
  Rivalta's (cervicofacial actinomycosis) 039.3
  Robles' (onchocerciasis) 125.3 *[360.13]*
  Roger's (congenital interventricular septal defect) 745.4
  Rokitansky's (*see also* Necrosis, liver) 570
  Romberg's 349.89
  Rosenthal's (factor XI deficiency) 286.2
  Rossbach's (hyperchlorhydria) 536.8
    psychogenic 306.4
  Roth (-Bernhardt) 355.1
  Runeberg's (progressive pernicious anemia) 281.0
  Rust's (tuberculous spondylitis) (*see also* Tuberculosis) 015.0 ● *[720.81]*
  Rustitskii's (multiple myeloma) (M9730/3) 203.0 ●
  Ruysch's (Hirschsprung's disease) 751.3
  Sachs (-Tay) 330.1
  sacroiliac NEC 724.6
  salivary gland or duct NEC 527.9
    inclusion 078.5
      streptococcal 034.0
    virus 078.5
  Sander's (paranoia) 297.1
  Sandhoff's 330.1
  sandworm 126.9
  Savill's (epidemic exfoliative dermatitis) 695.89
  Schamberg's (progressive pigmentary dermatosis) 709.09
  Schaumann's (sarcoidosis) 135
  Schenck's (sporotrichosis) 117.1
  Scheuermann's (osteochondrosis) 732.0
  Schilder (-Flatau) 341.1
  Schimmelbusch's 610.1
  Schlatter's tibia (tubercle) 732.4
  Schlatter-Osgood 732.4
  Schmorl's 722.30
    cervical 722.39
    lumbar, lumbosacral 722.32
    specified region NEC 722.39
    thoracic, thoracolumbar 722.31
  Scholz's 330.0
  Schönlein (-Henoch) (purpura rheumatica) 287.0
  Schottmüller's (*see also* Fever, paratyphoid) 002.9
  Schüller-Christian (chronic histiocytosis X) 277.89
  Schultz's (agranulocytosis) 288.09
  Schwalbe-Ziehen-Oppenheimer 333.6
  Schwartz-Jampel 359.23
  Schweninger-Buzzi (macular atrophy) 701.3
  sclera 379.19
  scrofulous (*see also* Tuberculosis) 017.2 ●
  scrotum 608.9
  sebaceous glands NEC 706.9
  Secretan's (posttraumatic edema) 782.3
  semilunar cartilage, cystic 717.5
  seminal vesicle 608.9
  Senear-Usher (pemphigus erythematosus) 694.4
  serum NEC 999.59
  Sever's (osteochondrosis calcaneum) 732.5
  sexually transmitted - *see* Disease, venereal
  Sézary's (reticulosis) (M9701/3) 202.2 ●
  Shaver's (bauxite pneumoconiosis) 503

Disease, diseased (Continued)
  Sheehan's (postpartum pituitary necrosis) 253.2
  shimamushi (scrub typhus) 081.2
  shipyard 077.1
  sickle-cell 282.60
    with
      crisis 282.62
      Hb-S disease 282.61
      other abnormal hemoglobin (Hb-D) (Hb-E) (Hb-G) (Hb-J) (Hb-K) (Hb-O) (Hb-P) (high fetal gene) (without crisis) 282.68
        with crisis 282.69
    elliptocytosis 282.60
    Hb-C (without crisis) 282.63
      with
        crisis 282.64
        vaso-occlusive pain 282.64
    Hb-S 282.61
      with
        crisis 282.62
        Hb-C (without crisis) 282.63
          with
            crisis 282.64
            vaso-occlusive pain 282.64
        other abnormal hemoglobin (Hb-D) (Hb-E) (Hb-G) (Hb-J) (Hb-K) (Hb-O) (Hb-P) (high fetal gene) (without crisis) 282.68
          with crisis 282.69
    spherocytosis 282.60
    thalassemia (without crisis) 282.41
      with
        crisis 282.42
        vaso-occlusive pain 282.42
  Siegal-Cattan-Mamou (periodic) 277.31
  silo fillers' 506.9
  Simian B 054.3
  Simmonds' (pituitary cachexia) 253.2
  Simons' (progressive lipodystrophy) 272.6
  Sinding-Larsen (juvenile osteopathia patellae) 732.4
  sinus - *see also* Sinusitis
    brain 437.9
    specified NEC 478.19
  Sirkari's 085.0
  sixth (*see also* Exanthem subitum) 058.10
  Sjögren (-Gougerot) 710.2
    with lung involvement 710.2 *[517.8]*
  Skevas-Zerfus 989.5
  skin NEC 709.9
    due to metabolic disorder 277.9
    specified type NEC 709.8
  sleeping (*see also* Narcolepsy) 347.00
    meaning sleeping sickness (*see also* Trypanosomiasis) 086.5
  small vessel 443.9
  Smith-Strang (oasthouse urine) 270.2
  Sneddon-Wilkinson (subcorneal pustular dermatosis) 694.1
  South African creeping 133.8
  Spencer's (epidemic vomiting) 078.82
  Spielmeyer-Stock 330.1
  Spielmeyer-Vogt 330.1
  spine, spinal 733.90
    combined system (*see also* Degeneration, combined) 266.2 *[336.2]*
      with pernicious anemia 281.0 *[336.2]*
    cord NEC 336.9
      congenital 742.9
    demyelinating NEC 341.8
    joint (*see also* Disease, joint, spine) 724.9
    tuberculous 015.0 ● *[730.8]* ●
  spinocerebellar 334.9
    specified NEC 334.8
  spleen (organic) (postinfectional) 289.50
    amyloid 277.39
    lardaceous 277.39
    polycystic 759.0
    specified NEC 289.59

Disease, diseased (Continued)
  sponge divers' 989.5
  Stanton's (melioidosis) 025
  Stargardt's 362.75
  Startle 759.89
  Steinert's 359.21
  Sternberg's - *see* Disease, Hodgkin's
  Stevens-Johnson (erythema multiforme exudativum) 695.13
  Sticker's (erythema infectiosum) 057.0
  Stieda's (calcification, knee joint) 726.62
  Still's (juvenile rheumatoid arthritis) 714.30
    adult onset 714.2
  Stiller's (asthenia) 780.79
  Stokes' (exophthalmic goiter) 242.0 ●
  Stokes-Adams (syncope with heart block) 426.9
  Stokvis (-Talma) (enterogenous cyanosis) 289.7
  stomach NEC (organic) 537.9
    functional 536.9
      psychogenic 306.4
    lardaceous 277.39
  stonemasons' 502
  storage
    glycogen (*see also* Disease, glycogen storage) 271.0
    lipid 272.7
    mucopolysaccharide 277.5
  striatopallidal system 333.90
    specified NEC 333.89
  Strümpell-Marie (ankylosing spondylitis) 720.0
  Stuart's (congenital factor X deficiency) (*see also* Defect, coagulation) 286.3
  Stuart-Prower (congenital factor X deficiency) (*see also* Defect, coagulation) 286.3
  Sturge (-Weber) (-Dimitri) (encephalocutaneous angiomatosis) 759.6
  Stuttgart 100.89
  Sudeck's 733.7
  supporting structures of teeth NEC 525.9
  suprarenal (gland) (capsule) 255.9
    hyperfunction 255.3
    hypofunction 255.41
  Sutton's 709.09
  Sutton and Gull's - *see* Hypertension, kidney
  sweat glands NEC 705.9
    specified type NEC 705.89
  sweating 078.2
  Sweeley-Klionsky 272.7
  Swift (-Feer) 985.0
  swimming pool (bacillus) 031.1
  swineherd's 100.89
  Sylvest's (epidemic pleurodynia) 074.1
  Symmers (follicular lymphoma) (M9690/3) 202.0 ●
  sympathetic nervous system (*see also* Neuropathy, peripheral, autonomic) 337.9
  synovium 727.9
  syphilitic - *see* Syphilis
  systemic tissue mast cell (M9741/3) 202.6 ●
  Taenzer's 757.4
  Takayasu's (pulseless) 446.7
  Talma's 728.85
  Tangier (familial high-density lipoprotein deficiency) 272.5
  Tarral-Besnier (pityriasis rubra pilaris) 696.4
  Tay-Sachs 330.1
  Taylor's 701.8
  tear duct 375.69
  teeth, tooth 525.9
    hard tissues 521.9
      specified NEC 521.89
    pulp NEC 522.9
  tendon 727.9
    inflammatory NEC 727.9
  terminal vessel 443.9

Disease, diseased (Continued)
- testis 608.9
- Thaysen-Gee (nontropical sprue) 579.0
- Thomsen's 359.22
- Thomson's (congenital poikiloderma) 757.33
- Thornwaldt's, Tornwaldt's (pharyngeal bursitis) 478.29
- throat 478.20
  - septic 034.0
- thromboembolic (see also Embolism) 444.9
- thymus (gland) 254.9
  - specified NEC 254.8
- thyroid (gland) NEC 246.9
  - heart (see also Hyperthyroidism) 242.9● [425.7]
  - lardaceous 277.39
  - specified NEC 246.8
- Tietze's 733.6
- Tommaselli's
  - correct substance properly administered 599.70
  - overdose or wrong substance given or taken 961.4
- tongue 529.9
- tonsils, tonsillar (and adenoids) (chronic) 474.9
  - specified NEC 474.8
- tooth, teeth 525.9
  - hard tissues 521.9
    - specified NEC 521.89
  - pulp NEC 522.9
- Tornwaldt's (pharyngeal bursitis) 478.29
- Tourette's 307.23
- trachea 519.19
- tricuspid - see Endocarditis, tricuspid
- triglyceride-storage, type I, II, III 272.7
- triple vessel - see Arteriosclerosis, coronary
- trisymptomatic, Gougerot's 709.1
- trophoblastic (see also Hydatidiform mole) 630
  - previous, affecting management of pregnancy V23.1
- tsutsugamushi (scrub typhus) 081.2
- tube (fallopian), noninflammatory 620.9
  - specified NEC 620.8
- tuberculous NEC (see also Tuberculosis) 011.9●
- tubo-ovarian
  - inflammatory (see also Salpingo-oophoritis) 614.2
  - noninflammatory 620.9
    - specified NEC 620.8
- tubotympanic, chronic (with anterior perforation of ear drum) 382.1
- tympanum 385.9
- Uhl's 746.84
- umbilicus (newborn) NEC 779.89
  - delayed separation 779.83
- Underwood's (sclerema neonatorum) 778.1
- undiagnosed 799.9
- Unna's (seborrheic dermatitis) 690.18
- unstable hemoglobin hemolytic 282.7
- Unverricht (-Lundborg) 345.1●
- Urbach-Oppenheim (necrobiosis lipoidica diabeticorum) 250.8● [709.3]
  - due to secondary diabetes 249.8● [709.3]
- Urbach-Wiethe (lipoid proteinosis) 272.8
- ureter 593.9
- urethra 599.9
  - specified type NEC 599.84
- urinary (tract) 599.9
  - bladder 596.9
    - specified NEC 596.89
  - maternal, affecting fetus or newborn 760.1
- Usher-Senear (pemphigus erythematosus) 694.4
- uterus (organic) 621.9
  - infective (see also Endometritis) 615.9
  - inflammatory (see also Endometritis) 615.9
  - noninflammatory 621.9
    - specified type NEC 621.8

Disease, diseased (Continued)
- uveal tract
  - anterior 364.9
  - posterior 363.9
- vagabonds' 132.1
- vagina, vaginal
  - inflammatory 616.10
  - noninflammatory 623.9
    - specified NEC 623.8
- Valsuani's (progressive pernicious anemia, puerperal) 648.2●
  - complicating pregnancy or puerperium 648.2●
- valve, valvular - see also Endocarditis
  - congenital NEC (see also Anomaly, heart, valve) 746.9
    - pulmonary 746.00
    - specified type NEC 746.89
- van Bogaert-Nijssen (-Peiffer) 330.0
- van Creveld-von Gierke (glycogenosis I) 271.0
- van den Bergh's (enterogenous cyanosis) 289.7
- van Neck's (juvenile osteochondrosis) 732.1
- Vaquez (-Osler) (polycythemia vera) (M9950/1) 238.4
- vascular 459.9
  - arteriosclerotic - see Arteriosclerosis
  - hypertensive - see Hypertension
  - obliterative 447.1
    - peripheral 443.9
  - occlusive 459.9
  - peripheral (occlusive) 443.9
    - in (due to) (with) diabetes mellitus 250.7● [443.81]
    - in (due to) (with) secondary diabetes 249.7● [443.81]
    - specified type NEC 443.89
- vas deferens 608.9
- vasomotor 443.9
- vasospastic 443.9
- vein 459.9
- venereal 099.9
  - chlamydial NEC 099.50
    - anus 099.52
    - bladder 099.53
    - cervix 099.53
    - epididymis 099.54
    - genitourinary NEC 099.55
      - lower 099.53
      - specified NEC 099.54
    - pelvic inflammatory disease 099.54
    - perihepatic 099.56
    - peritoneum 099.56
    - pharynx 099.51
    - rectum 099.52
    - specified site NEC 099.59
    - testis 099.54
    - vagina 099.53
    - vulva 099.53
  - fifth 099.1
  - sixth 099.1
  - complicating pregnancy, childbirth, or puerperium 647.2●
  - specified nature or type NEC 099.8
    - chlamydial - see Disease, venereal, chlamydial
- Verneuil's (syphilitic bursitis) 095.7
- Verse's (calcinosis intervertebralis) 275.49 [722.90]
- vertebra, vertebral NEC 733.90
  - disc - see Disease, Intervertebral disc
- vibration NEC 994.9
- Vidal's (lichen simplex chronicus) 698.3
- Vincent's (trench mouth) 101
- Virchow's 733.99
- virus (filterable) NEC 078.89
  - arbovirus NEC 066.9
  - arthropod-borne NEC 066.9
  - central nervous system NEC 049.9
    - specified type NEC 049.8

Disease, diseased (Continued)
- virus NEC (Continued)
  - complicating pregnancy, childbirth, or puerperium 647.6●
  - contact (with) V01.79
    - varicella V01.71
  - exposure to V01.79
    - varicella V01.71
  - Marburg 078.89
  - maternal
    - with fetal damage affecting management of pregnancy 655.3●
  - nonarthropod-borne NEC 078.89
    - central nervous system NEC 049.9
      - specified NEC 049.8
  - vaccination, prophylactic (against) V04.89
- vitreous 379.29
- vocal cords NEC 478.5
- Vogt's (Cecile) 333.71
- Vogt-Spielmeyer 330.1
- Volhard-Fahr (malignant nephrosclerosis) 403.00
- Volkmann's
  - acquired 958.6
- von Bechterew's (ankylosing spondylitis) 720.0
- von Economo's (encephalitis lethargica) 049.8
- von Eulenburg's (congenital paramyotonia) 359.29
- von Gierke's (glycogenosis I) 271.0
- von Graefe's 378.72
- von Hippel's (retinocerebral angiomatosis) 759.6
- von Hippel-Lindau (angiomatosis retinocerebellosa) 759.6
- von Jaksch's (pseudoleukemia infantum) 285.8
- von Recklinghausen's (M9540/1) 237.71
  - bone (osteitis fibrosa cystica) 252.01
- von Recklinghausen-Applebaum (hemochromatosis) (see also Hemochromatosis) 275.03
- von Willebrand (-Jürgens) (angiohemophilia) 286.4
- von Zambusch's (lichen sclerosus et atrophicus) 701.0
- Voorhoeve's (dyschondroplasia) 756.4
- Vrolik's (osteogenesis imperfecta) 756.51
- vulva
  - inflammatory 616.10
  - noninflammatory 624.9
    - specified NEC 624.8
- Wagner's (colloid milium) 709.3
- Waldenström's (osteochondrosis capital femoral) 732.1
- Wallgren's (obstruction of splenic vein with collateral circulation) 459.89
- Wardrop's (with lymphangitis) 681.9
  - finger 681.02
  - toe 681.11
- Wassilieff's (leptospiral jaundice) 100.0
- wasting NEC 799.4
  - due to malnutrition 261
  - paralysis 335.21
- Waterhouse-Friderichsen 036.3
- waxy (any site) 277.39
- Weber-Christian (nodular nonsuppurative panniculitis) 729.30
- Wegner's (syphilitic osteochondritis) 090.0
- Weil's (leptospiral jaundice) 100.0
  - of lung 100.0
- Weir Mitchell's (erythromelalgia) 443.82
- Werdnig-Hoffmann 335.0
- Werlhof's (see also Purpura, thrombocytopenic) 287.39
- Werner's 258.01
- Werner's (progeria adultorum) 259.8
- Werner-His (trench fever) 083.1
- Werner-Schultz (agranulocytosis) 288.09

Disease, diseased (Continued)
- Wernicke's (superior hemorrhagic polioencephalitis) 265.1
- Wernicke-Posadas 114.9
- Whipple's (intestinal lipodystrophy) 040.2
- whipworm 127.3
- white
  - blood cell 288.9
    - specified NEC 288.8
  - spot 701.0
- White's (congenital) (keratosis follicularis) 757.39
- Whitmore's (melioidosis) 025
- Widal-Abrami (acquired hemolytic jaundice) 283.9
- Wilkie's 557.1
- Wilkinson-Sneddon (subcorneal pustular dermatosis) 694.1
- Willis' (diabetes mellitus) (see also Diabetes) 250.0●
  - due to secondary diabetes 249.0●
- Wilson's (hepatolenticular degeneration) 275.1
- Wilson-Brocq (dermatitis exfoliativa) 695.89
- winter vomiting 078.82
- Wise's 696.2
- Wohlfart-Kugelberg-Welander 335.11
- Woillez's (acute idiopathic pulmonary congestion) 518.52
- Wolman's (primary familial xanthomatosis) 272.7
- wool-sorters' 022.1
- Zagari's (xerostomia) 527.7
- Zahorsky's (exanthem subitum) 058.10
- Ziehen-Oppenheim 333.6
- zoonotic, bacterial NEC 027.9
  - specified type NEC 027.8

Disfigurement (due to scar) 709.2
- head V48.6
- limb V49.4
- neck V48.7
- trunk V48.7

Disgerminoma - see Dysgerminoma
Disinsertion, retina 361.04
Disintegration, complete, of the body 799.89
- traumatic 869.1

Disk kidney 753.3
Dislocatable hip, congenital (see also Dislocation, hip, congenital) 754.30
Dislocation (articulation) (closed) (displacement) (simple) (subluxation) 839.8

> **Note:**
> "Closed" includes simple, complete, partial, uncomplicated, and unspecified dislocation.
>
> "Open" includes dislocation specified as infected or compound and dislocation with foreign body.
>
> "Chronic," "habitual," "old," or "recurrent" dislocations should be coded as indicated under the entry "Dislocation, recurrent"; and "pathological" as indicated under the entry "Dislocation, pathological."
>
> For late effect of dislocation see Late, effect, dislocation.

- with fracture - see Fracture, by site
- acromioclavicular (joint) (closed) 831.04
  - open 831.14
- anatomical site (closed)
  - specified NEC 839.69
    - open 839.79
  - unspecified or ill-defined 839.8
    - open 839.9
- ankle (scaphoid bone) (closed) 837.0
  - open 837.1

Dislocation (Continued)
- arm (closed) 839.8
  - open 839.9
- astragalus (closed) 837.0
  - open 837.1
- atlanto-axial (closed) 839.01
  - open 839.11
- atlas (closed) 839.01
  - open 839.11
- axis (closed) 839.02
  - open 839.12
- back (closed) 839.8
  - open 839.9
- Bell-Daly 723.8
- breast bone (closed) 839.61
  - open 839.71
- capsule, joint - see Dislocation, by site
- carpal (bone) - see Dislocation, wrist
- carpometacarpal (joint) (closed) 833.04
  - open 833.14
- cartilage (joint) - see also Dislocation, by site
  - knee - see Tear, meniscus
- cervical, cervicodorsal, or cervicothoracic (spine) (vertebra) - see Dislocation, vertebra, cervical
- chiropractic (see also Lesion, nonallopathic) 739.9
- chondrocostal - see Dislocation, costochondral
- chronic - see Dislocation, recurrent
- clavicle (closed) 831.04
  - open 831.14
- coccyx (closed) 839.41
  - open 839.51
- collar bone (closed) 831.04
  - open 831.14
- compound (open) NEC 839.9
- congenital NEC 755.8
  - hip (see also Dislocation, hip, congenital) 754.30
  - lens 743.37
  - rib 756.3
  - sacroiliac 755.69
  - spine NEC 756.19
  - vertebra 756.19
- coracoid (closed) 831.09
  - open 831.19
- costal cartilage (closed) 839.69
  - open 839.79
- costochondral (closed) 839.69
  - open 839.79
- cricoarytenoid articulation (closed) 839.69
  - open 839.79
- cricothyroid (cartilage) articulation (closed) 839.69
  - open 839.79
- dorsal vertebrae (closed) 839.21
  - open 839.31
- ear ossicle 385.23
- elbow (closed) 832.00
  - anterior (closed) 832.01
    - open 832.11
  - congenital 754.89
  - divergent (closed) 832.09
    - open 832.19
  - lateral (closed) 832.04
    - open 832.14
  - medial (closed) 832.03
    - open 832.13
  - open 832.10
  - posterior (closed) 832.02
    - open 832.12
  - recurrent 718.32
  - specified type NEC 832.09
    - open 832.19
- eye 360.81
  - lateral 376.36
- eyeball 360.81
  - lateral 376.36

Dislocation (Continued)
- femur
  - distal end (closed) 836.50
    - anterior 836.52
      - open 836.62
    - lateral 836.54
      - open 836.64
    - medial 836.53
      - open 836.63
    - open 836.60
    - posterior 836.51
      - open 836.61
  - proximal end (closed) 835.00
    - anterior (pubic) 835.03
      - open 835.13
    - obturator 835.02
      - open 835.12
    - open 835.10
    - posterior 835.01
      - open 835.11
- fibula
  - distal end (closed) 837.0
    - open 837.1
  - proximal end (closed) 836.59
    - open 836.69
- finger(s) (phalanx) (thumb) (closed) 834.00
  - interphalangeal (joint) 834.02
    - open 834.12
  - metacarpal (bone), distal end 834.01
    - open 834.11
  - metacarpophalangeal (joint) 834.01
    - open 834.11
  - open 834.10
  - recurrent 718.34
- foot (closed) 838.00
  - open 838.10
  - recurrent 718.37
- forearm (closed) 839.8
  - open 839.9
- fracture - see Fracture, by site
- glenoid (closed) 831.09
  - open 831.19
- habitual - see Dislocation, recurrent
- hand (closed) 839.8
  - open 839.9
- hip (closed) 835.00
  - anterior 835.03
    - obturator 835.02
      - open 835.12
    - open 835.13
  - congenital (unilateral) 754.30
    - with subluxation of other hip 754.35
    - bilateral 754.31
  - developmental 718.75
  - open 835.10
  - posterior 835.01
    - open 835.11
  - recurrent 718.35
- humerus (closed) 831.00
  - distal end (see also Dislocation, elbow) 832.00
  - open 831.10
  - proximal end (closed) 831.00
    - anterior (subclavicular) (subcoracoid) (subglenoid) (closed) 831.01
      - open 831.11
    - inferior (closed) 831.03
      - open 831.13
    - open 831.10
    - posterior (closed) 831.02
      - open 831.12
- implant - see Complications, mechanical
- incus 385.23
- infracoracoid (closed) 831.01
  - open 831.11
- innominate (pubic junction) (sacral junction) (closed) 839.69
  - acetabulum (see also Dislocation, hip) 835.00
  - open 839.79

SECTION 1 INDEX TO DISEASES AND INJURIES / Dislocation

Dislocation (Continued)
    interphalangeal (joint)
        finger or hand (closed) 834.02
            open 834.12
        foot or toe (closed) 838.06
            open 838.16
    jaw (cartilage) (meniscus) (closed) 830.0
        open 830.1
        recurrent 524.69
    joint NEC (closed) 839.8
        developmental 718.7 ●
        open 839.9
        pathological - see Dislocation, pathological
        recurrent - see Dislocation, recurrent
    knee (closed) 836.50
        anterior 836.51
            open 836.61
        congenital (with genu recurvatum) 754.41
        habitual 718.36
        lateral 836.54
            open 836.64
        medial 836.53
            open 836.63
        old 718.36
        open 836.60
        posterior 836.52
            open 836.62
        recurrent 718.36
        rotatory 836.59
            open 836.69
    lacrimal gland 375.16
    leg (closed) 839.8
        open 839.9
    lens (crystalline) (complete) (partial) 379.32
        anterior 379.33
        congenital 743.37
        ocular implant 996.53
        posterior 379.34
        traumatic 921.3
    ligament - see Dislocation, by site
    lumbar (vertebrae) (closed) 839.20
        open 839.30
    lumbosacral (vertebrae) (closed) 839.20
        congenital 756.19
        open 839.30
    mandible (closed) 830.0
        open 830.1
    maxilla (inferior) (closed) 830.0
        open 830.1
    meniscus (knee) - see also Tear, meniscus
        other sites - see Dislocation, by site
    metacarpal (bone)
        distal end (closed) 834.01
            open 834.11
        proximal end (closed) 833.05
            open 833.15
    metacarpophalangeal (joint) (closed) 834.01
        open 834.11
    metatarsal (bone) (closed) 838.04
        open 838.14
    metatarsophalangeal (joint) (closed) 838.05
        open 838.15
    midcarpal (joint) (closed) 833.03
        open 833.13
    midtarsal (joint) (closed) 838.02
        open 838.12
    Monteggia's - see Dislocation, hip
    multiple locations (except fingers only or toes only) (closed) 839.8
        open 839.9
    navicular (bone) foot (closed) 837.0
        open 837.1
    neck (see also Dislocation, vertebra, cervical) 839.00
    Nélaton's - see Dislocation, ankle
    nontraumatic (joint) - see Dislocation, pathological
    nose (closed) 839.69
        open 839.79
    not recurrent, not current injury - see Dislocation, pathological

Dislocation (Continued)
    occiput from atlas (closed) 839.01
        open 839.11
    old - see Dislocation, recurrent
    open (compound) NEC 839.9
    ossicle, ear 385.23
    paralytic (flaccid) (spastic) - see Dislocation, pathological
    patella (closed) 836.3
        congenital 755.64
        open 836.4
    pathological NEC 718.20
        ankle 718.27
        elbow 718.22
        foot 718.27
        hand 718.24
        hip 718.25
        knee 718.26
        lumbosacral joint 724.6
        multiple sites 718.29
        pelvic region 718.25
        sacroiliac 724.6
        shoulder (region) 718.21
        specified site NEC 718.28
        spine 724.8
            sacroiliac 724.6
        wrist 718.23
    pelvis (closed) 839.69
        acetabulum (see also Dislocation, hip) 835.00
        open 839.79
    phalanx
        foot or toe (closed) 838.09
            open 838.19
        hand or finger (see also Dislocation, finger) 834.00
    postpoliomyelitic - see Dislocation, pathological
    prosthesis, internal - see Complications, mechanical
    radiocarpal (joint) (closed) 833.02
        open 833.12
    radioulnar (joint)
        distal end (closed) 833.01
            open 833.11
        proximal end (see also Dislocation, elbow) 832.00
    radius
        distal end (closed) 833.00
            open 833.10
        proximal end (closed) 832.01
            open 832.11
    recurrent (see also Derangement, joint, recurrent) 718.3 ●
        elbow 718.32
        hip 718.35
        joint NEC 718.38
        knee 718.36
        lumbosacral (joint) 724.6
        patella 718.36
        sacroiliac 724.6
        shoulder 718.31
        temporomandibular 524.69
    rib (cartilage) (closed) 839.69
        congenital 756.3
        open 839.79
    sacrococcygeal (closed) 839.42
        open 839.52
    sacroiliac (joint) (ligament) (closed) 839.42
        congenital 755.69
        open 839.52
        recurrent 724.6
    sacrum (closed) 839.42
        open 839.52
    scaphoid (bone)
        ankle or foot (closed) 837.0
            open 837.1
        wrist (closed) (see also Dislocation, wrist) 833.00
            open 833.10

Dislocation (Continued)
    scapula (closed) 831.09
        open 831.19
    semilunar cartilage, knee - see Tear, meniscus
    septal cartilage (nose) (closed) 839.69
        open 839.79
    septum (nasal) (old) 470
    sesamoid bone - see Dislocation, by site
    shoulder (blade) (ligament) (closed) 831.00
        anterior (subclavicular) (subcoracoid) (subglenoid) (closed) 831.01
            open 831.11
        chronic 718.31
        inferior 831.03
            open 831.13
        open 831.10
        posterior (closed) 831.02
            open 831.12
        recurrent 718.31
    skull - see Injury, intracranial
    Smith's - see Dislocation, foot
    spine (articular process) (see also Dislocation, vertebra) (closed) 839.40
        atlanto-axial (closed) 839.01
            open 839.11
            recurrent 723.8
        cervical, cervicodorsal, cervicothoracic (closed) (see also Dislocation, vertebrae, cervical) 839.00
            open 839.10
            recurrent 723.8
        coccyx 839.41
            open 839.51
        congenital 756.19
        due to birth trauma 767.4
        open 839.50
        recurrent 724.9
        sacroiliac 839.42
            recurrent 724.6
        sacrum (sacrococcygeal) (sacroiliac) 839.42
            open 839.52
    spontaneous - see Dislocation, pathological
    sternoclavicular (joint) (closed) 839.61
        open 839.71
    sternum (closed) 839.61
        open 839.71
    subastragalar - see Dislocation, foot
    subglenoid (closed) 831.01
        open 831.11
    symphysis
        jaw (closed) 830.0
            open 830.1
        mandibular (closed) 830.0
            open 830.1
        pubis (closed) 839.69
            open 839.79
    tarsal (bone) (joint) 838.01
        open 838.11
    tarsometatarsal (joint) 838.03
        open 838.13
    temporomandibular (joint) (closed) 830.0
        open 830.1
        recurrent 524.69
    thigh
        distal end (see also Dislocation, femur, distal end) 836.50
        proximal end (see also Dislocation, hip) 835.00
    thoracic (vertebrae) (closed) 839.21
        open 839.31
    thumb(s) (see also Dislocation, finger) 834.00
    thyroid cartilage (closed) 839.69
        open 839.79
    tibia
        distal end (closed) 837.0
            open 837.1

Dislocation (Continued)
  tibia (Continued)
    proximal end (closed) 836.50
      anterior 836.51
        open 836.61
      lateral 836.54
        open 836.64
      medial 836.53
        open 836.63
      open 836.60
      posterior 836.52
        open 836.62
      rotatory 836.59
        open 836.69
  tibiofibular
    distal (closed) 837.0
      open 837.1
    superior (closed) 836.59
      open 836.69
  toe(s) (closed) 838.09
    open 838.19
  trachea (closed) 839.69
    open 839.79
  ulna
    distal end (closed) 833.09
      open 833.19
    proximal end - *see* Dislocation, elbow
  vertebra (articular process) (body) (closed) (traumatic) 839.40
    cervical, cervicodorsal or cervicothoracic (closed) 839.00
      first (atlas) 839.01
        open 839.11
      second (axis) 839.02
        open 839.12
      third 839.03
        open 839.13
      fourth 839.04
        open 839.14
      fifth 839.05
        open 839.15
      sixth 839.06
        open 839.16
      seventh 839.07
        open 839.17
      congenital 756.19
      multiple sites 839.08
        open 839.18
      open 839.10
    congenital 756.19
    dorsal 839.21
      open 839.31
      recurrent 724.9
    lumbar, lumbosacral 839.20
      open 839.30
    non-traumatic - *see* Displacement, intervertebral disc
    open NEC 839.50
    recurrent 724.9
    specified region NEC 839.49
      open 839.59
    thoracic 839.21
      open 839.31
  wrist (carpal bone) (scaphoid) (semilunar) (closed) 833.00
    carpometacarpal (joint) 833.04
      open 833.14
    metacarpal bone, proximal end 833.05
      open 833.15
    midcarpal (joint) 833.03
      open 833.13
    open 833.10
    radiocarpal (joint) 833.02
      open 833.12
    radioulnar (joint) 833.01
      open 833.11
    recurrent 718.33
    specified site NEC 833.09
      open 833.19
  xiphoid cartilage (closed) 839.61
    open 839.71

Dislodgement
  artificial skin graft 996.55
  decellularized allodermis graft 996.55
Disobedience, hostile (covert) (overt) (*see also* Disturbance, conduct) 312.0●
Disorder - *see also* Disease
  academic underachievement, childhood and adolescence 313.83
  accommodation 367.51
    drug-induced 367.89
    toxic 367.89
  adjustment (*see also* Reaction, adjustment) 309.9
    with
      anxiety 309.24
      anxiety and depressed mood 309.28
      depressed mood 309.0
      disturbance of conduct 309.3
      disturbance of emotions and conduct 309.4
  adrenal (capsule) (cortex) (gland) 255.9
    specified type NEC 255.8
  adrenogenital 255.2
  affective (*see also* Psychosis, affective) 296.90
    atypical 296.81
  aggressive, unsocialized (*see also* Disturbance, conduct) 312.0●
  alcohol, alcoholic (*see also* Alcohol) 291.9
    induced mood 291.89
  allergic - *see* Allergy
  amino acid (metabolic) (*see also* Disturbance, metabolism, amino acid) 270.9
    albinism 270.2
    alkaptonuria 270.2
    argininosuccinicaciduria 270.6
    beta-amino-isobutyricaciduria 277.2
    cystathioninuria 270.4
    cystinosis 270.0
    cystinuria 270.0
    glycinuria 270.0
    homocystinuria 270.4
    imidazole 270.5
    maple syrup (urine) disease 270.3
    neonatal, transitory 775.89
    oasthouse urine disease 270.2
    ochronosis 270.2
    phenylketonuria 270.1
    phenylpyruvic oligophrenia 270.1
    purine NEC 277.2
    pyrimidine NEC 277.2
    renal transport NEC 270.0
    specified type NEC 270.8
    transport NEC 270.0
      renal 270.0
    xanthinuria 277.2
  amnestic (*see also* Amnestic syndrome) 294.8
    alcohol-induced persisting 291.1
    drug-induced persisting 292.83
    in conditions classified elsewhere 294.0
  anaerobic glycolysis with anemia 282.3
  anxiety (*see also* Anxiety) 300.00
    due to or associated with physical condition 293.84
  arteriole 447.9
    specified type NEC 447.8
  artery 447.9
    specified type NEC 447.8
  articulation - *see* Disorder, joint
  Asperger's 299.8●
  attachment of infancy or early childhood 313.89
  attention deficit 314.00
    with hyperactivity 314.01
    predominantly
      combined hyperactive/inattentive 314.01
        hyperactive/impulsive 314.01
        inattentive 314.00
    residual type 314.8
  auditory processing disorder 388.45
    acquired 388.45
    developmental 315.32

Disorder (Continued)
  autistic 299.0●
  autoimmune NEC 279.49
    hemolytic (cold type) (warm type) 283.0
    parathyroid 252.1
    thyroid 245.2
  avoidant, childhood or adolescence 313.21
  balance
    acid-base 276.9
      mixed (with hypercapnia) 276.4
    electrolyte 276.9
    fluid 276.9
  behavior NEC (*see also* Disturbance, conduct) 312.9
    disruptive 312.9
  bilirubin excretion 277.4
  bipolar (affective) (alternating) 296.80

> Note: Use the following fifth-digit subclassification with categories 296.0–296.6:
>
> 0 unspecified
> 1 mild
> 2 moderate
> 3 severe, without mention of psychotic behavior
> 4 severe, specified as with psychotic behavior
> 5 in partial or unspecified remission
> 6 in full remission

    atypical 296.7
    specified type NEC 296.89
    type I 296.7
      most recent episode (or current)
        depressed 296.5●
        hypomanic 296.4●
        manic 296.4●
        mixed 296.6●
        unspecified 296.7
      single manic episode 296.0●
    type II (recurrent major depressive episodes with hypomania) 296.89
  bladder 596.9
    functional NEC 596.59
    specified NEC 596.89
  bleeding 286.9
  bone NEC 733.90
    specified NEC 733.99
  brachial plexus 353.0
  branched-chain amino-acid degradation 270.3
  breast 611.9
    puerperal, postpartum 676.3●
    specified NEC 611.89
  Briquet's 300.81
  bursa 727.9
    shoulder region 726.10
  carbohydrate metabolism, congenital 271.9
  cardiac, functional 427.9
    postoperative 997.1
    psychogenic 306.2
  cardiovascular, psychogenic 306.2
  cartilage NEC 733.90
    articular 718.00
      ankle 718.07
      elbow 718.02
      foot 718.07
      hand 718.04
      hip 718.05
      knee 717.9
      multiple sites 718.09
      pelvic region 718.05
      shoulder region 718.01
      specified
        site NEC 718.08
        type NEC 733.99
      wrist 718.03
  catatonic - *see* Catatonia
  central auditory processing 315.32
    acquired 388.45
    developmental 315.32

SECTION I INDEX TO DISEASES AND INJURIES / Disorder

Disorder (Continued)
   cervical region NEC 723.9
   cervical root (nerve) NEC 353.2
   character NEC (see also Disorder, personality) 301.9
   ciliary body 364.9
     specified NEC 364.89
   coagulation (factor) (see also Defect, coagulation) 286.9
     factor VIII (congenital) (functional) 286.0
     factor IX (congenital) (functional) 286.1
     neonatal, transitory 776.3
   coccyx 724.70
     specified NEC 724.79
   cognitive 294.9
   colon 569.9
     functional 564.9
     congenital 751.3
   communication 307.9
   conduct (see also Disturbance, conduct) 312.9
     adjustment reaction 309.3
     adolescent onset type 312.82
     childhood onset type 312.81
     compulsive 312.30
       specified type NEC 312.39
     hyperkinetic 314.2
     onset unspecified 312.89
     socialized (type) 312.20
       aggressive 312.23
       unaggressive 312.21
     specified NEC 312.89
   conduction, heart 426.9
     specified NEC 426.89
   conflict
     sexual orientation 302.0
   congenital
     glycosylation (CDG) 271.8
   convulsive (secondary) (see also Convulsions) 780.39
     due to injury at birth 767.0
     idiopathic 780.39
   coordination 781.3
   cornea NEC 371.89
     due to contact lens 371.82
   corticosteroid metabolism NEC 255.2
   cranial nerve - see Disorder, nerve, cranial
   cyclothymic 301.13
   degradation, branched-chain amino acid 270.3
   delusional 297.1
   dentition 520.6
   depersonalization 300.6
   depressive NEC 311
     atypical 296.82
     major (see also Psychosis, affective) 296.2●
       recurrent episode 296.3●
       single episode 296.2●
   development, specific 315.9
     associated with hyperkinesia 314.1
     coordination 315.4
     language 315.31
       and speech due to hearing loss 315.34
     learning 315.2
       arithmetical 315.1
       reading 315.00
     mixed 315.5
     motor coordination 315.4
     specified type NEC 315.8
     speech 315.39
       and language due to hearing loss 315.34
   diaphragm 519.4
   digestive 536.9
     fetus or newborn 777.9
       specified NEC 777.8
     psychogenic 306.4
   disintegrative childhood 299.1●
   dissociative 300.15
     identity 300.14
     nocturnal 307.47
   drug-related 292.9

Disorder (Continued)
   dysmorphic body 300.7
   dysthymic 300.4
   ear 388.9
     degenerative NEC 388.00
     external 380.9
       specified 380.89
     pinna 380.30
     specified type NEC 388.8
     vascular NEC 388.00
   eating NEC 307.50
   electrolyte NEC 276.9
     with
       abortion - see Abortion, by type, with metabolic disorder
       ectopic pregnancy (see also categories 633.0–633.9) 639.4
       molar pregnancy (see also categories 630–632) 639.4
     acidosis 276.2
       metabolic 276.2
       respiratory 276.2
     alkalosis 276.3
       metabolic 276.3
       respiratory 276.3
     following
       abortion 639.4
       ectopic or molar pregnancy 639.4
     neonatal, transitory NEC 775.5
   emancipation as adjustment reaction 309.22
   emotional (see also Disorder, mental, nonpsychotic) V40.9
   endocrine 259.9
     specified type NEC 259.8
   esophagus 530.9
     functional 530.5
     psychogenic 306.4
   explosive
     intermittent 312.34
     isolated 312.35
   expressive language 315.31
   eye 379.90
     globe - see Disorder, globe
     ill-defined NEC 379.99
     limited duction NEC 378.63
     specified NEC 379.8
   eyelid 374.9
     degenerative 374.50
     sensory 374.44
     specified type NEC 374.89
     vascular 374.85
   factitious (with combined psychological and physical signs and symptoms) (with predominantly physical signs and symptoms) 300.19
     with predominantly psychological signs and symptoms 300.16
   factor, coagulation (see also Defect, coagulation) 286.9
     VIII (congenital) (functional) 286.0
     IX (congenital) (functional) 286.1
   fascia 728.9
   fatty acid oxidation 277.85
   feeding - see Feeding
   female sexual arousal 302.72
   fluency 315.35
     adult onset 307.0
     childhood onset 315.35
     due to late effect of cerebrovascular accident 438.14
     in conditions classified elsewhere 784.52
   fluid NEC 276.9
   gastric (functional) 536.9
     motility 536.8
     psychogenic 306.4
     secretion 536.8
   gastrointestinal (functional) NEC 536.9
     newborn (neonatal) 777.9
       specified NEC 777.8
     psychogenic 306.4

Disorder (Continued)
   gender (child) 302.6
     adult 302.85
   gender identity (childhood) 302.6
     adolescents 302.85
     adults (-life) 302.85
   genitourinary system, psychogenic 306.50
   globe 360.9
     degenerative 360.20
       specified NEC 360.29
     specified type NEC 360.89
   hearing - see also Deafness
     conductive type (air) (see also Deafness, conductive) 389.00
     mixed conductive and sensorineural 389.20
       bilateral 389.22
       unilateral 389.21
     nerve
       bilateral 389.12
       unilateral 389.13
     perceptive (see also Deafness, perceptive) 389.10
     sensorineural type NEC (see also Deafness, sensorineural) 389.10
   heart action 427.9
     postoperative 997.1
   hematological, transient neonatal 776.9
     specified type NEC 776.8
   hematopoietic organs 289.9
   hemorrhagic NEC 287.9
     due to intrinsic circulating anticoagulants, antibodies, or inhibitors 286.59
     with
       acquired hemophilia 286.52
       antiphospholipid antibody 286.53
     specified type NEC 287.8
   hemostasis (see also Defect, coagulation) 286.9
   homosexual conflict 302.0
   hypomanic (chronic) 301.11
   identity
     childhood and adolescence 313.82
     gender 302.6
   immune mechanism (immunity) 279.9
     single complement (C_1–C_9) 279.8
     specified type NEC 279.8
   impulse control (see also Disturbance, conduct, compulsive) 312.30
   infant sialic acid storage 271.8
   integument, fetus or newborn 778.9
     specified type NEC 778.8
   interactional psychotic (childhood) (see also Psychosis, childhood) 299.1●
   intermittent explosive 312.34
   intervertebral disc 722.90
     cervical, cervicothoracic 722.91
     lumbar, lumbosacral 722.93
     thoracic, thoracolumbar 722.92
   intestinal 569.9
     functional NEC 564.9
       congenital 751.3
       postoperative 564.4
     psychogenic 306.4
   introverted, of childhood and adolescence 313.22
   involuntary emotional expression (IEED) 310.81
   iris 364.9
     specified NEC 364.89
   iron, metabolism 275.09
     specified type NEC 275.09
   isolated explosive 312.35
   joint NEC 719.90
     ankle 719.97
     elbow 719.92
     foot 719.97
     hand 719.94
     hip 719.95
     knee 719.96
     multiple sites 719.99

Disorder *(Continued)*
joint NEC *(Continued)*
pelvic region 719.95
psychogenic 306.0
shoulder (region) 719.91
specified site NEC 719.98
temporomandibular 524.60
sounds on opening or closing 524.64
specified NEC 524.69
wrist 719.93
kidney 593.9
functional 588.9
specified NEC 588.89
labyrinth, labyrinthine 386.9
specified type NEC 386.8
lactation 676.9●
language (developmental) (expressive) 315.31
mixed receptive-expressive 315.32
learning 315.9
ligament 728.9
ligamentous attachments, peripheral - *see also* Enthesopathy
spine 720.1
limb NEC 729.90
psychogenic 306.0
lipid
metabolism, congenital 272.9
storage 272.7
lipoprotein deficiency (familial) 272.5
low back NEC 724.9
psychogenic 306.0
lumbosacral
plexus 353.1
root (nerve) NEC 353.4
lymphoproliferative (chronic) NEC (M9970/1) 238.79
post-transplant (PTLD) 238.77
major depressive (*see also* Psychosis, affective) 296.2●
recurrent episode 296.3●
single episode 296.2●
male erectile 607.84
nonorganic origin 302.72
manic (*see also* Psychosis, affective) 296.0●
atypical 296.81
mathematics 315.1
meniscus NEC (*see also* Disorder, cartilage, articular) 718.0●
menopausal 627.9
specified NEC 627.8
menstrual 626.9
psychogenic 306.52
specified NEC 626.8
mental (nonpsychotic) 300.9
affecting management of pregnancy, childbirth, or puerperium 648.4●
drug-induced 292.9
hallucinogen persisting perception 292.89
specified type NEC 292.89
due to or associated with
alcoholism 291.9
drug consumption NEC 292.9
specified type NEC 292.89
physical condition NEC 293.9
induced by drug 292.9
specified type NEC 292.89
neurotic (*see also* Neurosis) 300.9
of infancy, childhood or adolescence 313.9
persistent
other
due to conditions classified elsewhere 294.8
unspecified
due to conditions classified elsewhere 294.9
presenile 310.1
psychotic NEC 290.10
previous, affecting management of pregnancy V23.89
psychoneurotic (*see also* Neurosis) 300.9

Disorder *(Continued)*
mental *(Continued)*
psychotic (*see also* Psychosis) 298.9
brief 298.8
senile 290.20
specific, following organic brain damage 310.9
cognitive or personality change of other type 310.1
frontal lobe syndrome 310.0
postconcussional syndrome 310.2
specified type NEC 310.89
transient
in conditions classified elsewhere 293.9
metabolism NEC 277.9
with
abortion - *see* Abortion, by type, with metabolic disorder
ectopic pregnancy (*see also* categories 633.0–633.9) 639.4
molar pregnancy (*see also* categories 630–632) 639.4
alkaptonuria 270.2
amino acid (*see also* Disorder, amino acid) 270.9
specified type NEC 270.8
ammonia 270.6
arginine 270.6
argininosuccinic acid 270.6
basal 794.7
bilirubin 277.4
calcium 275.40
carbohydrate 271.9
specified type NEC 271.8
cholesterol 272.9
citrulline 270.6
copper 275.1
corticosteroid 255.2
cystine storage 270.0
cystinuria 270.0
fat 272.9
fatty acid oxidation 277.85
following
abortion 639.4
ectopic or molar pregnancy 639.4
fructosemia 271.2
fructosuria 271.2
fucosidosis 271.8
galactose-1-phosphate uridyl transferase 271.1
glutamine 270.7
glycine 270.7
glycogen storage NEC 271.0
hepatorenal 271.0
hemochromatosis (*see also* Hemochromatosis) 275.03
in labor and delivery 669.0●
iron 275.09
lactose 271.3
lipid 272.9
specified type NEC 272.8
storage 272.7
lipoprotein - *see also* Hyperlipemia
deficiency (familial) 272.5
lysine 270.7
magnesium 275.2
mannosidosis 271.8
mineral 275.9
specified type NEC 275.8
mitochondrial 277.87
mucopolysaccharide 277.5
nitrogen 270.9
ornithine 270.6
oxalosis 271.8
pentosuria 271.8
phenylketonuria 270.1
phosphate 275.3
phosphorus 275.3
plasma protein 273.9
specified type NEC 273.8
porphyrin 277.1

Disorder *(Continued)*
metabolism NEC *(Continued)*
purine 277.2
pyrimidine 277.2
serine 270.7
sodium 276.9
specified type NEC 277.89
steroid 255.2
threonine 270.7
urea cycle 270.6
xylose 271.8
micturition NEC 788.69
psychogenic 306.53
misery and unhappiness, of childhood and adolescence 313.1
mitochondrial metabolism 277.87
mitral valve 424.0
mood (*see also* Disorder, bipolar) 296.90
alcohol-induced 291.89
episodic 296.90
specified NEC 296.99
in conditions classified elsewhere 293.83
motor tic 307.20
chronic 307.22
transient (childhood) 307.21
movement NEC 333.90
hysterical 300.11
medication-induced 333.90
periodic limb 327.51
sleep related unspecified 780.58
other organic 327.59
specified type NEC 333.99
stereotypic 307.3
mucopolysaccharide 277.5
muscle 728.9
psychogenic 306.0
specified type NEC 728.3
muscular attachments, peripheral - *see also* Enthesopathy
spine 720.1
musculoskeletal system NEC 729.90
psychogenic 306.0
myeloproliferative (chronic) NEC (M9960/1) 238.79
myoneural 358.9
due to lead 358.2
specified type NEC 358.8
toxic 358.2
myotonic 359.29
neck region NEC 723.9
nerve 349.9
abducens NEC 378.54
accessory 352.4
acoustic 388.5
auditory 388.5
auriculotemporal 350.8
axillary 353.0
cerebral - *see* Disorder, nerve, cranial
cranial 352.9
first 352.0
second 377.49
third
partial 378.51
total 378.52
fourth 378.53
fifth 350.9
sixth 378.54
seventh NEC 351.9
eighth 388.5
ninth 352.2
tenth 352.3
eleventh 352.4
twelfth 352.5
multiple 352.6
entrapment - *see* Neuropathy, entrapment
facial 351.9
specified NEC 351.8
femoral 355.2
glossopharyngeal NEC 352.2
hypoglossal 352.5
iliohypogastric 355.79

SECTION I INDEX TO DISEASES AND INJURIES / Disorder

Disorder (Continued)
- nerve (Continued)
  - ilioinguinal 355.79
  - intercostal 353.8
  - lateral
    - cutaneous of thigh 355.1
    - popliteal 355.3
  - lower limb NEC 355.8
  - medial, popliteal 355.4
  - median NEC 354.1
  - obturator 355.79
  - oculomotor
    - partial 378.51
    - total 378.52
  - olfactory 352.0
  - optic 377.49
    - hypoplasia 377.43
    - ischemic 377.41
    - nutritional 377.33
    - toxic 377.34
  - peroneal 355.3
  - phrenic 354.8
  - plantar 355.6
  - pneumogastric 352.3
  - posterior tibial 355.5
  - radial 354.3
  - recurrent laryngeal 352.3
  - root 353.9
    - specified NEC 353.8
  - saphenous 355.79
  - sciatic NEC 355.0
  - specified NEC 355.9
    - lower limb 355.79
    - upper limb 354.8
  - spinal 355.9
  - sympathetic NEC 337.9
  - trigeminal 350.9
    - specified NEC 350.8
  - trochlear 378.53
  - ulnar 354.2
  - upper limb NEC 354.9
  - vagus 352.3
- nervous system NEC 349.9
  - autonomic (peripheral) (see also Neuropathy, peripheral, autonomic) 337.9
  - cranial 352.9
  - parasympathetic (see also Neuropathy, peripheral, autonomic) 337.9
  - specified type NEC 349.89
  - sympathetic (see also Neuropathy, peripheral, autonomic) 337.9
  - vegetative (see also Neuropathy, peripheral, autonomic) 337.9
- neurohypophysis NEC 253.6
- neurological NEC 781.99
  - peripheral NEC 355.9
- neuromuscular NEC 358.9
  - hereditary NEC 359.1
  - specified NEC 358.8
  - toxic 358.2
- neurotic 300.9
  - specified type NEC 300.89
- neutrophil, polymorphonuclear (functional) 288.1
- nightmare 307.47
- night terror 307.46
- obsessive-compulsive 300.3
- oppositional defiant, childhood and adolescence 313.81
- optic
  - chiasm 377.54
    - associated with
      - inflammatory disorders 377.54
      - neoplasm NEC 377.52
      - pituitary 377.51
      - pituitary disorders 377.51
      - vascular disorders 377.53
  - nerve 377.49
  - radiations 377.63
  - tracts 377.63

Disorder (Continued)
- orbit 376.9
  - specified NEC 376.89
- orgasmic
  - female 302.73
  - male 302.74
- overanxious, of childhood and adolescence 313.0
- oxidation, fatty acid 277.85
- pancreas, internal secretion (other than diabetes mellitus) 251.9
  - specified type NEC 251.8
- panic 300.01
  - with agoraphobia 300.21
- papillary muscle NEC 429.81
- paranoid 297.9
  - induced 297.3
  - shared 297.3
- parathyroid 252.9
  - specified type NEC 252.8
- paroxysmal, mixed 780.39
- pentose phosphate pathway with anemia 282.2
- periodic limb movement 327.51
- peroxisomal 277.86
- personality 301.9
  - affective 301.10
  - aggressive 301.3
  - amoral 301.7
  - anancastic, anankastic 301.4
  - antisocial 301.7
  - asocial 301.7
  - asthenic 301.6
  - avoidant 301.82
  - borderline 301.83
  - compulsive 301.4
  - cyclothymic 301.13
  - dependent-passive 301.6
  - dyssocial 301.7
  - emotional instability 301.59
  - epileptoid 301.3
  - explosive 301.3
  - following organic brain damage 310.1
  - histrionic 301.50
  - hyperthymic 301.11
  - hypomanic (chronic) 301.11
  - hypothymic 301.12
  - hysterical 301.50
  - immature 301.89
  - inadequate 301.6
  - introverted 301.21
  - labile 301.59
  - moral deficiency 301.7
  - narcissistic 301.81
  - obsessional 301.4
  - obsessive-compulsive 301.4
  - overconscientious 301.4
  - paranoid 301.0
  - passive (-dependent) 301.6
  - passive-aggressive 301.84
  - pathological NEC 301.9
  - pseudosocial 301.7
  - psychopathic 301.9
  - schizoid 301.20
    - introverted 301.21
    - schizotypal 301.22
  - schizotypal 301.22
  - seductive 301.59
  - type A 301.4
  - unstable 301.59
- pervasive developmental 299.9 ●
  - childhood-onset 299.8 ●
  - specified NEC 299.8 ●
- phonological 315.39
- pigmentation, choroid (congenital) 743.53
- pinna 380.30
  - specified type NEC 380.39
- pituitary, thalamic 253.9
  - anterior NEC 253.4
  - iatrogenic 253.7

Disorder (Continued)
- pituitary, thalamic (Continued)
  - postablative 253.7
  - specified NEC 253.8
- pityriasis-like NEC 696.8
- platelets (blood) 287.1
- polymorphonuclear neutrophils (functional) 288.1
- porphyrin metabolism 277.1
- postmenopausal 627.9
  - specified type NEC 627.8
- post-transplant lymphoproliferative (PTLD) 238.77
- post-traumatic stress (PTSD) 309.81
- posttraumatic stress 309.81
  - acute 309.81
  - brief 309.81
  - chronic 309.81
- premenstrual dysphoric (PMDD) 625.4
- psoriatic-like NEC 696.8
- psychic, with diseases classified elsewhere 316
- psychogenic NEC (see also condition) 300.9
  - allergic NEC
    - respiratory 306.1
  - anxiety 300.00
    - atypical 300.00
    - generalized 300.02
  - appetite 307.59
  - articulation, joint 306.0
  - asthenic 300.5
  - blood 306.8
  - cardiovascular (system) 306.2
  - compulsive 300.3
  - cutaneous 306.3
  - depressive 300.4
  - digestive (system) 306.4
  - dysmenorrheic 306.52
  - dyspneic 306.1
  - eczematous 306.3
  - endocrine (system) 306.6
  - eye 306.7
  - feeding 307.59
  - functional NEC 306.9
  - gastric 306.4
  - gastrointestinal (system) 306.4
  - genitourinary (system) 306.50
  - heart (function) (rhythm) 306.2
  - hemic 306.8
  - hyperventilatory 306.1
  - hypochondriacal 300.7
  - hysterical 300.10
  - intestinal 306.4
  - joint 306.0
  - learning 315.2
  - limb 306.0
  - lymphatic (system) 306.8
  - menstrual 306.52
  - micturition 306.53
  - monoplegic NEC 306.0
  - motor 307.9
  - muscle 306.0
  - musculoskeletal 306.0
  - neurocirculatory 306.2
  - obsessive 300.3
  - occupational 300.89
  - organ or part of body NEC 306.9
  - organs of special sense 306.7
  - paralytic NEC 306.0
  - phobic 300.20
  - physical NEC 306.9
  - pruritic 306.3
  - rectal 306.4
  - respiratory (system) 306.1
  - rheumatic 306.0
  - sexual (function) 302.70
    - specified type NEC 302.79
  - sexual orientation conflict 302.0
  - skin (allergic) (eczematous) (pruritic) 306.3

Disorder (Continued)
  psychogenic NEC (Continued)
    sleep 307.40
      initiation or maintenance 307.41
        persistent 307.42
        transient 307.41
      movement 780.58
      sleep terror 307.46
      specified type NEC 307.49
    specified part of body NEC 306.8
    stomach 306.4
  psychomotor NEC 307.9
    hysterical 300.11
  psychoneurotic (see also Neurosis) 300.9
    mixed NEC 300.89
  psychophysiologic (see also Disorder, psychosomatic) 306.9
  psychosexual identity (childhood) 302.6
    adult-life 302.85
  psychosomatic NEC 306.9
    allergic NEC
      respiratory 306.1
    articulation, joint 306.0
    cardiovascular (system) 306.2
    cutaneous 306.3
    digestive (system) 306.4
    dysmenorrheic 306.52
    dyspneic 306.1
    endocrine (system) 306.6
    eye 306.7
    gastric 306.4
    gastrointestinal (system) 306.4
    genitourinary (system) 306.50
    heart (functional) (rhythm) 306.2
    hyperventilatory 306.1
    intestinal 306.4
    joint 306.0
    limb 306.0
    lymphatic (system) 306.8
    menstrual 306.52
    micturition 306.53
    monoplegic NEC 306.0
    muscle 306.0
    musculoskeletal 306.0
    neurocirculatory 306.2
    organs of special sense 306.7
    paralytic NEC 306.0
    pruritic 306.3
    rectal 306.4
    respiratory (system) 306.1
    rheumatic 306.0
    sexual (function) 302.70
      specified type NEC 302.79
    skin 306.3
    specified part of body NEC 306.8
    stomach 306.4
  psychotic (see also Psychosis) 298.9
    brief 298.8
  purine metabolism NEC 277.2
  pyrimidine metabolism NEC 277.2
  reactive attachment of infancy or early childhood 313.89
  reading, developmental 315.00
  reflex 796.1
  REM sleep behavior 327.42
  renal function, impaired 588.9
    specified type NEC 588.89
  renal transport NEC 588.89
  respiration, respiratory NEC 519.9
    due to
      aspiration of liquids or solids 508.9
      inhalation of fumes or vapors 506.9
      smoke inhalation 508.2
    psychogenic 306.1
  retina 362.9
    specified type NEC 362.89
  rumination 307.53
  sacroiliac joint NEC 724.6
  sacrum 724.6
  schizo-affective (see also Schizophrenia) 295.7

Disorder (Continued)
  schizoid, childhood or adolescence 313.22
  schizophreniform 295.4
  schizotypal personality 301.22
  secretion, thyrocalcitonin 246.0
  seizure 345.9
    recurrent 345.9
      epileptic - see Epilepsy
  semantic pragmatic 315.39
    with autism 299.0
  sense of smell 781.1
    psychogenic 306.7
  separation anxiety 309.21
  sexual (see also Deviation, sexual) 302.9
    aversion 302.79
    desire, hypoactive 302.71
    function, psychogenic 302.70
  shyness, of childhood and adolescence 313.21
  single complement (C_1–C_9) 279.8
  skin NEC 709.9
    fetus or newborn 778.9
      specified type 778.8
    psychogenic (allergic) (eczematous) (pruritic) 306.3
    specified type NEC 709.8
    vascular 709.1
  sleep 780.50
    with apnea - see Apnea, sleep
    alcohol induced 291.82
    arousal 307.46
      confusional 327.41
    circadian rhythm 327.30
      advanced sleep phase type 327.32
      alcohol induced 291.82
      delayed sleep phase type 327.31
      drug induced 292.85
      free running type 327.34
      in conditions classified elsewhere 327.37
      irregular sleep-wake type 327.33
      jet lag type 327.35
      other 327.39
      shift work type 327.36
    drug induced 292.85
    initiation or maintenance (see also Insomnia) 780.52
      nonorganic origin (transient) 307.41
        persistent 307.42
    nonorganic origin 307.40
      specified type NEC 307.49
    organic specified type NEC 327.8
    periodic limb movement 327.51
    specified NEC 780.59
    wake
      cycle - see Disorder, sleep, circadian rhythm
      schedule - see Disorder, sleep, circadian rhythm
  social, of childhood and adolescence 313.22
  soft tissue 729.90
    specified type NEC 729.99
  somatization 300.81
  somatoform (atypical) (undifferentiated) 300.82
    severe 300.81
    specified type NEC 300.89
  speech NEC 784.59
    nonorganic origin 307.9
  spine NEC 724.9
    ligamentous or muscular attachments, peripheral 720.1
  steroid metabolism NEC 255.2
  stomach (functional) (see also Disorder, gastric) 536.9
    psychogenic 306.4
  storage, iron 275.09
  stress (see also Reaction, stress, acute) 308.3
    posttraumatic
      acute 309.81
      brief 309.81
      chronic (motor or vocal) 309.81

Disorder (Continued)
  substitution 300.11
  suspected - see Observation
  synovium 727.9
  temperature regulation, fetus or newborn 778.4
  temporomandibular joint NEC 524.60
    sounds on opening or closing 524.64
    specified NEC 524.69
  tendon 727.9
    shoulder region 726.10
  thoracic root (nerve) NEC 353.3
  thyrocalcitonin secretion 246.0
  thyroid (gland) NEC 246.9
    specified type NEC 246.8
  tic 307.20
    chronic (motor or vocal) 307.22
    motor-verbal 307.23
    organic origin 333.1
    transient (of childhood) 307.21
  tooth NEC 525.9
    development NEC 520.9
      specified type NEC 520.8
    eruption 520.6
    specified type NEC 525.8
  Tourette's 307.23
  transport, carbohydrate 271.9
    specified type NEC 271.8
  tubular, phosphate-losing 588.0
  tympanic membrane 384.9
  unaggressive, unsocialized (see also Disturbance, conduct) 312.1
  undersocialized, unsocialized (see also Disturbance, conduct)
    aggressive (type) 312.0
    unaggressive (type) 312.1
  vision, visual NEC 368.9
    binocular NEC 368.30
    cortex 377.73
      associated with
        inflammatory disorders 377.73
        neoplasms 377.71
        vascular disorders 377.72
    pathway NEC 377.63
      associated with
        inflammatory disorders 377.63
        neoplasms 377.61
        vascular disorders 377.62
  vocal tic
    chronic 307.22
  wakefulness (see also Hypersomnia) 780.54
    nonorganic origin (transient) 307.43
      persistent 307.44
  written expression 315.2

Disorganized globe 360.29

Displacement, displaced

> Note: For acquired displacement of bones, cartilage, joints, tendons, due to injury, see also Dislocation.
>
> Displacements at ages under one year should be considered congenital, provided there is no indication the condition was acquired after birth.

  acquired traumatic of bone, cartilage, joint, tendon NEC (without fracture) (see also Dislocation) 839.8
    with fracture - see Fracture, by site
  adrenal gland (congenital) 759.1
  alveolus and teeth, vertical 524.75
  appendix, retrocecal (congenital) 751.5
  auricle (congenital) 744.29
  bladder (acquired) 596.89
    congenital 753.8
  brachial plexus (congenital) 742.8
  brain stem, caudal 742.4
  canaliculus lacrimalis 743.65
  cardia, through esophageal hiatus 750.6
  cerebellum, caudal 742.4
  cervix - see Displacement, uterus

Displacement, displaced (Continued)
- colon (congenital) 751.4
- device, implant, or graft - *see* Complications, mechanical
- epithelium
  - columnar of cervix 622.10
  - cuboidal, beyond limits of external os (uterus) 752.49
- esophageal mucosa into cardia of stomach, congenital 750.4
- esophagus (acquired) 530.89
  - congenital 750.4
- eyeball (acquired) (old) 376.36
  - congenital 743.8
  - current injury 871.3
  - lateral 376.36
- fallopian tube (acquired) 620.4
  - congenital 752.19
  - opening (congenital) 752.19
- gallbladder (congenital) 751.69
- gastric mucosa 750.7
  - into
    - duodenum 750.7
    - esophagus 750.7
    - Meckel's diverticulum, congenital 750.7
- globe (acquired) (lateral) (old) 376.36
  - current injury 871.3
- graft
  - artificial skin graft 996.55
  - decellularized allodermis graft 996.55
- heart (congenital) 746.87
  - acquired 429.89
- hymen (congenital) (upward) 752.49
- internal prosthesis NEC - *see* Complications, mechanical
- intervertebral disc (with neuritis, radiculitis, sciatica, or other pain) 722.2
  - with myelopathy 722.70
  - cervical, cervicodorsal, cervicothoracic 722.0
    - with myelopathy 722.71
    - due to major trauma - *see* Dislocation, vertebra, cervical
  - due to trauma - *see* Dislocation, vertebra
  - lumbar, lumbosacral 722.10
    - with myelopathy 722.73
    - due to major trauma - *see* Dislocation, vertebra, lumbar
  - thoracic, thoracolumbar 722.11
    - with myelopathy 722.72
    - due to major trauma - *see* Dislocation, vertebra, thoracic
- intrauterine device 996.32
- kidney (acquired) 593.0
  - congenital 753.3
- lacrimal apparatus or duct (congenital) 743.65
- macula (congenital) 743.55
- Meckel's diverticulum (congenital) 751.0
- nail (congenital) 757.5
  - acquired 703.8
- opening of Wharton's duct in mouth 750.26
- organ or site, congenital NEC - *see* Malposition, congenital
- ovary (acquired) 620.4
  - congenital 752.0
  - free in peritoneal cavity (congenital) 752.0
  - into hernial sac 620.4
- oviduct (acquired) 620.4
  - congenital 752.19
- parathyroid (gland) 252.8
- parotid gland (congenital) 750.26
- punctum lacrimale (congenital) 743.65
- sacroiliac (congenital) (joint) 755.69
  - current injury - *see* Dislocation, sacroiliac
  - old 724.6
- spine (congenital) 756.19
- spleen, congenital 759.0
- stomach (congenital) 750.7
  - acquired 537.89
- subglenoid (closed) 831.01
- sublingual duct (congenital) 750.26

Displacement, displaced (Continued)
- teeth, tooth 524.30
  - horizontal 524.33
  - vertical 524.34
- tongue (congenital) (downward) 750.19
- trachea (congenital) 748.3
- ureter or ureteric opening or orifice (congenital) 753.4
- uterine opening of oviducts or fallopian tubes 752.19
- uterus, uterine (*see also* Malposition, uterus) 621.6
  - congenital 752.39
- ventricular septum 746.89
  - with rudimentary ventricle 746.89
- xyphoid bone (process) 738.3

Disproportion 653.9●
- affecting fetus or newborn 763.1
- breast, reconstructed 612.1
  - between native and reconstructed 612.1
- caused by
  - conjoined twins 678.1●
  - contraction, pelvis (general) 653.1●
    - inlet 653.2●
    - midpelvic 653.8●
    - midplane 653.8●
    - outlet 653.3●
  - fetal
    - ascites 653.7●
    - hydrocephalus 653.6●
    - hydrops 653.7●
    - meningomyelocele 653.7●
    - sacral teratoma 653.7●
    - tumor 653.7●
  - hydrocephalic fetus 653.6●
  - pelvis, pelvic, abnormality (bony) NEC 653.0●
  - unusually large fetus 653.5●
- causing obstructed labor 660.1●
- cephalopelvic, normally formed fetus 653.4●
  - causing obstructed labor 660.1●
- fetal NEC 653.5●
  - causing obstructed labor 660.1●
- fetopelvic, normally formed fetus 653.4●
  - causing obstructed labor 660.1●
- mixed maternal and fetal origin, normally, formed fetus 653.4●
- pelvis, pelvic (bony) NEC 653.1●
  - causing obstructed labor 660.1●
- specified type NEC 653.8●

Disruption
- cesarean wound 674.1●
- family V61.09
  - due to
    - child in
      - care of non-parental family member V61.06
      - foster care V61.06
      - welfare custody V61.05
    - death of family member V61.07
    - divorce V61.03
    - estrangement V61.09
      - parent-child V61.04
    - extended absence of family member NEC V61.08
    - family member
      - on military deployment V61.01
      - return from military deployment V61.02
    - legal separation V61.03
- gastrointestinal anastomosis 997.49
- ligament(s) - *see also* Sprain
  - knee
    - current injury - *see* Dislocation, knee
    - old 717.89
      - capsular 717.85
      - collateral (medial) 717.82
        - lateral 717.81
      - cruciate (posterior) 717.84
        - anterior 717.83
      - specified site NEC 717.85

Disruption (Continued)
- marital V61.10
  - involving
    - divorce V61.03
    - estrangement V61.09
- operation wound (external) (*see also* Dehiscence) 998.32
  - internal 998.31
- organ transplant, anastomosis site - *see* Complications, transplant, organ, by site
- ossicles, ossicular chain 385.23
  - traumatic - *see* Fracture, skull, base
- parenchyma
  - liver (hepatic) - *see* Laceration, liver, major
  - spleen - *see* Laceration, spleen, parenchyma, massive
- phase-shift, of 24 hour sleep-wake cycle, unspecified 780.55
  - nonorganic origin 307.45
- sleep-wake cycle (24 hour), unspecified 780.55
  - circadian rhythm 327.33
  - nonorganic origin 307.45
- suture line (external) (*see also* Dehiscence) 998.32
  - internal 998.31
- wound 998.30
  - cesarean operation 674.1●
  - episiotomy 674.2●
  - operation (surgical) 998.32
    - cesarean 674.1●
    - internal 998.31
  - perineal (obstetric) 674.2●
  - uterine 674.1●

Disruptio uteri - *see also* Rupture, uterus
- complicating delivery - *see* Delivery, complicated, rupture, uterus

Dissatisfaction with
- employment V62.29
- school environment V62.3

Dissecting - *see* condition

Dissection
- aorta 441.00
  - abdominal 441.02
  - thoracic 441.01
  - thoracoabdominal 441.03
- artery, arterial
  - carotid 443.21
  - coronary 414.12
  - iliac 443.22
  - renal 443.23
  - specified NEC 443.29
  - vertebral 443.24
- vascular 459.9
- wound - *see* Wound, open, by site

Disseminated - *see* condition

Dissociated personality NEC 300.15

Dissociation
- auriculoventricular or atrioventricular (any degree) (AV) 426.89
  - with heart block 426.0
- interference 426.89
- isorhythmic 426.89
- rhythm
  - atrioventricular (AV) 426.89
  - interference 426.89

Dissociative
- identity disorder 300.14
- reaction NEC 300.15

Dissolution, vertebra (*see also* Osteoporosis) 733.00

Distention
- abdomen (gaseous) 787.3
- bladder 596.89
- cecum 569.89
- colon 569.89
- gallbladder 575.8
- gaseous (abdomen) 787.3
- intestine 569.89
- kidney 593.89

Distention (Continued)
  liver 573.9
  seminal vesicle 608.89
  stomach 536.8
    acute 536.1
      psychogenic 306.4
  ureter 593.5
  uterus 621.8
Distichia, distichiasis (eyelid) 743.63
Distoma hepaticum infestation 121.3
Distomiasis 121.9
  bile passages 121.3
    due to Clonorchis sinensis 121.1
  hemic 120.9
  hepatic (liver) 121.3
    due to Clonorchis sinensis (clonorchiasis) 121.1
  intestinal 121.4
  liver 121.3
    due to Clonorchis sinensis 121.1
  lung 121.2
  pulmonary 121.2
Distomolar (fourth molar) 520.1
  causing crowding 524.31
Disto-occlusion (division I) (division II) 524.22
Distortion (congenital)
  adrenal (gland) 759.1
  ankle (joint) 755.69
  anus 751.5
  aorta 747.29
  appendix 751.5
  arm 755.59
  artery (peripheral) NEC (*see also* Distortion, peripheral vascular system) 747.60
    cerebral 747.81
    coronary 746.85
    pulmonary 747.39
    retinal 743.58
    umbilical 747.5
  auditory canal 744.29
    causing impairment of hearing 744.02
  bile duct or passage 751.69
  bladder 753.8
  brain 742.4
  bronchus 748.3
  cecum 751.5
  cervix (uteri) 752.49
  chest (wall) 756.3
  clavicle 755.51
  clitoris 752.49
  coccyx 756.19
  colon 751.5
  common duct 751.69
  cornea 743.41
  cricoid cartilage 748.3
  cystic duct 751.69
  duodenum 751.5
  ear 744.29
    auricle 744.29
      causing impairment of hearing 744.02
    causing impairment of hearing 744.09
    external 744.29
      causing impairment of hearing 744.02
    inner 744.05
    middle, except ossicles 744.03
      ossicles 744.04
    ossicles 744.04
  endocrine (gland) NEC 759.2
  epiglottis 748.3
  Eustachian tube 744.24
  eye 743.8
    adnexa 743.69
  face bone(s) 756.0
  fallopian tube 752.19
  femur 755.69
  fibula 755.69
  finger(s) 755.59
  foot 755.67
  gallbladder 751.69

Distortion (Continued)
  genitalia, genital organ(s)
    female 752.89
      external 752.49
      internal NEC 752.89
    male 752.89
      penis 752.69
  glottis 748.3
  gyri 742.4
  hand bone(s) 755.59
  heart (auricle) (ventricle) 746.89
    valve (cusp) 746.89
  hepatic duct 751.69
  humerus 755.59
  hymen 752.49
  ileum 751.5
  intestine (large) (small) 751.5
    with anomalous adhesions, fixation or malrotation 751.4
  jaw NEC 524.89
  jejunum 751.5
  kidney 753.3
  knee (joint) 755.64
  labium (majus) (minus) 752.49
  larynx 748.3
  leg 755.69
  lens 743.36
  liver 751.69
  lumbar spine 756.19
    with disproportion (fetopelvic) 653.0●
      affecting fetus or newborn 763.1
      causing obstructed labor 660.1●
  lumbosacral (joint) (region) 756.19
  lung (fissures) (lobe) 748.69
  nerve 742.8
  nose 748.1
  organ
    of Corti 744.05
    of site not listed - *see* Anomaly, specified type NEC
  ossicles, ear 744.04
  ovary 752.0
  oviduct 752.19
  pancreas 751.7
  parathyroid (gland) 759.2
  patella 755.64
  peripheral vascular system NEC 747.60
    gastrointestinal 747.61
    lower limb 747.64
    renal 747.62
    spinal 747.82
    upper limb 747.63
  pituitary (gland) 759.2
  radius 755.59
  rectum 751.5
  rib 756.3
  sacroiliac joint 755.69
  sacrum 756.19
  scapula 755.59
  shoulder girdle 755.59
  site not listed - *see* Anomaly, specified type NEC
  skull bone(s) 756.0
    with
      anencephalus 740.0
      encephalocele 742.0
      hydrocephalus 742.3
        with spina bifida (*see also* Spina bifida) 741.0●
      microcephalus 742.1
  spinal cord 742.59
  spine 756.19
  spleen 759.0
  sternum 756.3
  thorax (wall) 756.3
  thymus (gland) 759.2
  thyroid (gland) 759.2
    cartilage 748.3
  tibia 755.69
  toe(s) 755.66
  tongue 750.19

Distortion (Continued)
  trachea (cartilage) 748.3
  ulna 755.59
  ureter 753.4
    causing obstruction 753.20
  urethra 753.8
    causing obstruction 753.6
  uterus 752.39
  vagina 752.49
  vein (peripheral) NEC (*see also* Distortion, peripheral vascular system) 747.60
    great 747.49
    portal 747.49
    pulmonary 747.49
  vena cava (inferior) (superior) 747.49
  vertebra 756.19
  visual NEC 368.15
    shape or size 368.14
  vulva 752.49
  wrist (bones) (joint) 755.59
Distress
  abdomen 789.0●
  colon 564.9
  emotional V40.9
  epigastric 789.0●
  fetal (syndrome) 768.4
    affecting management of pregnancy or childbirth 656.8●
    liveborn infant 768.4
      first noted
        before onset of labor 768.2
        during labor and delivery 768.3
    stillborn infant (death before onset of labor) 768.0
      death during labor 768.1
  gastrointestinal (functional) 536.9
    psychogenic 306.4
  intestinal (functional) NEC 564.9
    psychogenic 306.4
  intrauterine - *see* Distress, fetal
  leg 729.5
  maternal 669.0●
  mental V40.9
  respiratory 786.09
    acute (adult) 518.82
    adult syndrome (following trauma and surgery) 518.52
      specified NEC 518.82
    fetus or newborn 770.89
    syndrome (idiopathic) (newborn) 769
  stomach 536.9
    psychogenic 306.4
Distribution vessel, atypical NEC 747.60
  coronary artery 746.85
  spinal 747.82
Districhiasis 704.2
Disturbance - *see also* Disease
  absorption NEC 579.9
    calcium 269.3
    carbohydrate 579.8
    fat 579.8
    protein 579.8
    specified type NEC 579.8
    vitamin (*see also* Deficiency, vitamin) 269.2
  acid-base equilibrium 276.9
  activity and attention, simple, with hyperkinesis 314.01
  amino acid (metabolic) (*see also* Disorder, amino acid) 270.9
    imidazole 270.5
    maple syrup (urine) disease 270.3
    transport 270.0
  assimilation, food 579.9
  attention, simple 314.00
    with hyperactivity 314.01
  auditory, nerve, except deafness 388.5
  behavior (*see also* Disturbance, conduct) 312.9
  blood clotting (hypoproteinemia) (mechanism) (*see also* Defect, coagulation) 286.9
  central nervous system NEC 349.9

SECTION 1 INDEX TO DISEASES AND INJURIES / **Disturbance**

Disturbance (Continued)
- cerebral nerve NEC 352.9
- circulatory 459.9
- conduct 312.9
  - adjustment reaction 309.3
  - adolescent onset type 312.82
  - childhood onset type 312.81

> Note: Use the following fifth-digit subclassification with categories 312.0–312.2:
> 0 unspecified
> 1 mild
> 2 moderate
> 3 severe

- compulsive 312.30
  - intermittent explosive disorder 312.34
  - isolated explosive disorder 312.35
  - kleptomania 312.32
  - pathological gambling 312.31
  - pyromania 312.33
- hyperkinetic 314.2
- intermittent explosive 312.34
- isolated explosive 312.35
- mixed with emotions 312.4
- socialized (type) 312.20
  - aggressive 312.23
  - unaggressive 312.21
- specified type NEC 312.89
- undersocialized, unsocialized
  - aggressive (type) 312.0●
  - unaggressive (type) 312.1●
- coordination 781.3
- cranial nerve NEC 352.9
- deep sensibility - see Disturbance, sensation
- digestive 536.9
  - psychogenic 306.4
- electrolyte - see Imbalance, electrolyte
- emotions specific to childhood or adolescence 313.9
  - with
    - academic underachievement 313.83
    - anxiety and fearfulness 313.0
    - elective mutism 313.23
    - identity disorder 313.82
    - jealousy 313.3
    - misery and unhappiness 313.1
    - oppositional defiant disorder 313.81
    - overanxiousness 313.0
    - sensitivity 313.21
    - shyness 313.21
    - social withdrawal 313.22
    - withdrawal reaction 313.22
  - involving relationship problems 313.3
  - mixed 313.89
  - specified type NEC 313.89
- endocrine (gland) 259.9
  - neonatal, transitory 775.9
    - specified NEC 775.89
- equilibrium 780.4
- feeding (elderly) (infant) 783.3
  - newborn 779.31
  - nonorganic origin NEC 307.59
  - psychogenic NEC 307.59
- fructose metabolism 271.2
- gait 781.2
  - hysterical 300.11
- gastric (functional) 536.9
  - motility 536.8
  - psychogenic 306.4
  - secretion 536.8
- gastrointestinal (functional) 536.9
  - psychogenic 306.4
- habit, child 307.9
- hearing, except deafness 388.40
- heart, functional (conditions classifiable to 426, 427, 428)
  - due to presence of (cardiac) prosthesis 429.4

Disturbance (Continued)
- heart, functional (Continued)
  - postoperative (immediate) 997.1
    - long-term effect of cardiac surgery 429.4
  - psychogenic 306.2
- hormone 259.9
- innervation uterus, sympathetic, parasympathetic 621.8
- keratinization NEC
  - gingiva 523.10
  - lip 528.5
  - oral (mucosa) (soft tissue) 528.79
    - residual ridge mucosa
      - excessive 528.72
      - minimal 528.71
  - tongue 528.79
- labyrinth, labyrinthine (vestibule) 386.9
- learning, specific NEC 315.2
- memory (see also Amnesia) 780.93
  - mild, following organic brain damage 310.89
- mental (see also Disorder, mental) 300.9
  - associated with diseases classified elsewhere 316
- metabolism (acquired) (congenital) (see also Disorder, metabolism) 277.9
  - with
    - abortion - see Abortion, by type, with metabolic disorder
    - ectopic pregnancy (see also categories 633.0–633.9) 639.4
    - molar pregnancy (see also categories 630–632) 639.4
  - amino acid (see also Disorder, amino acid) 270.9
    - aromatic NEC 270.2
    - branched-chain 270.3
    - specified type NEC 270.8
    - straight-chain NEC 270.7
    - sulfur-bearing 270.4
    - transport 270.0
  - ammonia 270.6
  - arginine 270.6
  - argininosuccinic acid 270.6
  - carbohydrate NEC 271.9
  - cholesterol 272.9
  - citrulline 270.6
  - cystathionine 270.4
  - fat 272.9
  - following
    - abortion 639.4
    - ectopic or molar pregnancy 639.4
  - general 277.9
    - carbohydrate 271.9
    - iron 275.09
    - phosphate 275.3
    - sodium 276.9
  - glutamine 270.7
  - glycine 270.7
  - histidine 270.5
  - homocystine 270.4
  - in labor or delivery 669.0●
  - iron 275.09
  - isoleucine 270.3
  - leucine 270.3
  - lipoid 272.9
    - specified type NEC 272.8
  - lysine 270.7
  - methionine 270.4
  - neonatal, transitory 775.9
    - specified type NEC 775.89
  - nitrogen 788.99
  - ornithine 270.6
  - phosphate 275.3
  - phosphatides 272.7
  - serine 270.7
  - sodium NEC 276.9
  - threonine 270.7
  - tryptophan 270.2
  - tyrosine 270.2

Disturbance (Continued)
- metabolism (Continued)
  - urea cycle 270.6
  - valine 270.3
- motor 796.1
- nervous functional 799.21
- neuromuscular mechanism (eye) due to syphilis 094.84
- nutritional 269.9
  - nail 703.8
- ocular motion 378.87
  - psychogenic 306.7
- oculogyric 378.87
  - psychogenic 306.7
- oculomotor NEC 378.87
  - psychogenic 306.7
- olfactory nerve 781.1
- optic nerve NEC 377.49
- oral epithelium, including tongue 528.79
  - residual ridge mucosa
    - excessive 528.72
    - minimal 528.71
- personality (pattern) (trait) (see also Disorder, personality) 301.9
  - following organic brain damage 310.1
- polyglandular 258.9
- psychomotor 307.9
- pupillary 379.49
- reflex 796.1
- rhythm, heart 427.9
  - postoperative (immediate) 997.1
    - long-term effect of cardiac surgery 429.4
  - psychogenic 306.2
- salivary secretion 527.7
- sensation (cold) (heat) (localization) (tactile discrimination localization) (texture) (vibratory) NEC 782.0
  - hysterical 300.11
  - skin 782.0
  - smell 781.1
  - taste 781.1
- sensory (see also Disturbance, sensation) 782.0
  - innervation 782.0
- situational (transient) (see also Reaction, adjustment) 309.9
  - acute 308.3
- sleep 780.50
  - with apnea - see Apnea, sleep
  - initiation or maintenance (see also Insomnia) 780.52
    - nonorganic origin 307.41
  - nonorganic origin 307.40
    - specified type NEC 307.49
  - specified NEC 780.59
    - nonorganic origin 307.49
  - wakefulness (see also Hypersomnia) 780.54
    - nonorganic origin 307.43
- sociopathic 301.7
- speech NEC 784.59
  - developmental 315.39
    - associated with hyperkinesis 314.1
  - secondary to organic lesion 784.59
- stomach (functional) (see also Disturbance, gastric) 536.9
- sympathetic (nerve) (see also Neuropathy, peripheral, autonomic) 337.9
- temperature sense 782.0
  - hysterical 300.11
- tooth
  - eruption 520.6
  - formation 520.4
  - structure, hereditary NEC 520.5
- touch (see also Disturbance, sensation) 782.0
- vascular 459.9
  - arteriosclerotic - see Arteriosclerosis

Disturbance (Continued)
　vasomotor 443.9
　vasospastic 443.9
　vestibular labyrinth 386.9
　vision, visual NEC 368.9
　　psychophysical 368.16
　　specified NEC 368.8
　　subjective 368.10
　voice and resonance 784.40
　wakefulness (initiation or maintenance) (see also Hypersomnia) 780.54
　　nonorganic origin 307.43

Disulfiduria, beta-mercaptolactate-cysteine 270.0

Disuse atrophy, bone 733.7

Ditthomska syndrome 307.81

Diuresis 788.42

Divers'
　palsy or paralysis 993.3
　squeeze 993.3

Diverticula, diverticulosis, diverticulum (acute) (multiple) (perforated) (ruptured) 562.10
　with diverticulitis 562.11
　aorta (Kommerell's) 747.21
　appendix (noninflammatory) 543.9
　bladder (acquired) (sphincter) 596.3
　　congenital 753.8
　broad ligament 620.8
　bronchus (congenital) 748.3
　　acquired 494.0
　　　with acute exacerbation 494.1
　calyx, calyceal (kidney) 593.89
　cardia (stomach) 537.1
　cecum 562.10
　　with
　　　diverticulitis 562.11
　　　　with hemorrhage 562.13
　　　hemorrhage 562.12
　　congenital 751.5
　colon (acquired) 562.10
　　with
　　　diverticulitis 562.11
　　　　with hemorrhage 562.13
　　　hemorrhage 562.12
　　congenital 751.5
　duodenum 562.00
　　with
　　　diverticulitis 562.01
　　　　with hemorrhage 562.03
　　　hemorrhage 562.02
　　congenital 751.5
　epiphrenic (esophagus) 530.6
　esophagus (congenital) 750.4
　　acquired 530.6
　　epiphrenic 530.6
　　pulsion 530.6
　　traction 530.6
　　Zenker's 530.6
　Eustachian tube 381.89
　fallopian tube 620.8
　gallbladder (congenital) 751.69
　gastric 537.1
　heart (congenital) 746.89
　ileum 562.00
　　with
　　　diverticulitis 562.01
　　　　with hemorrhage 562.03
　　　hemorrhage 562.02
　intestine (large) 562.10
　　with
　　　diverticulitis 562.11
　　　　with hemorrhage 562.13
　　　hemorrhage 562.12
　　congenital 751.5
　　small 562.00
　　　with
　　　　diverticulitis 562.01
　　　　　with hemorrhage 562.03
　　　　hemorrhage 562.02
　　　congenital 751.5

Diverticula, diverticulosis (Continued)
　jejunum 562.00
　　with
　　　diverticulitis 562.01
　　　　with hemorrhage 562.03
　　　hemorrhage 562.02
　kidney (calyx) (pelvis) 593.89
　　with calculus 592.0
　Kommerell's 747.21
　laryngeal ventricle (congenital) 748.3
　Meckel's (displaced) (hypertrophic) 751.0
　midthoracic 530.6
　organ or site, congenital NEC - see Distortion
　pericardium (congenital) (cyst) 746.89
　　acquired (true) 423.8
　pharyngoesophageal (pulsion) 530.6
　pharynx (congenital) 750.27
　pulsion (esophagus) 530.6
　rectosigmoid 562.10
　　with
　　　diverticulitis 562.11
　　　　with hemorrhage 562.13
　　　hemorrhage 562.12
　　congenital 751.5
　rectum 562.10
　　with
　　　diverticulitis 562.11
　　　　with hemorrhage 562.13
　　　hemorrhage 562.12
　renal (calyces) (pelvis) 593.89
　　with calculus 592.0
　Rokitansky's 530.6
　seminal vesicle 608.0
　sigmoid 562.10
　　with
　　　diverticulitis 562.11
　　　　with hemorrhage 562.13
　　　hemorrhage 562.12
　　congenital 751.5
　small intestine 562.00
　　with
　　　diverticulitis 562.01
　　　　with hemorrhage 562.03
　　　hemorrhage 562.02
　stomach (cardia) (juxtacardia) (juxtapyloric) (acquired) 537.1
　　congenital 750.7
　subdiaphragmatic 530.6
　trachea (congenital) 748.3
　　acquired 519.19
　traction (esophagus) 530.6
　ureter (acquired) 593.89
　　congenital 753.4
　ureterovesical orifice 593.89
　urethra (acquired) 599.2
　　congenital 753.8
　ventricle, left (congenital) 746.89
　vesical (urinary) 596.3
　　congenital 753.8
　Zenker's (esophagus) 530.6

Diverticulitis (acute) (see also Diverticula) 562.11
　with hemorrhage 562.13
　bladder (urinary) 596.3
　cecum (perforated) 562.11
　　with hemorrhage 562.13
　colon (perforated) 562.11
　　with hemorrhage 562.13
　duodenum 562.01
　　with hemorrhage 562.03
　esophagus 530.6
　ileum (perforated) 562.01
　　with hemorrhage 562.03
　intestine (large) (perforated) 562.11
　　with hemorrhage 562.13
　　small 562.01
　　　with hemorrhage 562.03
　jejunum (perforated) 562.01
　　with hemorrhage 562.03
　Meckel's (perforated) 751.0
　pharyngoesophageal 530.6

Diverticulitis (Continued)
　rectosigmoid (perforated) 562.11
　　with hemorrhage 562.13
　rectum 562.11
　　with hemorrhage 562.13
　sigmoid (old) (perforated) 562.11
　　with hemorrhage 562.13
　small intestine (perforated) 562.01
　　with hemorrhage 562.03
　vesical (urinary) 596.3

Diverticulosis - see Diverticula

Division
　cervix uteri 622.8
　　external os into two openings by frenum 752.44
　　external (cervical) into two openings by frenum 752.44
　glans penis 752.69
　hymen 752.49
　labia minora (congenital) 752.49
　ligament (partial or complete) (current) - see also Sprain, by site
　　with open wound - see Wound, open, by site
　muscle (partial or complete) (current) - see also Sprain, by site
　　with open wound - see Wound, open, by site
　nerve - see Injury, nerve, by site
　penis glans 752.69
　spinal cord - see Injury, spinal, by site
　vein 459.9
　　traumatic - see Injury, vascular, by site

Divorce V61.03

Dix-Hallpike neurolabyrinthitis 386.12

Dizziness 780.4
　hysterical 300.11
　psychogenic 306.9

Doan-Wiseman syndrome (primary splenic neutropenia) 289.53

Dog bite - see Wound, open, by site

Döhle-Heller aortitis 093.1

Döhle body-panmyelopathic syndrome 288.2

Dolichocephaly, dolichocephalus 754.0

Dolichocolon 751.5

Dolichostenomelia 759.82

Donohue's syndrome (leprechaunism) 259.8

Donor
　blood V59.01
　　other blood components V59.09
　　stem cells V59.02
　　whole blood V59.01
　bone V59.2
　　marrow V59.3
　cornea V59.5
　egg (oocyte) (ovum) V59.70
　　over age 35 V59.73
　　　anonymous recipient V59.73
　　　designated recipient V59.74
　　under age 35 V59.71
　　　anonymous recipient V59.71
　　　designated recipient V59.72
　heart V59.8
　kidney V59.4
　liver V59.6
　lung V59.8
　lymphocyte V59.8
　organ V59.9
　　specified NEC V59.8
　potential, examination of V70.8
　skin V59.1
　specified organ or tissue NEC V59.8
　sperm V59.8
　stem cells V59.02
　tissue V59.9
　　specified type NEC V59.8

Donovanosis (granuloma venereum) 099.2

DOPS (diffuse obstructive pulmonary syndrome) 496

Double
- albumin 273.8
- aortic arch 747.21
- auditory canal 744.29
- auricle (heart) 746.82
- bladder 753.8
- external (cervical) os 752.44
- kidney with double pelvis (renal) 753.3
- larynx 748.3
- meatus urinarius 753.8
- organ or site NEC - see Accessory
- orifice
  - heart valve NEC 746.89
    - pulmonary 746.09
- outlet, right ventricle 745.11
- pelvis (renal) with double ureter 753.4
- penis 752.69
- tongue 750.13
- ureter (one or both sides) 753.4
  - with double pelvis (renal) 753.4
- urethra 753.8
- urinary meatus 753.8
- uterus (any degree) 752.2
  - with doubling of cervix and vagina 752.2
  - in pregnancy or childbirth 654.0 ●
    - affecting fetus or newborn 763.89
- vagina 752.47
  - with doubling of cervix and uterus 752.2
- vision 368.2
- vocal cords 748.3
- vulva 752.49
- whammy (syndrome) 360.81

Douglas' pouch, cul-de-sac - see condition
Down's disease or syndrome (mongolism) 758.0
Down-growth, epithelial (anterior chamber) 364.61
DPD (dihydropyrimidine dehydrogenase deficiency) 277.6
Dracontiasis 125.7
Dracunculiasis 125.7
Dracunculosis 125.7
Drainage
- abscess (spontaneous) - see Abscess
- anomalous pulmonary veins to hepatic veins or right atrium 747.41
- stump (amputation) (surgical) 997.62
- suprapubic, bladder 596.89

Dream state, hysterical 300.13
Drepanocytic anemia (see also Disease, sickle cell) 282.60
Dresbach's syndrome (elliptocytosis) 282.1
Dreschlera (infection) 118
- hawaiiensis 117.8

Dressler's syndrome (postmyocardial infarction) 411.0
Dribbling (post-void) 788.35
Drift, ulnar 736.09
Drinking (alcohol) - see also Alcoholism
- excessive, to excess NEC (see also Abuse, drugs, nondependent) 305.0 ●
  - bouts, periodic 305.0 ●
  - continual 303.9 ●
  - episodic 305.0 ●
  - habitual 303.9 ●
  - periodic 305.0 ●

Drip, postnasal (chronic) 784.91
- due to:
  - allergic rhinitis - see Rhinitis, allergic
  - common cold 460
  - gastroesophageal reflux - see Reflux, gastroesophageal
  - nasopharyngitis - see Nasopharyngitis
  - other known condition - code to condition
  - sinusitis - see Sinusitis

Drivers' license examination V70.3
Droop
- Cooper's 611.81
- facial 781.94

Drop
- finger 736.29
- foot 736.79
- hematocrit (precipitous) 790.01
- hemoglobin 790.01
- toe 735.8
- wrist 736.05

Dropped
- dead 798.1
- heart beats 426.6

Dropsy, dropsical (see also Edema) 782.3
- abdomen 789.59
- amnion (see also Hydramnios) 657 ●
- brain - see Hydrocephalus
- cardiac (see also Failure, heart) 428.0
- cardiorenal (see also Hypertension, cardiorenal) 404.90
- chest 511.9
- fetus or newborn 778.0
  - due to isoimmunization 773.3
- gangrenous (see also Gangrene) 785.4
- heart (see also Failure, heart) 428.0
- hepatic - see Cirrhosis, liver
- infantile - see Hydrops, fetalis
- kidney (see also Nephrosis) 581.9
- liver - see Cirrhosis, liver
- lung 514
- malarial (see also Malaria) 084.9
- neonatorum - see Hydrops, fetalis
- nephritic 581.9
- newborn - see Hydrops, fetalis
- nutritional 269.9
- ovary 620.8
- pericardium (see also Pericarditis) 423.9
- renal (see also Nephrosis) 581.9
- uremic - see Uremia

Drowned, drowning (near) 994.1
- lung 518.52

Drowsiness 780.09
Drug - see also condition
- addiction (see also Dependence) 304.9 ●
- adverse effect, correct substance properly administered 995.20
- allergy 995.27
- dependence (see also Dependence) 304.9 ●
- habit (see also Dependence) 304.9 ●
- hypersensitivity 995.27
- induced
  - circadian rhythm sleep disorder 292.85
  - hypersomnia 292.85
  - insomnia 292.85
  - mental disorder 292.9
    - anxiety 292.89
    - mood 292.84
    - sexual 292.89
    - sleep 292.85
    - specified type 292.89
  - parasomnia 292.85
  - persisting
    - amnestic disorder 292.83
    - dementia 292.82
  - psychotic disorder
    - with
      - delusions 292.11
      - hallucinations 292.12
  - sleep disorder 292.85
- intoxication 292.89
- overdose - see Table of Drugs and Chemicals
- poisoning - see Table of Drugs and Chemicals
- therapy (maintenance) status NEC
  - chemotherapy, antineoplastic V58.11
  - immunotherapy, antineoplastic V58.12
  - long-term (current) (prophylactic) use V58.69
    - antibiotics V58.62
    - anticoagulants V58.61
    - anti-inflammatories, non-steroidal (NSAID) V58.64
    - antiplatelets V58.63
    - antithrombotics V58.63
    - aspirin V58.66

Drug (Continued)
- therapy status NEC (Continued)
  - long-term use (Continued)
    - bisphosphonates V58.68
    - high-risk medications NEC V58.69
    - insulin V58.67
    - methadone for pain control V58.69
    - opiate analgesic V58.69
    - steroids V58.65
  - methadone 304.00
  - wrong substance given or taken in error - see Table of Drugs and Chemicals

Drunkenness (see also Abuse, drugs, nondependent) 305.0 ●
- acute in alcoholism (see also Alcoholism) 303.0 ●
- chronic (see also Alcoholism) 303.9 ●
- pathologic 291.4
- simple (acute) 305.0 ●
  - in alcoholism 303.0 ●
- sleep 307.47

Drusen
- optic disc or papilla 377.21
- retina (colloid) (hyaloid degeneration) 362.57
  - hereditary 362.77

Drusenfieber 075
Dry, dryness - see also condition
- eye 375.15
  - syndrome 375.15
- larynx 478.79
- mouth 527.7
- nose 478.19
- skin syndrome 701.1
- socket (teeth) 526.5
- throat 478.29

DSAP (disseminated superficial actinic porokeratosis) 692.75
DSTR (delayed serologic transfusion reaction)
- due to or resulting from incompatibility
  - ABO 999.69
  - non-ABO antigen (minor) (Duffy) (Kell) (Kidd) (Lewis) (M) (N) (P) (S) 999.79
  - Rh antigen (C) (c) (D) (E) (e) 999.74

Duane's retraction syndrome 378.71
Duane-Stilling-Türk syndrome (ocular retraction syndrome) 378.71
Dubin-Johnson disease or syndrome 277.4
Dubini's disease (electric chorea) 049.8
Dubois' abscess or disease 090.5
Duchenne's
- disease 094.0
  - locomotor ataxia 094.0
  - muscular dystrophy 359.1
  - pseudohypertrophy, muscles 359.1
- paralysis 335.22
- syndrome 335.22

Duchenne-Aran myelopathic, muscular atrophy (nonprogressive) (progressive) 335.21
Duchenne-Griesinger disease 359.1
Ducrey's
- bacillus 099.0
- chancre 099.0
- disease (chancroid) 099.0

Duct, ductus - see condition
Duengero 061
Duhring's disease (dermatitis herpetiformis) 694.0
Dukes (-Filatov) disease 057.8
Dullness
- cardiac (decreased) (increased) 785.3

Dumb ague (see also Malaria) 084.6
Dumbness (see also Aphasia) 784.3
Dumdum fever 085.0
Dumping syndrome (postgastrectomy) 564.2
- nonsurgical 536.8

Duodenitis (nonspecific) (peptic) 535.60
- with hemorrhage 535.61
- due to
  - strongyloides stercoralis 127.2

SECTION I INDEX TO DISEASES AND INJURIES / **Dysfunction**

Duodenocholangitis 575.8
Duodenum, duodenal - *see* condition
Duplay's disease, periarthritis, or syndrome 726.2
Duplex - *see also* Accessory
  kidney 753.3
  placenta - *see* Placenta, abnormal
  uterus 752.2
Duplication - *see also* Accessory
  anus 751.5
  aortic arch 747.21
  appendix 751.5
  biliary duct (any) 751.69
  bladder 753.8
  cecum 751.5
    and appendix 751.5
  cervical, cervix 752.44
  clitoris 752.49
  cystic duct 751.69
  digestive organs 751.8
  duodenum 751.5
  esophagus 750.4
  fallopian tube 752.19
  frontonasal process 756.0
  gallbladder 751.69
  ileum 751.5
  intestine (large) (small) 751.5
  jejunum 751.5
  kidney 753.3
  liver 751.69
  nose 748.1
  pancreas 751.7
  penis 752.69
  respiratory organs NEC 748.9
  salivary duct 750.22
  spinal cord (incomplete) 742.51
  stomach 750.7
  ureter 753.4
  vagina 752.47
  vas deferens 752.89
  vocal cords 748.3
Dupré's disease or syndrome (meningism) 781.6
Dupuytren's
  contraction 728.6
  disease (muscle contracture) 728.6
  fracture (closed) 824.4
    ankle (closed) 824.4
      open 824.5
    fibula (closed) 824.4
      open 824.5
    open 824.5
    radius (closed) 813.42
      open 813.52
  muscle contracture 728.6
Durand-Nicolas-Favre disease (climatic bubo) 099.1
Durotomy, incidental (inadvertent) (*see also* Tear, dural) 349.31
Duroziez's disease (congenital mitral stenosis) 746.5
Dust
  conjunctivitis 372.05
  reticulation (occupational) 504
Dutton's
  disease (trypanosomiasis) 086.9
  relapsing fever (West African) 087.1
Dwarf, dwarfism 259.4
  with infantilism (hypophyseal) 253.3
  achondroplastic 756.4
  Amsterdam 759.89
  bird-headed 759.89
  congenital 259.4
  constitutional 259.4
  hypophyseal 253.3
  infantile 259.4
  Levi type 253.3
  Lorain-Levi (pituitary) 253.3
  Lorain type (pituitary) 253.3
  metatropic 756.4

Dwarf, dwarfism (*Continued*)
  nephrotic-glycosuric, with hypophosphatemic rickets 270.0
  nutritional 263.2
  ovarian 758.6
  pancreatic 577.8
  pituitary 253.3
  polydystrophic 277.5
  primordial 253.3
  psychosocial 259.4
  renal 588.0
    with hypertension - *see* Hypertension, kidney
  Russell's (uterine dwarfism and craniofacial dysostosis) 759.89
Dyke-Young anemia or syndrome (acquired macrocytic hemolytic anemia) (secondary) (symptomatic) 283.9
Dynia abnormality (*see also* Defect, coagulation) 286.9
Dysacousis 388.40
Dysadrenocortism 255.9
  hyperfunction 255.3
  hypofunction 255.41
Dysarthria 784.51
  due to late effect of cerebrovascular disease (*see also* Late effect(s) (of) cerebrovascular disease) 438.13
Dysautonomia (*see also* Neuropathy, peripheral, autonomic) 337.9
  familial 742.8
Dysbarism 993.3
Dysbasia 719.7
  angiosclerotica intermittens 443.9
    due to atherosclerosis 440.21
  hysterical 300.11
  lordotica (progressiva) 333.6
  nonorganic origin 307.9
  psychogenic 307.9
Dysbetalipoproteinemia (familial) 272.2
Dyscalculia 315.1
Dyschezia (*see also* Constipation) 564.00
Dyschondroplasia (with hemangiomata) 756.4
  Voorhoeve's 756.4
Dyschondrosteosis 756.59
Dyschromia 709.00
Dyscollagenosis 710.9
Dyscoria 743.41
Dyscraniopyophalangy 759.89
Dyscrasia
  blood 289.9
    with antepartum hemorrhage 641.3 ●
    hemorrhage, subungual 287.8
    newborn NEC 776.9
    puerperal, postpartum 666.3 ●
  ovary 256.8
  plasma cell 273.9
  pluriglandular 258.9
  polyglandular 258.9
Dysdiadochokinesia 781.3
Dysectasia, vesical neck 596.89
Dysendocrinism 259.9
Dysentery, dysenteric (bilious) (catarrhal) (diarrhea) (epidemic) (gangrenous) (hemorrhagic) (infectious) (sporadic) (tropical) (ulcerative) 009.0
  abscess, liver (*see also* Abscess, amebic) 006.3
  amebic (*see also* Amebiasis) 006.9
    with abscess - *see* Abscess, amebic
    acute 006.0
    carrier (suspected) of V02.2
    chronic 006.1
  arthritis (*see also* Arthritis, due to, dysentery) 009.0 [711.3] ●
    bacillary 004.9 [711.3] ●
  asylum 004.9
  bacillary 004.9
    arthritis 004.9 [711.3] ●
    Boyd 004.2
    Flexner 004.1
    Schmitz (-Stutzer) 004.0

Dysentery, dysenteric (*Continued*)
  bacillary (*Continued*)
    Shiga 004.0
    Shigella 004.9
      group A 004.0
      group B 004.1
      group C 004.2
      group D 004.3
      specified type NEC 004.8
    Sonne 004.3
    specified type NEC 004.8
  bacterium 004.9
  balantidial 007.0
  Balantidium coli 007.0
  Boyd's 004.2
  Chilomastix 007.8
  Chinese 004.9
  choleriform 001.1
  coccidial 007.2
  Dientamoeba fragilis 007.8
  due to specified organism NEC - *see* Enteritis, due to, by organism
  Embadomonas 007.8
  Endolimax nana - *see* Dysentery, amebic
  Entamoba, entamebic - *see* Dysentery, amebic
  Flexner's 004.1
  Flexner-Boyd 004.2
  giardial 007.1
  Giardia lamblia 007.1
  Hiss-Russell 004.1
  lamblia 007.1
  leishmanial 085.0
  malarial (*see also* Malaria) 084.6
  metazoal 127.9
  Monilia 112.89
  protozoal NEC 007.9
  Russell's 004.8
  salmonella 003.0
  schistosomal 120.1
  Schmitz (-Stutzer) 004.0
  Shiga 004.0
  Shigella NEC (*see also* Dysentery, bacillary) 004.9
    boydii 004.2
    dysenteriae 004.0
      Schmitz 004.0
      Shiga 004.0
    flexneri 004.1
    group A 004.0
    group B 004.1
    group C 004.2
    group D 004.3
    Schmitz 004.0
    Shiga 004.0
    Sonnei 004.3
  Sonne 004.3
  strongyloidiasis 127.2
  trichomonal 007.3
  tuberculous (*see also* Tuberculosis) 014.8 ●
  viral (*see also* Enteritis, viral) 008.8
Dysequilibrium 780.4
Dysesthesia 782.0
  hysterical 300.11
Dysfibrinogenemia (congenital) (*see also* Defect, coagulation) 286.3
Dysfunction
  adrenal (cortical) 255.9
    hyperfunction 255.3
    hypofunction 255.41
  associated with sleep stages or arousal from sleep 780.56
    nonorganic origin 307.47
  bladder NEC 596.59
  bleeding, uterus 626.8
  brain, minimal (*see also* Hyperkinesia) 314.9
  cerebral 348.30
  colon 564.9
    psychogenic 306.4
  colostomy or enterostomy 569.62
  cystic duct 575.8

Dysfunction (Continued)
    diastolic 429.9
        with heart failure - see Failure, heart
        due to
            cardiomyopathy - see Cardiomyopathy
            hypertension - see Hypertension, heart
    endocrine NEC 259.9
    endometrium 621.8
    enteric stoma 569.62
    enterostomy 569.62
    erectile 607.84
        nonorganic origin 302.72
    esophagostomy 530.87
    Eustachian tube 381.81
    gallbladder 575.8
    gastrointestinal 536.9
    gland, glandular NEC 259.9
    heart 427.9
        postoperative (immediate) 997.1
            long-term effect of cardiac surgery 429.4
    hemoglobin 289.89
    hepatic 573.9
    hepatocellular NEC 573.9
    hypophysis 253.9
        hyperfunction 253.1
        hypofunction 253.2
        posterior lobe 253.6
            hypofunction 253.5
    kidney (see also Disease, renal) 593.9
    labyrinthine 386.50
        specified NEC 386.58
    liver 573.9
        constitutional 277.4
    minimal brain (child) (see also Hyperkinesia) 314.9
    ovary, ovarian 256.9
        hyperfunction 256.1
            estrogen 256.0
        hypofunction 256.39
            postablative 256.2
        postablative 256.2
        specified NEC 256.8
    papillary muscle 429.81
        with myocardial infarction 410.8●
    parathyroid 252.8
        hyperfunction 252.00
        hypofunction 252.1
    pineal gland 259.8
    pituitary (gland) 253.9
        hyperfunction 253.1
        hypofunction 253.2
        posterior 253.6
            hypofunction 253.5
    placental - see Placenta, insufficiency
    platelets (blood) 287.1
    polyglandular 258.9
        specified NEC 258.8
    psychosexual 302.70
        with
            dyspareunia (functional) (psychogenic) 302.76
            frigidity 302.72
            impotence 302.72
            inhibition
                orgasm
                    female 302.73
                    male 302.74
                sexual
                    desire 302.71
                    excitement 302.72
            premature ejaculation 302.75
            sexual aversion 302.79
            specified disorder NEC 302.79
            vaginismus 306.51
    pylorus 537.9
    rectum 564.9
        psychogenic 306.4
    segmental (see also Dysfunction, somatic) 739.9
    senile 797

Dysfunction (Continued)
    sexual 302.70
    sinoatrial node 427.81
    somatic 739.9
        abdomen 739.9
        acromioclavicular 739.7
        cervical 739.1
        cervicothoracic 739.1
        costochondral 739.8
        costovertebral 739.8
        extremities
            lower 739.6
            upper 739.7
        head 739.0
        hip 739.5
        lumbar, lumbosacral 739.3
        occipitocervical 739.0
        pelvic 739.5
        pubic 739.5
        rib cage 739.8
        sacral 739.4
        sacrococcygeal 739.4
        sacroiliac 739.4
        specified site NEC 739.9
        sternochondral 739.8
        sternoclavicular 739.7
        temporomandibular 739.0
        thoracic, thoracolumbar 739.2
    stomach 536.9
        psychogenic 306.4
    suprarenal 255.9
        hyperfunction 255.3
        hypofunction 255.41
    symbolic NEC 784.60
        specified type NEC 784.69
    systolic 429.9
        with heart failure - see Failure, heart
    temporomandibular (joint) (joint-pain-syndrome) NEC 524.60
        sounds on opening or closing 524.64
        specified NEC 524.69
    testicular 257.9
        hyperfunction 257.0
        hypofunction 257.2
        specified type NEC 257.8
    thymus 254.9
    thyroid 246.9
        complicating pregnancy, childbirth, or puerperium 648.1●
        hyperfunction - see Hyperthyroidism
        hypofunction - see Hypothyroidism
    uterus, complicating delivery 661.9●
        affecting fetus or newborn 763.7
        hypertonic 661.4●
        hypotonic 661.2●
            primary 661.0●
            secondary 661.1●
    velopharyngeal (acquired) 528.9
        congenital 750.29
    ventricular 429.9
        with congestive heart failure (see also Failure, heart) 428.0
        due to
            cardiomyopathy - see Cardiomyopathy
            hypertension - see Hypertension, heart
        left, reversible following sudden emotional stress 429.83
    vesicourethral NEC 596.59
    vestibular 386.50
        specified type NEC 386.58
Dysgammaglobulinemia 279.06
Dysgenesis
    gonadal (due to chromosomal anomaly) 758.6
        pure 752.7
    kidney(s) 753.0
    ovarian 758.6
    renal 753.0
    reticular 279.2
    seminiferous tubules 758.6
    tidal platelet 287.31

Dysgerminoma (M9060/3)
    specified site - see Neoplasm, by site, malignant
    unspecified site
        female 183.0
        male 186.9
Dysgeusia 781.1
Dysgraphia 781.3
Dyshidrosis 705.81
Dysidrosis 705.81
Dysinsulinism 251.8
Dyskaryotic cervical smear 795.09
Dyskeratosis (see also Keratosis) 701.1
    bullosa hereditaria 757.39
    cervix 622.10
    congenital 757.39
    follicularis 757.39
        vitamin A deficiency 264.8
    gingiva 523.8
    oral soft tissue NEC 528.79
    tongue 528.79
    uterus NEC 621.8
Dyskinesia 781.3
    biliary 575.8
    esophagus 530.5
    hysterical 300.11
    intestinal 564.89
    neuroleptic-induced tardive 333.85
    nonorganic origin 307.9
    orofacial 333.82
        due to drugs 333.85
    psychogenic 307.9
    subacute, due to drugs 333.85
    tardive (oral) 333.85
Dyslalia 784.59
    developmental 315.39
Dyslexia 784.61
    developmental 315.02
    secondary to organic lesion 784.61
Dyslipidemia 272.4
Dysmaturity (see also Immaturity) 765.1●
    lung 770.4
    pulmonary 770.4
Dysmenorrhea (essential) (exfoliative) (functional) (intrinsic) (membranous) (primary) (secondary) 625.3
    psychogenic 306.52
Dysmetabolic syndrome X 277.7
Dysmetria 781.3
Dysmorodystrophia mesodermalis congenita 759.82
Dysnomia 784.3
Dysorexia 783.0
    hysterical 300.11
Dysostosis
    cleidocranial, cleidocranialis 755.59
    craniofacial 756.0
    Fairbank's (idiopathic familial generalized osteophytosis) 756.50
    mandibularis 756.0
    mandibulofacial, incomplete 756.0
    multiplex 277.5
    orodigitofacial 759.89
Dyspareunia (female) 625.0
    male 608.89
    psychogenic 302.76
Dyspepsia (allergic) (congenital) (fermentative) (flatulent) (functional) (gastric) (gastrointestinal) (neurogenic) (occupational) (reflex) 536.8
    acid 536.8
    atonic 536.3
        psychogenic 306.4
    diarrhea 787.91
        psychogenic 306.4
    intestinal 564.89
        psychogenic 306.4
    nervous 306.4
    neurotic 306.4
    psychogenic 306.4

Dysphagia 787.20
　cervical 787.29
　functional 300.11
　hysterical 300.11
　nervous 300.11
　neurogenic 787.29
　oral phase 787.21
　oropharyngeal phase 787.22
　pharyngeal phase 787.23
　pharyngoesophageal phase 787.24
　psychogenic 306.4
　sideropenic 280.8
　spastica 530.5
　specified NEC 787.29
Dysphagocytosis, congenital 288.1
Dysphasia 784.59
Dysphonia 784.42
　clericorum 784.49
　functional 300.11
　hysterical 300.11
　psychogenic 306.1
　spastica 478.79
Dyspigmentation - see also Pigmentation
　eyelid (acquired) 374.52
Dyspituitarism 253.9
　hyperfunction 253.1
　hypofunction 253.2
　posterior lobe 253.6
Dysplasia - see also Anomaly
　alveolar capillary, with vein misalignment 516.64
　anus 569.44
　　intraepithelial neoplasia I (AIN I) (histologically confirmed) 569.44
　　intraepithelial neoplasia II (AIN II) (histologically confirmed) 569.44
　　intraepithelial neoplasia III (AIN III) 230.6
　　　anal canal 230.5
　　mild (histologically confirmed) 569.44
　　moderate (histologically confirmed) 569.44
　　severe 230.6
　　　anal canal 230.5
　artery
　　fibromuscular NEC 447.8
　　　carotid 447.8
　　　renal 447.3
　bladder 596.89
　bone (fibrous) NEC 733.29
　　diaphyseal, progressive 756.59
　　jaw 526.89
　　monostotic 733.29
　　polyostotic 756.54
　　solitary 733.29
　brain 742.9
　bronchopulmonary, fetus or newborn 770.7
　cervix (uteri) 622.10
　　cervical intraepithelial neoplasia I (CIN I) 622.11
　　cervical intraepithelial neoplasia II (CIN II) 622.12
　　cervical intraepithelial neoplasia III (CIN III) 233.1
　　CIN I 622.11
　　CIN II 622.12
　　CIN III 233.1
　　mild 622.11
　　moderate 622.12
　　severe 233.1
　chondroectodermal 756.55
　chondromatose 756.4
　colon 211.3
　craniocarpotarsal 759.89
　craniometaphyseal 756.89
　dentinal 520.5
　diaphyseal, progressive 756.59
　ectodermal (anhidrotic) (Bason) (Clouston's) (congenital) (Feinmesser) (hereditary) (hidrotic) (Marshall) (Robinson's) 757.31

Dysplasia (Continued)
　epiphysealis 756.9
　　multiplex 756.56
　　punctata 756.59
　epiphysis 756.9
　　multiple 756.56
　epithelial
　　epiglottis 478.79
　　uterine cervix 622.10
　erythroid NEC 289.89
　eye (see also Microphthalmos) 743.10
　familial metaphyseal 756.89
　fibromuscular, artery NEC 447.8
　　carotid 447.8
　　renal 447.3
　fibrous
　　bone NEC 733.29
　　diaphyseal, progressive 756.59
　　jaw 526.89
　　monostotic 733.29
　　polyostotic 756.54
　　solitary 733.29
　high grade, focal - see Neoplasm, by site, benign
　hip (congenital) 755.63
　　with dislocation (see also Dislocation, hip, congenital) 754.30
　hypohidrotic ectodermal 757.31
　joint 755.8
　kidney 753.15
　leg 755.69
　linguofacialis 759.89
　lung 748.5
　macular 743.55
　mammary (benign) (gland) 610.9
　　cystic 610.1
　　specified type NEC 610.8
　metaphyseal 756.9
　　familial 756.89
　monostotic fibrous 733.29
　muscle 756.89
　myeloid NEC 289.89
　nervous system (general) 742.9
　neuroectodermal 759.6
　oculoauriculovertebral 756.0
　oculodentodigital 759.89
　olfactogenital 253.4
　osteo-onycho-arthro (hereditary) 756.89
　periosteum 733.99
　polyostotic fibrous 756.54
　progressive diaphyseal 756.59
　prostate 602.3
　　intraepithelial neoplasia I [PIN I] 602.3
　　intraepithelial neoplasia II [PIN II] 602.3
　　intraepithelial neoplasia III [PIN III] 233.4
　renal 753.15
　renofacialis 753.0
　retinal NEC 743.56
　retrolental (see also Retinopathy of prematurity) 362.21
　skin 709.8
　spinal cord 742.9
　thymic, with immunodeficiency 279.2
　vagina 623.0
　　mild 623.0
　　moderate 623.0
　　severe 233.31
　vocal cord 478.5
　vulva 624.8
　　intraepithelial neoplasia I (VIN I) 624.01
　　intraepithelial neoplasia II (VIN II) 624.02
　　intraepithelial neoplasia III (VIN III) 233.32
　　mild 624.01
　　moderate 624.02
　　severe 233.32
　　VIN I 624.01
　　VIN II 624.02
　　VIN III 233.32

Dyspnea (nocturnal) (paroxysmal) 786.09
　asthmatic (bronchial) (see also Asthma) 493.9●
　　with bronchitis (see also Asthma) 493.9●
　　　chronic 493.2●
　cardiac (see also Failure, ventricular, left) 428.1
　cardiac (see also Failure, ventricular, left) 428.1
　functional 300.11
　hyperventilation 786.01
　hysterical 300.11
　Monday morning 504
　newborn 770.89
　psychogenic 306.1
　uremic - see Uremia
Dyspraxia 781.3
　syndrome 315.4
Dysproteinemia 273.8
　transient with copper deficiency 281.4
Dysprothrombinemia (constitutional) (see also Defect, coagulation) 286.3
Dysreflexia, autonomic 337.3
Dysrhythmia
　cardiac 427.9
　　postoperative (immediate) 997.1
　　　long-term effect of cardiac surgery 429.4
　　specified type NEC 427.89
　cerebral or cortical 348.30
Dyssecretosis, mucoserous 710.2
Dyssocial reaction, without manifest psychiatric disorder
　adolescent V71.02
　adult V71.01
　child V71.02
Dyssomnia NEC 780.56
　nonorganic origin 307.47
Dyssplenism 289.4
Dyssynergia
　biliary (see also Disease, biliary) 576.8
　cerebellaris myoclonica 334.2
　detrusor sphincter (bladder) 596.55
　ventricular 429.89
Dystasia, hereditary areflexic 334.3
Dysthymia 300.4
Dysthymic disorder 300.4
Dysthyroidism 246.9
Dystocia 660.9●
　affecting fetus or newborn 763.1
　cervical 661.2●
　　affecting fetus or newborn 763.7
　contraction ring 661.4●
　　affecting fetus or newborn 763.7
　fetal 660.9●
　　abnormal size 653.5●
　　　affecting fetus or newborn 763.1
　　deformity 653.7●
　maternal 660.9●
　　affecting fetus or newborn 763.1
　positional 660.0●
　　affecting fetus or newborn 763.1
　shoulder (girdle) 660.4●
　　affecting fetus or newborn 763.1
　uterine NEC 661.4●
　　affecting fetus or newborn 763.7
Dystonia
　acute
　　due to drugs 333.72
　　neuroleptic-induced acute 333.72
　deformans progressiva 333.6
　lenticularis 333.6
　musculorum deformans 333.6
　torsion (idiopathic) 333.6
　　acquired 333.79
　　fragments (of) 333.89
　　genetic 333.6
　　symptomatic 333.79
Dystonic
　movements 781.0
Dystopia kidney 753.3

Dystrophy, dystrophia 783.9
- adiposogenital 253.8
- asphyxiating thoracic 756.4
- Becker's type 359.22
- brevicollis 756.16
- Bruch's membrane 362.77
- cervical (sympathetic) NEC 337.09
- chondro-osseus with punctate epiphyseal dysplasia 756.59
- choroid (hereditary) 363.50
  - central (areolar) (partial) 363.53
    - total (gyrate) 363.54
  - circinate 363.53
  - circumpapillary (partial) 363.51
    - total 363.52
  - diffuse
    - partial 363.56
    - total 363.57
  - generalized
    - partial 363.56
    - total 363.57
  - gyrate
    - central 363.54
    - generalized 363.57
  - helicoid 363.52
  - peripapillary - see Dystrophy, choroid, circumpapillary
  - serpiginous 363.54
- cornea (hereditary) 371.50
  - anterior NEC 371.52
  - Cogan's 371.52
  - combined 371.57
  - crystalline 371.56
  - endothelial (Fuchs') 371.57
  - epithelial 371.50
    - juvenile 371.51
      - microscopic cystic 371.52
  - granular 371.53
  - lattice 371.54
  - macular 371.55
  - marginal (Terrien's) 371.48
  - Meesman's 371.51
  - microscopic cystic (epithelial) 371.52
  - nodular, Salzmann's 371.46
  - polymorphous 371.58
  - posterior NEC 371.58
  - ring-like 371.52

Dystrophy, dystrophia (Continued)
- cornea (Continued)
  - Salzmann's nodular 371.46
  - stromal NEC 371.56
- dermatochondrocorneal 371.50
- Duchenne's 359.1
- due to malnutrition 263.9
- Erb's 359.1
- familial
  - hyperplastic periosteal 756.59
  - osseous 277.5
- foveal 362.77
- Fuchs', cornea 371.57
- Gowers' muscular 359.1
- hair 704.2
- hereditary, progressive muscular 359.1
- hypogenital, with diabetic tendency 759.81
- Landouzy-Déjérine 359.1
- Leyden-Möbius 359.1
- mesodermalis congenita 759.82
- muscular 359.1
  - congenital (hereditary) 359.0
    - myotonic 359.22
  - distal 359.1
  - Duchenne's 359.1
  - Erb's 359.1
  - fascioscapulohumeral 359.1
  - Gowers' 359.1
  - hereditary (progressive) 359.1
  - Landouzy-Déjérine 359.1
  - limb-girdle 359.1
  - myotonic 359.21
  - progressive (hereditary) 359.1
    - Charcôt-Marie-Tooth 356.1
  - pseudohypertrophic (infantile) 359.1
- myocardium, myocardial (see also Degeneration, myocardial) 429.1
- myotonic 359.21
- myotonica 359.21
- nail 703.8
  - congenital 757.5
- neurovascular (traumatic) (see also Neuropathy, peripheral, autonomic) 337.9
- nutritional 263.9
- ocular 359.1
- oculocerebrorenal 270.8
- oculopharyngeal 359.1

Dystrophy, dystrophia (Continued)
- ovarian 620.8
- papillary (and pigmentary) 701.1
- pelvicrural atrophic 359.1
- pigmentary (see also Acanthosis) 701.2
- pituitary (gland) 253.8
- polyglandular 258.8
- posttraumatic sympathetic - see Dystrophy, sympathic
- progressive ophthalmoplegic 359.1
- reflex neuromuscular - see Dystrophy, sympathetic
- retina, retinal (hereditary) 362.70
  - albipunctate 362.74
  - Bruch's membrane 362.77
  - cone, progressive 362.75
  - hyaline 362.77
  - in
    - Bassen-Kornzweig syndrome 272.5 [362.72]
    - cerebroretinal lipidosis 330.1 [362.71]
    - Refsum's disease 356.3 [362.72]
    - systemic lipidosis 272.7 [362.71]
  - juvenile (Stargardt's) 362.75
  - pigmentary 362.74
  - pigment epithelium 362.76
  - progressive cone (-rod) 362.75
  - pseudoinflammatory foveal 362.77
  - rod, progressive 362.75
  - sensory 362.75
  - vitelliform 362.76
- Salzmann's nodular 371.46
- scapuloperoneal 359.1
- skin NEC 709.9
- sympathetic (posttraumatic) (reflex) 337.20
  - lower limb 337.22
  - specified site NEC 337.29
  - upper limb 337.21
- tapetoretinal NEC 362.74
- thoracic asphyxiating 756.4
- unguium 703.8
  - congenital 757.5
- vitreoretinal (primary) 362.73
  - secondary 362.66
- vulva 624.09

Dysuria 788.1
- psychogenic 306.53

E

Eagle-Barrett syndrome 756.71
Eales' disease (syndrome) 362.18
Ear - *see also* condition
   ache 388.70
      otogenic 388.71
      referred 388.72
   lop 744.29
   piercing V50.3
   swimmers' acute 380.12
   tank 380.12
   tropical 111.8 *[380.15]*
   wax 380.4
Earache 388.70
   otogenic 388.71
   referred 388.72
Early satiety 780.94
Eaton-Lambert syndrome (*see also* Syndrome, Lambert-Eaton) 358.30
Eberth's disease (typhoid fever) 002.0
Ebstein's
   anomaly or syndrome (downward displacement, tricuspid valve into right ventricle) 746.2
   disease (diabetes) 250.4 ● *[581.81]*
      due to secondary diabetes 249.4 ● *[581.81]*
Eccentro-osteochondrodysplasia 277.5
Ecchondroma (M9210/0) - *see* Neoplasm, bone, benign
Ecchondrosis (M9210/1) 238.0
Ecchordosis physaliphora 756.0
Ecchymosis (multiple) 459.89
   conjunctiva 372.72
   eye (traumatic) 921.0
   eyelids (traumatic) 921.1
   newborn 772.6
   spontaneous 782.7
   traumatic - *see* Contusion
ECD (Erdheim-Chester disease) 277.89
Echinococciasis - *see* Echinococcus
Echinococcosis - *see* Echinococcus
Echinococcus (infection) 122.9
   granulosus 122.4
      liver 122.0
      lung 122.1
      orbit 122.3 *[376.13]*
      specified site NEC 122.3
      thyroid 122.2
   liver NEC 122.8
      granulosus 122.0
      multilocularis 122.5
   lung NEC 122.9
      granulosus 122.1
      multilocularis 122.6
   multilocularis 122.7
      liver 122.5
      specified site NEC 122.6
   orbit 122.9 *[376.13]*
      granulosus 122.3 *[376.13]*
      multilocularis 122.6 *[376.13]*
   specified site NEC 122.9
      granulosus 122.3
      multilocularis 122.6 *[376.13]*
   thyroid NEC 122.9
      granulosus 122.2
      multilocularis 122.6
Echinorhynchiasis 127.7
Echinostomiasis 121.8
Echolalia 784.69
ECHO virus infection NEC 079.1
Eclampsia, eclamptic (coma) (convulsions) (delirium) 780.39
   female, child-bearing age NEC - *see* Eclampsia, pregnancy
   gravidarum - *see* Eclampsia, pregnancy
   male 780.39
   not associated with pregnancy or childbirth 780.39

Eclampsia, eclamptic (*Continued*)
   pregnancy, childbirth, or puerperium 642.6 ●
      with pre-existing hypertension 642.7 ●
      affecting fetus or newborn 760.0
   uremic 586
Eclipse blindness (total) 363.31
Economic circumstance affecting care V60.9
   specified type NEC V60.89
Economo's disease (encephalitis lethargica) 049.8
Ectasia, ectasis
   annuloaortic 424.1
   aorta (*see also* Ectasia, aortic) 447.70
      with aneurysm 441.9
      ruptured 441.5
   aortic 447.70
      with aneurysm 441.9
      abdominal 447.72
      thoracic 447.71
      thoracoabdominal 447.73
   breast 610.4
   capillary 448.9
   cornea (marginal) (postinfectional) 371.71
   duct (mammary) 610.4
   gastric antral vascular (GAVE) 537.82
      with hemorrhage 537.83
      without hemorrhage 537.82
   kidney 593.89
   mammary duct (gland) 610.4
   papillary 448.9
   renal 593.89
   salivary gland (duct) 527.8
   scar, cornea 371.71
   sclera 379.11
Ecthyma 686.8
   contagiosum 051.2
   gangrenosum 686.09
   infectiosum 051.2
Ectocardia 746.87
Ectodermal dysplasia, congenital 757.31
Ectodermosis erosiva plurioricifialis 695.19
Ectopic, ectopia (congenital) 759.89
   abdominal viscera 751.8
      due to defect in anterior abdominal wall 756.79
   ACTH syndrome 255.0
   adrenal gland 759.1
   anus 751.5
   auricular beats 427.61
   beats 427.60
   bladder 753.5
   bone and cartilage in lung 748.69
   brain 742.4
   breast tissue 757.6
   cardiac 746.87
   cerebral 742.4
   cordis 746.87
   endometrium 617.9
   gallbladder 751.69
   gastric mucosa 750.7
   gestation - *see* Pregnancy, ectopic
   heart 746.87
   hormone secretion NEC 259.3
   hyperparathyroidism 259.3
   kidney (crossed) (intrathoracic) (pelvis) 753.3
      in pregnancy or childbirth 654.4 ●
         causing obstructed labor 660.2 ●
   lens 743.37
   lentis 743.37
   mole - *see* Pregnancy, ectopic
   organ or site NEC - *see* Malposition, congenital
   ovary 752.0
   pancreas, pancreatic tissue 751.7
   pregnancy - *see* Pregnancy, ectopic
   pupil 364.75
   renal 753.3
   sebaceous glands of mouth 750.26

Ectopic, ectopia (*Continued*)
   secretion
      ACTH 255.0
      adrenal hormone 259.3
      adrenalin 259.3
      adrenocorticotropin 255.0
      antidiuretic hormone (ADH) 259.3
      epinephrine 259.3
      hormone NEC 259.3
      norepinephrine 259.3
      pituitary (posterior) 259.3
   spleen 759.0
   testis 752.51
   thyroid 759.2
   ureter 753.4
   ventricular beats 427.69
   vesicae 753.5
Ectrodactyly 755.4
   finger (*see also* Absence, finger, congenital) 755.29
   toe (*see also* Absence, toe, congenital) 755.39
Ectromelia 755.4
   lower limb 755.30
   upper limb 755.20
Ectropion 374.10
   anus 569.49
   cervix 622.0
      with mention of cervicitis 616.0
   cicatricial 374.14
   congenital 743.62
   eyelid 374.10
      cicatricial 374.14
      congenital 743.62
      mechanical 374.12
      paralytic 374.12
      senile 374.11
      spastic 374.13
   iris (pigment epithelium) 364.54
   lip (congenital) 750.26
      acquired 528.5
   mechanical 374.12
   paralytic 374.12
   rectum 569.49
   senile 374.11
   spastic 374.13
   urethra 599.84
   uvea 364.54
Eczema (acute) (allergic) (chronic) (erythematous) (fissum) (occupational) (rubrum) (squamous) 692.9
   asteatotic 706.8
   atopic 691.8
   contact NEC 692.9
   dermatitis NEC 692.9
   due to specified cause - *see* Dermatitis, due to
   dyshidrotic 705.81
   external ear 380.22
   flexural 691.8
   gouty 274.89
   herpeticum 054.0
   hypertrophicum 701.8
   hypostatic - *see* Varicose, vein
   impetiginous 684
   infantile (acute) (chronic) (due to any substance) (intertriginous) (seborrheic) 690.12
   intertriginous NEC 692.9
      infantile 690.12
   intrinsic 691.8
   lichenified NEC 692.9
   marginatum 110.3
   nummular 692.9
   pustular 686.8
   seborrheic 690.18
      infantile 690.12
   solare 692.72
   stasis (lower extremity) 454.1
      ulcerated 454.2
   vaccination, vaccinatum 999.0
   varicose (lower extremity) - *see* Varicose, vein
   verrucosum callosum 698.3

 deleted Deleted

Eczematoid, exudative 691.8
Eddowes' syndrome (brittle bones and blue sclera) 756.51
Edema, edematous 782.3
- with nephritis (see also Nephrosis) 581.9
- allergic 995.1
- angioneurotic (allergic) (any site) (with urticaria) 995.1
  - hereditary 277.6
- angiospastic 443.9
- Berlin's (traumatic) 921.3
- brain (cytotoxic) (vasogenic) 348.5
  - due to birth injury 767.8
  - fetus or newborn 767.8
- cardiac (see also Failure, heart) 428.0
- cardiovascular (see also Failure, heart) 428.0
- cerebral - see Edema, brain
- cerebrospinal vessel - see Edema, brain
- cervix (acute) (uteri) 622.8
  - puerperal, postpartum 674.8●
- chronic hereditary 757.0
- circumscribed, acute 995.1
  - hereditary 277.6
- complicating pregnancy (gestational) 646.1●
  - with hypertension - see Toxemia, of pregnancy
- conjunctiva 372.73
- connective tissue 782.3
- cornea 371.20
  - due to contact lenses 371.24
  - idiopathic 371.21
  - secondary 371.22
- cystoid macular 362.53
- due to
  - lymphatic obstruction - see Edema, lymphatic
  - salt retention 276.0
- epiglottis - see Edema, glottis
- essential, acute 995.1
  - hereditary 277.6
- extremities, lower - see Edema, legs
- eyelid NEC 374.82
- familial, hereditary (legs) 757.0
- famine 262
- fetus or newborn 778.5
- genital organs
  - female 629.89
  - male 608.86
- gestational 646.1●
  - with hypertension - see Toxemia, of pregnancy
- glottis, glottic, glottides (obstructive) (passive) 478.6
  - allergic 995.1
    - hereditary 277.6
  - due to external agent - see Condition, respiratory, acute, due to specified agent
- heart (see also Failure, heart) 428.0
  - newborn 779.89
- heat 992.7
- hereditary (legs) 757.0
- inanition 262
- infectious 782.3
- intracranial 348.5
  - due to injury at birth 767.8
- iris 364.89
- joint (see also Effusion, joint) 719.0●
- larynx (see also Edema, glottis) 478.6
- legs 782.3
  - due to venous obstruction 459.2
  - hereditary 757.0
- localized 782.3
  - due to venous obstruction 459.2
    - lower extremity 459.2
- lower extremities - see Edema, legs
- lung 514
  - acute 518.4
    - with heart disease or failure (see also Failure, ventricular, left) 428.1
      - congestive 428.0

Edema, edematous (Continued)
- lung (Continued)
  - acute (Continued)
    - chemical (due to fumes or vapors) 506.1
    - due to
      - external agent(s) NEC 508.9
        - specified NEC 508.8
      - fumes and vapors (chemical) (inhalation) 506.1
      - radiation 508.0
    - chemical (acute) 506.1
      - chronic 506.4
    - chronic 514
      - chemical (due to fumes or vapors) 506.4
      - due to
        - external agent(s) NEC 508.9
          - specified NEC 508.8
        - fumes or vapors (chemical) (inhalation) 506.4
        - radiation 508.1
    - due to
      - external agent 508.9
        - specified NEC 508.8
      - high altitude 993.2
      - near drowning 994.1
    - postoperative 518.4
    - terminal 514
- lymphatic 457.1
  - due to mastectomy operation 457.0
- macula 362.83
  - cystoid 362.53
  - diabetic 250.5● [362.07]
    - due to secondary diabetes 249.5● [362.07]
- malignant (see also Gangrene, gas) 040.0
- Milroy's 757.0
- nasopharynx 478.25
- neonatorum 778.5
- nutritional (newborn) 262
  - with dyspigmentation, skin and hair 260
- optic disc or nerve - see Papilledema
- orbit 376.33
  - circulatory 459.89
- palate (soft) (hard) 528.9
- pancreas 577.8
- penis 607.83
- periodic 995.1
  - hereditary 277.6
- pharynx 478.25
- pitting 782.3
- pulmonary - see Edema, lung
- Quincke's 995.1
  - hereditary 277.6
- renal (see also Nephrosis) 581.9
- retina (localized) (macular) (peripheral) 362.83
  - cystoid 362.53
  - diabetic 250.5● [362.07]
    - due to secondary diabetes 249.5● [362.07]
- salt 276.0
- scrotum 608.86
- seminal vesicle 608.86
- spermatic cord 608.86
- spinal cord 336.1
- starvation 262
- stasis - see also Hypertension, venous 459.30
- subconjunctival 372.73
- subglottic (see also Edema, glottis) 478.6
- supraglottic (see also Edema, glottis) 478.6
- testis 608.86
- toxic NEC 782.3
- traumatic NEC 782.3
- tunica vaginalis 608.86
- vas deferens 608.86
- vocal cord - see Edema, glottis
- vulva (acute) 624.8

Edentia (complete) (partial) (see also Absence, tooth) 520.0
- acquired (see also Edentulism) 525.40
  - due to
    - caries 525.13
    - extraction 525.10
    - periodontal disease 525.12
    - specified NEC 525.19
    - trauma 525.11
  - causing malocclusion 524.30
- congenital (deficiency of tooth buds) 520.0

Edentulism 525.40
- complete 525.40
  - class I 525.41
  - class II 525.42
  - class III 525.43
  - class IV 525.44
- partial 525.50
  - class I 525.51
  - class II 525.52
  - class III 525.53
  - class IV 525.54

Edsall's disease 992.2
Educational handicap V62.3
Edwards' syndrome 758.2
Effect, adverse NEC
- abnormal gravitational (G) forces or states 994.9
- air pressure - see Effect, adverse, atmospheric pressure
- altitude (high) - see Effect, adverse, high altitude
- anesthetic
  - in labor and delivery NEC 668.9●
    - affecting fetus or newborn 763.5
- antitoxin - see Complications, vaccination
- atmospheric pressure 993.9
  - due to explosion 993.4
  - high 993.3
  - low - see Effect, adverse, high altitude
  - specified effect NEC 993.8
- biological, correct substance properly administered (see also Effect, adverse, drug) 995.20
- blood (derivatives) (serum) (transfusion) - see Complications, transfusion
- chemical substance NEC 989.9
  - specified - see Table of Drugs and Chemicals
- cobalt, radioactive (see also Effect, adverse, radioactive substance) 990
- cold (temperature) (weather) 991.9
  - chilblains 991.5
  - frostbite - see Frostbite
  - specified effect NEC 991.8
- drugs and medicinals 995.20
  - correct substance properly administered 995.20
  - overdose or wrong substance given or taken 977.9
  - specified drug - see Table of Drugs and Chemicals
- electric current (shock) 994.8
  - burn - see Burn, by site
- electricity (electrocution) (shock) 994.8
  - burn - see Burn, by site
- exertion (excessive) 994.5
- exposure 994.9
  - exhaustion 994.4
- external cause NEC 994.9
- fallout (radioactive) NEC 990
- fluoroscopy NEC 990
- foodstuffs
  - allergic reaction (see also Allergy, food) 693.1
  - anaphylactic reaction or shock due to food NEC - see Anaphylactic reaction or shock, due to food

SECTION I INDEX TO DISEASES AND INJURIES / Elephantiasis

Effect, adverse NEC (Continued)
 foodstuffs (Continued)
  noxious 988.9
   specified type NEC (see also Poisoning, by name of noxious foodstuff) 988.8
 gases, fumes, or vapors - see Table of Drugs and Chemicals
 glue (airplane) sniffing 304.6 ●
 heat - see Heat
 high altitude NEC 993.2
  anoxia 993.2
  on
   ears 993.0
   sinuses 993.1
  polycythemia 289.0
 hot weather - see Heat
 hunger 994.2
 immersion, foot 991.4
 immunization - see Complications, vaccination
 immunological agents - see Complications, vaccination
 implantation (removable) of isotope or radium NEC 990
 infrared (radiation) (rays) NEC 990
  burn - see Burn, by site
  dermatitis or eczema 692.82
 infusion - see Complications, infusion
 ingestion or injection of isotope (therapeutic) NEC 990
 irradiation NEC (see also Effect, adverse, radiation) 990
 isotope (radioactive) NEC 990
 lack of care (child) (infant) (newborn) 995.52
  adult 995.84
 lightning 994.0
  burn - see Burn, by site
 Lirugin - see Complications, vaccination
 medicinal substance, correct, properly administered (see also Effect, adverse, drugs) 995.20
 mesothorium NEC 990
 motion 994.6
 noise, inner ear 388.10
 other drug, medicinal and biological substance 995.29
 overheated places - see Heat
 polonium NEC 990
 psychosocial, of work environment V62.1
 radiation (diagnostic) (fallout) (infrared) (natural source) (therapeutic) (tracer) (ultraviolet) (x-ray) NEC 990
  with pulmonary manifestations
   acute 508.0
   chronic 508.1
  dermatitis or eczema 692.82
   due to sun NEC (see also Dermatitis, due to, sun) 692.70
  fibrosis of lungs 508.1
  maternal with suspected damage to fetus affecting management of pregnancy 655.6 ●
  pneumonitis 508.0
 radioactive substance NEC 990
  dermatitis or eczema 692.82
 radioactivity NEC 990
 radiotherapy NEC 990
  dermatitis or eczema 692.82
 radium NEC 990
 reduced temperature 991.9
  frostbite - see Frostbite
  immersion, foot (hand) 991.4
  specified effect NEC 991.8
 roentgenography NEC 990
 roentgenoscopy NEC 990
 roentgen rays NEC 990
 serum (prophylactic) (therapeutic) NEC 999.59
 specified NEC 995.89
  external cause NEC 994.9

Effect, adverse NEC (Continued)
 strangulation 994.7
 submersion 994.1
 teletherapy NEC 990
 thirst 994.3
 transfusion - see Complications, transfusion
 ultraviolet (radiation) (rays) NEC 990
  burn - see also Burn, by site
   from sun (see also Sunburn) 692.71
  dermatitis or eczema 692.82
   due to sun NEC (see also Dermatitis, due to, sun) 692.70
 uranium NEC 990
 vaccine (any) - see Complications, vaccination
 weightlessness 994.9
 whole blood - see also Complications, transfusion
  overdose or wrong substance given (see also Table of Drugs and Chemicals) 964.7
 working environment V62.1
 x-rays NEC 990
  dermatitis or eczema 692.82
Effect, remote
 of cancer - see condition
Effects, late - see Late, effect (of)
Effluvium, telogen 704.02
Effort
 intolerance 306.2
 syndrome (aviators) (psychogenic) 306.2
Effusion
 amniotic fluid (see also Rupture, membranes, premature) 658.1 ●
 brain (serous) 348.5
 bronchial (see also Bronchitis) 490
 cerebral 348.5
 cerebrospinal (see also Meningitis) 322.9
  vessel 348.5
 chest - see Effusion, pleura
 intracranial 348.5
 joint 719.00
  ankle 719.07
  elbow 719.02
  foot 719.07
  hand 719.04
  hip 719.05
  knee 719.06
  multiple sites 719.09
  pelvic region 719.05
  shoulder (region) 719.01
  specified site NEC 719.08
  wrist 719.03
 meninges (see also Meningitis) 322.9
 pericardium, pericardial (see also Pericarditis) 423.9
  acute 420.90
 peritoneal (chronic) 568.82
 pleura, pleurisy, pleuritic, pleuropericardial 511.9
  bacterial, nontuberculous 511.1
  fetus or newborn 511.9
  malignant 511.81
  nontuberculous 511.9
   bacterial 511.1
   pneumococcal 511.1
   staphylococcal 511.1
   streptococcal 511.1
  traumatic 862.29
   with open wound 862.39
  tuberculous (see also Tuberculosis, pleura) 012.0 ●
   primary progressive 010.1 ●
 pulmonary - see Effusion, pleura
 spinal (see also Meningitis) 322.9
 thorax, thoracic - see Effusion, pleura
Egg (oocyte) (ovum)
 donor V59.70
  over age 35 V59.73
   anonymous recipient V59.73
   designated recipient V59.74

Egg (Continued)
 donor (Continued)
  under age 35 V59.71
   anonymous recipient V59.71
   designated recipient V59.72
Eggshell nails 703.8
 congenital 757.5
Ego-dystonic
 homosexuality 302.0
 lesbianism 302.0
 sexual orientation 302.0
Egyptian splenomegaly 120.1
Ehlers-Danlos syndrome 756.83
Ehrlichiosis 082.40
 chaffeensis 082.41
 specified type NEC 082.49
Eichstedt's disease (pityriasis versicolor) 111.0
EIN (endometrial intraepithelial neoplasia) 621.35
Eisenmenger's complex or syndrome (ventricular septal defect) 745.4
Ejaculation, semen
 painful 608.89
  psychogenic 306.59
 premature 302.75
 retrograde 608.87
Ekbom syndrome (restless legs) 333.94
Ekman's syndrome (brittle bones and blue sclera) 756.51
Elastic skin 756.83
 acquired 701.8
Elastofibroma (M8820/0) - see Neoplasm, connective tissue, benign
Elastoidosis
 cutanea nodularis 701.8
 cutis cystica et comedonica 701.8
Elastoma 757.39
 juvenile 757.39
 Miescher's (elastosis perforans serpiginosa) 701.1
Elastomyofibrosis 425.3
Elastosis 701.8
 atrophicans 701.8
 perforans serpiginosa 701.1
 reactive perforating 701.1
 senilis 701.8
 solar (actinic) 692.74
Elbow - see condition
Electric
 current, electricity, effects (concussion) (fatal) (nonfatal) (shock) 994.8
  burn - see Burn, by site
 feet (foot) syndrome 266.2
 shock from electroshock gun (taser) 994.8
Electrocution 994.8
Electrolyte imbalance 276.9
 with
  abortion - see Abortion, by type, with metabolic disorder
  ectopic pregnancy (see also categories 633.0–633.9) 639.4
  hyperemesis gravidarum (before 22 completed weeks' gestation) 643.1 ●
  molar pregnancy (see also categories 630–632) 639.4
 following
  abortion 639.4
  ectopic or molar pregnancy 639.4
Elephant man syndrome 237.71
Elephantiasis (nonfilarial) 457.1
 arabicum (see also Infestation, filarial) 125.9
 congenita hereditaria 757.0
 congenital (any site) 757.0
 due to
  Brugia (malayi) 125.1
  mastectomy operation 457.0
  Wuchereria (bancrofti) 125.0
   malayi 125.1
 eyelid 374.83
 filarial (see also Infestation, filarial) 125.9
 filariensis (see also Infestation, filarial) 125.9

SECTION I INDEX TO DISEASES AND INJURIES / Elephantiasis

Elephantiasis (Continued)
  gingival 523.8
  glandular 457.1
  graecorum 030.9
  lymphangiectatic 457.1
  lymphatic vessel 457.1
    due to mastectomy operation 457.0
  neuromatosa 237.71
  postmastectomy 457.0
  scrotum 457.1
  streptococcal 457.1
  surgical 997.99
    postmastectomy 457.0
  telangiectodes 457.1
  vulva (nonfilarial) 624.8
Elevated - see Elevation
  findings on laboratory examination - see
      Findings, abnormal, without diagnosis
      (examination) (laboratory test)
  GFR (glomerular filtration rate) - see
      Findings, abnormal, without diagnosis
      (examination) (laboratory test)
Elevation
  17-ketosteroids 791.9
  acid phosphatase 790.5
  alkaline phosphatase 790.5
  amylase 790.5
  antibody titers 795.79
  basal metabolic rate (BMR) 794.7
  blood pressure (see also Hypertension) 401.9
    reading (incidental) (isolated)
        (nonspecific), no diagnosis of
        hypertension 796.2
  blood sugar 790.29
  body temperature (of unknown origin) (see
      also Pyrexia) 780.60
  C-reactive protein (CRP) 790.95
  cancer antigen 125 [CA 125] 795.82
  carcinoembryonic antigen [CEA] 795.81
  cholesterol 272.0
    with high triglycerides 272.2
  conjugate, eye 378.81
  CRP (C-reactive protein) 790.95
  diaphragm, congenital 756.6
  GFR (glomerular filtration rate) - see
      Findings, abnormal, without diagnosis
      (examination) (laboratory test)
  glucose
    fasting 790.21
    tolerance test 790.22
  immunoglobulin level 795.79
  indolacetic acid 791.9
  lactic acid dehydrogenase (LDH) level 790.4
  leukocytes 288.60
  lipase 790.5
  lipoprotein a level 272.8
  liver function test (LFT) 790.6
    alkaline phosphatase 790.5
    aminotransferase 790.4
    bilirubin 782.4
    hepatic enzyme NEC 790.5
    lactate dehydrogenase 790.4
  lymphocytes 288.61
  prostate specific antigen (PSA) 790.93
  renin 790.99
    in hypertension (see also Hypertension,
        renovascular) 405.91
  Rh titer (see also Complications, transfusion)
      999.70
  scapula, congenital 755.52
  sedimentation rate 790.1
  SGOT 790.4
  SGPT 790.4
  transaminase 790.4
  triglycerides 272.1
    with high cholesterol 272.2
  vanillylmandelic acid 791.9
  venous pressure 459.89
  VMA 791.9
  white blood cell count 288.60
    specified NEC 288.69

Elliptocytosis (congenital) (hereditary) 282.1
  Hb-C (disease) 282.7
  hemoglobin disease 282.7
  sickle-cell (disease) 282.60
    trait 282.5
Ellis-van Creveld disease or syndrome
  (chondroectodermal dysplasia) 756.55
Ellison-Zollinger syndrome
  (gastric hypersecretion with pancreatic islet
  cell tumor) 251.5
Elongation, elongated (congenital) - see also
    Distortion
  bone 756.9
  cervix (uteri) 752.49
    acquired 622.6
    hypertrophic 622.6
  colon 751.5
  common bile duct 751.69
  cystic duct 751.69
  frenulum, penis 752.69
  labia minora, acquired 624.8
  ligamentum patellae 756.89
  petiolus (epiglottidis) 748.3
  styloid bone (process) 733.99
  tooth, teeth 520.2
  uvula 750.26
    acquired 528.9
Elschnig bodies or pearls 366.51
El Tor cholera 001.1
Emaciation (due to malnutrition) 261
Emancipation disorder 309.22
Embadomoniasis 007.8
Embarrassment heart, cardiac - see Disease,
    heart
Embedded
  fragment (status) - see Foreign body,
      retained
  root only 525.3
  splinter (status) - see Foreign body,
      retained
  tooth, teeth 520.6
Embolic - see condition
Embolism 444.9
  with
    abortion - see Abortion, by type, with
        embolism
    ectopic pregnancy (see also categories
        633.0–633.9) 639.6
    molar pregnancy (see also categories
        630–632) 639.6
  air (any site) 958.0
    with
      abortion - see Abortion, by type, with
          embolism
      ectopic pregnancy (see also categories
          633.0–633.9) 639.6
      molar pregnancy (see also categories
          630–632) 639.6
    due to implanted device - see
        Complications, due to (presence of)
        any device, implant, or graft
        classified to 996.0–996.5 NEC
    following
      abortion 639.6
      ectopic or molar pregnancy 639.6
      infusion, perfusion, or transfusion
          999.1
    in pregnancy, childbirth, or puerperium
        673.0●
    traumatic 958.0
  amniotic fluid (pulmonary) 673.1●
    with
      abortion - see Abortion, by type, with
          embolism
      ectopic pregnancy (see also categories
          633.0–633.9) 639.6
      molar pregnancy (see also categories
          630–632) 639.6
    following
      abortion 639.6
      ectopic or molar pregnancy 639.6

Embolism (Continued)
  aorta, aortic 444.1
    abdominal 444.09
      saddle 444.01
    bifurcation 444.09
      saddle 444.01
    thoracic 444.1
  artery 444.9
    auditory, internal 433.8●
    basilar (see also Occlusion, artery, basilar)
        433.0●
    bladder 444.89
    carotid (common) (internal) (see also
        Occlusion, artery, carotid) 433.1●
    cerebellar (anterior inferior) (posterior
        inferior) (superior) 433.8●
    cerebral (see also Embolism, brain) 434.1●
    choroidal (anterior) 433.8●
    communicating posterior 433.8●
    coronary (see also Infarct, myocardium)
        410.9●
      without myocardial infarction 411.81
    extremity 444.22
      lower 444.22
      upper 444.21
    hypophyseal 433.8●
    mesenteric (with gangrene) 557.0
    ophthalmic (see also Occlusion, retina)
        362.30
    peripheral 444.22
    pontine 433.8●
    precerebral NEC - see Occlusion, artery,
        precerebral
    pulmonary - see Embolism, pulmonary
  pyemic 449
    pulmonary 415.12
  renal 593.81
  retinal (see also Occlusion, retina) 362.30
  septic 449
    pulmonary 415.12
  specified site NEC 444.89
  vertebral (see also Occlusion, artery,
      vertebral) 433.2●
  auditory, internal 433.8●
  basilar (artery) (see also Occlusion, artery,
      basilar) 433.0●
  birth, mother - see Embolism, obstetrical
  blood-clot
    with
      abortion - see Abortion, by type, with
          embolism
      ectopic pregnancy (see also categories
          633.0–633.9) 639.6
      molar pregnancy (see also categories
          630–632) 639.6
    following
      abortion 639.6
      ectopic or molar pregnancy 639.6
    in pregnancy, childbirth, or puerperium
        673.2●
  brain 434.1●
    with
      abortion - see Abortion, by type, with
          embolism
      ectopic pregnancy (see also categories
          633.0–633.9) 639.6
      molar pregnancy (see also categories
          630–632) 639.6
    following
      abortion 639.6
      ectopic or molar pregnancy 639.6
    late effect - see Late effect(s) (of)
        cerebrovascular disease
    puerperal, postpartum, childbirth 674.0●
  capillary 448.9
  cardiac (see also Infarct, myocardium) 410.9●
  carotid (artery) (common) (internal) (see also
      Occlusion, artery, carotid) 433.1●
  cavernous sinus (venous) - see Embolism,
      intracranial venous sinus
  cerebral (see also Embolism, brain) 434.1●

Embolism (Continued)
  cholesterol - *see* Atheroembolism
  choroidal (anterior) (artery) 433.8 ●
  coronary (artery or vein) (systemic) (*see also*
      Infarct, myocardium) 410.9 ●
    without myocardial infarction 411.81
  due to (presence of) any device, implant, or
      graft classifiable to 996.0–996.5 - *see*
      Complications, due to (presence of)
      any device, implant, or graft classified
      to 996.0–996.5 NEC
  encephalomalacia (*see also* Embolism, brain)
      434.1 ●
  extremities 444.22
    lower 444.22
    upper 444.21
  eye 362.30
  fat (cerebral) (pulmonary) (systemic) 958.1
    with
      abortion - *see* Abortion, by type, with
          embolism
      ectopic pregnancy (*see also* categories
          633.0–633.9) 639.6
      molar pregnancy (*see also* categories
          630–632) 639.6
      complicating delivery or puerperium
          673.8 ●
    following
      abortion 639.6
      ectopic or molar pregnancy 639.6
    in pregnancy, childbirth, or the
        puerperium 673.8 ●
  femoral (artery) 444.22
    vein 453.6
      deep 453.41
  following
    abortion 639.6
    ectopic or molar pregnancy 639.6
    infusion, perfusion, or transfusion
      air 999.1
      thrombus 999.2
  heart (fatty) (*see also* Infarct, myocardium)
      410.9 ●
  hepatic (vein) 453.0
  iliac (artery) 444.81
  iliofemoral 444.81
  in pregnancy, childbirth, or puerperium
      (pulmonary) - *see* Embolism,
      obstetrical
  intestine (artery) (vein) (with gangrene) 557.0
  intracranial (*see also* Embolism, brain) 434.1 ●
    venous sinus (any) 325
      late effect - *see* category 326
      nonpyogenic 437.6
        in pregnancy or puerperium 671.5 ●
  kidney (artery) 593.81
  lateral sinus (venous) - *see* Embolism,
      intracranial venous sinus
  longitudinal sinus (venous) - *see* Embolism,
      intracranial venous sinus
  lower extremity 444.22
  lung (massive) - *see* Embolism, pulmonary
  meninges (*see also* Embolism, brain) 434.1 ●
  mesenteric (artery) (with gangrene) 557.0
  multiple NEC 444.9
  obstetrical (pulmonary) 673.2 ●
    air 673.0 ●
    amniotic fluid (pulmonary) 673.1 ●
    blood-clot 673.2 ●
    cardiac 674.8 ●
    fat 673.8 ●
    heart 674.8 ●
    pyemic 673.3 ●
    septic 673.3 ●
    specified NEC 674.8 ●
  ophthalmic (*see also* Occlusion, retina) 362.30
  paradoxical NEC 444.9
  penis 607.82
  peripheral arteries NEC 444.22
    lower 444.22
    upper 444.21

Embolism (Continued)
  pituitary 253.8
  popliteal (artery) 444.22
  portal (vein) 452
  postoperative NEC 997.2
    cerebral 997.02
    mesenteric artery 997.71
    other vessels 997.79
    peripheral vascular 997.2
    pulmonary 415.11
      septic 415.11
    renal artery 997.72
  precerebral artery (*see also* Occlusion, artery,
      precerebral) 433.9 ●
  puerperal - *see* Embolism, obstetrical
  pulmonary (acute) (artery) (vein) 415.19
    with
      abortion - *see* Abortion, by type, with
          embolism
      ectopic pregnancy (*see also* categories
          633.0–633.9) 639.6
      molar pregnancy (*see also* categories
          630–632) 639.6
    chronic 416.2
    following
      abortion 639.6
      ectopic or molar pregnancy 639.6
    healed or old V12.55
    iatrogenic 415.11
    in pregnancy, childbirth, or puerperium -
        see Embolism, obstetrical
    personal history of V12.55
    postoperative 415.11
    septic 415.12
  pyemic (multiple) (*see also* Septicemia) 415.12
    with
      abortion - *see* Abortion, by type, with
          embolism
      ectopic pregnancy (*see also* categories
          633.0–633.9) 639.6
      molar pregnancy (*see also* categories
          630–632) 639.6
    Aerobacter aerogenes 415.12
    enteric gram-negative bacilli 415.12
    Enterobacter aerogenes 415.12
    Escherichia coli 415.12
    following
      abortion 639.6
      ectopic or molar pregnancy 639.6
    Hemophilus influenzae 415.12
    pneumococcal 415.12
    Proteus vulgaris 415.12
    Pseudomonas (aeruginosa) 415.12
    puerperal, postpartum, childbirth (any
        organism) 673.3 ●
    Serratia 415.12
    specified organism NEC 415.12
    staphylococcal 415.12
      aureus 415.12
      specified organism NEC 415.12
    streptococcal 415.12
  renal (artery) 593.81
    vein 453.3
  retina, retinal (*see also* Occlusion, retina)
      362.30
  saddle
    abdominal aorta 444.01
    pulmonary artery 415.13
  septic 415.12
    arterial 449
  septicemic - *see* Embolism, pyemic
  sinus - *see* Embolism, intracranial venous
      sinus
  soap
    with
      abortion - *see* Abortion, by type, with
          embolism
      ectopic pregnancy (*see also* categories
          633.0–633.9) 639.6
      molar pregnancy (*see also* categories
          630–632) 639.6

Embolism (Continued)
  soap (Continued)
    following
      abortion 639.6
      ectopic or molar pregnancy 639.6
  spinal cord (nonpyogenic) 336.1
    in pregnancy or puerperium 671.5 ●
    pyogenic origin 324.1
      late effect - *see* category 326
  spleen, splenic (artery) 444.89
  thrombus (thromboembolism) following
      infusion, perfusion, or transfusion
      999.2
  upper extremity 444.21
  vein 453.9
    with inflammation or phlebitis - *see*
        Thrombophlebitis
    antecubital (acute) 453.81
      chronic 453.71
    axillary (acute) 453.84
      chronic 453.74
    basilic (acute) 453.81
      chronic 453.71
    brachial (acute) 453.82
      chronic 453.72
    brachiocephalic (acute) (innominate) 453.87
      chronic 453.77
    cephalic (acute) 453.81
      chronic 453.71
    cerebral (*see also* Embolism, brain) 434.1 ●
    coronary (*see also* Infarct, myocardium)
        410.9 ●
      without myocardial infarction 411.81
    hepatic 453.0
    internal jugular (acute) 453.86
      chronic 453.76
    lower extremity (superficial) 453.6
      deep 453.40
        acute 453.40
          calf 453.42
          distal (lower leg) 453.42
          femoral 453.41
          iliac 453.41
          lower leg 453.42
          peroneal 453.42
          popliteal 453.41
          proximal (upper leg) 453.41
          thigh 453.41
          tibial 453.42
        chronic 453.50
          calf 453.52
          distal (lower leg) 453.52
          femoral 453.51
          iliac 453.51
          lower leg 453.52
          peroneal 453.52
          popliteal 453.51
          proximal (upper leg) 453.51
          thigh 453.51
          tibial 453.52
      saphenous (greater) (lesser) 453.6
      superficial 453.6
    mesenteric (with gangrene) 557.0
    portal 452
    pulmonary - *see* Embolism, pulmonary
    radial (acute) 453.82
      chronic 453.72
    renal 453.3
    saphenous (greater) (lesser) 453.6
    specified NEC (acute) 453.89
      with inflammation or phlebitis - *see*
          Thrombophlebitis
      chronic 453.79
    subclavian (acute) 453.85
      chronic 453.75
    superior vena cava (acute) 453.87
      chronic 453.77
    thoracic (acute) 453.87
      chronic 453.77
    ulnar (acute) 453.82
      chronic 453.72

SECTION 1 INDEX TO DISEASES AND INJURIES / Embolism

Embolism (Continued)
  vein (Continued)
    upper extremity (acute) 453.83
      chronic 453.73
        deep 453.72
        superficial 453.71
      deep 453.82
      superficial 453.81
    vena cava
      inferior 453.2
      superior (acute) 453.87
        chronic 453.77
  vessels of brain (see also Embolism, brain) 434.1●

Embolization - see Embolism
Embolus - see Embolism
Embryoma (M9080/1) - see also Neoplasm, by site, uncertain behavior
  benign (M9080/0) - see Neoplasm, by site, benign
  kidney (M8960/3) 189.0
  liver (M8970/3) 155.0
  malignant (M9080/3) - see also Neoplasm, by site, malignant
  kidney (M8960/3) 189.0
  liver (M8970/3) 155.0
  testis (M9070/3) 186.9
    undescended 186.0
  testis (M9070/3) 186.9
    undescended 186.0

Embryonic
  circulation 747.9
  heart 747.9
  vas deferens 752.89

Embryopathia NEC 759.9
Embryotomy, fetal 763.89
Embryotoxon 743.43
  interfering with vision 743.42
Emesis - see also Vomiting
  bilious 787.04
  gravidarum - see Hyperemesis, gravidarum
Emissions, nocturnal (semen) 608.89
Emotional
  crisis - see Crisis, emotional
  disorder (see also Disorder, mental) 300.9
  instability (excessive) 301.3
  lability 799.24
  overlay - see Reaction, adjustment
  upset 300.9
Emotionality, pathological 301.3
Emotogenic disease (see also Disorder, psychogenic) 306.9
Emphysema (atrophic) (centriacinar) (centrilobular) (chronic) (diffuse) (essential) (hypertrophic) (interlobular) (lung) (obstructive) (panlobular) (paracicatricial) (paracinar) (postural) (pulmonary) (senile) (subpleural) (traction) (unilateral) (unilobular) (vesicular) 492.8
  with bronchitis
    chronic 491.20
      with
        acute bronchitis 491.22
        exacerbation (acute) 491.21
  bullous (giant) 492.0
  cellular tissue 958.7
    surgical 998.81
  compensatory 518.2
  congenital 770.2
  conjunctiva 372.89
  connective tissue 958.7
    surgical 998.81
  due to fumes or vapors 506.4
  eye 376.89
  eyelid 374.85
    surgical 998.81
    traumatic 958.7
  fetus or newborn (interstitial) (mediastinal) (unilobular) 770.2
  heart 416.9

Emphysema (Continued)
  interstitial 518.1
    congenital 770.2
    fetus or newborn 770.2
  laminated tissue 958.7
    surgical 998.81
  mediastinal 518.1
    fetus or newborn 770.2
  newborn (interstitial) (mediastinal) (unilobular) 770.2
  obstructive diffuse with fibrosis 492.8
  orbit 376.89
  subcutaneous 958.7
    due to trauma 958.7
    nontraumatic 518.1
    surgical 998.81
  surgical 998.81
  thymus (gland) (congenital) 254.8
  traumatic 958.7
  tuberculous (see also Tuberculosis, pulmonary) 011.9●

Employment examination (certification) V70.5
Empty sella (turcica) syndrome 253.8
Empyema (chest) (diaphragmatic) (double) (encapsulated) (general) (interlobar) (lung) (medial) (necessitatis) (perforating chest wall) (pleura) (pneumococcal) (residual) (sacculated) (streptococcal) (supradiaphragmatic) 510.9
  with fistula 510.0
  accessory sinus (chronic) (see also Sinusitis) 473.9
  acute 510.9
    with fistula 510.0
  antrum (chronic) (see also Sinusitis, maxillary) 473.0
  brain (any part) (see also Abscess, brain) 324.0
  ethmoidal (sinus) (chronic) (see also Sinusitis, ethmoidal) 473.2
  extradural (see also Abscess, extradural) 324.9
  frontal (sinus) (chronic) (see also Sinusitis, frontal) 473.1
  gallbladder (see also Cholecystitis, acute) 575.0
  mastoid (process) (acute) (see also Mastoiditis, acute) 383.00
  maxilla, maxillary 526.4
    sinus (chronic) (see also Sinusitis, maxillary) 473.0
  nasal sinus (chronic) (see also Sinusitis) 473.9
  sinus (accessory) (nasal) (see also Sinusitis) 473.9
  sphenoidal (chronic) (sinus) (see also Sinusitis, sphenoidal) 473.3
  subarachnoid (see also Abscess, extradural) 324.9
  subdural (see also Abscess, extradural) 324.9
  tuberculous (see also Tuberculosis, pleura) 012.0●
  ureter (see also Ureteritis) 593.89
  ventricular (see also Abscess, brain) 324.0

Enameloma 520.2
Encephalitis (bacterial) (chronic) (hemorrhagic) (idiopathic) (nonepidemic) (spurious) (subacute) 323.9
  acute - see also Encephalitis, viral
    disseminated (postinfectious) NEC 136.9 [323.61]
      postimmunization or postvaccination 323.51
    inclusional 049.8
    inclusion body 049.8
    necrotizing 049.8
  arboviral, arbovirus NEC 064
  arthropod-borne (see also Encephalitis, viral, arthropod-borne) 064
  Australian X 062.4
  Bwamba fever 066.3
  California (virus) 062.5
  Central European 063.2
  Czechoslovakian 063.2

Encephalitis (Continued)
  Dawson's (inclusion body) 046.2
  diffuse sclerosing 046.2
  due to
    actinomycosis 039.8 [323.41]
    cat-scratch disease 078.3 [323.01]
    human herpesvirus 6 058.21
    human herpesvirus 7 058.29
    human herpesvirus NEC 058.29
    human immunodeficiency virus [HIV] disease 042 [323.01]
    infectious mononucleosis 075 [323.01]
    malaria (see also Malaria) 084.6 [323.2]
    Negishi virus 064
    ornithosis 073.7 [323.01]
    other infection classified elsewhere 136.9 [323.41]
    prophylactic inoculation against smallpox 323.51
    rickettsiosis (see also Rickettsiosis) 083.9 [323.1]
    rubella 056.01
    toxoplasmosis (acquired) 130.0
      congenital (active) 771.2 [323.41]
    typhus (fever) (see also Typhus) 081.9 [323.1]
    vaccination (smallpox) 323.51
  Eastern equine 062.2
  endemic 049.8
  epidemic 049.8
  equine (acute) (infectious) (viral) 062.9
    eastern 062.2
    Venezuelan 066.2
    western 062.1
  Far Eastern 063.0
  following vaccination or other immunization procedure 323.51
  herpes 054.3
  human herpesvirus 6 058.21
  human herpesvirus 7 058.29
  human herpesvirus NEC 058.29
  Ilheus (virus) 062.8
  inclusion body 046.2
  infectious (acute) (virus) NEC 049.8
  influenzal (see also Influenza) 487.8 [323.41]
    lethargic 049.8
  Japanese (B type) 062.0
  La Crosse 062.5
  Langat 063.8
  late effect - see Late, effect, encephalitis
  lead 984.9 [323.71]
  lethargic (acute) (infectious) (influenzal) 049.8
  lethargica 049.8
  louping ill 063.1
  lupus 710.0 [323.81]
  lymphatica 049.0
  Mengo 049.8
  meningococcal 036.1
  mumps 072.2
  Murray Valley 062.4
  myoclonic 049.8
  Negishi virus 064
  otitic NEC 382.4 [323.41]
  parasitic NEC 123.9 [323.41]
  periaxialis (concentrica) (diffusa) 341.1
  postchickenpox 052.0
  postexanthematous NEC 057.9 [323.62]
  postimmunization 323.51
  postinfectious NEC 136.9 [323.62]
  postmeasles 055.0
  posttraumatic 323.81
  postvaccinal (smallpox) 323.51
  postvaricella 052.0
  postviral NEC 079.99 [323.62]
    postexanthematous 057.9 [323.62]
    specified NEC 057.8 [323.62]
  Powassan 063.8
  progressive subcortical (Binswanger's) 290.12
  Rasmussen 323.81

Encephalitis *(Continued)*
- Rio Bravo 049.8
- rubella 056.01
- Russian
  - autumnal 062.0
  - spring-summer type (taiga) 063.0
- saturnine 984.9 [323.71]
- Semliki Forest 062.8
- serous 048
- slow-acting virus NEC 046.8
- specified cause NEC 323.81
- St. Louis type 062.3
- subacute sclerosing 046.2
- subcorticalis chronica 290.12
- summer 062.0
- suppurative 324.0
- syphilitic 094.81
  - congenital 090.41
- tick-borne 063.9
- torula, torular 117.5 [323.41]
- toxic NEC 989.9 [323.71]
- toxoplasmic (acquired) 130.0
  - congenital (active) 771.2 [323.41]
- trichinosis 124 [323.41]
- Trypanosomiasis (see also Trypanosomiasis) 086.9 [323.2]
- tuberculous (see also Tuberculosis) 013.6 ●
- type B (Japanese) 062.0
- type C 062.3
- van Bogaert's 046.2
- Venezuelan 066.2
- Vienna type 049.8
- viral, virus 049.9
  - arthropod-borne NEC 064
    - mosquito-borne 062.9
      - Australian X disease 062.4
      - California virus 062.5
      - Eastern equine 062.2
      - Ilheus virus 062.8
      - Japanese (B type) 062.0
      - Murray Valley 062.4
      - specified type NEC 062.8
      - St. Louis 062.3
      - type B 062.0
      - type C 062.3
      - Western equine 062.1
    - tick-borne 063.9
      - biundulant 063.2
      - Central European 063.2
      - Czechoslovakian 063.2
      - diphasic meningoencephalitis 063.2
      - Far Eastern 063.0
      - Langat 063.8
      - louping ill 063.1
      - Powassan 063.8
      - Russian spring-summer (taiga) 063.0
      - specified type NEC 063.8
    - vector unknown 064
  - slow acting NEC 046.8
  - specified type NEC 049.8
- vaccination, prophylactic (against) V05.0
- von Economo's 049.8
- Western equine 062.1
- West Nile type 066.41

Encephalocele 742.0
- orbit 376.81

Encephalocystocele 742.0

Encephaloduroarteriomyosynangiosis (EDAMS) 437.5

Encephalomalacia (brain) (cerebellar) (cerebral) (cerebrospinal) (see also Softening, brain) 348.89
- due to
  - hemorrhage (see also Hemorrhage, brain) 431
  - recurrent spasm of artery 435.9
- embolic (cerebral) (see also Embolism, brain) 434.1 ●
- subcorticalis chronicus arteriosclerotica 290.12
- thrombotic (see also Thrombosis, brain) 434.0 ●

Encephalomeningitis - see Meningoencephalitis

Encephalomeningocele 742.0

Encephalomeningomyelitis - see Meningoencephalitis

Encephalomeningopathy (see also Meningoencephalitis) 349.9

Encephalomyelitis (chronic) (granulomatous) (myalgic, benign) (see also Encephalitis) 323.9
- abortive disseminated 049.8
- acute disseminated (ADEM) (postinfectious) 136.9 [323.61]
  - infectious 136.9 [323.61]
  - noninfectious 323.81
  - postimmunization 323.51
- due to
  - cat-scratch disease 078.3 [323.01]
  - infectious mononucleosis 075 [323.01]
  - ornithosis 073.7 [323.01]
  - vaccination (any) 323.51
- equine (acute) (infectious) 062.9
  - eastern 062.2
  - Venezuelan 066.2
  - western 062.1
- funicularis infectiosa 049.8
- late effect - see Late, effect, encephalitis
- Munch-Peterson's 049.8
- postchickenpox 052.0
- postimmunization 323.51
- postmeasles 055.0
- postvaccinal (smallpox) 323.51
- rubella 056.01
- specified cause NEC 323.81
- syphilitic 094.81
- West Nile 066.41

Encephalomyelocele 742.0

Encephalomyelomeningitis - see Meningoencephalitis

Encephalomyeloneuropathy 349.9

Encephalomyelopathy 349.9
- subacute necrotizing (infantile) 330.8

Encephalomyeloradiculitis (acute) 357.0

Encephalomyeloradiculoneuritis (acute) 357.0

Encephalomyeloradiculopathy 349.9

Encephalomyocarditis 074.23

Encephalopathia hyperbilirubinemica, newborn 774.7
- due to isoimmunization (conditions classifiable to 773.0–773.2) 773.4

Encephalopathy (acute) 348.30
- alcoholic 291.2
- anoxic - see Damage, brain, anoxic
- arteriosclerotic 437.0
  - late effect - see Late effect(s) (of) cerebrovascular disease
- bilirubin, newborn 774.7
  - due to isoimmunization 773.4
- congenital 742.9
- demyelinating (callosal) 341.8
- due to
  - birth injury (intracranial) 767.8
  - dialysis 294.8
    - transient 293.9
  - drugs - (see also Table of Drugs and Chemicals) 349.82
  - hyperinsulinism - see Hyperinsulinism
  - influenza (virus) (see also Influenza) 487.8
    - identified
      - avian 488.09
      - (novel) 2009 H1N1 488.19
  - lack of vitamin (see also Deficiency, vitamin) 269.2
  - nicotinic acid deficiency 291.2
  - serum (nontherapeutic) (therapeutic) 999.59
  - syphilis 094.81
  - trauma (postconcussional) 310.2
    - current (see also Concussion, brain) 850.9
      - with skull fracture - see Fracture, skull, by site, with intracranial injury
  - vaccination 323.51

Encephalopathy *(Continued)*
- hepatic 572.2
- hyperbilirubinemic, newborn 774.7
  - due to isoimmunization (conditions classifiable to 773.0–773.2) 773.4
- hypertensive 437.2
- hypoglycemic 251.2
- hypoxic - see also Damage, brain, anoxic
  - ischemic (HIE) 768.70
    - mild 768.71
    - moderate 768.72
    - severe 768.73
- infantile cystic necrotizing (congenital) 341.8
- lead 984.9 [323.71]
- leukopolio 330.0
- metabolic (see also Delirium) 348.31
  - drug induced 349.82
  - toxic 349.82
- necrotizing
  - hemorrhagic (acute) 323.61
  - subacute 330.8
- other specified type NEC 348.39
- pellagrous 265.2
- portal-systemic 572.2
- postcontusional 310.2
- posttraumatic 310.2
- saturnine 984.9 [323.71]
- septic 348.31
- spongiform, subacute (viral) 046.19
- subacute
  - necrotizing 330.8
  - spongiform 046.19
  - viral, spongiform 046.19
- subcortical progressive (Schilder) 341.1
  - chronic (Binswanger's) 290.12
- toxic 349.82
  - metabolic 349.82
- traumatic (postconcussional) 310.2
  - current (see also Concussion, brain) 850.9
    - with skull fracture - see Fracture, skull, by site, with intracranial injury
- vitamin B deficiency NEC 266.9
- Wernicke's (superior hemorrhagic polioencephalitis) 265.1

Encephalorrhagia (see also Hemorrhage, brain) 432.9
- healed or old V12.54
- late effect - see Late effect(s) (of) cerebrovascular disease

Encephalosis, posttraumatic 310.2

Enchondroma (M9220/0) - see also Neoplasm, bone, benign
- multiple, congenital 756.4

Enchondromatosis (cartilaginous) (congenital) (multiple) 756.4

Enchondroses, multiple (cartilaginous) (congenital) 756.4

Encopresis (see also Incontinence, feces) 787.60
- nonorganic origin 307.7

Encounter for - see also Admission for
- administrative purpose only V68.9
  - referral of patient without examination or treatment V68.81
  - specified purpose NEC V68.89
- chemotherapy, (oral) (intravenous), antineoplastic V58.11
- determination of fetal viability of pregnancy V23.87
- dialysis
  - extracorporeal (renal) V56.0
  - peritoneal V56.8
- disability examination V68.01
- end-of-life care V66.7
- hospice care V66.7
- immunizations (childhood) appropriate for age V20.2
- immunotherapy, antineoplastic V58.12
- joint prosthesis insertion following prior explantation of joint prosthesis V54.82
- palliative care V66.7
- paternity testing V70.4

Encounter for (Continued)
  radiotherapy V58.0
  respirator [ventilator] dependence
    during
      mechanical failure V46.14
      power failure V46.12
    for weaning V46.13
  routine infant and child vision and hearing
      testing V20.2
  school examination V70.3
    following surgery V67.09
  screening mammogram NEC V76.12
    for high-risk patient V76.11
  terminal care V66.7
  weaning from respirator [ventilator] V46.13
Encystment - see Cyst
End-of-life care V66.7
Endamebiasis - see Amebiasis
Endamoeba - see Amebiasis
Endarteritis (bacterial, subacute) (infective)
      (septic) 447.6
  brain, cerebral or cerebrospinal 437.4
    late effect - see Late effect(s) (of)
      cerebrovascular disease
  coronary (artery) - see Arteriosclerosis,
      coronary
  deformans - see Arteriosclerosis
  embolic (see also Embolism) 444.9
  obliterans - see also Arteriosclerosis
    pulmonary 417.8
  pulmonary 417.8
  retina 362.18
  senile - see Arteriosclerosis
  syphilitic 093.89
    brain or cerebral 094.89
    congenital 090.5
    spinal 094.89
  tuberculous (see also Tuberculosis) 017.9●
Endemic - see condition
Endocarditis (chronic) (indeterminate)
      (interstitial) (marantic) (nonbacterial
      thrombotic) (residual) (sclerotic)
      (sclerous) (senile) (valvular) 424.90
  with
    rheumatic fever (conditions classifiable to
        390)
      active - see Endocarditis, acute,
        rheumatic
      inactive or quiescent (with chorea)
        397.9
  acute or subacute 421.9
    rheumatic (aortic) (mitral) (pulmonary)
        (tricuspid) 391.1
      with chorea (acute) (rheumatic)
        (Sydenham's) 392.0
  aortic (heart) (nonrheumatic) (valve) 424.1
    with
      mitral (valve) disease 396.9
        active or acute 391.1
          with chorea (acute) (rheumatic)
            (Sydenham's) 392.0
      bacterial 421.0
      rheumatic fever (conditions classifiable
          to 390)
        active - see Endocarditis, acute,
          rheumatic
        inactive or quiescent (with chorea)
          395.9
          with mitral disease 396.9
    acute or subacute 421.9
    arteriosclerotic 424.1
    congenital 746.89
    hypertensive 424.1
    rheumatic (chronic) (inactive) 395.9
      with mitral (valve) disease 396.9
        active or acute 391.1
          with chorea (acute) (rheumatic)
            (Sydenham's) 392.0
        active or acute 391.1
          with chorea (acute) (rheumatic)
            (Sydenham's) 392.0

Endocarditis (Continued)
  aortic (Continued)
    specified cause, except rheumatic 424.1
    syphilitic 093.22
  arteriosclerotic or due to arteriosclerosis
      424.99
  atypical verrucous (Libman-Sacks) 710.0
      [424.91]
  bacterial (acute) (any valve) (chronic)
      (subacute) 421.0
  blastomycotic 116.0 [421.1]
  candidal 112.81
  congenital 425.3
  constrictive 421.0
  Coxsackie 074.22
  due to
    blastomycosis 116.0 [421.1]
    candidiasis 112.81
    Coxsackie (virus) 074.22
    disseminated lupus erythematosus 710.0
      [424.91]
    histoplasmosis (see also Histoplasmosis)
      115.94
    hypertension (benign) 424.99
    moniliasis 112.81
    prosthetic cardiac valve 996.61
    Q fever 083.0 [421.1]
    serratia marcescens 421.0
    typhoid (fever) 002.0 [421.1]
  fetal 425.3
  gonococcal 098.84
  hypertensive 424.99
  infectious or infective (acute) (any valve)
      (chronic) (subacute) 421.0
  lenta (acute) (any valve) (chronic) (subacute)
      421.0
  Libman-Sacks 710.0 [424.91]
  Loeffler's (parietal fibroplastic) 421.0
  malignant (acute) (any valve) (chronic)
      (subacute) 421.0
  meningococcal 036.42
  mitral (chronic) (double) (fibroid) (heart)
      (inactive) (valve) (with chorea)
      394.9
    with
      aortic (valve) disease 396.9
        active or acute 391.1
          with chorea (acute) (rheumatic)
            (Sydenham's) 392.0
      rheumatic fever (conditions classifiable
          to 390)
        active - see Endocarditis, acute,
          rheumatic
        inactive or quiescent (with chorea)
          394.9
          with aortic valve disease
            396.9
    active or acute 391.1
      with chorea (acute) (rheumatic)
        (Sydenham's) 392.0
    bacterial 421.0
    arteriosclerotic 424.0
    congenital 746.89
    hypertensive 424.0
    nonrheumatic 424.0
      acute or subacute 421.9
    syphilitic 093.21
  monilial 112.81
  mycotic (acute) (any valve) (chronic)
      (subacute) 421.0
  pneumococcic (acute) (any valve) (chronic)
      (subacute) 421.0
  pulmonary (chronic) (heart) (valve)
      424.3
    with
      rheumatic fever (conditions classifiable
          to 390)
        active - see Endocarditis, acute,
          rheumatic
        inactive or quiescent (with chorea)
          397.1

Endocarditis (Continued)
  pulmonary (Continued)
    acute or subacute 421.9
      rheumatic 391.1
        with chorea (acute) (rheumatic)
          (Sydenham's) 392.0
    arteriosclerotic or due to arteriosclerosis
      424.3
    congenital 746.09
    hypertensive or due to hypertension
        (benign) 424.3
    rheumatic (chronic) (inactive) (with
        chorea) 397.1
      active or acute 391.1
        with chorea (acute) (rheumatic)
          (Sydenham's) 392.0
    syphilitic 093.24
  purulent (acute) (any valve) (chronic)
      (subacute) 421.0
  rheumatic (chronic) (inactive) (with chorea)
      397.9
    active or acute (aortic) (mitral)
        (pulmonary) (tricuspid) 391.1
      with chorea (acute) (rheumatic)
        (Sydenham's) 392.0
  septic (acute) (any valve) (chronic)
      (subacute) 421.0
  specified cause, except rheumatic 424.99
  streptococcal (acute) (any valve) (chronic)
      (subacute) 421.0
  subacute - see Endocarditis, acute
  suppurative (any valve) (acute) (chronic)
      (subacute) 421.0
  syphilitic NEC 093.20
  toxic (see also Endocarditis, acute) 421.9
  tricuspid (chronic) (heart) (inactive)
      (rheumatic) (valve) (with chorea) 397.0
    with
      rheumatic fever (conditions classifiable
          to 390)
        active - see Endocarditis, acute,
          rheumatic
        inactive or quiescent (with chorea)
          397.0
    active or acute 391.1
      with chorea (acute) (rheumatic)
        (Sydenham's) 392.0
    arteriosclerotic 424.2
    congenital 746.89
    hypertensive 424.2
    nonrheumatic 424.2
      acute or subacute 421.9
    specified cause, except rheumatic 424.2
    syphilitic 093.23
  tuberculous (see also Tuberculosis) 017.9●
      [424.91]
  typhoid 002.0 [421.1]
  ulcerative (acute) (any valve) (chronic)
      (subacute) 421.0
  vegetative (acute) (any valve) (chronic)
      (subacute) 421.0
  verrucous (acute) (any valve) (chronic)
      (subacute) NEC 710.0 [424.91]
    nonbacterial 710.0 [424.91]
    nonrheumatic 710.0 [424.91]
Endocardium, endocardial - see also condition
  cushion defect 745.60
    specified type NEC 745.69
Endocervicitis (see also Cervicitis) 616.0
  due to
    intrauterine (contraceptive) device 996.65
  gonorrheal (acute) 098.15
    chronic or duration of 2 months or over
      098.35
  hyperplastic 616.0
  syphilitic 095.8
  trichomonal 131.09
  tuberculous (see also Tuberculosis) 016.7●
Endocrine - see condition
Endocrinopathy, pluriglandular 258.9
Endodontitis 522.0

Endomastoiditis (*see also* Mastoiditis) 383.9
Endometrioma 617.9
Endometriosis 617.9
  appendix 617.5
  bladder 617.8
  bowel 617.5
  broad ligament 617.3
  cervix 617.0
  colon 617.5
  cul-de-sac (Douglas') 617.3
  exocervix 617.0
  fallopian tube 617.2
  female genital organ NEC 617.8
  gallbladder 617.8
  in scar of skin 617.6
  internal 617.0
  intestine 617.5
  lung 617.8
  myometrium 617.0
  ovary 617.1
  parametrium 617.3
  pelvic peritoneum 617.3
  peritoneal (pelvic) 617.3
  rectovaginal septum 617.4
  rectum 617.5
  round ligament 617.3
  skin 617.6
  specified site NEC 617.8
  stromal (M8931/1) 236.0
  umbilicus 617.8
  uterus 617.0
    internal 617.0
  vagina 617.4
  vulva 617.8
Endometritis (nonspecific) (purulent) (septic) (suppurative) 615.9
  with
    abortion - *see* Abortion, by type, with sepsis
    ectopic pregnancy (*see also* categories 633.0-633.9) 639.0
    molar pregnancy (*see also* categories 630-632) 639.0
  acute 615.0
  blennorrhagic 098.16
    acute 098.16
    chronic or duration of 2 months or over 098.36
  cervix, cervical (*see also* Cervicitis) 616.0
    hyperplastic 616.0
  chronic 615.1
  complicating pregnancy 670.1 ●
    affecting fetus or newborn 760.8
    septic 670.2 ●
  decidual 615.9
  following
    abortion 639.0
    ectopic or molar pregnancy 639.0
  gonorrheal (acute) 098.16
    chronic or duration of 2 months or over 098.36
  hyperplastic (*see also* Hyperplasia, endometrium) 621.30
    cervix 616.0
  polypoid - *see* Endometritis, hyperplastic
  puerperal, postpartum, childbirth 670.1 ●
    septic 670.2 ●
  senile (atrophic) 615.9
  subacute 615.0
  tuberculous (*see also* Tuberculosis) 016.7 ●
Endometrium - *see* condition
Endomyocardiopathy, South African 425.2
Endomyocarditis - *see* Endocarditis
Endomyofibrosis 425.0
Endomyometritis (*see also* Endometritis) 615.9
Endopericarditis - *see* Endocarditis
Endoperineuritis - *see* Disorder, nerve
Endophlebitis (*see also* Phlebitis) 451.9
  leg 451.2
    deep (vessels) 451.19
    superficial (vessels) 451.0

Endophlebitis (*Continued*)
  portal (vein) 572.1
  retina 362.18
  specified site NEC 451.89
  syphilitic 093.89
Endophthalmia (*see also* Endophthalmitis) 360.00
  gonorrheal 098.42
Endophthalmitis (globe) (infective) (metastatic) (purulent) (subacute) 360.00
  acute 360.01
  bleb associated 379.63
  chronic 360.03
  parasitic 360.13
  phacoanaphylactic 360.19
  specified type NEC 360.19
  sympathetic 360.11
Endosalpingioma (M9111/1) 236.2
Endosalpingiosis 629.89
Endosteitis - *see* Osteomyelitis
Endothelioma, bone (M9260/3) - *see* Neoplasm, bone, malignant
Endotheliosis 287.8
  hemorrhagic infectional 287.8
Endotoxemia - *code to* condition
Endotoxic shock 785.52
  postoperative 998.02
Endotrachelitis (*see also* Cervicitis) 616.0
Enema rash 692.89
Engel-von Recklinghausen disease or syndrome (osteitis fibrosa cystica) 252.01
Engelmann's disease (diaphyseal sclerosis) 756.59
English disease (*see also* Rickets) 268.0
Engman's disease (infectious eczematoid dermatitis) 690.8
Engorgement
  breast 611.79
    newborn 778.7
    puerperal, postpartum 676.2 ●
  liver 573.9
  lung 514
  pulmonary 514
  retina, venous 362.37
  stomach 536.8
  venous, retina 362.37
Enlargement, enlarged - *see also* Hypertrophy
  abdomen 789.3 ●
  adenoids 474.12
    and tonsils 474.10
  alveolar process or ridge 525.8
  apertures of diaphragm (congenital) 756.6
  blind spot, visual field 368.42
  gingival 523.8
  heart, cardiac (*see also* Hypertrophy, cardiac) 429.3
  lacrimal gland, chronic 375.03
  liver (*see also* Hypertrophy, liver) 789.1
  lymph gland or node 785.6
  orbit 376.46
  organ or site, congenital NEC - *see* Anomaly, specified type NEC
  parathyroid (gland) 252.01
  pituitary fossa 793.0
  prostate (simple) (soft) 600.00
    with
      other lower urinary tract symptoms (LUTS) 600.01
      urinary
        obstruction 600.01
        retention 600.01
  sella turcica 793.0
  spleen (*see also* Splenomegaly) 789.2
    congenital 759.0
  thymus (congenital) (gland) 254.0
  thyroid (gland) (*see also* Goiter) 240.9
  tongue 529.8
  tonsils 474.11
    and adenoids 474.10
  uterus 621.2

Enophthalmos 376.50
  due to
    atrophy of orbital tissue 376.51
    surgery 376.52
    trauma 376.52
Enostosis 526.89
Entamebiasis - *see* Amebiasis
Entamebic - *see* Amebiasis
Entanglement, umbilical cord(s) 663.3 ●
  with compression 663.2 ●
  affecting fetus or newborn 762.5
  around neck with compression 663.1 ●
  twins in monoamniotic sac 663.2 ●
Enteralgia 789.0 ●
Enteric - *see* condition
Enteritis (acute) (catarrhal) (choleraic) (chronic) (congestive) (diarrheal) (exudative) (follicular) (hemorrhagic) (infantile) (lienteric) (noninfectious) (perforative) (phlegmonous) (presumed noninfectious) (pseudomembranous) 558.9
  adaptive 564.9
  aertrycke infection 003.0
  allergic 558.3
  amebic (*see also* Amebiasis) 006.9
    with abscess - *see* Abscess, amebic
    acute 006.0
      with abscess - *see* Abscess, amebic
      nondysenteric 006.2
    chronic 006.1
      with abscess - *see* Abscess, amebic
      nondysenteric 006.2
    nondysenteric 006.2
  anaerobic (cocci) (gram-negative) (gram-positive) (mixed) NEC 008.46
  bacillary NEC 004.9
  bacterial NEC 008.5
    specified NEC 008.49
  Bacteroides (fragilis) (melaninogeniscus) (oralis) 008.46
  Butyrivibrio (fibriosolvens) 008.46
  Campylobacter 008.43
  Candida 112.85
  Chilomastix 007.8
  choleriformis 001.1
  chronic 558.9
    ulcerative (*see also* Colitis, ulcerative) 556.9
  cicatrizing (chronic) 555.0
  Clostridium
    botulinum 005.1
    difficile 008.45
    haemolyticum 008.46
    novyi 008.46
    perfringens (C) (F) 008.46
    specified type NEC 008.46
  coccidial 007.2
  dietetic 558.9
  due to
    achylia gastrica 536.8
    adenovirus 008.62
    Aerobacter aerogenes 008.2
    anaerobes (*see also* Enteritis, anaerobic) 008.46
    Arizona (bacillus) 008.1
    astrovirus 008.66
    Bacillus coli - *see* Enteritis, E. coli
    bacteria NEC 008.5
      specified NEC 008.49
    Bacteroides (*see also* Enteritis, Bacteroides) 008.46
    Butyrivibrio (fibriosolvens) 008.46
    calicivirus 008.65
    Campylobacter 008.43
    Clostridium - *see* Enteritis, Clostridium
    Cockle agent 008.64
    Coxsackie (virus) 008.67
    Ditchling agent 008.64
    ECHO virus 008.67
    Enterobacter aerogenes 008.2
    enterococci 008.49

SECTION 1 INDEX TO DISEASES AND INJURIES / Enteritis

Enteritis (Continued)
- due to (Continued)
  - enterovirus NEC 008.67
  - Escherichia coli - see Enteritis, E. coli
  - Eubacterium 008.46
  - Fusobacterium (nucleatum) 008.46
  - gram-negative bacteria NEC 008.47
    - anaerobic NEC 008.46
  - Hawaii agent 008.63
  - irritating foods 558.9
  - Klebsiella aerogenes 008.47
  - Marin County agent 008.66
  - Montgomery County agent 008.63
  - noroviris 008.63
  - Norwalk-like agent 008.63
  - Norwalk virus 008.63
  - Otofuke agent 008.63
  - Paracolobactrum arizonae 008.1
  - paracolon bacillus NEC 008.47
    - Arizona 008.1
  - Paramatta agent 008.64
  - Peptococcus 008.46
  - Peptostreptococcus 008.46
  - Proprionibacterium 008.46
  - Proteus (bacillus) (mirabilis) (morganii) 008.3
  - Pseudomonas aeruginosa 008.42
  - Rotavirus 008.61
  - Sapporo agent 008.63
  - small round virus (SRV) NEC 008.64
    - featureless NEC 008.63
    - structured NEC 008.63
  - Snow Mountain (SM) agent 008.63
  - specified
    - bacteria NEC 008.49
    - organism, nonbacterial NEC 008.8
    - virus NEC 008.69
  - Staphylococcus 008.41
  - Streptococcus 008.49
    - anaerobic 008.46
  - Taunton agent 008.63
  - Torovirus 008.69
  - Treponema 008.46
  - Veillonella 008.46
  - virus 008.8
    - specified type NEC 008.69
  - Wollan (W) agent 008.64
  - Yersinia enterocolitica 008.44
- dysentery - see Dysentery
- E. coli 008.00
  - enterohemorrhagic 008.04
  - enteroinvasive 008.03
  - enteropathogenic 008.01
  - enterotoxigenic 008.02
  - specified type NEC 008.09
- El Tor 001.1
- embadomonial 007.8
- eosinophilic 558.41
- epidemic 009.0
- Eubacterium 008.46
- fermentative 558.9
- fulminant 557.0
- Fusobacterium (nucleatum) 008.46
- gangrenous (see also Enteritis, due to, by organism) 009.0
- giardial 007.1
- gram-negative bacteria NEC 008.47
  - anaerobic NEC 008.46
- infectious NEC (see also Enteritis, due to, by organism) 009.0
  - presumed 009.1
- influenzal (see also Influenza) 487.8
- ischemic 557.9
  - acute 557.0
  - chronic 557.1
  - due to mesenteric artery insufficiency 557.1
- membranous 564.9
- mucous 564.9
- myxomembranous 564.9

Enteritis (Continued)
- necrotic (see also Enteritis, due to, by organism) 009.0
- necroticans 005.2
- necrotizing of fetus or newborn (see also Enterocolitis, necrotizing, newborn) 777.50
- neurogenic 564.9
- newborn 777.8
  - necrotizing (see also Enterocolitis, necrotizing, newborn) 777.50
- parasitic NEC 129
- paratyphoid (fever) (see also Fever, paratyphoid) 002.9
- Peptococcus 008.46
- Peptostreptococcus 008.46
- Proprionibacterium 008.46
- protozoal NEC 007.9
- radiation 558.1
- regional (of) 555.9
  - intestine
    - large (bowel, colon, or rectum) 555.1
      - with small intestine 555.2
    - small (duodenum, ileum, or jejunum) 555.0
      - with large intestine 555.2
- Salmonella infection 003.0
- salmonellosis 003.0
- segmental (see also Enteritis, regional) 555.9
- septic (see also Enteritis, due to, by organism) 009.0
- Shigella 004.9
- simple 558.9
- spasmodic 564.9
- spastic 564.9
- staphylococcal 008.41
  - due to food 005.0
- streptococcal 008.49
  - anaerobic 008.46
- toxic 558.2
- Treponema (denticola) (macrodentium) 008.46
- trichomonal 007.3
- tuberculous (see also Tuberculosis) 014.8●
- typhosa 002.0
- ulcerative (chronic) (see also Colitis, ulcerative) 556.9
- Veillonella 008.46
- viral 008.8
  - adenovirus 008.62
  - enterovirus 008.67
  - specified virus NEC 008.69
- Yersinia enterocolitica 008.44
- zymotic 009.0

Enteroarticular syndrome 099.3
Enterobiasis 127.4
Enterobius vermicularis 127.4
Enterocele (see also Hernia) 553.9
- pelvis, pelvic (acquired) (congenital) 618.6
- vagina, vaginal (acquired) (congenital) 618.6

Enterocolitis - see also Enteritis
- fetus or newborn (see also Enterocolitis, necrotizing, newborn) 777.8
  - necrotizing 777.50
- fulminant 557.0
- granulomatous 555.2
- hemorrhagic (acute) 557.0
  - chronic 557.1
- necrotizing (acute) (membranous) 557.0
  - newborn 777.50
    - with
      - perforation 777.53
      - pneumatosis without perforation 777.52
      - pneumatosis and perforation 777.53
      - without pneumatosis, without perforation 777.51
    - stage I 777.51
    - stage II 777.52
    - stage III 777.53

Enterocolitis (Continued)
- primary necrotizing (see also Enterocolitis, necrotizing, newborn) 777.50
- pseudomembranous 008.45
  - newborn 008.45
- radiation 558.1
  - newborn (see also Enterocolitis, necrotizing, newborn) 777.50
- ulcerative 556.0

Enterocystoma 751.5
Enterogastritis - see Enteritis
Enterogenous cyanosis 289.7
Enterolith, enterolithiasis (impaction) 560.39
- with hernia - see also Hernia, by site, with obstruction
  - gangrenous - see Hernia, by site, with gangrene

Enteropathy 569.9
- exudative (of Gordon) 579.8
- gluten 579.0
- hemorrhagic, terminal 557.0
- protein-losing 579.8

Enteroperitonitis (see also Peritonitis) 567.9
Enteroptosis 569.89
Enterorrhagia 578.9
Enterospasm 564.9
- psychogenic 306.4

Enterostenosis (see also Obstruction, intestine) 560.9
Enterostomy status V44.4
- with complication 569.60

Enthesopathy 726.90
- ankle and tarsus 726.70
- elbow region 726.30
  - specified NEC 726.39
- hip 726.5
- knee 726.60
- peripheral NEC 726.8
- shoulder region 726.10
  - adhesive 726.0
- spinal 720.1
- wrist and carpus 726.4

Entrance, air into vein - see Embolism, air
Entrapment, nerve - see Neuropathy, entrapment

Entropion (eyelid) 374.00
- cicatricial 374.04
- congenital 743.62
- late effect of trachoma (healed) 139.1
- mechanical 374.02
- paralytic 374.02
- senile 374.01
- spastic 374.03

Enucleation of eye (current) (traumatic) 871.3
Enuresis 788.30
- habit disturbance 307.6
- nocturnal 788.36
  - psychogenic 307.6
- nonorganic origin 307.6
- psychogenic 307.6

Enzymopathy 277.9
Eosinopenia 288.59
Eosinophilia 288.3
- with
  - angiolymphoid hyperplasia (ALHE) 228.01
- allergic 288.3
- hereditary 288.3
- idiopathic 288.3
- infiltrative 518.3
- Loeffler's 518.3
- myalgia syndrome 710.5
- pulmonary (tropical) 518.3
- secondary 288.3
- tropical 518.3

Eosinophilic - see also condition
- fasciitis 728.89
- granuloma (bone) 277.89
- infiltration lung 518.3

Ependymitis (acute) (cerebral) (chronic) (granular) (see also Meningitis) 322.9

Ependymoblastoma (M9392/3)
   specified site - *see* Neoplasm, by site, malignant
   unspecified site 191.9
Ependymoma (epithelial) (malignant) (M9391/3)
   anaplastic type (M9392/3)
      specified site - *see* Neoplasm, by site, malignant
      unspecified site 191.9
   benign (M9391/0)
      specified site - *see* Neoplasm, by site, benign
      unspecified site 225.0
   myxopapillary (M9394/1) 237.5
   papillary (M9393/1) 237.5
      specified site - *see* Neoplasm, by site, malignant
      unspecified site 191.9
Ependymopathy 349.2
   spinal cord 349.2
Ephelides, ephelis 709.09
Ephemeral fever (*see also* Pyrexia) 780.60
Epiblepharon (congenital) 743.62
Epicanthus, epicanthic fold (congenital) (eyelid) 743.63
Epicondylitis (elbow) (lateral) 726.32
   medial 726.31
Epicystitis (*see also* Cystitis) 595.9
Epidemic - *see* condition
Epidermidalization, cervix - *see* condition
Epidermidization, cervix - *see* condition
Epidermis, epidermal - *see* condition
Epidermization, cervix - *see* condition
Epidermodysplasia verruciformis 078.19
Epidermoid
   cholesteatoma - *see* Cholesteatoma
   inclusion (*see also* Cyst, skin) 706.2
Epidermolysis
   acuta (combustiformis) (toxica) 695.15
   bullosa 757.39
   necroticans combustiformis 695.15
      due to drug
         correct substance properly administered 695.15
         overdose or wrong substance given or taken 977.9
            specified drug - *see* Table of Drugs and Chemicals
Epidermophytid - *see* Dermatophytosis
Epidermophytosis (infected) - *see* Dermatophytosis
Epidermosis, ear (middle) (*see also* Cholesteatoma) 385.30
Epididymis - *see* condition
Epididymitis (nonvenereal) 604.90
   with abscess 604.0
   acute 604.99
   blennorrhagic (acute) 098.0
      chronic or duration of 2 months or over 098.2
   caseous (*see also* Tuberculosis) 016.4●
   chlamydial 099.54
   diphtheritic 032.89 [604.91]
   filarial 125.9 [604.91]
   gonococcal (acute) 098.0
      chronic or duration of 2 months or over 098.2
   recurrent 604.99
   residual 604.99
   syphilitic 095.8 [604.91]
   tuberculous (*see also* Tuberculosis) 016.4●
Epididymo-orchitis (*see also* Epididymitis) 604.90
   with abscess 604.0
   chlamydial 099.54
   gonococcal (acute) 098.13
      chronic or duration of 2 months or over 098.33
Epidural - *see* condition
Epigastritis (*see also* Gastritis) 535.5●

Epigastrium, epigastric - *see* condition
Epigastrocele (*see also* Hernia, epigastric) 553.29
Epiglottiditis (acute) 464.30
   with obstruction 464.31
   chronic 476.1
   viral 464.30
      with obstruction 464.31
Epiglottis - *see* condition
Epiglottitis (acute) 464.30
   with obstruction 464.31
   chronic 476.1
   viral 464.30
      with obstruction 464.31
Epignathus 759.4
Epilepsia
   partialis continua (*see also* Epilepsy) 345.7●
   procursiva (*see also* Epilepsy) 345.8●
Epilepsy, epileptic (idiopathic) 345.9●

> Note: Use the following fifth-digit subclassifications with categories 345.0, 345.1, 345.4–345.9
>
> 0   without mention of intractable epilepsy
> 1   with intractable epilepsy
>   pharmacoresistant (pharmacologically resistant)
>   poorly controlled
>   refractory (medically)
>   treatment resistant

   abdominal 345.5●
   absence (attack) 345.0●
   akinetic 345.0●
      psychomotor 345.4●
   automatism 345.4●
   autonomic diencephalic 345.5●
   brain 345.9●
   Bravais-Jacksonian 345.5●
   cerebral 345.9●
   climacteric 345.9●
   clonic 345.1●
   clouded state 345.9●
   coma 345.3●
   communicating 345.4●
   complicating pregnancy, childbirth, or the puerperium 649.4●
   congenital 345.9●
   convulsions 345.9●
   cortical (focal) (motor) 345.5●
   cursive (running) 345.8●
   cysticercosis 123.1
   deterioration
      with behavioral disturbance 345.9● [294.11]
      without behavioral disturbance 345.9● [294.10]
   due to syphilis 094.89
   equivalent 345.5●
   fit 345.9●
   focal (motor) 345.5●
   gelastic 345.8●
   generalized 345.9●
      convulsive 345.1●
      flexion 345.1●
      nonconvulsive 345.0●
   grand mal (idiopathic) 345.1●
   Jacksonian (motor) (sensory) 345.5●
   Kojevnikoff's, Kojevnikov's, Kojewnikoff's 345.7●
   laryngeal 786.2
   limbic system 345.4●
   localization related (focal) (partial) and epileptic syndromes
      with
         complex partial seizures 345.4●
         simple partial seizures 345.5●
   major (motor) 345.1●
   minor 345.0●
   mixed (type) 345.9●
   motor partial 345.5●

Epilepsy, epileptic (Continued)
   musicogenic 345.1●
   myoclonus, myoclonic 345.1●
      progressive (familial) 345.1●
   nonconvulsive, generalized 345.0●
   parasitic NEC 123.9
   partial (focalized) 345.5●
      with
         impairment of consciousness 345.4●
            memory and ideational disturbances 345.4●
         without impairment of consciousness 345.5●
      abdominal type 345.5●
      motor type 345.5●
      psychomotor type 345.4●
      psychosensory type 345.4●
      secondarily generalized 345.4●
      sensory type 345.5●
      somatomotor type 345.5●
      somatosensory type 345.5●
      temporal lobe type 345.4●
      visceral type 345.5●
      visual type 345.5●
   peripheral 345.9●
   petit mal 345.0●
   photokinetic 345.8●
   progressive myoclonic (familial) 345.1●
   psychic equivalent 345.5●
   psychomotor 345.4●
   psychosensory 345.4●
   reflex 345.1●
   seizure 345.9●
   senile 345.9●
   sensory-induced 345.5●
   sleep (*see also* Narcolepsy) 347.00
   somatomotor type 345.5●
   somatosensory 345.5●
   specified type NEC 345.8●
   status (grand mal) 345.3
      focal motor 345.7●
      petit mal 345.2
      psychomotor 345.7●
      temporal lobe 345.7●
   symptomatic 345.9●
   temporal lobe 345.4●
   tonic (-clonic) 345.1●
   traumatic (injury unspecified) 907.0
      injury specified - *see* Late, effect (of) specified injury
   twilight 293.0
   uncinate (gyrus) 345.4●
   Unverricht (-Lundborg) (familial myoclonic) 345.1●
   visceral 345.5●
   visual 345.5●
Epileptiform
   convulsions 780.39
   seizure 780.39
Epiloia 759.5
Epimenorrhea 626.2
Epipharyngitis (*see also* Nasopharyngitis) 460
Epiphora 375.20
   due to
      excess lacrimation 375.21
      insufficient drainage 375.22
Epiphyseal arrest 733.91
   femoral head 732.2
Epiphyseolysis, epiphysiolysis (*see also* Osteochondrosis) 732.9
Epiphysitis (*see also* Osteochondrosis) 732.9
   juvenile 732.6
   marginal (Scheuermann's) 732.0
   os calcis 732.5
   syphilitic (congenital) 090.0
   vertebral (Scheuermann's) 732.0
Epiplocele (*see also* Hernia) 553.9
Epiploitis (*see also* Peritonitis) 567.9
Epiplosarcomphalocele (*see also* Hernia, umbilicus) 553.1

Episcleritis 379.00
  gouty 274.89 [379.09]
  nodular 379.02
  periodica fugax 379.01
    angioneurotic - see Edema, angioneurotic
  specified NEC 379.09
  staphylococcal 379.00
  suppurative 379.00
  syphilitic 095.0
  tuberculous (see also Tuberculosis) 017.3 [379.09]
Episode
  brain (see also Disease, cerebrovascular, acute) 436
  cerebral (see also Disease, cerebrovascular, acute) 436
  depersonalization (in neurotic state) 300.6
  hyporesponsive 780.09
  psychotic (see also Psychosis) 298.9
    organic, transient 293.9
  schizophrenic (acute) NEC (see also Schizophrenia) 295.4
Epispadias
  female 753.8
  male 752.62
Episplenitis 289.59
Epistaxis (multiple) 784.7
  hereditary 448.0
  vicarious menstruation 625.8
Epithelioma (malignant) (M8011/3) - see also Neoplasm, by site, malignant
  adenoides cysticum (M8100/0) - see Neoplasm, skin, benign
  basal cell (M8090/3) - see Neoplasm, skin, malignant
  benign (M8011/0) - see Neoplasm, by site, benign
  Bowen's (M8081/2) - see Neoplasm, skin, in situ
  calcifying (benign) (Malherbe's) (M8110/0) - see Neoplasm, skin, benign
  external site - see Neoplasm, skin, malignant
  intraepidermal, Jadassohn (M8096/0) - see Neoplasm, skin, benign
  squamous cell (M8070/3) - see Neoplasm, by site, malignant
Epitheliopathy
  pigment, retina 363.15
  posterior multifocal placoid (acute) 363.15
Epithelium, epithelial - see condition
Epituberculosis (allergic) (with atelectasis) (see also Tuberculosis) 010.8
Eponychia 757.5
Epstein's
  nephrosis or syndrome (see also Nephrosis) 581.9
  pearl (mouth) 528.4
Epstein-Barr infection (viral) 075
  chronic 780.79 [139.8]
Epulis (giant cell) (gingiva) 523.8
Equinia 024
Equinovarus (congenital) 754.51
  acquired 736.71
Equivalent
  angina 413.9
  convulsive (abdominal) (see also Epilepsy) 345.5
  epileptic (psychic) (see also Epilepsy) 345.5
Erb's
  disease 359.1
  palsy, paralysis (birth) (brachial) (newborn) 767.6
    spinal (spastic) syphilitic 094.89
  pseudohypertrophic muscular dystrophy 359.1
Erb (-Duchenne) paralysis (birth injury) (newborn) 767.6
Erb-Goldflam disease or syndrome 358.00
Erdheim-Chester disease (ECD) 277.89
Erdheim's syndrome (acromegalic macrospondylitis) 253.0

Erection, painful (persistent) 607.3
Ergosterol deficiency (vitamin D) 268.9
  with
    osteomalacia 268.2
    rickets (see also Rickets) 268.0
Ergotism (ergotized grain) 988.2
  from ergot used as drug (migraine therapy)
    correct substance properly administered 349.82
    overdose or wrong substance given or taken 975.0
Erichsen's disease (railway spine) 300.16
Erlacher-Blount syndrome (tibia vara) 732.4
Erosio interdigitalis blastomycetica 112.3
Erosion
  arteriosclerotic plaque - see Arteriosclerosis, by site
  artery NEC 447.2
    without rupture 447.8
  bone 733.99
  bronchus 519.19
  cartilage (joint) 733.99
  cervix (uteri) (acquired) (chronic) (congenital) 622.0
    with mention of cervicitis 616.0
  cornea (recurrent) (see also Keratitis) 371.42
    traumatic 918.1
  dental (idiopathic) (occupational) 521.30
    extending into
      dentine 521.32
      pulp 521.33
    generalized 521.35
    limited to enamel 521.31
    localized 521.34
  duodenum, postpyloric - see Ulcer, duodenum
  esophagus 530.89
  gastric 535.4
  implanted vaginal mesh
    in, into
      pelvic floor muscles 629.31
      surrounding organ(s) or tissue 629.31
  intestine 569.89
  lymphatic vessel 457.8
  pylorus, pyloric (ulcer) 535.4
  sclera 379.16
  spine, aneurysmal 094.89
  spleen 289.59
  stomach 535.4
  teeth (idiopathic) (occupational) (see also Erosion, dental) 521.30
    due to
      medicine 521.30
      persistent vomiting 521.30
  urethra 599.84
  uterus 621.8
  vaginal prosthetic materials NEC
    in, into
      pelvic floor muscles 629.31
      surrounding organ(s) or tissue 629.31
  vertebra 733.99
Erotomania 302.89
  Clerambault's 297.8
Error
  in diet 269.9
  refractive 367.9
    astigmatism (see also Astigmatism) 367.20
    drug-induced 367.89
    hypermetropia 367.0
    hyperopia 367.0
    myopia 367.1
    presbyopia 367.4
    toxic 367.89
Eructation 787.3
  nervous 306.4
  psychogenic 306.4
Eruption
  creeping 126.9
  drug - see Dermatitis, due to, drug
  Hutchinson, summer 692.72
  Kaposi's varicelliform 054.0

Eruption (Continued)
  napkin (psoriasiform) 691.0
  polymorphous
    light (sun) 692.72
    other source 692.82
  psoriasiform, napkin 691.0
  recalcitrant pustular 694.8
  ringed 695.89
  skin (see also Dermatitis) 782.1
    creeping (meaning hookworm) 126.9
    due to
      chemical(s) NEC 692.4
        internal use 693.8
      drug - see Dermatitis, due to, drug
      prophylactic inoculation or vaccination against disease - see Dermatitis, due to, vaccine
      smallpox vaccination NEC - see Dermatitis, due to, vaccine
    erysipeloid 027.1
    feigned 698.4
    Hutchinson, summer 692.72
    Kaposi's, varicelliform 054.0
      vaccinia 999.0
    lichenoid, axilla 698.3
    polymorphous, due to light 692.72
    toxic NEC 695.0
    vesicular 709.8
  teeth, tooth
    accelerated 520.6
    delayed 520.6
    difficult 520.6
    disturbance of 520.6
    in abnormal sequence 520.6
    incomplete 520.6
    late 520.6
    natal 520.6
    neonatal 520.6
    obstructed 520.6
    partial 520.6
    persistent primary 520.6
    premature 520.6
    prenatal 520.6
  vesicular 709.8
Erysipelas (gangrenous) (infantile) (newborn) (phlegmonous) (suppurative) 035
  external ear 035 [380.13]
  puerperal, postpartum, childbirth 670.8
Erysipelatoid (Rosenbach's) 027.1
Erysipeloid (Rosenbach's) 027.1
Erythema, erythematous (generalized) 695.9
  ab igne - see Burn, by site, first degree
  annulare (centrifugum) (rheumaticum) 695.0
  arthriticum epidemicum 026.1
  brucellum (see also Brucellosis) 023.9
  bullosum 695.19
  caloricum - see Burn, by site, first degree
  chronicum migrans 088.81
  circinatum 695.19
  diaper 691.0
  due to
    chemical (contact) NEC 692.4
      internal 693.8
    drug (internal use) 693.0
      contact 692.3
  elevatum diutinum 695.89
  endemic 265.2
  epidemic, arthritic 026.1
  figuratum perstans 695.0
  gluteal 691.0
  gyratum (perstans) (repens) 695.19
  heat - see Burn, by site, first degree
  ichthyosiforme congenitum 757.1
  induratum (primary) (scrofulosorum) (see also Tuberculosis) 017.1
    nontuberculous 695.2
  infantum febrile 057.8
  infectional NEC 695.9
  infectiosum 057.0
  inflammation NEC 695.9
  intertrigo 695.89

Erythema, erythematous (Continued)
  iris 695.10
  lupus (discoid) (localized) (see also Lupus, erythematosus) 695.4
  marginatum 695.0
    rheumaticum - see Fever, rheumatic
  medicamentosum - see Dermatitis, due to, drug
  migrans 529.1
    chronicum 088.81
  multiforme 695.10
    bullosum 695.19
    conjunctiva 695.19
    exudativum (Hebra) 695.19
    major 695.12
    minor 695.11
    pemphigoides 694.5
  napkin 691.0
  neonatorum 778.8
  nodosum 695.2
    tuberculous (see also Tuberculosis) 017.1●
  nummular, nummulare 695.19
  palmar 695.0
  palmaris hereditarium 695.0
  pernio 991.5
  perstans solare 692.72
  rash, newborn 778.8
  scarlatiniform (exfoliative) (recurrent) 695.0
  simplex marginatum 057.8
  solare (see also Sunburn) 692.71
  streptogenes 696.5
  toxic, toxicum NEC 695.0
    newborn 778.8
  tuberculous (primary) (see also Tuberculosis) 017.0●
  venenatum 695.0
Erythematosus - see condition
Erythematous - see condition
Erythermalgia (primary) 443.82
Erythralgia 443.82
Erythrasma 039.0
Erythredema 985.0
  polyneuritica 985.0
  polyneuropathy 985.0
Erythremia (acute) (M9841/3) 207.0●
  chronic (M9842/3) 207.1●
  secondary 289.0
Erythroblastopenia (acquired) 284.89
  congenital 284.01
Erythroblastophthisis 284.01
Erythroblastosis (fetalis) (newborn) 773.2
  due to
    ABO
      antibodies 773.1
      incompatibility, maternal/fetal 773.1
      isoimmunization 773.1
    Rh
      antibodies 773.0
      incompatibility, maternal/fetal 773.0
      isoimmunization 773.0
Erythrocyanosis (crurum) 443.89
Erythrocythemia - see Erythremia
Erythrocytopenia 285.9
Erythrocytosis (megalosplenic)
  familial 289.6
  oval, hereditary (see also Elliptocytosis) 282.1
  secondary 289.0
  stress 289.0
Erythroderma (see also Erythema) 695.9
  desquamativa (in infants) 695.89
  exfoliative 695.89
  ichthyosiform, congenital 757.1
  infantum 695.89
  maculopapular 696.2
  neonatorum 778.8
  psoriaticum 696.1
  secondary 695.9
Erythrodysesthesia, palmar plantar (PPE) 693.0
Erythrogenesis imperfecta 284.09
Erythroleukemia (M9840/3) 207.0●
Erythromelalgia 443.82

Erythromelia 701.8
Erythropenia 285.9
Erythrophagocytosis 289.9
Erythrophobia 300.23
Erythroplakia
  oral mucosa 528.79
  tongue 528.79
Erythroplasia (Queyrat) (M8080/2)
  specified site - see Neoplasm, skin, in situ
  unspecified site 233.5
Erythropoiesis, idiopathic ineffective 285.0
Escaped beats, heart 427.60
  postoperative 997.1
Escherichia coli (E. coli) - see Infection, Escherichia coli
Esoenteritis - see Enteritis
Esophagalgia 530.89
Esophagectasis 530.89
  due to cardiospasm 530.0
Esophagismus 530.5
Esophagitis (alkaline) (chemical) (chronic) (infectional) (necrotic) (peptic) (postoperative) (regurgitant) 530.10
  acute 530.12
  candidal 112.84
  eosinophilic 530.13
  reflux 530.11
  specified NEC 530.19
  tuberculous (see also Tuberculosis) 017.8●
  ulcerative 530.19
Esophagocele 530.6
Esophagodynia 530.89
Esophagomalacia 530.89
Esophagoptosis 530.89
Esophagospasm 530.5
Esophagostenosis 530.3
Esophagostomiasis 127.7
Esophagostomy
  complication 530.87
    infection 530.86
    malfunctioning 530.87
    mechanical 530.87
Esophagotracheal - see condition
Esophagus - see condition
Esophoria 378.41
  convergence, excess 378.84
  divergence, insufficiency 378.85
Esotropia (nonaccommodative) 378.00
  accommodative 378.35
  alternating 378.05
    with
      A pattern 378.06
      specified noncomitancy NEC 378.08
      V pattern 378.07
      X pattern 378.08
      Y pattern 378.08
    intermittent 378.22
  intermittent 378.20
    alternating 378.22
    monocular 378.21
  monocular 378.01
    with
      A pattern 378.02
      specified noncomitancy NEC 378.04
      V pattern 378.03
      X pattern 378.04
      Y pattern 378.04
    intermittent 378.21
Espundia 085.5
Essential - see condition
Esterapenia 289.89
Esthesioneuroblastoma (M9522/3) 160.0
Esthesioneurocytoma (M9521/3) 160.0
Esthesioneuroepithelioma (M9523/3) 160.0
Esthiomene 099.1
Estivo-autumnal
  fever 084.0
  malaria 084.0
Estrangement V61.09
Estriasis 134.0

Ethanolaminuria 270.8
Ethanolism (see also Alcoholism) 303.9●
Ether dependence, dependency (see also Dependence) 304.6●
Etherism (see also Dependence) 304.6●
Ethmoid, ethmoidal - see condition
Ethmoiditis (chronic) (nonpurulent) (purulent) (see also Sinusitis, ethmoidal) 473.2
  influenzal (see also Influenza) 487.1
  Woakes' 471.1
Ethylism (see also Alcoholism) 303.9●
Eulenburg's disease (congenital paramyotonia) 359.29
Eunuchism 257.2
Eunuchoidism 257.2
  hypogonadotropic 257.2
European blastomycosis 117.5
Eustachian - see condition
Euthyroid sick syndrome 790.94
Euthyroidism 244.9
Evaluation
  fetal lung maturity 659.8●
  for suspected condition (see also Observation) V71.9
    abuse V71.81
    exposure
      anthrax V71.82
      biologic agent NEC V71.83
      SARS V71.83
    neglect V71.81
    newborn - see Observation, suspected, condition, newborn
    specified condition NEC V71.89
  mental health V70.2
    requested by authority V70.1
  nursing care V63.8
  social service V63.8
Evans' syndrome (thrombocytopenic purpura) 287.32
Event, apparent life threatening in newborn and infant (ALTE) 799.82
Eventration
  colon into chest - see Hernia, diaphragm
  diaphragm (congenital) 756.6
Eversion
  bladder 596.89
  cervix (uteri) 622.0
    with mention of cervicitis 616.0
  foot NEC 736.79
    congenital 755.67
  lacrimal punctum 375.51
  punctum lacrimale (postinfectional) (senile) 375.51
  ureter (meatus) 593.89
  urethra (meatus) 599.84
  uterus 618.1
    complicating delivery 665.2●
      affecting fetus or newborn 763.89
    puerperal, postpartum 674.8●
Evidence
  of malignancy
    cytologic
      without histologic confirmation
        anus 796.76
        cervix 795.06
        vagina 795.16
Evisceration
  birth injury 767.8
  bowel (congenital) - see Hernia, ventral
  congenital (see also Hernia, ventral) 553.29
  operative wound 998.32
  traumatic NEC 869.1
    eye 871.3
Evulsion - see Avulsion
Ewing's
  angioendothelioma (M9260/3) - see Neoplasm, bone, malignant
  sarcoma (M9260/3) - see Neoplasm, bone, malignant
  tumor (M9260/3) - see Neoplasm, bone, malignant

Exaggerated lumbosacral angle (with
     impinging spine) 756.12
Examination (general) (routine) (of) (for) V70.9
   allergy V72.7
   annual V70.0
   cardiovascular preoperative V72.81
   cervical Papanicolaou smear V76.2
      as a part of routine gynecological
          examination V72.31
      to confirm findings of recent normal
          smear following initial abnormal
          smear V72.32
   child care (routine) V20.2
   clinical research investigation (normal
       control patient) (participant) V70.7
   dental V72.2
   developmental testing (child) (infant) V20.2
   donor (potential) V70.8
   ear V72.19
   eye V72.0
   following
      accident (motor vehicle) V71.4
      alleged rape or seduction (victim or
          culprit) V71.5
      inflicted injury (victim or culprit) NEC
          V71.6
      rape or seduction, alleged (victim or
          culprit) V71.5
      treatment (for) V67.9
         combined V67.6
         fracture V67.4
         involving high-risk medication NEC
             V67.51
         mental disorder V67.3
         specified condition NEC V67.59
   follow-up (routine) (following) V67.9
      cancer chemotherapy V67.2
      chemotherapy V67.2
      disease NEC V67.59
      high-risk medication NEC V67.51
      injury NEC V67.59
      population survey V70.6
      postpartum V24.2
      psychiatric V67.3
      psychotherapy V67.3
      radiotherapy V67.1
      specified surgery NEC V67.09
      surgery V67.00
         vaginal pap smear V67.01
   gynecological V72.31
      for contraceptive maintenance V25.40
         intrauterine device V25.42
         pill V25.41
         specified method NEC V25.49
   health (of)
      armed forces personnel V70.5
      checkup V70.0
      child, routine V20.2
      defined subpopulation NEC V70.5
      inhabitants of institutions V70.5
      occupational V70.5
      pre-employment screening V70.5
      preschool children V70.5
         for admission to school V70.3
      prisoners V70.5
         for entrance into prison V70.3
      prostitutes V70.5
      refugees V70.5
      school children V70.5
      students V70.5
   hearing V72.19
      following failed hearing screening
          V72.11
   infant
      8 to 28 days old V20.32
      over 28 days old, routine V20.2
      under 8 days old V20.31
   laboratory V72.60
      ordered as part of a routine general
          medical examination V72.62
      pre-operative V72.63

Examination (Continued)
   laboratory (Continued)
      pre-procedural V72.63
      specified NEC V72.69
   lactating mother V24.1
   medical (for) (of) V70.9
      administrative purpose NEC V70.3
      admission to
         old age home V70.3
         prison V70.3
         school V70.3
      adoption V70.3
      armed forces personnel V70.5
      at health care facility V70.0
      camp V70.3
      child, routine V20.2
      clinical research (control) (normal
          comparison) (participant) V70.7
      defined subpopulation NEC V70.5
      donor (potential) V70.8
      driving license V70.3
      general V70.9
         routine V70.0
         specified reason NEC V70.8
      immigration V70.3
      inhabitants of institutions V70.5
      insurance certification V70.3
      marriage V70.3
      medicolegal reasons V70.4
      naturalization V70.3
      occupational V70.5
      population survey V70.6
      pre-employment V70.5
      preschool children V70.5
         for admission to school V70.3
      prison V70.3
      prisoners V70.5
         for entrance into prison V70.3
      prostitutes V70.5
      refugees V70.5
      school children V70.5
      specified reason NEC V70.8
      sport competition V70.3
      students V70.5
   medicolegal reason V70.4
   pelvic (annual) (periodic) V72.31
   periodic (annual) (routine) V70.0
   postpartum
      immediately after delivery V24.0
      routine follow-up V24.2
   pregnancy (unconfirmed) (possible) V72.40
      negative result V72.41
      positive result V72.42
   prenatal V22.1
      first pregnancy V22.0
      high-risk pregnancy V23.9
         specified problem NEC V23.89
         to determine fetal viability V23.87
   preoperative V72.84
      cardiovascular V72.81
      respiratory V72.82
      specified NEC V72.83
   preprocedural V72.84
      cardiovascular V72.81
      general physical V72.83
      respiratory V72.82
      specified NEC V72.83
   prior to chemotherapy V72.83
   psychiatric V70.2
      follow-up not needing further care V67.3
      requested by authority V70.1
   radiological NEC V72.5
   respiratory preoperative V72.82
   screening - see Screening
   sensitization V72.7
   skin V72.7
      hypersensitivity V72.7
   special V72.9
   specified type or reason NEC V72.85
      preoperative V72.83
         specified NEC V72.83

Examination (Continued)
   teeth V72.2
   vaginal Papanicolaou smear V76.47
      following hysterectomy for malignant
          condition V67.01
   victim or culprit following
      alleged rape or seduction V71.5
      inflicted injury NEC V71.6
   vision V72.0
   well baby V20.2
Exanthem, exanthema (see also Rash) 782.1
   Boston 048
   epidemic, with meningitis 048
   lichenoid psoriasiform 696.2
   subitum 058.10
      due to
         human herpesvirus 6 058.11
         human herpesvirus 7 058.12
   viral, virus NEC 057.9
      specified type NEC 057.8
Excess, excessive, excessively
   alcohol level in blood 790.3
   carbohydrate tissue, localized 278.1
   carotene (dietary) 278.3
   cold 991.9
      specified effect NEC 991.8
   convergence 378.84
   crying 780.95
      of
         adolescent 780.95
         adult 780.95
         baby 780.92
         child 780.95
         infant (baby) 780.92
         newborn 780.92
   development, breast 611.1
   diaphoresis (see also Hyperhidrosis) 780.8
   distance, interarch 524.28
   divergence 378.85
   drinking (alcohol) NEC (see also Abuse,
       drugs, nondependent) 305.0●
      continual (see also Alcoholism) 303.9●
      habitual (see also Alcoholism) 303.9●
   eating 783.6
   eyelid fold (congenital) 743.62
   fat 278.02
      in heart (see also Degeneration,
          myocardial) 429.1
      tissue, localized 278.1
   foreskin 605
   gas 787.3
   gastrin 251.5
   glucagon 251.4
   heat (see also Heat) 992.9
   horizontal
      overjet 524.26
      overlap 524.26
   interarch distance 524.28
   intermaxillary vertical dimension 524.37
   interocclusal distance of teeth 524.37
   large
      colon 564.7
         congenital 751.3
      fetus or infant 766.0
         with obstructed labor 660.1●
         affecting management of pregnancy
             656.6●
         causing disproportion 653.5●
      newborn (weight of 4500 grams or more)
          766.0
      organ or site, congenital NEC - see
          Anomaly, specified type NEC
   lid fold (congenital) 743.62
   long
      colon 751.5
      organ or site, congenital NEC - see
          Anomaly, specified type NEC
   umbilical cord (entangled)
      affecting fetus or newborn 762.5
      in pregnancy or childbirth 663.3●
         with compression 663.2●

Excess, excessive, excessively (Continued)
  menstruation 626.2
  number of teeth 520.1
    causing crowding 524.31
  nutrients (dietary) NEC 783.6
  potassium (K) 276.7
  salivation (*see also* Ptyalism) 527.7
  secretion - *see also* Hypersecretion
    milk 676.6 ●
    sputum 786.4
    sweat (*see also* Hyperhidrosis) 780.8
  short
    organ or site, congenital NEC - *see*
      Anomaly, specified type NEC
    umbilical cord
      affecting fetus or newborn 762.6
      in pregnancy or childbirth 663.4 ●
  skin NEC 701.9
    eyelid 743.62
      acquired 374.30
  sodium (Na) 276.0
  spacing of teeth 524.32
  sputum 786.4
  sweating (*see also* Hyperhidrosis) 780.8
  tearing (ducts) (eye) (*see also* Epiphora) 375.20
  thirst 783.5
    due to deprivation of water 994.3
  tissue in reconstructed breast 612.0
  tuberosity 524.07
  vitamin
    A (dietary) 278.2
      administered as drug (chronic) (prolonged excessive intake) 278.2
      reaction to sudden overdose 963.5
    D (dietary) 278.4
      administered as drug (chronic) (prolonged excessive intake) 278.4
      reaction to sudden overdose 963.5
  weight 278.02
    gain 783.1
      of pregnancy 646.1 ●
    loss 783.21
Excitability, abnormal, under minor stress 309.29
Excitation
  catatonic (*see also* Schizophrenia) 295.2 ●
  psychogenic 298.1
  reactive (from emotional stress, psychological trauma) 298.1
Excitement
  manic (*see also* Psychosis, affective) 296.0 ●
    recurrent episode 296.1 ●
    single episode 296.0 ●
  mental, reactive (from emotional stress, psychological trauma) 298.1
  state, reactive (from emotional stress, psychological trauma) 298.1
Excluded pupils 364.76
Excoriation (traumatic) (*see also* Injury, superficial, by site) 919.8
  neurotic 698.4
Excyclophoria 378.44
Excyclotropia 378.33
Exencephalus, exencephaly 742.0
Exercise
  breathing V57.0
  remedial NEC V57.1
  therapeutic NEC V57.1
Exfoliation
  skin
    due to erythematous condition 695.50
      involving (percent of body surface)
        less than 10 percent 695.50
        10-19 percent 695.51
        20-29 percent 695.52
        30-39 percent 695.53

Exfoliation (Continued)
  skin (Continued)
    due to erythematous condition (Continued)
      involving (Continued)
        40-49 percent 695.54
        50-59 percent 695.55
        60-69 percent 695.56
        70-79 percent 695.57
        80-89 percent 695.58
        90 percent or more 695.59
  teeth
    due to systemic causes 525.0
Exfoliative - *see also* condition
  dermatitis 695.89
Exhaustion, exhaustive (physical NEC) 780.79
  battle (*see also* Reaction, stress, acute) 308.9
  cardiac (*see also* Failure, heart) 428.9
  delirium (*see also* Reaction, stress, acute) 308.9
  due to
    cold 991.8
    excessive exertion 994.5
    exposure 994.4
    overexertion 994.5
  fetus or newborn 779.89
  heart (*see also* Failure, heart) 428.9
  heat 992.5
    due to
      salt depletion 992.4
      water depletion 992.3
  manic (*see also* Psychosis, affective) 296.0 ●
    recurrent episode 296.1 ●
    single episode 296.0 ●
  maternal, complicating delivery 669.8 ●
    affecting fetus or newborn 763.89
  mental 300.5
  myocardium, myocardial (*see also* Failure, heart) 428.9
  nervous 300.5
  old age 797
  postinfectional NEC 780.79
  psychogenic 300.5
  psychosis (*see also* Reaction, stress, acute) 308.9
  senile 797
    dementia 290.0
Exhibitionism (sexual) 302.4
Exomphalos 756.72
Exophoria 378.42
  convergence, insufficiency 378.83
  divergence, excess 378.85
Exophthalmic
  cachexia 242.0 ●
  goiter 242.0 ●
  ophthalmoplegia 242.0 ● [376.22]
Exophthalmos 376.30
  congenital 743.66
  constant 376.31
  endocrine NEC 259.9 [376.22]
  hyperthyroidism 242.0 ● [376.21]
  intermittent NEC 376.34
  malignant 242.0 ● [376.21]
  pulsating 376.35
    endocrine NEC 259.9 [376.22]
  thyrotoxic 242.0 ● [376.21]
Exostosis 726.91
  cartilaginous (M9210/0) - *see* Neoplasm, bone, benign
  congenital 756.4
  ear canal, external 380.81
  gonococcal 098.89
  hip 726.5
  intracranial 733.3
  jaw (bone) 526.81
  luxurians 728.11
  multiple (cancellous) (congenital) (hereditary) 756.4

Exostosis (Continued)
  nasal bones 726.91
  orbit, orbital 376.42
  osteocartilaginous (M9210/0) - *see* Neoplasm, bone, benign
  spine 721.8
    with spondylosis - *see* Spondylosis
  syphilitic 095.5
  wrist 726.4
Exotropia 378.10
  alternating 378.15
    with
      A pattern 378.16
      specified noncomitancy NEC 378.18
      V pattern 378.17
      X pattern 378.18
      Y pattern 378.18
    intermittent 378.24
  intermittent 378.20
    alternating 378.24
    monocular 378.23
  monocular 378.11
    with
      A pattern 378.12
      specified noncomitancy NEC 378.14
      V pattern 378.13
      X pattern 378.14
      Y pattern 378.14
    intermittent 378.23
Explanation of
  investigation finding V65.4
  medication V65.4
Exposure (suspected) 994.9
  algae bloom V87.32
  cold 991.9
    specified effect NEC 991.8
  effects of 994.9
  exhaustion due to 994.4
  implanted vaginal mesh
    into vagina 629.32
    through vaginal wall 629.32
  to
    AIDS virus V01.79
    anthrax V01.81
    aromatic
      amines V87.11
      dyes V87.19
    arsenic V87.01
    asbestos V15.84
    benzene V87.12
    body fluids (hazardous) V15.85
    cholera V01.0
    chromium compounds V87.09
    communicable disease V01.9
      specified type NEC V01.89
    dyes V87.2
      aromatic V87.19
    Escherichia coli (E. coli) V01.83
    German measles V01.4
    gonorrhea V01.6
    hazardous
      aromatic compounds NEC V87.19
      body fluids V15.85
      chemicals NEC V87.2
      metals V87.09
      substances V87.39
    HIV V01.79
    human immunodeficiency virus V01.79
    lead V15.86
    meningococcus V01.84
    mold V87.31
    nickel dust V87.09
    parasitic disease V01.89
    poliomyelitis V01.2
    polycyclic aromatic hydrocarbons V87.19
    potentially hazardous body fluids V15.85
    rabies V01.5

Exposure *(Continued)*
 to *(Continued)*
  rubella V01.4
  SARS-associated coronavirus V01.82
  smallpox V01.3
  syphilis V01.6
  tuberculosis V01.1
  uranium V87.02
  varicella V01.71
  venereal disease V01.6
  viral disease NEC V01.79
   varicella V01.71
 vaginal prosthetic materials NEC
  into vagina 629.32
  through vaginal wall 629.32
Exsanguination, fetal 772.0
Exstrophy
 abdominal content 751.8
 bladder (urinary) 753.5
Extensive - *see* condition
Extra - *see also* Accessory
 rib 756.3
  cervical 756.2
Extraction
 with hook 763.89
  breech NEC 669.6●
   affecting fetus or newborn 763.0

Extraction *(Continued)*
 cataract postsurgical
  V45.61
 manual NEC 669.8●
  affecting fetus or newborn
   763.89
Extrasystole 427.60
 atrial 427.61
 postoperative 997.1
 ventricular 427.69
Extrauterine gestation or pregnancy -
  see Pregnancy, ectopic
Extravasation
 blood 459.0
  lower extremity 459.0
 chemotherapy, vesicant
  999.81
 chyle into mesentery 457.8
 pelvicalyceal 593.4
 pyelosinus 593.4
 urine 788.8
  from ureter 788.8
 vesicant
  agent NEC 999.82
  chemotherapy 999.81
Extremity - *see* condition
Extrophy - *see* Exstrophy

Extroversion
 bladder 753.5
 uterus 618.1
  complicating delivery 665.2●
   affecting fetus or newborn 763.89
  postpartal (old) 618.1
Extruded tooth 524.34
Extrusion
 alveolus and teeth 524.75
 breast implant (prosthetic) 996.54
 device, implant, or graft - *see* Complications, mechanical
 eye implant (ball) (globe) 996.59
 intervertebral disc - *see* Displacement, intervertebral disc
 lacrimal gland 375.43
 mesh (reinforcing) 996.59
 ocular lens implant 996.53
 prosthetic device NEC - *see* Complications, mechanical
 vitreous 379.26
Exudate, pleura - *see* Effusion, pleura
Exudates, retina 362.82
Exudative - *see* condition
Eye, eyeball, eyelid - *see* condition
Eyestrain 368.13
Eyeworm disease of Africa 125.2

F

Faber's anemia or syndrome (achlorhydric anemia) 280.9
Fabry's disease (angiokeratoma corporis diffusum) 272.7
Face, facial - *see* condition
Facet of cornea 371.44
Faciocephalalgia, autonomic (*see also* Neuropathy, peripheral, autonomic) 337.9
Facioscapulohumeral myopathy 359.1
Factitious disorder, illness - *see* Illness, factitious
Factor
   deficiency - *see* Deficiency, factor
   psychic, associated with diseases classified elsewhere 316
   risk-*see* problem
   V Leiden mutation 289.81
Fahr-Volhard disease (malignant nephrosclerosis) 403.00
Failure, failed
   adenohypophyseal 253.2
   attempted abortion (legal) (*see also* Abortion, failed) 638.9
   bone marrow (anemia) 284.9
      acquired (secondary) 284.89
      congenital 284.09
      idiopathic 284.9
   cardiac (*see also* Failure, heart) 428.9
      newborn 779.89
   cardiorenal (chronic) 428.9
      hypertensive (*see also* Hypertension, cardiorenal) 404.93
   cardiorespiratory 799.1
      specified during or due to a procedure 997.1
      long-term effect of cardiac surgery 429.4
   cardiovascular (chronic) 428.9
   cerebrovascular 437.8
   cervical dilatation in labor 661.0●
      affecting fetus or newborn 763.7
   circulation, circulatory 799.89
      fetus or newborn 779.89
      peripheral 785.50
         postoperative 998.00
   compensation - *see* Disease, heart
   congestive (*see also* Failure, heart) 428.0
   conscious sedation, during procedure 995.24
   coronary (*see also* Insufficiency, coronary) 411.89
   dental implant 525.79
      due to
         infection 525.71
         lack of attached gingiva 525.72
         occlusal trauma (caused by poor prosthetic design) 525.72
         parafunctional habits 525.72
         periodontal infection (periimplantitis) 525.72
         poor oral hygiene 525.72
         unintentional loading 525.71
      endosseous NEC 525.79
      mechanical 525.73
      osseointegration 525.71
         due to
            complications of systemic disease 525.71
            poor bone quality 525.71
            premature loading 525.71
         iatrogenic 525.71
         prior to intentional prosthetic loading 525.71
      post-osseointegration
         biological 525.72
            iatrogenic 525.72
         due to complications of systemic disease 525.72
         mechanical 525.73

Failure, failed (Continued)
   dental implant (Continued)
      pre-integration 525.71
      pre-osseointegration 525.71
   dental prosthesis causing loss of dental implant 525.73
   dental restoration
      marginal integrity 525.61
      periodontal anatomical integrity 525.65
   descent of head (at term) 652.5●
      affecting fetus or newborn 763.1
      in labor 660.0●
         affecting fetus or newborn 763.1
   device, implant, or graft - *see* Complications, mechanical
   engagement of head NEC 652.5●
      in labor 660.0●
   extrarenal 788.99
   fetal head to enter pelvic brim 652.5●
      affecting fetus or newborn 763.1
      in labor 660.0●
         affecting fetus or newborn 763.1
   forceps NEC 660.7●
      affecting fetus or newborn 763.1
   fusion (joint) (spinal) 996.49
   growth in childhood 783.43
   heart (acute) (sudden) 428.9
      with
         abortion - *see* Abortion, by type, with specified complication NEC
         acute pulmonary edema (*see also* Failure, ventricular, left) 428.1
            with congestion (*see also* Failure, heart) 428.0
         decompensation (*see also* Failure, heart) 428.0
         dilation - *see* Disease, heart
         ectopic pregnancy (*see also* categories 633.0–633.9) 639.8
         molar pregnancy (*see also* categories 630–632) 639.8
      arteriosclerotic 440.9
      combined left-right sided 428.0
      combined systolic and diastolic 428.40
         acute 428.41
         acute on chronic 428.43
         chronic 428.42
      compensated (*see also* Failure, heart) 428.0
      complicating
         abortion - *see* Abortion, by type, with specified complication NEC
         delivery (cesarean) (instrumental) 669.4●
         ectopic pregnancy (*see also* categories 633.0–633.9) 639.8
         molar pregnancy (*see also* categories 630–632) 639.8
         obstetric anesthesia or sedation 668.1●
         surgery 997.1
      congestive (compensated) (decompensated) (*see also* Failure, heart) 428.0
         with rheumatic fever (conditions classifiable to 390)
            active 391.8
            inactive or quiescent (with chorea) 398.91
      fetus or newborn 779.89
      hypertensive (*see also* Hypertension, heart) 402.91
         with renal disease (*see also* Hypertension, cardiorenal) 404.91
            with renal failure 404.93
         benign 402.11
         malignant 402.01
      rheumatic (chronic) (inactive) (with chorea) 398.91
         active or acute 391.8
            with chorea (Sydenham's) 392.0

Failure, failed (Continued)
   heart (Continued)
      decompensated (*see also* Failure, heart) 428.0
      degenerative (*see also* Degeneration, myocardial) 429.1
      diastolic 428.30
         acute 428.31
         acute on chronic 428.33
         chronic 428.32
      due to presence of (cardiac) prosthesis 429.4
      fetus or newborn 779.89
      following
         abortion 639.8
         cardiac surgery 429.4
         ectopic or molar pregnancy 639.8
      high output NEC 428.9
      hypertensive (*see also* Hypertension, heart) 402.91
         with renal disease (*see also* Hypertension, cardiorenal) 404.91
            with renal failure 404.93
         benign 402.11
         malignant 402.01
      left (ventricular) (*see also* Failure, ventricular, left) 428.1
         with right-sided failure (*see also* Failure, heart) 428.0
      low output (syndrome) NEC 428.9
      organic - *see* Disease, heart
      postoperative (immediate) 997.1
         long term effect of cardiac surgery 429.4
      rheumatic (chronic) (congestive) (inactive) 398.91
      right (secondary to left heart failure, conditions classifiable to 428.1) (ventricular) (*see also* Failure, heart) 428.0
      senile 797
      specified during or due to a procedure 997.1
         long-term effect of cardiac surgery 429.4
      systolic 428.20
         acute 428.21
         acute on chronic 428.23
         chronic 428.22
      thyrotoxic (*see also* Thyrotoxicosis) 242.9● [425.7]
      valvular - *see* Endocarditis
   hepatic 572.8
      acute 570
      due to a procedure 997.49
   hepatorenal 572.4
   hypertensive heart (*see also* Hypertension, heart) 402.91
      benign 402.11
      malignant 402.01
   induction (of labor) 659.1●
      abortion (legal) (*see also* Abortion, failed) 638.9
      affecting fetus or newborn 763.89
      by oxytocic drugs 659.1●
      instrumental 659.0●
      mechanical 659.0●
      medical 659.1●
      surgical 659.0●
   initial alveolar expansion, newborn 770.4
   involution, thymus (gland) 254.8
   kidney - *see* Failure, renal
   lactation 676.4●
   Leydig's cell, adult 257.2
   liver 572.8
      acute 570
   medullary 799.89
   mitral - *see* Endocarditis, mitral
   moderate sedation, during procedure 995.24

SECTION I INDEX TO DISEASES AND INJURIES / Failure, failed

Failure, failed (Continued)
  myocardium, myocardial (see also Failure, heart) 428.9
    chronic (see also Failure, heart) 428.0
    congestive (see also Failure, heart) 428.0
  ovarian (primary) 256.39
    iatrogenic 256.2
    postablative 256.2
    postirradiation 256.2
    postsurgical 256.2
  ovulation 628.0
  prerenal 788.99
  renal (kidney) 586
    with
      abortion - see Abortion, by type, with renal failure
      ectopic pregnancy (see also categories 633.0–633.9) 639.3
      edema (see also Nephrosis) 581.9
      hypertension (see also Hypertension, kidney) 403.91
      hypertensive heart disease (conditions classifiable to 402) 404.92
        with heart failure 404.93
        benign 404.12
          with heart failure 404.13
        malignant 404.02
          with heart failure 404.03
      molar pregnancy (see also categories 630–632) 639.3
      tubular necrosis (acute) 584.5
    acute 584.9
      with lesion of
        necrosis
          cortical (renal) 584.6
          medullary (renal) (papillary) 584.7
          tubular 584.5
        specified pathology NEC 584.8
    chronic 585.9
      hypertensive or with hypertension (see also Hypertension, kidney) 403.91
    due to a procedure 997.5
    following
      abortion 639.3
      crushing 958.5
      ectopic or molar pregnancy 639.3
      labor and delivery (acute) 669.3●
    hypertensive (see also Hypertension, kidney) 403.91
    puerperal, postpartum 669.3●
  respiration, respiratory 518.81
    acute 518.81
      following trauma and surgery 518.51
    acute and chronic 518.84
      following trauma and surgery 518.53
    center 348.89
      newborn 770.84
    chronic 518.83
      following trauma and surgery or shock 518.51
    newborn 770.84
  rotation
    cecum 751.4
    colon 751.4
    intestine 751.4
    kidney 753.3
  sedation, during procedure
    conscious 995.24
    moderate 995.24
  segmentation - see also Fusion
    fingers (see also Syndactylism, fingers) 755.11
    toes (see also Syndactylism, toes) 755.13
  seminiferous tubule, adult 257.2
  senile (general) 797
    with psychosis 290.20
  testis, primary (seminal) 257.2
  to progress 661.2●

Failure, failed (Continued)
  to thrive
    adult 783.7
    child 783.41
    newborn 779.34
  transplant 996.80
    bone marrow 996.85
    organ (immune or nonimmune cause) 996.80
      bone marrow 996.85
      heart 996.83
      intestines 996.87
      kidney 996.81
      liver 996.82
      lung 996.84
      pancreas 996.86
      specified NEC 996.89
    skin 996.52
      artificial 996.55
      decellularized allodermis 996.55
      temporary allograft or pigskin graft - *omit code*
    stem cell(s) 996.88
      from
        peripheral blood 996.88
        umbilical cord 996.88
  trial of labor NEC 660.6●
    affecting fetus or newborn 763.1
  tubal ligation 998.89
  urinary 586
  vacuum extraction
    abortion - see Abortion, failed
    delivery NEC 660.7●
      affecting fetus or newborn 763.1
  vasectomy 998.89
  ventouse NEC 660.7●
    affecting fetus or newborn 763.1
  ventricular (see also Failure, heart) 428.9
    left 428.1
      with rheumatic fever (conditions classifiable to 390)
        active 391.8
          with chorea 392.0
        inactive or quiescent (with chorea) 398.91
      hypertensive (see also Hypertension, heart) 402.91
        benign 402.11
        malignant 402.01
      rheumatic (chronic) (inactive) (with chorea) 398.91
        active or acute 391.8
          with chorea 392.0
    right (see also Failure, heart) 428.0
  vital centers, fetus or newborn 779.89
  weight gain in childhood 783.41
Fainting (fit) (spell) 780.2
Falciform hymen 752.49
Fall, maternal, affecting fetus or newborn 760.5
Fallen arches 734
Falling, any organ or part - see Prolapse
Fallopian
  insufflation
    fertility testing V26.21
    following sterilization reversal V26.22
  tube - see condition
Fallot's
  pentalogy 745.2
  tetrad or tetralogy 745.2
  triad or trilogy 746.09
Fallout, radioactive (adverse effect) NEC 990
False - see also condition
  bundle branch block 426.50
  bursa 727.89
  croup 478.75
  joint 733.82
  labor (pains) 644.1●
  opening, urinary, male 752.69
  passage, urethra (prostatic) 599.4

False (Continued)
  positive
    serological test for syphilis 795.6
    Wassermann reaction 795.6
  pregnancy 300.11
Family, familial - see also condition
  affected by
    family member
      currently on deployment (military) V61.01
      returned from deployment (military) (current or past conflict) V61.02
  disruption (see also Disruption, family) V61.09
  estrangement V61.09
  hemophagocytic
    lymphohistiocytosis 288.4
    reticulosis 288.4
  Li-Fraumeni (syndrome) V84.01
  planning advice V25.09
    natural
      procreative V26.41
      to avoid pregnancy V25.04
  problem V61.9
    specified circumstance NEC V61.8
  retinoblastoma (syndrome) 190.5
Famine 994.2
  edema 262
Fanconi's anemia (congenital pancytopenia) 284.09
Fanconi (-de Toni) (-Debré) syndrome (cystinosis) 270.0
Farber (-Uzman) syndrome or disease (disseminated lipogranulomatosis) 272.8
Farcin 024
Farcy 024
Farmers'
  lung 495.0
  skin 692.74
Farsightedness 367.0
Fascia - see condition
Fasciculation 781.0
Fasciculitis optica 377.32
Fasciitis 729.4
  eosinophilic 728.89
  necrotizing 728.86
  nodular 728.79
  perirenal 593.4
  plantar 728.71
  pseudosarcomatous 728.79
  traumatic (old) NEC 728.79
    current - see Sprain, by site
Fasciola hepatica infestation 121.3
Fascioliasis 121.3
Fasciolopsiasis (small intestine) 121.4
Fasciolopsis (small intestine) 121.4
Fast pulse 785.0
Fat
  embolism (cerebral) (pulmonary) (systemic) 958.1
    with
      abortion - see Abortion, by type, with embolism
      ectopic pregnancy (see also categories 633.0–633.9) 639.6
      molar pregnancy (see also categories 630–632) 639.6
      complicating delivery or puerperium 673.8●
      following
        abortion 639.6
        ectopic or molar pregnancy 639.6
      in pregnancy, childbirth, or the puerperium 673.8●
  excessive 278.02
    in heart (see also Degeneration, myocardial) 429.1
  general 278.02
  hernia, herniation 729.30
    eyelid 374.34
    knee 729.31

SECTION I INDEX TO DISEASES AND INJURIES / Fever

Fat *(Continued)*
   hernia, herniation *(Continued)*
      orbit 374.34
         retro-orbital 374.34
         retropatellar 729.31
         specified site NEC 729.39
      indigestion 579.8
      in stool 792.1
      localized (pad) 278.1
         heart *(see also* Degeneration, myocardial)
               429.1
         knee 729.31
         retropatellar 729.31
      necrosis - *see also* Fatty, degeneration
         breast (aseptic) (segmental) 611.3
         mesentery 567.82
         omentum 567.82
         peritoneum 567.82
      pad 278.1
Fatal familial insomnia (FFI) 046.72
Fatal syncope 798.1
Fatigue 780.79
   auditory deafness *(see also* Deafness) 389.9
   chronic, syndrome 780.71
   combat *(see also* Reaction, stress, acute) 308.9
   during pregnancy 646.8●
   general 780.79
      psychogenic 300.5
   heat (transient) 992.6
   muscle 729.89
   myocardium *(see also* Failure, heart) 428.9
   nervous 300.5
   neurosis 300.5
   operational 300.89
   postural 729.89
   posture 729.89
   psychogenic (general) 300.5
   senile 797
   syndrome NEC 300.5
      chronic 780.71
   undue 780.79
   voice 784.49
Fatness 278.02
Fatty - *see also* condition
   apron 278.1
   degeneration (diffuse) (general) NEC 272.8
      localized - *see* Degeneration, by site, fatty
      placenta - *see* Placenta, abnormal
   heart (enlarged) *(see also* Degeneration,
         myocardial) 429.1
   infiltration (diffuse) (general) *(see also*
         Degeneration, by site, fatty) 272.8
      heart (enlarged) *(see also* Degeneration,
            myocardial) 429.1
   liver 571.8
      alcoholic 571.0
   necrosis - *see* Degeneration, fatty
   phanerosis 272.8
Fauces - *see* condition
Fauchard's disease (periodontitis) 523.40
Faucitis 478.29
Faulty - *see also* condition
   position of teeth 524.30
Favism (anemia) 282.2
Favre-Racouchot disease (elastoidosis cutanea
      nodularis) 701.8
Favus 110.9
   beard 110.0
   capitis 110.0
   corporis 110.5
   eyelid 110.8
   foot 110.4
   hand 110.2
   scalp 110.0
   specified site NEC 110.8
Fear, fearfulness (complex) (reaction) 300.20
   child 313.0
   of
      animals 300.29
      closed spaces 300.29
      crowds 300.29

Fear, fearfulness *(Continued)*
   of *(Continued)*
      eating in public 300.23
      heights 300.29
      open spaces 300.22
         with panic attacks 300.21
      public speaking 300.23
      streets 300.22
         with panic attacks 300.21
      travel 300.22
         with panic attacks 300.21
      washing in public 300.23
   transient 308.0
Feared complaint unfounded V65.5
Febricula (continued) (simple) *(see also* Pyrexia)
      780.60
Febrile *(see also* Pyrexia) 780.60
   convulsion (simple) 780.31
      complex 780.32
   nonhemolytic transfusion reaction (FNHTR)
         780.66
   seizure (simple) 780.31
      atypical 780.32
      complex 780.32
      complicated 780.32
Febris *(see also* Fever) 780.60
   aestiva *(see also* Fever, hay) 477.9
   flava *(see also* Fever, yellow) 060.9
   melitensis 023.0
   pestis *(see also* Plague) 020.9
   puerperalis 672●
   recurrens *(see also* Fever, relapsing) 087.9
      pediculo vestimenti 087.0
   rubra 034.1
   typhoidea 002.0
   typhosa 002.0
Fecal - *see* condition
Fecalith (impaction) 560.32
   with hernia - *see also* Hernia, by site, with
         obstruction
      gangrenous - *see* Hernia, by site, with
            gangrene
   appendix 543.9
   congenital 777.1
Fede's disease 529.0
Feeble-minded 317
**Feeble rapid pulse due to shock following
      injury** 958.4
Feeding
   faulty (elderly) (infant) 783.3
      newborn 779.31
   formula check V20.2
   improper (elderly) (infant) 783.3
      newborn 779.31
   problem (elderly) (infant) 783.3
      newborn 779.31
      nonorganic origin 307.59
Feeling of foreign body in throat 784.99
Feer's disease 985.0
Feet - *see* condition
Feigned illness V65.2
Feil-Klippel syndrome (brevicollis) 756.16
Feinmesser's (hidrotic) ectodermal dysplasia
      757.31
Felix's disease (juvenile osteochondrosis, hip)
      732.1
Felon (any digit) (with lymphangitis) 681.01
   herpetic 054.6
Felty's syndrome (rheumatoid arthritis with
      splenomegaly and leukopenia) 714.1
Feminism in boys 302.6
Feminization, testicular 259.51
   with pseudohermaphroditism, male 259.51
Femoral hernia - *see* Hernia, femoral
Femora vara 736.32
Femur, femoral - *see* condition
Fenestrata placenta - *see* Placenta, abnormal
Fenestration, fenestrated - *see also* Imperfect,
      closure
   aorta-pulmonary 745.0
   aorticopulmonary 745.0

Fenestration, fenestrated *(Continued)*
   aortopulmonary 745.0
   cusps, heart valve NEC 746.89
      pulmonary 746.09
   hymen 752.49
   pulmonic cusps 746.09
Fenwick's disease 537.89
Fermentation (gastric) (gastrointestinal)
      (stomach) 536.8
   intestine 564.89
      psychogenic 306.4
   psychogenic 306.4
Fernell's disease (aortic aneurysm) 441.9
Fertile eunuch syndrome 257.2
Fertility, meaning multiparity - *see* Multiparity
Fetal
   alcohol syndrome 760.71
   anemia 678.0●
   thrombocytopenia 678.0●
   twin to twin transfusion 678.0●
Fetalis uterus 752.39
Fetid
   breath 784.99
   sweat 705.89
Fetishism 302.81
   transvestic 302.3
Fetomaternal hemorrhage
   affecting management of pregnancy 656.0●
   fetus or newborn 772.0
Fetus, fetal - *see also* condition
   papyraceous 779.89
   type lung tissue 770.4
Fever 780.60
   with chills 780.60
      in malarial regions *(see also* Malaria) 084.6
   abortus NEC 023.9
   aden 061
   African tick-borne 087.1
   American
      mountain tick 066.1
      spotted 082.0
   and ague *(see also* Malaria) 084.6
   aphthous 078.4
   arbovirus hemorrhagic 065.9
   Assam 085.0
   Australian A or Q 083.0
   Bangkok hemorrhagic 065.4
   biliary, Charcôt's intermittent - *see*
         Choledocholithiasis
   bilious, hemoglobinuric 084.8
   blackwater 084.8
   blister 054.9
   Bonvale Dam 780.79
   boutonneuse 082.1
   brain 323.9
      late effect - *see* category 326
   breakbone 061
   Bullis 082.8
   Bunyamwera 066.3
   Burdwan 085.0
   Bwamba (encephalitis) 066.3
   Cameroon *(see also* Malaria) 084.6
   Canton 081.9
   catarrhal (acute) 460
      chronic 472.0
   cat-scratch 078.3
   cerebral 323.9
      late effect - *see* category 326
   cerebrospinal (meningococcal) *(see also*
         Meningitis, cerebrospinal) 036.0
   Chagres 084.0
   Chandipura 066.8
   changuinola 066.0
   Charcôt's (biliary) (hepatic) (intermittent) *see*
         Choledocholithiasis
   Chikungunya (viral) 066.3
      hemorrhagic 065.4
   childbed 670.8●
   Chitral 066.0
   Colombo *(see also* Fever, paratyphoid) 002.9
   Colorado tick (virus) 066.1

Fever (Continued)
- congestive
  - malarial (see also Malaria) 084.6
  - remittent (see also Malaria) 084.6
- Congo virus 065.0
- continued 780.60
  - malarial 084.0
- Corsican (see also Malaria) 084.6
- Crimean hemorrhagic 065.0
- Cyprus (see also Brucellosis) 023.9
- dandy 061
- deer fly (see also Tularemia) 021.9
- dehydration, newborn 778.4
- dengue (virus) 061
  - hemorrhagic 065.4
- desert 114.0
- due to heat 992.0
- Dumdum 085.0
- enteric 002.0
- ephemeral (of unknown origin) (see also Pyrexia) 780.60
- epidemic, hemorrhagic of the Far East 065.0
- erysipelatous (see also Erysipelas) 035
- estivo-autumnal (malarial) 084.0
- etiocholanolone 277.31
- famine - see also Fever, relapsing
  - meaning typhus - see Typhus
- Far Eastern hemorrhagic 065.0
- five day 083.1
- Fort Bragg 100.89
- gastroenteric 002.0
- gastromalarial (see also Malaria) 084.6
- Gibraltar (see also Brucellosis) 023.9
- glandular 075
- Guama (viral) 066.3
- Haverhill 026.1
- hay (allergic) (with rhinitis) 477.9
  - with
    - asthma (bronchial) (see also Asthma) 493.0●
  - due to
    - dander, animal (cat) (dog) 477.2
    - dust 477.8
    - fowl 477.8
    - hair, animal (cat) (dog) 477.2
    - pollen, any plant or tree 477.0
    - specified allergen other than pollen 477.8
- heat (effects) 992.0
- hematuric, bilious 084.8
- hemoglobinuric (malarial) 084.8
  - bilious 084.8
- hemorrhagic (arthropod-borne) NEC 065.9
  - with renal syndrome 078.6
  - arenaviral 078.7
  - Argentine 078.7
  - Bangkok 065.4
  - Bolivian 078.7
  - Central Asian 065.0
  - chikungunya 065.4
  - Crimean 065.0
  - dengue (virus) 065.4
  - Ebola 065.8
  - epidemic 078.6
    - of Far East 065.0
  - Far Eastern 065.0
  - Junin virus 078.7
  - Korean 078.6
  - Kyasanur forest 065.2
  - Machupo virus 078.7
  - mite-borne NEC 065.8
  - mosquito-borne 065.4
  - Omsk 065.1
  - Philippine 065.4
  - Russian (Yaroslav) 078.6
  - Singapore 065.4
  - Southeast Asia 065.4
  - Thailand 065.4
  - tick-borne NEC 065.3

Fever (Continued)
- hepatic (see also Cholecystitis) 575.8
  - intermittent (Charcôt's) - see Choledocholithiasis
- herpetic (see also Herpes) 054.9
- hyalomma tick 065.0
- icterohemorrhagic 100.0
- inanition 780.60
  - newborn 778.4
- in conditions classified elsewhere 780.61
- infective NEC 136.9
- intermittent (bilious) (see also Malaria) 084.6
  - hepatic (Charcôt) - see Choledocholithiasis
  - of unknown origin (see also Pyrexia) 780.60
  - pernicious 084.0
- iodide
  - correct substance properly administered 780.60
  - overdose or wrong substance given or taken 975.5
- Japanese river 081.2
- jungle yellow 060.0
- Junin virus, hemorrhagic 078.7
- Katayama 120.2
- Kedani 081.2
- Kenya 082.1
- Korean hemorrhagic 078.6
- Lassa 078.89
- Lone Star 082.8
- lung - see Pneumonia
- Machupo virus, hemorrhagic 078.7
- malaria, malarial (see also Malaria) 084.6
- Malta (see also Brucellosis) 023.9
- Marseilles 082.1
- marsh (see also Malaria) 084.6
- Mayaro (viral) 066.3
- Mediterranean (see also Brucellosis) 023.9
  - familial 277.31
  - tick 082.1
- meningeal - see Meningitis
- metal fumes NEC 985.8
- Meuse 083.1
- Mexican - see Typhus, Mexican
- Mianeh 087.1
- miasmatic (see also Malaria) 084.6
- miliary 078.2
- milk, female 672●
- mill 504
- mite-borne hemorrhagic 065.8
- Monday 504
- mosquito-borne NEC 066.3
  - hemorrhagic NEC 065.4
- mountain 066.1
  - meaning
    - Rocky Mountain spotted 082.0
    - undulant fever (see also Brucellosis) 023.9
  - tick (American) 066.1
- Mucambo (viral) 066.3
- mud 100.89
- Neapolitan (see also Brucellosis) 023.9
- neutropenic 288.00
- newborn (environmentally-induced) 778.4
- nine-mile 083.0
- nonexanthematous tick 066.1
- North Asian tick-borne typhus 082.2
- Omsk hemorrhagic 065.1
- O'nyong nyong (viral) 066.3
- Oropouche (viral) 066.3
- Oroya 088.0
- paludal (see also Malaria) 084.6
- Panama 084.0
- pappataci 066.0
- paratyphoid 002.9
  - A 002.1
  - B (Schottmüller's) 002.2
  - C (Hirschfeld) 002.3
- parrot 073.9
- periodic 277.31
- pernicious, acute 084.0

Fever (Continued)
- persistent (of unknown origin) (see also Pyrexia) 780.60
- petechial 036.0
- pharyngoconjunctival 077.2
  - adenoviral type 3 077.2
- Philippine hemorrhagic 065.4
- phlebotomus 066.0
- Piry 066.8
- Pixuna (viral) 066.3
- Plasmodium ovale 084.3
- pleural (see also Pleurisy) 511.0
- pneumonic - see Pneumonia
- polymer fume 987.8
- postimmunization 780.63
- postoperative 780.62
  - due to infection 998.59
- posttransfusion 780.66
- postvaccination 780.63
- pretibial 100.89
- puerperal, postpartum 672●
- putrid - see Septicemia
- pyemic - see Septicemia
- Q 083.0
  - with pneumonia 083.0 [484.8]
- quadrilateral 083.0
- quartan (malaria) 084.2
- Queensland (coastal) 083.0
  - seven-day 100.89
- Quintan (A) 083.1
- quotidian 084.0
- rabbit (see also Tularemia) 021.9
- rat-bite 026.9
  - due to
    - Spirillum minor or minus 026.0
    - Spirochaeta morsus muris 026.0
    - Streptobacillus moniliformis 026.1
- recurrent - see Fever, relapsing
- relapsing 087.9
  - Carter's (Asiatic) 087.0
  - Dutton's (West African) 087.1
  - Koch's 087.9
  - louse-borne (epidemic) 087.0
  - Novy's (American) 087.1
  - Obermeyer's (European) 087.0
  - spirillum NEC 087.9
  - tick-borne (endemic) 087.1
- remittent (bilious) (congestive) (gastric) (see also Malaria) 084.6
- rheumatic (active) (acute) (chronic) (subacute) 390
  - with heart involvement 391.9
    - carditis 391.9
    - endocarditis (aortic) (mitral) (pulmonary) (tricuspid) 391.1
    - multiple sites 391.8
    - myocarditis 391.2
    - pancarditis, acute 391.8
    - pericarditis 391.0
    - specified type NEC 391.8
    - valvulitis 391.1
  - inactive or quiescent with
    - cardiac hypertrophy 398.99
    - carditis 398.90
    - endocarditis 397.9
      - aortic (valve) 395.9
        - with mitral (valve) disease 396.9
      - mitral (valve) 394.9
        - with aortic (valve) disease 396.9
      - pulmonary (valve) 397.1
      - tricuspid (valve) 397.0
    - heart conditions (classifiable to 429.3, 429.6, 429.9) 398.99
    - failure (congestive) (conditions classifiable to 428.0, 428.9) 398.91
    - left ventricular failure (conditions classifiable to 428.1) 398.91
    - myocardial degeneration (conditions classifiable to 429.1) 398.0

Fever (Continued)
　rheumatic (Continued)
　　inactive or quiescent with (Continued)
　　　myocarditis (conditions classifiable to 429.0) 398.0
　　　pancarditis 398.99
　　　pericarditis 393
　Rift Valley (viral) 066.3
　Rocky Mountain spotted 082.0
　rose 477.0
　Ross river (viral) 066.3
　Russian hemorrhagic 078.6
　sandfly 066.0
　San Joaquin (valley) 114.0
　Sao Paulo 082.0
　scarlet 034.1
　septic - see Septicemia
　seven-day 061
　　Japan 100.89
　　Queensland 100.89
　shin bone 083.1
　Singapore hemorrhagic 065.4
　solar 061
　sore 054.9
　South African tick-bite 087.1
　Southeast Asia hemorrhagic 065.4
　spinal - see Meningitis
　spirillary 026.0
　splenic (see also Anthrax) 022.9
　spotted (Rocky Mountain) 082.0
　　American 082.0
　　Brazilian 082.0
　　Colombian 082.0
　　meaning
　　　cerebrospinal meningitis 036.0
　　　typhus 082.9
　spring 309.23
　steroid
　　correct substance properly administered 780.60
　　overdose or wrong substance given or taken 962.0
　streptobacillary 026.1
　subtertian 084.0
　Sumatran mite 081.2
　sun 061
　swamp 100.89
　sweating 078.2
　swine 003.8
　sylvatic yellow 060.0
　Tahyna 062.5
　tertian - see Malaria, tertian
　Thailand hemorrhagic 065.4
　thermic 992.0
　three day 066.0
　　with Coxsackie exanthem 074.8
　tick
　　American mountain 066.1
　　Colorado 066.1
　　Kemerovo 066.1
　　Mediterranean 082.1
　　mountain 066.1
　　nonexanthematous 066.1
　　Quaranfil 066.1
　tick-bite NEC 066.1
　tick-borne NEC 066.1
　　hemorrhagic NEC 065.3
　transitory of newborn 778.4
　trench 083.1
　tsutsugamushi 081.2
　typhogastric 002.0
　typhoid (abortive) (ambulant) (any site) (hemorrhagic) (infection) (intermittent) (malignant) (rheumatic) 002.0
　typhomalarial (see also Malaria) 084.6
　typhus - see Typhus
　undulant (see also Brucellosis) 023.9
　unknown origin (see also Pyrexia) 780.60
　uremic - see Uremia
　uveoparotid 135
　valley (Coccidioidomycosis) 114.0

Fever (Continued)
　Venezuelan equine 066.2
　Volhynian 083.1
　Wesselsbron (viral) 066.3
　West
　　African 084.8
　　Nile (viral) 066.40
　　　with
　　　　cranial nerve disorders 066.42
　　　　encephalitis 066.41
　　　　optic neuritis 066.42
　　　　other complications 066.49
　　　　other neurologic manifestations 066.42
　　　　polyradiculitis 066.42
　Whitmore's 025
　Wolhynian 083.1
　worm 128.9
　Yaroslav hemorrhagic 078.6
　yellow 060.9
　　jungle 060.0
　　sylvatic 060.0
　　urban 060.1
　　vaccination, prophylactic (against) V04.4
　Zika (viral) 066.3
Fibrillation
　atrial (established) (paroxysmal) 427.31
　auricular (atrial) (established) 427.31
　cardiac (ventricular) 427.41
　coronary (see also Infarct, myocardium) 410.9●
　heart (ventricular) 427.41
　muscular 728.9
　postoperative 997.1
　ventricular 427.41
Fibrin
　ball or bodies, pleural (sac) 511.0
　chamber, anterior (eye) (gelatinous exudate) 364.04
Fibrinogenolysis (hemorrhagic) - see Fibrinolysis
Fibrinogenopenia (congenital) (hereditary) (see also Defect, coagulation) 286.3
　acquired 286.6
Fibrinolysis (acquired) (hemorrhagic) (pathologic) 286.6
　with
　　abortion - see Abortion, by type, with hemorrhage, delayed or excessive
　　ectopic pregnancy (see also categories 633.0–633.9) 639.1
　　molar pregnancy (see also categories 630–632) 639.1
　antepartum or intrapartum 641.3●
　　affecting fetus or newborn 762.1
　following
　　abortion 639.1
　　ectopic or molar pregnancy 639.1
　newborn, transient 776.2
　postpartum 666.3●
Fibrinopenia (hereditary) (see also Defect, coagulation) 286.3
　acquired 286.6
Fibrinopurulent - see condition
Fibrinous - see condition
Fibroadenoma (M9010/0)
　cellular intracanalicular (M9020/0) 217
　giant (intracanalicular) (M9020/0) 217
　intracanalicular (M9011/0)
　　cellular (M9020/0) 217
　　giant (M9020/0) 217
　　specified site - see Neoplasm, by site, benign
　　unspecified site 217
　juvenile (M9030/0) 217
　pericanicular (M9012/0)
　　specified site - see Neoplasm, by site, benign
　　unspecified site 217
　phyllodes (M9020/0) 217

Fibroadenoma (Continued)
　prostate 600.20
　　with
　　　other lower urinary tract symptoms (LUTS) 600.21
　　　urinary
　　　　obstruction 600.21
　　　　retention 600.21
　specified site - see Neoplasm, by site, benign
　unspecified site 217
Fibroadenosis, breast (chronic) (cystic) (diffuse) (periodic) (segmental) 610.2
Fibroangioma (M9160/0) - see also Neoplasm, by site, benign
　juvenile (M9160/0)
　　specified site - see Neoplasm, by site, benign
　　unspecified site 210.7
Fibrocellulitis progressiva ossificans 728.11
Fibrochondrosarcoma (M9220/3) - see Neoplasm, cartilage, malignant
Fibrocystic
　disease 277.00
　　bone NEC 733.29
　　breast 610.1
　　jaw 526.2
　　kidney (congenital) 753.19
　　liver 751.62
　　lung 518.89
　　　congenital 748.4
　　pancreas 277.00
　kidney (congenital) 753.19
Fibrodysplasia ossificans multiplex (progressiva) 728.11
Fibroelastosis (cordis) (endocardial) (endomyocardial) 425.3
Fibroid (tumor) (M8890/0) - see also Neoplasm, connective tissue, benign
　disease, lung (chronic) (see also Fibrosis, lung) 515
　heart (disease) (see also Myocarditis) 429.0
　induration, lung (chronic) (see also Fibrosis, lung) 515
　in pregnancy or childbirth 654.1●
　　affecting fetus or newborn 763.89
　　causing obstructed labor 660.2●
　　　affecting fetus or newborn 763.1
　liver - see Cirrhosis, liver
　lung (see also Fibrosis, lung) 515
　pneumonia (chronic) (see also Fibrosis, lung) 515
　uterus (M8890/0) (see also Leiomyoma, uterus) 218.9
Fibrolipoma (M8851/0) (see also Lipoma, by site) 214.9
Fibroliposarcoma (M8850/3) - see Neoplasm, connective tissue, malignant
Fibroma (M8810/0) - see also Neoplasm, connective tissue, benign
　ameloblastic (M9330/0) 213.1
　　upper jaw (bone) 213.0
　bone (nonossifying) 733.99
　　ossifying (M9262/0) - see Neoplasm, bone, benign
　cementifying (M9274/0) - see Neoplasm, bone, benign
　chondromyxoid (M9241/0) - see Neoplasm, bone, benign
　desmoplastic (M8823/1) - see Neoplasm, connective tissue, uncertain behavior
　facial (M8813/0) - see Neoplasm, connective tissue, benign
　invasive (M8821/1) - see Neoplasm, connective tissue, uncertain behavior
　molle (M8851/0) (see also Lipoma, by site) 214.9
　myxoid (M8811/0) - see Neoplasm, connective tissue, benign
　nasopharynx, nasopharyngeal (juvenile) (M9160/0) 210.7

SECTION 1 INDEX TO DISEASES AND INJURIES / Fibroma

Fibroma (Continued)
    nonosteogenic (nonossifying) - see Dysplasia, fibrous
    odontogenic (M9321/0) 213.1
        upper jaw (bone) 213.0
    ossifying (M9262/0) - see Neoplasm, bone, benign
    periosteal (M8812/0) - see Neoplasm, bone, benign
    prostate 600.20
        with
            other lower urinary tract symptoms (LUTS) 600.21
            urinary
                obstruction 600.21
                retention 600.21
    soft (M8851/0) (see also Lipoma, by site) 214.9

Fibromatosis 728.79
    abdominal (M8822/1) - see Neoplasm, connective tissue, uncertain behavior
    aggressive (M8821/1) - see Neoplasm, connective tissue, uncertain behavior
    congenital generalized (CGF) 759.89
    Dupuytren's 728.6
    gingival 523.8
    plantar fascia 728.71
    proliferative 728.79
    pseudosarcomatous (proliferative) (subcutaneous) 728.79
    subcutaneous pseudosarcomatous (proliferative) 728.79

Fibromyalgia 729.1

Fibromyoma (M8890/0) - see also Neoplasm, connective tissue, benign
    uterus (corpus) (see also Leiomyoma, uterus) 218.9
        in pregnancy or childbirth 654.1●
            affecting fetus or newborn 763.89
            causing obstructed labor 660.2●
                affecting fetus or newborn 763.1

Fibromyositis (see also Myositis) 729.1
    scapulohumeral 726.2

Fibromyxolipoma (M8852/0) (see also Lipoma, by site) 214.9

Fibromyxoma (M8811/0) - see Neoplasm, connective tissue, benign

Fibromyxosarcoma (M8811/3) - see Neoplasm, connective tissue, malignant

Fibro-odontoma, ameloblastic (M9290/0) 213.1
    upper jaw (bone) 213.0

Fibro-osteoma (M9262/0) - see Neoplasm, bone, benign

Fibroplasia, retrolental (see also Retinopathy of prematurity) 362.21

Fibropurulent - see condition

Fibrosarcoma (M8810/3) - see also Neoplasm, connective tissue, malignant
    ameloblastic (M9330/3) 170.1
        upper jaw (bone) 170.0
    congenital (M8814/3) - see Neoplasm, connective tissue, malignant
    fascial (M8813/3) - see Neoplasm, connective tissue, malignant
    infantile (M8814/3) - see Neoplasm, connective tissue, malignant
    odontogenic (M9330/3) 170.1
        upper jaw (bone) 170.0
    periosteal (M8812/3) - see Neoplasm, bone, malignant

Fibrosclerosis
    breast 610.3
    corpora cavernosa (penis) 607.89
    familial multifocal NEC 710.8
    multifocal (idiopathic) NEC 710.8
    penis (corpora cavernosa) 607.89

Fibrosis, fibrotic
    adrenal (gland) 255.8
    alveolar (diffuse) 516.31
    amnion 658.8●
    anal papillae 569.49

Fibrosis, fibrotic (Continued)
    anus 569.49
    appendix, appendiceal, noninflammatory 543.9
    arteriocapillary - see Arteriosclerosis
    bauxite (of lung) 503
    biliary 576.8
        due to Clonorchis sinensis 121.1
    bladder 596.89
        interstitial 595.1
        localized submucosal 595.1
        panmural 595.1
    bone, diffuse 756.59
    breast 610.3
    capillary - see also Arteriosclerosis
        lung (chronic) (see also Fibrosis, lung) 515
    cardiac (see also Myocarditis) 429.0
    cervix 622.8
    chorion 658.8●
    corpus cavernosum 607.89
    cystic (of pancreas) 277.00
        with
            manifestations
                gastrointestinal 277.03
                pulmonary 277.02
                specified NEC 277.09
            meconium ileus 277.01
            pulmonary exacerbation 277.02
    due to (presence of) any device, implant, or graft - see Complications, due to (presence of) any device, implant, or graft classified to 996.0–996.5 NEC
    ejaculatory duct 608.89
    endocardium (see also Endocarditis) 424.90
    endomyocardial (African) 425.0
    epididymis 608.89
    eye muscle 378.62
    graphite (of lung) 503
    heart (see also Myocarditis) 429.0
    hepatic - see also Cirrhosis, liver
        due to Clonorchis sinensis 121.1
    hepatolienal - see Cirrhosis, liver
    hepatosplenic - see Cirrhosis, liver
    infrapatellar fat pad 729.31
    interstitial pulmonary, newborn 770.7
    intrascrotal 608.89
    kidney (see also Sclerosis, renal) 587
    liver - see Cirrhosis, liver
    lung (atrophic) (capillary) (chronic) (confluent) (massive) (perialveolar) (peribronchial) 515
        with
            anthracosilicosis (occupational) 500
            anthracosis (occupational) 500
            asbestosis (occupational) 501
            bagassosis (occupational) 495.1
            bauxite 503
            berylliosis (occupational) 503
            byssinosis (occupational) 504
            calcicosis (occupational) 502
            chalicosis (occupational) 502
            dust reticulation (occupational) 504
            farmers' lung 495.0
            gannister disease (occupational) 502
            graphite 503
            pneumoconiosis (occupational) 505
            pneumosiderosis (occupational) 503
            siderosis (occupational) 503
            silicosis (occupational) 502
            tuberculosis (see also Tuberculosis) 011.4●
        diffuse (idiopathic) (interstitial) 516.31
        due to
            bauxite 503
            fumes or vapors (chemical) (inhalation) 506.4
            graphite 503
        following radiation 508.1
        postinflammatory 515
        silicotic (massive) (occupational) 502
        tuberculous (see also Tuberculosis) 011.4●

Fibrosis, fibrotic (Continued)
    lymphatic gland 289.3
    median bar 600.90
        with
            other lower urinary tract symptoms (LUTS) 600.91
            urinary
                obstruction 600.91
                retention 600.91
    mediastinum (idiopathic) 519.3
    meninges 349.2
    muscle NEC 728.2
        iatrogenic (from injection) 999.9
    myocardium, myocardial (see also Myocarditis) 429.0
    oral submucous 528.8
    ovary 620.8
    oviduct 620.8
    pancreas 577.8
        cystic 277.00
            with
                manifestations
                    gastrointestinal 277.03
                    pulmonary 277.02
                    specified NEC 277.09
                meconium ileus 277.01
                pulmonary exacerbation 277.02
    penis 607.89
    periappendiceal 543.9
    periarticular (see also Ankylosis) 718.5●
    pericardium 423.1
    perineum, in pregnancy or childbirth 654.8●
        affecting fetus or newborn 763.89
        causing obstructed labor 660.2●
            affecting fetus or newborn 763.1
    perineural NEC 355.9
        foot 355.6
    periureteral 593.89
    placenta - see Placenta, abnormal
    pleura 511.0
    popliteal fat pad 729.31
    preretinal 362.56
    prostate (chronic) 600.90
        with
            other lower urinary tract symptoms (LUTS) 600.91
            urinary
                obstruction 600.91
                retention 600.91
    pulmonary (chronic) (see also Fibrosis, lung) 515
        alveolar capillary block 516.8
        idiopathic 516.31
        interstitial
            diffuse (idiopathic) 516.31
            newborn 770.7
    radiation - see Effect, adverse, radiation
    rectal sphincter 569.49
    retroperitoneal, idiopathic 593.4
    sclerosing mesenteric (idiopathic) 567.82
    scrotum 608.89
    seminal vesicle 608.89
    senile 797
    skin NEC 709.2
    spermatic cord 608.89
    spleen 289.59
        bilharzial (see also Schistosomiasis) 120.9
    subepidermal nodular (M8832/0) - see Neoplasm, skin, benign
    submucous NEC 709.2
        oral 528.8
        tongue 528.8
    syncytium - see Placenta, abnormal
    testis 608.89
        chronic, due to syphilis 095.8
    thymus (gland) 254.8
    tunica vaginalis 608.89
    ureter 593.89
    urethra 599.84

Fibrosis, fibrotic *(Continued)*
    uterus (nonneoplastic) 621.8
        bilharzial *(see also* Schistosomiasis) 120.9
        neoplastic *(see also* Leiomyoma, uterus)
            218.9
    vagina 623.8
    valve, heart *(see also* Endocarditis) 424.90
    vas deferens 608.89
    vein 459.89
        lower extremities 459.89
    vesical 595.1
Fibrositis (periarticular) (rheumatoid) 729.0
    humeroscapular region 726.2
    nodular, chronic
        Jaccoud's 714.4
        rheumatoid 714.4
    ossificans 728.11
    scapulohumeral 726.2
Fibrothorax 511.0
Fibrotic - *see* Fibrosis
Fibrous - *see* condition
Fibroxanthoma (M8831/0) - *see also* Neoplasm,
        connective tissue, benign
    atypical (M8831/1) - *see* Neoplasm,
        connective tissue, uncertain behavior
    malignant (M8831/3) - *see* Neoplasm,
        connective tissue, malignant
Fibroxanthosarcoma (M8831/3) - *see* Neoplasm,
    connective tissue, malignant
Fiedler's
    disease (leptospiral jaundice) 100.0
    myocarditis or syndrome (acute isolated
        myocarditis) 422.91
Fiessinger-Leroy (-Reiter) syndrome 099.3
Fiessinger-Rendu syndrome (erythema
    muliforme exudativum) 695.19
Fifth disease (eruptive) 057.0
    venereal 099.1
Filaria, filarial - *see* Infestation, filarial
Filariasis *(see also* Infestation, filarial) 125.9
    bancroftian 125.0
    Brug's 125.1
    due to
        bancrofti 125.0
        Brugia (Wuchereria) (malayi) 125.1
        Loa loa 125.2
        malayi 125.1
        organism NEC 125.6
        Wuchereria (bancrofti) 125.0
            malayi 125.1
    Malayan 125.1
    ozzardi 125.5
    specified type NEC 125.6
Filatoff's, Filatov's, Filatow's disease
    (infectious mononucleosis) 075
File-cutters' disease 984.9
    specified type of lead - *see* Table of Drugs
        and Chemicals
Filling defect
    biliary tract 793.3
    bladder 793.5
    duodenum 793.4
    gallbladder 793.3
    gastrointestinal tract 793.4
    intestine 793.4
    kidney 793.5
    stomach 793.4
    ureter 793.5
Filtering bleb, eye (postglaucoma) (status)
    V45.69
    with complication or rupture 997.99
    postcataract extraction (complication) 997.99
Fimbrial cyst (congenital) 752.11
Fimbriated hymen 752.49
Financial problem affecting care V60.2
Findings, (abnormal), without diagnosis
    (examination) (laboratory test) 796.4
    17-ketosteroids, elevated 791.9
    acetonuria 791.6
    acid phosphatase 790.5
    albumin-globulin ratio 790.99

Findings *(Continued)*
    albuminuria 791.0
    alcohol in blood 790.3
    alkaline phosphatase 790.5
    amniotic fluid 792.3
    amylase 790.5
    antenatal screening 796.5
    antiphosphatidylglycerol antibody 795.79
    antiphosphatidylinositol antibody 795.79
    antiphosphatidylserine antibody 795.79
    anisocytosis 790.09
    anthrax, positive 795.31
    antibody titers, elevated 795.79
    anticardiolipin antibody 795.79
    antigen-antibody reaction 795.79
    antiphospholipid antibody 795.79
    bacteriuria 791.9
    ballistocardiogram 794.39
    bicarbonate 276.9
    bile in urine 791.4
    bilirubin 277.4
    bleeding time (prolonged) 790.92
    blood culture, positive 790.7
    blood gas level (arterial) 790.91
    blood sugar level 790.29
        high 790.29
            fasting glucose 790.21
            glucose tolerance test 790.22
        low 251.2
    C-reactive protein (CRP) 790.95
    calcium 275.40
    cancer antigen 125 [CA 125] 795.82
    carbonate 276.9
    carcinoembryonic antigen [CEA] 795.81
    casts, urine 791.7
    catecholamines 791.9
    cells, urine 791.7
    cerebrospinal fluid (color) (content)
        (pressure) 792.0
    cervical
        high risk human papillomavirus (HPV)
            DNA test positive 795.05
        low risk human papillomavirus (HPV)
            DNA test positive 795.09
        non-atypical endometrial cells 795.09
    chloride 276.9
    cholesterol 272.9
        high 272.0
            with high triglycerides 272.2
    chromosome analysis 795.2
    chyluria 791.1
    circulation time 794.39
    cloudy dialysis effluent 792.5
    cloudy urine 791.9
    coagulation study 790.92
    cobalt, blood 790.6
    color of urine (unusual) NEC 791.9
    copper, blood 790.6
    creatinine clearance 794.4
    crystals, urine 791.9
    culture, positive NEC 795.39
        blood 790.7
        HIV V08
        human immunodeficiency virus V08
        nose 795.39
            Staphylococcus - *see* Carrier
                (suspected) of, Staphylococcus
        skin lesion NEC 795.39
        spinal fluid 792.0
        sputum 795.39
        stool 792.1
        throat 795.39
        urine 791.9
        viral
            human immunodeficiency V08
        wound 795.39
    cytology specified site NEC 796.9
    echocardiogram 793.2
    echoencephalogram 794.01
    echogram NEC - *see* Findings, abnormal,
        structure

Findings *(Continued)*
    electrocardiogram (ECG) (EKG) 794.31
    electroencephalogram (EEG) 794.02
    electrolyte level, urinary 791.9
    electromyogram (EMG) 794.17
        ocular 794.14
    electro-oculogram (EOG) 794.12
    electroretinogram (ERG) 794.11
    enzymes, serum NEC 790.5
    fibrinogen titer coagulation study 790.92
    filling defect - *see* Filling defect
    function study NEC 794.9
        auditory 794.15
        bladder 794.9
        brain 794.00
        cardiac 794.30
        endocrine NEC 794.6
            thyroid 794.5
        kidney 794.4
        liver 794.8
        nervous system
            central 794.00
            peripheral 794.19
        oculomotor 794.14
        pancreas 794.9
        placenta 794.9
        pulmonary 794.2
        retina 794.11
        special senses 794.19
        spleen 794.9
        vestibular 794.16
    gallbladder, nonvisualization 793.3
    glucose 790.29
        elevated
            fasting 790.21
            tolerance test 790.22
    glycosuria 791.5
    heart
        shadow 793.2
        sounds 785.3
    hematinuria 791.2
    hematocrit
        drop (precipitous) 790.01
        elevated 282.7
        low 285.9
    hematologic NEC 790.99
    hematuria 599.70
    hemoglobin
        drop 790.01
        elevated 282.7
        low 285.9
    hemoglobinuria 791.2
    histological NEC 795.4
    hormones 259.9
    immunoglobulins, elevated 795.79
    indolacetic acid, elevated 791.9
    iron 790.6
    karyotype 795.2
    ketonuria 791.6
    lactic acid dehydrogenase (LDH) 790.4
    lead 790.6
    lipase 790.5
    lipids NEC 272.9
    lithium, blood 790.6
    liver function test 790.6
    lung field (shadow) 793.19
        coin lesion 793.11
    magnesium, blood 790.6
    mammogram 793.80
        calcification 793.89
        calculus 793.89
        dense breasts 793.82
        inconclusive 793.82
            due to dense breasts 793.82
        microcalcification 793.81
    mediastinal shift 793.2
    melanin, urine 791.9
    microbiologic NEC 795.39
    mineral, blood NEC 790.6
    myoglobinuria 791.3
    nasal swab, anthrax 795.31

SECTION I INDEX TO DISEASES AND INJURIES / Findings

Findings (Continued)
- neonatal screening 796.6
- nitrogen derivatives, blood 790.6
- nonvisualization of gallbladder 793.3
- nose culture, positive 795.39
- odor of urine (unusual) NEC 791.9
- oxygen saturation 790.91
- Papanicolaou (smear) 796.9
    - anus 796.70
        - with
            - atypical squamous cells
                - cannot exclude high grade squamous intraepithelial lesion (ASC-H) 796.72
                - of undetermined significance (ASC-US) 796.71
            - cytologic evidence of malignancy 796.76
            - high grade squamous intraepithelial lesion (HGSIL) 796.74
            - low grade squamous intraepithelial lesion (LGSIL) 796.73
        - glandular 796.70
        - specified finding NEC 796.79
    - cervix 795.00
        - with
            - atypical squamous cells
                - cannot exclude high grade squamous intraepithelial lesion (ASC-H) 795.02
                - of undetermined significance (ASC-US) 795.01
            - cytologic evidence of malignancy 795.06
            - high grade squamous intraepithelial lesion (HGSIL) 795.04
            - low grade squamous intraepithelial lesion (LGSIL) 795.03
            - non-atypical endometrial cells 795.09
        - dyskaryotic 795.09
        - non-atypical endometrial cells 795.09
        - nonspecific finding NEC 795.09
    - other site 796.9
    - vagina 795.10
        - with
            - atypical squamous cells
                - cannot exclude high grade squamous intraepithelial lesion (ASC-H) 795.12
                - of undetermined significance (ASC-US) 795.11
            - cytologic evidence of malignancy 795.16
            - high grade squamous intraepithelial lesion (HGSIL) 795.14
            - low grade squamous intraepithelial lesion (LGSIL) 795.13
        - glandular 795.10
        - specified NEC 795.19
- peritoneal fluid 792.9
- phonocardiogram 794.39
- phosphorus 275.3
- pleural fluid 792.9
- pneumoencephalogram 793.0
- PO_2-oxygen ratio 790.91
- poikilocytosis 790.09
- potassium
    - deficiency 276.8
    - excess 276.7
- PPD 795.51
- prostate specific antigen (PSA) 790.93
- protein, serum NEC 790.99
- proteinuria 791.0
- prothrombin time (prolonged) (partial) (PT) (PTT) 790.92
- pyuria 791.9

Findings (Continued)
- radiologic (x-ray) 793.99
    - abdomen 793.6
    - biliary tract 793.3
    - breast 793.89
        - abnormal mammogram NOS 793.80
        - mammographic
            - calcification 793.89
            - calculus 793.89
            - microcalcification 793.81
    - gastrointestinal tract 793.4
    - genitourinary organs 793.5
    - head 793.0
    - image test inconclusive due to excess body fat 793.91
    - intrathoracic organs NEC 793.2
    - lung 793.19
    - musculoskeletal 793.7
    - placenta 793.99
    - retroperitoneum 793.6
    - skin 793.99
    - skull 793.0
    - subcutaneous tissue 793.99
- red blood cell 790.09
    - count 790.09
    - morphology 790.09
    - sickling 790.09
    - volume 790.09
- saliva 792.4
- scan NEC 794.9
    - bladder 794.9
    - bone 794.9
    - brain 794.09
    - kidney 794.4
    - liver 794.8
    - lung 794.2
    - pancreas 794.9
    - placental 794.9
    - spleen 794.9
    - thyroid 794.5
- sedimentation rate, elevated 790.1
- semen 792.2
- serological (for)
    - human immunodeficiency virus (HIV)
        - inconclusive 795.71
        - positive V08
    - syphilis - see Findings, serology for syphilis
- serology for syphilis
    - false positive 795.6
    - positive 097.1
        - false 795.6
        - follow-up of latent syphilis - see Syphilis, latent
        - only finding - see Syphilis, latent
- serum 790.99
    - blood NEC 790.99
    - enzymes NEC 790.5
    - proteins 790.99
- SGOT 790.4
- SGPT 790.4
- sickling of red blood cells 790.09
- skin test, positive 795.79
    - tuberculin (without active tuberculosis) 795.51
- sodium 790.6
    - deficiency 276.1
    - excess 276.0
- specified NEC 796.9
- spermatozoa 792.2
- spinal fluid 792.0
    - culture, positive 792.0
- sputum culture, positive 795.39
    - for acid-fast bacilli 795.39
- stool NEC 792.1
    - bloody 578.1
        - occult 792.1
    - color 792.1
    - culture, positive 792.1
    - occult blood 792.1
- stress test 794.39

Findings (Continued)
- structure, body (echogram) (thermogram) (ultrasound) (x-ray) NEC 793.99
    - abdomen 793.6
    - breast 793.89
        - abnormal mammogram 793.80
        - mammographic
            - calcification 793.89
            - calculus 793.89
            - microcalcification 793.81
    - gastrointestinal tract 793.4
    - genitourinary organs 793.5
    - head 793.0
        - echogram (ultrasound) 794.01
    - intrathoracic organs NEC 793.2
    - lung 793.19
    - musculoskeletal 793.7
    - placenta 793.99
    - retroperitoneum 793.6
    - skin 793.99
    - subcutaneous tissue NEC 793.99
- synovial fluid 792.9
- thermogram - see Findings, abnormal, structure
- throat culture, positive 795.39
- thyroid (function) 794.5
    - metabolism (rate) 794.5
    - scan 794.5
    - uptake 794.5
- total proteins 790.99
- toxicology (drugs) (heavy metals) 796.0
- transaminase (level) 790.4
- triglycerides 272.9
    - high 272.1
        - with high cholesterol 272.2
- tuberculin skin test (without active tuberculosis) 795.51
- tumor markers NEC 795.89
- ultrasound - see also Findings, abnormal, structure
    - cardiogram 793.2
- uric acid, blood 790.6
- urine, urinary constituents 791.9
    - acetone 791.6
    - albumin 791.0
    - bacteria 791.9
    - bile 791.4
    - blood 599.70
    - casts or cells 791.7
    - chyle 791.1
    - culture, positive 791.9
    - glucose 791.5
    - hemoglobin 791.2
    - ketone 791.6
    - protein 791.0
    - pus 791.9
    - sugar 791.5
- vaginal
    - fluid 792.9
    - high risk human papillomavirus (HPV) DNA test positive 795.15
    - low risk human papillomavirus (HPV) DNA test positive 795.19
- vanillylmandelic acid, elevated 791.9
- vectorcardiogram (VCG) 794.39
- ventriculogram (cerebral) 793.0
- VMA, elevated 791.9
- Wassermann reaction
    - false positive 795.6
    - positive 097.1
        - follow-up of latent syphilis - see Syphilis, latent
        - only finding - see Syphilis, latent
- white blood cell 288.9
    - count 288.9
        - elevated 288.60
        - low 288.50
    - differential 288.9
    - morphology 288.9
- wound culture 795.39

Findings *(Continued)*
  xerography 793.89
  zinc, blood 790.6
Finger - *see* condition
Finnish type nephrosis (congenital) 759.89
Fire, St. Anthony's (*see also* Erysipelas) 035
Fish
  hook stomach 537.89
  meal workers' lung 495.8
Fisher's syndrome 357.0
Fissure, fissured
  abdominal wall (congenital) 756.79
  anus, anal 565.0
    congenital 751.5
  buccal cavity 528.9
  clitoris (congenital) 752.49
  ear, lobule (congenital) 744.29
  epiglottis (congenital) 748.3
  larynx 478.79
    congenital 748.3
  lip 528.5
    congenital (*see also* Cleft, lip) 749.10
  nipple 611.2
    puerperal, postpartum 676.1●
  palate (congenital) (*see also* Cleft, palate) 749.00
  postanal 565.0
  rectum 565.0
  skin 709.8
    streptococcal 686.9
  spine (congenital) (*see also* Spina bifida) 741.9●
  sternum (congenital) 756.3
  tongue (acquired) 529.5
    congenital 750.13
Fistula (sinus) 686.9
  abdomen (wall) 569.81
    bladder 596.2
    intestine 569.81
    ureter 593.82
    uterus 619.2
  abdominorectal 569.81
  abdominosigmoidal 569.81
  abdominothoracic 510.0
  abdominouterine 619.2
    congenital 752.39
  abdominovesical 596.2
  accessory sinuses (*see also* Sinusitis) 473.9
  actinomycotic - *see* Actinomycosis
  alveolar
    antrum (*see also* Sinusitis, maxillary) 473.0
    process 522.7
  anorectal 565.1
  antrobuccal (*see also* Sinusitis, maxillary) 473.0
  antrum (*see also* Sinusitis, maxillary) 473.0
  anus, anal (infectional) (recurrent) 565.1
    congenital 751.5
    tuberculous (*see also* Tuberculosis) 014.8●
  aortic sinus 747.29
  aortoduodenal 447.2
  appendix, appendicular 543.9
  arteriovenous (acquired) 447.0
    brain 437.3
      congenital 747.81
        ruptured (*see also* Hemorrhage, subarachnoid) 430
      ruptured (*see also* Hemorrhage, subarachnoid) 430
    cerebral 437.3
      congenital 747.81
    congenital (peripheral) 747.60
      brain - *see* Fistula, arteriovenous, brain, congenital
      coronary 746.85
      gastrointestinal 747.61
      lower limb 747.64
      pulmonary 747.39
      renal 747.62
      specified site NEC 747.69
      upper limb 747.63

Fistula *(Continued)*
  arteriovenous *(Continued)*
    coronary 414.19
      congenital 746.85
    heart 414.19
    pulmonary (vessels) 417.0
      congenital 747.39
    surgically created (for dialysis) V45.11
      complication NEC 996.73
        atherosclerosis - *see* Arteriosclerosis, extremities
        embolism 996.74
        infection or inflammation 996.62
        mechanical 996.1
        occlusion NEC 996.74
        thrombus 996.74
    traumatic - *see* Injury, blood vessel, by site
  artery 447.2
  aural 383.81
    congenital 744.49
  auricle 383.81
    congenital 744.49
  Bartholin's gland 619.8
  bile duct (*see also* Fistula, biliary) 576.4
  biliary (duct) (tract) 576.4
    congenital 751.69
  bladder (neck) (sphincter) 596.2
    into seminal vesicle 596.2
  bone 733.99
  brain 348.89
    arteriovenous - *see* Fistula, arteriovenous, brain
  branchial (cleft) 744.41
  branchiogenous 744.41
  breast 611.0
    puerperal, postpartum 675.1●
  bronchial 510.0
  bronchocutaneous, bronchomediastinal, bronchopleural, bronchopleuromediastinal (infective) 510.0
    tuberculous (*see also* Tuberculosis) 011.3●
  bronchoesophageal 530.84
    congenital 750.3
  buccal cavity (infective) 528.3
  canal, ear 380.89
  carotid-cavernous
    congenital 747.81
      with hemorrhage 430
    traumatic 900.82
      with hemorrhage (*see also* Hemorrhage, brain, traumatic) 853.0●
      late effect 908.3
  cecosigmoidal 569.81
  cecum 569.81
  cerebrospinal (fluid) 349.81
  cervical, lateral (congenital) 744.41
  cervicoaural (congenital) 744.49
  cervicosigmoidal 619.1
  cervicovesical 619.0
  cervix 619.8
  chest (wall) 510.0
  cholecystocolic (*see also* Fistula, gallbladder) 575.5
  cholecystocolonic (*see also* Fistula, gallbladder) 575.5
  cholecystoduodenal (*see also* Fistula, gallbladder) 575.5
  cholecystoenteric (*see also* Fistula, gallbladder) 575.5
  cholecystogastric (*see also* Fistula, gallbladder) 575.5
  cholecystointestinal (*see also* Fistula, gallbladder) 575.5
  choledochoduodenal 576.4
  cholocolic (*see also* Fistula, gallbladder) 575.5
  coccyx 685.1
    with abscess 685.0
  colon 569.81
  colostomy 569.69
  colovaginal (acquired) 619.1

Fistula *(Continued)*
  common duct (bile duct) 576.4
  congenital, NEC - *see* Anomaly, specified type NEC
  cornea, causing hypotony 360.32
  coronary, arteriovenous 414.19
    congenital 746.85
  costal region 510.0
  cul-de-sac, Douglas' 619.8
  cutaneous 686.9
  cystic duct (*see also* Fistula, gallbladder) 575.5
    congenital 751.69
  cystostomy 596.83
  dental 522.7
  diaphragm 510.0
    bronchovisceral 510.0
    pleuroperitoneal 510.0
    pulmonoperitoneal 510.0
  duodenum 537.4
  ear (canal) (external) 380.89
  enterocolic 569.81
  enterocutaneous 569.81
  enteroenteric 569.81
  entero-uterine 619.1
    congenital 752.39
  enterovaginal 619.1
    congenital 752.49
  enterovesical 596.1
  epididymis 608.89
    tuberculous (*see also* Tuberculosis) 016.4●
  esophagobronchial 530.89
    congenital 750.3
  esophagocutaneous 530.89
  esophagopleurocutaneous 530.89
  esophagotracheal 530.84
    congenital 750.3
  esophagus 530.89
    congenital 750.4
  ethmoid (*see also* Sinusitis, ethmoidal) 473.2
  eyeball (cornea) (sclera) 360.32
  eyelid 373.11
  fallopian tube (external) 619.2
  fecal 569.81
    congenital 751.5
  from periapical lesion 522.7
  frontal sinus (*see also* Sinusitis, frontal) 473.1
  gallbladder 575.5
    with calculus, cholelithiasis, stones (*see also* Cholelithiasis) 574.2●
    congenital 751.69
  gastric 537.4
  gastrocolic 537.4
    congenital 750.7
    tuberculous (*see also* Tuberculosis) 014.8●
  gastroenterocolic 537.4
  gastroesophageal 537.4
  gastrojejunal 537.4
  gastrojejunocolic 537.4
  genital
    organs
      female 619.9
        specified site NEC 619.8
      male 608.89
    tract-skin (female) 619.2
  hepatopleural 510.0
  hepatopulmonary 510.0
  horseshoe 565.1
  ileorectal 569.81
  ileosigmoidal 569.81
  ileostomy 569.69
  ileovesical 596.1
  ileum 569.81
  in ano 565.1
    tuberculous (*see also* Tuberculosis) 014.8●
  inner ear (*see also* Fistula, labyrinth) 386.40
  intestine 569.81
  intestinocolonic (abdominal) 569.81
  intestinoureteral 593.82
  intestinouterine 619.1
  intestinovaginal 619.1
    congenital 752.49

Fistula *(Continued)*
  intestinovesical 596.1
  involving female genital tract 619.9
    digestive-genital 619.1
    genital tract-skin 619.2
    specified site NEC 619.8
    urinary-genital 619.0
  ischiorectal (fossa) 566
  jejunostomy 569.69
  jejunum 569.81
  joint 719.80
    ankle 719.87
    elbow 719.82
    foot 719.87
    hand 719.84
    hip 719.85
    knee 719.86
    multiple sites 719.89
    pelvic region 719.85
    shoulder (region) 719.81
    specified site NEC 719.88
    tuberculous - *see* Tuberculosis, joint
    wrist 719.83
  kidney 593.89
  labium (majus) (minus) 619.8
  labyrinth, labyrinthine NEC 386.40
    combined sites 386.48
    multiple sites 386.48
    oval window 386.42
    round window 386.41
    semicircular canal 386.43
  lacrimal, lachrymal (duct) (gland) (sac) 375.61
  lacrimonasal duct 375.61
  laryngotracheal 748.3
  larynx 478.79
  lip 528.5
    congenital 750.25
  lumbar, tuberculous (*see also* Tuberculosis) 015.0● [730.8]●
  lung 510.0
  lymphatic (node) (vessel) 457.8
  mamillary 611.0
  mammary (gland) 611.0
    puerperal, postpartum 675.1●
  mastoid (process) (region) 383.1
  maxillary (*see also* Sinusitis, maxillary) 473.0
  mediastinal 510.0
  mediastinobronchial 510.0
  mediastinocutaneous 510.0
  middle ear 385.89
  mouth 528.3
  nasal 478.19
    sinus (*see also* Sinusitis) 473.9
  nasopharynx 478.29
  nipple - *see* Fistula, breast
  nose 478.19
  oral (cutaneous) 528.3
    maxillary (*see also* Sinusitis, maxillary) 473.0
    nasal (with cleft palate) (*see also* Cleft, palate) 749.00
  orbit, orbital 376.10
  oro-antral (*see also* Sinusitis, maxillary) 473.0
  oval window (internal ear) 386.42
  oviduct (external) 619.2
  palate (hard) 526.89
    soft 528.9
  pancreatic 577.8
  pancreaticoduodenal 577.8
  parotid (gland) 527.4
    region 528.3
  pelvoabdominointestinal 569.81
  penis 607.89
  perianal 565.1
  pericardium (pleura) (sac) (*see also* Pericarditis) 423.8
  pericecal 569.81
  perineal - *see* Fistula, perineum
  perineorectal 569.81
  perineosigmoidal 569.81

Fistula *(Continued)*
  perineo-urethroscrotal 608.89
  perineum, perineal (with urethral involvement) NEC 599.1
    tuberculous (*see also* Tuberculosis) 017.9●
    ureter 593.82
  perirectal 565.1
    tuberculous (*see also* Tuberculosis) 014.8●
  peritoneum (*see also* Peritonitis) 567.22
  periurethral 599.1
  pharyngo-esophageal 478.29
  pharynx 478.29
    branchial cleft (congenital) 744.41
  pilonidal (infected) (rectum) 685.1
    with abscess 685.0
  pleura, pleural, pleurocutaneous, pleuroperitoneal 510.0
    stomach 510.0
    tuberculous (*see also* Tuberculosis) 012.0●
  pleuropericardial 423.8
  postauricular 383.81
  postoperative, persistent 998.6
  preauricular (congenital) 744.46
  prostate 602.8
  pulmonary 510.0
    arteriovenous 417.0
      congenital 747.39
    tuberculous (*see also* Tuberculosis, pulmonary) 011.9●
  pulmonoperitoneal 510.0
  rectolabial 619.1
  rectosigmoid (intercommunicating) 569.81
  rectoureteral 593.82
  rectourethral 599.1
    congenital 753.8
  rectouterine 619.1
    congenital 752.39
  rectovaginal 619.1
    congenital 752.49
    old, postpartal 619.1
    tuberculous (*see also* Tuberculosis) 014.8●
  rectovesical 596.1
    congenital 753.8
  rectovesicovaginal 619.1
  rectovulvar 619.1
    congenital 752.49
  rectum (to skin) 565.1
    tuberculous (*see also* Tuberculosis) 014.8●
  renal 593.89
  retroauricular 383.81
  round window (internal ear) 386.41
  salivary duct or gland 527.4
    congenital 750.24
  sclera 360.32
  scrotum (urinary) 608.89
    tuberculous (*see also* Tuberculosis) 016.5●
  semicircular canals (internal ear) 386.43
  sigmoid 569.81
    vesicoabdominal 596.1
  sigmoidovaginal 619.1
    congenital 752.49
  skin 686.9
    ureter 593.82
    vagina 619.2
  sphenoidal sinus (*see also* Sinusitis, sphenoidal) 473.3
  splenocolic 289.59
  stercoral 569.81
  stomach 537.4
  sublingual gland 527.4
    congenital 750.24
  submaxillary
    gland 527.4
      congenital 750.24
    region 528.3
  thoracic 510.0
    duct 457.8
  thoracicoabdominal 510.0

Fistula *(Continued)*
  thoracicogastric 510.0
  thoracicointestinal 510.0
  thoracoabdominal 510.0
  thoracogastric 510.0
  thorax 510.0
  thyroglossal duct 759.2
  thyroid 246.8
  trachea (congenital) (external) (internal) 748.3
  tracheoesophageal 530.84
    congenital 750.3
    following tracheostomy 519.09
  traumatic
    arteriovenous (*see also* Injury, blood vessel, by site) 904.9
    brain - *see* Injury, intracranial
  tuberculous - *see* Tuberculosis, by site
  typhoid 002.0
  umbilical 759.89
  umbilico-urinary 753.8
  urachal, urachus 753.7
  ureter (persistent) 593.82
  ureteroabdominal 593.82
  ureterocervical 593.82
  ureterorectal 593.82
  ureterosigmoido-abdominal 593.82
  ureterovaginal 619.0
  ureterovesical 596.2
  urethra 599.1
    congenital 753.8
    tuberculous (*see also* Tuberculosis) 016.3●
  urethroperineal 599.1
  urethroperineovesical 596.2
  urethrorectal 599.1
    congenital 753.8
  urethroscrotal 608.89
  urethrovaginal 619.0
  urethrovesical 596.2
  urethrovesicovaginal 619.0
  urinary (persistent) (recurrent) 599.1
  uteroabdominal (anterior wall) 619.2
    congenital 752.39
  uteroenteric 619.1
  uterofecal 619.1
  uterointestinal 619.1
    congenital 752.39
  uterorectal 619.1
    congenital 752.39
  uteroureteric 619.0
  uterovaginal 619.8
  uterovesical 619.0
    congenital 752.39
  uterus 619.8
  vagina (wall) 619.8
    postpartal, old 619.8
  vaginocutaneous (postpartal) 619.2
  vaginoileal (acquired) 619.1
  vaginoperineal 619.2
  vesical NEC 596.2
  vesicoabdominal 596.2
  vesicocervicovaginal 619.0
  vesicocolic 596.1
  vesicocutaneous 596.2
  vesicoenteric 596.1
  vesicointestinal 596.1
  vesicometrorectal 619.1
  vesicoperineal 596.2
  vesicorectal 596.1
    congenital 753.8
  vesicosigmoidal 596.1
  vesicosigmoidovaginal 619.1
  vesicoureteral 596.2
  vesicoureterovaginal 619.0
  vesicourethral 596.2
  vesicourethrorectal 596.1
  vesicouterine 619.0
    congenital 752.39
  vesicovaginal 619.0
  vulvorectal 619.1
    congenital 752.49

Fit 780.39
    apoplectic (see also Disease, cerebrovascular, acute) 436
        late effect - see Late effect(s) (of) cerebrovascular disease
    epileptic (see also Epilepsy) 345.9●
    fainting 780.2
    hysterical 300.11
    newborn 779.0
Fitting (of)
    artificial
        arm (complete) (partial) V52.0
        breast V52.4
            implant exchange (different material) (different size) V52.4
        eye(s) V52.2
        leg(s) (complete) (partial) V52.1
    brain neuropacemaker V53.02
    cardiac pacemaker V53.31
    carotid sinus pacemaker V53.39
    cerebral ventricle (communicating) shunt V53.01
    colostomy belt V55.3
    contact lenses V53.1
    cystostomy device V53.6
    defibrillator, automatic implantable cardiac (with synchronous cardiac pacemaker) V53.32
    dentures V52.3
    device, unspecified type V53.90
        abdominal V53.59
        cardiac
            defibrillator, automatic implantable (with synchronous cardiac pacemaker) V53.32
            pacemaker V53.31
            specified NEC V53.39
        cerebral ventricle (communicating) shunt V53.01
        gastrointestinal NEC V53.59
        insulin pump V53.91
        intestinal V53.50
        intrauterine contraceptive
            insertion V25.11
            removal V25.12
                and reinsertion V25.13
            replacement V25.13
        nervous system V53.09
        orthodontic V53.4
        orthoptic V53.1
        other device V53.99
        prosthetic V52.9
            breast V52.4
            dental V52.3
            eye V52.2
            specified type NEC V52.8
        special senses V53.09
        substitution
            auditory V53.09
            nervous system V53.09
            visual V53.09
        urinary V53.6
    diaphragm (contraceptive) V25.02
    gastric lap band V53.51
    gastrointestinal appliance and device NEC V53.59
    glasses (reading) V53.1
    growth rod V54.02
    hearing aid V53.2
    ileostomy device V55.2
    intestinal appliance and device V53.50
    intrauterine contraceptive device
        insertion V25.11
        removal V25.12
            and reinsertion V25.13
        replacement V25.13
    neuropacemaker (brain) (peripheral nerve) (spinal cord) V53.02
    orthodontic device V53.4

Fitting (Continued)
    orthopedic (device) V53.7
        brace V53.7
        cast V53.7
        corset V53.7
        shoes V53.7
    pacemaker (cardiac) V53.31
        brain V53.02
        carotid sinus V53.39
        peripheral nerve V53.02
        spinal cord V53.02
    prosthesis V52.9
        arm (complete) (partial) V52.0
        breast V52.4
            implant exchange (different material) (different size) V52.4
        dental V52.3
        eye V52.2
        leg (complete) (partial) V52.1
        specified type NEC V52.8
    spectacles V53.1
    wheelchair V53.8
Fitz's syndrome (acute hemorrhagic pancreatitis) 577.0
Fitz-Hugh and Curtis syndrome 098.86
    due to
        Chlamydia trachomatis 099.56
        Neisseria gonorrhoeae (gonococcal peritonitis) 098.86
Fixation
    joint - see Ankylosis
    larynx 478.79
    pupil 364.76
    stapes 385.22
        deafness (see also Deafness, conductive) 389.04
    uterus (acquired) - see Malposition, uterus
    vocal cord 478.5
Flaccid - see also condition
    foot 736.79
    forearm 736.09
    palate, congenital 750.26
Flail
    chest 807.4
        newborn 767.3
    joint (paralytic) 718.80
        ankle 718.87
        elbow 718.82
        foot 718.87
        hand 718.84
        hip 718.85
        knee 718.86
        multiple sites 718.89
        pelvic region 718.85
        shoulder (region) 718.81
        specified site NEC 718.88
        wrist 718.83
Flajani (-Basedow) syndrome or disease (exophthalmic goiter) 242.0●
Flap, liver 572.8
Flare, anterior chamber (aqueous) (eye) 364.04
Flashback phenomena (drug) (hallucinogenic) 292.89
Flat
    chamber (anterior) (eye) 360.34
    chest, congenital 754.89
    electroencephalogram (EEG) 348.89
    foot (acquired) (fixed type) (painful) (postural) (spastic) 734
        congenital 754.61
            rocker bottom 754.61
            vertical talus 754.61
        rachitic 268.1
        rocker bottom (congenital) 754.61
        vertical talus, congenital 754.61
    organ or site, congenital NEC - see Anomaly, specified type NEC

Flat (Continued)
    pelvis 738.6
        with disproportion (fetopelvic) 653.2●
            affecting fetus or newborn 763.1
            causing obstructed labor 660.1●
                affecting fetus or newborn 763.1
        congenital 755.69
Flatau-Schilder disease 341.1
Flattening
    head, femur 736.39
    hip 736.39
    lip (congenital) 744.89
    nose (congenital) 754.0
        acquired 738.0
Flatulence 787.3
Flatus 787.3
    vaginalis 629.89
Flax dressers' disease 504
Flea bite - see Injury, superficial, by site
Fleischer (-Kayser) ring (corneal pigmentation) 275.1 [371.14]
Fleischner's disease 732.3
Fleshy mole 631.8
Flexibilitas cerea (see also Catalepsy) 300.11
Flexion
    cervix - see Flexion, uterus
    contracture, joint (see also Contraction, joint) 718.4●
    deformity, joint (see also Contraction, joint) 736.9
        hip, congenital (see also Subluxation, congenital, hip) 754.32
    uterus (see also Malposition, uterus) 621.6
Flexner's
    bacillus 004.1
    diarrhea (ulcerative) 004.1
    dysentery 004.1
Flexner-Boyd dysentery 004.2
Flexure - see condition
Floater, vitreous 379.24
Floating
    cartilage (joint) (see also Disorder, cartilage, articular) 718.0●
        knee 717.6
    gallbladder (congenital) 751.69
    kidney 593.0
        congenital 753.3
    liver (congenital) 751.69
    rib 756.3
    spleen 289.59
Flooding 626.2
Floor - see condition
Floppy
    infant NEC 781.99
    iris syndrome 364.81
    valve syndrome (mitral) 424.0
Flu - see also Influenza
    bird (see also Influenza, avian) 488.02
    gastric NEC 008.8
    swine - see Influenza, (novel) 2009 H1N1
Fluctuating blood pressure 796.4
Fluid
    abdomen 789.59
    chest (see also Pleurisy, with effusion) 511.9
    heart (see also Failure, heart) 428.0
    joint (see also Effusion, joint) 719.0●
    loss (acute) 276.50
        with
            hypernatremia 276.0
            hyponatremia 276.1
    lung - see also Edema, lung
        encysted 511.89
    peritoneal cavity 789.59
        malignant 789.51
    pleural cavity (see also Pleurisy, with effusion) 511.9
    retention 276.69
Flukes NEC (see also Infestation, fluke) 121.9
    blood NEC (see also Infestation, Schistosoma) 120.9
    liver 121.3

Fluor (albus) (vaginalis) 623.5
    trichomonal (Trichomonas vaginalis) 131.00
Fluorosis (dental) (chronic) 520.3
Flushing 782.62
    menopausal 627.2
Flush syndrome 259.2
Flutter
    atrial or auricular 427.32
    heart (ventricular) 427.42
        atrial 427.32
        impure 427.32
        postoperative 997.1
        ventricular 427.42
Flux (bloody) (serosanguineous) 009.0
FNHTR (febrile nonhemolytic transfusion reaction) 780.66
Focal - *see* condition
Fochier's abscess - *see* Abscess, by site
Focus, Assmann's (*see also* Tuberculosis) 011.0●
Fogo selvagem 694.4
Foix-Alajouanine syndrome 336.1
Folds, anomalous - *see also* Anomaly, specified type NEC
    Bowman's membrane 371.31
    Descemet's membrane 371.32
    epicanthic 743.63
    heart 746.89
    posterior segment of eye, congenital 743.54
Folie a deux 297.3
Follicle
    cervix (nabothian) (ruptured) 616.0
    graafian, ruptured, with hemorrhage 620.0
    nabothian 616.0
Folliclis (primary) (*see also* Tuberculosis) 017.0●
Follicular - *see also* condition
    cyst (atretic) 620.0
Folliculitis 704.8
    abscedens et suffodiens 704.8
    decalvans 704.09
    gonorrheal (acute) 098.0
        chronic or duration of 2 months or more 098.2
    keloid, keloidalis 706.1
    pustular 704.8
    ulerythematosa reticulata 701.8
Folliculosis, conjunctival 372.02
Følling's disease (phenylketonuria) 270.1
Follow-up (examination) (routine) (following) V67.9
    cancer chemotherapy V67.2
    chemotherapy V67.2
    fracture V67.4
    high-risk medication V67.51
    injury NEC V67.59
    postpartum
        immediately after delivery V24.0
        routine V24.2
    psychiatric V67.3
    psychotherapy V67.3
    radiotherapy V67.1
    specified condition NEC V67.59
    specified surgery NEC V67.09
    surgery V67.00
        vaginal pap smear V67.01
    treatment V67.9
        combined NEC V67.6
        fracture V67.4
        involving high-risk medication NEC V67.51
        mental disorder V67.3
        specified NEC V67.59
Fong's syndrome (hereditary osteoonychodysplasia) 756.89
Food
    allergy 693.1
    anaphylactic shock - *see* Anaphylactic reaction or shock, due to food

Food (*Continued*)
    asphyxia (from aspiration or inhalation) (*see also* Asphyxia, food) 933.1
    choked on (*see also* Asphyxia, food) 933.1
    deprivation 994.2
        specified kind of food NEC 269.8
    intoxication (*see also* Poisoning, food) 005.9
    lack of 994.2
    poisoning (*see also* Poisoning, food) 005.9
    refusal or rejection NEC 307.59
    strangulation or suffocation (*see also* Asphyxia, food) 933.1
    toxemia (*see also* Poisoning, food) 005.9
Foot - *see also* condition
    and mouth disease 078.4
    process disease 581.3
Foramen ovale (nonclosure) (patent) (persistent) 745.5
Forbes' (glycogen storage) disease 271.0
Forbes-Albright syndrome (nonpuerperal amenorrhea and lactation associated with pituitary tumor) 253.1
Forced birth or delivery NEC 669.8●
    affecting fetus or newborn NEC 763.89
Forceps
    delivery NEC 669.5●
    affecting fetus or newborn 763.2
Fordyce's disease (ectopic sebaceous glands) (mouth) 750.26
Fordyce-Fox disease (apocrine miliaria) 705.82
Forearm - *see* condition
Foreign body

> Note: For foreign body with open wound or other injury, *see* Wound, open, or the type of injury specified.

    accidentally left during a procedure 998.4
    anterior chamber (eye) 871.6
        magnetic 871.5
            retained or old 360.51
        retained or old 360.61
    ciliary body (eye) 871.6
        magnetic 871.5
            retained or old 360.52
        retained or old 360.62
    entering through orifice (current) (old)
        accessory sinus 932
        air passage (upper) 933.0
            lower 934.8
        alimentary canal 938
        alveolar process 935.0
        antrum (Highmore) 932
        anus 937
        appendix 936
        asphyxia due to (*see also* Asphyxia, food) 933.1
        auditory canal 931
        auricle 931
        bladder 939.0
        bronchioles 934.8
        bronchus (main) 934.1
        buccal cavity 935.0
        canthus (inner) 930.1
        cecum 936
        cervix (canal) uterine 939.1
        coil, ileocecal 936
        colon 936
        conjunctiva 930.1
        conjunctival sac 930.1
        cornea 930.0
        digestive organ or tract NEC 938
        duodenum 936
        ear (external) 931
        esophagus 935.1

Foreign body (*Continued*)
    entering through orifice (*Continued*)
        eye (external) 930.9
            combined sites 930.8
            intraocular - *see* Foreign body, by site
            specified site NEC 930.8
        eyeball 930.8
            intraocular - *see* Foreign body, intraocular
        eyelid 930.1
            retained or old 374.86
        frontal sinus 932
        gastrointestinal tract 938
        genitourinary tract 939.9
        globe 930.8
            penetrating 871.6
                magnetic 871.5
                    retained or old 360.50
                retained or old 360.60
        gum 935.0
        Highmore's antrum 932
        hypopharynx 933.0
        ileocecal coil 936
        ileum 936
        inspiration (of) 933.1
        intestine (large) (small) 936
        lacrimal apparatus, duct, gland, or sac 930.2
        larynx 933.1
        lung 934.8
        maxillary sinus 932
        mouth 935.0
        nasal sinus 932
        nasopharynx 933.0
        nose (passage) 932
        nostril 932
        oral cavity 935.0
        palate 935.0
        penis 939.3
        pharynx 933.0
        pyriform sinus 933.0
        rectosigmoid 937
            junction 937
        rectum 937
        respiratory tract 934.9
            specified part NEC 934.8
        sclera 930.1
        sinus 932
            accessory 932
            frontal 932
            maxillary 932
            nasal 932
            pyriform 933.0
        small intestine 936
        stomach (hairball) 935.2
        suffocation by (*see also* Asphyxia, food) 933.1
        swallowed 938
            tongue 933.0
        tear ducts or glands 930.2
        throat 933.0
        tongue 935.0
            swallowed 933.0
        tonsil, tonsillar 933.0
            fossa 933.0
        trachea 934.0
        ureter 939.0
        urethra 939.0
        uterus (any part) 939.1
        vagina 939.2
        vulva 939.2
        wind pipe 934.0
    feeling of, in throat 784.99
    granuloma (old) 728.82
        bone 733.99
        in operative wound (inadvertently left) 998.4
            due to surgical material intentionally left - *see* Complications, due to (presence of) any device, implant, or graft classified to 996.0–996.5 NEC

Foreign body (Continued)
granuloma (Continued)
muscle 728.82
skin 709.4
soft tissue NEC 709.4
subcutaneous tissue 709.4
in
bone (residual) 733.99
open wound - see Wound, open, by site complicated
soft tissue (residual) 729.6
inadvertently left in operation wound (causing adhesions, obstruction, or perforation) 998.4
ingestion, ingested NEC 938
inhalation or inspiration (see also Asphyxia, food) 933.1
internal organ, not entering through an orifice - see Injury, internal, by site, with open wound
intraocular (nonmagnetic) 871.6
combined sites 871.6
magnetic 871.5
retained or old 360.59
retained or old 360.69
magnetic 871.5
retained or old 360.50
retained or old 360.60
specified site NEC 871.6
magnetic 871.5
retained or old 360.59
retained or old 360.69
iris (nonmagnetic) 871.6
magnetic 871.5
retained or old 360.52
retained or old 360.62
lens (nonmagnetic) 871.6
magnetic 871.5
retained or old 360.53
retained or old 360.63
lid, eye 930.1
ocular muscle 870.4
retained or old 376.6
old or residual
bone 733.99
eyelid 374.86
middle ear 385.83
muscle 729.6
ocular 376.6
retrobulbar 376.6
skin 729.6
with granuloma 709.4
soft tissue 729.6
with granuloma 709.4
subcutaneous tissue 729.6
with granuloma 709.4
operation wound, left accidentally 998.4
orbit 870.4
retained or old 376.6
posterior wall, eye 871.6
magnetic 871.5
retained or old 360.55
retained or old 360.65
respiratory tree 934.9
specified site NEC 934.8
retained (old) (nonmagnetic) (in) V90.9
anterior chamber (eye) 360.61
magnetic 360.51
ciliary body 360.62
magnetic 360.52
eyelid 374.86
fragment(s)
acrylics V90.2
animal quills V90.31
animal spines V90.31
cement V90.83
concrete V90.83
crystalline V90.83
depleted
isotope V90.09
uranium V90.01

Foreign body (Continued)
retained (Continued)
fragment(s) (Continued)
diethylhexylphthalates V90.2
glass V90.81
isocyanate V90.2
metal V90.10
magnetic V90.11
nonmagnetic V90.12
organic NEC V90.39
plastic V90.2
radioactive
nontherapeutic V90.09
specified NEC V90.09
stone V90.83
tooth V90.32
wood V90.33
globe 360.60
magnetic 360.50
intraocular 360.60
magnetic 360.50
specified site NEC 360.69
magnetic 360.59
iris 360.62
magnetic 360.52
lens 360.63
magnetic 360.53
muscle 729.6
orbit 376.6
posterior wall of globe 360.65
magnetic 360.55
retina 360.65
magnetic 360.55
retrobulbar 376.6
skin 729.6
with granuloma 709.4
soft tissue 729.6
with granuloma 709.4
specified NEC V90.89
subcutaneous tissue 729.6
with granuloma 709.4
vitreous 360.64
magnetic 360.54
retina 871.6
magnetic 871.5
retained or old 360.55
retained or old 360.65
superficial, without major open wound (see also Injury, superficial, by site) 919.6
swallowed NEC 938
throat, feeling of 784.99
vitreous (humor) 871.6
magnetic 871.5
retained or old 360.54
retained or old 360.64
Forking, aqueduct of Sylvius 742.3
with spina bifida (see also Spina bifida) 741.0●
Formation
bone in scar tissue (skin) 709.3
connective tissue in vitreous 379.25
Elschnig pearls (postcataract extraction) 366.51
hyaline in cornea 371.49
sequestrum in bone (due to infection) (see also Osteomyelitis) 730.1●
valve
colon, congenital 751.5
ureter (congenital) 753.29
Formication 782.0
Fort Bragg fever 100.89
Fossa - see also condition
pyriform - see condition
Foster care (status) V60.81
Foster-Kennedy syndrome 377.04
Fothergill's
disease, meaning scarlatina anginosa 034.1
neuralgia (see also Neuralgia, trigeminal) 350.1
Foul breath 784.99

Found dead (cause unknown) 798.9
Foundling V20.0
Fournier's disease (idiopathic gangrene) 608.83
female 616.89
Fourth
cranial nerve - see condition
disease 057.8
molar 520.1
Foville's syndrome 344.89
Fox's
disease (apocrine miliaria) 705.82
impetigo (contagiosa) 684
Fox-Fordyce disease (apocrine miliaria) 705.82
Fracture (abduction) (adduction) (avulsion) (compression) (crush) (dislocation) (oblique) (separation) (closed) 829.0

> Note: For fracture of any of the following sites with fracture of other bones - see Fracture, multiple.
>
> "Closed" includes the following descriptions of fractures, with or without delayed healing, unless they are specified as open or compound:
>
> comminuted
> depressed
> elevated
> fissured
> greenstick
> impacted
> linear
> simple
> slipped epiphysis
> spiral
> unspecified
>
> "Open" includes the following descriptions of fractures, with or without delayed healing:
>
> compound
> infected
> missile
> puncture
> with foreign body
>
> For late effect of fracture, see Late, effect, fracture, by site.

with
internal injuries in same region (conditions classifiable to 860–869) - see also Injury, internal, by site
pelvic region - see Fracture, pelvis
acetabulum (with visceral injury) (closed) 808.0
open 808.1
acromion (process) (closed) 811.01
open 811.11
alveolus (closed) 802.8
open 802.9
ankle (malleolus) (closed) 824.8
bimalleolar (Dupuytren's) (Pott's) 824.4
open 824.5
bone 825.21
open 825.31
lateral malleolus only (fibular) 824.2
open 824.3
medial malleolus only (tibial) 824.0
open 824.1
open 824.9
pathologic 733.16
talus 825.21
open 825.31
trimalleolar 824.6
open 824.7
antrum - see Fracture, skull, base
arm (closed) 818.0
and leg(s) (any bones) 828.0
open 828.1

SECTION I INDEX TO DISEASES AND INJURIES / Fracture

Fracture (Continued)
  arm (Continued)
    both (any bones) (with rib(s)) (with sternum) 819.0
      open 819.1
    lower 813.80
      open 813.90
      open 818.1
    upper - see Fracture, humerus
  astragalus (closed) 825.21
    open 825.31
  atlas - see Fracture, vertebra, cervical, first
  axis - see Fracture, vertebra, cervical, second
  back - see Fracture, vertebra, by site
  Barton's - see Fracture, radius, lower end
  basal (skull) - see Fracture, skull, base
  Bennett's (closed) 815.01
    open 815.11
  bimalleolar (closed) 824.4
    open 824.5
  bone (closed) NEC 829.0
    birth injury NEC 767.3
    open 829.1
    pathological NEC (see also Fracture, pathologic) 733.10
    stress NEC (see also Fracture, stress) 733.95
  boot top - see Fracture, fibula
  boxers' - see Fracture, metacarpal bone(s)
  breast bone - see Fracture, sternum
  buckle - see Fracture, torus
  bucket handle (semilunar cartilage) - see Tear, meniscus
  burst - see Fracture, traumatic, by site
  bursting - see Fracture, phalanx, hand, distal
  calcaneus (closed) 825.0
    open 825.1
  capitate (bone) (closed) 814.07
    open 814.17
  capitellum (humerus) (closed) 812.49
    open 812.59
  carpal bone(s) (wrist NEC) (closed) 814.00
    open 814.10
    specified site NEC 814.09
      open 814.19
  cartilage, knee (semilunar) - see Tear, meniscus
  cervical - see Fracture, vertebra, cervical
  chauffeur's - see Fracture, ulna, lower end
  chisel - see Fracture, radius, upper end
  chronic - see Fracture, pathologic
  clavicle (interligamentous part) (closed) 810.00
    acromial end 810.03
      open 810.13
    due to birth trauma 767.2
    open 810.10
    shaft (middle third) 810.02
      open 810.12
    sternal end 810.01
      open 810.11
  clayshovelers' - see Fracture, vertebra, cervical
  coccyx - see also Fracture, vertebra, coccyx
    complicating delivery 665.6●
  collar bone - see Fracture, clavicle
  Colles' (reversed) (closed) 813.41
    open 813.51
  comminuted - see Fracture, by site
  compression - see also Fracture, by site
    nontraumatic - see Fracture, pathologic
  congenital 756.9
  coracoid process (closed) 811.02
    open 811.12
  coronoid process (ulna) (closed) 813.02
    mandible (closed) 802.23
      open 802.33
    open 813.12
  corpus cavernosum penis 959.13
  costochondral junction - see Fracture, rib
  costosternal junction - see Fracture, rib
  cranium - see Fracture, skull, by site

Fracture (Continued)
  cricoid cartilage (closed) 807.5
    open 807.6
  cuboid (ankle) (closed) 825.23
    open 825.33
  cuneiform
    foot (closed) 825.24
      open 825.34
    wrist (closed) 814.03
      open 814.13
  dental implant 525.73
  dental restorative material
    with loss of material 525.64
    without loss of material 525.63
  due to
    birth injury - see Birth injury, fracture
    gunshot - see Fracture, by site, open
    neoplasm - see Fracture, pathologic
    osteoporosis - see Fracture, pathologic
  Dupuytren's (ankle) (fibula) (closed) 824.4
    open 824.5
    radius 813.42
      open 813.52
  Duverney's - see Fracture, ilium
  elbow - see also Fracture, humerus, lower end
    olecranon (process) (closed) 813.01
      open 813.11
    supracondylar (closed) 812.41
      open 812.51
  ethmoid (bone) (sinus) - see Fracture, skull, base
  face bone(s) (closed) NEC 802.8
    with
      other bone(s) - see Fracture, multiple, skull
      skull - see also Fracture, skull
        involving other bones - see Fracture, multiple, skull
    open 802.9
  fatigue - see Fracture, march
  femur, femoral (closed) 821.00
    cervicotrochanteric 820.03
      open 820.13
    condyles, epicondyles 821.21
      open 821.31
    distal end - see Fracture, femur, lower end
    epiphysis (separation)
      capital 820.01
        open 820.11
      head 820.01
        open 820.11
      lower 821.22
        open 821.32
      trochanteric 820.01
        open 820.11
      upper 820.01
        open 820.11
    head 820.09
      open 820.19
    lower end or extremity (distal end) (closed) 821.20
      condyles, epicondyles 821.21
        open 821.31
      epiphysis (separation) 821.22
        open 821.32
      multiple sites 821.29
        open 821.39
      open 821.30
      specified site NEC 821.29
        open 821.39
      supracondylar 821.23
        open 821.33
      T-shaped 821.21
        open 821.31
    neck (closed) 820.8
      base (cervicotrochanteric) 820.03
        open 820.13
      extracapsular 820.20
        open 820.30
      intertrochanteric (section) 820.21
        open 820.31

Fracture (Continued)
  femur, femoral (Continued)
    neck (Continued)
      intracapsular 820.00
        open 820.10
      intratrochanteric 820.21
        open 820.31
      midcervical 820.02
        open 820.12
      open 820.9
      pathologic 733.14
        specified part NEC 733.15
      specified site NEC 820.09
        open 820.19
      stress 733.96
      transcervical 820.02
        open 820.12
      transtrochanteric 820.20
        open 820.30
    open 821.10
    pathologic 733.14
      specified part NEC 733.15
    peritrochanteric (section) 820.20
      open 820.30
    shaft (lower third) (middle third) (upper third) 821.01
      open 821.11
      stress 733.97
    subcapital 820.09
      open 820.19
    subtrochanteric (region) (section) 820.22
      open 820.32
    supracondylar 821.23
      open 821.33
    transepiphyseal 820.01
      open 820.11
    trochanter (greater) (lesser) (see also Fracture, femur, neck, by site) 820.20
      open 820.30
    T-shaped, into knee joint 821.21
      open 821.31
    upper end 820.8
      open 820.9
  fibula (closed) 823.81
    with tibia 823.82
      open 823.92
    distal end 824.8
      open 824.9
    epiphysis
      lower 824.8
        open 824.9
      upper - see Fracture, fibula, upper end
    head - see Fracture, fibula, upper end
    involving ankle 824.2
      open 824.3
    lower end or extremity 824.8
      open 824.9
    malleolus (external) (lateral) 824.2
      open 824.3
    open NEC 823.91
    pathologic 733.16
    proximal end - see Fracture, fibula, upper end
    shaft 823.21
      with tibia 823.22
        open 823.32
      open 823.31
    stress 733.93
    torus 823.41
      with tibia 823.42
    upper end or extremity (epiphysis) (head) (proximal end) (styloid) 823.01
      with tibia 823.02
        open 823.12
      open 823.11
  finger(s), of one hand (closed) (see also Fracture, phalanx, hand) 816.00
    with
      metacarpal bone(s), of same hand 817.0
        open 817.1

SECTION I INDEX TO DISEASES AND INJURIES / Fracture

Fracture *(Continued)*
  finger(s), of one hand *(Continued)*
    with *(Continued)*
      thumb of same hand 816.03
        open 816.13
      open 816.10
  foot, except toe(s) alone (closed) 825.20
    open 825.30
  forearm (closed) NEC 813.80
    lower end (distal end) (lower epiphysis) 813.40
      open 813.50
    open 813.90
    shaft 813.20
      open 813.30
    upper end (proximal end) (upper epiphysis) 813.00
      open 813.10
  fossa, anterior, middle, or posterior - *see* Fracture, skull, base
  frontal (bone) - *see also* Fracture, skull, vault
    sinus - *see* Fracture, skull, base
  Galeazzi's - *see* Fracture, radius, lower end
  glenoid (cavity) (fossa) (scapula) (closed) 811.03
    open 811.13
  Gosselin's - *see* Fracture, ankle
  greenstick - *see* Fracture, by site
  grenade-throwers' - *see* Fracture, humerus, shaft
  gutter - *see* Fracture, skull, vault
  hamate (closed) 814.08
    open 814.18
  hand, one (closed) 815.00
    carpals 814.00
      open 814.10
      specified site NEC 814.09
        open 814.19
    metacarpals 815.00
      open 815.10
    multiple, bones of one hand 817.0
      open 817.1
    open 815.10
    phalanges (*see also* Fracture, phalanx, hand) 816.00
      open 816.10
  healing
    aftercare (*see also* Aftercare, fracture) V54.89
    change of cast V54.89
    complications - *see* condition
    convalescence V66.4
    removal of
      cast V54.89
      fixation device
        external V54.89
        internal V54.01
  heel bone (closed) 825.0
    open 825.1
  Hill-Sachs 812.09
  hip (closed) (*see also* Fracture, femur, neck) 820.8
    open 820.9
    pathologic 733.14
  humerus (closed) 812.20
    anatomical neck 812.02
      open 812.12
    articular process (*see also* Fracture humerus, condyle(s)) 812.44
      open 812.54
    capitellum 812.49
      open 812.59
    condyle(s) 812.44
      lateral (external) 812.42
        open 812.52
      medial (internal epicondyle) 812.43
        open 812.53
      open 812.54
    distal end - *see* Fracture, humerus, lower end

Fracture *(Continued)*
  humerus *(Continued)*
    epiphysis
      lower (*see also* Fracture, humerus, condyle(s)) 812.44
        open 812.54
      upper 812.09
        open 812.19
    external condyle 812.42
      open 812.52
    great tuberosity 812.03
      open 812.13
    head 812.09
      open 812.19
    internal epicondyle 812.43
      open 812.53
    lesser tuberosity 812.09
      open 812.19
    lower end or extremity (distal end) (*see also* Fracture, humerus, by site) 812.40
      multiple sites NEC 812.49
        open 812.59
      open 812.50
      specified site NEC 812.49
        open 812.59
    neck 812.01
      open 812.11
    open 812.30
    pathologic 733.11
    proximal end - *see* Fracture, humerus, upper end
    shaft 812.21
      open 812.31
    supracondylar 812.41
      open 812.51
    surgical neck 812.01
      open 812.11
    trochlea 812.49
      open 812.59
    T-shaped 812.44
      open 812.54
    tuberosity - *see* Fracture, humerus, upper end
    upper end or extremity (proximal end) (*see also* Fracture, humerus, by site) 812.00
      open 812.10
      specified site NEC 812.09
        open 812.19
  hyoid bone (closed) 807.5
    open 807.6
  hyperextension - *see* Fracture, radius, lower end
  ilium (with visceral injury) (closed) 808.41
    open 808.51
  impaction, impacted - *see* Fracture, by site
  incus - *see* Fracture, skull, base
  innominate bone (with visceral injury) (closed) 808.49
    open 808.59
  instep, of one foot (closed) 825.20
    with toe(s) of same foot 827.0
      open 827.1
    open 825.30
  insufficiency - *see* Fracture, pathologic, by site
  internal
    ear - *see* Fracture, skull, base
    semilunar cartilage, knee - *see* Tear, meniscus, medial
  intertrochanteric - *see* Fracture, femur, neck, intertrochanteric
  ischium (with visceral injury) (closed) 808.42
    open 808.52
  jaw (bone) (lower) (closed) (*see also* Fracture, mandible) 802.20
    angle 802.25
      open 802.35
    open 802.30
    upper - *see* Fracture, maxilla

Fracture *(Continued)*
  knee
    cap (closed) 822.0
      open 822.1
    cartilage (semilunar) - *see* Tear, meniscus
  labyrinth (osseous) - *see* Fracture, skull, base
  larynx (closed) 807.5
    open 807.6
  late effect - *see* Late, effects (of), fracture
  Le Fort's - *see* Fracture, maxilla
  leg (closed) 827.0
    with rib(s) or sternum 828.0
      open 828.1
    both (any bones) 828.0
      open 828.1
    lower - *see* Fracture, tibia
    open 827.1
    upper - *see* Fracture, femur
  limb
    lower (multiple) (closed) NEC 827.0
      open 827.1
    upper (multiple) (closed) NEC 818.0
      open 818.1
  long bones, due to birth trauma - *see* Birth injury, fracture
  lumbar - *see* Fracture, vertebra, lumbar
  lunate bone (closed) 814.02
    open 814.12
  malar bone (closed) 802.4
    open 802.5
  Malgaigne's (closed) 808.43
    open 808.53
  malleolus (closed) 824.8
    bimalleolar 824.4
      open 824.5
    lateral 824.2
      and medial - *see also* Fracture, malleolus, bimalleolar
        with lip of tibia - *see* Fracture, malleolus, trimalleolar
      open 824.3
    medial (closed) 824.0
      and lateral - *see also* Fracture, malleolus, bimalleolar
        with lip of tibia - *see* Fracture, malleolus, trimalleolar
      open 824.1
    open 824.9
    trimalleolar (closed) 824.6
      open 824.7
  malleus - *see* Fracture, skull, base
  malunion 733.81
  mandible (closed) 802.20
    angle 802.25
      open 802.35
    body 802.28
      alveolar border 802.27
        open 802.37
      open 802.38
      symphysis 802.26
        open 802.36
    condylar process 802.21
      open 802.31
    coronoid process 802.23
      open 802.33
    multiple sites 802.29
      open 802.39
    open 802.30
    ramus NEC 802.24
      open 802.34
    subcondylar 802.22
      open 802.32
  manubrium - *see* Fracture, sternum
  march 733.95
    femoral neck 733.96
    fibula 733.93
    metatarsals 733.94
    pelvis 733.98
    shaft of femur 733.97
    tibia 733.93

SECTION 1 INDEX TO DISEASES AND INJURIES / Fracture

Fracture (Continued)
- maxilla, maxillary (superior) (upper jaw) (closed) 802.4
  - inferior - see Fracture, mandible
  - open 802.5
- meniscus, knee - see Tear, meniscus
- metacarpus, metacarpal (bone(s)), of one hand (closed) 815.00
  - with phalanx, phalanges, hand (finger(s)) (thumb) of same hand 817.0
    - open 817.1
  - base 815.02
    - first metacarpal 815.01
      - open 815.11
    - open 815.12
    - thumb 815.01
      - open 815.11
  - multiple sites 815.09
    - open 815.19
  - neck 815.04
    - open 815.14
  - open 815.10
  - shaft 815.03
    - open 815.13
- metatarsus, metatarsal (bone(s)), of one foot (closed) 825.25
  - with tarsal bone(s) 825.29
    - open 825.39
  - open 825.35
- Monteggia's (closed) 813.03
  - open 813.13
- Moore's - see Fracture, radius, lower end
- multangular bone (closed)
  - larger 814.05
    - open 814.15
  - smaller 814.06
    - open 814.16
- multiple (closed) 829.0

> Note: Multiple fractures of sites classifiable to the same three- or four-digit category are coded to that category, except for sites classifiable to 810–818 or 820–827 in different limbs.
>
> Multiple fractures of sites classifiable to different fourth-digit subdivisions within the same three-digit category should be dealt with according to coding rules.
>
> Multiple fractures of sites classifiable to different three-digit categories (identifiable from the listing under "Fracture"), and of sites classifiable to 810–818 or 820–827 in different limbs should be coded according to the following list, which should be referred to in the following priority order: skull or face bones, pelvis or vertebral column, legs, arms.

- arm (multiple bones in same arm except in hand alone) (sites classifiable to 810–817 with sites classifiable to a different three-digit category in 810–817 in same arm) (closed) 818.0
  - open 818.1
- arms, both or arm(s) with rib(s) or sternum (sites classifiable to 810–818 with sites classifiable to same range of categories in other limb or to 807) (closed) 819.0
  - open 819.1
- bones of trunk NEC (closed) 809.0
  - open 809.1
- hand, metacarpal bone(s) with phalanx or phalanges of same hand (sites classifiable to 815 with sites classifiable to 816 in same hand) (closed) 817.0
  - open 817.1

Fracture (Continued)
- multiple (Continued)
  - leg (multiple bones in same leg) (sites classifiable to 820–826 with sites classifiable to a different three-digit category in that range in same leg) (closed) 827.0
    - open 827.1
  - legs, both or leg(s) with arm(s), rib(s), or sternum (sites classifiable to 820–827 with sites classifiable to same range of categories in other leg or to 807 or 810–819) (closed) 828.0
    - open 828.1
  - open 829.1
  - pelvis with other bones except skull or face bones (sites classifiable to 808 with sites classifiable to 805–807 or 810–829) (closed) 809.0
    - open 809.1
  - skull, specified or unspecified bones, or face bone(s) with any other bone(s) (sites classifiable to 800–803 with sites classifiable to 805–829) (closed) 804.0 ●

> Note: Use the following fifth-digit subclassification with categories 800, 801, 803, and 804:
> 0 unspecified state of consciousness
> 1 with no loss of consciousness
> 2 with brief [less than one hour] loss of consciousness
> 3 with moderate [1–24 hours] loss of consciousness
> 4 with prolonged [more than 24 hours] loss of consciousness and return to pre-existing conscious level
> 5 with prolonged [more than 24 hours] loss of consciousness, without return to pre-existing conscious level
>
> Use fifth-digit 5 to designate when a patient is unconscious and dies before regaining consciousness, regardless of the duration of the loss of consciousness
>
> 6 with loss of consciousness of unspecified duration
> 9 with concussion, unspecified

- with
  - contusion, cerebral 804.1 ●
  - epidural hemorrhage 804.2 ●
  - extradural hemorrhage 804.2 ●
  - hemorrhage (intracranial) NEC 804.3 ●
  - intracranial injury NEC 804.4 ●
  - laceration, cerebral 804.1 ●
  - subarachnoid hemorrhage 804.2 ●
  - subdural hemorrhage 804.2 ●
- open 804.5 ●
  - with
    - contusion, cerebral 804.6 ●
    - epidural hemorrhage 804.7 ●
    - extradural hemorrhage 804.7 ●
    - hemorrhage (intracranial) NEC 804.8 ●
    - intracranial injury NEC 804.9 ●
    - laceration, cerebral 804.6 ●
    - subarachnoid hemorrhage 804.7 ●
    - subdural hemorrhage 804.7 ●
- vertebral column with other bones, except skull or face bones (sites classifiable to 805 or 806 with sites classifiable to 807–808 or 810–829) (closed) 809.0
  - open 809.1

Fracture (Continued)
- nasal (bone(s)) (closed) 802.0
  - open 802.1
  - sinus - see Fracture, skull, base
- navicular
  - carpal (wrist) (closed) 814.01
    - open 814.11
  - tarsal (ankle) (closed) 825.22
    - open 825.32
- neck - see Fracture, vertebra, cervical
- neural arch - see Fracture, vertebra, by site
- nonunion 733.82
- nose, nasal, (bone) (septum) (closed) 802.0
  - open 802.1
- occiput - see Fracture, skull, base
- odontoid process - see Fracture, vertebra, cervical
- olecranon (process) (ulna) (closed) 813.01
  - open 813.11
- open 829.1
- orbit, orbital (bone) (region) (closed) 802.8
  - floor (blow-out) 802.6
    - open 802.7
  - open 802.9
  - roof - see Fracture, skull, base
  - specified part NEC 802.8
    - open 802.9
- os
  - calcis (closed) 825.0
    - open 825.1
  - magnum (closed) 814.07
    - open 814.17
  - pubis (with visceral injury) (closed) 808.2
    - open 808.3
  - triquetrum (closed) 814.03
    - open 814.13
- osseous
  - auditory meatus - see Fracture, skull, base
  - labyrinth - see Fracture, skull, base
- ossicles, auditory (incus) (malleus) (stapes) - see Fracture, skull, base
- osteoporotic - see Fracture, pathologic
- palate (closed) 802.8
  - open 802.9
- paratrooper - see Fracture, tibia, lower end
- parietal bone - see Fracture, skull, vault
- parry - see Fracture, Monteggia's
- patella (closed) 822.0
  - open 822.1
- pathologic (cause unknown) 733.10
  - ankle 733.16
  - femur (neck) 733.14
    - specified NEC 733.15
  - fibula 733.16
  - hip 733.14
  - humerus 733.11
  - radius (distal) 733.12
  - specified site NEC 733.19
  - tibia 733.16
  - ulna 733.12
  - vertebrae (collapse) 733.13
  - wrist 733.12
- pedicle (of vertebral arch) - see Fracture, vertebra, by site
- pelvis, pelvic (bone(s)) (with visceral injury) (closed) 808.8
  - multiple
    - with
      - disruption of pelvic circle 808.43
        - open 808.53
      - disruption of pelvic ring 808.43
        - open 808.53
    - without
      - disruption of pelvic circle 808.44
        - open 808.54
      - disruption of pelvic ring 808.44
        - open 808.54
  - open 808.9
  - rim (closed) 808.49
    - open 808.59
  - stress 733.98

Fracture *(Continued)*
- peritrochanteric (closed) 820.20
  - open 820.30
- phalanx, phalanges, of one
  - foot (closed) 826.0
    - with bone(s) of same lower limb 827.0
      - open 827.1
    - open 826.1
  - hand (closed) 816.00
    - with metacarpal bone(s) of same hand 817.0
      - open 817.1
    - distal 816.02
      - open 816.12
    - middle 816.01
      - open 816.11
    - multiple sites NEC 816.03
      - open 816.13
    - open 816.10
    - proximal 816.01
      - open 816.11
- pisiform (closed) 814.04
  - open 814.14
- pond - *see* Fracture, skull, vault
- Pott's (closed) 824.4
  - open 824.5
- prosthetic device, internal - *see* Complications, mechanical
- pubis (with visceral injury) (closed) 808.2
  - open 808.3
- Quervain's (closed) 814.01
  - open 814.11
- radius (alone) (closed) 813.81
  - with ulna NEC 813.83
    - open 813.93
  - distal end - *see* Fracture, radius, lower end
  - epiphysis
    - lower - *see* Fracture, radius, lower end
    - upper - *see* Fracture, radius, upper end
  - head - *see* Fracture, radius, upper end
  - lower end or extremity (distal end) (lower epiphysis) 813.42
    - with ulna (lower end) 813.44
      - open 813.54
    - open 813.52
    - torus 813.45
      - with ulna 813.47
  - neck - *see* Fracture, radius, upper end
  - open NEC 813.91
  - pathologic 733.12
  - proximal end - *see* Fracture, radius, upper end
  - shaft (closed) 813.21
    - with ulna (shaft) 813.23
      - open 813.33
    - open 813.31
  - upper end 813.07
    - with ulna (upper end) 813.08
      - open 813.18
    - epiphysis 813.05
      - open 813.15
    - head 813.05
      - open 813.15
    - multiple sites 813.07
      - open 813.17
    - neck 813.06
      - open 813.16
    - open 813.17
    - specified site NEC 813.07
      - open 813.17
- ramus
  - inferior or superior (with visceral injury) (closed) 808.2
    - open 808.3
  - ischium - *see* Fracture, ischium
  - mandible 802.24
    - open 802.34

Fracture *(Continued)*
- rib(s) (closed) 807.0 ●

> Note: Use the following fifth-digit subclassification with categories 807.0–807.1:
>
> 0 rib(s), unspecified
> 1 one rib
> 2 two ribs
> 3 three ribs
> 4 four ribs
> 5 five ribs
> 6 six ribs
> 7 seven ribs
> 8 eight or more ribs
> 9 multiple ribs, unspecified

  - with flail chest (open) 807.4
    - open 807.1 ●
- root, tooth 873.63
  - complicated 873.73
- sacrum - *see* Fracture, vertebra, sacrum
- scaphoid
  - ankle (closed) 825.22
    - open 825.32
  - wrist (closed) 814.01
    - open 814.11
- scapula (closed) 811.00
  - acromial, acromion (process) 811.01
    - open 811.11
  - body 811.09
    - open 811.19
  - coracoid process 811.02
    - open 811.12
  - glenoid (cavity) (fossa) 811.03
    - open 811.13
  - neck 811.03
    - open 811.13
  - open 811.10
- semilunar
  - bone, wrist (closed) 814.02
    - open 814.12
  - cartilage (interior) (knee) - *see* Tear, meniscus
- sesamoid bone - *see* Fracture, by site
- Shepherd's (closed) 825.21
  - open 825.31
- shoulder - *see also* Fracture, humerus, upper end
  - blade - *see* Fracture, scapula
- silverfork - *see* Fracture, radius, lower end
- sinus (ethmoid) (frontal) (maxillary) (nasal) (sphenoidal) - *see* Fracture, skull, base
- Skillern's - *see* Fracture, radius, shaft
- skull (multiple NEC) (with face bones) (closed) 803.0 ●

> Note: Use the following fifth-digit subclassification with categories 800, 801, 803, and 804:
>
> 0 unspecified state of consciousness
> 1 with no loss of consciousness
> 2 with brief [less than one hour] loss of consciousness
> 3 with moderate [1-24 hours] loss of consciousness
> 4 with prolonged [more than 24 hours] loss of consciousness and return to pre-existing conscious level
> 5 with prolonged [more than 24 hours] loss of consciousness, without return to pre-existing conscious level
>
> Use fifth-digit 5 to designate when a patient is unconscious and dies before regaining consciousness, regardless of the duration of the loss of consciousness
>
> 6 with loss of consciousness of unspecified duration
> 9 with concussion, unspecified

Fracture *(Continued)*
- skull *(Continued)*
  - with
    - contusion, cerebral 803.1 ●
    - epidural hemorrhage 803.2 ●
    - extradural hemorrhage 803.2 ●
    - hemorrhage (intracranial) NEC 803.3 ●
    - intracranial injury NEC 803.4 ●
    - laceration, cerebral 803.1 ●
    - other bones - *see* Fracture, multiple, skull
    - subarachnoid hemorrhage 803.2 ●
    - subdural hemorrhage 803.2 ●
  - base (antrum) (ethmoid bone) (fossa) (internal ear) (nasal sinus) (occiput) (sphenoid) (temporal bone) (closed) 801.0 ●
    - with
      - contusion, cerebral 801.1 ●
      - epidural hemorrhage 801.2 ●
      - extradural hemorrhage 801.2 ●
      - hemorrhage (intracranial) NEC 801.3 ●
      - intracranial injury NEC 801.4 ●
      - laceration, cerebral 801.1 ●
      - subarachnoid hemorrhage 801.2 ●
      - subdural hemorrhage 801.2 ●
    - open 801.5 ●
      - with
        - contusion, cerebral 801.6 ●
        - epidural hemorrhage 801.7 ●
        - extradural hemorrhage 801.7 ●
        - hemorrhage (intracranial) NEC 801.8 ●
        - intracranial injury NEC 801.9 ●
        - laceration, cerebral 801.6 ●
        - subarachnoid hemorrhage 801.7 ●
        - subdural hemorrhage 801.7 ●
  - birth injury 767.3
  - face bones - *see* Fracture, face bones
  - open 803.5 ●
    - with
      - contusion, cerebral 803.6 ●
      - epidural hemorrhage 803.7 ●
      - extradural hemorrhage 803.7 ●
      - hemorrhage (intracranial) NEC 803.8 ●
      - intracranial injury NEC 803.9 ●
      - laceration, cerebral 803.6 ●
      - subarachnoid hemorrhage 803.7 ●
      - subdural hemorrhage 803.7 ●
  - vault (frontal bone) (parietal bone) (vertex) (closed) 800.0 ●
    - with
      - contusion, cerebral 800.1 ●
      - epidural hemorrhage 800.2 ●
      - extradural hemorrhage 800.2 ●
      - hemorrhage (intracranial) NEC 800.3 ●
      - intracranial injury NEC 800.4 ●
      - laceration, cerebral 800.1 ●
      - subarachnoid hemorrhage 800.2 ●
      - subdural hemorrhage 800.2 ●
    - open 800.5 ●
      - with
        - contusion, cerebral 800.6 ●
        - epidural hemorrhage 800.7 ●
        - extradural hemorrhage 800.7 ●
        - hemorrhage (intracranial) NEC 800.8 ●
        - intracranial injury NEC 800.9 ●
        - laceration, cerebral 800.6 ●
        - subarachnoid hemorrhage 800.7 ●
        - subdural hemorrhage 800.7 ●
- Smith's 813.41
  - open 813.51
- sphenoid (bone) (sinus) - *see* Fracture, skull, base

SECTION I INDEX TO DISEASES AND INJURIES / Fracture

Fracture (Continued)
  spine - *see also* Fracture, vertebra, by site due to birth trauma 767.4
  spinous process - *see* Fracture, vertebra, by site
  spontaneous - *see* Fracture, pathologic
  sprinters' - *see* Fracture, ilium
  stapes - *see* Fracture, skull, base
  stave - *see also* Fracture, metacarpus, metacarpal bone(s)
    spine - *see* Fracture, tibia, upper end
  sternum (closed) 807.2
    with flail chest (open) 807.4
    open 807.3
  Stieda's - *see* Fracture, femur, lower end
  stress 733.95
    femoral neck 733.96
    fibula 733.93
    metatarsals 733.94
    pelvis 733.98
    shaft of femur 733.97
    specified site NEC 733.95
    tibia 733.93
  styloid process
    metacarpal (closed) 815.02
      open 815.12
    radius - *see* Fracture, radius, lower end
    temporal bone - *see* Fracture, skull, base
    ulna - *see* Fracture, ulna, lower end
  supracondylar, elbow 812.41
    open 812.51
  symphysis pubis (with visceral injury) (closed) 808.2
    open 808.3
  talus (ankle bone) (closed) 825.21
    open 825.31
  tarsus, tarsal bone(s) (with metatarsus) of one foot (closed) NEC 825.29
    open 825.39
  temporal bone (styloid) - *see* Fracture, skull, base
  tendon - *see* Sprain, by site
  thigh - *see* Fracture, femur, shaft
  thumb (and finger(s)) of one hand (closed) (*see also* Fracture, phalanx, hand) 816.00
    with metacarpal bone(s) of same hand 817.0
      open 817.1
    metacarpal(s) - *see* Fracture, metacarpus
    open 816.10
  thyroid cartilage (closed) 807.5
    open 807.6
  tibia (closed) 823.80
    with fibula 823.82
      open 823.92
    condyles - *see* Fracture, tibia, upper end
    distal end 824.8
      open 824.9
    epiphysis
      lower 824.8
        open 824.9
      upper - *see* Fracture, tibia, upper end
    head (involving knee joint) - *see* Fracture, tibia, upper end
    intercondyloid eminence - *see* Fracture, tibia, upper end
    involving ankle 824.0
      open 824.1
    lower end or extremity (anterior lip) (posterior lip) 824.8
      open 824.9
    malleolus (internal) (medial) 824.0
      open 824.1
    open NEC 823.90
    pathologic 733.16
    proximal end - *see* Fracture, tibia, upper end
    shaft 823.20
      with fibula 823.22
        open 823.32
      open 823.30

Fracture (Continued)
  tibia (Continued)
    spine - *see* Fracture, tibia, upper end
    stress 733.93
    torus 823.40
      with fibula 823.42
    tuberosity - *see* Fracture, tibia, upper end
    upper end or extremity (condyle) (epiphysis) (head) (spine) (proximal end) (tuberosity) 823.00
      with fibula 823.02
        open 823.12
      open 823.10
  toe(s), of one foot (closed) 826.0
    with bone(s) of same lower limb 827.0
      open 827.1
    open 826.1
  tooth (root) 873.63
    complicated 873.73
  torus
    fibula 823.41
      with tibia 823.42
    humerus 812.49
    radius (alone) 813.45
      with ulna 813.47
    tibia 823.40
      with fibula 823.42
    ulna (alone) 813.46
      with radius 813.47
  trachea (closed) 807.5
    open 807.6
  transverse process - *see* Fracture, vertebra, by site
  trapezium (closed) 814.05
    open 814.15
  trapezoid bone (closed) 814.06
    open 814.16
  trimalleolar (closed) 824.6
    open 824.7
  triquetral (bone) (closed) 814.03
    open 814.13
  trochanter (greater) (lesser) (closed) (*see also* Fracture, femur, neck, by site) 820.20
    open 820.30
  trunk (bones) (closed) 809.0
    open 809.1
  tuberosity (external) - *see* Fracture, by site
  ulna (alone) (closed) 813.82
    with radius NEC 813.83
      open 813.93
    coronoid process (closed) 813.02
      open 813.12
    distal end - *see* Fracture, ulna, lower end
    epiphysis
      lower - *see* Fracture, ulna, lower end
      upper - *see* Fracture, ulna, upper, end
    head - *see* Fracture, ulna, lower end
    lower end (distal end) (head) (lower epiphysis) (styloid process) 813.43
      with radius (lower end) 813.44
        open 813.54
      open 813.53
    olecranon process (closed) 813.01
      open 813.11
    open NEC 813.92
    pathologic 733.12
    proximal end - *see* Fracture, ulna, upper end
    shaft 813.22
      with radius (shaft) 813.23
        open 813.33
      open 813.32
    styloid process - *see* Fracture, ulna, lower end
    torus 813.46
      with radius 813.47
    transverse - *see* Fracture, ulna, by site

Fracture (Continued)
  ulna (Continued)
    upper end (epiphysis) 813.04
      with radius (upper end) 813.08
        open 813.18
      multiple sites 813.04
        open 813.14
      open 813.14
      specified site NEC 813.04
        open 813.14
  unciform (closed) 814.08
    open 814.18
  vertebra, vertebral (back) (body) (column) (neural arch) (pedicle) (spine) (spinous process) (transverse process) (closed) 805.8
    with
      hematomyelia - *see* Fracture, vertebra, by site, with spinal cord injury
      injury to
        cauda equina - *see* Fracture, vertebra, sacrum, with spinal cord injury
        nerve - *see* Fracture, vertebra, by site, with spinal cord injury
      paralysis - *see* Fracture, vertebra, by site, with spinal cord injury
      paraplegia - *see* Fracture, vertebra, by site, with spinal cord injury
      quadriplegia - *see* Fracture, vertebra, by site, with spinal cord injury
      spinal concussion - *see* Fracture, vertebra, by site, with spinal cord injury
      spinal cord injury (closed) NEC 806.8

> Note: Use the following fifth-digit subclassification with categories 806.0–806.3:
>
> C_1–C_4 or unspecified level and D_1–D_6 (T_1–T_6) or unspecified level with:
>
> 0   unspecified spinal cord injury
> 1   complete lesion of cord
> 2   anterior cord syndrome
> 3   central cord syndrome
> 4   specified injury NEC
>
> level and D_1–D_{12} level with:
>
> 5   unspecified spinal cord injury
> 6   complete lesion of cord
> 7   anterior cord syndrome
> 8   central cord syndrome
> 9   specified injury NEC

        cervical 806.0●
          open 806.1●
        chronic 733.13
        dorsal, dorsolumbar 806.2●
          open 806.3●
        open 806.9
        thoracic, thoracolumbar 806.2●
          open 806.3●
    atlanto-axial - *see* Fracture, vertebra, cervical
    cervical (hangman) (teardrop) (closed) 805.00
      with spinal cord injury - *see* Fracture, vertebra, with spinal cord injury, cervical
      first (atlas) 805.01
        open 805.11
      second (axis) 805.02
        open 805.12
      third 805.03
        open 805.13
      fourth 805.04
        open 805.14
      fifth 805.05
        open 805.15
      sixth 805.06
        open 805.16

Fracture *(Continued)*
  vertebra, vertebral *(Continued)*
    cervical *(Continued)*
      seventh 805.07
        open 805.17
      multiple sites 805.08
        open 805.18
      open 805.10
    coccyx (closed) 805.6
      with spinal cord injury (closed) 806.60
        cauda equina injury 806.62
          complete lesion 806.61
            open 806.71
          open 806.72
        open 806.70
        specified type NEC 806.69
          open 806.79
      open 805.7
    collapsed 733.13
    compression, not due to trauma 733.13
    dorsal (closed) 805.2
      with spinal cord injury - see Fracture, vertebra, with spinal cord injury, dorsal
      open 805.3
    dorsolumbar (closed) 805.2
      with spinal cord injury - see Fracture, vertebra, with spinal cord injury, dorsal
      open 805.3
    due to osteoporosis 733.13
    fetus or newborn 767.4
    lumbar (closed) 805.4
      with spinal cord injury (closed) 806.4
        open 806.5
      open 805.5
    nontraumatic 733.13
    open NEC 805.9
    pathologic (any site) 733.13
    sacrum (closed) 805.6
      with spinal cord injury 806.60
        cauda equina injury 806.62
          complete lesion 806.61
            open 806.71
          open 806.72
        open 806.70
        specified type NEC 806.69
          open 806.79
      open 805.7
    site unspecified (closed) 805.8
      with spinal cord injury (closed) 806.8
        open 806.9
      open 805.9
    stress (any site) 733.95
    thoracic (closed) 805.2
      with spinal cord injury - see Fracture, vertebra, with spinal cord injury, thoracic
      open 805.3
    vertex - see Fracture, skull, vault
    vomer (bone) 802.0
      open 802.1
    Wagstaffe's - see Fracture, ankle
    wrist (closed) 814.00
      open 814.10
      pathologic 733.12
    xiphoid (process) - see Fracture, sternum
    zygoma (zygomatic arch) (closed) 802.4
      open 802.5
Fragile X syndrome 759.83
Fragilitas
  crinium 704.2
  hair 704.2
  ossium 756.51
    with blue sclera 756.51
  unguium 703.8
    congenital 757.5
Fragility
  bone 756.51
    with deafness and blue sclera 756.51
  capillary (hereditary) 287.8

Fragility *(Continued)*
  hair 704.2
  nails 703.8
Fragmentation - see Fracture, by site
Frailty 797
Frambesia, frambesial (tropica) *(see also* Yaws) 102.9
  initial lesion or ulcer 102.0
  primary 102.0
Frambeside
  gummatous 102.4
  of early yaws 102.2
Frambesioma 102.1
Franceschetti's syndrome (mandibulofacial dysostosis) 756.0
Francis' disease *(see also* Tularemia) 021.9
Frank's essential thrombocytopenia *(see also* Purpura, thrombocytopenic) 287.39
Franklin's disease (heavy chain) 273.2
Fraser's syndrome 759.89
Freckle 709.09
  malignant melanoma in (M8742/3) - see Melanoma
  melanotic (of Hutchinson) (M8742/2) - see Neoplasm, skin, in situ
  retinal 239.81
Freeman-Sheldon syndrome 759.89
Freezing 991.9
  specified effect NEC 991.8
Frei's disease (climatic bubo) 099.1
Freiberg's
  disease (osteochondrosis, second metatarsal) 732.5
  infraction of metatarsal head 732.5
  osteochondrosis 732.5
Fremitus, friction, cardiac 785.3
Frenulum linguae 750.0
Frenum
  external os 752.44
  tongue 750.0
Frequency (urinary) NEC 788.41
  micturition 788.41
  nocturnal 788.43
  polyuria 788.42
  psychogenic 306.53
Frey's syndrome (auriculotemporal syndrome) 705.22
Friction
  burn *(see also* Injury, superficial, by site) 919.0
  fremitus, cardiac 785.3
  precordial 785.3
  sounds, chest 786.7
Friderichsen-Waterhouse syndrome or disease 036.3
Friedländer's
  B (bacillus) NEC *(see also* condition) 041.3
    sepsis or septicemia 038.49
  disease (endarteritis obliterans) - see Arteriosclerosis
Friedreich's
  ataxia 334.0
  combined systemic disease 334.0
  disease 333.2
    combined systemic 334.0
  myoclonia 333.2
  sclerosis (spinal cord) 334.0
Friedrich-Erb-Arnold syndrome (acropachyderma) 757.39
Frigidity 302.72
  psychic or psychogenic 302.72
Fröhlich's disease or syndrome (adiposogenital dystrophy) 253.8
Froin's syndrome 336.8
Frommel's disease 676.6●
Frommel-Chiari syndrome 676.6●
Frontal - see also condition
  lobe syndrome 310.0
Frostbite 991.3
  face 991.0
  foot 991.2

Frostbite *(Continued)*
  hand 991.1
  specified site NEC 991.3
Frotteurism 302.89
Frozen 991.9
  pelvis 620.8
  shoulder 726.0
Fructosemia 271.2
Fructosuria (benign) (essential) 271.2
Fuchs'
  black spot (myopic) 360.21
  corneal dystrophy (endothelial) 371.57
  heterochromic cyclitis 364.21
Fucosidosis 271.8
Fugue 780.99
  dissociative 300.13
  hysterical (dissociative) 300.13
  reaction to exceptional stress (transient) 308.1
Fukuhara syndrome 277.87
Fuller Albright's syndrome (osteitis fibrosa disseminata) 756.59
Fuller's earth disease 502
Fulminant, fulminating - see condition
Functional - see condition
Functioning
  borderline intellectual V62.89
Fundus - see also condition
  flavimaculatus 362.76
Fungemia 117.9
Fungus, fungous
  cerebral 348.89
  disease NEC 117.9
  infection - see Infection, fungus
  testis *(see also* Tuberculosis) 016.5● [608.81]
Funiculitis (acute) 608.4
  chronic 608.4
  endemic 608.4
  gonococcal (acute) 098.14
    chronic or duration of 2 months or over 098.34
  tuberculous *(see also* Tuberculosis) 016.5●
FUO *(see also* Pyrexia) 780.60
Funnel
  breast (acquired) 738.3
    congenital 754.81
    late effect of rickets 268.1
  chest (acquired) 738.3
    congenital 754.81
    late effect of rickets 268.1
  pelvis (acquired) 738.6
    with disproportion (fetopelvic) 653.3●
      affecting fetus or newborn 763.1
      causing obstructed labor 660.1●
        affecting fetus or newborn 763.1
    congenital 755.69
    tuberculous *(see also* Tuberculosis) 016.9●
Furfur 690.18
  microsporon 111.0
Furor, paroxysmal (idiopathic) *(see also* Epilepsy) 345.8●
Furriers' lung 495.8
Furrowed tongue 529.5
  congenital 750.13
Furrowing nail(s) (transverse) 703.8
  congenital 757.5
Furuncle 680.9
  abdominal wall 680.2
  ankle 680.6
  anus 680.5
  arm (any part, above wrist) 680.3
  auditory canal, external 680.0
  axilla 680.3
  back (any part) 680.2
  breast 680.2
  buttock 680.5
  chest wall 680.2
  corpus cavernosum 607.2
  ear (any part) 680.0
  eyelid 373.13
  face (any part, except eye) 680.0
  finger (any) 680.4

Furuncle (Continued)
- flank 680.2
- foot (any part) 680.7
- forearm 680.3
- gluteal (region) 680.5
- groin 680.2
- hand (any part) 680.4
- head (any part, except face) 680.8
- heel 680.7
- hip 680.6
- kidney (see also Abscess, kidney) 590.2
- knee 680.6
- labium (majus) (minus) 616.4
- lacrimal
    - gland (see also Dacryoadenitis) 375.00
    - passages (duct) (sac) (see also Dacryocystitis) 375.30
- leg, any part except foot 680.6
- malignant 022.0
- multiple sites 680.9
- neck 680.1
- nose (external) (septum) 680.0
- orbit 376.01
- partes posteriores 680.5
- pectoral region 680.2
- penis 607.2
- perineum 680.2
- pinna 680.0
- scalp (any part) 680.8
- scrotum 608.4
- seminal vesicle 608.0
- shoulder 680.3
- skin NEC 680.9
- specified site NEC 680.8
- spermatic cord 608.4
- temple (region) 680.0
- testis 604.90
- thigh 680.6
- thumb 680.4
- toe (any) 680.7
- trunk 680.2

Furuncle (Continued)
- tunica vaginalis 608.4
- umbilicus 680.2
- upper arm 680.3
- vas deferens 608.4
- vulva 616.4
- wrist 680.4

Furunculosis (see also Furuncle) 680.9
- external auditory meatus 680.0 [380.13]

Fusarium (infection) 118

Fusion, fused (congenital)
- anal (with urogenital canal) 751.5
- aorta and pulmonary artery 745.0
- astragaloscaphoid 755.67
- atria 745.5
- atrium and ventricle 745.69
- auditory canal 744.02
- auricles, heart 745.5
- binocular, with defective stereopsis 368.33
- bone 756.9
- cervical spine - see Fusion, spine
- choanal 748.0
- commissure, mitral valve 746.5
- cranial sutures, premature 756.0
- cusps, heart valve NEC 746.89
    - mitral 746.5
    - tricuspid 746.89
- ear ossicles 744.04
- fingers (see also Syndactylism, fingers) 755.11
- hymen 752.42
- hymeno-urethral 599.89
    - causing obstructed labor 660.1●
        - affecting fetus or newborn 763.1
- joint (acquired) - see also Ankylosis
    - congenital 755.8
- kidneys (incomplete) 753.3
- labium (majus) (minus) 752.49
- larynx and trachea 748.3
- limb 755.8
    - lower 755.69
    - upper 755.59

Fusion, fused (Continued)
- lobe, lung 748.5
- lumbosacral (acquired) 724.6
    - congenital 756.15
    - surgical V45.4
- nares (anterior) (posterior) 748.0
- nose, nasal 748.0
- nostril(s) 748.0
- organ or site NEC - see Anomaly, specified type NEC
- ossicles 756.9
    - auditory 744.04
- pulmonary valve segment 746.02
- pulmonic cusps 746.02
- ribs 756.3
- sacroiliac (acquired) (joint) 724.6
    - congenital 755.69
    - surgical V45.4
- skull, imperfect 756.0
- spine (acquired) 724.9
    - arthrodesis status V45.4
    - congenital (vertebra) 756.15
    - postoperative status V45.4
- sublingual duct with submaxillary duct at opening in mouth 750.26
- talonavicular (bar) 755.67
- teeth, tooth 520.2
- testes 752.89
- toes (see also Syndactylism, toes) 755.13
- trachea and esophagus 750.3
- twins 759.4
- urethral-hymenal 599.89
- vagina 752.49
- valve cusps - see Fusion, cusps, heart valve
- ventricles, heart 745.4
- vertebra (arch) - see Fusion, spine
- vulva 752.49

Fusospirillosis (mouth) (tongue) (tonsil) 101

Fussy infant (baby) 780.91

G

Gafsa boil 085.1
Gain, weight (abnormal) (excessive) (see also Weight, gain) 783.1
Gaisböck's disease or syndrome (polycythemia hypertonica) 289.0
Gait
    abnormality 781.2
        hysterical 300.11
    ataxic 781.2
        hysterical 300.11
    disturbance 781.2
        hysterical 300.11
    paralytic 781.2
    scissor 781.2
    spastic 781.2
    staggering 781.2
        hysterical 300.11
Galactocele (breast) (infected) 611.5
    puerperal, postpartum 676.8 ●
Galactophoritis 611.0
    puerperal, postpartum 675.2 ●
Galactorrhea 676.6 ●
    not associated with childbirth 611.6
Galactosemia (classic) (congenital) 271.1
Galactosuria 271.1
Galacturia 791.1
    bilharziasis 120.0
Galen's vein - see condition
Gallbladder - see also condition
    acute (see also Disease, gallbladder) 575.0
Gall duct - see condition
Gallop rhythm 427.89
Gallstone (cholemic) (colic) (impacted) - see also Cholelithiasis
    causing intestinal obstruction 560.31
Gambling, pathological 312.31
Gammaloidosis 277.39
Gammopathy 273.9
    macroglobulinemia 273.3
    monoclonal (benign) (essential) (idiopathic) (with lymphoplasmacytic dyscrasia) 273.1
Gamna's disease (siderotic splenomegaly) 289.51
Gampsodactylia (congenital) 754.71
Gamstorp's disease (adynamia episodica hereditaria) 359.3
Gandy-Nanta disease (siderotic splenomegaly) 289.51
Gang activity, without manifest psychiatric disorder V71.09
    adolescent V71.02
    adult V71.01
    child V71.02
Gangliocytoma (M9490/0) - see Neoplasm, connective tissue, benign
Ganglioglioma (M9505/1) - see Neoplasm, by site, uncertain behavior
Ganglion 727.43
    joint 727.41
    of yaws (early) (late) 102.6
    periosteal (see also Periostitis) 730.3 ●
    tendon sheath (compound) (diffuse) 727.42
    tuberculous (see also Tuberculosis) 015.9 ●
Ganglioneuroblastoma (M9490/3) - see Neoplasm, connective tissue, malignant
Ganglioneuroma (M9490/0) - see Neoplasm, connective tissue, benign
    malignant (M9490/3) - see Neoplasm, connective tissue, malignant
Ganglioneuromatosis (M9491/0) - see Neoplasm, connective tissue, benign
Ganglionitis
    fifth nerve (see also Neuralgia, trigeminal) 350.1
    gasserian 350.1
    geniculate 351.1
        herpetic 053.11
        newborn 767.5

Ganglionitis (Continued)
    herpes zoster 053.11
    herpetic geniculate (Hunt's syndrome) 053.11
Gangliosidosis 330.1
Gangosa 102.5
Gangrene, gangrenous (anemia) (artery) (cellulitis) (dermatitis) (dry) (infective) (moist) (pemphigus) (septic) (skin) (stasis) (ulcer) 785.4
    with
        arteriosclerosis (native artery) 440.24
            bypass graft 440.30
                autologous vein 440.31
                nonautologous biological 440.32
        diabetes (mellitus) 250.7 ● [785.4]
            due to secondary diabetes 249.7 ● [785.4]
    abdomen (wall) 785.4
    adenitis 683
    alveolar 526.5
    angina 462
        diphtheritic 032.0
    anus 569.49
    appendices epiploicae - see Gangrene, mesentery
    appendix - see Appendicitis, acute
    arteriosclerotic - see Arteriosclerosis, with, gangrene
    auricle 785.4
    Bacillus welchii (see also Gangrene, gas) 040.0
    bile duct (see also Cholangitis) 576.8
    bladder 595.89
    bowel - see Gangrene, intestine
    cecum - see Gangrene, intestine
    Clostridium perfringens or welchii (see also Gangrene, gas) 040.0
    colon - see Gangrene, intestine
    connective tissue 785.4
    cornea 371.40
    corpora cavernosa (infective) 607.2
        noninfective 607.89
    cutaneous, spreading 785.4
    decubital (see also Ulcer, pressure) 707.00 [785.4]
    diabetic (any site) 250.7 ● [785.4]
        due to secondary diabetes 249.7 ● [785.4]
    dropsical 785.4
    emphysematous (see also Gangrene, gas) 040.0
    epidemic (ergotized grain) 988.2
    epididymis (infectional) (see also Epididymitis) 604.99
    erysipelas (see also Erysipelas) 035
    extremity (lower) (upper) 785.4
    gallbladder or duct (see also Cholecystitis, acute) 575.0
    gas (bacillus) 040.0
        with
            abortion - see Abortion, by type, with sepsis
            ectopic pregnancy (see also categories 633.0–633.9) 639.0
            molar pregnancy (see also categories 630–632) 639.0
        following
            abortion 639.0
            ectopic or molar pregnancy 639.0
        puerperal, postpartum, childbirth 670.8 ●
    glossitis 529.0
    gum 523.8
    hernia - see Hernia, by site, with gangrene
    hospital noma 528.1
    intestine, intestinal (acute) (hemorrhagic) (massive) 557.0
        with
            hernia - see Hernia, by site, with gangrene
            mesenteric embolism or infarction 557.0
            obstruction (see also Obstruction, intestine) 560.9

Gangrene, gangrenous (Continued)
    laryngitis 464.00
        with obstruction 464.01
    liver 573.8
    lung 513.0
        spirochetal 104.8
    lymphangitis 457.2
    Meleney's (cutaneous) 686.09
    mesentery 557.0
        with
            embolism or infarction 557.0
                intestinal obstruction (see also Obstruction, intestine) 560.9
    mouth 528.1
    noma 528.1
    orchitis 604.90
    ovary (see also Salpingo-oophoritis) 614.2
    pancreas 577.0
    penis (infectional) 607.2
        noninfective 607.89
    perineum 785.4
    pharynx 462
        septic 034.0
    pneumonia 513.0
    Pott's 440.24
    presenile 443.1
    pulmonary 513.0
    pulp, tooth 522.1
    quinsy 475
    Raynaud's (symmetric gangrene) 443.0 [785.4]
    rectum 569.49
    retropharyngeal 478.24
    rupture - see Hernia, by site, with gangrene
    scrotum 608.4
        noninfective 608.83
    senile 440.24
    sore throat 462
    spermatic cord 608.4
        noninfective 608.89
    spine 785.4
    spirochetal NEC 104.8
    spreading cutaneous 785.4
    stomach 537.89
    stomatitis 528.1
    symmetrical 443.0 [785.4]
    testis (infectional) (see also Orchitis) 604.99
        noninfective 608.89
    throat 462
        diphtheritic 032.0
    thyroid (gland) 246.8
    tonsillitis (acute) 463
    tooth (pulp) 522.1
    tuberculous NEC (see also Tuberculosis) 011.9 ●
    tunica vaginalis 608.4
        noninfective 608.89
    umbilicus 785.4
    uterus (see also Endometritis) 615.9
    uvulitis 528.3
    vas deferens 608.4
        noninfective 608.89
    vulva (see also Vulvitis) 616.10
Gannister disease (occupational) 502
    with tuberculosis - see Tuberculosis, pulmonary
Ganser's syndrome, hysterical 300.16
Gardner-Diamond syndrome (autoerythrocyte sensitization) 287.2
Gargoylism 277.5
Garré's
    disease (see also Osteomyelitis) 730.1 ●
    osteitis (sclerosing) (see also Osteomyelitis) 730.1 ●
    osteomyelitis (see also Osteomyelitis) 730.1 ●
Garrod's pads, knuckle 728.79
Gartner's duct
    cyst 752.41
    persistent 752.41

 New   ◀▥ Revised   ~~deleted~~ Deleted   ● Use Additional Digit(s)   Omit code

SECTION 1 INDEX TO DISEASES AND INJURIES / Gas

Gas 787.3
- asphyxia, asphyxiation, inhalation, poisoning, suffocation NEC 987.9
  - specified gas - see Table of Drugs and Chemicals
- bacillus gangrene or infection - see Gas, gangrene
- cyst, mesentery 568.89
- excessive 787.3
- gangrene 040.0
  - with
    - abortion - see Abortion, by type, with sepsis
    - ectopic pregnancy (see also categories 633.0–633.9) 639.0
    - molar pregnancy (see also categories 630–632) 639.0
  - following
    - abortion 639.0
    - ectopic or molar pregnancy 639.0
  - puerperal, postpartum, childbirth 670.8●
- on stomach 787.3
- pains 787.3

Gastradenitis 535.0●
Gastralgia 536.8
- psychogenic 307.89
Gastrectasis, gastrectasia 536.1
- psychogenic 306.4
Gastric - see condition
Gastrinoma (M8153/1)
- malignant (M8153/3)
  - pancreas 157.4
  - specified site NEC - see Neoplasm, by site, malignant
  - unspecified site 157.4
- specified site - see Neoplasm, by site, uncertain behavior
- unspecified site 235.5
Gastritis 535.5●

Note: Use the following fifth-digit subclassification for category 535:
- 0 without mention of hemorrhage
- 1 with hemorrhage

- acute 535.0●
- alcoholic 535.3●
- allergic 535.4●
- antral 535.4●
- atrophic 535.1●
- atrophic-hyperplastic 535.1●
- bile-induced 535.4●
- catarrhal 535.0●
- chronic (atrophic) 535.1●
- cirrhotic 535.4●
- corrosive (acute) 535.4●
- dietetic 535.4●
- due to diet deficiency 269.9 [535.4]●
- eosinophilic 535.7●
- erosive 535.4●
- follicular 535.4●
  - chronic 535.1●
- giant hypertrophic 535.2●
- glandular 535.4●
  - chronic 535.1●
- hypertrophic (mucosa) 535.2●
  - chronic giant 211.1
- irritant 535.4●
- nervous 306.4
- phlegmonous 535.0●
- psychogenic 306.4
- sclerotic 535.4●
- spastic 536.8
- subacute 535.0●
- superficial 535.4●
- suppurative 535.0●
- toxic 535.4●
- tuberculous (see also Tuberculosis) 017.9●
Gastrocarcinoma (M8010/3) 151.9
Gastrocolic - see condition

Gastrocolitis - see Enteritis
Gastrodisciasis 121.8
Gastroduodenitis (see also Gastritis) 535.5●
- catarrhal 535.0●
- infectional 535.0●
- virus, viral 008.8
  - specified type NEC 008.69
Gastrodynia 536.8
Gastroenteritis (acute) (catarrhal) (congestive) (hemorrhagic) (noninfectious) (see also Enteritis) 558.9
- aertrycke infection 003.0
- allergic 558.3
- chronic 558.9
  - ulcerative (see also Colitis, ulcerative) 556.9
- dietetic 558.9
- due to
  - antineoplastic chemotherapy 558.9
  - food poisoning (see also Poisoning, food) 005.9
  - radiation 558.1
- eosinophilic 558.41
- epidemic 009.0
- functional 558.9
- infectious (see also Enteritis, due to, by organism) 009.0
  - presumed 009.1
- salmonella 003.0
- septic (see also Enteritis, due to, by organism) 009.0
- toxic 558.2
- tuberculous (see also Tuberculosis) 014.8●
- ulcerative (see also Colitis, ulcerative) 556.9
- viral NEC 008.8
  - specified type NEC 008.69
- zymotic 009.0
Gastroenterocolitis - see Enteritis
Gastroenteropathy, protein-losing 579.8
Gastroenteroptosis 569.89
Gastroesophageal laceration-hemorrhage syndrome 530.7
Gastroesophagitis 530.19
Gastrohepatitis (see also Gastritis) 535.5●
Gastrointestinal - see condition
Gastrojejunal - see condition
Gastrojejunitis (see also Gastritis) 535.5●
Gastrojejunocolic - see condition
Gastroliths 537.89
Gastromalacia 537.89
Gastroparalysis 536.3
- diabetic 250.6● [536.3]
  - due to secondary diabetes 249.6● [536.3]
Gastroparesis 536.3
- diabetic 250.6● [536.3]
  - due to secondary diabetes 249.6● [536.3]
Gastropathy 537.9
- congestive portal 537.89
- erythematous 535.5●
- exudative 579.8
- portal hypertensive 537.89
Gastroptosis 537.5
Gastrorrhagia 578.0
Gastrorrhea 536.8
- psychogenic 306.4
Gastroschisis (congenital) 756.73
- acquired 569.89
Gastrospasm (neurogenic) (reflex) 536.8
- neurotic 306.4
- psychogenic 306.4
Gastrostaxis 578.0
Gastrostenosis 537.89
Gastrostomy
- attention to V55.1
- complication 536.40
  - specified type 536.49
- infection 536.41
- malfunctioning 536.42
- status V44.1

Gastrosuccorrhea (continuous) (intermittent) 536.8
- neurotic 306.4
- psychogenic 306.4
Gaucher's
- disease (adult) (cerebroside lipidosis) (infantile) 272.7
- hepatomegaly 272.7
- splenomegaly (cerebroside lipidosis) 272.7
GAVE (gastric antral vascular ectasia) 537.82
- with hemorrhage 537.83
- without hemorrhage 537.82
Gayet's disease (superior hemorrhagic polioencephalitis) 265.1
Gayet-Wernicke's syndrome (superior hemorrhagic polioencephalitis) 265.1
Gee (-Herter) (-Heubner) (-Thaysen) disease or syndrome (nontropical sprue) 579.0
Gélineau's syndrome (see also Narcolepsy) 347.00
Gemination, teeth 520.2
Gemistocytoma (M9411/3)
- specified site - see Neoplasm, by site, malignant
- unspecified site 191.9
General, generalized - see condition
Genetic
- susceptibility to
  - MEN (multiple endocrine neoplasia) V84.81
  - neoplasia
    - multiple endocrine (MEN) V84.81
  - neoplasm
    - malignant, of
      - breast V84.01
      - endometrium V84.04
      - other V84.09
      - ovary V84.02
      - prostate V84.03
    - specified disease NEC V84.89
Genital - see condition
- warts 078.11
Genito-anorectal syndrome 099.1
Genitourinary system - see condition
Genu
- congenital 755.64
- extrorsum (acquired) 736.42
  - congenital 755.64
  - late effects of rickets 268.1
- introrsum (acquired) 736.41
  - congenital 755.64
  - late effects of rickets 268.1
- rachitic (old) 268.1
- recurvatum (acquired) 736.5
  - congenital 754.40
    - with dislocation of knee 754.41
  - late effects of rickets 268.1
- valgum (acquired) (knock-knee) 736.41
  - congenital 755.64
  - late effects of rickets 268.1
- varum (acquired) (bowleg) 736.42
  - congenital 755.64
  - late effect of rickets 268.1
Geographic tongue 529.1
Geophagia 307.52
Geotrichosis 117.9
- intestine 117.9
- lung 117.9
- mouth 117.9
Gephyrophobia 300.29
Gerbode defect 745.4
GERD (gastroesophageal reflux disease) 530.81
Gerhardt's
- disease (erythromelalgia) 443.82
- syndrome (vocal cord paralysis) 478.30
Gerlier's disease (epidemic vertigo) 078.81
German measles 056.9
- exposure to V01.4
Germinoblastoma (diffuse) (M9614/3) 202.8●
- follicular (M9692/3) 202.0●

SECTION 1 INDEX TO DISEASES AND INJURIES / Glaucoma

Germinoma (M9064/3) - see Neoplasm, by site, malignant
Gerontoxon 371.41
Gerstmann-Sträussler-Scheinker syndrome (GSS) 046.71
Gerstmann's syndrome (finger agnosia) 784.69
Gestation (period) - see also Pregnancy
  ectopic NEC (see also Pregnancy, ectopic) 633.90
    with intrauterine pregnancy 633.91
  multiple
    placenta status
      quadruplet
        two or more monoamniotic fetuses V91.22
        two or more monochorionic fetuses V91.21
        unable to determine number of placenta and number of amniotic sacs V91.29
        unspecified number of placenta and unspecified number of amniotic sacs V91.20
      specified (greater than quadruplets) NEC
        two or more monoamniotic fetuses V91.92
        two or more monochorionic fetuses V91.91
        unable to determine number of placenta and number of amniotic sacs V91.99
        unspecified number of placenta and unspecified number of amniotic sacs V91.90
      triplet
        two or more monoamniotic fetuses V91.12
        two or more monochorionic fetuses V91.11
        unable to determine number of placenta and number of amniotic sacs V91.19
        unspecified number of placenta, unspecified number of amniotic sacs V91.10
      twin
        dichorionic/diamniotic (two placentae, two amniotic sacs) V91.03
        monochorionic/diamniotic (one placenta, two amniotic sacs) V91.02
        monochorionic/monoamniotic (one placenta, one amniotic sac) V91.01
        unable to determine number of placenta and number of amniotic sacs V91.09
        unspecified number of placenta, unspecified number of amniotic sacs V91.00
Gestational proteinuria 646.2●
  with hypertension - see Toxemia, of pregnancy
Ghon tubercle primary infection (see also Tuberculosis) 010.0●
Ghost
  teeth 520.4
  vessels, cornea 370.64
Ghoul hand 102.3
Gianotti Crosti syndrome 057.8
  due to known virus - see Infection, virus
  due to unknown virus 057.8
Giant
  cell
    epulis 523.8
      peripheral (gingiva) 523.8
    tumor, tendon sheath 727.02
  colon (congenital) 751.3
  esophagus (congenital) 750.4

Giant (Continued)
  kidney 753.3
  urticaria 995.1
    hereditary 277.6
Giardia lamblia infestation 007.1
Giardiasis 007.1
Gibert's disease (pityriasis rosea) 696.3
Gibraltar fever - see Brucellosis
Giddiness 780.4
  hysterical 300.11
  psychogenic 306.9
Gierke's disease (glycogenosis I) 271.0
Gigantism (cerebral) (hypophyseal) (pituitary) 253.0
Gilbert's disease or cholemia (familial nonhemolytic jaundice) 277.4
Gilchrist's disease (North American blastomycosis) 116.0
Gilford (-Hutchinson) disease or syndrome (progeria) 259.8
Gilles de la Tourette's disease (motor-verbal tic) 307.23
Gillespie's syndrome (dysplasia oculodentodigitalis) 759.89
Gingivitis 523.10
  acute 523.00
    necrotizing 101
    non-plaque induced 523.01
    plaque induced 523.00
  catarrhal 523.00
  chronic 523.10
    non-plaque induced 523.11
  desquamative 523.10
  expulsiva 523.40
  hyperplastic 523.10
  marginal, simple 523.10
  necrotizing, acute 101
  non-plaque induced 523.11
  pellagrous 265.2
  plaque induced 523.10
  ulcerative 523.10
    acute necrotizing 101
  Vincent's 101
Gingivoglossitis 529.0
Gingivopericementitis 523.40
Gingivosis 523.10
Gingivostomatitis 523.10
  herpetic 054.2
Giovannini's disease 117.9
GISA (glycopeptide intermediate staphylococcus aureus) V09.8
Gland, glandular - see condition
Glanders 024
Glanzmann (-Naegeli) disease or thrombasthenia 287.1
Glassblowers' disease 527.1
Glaucoma (capsular) (inflammatory) (noninflammatory) (primary) 365.9
  with increased episcleral venous pressure 365.82
  absolute 360.42
  acute 365.22
    narrow angle 365.22
    secondary 365.60
  angle closure 365.20
    acute 365.22
    attack 365.22
    chronic 365.23
    crisis 365.22
    intermittent 365.21
    interval 365.21
    primary 365.20
      chronic 365.23
    residual stage 365.24
    subacute 365.21
  angle recession 365.65
  borderline 365.00
  chronic 365.11
    noncongestive 365.11
    open angle 365.11
    simple 365.11

Glaucoma (Continued)
  closed angle - see Glaucoma, angle closure
  congenital 743.20
    associated with other eye anomalies 743.22
    simple 743.21
  congestive - see Glaucoma, narrow angle
  corticosteroid-induced (glaucomatous stage) 365.31
    residual stage 365.32
  exfoliation 365.52
  hemorrhagic 365.60
  hypersecretion 365.81
  in or with
    aniridia 365.42
    Axenfeld's anomaly 365.41
    congenital syndromes NEC 759.89 [365.44]
    disorder of lens NEC 365.59
    inflammation, ocular 365.62
    iris
      anomalies NEC 365.42
      atrophy, essential 365.42
      bombé 365.61
    microcornea 365.43
    neurofibromatosis 237.71 [365.44]
    ocular
      cysts NEC 365.64
      disorders NEC 365.60
      trauma 365.65
      tumors NEC 365.64
    pupillary block or seclusion 365.61
    Rieger's anomaly or syndrome 365.41
    seclusion of pupil 365.61
    Sturge-Weber (-Dimitri) syndrome 759.6 [365.44]
    systemic syndrome NEC 365.44
    tumor of globe 365.64
    vascular disorders NEC 365.63
  infantile 365.14
    congenital 743.20
      associated with other eye anomalies 743.22
      simple 743.21
  inflammatory 365.62
  juvenile 365.14
  low tension 365.12
  malignant 365.83
  narrow angle (primary) 365.20
    acute 365.22
    chronic 365.23
    intermittent 365.21
    interval 365.21
    residual stage 365.24
    subacute 365.21
  neovascular 365.63
  newborn 743.20
    associated with other eye anomalies 743.22
    simple 743.21
  noncongestive (chronic) 365.11
  nonobstructive (chronic) 365.11
  normal tension 365.12
  obstructive 365.60
    due to lens changes 365.59
  open angle 365.10
    with
      abnormal optic disc appearance or asymmetry 365.01
      borderline findings
        high risk 365.05
        intraocular pressure 365.01
        low risk 365.01
      cupping of optic discs 365.01
      thin central corneal thickness (pachymetry) 365.01
    primary 365.11
    residual stage 365.15
    high risk 365.05
    low risk 365.01
  phacoanaphylactic 365.59

◀ New ◀║ Revised ~~deleted~~ Deleted ● Use Additional Digit(s) Omit code

Glaucoma (Continued)
phacolytic 365.51
phacomorphic
    acute 365.22
    borderline 365.06
pigment dispersion 365.13
pigmentary 365.13
postinfectious 365.60
pseudoexfoliation 365.52
secondary NEC 365.60
    due to
        steroids 365.31
        surgery 365.60
simple (chronic) 365.11
simplex 365.11
stage
    advanced 365.73
    early 365.71
    end-stage 365.73
    indeterminate 365.74
    mild 365.71
    moderate 365.72
    severe 365.73
    unspecified 365.70
steroid
    induced 365.31
    responders 365.03
suspect 365.00
    primary angle closure 365.02
syphilitic 095.8
traumatic NEC 365.65
    newborn 767.8
uveitic 365.62
wide angle (see also Glaucoma, open angle) 365.10

Glaucomatous flecks (subcapsular) 366.31
Glazed tongue 529.4
Gleet 098.2
Glénard's disease or syndrome (enteroptosis) 569.89
Glinski-Simmonds syndrome (pituitary cachexia) 253.2
Glioblastoma (multiforme) (M9440/3)
    with sarcomatous component (M9442/3)
        specified site - see Neoplasm, by site, malignant
        unspecified site 191.9
    giant cell (M9441/3)
        specified site - see Neoplasm, by site, malignant
        unspecified site 191.9
    specified site - see Neoplasm, by site, malignant
    unspecified site 191.9
Glioma (malignant) (M9380/3)
    astrocytic (M9400/3)
        specified site - see Neoplasm, by site, malignant
        unspecified site 191.9
    mixed (M9382/3)
        specified site - see Neoplasm, by site, malignant
        unspecified site 191.9
    nose 748.1
    specified site NEC - see Neoplasm, by site, malignant
    subependymal (M9383/1) 237.5
    unspecified site 191.9
Gliomatosis cerebri (M9381/3) 191.0
Glioneuroma (M9505/1) - see Neoplasm, by site, uncertain behavior
Gliosarcoma (M9380/3)
    specified site - see Neoplasm, by site, malignant
    unspecified site 191.9
Gliosis (cerebral) 349.89
    spinal 336.0
Glisson's
    cirrhosis - see Cirrhosis, portal
    disease (see also Rickets) 268.0
Glissonitis 573.3

Globinuria 791.2
Globus 306.4
    hystericus 300.11
Glomangioma (M8712/0) (see also Hemangioma) 228.00
Glomangiosarcoma (M8710/3) - see Neoplasm, connective tissue, malignant
Glomerular nephritis (see also Nephritis) 583.9
Glomerulitis (see also Nephritis) 583.9
Glomerulonephritis (see also Nephritis) 583.9
    with
        edema (see also Nephrosis) 581.9
        lesion of
            exudative nephritis 583.89
            interstitial nephritis (diffuse) (focal) 583.89
            necrotizing glomerulitis 583.4
                acute 580.4
                chronic 582.4
            renal necrosis 583.9
                cortical 583.6
                medullary 583.7
            specified pathology NEC 583.89
                acute 580.89
                chronic 582.89
        necrosis, renal 583.9
            cortical 583.6
            medullary (papillary) 583.7
        specified pathology or lesion NEC 583.89
    acute 580.9
        with
            exudative nephritis 580.89
            interstitial nephritis (diffuse) (focal) 580.89
            necrotizing glomerulitis 580.4
            extracapillary with epithelial crescents 580.4
            poststreptococcal 580.0
            proliferative (diffuse) 580.0
            rapidly progressive 580.4
            specified pathology NEC 580.89
    arteriolar (see also Hypertension, kidney) 403.90
    arteriosclerotic (see also Hypertension, kidney) 403.90
    ascending (see also Pyelitis) 590.80
    basement membrane NEC 583.89
        with
            pulmonary hemorrhage (Goodpasture's syndrome) 446.21 [583.81]
    chronic 582.9
        with
            exudative nephritis 582.89
            interstitial nephritis (diffuse) (focal) 582.89
            necrotizing glomerulitis 582.4
            specified pathology or lesion NEC 582.89
        endothelial 582.2
        extracapillary with epithelial crescents 582.4
        hypocomplementemic persistent 582.2
        lobular 582.2
        membranoproliferative 582.2
        membranous 582.1
            and proliferative (mixed) 582.2
            sclerosing 582.1
        mesangiocapillary 582.2
        mixed membranous and proliferative 582.2
        proliferative (diffuse) 582.0
        rapidly progressive 582.4
        sclerosing 582.1
    cirrhotic - see Sclerosis, renal
    desquamative - see Nephrosis
    due to or associated with
        amyloidosis 277.39 [583.81]
            with nephrotic syndrome 277.39 [581.81]
            chronic 277.39 [582.81]

Glomerulonephritis (Continued)
    due to or associated with (Continued)
        diabetes mellitus 250.4● [583.81]
            due to secondary diabetes 249.4● [581.81]
            with nephrotic syndrome 250.4● [581.81]
                due to secondary diabetes 249.4● [581.81]
        diphtheria 032.89 [580.81]
        gonococcal infection (acute) 098.19 [583.81]
            chronic or duration of 2 months or over 098.39 [583.81]
        infectious hepatitis 070.9 [580.81]
        malaria (with nephrotic syndrome) 084.9 [581.81]
        mumps 072.79 [580.81]
        polyarteritis (nodosa) (with nephrotic syndrome) 446.0 [581.81]
        specified pathology NEC 583.89
            acute 580.89
            chronic 582.89
        streptotrichosis 039.8 [583.81]
        subacute bacterial endocarditis 421.0 [580.81]
        syphilis (late) 095.4
            congenital 090.5 [583.81]
            early 091.69 [583.81]
        systemic lupus erythematosus 710.0 [583.81]
            with nephrotic syndrome 710.0 [581.81]
            chronic 710.0 [582.81]
        tuberculosis (see also Tuberculosis) 016.0● [583.81]
        typhoid fever 002.0 [580.81]
    extracapillary with epithelial crescents 583.4
        acute 580.4
        chronic 582.4
    exudative 583.89
        acute 580.89
        chronic 582.89
    focal (see also Nephritis) 583.9
        embolic 580.4
    granular 582.89
    granulomatous 582.89
    hydremic (see also Nephrosis) 581.9
    hypocomplementemic persistent 583.2
        with nephrotic syndrome 581.2
        chronic 582.2
    immune complex NEC 583.89
    infective (see also Pyelitis) 590.80
    interstitial (diffuse) (focal) 583.89
        with nephrotic syndrome 581.89
        acute 580.89
        chronic 582.89
    latent or quiescent 582.9
    lobular 583.2
        with nephrotic syndrome 581.2
        chronic 582.2
    membranoproliferative 583.2
        with nephrotic syndrome 581.2
        chronic 582.2
    membranous 583.1
        with nephrotic syndrome 581.1
        and proliferative (mixed) 583.2
            with nephrotic syndrome 581.2
            chronic 582.2
        chronic 582.1
        sclerosing 582.1
            with nephrotic syndrome 581.1
    mesangiocapillary 583.2
        with nephrotic syndrome 581.2
        chronic 582.2
    minimal change 581.3
    mixed membranous and proliferative 583.2
        with nephrotic syndrome 581.2
        chronic 582.2

Glomerulonephritis (Continued)
  necrotizing 583.4
    acute 580.4
    chronic 582.4
  nephrotic (see also Nephrosis) 581.9
  old - see Glomerulonephritis, chronic
  parenchymatous 581.89
  poststreptococcal 580.0
  proliferative (diffuse) 583.0
    with nephrotic syndrome 581.0
      acute 580.0
      chronic 582.0
  purulent (see also Pyelitis) 590.80
  quiescent - see Nephritis, chronic
  rapidly progressive 583.4
    acute 580.4
    chronic 582.4
  sclerosing membranous (chronic) 582.1
    with nephrotic syndrome 581.1
  septic (see also Pyelitis) 590.80
  specified pathology or lesion NEC 583.89
    with nephrotic syndrome 581.89
      acute 580.89
      chronic 582.89
  suppurative (acute) (disseminated) (see also Pyelitis) 590.80
  toxic - see Nephritis, acute
  tubal, tubular - see Nephrosis, tubular
  type II (Ellis) - see Nephrosis
  vascular - see Hypertension, kidney
Glomerulosclerosis (see also Sclerosis, renal) 587
  focal 582.1
    with nephrotic syndrome 581.1
  intercapillary (nodular) (with diabetes) 250.4 ● [581.81]
    due to secondary diabetes 249.4 ● [581.81]
Glossagra 529.6
Glossalgia 529.6
Glossitis 529.0
  areata exfoliativa 529.1
  atrophic 529.4
  benign migratory 529.1
  gangrenous 529.0
  Hunter's 529.4
  median rhomboid 529.2
  Moeller's 529.4
  pellagrous 265.2
Glossocele 529.8
Glossodynia 529.6
  exfoliativa 529.4
Glossoncus 529.8
Glossophytia 529.3
Glossoplegia 529.8
Glossoptosis 529.8
Glossopyrosis 529.6
Glossotrichia 529.3
Glossy skin 701.9
Glottis - see condition
Glottitis - see Glossitis
Glucagonoma (M8152/0)
  malignant (M8152/3)
    pancreas 157.4
    specified site NEC - see Neoplasm, by site, malignant
    unspecified site 157.4
  pancreas 211.7
  specified site NEC - see Neoplasm, by site, benign
  unspecified site 211.7
Glucoglycinuria 270.7
Glue ear syndrome 381.20
Glue sniffing (airplane glue) (see also Dependence) 304.6 ●
Glycinemia (with methylmalonic acidemia) 270.7
Glycinuria (renal) (with ketosis) 270.0
Glycogen
  infiltration (see also Disease, glycogen storage) 271.0
  storage disease (see also Disease, glycogen storage) 271.0

Glycogenosis (see also Disease, glycogen storage) 271.0
  cardiac 271.0 [425.7]
  Cori, types I-VII 271.0
  diabetic, secondary 250.8 ● [259.8]
    due to secondary diabetes 249.8 ● [259.8]
  diffuse (with hepatic cirrhosis) 271.0
  generalized 271.0
  glucose-6-phosphatase deficiency 271.0
  hepatophosphorylase deficiency 271.0
  hepatorenal 271.0
  myophosphorylase deficiency 271.0
  pulmonary interstitial 516.62
Glycopenia 251.2
Glycopeptide
  intermediate staphylococcus aureus (GISA) V09.8
  resistant
    enterococcus V09.8
    staphylococcus aureus (GRSA) V09.8
Glycoprolinuria 270.8
Glycosuria 791.5
  renal 271.4
Gnathostoma (spinigerum) (infection) (infestation) 128.1
  wandering swellings from 128.1
Gnathostomiasis 128.1
Goiter (adolescent) (colloid) (diffuse) (dipping) (due to iodine deficiency) (endemic) (euthyroid) (heart) (hyperplastic) (internal) (intrathoracic) (juvenile) (mixed type) (nonendemic) (parenchymatous) (plunging) (sporadic) (subclavicular) (substernal) 240.9
  with
    hyperthyroidism (recurrent) (see also Goiter, toxic) 242.0 ●
    thyrotoxicosis (see also Goiter, toxic) 242.0 ●
  adenomatous (see also Goiter, nodular) 241.9
  cancerous (M8000/3) 193
  complicating pregnancy, childbirth, or puerperium 648.1 ●
  congenital 246.1
  cystic (see also Goiter, nodular) 241.9
  due to enzyme defect in synthesis of thyroid hormone (butane-insoluble iodine) (coupling) (deiodinase) (iodide trapping or organification) (iodotyrosine dehalogenase) (peroxidase) 246.1
  dyshormonogenic 246.1
  exophthalmic (see also Goiter, toxic) 242.0 ●
  familial (with deaf-mutism) 243
  fibrous 245.3
  lingual 759.2
  lymphadenoid 245.2
  malignant (M8000/3) 193
  multinodular (nontoxic) 241.1
    toxic or with hyperthyroidism (see also Goiter, toxic) 242.2 ●
  nodular (nontoxic) 241.9
    with
      hyperthyroidism (see also Goiter, toxic) 242.3 ●
      thyrotoxicosis (see also Goiter, toxic) 242.3 ●
    endemic 241.9
    exophthalmic (diffuse) (see also Goiter, toxic) 242.0 ●
    multinodular (nontoxic) 241.1
    sporadic 241.9
    toxic (see also Goiter, toxic) 242.3 ●
    uninodular (nontoxic) 241.0
  nontoxic (nodular) 241.9
    multinodular 241.1
    uninodular 241.0
  pulsating (see also Goiter, toxic) 242.0 ●
  simple 240.0

Goiter (Continued)
  toxic 242.0 ●

> Note: Use the following fifth-digit subclassification with category 242:
>
> 0 without mention of thyrotoxic crisis or storm
> 1 with mention of thyrotoxic crisis or storm

  adenomatous 242.3 ●
    multinodular 242.2 ●
    uninodular 242.1 ●
  multinodular 242.2 ●
  nodular 242.3 ●
    multinodular 242.2 ●
    uninodular 242.1 ●
  uninodular 242.1 ●
  uninodular (nontoxic) 241.0
    toxic or with hyperthyroidism (see also Goiter, toxic) 242.1 ●
Goldberg (-Maxwell) (-Morris) syndrome (testicular feminization) 259.51
Goldblatt's
  hypertension 440.1
  kidney 440.1
Goldenhar's syndrome (oculoauriculovertebral dysplasia) 756.0
Goldflam-Erb disease or syndrome 358.00
Goldscheider's disease (epidermolysis bullosa) 757.39
Goldstein's disease (familial hemorrhagic telangiectasia) 448.0
Golfer's elbow 726.32
Goltz-Gorlin syndrome (dermal hypoplasia) 757.39
Gonadoblastoma (M9073/1)
  specified site - see Neoplasm, by site, uncertain behavior
  unspecified site
    female 236.2
    male 236.4
Gonecystitis (see also Vesiculitis) 608.0
Gongylonemiasis 125.6
  mouth 125.6
Goniosynechiae 364.73
Gonococcemia 098.89
Gonococcus, gonococcal (disease) (infection) (see also condition) 098.0
  anus 098.7
  bursa 098.52
  chronic NEC 098.2
  complicating pregnancy, childbirth, or puerperium 647.1 ●
    affecting fetus or newborn 760.2
  conjunctiva, conjunctivitis (neonatorum) 098.40
  dermatosis 098.89
  endocardium 098.84
  epididymo-orchitis 098.13
    chronic or duration of 2 months or over 098.33
  eye (newborn) 098.40
  fallopian tube (chronic) 098.37
    acute 098.17
  genitourinary (acute) (organ) (system) (tract) (see also Gonorrhea) 098.0
    lower 098.0
      chronic 098.2
    upper 098.10
      chronic 098.30
  heart NEC 098.85
  joint 098.50
  keratoderma 098.81
  keratosis (blennorrhagica) 098.81
  lymphatic (gland) (node) 098.89
  meninges 098.82
  orchitis (acute) 098.13
    chronic or duration of 2 months or over 098.33

Gonococcus, gonococcal (Continued)
  pelvis (acute) 098.19
    chronic or duration of 2 months or over 098.39
  pericarditis 098.83
  peritonitis 098.86
  pharyngitis 098.6
  pharynx 098.6
  proctitis 098.7
  pyosalpinx (chronic) 098.37
    acute 098.17
  rectum 098.7
  septicemia 098.89
  skin 098.89
  specified site NEC 098.89
  synovitis 098.51
  tendon sheath 098.51
  throat 098.6
  urethra (acute) 098.0
    chronic or duration of 2 months or over 098.2
  vulva (acute) 098.0
    chronic or duration of 2 months or over 098.2
Gonocytoma (M9073/1)
  specified site - see Neoplasm, by site, uncertain behavior
  unspecified site
    female 236.2
    male 236.4
Gonorrhea 098.0
  acute 098.0
  Bartholin's gland (acute) 098.0
    chronic or duration of 2 months or over 098.2
  bladder (acute) 098.11
    chronic or duration of 2 months or over 098.31
  carrier (suspected of) V02.7
  cervix (acute) 098.15
    chronic or duration of 2 months or over 098.35
  chronic 098.2
  complicating pregnancy, childbirth, or puerperium 647.1●
    affecting fetus or newborn 760.2
  conjunctiva, conjunctivitis (neonatorum) 098.40
  contact V01.6
  Cowper's gland (acute) 098.0
    chronic or duration of 2 months or over 098.2
  duration of 2 months or over 098.2
  exposure to V01.6
  fallopian tube (chronic) 098.37
    acute 098.17
  genitourinary (acute) (organ) (system) (tract) 098.0
    chronic 098.2
    duration of 2 months or over 098.2
  kidney (acute) 098.19
    chronic or duration of 2 months or over 098.39
  ovary (acute) 098.19
    chronic or duration of 2 months or over 098.39
  pelvis (acute) 098.19
    chronic or duration of 2 months or over 098.39
  penis (acute) 098.0
    chronic or duration of 2 months or over 098.2
  prostate (acute) 098.12
    chronic or duration of 2 months or over 098.32
  seminal vesicle (acute) 098.14
    chronic or duration of 2 months or over 098.34
  specified site NEC - see Gonococcus

Gonorrhea (Continued)
  spermatic cord (acute) 098.14
    chronic or duration of 2 months or over 098.34
  urethra (acute) 098.0
    chronic or duration of 2 months or over 098.2
  vagina (acute) 098.0
    chronic or duration of 2 months or over 098.2
  vas deferens (acute) 098.14
    chronic or duration of 2 months or over 098.34
  vulva (acute) 098.0
    chronic or duration of 2 months or over 098.2
Goodpasture's syndrome (pneumorenal) 446.21
Good's syndrome 279.06
Gopalan's syndrome (burning feet) 266.2
Gordon's disease (exudative enteropathy) 579.8
Gorlin-Chaudhry-Moss syndrome 759.89
Gougerot's syndrome (trisymptomatic) 709.1
Gougerot-Blum syndrome (pigmented purpuric lichenoid dermatitis) 709.1
Gougerot-Carteaud disease or syndrome (confluent reticulate papillomatosis) 701.8
Gougerot-Hailey-Hailey disease (benign familial chronic pemphigus) 757.39
Gougerot (-Houwer)-Sjögren syndrome (keratoconjunctivitis sicca) 710.2
Gouley's syndrome (constrictive pericarditis) 423.2
Goundou 102.6
Gout, gouty 274.9
  with
    specified manifestations NEC 274.89
    tophi (tophus) 274.03
  acute 274.01
  arthritis 274.00
    acute 274.01
  arthropathy 274.00
    acute 274.01
    chronic (without mention of tophus (tophi)) 274.02
      with tophus (tophi) 274.03
  attack 274.01
  chronic 274.02
    tophaceous 274.03
  degeneration, heart 274.82
  diathesis 274.9
  eczema 274.89
  episcleritis 274.89 [379.09]
  external ear (tophus) 274.81
  flare 274.01
  glomerulonephritis 274.10
  iritis 274.89 [364.11]
  joint 274.00
  kidney 274.10
  lead 984.9
    specified type of lead - see Table of Drugs and Chemicals
  nephritis 274.10
  neuritis 274.89 [357.4]
  phlebitis 274.89 [451.9]
  rheumatic 714.0
  saturnine 984.9
    specified type of lead - see Table of Drugs and Chemicals
  spondylitis 274.00
  synovitis 274.00
  syphilitic 095.8
  tophi 274.03
    ear 274.81
    heart 274.82
    specified site NEC 274.82
Gowers'
  muscular dystrophy 359.1
  syndrome (vasovagal attack) 780.2
Gowers-Paton-Kennedy syndrome 377.04
Gradenigo's syndrome 383.02

Graft-versus-host disease 279.50
  due to organ transplant NEC - see Complications, transplant, organ
Graham Steell's murmur (pulmonic regurgitation) (see also Endocarditis, pulmonary) 424.3
Grain-handlers' disease or lung 495.8
Grain mite (itch) 133.8
Grand
  mal (idiopathic) (see also Epilepsy) 345.1●
    hysteria of Charcôt 300.11
    nonrecurrent or isolated 780.39
  multipara
    affecting management of labor and delivery 659.4●
    status only (not pregnant) V61.5
Granite workers' lung 502
Granular - see also condition
  inflammation, pharynx 472.1
  kidney (contracting) (see also Sclerosis, renal) 587
  liver - see Cirrhosis, liver
  nephritis - see Nephritis
Granulation tissue, abnormal - see also Granuloma
  abnormal or excessive 701.5
  postmastoidectomy cavity 383.33
  postoperative 701.5
  skin 701.5
Granulocytopenia, granulocytopenic (primary) 288.00
  malignant 288.09
Granuloma NEC 686.1
  abdomen (wall) 568.89
    skin (pyogenicum) 686.1
      from residual foreign body 709.4
  annulare 695.89
  anus 569.49
  apical 522.6
  appendix 543.9
  aural 380.23
  beryllium (skin) 709.4
    lung 503
  bone (see also Osteomyelitis) 730.1●
    eosinophilic 277.89
    from residual foreign body 733.99
  canaliculus lacrimalis 375.81
  cerebral 348.89
  cholesterin, middle ear 385.82
  coccidioidal (progressive) 114.3
    lung 114.4
    meninges 114.2
    primary (lung) 114.0
  colon 569.89
  conjunctiva 372.61
  dental 522.6
  ear, middle (cholesterin) 385.82
    with otitis media - see Otitis media
  eosinophilic 277.89
    bone 277.89
    lung 277.89
    oral mucosa 528.9
  exuberant 701.5
  eyelid 374.89
  facial
    lethal midline 446.3
    malignant 446.3
  faciale 701.8
  fissuratum (gum) 523.8
  foot NEC 686.1
  foreign body (in soft tissue) NEC 728.82
    bone 733.99
    in operative wound 998.4
    muscle 728.82
    skin 709.4
    subcutaneous tissue 709.4
  fungoides 202.1●
  gangraenescens 446.3
  giant cell (central) (jaw) (reparative) 526.3
    gingiva 523.8
    peripheral (gingiva) 523.8
  gland (lymph) 289.3

Granuloma NEC *(Continued)*
  Hodgkin's (M9661/3) 201.1●
  ileum 569.89
  infectious NEC 136.9
  inguinale (Donovan) 099.2
    venereal 099.2
  intestine 569.89
  iridocyclitis 364.10
  jaw (bone) 526.3
    reparative giant cell 526.3
  kidney *(see also* Infection, kidney) 590.9
  lacrimal sac 375.81
  larynx 478.79
  lethal midline 446.3
  lipid 277.89
  lipoid 277.89
  liver 572.8
  lung (infectious) *(see also* Fibrosis, lung) 515
    coccidioidal 114.4
    eosinophilic 277.89
  lymph gland 289.3
  Majocchi's 110.6
  malignant, face 446.3
  mandible 526.3
  mediastinum 519.3
  midline 446.3
  monilial 112.3
  muscle 728.82
    from residual foreign body 728.82
  nasal sinus *(see also* Sinusitis) 473.9
  operation wound 998.59
    foreign body 998.4
    stitch (external) 998.89
      internal wound 998.89
    talc 998.7
  oral mucosa, eosinophilic or pyogenic 528.9
  orbit, orbital 376.11
  paracoccidioidal 116.1
  penis, venereal 099.2
  periapical 522.6
  peritoneum 568.89
    due to ova of helminths NEC *(see also* Helminthiasis) 128.9
  postmastoidectomy cavity 383.33
  postoperative - *see* Granuloma, operation wound
  prostate 601.8
  pudendi (ulcerating) 099.2
  pudendorum (ulcerative) 099.2
  pulp, internal (tooth) 521.49
  pyogenic, pyogenicum (skin) 686.1
    maxillary alveolar ridge 522.6
    oral mucosa 528.9
  rectum 569.49
  reticulohistiocytic 277.89
  rubrum nasi 705.89
  sarcoid 135
  Schistosoma 120.9
  septic (skin) 686.1
  silica (skin) 709.4
  sinus (accessory) (infectional) (nasal) *(see also* Sinusitis) 473.9
  skin (pyogenicum) 686.1
    from foreign body or material 709.4
  sperm 608.89
  spine
    syphilitic (epidural) 094.89
    tuberculous *(see also* Tuberculosis) 015.0● [730.88]
  stitch (postoperative) 998.89
    internal wound 998.89
  suppurative (skin) 686.1
  suture (postoperative) 998.89
    internal wound 998.89
  swimming pool 031.1
  talc 728.82
    in operation wound 998.7
  telangiectaticum (skin) 686.1
  tracheostomy 519.09
  trichophyticum 110.6
  tropicum 102.4
  umbilicus 686.1
    newborn 771.4

Granuloma NEC *(Continued)*
  urethra 599.84
  uveitis 364.10
  vagina 099.2
  venereum 099.2
  vocal cords 478.5
  Wegener's (necrotizing respiratory granulomatosis) 446.4
Granulomatosis NEC 686.1
  disciformis chronica et progressiva 709.3
  infantiseptica 771.2
  lipoid 277.89
  lipophagic, intestinal 040.2
  miliary 027.0
  necrotizing, respiratory 446.4
  progressive, septic 288.1
  Wegener's (necrotizing respiratory) 446.4
Granulomatous tissue - *see* Granuloma
Granulosis rubra nasi 705.89
Graphite fibrosis (of lung) 503
Graphospasm 300.89
  organic 333.84
Grating scapula 733.99
Gravel (urinary) *(see also* Calculus) 592.9
Graves' disease (exophthalmic goiter) *(see also* Goiter, toxic) 242.0●
Gravis - *see* condition
Grawitz's tumor (hypernephroma) (M8312/3) 189.0
Grayness, hair (premature) 704.3
  congenital 757.4
Gray or grey syndrome (chloramphenicol) (newborn) 779.4
Greenfield's disease 330.0
Green sickness 280.9
Greenstick fracture - *see* Fracture, by site
Greig's syndrome (hypertelorism) 756.0
Grief 309.0
Griesinger's disease *(see also* Ancylostomiasis) 126.9
Grinders'
  asthma 502
  lung 502
  phthisis *(see also* Tuberculosis) 011.4●
Grinding, teeth 306.8
Grip
  Dabney's 074.1
  devil's 074.1
Grippe, grippal - *see* Influenza
  Balkan 083.0
  intestinal *(see also* Influenza) 487.8
  summer 074.8
Grippy cold *(see also* Influenza) 487.1
Grisel's disease 723.5
Groin - *see* condition
Grooved
  nails (transverse) 703.8
  tongue 529.5
    congenital 750.13
Ground itch 126.9
Growing pains, children 781.99
Growth (fungoid) (neoplastic) (new) (M8000/1) - *see also* Neoplasm, by site, unspecified nature
  adenoid (vegetative) 474.12
  benign (M8000/0) - *see* Neoplasm, by site, benign
  fetal, poor 764.9●
    affecting management of pregnancy 656.5●
  malignant (M8000/3) - *see* Neoplasm, by site, malignant
  rapid, childhood V21.0
  secondary (M8000/6) - *see* Neoplasm, by site, malignant, secondary
GRSA (glycopeptide resistant staphylococcus aureus) V09.8
Gruber's hernia - *see* Hernia, Gruber's
Gruby's disease (tinea tonsurans) 110.0
GSS (Gerstmann-Sträussler-Scheinker syndrome) 046.71
G-trisomy 758.0
Guama fever 066.3

Gubler (-Millard) paralysis or syndrome 344.89
Guérin-Stern syndrome (arthrogryposis multiplex congenita) 754.89
Guertin's disease (electric chorea) 049.8
Guillain-Barré disease or syndrome 357.0
Guinea worms (infection) (infestation) 125.7
Guinon's disease (motor-verbal tic) 307.23
Gull's disease (thyroid atrophy with myxedema) 244.8
Gull and Sutton's disease - *see* Hypertension, kidney
Gum - *see* condition
Gumboil 522.7
Gumma (syphilitic) 095.9
  artery 093.89
    cerebral or spinal 094.89
  bone 095.5
    of yaws (late) 102.6
  brain 094.89
  cauda equina 094.89
  central nervous system NEC 094.9
  ciliary body 095.8 *[364.11]*
  congenital 090.5
    testis 090.5
  eyelid 095.8 *[373.5]*
  heart 093.89
  intracranial 094.89
  iris 095.8 *[364.11]*
  kidney 095.4
  larynx 095.8
  leptomeninges 094.2
  liver 095.3
  meninges 094.2
  myocardium 093.82
  nasopharynx 095.8
  neurosyphilitic 094.9
  nose 095.8
  orbit 095.8
  palate (soft) 095.8
  penis 095.8
  pericardium 093.81
  pharynx 095.8
  pituitary 095.8
  scrofulous *(see also* Tuberculosis) 017.0●
  skin 095.8
  specified site NEC 095.8
  spinal cord 094.89
  tongue 095.8
  tonsil 095.8
  trachea 095.8
  tuberculous *(see also* Tuberculosis) 017.0●
  ulcerative due to yaws 102.4
  ureter 095.8
  yaws 102.4
    bone 102.6
Gunn's syndrome (jaw-winking syndrome) 742.8
Gunshot wound - *see also* Wound, open, by site
  fracture - *see* Fracture, by site, open
  internal organs (abdomen, chest, or pelvis) - *see* Injury, internal, by site, with open wound
  intracranial - *see* Laceration, brain, with open intracranial wound
Günther's disease or syndrome (congenital erythropoietic porphyria) 277.1
Gustatory hallucination 780.1
Gynandrism 752.7
Gynandroblastoma (M8632/1)
  specified site - *see* Neoplasm, by site, uncertain behavior
  unspecified site
    female 236.2
    male 236.4
Gynandromorphism 752.7
Gynatresia (congenital) 752.49
Gynecoid pelvis, male 738.6
Gynecological examination V72.31
  for contraceptive maintenance V25.40
Gynecomastia 611.1
Gynephobia 300.29
Gyrate scalp 757.39

H

Haas' disease (osteochondrosis head of humerus) 732.3
Habermann's disease (acute parapsoriasis varioliformis) 696.2
Habit, habituation
 chorea 307.22
 disturbance, child 307.9
 drug (see also Dependence) 304.9●
 laxative (see also Abuse, drugs, nondependent) 305.9●
 spasm 307.20
  chronic 307.22
  transient (of childhood) 307.21
 tic 307.20
  chronic 307.22
  transient (of childhood) 307.21
 use of
  nonprescribed drugs (see also Abuse, drugs, nondependent) 305.9●
  patent medicines (see also Abuse, drugs, nondependent) 305.9●
 vomiting 536.2
Hadfield-Clarke syndrome (pancreatic infantilism) 577.8
Haff disease 985.1
Hag teeth, tooth 524.39
Hageman factor defect, deficiency, or disease (see also Defect, coagulation) 286.3
Haglund's disease (osteochondrosis os tibiale externum) 732.5
Haglund-Läwen-Fründ syndrome 717.89
Hagner's disease (hypertrophic pulmonary osteoarthropathy) 731.2
Hailey-Hailey disease (benign familial chronic pemphigus) 757.39
Hair - see also condition
 plucking 307.9
Hairball in stomach 935.2
Hairy black tongue 529.3
Half vertebra 756.14
Halitosis 784.99
Hallermann-Streiff syndrome 756.0
Hallervorden-Spatz disease or syndrome 333.0
Hallopeau's
 acrodermatitis (continua) 696.1
 disease (lichen sclerosis et atrophicus) 701.0
Hallucination (auditory) (gustatory) (olfactory) (tactile) 780.1
 alcohol-induced 291.3
 drug-induced 292.12
 visual 368.16
Hallucinosis 298.9
 alcohol-induced (acute) 291.3
 drug-induced 292.12
Hallus - see Hallux
Hallux 735.9
 limitus 735.8
 malleus (acquired) 735.3
 rigidus (acquired) 735.2
  congenital 755.66
  late effects of rickets 268.1
 valgus (acquired) 735.0
  congenital 755.66
 varus (acquired) 735.1
  congenital 755.66
Halo, visual 368.15
Hamartoblastoma 759.6
Hamartoma 759.6
 epithelial (gingival), odontogenic, central, or peripheral (M9321/0) 213.1
  upper jaw (bone) 213.0
 vascular 757.32
Hamartosis, hamartoses NEC 759.6
Hamman's disease or syndrome (spontaneous mediastinal emphysema) 518.1
Hamman-Rich syndrome (diffuse interstitial pulmonary fibrosis) 516.33

Hammer toe (acquired) 735.4
 congenital 755.66
 late effects of rickets 268.1
Hand - see condition
Hand-Schüller-Christian disease or syndrome (chronic histiocytosis x) 277.89
Hand-foot syndrome 693.0
Hanging (asphyxia) (strangulation) (suffocation) 994.7
Hangnail (finger) (with lymphangitis) 681.02
Hangover (alcohol) (see also Abuse, drugs, nondependent) 305.0●
Hanot's cirrhosis or disease - see Cirrhosis, biliary
Hanot-Chauffard (-Troisier) syndrome (bronze diabetes) 275.01
Hansen's disease (leprosy) 030.9
 benign form 030.1
 malignant form 030.0
Harada's disease or syndrome 363.22
Hard chancre 091.0
Hard firm prostate 600.10
 with
  urinary
   obstruction 600.11
   retention 600.11
Hardening
 artery - see Arteriosclerosis
 brain 348.89
 liver 571.8
Hare's syndrome (M8010/3) (carcinoma, pulmonary apex) 162.3
Harelip (see also Cleft, lip) 749.10
Harkavy's syndrome 446.0
Harlequin (fetus) 757.1
 color change syndrome 779.89
Harley's disease (intermittent hemoglobinuria) 283.2
Harris'
 lines 733.91
 syndrome (organic hyperinsulinism) 251.1
Hart's disease or syndrome (pellagra-cerebellar ataxia-renal aminoaciduria) 270.0
Hartmann's pouch (abnormal sacculation of gallbladder neck) 575.8
 of intestine V44.3
  attention to V55.3
Hartnup disease (pellagra-cerebellar ataxia-renal aminoaciduria) 270.0
Harvester lung 495.0
Hashimoto's disease or struma (struma lymphomatosa) 245.2
Hassall-Henle bodies (corneal warts) 371.41
Haut mal (see also Epilepsy) 345.1●
Haverhill fever 026.1
Hawaiian wood rose dependence 304.5●
Hawkins' keloid 701.4
Hay
 asthma (see also Asthma) 493.0●
 fever (allergic) (with rhinitis) 477.9
  with asthma (bronchial) (see also Asthma) 493.0●
  allergic, due to grass, pollen, ragweed, or tree 477.0
  conjunctivitis 372.05
  due to
   dander, animal (cat) (dog) 477.2
   dust 477.8
   fowl 477.8
   hair, animal (cat) (dog) 477.2
   pollen 477.0
   specified allergen other than pollen 477.8
Hayem-Faber syndrome (achlorhydric anemia) 280.9
Hayem-Widal syndrome (acquired hemolytic jaundice) 283.9
Haygarth's nodosities 715.04
Hazard-Crile tumor (M8350/3) 193

Hb (abnormal)
 disease - see Disease, hemoglobin
 trait - see Trait
H disease 270.0
Head - see also condition
 banging 307.3
Headache 784.0
 allergic 339.00
 associated with sexual activity 339.82
 cluster 339.00
  chronic 339.02
  episodic 339.01
 daily
  chronic 784.0
  new persistent (NPDH) 339.42
 drug induced 339.3
 due to
  loss, spinal fluid 349.0
  lumbar puncture 349.0
  saddle block 349.0
 emotional 307.81
 histamine 339.00
 hypnic 339.81
 lumbar puncture 349.0
 medication overuse 339.3
 menopausal 627.2
 menstrual 346.4●
 migraine 346.9●
 nasal septum 784.0
 nonorganic origin 307.81
 orgasmic 339.82
 postspinal 349.0
 post-traumatic 339.20
  acute 339.21
  chronic 339.22
 premenstrual 346.4●
 preorgasmic 339.82
 primary
  cough 339.83
  exertional 339.84
  stabbing 339.85
  thunderclap 339.43
 psychogenic 307.81
 psychophysiologic 307.81
 rebound 339.3
 short lasting unilateral neuralgiform with conjunctival injection and tearing (SUNCT) 339.05
 sick 346.9●
 spinal 349.0
  complicating labor and delivery 668.8●
  postpartum 668.8●
 spinal fluid loss 349.0
 syndrome
  cluster 339.00
  complicated NEC 339.44
  periodic in child or adolescent 346.2●
  specified NEC 339.89
 tension 307.81
  type 339.10
   chronic 339.12
   episodic 339.11
 vascular 784.0
  migraine type 346.9●
 vasomotor 346.9●
Health
 advice V65.4
 audit V70.0
 checkup V70.0
 education V65.4
 hazard (see also History of) V15.9
  falling V15.88
  specified cause NEC V15.89
 instruction V65.4
 services provided because (of)
  boarding school residence V60.6
  holiday relief for person providing home care V60.5
  inadequate
   housing V60.1
   resources V60.2

SECTION 1 INDEX TO DISEASES AND INJURIES / Hematogenous

Health *(Continued)*
  services provided because *(Continued)*
    lack of housing V60.0
    no care available in home V60.4
    person living alone V60.3
    poverty V60.3
    residence in institution V60.6
    specified cause NEC V60.89
    vacation relief for person providing home care V60.5
Healthy
  donor *(see also* Donor) V59.9
  infant or child
    accompanying sick mother V65.0
    receiving care V20.1
  person
    accompanying sick relative V65.0
    admitted for sterilization V25.2
    receiving prophylactic inoculation or vaccination *(see also* Vaccination, prophylactic) V05.9
Hearing
  conservation and treatment V72.12
  examination V72.19
    following failed hearing screening V72.11
Heart - *see* condition
Heartburn 787.1
  psychogenic 306.4
Heat (effects) 992.9
  apoplexy 992.0
  burn - *see also* Burn, by site
    from sun *(see also* Sunburn) 692.71
  collapse 992.1
  cramps 992.2
  dermatitis or eczema 692.89
  edema 992.7
  erythema - *see* Burn, by site
  excessive 992.9
    specified effect NEC 992.8
  exhaustion 992.5
    anhydrotic 992.3
    due to
      salt (and water) depletion 992.4
      water depletion 992.3
  fatigue (transient) 992.6
  fever 992.0
  hyperpyrexia 992.0
  prickly 705.1
  prostration - *see* Heat, exhaustion
  pyrexia 992.0
  rash 705.1
  specified effect NEC 992.8
  stroke 992.0
  sunburn *(see also* Sunburn) 692.71
  syncope 992.1
Heavy-chain disease 273.2
Heavy-for-dates (fetus or infant) 766.1
  4500 grams or more 766.0
  exceptionally 766.0
Hebephrenia, hebephrenic (acute) *(see also* Schizophrenia) 295.1●
  dementia (praecox) *(see also* Schizophrenia) 295.1●
  schizophrenia *(see also* Schizophrenia) 295.1●
Heberden's
  disease or nodes 715.04
  syndrome (angina pectoris) 413.9
Hebra's disease
  dermatitis exfoliativa 695.89
  erythema multiforme exudativum 695.19
  pityriasis 695.89
    maculata et circinata 696.3
    rubra 695.89
      pilaris 696.4
  prurigo 698.2
Hebra, nose 040.1
Hedinger's syndrome (malignant carcinoid) 259.2
Heel - *see* condition
Heerfordt's disease or syndrome (uveoparotitis) 135

Hegglin's anomaly or syndrome 288.2
Heidenhain's disease 290.10
  with dementia 290.10
Heilmeyer-Schoner disease (M9842/3) 207.1●
Heine-Medin disease *(see also* Poliomyelitis) 045.9●
Heinz-body anemia, congenital 282.7
Heller's disease or syndrome (infantile psychosis) *(see also* Psychosis, childhood) 299.1●
H.E.L.L.P. 642.5●
Helminthiasis *(see also* Infestation, by specific parasite) 128.9
  Ancylostoma *(see also* Ancylostoma) 126.9
  intestinal 127.9
    mixed types (types classifiable to more than one of the categories 120.0–127.7) 127.8
    specified type 127.7
  mixed types (intestinal) (types classifiable to more than one of the categories 120.0–127.7) 127.8
  Necator americanus 126.1
  specified type NEC 128.8
  Trichinella 124
Heloma 700
Hemangioblastoma (M9161/1) - *see also* Neoplasm, connective tissue, uncertain behavior
  malignant (M9161/3) - *see* Neoplasm, connective tissue, malignant
Hemangioblastomatosis, cerebelloretinal 759.6
Hemangioendothelioma (M9130/1) - *see also* Neoplasm, by site, uncertain behavior
  benign (M9130/0) 228.00
  bone (diffuse) (M9130/3) - *see* Neoplasm, bone, malignant
  malignant (M9130/3) - *see* Neoplasm, connective tissue, malignant
  nervous system (M9130/0) 228.09
Hemangioendotheliosarcoma (M9130/3) - *see* Neoplasm, connective tissue, malignant
Hemangiofibroma (M9160/0) - *see* Neoplasm, by site, benign
Hemangiolipoma (M8861/0) - *see* Lipoma
Hemangioma (M9120/0) 228.00
  arteriovenous (M9123/0) - *see* Hemangioma, by site
  brain 228.02
  capillary (M9131/0) - *see* Hemangioma, by site
  cavernous (M9121/0) - *see* Hemangioma, by site
  central nervous system NEC 228.09
  choroid 228.09
  heart 228.09
  infantile (M9131/0) - *see* Hemangioma, by site
  intra-abdominal structures 228.04
  intracranial structures 228.02
  intramuscular (M9132/0) - *see* Hemangioma, by site
  iris 228.09
  juvenile (M9131/0) - *see* Hemangioma, by site
  malignant (M9120/3) - *see* Neoplasm, connective tissue, malignant
  meninges 228.09
    brain 228.02
    spinal cord 228.09
  peritoneum 228.04
  placenta - *see* Placenta, abnormal
  plexiform (M9131/0) - *see* Hemangioma, by site
  racemose (M9123/0) - *see* Hemangioma, by site
  retina 228.03
  retroperitoneal tissue 228.04
  sclerosing (M8832/0) - *see* Neoplasm, skin, benign

Hemangioma *(Continued)*
  simplex (M9131/0) - *see* Hemangioma, by site
  skin and subcutaneous tissue 228.01
  specified site NEC 228.09
  spinal cord 228.09
  venous (M9122/0) - *see* Hemangioma, by site
  verrucous keratotic (M9142/0) - *see* Hemangioma, by site
Hemangiomatosis (systemic) 757.32
  involving single site - *see* Hemangioma
Hemangiopericytoma (M9150/1) - *see also* Neoplasm, connective tissue, uncertain behavior
  benign (M9150/0) - *see* Neoplasm, connective tissue, benign
  malignant (M9150/3) - *see* Neoplasm, connective tissue, malignant
Hemangiosarcoma (M9120/3) - *see* Neoplasm, connective tissue, malignant
Hemarthrosis (nontraumatic) 719.10
  ankle 719.17
  elbow 719.12
  foot 719.17
  hand 719.14
  hip 719.15
  knee 719.16
  multiple sites 719.19
  pelvic region 719.15
  shoulder (region) 719.11
  specified site NEC 719.18
  traumatic - *see* Sprain, by site
  wrist 719.13
Hematemesis 578.0
  with ulcer - *see* Ulcer, by site, with hemorrhage
  due to S. japonicum 120.2
  Goldstein's (familial hemorrhagic telangiectasia) 448.0
  newborn 772.4
    due to swallowed maternal blood 777.3
Hematidrosis 705.89
Hematinuria *(see also* Hemoglobinuria) 791.2
  malarial 084.8
  paroxysmal 283.2
Hematite miners' lung 503
Hematobilia 576.8
Hematocele (congenital) (diffuse) (idiopathic) 608.83
  broad ligament 620.7
  canal of Nuck 629.0
  cord, male 608.83
  fallopian tube 620.8
  female NEC 629.0
  ischiorectal 569.89
  male NEC 608.83
  ovary 629.0
  pelvis, pelvic
    female 629.0
      with ectopic pregnancy *(see also* Pregnancy, ectopic) 633.90
        with intrauterine pregnancy 633.91
    male 608.83
  periuterine 629.0
  retrouterine 629.0
  scrotum 608.83
  spermatic cord (diffuse) 608.83
  testis 608.84
  traumatic - *see* Injury, internal, pelvis
  tunica vaginalis 608.83
  uterine ligament 629.0
  uterus 621.4
  vagina 623.6
  vulva 624.5
Hematocephalus 742.4
Hematochezia *(see also* Melena) 578.1
Hematochyluria *(see also* Infestation, filarial) 125.9
Hematocolpos 626.8
Hematocornea 371.12
Hematogenous - *see* condition

 New   Revised   deleted Deleted   ● Use Additional Digit(s)   Omit code   237

SECTION I INDEX TO DISEASES AND INJURIES / Hematoma

Hematoma (skin surface intact) (traumatic) - *see also* Contusion

> Note: Hematomas are coded according to origin and the nature and site of the hematoma or the accompanying injury. Hematomas of unspecified origin are coded as injuries of the sites involved, except:
> (a) hematomas of genital organs which are coded as diseases of the organ involved unless they complicate pregnancy or delivery
> (b) hematomas of the eye which are coded as diseases of the eye.
>
> For late effect of hematoma classifiable to 920–924 *see* Late, effect, contusion.

   with
      crush injury - *see* Crush
      fracture - *see* Fracture, by site
      injury of internal organs - *see also* Injury, internal, by site
         kidney - *see* Hematoma, kidney, traumatic
         liver - *see* Hematoma, liver, traumatic
         spleen - *see* Hematoma, spleen
      nerve injury - *see* Injury, nerve
      open wound - *see* Wound, open, by site
      skin surface intact - *see* Contusion
   abdomen (wall) - *see* Contusion, abdomen
   amnion 658.8●
   aorta, dissecting 441.00
      abdominal 441.02
      thoracic 441.01
      thoracoabdominal 441.03
   aortic intramural - *see* Dissection, aorta
   arterial (complicating trauma) 904.9
      specified site - *see* Injury, blood vessel, by site
   auricle (ear) 380.31
   birth injury 767.8
      skull 767.19
   brain (traumatic) 853.0●

> Note: Use the following fifth-digit subclassification with categories 851–854:
> 0 unspecified state of consciousness
> 1 with no loss of consciousness
> 2 with brief [less than one hour] loss of consciousness
> 3 with moderate [1–24 hours] loss of consciousness
> 4 with prolonged [more than 24 hours] loss of consciousness and return to pre-existing conscious level
> 5 with prolonged [more than 24 hours] loss of consciousness, without return to pre-existing conscious level
>
> Use fifth-digit 5 to designate when a patient is unconscious and dies before regaining consciousness, regardless of the duration of the loss of consciousness
>
> 6 with loss of consciousness of unspecified duration
> 9 with concussion, unspecified

      with
         cerebral
            contusion - *see* Contusion, brain
            laceration - *see* Laceration, brain
         open intracranial wound 853.1●
         skull fracture - *see* Fracture, skull, by site
      extradural or epidural 852.4●
         with open intracranial wound 852.5●
         fetus or newborn 767.0
         nontraumatic 432.0

Hematoma (Continued)
   brain (Continued)
      fetus or newborn NEC 767.0
      nontraumatic (*see also* Hemorrhage, brain) 431
         epidural or extradural 432.0
         newborn NEC 772.8
         subarachnoid, arachnoid, or meningeal (*see also* Hemorrhage, subarachnoid) 430
         subdural (*see also* Hemorrhage, subdural) 432.1
      subarachnoid, arachnoid, or meningeal 852.0●
         with open intracranial wound 852.1●
         fetus or newborn 772.2
         nontraumatic (*see also* Hemorrhage, subarachnoid) 430
      subdural 852.2●
         with open intracranial wound 852.3●
         fetus or newborn (localized) 767.0
         nontraumatic (*see also* Hemorrhage, subdural) 432.1
   breast (nontraumatic) 611.89
   broad ligament (nontraumatic) 620.7
      complicating delivery 665.7●
      traumatic - *see* Injury, internal, broad ligament
   calcified NEC 959.9
   capitis 920
      due to birth injury 767.19
      newborn 767.19
   cerebral - *see* Hematoma, brain
   cesarean section wound 674.3●
   chorion - *see* Placenta, abnormal
   complicating delivery (perineum) (vulva) 664.5●
      pelvic 665.7●
      vagina 665.7●
   corpus
      cavernosum (nontraumatic) 607.82
      luteum (nontraumatic) (ruptured) 620.1
   dura (mater) - *see* Hematoma, brain, subdural
   epididymis (nontraumatic) 608.83
   epidural (traumatic) - *see also* Hematoma, brain, extradural
      spinal - *see* Injury, spinal, by site
   episiotomy 674.3●
   external ear 380.31
   extradural - *see also* Hematoma, brain, extradural
      fetus or newborn 767.0
      nontraumatic 432.0
         fetus or newborn 767.0
   fallopian tube 620.8
   genital organ (nontraumatic)
      female NEC 629.89
      male NEC 608.83
      traumatic (external site) 922.4
         internal - *see* Injury, internal, genital organ
   graafian follicle (ruptured) 620.0
   internal organs (abdomen, chest, or pelvis) - *see also* Injury, internal, by site
      kidney - *see* Hematoma, kidney, traumatic
      liver - *see* Hematoma, liver, traumatic
      spleen - *see* Hematoma, spleen
   intracranial - *see* Hematoma, brain
   kidney, cystic 593.81
      traumatic 866.01
         with open wound into cavity 866.11
   labia (nontraumatic) 624.5
   lingual (and other parts of neck, scalp, or face, except eye) 920
   liver (subcapsular) 573.8
      birth injury 767.8
      fetus or newborn 767.8

Hematoma (Continued)
   liver (Continued)
      traumatic NEC 864.01
         with
            laceration - *see* Laceration, liver
            open wound into cavity 864.11
   mediastinum - *see* Injury, internal, mediastinum
   meninges, meningeal (brain) - *see also* Hematoma, brain, subarachnoid
      spinal - *see* Injury, spinal, by site
   mesosalpinx (nontraumatic) 620.8
      traumatic - *see* Injury, internal, pelvis
   muscle (traumatic) - *see* Contusion, by site
      nontraumatic 729.92
   nasal (septum) (and other part(s) of neck, scalp, or face, except eye) 920
   obstetrical surgical wound 674.3●
   orbit, orbital (nontraumatic) 376.32
      traumatic 921.2
   ovary (corpus luteum) (nontraumatic) 620.1
      traumatic - *see* Injury, internal, ovary
   pelvis (female) (nontraumatic) 629.89
      complicating delivery 665.7●
      male 608.83
      traumatic - *see also* Injury, internal, pelvis
         specified organ NEC (*see also* Injury, internal, pelvis) 867.6
   penis (nontraumatic) 607.82
   pericranial (and neck, or face any part, except eye) 920
      due to injury at birth 767.19
   perineal wound (obstetrical) 674.3●
      complicating delivery 664.5●
   perirenal, cystic 593.81
   pinna 380.31
   placenta - *see* Placenta, abnormal
   postoperative 998.12
   retroperitoneal (nontraumatic) 568.81
      traumatic - *see* Injury, internal, retroperitoneum
   retropubic, male 568.81
   scalp (and neck, or face any part, except eye) 920
      fetus or newborn 767.19
   scrotum (nontraumatic) 608.83
      traumatic 922.4
   seminal vesicle (nontraumatic) 608.83
      traumatic - *see* Injury, internal, seminal, vesicle
   soft tissue, nontraumatic 729.92
   spermatic cord - *see also* Injury, internal, spermatic cord
      nontraumatic 608.83
   spinal (cord) (meninges) - *see also* Injury, spinal, by site
      fetus or newborn 767.4
      nontraumatic 336.1
   spleen 865.01
      with
         laceration - *see* Laceration, spleen
         open wound into cavity 865.11
   sternocleidomastoid, birth injury 767.8
   sternomastoid, birth injury 767.8
   subarachnoid - *see also* Hematoma, brain, subarachnoid
      fetus or newborn 772.2
      nontraumatic (*see also* Hemorrhage, subarachnoid) 430
      newborn 772.2
   subdural - *see also* Hematoma, brain, subdural
      fetus or newborn (localized) 767.0
      nontraumatic (*see also* Hemorrhage, subdural) 432.1
   subperiosteal (syndrome) 267
      traumatic - *see* Hematoma, by site
   superficial, fetus or newborn 772.6
   syncytium - *see* Placenta, abnormal

Hematoma *(Continued)*
  testis (nontraumatic) 608.83
    birth injury 767.8
    traumatic 922.4
  tunica vaginalis (nontraumatic) 608.83
  umbilical cord 663.6 ●
    affecting fetus or newborn 762.6
  uterine ligament (nontraumatic) 620.7
    traumatic - *see* Injury, internal, pelvis
  uterus 621.4
    traumatic - *see* Injury, internal, pelvis
  vagina (nontraumatic) (ruptured) 623.6
    complicating delivery 665.7 ●
    traumatic 922.4
  vas deferens (nontraumatic) 608.83
    traumatic - *see* Injury, internal, vas deferens
  vitreous 379.23
  vocal cord 920
  vulva (nontraumatic) 624.5
    complicating delivery 664.5 ●
    fetus or newborn 767.8
    traumatic 922.4
Hematometra 621.4
Hematomyelia 336.1
  with fracture of vertebra (*see also* Fracture, vertebra, by site, with spinal cord injury) 806.8
  fetus or newborn 767.4
Hematomyelitis 323.9
  late effect - *see* category 326
Hematoperitoneum (*see also* Hemoperitoneum) 568.81
Hematopneumothorax (*see also* Hemothorax) 511.89
Hematopoiesis, cyclic 288.02
Hematoporphyria (acquired) (congenital) 277.1
Hematoporphyrinuria (acquired) (congenital) 277.1
Hematorachis, hematorrhachis 336.1
  fetus or newborn 767.4
Hematosalpinx 620.8
  with
    ectopic pregnancy (*see also* categories 633.0–633.9) 639.2
    molar pregnancy (*see also* categories 630–632) 639.2
    infectional (*see also* Salpingo-oophoritis) 614.2
Hematospermia 608.82
Hematothorax (*see also* Hemothorax) 511.89
Hematotympanum 381.03
Hematuria (benign) (essential) (idiopathic) 599.70
  due to S. hematobium 120.0
  endemic 120.0
  gross 599.71
  intermittent 599.70
  malarial 084.8
  microscopic 599.72
  paroxysmal 599.70
  sulfonamide
    correct substance properly administered 599.70
    overdose or wrong substance given or taken 961.0
  tropical (bilharziasis) 120.0
  tuberculous (*see also* Tuberculosis) 016.9 ●
Hematuric bilious fever 084.8
Hemeralopia 368.10
Hemiabiotrophy 799.89
Hemi-akinesia 781.8
Hemianalgesia (*see also* Disturbance, sensation) 782.0
Hemianencephaly 740.0
Hemianesthesia (*see also* Disturbance, sensation) 782.0

Hemianopia, hemianopsia (altitudinal) (homonymous) 368.46
  binasal 368.47
  bitemporal 368.47
  heteronymous 368.47
  syphilitic 095.8
Hemiasomatognosia 307.9
Hemiathetosis 781.0
Hemiatrophy 799.89
  cerebellar 334.8
  face 349.89
    progressive 349.89
  fascia 728.9
  leg 728.2
  tongue 529.8
Hemiballism (us) 333.5
Hemiblock (cardiac) (heart) (left) 426.2
Hemicardia 746.89
Hemicephalus, hemicephaly 740.0
Hemichorea 333.5
Hemicrania 346.9 ●
  congenital malformation 740.0
  continua 339.41
  paroxysmal 339.03
    chronic 339.04
    episodic 339.03
Hemidystrophy - *see* Hemiatrophy
Hemiectromelia 755.4
Hemihypalgesia (*see also* Disturbance, sensation) 782.0
Hemihypertrophy (congenital) 759.89
  cranial 756.0
Hemihypesthesia (*see also* Disturbance, sensation) 782.0
Hemi-inattention 781.8
Hemimelia 755.4
  lower limb 755.30
    paraxial (complete) (incomplete) (intercalary) (terminal) 755.32
      fibula 755.37
      tibia 755.36
    transverse (complete) (partial) 755.31
  upper limb 755.20
    paraxial (complete) (incomplete) (intercalary) (terminal) 755.22
      radial 755.26
      ulnar 755.27
    transverse (complete) (partial) 755.21
Hemiparalysis (*see also* Hemiplegia) 342.9 ●
Hemiparesis (*see also* Hemiplegia) 342.9 ●
Hemiparesthesia (*see also* Disturbance, sensation) 782.0
Hemiplegia 342.9 ●
  acute (*see also* Disease, cerebrovascular, acute) 436
  alternans facialis 344.89
  apoplectic (*see also* Disease, cerebrovascular, acute) 436
    late effect or residual
      affecting
        dominant side 438.21
        nondominant side 438.22
        unspecified side 438.20
  arteriosclerotic 437.0
    late effect or residual
      affecting
        dominant side 438.21
        nondominant side 438.22
        unspecified side 438.20
  ascending (spinal) NEC 344.89
  attack (*see also* Disease, cerebrovascular, acute) 436
  brain, cerebral (current episode) 437.8
    congenital 343.1
  cerebral - *see* Hemiplegia, brain
  congenital (cerebral) (spastic) (spinal) 343.1
  conversion neurosis (hysterical) 300.11
  cortical - *see* Hemiplegia, brain

Hemiplegia *(Continued)*
  due to
    arteriosclerosis 437.0
      late effect or residual
        affecting
          dominant side 438.21
          nondominant side 438.22
          unspecified side 438.20
    cerebrovascular lesion (*see also* Disease, cerebrovascular, acute) 436
      late effect
        affecting
          dominant side 438.21
          nondominant side 438.22
          unspecified side 438.20
  embolic (current) (*see also* Embolism, brain) 434.1 ●
    late effect
      affecting
        dominant side 438.21
        nondominant side 438.22
        unspecified side 438.20
  flaccid 342.0 ●
  hypertensive (current episode) 437.8
  infantile (postnatal) 343.4
  late effect
    birth injury, intracranial or spinal 343.4
    cerebrovascular lesion - *see* Late effect(s) (of) cerebrovascular disease
    viral encephalitis 139.0
  middle alternating NEC 344.89
  newborn NEC 767.0
  seizure (current episode) (*see also* Disease, cerebrovascular, acute) 436
  spastic 342.1 ●
    congenital or infantile 343.1
  specified NEC 342.8 ●
  thrombotic (current) (*see also* Thrombosis, brain) 434.0 ●
    late effect - *see* Late effect(s) (of) cerebrovascular disease
Hemisection, spinal cord - *see* Fracture, vertebra, by site, with spinal cord injury
Hemispasm 781.0
  facial 781.0
Hemispatial neglect 781.8
Hemisporosis 117.9
Hemitremor 781.0
Hemivertebra 756.14
Hemobilia 576.8
Hemocholecyst 575.8
Hemochromatosis (acquired) (liver) (myocardium) (secondary) 275.03
  with refractory anemia 238.72
  diabetic 275.03
  due to repeated red blood cell transfusions 275.02
  hereditary 275.01
  primary idiopathic 275.01
  specified NEC 275.03
  transfusion associated (red blood cell) 275.02
Hemodialysis V56.0
Hemoglobin - *see also* condition
  abnormal (disease) - *see* Disease, hemoglobin
  AS genotype 282.5
  fetal, hereditary persistence 282.7
  H Constant Spring 282.43
  H disease 282.43
  high-oxygen-affinity 289.0
  low NEC 285.9
  S (Hb-S), heterozygous 282.5
Hemoglobinemia 283.2
  due to blood transfusion NEC 999.89
    bone marrow 996.85
  paroxysmal 283.2

SECTION 1 INDEX TO DISEASES AND INJURIES / Hemoglobinopathy

Hemoglobinopathy (mixed) (see also Disease, hemoglobin) 282.7
- with thalassemia 282.49
- sickle-cell 282.60
  - with thalassemia (without crisis) 282.41
    - with
      - crisis 282.42
      - vaso-occlusive pain 282.42

Hemoglobinuria, hemoglobinuric 791.2
- with anemia, hemolytic, acquired (chronic) NEC 283.2
- cold (agglutinin) (paroxysmal) (with Raynaud's syndrome) 283.2
- due to
  - exertion 283.2
  - hemolysis (from external causes) NEC 283.2
- exercise 283.2
- fever (malaria) 084.8
- infantile 791.2
- intermittent 283.2
- malarial 084.8
- march 283.2
- nocturnal (paroxysmal) 283.2
- paroxysmal (cold) (nocturnal) 283.2

Hemolymphangioma (M9175/0) 228.1

Hemolysis
- fetal - see Jaundice, fetus or newborn
- intravascular (disseminated) NEC 286.6
  - with
    - abortion - see Abortion, by type, with hemorrhage, delayed or excessive
    - ectopic pregnancy (see also categories 633.0–633.9) 639.1
      - hemorrhage of pregnancy 641.3●
        - affecting fetus or newborn 762.1
    - molar pregnancy (see also categories 630–632) 639.1
  - acute 283.2
  - following
    - abortion 639.1
    - ectopic or molar pregnancy 639.1
- neonatal - see Jaundice, fetus or newborn
- transfusion NEC 999.89
  - bone marrow 996.85

Hemolytic - see also condition
- anemia - see Anemia, hemolytic
- uremic syndrome 283.11

Hemometra 621.4

Hemopericardium (with effusion) 423.0
- newborn 772.8
- traumatic (see also Hemothorax, traumatic) 860.2
  - with open wound into thorax 860.3

Hemoperitoneum 568.81
- infectional (see also Peritonitis) 567.29
- traumatic - see Injury, internal, peritoneum

Hemophagocytic syndrome 288.4
- infection-associated 288.4

Hemophilia (familial) (hereditary) 286.0
- A 286.0
  - carrier (asymptomatic) V83.01
    - symptomatic V83.02
- acquired 286.52
- autoimmune 286.52
- B (Leyden) 286.1
- C 286.2
- calcipriva (see also Fibrinolysis) 286.7
- classical 286.0
- nonfamilial 286.7
- secondary 286.52
- vascular 286.4

Hemophilus influenzae NEC 041.5
- arachnoiditis (basic) (brain) (spinal) 320.0
  - late effect - see category 326
- bronchopneumonia 482.2
- cerebral ventriculitis 320.0
  - late effect - see category 326
- cerebrospinal inflammation 320.0
  - late effect - see category 326

Hemophilus influenzae NEC (Continued)
- infection NEC 041.5
- leptomeningitis 320.0
  - late effect - see category 326
- meningitis (cerebral) (cerebrospinal) (spinal) 320.0
  - late effect - see category 326
- meningomyelitis 320.0
  - late effect - see category 326
- pachymeningitis (adhesive) (fibrous) (hemorrhagic) (hypertrophic) (spinal) 320.0
  - late effect - see category 326
- pneumonia (broncho-) 482.2

Hemophthalmos 360.43

Hemopneumothorax (see also Hemothorax) 511.89
- traumatic 860.4
  - with open wound into thorax 860.5

Hemoptysis 786.30
- due to Paragonimus (westermani) 121.2
- newborn 770.3
- specified NEC 786.39
- tuberculous (see also Tuberculosis, pulmonary) 011.9●

Hemorrhage, hemorrhagic (nontraumatic) 459.0
- abdomen 459.0
- accidental (antepartum) 641.2●
  - affecting fetus or newborn 762.1
- adenoid 474.8
- adrenal (capsule) (gland) (medulla) 255.41
  - newborn 772.5
- after labor - see Hemorrhage, postpartum
- alveolar
  - lung, newborn 770.3
  - process 525.8
- alveolus 525.8
- amputation stump (surgical) 998.11
  - secondary, delayed 997.69
- anemia (chronic) 280.0
  - acute 285.1
- antepartum - see Hemorrhage, pregnancy
- anus (sphincter) 569.3
- apoplexy (stroke) 432.9
- arachnoid - see Hemorrhage, subarachnoid
- artery NEC 459.0
  - brain (see also Hemorrhage, brain) 431
  - middle meningeal - see Hemorrhage, subarachnoid
- basilar (ganglion) (see also Hemorrhage, brain) 431
- bladder 596.89
- blood dyscrasia 289.9
- bowel 578.9
  - newborn 772.4
- brain (miliary) (nontraumatic) 431
  - with
    - birth injury 767.0
    - arachnoid - see Hemorrhage, subarachnoid
    - due to
      - birth injury 767.0
      - rupture of aneurysm (congenital) (see also Hemorrhage, subarachnoid) 430
      - mycotic 431
      - syphilis 094.89
    - epidural or extradural - see Hemorrhage, extradural
    - fetus or newborn (anoxic) (hypoxic) (due to birth trauma) (nontraumatic) 767.0
    - intraventricular 772.10
      - grade I 772.11
      - grade II 772.12
      - grade III 772.13
      - grade IV 772.14
    - iatrogenic 997.02
    - postoperative 997.02
    - puerperal, postpartum, childbirth 674.0●

Hemorrhage, hemorrhagic (Continued)
- brain (Continued)
  - stem 431
  - subarachnoid, arachnoid, or meningeal - see Hemorrhage, subarachnoid
  - subdural - see Hemorrhage, subdural
  - traumatic NEC 853.0●

> Note: Use the following fifth-digit subclassification with categories 851–854:
> 0 unspecified state of consciousness
> 1 with no loss of consciousness
> 2 with brief [less than one hour] loss of consciousness
> 3 with moderate [1–24 hours] loss of consciousness
> 4 with prolonged [more than 24 hours] loss of consciousness and return to pre-existing conscious level
> 5 with prolonged [more than 24 hours] loss of consciousness, without return to pre-existing conscious level
>
> Use fifth-digit 5 to designate when a patient is unconscious and dies before regaining consciousness, regardless of the duration of the loss of consciousness
>
> 6 with loss of consciousness of unspecified duration
> 9 with concussion, unspecified

- with
  - cerebral
    - contusion - see Contusion, brain
    - laceration - see Laceration, brain
  - open intracranial wound 853.1●
  - skull fracture - see Fracture, skull, by site
  - extradural or epidural 852.4●
    - with open intracranial wound 852.5●
  - subarachnoid 852.0●
    - with open intracranial wound 852.1●
  - subdural 852.2●
    - with open intracranial wound 852.3●
- breast 611.79
- bronchial tube - see Hemorrhage, lung
- bronchopulmonary - see Hemorrhage, lung
- bronchus (cause unknown) (see also Hemorrhage, lung) 786.30
- bulbar (see also Hemorrhage, brain) 431
- bursa 727.89
- capillary 448.9
  - primary 287.8
- capsular - see Hemorrhage, brain
- cardiovascular 429.89
- cecum 578.9
- cephalic (see also Hemorrhage, brain) 431
- cerebellar (see also Hemorrhage, brain) 431
- cerebellum (see also Hemorrhage, brain) 431
- cerebral (see also Hemorrhage, brain) 431
  - fetus or newborn (anoxic) (traumatic) 767.0
- cerebromeningeal (see also Hemorrhage, brain) 431
- cerebrospinal (see also Hemorrhage, brain) 431
- cerebrovascular accident - see Hemorrhage, brain
- cerebrum (see also Hemorrhage, brain) 431
- cervix (stump) (uteri) 622.8
- cesarean section wound 674.3●
- chamber, anterior (eye) 364.41
- childbirth - see Hemorrhage, complicating, delivery

SECTION I INDEX TO DISEASES AND INJURIES / Hemorrhage, hemorrhagic

Hemorrhage, hemorrhagic (Continued)
  choroid 363.61
    expulsive 363.62
  ciliary body 364.41
  cochlea 386.8
  colon - see Hemorrhage, intestine
  complicating
    delivery 641.9●
      affecting fetus or newborn 762.1
      associated with
        afibrinogenemia 641.3●
          affecting fetus or newborn 763.89
        coagulation defect 641.3●
          affecting fetus or newborn 763.89
        hyperfibrinolysis 641.3●
          affecting fetus or newborn 763.89
        hypofibrinogenemia 641.3●
          affecting fetus or newborn 763.89
      due to
        low-lying placenta 641.1●
          affecting fetus or newborn 762.0
        placenta previa 641.1●
          affecting fetus or newborn 762.0
        premature separation of placenta 641.2●
          affecting fetus or newborn 762.1
        retained
          placenta 666.0●
          secundines 666.2●
        trauma 641.8●
          affecting fetus or newborn 763.89
        uterine leiomyoma 641.8●
          affecting fetus or newborn 763.89
  complication(s)
    of dental implant placement 525.71
    surgical procedure 998.11
  concealed NEC 459.0
  congenital 772.9
    conjunctiva 372.72
      newborn 772.8
  cord, newborn 772.0
    slipped ligature 772.3
    stump 772.3
  corpus luteum (ruptured) 620.1
  cortical (see also Hemorrhage, brain) 431
  cranial 432.9
  cutaneous 782.7
    newborn 772.6
  cyst, pancreas 577.2
  cystitis - see Cystitis
  delayed
    with
      abortion - see Abortion, by type, with hemorrhage, delayed or excessive
      ectopic pregnancy (see also categories 633.0–633.9) 639.1
      molar pregnancy (see also categories 630–632) 639.1
    following
      abortion 639.1
      ectopic or molar pregnancy 639.1
    postpartum 666.2●
  diathesis (familial) 287.9
    newborn 776.0
  disease 287.9
    newborn 776.0
    specified type NEC 287.8
  disorder 287.9
    due to intrinsic circulating anticoagulants, antibodies, or inhibitors 286.59
      with
        acquired hemophilia 286.52
        antiphospholipid antibody 286.53
    specified type NEC 287.8
  due to
    any device, implant, or graft (presence of)
      classifiable to 996.0–996.5 - see Complications, due to (presence of) any device, implant, or graft classified to 996.0–996.5 NEC

Hemorrhage, hemorrhagic (Continued)
  due to (Continued)
    intrinsic circulating anticoagulant, antibodies, or inhibitors 286.59
      with
        acquired hemophilia 286.52
        antiphospholipid antibody 286.53
  duodenum, duodenal 537.89
    ulcer - see Ulcer, duodenum, with hemorrhage
  dura mater - see Hemorrhage, subdural
  endotracheal - see Hemorrhage, lung
  epicranial subaponeurotic (massive) 767.11
  epidural - see Hemorrhage, extradural
  episiotomy 674.3●
  esophagus 530.82
    varix (see also Varix, esophagus, bleeding) 456.0
  excessive
    with
      abortion - see Abortion, by type, with hemorrhage, delayed or excessive
      ectopic pregnancy (see also categories 633.0–633.9) 639.1
      molar pregnancy (see also categories 630–632) 639.1
    following
      abortion 639.1
      ectopic or molar pregnancy 639.1
  external 459.0
  extradural (traumatic) - see Hemorrhage, brain, traumatic, extradural
    birth injury 767.0
    fetus or newborn (anoxic) (traumatic) 767.0
    nontraumatic 432.0
  eye 360.43
    chamber (anterior) (aqueous) 364.41
    fundus 362.81
  eyelid 374.81
  fallopian tube 620.8
  fetomaternal 772.0
    affecting management of pregnancy or puerperium 656.0●
  fetus, fetal, affecting newborn 772.0
    from
      cut end of co-twin's cord 772.0
      placenta 772.0
      ruptured cord 772.0
      vasa previa 772.0
    into
      co-twin 772.0
      mother's circulation 772.0
        affecting management of pregnancy or puerperium 656.0●
  fever (see also Fever, hemorrhagic) 065.9
    with renal syndrome 078.6
    arthropod-borne NEC 065.9
    Bangkok 065.4
    Crimean 065.0
    dengue virus 065.4
    epidemic 078.6
    Junin virus 078.7
    Korean 078.6
    Machupo virus 078.7
    mite-borne 065.8
    mosquito-borne 065.4
    Philippine 065.4
    Russian (Yaroslav) 078.7
    Singapore 065.4
    Southeast Asia 065.4
    Thailand 065.4
    tick-borne NEC 065.3
  fibrinogenolysis (see also Fibrinolysis) 286.6
  fibrinolytic (acquired) (see also Fibrinolysis) 286.6
  fontanel 767.19
  from tracheostomy stoma 519.09
  fundus, eye 362.81

Hemorrhage, hemorrhagic (Continued)
  funis
    affecting fetus or newborn 772.0
    complicating delivery 663.8●
  gastric (see also Hemorrhage, stomach) 578.9
  gastroenteric 578.9
    newborn 772.4
  gastrointestinal (tract) 578.9
    newborn 772.4
  genitourinary (tract) NEC 599.89
  gingiva 523.8
  globe 360.43
  gravidarum - see Hemorrhage, pregnancy
  gum 523.8
  heart 429.89
  hypopharyngeal (throat) 784.8
  intermenstrual 626.6
    irregular 626.6
    regular 626.5
  internal (organs) 459.0
    capsule (see also Hemorrhage brain) 431
    ear 386.8
    newborn 772.8
  intestine 578.9
    congenital 772.4
    newborn 772.4
  into
    bladder wall 596.7
    bursa 727.89
    corpus luysii (see also Hemorrhage, brain) 431
  intra-abdominal 459.0
    during or following surgery 998.11
  intra-alveolar, newborn (lung) 770.3
  intracerebral (see also Hemorrhage, brain) 431
  intracranial NEC 432.9
    puerperal, postpartum, childbirth 674.0●
    traumatic - see Hemorrhage, brain, traumatic
  intramedullary NEC 336.1
  intraocular 360.43
  intraoperative 998.11
  intrapartum - see Hemorrhage, complicating, delivery
  intrapelvic
    female 629.89
    male 459.0
  intraperitoneal 459.0
  intrapontine (see also Hemorrhage, brain) 431
  intrauterine 621.4
    complicating delivery - see Hemorrhage, complicating, delivery
    in pregnancy or childbirth - see Hemorrhage, pregnancy
    postpartum (see also Hemorrhage, postpartum) 666.1●
  intraventricular (see also Hemorrhage, brain) 431
    fetus or newborn (anoxic) (traumatic) 772.10
      grade I 772.11
      grade II 772.12
      grade III 772.13
      grade IV 772.14
  intravesical 596.7
  iris (postinfectional) (postinflammatory) (toxic) 364.41
  joint (nontraumatic) 719.10
    ankle 719.17
    elbow 719.12
    foot 719.17
    forearm 719.13
    hand 719.14
    hip 719.15
    knee 719.16
    lower leg 719.16
    multiple sites 719.19
    pelvic region 719.15
    shoulder (region) 719.11
    specified site NEC 719.18
    thigh 719.15

241

SECTION I INDEX TO DISEASES AND INJURIES / Hemorrhage, hemorrhagic

Hemorrhage, hemorrhagic *(Continued)*
- joint *(Continued)*
  - upper arm 719.12
  - wrist 719.13
- kidney 593.81
- knee (joint) 719.16
- labyrinth 386.8
- leg NEC 459.0
- lenticular striate artery *(see also* Hemorrhage, brain) 431
- ligature, vessel 998.11
- liver 573.8
- lower extremity NEC 459.0
- lung 786.30
  - newborn 770.3
  - tuberculous *(see also* Tuberculosis, pulmonary) 011.9
- malaria 084.8
- marginal sinus 641.2
- massive subaponeurotic, birth injury 767.11
- maternal, affecting fetus or newborn 762.1
- mediastinum 786.30
- medulla *(see also* Hemorrhage, brain) 431
- membrane (brain) *(see also* Hemorrhage, subarachnoid) 430
  - spinal cord - *see* Hemorrhage, spinal cord
- meninges, meningeal (brain) (middle) *(see also* Hemorrhage, subarachnoid) 430
  - spinal cord - *see* Hemorrhage, spinal cord
- mesentery 568.81
- metritis 626.8
- midbrain *(see also* Hemorrhage, brain) 431
- mole 631.8
- mouth 528.9
- mucous membrane NEC 459.0
  - newborn 772.8
- muscle 728.89
- nail (subungual) 703.8
- nasal turbinate 784.7
  - newborn 772.8
- nasopharynx 478.29
- navel, newborn 772.3
- newborn 772.9
  - adrenal 772.5
  - alveolar (lung) 770.3
  - brain (anoxic) (hypoxic) (due to birth trauma) 767.0
  - cerebral (anoxic) (hypoxic) (due to birth trauma) 767.0
  - conjunctiva 772.8
  - cutaneous 772.6
  - diathesis 776.0
  - due to vitamin K deficiency 776.0
  - epicranial subaponeurotic (massive) 767.11
  - gastrointestinal 772.4
  - internal (organs) 772.8
  - intestines 772.4
  - intra-alveolar (lung) 770.3
  - intracranial (from any perinatal cause) 767.0
  - intraventricular (from any perinatal cause) 772.10
    - grade I 772.11
    - grade II 772.12
    - grade III 772.13
    - grade IV 772.14
  - lung 770.3
  - pulmonary (massive) 770.3
  - spinal cord, traumatic 767.4
  - stomach 772.4
  - subaponeurotic (massive) 767.11
  - subarachnoid (from any perinatal cause) 772.2
  - subconjunctival 772.8
  - subgaleal 767.11
  - umbilicus 772.0
    - slipped ligature 772.3
    - vasa previa 772.0
- nipple 611.79

Hemorrhage, hemorrhagic *(Continued)*
- nose 784.7
  - newborn 772.8
- obstetrical surgical wound 674.3
- omentum 568.89
  - newborn 772.4
- optic nerve (sheath) 377.42
- orbit 376.32
- ovary 620.1
- oviduct 620.8
- pancreas 577.8
- parathyroid (gland) (spontaneous) 252.8
- parturition - *see* Hemorrhage, complicating, delivery
- penis 607.82
- pericardium, pericarditis 423.0
- perineal wound (obstetrical) 674.3
- peritoneum, peritoneal 459.0
- peritonsillar tissue 474.8
  - after operation on tonsils 998.11
  - due to infection 475
- petechial 782.7
- pituitary (gland) 253.8
- placenta NEC 641.9
  - affecting fetus or newborn 762.1
  - from surgical or instrumental damage 641.8
    - affecting fetus or newborn 762.1
  - previa 641.1
    - affecting fetus or newborn 762.0
- pleura - *see* Hemorrhage, lung
- polioencephalitis, superior 265.1
- polymyositis - *see* Polymyositis
- pons *(see also* Hemorrhage, brain) 431
- pontine *(see also* Hemorrhage, brain) 431
- popliteal 459.0
- postcoital 626.7
- postextraction (dental) 998.11
- postmenopausal 627.1
- postnasal 784.7
- postoperative 998.11
- postpartum (atonic) (following delivery of placenta) 666.1
  - delayed or secondary (after 24 hours) 666.2
  - retained placenta 666.0
  - third stage 666.0
- pregnancy (concealed) 641.9
  - accidental 641.2
    - affecting fetus or newborn 762.1
  - affecting fetus or newborn 762.1
  - before 22 completed weeks' gestation 640.9
    - affecting fetus or newborn 762.1
  - due to
    - abruptio placenta 641.2
      - affecting fetus or newborn 762.1
    - afibrinogenemia or other coagulation defect (conditions classifiable to 286.0–286.9) 641.3
      - affecting fetus or newborn 762.1
    - coagulation defect 641.3
      - affecting fetus or newborn 762.1
    - hyperfibrinolysis 641.3
      - affecting fetus or newborn 762.1
    - hypofibrinogenemia 641.3
      - affecting fetus or newborn 762.1
    - leiomyoma, uterus 641.8
      - affecting fetus or newborn 762.1
    - low-lying placenta 641.1
      - affecting fetus or newborn 762.1
    - marginal sinus (rupture) 641.2
      - affecting fetus or newborn 762.1
    - placenta previa 641.1
      - affecting fetus or newborn 762.0
    - premature separation of placenta (normally implanted) 641.2
      - affecting fetus or newborn 762.1
    - threatened abortion 640.0
      - affecting fetus or newborn 762.1

Hemorrhage, hemorrhagic *(Continued)*
- pregnancy *(Continued)*
  - due to *(Continued)*
    - trauma 641.8
      - affecting fetus or newborn 762.1
    - early (before 22 completed weeks' gestation) 640.9
      - affecting fetus or newborn 762.1
    - previous, affecting management of pregnancy or childbirth V23.49
    - unavoidable - *see* Hemorrhage, pregnancy, due to placenta previa
  - prepartum (mother) - *see* Hemorrhage, pregnancy
- preretinal, cause unspecified 362.81
- prostate 602.1
- puerperal *(see also* Hemorrhage, postpartum) 666.1
- pulmonary *(see also* Hemorrhage, lung) 786.30
  - acute idiopathic in infants (AIPHI) (over 28 days old) 786.31
  - newborn (massive) 770.3
  - renal syndrome 446.21
- purpura (primary) *(see also* Purpura, thrombocytopenic) 287.39
- rectum (sphincter) 569.3
- recurring, following initial hemorrhage at time of injury 958.2
- renal 593.81
  - pulmonary syndrome 446.21
- respiratory tract *(see also* Hemorrhage, lung) 786.30
- retina, retinal (deep) (superficial) (vessels) 362.81
  - diabetic 250.5 [362.01]
    - due to secondary diabetes 249.5 [362.01]
  - due to birth injury 772.8
- retrobulbar 376.89
- retroperitoneal 459.0
- retroplacental *(see also* Placenta, separation) 641.2
- scalp 459.0
  - due to injury at birth 767.19
- scrotum 608.83
- secondary (nontraumatic) 459.0
  - following initial hemorrhage at time of injury 958.2
- seminal vesicle 608.83
- skin 782.7
  - newborn 772.6
- spermatic cord 608.83
- spinal (cord) 336.1
  - aneurysm (ruptured) 336.1
    - syphilitic 094.89
  - due to birth injury 767.4
  - fetus or newborn 767.4
- spleen 289.59
- spontaneous NEC 459.0
  - petechial 782.7
- stomach 578.9
  - newborn 772.4
  - ulcer - *see* Ulcer, stomach, with hemorrhage
- subaponeurotic, newborn 767.11
  - massive (birth injury) 767.11
- subarachnoid (nontraumatic) 430
  - fetus or newborn (anoxic) (traumatic) 772.2
  - puerperal, postpartum, childbirth 674.0
  - traumatic - *see* Hemorrhage, brain, traumatic, subarachnoid
- subconjunctival 372.72
  - due to birth injury 772.8
  - newborn 772.8
- subcortical *(see also* Hemorrhage, brain) 431
- subcutaneous 782.7
- subdiaphragmatic 459.0

Hemorrhage, hemorrhagic (Continued)
  subdural (nontraumatic) 432.1
    due to birth injury 767.0
      fetus or newborn (anoxic) (hypoxic) (due to birth trauma) 767.0
      puerperal, postpartum, childbirth 674.0●
      spinal 336.1
      traumatic - see Hemorrhage, brain, traumatic, subdural
  subgaleal 767.11
  subhyaloid 362.81
  subperiosteal 733.99
  subretinal 362.81
  subtentorial (see also Hemorrhage, subdural) 432.1
  subungual 703.8
    due to blood dyscrasia 287.8
  suprarenal (capsule) (gland) 255.41
    fetus or newborn 772.5
  tentorium (traumatic) - see also Hemorrhage, brain, traumatic
    fetus or newborn 767.0
    nontraumatic - see Hemorrhage, subdural
  testis 608.83
  thigh 459.0
  third stage 666.0●
  thorax - see Hemorrhage, lung
  throat 784.8
  thrombocythemia 238.71
  thymus (gland) 254.8
  thyroid (gland) 246.3
    cyst 246.3
  tongue 529.8
  tonsil 474.8
    postoperative 998.11
  tooth socket (postextraction) 998.11
  trachea - see Hemorrhage, lung
  traumatic - see also nature of injury
    brain - see Hemorrhage, brain, traumatic
    recurring or secondary (following initial hemorrhage at time of injury) 958.2
  tuberculous NEC (see also Tuberculosis, pulmonary) 011.9●
  tunica vaginalis 608.83
  ulcer - see Ulcer, by site, with hemorrhage
  umbilicus, umbilical cord 772.0
    after birth, newborn 772.3
    complicating delivery 663.8●
      affecting fetus or newborn 772.0
    slipped ligature 772.3
    stump 772.3
  unavoidable (due to placenta previa) 641.1●
    affecting fetus or newborn 762.0
  upper extremity 459.0
  urethra (idiopathic) 599.84
  uterus, uterine (abnormal) 626.9
    climacteric 627.0
    complicating delivery - see Hemorrhage, complicating, delivery
    due to
      intrauterine contraceptive device 996.76
      perforating uterus 996.32
    functional or dysfunctional 626.8
    in pregnancy - see Hemorrhage, pregnancy
    intermenstrual 626.6
      irregular 626.6
      regular 626.5
    postmenopausal 627.1
    postpartum (see also Hemorrhage, postpartum) 666.1●
    prepubertal 626.8
    pubertal 626.3
    puerperal (immediate) 666.1●
  vagina 623.8
  vasa previa 663.5●
    affecting fetus or newborn 772.0
  vas deferens 608.83
  ventricular (see also Hemorrhage, brain) 431
  vesical 596.89

Hemorrhage, hemorrhagic (Continued)
  viscera 459.0
    newborn 772.8
  vitreous (humor) (intraocular) 379.23
  vocal cord 478.5
  vulva 624.8
Hemorrhoids (anus) (rectum) (without complication) 455.6
  bleeding, prolapsed, strangulated, or ulcerated NEC 455.8
    external 455.5
    internal 455.2
  complicated NEC 455.8
  complicating pregnancy and puerperium 671.8●
  external 455.3
    with complication NEC 455.5
      bleeding, prolapsed, strangulated, or ulcerated 455.5
      thrombosed 455.4
  internal 455.0
    with complication NEC 455.2
      bleeding, prolapsed, strangulated, or ulcerated 455.2
      thrombosed 455.1
  residual skin tag 455.9
  sentinel pile 455.9
  thrombosed NEC 455.7
    external 455.4
    internal 455.1
Hemosalpinx 620.8
Hemosiderosis 275.09
  dietary 275.09
  pulmonary (idiopathic) 275.09 [516.1]
  transfusion NEC 275.02
    bone marrow 996.85
Hemospermia 608.82
Hemothorax 511.89
  bacterial, nontuberculous 511.1
  newborn 772.8
  nontuberculous 511.89
    bacterial 511.1
  pneumococcal 511.1
  postoperative 998.11
  staphylococcal 511.1
  streptococcal 511.1
  traumatic 860.2
    with
      open wound into thorax 860.3
      pneumothorax 860.4
        with open wound into thorax 860.5
  tuberculous (see also Tuberculosis, pleura) 012.0●
Hemotympanum 385.89
Hench-Rosenberg syndrome (palindromic arthritis) (see also Rheumatism, palindromic) 719.3●
Henle's warts 371.41
Henoch (-Schönlein)
  disease or syndrome (allergic purpura) 287.0
  purpura (allergic) 287.0
Henpue, henpuye 102.6
Heparin-induced thrombocytopenia (HIT) 289.84
Heparitinuria 277.5
Hepar lobatum 095.3
Hepatalgia 573.8
Hepatic - see also condition
  flexure syndrome 569.89
Hepatitis 573.3
  acute (see also Necrosis, liver) 570
    alcoholic 571.1
    infective 070.1
      with hepatic coma 070.0
  alcoholic 571.1
  amebic - see Abscess, liver, amebic
  anicteric (acute) - see Hepatitis, viral
  antigen-associated (HAA) - see Hepatitis, viral, type B
  Australian antigen (positive) - see Hepatitis, viral, type B

Hepatitis (Continued)
  autoimmune 571.42
  catarrhal (acute) 070.1
    with hepatic coma 070.0
    chronic 571.40
    newborn 070.1
      with hepatic coma 070.0
  chemical 573.3
  cholangiolitic 573.8
  cholestatic 573.8
  chronic 571.40
    active 571.49
      viral - see Hepatitis, viral
    aggressive 571.49
    persistent 571.41
    viral - see Hepatitis, viral
  cytomegalic inclusion virus 078.5 [573.1]
  diffuse 573.3
  "dirty needle" - see Hepatitis, viral
  drug-induced 573.3
  due to
    Coxsackie 074.8 [573.1]
    cytomegalic inclusion virus 078.5 [573.1]
    infectious mononucleosis 075 [573.1]
    malaria 084.9 [573.2]
    mumps 072.71
    secondary syphilis 091.62
    toxoplasmosis (acquired) 130.5
      congenital (active) 771.2
  epidemic - see Hepatitis, viral, type A
  fetus or newborn 774.4
  fibrous (chronic) 571.49
    acute 570
  from injection, inoculation, or transfusion (blood) (other substance) (plasma) (serum) (onset within 8 months after administration) - see Hepatitis, viral
  fulminant (viral) (see also Hepatitis, viral) 070.9
    with hepatic coma 070.6
    type A 070.1
      with hepatic coma 070.0
    type B - see Hepatitis, viral, type B
  giant cell (neonatal) 774.4
  hemorrhagic 573.8
  history of
    B V12.09
    C V12.09
  homologous serum - see Hepatitis, viral
  hypertrophic (chronic) 571.49
    acute 570
  infectious, infective (acute) (chronic) (subacute) 070.1
    with hepatic coma 070.0
  inoculation - see Hepatitis, viral
  interstitial (chronic) 571.49
    acute 570
  lupoid 571.49
  malarial 084.9 [573.2]
  malignant (see also Necrosis, liver) 570
  neonatal (toxic) 774.4
  newborn 774.4
  parenchymatous (acute) (see also Necrosis, liver) 570
  peliosis 573.3
  persistent, chronic 571.41
  plasma cell 571.49
  postimmunization - see Hepatitis, viral
  postnecrotic 571.49
  posttransfusion - see Hepatitis, viral
  recurrent 571.49
  septic 573.3
  serum - see Hepatitis, viral
    carrier (suspected of) V02.61
  subacute (see also Necrosis, liver) 570
  suppurative (diffuse) 572.0
  syphilitic (late) 095.3
    congenital (early) 090.0 [573.2]
    late 090.5 [573.2]
  secondary 091.62

SECTION 1 INDEX TO DISEASES AND INJURIES / Hepatitis

Hepatitis (Continued)
  toxic (noninfectious) 573.3
    fetus or newborn 774.4
  tuberculous (see also Tuberculosis) 017.9●
  viral (acute) (anicteric) (cholangiolitic)
      (cholestatic) (chronic) (subacute) 070.9
    with hepatic coma 070.6
    AU-SH type virus - see Hepatitis, viral,
        type B
    Australian antigen - see Hepatitis, viral,
        type B
    B-antigen - see Hepatitis, viral, type B
    Coxsackie 074.8 [573.1]
    cytomegalic inclusion 078.5 [573.1]
    IH (virus) - see Hepatitis, viral, type A
    infectious hepatitis virus - see Hepatitis,
        viral, type A
    serum hepatitis virus - see Hepatitis, viral,
        type B
    SH - see Hepatitis, viral, type B
    specified type NEC 070.59
      with hepatic coma 070.49
    type A 070.1
      with hepatic coma 070.0
    type B (acute) 070.30
      with
        hepatic coma 070.20
      carrier status V02.61
      chronic 070.32
        with
          hepatic coma 070.22
            with hepatitis delta 070.23
          hepatitis delta 070.33
            with hepatic coma 070.23
          with hepatitis delta 070.21
        hepatitis delta 070.31
          with hepatic coma 070.21
    type C
      acute 070.51
        with hepatic coma 070.41
      carrier status V02.62
      chronic 070.54
        with hepatic coma 070.44
      in remission 070.54
      unspecified 070.70
        with hepatic coma 070.71
    type delta (with hepatitis B carrier state)
        070.52
      with
        active hepatitis B disease - see
            Hepatitis, viral, type B
        hepatic coma 070.42
    type E 070.53
      with hepatic coma 070.43
    vaccination and inoculation
        (prophylactic) V05.3
  Waldenström's (lupoid hepatitis) 571.49
Hepatization, lung (acute) - see also Pneumonia,
    lobar
  chronic (see also Fibrosis, lung) 515
Hepatoblastoma (M8970/3) 155.0
Hepatocarcinoma (M8170/3) 155.0
Hepatocholangiocarcinoma (M8180/3) 155.0
Hepatocholangioma, benign (M8180/0) 211.5
Hepatocholangitis 573.8
Hepatocystitis (see also Cholecystitis) 575.10
Hepatodystrophy 570
Hepatolenticular degeneration 275.1
Hepatolithiasis - see Choledocholithiasis
Hepatoma (malignant) (M8170/3) 155.0
  benign (M8170/0) 211.5
  congenital (M8970/3) 155.0
  embryonal (M8970/3) 155.0
Hepatomegalia glycogenica diffusa 271.0
Hepatomegaly (see also Hypertrophy, liver)
    789.1
  congenital 751.69
    syphilitic 090.0
  due to Clonorchis sinensis 121.1
  Gaucher's 272.7
  syphilitic (congenital) 090.0

Hepatoptosis 573.8
Hepatorrhexis 573.8
Hepatosis, toxic 573.8
Hepatosplenomegaly 571.8
  due to S. japonicum 120.2
  hyperlipemic (Bürger-Grutz type) 272.3
Herald patch 696.3
Hereditary - see condition
Heredodegeneration 330.9
  macular 362.70
Heredopathia atactica polyneuritiformis
    356.3
Heredosyphilis (see also Syphilis, congenital)
    090.9
Hermaphroditism (true) 752.7
  with specified chromosomal anomaly - see
      Anomaly, chromosomes, sex
Hernia, hernial (acquired) (recurrent)
    553.9
  with
    gangrene (obstructed) NEC 551.9
    obstruction NEC 552.9
      and gangrene 551.9
  abdomen (wall) - see Hernia, ventral
  abdominal, specified site NEC 553.8
    with
      gangrene (obstructed) 551.8
      obstruction 552.8
        and gangrene 551.8
  appendix 553.8
    with
      gangrene (obstructed) 551.8
      obstruction 552.8
        and gangrene 551.8
  bilateral (inguinal) - see Hernia, inguinal
  bladder (sphincter)
    congenital (female) (male) 756.71
    female (see also Cystocele, female)
        618.01
    male 596.89
  brain 348.4
    congenital 742.0
  broad ligament 553.8
  cartilage, vertebral - see Displacement,
      intervertebral disc
  cerebral 348.4
    congenital 742.0
    endaural 742.0
  ciliary body 364.89
    traumatic 871.1
  colic 553.9
    with
      gangrene (obstructed) 551.9
      obstruction 552.9
        and gangrene 551.9
  colon 553.9
    with
      gangrene (obstructed) 551.9
      obstruction 552.9
        and gangrene 551.9
  colostomy (stoma) 569.69
  Cooper's (retroperitoneal) 553.8
    with
      gangrene (obstructed) 551.8
      obstruction 552.8
        and gangrene 551.8
  crural - see Hernia, femoral
  cystostomy 596.83
  diaphragm, diaphragmatic 553.3
    with
      gangrene (obstructed) 551.3
      obstruction 552.3
        and gangrene 551.3
    congenital 756.6
    due to gross defect of diaphragm
        756.6
    traumatic 862.0
      with open wound into cavity 862.1
  direct (inguinal) - see Hernia, inguinal
  disc, intervertebral - see Displacement,
      intervertebral disc

Hernia, hernial (Continued)
  diverticulum, intestine 553.9
    with
      gangrene (obstructed) 551.9
      obstruction 552.9
        and gangrene 551.9
  double (inguinal) - see Hernia, inguinal
  due to adhesion with obstruction 552.9
  duodenojejunal 553.8
    with
      gangrene (obstructed) 551.8
      obstruction 552.8
        and gangrene 551.8
  en glissade - see Hernia, inguinal
  enterostomy (stoma) 569.69
  epigastric 553.29
    with
      gangrene (obstruction) 551.29
      obstruction 552.29
        and gangrene 551.29
    recurrent 553.21
      with
        gangrene (obstructed)
            551.21
        obstruction 552.21
          and gangrene 551.21
  esophageal hiatus (sliding) 553.3
    with
      gangrene (obstructed) 551.3
      obstruction 552.3
        and gangrene 551.3
    congenital 750.6
  external (inguinal) - see Hernia, inguinal
  fallopian tube 620.4
  fascia 728.89
  fat 729.30
    eyelid 374.34
    orbital 374.34
    pad 729.30
      eye, eyelid 374.34
      knee 729.31
      orbit 374.34
      popliteal (space) 729.31
      specified site NEC 729.39
  femoral (unilateral) 553.00
    with
      gangrene (obstructed) 551.00
      obstruction 552.00
        with gangrene 551.00
    bilateral 553.02
      gangrenous (obstructed) 551.02
      obstructed 552.02
        with gangrene 551.02
      recurrent 553.03
        gangrenous (obstructed)
            551.03
        obstructed 552.03
          with gangrene 551.03
    recurrent (unilateral) 553.01
      bilateral 553.03
        gangrenous (obstructed)
            551.03
        obstructed 552.03
          with gangrene 551.03
      gangrenous (obstructed) 551.01
      obstructed 552.01
        with gangrene 551.01
  foramen
    Bochdalek 553.3
      with
        gangrene (obstructed) 551.3
        obstruction 552.3
          and gangrene 551.3
      congenital 756.6
    magnum 348.4
    Morgagni, Morgagnian 553.3
      with
        gangrene 551.3
        obstruction 552.3
          and gangrene 551.3
      congenital 756.6

Hernia, hernial *(Continued)*
   funicular (umbilical) 553.1
      with
         gangrene (obstructed) 551.1
         obstruction 552.1
            and gangrene 551.1
      spermatic cord - *see* Hernia, inguinal
   gangrenous - *see* Hernia, by site, with gangrene
   gastrointestinal tract 553.9
      with
         gangrene (obstructed) 551.9
         obstruction 552.9
            and gangrene 551.9
   gluteal - *see* Hernia, femoral
   Gruber's (internal mesogastric) 553.8
      with
         gangrene (obstructed) 551.8
         obstruction 552.8
            and gangrene 551.8
   Hesselbach's 553.8
      with
         gangrene (obstructed) 551.8
         obstruction 552.8
            and gangrene 551.8
   hiatal (esophageal) (sliding) 553.3
      with
         gangrene (obstructed) 551.3
         obstruction 552.3
            and gangrene 551.3
      congenital 750.6
   incarcerated (*see also* Hernia, by site, with obstruction) 552.9
      gangrenous (*see also* Hernia, by site, with gangrene) 551.9
   incisional 553.21
      with
         gangrene (obstructed) 551.21
         obstruction 552.21
            and gangrene 551.21
      lumbar - *see* Hernia, lumbar
      recurrent 553.21
         with
            gangrene (obstructed) 551.21
            obstruction 552.21
               and gangrene 551.21
   indirect (inguinal) - *see* Hernia, inguinal
   infantile - *see* Hernia, inguinal
   infrapatellar fat pad 729.31
   inguinal (direct) (double) (encysted) (external) (funicular) (indirect) (infantile) (internal) (interstitial) (oblique) (scrotal) (sliding) 550.9●

> Note: Use the following fifth-digit subclassification with category 550:
>
> 0   unilateral or unspecified (not specified as recurrent)
> 1   unilateral or unspecified, recurrent
> 2   bilateral (not specified as recurrent)
> 3   bilateral, recurrent

      with
         gangrene (obstructed) 550.0●
         obstruction 550.1●
            and gangrene 550.0●
   internal 553.8
      with
         gangrene (obstructed) 551.8
         obstruction 552.8
            and gangrene 551.8
      inguinal - *see* Hernia, inguinal
   interstitial 553.9
      with
         gangrene (obstructed) 551.9
         obstruction 552.9
            and gangrene 551.9
      inguinal - *see* Hernia, inguinal
   intervertebral cartilage or disc - *see* Displacement, intervertebral disc

Hernia, hernial *(Continued)*
   intestine, intestinal 553.9
      with
         gangrene (obstructed) 551.9
         obstruction 552.9
            and gangrene 551.9
   intra-abdominal 553.9
      with
         gangrene (obstructed) 551.9
         obstruction 552.9
            and gangrene 551.9
   intraparietal 553.9
      with
         gangrene (obstructed) 551.9
         obstruction 552.9
            and gangrene 551.9
   iris 364.89
      traumatic 871.1
   irreducible (*see also* Hernia, by site, with obstruction) 552.9
      gangrenous (with obstruction) (*see also* Hernia, by site, with gangrene) 551.9
   ischiatic 553.8
      with
         gangrene (obstructed) 551.8
         obstruction 552.8
            and gangrene 551.8
   ischiorectal 553.8
      with
         gangrene (obstructed) 551.8
         obstruction 552.8
            and gangrene 551.8
   lens 379.32
      traumatic 871.1
   linea
      alba - *see* Hernia, epigastric
      semilunaris - *see* Hernia, spigelian
   Littre's (diverticular) 553.9
      with
         gangrene (obstructed) 551.9
         obstruction 552.9
            and gangrene 551.9
   lumbar 553.8
      with
         gangrene (obstructed) 551.8
         obstruction 552.8
            and gangrene 551.8
      intervertebral disc 722.10
   lung (subcutaneous) 518.89
      congenital 748.69
   mediastinum 519.3
   mesenteric (internal) 553.8
      with
         gangrene (obstructed) 551.8
         obstruction 552.8
            and gangrene 551.8
   mesocolon 553.8
      with
         gangrene (obstructed) 551.8
         obstruction 552.8
            and gangrene 551.8
   muscle (sheath) 728.89
   nucleus pulposus - *see* Displacement, intervertebral disc
   oblique (inguinal) - *see* Hernia, inguinal
   obstructive (*see also* Hernia, by site, with obstruction) 552.9
      gangrenous (with obstruction) (*see also* Hernia, by site, with gangrene) 551.9
   obturator 553.8
      with
         gangrene (obstructed) 551.8
         obstruction 552.8
            and gangrene 551.8
   omental 553.8
      with
         gangrene (obstructed) 551.8
         obstruction 552.8
            and gangrene 551.8

Hernia, hernial *(Continued)*
   orbital fat (pad) 374.34
   ovary 620.4
   oviduct 620.4
   paracolostomy (stoma) 569.69
   paraduodenal 553.8
      with
         gangrene (obstructed) 551.8
         obstruction 552.8
            and gangrene 551.8
   paraesophageal 553.3
      with
         gangrene (obstructed) 551.3
         obstruction 552.3
            and gangrene 551.3
      congenital 750.6
   parahiatal 553.3
      with
         gangrene (obstructed) 551.3
         obstruction 552.3
            and gangrene 551.3
   paraumbilical 553.1
      with
         gangrene (obstructed) 551.1
         obstruction 552.1
            and gangrene 551.1
   parietal 553.9
      with
         gangrene (obstructed) 551.9
         obstruction 552.9
            and gangrene 551.9
   perineal 553.8
      with
         gangrene (obstructed) 551.8
         obstruction 552.8
            and gangrene 551.8
   peritoneal sac, lesser 553.8
      with
         gangrene (obstructed) 551.8
         obstruction 552.8
            and gangrene 551.8
   popliteal fat pad 729.31
   postoperative 553.21
      with
         gangrene (obstructed) 551.21
         obstruction 552.21
            and gangrene 551.21
   pregnant uterus 654.4●
   prevesical 596.89
   properitoneal 553.8
      with
         gangrene (obstructed) 551.8
         obstruction 552.8
            and gangrene 551.8
   pudendal 553.8
      with
         gangrene (obstructed) 551.8
         obstruction 552.8
            and gangrene 551.8
   rectovaginal 618.6
   retroperitoneal 553.8
      with
         gangrene (obstructed) 551.8
         obstruction 552.8
            and gangrene 551.8
   Richter's (parietal) 553.9
      with
         gangrene (obstructed) 551.9
         obstruction 552.9
            and gangrene 551.9
   Rieux's, Riex's (retrocecal) 553.8
      with
         gangrene (obstructed) 551.8
         obstruction 552.8
            and gangrene 551.8
   sciatic 553.8
      with
         gangrene (obstructed) 551.8
         obstruction 552.8
            and gangrene 551.8
   scrotum, scrotal - *see* Hernia, inguinal

Hernia, hernial (Continued)
- sliding (inguinal) - *see also* Hernia, inguinal
- hiatus - *see* Hernia, hiatal
- spigelian 553.29
  - with
    - gangrene (obstructed) 551.29
    - obstruction 552.29
      - and gangrene 551.29
- spinal (*see also* Spina bifida) 741.9●
  - with hydrocephalus 741.0●
- strangulated (*see also* Hernia, by site, with obstruction) 552.9
  - gangrenous (with obstruction) (*see also* Hernia, by site, with gangrene) 551.9
- supraumbilicus (linea alba) - *see* Hernia, epigastric
- tendon 727.9
- testis (nontraumatic) 550.9●
  - meaning
    - scrotal hernia 550.9●
  - symptomatic late syphilis 095.8
- Treitz's (fossa) 553.8
  - with
    - gangrene (obstructed) 551.8
    - obstruction 552.8
      - and gangrene 551.8
- tunica
  - albuginea 608.89
  - vaginalis 752.89
- umbilicus, umbilical 553.1
  - with
    - gangrene (obstructed) 551.1
    - obstruction 552.1
      - and gangrene 551.1
- ureter 593.89
  - with obstruction 593.4
- uterus 621.8
  - pregnant 654.4●
- vaginal (posterior) 618.6
- Velpeau's (femoral) (*see also* Hernia, femoral) 553.00
- ventral 553.20
  - with
    - gangrene (obstructed) 551.20
    - obstruction 552.20
      - and gangrene 551.20
  - incisional 553.21
  - recurrent 553.21
    - with
      - gangrene (obstructed) 551.21
      - obstruction 552.21
        - and gangrene 551.21
- vesical
  - congenital (female) (male) 756.71
  - female (*see also* Cystocele, female) 618.01
  - male 596.89
- vitreous (into anterior chamber) 379.21
  - traumatic 871.1

Herniation - *see also* Hernia
- brain (stem) 348.4
- cerebral 348.4
- gastric mucosa (into duodenal bulb) 537.89
- mediastinum 519.3
- nucleus pulposus - *see* Displacement, intervertebral disc

Herpangina 074.0
Herpes, herpetic 054.9
- auricularis (zoster) 053.71
  - simplex 054.73
- blepharitis (zoster) 053.20
  - simplex 054.41
- circinate 110.5
- circinatus 110.5
  - bullous 694.5
- conjunctiva (simplex) 054.43
  - zoster 053.21
- cornea (simplex) 054.43
  - disciform (simplex) 054.43
  - zoster 053.21
- encephalitis 054.3

Herpes, herpetic (Continued)
- eye (zoster) 053.29
  - simplex 054.40
- eyelid (zoster) 053.20
  - simplex 054.41
- febrilis 054.9
- fever 054.9
- geniculate ganglionitis 053.11
- genital, genitalis 054.10
  - specified site NEC 054.19
- gestationis 646.8●
- gingivostomatitis 054.2
- iridocyclitis (simplex) 054.44
  - zoster 053.22
- iris (any site) 695.10
- iritis (simplex) 054.44
- keratitis (simplex) 054.43
  - dendritic 054.42
  - disciform 054.43
  - interstitial 054.43
    - zoster 053.21
- keratoconjunctivitis (simplex) 054.43
  - zoster 053.21
- labialis 054.9
  - meningococcal 036.89
- lip 054.9
- meningitis (simplex) 054.72
  - zoster 053.0
- ophthalmicus (zoster) 053.20
  - simplex 054.40
- otitis externa (zoster) 053.71
  - simplex 054.73
- penis 054.13
- perianal 054.10
- pharyngitis 054.79
- progenitalis 054.10
- scrotum 054.19
- septicemia 054.5
- simplex 054.9
  - complicated 054.8
    - ophthalmic 054.40
      - specified NEC 054.49
    - specified NEC 054.79
  - congenital 771.2
  - external ear 054.73
  - keratitis 054.43
    - dendritic 054.42
  - meningitis 054.72
  - myelitis 054.74
  - neuritis 054.79
  - specified complication NEC 054.79
    - ophthalmic 054.49
  - visceral 054.71
- stomatitis 054.2
- tonsurans 110.0
  - maculosus (of Hebra) 696.3
- visceral 054.71
- vulva 054.12
- vulvovaginitis 054.11
- whitlow 054.6
- zoster 053.9
  - auricularis 053.71
  - complicated 053.8
    - specified NEC 053.79
  - conjunctiva 053.21
  - cornea 053.21
  - ear 053.71
  - eye 053.29
  - geniculate 053.11
  - keratitis 053.21
    - interstitial 053.21
  - myelitis 053.14
  - neuritis 053.10
  - ophthalmicus(a) 053.20
  - oticus 053.71
  - otitis externa 053.71
  - specified complication NEC 053.79
  - specified site NEC 053.9
- zosteriform, intermediate type 053.9

Herrick's
- anemia (hemoglobin S disease) 282.61
- syndrome (hemoglobin S disease) 282.61

Hers' disease (glycogenosis VI) 271.0
Herter's infantilism (nontropical sprue) 579.0
Herter (-Gee) disease or syndrome (nontropical sprue) 579.0
Herxheimer's disease (diffuse idiopathic cutaneous atrophy) 701.8
Herxheimer's reaction 995.91
Hesitancy, urinary 788.64
Hesselbach's hernia - *see* Hernia, Hesselbach's
Heterochromia (congenital) 743.46
- acquired 364.53
- cataract 366.33
- cyclitis 364.21
- hair 704.3
- iritis 364.21
- retained metallic foreign body 360.62
  - magnetic 360.52
- uveitis 364.21

Heterophoria 378.40
- alternating 378.45
- vertical 378.43

Heterophyes, small intestine 121.6
Heterophyiasis 121.6
Heteropsia 368.8
Heterotopia, heterotopic - *see also* Malposition, congenital
- cerebralis 742.4
- pancreas, pancreatic 751.7
- spinalis 742.59

Heterotropia 378.30
- intermittent 378.20
  - vertical 378.31
- vertical (constant) (intermittent) 378.31

Heubner's disease 094.89
Heubner-Herter disease or syndrome (nontropical sprue) 579.0
Hexadactylism 755.00
Heyd's syndrome (hepatorenal) 572.4
HGSIL (high grade squamous intraepithelial lesion) (cytologic finding) (Pap smear finding)
- anus 796.74
- cervix 795.04
  - biopsy finding - *code to* CIN II or CIN III
- vagina 795.14

Hibernoma (M8880/0) - *see* Lipoma
Hiccough 786.8
- epidemic 078.89
- psychogenic 306.1

Hiccup (*see also* Hiccough) 786.8
Hicks (-Braxton) contractures 644.1●
Hidden penis 752.65
Hidradenitis (axillaris) (suppurative) 705.83
Hidradenoma (nodular) (M8400/0) - *see also* Neoplasm, skin, benign
- clear cell (M8402/0) - *see* Neoplasm, skin, benign
- papillary (M8405/0) - *see* Neoplasm, skin, benign

Hidrocystoma (M8404/0) - *see* Neoplasm, skin, benign
HIE (hypoxic-ischemic encephalopathy) 768.70
- mild 768.71
- moderate 768.72
- severe 768.73

High
- A_2 anemia 282.46
- altitude effects 993.2
  - anoxia 993.2
  - on
    - ears 993.0
    - sinuses 993.1
  - polycythemia 289.0
- arch
  - foot 755.67
  - palate 750.26

High (Continued)
    artery (arterial) tension (see also
            Hypertension) 401.9
        without diagnosis of hypertension 796.2
    basal metabolic rate (BMR) 794.7
    blood pressure (see also Hypertension) 401.9
        borderline 796.2
            incidental reading (isolated) (nonspecific),
                no diagnosis of hypertension 796.2
    cholesterol 272.0
        with high triglycerides 272.2
    compliance bladder 596.4
    diaphragm (congenital) 756.6
    frequency deafness (congenital) (regional)
            389.8
    head at term 652.5●
        affecting fetus or newborn 763.1
    output failure (cardiac) (see also Failure,
            heart) 428.9
    oxygen-affinity hemoglobin 289.0
    palate 750.26
    risk
        behavior -see problem
        family situation V61.9
            specified circumstance NEC V61.8
        human papillomavirus (HPV) DNA test
                positive
            anal 796.75
            cervical 795.05
            vaginal 795.15
        individual NEC V62.89
        infant NEC V20.1
        patient taking drugs (prescribed) V67.51
            nonprescribed (see also Abuse, drugs,
                nondependent) 305.9●
        pregnancy V23.9
            inadequate prenatal care V23.7
            inconclusive fetal viability V23.87
            specified problem NEC V23.89
    temperature (of unknown origin) (see also
            Pyrexia) 780.60
    thoracic rib 756.3
    triglycerides 272.1
        with high cholesterol 272.2
Hildenbrand's disease (typhus) 081.9
Hilger's syndrome 337.09
Hill diarrhea 579.1
Hilliard's lupus (see also Tuberculosis) 017.0●
Hilum - see condition
Hip - see condition
Hippel's disease (retinocerebral angiomatosis)
        759.6
Hippus 379.49
Hirschfeld's disease (acute diabetes mellitus)
        (see also Diabetes) 250.0●
    due to secondary diabetes 249.0●
Hirschsprung's disease or megacolon
        (congenital) 751.3
Hirsuties (see also Hypertrichosis) 704.1
Hirsutism (see also Hypertrichosis) 704.1
Hirudiniasis (external) (internal) 134.2
His-Werner disease (trench fever) 083.1
Hiss-Russell dysentery 004.1
Histamine cephalgia 339.00
Histidinemia 270.5
Histidinuria 270.5
Histiocytic syndromes 288.4
Histiocytoma (M8832/0) - see also Neoplasm,
        skin, benign
    fibrous (M8830/0) - see also Neoplasm, skin,
            benign
        atypical (M8830/1) - see Neoplasm,
                connective tissue, uncertain
                behavior
        malignant (M8830/3) - see Neoplasm,
                connective tissue, malignant
Histiocytosis (acute) (chronic) (subacute) 277.89
    acute differentiated progressive (M9722/3)
            202.5●
    adult pulmonary Langerhans cell (PLCH)
            516.5

Histiocytosis (Continued)
    cholesterol 277.89
    essential 277.89
    lipid, lipoid (essential) 272.7
    lipochrome (familial) 288.1
    malignant (M9720/3) 202.3●
    non-Langerhans cell 277.89
    polyostotic sclerosing 277.89
    X (chronic) 277.89
        acute (progressive) (M9722/3) 202.5●
Histoplasmosis 115.90
    with
        endocarditis 115.94
        meningitis 115.91
        pericarditis 115.93
        pneumonia 115.95
        retinitis 115.92
        specified manifestation NEC 115.99
    African (due to Histoplasma duboisii) 115.10
        with
            endocarditis 115.14
            meningitis 115.11
            pericarditis 115.13
            pneumonia 115.15
            retinitis 115.12
            specified manifestation NEC 115.19
    American (due to Histoplasma capsulatum)
            115.00
        with
            endocarditis 115.04
            meningitis 115.01
            pericarditis 115.03
            pneumonia 115.05
            retinitis 115.02
            specified manifestation NEC 115.09
    Darling's - see Histoplasmosis, American
    large form (see also Histoplasmosis, African)
            115.10
    lung 115.05
    small form (see also Histoplasmosis,
            American) 115.00
History (personal) of
    abuse
        emotional V15.42
        neglect V15.42
        physical V15.41
        sexual V15.41
    affective psychosis V11.1
    alcoholism V11.3
        specified as drinking problem (see also
                Abuse, drugs, nondependent)
                305.0●
    allergy (to) V15.09
        analgesic agent NEC V14.6
        anesthetic NEC V14.4
        antibiotic agent NEC V14.1
            penicillin V14.0
        anti-infective agent NEC V14.3
        arachnid bite V15.06
        diathesis V15.09
        drug V14.9
            specified type NEC V14.8
        eggs V15.03
        food additives V15.05
        insect bite V15.06
        latex V15.07
        medicinal agents V14.9
            specified type NEC V14.8
        milk products V15.02
        narcotic agent NEC V14.5
        nuts V15.05
            peanuts V15.01
        penicillin V14.0
        radiographic dye V15.08
        seafood V15.04
        serum V14.7
        specified food NEC V15.05
        specified nonmedicinal agents NEC
                V15.09
        spider bite V15.06
        sulfa V14.2

History (Continued)
    allergy (Continued)
        sulfonamides V14.2
        therapeutic agent NEC V15.09
        vaccine V14.7
    anaphylactic reaction or shock
            V13.81
    anaphylaxis V13.81
    anemia V12.3
    arrest, sudden cardiac V12.53
    arthritis V13.4
    attack, transient ischemic (TIA) V12.54
    benign neoplasm of brain V12.41
    blood disease V12.3
    calculi, urinary V13.01
    cardiovascular disease V12.50
        myocardial infarction 412
    chemotherapy, antineoplastic V87.41
    child abuse V15.41
    cigarette smoking V15.82
    circulatory system disease V12.50
        myocardial infarction 412
    cleft lip and palate, corrected V13.64
    combat and operational stress reaction
            V11.4
    congenital malformation (corrected)
        circulatory system V13.65
        digestive system V13.67
        ear V13.64
        eye V13.64
        face V13.64
        genitourinary system V13.62
        heart V13.65
        integument V13.68
        limbs V13.68
        musculoskeletal V13.68
        neck V13.64
        nervous system V13.63
        respiratory system V13.66
        specified type NEC V13.69
    contraception V15.7
    death, sudden, successfully resuscitated
            V12.53
    deficit
        prolonged reversible ischemic neurologic
                (PRIND) V12.54
        reversible ischemic neurologic (RIND)
                V12.54
    diathesis, allergic V15.09
    digestive system disease V12.70
        peptic ulcer V12.71
        polyps, colonic V12.72
        specified NEC V12.79
    disease (of) V13.9
        blood V12.3
        blood-forming organs V12.3
        cardiovascular system V12.50
        circulatory system V12.50
            specified NEC V12.59
        digestive system V12.70
            peptic ulcer V12.71
            polyps, colonic V12.72
            specified NEC V12.79
        infectious V12.00
            malaria V12.03
            methicillin resistant Staphylococcus
                    aureus (MRSA) V12.04
            MRSA (methicillin resistant
                    Staphylococcus aureus)
                    V12.04
            poliomyelitis V12.02
            specified NEC V12.09
            tuberculosis V12.01
        parasitic V12.00
            specified NEC V12.09
        respiratory system V12.60
            pneumonia V12.61
            specified NEC V12.69
        skin V13.3
            specified site NEC V13.89
            subcutaneous tissue V13.3

SECTION 1 INDEX TO DISEASES AND INJURIES / History

History (Continued)
   disease (Continued)
      trophoblastic V13.1
         affecting management of pregnancy V23.1
     disorder (of) V13.9
       endocrine V12.29
         gestational diabetes V12.21
       genital system V13.29
       hematological V12.3
       immunity V12.29
       mental V11.9
         affective type V11.1
         manic-depressive V11.1
         neurosis V11.2
         schizophrenia V11.0
         specified type NEC V11.8
       metabolic V12.29
       musculoskeletal NEC V13.59
       nervous system V12.40
         specified type NEC V12.49
       obstetric V13.29
         affecting management of current pregnancy V23.49
           ectopic pregnancy V23.42
           pre-term labor V23.41
         pre-term labor V13.21
       sense organs V12.40
         specified type NEC V12.49
       specified site NEC V13.89
       urinary system V13.00
         calculi V13.01
         infection V13.02
         nephrotic syndrome V13.03
         specified NEC V13.09
   drug use
     nonprescribed (see also Abuse, drugs, nondependent) 305.9●
     patent (see also Abuse, drugs, nondependent) 305.9●
   dysplasia
     cervical (conditions classifiable to 622.10–622.12) V13.22
     vaginal (conditions classifiable to 623.0) V13.23
     vulvar (conditions classifiable to 624.01-624.02) V13.24
   effect NEC of external cause V15.89
   embolism V12.51
     pulmonary V12.55
   emotional abuse V15.42
   encephalitis V12.42
   endocrine disorder V12.29
     gestational diabetes V12.21
   estrogen therapy V87.43
   extracorporeal membrane oxygenation (ECMO) V15.87
   failed
     conscious sedation V15.80
     moderate sedation V15.80
   falling V15.88
   family
     allergy V19.6
     anemia V18.2
     arteriosclerosis V17.49
     arthritis V17.7
     asthma V17.5
     blindness V19.0
     blood disorder NEC V18.3
     cardiovascular disease V17.49
     carrier, genetic disease V18.9
     cerebrovascular disease V17.1
     chronic respiratory condition NEC V17.6
     colonic polyps V18.51
     congenital anomalies V19.5
     consanguinity V19.7
     coronary artery disease V17.3
     cystic fibrosis V18.19
     deafness V19.2
     diabetes mellitus V18.0
     digestive disorders V18.59

History (Continued)
   family (Continued)
     disabilities, intellectual V18.4
     disease or disorder (of)
       allergic V19.6
       blood NEC V18.3
       cardiovascular NEC V17.49
       cerebrovascular V17.1
       colonic polyps V18.51
       coronary artery V17.3
       death, sudden cardiac (SCD) V17.41
       digestive V18.59
       ear NEC V19.3
       endocrine V18.19
         multiple neoplasia (MEN) syndrome V18.11
       eye NEC V19.19
         glaucoma V19.11
       genitourinary NEC V18.7
       glaucoma V19.11
       hypertensive V17.49
       infectious V18.8
       ischemic heart V17.3
       kidney V18.69
         polycystic V18.61
       mental V17.0
       metabolic V18.19
       musculoskeletal NEC V17.89
         osteoporosis V17.81
       neurological NEC V17.2
       parasitic V18.8
       psychiatric condition V17.0
       skin condition V19.4
     ear disorder NEC V19.3
     endocrine disease V18.19
       multiple neoplasia (MEN) syndrome V18.11
     epilepsy V17.2
     eye disorder NEC V19.19
       glaucoma V19.11
     genetic disease carrier V18.9
     genitourinary disease NEC V18.7
     glaucoma V19.11
     glomerulonephritis V18.69
     gout V18.19
     hay fever V17.6
     hearing loss V19.2
     hematopoietic neoplasia V16.7
     Hodgkin's disease V16.7
     Huntington's chorea V17.2
     hydrocephalus V19.5
     hypertension V17.49
     infarction, myocardial V17.3
     infectious disease V18.8
     intellectual disabilities V18.4
     ischemic heart disease V17.3
     kidney disease V18.69
       polycystic V18.61
     leukemia V16.6
     lymphatic malignant neoplasia NEC V16.7
     malignant neoplasm (of) NEC V16.9
       anorectal V16.0
       anus V16.0
       appendix V16.0
       bladder V16.52
       bone V16.8
       brain V16.8
       breast V16.3
         male V16.8
       bronchus V16.1
       cecum V16.0
       cervix V16.49
       colon V16.0
       duodenum V16.0
       esophagus V16.0
       eye V16.8
       gallbladder V16.0
       gastrointestinal tract V16.0
       genital organs V16.40
       hemopoietic NEC V16.7

History (Continued)
   family (Continued)
     malignant neoplasm NEC (Continued)
       ileum V16.0
       ilium V16.8
       intestine V16.0
       intrathoracic organs NEC V16.2
       kidney V16.51
       larynx V16.2
       liver V16.0
       lung V16.1
       lymphatic NEC V16.7
       ovary V16.41
       oviduct V16.41
       pancreas V16.0
       penis V16.49
       prostate V16.42
       rectum V16.0
       respiratory organs NEC V16.2
       skin V16.8
       specified site NEC V16.8
       stomach V16.0
       testis V16.43
       trachea V16.1
       ureter V16.59
       urethra V16.59
       urinary organs V16.59
       uterus V16.49
       vagina V16.49
       vulva V16.49
     MEN (multiple endocrine neoplasia syndrome) V18.11
     mental retardation - see History, family, intellectual disabilities
     metabolic disease NEC V18.19
     mongolism V19.5
     multiple
       endocrine neoplasia (MEN) syndrome V18.11
       myeloma V16.7
     musculoskeletal disease NEC V17.89
       osteoporosis V17.81
     myocardial infarction V17.3
     nephritis V18.69
     nephrosis V18.69
       osteoporosis V17.81
     parasitic disease V18.8
     polycystic kidney disease V18.61
     psychiatric disorder V17.0
     psychosis V17.0
     retinitis pigmentosa V19.19
     schizophrenia V17.0
     skin conditions V19.4
     specified condition NEC V19.8
     stroke (cerebrovascular) V17.1
     sudden cardiac death (SCD) V17.41
     visual loss V19.0
   foreign body fully removed V15.53
   fracture, healed
     pathologic V13.51
     stress V13.52
     traumatic V15.51
   genital system disorder V13.29
     pre-term labor V13.21
   gestational diabetes V12.21
   health hazard V15.9
     falling V15.88
     specified cause NEC V15.89
   hepatitis
     B V12.09
     C V12.09
   Hodgkin's disease V10.72
   hypospadias (corrected) V13.61
   immunity disorder V12.29
   immunosuppression therapy V87.46
   infarction, cerebral, without residual deficits V12.54
   infection
     central nervous system V12.42
     urinary (tract) V13.02

History (Continued)
  infectious disease V12.00
    malaria V12.03
    methicillin resistant Staphylococcus aureus (MRSA) V12.04
    MRSA (methicillin resistant Staphylococcus aureus) V12.04
    poliomyelitis V12.02
    specified NEC V12.09
    tuberculosis V12.01
  injury NEC V15.59
    traumatic brain V15.52
  insufficient prenatal care V23.7
  in utero procedure
    during pregnancy V15.21
    while a fetus V15.22
  irradiation V15.3
  leukemia V10.60
    lymphoid V10.61
    monocytic V10.63
    myeloid V10.62
    specified type NEC V10.69
  little or no prenatal care V23.7
  low birth weight (see also Status, low birth weight) V21.30
  lymphosarcoma V10.71
  malaria V12.03
  malignant carcinoid tumor V10.91
  malignant neoplasm (of) V10.90
    accessory sinus V10.22
    adrenal V10.88
    anus V10.06
    bile duct V10.09
    bladder V10.51
    bone V10.81
    brain V10.85
    breast V10.3
    bronchus V10.11
    cervix uteri V10.41
    colon V10.05
    connective tissue NEC V10.89
    corpus uteri V10.42
    digestive system V10.00
      specified part NEC V10.09
    duodenum V10.09
    endocrine gland NEC V10.88
    epididymis V10.48
    esophagus V10.03
    eye V10.84
    fallopian tube V10.44
    female genital organ V10.40
      specified site NEC V10.44
    gallbladder V10.09
    gastrointestinal tract V10.00
    gum V10.02
    hematopoietic NEC V10.79
    hypopharynx V10.02
    ileum V10.09
    intrathoracic organs NEC V10.20
    jejunum V10.09
    kidney V10.52
    large intestine V10.05
    larynx V10.21
    lip V10.02
    liver V10.07
    lung V10.11
    lymphatic NEC V10.79
    lymph glands or nodes NEC V10.79
    male genital organ V10.45
      specified site NEC V10.49
    mediastinum V10.29
    melanoma (of skin) V10.82
    middle ear V10.22
    mouth V10.02
      specified part NEC V10.02
    nasal cavities V10.22
    nasopharynx V10.02
    nervous system NEC V10.86
    nose V10.22
    oropharynx V10.02
    ovary V10.43

History (Continued)
  malignant neoplasm (Continued)
    pancreas V10.09
    parathyroid V10.88
    penis V10.49
    pharynx V10.02
    pineal V10.88
    pituitary V10.88
    placenta V10.44
    pleura V10.29
    prostate V10.46
    rectosigmoid junction V10.06
    rectum V10.06
    renal pelvis V10.53
    respiratory organs NEC V10.20
    salivary gland V10.02
    skin V10.83
      melanoma V10.82
    small intestine NEC V10.09
    soft tissue NEC V10.89
    specified site NEC V10.89
    stomach V10.04
    testis V10.47
    thymus V10.29
    thyroid V10.87
    tongue V10.01
    trachea V10.12
    ureter V10.59
    urethra V10.59
    urinary organ V10.50
    uterine adnexa V10.44
    uterus V10.42
    vagina V10.44
    vulva V10.44
  malignant neuroendocrine tumor V10.91
  manic-depressive psychosis V11.1
  meningitis V12.42
  mental disorder V11.9
    affective type V11.1
    manic-depressive V11.1
    neurosis V11.2
    schizophrenia V11.0
    specified type NEC V11.8
  Merkel cell carcinoma V10.91
  metabolic disorder V12.29
  methicillin resistant Staphylococcus aureus (MRSA) V12.04
  MRSA (methicillin resistant Staphylococcus aureus) V12.04
  musculoskeletal disorder NEC V13.59
  myocardial infarction 412
  neglect (emotional) V15.42
  nephrotic syndrome V13.03
  nervous system disorder V12.40
    specified type NEC V12.49
  neurosis V11.2
  noncompliance with medical treatment V15.81
  nutritional deficiency V12.1
  obstetric disorder V13.29
    affecting management of current pregnancy V23.49
      ectopic pregnancy V23.42
      pre-term labor V23.41
    pre-term labor V13.21
  parasitic disease V12.00
    specified NEC V12.09
  perinatal problems V13.7
    low birth weight (see also Status, low birth weight) V21.30
  physical abuse V15.41
  poisoning V15.6
  poliomyelitis V12.02
  polyps, colonic V12.72
  poor obstetric V13.29
    affecting management of current pregnancy V23.49
      ectopic pregnancy V23.42
      pre-term labor V23.41
    pre-term labor V13.21

History (Continued)
  prolonged reversible ischemic neurologic deficit (PRIND) V12.54
  psychiatric disorder V11.9
    affective type V11.1
    manic-depressive V11.1
    neurosis V11.2
    schizophrenia V11.0
    specified type NEC V11.8
  psychological trauma V15.49
    emotional abuse V15.42
    neglect V15.42
    physical abuse V15.41
    rape V15.41
  psychoneurosis V11.2
  radiation therapy V15.3
  rape V15.41
  respiratory system disease V12.60
    pneumonia V12.61
    specified NEC V12.69
  reticulosarcoma V10.71
  return from military deployment V62.22
  reversible ischemic neurologic deficit (RIND) V12.54
  schizophrenia V11.0
  skin disease V13.3
  smoking (tobacco) V15.82
  steroid therapy V87.45
    inhaled V87.44
    systemic V87.45
  stroke without residual deficits V12.54
  subcutaneous tissue disease V13.3
  sudden
    cardiac
      arrest V12.53
      death (successfully resuscitated) V12.53
  surgery to
    great vessels V15.1
    heart V15.1
    in utero
      during pregnancy V15.21
      while a fetus V15.22
    organs NEC V15.29
  syndrome, nephrotic V13.03
  therapy
    antineoplastic drug V87.41
    drug NEC V87.49
    estrogen V87.43
    immunosuppression V87.46
    monoclonal drug V87.42
    steroid V87.45
      inhaled V87.44
      systemic V87.45
  thrombophlebitis V12.52
  thrombosis V12.51
    pulmonary V12.55
  tobacco use V15.82
  trophoblastic disease V13.1
    affecting management of pregnancy V23.1
  tuberculosis V12.01
  ulcer, peptic V12.71
  urinary system disorder V13.00
    calculi V13.01
    infection V13.02
    nephrotic syndrome V13.03
    specified NEC V13.09
HIT (heparin-induced thrombocytopenia) 289.84
HIV infection (disease) (illness) - see Human immunodeficiency virus (disease) (illness) (infection)
Hives (bold) (see also Urticaria) 708.9
Hoarseness 784.42
Hobnail liver - see Cirrhosis, portal
Hobo, hoboism V60.0

SECTION I INDEX TO DISEASES AND INJURIES / Hodgkin's

Hodgkin's
- disease (M9650/3) 201.9
  - lymphocytic
    - depletion (M9653/3) 201.7
      - diffuse fibrosis (M9654/3) 201.7
      - reticular type (M9655/3) 201.7
    - predominance (M9651/3) 201.4
  - lymphocytic-histiocytic predominance (M9651/3) 201.4
  - mixed cellularity (M9652/3) 201.6
  - nodular sclerosis (M9656/3) 201.5
    - cellular phase (M9657/3) 201.5
  - granuloma (M9661/3) 201.1
  - lymphogranulomatosis (M9650/3) 201.9
  - lymphoma (M9650/3) 201.9
  - lymphosarcoma (M9650/3) 201.9
  - paragranuloma (M9660/3) 201.0
  - sarcoma (M9662/3) 201.2

Hodgson's disease (aneurysmal dilatation of aorta) 441.9
- ruptured 441.5

Hodi-potsy 111.0
Hoffa (-Kastert) disease or syndrome (liposynovitis prepatellaris) 272.8
Hoffmann's syndrome 244.9 [359.5]
Hoffmann-Bouveret syndrome (paroxysmal tachycardia) 427.2
Hole
- macula 362.54
- optic disc, crater-like 377.22
- retina (macula) 362.54
  - round 361.31
    - with detachment 361.01

Holla disease (see also Spherocytosis) 282.0
Holländer-Simons syndrome (progressive lipodystrophy) 272.6
Hollow foot (congenital) 754.71
- acquired 736.73

Holmes' syndrome (visual disorientation) 368.16
Holoprosencephaly 742.2
- due to
  - trisomy 13 758.1
  - trisomy 18 758.2

Holthouse's hernia - see Hernia, inguinal
Homesickness 309.89
Homicidal ideation V62.85
Homocystinemia 270.4
Homocystinuria 270.4
Homologous serum jaundice (prophylactic) (therapeutic) - see Hepatitis, viral
Homosexuality - omit code
- ego-dystonic 302.0
- pedophilic 302.2
- problems with 302.0

Homozygous Hb-S disease 282.61
Honeycomb lung 518.89
- congenital 748.4

Hong Kong ear 117.3
HOOD (hereditary osteo-onychodysplasia) 756.89
Hooded
- clitoris 752.49
- penis 752.69

Hookworm (anemia) (disease) (infestation) - see Ancylostomiasis
Hoppe-Goldflam syndrome 358.00
Hordeolum (external) (eyelid) 373.11
- internal 373.12

Horn
- cutaneous 702.8
  - cheek 702.8
  - eyelid 702.8
  - penis 702.8
- iliac 756.89
- nail 703.8
  - congenital 757.5
- papillary 700

Horner's
- syndrome (see also Neuropathy, peripheral, autonomic) 337.9
  - traumatic 954.0
- teeth 520.4

Horseshoe kidney (congenital) 753.3
Horton's
- disease (temporal arteritis) 446.5
- headache or neuralgia 339.00

Hospice care V66.7
Hospitalism (in children) NEC 309.83
Hourglass contraction, contracture
- bladder 596.89
- gallbladder 575.2
  - congenital 751.69
- stomach 536.8
  - congenital 750.7
  - psychogenic 306.4
- uterus 661.4
  - affecting fetus or newborn 763.7

Household circumstance affecting care V60.9
- specified type NEC V60.89

Housemaid's knee 727.2
Housing circumstance affecting care V60.9
- specified type NEC V60.89

HTR (hemolytic transfusion reaction)
- due to or resulting from incompatibility
  - ABO 999.61
    - acute 999.62
    - delayed 999.63
  - non-ABO antigen (minor) (Duffy) (Kell) (Kidd) (Lewis) (M) (N) (P) (S) 999.76
    - acute 999.77
    - delayed 999.78
  - Rh antigen (C) (c) (D) (E) (e) 999.71
    - acute 999.72
    - delayed 999.73

Huchard's disease (continued arterial hypertension) 401.9
Hudson-Stähli lines 371.11
Huguier's disease (uterine fibroma) 218.9
Hum, venous - omit code
Human bite (open wound) - (see also Wound, open, by site)
- intact skin surface - see Contusion

Human immunodeficiency virus (disease) (illness) 042
- infection V08
- with symptoms, symptomatic 042

Human immunodeficiency virus-2 infection 079.53
Human immunovirus (disease) (illness) (infection) - see Human immunodeficiency virus (disease) (illness) (infection)
Human papillomavirus 079.4
- high risk, DNA test positive
  - anal 796.75
  - cervical 795.05
  - vaginal 795.15
- low risk, DNA test positive
  - anal 796.79
  - cervical 795.09
  - vaginal 795.19

Human parvovirus 079.83
Human T-cell lymphotrophic virus I infection 079.51
Human T-cell lymphotrophic virus II infection 079.52
Human T-cell lymphotropic virus-III (disease) (illness) (infection) - see Human immunodeficiency virus (disease) (illness) (infection)
HTLV-I infection 079.51
HTLV-II infection 079.52
HTLV-III (disease) (illness) (infection) - see Human immunodeficiency virus (disease) (illness) (infection)
HTLV-III/LAV (disease) (illness) (infection) - see Human immunodeficiency virus (disease) (illness) (infection)

Humpback (acquired) 737.9
- congenital 756.19

Hunchback (acquired) 737.9
- congenital 756.19

Hunger 994.2
- air, psychogenic 306.1
- disease 251.1

Hungry bone syndrome 275.5
Hunner's ulcer (see also Cystitis) 595.1
Hunt's
- neuralgia 053.11
- syndrome (herpetic geniculate ganglionitis) 053.11
- dyssynergia cerebellaris myoclonica 334.2

Hunter's glossitis 529.4
Hunter (-Hurler) syndrome (mucopolysaccharidosis II) 277.5
Hunterian chancre 091.0
Huntington's
- chorea 333.4
- disease 333.4

Huppert's disease (multiple myeloma) (M9730/3) 203.0
Hurler (-Hunter) disease or syndrome (mucopolysaccharidosis II) 277.5
Hürthle cell
- adenocarcinoma (M8290/3) 193
- adenoma (M8290/0) 226
- carcinoma (M8290/3) 193
- tumor (M8290/0) 226

Hutchinson's
- disease meaning
  - angioma serpiginosum 709.1
  - cheiropompholyx 705.81
  - prurigo estivalis 692.72
  - summer eruption, or summer prurigo 692.72
- incisors 090.5
- melanotic freckle (M8742/2) - see also Neoplasm, skin, in situ
  - malignant melanoma in (M8742/3) - see Melanoma
- teeth or incisors (congenital syphilis) 090.5

Hutchinson-Boeck disease or syndrome (sarcoidosis) 135
Hutchinson-Gilford disease or syndrome (progeria) 259.8
Hyaline
- degeneration (diffuse) (generalized) 728.9
- localized - see Degeneration, by site
- membrane (disease) (lung) (newborn) 769

Hyalinosis cutis et mucosae 272.8
Hyalin plaque, sclera, senile 379.16
Hyalitis (asteroid) 379.22
- syphilitic 095.8

Hydatid
- cyst or tumor - see also Echinococcus
  - fallopian tube 752.11
- mole - see Hydatidiform mole
- Morgagni (congenital) 752.89
  - fallopian tube 752.11

Hydatidiform mole (benign) (complicating pregnancy) (delivered) (undelivered) 630
- invasive (M9100/1) 236.1
- malignant (M9100/1) 236.1
- previous, affecting management of pregnancy V23.1

Hydatidosis - see Echinococcus
Hyde's disease (prurigo nodularis) 698.3
Hydradenitis 705.83
Hydradenoma (M8400/0) - see Hidradenoma
Hydralazine lupus or syndrome
- correct substance properly administered 695.4
- overdose or wrong substance given or taken 972.6

Hydramnios 657
- affecting fetus or newborn 761.3

Hydrancephaly 742.3
    with spina bifida (see also Spina bifida) 741.0●
Hydranencephaly 742.3
    with spina bifida (see also Spina bifida) 741.0●
Hydrargyrism NEC 985.0
Hydrarthrosis (see also Effusion, joint) 719.0●
    gonococcal 098.50
    intermittent (see also Rheumatism, palindromic) 719.3●
    of yaws (early) (late) 102.6
    syphilitic 095.8
        congenital 090.5
Hydremia 285.9
Hydrencephalocele (congenital) 742.0
Hydrencephalomeningocele (congenital) 742.0
Hydroa 694.0
    aestivale 692.72
    gestationis 646.8●
    herpetiformis 694.0
    pruriginosa 694.0
    vacciniforme 692.72
Hydroadenitis 705.83
Hydrocalycosis (see also Hydronephrosis) 591
    congenital 753.29
Hydrocalyx (see also Hydronephrosis) 591
Hydrocele (calcified) (chylous) (idiopathic) (infantile) (inguinal canal) (recurrent) (senile) (spermatic cord) (testis) (tunica vaginalis) 603.9
    canal of Nuck (female) 629.1
        male 603.9
    congenital 778.6
    encysted 603.0
        congenital 778.6
    female NEC 629.89
    infected 603.1
    round ligament 629.89
    specified type NEC 603.8
        congenital 778.6
    spinalis (see also Spina bifida) 741.9●
    vulva 624.8
Hydrocephalic fetus
    affecting management or pregnancy 655.0●
    causing disproportion 653.6●
        with obstructed labor 660.1●
            affecting fetus or newborn 763.1
Hydrocephalus (acquired) (external) (internal) (malignant) (noncommunicating) (obstructive) (recurrent) 331.4
    aqueduct of Sylvius stricture 742.3
        with spina bifida (see also Spina bifida) 741.0●
    chronic 742.3
        with spina bifida (see also Spina bifida) 741.0●
    communicating 331.3
    congenital (external) (internal) 742.3
        with spina bifida (see also Spina bifida) 741.0●
    due to
        stricture of aqueduct of Sylvius 742.3
            with spina bifida (see also Spina bifida) 741.0●
        toxoplasmosis (congenital) 771.2
    fetal affecting management of pregnancy 655.0●
    foramen Magendie block (acquired) 331.3
        congenital 742.3
            with spina bifida (see also Spina bifida) 741.0●
    newborn 742.3
        with spina bifida (see also Spina bifida) 741.0●
    normal pressure 331.5
        idiopathic (INPH) 331.5
        secondary 331.3
    otitic 348.2
    syphilitic, congenital 090.49
    tuberculous (see also Tuberculosis) 013.8●

Hydrocolpos (congenital) 623.8
Hydrocystoma (M8404/0) - see Neoplasm, skin, benign
Hydroencephalocele (congenital) 742.0
Hydroencephalomeningocele (congenital) 742.0
Hydrohematopneumothorax (see also Hemothorax) 511.89
Hydromeningitis - see Meningitis
Hydromeningocele (spinal) (see also Spina bifida) 741.9●
    cranial 742.0
Hydrometra 621.8
Hydrometrocolpos 623.8
Hydromicrocephaly 742.1
Hydromphalus (congenital) (since birth) 757.39
Hydromyelia 742.53
Hydromyelocele (see also Spina bifida) 741.9●
Hydronephrosis 591
    atrophic 591
    congenital 753.29
    due to S. hematobium 120.0
    early 591
    functionless (infected) 591
    infected 591
    intermittent 591
    primary 591
    secondary 591
    tuberculous (see also Tuberculosis) 016.0●
Hydropericarditis (see also Pericarditis) 423.9
Hydropericardium (see also Pericarditis) 423.9
Hydroperitoneum 789.59
Hydrophobia 071
Hydrophthalmos (see also Buphthalmia) 743.20
Hydropneumohemothorax (see also Hemothorax) 511.89
Hydropneumopericarditis (see also Pericarditis) 423.9
Hydropneumopericardium (see also Pericarditis) 423.9
Hydropneumothorax 511.89
    nontuberculous 511.89
        bacterial 511.1
        pneumococcal 511.1
        staphylococcal 511.1
        streptococcal 511.1
    traumatic 860.0
        with open wound into thorax 860.1
    tuberculous (see also Tuberculosis, pleura) 012.0●
Hydrops 782.3
    abdominis 789.59
    amnii (complicating pregnancy) (see also Hydramnios) 657●
    articulorum intermittens (see also Rheumatism, palindromic) 719.3●
    cardiac (see also Failure, heart) 428.0
    congenital - see Hydrops, fetalis
    endolymphatic (see also Disease, Ménière's) 386.00
    fetal, fetalis or newborn 778.0
        due to
            alpha thalassemia 282.43
            isoimmunization 773.3
        not due to isoimmunization 778.0
    gallbladder 575.3
    idiopathic (fetus or newborn) 778.0
    joint (see also Effusion, joint) 719.0●
    labyrinth (see also Disease, Ménière's) 386.00
    meningeal NEC 331.4
    nutritional 262
    pericardium - see Pericarditis
    pleura (see also Hydrothorax) 511.89
    renal (see also Nephrosis) 581.9
    spermatic cord (see also Hydrocele) 603.9
Hydropyonephrosis (see also Pyelitis) 590.80
    chronic 590.00
Hydrorachis 742.53
Hydrorrhea (nasal) 478.19
    gravidarum 658.1●
    pregnancy 658.1●

Hydrosadenitis 705.83
Hydrosalpinx (fallopian tube) (follicularis) 614.1
Hydrothorax (double) (pleural) 511.89
    chylous (nonfilarial) 457.8
        filaria (see also Infestation, filarial) 125.9
    nontuberculous 511.89
        bacterial 511.1
        pneumococcal 511.1
        staphylococcal 511.1
        streptococcal 511.1
    traumatic 862.29
        with open wound into thorax 862.39
    tuberculous (see also Tuberculosis, pleura) 012.0●
Hydroureter 593.5
    congenital 753.22
Hydroureteronephrosis (see also Hydronephrosis) 591
Hydrourethra 599.84
Hydroxykynureninuria 270.2
Hydroxyprolinemia 270.8
Hydroxyprolinuria 270.8
Hygroma (congenital) (cystic) (M9173/0) 228.1
    prepatellar 727.3
    subdural - see Hematoma, subdural
Hymen - see condition
Hymenolepiasis (diminuta) (infection) (infestation) (nana) 123.6
Hymenolepsis (diminuta) (infection) (infestation) (nana) 123.6
Hypalgesia (see also Disturbance, sensation) 782.0
Hyperabduction syndrome 447.8
Hyperacidity, gastric 536.8
    psychogenic 306.4
Hyperactive, hyperactivity 314.01
    basal cell, uterine cervix 622.10
    bladder 596.51
    bowel (syndrome) 564.9
        sounds 787.5
    cervix epithelial (basal) 622.10
    child 314.01
    colon 564.9
    gastrointestinal 536.8
        psychogenic 306.4
    intestine 564.9
    labyrinth (unilateral) 386.51
        with loss of labyrinthine reactivity 386.58
        bilateral 386.52
    nasal mucous membrane 478.19
    stomach 536.8
    thyroid (gland) (see also Thyrotoxicosis) 242.9●
Hyperacusis 388.42
Hyperadrenalism (cortical) 255.3
    medullary 255.6
Hyperadrenocorticism 255.3
    congenital 255.2
    iatrogenic
        correct substance properly administered 255.3
        overdose or wrong substance given or taken 962.0
Hyperaffectivity 301.11
Hyperaldosteronism (atypical) (hyperplastic) (normoaldosteronal) (nor-motensive) (primary) 255.10
    secondary 255.14
Hyperalgesia (see also Disturbance, sensation) 782.0
Hyperalimentation 783.6
    carotene 278.3
    specified NEC 278.8
    vitamin A 278.2
    vitamin D 278.4
Hyperaminoaciduria 270.9
    arginine 270.6
    citrulline 270.6
    cystine 270.0
    glycine 270.0

SECTION I INDEX TO DISEASES AND INJURIES / Hyperaminoaciduria

Hyperaminoaciduria *(Continued)*
   lysine 270.7
   ornithine 270.6
   renal (types I, II, III) 270.0
Hyperammonemia (congenital) 270.6
Hyperamnesia 780.99
Hyperamylasemia 790.5
Hyperaphia 782.0
Hyperazotemia 791.9
Hyperbetalipoproteinemia (acquired)
      (essential) (familial) (hereditary)
      (primary) (secondary) 272.0
   with prebetalipoproteinemia 272.2
Hyperbilirubinemia 782.4
   congenital 277.4
   constitutional 277.4
   neonatal (transient) *(see also* Jaundice, fetus
      or newborn) 774.6
   of prematurity 774.2
Hyperbilirubinemica encephalopathia,
   newborn 774.7
   due to isoimmunization 773.4
Hypercalcemia, hypercalcemic (idiopathic)
   275.42
   nephropathy 588.89
Hypercalcinuria 275.40
Hypercapnia 786.09
   with mixed acid-based disorder 276.4
   fetal, affecting newborn 770.89
Hypercarotinemia 278.3
Hypercementosis 521.5
Hyperchloremia 276.9
Hyperchlorhydria 536.8
   neurotic 306.4
   psychogenic 306.4
Hypercholesterinemia - *see*
   Hypercholesterolemia
Hypercholesterolemia 272.0
   with hyperglyceridemia, endogenous
      272.2
   essential 272.0
   familial 272.0
   hereditary 272.0
   primary 272.0
   pure 272.0
Hypercholesterolosis 272.0
Hyperchylia gastrica 536.8
   psychogenic 306.4
Hyperchylomicronemia (familial) (with
   hyperbetalipoproteinemia) 272.3
Hypercoagulation syndrome (primary)
   289.81
   secondary 289.82
Hypercorticosteronism
   correct substance properly administered
      255.3
   overdose or wrong substance given or taken
      962.0
Hypercortisonism
   correct substance properly administered
      255.3
   overdose or wrong substance given or taken
      962.0
Hyperdynamic beta-adrenergic state or
   syndrome (circulatory) 429.82
Hyperekplexia 759.89
Hyperelectrolytemia 276.9
Hyperemesis 536.2
   arising during pregnancy - *see* Hyperemesis,
      gravidarum
   gravidarum (mild) (before 22 completed
      weeks' gestation) 643.0●
      with
         carbohydrate depletion 643.1●
         dehydration 643.1●
         electrolyte imbalance 643.1●
         metabolic disturbance 643.1●
      affecting fetus or newborn 761.8
      severe (with metabolic disturbance)
         643.1●
   psychogenic 306.4

Hyperemia (acute) 780.99
   anal mucosa 569.49
   bladder 596.7
   cerebral 437.8
   conjunctiva 372.71
   ear, internal, acute 386.30
   enteric 564.89
   eye 372.71
   eyelid (active) (passive) 374.82
   intestine 564.89
   iris 364.41
   kidney 593.81
   labyrinth 386.30
   liver (active) (passive) 573.8
   lung 514
   ovary 620.8
   passive 780.99
   pulmonary 514
   renal 593.81
   retina 362.89
   spleen 289.59
   stomach 537.89
Hyperesthesia (body surface) *(see also*
   Disturbance, sensation) 782.0
   larynx (reflex) 478.79
      hysterical 300.11
   pharynx (reflex) 478.29
Hyperestrinism 256.0
Hyperestrogenism 256.0
Hyperestrogenosis 256.0
Hyperexplexia 759.89
Hyperextension, joint 718.80
   ankle 718.87
   elbow 718.82
   foot 718.87
   hand 718.84
   hip 718.85
   knee 718.86
   multiple sites 718.89
   pelvic region 718.85
   shoulder (region) 718.81
   specified site NEC 718.88
   wrist 718.83
Hyperfibrinolysis - *see* Fibrinolysis
Hyperfolliculinism 256.0
Hyperfructosemia 271.2
Hyperfunction
   adrenal (cortex) 255.3
      androgenic, acquired benign
         255.3
      medulla 255.6
      virilism 255.2
   corticoadrenal NEC 255.3
   labyrinth - *see* Hyperactive, labyrinth
   medulloadrenal 255.6
   ovary 256.1
      estrogen 256.0
   pancreas 577.8
   parathyroid (gland) 252.00
   pituitary (anterior) (gland) (lobe)
      253.1
   testicular 257.0
Hypergammaglobulinemia 289.89
   monoclonal, benign (BMH) 273.1
   polyclonal 273.0
   Waldenström's 273.0
Hyperglobulinemia 273.8
Hyperglycemia 790.29
   maternal
      affecting fetus or newborn 775.0
      manifest diabetes in infant 775.1
   postpancreatectomy (complete) (partial)
      251.3
Hyperglyceridemia 272.1
   endogenous 272.1
   essential 272.1
   familial 272.1
   hereditary 272.1
   mixed 272.3
   pure 272.1
Hyperglycinemia 270.7

Hypergonadism
   ovarian 256.1
   testicular (infantile) (primary) 257.0
Hyperheparinemia *(see also* Circulating,
   intrinsic anticoagulants) 287.5
Hyperhidrosis, hyperidrosis 705.21
   axilla 705.21
   face 705.21
   focal (localized) 705.21
      primary 705.21
         axilla 705.21
         face 705.21
         palms 705.21
         soles 705.21
      secondary 705.22
         axilla 705.22
         face 705.22
         palms 705.22
         soles 705.22
   generalized 780.8
   palms 705.21
   psychogenic 306.3
   secondary 780.8
   soles 705.21
Hyperhistidinemia 270.5
Hyperinsulinism (ectopic) (functional)
   (organic) NEC 251.1
   iatrogenic 251.0
   reactive 251.2
   spontaneous 251.2
   therapeutic misadventure (from
      administration of insulin) 962.3
Hyperiodemia 276.9
Hyperirritability (cerebral), in newborn 779.1
Hyperkalemia 276.7
Hyperkeratosis *(see also* Keratosis) 701.1
   cervix 622.2
   congenital 757.39
   cornea 371.89
   due to yaws (early) (late) (palmar or plantar)
      102.3
   eccentrica 757.39
   figurata centrifuga atrophica 757.39
   follicularis 757.39
      in cutem penetrans 701.1
   limbic (cornea) 371.89
   palmoplantaris climacterica 701.1
   pinta (carate) 103.1
   senile (with pruritus) 702.0
   tongue 528.79
   universalis congenita 757.1
   vagina 623.1
   vocal cord 478.5
   vulva 624.09
Hyperkinesia, hyperkinetic (disease) (reaction)
   (syndrome) 314.9
   with
      attention deficit - *see* Disorder, attention
         deficit
      conduct disorder 314.2
      developmental delay 314.1
      simple disturbance of activity and
         attention 314.01
      specified manifestation NEC 314.8
   heart (disease) 429.82
   of childhood or adolescence NEC 314.9
Hyperlacrimation *(see also* Epiphora) 375.20
Hyperlipemia *(see also* Hyperlipidemia) 272.4
Hyperlipidemia 272.4
   carbohydrate-induced 272.1
   combined 272.2
   endogenous 272.1
   exogenous 272.3
   fat-induced 272.3
   group
      A 272.0
      B 272.1
      C 272.2
      D 272.3
   mixed 272.2
   specified type NEC 272.4

Hyperlipidosis 272.7
  hereditary 272.7
Hyperlipoproteinemia (acquired) (essential)
    (familial) (hereditary) (primary)
    (secondary) 272.4
  Fredrickson type
    I 272.3
    IIA 272.0
    IIB 272.2
    III 272.2
    IV 272.1
    V 272.3
  low-density-lipoid-type (LDL) 272.0
  very-low-density-lipoid-type [VLDL]
    272.1
Hyperlucent lung, unilateral 492.8
Hyperluteinization 256.1
Hyperlysinemia 270.7
Hypermagnesemia 275.2
  neonatal 775.5
Hypermaturity (fetus or newborn)
  post-term infant 766.21
  prolonged gestation infant 766.22
Hypermenorrhea 626.2
Hypermetabolism 794.7
Hypermethioninemia 270.4
Hypermetropia (congenital) 367.0
Hypermobility
  cecum 564.9
  coccyx 724.71
  colon 564.9
    psychogenic 306.4
  ileum 564.89
  joint (acquired) 718.80
    ankle 718.87
    elbow 718.82
    foot 718.87
    hand 718.84
    hip 718.85
    knee 718.86
    multiple sites 718.89
    pelvic region 718.85
    shoulder (region) 718.81
    specified site NEC 718.88
    wrist 718.83
  kidney, congenital 753.3
  meniscus (knee) 717.5
  scapula 718.81
  stomach 536.8
    psychogenic 306.4
  syndrome 728.5
  testis, congenital 752.52
  urethral 599.81
Hypermotility
  gastrointestinal 536.8
  intestine 564.9
    psychogenic 306.4
  stomach 536.8
Hypernasality 784.43
Hypernatremia 276.0
  with water depletion 276.0
Hypernephroma (M8312/3) 189.0
Hyperopia 367.0
Hyperorexia 783.6
Hyperornithinemia 270.6
Hyperosmia (see also Disturbance, sensation)
    781.1
Hyperosmolality 276.0
Hyperosteogenesis 733.99
Hyperostosis 733.99
  calvarial 733.3
  cortical 733.3
    infantile 756.59
  frontal, internal of skull 733.3
  interna frontalis 733.3
  monomelic 733.99
  skull 733.3
    congenital 756.0
  vertebral 721.8
    with spondylosis - see Spondylosis
    ankylosing 721.6

Hyperovarianism 256.1
Hyperovarism, hyperovaria 256.1
Hyperoxaluria (primary) 271.8
Hyperoxia 987.8
Hyperparathyroidism 252.00
  ectopic 259.3
  other 252.08
  primary 252.01
  secondary (of renal origin) 588.81
    non-renal 252.02
  tertiary 252.08
Hyperpathia (see also Disturbance, sensation)
    782.0
  psychogenic 307.80
Hyperperistalsis 787.4
  psychogenic 306.4
Hyperpermeability, capillary 448.9
Hyperphagia 783.6
Hyperphenylalaninemia 270.1
Hyperphoria 378.40
  alternating 378.45
Hyperphosphatemia 275.3
Hyperpiesia (see also Hypertension) 401.9
Hyperpiesis (see also Hypertension) 401.9
Hyperpigmentation - see Pigmentation
Hyperpinealism 259.8
Hyperpipecolatemia 270.7
Hyperpituitarism 253.1
Hyperplasia, hyperplastic
  adenoids (lymphoid tissue) 474.12
    and tonsils 474.10
  adrenal (capsule) (cortex) (gland) 255.8
    with
      sexual precocity (male) 255.2
      virilism, adrenal 255.2
      virilization (female) 255.2
    congenital 255.2
    due to excess ACTH (ectopic) (pituitary)
      255.0
    medulla 255.8
  alpha cells (pancreatic)
    with
      gastrin excess 251.5
      glucagon excess 251.4
  angiolymphoid, with eosinophilia (ALHE)
    228.01
  appendix (lymphoid) 543.0
  artery, fibromuscular NEC 447.8
    carotid 447.8
    renal 447.3
  bone 733.99
    marrow 289.9
  breast (see also Hypertrophy, breast) 611.1
    ductal 610.8
      atypical 610.8
  carotid artery 447.8
  cementation, cementum (teeth) (tooth) 521.5
  cervical gland 785.6
  cervix (uteri) 622.10
    basal cell 622.10
    congenital 752.49
    endometrium 622.10
    polypoid 622.10
  chin 524.05
  clitoris, congenital 752.49
  dentin 521.5
  endocervicitis 616.0
  endometrium, endometrial (adenomatous)
      (atypical) (cystic) (glandular)
      (polypoid) (uterus) 621.30
    with atypia 621.33
    without atypia
      complex 621.32
      simple 621.31
    benign 621.34
    cervix 622.10
  epithelial 709.8
    focal, oral, including tongue 528.79
    mouth (focal) 528.79
    nipple 611.89
    skin 709.8

Hyperplasia, hyperplastic (Continued)
  epithelial (Continued)
    tongue (focal) 528.79
    vaginal wall 623.0
  erythroid 289.9
  fascialis ossificans (progressiva) 728.11
  fibromuscular, artery NEC 447.8
    carotid 447.8
    renal 447.3
  genital
    female 629.89
    male 608.89
  gingiva 523.8
  glandularis
    cystica uteri 621.30
    endometrium (uterus) 621.30
    interstitialis uteri 621.30
  granulocytic 288.69
  gum 523.8
  hymen, congenital 752.49
  islands of Langerhans 251.1
  islet cell (pancreatic) 251.9
    alpha cells
      with excess
        gastrin 251.5
        glucagon 251.4
      beta cells 251.1
  juxtaglomerular (complex) (kidney) 593.89
  kidney (congenital) 753.3
  liver (congenital) 751.69
  lymph node (gland) 785.6
  lymphoid (diffuse) (nodular) 785.6
    appendix 543.0
    intestine 569.89
  mandibular 524.02
    alveolar 524.72
    unilateral condylar 526.89
  Marchand multiple nodular (liver) - see
      Cirrhosis, postnecrotic
  maxillary 524.01
    alveolar 524.71
  medulla, adrenal 255.8
  myometrium, myometrial 621.2
  neuroendocrine cell, of infancy 516.61
  nose (lymphoid) (polypoid) 478.19
  oral soft tissue (inflammatory) (irritative)
      (mucosa) NEC 528.9
    gingiva 523.8
    tongue 529.8
  organ or site, congenital NEC - see Anomaly,
      specified type NEC
  ovary 620.8
  palate, papillary 528.9
  pancreatic islet cells 251.9
    alpha
      with excess
        gastrin 251.5
        glucagon 251.4
      beta 251.1
  parathyroid (gland) 252.01
  persistent, vitreous (primary) 743.51
  pharynx (lymphoid) 478.29
  prostate 600.90
    with
      other lower urinary tract symptoms
        (LUTS) 600.91
      urinary
        obstruction 600.91
        retention 600.91
    adenofibromatous 600.20
      with
        other lower urinary tract
          symptoms (LUTS) 600.21
        urinary
          obstruction 600.21
          retention 600.21
    nodular 600.10
      with
        urinary
          obstruction 600.11
          retention 600.11

Hyperplasia, hyperplastic (Continued)
  renal artery (fibromuscular) 447.3
  reticuloendothelial (cell) 289.9
  salivary gland (any) 527.1
  Schimmelbusch's 610.1
  suprarenal (capsule) (gland) 255.8
  thymus (gland) (persistent) 254.0
  thyroid (see also Goiter) 240.9
    primary 242.0●
    secondary 242.2●
  tonsil (lymphoid tissue) 474.11
    and adenoids 474.10
  urethrovaginal 599.89
  uterus, uterine (myometrium) 621.2
    endometrium (see also Hyperplasia, endometrium) 621.30
  vitreous (humor), primary persistent 743.51
  vulva 624.3
  zygoma 738.11
Hyperpnea (see also Hyperventilation) 786.01
Hyperpotassemia 276.7
Hyperprebetalipoproteinemia 272.1
  with chylomicronemia 272.3
  familial 272.1
Hyperprolactinemia 253.1
Hyperprolinemia 270.8
Hyperproteinemia 273.8
Hyperprothrombinemia 289.89
Hyperpselaphesia 782.0
Hyperpyrexia 780.60
  heat (effects of) 992.0
  malarial (see also Malaria) 084.6
  malignant, due to anesthetic 995.86
  rheumatic - see Fever, rheumatic
  unknown origin (see also Pyrexia) 780.60
Hyperreactor, vascular 780.2
Hyperreflexia 796.1
  bladder, autonomic 596.54
    with cauda equina 344.61
  detrusor 344.61
Hypersalivation (see also Ptyalism) 527.7
Hypersarcosinemia 270.8

Hypersecretion
  ACTH 255.3
  androgens (ovarian) 256.1
  calcitonin 246.0
  corticoadrenal 255.3
  cortisol 255.0
  estrogen 256.0
  gastric 536.8
    psychogenic 306.4
  gastrin 251.5
  glucagon 251.4
  hormone
    ACTH 255.3
    anterior pituitary 253.1
    growth NEC 253.0
    ovarian androgen 256.1
    testicular 257.0
    thyroid stimulating 242.8●
  insulin - see Hyperinsulinism
  lacrimal glands (see also Epiphora) 375.20
  medulloadrenal 255.6
  milk 676.6●
  ovarian androgens 256.1
  pituitary (anterior) 253.1
  salivary gland (any) 527.7
  testicular hormones 257.0
  thyrocalcitonin 246.0
  upper respiratory 478.9
Hypersegmentation, hereditary 288.2
  eosinophils 288.2
  neutrophil nuclei 288.2
Hypersensitive, hypersensitiveness, hypersensitivity - see also Allergy
  angiitis 446.20
    specified NEC 446.29
  carotid sinus 337.01
  colon 564.9
    psychogenic 306.4
  DNA (deoxyribonucleic acid) NEC 287.2
  drug (see also Allergy, drug) 995.27
  due to correct medical substance properly administered 995.27

Hypersensitive, hypersensitiveness, hypersensitivity (Continued)
  esophagus 530.89
  insect bites - see Injury, superficial, by site
  labyrinth 386.58
  pain (see also Disturbance, sensation) 782.0
  pneumonitis NEC 495.9
  reaction (see also Allergy) 995.3
    upper respiratory tract NEC 478.8
  stomach (allergic) (nonallergic) 536.8
    psychogenic 306.4
Hypersomatotropism (classic) 253.0
Hypersomnia, unspecified 780.54
  with sleep apnea, unspecified 780.53
  alcohol induced 291.82
  drug induced 292.85
  due to
    medical condition classified elsewhere 327.14
    mental disorder 327.15
  idiopathic
    with long sleep time 327.11
    without long sleep time 327.12
  menstrual related 327.13
  nonorganic origin 307.43
    persistent (primary) 307.44
    transient 307.43
  organic 327.10
  other 327.19
  primary 307.44
  recurrent 327.13
Hypersplenia 289.4
Hypersplenism 289.4
Hypersteatosis 706.3
Hyperstimulation, ovarian 256.1
Hypersuprarenalism 255.3
Hypersusceptibility - see Allergy
Hyper-TBG-nemia 246.8
Hypertelorism 756.0
  orbit, orbital 376.41
Hypertension, hypertensive - see table on pages 255–258

SECTION I INDEX TO DISEASES AND INJURIES / Hypertension, hypertensive

OGCR Section I.C.7.a.1
Assign hypertension (arterial) (essential) (systemic) (NOS) to category code 401 with appropriate fourth digit to indicate malignant (.0), benign (.1), or unspecified (.9). Do not use either .0 malignant or .1 benign unless medical record documentation supports such a designation.

	Malignant	Benign	Unspecified
Hypertension, hypertensive (arterial) (arteriolar) (crisis) (degeneration) (disease) (essential) (fluctuating) (idiopathic) (intermittent) (labile) (low renin) (orthostatic) (paroxysmal) (primary) (systemic) (uncontrolled) (vascular)	401.0	401.1	401.9
with			
chronic kidney disease	—	—	—
stage I through stage IV, or unspecified	403.00	403.10	403.90
stage V or end stage renal disease	403.01	403.11	403.91
heart involvement (conditions classifiable to 429.0–429.3, 429.8, 429.9 due to hypertension) (see also Hypertension, heart)	402.00	402.10	402.90
with kidney involvement - see Hypertension, cardiorenal			
renal (kidney) involvement (only conditions classifiable to 585, 587) (excludes conditions classifiable to 584) (see also Hypertension, kidney)	403.00	403.10	403.90
with heart involvement - see Hypertension, cardiorenal failure (and sclerosis) (see also Hypertension, kidney)	403.01	403.11	403.91
sclerosis without failure (see also Hypertension, kidney)	403.00	403.10	403.90
accelerated (see also Hypertension, by type, malignant)	401.0	—	—
antepartum - see Hypertension, complicating pregnancy, childbirth, or the puerperium			
borderline	—	—	796.2
cardiorenal (disease)	404.00	404.10	404.90
with			
chronic kidney disease	—	—	—
stage I through stage IV, or unspecified	404.00	404.10	404.90
and heart failure	404.01	404.11	404.91
stage V or end stage renal disease	404.02	404.12	404.92
and heart failure	404.03	404.13	404.93
heart failure	404.01	404.11	404.91
and chronic kidney disease	404.01	404.11	404.91
stage I through stage IV or unspecified	404.01	404.11	404.91
stage V or end stage renal disease	404.03	404.13	404.93
cardiovascular disease (arteriosclerotic) (sclerotic)	402.00	402.10	402.90
with			
heart failure	402.01	402.11	402.91
renal involvement (conditions classifiable to 403) (see also Hypertension, cardiorenal)	404.00	404.10	404.90
cardiovascular renal (disease) (sclerosis) (see also Hypertension, cardiorenal)	404.00	404.10	404.90
cerebrovascular disease NEC	437.2	437.2	437.2
complicating pregnancy, childbirth, or the puerperium	642.2●	642.0●	642.9●
with			
albuminuria (and edema) (mild)	—	—	642.4●
severe	—	—	642.5●
chronic kidney disease	642.2●	642.2●	642.2●
and heart disease	642.2●	642.2●	642.2●
edema (mild)	—	—	642.4●
severe	—	—	642.5●
heart disease	642.2●	642.2●	642.2●
and chronic kidney disease	642.2●	642.2●	642.2●

◀ New   Revised   ~~deleted~~ Deleted   ● Use Additional Digit(s)   ▨ Omit code

	Malignant	Benign	Unspecified
Hypertension, hypertensive *(Continued)*			
complicating pregnancy, childbirth, or the puerperium *(Continued)*			
with *(Continued)*			
renal disease	642.2●	642.2●	642.2●
and heart disease	642.2●	642.2●	642.2●
chronic	642.2●	642.0●	642.0●
with pre-eclampsia or eclampsia	642.7●	642.7●	642.7●
fetus or newborn	760.0	760.0	760.0
essential	—	642.0●	642.0●
with pre-eclampsia or eclampsia	—	642.7●	642.7●
fetus or newborn	760.0	760.0	760.0
fetus or newborn	760.0	760.0	760.0
gestational	—	—	642.3●
pre-existing	642.2●	642.0●	642.0●
with pre-eclampsia or eclampsia	642.7●	642.7●	642.7●
fetus or newborn	760.0	760.0	760.0
secondary to renal disease	642.1●	642.1●	642.1●
with pre-eclampsia or eclampsia	642.7●	642.7●	642.7●
fetus or newborn	760.0	760.0	760.0
transient	—	—	642.3●
due to			
aldosteronism, primary	405.09	405.19	405.99
brain tumor	405.09	405.19	405.99
bulbar poliomyelitis	405.09	405.19	405.99
calculus			
kidney	405.09	405.19	405.99
ureter	405.09	405.19	405.99
coarctation, aorta	405.09	405.19	405.99
Cushing's disease	405.09	405.19	405.99
glomerulosclerosis *(see also* Hypertension, kidney)	403.00	403.10	403.90
periarteritis nodosa	405.09	405.19	405.99
pheochromocytoma	405.09	405.19	405.99
polycystic kidney(s)	405.09	405.19	405.99
polycythemia	405.09	405.19	405.99
porphyria	405.09	405.19	405.99
pyelonephritis	405.09	405.19	405.99
renal (artery)			
aneurysm	405.01	405.11	405.91
anomaly	405.01	405.11	405.91
embolism	405.01	405.11	405.91
fibromuscular hyperplasia	405.01	405.11	405.91
occlusion	405.01	405.11	405.91
stenosis	405.01	405.11	405.91
thrombosis	405.01	405.11	405.91

SECTION I INDEX TO DISEASES AND INJURIES / Hypertension, hypertensive

	Malignant	Benign	Unspecified
Hypertension, hypertensive *(Continued)*			
encephalopathy	437.2	437.2	437.2
gestational (transient) NEC	—	—	642.3 ●
Goldblatt's	440.1	440.1	440.1
heart (disease) (conditions classifiable to 429.0–429.3, 429.8, 429.9 due to hypertension)	402.00	402.10	402.90
with			
heart failure	402.01	402.11	402.91
hypertensive kidney disease (conditions classifiable to 403) (*see also* Hypertension, cardiorenal)	404.00	404.10	404.90
renal sclerosis (*see also* Hypertension, cardiorenal)	404.00	404.10	404.90
intracranial, benign	—	348.2	—
intraocular	—	—	365.04
kidney	403.00	403.10	403.90
with			
chronic kidney disease	—	—	—
stage I through stage IV, or unspecified	403.00	403.10	403.90
stage V or end stage renal disease	403.01	403.11	403.91
heart involvement (conditions classifiable to 429.0–429.3, 429.8, 429.9 due to hypertension) (*see also* Hypertension, cardiorenal)	404.00	404.10	404.90
hypertensive heart (disease) (conditions classifiable to 402) (*see also* Hypertension, cardiorenal)	404.00	404.10	404.90
lesser circulation	—	—	416.0
necrotizing	401.0	—	—
pancreatic duct - *code to* underlying condition			
with			
chronic pancreatitis	—	—	577.11
ocular			365.04
portal (due to chronic liver disease)	—	—	572.3
postoperative			997.91
psychogenic	—	—	306.2
puerperal, postpartum - *see* Hypertension, complicating pregnancy, childbirth, or the puerperium			
pulmonary (artery) (secondary)	—	—	416.8
with			
cor pulmonale (chronic)	—	—	416.8
acute	—	—	415.0
right heart ventricular strain/failure	—	—	416.8
acute	—	—	415.0
idiopathic	—	—	416.0
primary	—	—	416.0
of newborn	—	—	747.83
secondary	—	—	416.8

◄ New   ◄◄ Revised   ~~deleted~~ Deleted   Use Additional Digit(s)   Omit code

SECTION I INDEX TO DISEASES AND INJURIES / Hypertension, hypertensive

	Malignant	Benign	Unspecified
Hypertension, hypertensive *(Continued)*			
renal (disease) *(see also* Hypertension, kidney)	403.00	403.10	403.90
renovascular NEC	405.01	405.11	405.91
secondary NEC	405.09	405.19	405.99
due to			
aldosteronism, primary	405.09	405.19	405.99
brain tumor	405.09	405.19	405.99
bulbar poliomyelitis	405.09	405.19	405.99
calculus			
kidney	405.09	405.19	405.99
ureter	405.09	405.19	405.99
coarctation, aorta	405.09	405.19	405.99
Cushing's disease	405.09	405.19	405.99
glomerulosclerosis *(see also* Hypertension, kidney)	403.00	403.10	403.90
periarteritis nodosa	405.09	405.19	405.99
pheochromocytoma	405.09	405.19	405.99
polycystic kidney(s)	405.09	405.19	405.99
polycythemia	405.09	405.19	405.99
porphyria	405.09	405.19	405.99
pyelonephritis	405.09	405.19	405.99
renal (artery)			
aneurysm	405.01	405.11	405.91
anomaly	405.01	405.11	405.91
embolism	405.01	405.11	405.91
fibromuscular hyperplasia	405.01	405.11	405.91
occlusion	405.01	405.11	405.91
stenosis	405.01	405.11	405.91
thrombosis	405.01	405.11	405.91
transient	—	—	796.2
of pregnancy	—	—	642.3●
venous, chronic (asymptomatic) (idiopathic)	—	—	459.30
with			
complication, NEC	—	—	459.39
inflammation	—	—	459.32
with ulcer	—	—	459.33
ulcer	—	—	459.31
with inflammation	—	—	459.33
due to			
deep vein thrombosis *(see also* Syndrome, postphlebitic)	—	—	459.10

Hypertensive urgency - *see* Hypertension
Hyperthecosis, ovary 256.8
Hyperthermia (of unknown origin) (*see also* Pyrexia) 780.60
    malignant (due to anesthesia) 995.86
    newborn 778.4
Hyperthymergasia (*see also* Psychosis, affective) 296.0●
    reactive (from emotional stress, psychological trauma) 298.1
    recurrent episode 296.1●
    single episode 296.0●
Hyperthymism 254.8
Hyperthyroid (recurrent) - *see* Hyperthyroidism
Hyperthyroidism (latent) (preadult) (recurrent) (without goiter) 242.9●

> Note: Use the following fifth-digit subclassification with category 242:
> 0 without mention of thyrotoxic crisis or storm
> 1 with mention of thyrotoxic crisis or storm

    with
        goiter (diffuse) 242.0●
            adenomatous 242.3●
                multinodular 242.2●
                uninodular 242.1●
            nodular 242.3●
                multinodular 242.2●
                uninodular 242.1●
        thyroid nodule 242.1●
    complicating pregnancy, childbirth, or puerperium 648.1●
    neonatal (transient) 775.3
Hypertonia - *see* Hypertonicity
Hypertonicity
    bladder 596.51
    fetus or newborn 779.89
    gastrointestinal (tract) 536.8
    infancy 779.89
        due to electrolyte imbalance 779.89
    muscle 728.85
    stomach 536.8
        psychogenic 306.4
    uterus, uterine (contractions) 661.4●
        affecting fetus or newborn 763.7
Hypertony - *see* Hypertonicity
Hypertransaminemia 790.4
Hypertrichosis 704.1
    congenital 757.4
    eyelid 374.54
    lanuginosa 757.4
        acquired 704.1
Hypertriglyceridemia, essential 272.1
Hypertrophy, hypertrophic
    adenoids (infectional) 474.12
        and tonsils (faucial) (infective) (lingual) (lymphoid) 474.10
    adrenal 255.8
    alveolar process or ridge 525.8
    anal papillae 569.49
    apocrine gland 705.82
    artery NEC 447.8
        carotid 447.8
        congenital (peripheral) NEC 747.60
            gastrointestinal 747.61
            lower limb 747.64
            renal 747.62
            specified NEC 747.69
            spinal 747.82
            upper limb 747.63
        renal 447.3
    arthritis (chronic) (*see also* Osteoarthrosis) 715.9●
        spine (*see also* Spondylosis) 721.90
    arytenoid 478.79
    asymmetrical (heart) 429.9
    auricular - *see* Hypertrophy, cardiac
    Bartholin's gland 624.8
    bile duct 576.8

Hypertrophy, hypertrophic (*Continued*)
    bladder (sphincter) (trigone) 596.89
    blind spot, visual field 368.42
    bone 733.99
    brain 348.89
    breast 611.1
        cystic 610.1
        fetus or newborn 778.7
        fibrocystic 610.1
        massive pubertal 611.1
        puerperal, postpartum 676.3●
        senile (parenchymatous) 611.1
    cardiac (chronic) (idiopathic) 429.3
        with
            rheumatic fever (conditions classifiable to 390)
                active 391.8
                    with chorea 392.0
                inactive or quiescent (with chorea) 398.99
        congenital NEC 746.89
        fatty (*see also* Degeneration, myocardial) 429.1
        hypertensive (*see also* Hypertension, heart) 402.90
        rheumatic (with chorea) 398.99
            active or acute 391.8
                with chorea 392.0
        valve (*see also* Endocarditis) 424.90
            congenital NEC 746.89
    cartilage 733.99
    cecum 569.89
    cervix (uteri) 622.6
        congenital 752.49
        elongation 622.6
    clitoris (cirrhotic) 624.2
        congenital 752.49
    colon 569.89
        congenital 751.3
    conjunctiva, lymphoid 372.73
    cornea 371.89
    corpora cavernosa 607.89
    duodenum 537.89
    endometrium (uterus) (*see also* Hyperplasia, endometrium) 621.30
        cervix 622.6
    epididymis 608.89
    esophageal hiatus (congenital) 756.6
        with hernia - *see* Hernia, diaphragm
    eyelid 374.30
    falx, skull 733.99
    fat pad 729.30
        infrapatellar 729.31
        knee 729.31
        orbital 374.34
        popliteal 729.31
        prepatellar 729.31
        retropatellar 729.31
        specified site NEC 729.39
    foot (congenital) 755.67
    frenum, frenulum (tongue) 529.8
        linguae 529.8
        lip 528.5
    gallbladder or cystic duct 575.8
    gastric mucosa 535.2●
    gingiva 523.8
    gland, glandular (general) NEC 785.6
    gum (mucous membrane) 523.8
    heart (idiopathic) - *see also* Hypertrophy, cardiac
        valve - *see also* Endocarditis
            congenital NEC 746.89
    hemifacial 754.0
    hepatic - *see* Hypertrophy, liver
    hiatus (esophageal) 756.6
    hilus gland 785.6
    hymen, congenital 752.49
    ileum 569.89
    infrapatellar fat pad 729.31
    intestine 569.89
    jejunum 569.89

Hypertrophy, hypertrophic (*Continued*)
    kidney (compensatory) 593.1
        congenital 753.3
    labial frenulum 528.5
    labium (majus) (minus) 624.3
    lacrimal gland, chronic 375.03
    ligament 728.9
        spinal 724.8
    linguae frenulum 529.8
    lingual tonsil (infectional) 474.11
    lip (frenum) 528.5
        congenital 744.81
    liver 789.1
        acute 573.8
        cirrhotic - *see* Cirrhosis, liver
        congenital 751.69
        fatty - *see* Fatty, liver
    lymph gland 785.6
        tuberculous - *see* Tuberculosis, lymph gland
    mammary gland - *see* Hypertrophy, breast
    maxillary frenulum 528.5
    Meckel's diverticulum (congenital) 751.0
    medial meniscus, acquired 717.3
    median bar 600.90
        with
            other lower urinary tract symptoms (LUTS) 600.91
            urinary
                obstruction 600.91
                retention 600.91
    mediastinum 519.3
    meibomian gland 373.2
    meniscus, knee, congenital 755.64
    metatarsal head 733.99
    metatarsus 733.99
    mouth 528.9
    mucous membrane
        alveolar process 523.8
        nose 478.19
        turbinate (nasal) 478.0
    muscle 728.9
    muscular coat, artery NEC 447.8
        carotid 447.8
        renal 447.3
    myocardium (*see also* Hypertrophy, cardiac) 429.3
        idiopathic 425.18
    myometrium 621.2
    nail 703.8
        congenital 757.5
    nasal 478.19
        alae 478.19
        bone 738.0
        cartilage 478.19
        mucous membrane (septum) 478.19
        sinus (*see also* Sinusitis) 473.9
        turbinate 478.0
    nasopharynx, lymphoid (infectional) (tissue) (wall) 478.29
    neck, uterus 622.6
    nipple 611.1
    normal aperture diaphragm (congenital) 756.6
    nose (*see also* Hypertrophy, nasal) 478.19
    orbit 376.46
    organ or site, congenital NEC - *see* Anomaly, specified type NEC
    osteoarthropathy (pulmonary) 731.2
    ovary 620.8
    palate (hard) 526.89
        soft 528.9
    pancreas (congenital) 751.7
    papillae
        anal 569.49
        tongue 529.3
    parathyroid (gland) 252.01
    parotid gland 527.1
    penis 607.89
    phallus 607.89
        female (clitoris) 624.2
    pharyngeal tonsil 474.12
    pharyngitis 472.1

Hypertrophy, hypertrophic (Continued)
  pharynx 478.29
    lymphoid (infectional) (tissue) (wall) 478.29
  pituitary (fossa) (gland) 253.8
  popliteal fat pad 729.31
  preauricular (lymph) gland (Hampstead) 785.6
  prepuce (congenital) 605
    female 624.2
  prostate (asymptomatic) (early) (recurrent) 600.90
    with
      other lower urinary tract symptoms (LUTS) 600.91
      urinary
        obstruction 600.91
        retention 600.91
    adenofibromatous 600.20
      with
        other lower urinary tract symptoms (LUTS) 600.21
        urinary
          obstruction 600.21
          retention 600.21
    benign 600.00
      with
        other lower urinary tract symptoms (LUTS) 600.01
        urinary
          obstruction 600.01
          retention 600.01
    congenital 752.89
  pseudoedematous hypodermal 757.0
  pseudomuscular 359.1
  pylorus (muscle) (sphincter) 537.0
    congenital 750.5
    infantile 750.5
  rectal sphincter 569.49
  rectum 569.49
  renal 593.1
  rhinitis (turbinate) 472.0
  salivary duct or gland 527.1
    congenital 750.26
  scaphoid (tarsal) 733.99
  scar 701.4
  scrotum 608.89
  sella turcica 253.8
  seminal vesicle 608.89
  sigmoid 569.89
  skin condition NEC 701.9
  spermatic cord 608.89
  spinal ligament 724.8
  spleen - *see* Splenomegaly
  spondylitis (spine) (*see also* Spondylosis) 721.90
  stomach 537.89
  subaortic stenosis (idiopathic) 425.11
  sublingual gland 527.1
    congenital 750.26
  submaxillary gland 527.1
  suprarenal (gland) 255.8
  tendon 727.9
  testis 608.89
    congenital 752.89
  thymic, thymus (congenital) (gland) 254.0
  thyroid (gland) (*see also* Goiter) 240.9
    primary 242.0●
    secondary 242.2●
  toe (congenital) 755.65
    acquired 735.8
  tongue 529.8
    congenital 750.15
    frenum 529.8
    papillae (foliate) 529.3
  tonsil (faucial) (infective) (lingual) (lymphoid) 474.11
    with
      adenoiditis 474.01
      tonsillitis 474.00
        and adenoiditis 474.02
    and adenoids 474.10
  tunica vaginalis 608.89

Hypertrophy, hypertrophic (Continued)
  turbinate (mucous membrane) 478.0
  ureter 593.89
  urethra 599.84
  uterus 621.2
    puerperal, postpartum 674.8●
  uvula 528.9
  vagina 623.8
  vas deferens 608.89
  vein 459.89
  ventricle, ventricular (heart) (left) (right) - *see also* Hypertrophy, cardiac
    congenital 746.89
    due to hypertension (left) (right) (*see also* Hypertension, heart) 402.90
      benign 402.10
      malignant 402.00
    right with ventricular septal defect, pulmonary stenosis or atresia, and dextraposition of aorta 745.2
  verumontanum 599.89
  vesical 596.89
  vocal cord 478.5
  vulva 624.3
    stasis (nonfilarial) 624.3
Hypertropia (intermittent) (periodic) 378.31
Hypertyrosinemia 270.2
Hyperuricemia 790.6
Hypervalinemia 270.3
Hyperventilation (tetany) 786.01
  hysterical 300.11
  psychogenic 306.1
  syndrome 306.1
Hyperviscidosis 277.00
Hyperviscosity (of serum) (syndrome) NEC 273.3
  polycythemic 289.0
  sclerocythemic 282.8
Hypervitaminosis (dietary) NEC 278.8
  A (dietary) 278.2
  D (dietary) 278.4
  from excessive administration or use of vitamin preparations (chronic) 278.8
    reaction to sudden overdose 963.5
    vitamin A 278.2
      reaction to sudden overdose 963.5
    vitamin D 278.4
      reaction to sudden overdose 963.5
    vitamin K
      correct substance properly administered 278.8
      overdose or wrong substance given or taken 964.3
Hypervolemia 276.69
Hypesthesia (*see also* Disturbance, sensation) 782.0
  cornea 371.81
Hyphema (anterior chamber) (ciliary body) (iris) 364.41
  traumatic 921.3
Hyphemia - *see* Hyphema
Hypoacidity, gastric 536.8
  psychogenic 306.4
Hypoactive labyrinth (function) - *see* Hypofunction, labyrinth
Hypoadrenalism 255.41
  tuberculous (*see also* Tuberculosis) 017.6●
Hypoadrenocorticism 255.41
  pituitary 253.4
Hypoalbuminemia 273.8
Hypoaldosteronism 255.42
Hypoalphalipoproteinemia 272.5
Hypobarism 993.2
Hypobaropathy 993.2
Hypobetalipoproteinemia (familial) 272.5
Hypocalcemia 275.41
  cow's milk 775.4
  dietary 269.3
  neonatal 775.4
  phosphate-loading 775.4
Hypocalcification, teeth 520.4
Hypochloremia 276.9

Hypochlorhydria 536.8
  neurotic 306.4
  psychogenic 306.4
Hypocholesteremia 272.5
Hypochondria (reaction) 300.7
Hypochondriac 300.7
Hypochondriasis 300.7
Hypochromasia blood cells 280.9
Hypochromic anemia 280.9
  due to blood loss (chronic) 280.0
    acute 285.1
  microcytic 280.9
Hypocoagulability (*see also* Defect, coagulation) 286.9
Hypocomplementemia 279.8
Hypocythemia (progressive) 284.9
Hypodontia (*see also* Anodontia) 520.0
Hypoeosinophilia 288.59
Hypoesthesia (*see also* Disturbance, sensation) 782.0
  cornea 371.81
  tactile 782.0
Hypoestrinism 256.39
Hypoestrogenism 256.39
Hypoferremia 280.9
  due to blood loss (chronic) 280.0
Hypofertility
  female 628.9
  male 606.1
Hypofibrinogenemia 286.3
  acquired 286.6
  congenital 286.3
Hypofunction
  adrenal (gland) 255.41
    cortex 255.41
    medulla 255.5
    specified NEC 255.5
  cerebral 331.9
  corticoadrenal NEC 255.41
  intestinal 564.89
  labyrinth (unilateral) 386.53
    with loss of labyrinthine reactivity 386.55
    bilateral 386.54
      with loss of labyrinthine reactivity 386.56
  Leydig cell 257.2
  ovary 256.39
    postablative 256.2
  pituitary (anterior) (gland) (lobe) 253.2
    posterior 253.5
  testicular 257.2
    iatrogenic 257.1
    postablative 257.1
    postirradiation 257.1
    postsurgical 257.1
Hypogammaglobulinemia 279.00
  acquired primary 279.06
  non-sex-linked, congenital 279.06
  sporadic 279.06
  transient of infancy 279.09
Hypogenitalism (congenital) (female) (male) 752.89
  penis 752.69
Hypoglycemia (spontaneous) 251.2
  coma 251.0
    diabetic 250.3●
      due to secondary diabetes 249.3●
  diabetic 250.8●
    due to secondary diabetes 249.8●
  due to insulin 251.0
    therapeutic misadventure 962.3
  familial (idiopathic) 251.2
  following gastrointestinal surgery 579.3
  infantile (idiopathic) 251.2
  in infant of diabetic mother 775.0
  leucine-induced 270.3
  neonatal 775.6
  reactive 251.2
  specified NEC 251.1
Hypoglycemic shock 251.0
  diabetic 250.8●
    due to secondary diabetes 249.8●

Hypoglycemic shock (Continued)
- due to insulin 251.0
- functional (syndrome) 251.1

Hypogonadism
- female 256.39
- gonadotrophic (isolated) 253.4
- hypogonadotropic (isolated) (with anosmia) 253.4
- isolated 253.4
- male 257.2
  - hereditary familial (Reifenstein's syndrome) 259.52
- ovarian (primary) 256.39
- pituitary (secondary) 253.4
- testicular (primary) (secondary) 257.2

Hypohidrosis 705.0
Hypohidrotic ectodermal dysplasia 757.31
Hypoidrosis 705.0
Hypoinsulinemia, postsurgical 251.3
- postpancreatectomy (complete) (partial) 251.3

Hypokalemia 276.8
Hypokinesia 780.99
Hypoleukia splenica 289.4
Hypoleukocytosis 288.50
Hypolipidemia 272.5
Hypolipoproteinemia 272.5
Hypomagnesemia 275.2
- neonatal 775.4

Hypomania, hypomanic reaction (see also Psychosis, affective) 296.0 ●
- recurrent episode 296.1 ●
- single episode 296.0 ●

Hypomastia (congenital) 611.82
Hypomenorrhea 626.1
Hypometabolism 783.9
Hypomotility
- gastrointestinal tract 536.8
  - psychogenic 306.4
- intestine 564.89
  - psychogenic 306.4
- stomach 536.8
  - psychogenic 306.4

Hyponasality 784.44
Hyponatremia 276.1
Hypo-ovarianism 256.39
Hypo-ovarism 256.39
Hypoparathyroidism (idiopathic) (surgically induced) 252.1
- neonatal 775.4

Hypoperfusion (in)
- newborn 779.89

Hypopharyngitis 462
Hypophoria 378.40
Hypophosphatasia 275.3
Hypophosphatemia (acquired) (congenital) (familial) 275.3
- renal 275.3

Hypophyseal, hypophysis - see also condition
- dwarfism 253.3
- gigantism 253.0
- syndrome 253.8

Hypophyseothalamic syndrome 253.8
Hypopiesis - see Hypotension
Hypopigmentation 709.00
- eyelid 374.53

Hypopinealism 259.8
Hypopituitarism (juvenile) (syndrome) 253.2
- due to
  - hormone therapy 253.7
  - hypophysectomy 253.7
  - radiotherapy 253.7
- postablative 253.7
- postpartum hemorrhage 253.2

Hypoplasia, hypoplasis 759.89
- adrenal (gland) 759.1
- alimentary tract 751.8
  - lower 751.2
  - upper 750.8
- angiolymphoid, with eosinophilia (ALHE) 228.01
- anus, anal (canal) 751.2

Hypoplasia, hypoplasis (Continued)
- aorta 747.22
- aortic
  - arch (tubular) 747.10
  - orifice or valve with hypoplasia of ascending aorta and defective development of left ventricle (with mitral valve atresia) 746.7
- appendix 751.2
- areola 757.6
- arm (see also Absence, arm, congenital) 755.20
- artery (congenital) (peripheral) 747.60
  - brain 747.81
  - cerebral 747.81
  - coronary 746.85
  - gastrointestinal 747.61
  - lower limb 747.64
  - pulmonary 747.31
  - renal 747.62
  - retinal 743.58
  - specified NEC 747.69
  - spinal 747.82
  - umbilical 747.5
  - upper limb 747.63
- auditory canal 744.29
  - causing impairment of hearing 744.02
- biliary duct (common) or passage 751.61
- bladder 753.8
- bone NEC 756.9
  - face 756.0
  - malar 756.0
  - mandible 524.04
    - alveolar 524.74
  - marrow 284.9
    - acquired (secondary) 284.89
    - congenital 284.09
    - idiopathic 284.9
  - maxilla 524.03
    - alveolar 524.73
  - skull (see also Hypoplasia, skull) 756.0
- brain 742.1
  - gyri 742.2
  - specified part 742.2
- breast (areola) 611.82
- bronchus (tree) 748.3
- cardiac 746.89
  - valve - see Hypoplasia, heart, valve
  - vein 746.89
- carpus (see also Absence, carpal, congenital) 755.28
- cartilaginous 756.9
- cecum 751.2
- cementum 520.4
  - hereditary 520.5
- cephalic 742.1
- cerebellum 742.2
- cervix (uteri) 752.43
- chin 524.06
- clavicle 755.51
- coccyx 756.19
- colon 751.2
- corpus callosum 742.2
- cricoid cartilage 748.3
- dermal, focal (Goltz) 757.39
- digestive organ(s) or tract NEC 751.8
  - lower 751.2
  - upper 750.8
- ear 744.29
  - auricle 744.23
  - lobe 744.29
  - middle, except ossicles 744.03
    - ossicles 744.04
  - ossicles 744.04
- enamel of teeth (neonatal) (postnatal) (prenatal) 520.4
  - hereditary 520.5
- endocrine (gland) NEC 759.2
- endometrium 621.8
- epididymis 752.89
- epiglottis 748.3
- erythroid, congenital 284.01
- erythropoietic, chronic acquired 284.81

Hypoplasia, hypoplasis (Continued)
- esophagus 750.3
- Eustachian tube 744.24
- eye (see also Microphthalmos) 743.10
  - lid 743.62
- face 744.89
  - bone(s) 756.0
- fallopian tube 752.19
- femur (see also Absence, femur, congenital) 755.34
- fibula (see also Absence, fibula, congenital) 755.37
- finger (see also Absence, finger, congenital) 755.29
- focal dermal 757.39
- foot 755.31
- gallbladder 751.69
- genitalia, genital organ(s)
  - female 752.89
    - external 752.49
    - internal NEC 752.89
  - in adiposogenital dystrophy 253.8
  - male 752.89
    - penis 752.69
- glottis 748.3
- hair 757.4
- hand 755.21
- heart 746.89
  - left (complex) (syndrome) 746.7
  - valve NEC 746.89
    - pulmonary 746.01
- humerus (see also Absence, humerus, congenital) 755.24
- hymen 752.49
- intestine (small) 751.1
  - large 751.2
- iris 743.46
- jaw 524.09
- kidney(s) 753.0
- labium (majus) (minus) 752.49
- labyrinth, membranous 744.05
- lacrimal duct (apparatus) 743.65
- larynx 748.3
- leg (see also Absence, limb, congenital, lower) 755.30
- limb 755.4
  - lower (see also Absence, limb, congenital, lower) 755.30
  - upper (see also Absence, limb, congenital, upper) 755.20
- liver 751.69
- lung (lobe) 748.5
- mammary (areolar) 611.82
- mandibular 524.04
  - alveolar 524.74
  - unilateral condylar 526.89
- maxillary 524.03
  - alveolar 524.73
- medullary 284.9
- megakaryocytic 287.30
- metacarpus (see also Absence, metacarpal, congenital) 755.28
- metatarsus (see also Absence, metatarsal, congenital) 755.38
- muscle 756.89
  - eye 743.69
- myocardium (congenital) (Uhl's anomaly) 746.84
- nail(s) 757.5
- nasolacrimal duct 743.65
- nervous system NEC 742.8
- neural 742.8
- nose, nasal 748.1
- ophthalmic (see also Microphthalmos) 743.10
- optic nerve 377.43
- organ
  - of Corti 744.05
  - or site NEC - see Anomaly, by site
- osseous meatus (ear) 744.03
- ovary 752.0
- oviduct 752.19
- pancreas 751.7

Hypoplasia, hypoplasis (Continued)
  parathyroid (gland) 759.2
  parotid gland 750.26
  patella 755.64
  pelvis, pelvic girdle 755.69
  penis 752.69
  peripheral vascular system (congenital) NEC 747.60
    gastrointestinal 747.61
    lower limb 747.64
    renal 747.62
    specified NEC 747.69
    spinal 747.82
    upper limb 747.63
  pituitary (gland) 759.2
  pulmonary 748.5
    arteriovenous 747.32
    artery 747.31
    valve 746.01
  punctum lacrimale 743.65
  radioulnar (see also Absence, radius, congenital, with ulna) 755.25
  radius (see also Absence, radius, congenital) 755.26
  rectum 751.2
  respiratory system NEC 748.9
  rib 756.3
  sacrum 756.19
  scapula 755.59
  shoulder girdle 755.59
  skin 757.39
  skull (bone) 756.0
    with
      anencephalus 740.0
      encephalocele 742.0
      hydrocephalus 742.3
        with spina bifida (see also Spina bifida) 741.0●
      microcephalus 742.1
  spinal (cord) (ventral horn cell) 742.59
    vessel 747.82
  spine 756.19
  spleen 759.0
  sternum 756.3
  tarsus (see also Absence, tarsal, congenital) 755.38
  testis, testicle 752.89
  thymus (gland) 279.11
  thyroid (gland) 243
    cartilage 748.3
  tibiofibular (see also Absence, tibia, congenital, with fibula) 755.35
  toe (see also Absence, toe, congenital) 755.39
  tongue 750.16
  trachea (cartilage) (rings) 748.3
  Turner's (tooth) 520.4
  ulna (see also Absence, ulna, congenital) 755.27
  umbilical artery 747.5
  ureter 753.29
  uterus 752.32
  vagina 752.45
  vascular (peripheral) NEC (see also Hypoplasia, peripheral vascular system) 747.60
    brain 747.81
  vein(s) (peripheral) NEC (see also Hypoplasia, peripheral vascular system) 747.60
    brain 747.81
    cardiac 746.89
    great 747.49
    portal 747.49
    pulmonary 747.49
  vena cava (inferior) (superior) 747.49
  vertebra 756.19
  vulva 752.49
  zonule (ciliary) 743.39
  zygoma 738.12
Hypopotassemia 276.8
Hypoproaccelerinemia (see also Defect, coagulation) 286.3
Hypoproconvertinemia (congenital) (see also Defect, coagulation) 286.3
Hypoproteinemia (essential) (hypermetabolic) (idiopathic) 273.8
Hypoproteinosis 260
Hypoprothrombinemia (congenital) (hereditary) (idiopathic) (see also Defect, coagulation) 286.3
  acquired 286.7
  newborn 776.3
Hypopselaphesia 782.0
Hypopyon (anterior chamber) (eye) 364.05
  iritis 364.05
  ulcer (cornea) 370.04
Hypopyrexia 780.99
Hyporeflex 796.1
Hyporeninemia, extreme 790.99
  in primary aldosteronism 255.10
Hyporesponsive episode 780.09
Hyposecretion
  ACTH 253.4
  ovary 256.39
    postablative 256.2
  salivary gland (any) 527.7
Hyposegmentation of neutrophils, hereditary 288.2
Hyposiderinemia 280.9
Hyposmolality 276.1
  syndrome 276.1
Hyposomatotropism 253.3
Hyposomnia, unspecified (see also Insomnia) 780.52
  with sleep apnea, unspecified 780.51
Hypospadias (male) 752.61
  female 753.8
Hypospermatogenesis 606.1
Hyposphagma 372.72
Hyposplenism 289.59
Hypostasis, pulmonary 514
Hypostatic - see condition
Hyposthenuria 593.89
Hyposuprarenalism 255.41
Hypo-TBG-nemia 246.8
Hypotension (arterial) (constitutional) 458.9
  chronic 458.1
  iatrogenic 458.29
  maternal, syndrome (following labor and delivery) 669.2●
  of hemodialysis 458.21
  orthostatic (chronic) 458.0
    dysautonomic-dyskinetic syndrome 333.0
  permanent idiopathic 458.1
  postoperative 458.29
  postural 458.0
  specified type NEC 458.8
  transient 796.3
Hypothermia (accidental) 991.6
  anesthetic 995.89
  associated with low environmental temperature 991.6
  newborn NEC 778.3
  not associated with low environmental temperature 780.65
Hypothymergasia (see also Psychosis, affective) 296.2●
  recurrent episode 296.3●
  single episode 296.2●
Hypothyroidism (acquired) 244.9
  complicating pregnancy, childbirth, or puerperium 648.1●
  congenital 243
  due to
    ablation 244.1
      radioactive iodine 244.1
      surgical 244.0
    iodine (administration) (ingestion) 244.2
      radioactive 244.1
    irradiation therapy 244.1
    p-aminosalicylic acid (PAS) 244.3
    phenylbutazone 244.3
    resorcinol 244.3
Hypothyroidism (Continued)
  due to (Continued)
    specified cause NEC 244.8
    surgery 244.0
  goitrous (sporadic) 246.1
  iatrogenic NEC 244.3
  iodine 244.2
  pituitary 244.8
  postablative NEC 244.1
  postsurgical 244.0
  primary 244.9
  secondary NEC 244.8
  specified cause NEC 244.8
  sporadic goitrous 246.1
Hypotonia, hypotonicity, hypotony 781.3
  benign congenital 358.8
  bladder 596.4
  congenital 779.89
    benign 358.8
  eye 360.30
    due to
      fistula 360.32
      ocular disorder NEC 360.33
      following loss of aqueous or vitreous 360.33
    primary 360.31
  infantile muscular (benign) 359.0
  muscle 728.9
  uterus, uterine (contractions) - see Inertia, uterus
Hypotrichosis 704.09
  congenital 757.4
  lid (congenital) 757.4
    acquired 374.55
  postinfectional NEC 704.09
Hypotropia 378.32
Hypoventilation 786.09
  congenital central alveolar syndrome 327.25
  idiopathic sleep related nonobstructive alveolar 327.24
  obesity 278.03
  sleep related, in conditions classifiable elsewhere 327.26
Hypovitaminosis (see also Deficiency, vitamin) 269.2
Hypovolemia 276.52
  surgical shock 998.09
  traumatic (shock) 958.4
Hypoxemia (see also Anoxia) 799.02
  sleep related, in conditions classifiable elsewhere 327.26
Hypoxia (see also Anoxia) 799.02
  cerebral 348.1
    during or resulting from a procedure 997.01
    newborn 770.88
      mild or moderate 768.6
      severe 768.5
  fetal, affecting newborn 770.88
  intrauterine - see Distress, fetal
  myocardial (see also Insufficiency, coronary) 411.89
    arteriosclerotic - see Arteriosclerosis, coronary
  newborn 770.88
  sleep related 327.24
Hypoxic-ischemic encephalopathy (HIE) 768.70
  mild 768.71
  moderate 768.72
  severe 768.73
Hypsarrhythmia (see also Epilepsy) 345.6●
Hysteralgia, pregnant uterus 646.8●
Hysteria, hysterical 300.10
  anxiety 300.20
  Charcôt's gland 300.11
  conversion (any manifestation) 300.11
  dissociative type NEC 300.15
  psychosis, acute 298.1
Hysteroepilepsy 300.11
Hysterotomy, affecting fetus or newborn 763.89

I

Iatrogenic syndrome of excess cortisol 255.0
IBM (inclusion body myositis) 359.71
Iceland disease (epidemic neuromyasthenia) 049.8
Ichthyosis (congenita) 757.1
    acquired 701.1
    fetalis gravior 757.1
    follicularis 757.1
    hystrix 757.39
    lamellar 757.1
    lingual 528.6
    palmaris and plantaris 757.39
    simplex 757.1
    vera 757.1
    vulgaris 757.1
Ichthyotoxism 988.0
    bacterial (*see also* Poisoning, food) 005.9
Icteroanemia, hemolytic (acquired) 283.9
    congenital (*see also* Spherocytosis) 282.0
Icterus (*see also* Jaundice) 782.4
    catarrhal - *see* Icterus, infectious
    conjunctiva 782.4
        newborn 774.6
    epidemic - *see* Icterus, infectious
    febrilis - *see* Icterus, infectious
    fetus or newborn - *see* Jaundice, fetus or newborn
    gravis (*see also* Necrosis, liver) 570
        complicating pregnancy 646.7 ●
            affecting fetus or newborn 760.8
        fetus or newborn NEC 773.0
        obstetrical 646.7 ●
            affecting fetus or newborn 760.8
    hematogenous (acquired) 283.9
    hemolytic (acquired) 283.9
        congenital (*see also* Spherocytosis) 282.0
    hemorrhagic (acute) 100.0
        leptospiral 100.0
        newborn 776.0
        spirochetal 100.0
    infectious 070.1
        with hepatic coma 070.0
        leptospiral 100.0
        spirochetal 100.0
    intermittens juvenilis 277.4
    malignant (*see also* Necrosis, liver) 570
    neonatorum (*see also* Jaundice, fetus or newborn) 774.6
    pernicious (*see also* Necrosis, liver) 570
    spirochetal 100.0
Ictus solaris, solis 992.0
Id reaction (due to bacteria) 692.89
Ideation
    homicidal V62.85
    suicidal V62.84
Identity disorder 313.82
    dissociative 300.14
    gender role (child) 302.6
        adult 302.85
    psychosexual (child) 302.6
        adult 302.85
Idioglossia 307.9
Idiopathic - *see* condition
Idiosyncrasy (*see also* Allergy) 995.3
    drug, medicinal substance, and biological - *see* Allergy, drug
Idiot, idiocy (congenital) 318.2
    amaurotic (Bielschowsky) (-Jansky) (family) (infantile (late)) (juvenile (late)) (Vogt-Spielmeyer) 330.1
    microcephalic 742.1
    Mongolian 758.0
    oxycephalic 756.0
IEED (involuntary emotional expression disorder) 310.81
IFIS (intraoperative floppy iris syndrome) 364.81
IgE asthma 493.0 ●

Ileitis (chronic) (*see also* Enteritis) 558.9
    infectious 009.0
    noninfectious 558.9
    regional (ulcerative) 555.0
        with large intestine 555.2
    segmental 555.0
        with large intestine 555.2
    terminal (ulcerative) 555.0
        with large intestine 555.2
Ileocolitis (*see also* Enteritis) 558.9
    infectious 009.0
    regional 555.2
    ulcerative 556.1
Ileostomy status V44.2 ●
    with complication 569.60
Ileotyphus 002.0
Ileum - *see* condition
Ileus (adynamic) (bowel) (colon) (inhibitory) (intestine) (neurogenic) (paralytic) 560.1
    arteriomesenteric duodenal 537.2
    due to gallstone (in intestine) 560.31
    duodenal, chronic 537.2
    following gastrointestinal surgery 997.49
    gallstone 560.31
    mechanical (*see also* Obstruction, intestine) 560.9
    meconium 777.1
        due to cystic fibrosis 277.01
    myxedema 564.89
    postoperative 997.49
    transitory, newborn 777.4
Iliac - *see* condition
Iliotibial band friction syndrome 728.89
Ill, louping 063.1
Illegitimacy V61.6
Illness - *see also* Disease
    factitious 300.19
        with
            combined psychological and physical signs and symptoms 300.19
            physical symptoms 300.19
            predominantly
                physical signs and symptoms 300.19
                psychological symptoms 300.16
        chronic (with physical symptoms) 301.51
    heart - *see* Disease, heart
    manic-depressive (*see also* Psychosis, affective) 296.80
    mental (*see also* Disorder, mental) 300.9
Imbalance 781.2
    autonomic (*see also* Neuropathy, peripheral, autonomic) 337.9
    electrolyte 276.9
        with
            abortion - *see* Abortion, by type, with metabolic disorder
            ectopic pregnancy (*see also* categories 633.0–633.9) 639.4
            hyperemesis gravidarum (before 22 completed weeks' gestation) 643.1 ●
            molar pregnancy (*see also* categories 630–632) 639.4
        following
            abortion 639.4
            ectopic or molar pregnancy 639.4
        neonatal, transitory NEC 775.5
    endocrine 259.9
    eye muscle NEC 378.9
        heterophoria - *see* Heterophoria
    glomerulotubular NEC 593.89
    hormone 259.9
    hysterical (*see also* Hysteria) 300.10
    labyrinth NEC 386.50
    posture 729.90
    sympathetic (*see also* Neuropathy, peripheral, autonomic) 337.9
Imbecile, imbecility 318.0
    moral 301.7
    old age 290.9

Imbecile, imbecility (*Continued*)
    senile 290.9
    specified IQ - *see* IQ
    unspecified IQ 318.0
Imbedding, intrauterine device 996.32
Imbibition, cholesterol (gallbladder) 575.6
Imerslund (-Gräsbeck) syndrome (anemia due to familial selective vitamin B_{12} malabsorption) 281.1
Iminoacidopathy 270.8
Iminoglycinuria, familial 270.8
Immature - *see also* Immaturity
    personality 301.89
Immaturity 765.1 ●
    extreme 765.0 ●
    fetus or infant light-for-dates - *see* Light-for-dates
    lung, fetus or newborn 770.4
    organ or site NEC - *see* Hypoplasia
    pulmonary, fetus or newborn 770.4
    reaction 301.89
    sexual (female) (male) 259.0
Immersion 994.1
    foot 991.4
    hand 991.4
Immobile, immobility
    complete
        due to severe physical disability or frality 780.72
    intestine 564.89
    joint - *see* Ankylosis
    syndrome (paraplegic) 728.3
Immunization
    ABO
        affecting management of pregnancy 656.2 ●
        fetus or newborn 773.1
    complication - *see* Complications, vaccination
    Rh factor
        affecting management of pregnancy 656.1 ●
        fetus or newborn 773.0
        from transfusion (*see also* Complications, transfusion) 999.70
Immunodeficiency 279.3
    with
        adenosine-deaminase deficiency 279.2
        defect, predominant
            B-cell 279.00
            T-cell 279.10
        hyperimmunoglobulinemia 279.2
        lymphopenia, hereditary 279.2
        thrombocytopenia and eczema 279.12
        thymic
            aplasia 279.2
            dysplasia 279.2
    autosomal recessive, Swiss-type 279.2
    common variable 279.06
    severe combined (SCID) 279.2
    to Rh factor
        affecting management of pregnancy 656.1 ●
        fetus or newborn 773.0
    X-linked, with increased IgM 279.05
Immunotherapy, prophylactic V07.2
    antineoplastic V58.12
Impaction, impacted
    bowel, colon, rectum 560.30
        with hernia - *see also* Hernia, by site, with, obstruction
            gangrenous - *see* Hernia, by site, with gangrene
        by
            calculus 560.32
            gallstone 560.31
        fecal 560.32
        specified type NEC 560.32
    calculus - *see* Calculus
    cerumen (ear) (external) 380.4
    cuspid 520.6
    dental 520.6

SECTION I INDEX TO DISEASES AND INJURIES / Impaction, impacted

Impaction, impacted (Continued)
- fecal, feces 560.32
  - with hernia - see also Hernia, by site, with obstruction
    - gangrenous - see Hernia, by site, with gangrene
- fracture - see Fracture, by site
- gallbladder - see Cholelithiasis
- gallstone(s) - see Cholelithiasis
  - in intestine (any part) 560.31
- intestine(s) 560.30
  - with hernia - see also Hernia, by site, with obstruction
    - gangrenous - see Hernia, by site, with gangrene
  - by
    - calculus 560.32
    - gallstone 560.31
  - fecal 560.32
  - specified type NEC 560.32
- intrauterine device (IUD) 996.32
- molar 520.6
- shoulder 660.4●
  - affecting fetus or newborn 763.1
- tooth, teeth 520.6
- turbinate 733.99

Impaired, impairment (function)
- arm V49.1
  - movement, involving
    - musculoskeletal system V49.1
    - nervous system V49.2
- auditory discrimination 388.43
- back V48.3
- body (entire) V49.89
- cognitive, mild, so stated 331.83
- combined visual hearing V49.85
- dual sensory V49.85
- glucose
  - fasting 790.21
  - tolerance test (oral) 790.22
- hearing (see also Deafness) 389.9
  - combined with visual impairment V49.85
- heart - see Disease, heart
- kidney (see also Disease, renal) 593.9
  - disorder resulting from 588.9
    - specified NEC 588.89
- leg V49.1
  - movement, involving
    - musculoskeletal system V49.1
    - nervous system V49.2
- limb V49.1
  - movement, involving
    - musculoskeletal system V49.1
    - nervous system V49.2
- liver 573.8
- mastication 524.9
- mild cognitive, so stated 331.83
- mobility
  - ear ossicles NEC 385.22
  - incostapedial joint 385.22
  - malleus 385.21
- myocardium, myocardial (see also Insufficiency, myocardial) 428.0
- neuromusculoskeletal NEC V49.89
  - back V48.3
  - head V48.2
  - limb V49.2
  - neck V48.3
  - spine V48.3
  - trunk V48.3
- rectal sphincter 787.99
- renal (see also Disease, renal) 593.9
  - disorder resulting from 588.9
    - specified NEC 588.89
- spine V48.3
- vision NEC 369.9
  - both eyes NEC 369.3
    - combined with hearing impairment V49.85

Impaired, impairment (Continued)
- vision NEC (Continued)
  - moderate 369.74
    - both eyes 369.25
      - with impairment of lesser eye (specified as)
        - blind, not further specified 369.15
        - low vision, not further specified 369.23
        - near-total 369.17
        - profound 369.18
        - severe 369.24
        - total 369.16
    - one eye 369.74
      - with vision of other eye (specified as)
        - near-normal 369.75
        - normal 369.76
  - near-total 369.64
    - both eyes 369.04
      - with impairment of lesser eye (specified as)
        - blind, not further specified 369.02
        - total 369.03
    - one eye 369.64
      - with vision of other eye (specified as)
        - near-normal 369.65
        - normal 369.66
  - one eye 369.60
    - with low vision of other eye 369.10
  - profound 369.67
    - both eyes 369.08
      - with impairment of lesser eye (specified as)
        - blind, not further specified 369.05
        - near-total 369.07
        - total 369.06
    - one eye 369.67
      - with vision of other eye (specified as)
        - near-normal 369.68
        - normal 369.69
  - severe 369.71
    - both eyes 369.22
      - with impairment of lesser eye (specified as)
        - blind, not further specified 369.11
        - low vision, not further specified 369.21
        - near-total 369.13
        - profound 369.14
        - total 369.12
    - one eye 369.71
      - with vision of other eye (specified as)
        - near-normal 369.72
        - normal 369.73
  - total
    - both eyes 369.01
    - one eye 369.61
      - with vision of other eye (specified as)
        - near-normal 369.62
        - normal 369.63

Impaludism - see Malaria
Impediment, speech NEC 784.59
- psychogenic 307.9
- secondary to organic lesion 784.59

Impending
- cerebrovascular accident or attack 435.9
- coronary syndrome 411.1
- delirium tremens 291.0
- myocardial infarction 411.1

Imperception, auditory (acquired) (congenital) 389.9

Imperfect
- aeration, lung (newborn) 770.5
- closure (congenital)
  - alimentary tract NEC 751.8
    - lower 751.5
    - upper 750.8
  - atrioventricular ostium 745.69
  - atrium (secundum) 745.5
    - primum 745.61
  - branchial cleft or sinus 744.41
  - choroid 743.59
  - cricoid cartilage 748.3
  - cusps, heart valve NEC 746.89
    - pulmonary 746.09
  - ductus
    - arteriosus 747.0
    - Botalli 747.0
  - ear drum 744.29
    - causing impairment of hearing 744.03
  - endocardial cushion 745.60
  - epiglottis 748.3
  - esophagus with communication to bronchus or trachea 750.3
  - Eustachian valve 746.89
  - eyelid 743.62
  - face, facial (see also Cleft, lip) 749.10
  - foramen
    - Botalli 745.5
    - ovale 745.5
  - genitalia, genital organ(s) or system
    - female 752.89
      - external 752.49
      - internal NEC 752.89
      - uterus 752.39
    - male 752.89
      - penis 752.69
  - glottis 748.3
  - heart valve (cusps) NEC 746.89
  - interatrial ostium or septum 745.5
  - interauricular ostium or septum 745.5
  - interventricular ostium or septum 745.4
  - iris 743.46
  - kidney 753.3
  - larynx 748.3
  - lens 743.36
  - lip (see also Cleft, lip) 749.10
  - nasal septum or sinus 748.1
  - nose 748.1
  - omphalomesenteric duct 751.0
  - optic nerve entry 743.57
  - organ or site NEC - see Anomaly, specified type, by site
  - ostium
    - interatrial 745.5
    - interauricular 745.5
    - interventricular 745.4
  - palate (see also Cleft, palate) 749.00
  - preauricular sinus 744.46
  - retina 743.56
  - roof of orbit 742.0
  - sclera 743.47
  - septum
    - aortic 745.0
    - aorticopulmonary 745.0
    - atrial (secundum) 745.5
      - primum 745.61
    - between aorta and pulmonary artery 745.0
    - heart 745.9
    - interatrial (secundum) 745.5
      - primum 745.61
    - interauricular (secundum) 745.5
      - primum 745.61
    - interventricular 745.4
      - with pulmonary stenosis or atresia, dextraposition of aorta, and hypertrophy of right ventricle 745.2
      - in tetralogy of Fallot 745.2
    - nasal 748.1

Imperfect *(Continued)*
  closure *(Continued)*
    septum *(Continued)*
      ventricular 745.4
        with pulmonary stenosis or atresia, dextraposition of aorta, and hypertrophy of right ventricle 745.2
        in tetralogy of Fallot 745.2
    skull 756.0
      with
        anencephalus 740.0
        encephalocele 742.0
        hydrocephalus 742.3
          with spina bifida *(see also* Spina bifida) 741.0 ●
        microcephalus 742.1
    spine (with meningocele) *(see also* Spina bifida) 741.90
    thyroid cartilage 748.3
    trachea 748.3
    tympanic membrane 744.29
      causing impairment of hearing 744.03
    uterus (with communication to bladder, intestine, or rectum) 752.39
    uvula 749.02
      with cleft lip *(see also* Cleft, palate, with cleft lip) 749.20
    vitelline duct 751.0
  development - *see* Anomaly, by site
  erection 607.84
  fusion - *see* Imperfect, closure
  inflation lung (newborn) 770.5
  intestinal canal 751.5
  poise 729.90
  rotation - *see* Malrotation
  septum, ventricular 745.4
Imperfectly descended testis 752.51
Imperforate (congenital) - *see also* Atresia
  anus 751.2
  bile duct 751.61
  cervix (uteri) 752.49
  esophagus 750.3
  hymen 752.42
  intestine (small) 751.1
    large 751.2
  jejunum 751.1
  pharynx 750.29
  rectum 751.2
  salivary duct 750.23
  urethra 753.6
  urinary meatus 753.6
  vagina 752.49
Impervious (congenital) - *see also* Atresia
  anus 751.2
  bile duct 751.61
  esophagus 750.3
  intestine (small) 751.1
    large 751.5
  rectum 751.2
  urethra 753.6
Impetiginization of other dermatoses 684
Impetigo (any organism) (any site) (bullous) (circinate) (contagiosa) (neonatorum) (simplex) 684
  Bockhart's (superficial folliculitis) 704.8
  external ear 684 *[380.13]*
  eyelid 684 *[373.5]*
  Fox's (contagiosa) 684
  furfuracea 696.5
  herpetiformis 694.3
    nonobstetrical 694.3
  staphylococcal infection 684
  ulcerative 686.8
  vulgaris 684
Impingement, soft tissue between teeth 524.89
  anterior 524.81
  posterior 524.82
Implant, endometrial 617.9

Implantation
  anomalous - *see also* Anomaly, specified type, by site
    ureter 753.4
  cyst
    external area or site (skin) NEC 709.8
    iris 364.61
    vagina 623.8
    vulva 624.8
  dermoid (cyst)
    external area or site (skin) NEC 709.8
    iris 364.61
    vagina 623.8
    vulva 624.8
  placenta, low or marginal - *see* Placenta previa
Impotence (sexual) 607.84
  organic origin NEC 607.84
  psychogenic 302.72
Impoverished blood 285.9
Impression, basilar 756.0
Imprisonment V62.5
Improper
  development, infant 764.9 ●
Improperly tied umbilical cord (causing hemorrhage) 772.3
Impulses, obsessional 300.3
Impulsive 799.23
  neurosis 300.3
Impulsiveness 799.23
Inaction, kidney (*see also* Disease, renal) 593.9
Inactive - *see* condition
Inadequate, inadequacy
  aesthetics of dental restoration 525.67
  biologic 301.6
  cardiac and renal - *see* Hypertension, cardiorenal
  constitutional 301.6
  development
    child 783.40
    fetus 764.9 ●
      affecting management of pregnancy 656.5 ●
    genitalia
      after puberty NEC 259.0
      congenital - *see* Hypoplasia, genitalia
    lungs 748.5
    organ or site NEC - *see* Hypoplasia, by site
  dietary 269.9
  distance, interarch 524.28
  education V62.3
  environment
    economic problem V60.2
    household condition NEC V60.1
    poverty V60.2
    unemployment V62.0
  functional 301.6
  household care, due to
    family member
      handicapped or ill V60.4
      temporarily away from home V60.4
      on vacation V60.5
    technical defects in home V60.1
    temporary absence from home of person rendering care V60.4
  housing (heating) (space) V60.1
  interarch distance 524.28
  material resources V60.2
  mental (*see also* Disability, intellectual) 319
  nervous system 799.29
  personality 301.6
  prenatal care in current pregnancy V23.7
  pulmonary
    function 786.09
      newborn 770.89
    ventilation, newborn 770.89

Inadequate, inadequacy *(Continued)*
  respiration 786.09
    newborn 770.89
  sample
    cytology
      anal 796.78
      cervical 795.08
      vaginal 795.18
  social 301.6
Inanition 263.9
  with edema 262
  due to
    deprivation of food 994.2
    malnutrition 263.9
  fever 780.60
Inappropriate
  change in quantitative human chorionic gonadotropin (hCG) in early pregnancy 631.0
  level of quantitative human chorionic gonadotropin (hCG) for gestational age in early pregnancy 631.0
  secretion
    ACTH 255.0
    antidiuretic hormone (ADH) (excessive) 253.6
    deficiency 253.5
    ectopic hormone NEC 259.3
    pituitary (posterior) 253.6
Inattention after or at birth 995.52
Inborn errors of metabolism - *see* Disorder, metabolism
Incarceration, incarcerated
  bubonocele - *see also* Hernia, inguinal, with obstruction
    gangrenous - *see* Hernia, inguinal, with gangrene
  colon (by hernia) - *see also* Hernia, by site with obstruction
    gangrenous - *see* Hernia, by site, with gangrene
  enterocele 552.9
    gangrenous 551.9
  epigastrocele 552.29
    gangrenous 551.29
  epiplocele 552.9
    gangrenous 551.9
  exomphalos 552.1
    gangrenous 551.1
  fallopian tube 620.8
  hernia - *see also* Hernia, by site, with obstruction
    gangrenous - *see* Hernia, by site, with gangrene
  iris, in wound 871.1
  lens, in wound 871.1
  merocele (*see also* Hernia, femoral, with obstruction) 552.00
  omentum (by hernia) - *see also* Hernia, by site, with obstruction
    gangrenous - *see* Hernia, by site, with gangrene
  omphalocele 756.72
  rupture (meaning hernia) (*see also* Hernia, by site, with obstruction) 552.9
    gangrenous (*see also* Hernia, by site, with gangrene) 551.9
  sarcoepiplocele 552.9
    gangrenous 551.9
  sarcoepiplomphalocele 552.1
    with gangrene 551.1
  uterus 621.8
    gravid 654.3 ●
      causing obstructed labor 660.2 ●
        affecting fetus or newborn 763.1
Incident, cerebrovascular (*see also* Disease, cerebrovascular, acute) 436
Incineration (entire body) (from fire, conflagration, electricity, or lightning) - *see* Burn, multiple, specified sites

SECTION I INDEX TO DISEASES AND INJURIES / Incised wound

Incised wound
   external - *see* Wound, open, by site
   internal organs (abdomen, chest, or pelvis) - *see* Injury, internal, by site, with open wound

Incision, incisional
   hernia - *see* Hernia, incisional
   surgical, complication - *see* Complications, surgical procedures
   traumatic
     external - *see* Wound, open, by site
     internal organs (abdomen, chest, or pelvis) - *see* Injury, internal, by site, with open wound

Inclusion
   azurophilic leukocytic 288.2
   blennorrhea (neonatal) (newborn) 771.6
   cyst - *see* Cyst, skin
   gallbladder in liver (congenital) 751.69

Incompatibility
   ABO
     affecting management of pregnancy 656.2●
     fetus or newborn 773.1
     infusion or transfusion reaction (*see also* Complications, transfusion) 999.60
   blood (group) (Duffy) (E) (K(ell)) (Kidd) (Lewis) (M) (N) (P) (S) NEC
     affecting management of pregnancy 656.2●
     fetus or newborn 773.2
     infusion or transfusion reaction (*see also* Complications, transfusion) 999.75
   contour of existing restoration of tooth with oral health 525.65
   marital V61.10
     involving
       divorce V61.03
       estrangement V61.09
   non-ABO (*see also* Complications, transfusion) 999.75
   Rh (antigen) (C) (c) (D) (E) (e) (blood group) (factor)
     affecting management of pregnancy 656.1●
     fetus or newborn 773.0
     infusion or transfusion reaction (*see also* Complications, transfusion) 999.70
   Rhesus - *see* Incompatibility, Rh

Incompetency, incompetence, incompetent
   annular
     aortic (valve) (*see also* Insufficiency, aortic) 424.1
     mitral (valve) - (*see also* Insufficiency, mitral) 424.0
     pulmonary valve (heart) (*see also* Endocarditis, pulmonary) 424.3
   aortic (valve) (*see also* Insufficiency, aortic) 424.1
     syphilitic 093.22
   cardiac (orifice) 530.0
     valve - *see* Endocarditis
   cervix, cervical (os) 622.5
     in pregnancy 654.5●
       affecting fetus or newborn 761.0
   chronotropic 426.89
     with
       autonomic dysfunction 337.9
       ischemic heart disease 414.9
       left ventricular dysfunction 429.89
       sinus node dysfunction 427.81
   esophagogastric (junction) (sphincter) 530.0
   heart valve, congenital 746.89
   mitral (valve) - *see* Insufficiency, mitral
   papillary muscle (heart) 429.81
   pelvic fundus
     pubocervical tissue 618.81
     rectovaginal tissue 618.82

Incompetency, incompetence, incompetent (*Continued*)
   pulmonary valve (heart) (*see also* Endocarditis, pulmonary) 424.3
     congenital 746.09
   tricuspid (annular) (rheumatic) (valve) (*see also* Endocarditis, tricuspid) 397.0
   valvular - *see* Endocarditis
   vein, venous (saphenous) (varicose) (*see also* Varicose, vein) 454.9
   velopharyngeal (closure)
     acquired 528.9
     congenital 750.29

Incomplete - *see also* condition
   bladder emptying 788.21
   defecation 787.61
   expansion lungs (newborn) 770.5
   gestation (liveborn) - *see* Immaturity
   rotation - *see* Malrotation

Inconclusive
   image test due to excess body fat 793.91
   mammogram, mammography 793.82
     due to dense breasts 793.82

Incontinence 788.30
   without sensory awareness 788.34
   anal sphincter 787.60
   continuous leakage 788.37
   feces, fecal 787.60
     due to hysteria 300.11
     nonorganic origin 307.7
   hysterical 300.11
   mixed (male) (female) (urge and stress) 788.33
   overflow 788.38
   paradoxical 788.39
   rectal 787.60
   specified NEC 788.39
   stress (female) 625.6
     male NEC 788.32
   urethral sphincter 599.84
   urge 788.31
     and stress (male) (female) 788.33
   urine 788.30
     active 788.30
     due to
       cognitive impairment 788.91
       severe physical disability 788.91
       immobility 788.91
     functional 788.91
     male 788.30
       stress 788.32
       and urge 788.33
     neurogenic 788.39
     nonorganic origin 307.6
     stress (female) 625.6
       male NEC 788.32
     urge 788.31
       and stress 788.33

Incontinentia pigmenti 757.33

Incoordinate
   uterus (action) (contractions) 661.4●
     affecting fetus or newborn 763.7

Incoordination
   esophageal-pharyngeal (newborn) 787.24
   muscular 781.3
   papillary muscle 429.81

Increase, increased
   abnormal, in development 783.9
   androgens (ovarian) 256.1
   anticoagulants (antithrombin) (anti-II) (anti-VIIIa) (anti-IXa) (anti-XIa) (prothrombin) (*see also* Anticoagulants) 286.59
   anti-IIa 287.8
   anti-Xa 287.8
   extrinsic 287.8
   postpartum 666.3●
   cold sense (*see also* Disturbance, sensation) 782.0
   estrogen 256.0

Increase, increased (*Continued*)
   function
     adrenal (cortex) 255.3
       medulla 255.6
     pituitary (anterior) (gland) (lobe) 253.1
       posterior 253.6
   heat sense (*see also* Disturbance, sensation) 782.0
   intracranial pressure 781.99
     injury at birth 767.8
   light reflex of retina 362.13
   permeability, capillary 448.9
   pressure
     intracranial 781.99
       injury at birth 767.8
     intraocular 365.00
   pulsations 785.9
   pulse pressure 785.9
   sphericity, lens 743.36
   splenic activity 289.4
   venous pressure 459.89
     portal 572.3

Incrustation, cornea, lead, or zinc 930.0
Incyclophoria 378.44
Incyclotropia 378.33
Indeterminate sex 752.7
India rubber skin 756.83
Indicanuria 270.2
Indigestion (bilious) (functional) 536.8
   acid 536.8
   catarrhal 536.8
   due to decomposed food NEC 005.9
   fat 579.8
   nervous 306.4
   psychogenic 306.4

Indirect - *see* condition
Indolent bubo NEC 099.8
Induced
   abortion - *see* Abortion, induced
   birth, affecting fetus or newborn 763.89
   delivery - *see* Delivery
   labor - *see* Delivery

Induration, indurated
   brain 348.89
   breast (fibrous) 611.79
     puerperal, postpartum 676.3●
   broad ligament 620.8
   chancre 091.0
     anus 091.1
     congenital 090.0
     extragenital NEC 091.2
   corpora cavernosa (penis) (plastic) 607.89
   liver (chronic) 573.8
     acute 573.8
   lung (black) (brown) (chronic) (fibroid) (*see also* Fibrosis, lung) 515
     essential brown 275.09 [516.1]
   penile 607.89
   phlebitic - *see* Phlebitis
   skin 782.8
   stomach 537.89

Induratio penis plastica 607.89
Industrial - *see* condition
Inebriety (*see also* Abuse, drugs, nondependent) 305.0●
Inefficiency
   kidney (*see also* Disease, renal) 593.9
   thyroid (acquired) (gland) 244.9

Inelasticity, skin 782.8
Inequality, leg (acquired) (length) 736.81
   congenital 755.30
Inertia
   bladder 596.4
     neurogenic 596.54
       with cauda equina syndrome 344.61
   stomach 536.8
     psychogenic 306.4
   uterus, uterine 661.2●
     affecting fetus or newborn 763.7
     primary 661.0●
     secondary 661.1●

Inertia (Continued)
vesical 596.4
neurogenic 596.54
with cauda equina 344.61
Infant - *see also* condition
excessive crying of 780.92
fussy (baby) 780.91
held for adoption V68.89
newborn - *see* Newborn
post-term (gestation period over 40 completed weeks to 42 completed weeks) 766.21
prolonged gestation of (period over 42 completed weeks) 766.22
syndrome of diabetic mother 775.0
"Infant Hercules" syndrome 255.2
Infantile - *see also* condition
genitalia, genitals 259.0
in pregnancy or childbirth NEC 654.4●
affecting fetus or newborn 763.89
causing obstructed labor 660.2●
affecting fetus or newborn 763.1
heart 746.9
kidney 753.3
lack of care 995.52
macula degeneration 362.75
melanodontia 521.05
os, uterus (*see also* Infantile, genitalia) 259.0
pelvis 738.6
with disproportion (fetopelvic) 653.1●
affecting fetus or newborn 763.1
causing obstructed labor 660.1●
affecting fetus or newborn 763.1
penis 259.0
testis 257.2
uterus (*see also* Infantile, genitalia)259.0
vulva 752.49
Infantilism 259.9
with dwarfism (hypophyseal) 253.3
Brissaud's (infantile myxedema) 244.9
celiac 579.0
Herter's (nontropical sprue) 579.0
hypophyseal 253.3
hypothalamic (with obesity) 253.8
idiopathic 259.9
intestinal 579.0
pancreatic 577.8
pituitary 253.3
renal 588.0
sexual (with obesity) 259.0
Infants, healthy liveborn - *see* Newborn
Infarct, infarction
adrenal (capsule) (gland) 255.41
amnion 658.8●
anterior (with contiguous portion of intraventricular septum) NEC (*see also* Infarct, myocardium) 410.1●
appendices epiploicae 557.0
bowel 557.0
brain (stem) 434.91
embolic (*see also* Embolism, brain) 434.11
healed or old without residuals V12.54
iatrogenic 997.02
lacunar 434.91
late effect - *see* Late effect(s) (of) cerebrovascular disease
postoperative 997.02
puerperal, postpartum, childbirth 674.0●
thrombotic (*see also* Thrombosis, brain) 434.01
breast 611.89
Brewer's (kidney) 593.81
cardiac (*see also* Infarct, myocardium) 410.9●
cerebellar (*see also* Infarct, brain) 434.91
embolic (*see also* Embolism, brain) 434.11
cerebral (*see also* Infarct, brain) 434.91
aborted 434.91
embolic (*see also* Embolism, brain) 434.11
thrombotic (*see also* Infarct, brain) 434.01
chorion 658.8●

Infarct, infarction (Continued)
colon (acute) (agnogenic) (embolic) (hemorrhagic) (nonocclusive) (nonthrombotic) (occlusive) (segmental) (thrombotic) (with gangrene) 557.0
coronary artery (*see also* Infarct, myocardium) 410.9●
cortical 434.87
embolic (*see also* Embolism) 444.9
fallopian tube 620.8
gallbladder 575.8
heart (*see also* Infarct, myocardium) 410.9●
hepatic 573.4
hypophysis (anterior lobe) 253.8
impending (myocardium) 411.1
intestine (acute) (agnogenic) (embolic) (hemorrhagic) (nonocclusive) (nonthrombotic) (occlusive) (thrombotic) (with gangrene) 557.0
kidney 593.81
lacunar 434.91
liver 573.4
lung (embolic) (thrombotic) 415.19
with
abortion - *see* Abortion, by type, with, embolism
ectopic pregnancy (*see also* categories 633.0–633.9) 639.6
molar pregnancy (*see also* categories 630–632) 639.6
following
abortion 639.6
ectopic or molar pregnancy 639.6
iatrogenic 415.11
in pregnancy, childbirth, or puerperium - *see* Embolism, obstetrical
postoperative 415.11
septic 415.12
lymph node or vessel 457.8
medullary (brain) - *see* Infarct, brain
meibomian gland (eyelid) 374.85
mesentery, mesenteric (embolic) (thrombotic) (with gangrene) 557.0
midbrain - *see* Infarct, brain
myocardium, myocardial (acute or with a stated duration of 8 weeks or less) (with hypertension) 410.9●

> Note: Use the following fifth-digit subclassification with category 410:
> 0 episode unspecified
> 1 initial episode
> 2 subsequent episode without recurrence

with symptoms after 8 weeks from date of infarction 414.8
anterior (wall) (with contiguous portion of intraventricular septum) NEC 410.1●
anteroapical (with contiguous portion of intraventricular septum) 410.1●
anterolateral (wall) 410.0●
anteroseptal (with contiguous portion of intraventricular septum) 410.1●
apical-lateral 410.5●
atrial 410.8●
basal-lateral 410.5●
chronic (with symptoms after 8 weeks from date of infarction) 414.8
diagnosed on ECG, but presenting no symptoms 412
diaphragmatic wall (with contiguous portion of intraventricular septum) 410.4●
healed or old, currently presenting no symptoms 412
high lateral 410.5●
impending 411.1

Infarct, infarction (Continued)
myocardium, myocardial (Continued)
inferior (wall) (with contiguous portion of intraventricular septum) 410.4●
inferolateral (wall) 410.2●
inferoposterior wall 410.3●
intraoperative 997.1
lateral wall 410.5●
non-Q wave 410.7●
non-ST elevation (NSTEMI) 410.7●
nontransmural 410.7●
papillary muscle 410.8●
past (diagnosed on ECG or other special investigation, but currently presenting no symptoms) 412
with symptoms NEC 414.8
posterior (strictly) (true) (wall) 410.6●
posterobasal 410.6●
posteroinferior 410.3●
posterolateral 410.5●
postprocedural 997.1
previous, currently presenting no symptoms 412
Q wave (*see also* Infarct, myocardium, by site) 410.9●
septal 410.8●
specified site NEC 410.8●
ST elevation (STEMI) 410.9●
anterior (wall) 410.1●
anterolateral (wall) 410.0●
inferior (wall) 410.4●
inferolateral (wall) 410.2●
inferoposterior wall 410.3●
lateral wall 410.5●
posterior (strictly) (true) (wall) 410.6●
specified site NEC 410.8●
subendocardial 410.7●
syphilitic 093.82
non-ST elevation myocardial infarction (NSTEMI) 410.7●
nontransmural 410.7●
omentum 557.0
ovary 620.8
pancreas 577.8
papillary muscle (*see also* Infarct, myocardium) 410.8●
parathyroid gland 252.8
pituitary (gland) 253.8
placenta (complicating pregnancy) 656.7●
affecting fetus or newborn 762.2
pontine - *see* Infarct, brain
posterior NEC (*see also* Infarct, myocardium) 410.6●
prostate 602.8
pulmonary (artery) (hemorrhagic) (vein) 415.19
with
abortion - *see* Abortion, by type, with embolism
ectopic pregnancy (*see also* categories 633.0–633.9) 639.6
molar pregnancy (*see also* categories 630–632) 639.6
following
abortion 639.6
ectopic or molar pregnancy 639.6
iatrogenic 415.11
in pregnancy, childbirth, or puerperium - *see* Embolism, obstetrical
postoperative 415.11
septic 415.12
renal 593.81
embolic or thrombotic 593.81
retina, retinal 362.84
with occlusion - *see* Occlusion, retina
spinal (acute) (cord) (embolic) (nonembolic) 336.1
spleen 289.59
embolic or thrombotic 444.89
subchorionic - *see* Infarct, placenta

SECTION I INDEX TO DISEASES AND INJURIES / Infarct, infarction

Infarct, infarction (Continued)
   subendocardial (see also Infarct, myocardium) 410.7●
   suprarenal (capsule) (gland) 255.41
   syncytium - see Infarct, placenta
   testis 608.83
   thrombotic (see also Thrombosis) 453.9
      artery, arterial - see Embolism
   thyroid (gland) 246.3
   ventricle (heart) (see also Infarct, myocardium) 410.9●
Infecting - see condition
Infection, infected, infective (opportunistic) 136.9
   with
      influenza viruses occurring in pigs or other animals - see Influenza, due to identified, novel influenza A virus
      lymphangitis - see Lymphangitis
   abortion - see Abortion, by type, with, sepsis
   abscess (skin) - see Abscess, by site
   Absidia 117.7
   acanthamoeba 136.21
   Acanthocheilonema (perstans) 125.4
      streptocerca 125.6
   accessory sinus (chronic) (see also Sinusitis) 473.9
   Achorion - see Dermatophytosis
   Acremonium falciforme 117.4
   acromioclavicular (joint) 711.91
   Actinobacillus
      lignieresii 027.8
      mallei 024
      muris 026.1
   Actinomadura - see Actinomycosis
   Actinomyces (israelii) - see also Actinomycosis
      muris-ratti 026.1
   Actinomycetales (Actinomadura) (Actinomyces) (Nocardia) (Streptomyces) - see Actinomycosis
   actinomycotic NEC (see also Actinomycosis) 039.9
   adenoid (chronic) 474.01
      acute 463
      and tonsil (chronic) 474.02
         acute or subacute 463
   adenovirus NEC 079.0
      in diseases classified elsewhere - see category 079
      unspecified nature or site 079.0
   Aerobacter aerogenes NEC 041.85
      enteritis 008.2
   Aerogenes capsulatus (see also Gangrene, gas) 040.0
   aertrycke (see also Infection, Salmonella) 003.9
   Ajellomyces dermatitidis 116.0
   alimentary canal NEC (see also Enteritis, due to, by organism) 009.0
   Allescheria boydii 117.6
   Alternaria 118
   alveolus, alveolar (process) (pulpal origin) 522.4
   ameba, amebic (histolytica) (see also Amebiasis) 006.9
      acute 006.0
      chronic 006.1
      free-living 136.29
      hartmanni 007.8
      specified
         site NEC 006.8
         type NEC 007.8
   amniotic fluid or cavity 658.4●
      affecting fetus or newborn 762.7
   anaerobes (cocci) (gram-negative) (gram-positive) (mixed) NEC 041.84
   anal canal 569.49
   Ancylostoma braziliense 126.2

Infection, infected, infective (Continued)
   Angiostrongylus cantonensis 128.8
   anisakiasis 127.1
   Anisakis larva 127.1
   anthrax (see also Anthrax) 022.9
   antrum (chronic) (see also Sinusitis, maxillary) 473.0
   anus (papillae) (sphincter) 569.49
   arbor virus NEC 066.9
   arbovirus NEC 066.9
   argentophil-rod 027.0
   Ascaris lumbricoides 127.0
   ascomycetes 117.4
   Aspergillus (flavus) (fumigatus) (terreus) 117.3
   atypical
      acid-fast (bacilli) (see also Mycobacterium, atypical) 031.9
      mycobacteria (see also Mycobacterium, atypical) 031.9
   auditory meatus (circumscribed) (diffuse) (external) (see also Otitis, externa) 380.10
   auricle (ear) (see also Otitis, externa) 380.10
   axillary gland 683
   Babesiasis 088.82
   Babesiosis 088.82
   Bacillus NEC 041.89
      abortus 023.1
      anthracis (see also Anthrax) 022.9
      cereus (food poisoning) 005.89
      coli - see Infection, Escherichia coli
      coliform NEC 041.85
      Ducrey's (any location) 099.0
      Flexner's 004.1
      Friedländer's NEC 041.3
      fusiformis 101
      gas (gangrene) (see also Gangrene, gas) 040.0
      mallei 024
      melitensis 023.0
      paratyphoid, paratyphosus 002.9
         A 002.1
         B 002.2
         C 002.3
      Schmorl's 040.3
      Shiga 004.0
      suipestifer (see also Infection, Salmonella) 003.9
      swimming pool 031.1
      typhosa 002.0
      welchii (see also Gangrene, gas) 040.0
      Whitmore's 025
   bacterial NEC 041.9
      specified NEC 041.89
         anaerobic NEC 041.84
         gram-negative NEC 041.85
            anaerobic NEC 041.84
   Bacterium
      paratyphosum 002.9
         A 002.1
         B 002.2
         C 002.3
      typhosum 002.9
   Bacteroides (fragilis) (melaninogenicus) (oralis) NEC 041.82
   Balantidium coli 007.0
   Bartholin's gland 616.89
   Basidiobolus 117.7
   Bedsonia 079.98
      specified NEC 079.88
   bile duct 576.1
   bladder (see also Cystitis) 595.9
   Blastomyces, blastomycotic 116.0
      brasiliensis 116.1
      dermatitidis 116.0
      European 117.5
      loboi 116.2
      North American 116.0
      South American 116.1

Infection, infected, infective (Continued)
   bleb
      postprocedural 379.60
         stage 1 379.61
         stage 2 379.62
         stage 3 379.63
   blood stream - see also Septicemia
      catheter-related (CRBSI) 999.31
      central line-associated (CLABSI) 999.32
      due to central venous catheter 999.32
   bone 730.9●
      specified - see Osteomyelitis
   Bordetella 033.9
      bronchiseptica 033.8
      parapertussis 033.1
      pertussis 033.0
   Borrelia
      bergdorfi 088.81
      vincentii (mouth) (pharynx) (tonsil) 101
   bovine stomatitis 059.11
   brain (see also Encephalitis) 323.9
      late effect - see category 326
      membranes - (see also Meningitis) 322.9
      septic 324.0
         late effect - see category 326
         meninges (see also Meningitis) 320.9
   branchial cyst 744.42
   breast 611.0
      puerperal, postpartum 675.2●
         with nipple 675.9●
            specified type NEC 675.8●
         nonpurulent 675.2●
         purulent 675.1●
   bronchus (see also Bronchitis) 490
      fungus NEC 117.9
   Brucella 023.9
      abortus 023.1
      canis 023.3
      melitensis 023.0
      mixed 023.8
      suis 023.2
   Brugia (Wuchereria) malayi 125.1
   bursa - see Bursitis
   buttocks (skin) 686.9
   Candida (albicans) (tropicalis) (see also Candidiasis) 112.9
      congenital 771.7
   Candiru 136.8
   Capillaria
      hepatica 128.8
      philippinensis 127.5
   cartilage 733.99
   cat liver fluke 121.0
   catheter-related bloodstream (CRBSI) 999.31
   cellulitis - see Cellulitis, by site
   central line-associated 999.31
      bloodstream 999.32
   Cephalosporum falciforme 117.4
   Cercomonas hominis (intestinal) 007.3
   cerebrospinal (see also Meningitis) 322.9
      late effect - see category 326
   cervical gland 683
   cervix (see also Cervicitis) 616.0
   cesarean section wound 674.3●
   Chilomastix (intestinal) 007.8
   Chlamydia 079.98
      specified NEC 079.88
   Cholera (see also Cholera) 001.9
   chorionic plate 658.8●
   Cladosporium
      bantianum 117.8
      carrionii 117.2
      mansoni 111.1
      trichoides 117.8
      wernecki 111.1
   Clonorchis (sinensis) (liver) 121.1
   Clostridium (haemolyticum) (novyi) NEC 041.84
      botulinum 005.1
      histolyticum (see also Gangrene, gas) 040.0
      oedematiens (see also Gangrene, gas) 040.0

Infection, infected, infective *(Continued)*
  Clostridium NEC *(Continued)*
    perfringens 041.83
      due to food 005.2
    septicum *(see also* Gangrene, gas*)* 040.0
    sordellii *(see also* Gangrene, gas*)* 040.0
    welchii *(see also* Gangrene, gas*)* 040.0
      due to food 005.2
  Coccidioides (immitis) *(see also* Coccidioidomycosis) 114.9
  coccus NEC 041.89
  colon *(see also* Enteritis, due to, by organism) 009.0
    bacillus - *see* Infection, Escherichia coli
  colostomy or enterostomy 569.61
  common duct 576.1
  complicating pregnancy, childbirth, or puerperium NEC 647.9●
    affecting fetus or newborn 760.2
  Condiobolus 117.7
  congenital NEC 771.89
    Candida albicans 771.7
    chronic 771.2
    Cytomegalovirus 771.1
    hepatitis, viral 771.2
    herpes simplex 771.2
    listeriosis 771.2
    malaria 771.2
    poliomyelitis 771.2
    rubella 771.0
    toxoplasmosis 771.2
    tuberculosis 771.2
    urinary (tract) 771.82
    vaccinia 771.2
  coronavirus 079.89
    SARS-associated 079.82
  corpus luteum *(see also* Salpingo-oophoritis) 614.2
  Corynebacterium diphtheriae - *see* Diphtheria
  cotia virus 059.8
  Coxsackie *(see also* Coxsackie) 079.2
    endocardium 074.22
    heart NEC 074.20
    in diseases classified elsewhere - *see* category 079
    meninges 047.0
    myocardium 074.23
    pericardium 074.21
    pharynx 074.0
    specified disease NEC 074.8
    unspecified nature or site 079.2
  Cryptococcus neoformans 117.5
  Cryptosporidia 007.4
  Cunninghamella 117.7
  cyst - *see* Cyst
  Cysticercus cellulosae 123.1
  cystostomy 596.83
  cytomegalovirus 078.5
    congenital 771.1
  dental (pulpal origin) 522.4
  deuteromycetes 117.4
  Dicrocoelium dendriticum 121.8
  Dipetalonema (perstans) 125.4
    streptocerca 125.6
  diphtherial - *see* Diphtheria
  Diphyllobothrium (adult) (latum) (pacificum) 123.4
    larval 123.5
  Diplogonoporus (grandis) 123.8
  Dipylidium (caninum) 123.8
  Dirofilaria 125.6
  dog tapeworm 123.8
  Dracunculus medinensis 125.7
  Dreschlera 118
    hawaiiensis 117.8
  Ducrey's bacillus (any site) 099.0

Infection, infected, infective *(Continued)*
  due to or resulting from
    central venous catheter *(see also* Complications, due to, catheter, central venous) 999.31
      bloodstream 999.32
      localized 999.33
    device, implant, or graft (any) (presence of) - *see* Complications, infection and inflammation, due to (presence of) any device, implant, or graft classified to 996.0–996.5 NEC
    injection, inoculation, infusion, transfusion, or vaccination (prophylactic) (therapeutic) 999.39
    blood and blood products acute 999.34
    injury NEC - *see* Wound, open, by site, complicated
    surgery 998.59
  duodenum 535.6●
  ear - *see also* Otitis
    external *(see also* Otitis, externa) 380.10
    inner *(see also* Labyrinthitis) 386.30
    middle - *see* Otitis, media
  Eaton's agent NEC 041.81
  Eberthella typhosa 002.0
  Ebola 078.89
  echinococcosis 122.9
  Echinococcus *(see also* Echinococcus) 122.9
  Echinostoma 121.8
  ECHO virus 079.1
    in diseases classified elsewhere - *see* category 079
    unspecified nature or site 079.1
  Ehrlichiosis 082.40
    chaffeensis 082.41
    specified type NEC 082.49
  Endamoeba - *see* Infection, ameba
  endocardium *(see also* Endocarditis) 421.0
  endocervix *(see also* Cervicitis) 616.0
  Entamoeba - *see* Infection, ameba
  enteric *(see also* Enteritis, due to, by organism) 009.0
  Enterobacter aerogenes NEC 041.85
  Enterobacter sakazakii 041.85
  Enterobius vermicularis 127.4
  enterococcus NEC 041.04
  enterovirus NEC 079.89
    central nervous system NEC 048
    enteritis 008.67
    meningitis 047.9
  Entomophthora 117.7
  Epidermophyton - *see* Dermatophytosis
  epidermophytosis - *see* Dermatophytosis
  episiotomy 674.3●
  Epstein-Barr virus 075
    chronic 780.79 [139.8]
  erysipeloid 027.1
  Erysipelothrix (insidiosa) (rhusiopathiae) 027.1
  erythema infectiosum 057.0
  Escherichia coli (E. coli) 041.49
    enteritis - *see* Enteritis, E. coli
    generalized 038.42
    intestinal - *see* Enteritis, E. coli
    non-Shiga toxin-producing 041.49
    Shiga toxin-producing (STEC) 041.43
      with
        unspecified O group 041.43
      non-O157 (with known O group) 041.42
      O157 (with confirmation of Shiga toxin when H antigen is unknown, or is not H7) 041.41
      O157:H- (nonmotile) with confirmation of Shiga toxin 041.41
      O157:H7 with or without confirmation of Shiga toxin-production 041.41
      specified NEC 041.42
  esophagostomy 530.86

Infection, infected, infective *(Continued)*
  ethmoidal (chronic) (sinus) *(see also* Sinusitis, ethmoidal) 473.2
  Eubacterium 041.84
  Eustachian tube (ear) 381.50
    acute 381.51
    chronic 381.52
  exanthema subitum *(see also* Exanthem subitum) 058.10
  exit site 999.33
  external auditory canal (meatus) *(see also* Otitis, externa) 380.10
  eye NEC 360.00
  eyelid 373.9
    specified NEC 373.8
  fallopian tube *(see also* Salpingo-oophoritis) 614.2
  fascia 728.89
  Fasciola
    gigantica 121.3
    hepatica 121.3
  Fasciolopsis (buski) 121.4
  fetus (intra-amniotic) - *see* Infection, congenital
  filarial - *see* Infestation, filarial
  finger (skin) 686.9
    abscess (with lymphangitis) 681.00
      pulp 681.01
    cellulitis (with lymphangitis) 681.00
    distal closed space (with lymphangitis) 681.00
    nail 681.02
      fungus 110.1
  fish tapeworm 123.4
    larval 123.5
  flagellate, intestinal 007.9
  fluke - *see* Infestation, fluke
  focal
    teeth (pulpal origin) 522.4
    tonsils 474.00
      and adenoids 474.02
  Fonsecaea
    compactum 117.2
    pedrosoi 117.2
  food *(see also* Poisoning, food) 005.9
  foot (skin) 686.9
    fungus 110.4
  Francisella tularensis *(see also* Tularemia) 021.9
  frontal sinus (chronic) *(see also* Sinusitis, frontal) 473.1
  fungus NEC 117.9
    beard 110.0
    body 110.5
    dermatiacious NEC 117.8
    foot 110.4
    groin 110.3
    hand 110.2
    nail 110.1
    pathogenic to compromised host only 118
    perianal (area) 110.3
    scalp 110.0
    scrotum 110.8
    skin 111.9
      foot 110.4
      hand 110.2
    toenails 110.1
    trachea 117.9
  Fusarium 118
  Fusobacterium 041.84
  gallbladder *(see also* Cholecystitis, acute) 575.0
  Gardnerella vaginalis 041.89
  gas bacillus *(see also* Gas, gangrene) 040.0
  gastric *(see also* Gastritis) 535.5●
  Gastrodiscoides hominis 121.8
  gastroenteric *(see also* Enteritis, due to, by organism) 009.0
  gastrointestinal *(see also* Enteritis, due to, by organism) 009.0
  gastrostomy 536.41

SECTION 1 INDEX TO DISEASES AND INJURIES / Infection, infected, infective

Infection, infected, infective (Continued)
  generalized NEC (see also Septicemia) 038.9
  genital organ or tract NEC
    female 614.9
      with
        abortion - see Abortion, by type, with sepsis
        ectopic pregnancy (see also categories 633.0–633.9) 639.0
        molar pregnancy (see also categories 630–632) 639.0
      complicating pregnancy 646.6●
        affecting fetus or newborn 760.8
      following
        abortion 639.0
        ectopic or molar pregnancy 639.0
      puerperal, postpartum, childbirth 670.8●
        minor or localized 646.6●
          affecting fetus or newborn 760.8
    male 608.4
  genitourinary tract NEC 599.0
  Ghon tubercle, primary (see also Tuberculosis) 010.0●
  Giardia lamblia 007.1
  gingival (chronic) 523.10
    acute 523.00
    Vincent's 101
  glanders 024
  Glenosporopsis amazonica 116.2
  Gnathostoma spinigerum 128.1
  Gongylonema 125.6
  gonococcal NEC (see also Gonococcus) 098.0
  gram-negative bacilli NEC 041.85
    anaerobic 041.84
  guinea worm 125.7
  gum (see also Infection, gingival) 523.10
  Hantavirus 079.81
  heart 429.89
  Helicobacter pylori [H. pylori] 041.86
    helminths NEC 128.9
    intestinal 127.9
      mixed (types classifiable to more than one category in 120.0–127.7) 127.8
      specified type NEC 127.7
    specified type NEC 128.8
  Hemophilus influenzae NEC 041.5
    generalized 038.41
  Herpes (simplex) (see also Herpes, simplex) 054.9
    congenital 771.2
    zoster (see also Herpes, zoster) 053.9
      eye NEC 053.29
  Heterophyes heterophyes 121.6
  Histoplasma (see also Histoplasmosis) 115.90
    capsulatum (see also Histoplasmosis, American) 115.00
    duboisii (see also Histoplasmosis, African) 115.10
  HIV V08
    with symptoms, symptomatic 042
  hookworm (see also Ancylostomiasis) 126.9
  human herpesvirus 6 058.81
  human herpesvirus 7 058.82
  human herpesvirus 8 058.89
  human herpesvirus NEC 058.89
  human immunodeficiency virus V08
    with symptoms, symptomatic 042
  human papillomavirus 079.4
  hydrocele 603.1
  hydronephrosis 591
  Hymenolepis 123.6
  hypopharynx 478.29
  inguinal glands 683
    due to soft chancre 099.0
  insertion site 999.33
  intestine, intestinal (see also Enteritis, due to, by organism) 009.0
  intrauterine (see also Endometritis) 615.9
    complicating delivery 646.6●

Infection, infected, infective (Continued)
  isospora belli or hominis 007.2
  Japanese B encephalitis 062.0
  jaw (bone) (acute) (chronic) (lower) (subacute) (upper) 526.4
  joint - see Arthritis, infectious or infective
  Kaposi's sarcoma-associated herpesvirus 058.89
  kidney (cortex) (hematogenous) 590.9
    with
      abortion - see Abortion, by type, with urinary tract infection
      calculus 592.0
      ectopic pregnancy (see also categories 633.0–633.9) 639.8
      molar pregnancy (see also categories 630–632) 639.8
    complicating pregnancy or puerperium 646.6●
      affecting fetus or newborn 760.1
    following
      abortion 639.8
      ectopic or molar pregnancy 639.8
    pelvis and ureter 590.3
  Klebsiella pneumoniae NEC 041.3
  knee (skin) NEC 686.9
    joint - see Arthritis, infectious
  Koch's (see also Tuberculosis, pulmonary) 011.9●
  labia (majora) (minora) (see also Vulvitis) 616.10
  lacrimal
    gland (see also Dacryoadenitis) 375.00
    passages (duct) (sac) (see also Dacryocystitis) 375.30
  larynx NEC 478.79
  leg (skin) NEC 686.9
  Leishmania (see also Leishmaniasis) 085.9
    braziliensis 085.5
    donovani 085.0
    Ethiopica 085.3
    furunculosa 085.1
    infantum 085.0
    Mexicana 085.4
    tropica (minor) 085.1
      major 085.2
  Leptosphaeria senegalensis 117.4
  Leptospira (see also Leptospirosis) 100.9
    australis 100.89
    bataviae 100.89
    pyrogenes 100.89
    specified type NEC 100.89
  leptospirochetal NEC (see also Leptospirosis) 100.9
  Leptothrix - see Actinomycosis
  Listeria monocytogenes (listeriosis) 027.0
    congenital 771.2
  liver fluke - see Infestation, fluke, liver
  Loa loa 125.2
    eyelid 125.2 [373.6]
  Loboa loboi 116.2
  local, skin (staphylococcal) (streptococcal) NEC 686.9
    abscess - see Abscess, by site
    cellulitis - see Cellulitis, by site
    ulcer (see also Ulcer, skin) 707.9
  Loefflerella
    mallei 024
    whitmori 025
  lung 518.89
    atypical Mycobacterium 031.0
    tuberculous (see also Tuberculosis, pulmonary) 011.9●
    basilar 518.89
    chronic 518.89
    fungus NEC 117.9
    spirochetal 104.8
    virus - see Pneumonia, virus
  lymph gland (axillary) (cervical) (inguinal) 683
    mesenteric 289.2

Infection, infected, infective (Continued)
  lymphoid tissue, base of tongue or posterior pharynx, NEC 474.00
  Madurella
    grisea 117.4
    mycetomii 117.4
  major
    with
      abortion - see Abortion, by type, with sepsis
      ectopic pregnancy (see also categories 633.0–633.9) 639.0
      molar pregnancy (see also categories 630–632) 639.0
    following
      abortion 639.0
      ectopic or molar pregnancy 639.0
    puerperal, postpartum, childbirth 670.0●
  malarial - see Malaria
  Malassezia furfur 111.0
  Malleomyces
    mallei 024
    pseudomallei 025
  mammary gland 611.0
    puerperal, postpartum 675.2●
  Mansonella (ozzardi) 125.5
  mastoid (suppurative) - see Mastoiditis
  maxilla, maxillary 526.4
    sinus (chronic) (see also Sinusitis, maxillary) 473.0
  mediastinum 519.2
  medina 125.7
  meibomian
    cyst 373.12
    gland 373.12
  melioidosis 025
  meninges (see also Meningitis) 320.9
  meningococcal (see also condition) 036.9
    brain 036.1
    cerebrospinal 036.0
    endocardium 036.42
    generalized 036.2
    meninges 036.0
    meningococcemia 036.2
    specified site NEC 036.89
  mesenteric lymph nodes or glands NEC 289.2
  Metagonimus 121.5
  metatarsophalangeal 711.97
  methicillin
    resistant Staphylococcus aureus (MRSA) 041.12
    susceptible Staphylococcus aureus (MSSA) 041.11
  microorganism resistant to drugs - see Resistance (to), drugs by microorganisms
  Microsporidia 136.8
  microsporum, microsporic - see Dermatophytosis
  mima polymorpha NEC 041.85
  mixed flora NEC 041.89
  Monilia (see also Candidiasis) 112.9
    neonatal 771.7
  monkeypox 059.01
  Monosporium apiospermum 117.6
  mouth (focus) NEC 528.9
    parasitic 136.9
  MRSA (methicillin resistant Staphylococcus aureus) 041.12
  MSSA (methicillin susceptible Staphylococcus aureus) 041.11
  Mucor 117.7
  muscle NEC 728.89
  mycelium NEC 117.9
  mycetoma
    actinomycotic NEC (see also Actinomycosis) 039.9
    mycotic NEC 117.4
  Mycobacterium, mycobacterial (see also Mycobacterium) 031.9

Infection, infected, infective (Continued)
Mycoplasma NEC 041.81
mycotic NEC 117.9
   pathogenic to compromised host only 118
   skin NEC 111.9
   systemic 117.9
myocardium NEC 422.90
nail (chronic) (with lymphangitis) 681.9
   finger 681.02
     fungus 110.1
   ingrowing 703.0
   toe 681.11
     fungus 110.1
nasal sinus (chronic (see also Sinusitis) 473.9
nasopharynx (chronic) 478.29
   acute 460
navel 686.9
   newborn 771.4
Neisserian - see Gonococcus
Neotestudina rosatii 117.4
newborn, generalized 771.89
nipple 611.0
   puerperal, postpartum 675.0
     with breast 675.9
       specified type NEC 675.8
Nocardia - see Actinomycosis
nose 478.19
nostril 478.19
obstetrical surgical wound 674.3
Oesophagostomum (apiostomum) 127.7
Oestrus ovis 134.0
Oidium albicans (see also Candidiasis) 112.9
Onchocerca (volvulus) 125.3
   eye 125.3 [360.13]
   eyelid 125.3 [373.6]
operation wound 998.59
Opisthorchis (felineus) (tenuicollis)
     (viverrini) 121.0
orbit 376.00
   chronic 376.10
orthopoxvirus 059.00
   specified NEC 059.09
ovary (see also Salpingo-oophoritis) 614.2
Oxyuris vermicularis 127.4
pancreas 577.0
Paracoccidioides brasiliensis 116.1
Paragonimus (westermani) 121.2
parainfluenza virus 079.89
parameningococcus NEC 036.9
   with meningitis 036.0
parapoxvirus 059.10
   specified NEC 059.19
parasitic NEC 136.9
paratyphoid 002.9
   type A 002.1
   type B 002.2
   type C 002.3
paraurethral ducts 597.89
parotid gland 527.2
Pasteurella NEC 027.2
   multocida (cat-bite) (dog-bite) 027.2
   pestis (see also Plague) 020.9
   pseudotuberculosis 027.2
   septica (cat-bite) (dog-bite) 027.2
   tularensis (see also Tularemia) 021.9
pelvic, female (see also Disease, pelvis,
     inflammatory) 614.9
penis (glans) (retention) NEC 607.2
   herpetic 054.13
Peptococcus 041.84
Peptostreptococcus 041.84
periapical (pulpal origin) 522.4
peridental 523.30
perineal wound (obstetrical) 674.3
periodontal 523.31
periorbital 376.00
   chronic 376.10
perirectal 569.49
perirenal (see also Infection, kidney) 590.9
peritoneal (see also Peritonitis) 567.9
periureteral 593.89

Infection, infected, infective (Continued)
periurethral 597.89
Petriellidium boydii 117.6
pharynx 478.29
   Coxsackie virus 074.0
   phlegmonous 462
   posterior, lymphoid 474.00
Phialophora
   gougerotii 117.8
   jeanselmei 117.8
   verrucosa 117.2
Piedraia hortai 111.3
pinna, acute 380.11
pinta 103.9
   intermediate 103.1
   late 103.2
   mixed 103.3
   primary 103.0
pinworm 127.4
pityrosporum furfur 111.0
pleuropneumonia-like organisms NEC
     (PPLO) 041.81
pneumococcal NEC 041.2
   generalized (purulent) 038.2
Pneumococcus NEC 041.2
port 999.33
postoperative wound 998.59
posttraumatic NEC 958.3
postvaccinal 999.39
poxvirus 059.9
   specified NEC 059.8
prepuce NEC 607.1
Proprionibacterium 041.84
prostate (capsule) (see also Prostatitis) 601.9
Proteus (mirabilis) (morganii) (vulgaris)
     NEC 041.6
   enteritis 008.3
protozoal NEC 136.8
   intestinal NEC 007.9
Pseudomonas NEC 041.7
   mallei 024
   pneumonia 482.1
   pseudomallei 025
psittacosis 073.9
puerperal, postpartum (major) 670.0
   minor 646.6
pulmonary - see Infection, lung
purulent - see Abscess
putrid, generalized - see Septicemia
pyemic - see Septicemia
Pyrenochaeta romeroi 117.4
Q fever 083.0
rabies 071
rectum (sphincter) 569.49
renal (see also Infection, kidney) 590.9
   pelvis and ureter 590.3
reservoir 999.33
resistant to drugs - see Resistance (to), drugs
     by microorganisms
respiratory 519.8
   chronic 519.8
   influenzal (acute) (upper) (see also
     Influenza) 487.1
   lung 518.89
   rhinovirus 460
   syncytial virus 079.6
   upper (acute) (infectious) NEC 465.9
     with flu, grippe, or influenza (see also
       Influenza) 487.1
     influenzal (see also Influenza) 487.1
     multiple sites NEC 465.8
     streptococcal 034.0
     viral NEC 465.9
respiratory syncytial virus (RSV) 079.6
resulting from presence of shunt or other
     internal prosthetic device - see
     Complications, infection and
     inflammation, due to (presence of) any
     device, implant, or graft classified to
     996.0–996.5 NEC
retroperitoneal 567.39

Infection, infected, infective (Continued)
retrovirus 079.50
   human immunodeficiency virus type 2
     (HIV 2) 079.53
   human T-cell lymphotrophic virus type I
     (HTLV-I) 079.51
   human T-cell lymphotrophic virus type II
     (HTLV-II) 079.52
   specified NEC 079.59
Rhinocladium 117.1
Rhinosporidium (seeberi) 117.0
rhinovirus
   in diseases classified elsewhere - see
     category 079
   unspecified nature or site 079.3
Rhizopus 117.7
rickettsial 083.9
rickettsialpox 083.2
rubella (see also Rubella) 056.9
   congenital 771.0
Saccharomyces (see also Candidiasis)
     112.9
Saksenaea 117.7
salivary duct or gland (any) 527.2
Salmonella (aertrycke) (callinarum)
     (choleraesuis) (enteritidis) (suipestifer)
     (typhimurium) 003.9
   with
     arthritis 003.23
     gastroenteritis 003.0
     localized infection 003.20
       specified type NEC 003.29
     meningitis 003.21
     osteomyelitis 003.24
     pneumonia 003.22
     septicemia 003.1
     specified manifestation NEC 003.8
   due to food (poisoning) (any serotype)
     (see also Poisoning, food, due to,
     Salmonella)
   hirschfeldii 002.3
   localized 003.20
     specified type NEC 003.29
   paratyphi 002.9
     A 002.1
     B 002.2
     C 002.3
   schottmuelleri 002.2
   specified type NEC 003.8
   typhi 002.0
   typhosa 002.0
saprophytic 136.8
Sarcocystis, lindemanni 136.5
SARS-associated coronavirus 079.82
scabies 133.0
Schistosoma - see Infestation, Schistosoma
Schmorl's bacillus 040.3
scratch or other superficial injury - see Injury,
     superficial, by site
scrotum (acute) NEC 608.4
sealpox 059.12
secondary, burn or open wound (dislocation)
     (fracture) 958.3
seminal vesicle (see also Vesiculitis) 608.0
septic
   generalized - see Septicemia
   localized, skin (see also Abscess) 682.9
septicemic - see Septicemia
seroma 998.51
Serratia (marcescens) 041.85
   generalized 038.44
sheep liver fluke 121.3
Shigella 004.9
   boydii 004.2
   dysenteriae 004.0
   Flexneri 004.1
   group
     A 004.0
     B 004.1
     C 004.2
     D 004.3

Infection, infected, infective (Continued)
- Shigella (Continued)
  - Schmitz (-Stutzer) 004.0
  - Schmitzii 004.0
  - Shiga 004.0
  - Sonnei 004.3
  - specified type NEC 004.8
- Sin Nombre virus 079.81
- sinus (see also Sinusitis) 473.9
  - pilonidal 685.1
    - with abscess 685.0
  - skin NEC 686.9
- Skene's duct or gland (see also Urethritis) 597.89
- skin (local) (staphylococcal) (streptococcal) NEC 686.9
  - abscess - see Abscess, by site
  - cellulitis - see Cellulitis, by site
  - due to fungus 111.9
    - specified type NEC 111.8
  - mycotic 111.9
    - specified type NEC 111.8
  - ulcer (see also Ulcer, skin) 707.9
- slow virus 046.9
  - specified condition NEC 046.8
- Sparganum (mansoni) (proliferum) 123.5
- spermatic cord NEC 608.4
- sphenoidal (chronic) (sinus) (see also Sinusitis, sphenoidal) 473.3
- Spherophorus necrophorus 040.3
- spinal cord NEC (see also Encephalitis) 323.9
  - abscess 324.1
    - late effect - see category 326
  - late effect - see category 326
  - meninges - see Meningitis
  - streptococcal 320.2
- Spirillum
  - minus or minor 026.0
  - morsus muris 026.0
  - obermeieri 087.0
- spirochetal NEC 104.9
  - lung 104.8
  - specified nature or site NEC 104.8
- spleen 289.59
- Sporothrix schenckii 117.1
- Sporotrichum (schenckii) 117.1
- Sporozoa 136.8
- staphylococcal NEC 041.10
  - aureus 041.11
    - methicillin
      - resistant (MRSA) 041.12
      - susceptible MSSA) 041.11
  - food poisoning 005.0
  - generalized (purulent) 038.10
    - aureus 038.11
      - methicillin
        - resistant 038.12
        - susceptible 038.11
    - specified organism NEC 038.19
  - pneumonia 482.40
    - aureus 482.41
      - methicillin
        - resistant (MRSA) 482.42
        - susceptible (MSSA) 482.41
    - MRSA (methicillin resistant staphylococcus aureus) 482.42
    - MSSA (methicillin susceptible staphylococcus aureus) 482.41
    - specified type NEC 482.49
  - septicemia 038.10
    - aureus 038.11
      - methicillin
        - resistant (MRSA) 038.12
        - susceptible (MSSA) 038.11
    - MRSA (methicillin resistant staphylococcus aureus) 038.12
    - MSSA (methicillin susceptible staphylococcus aureus) 038.11
    - specified organism NEC 038.19
  - specified NEC 041.19

Infection, infected, infective (Continued)
- steatoma 706.2
- Stellantchasmus falcatus 121.6
- Streptobacillus moniliformis 026.1
- streptococcal NEC 041.00
  - generalized (purulent) 038.0
  - group
    - A 041.01
    - B 041.02
    - C 041.03
    - D [enterococcus] 041.04
    - G 041.05
  - pneumonia - see Pneumonia, streptococcal
  - septicemia 038.0
  - sore throat 034.0
  - specified NEC 041.09
- Streptomyces - see Actinomycosis
- streptotrichosis - see Actinomycosis
- Strongyloides (stercoralis) 127.2
- stump (amputation) (posttraumatic) (surgical) 997.62
  - traumatic - see Amputation, traumatic, by site, complicated
- subcutaneous tissue, local NEC 686.9
- submaxillary region 528.9
- suipestifer (see also Infection, Salmonella) 003.9
- swimming pool bacillus 031.1
- syphilitic - see Syphilis
- systemic - see Septicemia
- Taenia - see Infestation, Taenia
- Taeniarhynchus saginatus 123.2
- tanapox 059.21
- tapeworm - see Infestation, tapeworm
- tendon (sheath) 727.89
- Ternidens diminutus 127.7
- testis (see also Orchitis) 604.90
- thigh (skin) 686.9
- threadworm 127.4
- throat 478.29
  - pneumococcal 462
  - staphylococcal 462
  - streptococcal 034.0
  - viral NEC (see also Pharyngitis) 462
- thumb (skin) 686.9
  - abscess (with lymphangitis) 681.00
    - pulp 681.01
  - cellulitis (with lymphangitis) 681.00
  - nail 681.02
- thyroglossal duct 529.8
- toe (skin) 686.9
  - abscess (with lymphangitis) 681.10
  - cellulitis (with lymphangitis) 681.10
  - nail 681.11
    - fungus 110.1
- tongue NEC 529.0
  - parasitic 112.0
- tonsil (faucial) (lingual) (pharyngeal) 474.00
  - acute or subacute 463
  - and adenoid 474.02
  - tag 474.00
- tooth, teeth 522.4
  - periapical (pulpal origin) 522.4
  - peridental 523.30
  - periodontal 523.31
  - pulp 522.0
  - socket 526.5
- TORCH - see Infection, congenital NEC
  - without active infection 760.2
- Torula histolytica 117.5
- Toxocara (cani) (cati) (felis) 128.0
- Toxoplasma gondii (see also Toxoplasmosis) 130.9
- trachea, chronic 491.8
  - fungus 117.9
- traumatic NEC 958.3
- trematode NEC 121.9
- trench fever 083.1
- Treponema
  - denticola 041.84
  - macrodenticum 041.84
  - pallidum (see also Syphilis) 097.9

Infection, infected, infective (Continued)
- Trichinella (spiralis) 124
- Trichomonas 131.9
  - bladder 131.09
  - cervix 131.09
  - hominis 007.3
  - intestine 007.3
  - prostate 131.03
  - specified site NEC 131.8
  - urethra 131.02
  - urogenitalis 131.00
  - vagina 131.01
  - vulva 131.01
- Trichophyton, trichophytid - see Dermatophytosis
- Trichosporon (beigelii) cutaneum 111.2
- Trichostrongylus 127.6
- Trichuris (trichiuria) 127.3
- Trombicula (irritans) 133.8
- Trypanosoma (see also Trypanosomiasis) 086.9
  - cruzi 086.2
- tubal (see also Salpingo-oophoritis) 614.2
- tuberculous NEC (see also Tuberculosis) 011.9●
- tubo-ovarian (see also Salpingo-oophoritis) 614.2
- tunica vaginalis 608.4
- tunnel 999.33
- tympanic membrane - see Myringitis
- typhoid (abortive) (ambulant) (bacillus) 002.0
- typhus 081.9
  - flea-borne (endemic) 081.0
  - louse-borne (epidemic) 080
  - mite-borne 081.2
  - recrudescent 081.1
  - tick-borne 082.9
    - African 082.1
    - North Asian 082.2
- umbilicus (septic) 686.9
  - newborn NEC 771.4
- ureter 593.89
- urethra (see also Urethritis) 597.80
- urinary (tract) NEC 599.0
  - with
    - abortion - see Abortion, by type, with urinary tract infection
    - ectopic pregnancy (see also categories 633.0–633.9) 639.8
    - molar pregnancy (see also categories 630–632) 639.8
  - candidal 112.2
  - complicating pregnancy, childbirth, or puerperium 646.6●
    - affecting fetus or newborn 760.1
  - asymptomatic 646.5●
    - affecting fetus or newborn 760.1
  - diplococcal (acute) 098.0
    - chronic 098.2
  - due to Trichomonas (vaginalis) 131.00
  - following
    - abortion 639.8
    - ectopic or molar pregnancy 639.8
  - gonococcal (acute) 098.0
    - chronic or duration of 2 months or over 098.2
  - newborn 771.82
  - trichomonal 131.00
  - tuberculous (see also Tuberculosis) 016.3●
- uterus, uterine (see also Endometritis) 615.9
- utriculus masculinus NEC 597.89
- vaccination 999.39
- vagina (granulation tissue) (wall) (see also Vaginitis) 616.10
- varicella 052.9
- varicose veins - see Varicose, veins
- variola 050.9
  - major 050.0
  - minor 050.1
- vas deferens NEC 608.4

Infection, infected, infective (Continued)
Veillonella 041.84
verumontanum 597.89
vesical (see also Cystitis) 595.9
Vibrio
    cholerae 001.0
        El Tor 001.1
    parahaemolyticus (food poisoning) 005.4
    vulnificus 041.85
Vincent's (gums) (mouth) (tonsil) 101
virus, viral 079.99
    adenovirus
        in diseases classified elsewhere - see category 079
        unspecified nature or site 079.0
    central nervous system NEC 049.9
        enterovirus 048
            meningitis 047.9
                specified type NEC 047.8
        slow virus 046.9
            specified condition NEC 046.8
    chest 519.8
    conjunctivitis 077.99
        specified type NEC 077.89
    coronavirus 079.89
        SARS-associated 079.82
    Coxsackie (see also Infection, Coxsackie) 079.2
    Ebola 065.8
    ECHO
        in diseases classified elsewhere - see category 079
        unspecified nature or site 079.1
    encephalitis 049.9
        arthropod-borne NEC 064
        tick-borne 063.9
            specified type NEC 063.8
    enteritis NEC (see also Enteritis, viral) 008.8
    exanthem NEC 057.9
    Hantavirus 079.81
    human papilloma 079.4
    in diseases classified elsewhere - see category 079
    intestine (see also Enteritis, viral) 008.8
    lung - see Pneumonia, viral
    respiratory syncytial (RSV) 079.6
    Retrovirus 079.50
    rhinovirus
        in diseases classified elsewhere - see category 079
        unspecified nature or site 079.3
    salivary gland disease 078.5
    slow 046.9
        specified condition NEC 046.8
    specified type NEC 079.89
        in diseases classified elsewhere - see category 079
    unspecified nature or site 079.99
    warts 078.10
        specified NEC 078.19
    yaba monkey tumor 059.22
vulva (see also Vulvitis) 616.10
whipworm 127.3
Whitmore's bacillus 025
wound (local) (posttraumatic) NEC 958.3
    with
        dislocation - see Dislocation, by site, open
        fracture - see Fracture, by site, open
        open wound - see Wound, open, by site, complicated
    postoperative 998.59
    surgical 998.59
Wuchereria 125.0
    bancrofti 125.0
    malayi 125.1
yaba monkey tumor virus 059.22
yatapoxvirus 059.20
yaws - see Yaws
yeast (see also Candidiasis) 112.9

Infection, infected, infective (Continued)
yellow fever (see also Fever, yellow) 060.9
Yersinia pestis (see also Plague) 020.9
Zeis' gland 373.12
zoonotic bacterial NEC 027.9
Zopfia senegalensis 117.4
Infective, infectious - see condition
Inferiority complex 301.9
    constitutional psychopathic 301.9
Infertility
    female 628.9
        age related 628.8
        associated with
            adhesions, peritubal 614.6 [628.2]
            anomaly
                cervical mucus 628.4
                congenital
                      cervix 628.4
                      fallopian tube 628.2
                      uterus 628.3
                      vagina 628.4
            anovulation 628.0
            dysmucorrhea 628.4
            endometritis, tuberculous (see also Tuberculosis) 016.7● [628.3]
            Stein-Leventhal syndrome 256.4 [628.0]
        due to
            adiposogenital dystrophy 253.8 [628.1]
            anterior pituitary disorder NEC 253.4 [628.1]
                hyperfunction 253.1 [628.1]
            cervical anomaly 628.4
            fallopian tube anomaly 628.2
            ovarian failure 256.39 [628.0]
            Stein-Leventhal syndrome 256.4 [628.0]
            uterine anomaly 628.3
            vaginal anomaly 628.4
        nonimplantation 628.3
        origin
            cervical 628.4
            pituitary-hypothalamus NEC 253.8 [628.1]
                anterior pituitary NEC 253.4 [628.1]
                      hyperfunction NEC 253.1 [628.1]
                dwarfism 253.3 [628.1]
                panhypopituitarism 253.2 [628.1]
            specified NEC 628.8
            tubal (block) (occlusion) (stenosis) 628.2
                adhesions 614.6 [628.2]
            uterine 628.3
            vaginal 628.4
        previous, requiring supervision of pregnancy V23.0
    male 606.9
        absolute 606.0
        due to
            azoospermia 606.0
            drug therapy 606.8
            extratesticular cause NEC 606.8
            germinal cell
                aplasia 606.0
                desquamation 606.1
            hypospermatogenesis 606.1
            infection 606.8
            obstruction, afferent ducts 606.8
            oligospermia 606.1
            radiation 606.8
            spermatogenic arrest (complete) 606.0
                incomplete 606.1
            systemic disease 606.8
Infestation 134.9
    Acanthocheilonema (perstans) 125.4
        streptocerca 125.6
    Acariasis 133.9
        demodex folliculorum 133.8
        sarcoptes scabiei 133.0
        trombiculae 133.8
    Agamofilaria streptocerca 125.6

Infestation (Continued)
Ancylostoma, Ankylostoma 126.9
    americanum 126.1
    braziliense 126.2
    canium 126.8
    ceylanicum 126.3
    duodenale 126.0
    new world 126.1
    old world 126.0
Angiostrongylus cantonensis 128.8
anisakiasis 127.1
Anisakis larva 127.1
arthropod NEC 134.1
Ascaris lumbricoides 127.0
Bacillus fusiformis 101
Balantidium coli 007.0
beef tapeworm 123.2
Bothriocephalus (latus) 123.4
    larval 123.5
broad tapeworm 123.4
    larval 123.5
Brugia malayi 125.1
Candiru 136.8
Capillaria
    hepatica 128.8
    philippinensis 127.5
cat liver fluke 121.0
Cercomonas hominis (intestinal) 007.3
cestodes 123.9
    specified type NEC 123.8
chigger 133.8
chigoe 134.1
Chilomastix 007.8
Clonorchis (sinensis) (liver) 121.1
coccidia 007.2
complicating pregnancy, childbirth, or puerperium 647.9●
    affecting fetus or newborn 760.8
Cysticercus cellulosae 123.1
Demodex folliculorum 133.8
Dermatobia (hominis) 134.0
Dibothriocephalus (latus) 123.4
    larval 123.5
Dicrocoelium dendriticum 121.8
Diphyllobothrium (adult) (intestinal) (latum) (pacificum) 123.4
    larval 123.5
Diplogonoporus (grandis) 123.8
Dipylidium (caninum) 123.8
Distoma hepaticum 121.3
dog tapeworm 123.8
Dracunculus medinensis 125.7
dragon worm 125.7
dwarf tapeworm 123.6
Echinococcus (see also Echinococcus) 122.9
Echinostoma ilocanum 121.8
Embadomonas 007.8
Endamoeba (histolytica) - see Infection, ameba
Entamoeba (histolytica) - see Infection, ameba
Enterobius vermicularis 127.4
Epidermophyton - see Dermatophytosis
eyeworm 125.2
Fasciola
    gigantica 121.3
    hepatica 121.3
Fasciolopsis (buski) (small intestine) 121.4
filarial 125.9
    due to
        acanthocheilonema (perstans) 125.4
            streptocerca 125.6
        Brugia (Wuchereria) malayi 125.1
        Dracunculus medinensis 125.7
        guinea worms 125.7
        Mansonella (ozzardi) 125.5
        Onchocerca volvulus 125.3
            eye 125.3 [360.13]
            eyelid 125.3 [373.6]
        Wuchereria (bancrofti) 125.0
            malayi 125.1
    specified type NEC 125.6

Infestation (Continued)
- fish tapeworm 123.4
  - larval 123.5
- fluke 121.9
  - blood NEC (see also Schistosomiasis) 120.9
  - cat liver 121.0
  - intestinal (giant) 121.4
  - liver (sheep) 121.3
    - cat 121.0
    - Chinese 121.1
    - clonorchiasis 121.1
    - fascioliasis 121.3
    - Oriental 121.1
  - lung (oriental) 121.2
  - sheep liver 121.3
- fly larva 134.0
- Gasterophilus (intestinalis) 134.0
- Gastrodiscoides hominis 121.8
- Giardia lamblia 007.1
- Gnathostoma (spinigerum) 128.1
- Gongylonema 125.6
- guinea worm 125.7
- helminth NEC 128.9
  - intestinal 127.9
    - mixed (types classifiable to more than one category in 120.0–127.7) 127.8
    - specified type NEC 127.7
  - specified type NEC 128.8
- Heterophyes heterophyes (small intestine) 121.6
- hookworm (see also Infestation, ancylostoma) 126.9
- Hymenolepis (diminuta) (nana) 123.6
- intestinal NEC 129
- leeches (aquatic) (land) 134.2
- Leishmania - see Leishmaniasis
- lice (see also Infestation, pediculus) 132.9
- Linguatulidae, linguatula (pentastoma) (serrata) 134.1
- Loa loa 125.2
  - eyelid 125.2 [373.6]
- louse (see also Infestation, pediculus) 132.9
  - body 132.1
  - head 132.0
  - pubic 132.2
- maggots 134.0
- Mansonella (ozzardi) 125.5
- medina 125.7
- Metagonimus yokogawai (small intestine) 121.5
- Microfilaria streptocerca 125.3
  - eye 125.3 [360.13]
  - eyelid 125.3 [373.6]
- Microsporon furfur 111.0
- microsporum - see Dermatophytosis
- mites 133.9
  - scabic 133.0
  - specified type NEC 133.8
- Monilia (albicans) (see also Candidiasis) 112.9
  - vagina 112.1
  - vulva 112.1
- mouth 112.0
- Necator americanus 126.1
- nematode (intestinal) 127.9
  - Ancylostoma (see also Ancylostoma) 126.9
  - Ascaris lumbricoides 127.0
  - conjunctiva NEC 128.9
  - Dioctophyma 128.8
  - Enterobius vermicularis 127.4
  - Gnathostoma spinigerum 128.1
  - Oesophagostomum (apiostomum) 127.7
  - Physaloptera 127.4
  - specified type NEC 127.7
  - Strongyloides stercoralis 127.2
  - Ternidens diminutus 127.7
  - Trichinella spiralis 124
  - Trichostrongylus 127.6
  - Trichuris (trichiuria) 127.3
- Oesophagostomum (apiostomum) 127.7
- Oestrus ovis 134.0

Infestation (Continued)
- Onchocerca (volvulus) 125.3
  - eye 125.3 [360.13]
  - eyelid 125.3 [373.6]
- Opisthorchis (felineus) (tenuicollis) (viverrini) 121.0
- Oxyuris vermicularis 127.4
- Paragonimus (westermani) 121.2
- parasite, parasitic NEC 136.9
  - eyelid 134.9 [373.6]
  - intestinal 129
  - mouth 112.0
  - orbit 376.13
  - skin 134.9
  - tongue 112.0
- pediculus 132.9
  - capitis (humanus) (any site) 132.0
  - corporis (humanus) (any site) 132.1
  - eyelid 132.0 [373.6]
  - mixed (classifiable to more than one category in 132.0–132.2) 132.3
  - pubis (any site) 132.2
- phthirus (pubis) (any site) 132.2
  - with any infestation classifiable to 132.0 and 132.1 132.3
- pinworm 127.4
- pork tapeworm (adult) 123.0
- protozoal NEC 136.8
- pubic louse 132.2
- rat tapeworm 123.6
- red bug 133.8
- roundworm (large) NEC 127.0
- sand flea 134.1
- saprophytic NEC 136.8
- Sarcoptes scabiei 133.0
- scabies 133.0
- Schistosoma 120.9
  - bovis 120.8
  - cercariae 120.3
  - hematobium 120.0
  - intercalatum 120.8
  - japonicum 120.2
  - mansoni 120.1
  - mattheii 120.8
  - specified
    - site - see Schistosomiasis
    - type NEC 120.8
  - spindale 120.8
- screw worms 134.0
- skin NEC 134.9
- Sparganum (mansoni) (proliferum) 123.5
  - larval 123.5
- specified type NEC 134.8
- Spirometra larvae 123.5
- Sporozoa NEC 136.8
- Stellantchasmus falcatus 121.6
- Strongyloides 127.2
- Strongylus (gibsoni) 127.7
- Taenia 123.3
  - diminuta 123.6
  - Echinococcus (see also Echinococcus) 122.9
  - mediocanellata 123.2
  - nana 123.6
  - saginata (mediocanellata) 123.2
  - solium (intestinal form) 123.0
    - larval form 123.1
- Taeniarhynchus saginatus 123.2
- tapeworm 123.9
  - beef 123.2
  - broad 123.4
    - larval 123.5
  - dog 123.8
  - dwarf 123.6
  - fish 123.4
    - larval 123.5
  - pork 123.0
  - rat 123.6
- Ternidens diminutus 127.7
- Tetranychus molestissimus 133.8
- threadworm 127.4
- tongue 112.0

Infestation (Continued)
- Toxocara (cani) (cati) (felis) 128.0
- trematode(s) NEC 121.9
- Trichina spiralis 124
- Trichinella spiralis 124
- Trichocephalus 127.3
- Trichomonas 131.9
  - bladder 131.09
  - cervix 131.09
  - intestine 007.3
  - prostate 131.03
  - specified site NEC 131.8
  - urethra (female) (male) 131.02
  - urogenital 131.00
  - vagina 131.01
  - vulva 131.01
- Trichophyton - see Dermatophytosis
- Trichostrongylus instabilis 127.6
- Trichuris (trichiuria) 127.3
- Trombicula (irritans) 133.8
- Trypanosoma - see Trypanosomiasis
- Tunga penetrans 134.1
- Uncinaria americana 126.1
- whipworm 127.3
- worms NEC 128.9
  - intestinal 127.9
- Wuchereria 125.0
  - bancrofti 125.0
  - malayi 125.1

Infiltrate, infiltration
- with an iron compound 275.09
- amyloid (any site) (generalized) 277.39
- calcareous (muscle) NEC 275.49
  - localized - see Degeneration, by site
- calcium salt (muscle) 275.49
- chemotherapy, vesicant 999.81
- corneal (see also Edema, cornea) 371.20
- eyelid 373.9
- fatty (diffuse) (generalized) 272.8
  - localized - see Degeneration, by site, fatty
- glycogen, glycogenic (see also Disease, glycogen storage) 271.0
- heart, cardiac
  - fatty (see also Degeneration, myocardial) 429.1
  - glycogenic 271.0 [425.7]
- inflammatory in vitreous 379.29
- kidney (see also Disease, renal) 593.9
- leukemic (M9800/3) - see Leukemia
- liver 573.8
  - fatty - see Fatty, liver
  - glycogen (see also Disease, glycogen storage) 271.0
- lung (see also Infiltrate, pulmonary) 793.19
  - eosinophilic 518.3
  - x-ray finding only 793.19
- lymphatic (see also Leukemia, lymphatic) 204.9
- gland, pigmentary 289.3
- muscle, fatty 728.9
- myelogenous (see also Leukemia, myeloid) 205.9
- myocardium, myocardial
  - fatty (see also Degeneration, myocardial) 429.1
  - glycogenic 271.0 [425.7]
- pulmonary 793.19
  - with
    - eosinophilia 518.3
    - pneumonia - see Pneumonia, by type
  - x-ray finding only 793.19
- Ranke's primary (see also Tuberculosis) 010.0
- skin, lymphocytic (benign) 709.8
- thymus (gland) (fatty) 254.8
- urine 788.8
- vesicant
  - agent NEC 999.82
  - chemotherapy 999.81
- vitreous humor 379.29

Infirmity 799.89
  senile 797
Inflammation, inflamed, inflammatory (with exudation)
  abducens (nerve) 378.54
  accessory sinus (chronic) (*see also* Sinusitis) 473.9
  adrenal (gland) 255.8
  alimentary canal - *see* Enteritis
  alveoli (teeth) 526.5
    scorbutic 267
  amnion - *see* Amnionitis
  anal canal 569.49
  antrum (chronic) (*see also* Sinusitis, maxillary) 473.0
  anus 569.49
  appendix (*see also* Appendicitis) 541
  arachnoid - *see* Meningitis
  areola 611.0
    puerperal, postpartum 675.0●
  areolar tissue NEC 686.9
  artery - *see* Arteritis
  auditory meatus (external) (*see also* Otitis, externa) 380.10
  Bartholin's gland 616.89
  bile duct or passage 576.1
  bladder (*see also* Cystitis) 595.9
  bleb
    postprocedural 379.60
      stage 1 379.61
      stage 2 379.62
      stage 3 379.63
  bone - *see* Osteomyelitis
  bowel (*see also* Enteritis) 558.9
  brain (*see also* Encephalitis) 323.9
    late effect - *see* category 326
    membrane - *see* Meningitis
  breast 611.0
    puerperal, postpartum 675.2●
  broad ligament (*see also* Disease, pelvis, inflammatory) 614.4
    acute 614.3
  bronchus - *see* Bronchitis
  bursa - *see* Bursitis
  capsule
    liver 573.3
    spleen 289.59
  catarrhal (*see also* Catarrh) 460
    vagina 616.10
  cecum (*see also* Appendicitis) 541
  cerebral (*see also* Encephalitis) 323.9
    late effect - *see* category 326
    membrane - *see* Meningitis
  cerebrospinal (*see also* Meningitis) 322.9
    late effect - *see* category 326
    meningococcal 036.0
    tuberculous (*see also* Tuberculosis) 013.6●
  cervix (uteri) (*see also* Cervicitis) 616.0
  chest 519.9
  choroid NEC (*see also* Choroiditis) 363.20
  cicatrix (tissue) - *see* Cicatrix
  colon (*see also* Enteritis) 558.9
    granulomatous 555.1
    newborn 558.9
  connective tissue (diffuse) NEC 728.9
  cornea (*see also* Keratitis) 370.9
    with ulcer (*see also* Ulcer, cornea) 370.00
  corpora cavernosa (penis) 607.2
  cranial nerve - *see* Disorder, nerve, cranial
  diarrhea - *see* Diarrhea
  disc (intervertebral) (space) 722.90
    cervical, cervicothoracic 722.91
    lumbar, lumbosacral 722.93
    thoracic, thoracolumbar 722.92
  Douglas' cul-de-sac or pouch (chronic) (*see also* Disease, pelvis, inflammatory) 614.4
    acute 614.3

Inflammation, inflamed, inflammatory
(Continued)
  due to (presence of) any device, implant, or graft classifiable to 996.0–996.5 - *see* Complications, infection and inflammation, due to (presence of) any device, implant, or graft classified to 996.0–996.5 NEC
  duodenum 535.6●
  dura mater - *see* Meningitis
  ear - *see also* Otitis
    external (*see also* Otitis, externa) 380.10
    inner (*see also* Labyrinthitis) 386.30
    middle - *see* Otitis media
  esophagus 530.10
  ethmoidal (chronic) (sinus) (*see also* Sinusitis, ethmoidal) 473.2
  Eustachian tube (catarrhal) 381.50
    acute 381.51
    chronic 381.52
  extrarectal 569.49
  eye 379.99
  eyelid 373.9
    specified NEC 373.8
  fallopian tube (*see also* Salpingo-oophoritis) 614.2
  fascia 728.9
  fetal membranes (acute) 658.4●
    affecting fetus or newborn 762.7
  follicular, pharynx 472.1
  frontal (chronic) (sinus) (*see also* Sinusitis, frontal) 473.1
  gallbladder (*see also* Cholecystitis, acute) 575.0
  gall duct (*see also* Cholecystitis) 575.10
  gastrointestinal (*see also* Enteritis) 558.9
  genital organ (diffuse) (internal)
    female 614.9
      with
        abortion - *see* Abortion, by type, with sepsis
        ectopic pregnancy (*see also* categories 633.0–633.9) 639.0
        molar pregnancy (*see also* categories 630–632) 639.0
      complicating pregnancy, childbirth, or puerperium 646.6●
        affecting fetus or newborn 760.8
      following
        abortion 639.0
        ectopic or molar pregnancy 639.0
    male 608.4
  gland (lymph) (*see also* Lymphadenitis) 289.3
  glottis (*see also* Laryngitis) 464.00
    with obstruction 464.01
  granular, pharynx 472.1
  gum 523.10
  heart (*see also* Carditis) 429.89
  hepatic duct 576.8
  hernial sac - *see* Hernia, by site
  ileum (*see also* Enteritis) 558.9
    terminal or regional 555.0
      with large intestine 555.2
  intervertebral disc 722.90
    cervical, cervicothoracic 722.91
    lumbar, lumbosacral 722.93
    thoracic, thoracolumbar 722.92
  intestine (*see also* Enteritis) 558.9
  jaw (acute) (bone) (chronic) (lower) (suppurative) (upper) 526.4
  jejunum - *see* Enteritis
  joint NEC (*see also* Arthritis) 716.9●
    sacroiliac 720.2
  kidney (*see also* Nephritis) 583.9
  knee (joint) 716.66
    tuberculous (active) (*see also* Tuberculosis) 015.2●
  labium (majus) (minus) (*see also* Vulvitis) 616.10

Inflammation, inflamed, inflammatory
(Continued)
  lacrimal
    gland (*see also* Dacryoadenitis) 375.00
    passages (duct) (sac) (*see also* Dacryocystitis) 375.30
  larynx (*see also* Laryngitis) 464.00
    with obstruction 464.01
    diphtheritic 032.3
  leg NEC 686.9
  lip 528.5
  liver (capsule) (*see also* Hepatitis) 573.3
    acute 570
    chronic 571.40
    suppurative 572.0
  lung (acute) (*see also* Pneumonia) 486
    chronic (interstitial) 518.89
  lymphatic vessel (*see also* Lymphangitis) 457.2
  lymph node or gland (*see also* Lymphadenitis) 289.3
  mammary gland 611.0
    puerperal, postpartum 675.2●
  maxilla, maxillary 526.4
    sinus (chronic) (*see also* Sinusitis, maxillary) 473.0
  membranes of brain or spinal cord - *see* Meningitis
  meninges - *see* Meningitis
  mouth 528.00
  muscle 728.9
  myocardium (*see also* Myocarditis) 429.0
  nasal sinus (chronic) (*see also* Sinusitis) 473.9
  nasopharynx - *see* Nasopharyngitis
  navel 686.9
    newborn NEC 771.4
  nerve NEC 729.2
  nipple 611.0
    puerperal, postpartum 675.0●
  nose 478.19
    suppurative 472.0
  oculomotor nerve 378.51
  optic nerve 377.30
  orbit (chronic) 376.10
    acute 376.00
    chronic 376.10
  ovary (*see also* Salpingo-oophoritis) 614.2
  oviduct (*see also* Salpingo-oophoritis) 614.2
  pancreas - *see* Pancreatitis
  parametrium (chronic) (*see also* Disease, pelvis, inflammatory) 614.4
    acute 614.3
  parotid region 686.9
    gland 527.2
  pelvis, female (*see also* Disease, pelvis, inflammatory) 614.9
  penis (corpora cavernosa) 607.2
  perianal 569.49
  pericardium (*see also* Pericarditis) 423.9
  perineum (female) (male) 686.9
  perirectal 569.49
  peritoneum (*see also* Peritonitis) 567.9
  periuterine (*see also* Disease, pelvis, inflammatory) 614.9
  perivesical (*see also* Cystitis) 595.9
  petrous bone (*see also* Petrositis) 383.20
  pharynx (*see also* Pharyngitis) 462
    follicular 472.1
    granular 472.1
  pia mater - *see* Meningitis
  pleura - *see* Pleurisy
  postmastoidectomy cavity 383.30
    chronic 383.33
  pouch, internal ileoanal 569.71
  prostate (*see also* Prostatitis) 601.9
  rectosigmoid - *see* Rectosigmoiditis
  rectum (*see also* Proctitis) 569.49

SECTION I INDEX TO DISEASES AND INJURIES / Inflammation, inflamed, inflammatory

Inflammation, inflamed, inflammatory
(Continued)
  respiratory, upper (see also Infection, respiratory, upper) 465.9
    chronic, due to external agent - see Condition, respiratory, chronic, due to, external agent
    due to
      fumes or vapors (chemical) (inhalation) 506.2
      radiation 508.1
  retina (see also Retinitis) 363.20
  retrocecal (see also Appendicitis) 541
  retroperitoneal (see also Peritonitis) 567.9
  salivary duct or gland (any) (suppurative) 527.2
  scorbutic, alveoli, teeth 267
  scrotum 608.4
  sigmoid - see Enteritis
  sinus (see also Sinusitis) 473.9
  Skene's duct or gland (see also Urethritis) 597.89
  skin 686.9
  spermatic cord 608.4
  sphenoidal (sinus) (see also Sinusitis, sphenoidal) 473.3
  spinal
    cord (see also Encephalitis) 323.9
      late effect - see category 326
    membrane - see Meningitis
    nerve - see Disorder, nerve
  spine (see also Spondylitis) 720.9
  spleen (capsule) 289.59
  stomach - see Gastritis
  stricture, rectum 569.49
  subcutaneous tissue NEC 686.9
  suprarenal (gland) 255.8
  synovial (fringe) (membrane) - see Bursitis
  tendon (sheath) NEC 726.90
  testis (see also Orchitis) 604.90
  thigh 686.9
  throat (see also Sore throat) 462
  thymus (gland) 254.8
  thyroid (gland) (see also Thyroiditis) 245.9
  tongue 529.0
  tonsil - see Tonsillitis
  trachea - see Tracheitis
  trochlear nerve 378.53
  tubal (see also Salpingo-oophoritis) 614.2
  tuberculous NEC (see also Tuberculosis) 011.9●
  tubo-ovarian (see also Salpingo-oophoritis) 614.2
  tunica vaginalis 608.4
  tympanic membrane - see Myringitis
  umbilicus, umbilical 686.9
    newborn NEC 771.4
  uterine ligament (see also Disease, pelvis, inflammatory) 614.4
    acute 614.3
  uterus (catarrhal) (see also Endometritis) 615.9
  uveal tract (anterior) (see also Iridocyclitis) 364.3
    posterior - see Chorioretinitis
    sympathetic 360.11
  vagina (see also Vaginitis) 616.10
  vas deferens 608.4
  vein (see also Phlebitis) 451.9
    thrombotic 451.9
      cerebral (see also Thrombosis, brain) 434.0●
      leg 451.2
        deep (vessels) NEC 451.19
        superficial (vessels) 451.0
      lower extremity 451.2
        deep (vessels) NEC 451.19
        superficial (vessels) 451.0
  vocal cord 478.5
  vulva (see also Vulvitis) 616.10
Inflation, lung imperfect (newborn) 770.5

Influenza, influenzal 487.1
  with
    bronchitis 487.1
    bronchopneumonia 487.0
    cold (any type) 487.1
    digestive manifestations 487.8
    hemoptysis 487.1
    involvement of
      gastrointestinal tract 487.8
      nervous system 487.8
    laryngitis 487.1
    manifestations NEC 487.8
      respiratory 487.1
        pneumonia 487.0
    pharyngitis 487.1
    pneumonia (any form classifiable to 480-483, 485-486) 487.0
    respiratory manifestations NEC 487.1
    sinusitis 487.1
    sore throat 487.1
    tonsillitis 487.1
    tracheitis 487.1
    upper respiratory infection (acute) 487.1
  A/H5N1 (see also Influenza, avian) 488.02
  abdominal 487.8
  Asian 487.1
  avian 488.02
    with involvement of gastrointestinal tract 488.09
    bronchopneumonia 488.01
    laryngitis 488.02
    manifestations NEC 488.09
      respiratory 488.02
    pharyngitis 488.02
    pneumonia (any form classifiable to 480-483, 485-486) 488.01
    respiratory infection (acute) (upper) 488.02
  bronchial 487.1
  bronchopneumonia 487.0
  catarrhal 487.1
  due to identified
    animal origin influenza virus - see Influenza, due to identified, novel influenza A virus
    avian influenza virus 488.02
      with
        manifestations NEC 488.09
          respiratory 488.02
        pneumonia (any form classifiable to 480-483, 485-486) 488.01
    (novel) 2009 H1N1 influenza virus 488.12
      with
        manifestations NEC 488.19
          respiratory 488.12
        pneumonia 488.11
    novel influenza A virus 488.82
      with
        encephalopathy 488.89
        involvement of gastrointestinal tract 488.89
        laryngitis 488.82
        manifestations NEC 488.89
          respiratory (acute) (upper) 488.82
        pharyngitis 488.82
        pneumonia 488.81
  epidemic 487.1
  gastric 487.8
  intestinal 487.8
  laryngitis 487.1
  maternal affecting fetus or newborn 760.2
    manifest influenza in infant 771.2
  (novel) 2009 H1N1 488.12
    with involvement of gastrointestinal tract 488.19
    bronchopneumonia 488.11
    laryngitis 488.12
    manifestations NEC 488.19
      respiratory 488.12
    pharyngitis 488.12

Influenza, influenzal (Continued)
  (novel) 2009 H1N1 (Continued)
    pneumonia (any form classifiable to 480-483, 485-486) 488.11
    respiratory infection (acute) (upper) 488.12
  novel A/H1N1 (see also Influenza, (novel) 2009 H1N1) 488.12
  novel influenza A viruses not previously found in humans - see Influenza, due to identified, novel influenza A virus
  pharyngitis 487.1
  pneumonia (any form) 487.0
  respiratory (upper) 487.1
  specified NEC 487.1
  stomach 487.8
  vaccination, prophylactic (against) V04.81
Influenza-like disease (see also Influenza) 487.1
Infraction, Freiberg's (metatarsal head) 732.5
Infraeruption, teeth 524.34
Infusion complication, misadventure, or reaction - see Complication, infusion
Ingestion
  chemical - see Table of Drugs and Chemicals
  drug or medicinal substance
    overdose or wrong substance given or taken 977.9
      specified drug - see Table of Drugs and Chemicals
  foreign body NEC (see also Foreign body) 938
Ingrowing
  hair 704.8
  nail (finger) (toe) (infected) 703.0
Inguinal - see also condition
  testis 752.51
Inhalation
  carbon monoxide 986
  flame
    mouth 947.0
    lung 947.1
  food or foreign body (see also Asphyxia, food or foreign body) 933.1
  gas, fumes, or vapor (noxious) 987.9
    specified agent - see Table of Drugs and Chemicals
  liquid or vomitus (see also Asphyxia, food or foreign body) 933.1
    lower respiratory tract NEC 934.9
  meconium (fetus or newborn) 770.11
    with respiratory symptoms 770.12
  mucus (see also Asphyxia, mucus) 933.1
  oil (causing suffocation) (see also Asphyxia, food or foreign body) 933.1
  pneumonia - see Pneumonia, aspiration
  smoke 508.2
  steam 987.9
  stomach contents or secretions (see also Asphyxia, food or foreign body) 933.1
    in labor and delivery 668.0●
Inhibition, inhibited
  academic as adjustment reaction 309.23
  orgasm
    female 302.73
    male 302.74
  sexual
    desire 302.71
    excitement 302.72
  work as adjustment reaction 309.23
Inhibitor
  autoimmune, to clotting factors 286.52
  systemic lupus erythematosus (presence of) 795.79
    with
      hemorrhagic disorder 286.53
      hypercoagulable state 289.81
Iniencephalus, iniencephaly 740.2
Injected eye 372.74

SECTION 1 INDEX TO DISEASES AND INJURIES / Injury

Injury 959.9

> Note: For abrasion, insect bite (nonvenomous), blister, or scratch, see Injury, superficial.
>
> For laceration, traumatic rupture, tear, or penetrating wound of internal organs, such as heart, lung, liver, kidney, pelvic organs, whether or not accompanied by open wound in the same region, see Injury, internal.
>
> For nerve injury, see Injury, nerve.
>
> For late effect of injuries classifiable to 850–854, 860–869, 900–919, 950–959, see Late, effect, injury, by type.

abdomen, abdominal (viscera) - see also Injury, internal, abdomen
  muscle or wall 959.12
acoustic, resulting in deafness 951.5
adenoid 959.09
adrenal (gland) - see Injury, internal, adrenal
alveolar (process) 959.09
ankle (and foot) (and knee) (and leg, except thigh) 959.7
anterior chamber, eye 921.3
anus 959.19
aorta (thoracic) 901.0
  abdominal 902.0
appendix - see Injury, internal, appendix
arm, upper (and shoulder) 959.2
artery (complicating trauma) (see also Injury, blood vessel, by site) 904.9
  cerebral or meningeal (see also Hemorrhage, brain, traumatic, subarachnoid) 852.0●
auditory canal (external) (meatus) 959.09
auricle, auris, ear 959.09
axilla 959.2
back 959.19
bile duct - see Injury, internal, bile duct
birth - see also Birth, injury
  canal NEC, complicating delivery 665.9●
bladder (sphincter) - see Injury, internal, bladder
blast (air) (hydraulic) (immersion) (underwater) NEC 869.0
  with open wound into cavity NEC 869.1
  abdomen or thorax - see Injury, internal, by site
  brain - see Concussion, brain
  ear (acoustic nerve trauma) 951.5
    with perforation of tympanic membrane - see Wound, open, ear, drum
blood vessel NEC 904.9
  abdomen 902.9
    multiple 902.87
    specified NEC 902.89
  aorta (thoracic) 901.0
    abdominal 902.0
  arm NEC 903.9
  axillary 903.00
    artery 903.1
    vein 903.02
  azygos vein 901.89
  basilic vein 903.1
  brachial (artery) (vein) 903.1
  bronchial 901.89
  carotid artery 900.00
    common 900.01
    external 900.02
    internal 900.03
  celiac artery 902.20
    specified branch NEC 902.24
  cephalic vein (arm) 903.1
  colica dextra 902.26
  cystic
    artery 902.24
    vein 902.39

Injury (Continued)
  blood vessel NEC (Continued)
    deep plantar 904.6
    digital (artery) (vein) 903.5
    due to accidental puncture or laceration during procedure 998.2
    extremity
      lower 904.8
        multiple 904.7
        specified NEC 904.7
      upper 903.9
        multiple 903.8
        specified NEC 903.8
    femoral
      artery (superficial) 904.1
        above profunda origin 904.0
        common 904.0
      vein 904.2
    gastric
      artery 902.21
      vein 902.39
    head 900.9
      intracranial - see Injury, intracranial
      multiple 900.82
      specified NEC 900.89
    hemiazygos vein 901.89
    hepatic
      artery 902.22
      vein 902.11
    hypogastric 902.59
      artery 902.51
      vein 902.52
    ileocolic
      artery 902.26
      vein 902.31
    iliac 902.50
      artery 902.53
      specified branch NEC 902.59
      vein 902.54
    innominate
      artery 901.1
      vein 901.3
    intercostal (artery) (vein) 901.81
    jugular vein (external) 900.81
      internal 900.1
    leg NEC 904.8
    mammary (artery) (vein) 901.82
    mesenteric
      artery 902.20
        inferior 902.27
        specified branch NEC 902.29
        superior (trunk) 902.25
          branches, primary 902.26
      vein 902.39
        inferior 902.32
        superior (and primary subdivisions) 902.31
    neck 900.9
      multiple 900.82
      specified NEC 900.89
    ovarian 902.89
      artery 902.81
      vein 902.82
    palmar artery 903.4
    pelvis 902.9
      multiple 902.87
      specified NEC 902.89
    plantar (deep) (artery) (vein) 904.6
    popliteal 904.40
      artery 904.41
      vein 904.42
    portal 902.33
    pulmonary 901.40
      artery 901.41
      vein 901.42
    radial (artery) (vein) 903.2
    renal 902.40
      artery 902.41
      specified NEC 902.49
      vein 902.42

Injury (Continued)
  blood vessel NEC (Continued)
    saphenous
      artery 904.7
      vein (greater) (lesser) 904.3
    splenic
      artery 902.23
      vein 902.34
    subclavian
      artery 901.1
      vein 901.3
    suprarenal 902.49
    thoracic 901.9
      multiple 901.83
      specified NEC 901.89
    tibial 904.50
      artery 904.50
        anterior 904.51
        posterior 904.53
      vein 904.50
        anterior 904.52
        posterior 904.54
    ulnar (artery) (vein) 903.3
    uterine 902.59
      artery 902.55
      vein 902.56
    vena cava
      inferior 902.10
        specified branches NEC 902.19
      superior 901.2
  brachial plexus 953.4
    newborn 767.6
  brain (traumatic) NEC (see also Injury, intracranial) 854.0●
    due to fracture of skull - see Fracture, skull, by site
  breast 959.19
  broad ligament - see Injury, internal, broad ligament
  bronchus, bronchi - see Injury, internal, bronchus
  brow 959.09
  buttock 959.19
  canthus, eye 921.1
  cathode ray 990
  cauda equina 952.4
    with fracture, vertebra - see Fracture, vertebra, sacrum
  cavernous sinus (see also Injury, intracranial) 854.0●
  cecum - see Injury, internal, cecum
  celiac ganglion or plexus 954.1
  cerebellum (see also Injury, intracranial) 854.0●
  cervix (uteri) - see Injury, internal, cervix
  cheek 959.09
  chest - see Injury, internal, chest
    wall 959.11
  childbirth - see also Birth, injury
    maternal NEC 665.9●
  chin 959.09
  choroid (eye) 921.3
  clitoris 959.14
  coccyx 959.19
    complicating delivery 665.6●
  colon - see Injury, internal, colon
  common duct - see Injury, internal, common duct
  conjunctiva 921.1
    superficial 918.2
  cord
    spermatic - see Injury, internal, spermatic cord
    spinal - see Injury, spinal, by site
  cornea 921.3
    abrasion 918.1
      due to contact lens 371.82
    penetrating - see Injury, eyeball, penetrating
    superficial 918.1
      due to contact lens 371.82

SECTION I INDEX TO DISEASES AND INJURIES / Injury

Injury (Continued)
- cortex (cerebral) (see also Injury, intracranial) 854.0●
  - visual 950.3
- costal region 959.11
- costochondral 959.11
- cranial
  - bones - see Fracture, skull, by site
  - cavity (see also Injury, intracranial) 854.0●
  - nerve - see Injury, nerve, cranial
- crushing - see Crush
- cutaneous sensory nerve
  - lower limb 956.4
  - upper limb 955.5
- deep tissue - see Contusion, by site
  - meaning pressure ulcer 707.25
- delivery - see also Birth, injury
  - maternal NEC 665.9●
- Descemet's membrane - see Injury, eyeball, penetrating
- diaphragm - see Injury, internal, diaphragm
- diffuse axonal - see Injury, intracranial
- duodenum - see Injury, internal, duodenum
- ear (auricle) (canal) (drum) (external) 959.09
- elbow (and forearm) (and wrist) 959.3
- epididymis 959.14
- epigastric region 959.12
- epiglottis 959.09
- epiphyseal, current - see Fracture, by site
- esophagus - see Injury, internal, esophagus
- Eustachian tube 959.09
- extremity (lower) (upper) NEC 959.8
- eye 921.9
  - penetrating eyeball - see Injury, eyeball, penetrating
  - superficial 918.9
- eyeball 921.3
  - penetrating 871.7
    - with
      - partial loss (of intraocular tissue) 871.2
      - prolapse or exposure (of intraocular tissue) 871.1
      - without prolapse 871.0
      - foreign body (nonmagnetic) 871.6
        - magnetic 871.5
  - superficial 918.9
- eyebrow 959.09
- eyelid(s) 921.1
  - laceration - see Laceration, eyelid
  - superficial 918.0
- face (and neck) 959.09
- fallopian tube - see Injury, internal, fallopian tube
- fingers(s) (nail) 959.5
- flank 959.19
- foot (and ankle) (and knee) (and leg, except thigh) 959.7
- forceps NEC 767.9
  - scalp 767.19
- forearm (and elbow) (and wrist) 959.3
- forehead 959.09
- gallbladder - see Injury, internal, gallbladder
- gasserian ganglion 951.2
- gastrointestinal tract - see Injury, internal, gastrointestinal tract
- genital organ(s)
  - with
    - abortion - see Abortion, by type, with, damage to pelvic organs
    - ectopic pregnancy (see also categories 633.0–633.9) 639.2
    - molar pregnancy (see also categories 630–632) 639.2
  - external 959.14
    - fracture of corpus cavernosum penis 959.13
  - following
    - abortion 639.2
    - ectopic or molar pregnancy 639.2

Injury (Continued)
- genital organ(s) (Continued)
  - internal - see Injury, internal, genital organs
  - obstetrical trauma NEC 665.9●
    - affecting fetus or newborn 763.89
- gland
  - lacrimal 921.1
    - laceration 870.8
  - parathyroid 959.09
  - salivary 959.09
  - thyroid 959.09
- globe (eye) (see also Injury, eyeball) 921.3
- grease gun - see Wound, open, by site, complicated
- groin 959.19
- gum 959.09
- hand(s) (except fingers) 959.4
- head NEC 959.01
  - with
    - loss of consciousness 850.5
    - skull fracture - see Fracture, skull, by site
- heart - see Injury, internal, heart
- heel 959.7
- hip (and thigh) 959.6
- hymen 959.14
- hyperextension (cervical) (vertebra) 847.0
- ileum - see Injury, internal, ileum
- iliac region 959.19
- infrared rays NEC 990
- instrumental (during surgery) 998.2
  - birth injury - see Birth, injury
  - nonsurgical (see also Injury, by site) 959.9
  - obstetrical 665.9●
    - affecting fetus or newborn 763.89
    - bladder 665.5●
    - cervix 665.3●
    - high vaginal 665.4●
    - perineal NEC 664.9●
    - urethra 665.5●
    - uterus 665.5●
- internal 869.0

> Note: For injury of internal organ(s) by foreign body entering through a natural orifice (e.g., inhaled, ingested, or swallowed)-see Foreign body, entering through orifice.
>
> For internal injury of any of the following sites with internal injury of any other of the sites-see Injury, internal, multiple.

- with
  - fracture
    - pelvis - see Fracture, pelvis
    - specified site, except pelvis - see Injury, internal, by site
  - open wound into cavity 869.1
  - abdomen, abdominal (viscera) NEC 868.00
    - with
      - fracture, pelvis - see Fracture, pelvis
      - open wound into cavity 868.10
    - specified site NEC 868.09
      - with open wound into cavity 868.19
  - adrenal (gland) 868.01
    - with open wound into cavity 868.11
  - aorta (thoracic) 901.0
    - abdominal 902.0
  - appendix 863.85
    - with open wound into cavity 863.95
  - bile duct 868.02
    - with open wound into cavity 868.12
  - bladder (sphincter) 867.0
    - with
      - abortion - see Abortion, by type, with, damage to pelvic organs
      - ectopic pregnancy (see also categories 633.0–633.9) 639.2

Injury (Continued)
- internal (Continued)
  - bladder (Continued)
    - with (Continued)
      - molar pregnancy (see also categories 630–632) 639.2
      - open wound into cavity 867.1
    - following
      - abortion 639.2
      - ectopic or molar pregnancy 639.2
    - obstetrical trauma 665.5●
      - affecting fetus or newborn 763.89
  - blood vessel - see Injury, blood vessel, by site
  - broad ligament 867.6
    - with open wound into cavity 867.7
  - bronchus, bronchi 862.21
    - with open wound into cavity 862.31
  - cecum 863.89
    - with open wound into cavity 863.99
  - cervix (uteri) 867.4
    - with
      - abortion - see Abortion, by type, with damage to pelvic organs
      - ectopic pregnancy (see also categories 633.0–633.9) 639.2
      - molar pregnancy (see also categories 630–632) 639.2
      - open wound into cavity 867.5
    - following
      - abortion 639.2
      - ectopic or molar pregnancy 639.2
    - obstetrical trauma 665.3●
      - affecting fetus or newborn 763.89
  - chest (see also Injury, internal, intrathoracic organs) 862.8
    - with open wound into cavity 862.9
  - colon 863.40
    - with
      - open wound into cavity 863.50
      - rectum 863.46
        - with open wound into cavity 863.56
    - ascending (right) 863.41
      - with open wound into cavity 863.51
    - descending (left) 863.43
      - with open wound into cavity 863.53
    - multiple sites 863.46
      - with open wound into cavity 863.56
    - sigmoid 863.44
      - with open wound into cavity 863.54
    - specified site NEC 863.49
      - with open wound into cavity 863.59
    - transverse 863.42
      - with open wound into cavity 863.52
  - common duct 868.02
    - with open wound into cavity 868.12
  - complicating delivery 665.9●
    - affecting fetus or newborn 763.89
  - diaphragm 862.0
    - with open wound into cavity 862.1
  - duodenum 863.21
    - with open wound into cavity 863.31
  - esophagus (intrathoracic) 862.22
    - with open wound into cavity 862.32
    - cervical region 874.4
      - complicated 874.5
  - fallopian tube 867.6
    - with open wound into cavity 867.7
  - gallbladder 868.02
    - with open wound into cavity 868.12
  - gastrointestinal tract NEC 863.80
    - with open wound into cavity 863.90
  - genital organ NEC 867.6
    - with open wound into cavity 867.7
  - heart 861.00
    - with open wound into thorax 861.10
  - ileum 863.29
    - with open wound into cavity 863.39

Injury (Continued)
  internal (Continued)
    intestine NEC 863.89
      with open wound into cavity 863.99
      large NEC 863.40
        with open wound into cavity 863.50
      small NEC 863.20
        with open wound into cavity 863.30
    intra-abdominal (organ) 868.00
      with open wound into cavity 868.10
      multiple sites 868.09
        with open wound into cavity 868.19
      specified site NEC 868.09
        with open wound into cavity 868.19
    intrathoracic organs (multiple) 862.8
      with open wound into cavity 862.9
      diaphragm (only) - see Injury, internal, diaphragm
      heart (only) - see Injury, internal, heart
      lung (only) - see Injury, internal, lung
      specified site NEC 862.29
        with open wound into cavity 862.39
    intrauterine (see also Injury, internal, uterus) 867.4
      with open wound into cavity 867.5
    jejunum 863.29
      with open wound into cavity 863.39
    kidney (subcapsular) 866.00
      with
        disruption of parenchyma (complete) 866.03
          with open wound into cavity 866.13
        hematoma (without rupture of capsule) 866.01
          with open wound into cavity 866.11
        laceration 866.02
          with open wound into cavity 866.12
        open wound into cavity 866.10
    liver 864.00
      with
        contusion 864.01
          with open wound into cavity 864.11
        hematoma 864.01
          with open wound into cavity 864.11
        laceration 864.05
          with open wound into cavity 864.15
          major (disruption of hepatic parenchyma) 864.04
            with open wound into cavity 864.14
          minor (capsule only) 864.02
            with open wound into cavity 864.12
          moderate (involving parenchyma) 864.03
            with open wound into cavity 864.13
          multiple 864.04
          stellate 864.04
            with open wound into cavity 864.14
        open wound into cavity 864.10
    lung 861.20
      with open wound into thorax 861.30
      aspiration 507.0
      hemopneumothorax - see Hemopneumothorax, traumatic
      hemothorax - see Hemothorax, traumatic
      pneumohemothorax - see Pneumohemothorax, traumatic
      pneumothorax - see Pneumothorax, traumatic
      transfusion related, acute (TRALI) 518.7
    mediastinum 862.29
      with open wound into cavity 862.39
    mesentery 863.89
      with open wound into cavity 863.99
    mesosalpinx 867.6
      with open wound into cavity 867.7
    multiple 869.0

> Note: Multiple internal injuries of sites classifiable to the same three- or four-digit category should be classified to that category.
>
> Multiple injuries classifiable to different fourth-digit subdivisions of 861.-(heart and lung injuries) should be dealt with according to coding rules.

      internal 869.0
        with open wound into cavity 869.1
      intra-abdominal organ (sites classifiable to 863–868)
        with
          intrathoracic organ(s) (sites classifiable to 861–862) 869.0
            with open wound into cavity 869.1
          other intra-abdominal organ(s) (sites classifiable to 863–868, except where classifiable to the same three-digit category) 868.09
            with open wound into cavity 868.19
      intrathoracic organ (sites classifiable to 861–862)
        with
          intra-abdominal organ(s) (sites classifiable to 863–868) 869.0
            with open wound into cavity 869.1
          other intrathoracic organs(s) (sites classifiable to 861–862, except where classifiable to the same three-digit category) 862.8
            with open wound into cavity 862.9
    myocardium - see Injury, internal, heart
    ovary 867.6
      with open wound into cavity 867.7
    pancreas (multiple sites) 863.84
      with open wound into cavity 863.94
      body 863.82
        with open wound into cavity 863.92
      head 863.81
        with open wound into cavity 863.91
      tail 863.83
        with open wound into cavity 863.93
    pelvis, pelvic (organs) (viscera) 867.8
      with
        fracture, pelvis - see Fracture, pelvis
        open wound into cavity 867.9
      specified site NEC 867.6
        with open wound into cavity 867.7
    peritoneum 868.03
      with open wound into cavity 868.13
    pleura 862.29
      with open wound into cavity 862.39
    prostate 867.6
      with open wound into cavity 867.7
    rectum 863.45
      with
        colon 863.46
          with open wound into cavity 863.56
        open wound into cavity 863.55
    retroperitoneum 868.04
      with open wound into cavity 868.14
    round ligament 867.6
      with open wound into cavity 867.7
    seminal vesicle 867.6
      with open wound into cavity 867.7
    spermatic cord 867.6
      with open wound into cavity 867.7
      scrotal - see Wound, open, spermatic cord
    spleen 865.00
      with
        disruption of parenchyma (massive) 865.04
          with open wound into cavity 865.14
        hematoma (without rupture of capsule) 865.01
          with open wound into cavity 865.11
        open wound into cavity 865.10
        tear, capsular 865.02
          with open wound into cavity 865.12
          extending into parenchyma 865.03
            with open wound into cavity 865.13
    stomach 863.0
      with open wound into cavity 863.1
    suprarenal gland (multiple) 868.01
      with open wound into cavity 868.11
    thorax, thoracic (cavity) (organs) (multiple) (see also Injury, internal, intrathoracic organs) 862.8
      with open wound into cavity 862.9
    thymus (gland) 862.29
      with open wound into cavity 862.39
    trachea (intrathoracic) 862.29
      with open wound into cavity 862.39
      cervical region (see also Wound, open, trachea) 874.02
    ureter 867.2
      with open wound into cavity 867.3
    urethra (sphincter) 867.0
      with
        abortion - see Abortion, by type, with, damage to pelvic organs
        ectopic pregnancy (see also categories 633.0–633.9) 639.2
        molar pregnancy (see also categories 630–632) 639.2
        open wound into cavity 867.1
      following
        abortion 639.2
        ectopic or molar pregnancy 639.2
      obstetrical trauma 665.5●
        affecting fetus or newborn 763.89
    uterus 867.4
      with
        abortion - see Abortion, by type, with, damage to pelvic organs
        ectopic pregnancy (see also categories 633.0–633.9) 639.2
        molar pregnancy (see also categories 630–632) 639.2
        open wound into cavity 867.5
      following
        abortion 639.2
        ectopic or molar pregnancy 639.2
      obstetrical trauma NEC 665.5●
        affecting fetus or newborn 763.89
    vas deferens 867.6
      with open wound into cavity 867.7
    vesical (sphincter) 867.0
      with open wound into cavity 867.1

SECTION I INDEX TO DISEASES AND INJURIES / Injury

Injury (Continued)
- internal (Continued)
  - viscera (abdominal) (see also Injury, internal, multiple) 868.00
    - with
      - fracture, pelvis - see Fracture, pelvis
      - open wound into cavity 868.10
    - thoracic NEC (see also Injury, internal, intrathoracic organs) 862.8
      - with open wound into cavity 862.9
- interscapular region 959.19
- intervertebral disc 959.19
- intestine - see Injury, internal, intestine
- intra-abdominal (organs) NEC - see Injury, internal, intra-abdominal
- intracranial (traumatic) 854.0●

> Note: Use the following fifth-digit subclassification with categories 851–854:
> 0 unspecified state of consciousness
> 1 with no loss of consciousness
> 2 with brief [less than one hour] loss of consciousness
> 3 with moderate [1–24 hours] loss of consciousness
> 4 with prolonged [more than 24 hours] loss of consciousness and return to pre-existing conscious level
> 5 with prolonged [more than 24 hours] loss of consciousness, without return to pre-existing conscious level
>
> Use fifth-digit 5 to designate when a patient is unconscious and dies before regaining consciousness, regardless of the duration of the loss of consciousness
>
> 6 with loss of consciousness of unspecified duration
> 9 with concussion, unspecified

- with
  - open intracranial wound 854.1●
  - skull fracture - see Fracture, skull, by site
- contusion 851.8●
  - with open intracranial wound 851.9●
  - brain stem 851.4●
    - with open intracranial wound 851.5●
  - cerebellum 851.4●
    - with open intracranial wound 851.5●
  - cortex (cerebral) 851.0●
    - with open intracranial wound 851.2●
- hematoma - see Injury, intracranial, hemorrhage
- hemorrhage 853.0●
  - with
    - laceration - see Injury, intracranial, laceration
    - open intracranial wound 853.1●
  - extradural 852.4●
    - with open intracranial wound 852.5●
  - subarachnoid 852.0●
    - with open intracranial wound 852.1●
  - subdural 852.2●
    - with open intracranial wound 852.3●
- laceration 851.8●
  - with open intracranial wound 851.9●
  - brain stem 851.6●
    - with open intracranial wound 851.7●

Injury (Continued)
- intracranial (Continued)
  - contusion (Continued)
    - laceration (Continued)
      - cerebellum 851.6●
        - with open intracranial wound 851.7●
      - cortex (cerebral) 851.2●
        - with open intracranial wound 851.3●
- intraocular - see Injury, eyeball, penetrating
- intrathoracic organs (multiple) - see Injury, internal, intrathoracic organs
- intrauterine - see Injury, internal, intrauterine
- iris 921.3
  - penetrating - see Injury, eyeball, penetrating
- jaw 959.09
- jejunum - see Injury, internal, jejunum
- joint NEC 959.9
  - old or residual 718.80
    - ankle 718.87
    - elbow 718.82
    - foot 718.87
    - hand 718.84
    - hip 718.85
    - knee 718.86
    - multiple sites 718.89
    - pelvic region 718.85
    - shoulder (region) 718.81
    - specified site NEC 718.88
    - wrist 718.83
- kidney - see Injury, internal, kidney
  - acute (nontraumatic) 584.9
- knee (and ankle) (and foot) (and leg, except thigh) 959.7
- labium (majus) (minus) 959.14
- labyrinth, ear 959.09
- lacrimal apparatus, gland, or sac 921.1
  - laceration 870.8
- larynx 959.09
- late effect - see Late, effects (of), injury
- leg, except thigh (and ankle) (and foot) (and knee) 959.7
  - upper or thigh 959.6
- lens, eye 921.3
  - penetrating - see Injury, eyeball, penetrating
- lid, eye - see Injury, eyelid
- lip 959.09
- liver - see Injury, internal, liver
- lobe, parietal - see Injury, intracranial
- lumbar (region) 959.19
  - plexus 953.5
- lumbosacral (region) 959.19
  - plexus 953.5
- lung - see Injury, internal, lung
- malar region 959.09
- mastoid region 959.09
- maternal, during pregnancy, affecting fetus or newborn 760.5
- maxilla 959.09
- mediastinum - see Injury, internal, mediastinum
- membrane
  - brain (see also Injury, intracranial) 854.0●
  - tympanic 959.09
- meningeal artery - see Hemorrhage, brain, traumatic, subarachnoid
- meninges (cerebral) - see Injury, intracranial
- mesenteric
  - artery - see Injury, blood vessel, mesenteric, artery
  - plexus, inferior 954.1
  - vein - see Injury, blood vessel, mesenteric, vein
- mesentery - see Injury, internal, mesentery
- mesosalpinx - see Injury, internal, mesosalpinx
- middle ear 959.09
- midthoracic region 959.11

Injury (Continued)
- mouth 959.09
- multiple (sites not classifiable to the same four-digit category in 959.0–959.7) 959.8
  - internal 869.0
    - with open wound into cavity 869.1
- musculocutaneous nerve 955.4
- nail
  - finger 959.5
  - toe 959.7
- nasal (septum) (sinus) 959.09
- nasopharynx 959.09
- neck (and face) 959.09
- nerve 957.9
  - abducens 951.3
  - abducent 951.3
  - accessory 951.6
  - acoustic 951.5
  - ankle and foot 956.9
  - anterior crural, femoral 956.1
  - arm (see also Injury, nerve, upper limb) 955.9
  - auditory 951.5
  - axillary 955.0
  - brachial plexus 953.4
  - cervical sympathetic 954.0
  - cranial 951.9
    - first or olfactory 951.8
    - second or optic 950.0
    - third or oculomotor 951.0
    - fourth or trochlear 951.1
    - fifth or trigeminal 951.2
    - sixth or abducens 951.3
    - seventh or facial 951.4
    - eighth, acoustic, or auditory 951.5
    - ninth or glossopharyngeal 951.8
    - tenth, pneumogastric, or vagus 951.8
    - eleventh or accessory 951.6
    - twelfth or hypoglossal 951.7
    - newborn 767.7
  - cutaneous sensory
    - lower limb 956.4
    - upper limb 955.5
  - digital (finger) 955.6
    - toe 956.5
  - facial 951.4
    - newborn 767.5
  - femoral 956.1
  - finger 955.9
  - foot and ankle 956.9
  - forearm 955.9
  - glossopharyngeal 951.8
  - hand and wrist 955.9
  - head and neck, superficial 957.0
  - hypoglossal 951.7
  - involving several parts of body 957.8
  - leg (see also Injury, nerve, lower limb) 956.9
  - lower limb 956.9
    - multiple 956.8
    - specified site NEC 956.5
  - lumbar plexus 953.5
  - lumbosacral plexus 953.5
  - median 955.1
    - forearm 955.1
    - wrist and hand 955.1
  - multiple (in several parts of body) (sites not classifiable to the same three-digit category) 957.8
  - musculocutaneous 955.4
  - musculospiral 955.3
    - upper arm 955.3
  - oculomotor 951.0
  - olfactory 951.8
  - optic 950.0
  - pelvic girdle 956.9
    - multiple sites 956.8
    - specified site NEC 956.5

Injury (Continued)
- nerve (Continued)
  - peripheral 957.9
    - multiple (in several regions) (sites not classifiable to the same three-digit category) 957.8
    - specified site NEC 957.1
  - peroneal 956.3
    - ankle and foot 956.3
    - lower leg 956.3
  - plantar 956.5
  - plexus 957.9
    - celiac 954.1
    - mesenteric, inferior 954.1
    - spinal 953.9
      - brachial 953.4
      - lumbosacral 953.5
      - multiple sites 953.8
    - sympathetic NEC 954.1
  - pneumogastric 951.8
  - radial 955.3
    - wrist and hand 955.3
  - sacral plexus 953.5
  - sciatic 956.0
    - thigh 956.0
  - shoulder girdle 955.9
    - multiple 955.8
    - specified site NEC 955.7
  - specified site NEC 957.1
  - spinal 953.9
    - plexus - see Injury, nerve, plexus, spinal
    - root 953.9
      - cervical 953.0
      - dorsal 953.1
      - lumbar 953.2
      - multiple sites 953.8
      - sacral 953.3
  - splanchnic 954.1
  - sympathetic NEC 954.1
    - cervical 954.0
  - thigh 956.9
  - tibial 956.5
    - ankle and foot 956.2
    - lower leg 956.5
    - posterior 956.2
  - toe 956.9
  - trigeminal 951.2
  - trochlear 951.1
  - trunk, excluding shoulder and pelvic girdles 954.9
    - specified site NEC 954.8
    - sympathetic NEC 954.1
  - ulnar 955.2
    - forearm 955.2
    - wrist (and hand) 955.2
  - upper limb 955.9
    - multiple 955.8
    - specified site NEC 955.7
  - vagus 951.8
  - wrist and hand 955.9
- nervous system, diffuse 957.8
- nose (septum) 959.09
- obstetrical NEC 665.9●
  - affecting fetus or newborn 763.89
- occipital (region) (scalp) 959.09
  - lobe (see also Injury, intracranial) 854.0●
- optic 950.9
  - chiasm 950.1
  - cortex 950.3
  - nerve 950.0
  - pathways 950.2
- orbit, orbital (region) 921.2
  - penetrating 870.3
    - with foreign body 870.4
- ovary - see Injury, internal, ovary
- paint-gun - see Wound, open, by site, complicated
- palate (soft) 959.09
- pancreas - see Injury, internal, pancreas
- parathyroid (gland) 959.09

Injury (Continued)
- parietal (region) (scalp) 959.09
  - lobe - see Injury, intracranial
- pelvic
  - floor 959.19
    - complicating delivery 664.1●
      - affecting fetus or newborn 763.89
  - joint or ligament, complicating delivery 665.6●
    - affecting fetus or newborn 763.89
  - organs - see also Injury, internal, pelvis
    - with
      - abortion - see Abortion, by type, with damage to pelvic organs
      - ectopic pregnancy (see also categories 633.0–633.9) 639.2
      - molar pregnancy (see also categories 633.0–633.9) 639.2
    - following
      - abortion 639.2
      - ectopic or molar pregnancy 639.2
    - obstetrical trauma 665.5●
      - affecting fetus or newborn 763.89
- pelvis 959.19
- penis 959.14
  - fracture of corpus cavernosum 959.13
- perineum 959.14
- peritoneum - see Injury, internal, peritoneum
- periurethral tissue
  - with
    - abortion - see Abortion, by type, with damage to pelvic organs
    - ectopic pregnancy (see also categories 633.0–633.9) 639.2
    - molar pregnancy (see also categories 630–632) 639.2
  - complicating delivery 664.8●
    - affecting fetus or newborn 763.89
  - following
    - abortion 639.2
    - ectopic or molar pregnancy 639.2
- phalanges
  - foot 959.7
  - hand 959.5
- pharynx 959.09
- pleura - see Injury, internal, pleura
- popliteal space 959.7
- post-cardiac surgery (syndrome) 429.4
- prepuce 959.14
- prostate - see Injury, internal, prostate
- pubic region 959.19
- pudenda 959.14
- radiation NEC 990
- radioactive substance or radium NEC 990
- rectovaginal septum 959.14
- rectum - see Injury, internal, rectum
- retina 921.3
  - penetrating - see Injury, eyeball, penetrating
- retroperitoneal - see Injury, internal, retroperitoneum
- roentgen rays NEC 990
- round ligament - see Injury, internal, round ligament
- sacral (region) 959.19
  - plexus 953.5
- sacroiliac ligament NEC 959.19
- sacrum 959.19
- salivary ducts or glands 959.09
- scalp 959.09
  - due to birth trauma 767.19
  - fetus or newborn 767.19
- scapular region 959.2
- sclera 921.3
  - penetrating - see Injury, eyeball, penetrating
  - superficial 918.2
- scrotum 959.14
- seminal vesicle - see Injury, internal, seminal vesicle
- shoulder (and upper arm) 959.2

Injury (Continued)
- sinus
  - cavernous (see also Injury, intracranial) 854.0●
  - nasal 959.09
- skeleton NEC, birth injury 767.3
- skin NEC 959.9
- skull - see Fracture, skull, by site
- soft tissue (of external sites) (severe) - see Wound, open, by site
- specified site NEC 959.8
- spermatic cord - see Injury, internal, spermatic cord
- spinal (cord) 952.9
  - with fracture, vertebra - see Fracture, vertebra, by site, with spinal cord injury
  - cervical (C_1–C_4) 952.00
    - with
      - anterior cord syndrome 952.02
      - central cord syndrome 952.03
      - complete lesion of cord 952.01
      - incomplete lesion NEC 952.04
      - posterior cord syndrome 952.04
    - C_5–C_7 level 952.05
      - with
        - anterior cord syndrome 952.07
        - central cord syndrome 952.08
        - complete lesion of cord 952.06
        - incomplete lesion NEC 952.09
        - posterior cord syndrome 952.09
      - specified type NEC 952.09
    - specified type NEC 952.04
  - dorsal (D_1–D_6) (T_1–T_6) (thoracic) 952.10
    - with
      - anterior cord syndrome 952.12
      - central cord syndrome 952.13
      - complete lesion of cord 952.11
      - incomplete lesion NEC 952.14
      - posterior cord syndrome 952.14
    - D_7–D_{12} level (T_7–T_{12}) 952.15
      - with
        - anterior cord syndrome 952.17
        - central cord syndrome 952.18
        - complete lesion of cord 952.16
        - incomplete lesion NEC 952.19
        - posterior cord syndrome 952.19
      - specified type NEC 952.19
    - specified type NEC 952.14
  - lumbar 952.2
  - multiple sites 952.8
  - nerve (root) NEC - see Injury, nerve, spinal, root
  - plexus 953.9
    - brachial 953.4
    - lumbosacral 953.5
    - multiple sites 953.8
  - sacral 952.3
  - thoracic (see also Injury, spinal, dorsal) 952.10
- spleen - see Injury, internal, spleen
- stellate ganglion 954.1
- sternal region 959.11
- stomach - see Injury, internal, stomach
- subconjunctival 921.1
- subcutaneous 959.9
- subdural - see Injury, intracranial
- submaxillary region 959.09
- submental region 959.09
- subungual
  - fingers 959.5
  - toes 959.7

SECTION I INDEX TO DISEASES AND INJURIES / Injury

Injury (Continued)
  superficial 919

> Note: Use the following fourth-digit subdivisions with categories 910–919:
>
> .0 abrasion or friction burn without mention of infection
> .1 abrasion or friction burn, infected
> .2 blister without mention of infection
> .3 blister, infected
> .4 insect bite, nonvenomous, without mention of infection
> .5 insect bite, nonvenomous, infected
> .6 superficial foreign body (splinter) without major open wound and without mention of infection
> .7 superficial foreign body (splinter) without major open wound, infected
> .8 other and unspecified superficial injury without mention of infection
> .9 other and unspecified superficial injury, infected
>
> For late effects of superficial injury, see category 906.2.

    abdomen, abdominal (muscle) (wall) (and other part(s) of trunk) 911
    ankle (and hip, knee, leg, or thigh) 916
    anus (and other part(s) of trunk) 911
    arm 913
      upper (and shoulder) 912
    auditory canal (external) (meatus) (and other part(s) of face, neck, or scalp, except eye) 910
    axilla (and upper arm) 912
    back (and other part(s) of trunk) 911
    breast (and other part(s) of trunk) 911
    brow (and other part(s) of face, neck, or scalp, except eye) 910
    buttock (and other part(s) of trunk) 911
    canthus, eye 918.0
    cheek(s) (and other part(s) of face, neck, or scalp, except eye) 910
    chest wall (and other part(s) of trunk) 911
    chin (and other part(s) of face, neck, or scalp, except eye) 910
    clitoris (and other part(s) of trunk) 911
    conjunctiva 918.2
    cornea 918.1
      due to contact lens 371.82
    costal region (and other part(s) of trunk) 911
    ear(s) (auricle) (canal) (drum) (external) (and other part(s) of face, neck, or scalp, except eye) 910
    elbow (and forearm) (and wrist) 913
    epididymis (and other part(s) of trunk) 911
    epigastric region (and other part(s) of trunk) 911
    epiglottis (and other part(s) of face, neck, or scalp, except eye) 910
    eye(s) (and adnexa) NEC 918.9
    eyelid(s) (and periocular area) 918.0
    face (any part(s), except eye) (and neck or scalp) 910
    finger(s) (nail) (any) 915
    flank (and other part(s) of trunk) 911
    foot (phalanges) (and toe(s)) 917
    forearm (and elbow) (and wrist) 913
    forehead (and other part(s) of face, neck, or scalp, except eye) 910
    globe (eye) 918.9
    groin (and other part(s) of trunk) 911
    gum(s) (and other part(s) of face, neck, or scalp, except eye) 910
    hand(s) (except fingers alone) 914

Injury (Continued)
  superficial (Continued)
    head (and other part(s) of face, neck, or scalp, except eye) 910
    heel (and foot or toe) 917
    hip (and ankle, knee, leg, or thigh) 916
    iliac region (and other part(s) of trunk) 911
    interscapular region (and other part(s) of trunk) 911
    iris 918.9
    knee (and ankle, hip, leg, or thigh) 916
    labium (majus) (minus) (and other part(s) of trunk) 911
    lacrimal (apparatus) (gland) (sac) 918.0
    leg (lower) (upper) (and ankle, hip, knee, or thigh) 916
    lip(s) (and other part(s) of face, neck, or scalp, except eye) 910
    lower extremity (except foot) 916
    lumbar region (and other part(s) of trunk) 911
    malar region (and other part(s) of face, neck, or scalp, except eye) 910
    mastoid region (and other part(s) of face, neck, or scalp, except eye) 910
    midthoracic region (and other part(s) of trunk) 911
    mouth (and other part(s) of face, neck, or scalp, except eye) 910
    multiple sites (not classifiable to the same three-digit category) 919
    nasal (septum) (and other part(s) of face, neck, or scalp, except eye) 910
    neck (and face or scalp, any part(s), except eye) 910
    nose (septum) (and other part(s) of face, neck, or scalp, except eye) 910
    occipital region (and other part(s) of face, neck, or scalp, except eye) 910
    orbital region 918.0
    palate (soft) (and other part(s) of face, neck, or scalp, except eye) 910
    parietal region (and other part(s) of face, neck, or scalp, except eye) 910
    penis (and other part(s) of trunk) 911
    perineum (and other part(s) of trunk) 911
    periocular area 918.0
    pharynx (and other part(s) of face, neck, or scalp, except eye) 910
    popliteal space (and ankle, hip, leg, or thigh) 916
    prepuce (and other part(s) of trunk) 911
    pubic region (and other part(s) of trunk) 911
    pudenda (and other part(s) of trunk) 911
    sacral region (and other part(s) of trunk) 911
    salivary (ducts) (glands) (and other part(s) of face, neck, or scalp, except eye) 910
    scalp (and other part(s) of face or neck, except eye) 910
    scapular region (and upper arm) 912
    sclera 918.2
    scrotum (and other part(s) of trunk) 911
    shoulder (and upper arm) 912
    skin NEC 919
    specified site(s) NEC 919
    sternal region (and other part(s) of trunk) 911
    subconjunctival 918.2
    subcutaneous NEC 919
    submaxillary region (and other part(s) of face, neck, or scalp, except eye) 910
    submental region (and other part(s) of face, neck, or scalp, except eye) 910
    supraclavicular fossa (and other part(s) of face, neck, or scalp, except eye) 910
    supraorbital 918.0

Injury (Continued)
  superficial (Continued)
    temple (and other part(s) of face, neck, or scalp, except eye) 910
    temporal region (and other part(s) of face, neck, or scalp, except eye) 910
    testis (and other part(s) of trunk) 911
    thigh (and ankle, hip, knee, or leg) 916
    thorax, thoracic (external) (and other part(s) of trunk) 911
    throat (and other part(s) of face, neck, or scalp, except eye) 910
    thumb(s) (nail) 915
    toe(s) (nail) (subungual) (and foot) 917
    tongue (and other part(s) of face, neck, or scalp, except eye) 910
    tooth, teeth (see also Abrasion, dental) 521.20
    trunk (any part(s)) 911
    tunica vaginalis (and other part(s) of trunk) 911
    tympanum, tympanic membrane (and other part(s) of face, neck, or scalp, except eye) 910
    upper extremity NEC 913
    uvula (and other part(s) of face, neck, or scalp, except eye) 910
    vagina (and other part(s) of trunk) 911
    vulva (and other part(s) of trunk) 911
    wrist (and elbow) (and forearm) 913
  supraclavicular fossa 959.19
  supraorbital 959.09
  surgical complication (external or internal site) 998.2
  symphysis pubis 959.19
    complicating delivery 665.6●
      affecting fetus or newborn 763.89
  temple 959.09
  temporal region 959.09
  testis 959.14
  thigh (and hip) 959.6
  thorax, thoracic (external) 959.11
    cavity - see Injury, internal, thorax
    internal - see Injury, internal, intrathoracic organs
  throat 959.09
  thumb(s) (nail) 959.5
  thymus - see Injury, internal, thymus
  thyroid (gland) 959.09
  toe (nail) (any) 959.7
  tongue 959.09
  tonsil 959.09
  tooth NEC 873.63
    complicated 873.73
  trachea - see Injury, internal, trachea
  trunk 959.19
  tunica vaginalis 959.14
  tympanum, tympanic membrane 959.09
  ultraviolet rays NEC 990
  ureter - see Injury, internal, ureter
  urethra (sphincter) - see Injury, internal, urethra
  uterus - see Injury, internal, uterus
  uvula 959.09
  vagina 959.14
  vascular - see Injury, blood vessel
  vas deferens - see Injury, internal, vas deferens
  vein (see also Injury, blood vessel, by site) 904.9
  vena cava
    inferior 902.10
    superior 901.2
  vesical (sphincter) - see Injury, internal, vesical
  viscera (abdominal) - see Injury, internal, viscera
    with fracture, pelvis - see Fracture, pelvis
  visual 950.9
    cortex 950.3
  vitreous (humor) 871.2

Injury (Continued)
  vulva 959.14
  whiplash (cervical spine) 847.0
  wringer - *see* Crush, by site
  wrist (and elbow) (and forearm) 959.3
  x-ray NEC 990
Inoculation - *see also* Vaccination
  complication or reaction - *see* Complication, vaccination
INPH (idiopathic normal pressure hydrocephalus) 331.5
Insanity, insane (*see also* Psychosis) 298.9
  adolescent (*see also* Schizophrenia) 295.9●
  alternating (*see also* Psychosis, affective, circular) 296.7
  confusional 298.9
    acute 293.0
    subacute 293.1
  delusional 298.9
  paralysis, general 094.1
    progressive 094.1
  paresis, general 094.1
  senile 290.20
Insect
  bite - *see* Injury, superficial, by site
  venomous, poisoning by 989.5
Insemination, artificial V26.1
Insensitivity
  adrenocorticotropin hormone (ACTH) 255.41
  androgen 259.50
    complete 259.51
    partial 259.52
Insertion
  cord (umbilical) lateral or velamentous 663.8●
    affecting fetus or newborn 762.6
  intrauterine contraceptive device V25.11
  placenta, vicious - *see* Placenta, previa
  subdermal implantable contraceptive V25.5
  velamentous, umbilical cord 663.8●
    affecting fetus or newborn 762.6
Insolation 992.0
  meaning sunstroke 992.0
Insomnia, unspecified 780.52
  with sleep apnea, unspecified 780.51
  adjustment 307.41
  alcohol induced 291.82
  behavioral, of childhood V69.5
  drug induced 292.85
  due to
    medical condition classified elsewhere 327.01
    mental disorder 327.02
  fatal familial (FFI) 046.72
  idiopathic 307.42
  nonorganic origin 307.41
    persistent (primary) 307.42
    transient 307.41
  organic 327.00
    other 327.09
  paradoxical 307.42
  primary 307.42
  psychophysiological 307.42
  subjective complaint 307.49
Inspiration
  food or foreign body (*see also* Asphyxia, food or foreign body) 933.1
  mucus (*see also* Asphyxia, mucus) 933.1
Inspissated bile syndrome, newborn 774.4
Instability
  detrusor 596.59
  emotional (excessive) 301.3
  joint (posttraumatic) 718.80
    ankle 718.87
    elbow 718.82
    foot 718.87
    hand 718.84
    hip 718.85
    knee 718.86
    lumbosacral 724.6
    multiple sites 718.89

Instability (Continued)
  joint (Continued)
    pelvic region 718.85
    sacroiliac 724.6
    shoulder (region) 718.81
    specified site NEC 718.88
    wrist 718.83
  lumbosacral 724.6
  nervous 301.89
  personality (emotional) 301.59
  thyroid, paroxysmal 242.9●
  urethral 599.83
  vasomotor 780.2
Insufficiency, insufficient
  accommodation 367.4
  adrenal (gland) (acute) (chronic) 255.41
    medulla 255.5
    primary 255.41
    specified site NEC 255.5
  adrenocortical 255.41
  anterior (occlusal) guidance 524.54
  anus 569.49
  aortic (valve) 424.1
    with
      mitral (valve) disease 396.1
        insufficiency, incompetence, or regurgitation 396.3
        stenosis or obstruction 396.1
      stenosis or obstruction 424.1
        with mitral (valve) disease 396.8
    congenital 746.4
    rheumatic 395.1
      with
        mitral (valve) disease 396.1
          insufficiency, incompetence, or regurgitation 396.3
          stenosis or obstruction 396.1
        stenosis or obstruction 395.2
          with mitral (valve) disease 396.8
    specified cause NEC 424.1
    syphilitic 093.22
  arterial 447.1
    basilar artery 435.0
    carotid artery 435.8
    cerebral 437.1
    coronary (acute or subacute) 411.89
    mesenteric 557.1
    peripheral 443.9
    precerebral 435.9
    vertebral artery 435.1
    vertebrobasilar 435.3
  arteriovenous 459.9
  basilar artery 435.0
  biliary 575.8
  cardiac (*see also* Insufficiency, myocardial) 428.0
    complicating surgery 997.1
    due to presence of (cardiac) prosthesis 429.4
    postoperative 997.1
      long-term effect of cardiac surgery 429.4
    specified during or due to a procedure 997.1
      long-term effect of cardiac surgery 429.4
  cardiorenal (*see also* Hypertension, cardiorenal) 404.90
  cardiovascular (*see also* Disease, cardiovascular) 429.2
    renal (*see also* Hypertension, cardiorenal) 404.90
  carotid artery 435.8
  cerebral (vascular) 437.9
  cerebrovascular 437.9
    with transient focal neurological signs and symptoms 435.9
    acute 437.1
      with transient focal neurological signs and symptoms 435.9

Insufficiency, insufficient (Continued)
  circulatory NEC 459.9
    fetus or newborn 779.89
  convergence 378.83
  coronary (acute or subacute) 411.89
    chronic or with a stated duration of over 8 weeks 414.8
  corticoadrenal 255.41
  dietary 269.9
  divergence 378.85
  food 994.2
  gastroesophageal 530.89
  gonadal
    ovary 256.39
    testis 257.2
  gonadotropic hormone secretion 253.4
  heart - *see also* Insufficiency, myocardial
    fetus or newborn 779.89
    valve (*see also* Endocarditis) 424.90
      congenital NEC 746.89
  hepatic 573.8
  idiopathic autonomic 333.0
  interocclusal distance of teeth (ridge) 524.36
  kidney
    acute 593.9
    chronic 585.9
  labyrinth, labyrinthine (function) 386.53
    bilateral 386.54
    unilateral 386.53
  lacrimal 375.15
  liver 573.8
  lung (acute) (*see also* Insufficiency, pulmonary) 518.82
    following trauma and surgery 518.52
    newborn 770.89
  mental (congenital) (*see also* Disability, intellectual) 319
  mesenteric 557.1
  mitral (valve) 424.0
    with
      aortic (valve) disease 396.3
        insufficiency, incompetence, or regurgitation 396.3
        stenosis or obstruction 396.2
      obstruction or stenosis 394.2
        with aortic valve disease 396.8
    congenital 746.6
    rheumatic 394.1
      with
        aortic (valve) disease 396.3
          insufficiency, incompetence, or regurgitation 396.3
          stenosis or obstruction 396.2
        obstruction or stenosis 394.2
          with aortic valve disease 396.8
      active or acute 391.1
        with chorea, rheumatic (Sydenham's) 392.0
    specified cause, except rheumatic 424.0
  muscle
    heart - *see* Insufficiency, myocardial
    ocular (*see also* Strabismus) 378.9
  myocardial, myocardium (with arteriosclerosis) 428.0
    with rheumatic fever (conditions classifiable to 390)
      active, acute, or subacute 391.2
        with chorea 392.0
      inactive or quiescent (with chorea) 398.0
    congenital 746.89
    due to presence of (cardiac) prosthesis 429.4
    fetus or newborn 779.89
    following cardiac surgery 429.4
    hypertensive (*see also* Hypertension, heart) 402.91
      benign 402.11
      malignant 402.01

SECTION I INDEX TO DISEASES AND INJURIES / Insufficiency, insufficient

Insufficiency, insufficient *(Continued)*
  myocardial, myocardium *(Continued)*
    postoperative 997.1
      long-term effect of cardiac surgery 429.4
    rheumatic 398.0
      active, acute, or subacute 391.2
        with chorea (Sydenham's) 392.0
    syphilitic 093.82
  nourishment 994.2
  organic 799.89
  ovary 256.39
    postablative 256.2
  pancreatic 577.8
  parathyroid (gland) 252.1
  peripheral vascular (arterial) 443.9
  pituitary (anterior) 253.2
    posterior 253.5
  placental - *see* Placenta, insufficiency
  platelets 287.5
  prenatal care in current pregnancy V23.7
  progressive pluriglandular 258.9
  pseudocholinesterase 289.89
  pulmonary (acute) 518.82
    following
      shock 518.52
      surgery 518.52
      trauma 518.52
    newborn 770.89
    valve (*see also* Endocarditis, pulmonary) 424.3
      congenital 746.09
  pyloric 537.0
  renal 593.9
    acute 593.9
    chronic 585.9
    due to a procedure 997.5
  respiratory 786.09
    acute 518.82
      following trauma and surgery 518.52
    newborn 770.89
  rotation - *see* Malrotation
  suprarenal 255.41
    medulla 255.5
  tarso-orbital fascia, congenital 743.66
  tear film 375.15
  testis 257.2
  thyroid (gland) (acquired) - *see also* Hypothyroidism
    congenital 243
  tricuspid (*see also* Endocarditis, tricuspid) 397.0
    congenital 746.89
    syphilitic 093.23
  urethral sphincter 599.84
  valve, valvular (heart) (*see also* Endocarditis) 424.90
  vascular 459.9
    intestine NEC 557.9
    mesenteric 557.1
    peripheral 443.9
    renal (*see also* Hypertension, kidney) 403.90
  velopharyngeal
    acquired 528.9
    congenital 750.29
  venous (peripheral) 459.81
  ventricular - *see* Insufficiency, myocardial
  vertebral artery 435.1
  vertebrobasilar artery 435.3
  weight gain during pregnancy 646.8 ●
  zinc 269.3
Insufflation
  fallopian
    fertility testing V26.21
    following sterilization reversal V26.22
  meconium 770.11
    with respiratory symptoms 770.12
Insular - *see* condition

Insulinoma (M8151/0)
  malignant (M8151/3)
    pancreas 157.4
    specified site - *see* Neoplasm, by site, malignant
    unspecified site 157.4
  pancreas 211.7
  specified site - *see* Neoplasm, by site, benign
  unspecified site 211.7
Insuloma - *see* Insulinoma
Insult
  brain 437.9
    acute 436
  cerebral 437.9
    acute 436
  cerebrovascular 437.9
    acute 436
  vascular NEC 437.9
    acute 436
Insurance examination (certification) V70.3
Intemperance (*see also* Alcoholism) 303.9 ●
Interception of pregnancy (menstrual extraction) V25.3
Interference
  balancing side 524.56
  non-working side 524.56
Intermenstrual
  bleeding 626.6
    irregular 626.6
    regular 626.5
  hemorrhage 626.6
    irregular 626.6
    regular 626.5
  pain(s) 625.2
Intermittent - *see* condition
Internal - *see* condition
Interproximal wear 521.10
Interrogation
  cardiac defibrillator (automatic) (implantable) V53.32
  cardiac pacemaker V53.31
  cardiac (event) (loop) recorder V53.39
  infusion pump (implanted) (intrathecal) V53.09
  neurostimulator V53.02
Interruption
  aortic arch 747.11
  bundle of His 426.50
  fallopian tube (for sterilization) V25.2
  phase-shift, sleep cycle 307.45
  repeated REM-sleep 307.48
  sleep
    due to perceived environmental disturbances 307.48
    phase-shift, of 24-hour sleep-wake cycle 307.45
    repeated REM-sleep type 307.48
  vas deferens (for sterilization) V25.2
Intersexuality 752.7
Interstitial - *see* condition
Intertrigo 695.89
  labialis 528.5
Intervertebral disc - *see* condition
Intestine, intestinal - *see also* condition
  flu 487.8
Intolerance
  carbohydrate NEC 579.8
  cardiovascular exercise, with pain (at rest) (with less than ordinary activity) (with ordinary activity) V47.2
  cold 780.99
  dissacharide (hereditary) 271.3
  drug
    correct substance properly administered 995.27
    wrong substance given or taken in error 977.9
      specified drug - *see* Table of Drugs and Chemicals
  effort 306.2
  fat NEC 579.8

Intolerance *(Continued)*
  foods NEC 579.8
  fructose (hereditary) 271.2
  glucose (-galactose) (congenital) 271.3
  gluten 579.0
  lactose (hereditary) (infantile) 271.3
  lysine (congenital) 270.7
  milk NEC 579.8
  protein (familial) 270.7
  starch NEC 579.8
  sucrose (-isomaltose) (congenital) 271.3
Intoxicated NEC (*see also* Alcoholism) 305.0 ●
Intoxication
  acid 276.2
  acute
    alcoholic 305.0 ●
      with alcoholism 303.0 ●
      hangover effects 305.0 ●
    caffeine 305.9 ●
    hallucinogenic (*see also* Abuse, drugs, nondependent) 305.3 ●
  alcohol (acute) 305.0 ●
    with alcoholism 303.0 ●
    hangover effects 305.0 ●
    idiosyncratic 291.4
    pathological 291.4
  alimentary canal 558.2
  ammonia (hepatic) 572.2
  caffeine 305.9 ●
  chemical - *see also* Table of Drugs and Chemicals
    via placenta or breast milk 760.70
      alcohol 760.71
      anticonvulsants 760.77
      antifungals 760.74
      anti-infective agents 760.74
      antimetabolics 760.78
      cocaine 760.75
      "crack" 760.75
      hallucinogenic agents NEC 760.73
      medicinal agents NEC 760.79
      narcotics 760.72
      obstetric anesthetic or analgesic drug 763.5
      specified agent NEC 760.79
      suspected, affecting management of pregnancy 655.5 ●
  cocaine, through placenta or breast milk 760.75
  delirium
    alcohol 291.0
    drug 292.81
  drug 292.89
    with delirium 292.81
    correct substance properly administered (*see also* Allergy, drug) 995.27
    newborn 779.4
    obstetric anesthetic or sedation 668.9 ●
      affecting fetus or newborn 763.5
    overdose or wrong substance given or taken - *see* Table of Drugs and Chemicals
    pathologic 292.2
    specific to newborn 779.4
    via placenta or breast milk 760.70
      alcohol 760.71
      anticonvulsants 760.77
      antifungals 760.74
      anti-infective agents 760.74
      antimetabolics 760.78
      cocaine 760.75
      "crack" 760.75
      hallucinogenic agents 760.73
      medicinal agents NEC 760.79
      narcotics 760.72
      obstetric anesthetic or analgesic drug 763.5
      specified agent NEC 760.79
      suspected, affecting management of pregnancy 655.5 ●

Intoxication (Continued)
  enteric - see Intoxication, intestinal
  fetus or newborn, via placenta or breast milk 760.70
    alcohol 760.71
    anticonvulsants 760.77
    antifungals 760.74
    anti-infective agents 760.74
    antimetabolics 760.78
    cocaine 760.75
    "crack" 760.75
    hallucinogenic agents 760.73
    medicinal agents NEC 760.79
    narcotics 760.72
    obstetric anesthetic or analgesic drug 763.5
    specified agent NEC 760.79
    suspected, affecting management of pregnancy 655.5●
  food - see Poisoning, food
  gastrointestinal 558.2
  hallucinogenic (acute) 305.3●
  hepatocerebral 572.2
  idiosyncratic alcohol 291.4
  intestinal 569.89
    due to putrefaction of food 005.9
  methyl alcohol (see also Alcoholism) 305.0●
    with alcoholism 303.0●
  non-foodborne due to toxins of Clostridium botulinum [C. botulinum] - see Botulism
  pathologic 291.4
    drug 292.2
  potassium (K) 276.7
  septic
    with
      abortion - see Abortion, by type, with sepsis
      ectopic pregnancy (see also categories 633.0–633.9) 639.0
      molar pregnancy (see also categories 630–632) 639.0
    during labor 659.3●
    following
      abortion 639.0
      ectopic or molar pregnancy 639.0
    generalized - see Septicemia
    puerperal, postpartum, childbirth 670.2●
  serum (prophylactic) (therapeutic) 999.59
  uremic - see Uremia
  water 276.69
Intracranial - see condition
Intrahepatic gallbladder 751.69
Intraligamentous - see also condition
  pregnancy - see Pregnancy, cornual
Intraocular - see also condition
  sepsis 360.00
Intrathoracic - see also condition
  kidney 753.3
  stomach - see Hernia, diaphragm
Intrauterine contraceptive device
  checking V25.42
  insertion V25.11
  in situ V45.51
  management V25.42
  prescription V25.02
    repeat V25.42
  reinsertion V25.13
  removal V25.12
    and reinsertion V25.13
  replacement V25.13
Intraventricular - see condition
Intrinsic deformity - see Deformity
Intruded tooth 524.34
Intrusion, repetitive, of sleep (due to environmental disturbances) (with atypical polysomnographic features) 307.48
Intumescent, lens (eye) NEC 366.9
  senile 366.12

Intussusception (colon) (enteric) (intestine) (rectum) 560.0
  appendix 543.9
  congenital 751.5
  fallopian tube 620.8
  ileocecal 560.0
  ileocolic 560.0
  ureter (obstruction) 593.4
Invagination
  basilar 756.0
  colon or intestine 560.0
Invalid (since birth) 799.89
Invalidism (chronic) 799.89
Inversion
  albumin-globulin (A-G) ratio 273.8
  bladder 596.89
  cecum (see also Intussusception) 560.0
  cervix 622.8
  nipple 611.79
    congenital 757.6
    puerperal, postpartum 676.3●
  optic papilla 743.57
  organ or site, congenital NEC - see Anomaly, specified type NEC
  sleep rhythm 327.39
    nonorganic origin 307.45
  testis (congenital) 752.51
  uterus (postinfectional) (postpartal, old) 621.7
    chronic 621.7
    complicating delivery 665.2●
      affecting fetus or newborn 763.89
  vagina - see Prolapse, vagina
Investigation
  allergens V72.7
  clinical research (control) (normal comparison) (participant) V70.7
Inviability - see Immaturity
Involuntary movement, abnormal 781.0
Involution, involutional - see also condition
  breast, cystic or fibrocystic 610.1
  depression (see also Psychosis, affective) 296.2●
    recurrent episode 296.3●
    single episode 296.2●
  melancholia (see also Psychosis, affective) 296.2●
    recurrent episode 296.3●
    single episode 296.2●
  ovary, senile 620.3
  paranoid state (reaction) 297.2
  paraphrenia (climacteric) (menopause) 297.2
  psychosis 298.8
  thymus failure 254.8
IQ
  under 20 318.2
  20–34 318.1
  35–49 318.0
  50–70 317
IRDS 769
Irideremia 743.45
Iridis rubeosis 364.42
  diabetic 250.5● [364.42]
    due to secondary diabetes 249.5● [364.42]
Iridochoroiditis (panuveitis) 360.12
Iridocyclitis NEC 364.3
  acute 364.00
    primary 364.01
    recurrent 364.02
  chronic 364.10
    in
      lepromatous leprosy 030.0 [364.11]
      sarcoidosis 135 [364.11]
      tuberculosis (see also Tuberculosis) 017.3● [364.11]
  due to allergy 364.04
  endogenous 364.01
  gonococcal 098.41
  granulomatous 364.10
  herpetic (simplex) 054.44
    zoster 053.22
  hypopyon 364.05
  lens induced 364.23

Iridocyclitis NEC (Continued)
  nongranulomatous 364.00
  primary 364.01
  recurrent 364.02
  rheumatic 364.10
  secondary 364.04
    infectious 364.03
    noninfectious 364.04
  subacute 364.00
    primary 364.01
    recurrent 364.02
  sympathetic 360.11
  syphilitic (secondary) 091.52
  tuberculous (chronic) (see also Tuberculosis) 017.3● [364.11]
Iridocyclochoroiditis (panuveitis) 360.12
Iridodialysis 364.76
Iridodonesis 364.89
Iridoplegia (complete) (partial) (reflex) 379.49
Iridoschisis 364.52
IRIS (Immune Reconstitution Inflammatory Syndrome) 995.90
Iris - see condition
Iritis 364.3
  acute 364.00
    primary 364.01
    recurrent 364.02
  chronic 364.10
    in
      sarcoidosis 135 [364.11]
      tuberculosis (see also Tuberculosis) 017.3● [364.11]
  diabetic 250.5● [364.42]
    due to secondary diabetes 249.5● [364.42]
  due to
    allergy 364.04
    herpes simplex 054.44
    leprosy 030.0 [364.11]
  endogenous 364.01
  gonococcal 098.41
  gouty 274.89 [364.11]
  granulomatous 364.10
  hypopyon 364.05
  lens induced 364.23
  nongranulomatous 364.00
  papulosa 095.8 [364.11]
  primary 364.01
  recurrent 364.02
  rheumatic 364.10
  secondary 364.04
    infectious 364.03
    noninfectious 364.04
  subacute 364.00
    primary 364.01
    recurrent 364.02
  sympathetic 360.11
  syphilitic (secondary) 091.52
    congenital 090.0 [364.11]
    late 095.8 [364.11]
  tuberculous (see also Tuberculosis) 017.3● [364.11]
  uratic 274.89 [364.11]
Iron
  deficiency anemia 280.9
  metabolism disease 275.09
  storage disease 275.09
Iron-miners' lung 503
Irradiated enamel (tooth, teeth) 521.89
Irradiation
  burn - see Burn, by site
  effects, adverse 990
Irreducible, irreducibility - see condition
Irregular, irregularity
  action, heart 427.9
  alveolar process 525.8
  bleeding NEC 626.4
  breathing 786.09
  colon 569.89
  contour
    of cornea 743.41
      acquired 371.70
    reconstructed breast 612.0

Irregular, irregularity (Continued)
- dentin in pulp 522.3
- eye movements NEC 379.59
- menstruation (cause unknown) 626.4
- periods 626.4
- prostate 602.9
- pupil 364.75
- respiratory 786.09
- septum (nasal) 470
- shape, organ or site, congenital NEC - see Distortion
- sleep-wake rhythm (non-24-hour) 327.39
  - nonorganic origin 307.45
- vertebra 733.99

Irritability 799.22
- bladder 596.89
  - neurogenic 596.54
    - with cauda equina syndrome 344.61
- bowel (syndrome) 564.1
- bronchial (see also Bronchitis) 490
- cerebral, newborn 779.1
- colon 564.1
  - psychogenic 306.4
- duodenum 564.89
- heart (psychogenic) 306.2
- ileum 564.89
- jejunum 564.89
- myocardium 306.2
- nervousness 799.21
- rectum 564.89
- stomach 536.9
  - psychogenic 306.4
- sympathetic (nervous system) (see also Neuropathy, peripheral, autonomic) 337.9
- urethra 599.84
- ventricular (heart) (psychogenic) 306.2

Irritable (see also Irritability) 799.22

Irritation
- anus 569.49
- axillary nerve 353.0
- bladder 596.89
- brachial plexus 353.0
- brain (traumatic) (see also Injury, intracranial) 854.0●
  - nontraumatic - see Encephalitis
- bronchial (see also Bronchitis) 490
- cerebral (traumatic) (see also Injury, intracranial) 854.0●
  - nontraumatic - see Encephalitis
- cervical plexus 353.2
- cervix (see also Cervicitis) 616.0
- choroid, sympathetic 360.11
- cranial nerve - see Disorder, nerve, cranial
- digestive tract 536.9
  - psychogenic 306.4
- gastric 536.9
  - psychogenic 306.4
- gastrointestinal (tract) 536.9
  - functional 536.9
  - psychogenic 306.4
- globe, sympathetic 360.11
- intestinal (bowel) 564.9
- labyrinth 386.50
- lumbosacral plexus 353.1
- meninges (traumatic) (see also Injury, intracranial) 854.0●
  - nontraumatic - see Meningitis
- myocardium 306.2
- nerve - see Disorder, nerve
- nervous 799.21
- nose 478.19
- penis 607.89
- perineum 709.9
- peripheral
  - autonomic nervous system (see also Neuropathy, peripheral, autonomic) 337.9
  - nerve - see Disorder, nerve
- peritoneum (see also Peritonitis) 567.9
- pharynx 478.29

Irritation (Continued)
- plantar nerve 355.6
- spinal (cord) (traumatic) - see also Injury, spinal, by site
  - nerve - see also Disorder, nerve
    - root NEC 724.9
    - traumatic - see Injury, nerve, spinal
  - nontraumatic - see Myelitis
- stomach 536.9
  - psychogenic 306.4
- sympathetic nerve NEC (see also Neuropathy, peripheral, autonomic) 337.9
- ulnar nerve 354.2
- vagina 623.9

Isambert's disease 012.3●
Ischemia, ischemic 459.9
- basilar artery (with transient neurologic deficit) 435.0
- bone NEC 733.40
- bowel (transient) 557.9
  - acute 557.0
  - chronic 557.1
  - due to mesenteric artery insufficiency 557.1
- brain - see also Ischemia, cerebral
  - recurrent focal 435.9
- cardiac (see also Ischemia, heart) 414.9
- cardiomyopathy 414.8
- carotid artery (with transient neurologic deficit) 435.8
- cerebral (chronic) (generalized) 437.1
  - arteriosclerotic 437.0
  - intermittent (with transient neurologic deficit) 435.9
  - newborn 779.2
  - puerperal, postpartum, childbirth 674.0●
  - recurrent focal (with transient neurologic deficit) 435.9
  - transient (with transient neurologic deficit) 435.9
- colon 557.9
  - acute 557.0
  - chronic 557.1
  - due to mesenteric artery insufficiency 557.1
- coronary (chronic) (see also Ischemia, heart) 414.9
- demand 411.89
- heart (chronic or with a stated duration of over 8 weeks) 414.9
  - acute or with a stated duration of 8 weeks or less (see also Infarct, myocardium) 410.9●
    - without myocardial infarction 411.89
      - with coronary (artery) occlusion 411.81
  - subacute 411.89
- intestine (transient) 557.9
  - acute 557.0
  - chronic 557.1
  - due to mesenteric artery insufficiency 557.1
- kidney 593.81
- labyrinth 386.50
- muscles, leg 728.89
- myocardium, myocardial (chronic or with a stated duration of over 8 weeks) 414.8
  - acute (see also Infarct, myocardium) 410.9●
    - without myocardial infarction 411.89
      - with coronary (artery) occlusion 411.81
- renal 593.81
- retina, retinal 362.84
- small bowel 557.9
  - acute 557.0
  - chronic 557.1
  - due to mesenteric artery insufficiency 557.1
- spinal cord 336.1
- subendocardial (see also Insufficiency, coronary) 411.89
- supply (see also Angina) 414.9
- vertebral artery (with transient neurologic deficit) 435.1

Ischialgia (see also Sciatica) 724.3
Ischiopagus 759.4
Ischium, ischial - see condition
Ischomenia 626.8
Ischuria 788.5
Iselin's disease or osteochondrosis 732.5
Islands of
- parotid tissue in
  - lymph nodes 750.26
  - neck structures 750.26
- submaxillary glands in
  - fascia 750.26
  - lymph nodes 750.26
  - neck muscles 750.26

Islet cell tumor, pancreas (M8150/0) 211.7
Isoimmunization NEC (see also Incompatibility) 656.2●
- anti-E 656.2●
- fetus or newborn 773.2
  - ABO blood groups 773.1
  - Rhesus (Rh) factor 773.0

Isolation V07.0
- social V62.4

Isosporosis 007.2
Issue
- medical certificate NEC V68.09
  - cause of death V68.09
  - disability examination V68.01
  - fitness V68.09
  - incapacity V68.09
- repeat prescription NEC V68.1
  - appliance V68.1
  - contraceptive V25.40
    - device NEC V25.49
      - intrauterine V25.42
      - specified type NEC V25.49
    - pill V25.41
  - glasses V68.1
  - medicinal substance V68.1

Itch (see also Pruritus) 698.9
- bakers' 692.89
- barbers' 110.0
- bricklayers' 692.89
- cheese 133.8
- clam diggers' 120.3
- coolie 126.9
- copra 133.8
- Cuban 050.1
- dew 126.9
- dhobie 110.3
- eye 379.99
- filarial (see also Infestation, filarial) 125.9
- grain 133.8
- grocers' 133.8
- ground 126.9
- harvest 133.8
- jock 110.3
- Malabar 110.9
  - beard 110.0
  - foot 110.4
  - scalp 110.0
- meaning scabies 133.0
- Norwegian 133.0
- perianal 698.0
- poultrymen's 133.8
- sarcoptic 133.0
- scrub 134.1
- seven year V61.10
  - meaning scabies 133.0
- straw 133.8
- swimmers' 120.3
- washerwoman's 692.4
- water 120.3
- winter 698.8

Itsenko-Cushing syndrome (pituitary basophilism) 255.0
Ivemark's syndrome (asplenia with congenital heart disease) 759.0
Ivory bones 756.52
Ixodes 134.8
Ixodiasis 134.8

J

Jaccoud's nodular fibrositis, chronic (Jaccoud's syndrome) 714.4
Jackson's
    membrane 751.4
    paralysis or syndrome 344.89
    veil 751.4
Jacksonian
    epilepsy (see also Epilepsy) 345.5●
    seizures (focal) (see also Epilepsy) 345.5●
Jacob's ulcer (M8090/3) - see Neoplasm, skin, malignant, by site
Jacquet's dermatitis (diaper dermatitis) 691.0
Jadassohn's
    blue nevus (M8780/0) - see Neoplasm, skin, benign
    disease (maculopapular erythroderma) 696.2
    intraepidermal epithelioma (M8096/0) - see Neoplasm, skin, benign
Jadassohn-Lewandowski syndrome (pachyonychia congenita) 757.5
Jadassohn-Pellizari's disease (anetoderma) 701.3
Jadassohn-Tièche nevus (M8780/0) - see Neoplasm, skin, benign
Jaffe-Lichtenstein (-Uehlinger) syndrome 252.01
Jahnke's syndrome (encephalocutaneous angiomatosis) 759.6
Jakob-Creutzfeldt disease (CJD) (syndrome) 046.19
    with dementia
        with behavioral disturbance 046.19 [294.11]
        without behavioral disturbance 046.19 [294.10]
    familial 046.19
    iatrogenic 046.19
    specified NEC 046.19
    sporadic 046.19
    variant (vCJD) 046.11
        with dementia
            with behavioral disturbance 046.11 [294.11]
            without behavioral disturbance 046.11 [294.10]
Jaksch (-Luzet) disease or syndrome (pseudoleukemia infantum) 285.8
Jamaican
    neuropathy 349.82
    paraplegic tropical ataxic-spastic syndrome 349.82
Janet's disease (psychasthenia) 300.89
Janiceps 759.4
Jansky-Bielschowsky amaurotic familial idiocy 330.1
Japanese
    B-type encephalitis 062.0
    river fever 081.2
    seven-day fever 100.89
Jaundice (yellow) 782.4
    acholuric (familial) (splenomegalic) (see also Spherocytosis) 282.0
        acquired 283.9
    breast milk 774.39
    catarrhal (acute) 070.1
        with hepatic coma 070.0
        chronic 571.9
        epidemic - see Jaundice, epidemic
    cholestatic (benign) 782.4
    chronic idiopathic 277.4

Jaundice (Continued)
    epidemic (catarrhal) 070.1
        with hepatic coma 070.0
        leptospiral 100.0
        spirochetal 100.0
    febrile (acute) 070.1
        with hepatic coma 070.0
        leptospiral 100.0
        spirochetal 100.0
    fetus or newborn 774.6
        due to or associated with
            ABO
                antibodies 773.1
                incompatibility, maternal/fetal 773.1
                isoimmunization 773.1
            absence or deficiency of enzyme system for bilirubin conjugation (congenital) 774.39
            blood group incompatibility NEC 773.2
            breast milk inhibitors to conjugation 774.39
            associated with preterm delivery 774.2
            bruising 774.1
            Crigler-Najjar syndrome 277.4 [774.31]
            delayed conjugation 774.30
                associated with preterm delivery 774.2
            development 774.39
            drugs or toxins transmitted from mother 774.1
            G-6-PD deficiency 282.2 [774.0]
            galactosemia 271.1 [774.5]
            Gilbert's syndrome 277.4 [774.31]
            hepatocellular damage 774.4
            hereditary hemolytic anemia (see also Anemia, hemolytic) 282.9 [774.0]
            hypothyroidism, congenital 243 [774.31]
            incompatibility, maternal/fetal NEC 773.2
            infection 774.1
            inspissated bile syndrome 774.4
            isoimmunization NEC 773.2
            mucoviscidosis 277.01 [774.5]
            obliteration of bile duct, congenital 751.61 [774.5]
            polycythemia 774.1
            preterm delivery 774.2
            red cell defect 282.9 [774.0]
            Rh
                antibodies 773.0
                incompatibility, maternal/fetal 773.0
                isoimmunization 773.0
            spherocytosis (congenital) 282.0 [774.0]
            swallowed maternal blood 774.1
        physiological NEC 774.6
    from injection, inoculation, infusion, or transfusion (blood) (plasma) (serum) (other substance) (onset within 8 months after administration) - see Hepatitis, viral
    Gilbert's (familial nonhemolytic) 277.4
    hematogenous 283.9
    hemolytic (acquired) 283.9
        congenital (see also Spherocytosis) 282.0
    hemorrhagic (acute) 100.0
        leptospiral 100.0
        newborn 776.0
        spirochetal 100.0

Jaundice (Continued)
    hepatocellular 573.8
    homologous (serum) - see Hepatitis, viral
    idiopathic, chronic 277.4
    infectious (acute) (subacute) 070.1
        with hepatic coma 070.0
        leptospiral 100.0
        spirochetal 100.0
    leptospiral 100.0
    malignant (see also Necrosis, liver) 570
    newborn (physiological) (see also Jaundice, fetus or newborn) 774.6
    nonhemolytic, congenital familial (Gilbert's) 277.4
    nuclear, newborn (see also Kernicterus of newborn) 774.7
    obstructive NEC (see also Obstruction, biliary) 576.8
    postimmunization - see Hepatitis, viral
    posttransfusion - see Hepatitis, viral
    regurgitation (see also Obstruction, biliary) 576.8
    serum (homologous) (prophylactic) (therapeutic) - see Hepatitis, viral
    spirochetal (hemorrhagic) 100.0
    symptomatic 782.4
        newborn 774.6
Jaw - see condition
Jaw-blinking 374.43
    congenital 742.8
Jaw-winking phenomenon or syndrome 742.8
Jealousy
    alcoholic 291.5
    childhood 313.3
    sibling 313.3
Jejunitis (see also Enteritis) 558.9
Jejunostomy status V44.4
Jejunum, jejunal - see condition
Jensen's disease 363.05
Jericho boil 085.1
Jerks, myoclonic 333.2
Jervell-Lange-Nielsen syndrome 426.82
Jeune's disease or syndrome (asphyxiating thoracic dystrophy) 756.4
Jigger disease 134.1
Job's syndrome (chronic granulomatous disease) 288.1
Jod-Basedow phenomenon 242.8●
Johnson-Stevens disease (erythema multiforme exudativum) 695.13
Joint - see also condition
    Charcôt's 094.0 [713.5]
    false 733.82
    flail - see Flail, joint
    mice - see Loose, body, joint, by site
    sinus to bone 730.9●
    von Gies' 095.8
Jordan's anomaly or syndrome 288.2
Josephs-Diamond-Blackfan anemia (congenital hypoplastic) 284.01
Joubert syndrome 759.89
Jumpers' knee 727.2
Jungle yellow fever 060.0
Jungling's disease (sarcoidosis) 135
Junin virus hemorrhagic fever 078.7
Juvenile - see also condition
    delinquent 312.9
        group (see also Disturbance, conduct) 312.2●
        neurotic 312.4

K

Kabuki syndrome 759.89
Kahler (-Bozzolo) **disease** (multiple myeloma) (M9730/3) 203.0 ●
Kakergasia 300.9
Kakke 265.0
Kala-azar (Indian) (infantile) (Mediterranean) (Sudanese) 085.0
Kalischer's syndrome (encephalocutaneous angiomatosis) 759.6
Kallmann's syndrome (hypogonadotropic hypogonadism with anosmia) 253.4
Kanner's syndrome (autism) (see also Psychosis, childhood) 299.0 ●
Kaolinosis 502
Kaposi's
  disease 757.33
    lichen ruber 696.4
      acuminatus 696.4
      moniliformis 697.8
    xeroderma pigmentosum 757.33
  sarcoma (M9140/3) 176.9
    adipose tissue 176.1
    aponeurosis 176.1
    artery 176.1
    associated herpesvirus infection 058.89
    blood vessel 176.1
    bursa 176.1
    connective tissue 176.1
    external genitalia 176.8
    fascia 176.1
    fatty tissue 176.1
    fibrous tissue 176.1
    gastrointestinal tract NEC 176.3
    ligament 176.1
    lung 176.4
    lymph
      gland(s) 176.5
      node(s) 176.5
    lymphatic(s) NEC 176.1
    muscle (skeletal) 176.1
    oral cavity NEC 176.8
    palate 176.2
    scrotum 176.8
    skin 176.0
    soft tissue 176.1
    specified site NEC 176.8
    subcutaneous tissue 176.1
    synovia 176.1
    tendon (sheath) 176.1
    vein 176.1
    vessel 176.1
    viscera NEC 176.9
    vulva 176.8
  varicelliform eruption 054.0
  vaccinia 999.0
Kartagener's syndrome or triad (sinusitis, bronchiectasis, situs inversus) 759.3
Kasabach-Merritt syndrome (capillary hemangioma associated with thrombocytopenic purpura) 287.39
Kaschin-Beck disease (endemic polyarthritis) - see Disease, Kaschin-Beck
Kast's syndrome (dyschondroplasia with hemangiomas) 756.4
Katatonia- see Catatonia
Katayama disease or fever 120.2
Kathisophobia 781.0
Kawasaki disease 446.1
Kayser-Fleischer ring (cornea) (pseudosclerosis) 275.1 [371.14]
Kaznelson's syndrome (congenital hypoplastic anemia) 284.01
Kearns-Sayre syndrome 277.87
Kedani fever 081.2
Kelis 701.4
Kelly (-Patterson) syndrome (sideropenic dysphagia) 280.8

Keloid, cheloid 701.4
  Addison's (morphea) 701.0
  cornea 371.00
  Hawkins' 701.4
  scar 701.4
Keloma 701.4
Kenya fever 082.1
Keratectasia 371.71
  congenital 743.41
Keratinization NEC
  alveolar ridge mucosa
    excessive 528.72
    minimal 528.71
Keratitis (nodular) (nonulcerative) (simple) (zonular) NEC 370.9
  with ulceration (see also Ulcer, cornea) 370.00
  actinic 370.24
  arborescens 054.42
  areolar 370.22
  bullosa 370.8
  deep - see Keratitis, interstitial
  dendritic(a) 054.42
  desiccation 370.34
  diffuse interstitial 370.52
  disciform(is) 054.43
    varicella 052.7 [370.44]
  epithelialis vernalis 372.13 [370.32]
  exposure 370.34
  filamentary 370.23
  gonococcal (congenital) (prenatal) 098.43
  herpes, herpetic (simplex) NEC 054.43
    zoster 053.21
  hypopyon 370.04
  in
    chickenpox 052.7 [370.44]
    exanthema (see also Exanthem) 057.9 [370.44]
    paravaccinia (see also Paravaccinia) 051.9 [370.44]
    smallpox (see also Smallpox) 050.9 [370.44]
    vernal conjunctivitis 372.13 [370.32]
  interstitial (nonsyphilitic) 370.50
    with ulcer (see also Ulcer, cornea) 370.00
    diffuse 370.52
    herpes, herpetic (simplex) 054.43
      zoster 053.21
    syphilitic (congenital) (hereditary) 090.3
    tuberculous (see also Tuberculosis) 017.3 ● [370.59]
  lagophthalmic 370.34
  macular 370.22
  neuroparalytic 370.35
  neurotrophic 370.35
  nummular 370.22
  oyster-shuckers' 370.8
  parenchymatous - see Keratitis, interstitial
  petrificans 370.8
  phlyctenular 370.31
  postmeasles 055.71
  punctata, punctate 370.21
    leprosa 030.0 [370.21]
    profunda 090.3
    superficial (Thygeson's) 370.21
  purulent 370.8
  pustuliformis profunda 090.3
  rosacea 695.3 [370.49]
  sclerosing 370.54
  specified type NEC 370.8
  stellate 370.22
  striate 370.22
  superficial 370.20
    with conjunctivitis (see also Keratoconjunctivitis) 370.40
    punctate (Thygeson's) 370.21
  suppurative 370.8
  syphilitic (congenital) (prenatal) 090.3
  trachomatous 076.1
    late effect 139.1
  tuberculous (phlyctenular) (see also Tuberculosis) 017.3 ● [370.31]
  ulcerated (see also Ulcer, cornea) 370.00

Keratitis (Continued)
  vesicular 370.8
  welders' 370.24
  xerotic (see also Keratomalacia) 371.45
    vitamin A deficiency 264.4
Keratoacanthoma 238.2
Keratocele 371.72
Keratoconjunctivitis (see also Keratitis) 370.40
  adenovirus type 8 077.1
  epidemic 077.1
  exposure 370.34
  gonococcal 098.43
  herpetic (simplex) 054.43
    zoster 053.21
  in
    chickenpox 052.7 [370.44]
    exanthema (see also Exanthem) 057.9 [370.44]
    paravaccinia (see also Paravaccinia) 051.9 [370.44]
    smallpox (see also Smallpox) 050.9 [370.44]
  infectious 077.1
  neurotrophic 370.35
  phlyctenular 370.31
  postmeasles 055.71
  shipyard 077.1
  sicca (Sjögren's syndrome) 710.2
    not in Sjögren's syndrome 370.33
  specified type NEC 370.49
  tuberculous (phlyctenular) (see also Tuberculosis) 017.3 ● [370.31]
Keratoconus 371.60
  acute hydrops 371.62
  congenital 743.41
  stable 371.61
Keratocyst (dental) 526.0
Keratoderma, keratodermia (congenital) (palmaris et plantaris) (symmetrical) 757.39
  acquired 701.1
  blennorrhagica 701.1
    gonococcal 098.81
  climacterium 701.1
  eccentrica 757.39
  gonorrheal 098.81
  punctata 701.1
  tylodes, progressive 701.1
Keratodermatocele 371.72
Keratoglobus 371.70
  congenital 743.41
    associated with buphthalmos 743.22
Keratohemia 371.12
Keratoiritis (see also Iridocyclitis) 364.3
  syphilitic 090.3
  tuberculous (see also Tuberculosis) 017.3 ● [364.11]
Keratolysis exfoliativa (congenital) 757.39
  acquired 695.89
  neonatorum 757.39
Keratoma 701.1
  congenital 757.39
  malignum congenitale 757.1
  palmaris et plantaris hereditarium 757.39
  senile 702.0
Keratomalacia 371.45
  vitamin A deficiency 264.4
Keratomegaly 743.41
Keratomycosis 111.1
  nigricans (palmaris) 111.1
Keratopathy 371.40
  band (see also Keratitis) 371.43
  bullous (see also Keratitis) 371.23
  degenerative (see also Degeneration, cornea) 371.40
  hereditary (see also Dystrophy, cornea) 371.50
  discrete colliquative 371.49
Keratoscleritis, tuberculous (see also Tuberculosis) 017.3 ● [370.31]

Keratosis 701.1
 actinic 702.0
 arsenical 692.4
 blennorrhagica 701.1
  gonococcal 098.81
 congenital (any type) 757.39
 ear (middle) (see also Cholesteatoma) 385.30
 female genital (external) 629.89
 follicular, vitamin A deficiency 264.8
 follicularis 757.39
  acquired 701.1
  congenital (acneiformis) (Siemens') 757.39
  spinulosa (decalvans) 757.39
  vitamin A deficiency 264.8
 gonococcal 098.81
 larynx, laryngeal 478.79
 male genital (external) 608.89
 middle ear (see also Cholesteatoma) 385.30
 nigricans 701.2
  congenital 757.39
 obturans 380.21
 oral epithelium
  residual ridge mucosa
   excessive 528.72
   minimal 528.71
 palmaris et plantaris (symmetrical) 757.39
 penile 607.89
 pharyngeus 478.29
 pilaris 757.39
  acquired 701.1
 punctata (palmaris et plantaris) 701.1
 scrotal 608.89
 seborrheic 702.19
  inflamed 702.11
 senilis 702.0
 solar 702.0
 suprafollicularis 757.39
 tonsillaris 478.29
 vagina 623.1
 vegetans 757.39
 vitamin A deficiency 264.8
Kerato-uveitis (see also Iridocyclitis) 364.3
Keraunoparalysis 994.0
Kerion (celsi) 110.0
Kernicterus of newborn (not due to
   isoimmunization) 774.7
 due to isoimmunization (conditions
    classifiable to 773.0–773.2) 773.4
Ketoacidosis 276.2
 diabetic 250.1 ●
  due to secondary diabetes 249.1 ●
Ketonuria 791.6
 branched-chain, intermittent 270.3
Ketosis 276.2
 diabetic 250.1 ●
  due to secondary diabetes 249.1 ●
Kidney - see condition
Kienböck's
 disease 732.3
  adult 732.8
 osteochondrosis 732.3
Kimmelstiel (-Wilson) disease or syndrome
   (intercapillary glomerulosclerosis) 250.4 ●
   [581.81]
 due to secondary diabetes 249.4 ● [581.81]
Kink, kinking
 appendix 543.9
 artery 447.1
 cystic duct, congenital 751.61
 hair (acquired) 704.2
 ileum or intestine (see also Obstruction,
    intestine) 560.9
 Lane's (see also Obstruction, intestine) 560.9
 organ or site, congenital NEC - see Anomaly,
    specified type NEC, by site
 ureter (pelvic junction) 593.3
  congenital 753.20
 vein(s) 459.2
  caval 459.2
  peripheral 459.2

Kinnier Wilson's disease (hepatolenticular
   degeneration) 275.1
Kissing
 osteophytes 721.5
 spine 721.5
 vertebra 721.5
Klauder's syndrome (erythema multiforme
   exudativum) 695.19
Klebs' disease (see also Nephritis) 583.9
Klein-Waardenburg syndrome (ptosis-
   epicanthus) 270.2
Kleine-Levin syndrome 327.13
Kleptomania 312.32
Klinefelter's syndrome 758.7
Klinger's disease 446.4
Klippel's disease 723.8
Klippel-Feil disease or syndrome (brevicollis)
   756.16
Klippel-Trenaunay syndrome 759.89
Klumpke (-Déjérine) palsy, paralysis (birth)
   (newborn) 767.6
Klüver-Bucy (-Terzian) syndrome 310.0
Knee - see condition
Knifegrinders' rot (see also Tuberculosis)
   011.4 ●
Knock-knee (acquired) 736.41
 congenital 755.64
Knot
 intestinal, syndrome (volvulus) 560.2
 umbilical cord (true) 663.2 ●
  affecting fetus or newborn 762.5
Knots, surfer 919.8
 infected 919.9
Knotting (of)
 hair 704.2
 intestine 560.2
Knuckle pads (Garrod's) 728.79
Köbner's disease (epidermolysis bullosa)
   757.39
Koch's
 infection (see also Tuberculosis, pulmonary)
    011.9 ●
 relapsing fever 087.9
Koch-Weeks conjunctivitis 372.03
Koenig-Wichman disease (pemphigus)
   694.4
Köhler's disease (osteochondrosis) 732.5
 first (osteochondrosis juvenilis) 732.5
 second (Freiburg's infarction, metatarsal
    head) 732.5
 patellar 732.4
 tarsal navicular (bone) (osteoarthrosis
    juvenilis) 732.5
Köhler-Mouchet disease (osteoarthrosis
   juvenilis) 732.5
Köhler-Pellegrini-Stieda disease or syndrome
   (calcification, knee joint) 726.62
Koilonychia 703.8
 congenital 757.5
Kojevnikov's, Kojewnikoff's epilepsy (see also
   Epilepsy) 345.7 ●
König's
 disease (osteochondritis dissecans) 732.7
 syndrome 564.89
Koniophthisis (see also Tuberculosis) 011.4 ●
Koplik's spots 055.9
Kopp's asthma 254.8
Korean hemorrhagic fever 078.6
Korsakoff (-Wernicke) disease, psychosis, or
   syndrome (nonalcoholic) 294.0
 alcoholic 291.1
Korsakov's disease - see Korsakoff's disease
Korsakow's disease - see Korsakoff's disease
Kostmann's disease or syndrome (infantile
   genetic agranulocytosis) 288.01
Krabbe's
 disease (leukodystrophy) 330.0
 syndrome
  congenital muscle hypoplasia 756.89
  cutaneocerebral angioma 759.6

Kraepelin-Morel disease (see also
   Schizophrenia) 295.9 ●
Kraft-Weber-Dimitri disease 759.6
Kraurosis
 ani 569.49
 penis 607.0
 vagina 623.8
 vulva 624.09
Kreotoxism 005.9
Krukenberg's
 spindle 371.13
 tumor (M8490/6) 198.6
Kufs' disease 330.1
Kugelberg-Welander disease 335.11
Kuhnt-Junius degeneration or disease
   362.52
Kulchitsky's cell carcinoma (carcinoid tumor of
   intestine) 259.2
Kümmell's disease or spondylitis 721.7
Kundrat's disease (lymphosarcoma) 200.1 ●
Kunekune - see Dermatophytosis
Kunkel syndrome (lupoid hepatitis)
   571.49
Kupffer cell sarcoma (M9124/3) 155.0
Kuru 046.0
Kussmaul's
 coma (diabetic) 250.3 ●
  due to secondary diabetes 249.3 ●
 disease (polyarteritis nodosa) 446.0
 respiration (air hunger) 786.09
Kwashiorkor (marasmus type) 260
Kyasanur Forest disease 065.2
Kyphoscoliosis, kyphoscoliotic (acquired)
   (see also Scoliosis) 737.30
 congenital 756.19
 due to radiation 737.33
 heart (disease) 416.1
 idiopathic 737.30
  infantile
   progressive 737.32
   resolving 737.31
 late effect of rickets 268.1 [737.43]
 specified NEC 737.39
 thoracogenic 737.34
 tuberculous (see also Tuberculosis) 015.0 ●
    [737.43]
Kyphosis, kyphotic (acquired) (postural)
   737.10
 adolescent postural 737.0
 congenital 756.19
 dorsalis juvenilis 732.0
 due to or associated with
  Charcôt-Marie-Tooth disease 356.1
     [737.41]
  mucopolysaccharidosis 277.5 [737.41]
  neurofibromatosis 237.71 [737.41]
  osteitis
   deformans 731.0 [737.41]
   fibrosa cystica 252.01 [737.41]
  osteoporosis (see also Osteoporosis) 733.0
     [737.41]
  poliomyelitis (see also Poliomyelitis) 138
     [737.41]
  radiation 737.11
  tuberculosis (see also Tuberculosis) 015.0 ●
     [737.41]
 Kümmell's 721.7
 late effect of rickets 268.1 [737.41]
 Morquio-Brailsford type (spinal) 277.5
    [737.41]
 pelvis 738.6
 postlaminectomy 737.12
 specified cause NEC 737.19
 syphilitic, congenital 090.5 [737.41]
 tuberculous (see also Tuberculosis) 015.0 ●
    [737.41]
Kyrle's disease (hyperkeratosis follicularis in
   cutem penetrans) 701.1

 New   Revised   deleted Deleted   ● Use Additional Digit(s)   Omit code

SECTION I INDEX TO DISEASES AND INJURIES / Labia, labium

L

Labia, labium - *see* condition
Labiated hymen 752.49
Labile
  blood pressure 796.2
  emotions, emotionality 301.3
  vasomotor system 443.9
Lability, emotional 799.24
Labioglossal paralysis 335.22
Labium leporinum (*see also* Cleft, lip) 749.10
Labor (*see also* Delivery)
  with complications - *see* Delivery, complicated
  abnormal NEC 661.9●
    affecting fetus or newborn 763.7
  arrested active phase 661.1●
    affecting fetus or newborn 763.7
  desultory 661.2●
    affecting fetus or newborn 763.7
  dyscoordinate 661.4●
    affecting fetus or newborn 763.7
  early onset (22–36 weeks gestation) 644.2●
  failed
    induction 659.1●
      mechanical 659.0●
      medical 659.1●
      surgical 659.0●
    trial (vaginal delivery) 660.6●
  false 644.1●
  forced or induced, affecting fetus or newborn 763.89
  hypertonic 661.4●
    affecting fetus or newborn 763.7
  hypotonic 661.2●
    affecting fetus or newborn 763.7
    primary 661.0●
      affecting fetus or newborn 763.7
    secondary 661.1●
      affecting fetus or newborn 763.7
  incoordinate 661.4●
    affecting fetus or newborn 763.7
  irregular 661.2●
    affecting fetus or newborn 763.7
  long - *see* Labor, prolonged
  missed (at or near term) 656.4●
  obstructed NEC 660.9●
    affecting fetus or newborn 763.1
    due to female genital mutilation 660.8●
    specified cause NEC 660.8●
      affecting fetus or newborn 763.1
  pains, spurious 644.1●
  precipitate 661.3●
    affecting fetus or newborn 763.6
  premature 644.2●
    threatened 644.0●
  prolonged or protracted 662.1●
    affecting fetus or newborn 763.89
    first stage 662.0●
      affecting fetus or newborn 763.89
    second stage 662.2●
      affecting fetus or newborn 763.89
  threatened NEC 644.1●
  undelivered 644.1●
Labored breathing (*see also* Hyperventilation) 786.09
Labyrinthitis (inner ear) (destructive) (latent) 386.30
  circumscribed 386.32
  diffuse 386.31
  focal 386.32
  purulent 386.33
  serous 386.31
  suppurative 386.33
  syphilitic 095.8
  toxic 386.34
  viral 386.35
Laceration - *see also* Wound, open, by site
  accidental, complicating surgery 998.2
  Achilles tendon 845.09
    with open wound 892.2

Laceration (*Continued*)
  anus (sphincter) 879.6
    with
      abortion - *see* Abortion, by type, with damage to pelvic organs
      ectopic pregnancy (*see also* categories 633.0–633.9) 639.2
      molar pregnancy (*see also* categories 630–632) 639.2
    complicated 879.7
    complicating delivery (healed) (old) 654.8●
      with laceration of anal or rectal mucosa 664.3●
      not associated with third-degree perineal laceration 664.6●
    following
      abortion 639.2
      ectopic or molar pregnancy 639.2
    nontraumatic, nonpuerperal (healed) (old) 569.43
  bladder (urinary)
    with
      abortion - *see* Abortion, by type, with damage to pelvic organs
      ectopic pregnancy (*see also* categories 633.0–633.9) 639.2
      molar pregnancy (*see also* categories 630–632) 639.2
    following
      abortion 639.2
      ectopic or molar pregnancy 639.2
    obstetrical trauma 665.5●
  blood vessel - *see* Injury, blood vessel, by site
  bowel
    with
      abortion - *see* Abortion, by type, with damage to pelvic organs
      ectopic pregnancy (*see also* categories 633.0–633.9) 639.2
      molar pregnancy (*see also* categories 630–632) 639.2
    following
      abortion 639.2
      ectopic or molar pregnancy 639.2
    obstetrical trauma 665.5●
  brain (cerebral) (membrane) (with hemorrhage) 851.8●

> Note: Use the following fifth-digit subclassification with categories 851–854:
>
> 0 unspecified state of consciousness
> 1 with no loss of consciousness
> 2 with brief [less than one hour] loss of consciousness
> 3 with moderate [1–24 hours] loss of consciousness
> 4 with prolonged [more than 24 hours] loss of consciousness and return to pre-existing conscious level
> 5 with prolonged [more than 24 hours] loss of consciousness, without return to pre-existing conscious level
>
> Use fifth-digit 5 to designate when a patient is unconscious and dies before regaining consciousness, regardless of the duration of the loss of consciousness
>
> 6 with loss of consciousness of unspecified duration
> 9 with concussion, unspecified

  with
    open intracranial wound 851.9●
    skull fracture - *see* Fracture, skull, by site
  cerebellum 851.6●
    with open intracranial wound 851.7●

Laceration (*Continued*)
  brain (*Continued*)
    cortex 851.2●
      with open intracranial wound 851.3●
    during birth 767.0
    stem 851.6●
      with open intracranial wound 851.7●
  broad ligament
    with
      abortion - *see* Abortion, by type, with damage to pelvic organs
      ectopic pregnancy (*see also* categories 633.0–633.9) 639.2
      molar pregnancy (*see also* categories 630–632) 639.2
    following
      abortion 639.2
      ectopic or molar pregnancy 639.2
    nontraumatic 620.6
    obstetrical trauma 665.6●
    syndrome (nontraumatic) 620.6
  capsule, joint - *see* Sprain, by site
  cardiac - *see* Laceration, heart
  causing eversion of cervix uteri (old) 622.0
  central, complicating delivery 664.4●
  cerebellum - *see* Laceration, brain, cerebellum
  cerebral - *see also* Laceration, brain
    during birth 767.0
  cervix (uteri)
    with
      abortion - *see* Abortion, by type, with damage to pelvic organs
      ectopic pregnancy (*see also* categories 633.0–633.9) 639.2
      molar pregnancy (*see also* categories 630–632) 639.2
    following
      abortion 639.2
      ectopic or molar pregnancy 639.2
    nonpuerperal, nontraumatic 622.3
    obstetrical trauma (current) 665.3●
    old (postpartal) 622.3
    traumatic - *see* Injury, internal, cervix
  chordae heart 429.5
  complicated 879.9
  cornea - *see* Laceration, eyeball
    superficial 918.1
  cortex (cerebral) - *see* Laceration, brain, cortex
  esophagus 530.89
  eye(s) - *see* Laceration, ocular
  eyeball NEC 871.4
    with prolapse or exposure of intraocular tissue 871.1
    penetrating - *see* Penetrating wound, eyeball
    specified as without prolapse of intraocular tissue 871.0
  eyelid NEC 870.8
    full thickness 870.1
      involving lacrimal passages 870.2
    skin (and periocular area) 870.0
      penetrating - *see* Penetrating wound, orbit
  fourchette
    with
      abortion - *see* Abortion, by type, with damage to pelvic organs
      ectopic pregnancy (*see also* categories 633.0–633.9) 639.2
      molar pregnancy (*see also* categories 630–632) 639.2
    complicating delivery 664.0●
    following
      abortion 639.2
      ectopic or molar pregnancy 639.2
  heart (without penetration of heart chambers) 861.02
    with
      open wound into thorax 861.12
      penetration of heart chambers 861.03
        with open wound into thorax 861.13

Laceration (Continued)
- hernial sac - see Hernia, by site
- internal organ (abdomen) (chest) (pelvis) NEC - see Injury, internal, by site
- kidney (parenchyma) 866.02
  - with
    - complete disruption of parenchyma (rupture) 866.03
      - with open wound into cavity 866.13
    - open wound into cavity 866.12
- labia
  - complicating delivery 664.0●
- ligament - see also Sprain, by site
  - with open wound - see Wound, open, by site
- liver 864.05
  - with open wound into cavity 864.15
  - major (disruption of hepatic parenchyma) 864.04
    - with open wound into cavity 864.14
  - minor (capsule only) 864.02
    - with open wound into cavity 864.12
  - moderate (involving parenchyma without major disruption) 864.03
    - with open wound into cavity 864.13
  - multiple 864.04
    - with open wound into cavity 864.14
  - stellate 864.04
    - with open wound into cavity 864.14
- lung 861.22
  - with open wound into thorax 861.32
- meninges - see Laceration, brain
- meniscus (knee) (see also Tear, meniscus) 836.2
  - old 717.5
  - site other than knee - see also Sprain, by site
    - old NEC (see also Disorder, cartilage, articular) 718.0●
- muscle - see also Sprain, by site
  - with open wound - see Wound, open, by site
- myocardium - see Laceration, heart
- nerve - see Injury, nerve, by site
- ocular NEC (see also Laceration, eyeball) 871.4
  - adnexa NEC 870.8
    - penetrating 870.3
      - with foreign body 870.4
- orbit (eye) 870.8
  - penetrating 870.3
    - with foreign body 870.4
- pelvic
  - floor (muscles)
    - with
      - abortion - see Abortion, by type, with damage to pelvic organs
      - ectopic pregnancy (see also categories 633.0–633.9) 639.2
      - molar pregnancy (see also categories 630–632) 639.2
    - complicating delivery 664.1●
    - following
      - abortion 639.2
      - ectopic or molar pregnancy 639.2
    - nonpuerperal 618.7
    - old (postpartal) 618.7
  - organ NEC
    - with
      - abortion - see Abortion, by type, with damage to pelvic organs
      - ectopic pregnancy (see also categories 633.0–633.9) 639.2
      - molar pregnancy (see also categories 630–632) 639.2
    - complicating delivery 665.5●
      - affecting fetus or newborn 763.89
    - following
      - abortion 639.2
      - ectopic or molar pregnancy 639.2
    - obstetrical trauma 665.5●

Laceration (Continued)
- perineum, perineal (old) (postpartal) 618.7
  - with
    - abortion - see Abortion, by type, with damage to pelvic floor
    - ectopic pregnancy (see also categories 633.0–633.9) 639.2
    - molar pregnancy (see also categories 630–632) 639.2
  - complicating delivery 664.4●
    - first degree 664.0●
    - second degree 664.1●
    - third degree 664.2●
    - fourth degree 664.3●
    - central 664.4●
    - involving
      - anal sphincter (healed) (old) 654.8●
      - fourchette 664.0●
      - hymen 664.0●
      - labia 664.0●
      - not associated with third-degree perineal laceration 664.6●
      - pelvic floor 664.1●
      - perineal muscles 664.1●
      - rectovaginal with septum 664.2●
        - with anal mucosa 664.3●
      - skin 664.0●
      - sphincter (anal) (healed) (old) 654.8●
        - with anal mucosa 664.3●
        - not associated with third-degree perineal laceration 664.6●
      - vagina 664.0●
      - vaginal muscles 664.1●
      - vulva 664.0●
    - secondary 674.2●
  - following
    - abortion 639.2
    - ectopic or molar pregnancy 639.2
  - male 879.6
    - complicated 879.7
  - muscles, complicating delivery 664.1●
  - nonpuerperal, current injury 879.6
    - complicated 879.7
  - secondary (postpartal) 674.2●
- peritoneum
  - with
    - abortion - see Abortion, by type, with damage to pelvic organs
    - ectopic pregnancy (see also categories 633.0–633.9) 639.2
    - molar pregnancy (see also categories 630–632) 639.2
  - following
    - abortion 639.2
    - ectopic or molar pregnancy 639.2
  - obstetrical trauma 665.5●
- periurethral tissue
  - with
    - abortion - see Abortion, by type, with damage to pelvic organs
    - ectopic pregnancy (see also categories 633.0–633.9) 639.2
    - molar pregnancy (see also categories 630–632) 639.2
  - following
    - abortion 639.2
    - ectopic or molar pregnancy 639.2
  - obstetrical trauma 664.8●
- rectovaginal (septum)
  - with
    - abortion - see Abortion, by type, with damage to pelvic organs
    - ectopic pregnancy (see also categories 633.0–633.9) 639.2
    - molar pregnancy (see also categories 630–632) 639.2
  - complicating delivery 665.4●
    - with perineum 664.2●
      - involving anal or rectal mucosa 664.3●

Laceration (Continued)
- rectovaginal (Continued)
  - following
    - abortion 639.2
    - ectopic or molar pregnancy 639.2
  - nonpuerperal 623.4
  - old (postpartal) 623.4
- spinal cord (meninges) - see also Injury, spinal, by site
  - due to injury at birth 767.4
  - fetus or newborn 767.4
- spleen 865.09
  - with
    - disruption of parenchyma (massive) 865.04
      - with open wound into cavity 865.14
    - open wound into cavity 865.19
    - capsule (without disruption of parenchyma) 865.02
      - with open wound into cavity 865.12
    - parenchyma 865.03
      - with open wound into cavity 865.13
      - massive disruption (rupture) 865.04
        - with open wound into cavity 865.14
- tendon 848.9
  - with open wound - see Wound, open, by site
  - Achilles 845.09
    - with open wound 892.2
  - lower limb NEC 844.9
    - with open wound NEC 894.2
  - upper limb NEC 840.9
    - with open wound NEC 884.2
- tentorium cerebelli - see Laceration, brain, cerebellum
- tongue 873.64
  - complicated 873.74
- urethra
  - with
    - abortion - see Abortion, by type, with damage to pelvic organs
    - ectopic pregnancy (see also categories 633.0–633.9) 639.2
    - molar pregnancy (see also categories 630–632) 639.2
  - following
    - abortion 639.2
    - ectopic or molar pregnancy 639.2
  - nonpuerperal, nontraumatic 599.84
  - obstetrical trauma 665.5●
- uterus
  - with
    - abortion - see Abortion, by type, with damage to pelvic organs
    - ectopic pregnancy (see also categories 633.0–633.9) 639.2
    - molar pregnancy (see also categories 630–632) 639.2
  - following
    - abortion 639.2
    - ectopic or molar pregnancy 639.2
  - nonpuerperal, nontraumatic 621.8
  - obstetrical trauma NEC 665.5●
  - old (postpartal) 621.8
- vagina
  - with
    - abortion - see Abortion, by type, with damage to pelvic organs
    - ectopic pregnancy (see also categories 633.0–633.9) 639.2
    - molar pregnancy (see also categories 630–632) 639.2
    - perineal involvement, complicating delivery 664.0●
  - complicating delivery 665.4●
    - first degree 664.0●
    - second degree 664.1●
    - third degree 664.2●
    - fourth degree 664.3●
    - high 665.4●
    - muscles 664.1●

SECTION I INDEX TO DISEASES AND INJURIES / Laceration

Laceration (Continued)
- vagina (Continued)
  - complicating delivery (Continued)
    - sulcus 665.4●
    - wall 665.4●
  - following
    - abortion 639.2
    - ectopic or molar pregnancy 639.2
  - nonpuerperal, nontraumatic 623.4
  - old (postpartal) 623.4
- valve, heart - see Endocarditis
- vulva
  - with
    - abortion - see Abortion, by type, with damage to pelvic organs
    - ectopic pregnancy (see also categories 633.0–633.9) 639.2
    - molar pregnancy (see also categories 630–632) 639.2
  - complicating delivery 664.0●
  - following
    - abortion 639.2
    - ectopic or molar pregnancy 639.2
  - nonpuerperal, nontraumatic 624.4
  - old (postpartal) 624.4

Lachrymal - see condition
Lachrymonasal duct - see condition
Lack of
- adequate intermaxillary vertical dimension 524.36
- appetite (see also Anorexia) 783.0
- care
  - in home V60.4
  - of adult 995.84
  - of infant (at or after birth) 995.52
- coordination 781.3
- development - see also Hypoplasia
  - physiological in childhood 783.40
- education V62.3
- energy 780.79
- financial resources V60.2
- food 994.2
  - in environment V60.89
- growth in childhood 783.43
- heating V60.1
- housing (permanent) (temporary) V60.0
  - adequate V60.1
- material resources V60.2
- medical attention 799.89
- memory (see also Amnesia) 780.93
  - mild, following organic brain damage 310.89
- ovulation 628.0
- person able to render necessary care V60.4
- physical exercise V69.0
- physiologic development in childhood 783.40
- posterior occlusal support 524.57
- prenatal care in current pregnancy V23.7
- shelter V60.0
- sleep V69.4
- water 994.3

Lacrimal - see condition
Lacrimation, abnormal (see also Epiphora) 375.20
Lacrimonasal duct - see condition
Lactation, lactating (breast) (puerperal) (postpartum)
- defective 676.4●
- disorder 676.9●
  - specified type NEC 676.8●
- excessive 676.6●
- failed 676.4●
- mastitis NEC 675.2●
- mother (care and/or examination) V24.1
- nonpuerperal 611.6
- suppressed 676.5●

Lacticemia 271.3
- excessive 276.2

Lactosuria 271.3
Lacunar skull 756.0
Laennec's cirrhosis (alcoholic) 571.2
- nonalcoholic 571.5

Lafora's disease 333.2
Lag, lid (nervous) 374.41
Lagleyze-von Hippel disease (retinocerebral angiomatosis) 759.6
Lagophthalmos (eyelid) (nervous) 374.20
- cicatricial 374.23
- keratitis (see also Keratitis) 370.34
- mechanical 374.22
- paralytic 374.21

La grippe - see Influenza
Lahore sore 085.1
Lakes, venous (cerebral) 437.8
Laki-Lorand factor deficiency (see also Defect, coagulation) 286.3
Lalling 307.9
Lambliasis 007.1
Lame back 724.5
Lancereaux's diabetes (diabetes mellitus with marked emaciation) 250.8● [261]
- due to secondary diabetes 249.8● [261]

Landau-Kleffner syndrome 345.8●
Landouzy-Déjérine dystrophy (fascioscapulohumeral atrophy) 359.1
Landry's disease or paralysis 357.0
Landry-Guillain-Barré syndrome 357.0
Lane's
- band 751.4
- disease 569.89
- kink (see also Obstruction, intestine) 560.9

Langdon Down's syndrome (mongolism) 758.0
Language abolition 784.69
Lanugo (persistent) 757.4
Laparoscopic surgical procedure converted to open procedure V64.41
Lardaceous
- degeneration (any site) 277.39
- disease 277.39
- kidney 277.39 [583.81]
- liver 277.39

Large
- baby (regardless of gestational age) 766.1
  - exceptionally (weight of 4500 grams or more) 766.0
  - of diabetic mother 775.0
- ear 744.22
- fetus - see also Oversize, fetus
  - causing disproportion 653.5●
    - with obstructed labor 660.1●
  - for dates
    - fetus or newborn (regardless of gestational age) 766.1
      - affecting management of pregnancy 656.6●
    - exceptionally (weight of 4500 grams or more) 766.0
- physiological cup 743.57
- stature 783.9
- waxy liver 277.39
- white kidney - see Nephrosis

Larsen's syndrome (flattened facies and multiple congenital dislocations) 755.8
Larsen-Johansson disease (juvenile osteopathia patellae) 732.4
Larva migrans
- cutaneous NEC 126.9
  - ancylostoma 126.9
- of Diptera in vitreous 128.0
- visceral NEC 128.0

Laryngeal - see also condition
- syncope 786.2

Laryngismus (acute) (infectious) (stridulous) 478.75
- congenital 748.3
- diphtheritic 032.3

Laryngitis (acute) (edematous) (fibrinous) (gangrenous) (infective) (infiltrative) (malignant) (membranous) (phlegmonous) (pneumococcal) (pseudomembranous) (septic) (subglottic) (suppurative) (ulcerative) (viral) 464.00
- with
  - influenza, flu, or grippe (see also Influenza) 487.1
  - obstruction 464.01
  - tracheitis (see also Laryngotracheitis) 464.20
    - with obstruction 464.21
    - acute 464.20
      - with obstruction 464.21
    - chronic 476.1
- atrophic 476.0
- Borrelia vincentii 101
- catarrhal 476.0
- chronic 476.0
  - with tracheitis (chronic) 476.1
  - due to external agent - see Condition, respiratory, chronic, due to
- diphtheritic (membranous) 032.3
- due to external agent - see Inflammation, respiratory, upper, due to
- H. influenzae 464.00
  - with obstruction 464.01
- Hemophilus influenzae 464.00
  - with obstruction 464.01
- hypertrophic 476.0
- influenzal (see also Influenza) 487.1
- pachydermic 478.79
- sicca 476.0
- spasmodic 478.75
  - acute 464.00
    - with obstruction 464.01
- streptococcal 034.0
- stridulous 478.75
- syphilitic 095.8
  - congenital 090.5
- tuberculous (see also Tuberculosis, larynx) 012.3●
- Vincent's 101

Laryngocele (congenital) (ventricular) 748.3
Laryngofissure 478.79
- congenital 748.3

Laryngomalacia (congenital) 748.3
Laryngopharyngitis (acute) 465.0
- chronic 478.9
- due to external agent - see Condition, respiratory, chronic, due to
- due to external agent - see Inflammation, respiratory, upper, due to
- septic 034.0

Laryngoplegia (see also Paralysis, vocal cord) 478.30
Laryngoptosis 478.79
Laryngospasm 478.75
- due to external agent - see Condition, respiratory, acute, due to

Laryngostenosis 478.74
- congenital 748.3

Laryngotracheitis (acute) (infectional) (viral) (see also Laryngitis) 464.20
- with obstruction 464.21
- atrophic 476.1
- Borrelia vincentii 101
- catarrhal 476.1
- chronic 476.1
  - due to external agent - see Condition, respiratory, chronic, due to
- diphtheritic (membranous) 032.3
- due to external agent - see Inflammation, respiratory, upper, due to
- H. influenzae 464.20
  - with obstruction 464.21
- hypertrophic 476.1
- influenzal (see also Influenza) 487.1
- pachydermic 478.75
- sicca 476.1

Laryngotracheitis *(Continued)*
  spasmodic 478.75
    acute 464.20
      with obstruction 464.21
  streptococcal 034.0
  stridulous 478.75
  syphilitic 095.8
    congenital 090.5
  tuberculous (*see also* Tuberculosis, larynx)
    012.3 ●
  Vincent's 101
Laryngotracheobronchitis (*see also* Bronchitis)
    490
  acute 466.0
  chronic 491.8
  viral 466.0
Laryngotracheobronchopneumonitis - *see*
    Pneumonia, broncho-
Larynx, laryngeal - *see* condition
Lasègue's disease (persecution mania) 297.9
Lassa fever 078.89
Lassitude (*see also* Weakness) 780.79
Late - *see also* condition
  effect(s) (of) - *see also* condition
    abscess
      intracranial or intraspinal (conditions
          classifiable to 324) - *see* category
          326
    adverse effect of drug, medicinal or
        biological substance 909.5
    allergic reaction 909.9
    amputation
      postoperative (late) 997.60
      traumatic (injury classifiable to
          885–887 and 895–897) 905.9
    burn (injury classifiable to 948–949) 906.9
      extremities NEC (injury classifiable to
          943 or 945) 906.7
        hand or wrist (injury classifiable to
            944) 906.6
      eye (injury classifiable to 940) 906.5
      face, head, and neck (injury classifiable
          to 941) 906.5
      specified site NEC (injury classifiable
          to 942 and 946–947) 906.8
    cerebrovascular disease (conditions
        classifiable to 430–437) 438.9
      with
        alterations of sensations 438.6
        aphasia 438.11
        apraxia 438.81
        ataxia 438.84
        cognitive deficits 438.0
        disturbances of vision 438.7
        dysarthria 438.13
        dysphagia 438.82
        dysphasia 438.12
        facial droop 438.83
        facial weakness 438.83
        fluency disorder 438.14
        hemiplegia/hemiparesis
          affecting
            dominant side 438.21
            nondominant side 438.22
            unspecified side 438.20
        monoplegia of lower limb
          affecting
            dominant side 438.41
            nondominant side 438.42
            unspecified side 438.40
        monoplegia of upper limb
          affecting
            dominant side 438.31
            nondominant side 438.32
            unspecified side 438.30
        paralytic syndrome NEC
          affecting
            bilateral 438.53
            dominant side 438.51
            nondominant side 438.52
            unspecified side 438.50

Late *(Continued)*
  effect(s) *(Continued)*
    cerebrovascular disease *(Continued)*
      with *(Continued)*
        speech and language deficit
            438.10
          specified type NEC 438.19
        stuttering 438.14
        vertigo 438.85
      specified type NEC 438.89
    childbirth complication(s) 677
    complication(s) of
      childbirth 677
      delivery 677
      pregnancy 677
      puerperium 677
      surgical and medical care (conditions
          classifiable to 996–999) 909.3
      trauma (conditions classifiable to 958)
          908.6
    contusion (injury classifiable to 920–924)
        906.3
    crushing (injury classifiable to 925–929)
        906.4
    delivery complication(s) 677
    dislocation (injury classifiable to 830–839)
        905.6
    encephalitis or encephalomyelitis
        (conditions classifiable to 323) - *see*
        category 326
      in infectious diseases 139.8
        viral (conditions classifiable to
            049.8, 049.9, 062–064) 139.0
    external cause NEC (conditions
        classifiable to 995) 909.9
      certain conditions classifiable to
          categories 991–994 909.4
    foreign body in orifice (injury classifiable
        to 930–939) 908.5
    fracture (multiple) (injury classifiable to
        828–829) 905.5
      extremity
        lower (injury classifiable to
            821–827) 905.4
          neck of femur (injury classifiable
              to 820) 905.3
        upper (injury classifiable to
            810–819) 905.2
      face and skull (injury classifiable to
          800–804) 905.0
      skull and face (injury classifiable to
          800–804) 905.0
      spine and trunk (injury classifiable to
          805 and 807–809) 905.1
        with spinal cord lesion (injury
            classifiable to 806) 907.2
    infection
      pyogenic, intracranial - *see* category
          326
    infectious diseases (conditions classifiable
        to 001–136) NEC 139.8
    injury (injury classifiable to 959)
        908.9
      blood vessel 908.3
        abdomen and pelvis (injury
            classifiable to 902) 908.4
        extremity (injury classifiable to
            903–904) 908.3
        head and neck (injury classifiable to
            900) 908.3
        intracranial (injury classifiable to
            850–854) 907.0
          with skull fracture 905.0
        thorax (injury classifiable to 901)
            908.4
        internal organ NEC (injury classifiable
            to 867 and 869) 908.2
          abdomen (injury classifiable to
              863–866 and 868) 908.1
          thorax (injury classifiable to
              860–862) 908.0

Late *(Continued)*
  effect(s) *(Continued)*
    injury *(Continued)*
      intracranial (injury classifiable to
          850–854) 907.0
        with skull fracture (injury
            classifiable to 800–801 and
            803–804) 905.0
      nerve NEC (injury classifiable to 957)
          907.9
        cranial (injury classifiable to
            950–951) 907.1
        peripheral NEC (injury classifiable
            to 957) 907.9
          lower limb and pelvic girdle
              (injury classifiable to 956)
              907.5
          upper limb and shoulder girdle
              (injury classifiable to 955)
              907.4
        roots and plexus(es), spinal (injury
            classifiable to 953) 907.3
        trunk (injury classifiable to 954)
            907.3
      spinal
        cord (injury classifiable to 806 and
            952) 907.2
        nerve root(s) and plexus(es) (injury
            classifiable to 953) 907.3
      superficial (injury classifiable to
          910–919) 906.2
      tendon (tendon injury classifiable to
          840–848, 880–884 with .2, and
          890–894 with .2) 905.8
    meningitis
      bacterial (conditions classifiable to
          320) - *see* category 326
      unspecified cause (conditions
          classifiable to 322) - *see* category
          326
    myelitis (*see also* Late, effect(s) (of),
        encephalitis) - *see* category 326
    parasitic diseases (conditions classifiable
        to 001–136 NEC) 139.8
    phlebitis or thrombophlebitis of
        intracranial venous sinuses
        (conditions classifiable to 325) - *see*
        category 326
    poisoning due to drug, medicinal or
        biological substance (conditions
        classifiable to 960–979) 909.0
    poliomyelitis, acute (conditions
        classifiable to 045) 138
    pregnancy complication(s) 677
    puerperal complication(s) 677
    radiation (conditions classifiable to 990)
        909.2
    rickets 268.1
    sprain and strain without mention of
        tendon injury (injury classifiable to
        840–848, except tendon injury) 905.7
      tendon involvement 905.8
    toxic effect of
      drug, medicinal or biological substance
          (conditions classifiable to
          960–979) 909.0
      nonmedical substance (conditions
          classifiable to 980–989) 909.1
    trachoma (conditions classifiable to 076)
        139.1
    tuberculosis 137.0
      bones and joints (conditions
          classifiable to 015) 137.3
      central nervous system (conditions
          classifiable to 013) 137.1
      genitourinary (conditions classifiable
          to 016) 137.2
      pulmonary (conditions classifiable to
          010–012) 137.0
      specified organs NEC (conditions
          classifiable to 014, 017–018) 137.4

Late (Continued)
  effect(s) (Continued)
    viral encephalitis (conditions classifiable to 049.8, 049.9, 062–064) 139.0
    wound, open
      extremity (injury classifiable to 880–884 and 890–894, except .2) 906.1
      tendon (injury classifiable to 880–884 with .2 and 890–894 with .2) 905.8
      head, neck, and trunk (injury classifiable to 870–879) 906.0
    infant
      post-term (gestation period over 40 completed weeks to 42 completed weeks) 766.21
      prolonged gestation (period over 42 completed weeks) 766.22
Latent - see condition
Lateral - see condition
Laterocession - see Lateroversion
Lateroflexion - see Lateroversion
Lateroversion
  cervix - see Lateroversion, uterus
  uterus, uterine (cervix) (postinfectional) (postpartal, old) 621.6
    congenital 752.39
    in pregnancy or childbirth 654.4●
      affecting fetus or newborn 763.89
Lathyrism 988.2
Launois' syndrome (pituitary gigantism) 253.0
Launois-Bensaude's lipomatosis 272.8
Launois-Cleret syndrome (adiposogenital dystrophy) 253.8
Laurence-Moon-Biedl syndrome (obesity, polydactyly, and intellectual disabilities) 759.89
LAV (disease) (illness) (infection) - see Human immunodeficiency virus (disease) (illness) (infection)
LAV/HTLV-III (disease) (illness) (infection) - see Human immunodeficiency virus (disease) (illness) (infection)
Lawford's syndrome (encephalocutaneous angiomatosis) 759.6
Lax, laxity - see also Relaxation
  ligament 728.4
  skin (acquired) 701.8
    congenital 756.83
Laxative habit (see also Abuse, drugs, nondependent) 305.9●
Lazy leukocyte syndrome 288.09
LCAD (long chain/very long chain acyl CoA dehydrogenase deficiency, VLCAD) 277.85
LCHAD (long chain 3-hydroxyacyl CoA dehydrogenase deficiency) 277.85
Lead - see also condition
  exposure (suspected) to V15.86
  incrustation of cornea 371.15
  poisoning 984.9
    specified type of lead - see Table of Drugs and Chemicals
Lead miners' lung 503
Leakage
  amniotic fluid 658.1●
    with delayed delivery 658.2●
      affecting fetus or newborn 761.1
  bile from drainage tube (T tube) 997.49
  blood (microscopic), fetal, into maternal circulation 656.0●
    affecting management of pregnancy or puerperium 656.0●
  device, implant, or graft - see Complications, mechanical
  spinal fluid at lumbar puncture site 997.09
  urine, continuous 788.37
Leaky heart - see Endocarditis
Learning defect, specific NEC (strephosymbolia) 315.2

Leather bottle stomach (M8142/3) 151.9
Leber's
  congenital amaurosis 362.76
  optic atrophy (hereditary) 377.16
Lederer's anemia or disease (acquired infectious hemolytic anemia) 283.19
Lederer-Brill syndrome (acquired infectious hemolytic anemia) 283.19
Leeches (aquatic) (land) 134.2
Left-sided neglect 781.8
Leg - see condition
Legal investigation V62.5
Legg (-Calvé)-Perthes disease or syndrome (osteochondrosis, femoral capital) 732.1
Legionnaires' disease 482.84
Leigh's disease 330.8
Leiner's disease (exfoliative dermatitis) 695.89
Leiofibromyoma (M8890/0) - see also Leiomyoma
  uterus (cervix) (corpus) (see also Leiomyoma, uterus) 218.9
Leiomyoblastoma (M8891/1) - see Neoplasm, connective tissue, uncertain behavior
Leiomyofibroma (M8890/0) - see also Neoplasm, connective tissue, benign
  uterus (cervix) (corpus) (see also Leiomyoma, uterus) 218.9
Leiomyoma (M8890/0) - see also Neoplasm, connective tissue, benign
  bizarre (M8893/0) - see Neoplasm, connective tissue, benign
  cellular (M8892/1) - see Neoplasm, connective tissue, uncertain behavior
  epithelioid (M8891/1) - see Neoplasm, connective tissue, uncertain behavior
  prostate (polypoid) 600.20
    with
      other lower urinary tract symptoms (LUTS) 600.21
      urinary
        obstruction 600.21
        retention 600.21
  uterus (cervix) (corpus) 218.9
    interstitial 218.1
    intramural 218.1
    submucous 218.0
    subperitoneal 218.2
    subserous 218.2
  vascular (M8894/0) - see Neoplasm, connective tissue, benign
Leiomyomatosis (intravascular) (M8890/1) - see Neoplasm, connective tissue, uncertain behavior
Leiomyosarcoma (M8890/3) - see also Neoplasm, connective tissue, malignant
  epithelioid (M8891/3) - see Neoplasm, connective tissue, malignant
Leishmaniasis 085.9
  American 085.5
    cutaneous 085.4
    mucocutaneous 085.5
  Asian desert 085.2
  Brazilian 085.5
  cutaneous 085.9
    acute necrotizing 085.2
    American 085.4
    Asian desert 085.2
    diffuse 085.3
    dry form 085.1
    Ethiopian 085.3
    eyelid 085.5 [373.6]
    late 085.1
    lepromatous 085.3
    recurrent 085.1
    rural 085.2
    ulcerating 085.1
    urban 085.1
    wet form 085.2
    zoonotic form 085.2
  dermal - see also Leishmaniasis, cutaneous
    post kala-azar 085.0

Leishmaniasis (Continued)
  eyelid 085.5 [373.6]
  infantile 085.0
  Mediterranean 085.0
  mucocutaneous (American) 085.5
  naso-oral 085.5
  nasopharyngeal 085.5
  Old World 085.1
  tegumentaria diffusa 085.4
  vaccination, prophylactic (against) V05.2
  visceral (Indian) 085.0
Leishmanoid, dermal - see also Leishmaniasis, cutaneous
  post kala-azar 085.0
Leloir's disease 695.4
Lemiere syndrome 451.89
Lenegre's disease 426.0
Lengthening, leg 736.81
Lennox-Gastaut syndrome 345.0●
  with tonic seizures 345.1●
Lennox's syndrome (see also Epilepsy) 345.0●
Lens - see condition
Lenticonus (anterior) (posterior) (congenital) 743.36
Lenticular degeneration, progressive 275.1
Lentiglobus (posterior) (congenital) 743.36
Lentigo (congenital) 709.09
  juvenile 709.09
  Maligna (M8742/2) - see also Neoplasm, skin, in situ
    melanoma (M8742/3) - see Melanoma
  senile 709.09
Leonine leprosy 030.0
Leontiasis
  ossium 733.3
  syphilitic 095.8
    congenital 090.5
Léopold-Lévi's syndrome (paroxysmal thyroid instability) 242.9●
Lepore hemoglobin syndrome 282.45
Lepothrix 039.0
Lepra 030.9
  Willan's 696.1
Leprechaunism 259.8
Lepromatous leprosy 030.0
Leprosy 030.9
  anesthetic 030.1
  beriberi 030.1
  borderline (group B) (infiltrated) (neuritic) 030.3
  cornea (see also Leprosy, by type) 030.9 [371.89]
  dimorphous (group B) (infiltrated) (lepromatous) (neuritic) (tuberculoid) 030.3
  eyelid 030.0 [373.4]
  indeterminate (group I) (macular) (neuritic) (uncharacteristic) 030.2
  leonine 030.0
  lepromatous (diffuse) (infiltrated) (macular) (neuritic) (nodular) (type L) 030.0
  macular (early) (neuritic) (simple) 030.2
  maculoanesthetic 030.1
  mixed 030.0
  neuro 030.1
  nodular 030.0
  primary neuritic 030.3
  specified type or group NEC 030.8
  tubercular 030.1
  tuberculoid (macular) (maculoanesthetic) (major) (minor) (neuritic) (type T) 030.1
Leptocytosis, hereditary 282.40
Leptomeningitis (chronic) (circumscribed) (hemorrhagic) (nonsuppurative) (see also Meningitis) 322.9
  aseptic 047.9
    adenovirus 049.1
    Coxsackie virus 047.0
    ECHO virus 047.1
    enterovirus 047.9
    lymphocytic choriomeningitis 049.0

Leptomeningitis (Continued)
  epidemic 036.0
  late effect - see category 326
  meningococcal 036.0
  pneumococcal 320.1
  syphilitic 094.2
  tuberculous (see also Tuberculosis, meninges) 013.0●
Leptomeningopathy (see also Meningitis) 322.9
Leptospiral - see condition
Leptospirochetal - see condition
Leptospirosis 100.9
  autumnalis 100.89
  canicula 100.89
  grippotyphosa 100.89
  hebdomadis 100.89
  icterohemorrhagica 100.0
  nanukayami 100.89
  pomona 100.89
  Weil's disease 100.0
Leptothricosis - see Actinomycosis
Leptothrix infestation - see Actinomycosis
Leptotricosis - see Actinomycosis
Leptus dermatitis 133.8
Léris pleonosteosis 756.89
Léri-Weill syndrome 756.59
Leriche's syndrome (aortic bifurcation occlusion) 444.09
Lermoyez's syndrome (see also Disease, Ménière's) 386.00
Lesbianism - *omit code*
  ego-dystonic 302.0
  problems with 302.0
Lesch-Nyhan syndrome (hypoxanthine-guanine-phosphoribosyltransferase deficiency) 277.2
Lesion(s)
  abducens nerve 378.54
  alveolar process 525.8
  anorectal 569.49
  aortic (valve) - see Endocarditis, aortic
  auditory nerve 388.5
  basal ganglion 333.90
  bile duct (see also Disease, biliary) 576.8
  bladder 596.9
  bone 733.90
  brachial plexus 353.0
  brain 348.89
    congenital 742.9
    vascular (see also Lesion, cerebrovascular) 437.9
      degenerative 437.1
      healed or old without residuals V12.54
      hypertensive 437.2
      late effect - see Late effect(s) (of) cerebrovascular disease
  buccal 528.9
  calcified - see Calcification
  canthus 373.9
  carate - see Pinta, lesions
  cardia 537.89
  cardiac - see also Disease, heart
    congenital 746.9
    valvular - see Endocarditis
  cauda equina 344.60
    with neurogenic bladder 344.61
  cecum 569.89
  cerebral - see Lesion, brain
  cerebrovascular (see also Disease, cerebrovascular NEC) 437.9
    degenerative 437.1
    healed or old without residuals V12.54
    hypertensive 437.2
    specified type NEC 437.8
  cervical root (nerve) NEC 353.2
  chiasmal 377.54
    associated with
      inflammatory disorders 377.54
      neoplasm NEC 377.52
        pituitary 377.51

Lesion(s) (Continued)
  chiasmal (Continued)
    associated with (Continued)
      pituitary disorders 377.51
      vascular disorders 377.53
  chorda tympani 351.8
  coin, lung 793.11
  colon 569.89
  congenital - see Anomaly
  conjunctiva 372.9
  coronary artery (see also Ischemia, heart) 414.9
  cranial nerve 352.9
    first 352.0
    second 377.49
    third
      partial 378.51
      total 378.52
    fourth 378.53
    fifth 350.9
    sixth 378.54
    seventh 351.9
    eighth 388.5
    ninth 352.2
    tenth 352.3
    eleventh 352.4
    twelfth 352.5
  cystic - see Cyst
  degenerative - see Degeneration
  dermal (skin) 709.9
  Dieulafoy (hemorrhagic)
    of
      duodenum 537.84
      intestine 569.86
      stomach 537.84
  duodenum 537.89
    with obstruction 537.3
  eyelid 373.9
  gasserian ganglion 350.8
  gastric 537.89
  gastroduodenal 537.89
  gastrointestinal 569.89
  glossopharyngeal nerve 352.2
  heart (organic) - see also Disease, heart
    vascular - see Disease, cardiovascular
  helix (ear) 709.9
  high grade myelodysplastic syndrome 238.73
  hyperchromic, due to pinta (carate) 103.1
  hyperkeratotic (see also Hyperkeratosis) 701.1
  hypoglossal nerve 352.5
  hypopharynx 478.29
  hypothalamic 253.9
  ileocecal coil 569.89
  ileum 569.89
  iliohypogastric nerve 355.79
  ilioinguinal nerve 355.79
  in continuity - see Injury, nerve, by site
  inflammatory - see Inflammation
  intestine 569.89
  intracerebral - see Lesion, brain
  intrachiasmal (optic) (see also Lesion, chiasmal) 377.54
  intracranial, space-occupying NEC 784.2
  joint 719.90
    ankle 719.97
    elbow 719.92
    foot 719.97
    hand 719.94
    hip 719.95
    knee 719.96
    multiple sites 719.99
    pelvic region 719.95
    sacroiliac (old) 724.6
    shoulder (region) 719.91
    specified site NEC 719.98
    wrist 719.93
  keratotic (see also Keratosis) 701.1
  kidney (see also Disease, renal) 593.9
  laryngeal nerve (recurrent) 352.3
  leonine 030.0
  lip 528.5

Lesion(s) (Continued)
  liver 573.8
  low grade myelodysplastic syndrome 238.72
  lumbosacral
    plexus 353.1
    root (nerve) NEC 353.4
  lung 518.89
    coin 793.11
  maxillary sinus 473.0
  mitral - see Endocarditis, mitral
  Morel Lavallée - see Hematoma, by site
  motor cortex 348.89
  nerve (see also Disorder, nerve) 355.9
  nervous system 349.9
    congenital 742.9
  nonallopathic NEC 739.9
    in region (of)
      abdomen 739.9
      acromioclavicular 739.7
      cervical, cervicothoracic 739.1
      costochondral 739.8
      costovertebral 739.8
      extremity
        lower 739.6
        upper 739.7
      head 739.0
      hip 739.5
      lower extremity 739.6
      lumbar, lumbosacral 739.3
      occipitocervical 739.0
      pelvic 739.5
      pubic 739.5
      rib cage 739.8
      sacral, sacrococcygeal, sacroiliac 739.4
      sternochondral 739.8
      sternoclavicular 739.7
      thoracic, thoracolumbar 739.2
      upper extremity 739.7
  nose (internal) 478.19
  obstructive - see Obstruction
  obturator nerve 355.79
  occlusive
    artery - see Embolism, artery
    organ or site NEC - see Disease, by site
  osteolytic 733.90
  paramacular, of retina 363.32
  peptic 537.89
  periodontal, due to traumatic occlusion 523.8
  perirectal 569.49
  peritoneum (granulomatous) 568.89
  pigmented (skin) 709.00
  pinta - see Pinta, lesions
  polypoid - see Polyp
  prechiasmal (optic) (see also Lesion, chiasmal) 377.54
  primary - see also Syphilis, primary
    carate 103.0
    pinta 103.0
    yaws 102.0
  pulmonary 518.89
    valve (see also Endocarditis, pulmonary) 424.3
  pylorus 537.89
  radiation NEC 990
  radium NEC 990
  rectosigmoid 569.89
  retina, retinal - see also Retinopathy
    vascular 362.17
  retroperitoneal 568.89
  romanus 720.1
  sacroiliac (joint) 724.6
  salivary gland 527.8
    benign lymphoepithelial 527.8
  saphenous nerve 355.79
  secondary - see Syphilis, secondary
  sigmoid 569.89
  sinus (accessory) (nasal) (see also Sinusitis) 473.9
  skin 709.9
    suppurative 686.00
  SLAP (superior glenoid labrum) 840.7

SECTION 1 INDEX TO DISEASES AND INJURIES / Lesion(s)

Lesion(s) *(Continued)*
- space-occupying, intracranial NEC 784.2
- spinal cord 336.9
  - congenital 742.9
  - traumatic (complete) (incomplete) (transverse) - *see also* Injury, spinal, by site
    - with
      - broken
        - back - *see* Fracture, vertebra, by site, with spinal cord injury
        - neck - *see* Fracture, vertebra, cervical, with spinal cord injury
      - fracture, vertebra - *see* Fracture, vertebra, by site, with spinal cord injury
- spleen 289.50
- stomach 537.89
- superior glenoid labrum (SLAP) 840.7
- syphilitic - *see* Syphilis
- tertiary - *see* Syphilis, tertiary
- thoracic root (nerve) 353.3
- tonsillar fossa 474.9
- tooth, teeth 525.8
  - white spot 521.01
- traumatic NEC (*see also* nature and site of injury) 959.9
- tricuspid (valve) - *see* Endocarditis, tricuspid
- trigeminal nerve 350.9
- ulcerated or ulcerative - *see* Ulcer
- uterus NEC 621.9
- vagina 623.8
- vagus nerve 352.3
- valvular - *see* Endocarditis
- vascular 459.9
  - affecting central nervous system (*see also* Lesion, cerebrovascular) 437.9
  - following trauma (*see also* Injury, blood vessel, by site) 904.9
  - retina 362.17
  - traumatic - *see* Injury, blood vessel, by site
  - umbilical cord 663.6●
    - affecting fetus or newborn 762.6
- visual
  - cortex NEC (*see also* Disorder, visual, cortex) 377.73
  - pathway NEC (*see also* Disorder, visual, pathway) 377.63
- warty - *see* Verruca
- white spot, on teeth 521.01
- x-ray NEC 990

Lethargic - *see* condition
Lethargy 780.79
Letterer-Siwe disease (acute histiocytosis X) (M9722/3) 202.5●
Leucinosis 270.3
Leucocoria 360.44
Leucosarcoma (M9850/3) 207.8●
Leukasmus 270.2
Leukemia, leukemic (congenital) (M9800/3) 208.9●

Note: Use the following fifth-digit subclassification for categories 203–208:
- 0 without mention of having achieved remission
      failed remission
- 1 with remission
- 2 in relapse

- acute NEC (M9801/3) 208.0●
- aleukemic NEC (M9804/3) 208.8●
  - granulocytic (M9864/3) 205.8●
- basophilic (M9870/3) 205.1●
- blast (cell) (M9801/3) 208.0●
- blastic (M9801/3) 208.0●
  - granulocytic (M9861/3) 205.0●
- chronic NEC (M9803/3) 208.1●
- compound (M9810/3) 207.8●

Leukemia, leukemic *(Continued)*
- eosinophilic (M9880/3) 205.1●
- giant cell (M9910/3) 207.2●
- granulocytic (M9860/3) 205.9●
  - acute (M9861/3) 205.0●
  - aleukemic (M9864/3) 205.8●
  - blastic (M9861/3) 205.0●
  - chronic (M9863/3) 205.1●
  - subacute (M9862/3) 205.2●
  - subleukemic (M9864/3) 205.8●
- hairy cell (M9940/3) 202.4●
- hemoblastic (M9801/3) 208.0●
- histiocytic (M9890/3) 206.9●
- lymphatic (M9820/3) 204.9●
  - acute (M9821/3) 204.0●
  - aleukemic (M9824/3) 204.8●
  - chronic (M9823/3) 204.1●
  - subacute (M9822/3) 204.2●
  - subleukemic (M9824/3) 204.8●
- lymphoblastic (M9821/3) 204.0●
- lymphocytic (M9820/3) 204.9●
  - acute (M9821/3) 204.0●
  - aleukemic (M9824/3) 204.8●
  - chronic (M9823/3) 204.1●
  - granular
    - large T-cell 204.8●
  - subacute (M9822/3) 204.2●
  - subleukemic (M9824/3) 204.8●
- lymphogenous (M9820/3) - *see* Leukemia, lymphoid
- lymphoid (M9820/3) 204.9●
  - acute (M9821/3) 204.0●
  - aleukemic (M9824/3) 204.8●
  - blastic (M9821/3) 204.0●
  - chronic (M9823/3) 204.1●
  - subacute (M9822/3) 204.2●
  - subleukemic (M9824/3) 204.8●
- lymphosarcoma cell (M9850/3) 207.8●
- mast cell (M9900/3) 207.8●
- megakaryocytic (M9910/3) 207.2●
- megakaryocytoid (M9910/3) 207.2●
- mixed (cell) (M9810/3) 207.8●
- monoblastic (M9891/3) 206.0●
- monocytic (Schilling-type) (M9890/3) 206.9●
  - acute (M9891/3) 206.0●
  - aleukemic (M9894/3) 206.8●
  - chronic (M9893/3) 206.1●
  - Naegeli-type (M9863/3) 205.1●
  - subacute (M9892/3) 206.2●
  - subleukemic (M9894/3) 206.8●
- monocytoid (M9890/3) 206.9●
  - acute (M9891/3) 206.0●
  - aleukemic (M9894/3) 206.8●
  - chronic (M9893/3) 206.1●
  - myelogenous (M9863/3) 205.1●
  - subacute (M9892/3) 206.2●
  - subleukemic (M9894/3) 206.8●
- monomyelocytic (M9860/3) - *see* Leukemia, myelomonocytic
- myeloblastic (M9861/3) 205.0●
- myelocytic (M9863/3) 205.1●
  - acute (M9861/3) 205.0●
- myelogenous (M9860/3) 205.9●
  - acute (M9861/3) 205.0●
  - aleukemic (M9864/3) 205.8●
  - chronic (M9863/3) 205.1●
  - monocytoid (M9863/3) 205.1●
  - subacute (M9862/3) 205.2●
  - subleukemic (M9864) 205.8●
- myeloid (M9860/3) 205.9●
  - acute (M9861/3) 205.0●
  - aleukemic (M9864/3) 205.8●
  - chronic (M9863/3) 205.1●
  - subacute (M9862/3) 205.2●
  - subleukemic (M9864/3) 205.8●
- myelomonocytic (M9860/3) 205.9●
  - acute (M9861/3) 205.0●
  - chronic (M9863/3) 205.1●
- Naegeli-type monocytic (M9863/3) 205.1●
- neutrophilic (M9865/3) 205.1●
- plasma cell (M9830/3) 203.1●

Leukemia, leukemic *(Continued)*
- plasmacytic (M9830/3) 203.1●
- prolymphocytic (M9825/3) - *see* Leukemia, lymphoid
- promyelocytic, acute (M9866/3) 205.0●
- Schilling-type monocytic (M9890/3) - *see* Leukemia, monocytic
- stem cell (M9801/3) 208.0●
- subacute NEC (M9802/3) 208.2●
- subleukemic NEC (M9804/3) 208.8●
- thrombocytic (M9910/3) 207.2●
- undifferentiated (M9801/3) 208.0●

Leukemoid reaction (basophilic) (lymphocytic) (monocytic) (myelocytic) (neutrophilic) 288.62
Leukoaraiosis (hypertensive) 437.1
Leukoariosis - *see* Leukoaraiosis
Leukoclastic vasculitis 446.29
Leukocoria 360.44
Leukocythemia - *see* Leukemia
Leukocytopenia 288.50
Leukocytosis 288.60
- basophilic 288.8
- eosinophilic 288.3
- lymphocytic 288.8
- monocytic 288.8
- neutrophilic 288.8

Leukoderma 709.09
- syphilitic 091.3
- late 095.8

Leukodermia (*see also* Leukoderma) 709.09
Leukodystrophy (cerebral) (globoid cell) (metachromatic) (progressive) (sudanophilic) 330.0
Leukoedema, mouth or tongue 528.79
Leukoencephalitis
- acute hemorrhagic (postinfectious) NEC 136.9 [323.61]
  - postimmunization or postvaccinal 323.51
- subacute sclerosing 046.2
  - van Bogaert's 046.2
- van Bogaert's (sclerosing) 046.2

Leukoencephalopathy (*see also* Encephalitis) 323.9
- acute necrotizing hemorrhagic (postinfectious) 136.9 [323.61]
  - postimmunization or postvaccinal 323.51
- arteriosclerotic 437.0
- Binswanger's 290.12
- metachromatic 330.0
- multifocal (progressive) 046.3
- progressive multifocal 046.3
- reversible, posterior 348.5

Leukoerythroblastosis 289.9
Leukoerythrosis 289.0
Leukokeratosis (*see also* Leukoplakia) 702.8
- mouth 528.6
- nicotina palati 528.79
- tongue 528.6

Leukokoria 360.44
Leukokraurosis vulva, vulvae 624.09
Leukolymphosarcoma (M9850/3) 207.8●
Leukoma (cornea) (interfering with central vision) 371.03
- adherent 371.04

Leukomalacia, periventricular 779.7
Leukomelanopathy, hereditary 288.2
Leukonychia (punctata) (striata) 703.8
- congenital 757.5

Leukopathia
- unguium 703.8
  - congenital 757.5

Leukopenia 288.50
- basophilic 288.59
- cyclic 288.02
- eosinophilic 288.59
- familial 288.59
- malignant (*see also* Agranulocytosis) 288.09
- periodic 288.02
- transitory neonatal 776.7

Leukopenic - see condition
Leukoplakia 702.8
    anus 569.49
    bladder (postinfectional) 596.89
    buccal 528.6
    cervix (uteri) 622.2
    esophagus 530.83
    gingiva 528.6
    kidney (pelvis) 593.89
    larynx 478.79
    lip 528.6
    mouth 528.6
    oral soft tissue (including tongue) (mucosa) 528.6
    palate 528.6
    pelvis (kidney) 593.89
    penis (infectional) 607.0
    rectum 569.49
    syphilitic 095.8
    tongue 528.6
    tonsil 478.29
    ureter (postinfectional) 593.89
    urethra (postinfectional) 599.84
    uterus 621.8
    vagina 623.1
    vesical 596.89
    vocal cords 478.5
    vulva 624.09
Leukopolioencephalopathy 330.0
Leukorrhea (vagina) 623.5
    due to Trichomonas (vaginalis) 131.00
    trichomonal (Trichomonas vaginalis) 131.00
Leukosarcoma (M9850/3) 207.8●
Leukosis (M9800/3) - see Leukemia
Lev's disease or syndrome (acquired complete heart block) 426.0
Levi's syndrome (pituitary dwarfism) 253.3
Levocardia (isolated) 746.87
    with situs inversus 759.3
Levulosuria 271.2
Lewandowski's disease (primary) (see also Tuberculosis) 017.0●
Lewandowski-Lutz disease (epidermodysplasia verruciformis) 078.19
Lewy body dementia 331.82
Lewy body disease 331.82
Leyden's disease (periodic vomiting) 536.2
Leyden-Möbius dystrophy 359.1
Leydig cell
    carcinoma (M8650/3)
        specified site - see Neoplasm, by site, malignant
        unspecified site
            female 183.0
            male 186.9
    tumor (M8650/1)
        benign (M8650/0)
            specified site - see Neoplasm, by site, benign
            unspecified site
                female 220
                male 222.0
        malignant (M8650/3)
            specified site - see Neoplasm, by site, malignant
            unspecified site
                female 183.0
                male 186.9
        specified site - see Neoplasm, by site, uncertain behavior
        unspecified site
            female 236.2
            male 236.4
Leydig-Sertoli cell tumor (M8631/0)
    specified site - see Neoplasm, by site, benign
    unspecified site
        female 220
        male 222.0

LGSIL (low grade squamous intraepithelial lesion)
    anus 796.73
    cervix 795.03
    vagina 795.13
Liar, pathologic 301.7
Libman-Sacks disease or syndrome 710.0 [424.91]
Lice (infestation) 132.9
    body (pediculus corporis) 132.1
    crab 132.2
    head (pediculus capitis) 132.0
    mixed (classifiable to more than one of the categories 132.0–132.2) 132.3
    pubic (pediculus pubis) 132.2
Lichen 697.9
    albus 701.0
    annularis 695.89
    atrophicus 701.0
    corneus obtusus 698.3
    myxedematous 701.8
    nitidus 697.1
    pilaris 757.39
        acquired 701.1
    planopilaris 697.0
    planus (acute) (chronicus) (hypertrophic) (verrucous) 697.0
        morphoeicus 701.0
        sclerosus (et atrophicus) 701.0
    ruber 696.4
        acuminatus 696.4
        moniliformis 697.8
        obtusus corneus 698.3
        of Wilson 697.0
        planus 697.0
    sclerosus (et atrophicus) 701.0
    scrofulosus (primary) (see also Tuberculosis) 017.0●
    simplex (Vidal's) 698.3
        chronicus 698.3
        circumscriptus 698.3
    spinulosus 757.39
        mycotic 117.9
    striata 697.8
    urticatus 698.2
Lichenification 698.3
    nodular 698.3
Lichenoides tuberculosis (primary) (see also Tuberculosis) 017.0
Lichtheim's disease or syndrome (subacute combined sclerosis with pernicious anemia) 281.0 [336.2]
Lien migrans 289.59
Lientery (see also Diarrhea) 787.91
    infectious 009.2
Life circumstance problem NEC V62.89
Li-Fraumeni cancer syndrome V84.01
Ligament - see condition
Light-for-dates (infant) 764.0●
    with signs of fetal malnutrition 764.1●
    affecting management of pregnancy 656.5●
Light-headedness 780.4
Lightning (effects) (shock) (stroke) (struck by) 994.0
    burn - see Burn, by site
    foot 266.2
Lightwood's disease or syndrome (renal tubular acidosis) 588.89
Lignac's disease (cystinosis) 270.0
Lignac (-de Toni) (-Fanconi) (-Debré) syndrome (cystinosis) 270.0
Lignac (-Fanconi) syndrome (cystinosis) 270.0
Ligneous thyroiditis 245.3
Likoff's syndrome (angina in menopausal women) 413.9
Limb - see condition
Limitation of joint motion (see also Stiffness, joint) 719.5●
    sacroiliac 724.6
Limit dextrinosis 271.0

Limited
    cardiac reserve - see Disease, heart
    duction, eye NEC 378.63
    mandibular range of motion 524.52
Lindau's disease (retinocerebral angiomatosis) 759.6
Lindau (-von Hippel) disease (angiomatosis retinocerebellosa) 759.6
Linea corneae senilis 371.41
Lines
    Beau's (transverse furrows on fingernails) 703.8
    Harris' 733.91
    Hudson-Stähli 371.11
    Stähli's 371.11
Lingua
    geographical 529.1
    nigra (villosa) 529.3
    plicata 529.5
        congenital 750.13
    tylosis 528.6
Lingual (tongue) - see also condition
    thyroid 759.2
Linitis (gastric) 535.4●
    plastica (M8142/3) 151.9
Lioderma essentialis (cum melanosis et telangiectasia) 757.33
Lip - see also condition
    biting 528.9
Lipalgia 272.8
Lipedema - see Edema
Lipemia (see also Hyperlipidemia) 272.4
    retina, retinalis 272.3
Lipidosis 272.7
    cephalin 272.7
    cerebral (infantile) (juvenile) (late) 330.1
    cerebroretinal 330.1 [362.71]
    cerebroside 272.7
    cerebrospinal 272.7
    chemically-induced 272.7
    cholesterol 272.7
    diabetic 250.8● [272.7]
        due to secondary diabetes 249.8● [272.7]
    dystopic (hereditary) 272.7
    glycolipid 272.7
    hepatosplenomegalic 272.3
    hereditary, dystopic 272.7
    sulfatide 330.0
Lipoadenoma (M8324/0 - see Neoplasm, by site, benign
Lipoblastoma (M8881/0) - see Lipoma, by site
Lipoblastomatosis (M8881/0) - see Lipoma, by site
Lipochondrodystrophy 277.5
Lipochrome histiocytosis (familial) 288.1
Lipodermatosclerosis 729.39
Lipodystrophia progressiva 272.6
Lipodystrophy (progressive) 272.6
    insulin 272.6
    intestinal 040.2
    mesenteric 567.82
Lipofibroma (M8851/0) - see Lipoma, by site
Lipoglycoproteinosis 272.8
Lipogranuloma, sclerosing 709.8
Lipogranulomatosis (disseminated) 272.8
    kidney 272.8
Lipoid - see also condition
    histiocytosis 272.7
        essential 272.7
    nephrosis (see also Nephrosis) 581.3
    proteinosis of Urbach 272.8
Lipoidemia (see also Hyperlipidemia) 272.4
Lipoidosis (see also Lipidosis) 272.7
Lipoma (M8850/0) 214.9
    breast (skin) 214.1
    face 214.0
    fetal (M8881/0) - see also Lipoma, by site
        fat cell (M8880/0) - see Lipoma, by site
    infiltrating (M8856/0) - see Lipoma, by site
    intra-abdominal 214.3

SECTION 1 INDEX TO DISEASES AND INJURIES / Lipoma

Lipoma (Continued)
- intramuscular (M8856/0) - see Lipoma, by site
- intrathoracic 214.2
- kidney 214.3
- mediastinum 214.2
- muscle 214.8
- peritoneum 214.3
- retroperitoneum 214.3
- skin 214.1
  - face 214.0
- spermatic cord 214.4
- spindle cell (M8857/0) - see Lipoma, by site
- stomach 214.3
- subcutaneous tissue 214.1
  - face 214.0
- thymus 214.2
- thyroid gland 214.2

Lipomatosis (dolorosa) 272.8
- epidural 214.8
- fetal (M8881/0) - see Lipoma, by site
- Launois-Bensaude's 272.8

Lipomyohemangioma (M8860/0)
- specified site - see Neoplasm, connective tissue, benign
- unspecified site 223.0

Lipomyoma (M8860/0)
- specified site - see Neoplasm, connective tissue, benign
- unspecified site 223.0

Lipomyxoma (M8852/0) - see Lipoma, by site

Lipomyxosarcoma (M8852/3) - see Neoplasm, connective tissue, malignant

Lipophagocytosis 289.89

Lipoproteinemia (alpha) 272.4
- broad-beta 272.2
- floating-beta 272.2
- hyper-pre-beta 272.1

Lipoproteinosis (Rossle-Urbach-Wiethe) 272.8

Liposarcoma (M8850/3) - see also Neoplasm, connective tissue, malignant
- differentiated type (M8851/3) - see Neoplasm, connective tissue, malignant
- embryonal (M8852/3) - see Neoplasm, connective tissue, malignant
- mixed type (M8855/3) - see Neoplasm, connective tissue, malignant
- myxoid (M8852/3) - see Neoplasm, connective tissue, malignant
- pleomorphic (M8854/3) - see Neoplasm, connective tissue, malignant
- round cell (M8853/3) - see Neoplasm, connective tissue, malignant
- well differentiated type (M8851/3) - see Neoplasm, connective tissue, malignant

Liposynovitis prepatellaris 272.8

Lipping
- cervix 622.0
- spine (see also Spondylosis) 721.90
- vertebra (see also Spondylosis) 721.90

Lip pits (mucus), congenital 750.25

Lipschütz disease or ulcer 616.50

Lipuria 791.1
- bilharziasis 120.0

Liquefaction, vitreous humor 379.21

Lisping 307.9

Lissauer's paralysis 094.1

Lissencephalia, lissencephaly 742.2

Listerellose 027.0

Listeriose 027.0

Listeriosis 027.0
- congenital 771.2
- fetal 771.2
- suspected fetal damage affecting management of pregnancy 655.4●

Listlessness 780.79

Lithemia 790.6

Lithiasis - see also Calculus
- hepatic (duct) - see Choledocholithiasis
- urinary 592.9

Lithopedion 779.9
- affecting management of pregnancy 656.8●

Lithosis (occupational) 502
- with tuberculosis - see Tuberculosis, pulmonary

Lithuria 791.9

Litigation V62.5

Little
- league elbow 718.82
- stroke syndrome 435.9

Little's disease - see Palsy, cerebral

Littre's
- gland - see condition
- hernia - see Hernia, Littre's

Littritis (see also Urethritis) 597.89

Livedo 782.61
- annularis 782.61
- racemose 782.61
- reticularis 782.61

Live flesh 781.0

Liver - see also condition
- donor V59.6

Livida, asphyxia
- newborn 768.6

Living
- alone V60.3
- with handicapped person V60.4

Lloyd's syndrome 258.1

Loa loa 125.2

Loasis 125.2

Lobe, lobar - see condition

Lobo's disease or blastomycosis 116.2

Lobomycosis 116.2

Lobotomy syndrome 310.0

Lobstein's disease (brittle bones and blue sclera) 756.51

Lobster-claw hand 755.58

Lobulation (congenital) - see also Anomaly, specified type NEC, by site
- kidney, fetal 753.3
- liver, abnormal 751.69
- spleen 759.0

Lobule, lobular - see condition

Local, localized - see condition

Locked bowel or intestine (see also Obstruction, intestine) 560.9

Locked-in state 344.81

Locked twins 660.5●
- affecting fetus or newborn 763.1

Locking
- joint (see also Derangement, joint) 718.90
- knee 717.9

Lockjaw (see also Tetanus) 037

Locomotor ataxia (progressive) 094.0

Löffler's
- endocarditis 421.0
- eosinophilia or syndrome 518.3
- pneumonia 518.3
- syndrome (eosinophilic pneumonitis) 518.3

Löfgren's syndrome (sarcoidosis) 135

Loiasis 125.2
- eyelid 125.2 [373.6]

Loneliness V62.89

Lone Star fever 082.8

Long labor 662.1●
- affecting fetus or newborn 763.89
- first stage 662.0●
- second stage 662.2●

Longitudinal stripes or grooves, nails 703.8
- congenital 757.5

Long-term (current) (prophylactic) **drug use** V58.69
- antibiotics V58.62
- anticoagulants V58.61
- anti-inflammatories, non-steroidal (NSAID) V58.64
- antiplatelets/antithrombotics V58.63
- aspirin V58.66

Long-term drug use (Continued)
- bisphosphonates V58.68
- high-risk medications NEC V58.69
- insulin V58.67
- methadone for pain control V58.69
- opiate analgesic V58.69
- pain killers V58.69
  - anti-inflammatories, non-steroidal (NSAID) V58.64
  - aspirin V58.66
- steroids V58.65
- tamoxifen V07.51

Loop
- intestine (see also Volvulus) 560.2
- intrascleral nerve 379.29
- vascular on papilla (optic) 743.57

Loose - see also condition
- body
  - in tendon sheath 727.82
  - joint 718.10
    - ankle 718.17
    - elbow 718.12
    - foot 718.17
    - hand 718.14
    - hip 718.15
    - knee 717.6
    - multiple sites 718.19
    - pelvic region 718.15
    - prosthetic implant - see Complications, mechanical
    - shoulder (region) 718.11
    - specified site NEC 718.18
    - wrist 718.13
- cartilage (joint) (see also Loose, body, joint) 718.1●
  - knee 717.6
- facet (vertebral) 724.9
- prosthetic implant - see Complications, mechanical
- sesamoid, joint (see also Loose, body, joint) 718.1●
- tooth, teeth 525.8

Loosening epiphysis 732.9

Looser (-Debray)-Milkman syndrome (osteomalacia with pseudofractures) 268.2

Lop ear (deformity) 744.29

Lorain's disease or syndrome (pituitary dwarfism) 253.3

Lorain-Levi syndrome (pituitary dwarfism) 253.3

Lordosis (acquired) (postural) 737.20
- congenital 754.2
- due to or associated with
  - Charcôt-Marie-Tooth disease 356.1 [737.42]
  - mucopolysaccharidosis 277.5 [737.42]
  - neurofibromatosis 237.71 [737.42]
  - osteitis
    - deformans 731.0 [737.42]
    - fibrosa cystica 252.01 [737.42]
  - osteoporosis (see also Osteoporosis) 733.00 [737.42]
  - poliomyelitis (see also Poliomyelitis) 138 [737.42]
  - tuberculosis (see also Tuberculosis) 015.0● [737.42]
- late effect of rickets 268.1 [737.42]
- postlaminectomy 737.21
- postsurgical NEC 737.22
- rachitic 268.1 [737.42]
- specified NEC 737.29
- tuberculous (see also Tuberculosis) 015.0● [737.42]

Loss
- appetite 783.0
  - hysterical 300.11
  - nonorganic origin 307.59
  - psychogenic 307.59
- blood - see Hemorrhage
- central vision 368.41

Loss (Continued)
consciousness 780.09
  transient 780.2
control, sphincter, rectum 787.60
  nonorganic origin 307.7
ear ossicle, partial 385.24
elasticity, skin 782.8
extremity or member, traumatic, current - *see* Amputation, traumatic
fluid (acute) 276.50
  with
    hypernatremia 276.0
    hyponatremia 276.1
    fetus or newborn 775.5
hair 704.00
hearing - *see also* Deafness
  central 389.14
  conductive (air) 389.00
    with sensorineural hearing loss 389.20
      bilateral 389.22
      unilateral 389.21
    bilateral 389.06
    combined types 389.08
    external ear 389.01
    inner ear 389.04
    middle ear 389.03
    multiple types 389.08
    tympanic membrane 389.02
    unilateral 389.05
  mixed conductive and sensorineural 389.20
    bilateral 389.22
    unilateral 389.21
  mixed type 389.20
    bilateral 389.22
    unilateral 389.21
  nerve
    bilateral 389.12
    unilateral 389.13
  neural
    bilateral 389.12
    unilateral 389.13
  noise-induced 388.12
  perceptive NEC (*see also* Loss, hearing, sensorineural) 389.10
  sensorineural 389.10
    with conductive hearing loss 389.20
      bilateral 389.22
      unilateral 389.21
    asymmetrical 389.16
    bilateral 389.18
    central 389.14
    neural
      bilateral 389.12
      unilateral 389.13
    sensory
      bilateral 389.11
      unilateral 389.17
    unilateral 389.15
  sensory
    bilateral 389.11
    unilateral 389.17
  specified type NEC 389.8
  sudden NEC 388.2
height 781.91
labyrinthine reactivity (unilateral) 386.55
  bilateral 386.56
memory (*see also* Amnesia) 780.93
  mild, following organic brain damage 310.89
mind (*see also* Psychosis) 298.9
occusal vertical dimension 524.37
organ or part - *see* Absence, by site, acquired
recurrent pregnancy - *see* Pregnancy, management affected by, abortion, habitual
sensation 782.0

Loss (Continued)
sense of
  smell (*see also* Disturbance, sensation) 781.1
  taste (*see also* Disturbance, sensation) 781.1
  touch (*see also* Disturbance, sensation) 781.1
sight (acquired) (complete) (congenital) - *see* Blindness
spinal fluid
  headache 349.0
substance of
  bone (*see also* Osteoporosis) 733.00
  cartilage 733.99
    ear 380.32
  vitreous (humor) 379.26
tooth, teeth
  acquired 525.10
    due to
      caries 525.13
      extraction 525.10
      periodontal disease 525.12
      specified NEC 525.19
      trauma 525.11
vision, visual (*see also* Blindness) 369.9
  both eyes (*see also* Blindness, both eyes) 369.3
  complete (*see also* Blindness, both eyes) 369.00
  one eye 369.8
  sudden 368.11
  transient 368.12
vitreous 379.26
voice (*see also* Aphonia) 784.41
weight (cause unknown) 783.21
Lou Gehrig's disease 335.20
Louis-Bar syndrome (ataxia-telangiectasia) 334.8
Louping ill 063.1
Lousiness - *see* Lice
Low
back syndrome 724.2
basal metabolic rate (BMR) 794.7
birthweight 765.1●
  extreme (less than 1000 grams) 765.0●
  for gestational age 764.0●
  status (*see also* Status, low birth weight) V21.30
bladder compliance 596.52
blood pressure (*see also* Hypotension) 458.9
  reading (incidental) (isolated) (nonspecific) 796.3
cardiac reserve - *see* Disease, heart
compliance bladder 596.52
frequency deafness - *see* Disorder, hearing
function - *see also* Hypofunction
  kidney (*see also* Disease, renal) 593.9
  liver 573.9
hemoglobin 285.9
implantation, placenta - *see* Placenta, previa
insertion, placenta - *see* Placenta, previa
lying
  kidney 593.0
  organ or site, congenital - *see* Malposition, congenital
  placenta - *see* Placenta, previa
output syndrome (cardiac) (*see also* Failure, heart) 428.9
platelets (blood) (*see also* Thrombocytopenia) 287.5
reserve, kidney (*see also* Disease, renal) 593.9
risk
  human papillomavirus (HPV) DNA test positive
    anal 796.79
    cervical 795.09
    vaginal 795.19
salt syndrome 593.9
tension glaucoma 365.12

Low (Continued)
vision 369.9
  both eyes 369.20
  one eye 369.70
Lowe (-Terrey-MacLachlan) syndrome (oculocerebrorenal dystrophy) 270.8
Lower extremity - *see* condition
Lown (-Ganong)-Levine syndrome (short P-R interval, normal QRS complex, and paroxysmal supraventricular tachycardia) 426.81
LSD reaction (*see also* Abuse, drugs, nondependent) 305.3●
L-shaped kidney 753.3
Lucas-Championnière disease (fibrinous bronchitis) 466.0
Lucey-Driscoll syndrome (jaundice due to delayed conjugation) 774.30
Ludwig's
angina 528.3
disease (submaxillary cellulitis) 528.3
Lues (venerea), luetic - *see* Syphilis
Luetscher's syndrome (dehydration) 276.51
Lumbago 724.2
  due to displacement, intervertebral disc 722.10
Lumbalgia 724.2
  due to displacement, intervertebral disc 722.10
Lumbar - *see* condition
Lumbarization, vertebra 756.15
Lumbermen's itch 133.8
Lump - *see also* Mass
  abdominal 789.3●
  breast 611.72
  chest 786.6
  epigastric 789.3●
  head 784.2
  kidney 753.3
  liver 789.1
  lung 786.6
  mediastinal 786.6
  neck 784.2
  nose or sinus 784.2
  pelvic 789.3●
  skin 782.2
  substernal 786.6
  throat 784.2
  umbilicus 789.3●
Lunacy (*see also* Psychosis) 298.9
Lunatomalacia 732.3
Lung - *see also* condition
  donor V59.8
  drug addict's 417.8
  mainliners' 417.8
  vanishing 492.0
Lupoid (miliary) of Boeck 135
Lupus 710.0
anticoagulant 795.79
  with
    hemorrhagic disorder 286.53
    hypercoagulable state 289.81
Cazenave's (erythematosus) 695.4
discoid (local) 695.4
disseminated 710.0
erythematodes (discoid) (local) 695.4
erythematosus (discoid) (local) 695.4
  disseminated 710.0
  eyelid 373.34
  systemic 710.0
    with
      encephalitis 710.0 [323.81]
      lung involvement 710.0 [517.8]
      inhibitor (presence of) 795.79
        with hypercoagulable state 289.81
exedens 017.0●
eyelid (*see also* Tuberculosis) 017.0● [373.4]
Hilliard's 017.0●

Lupus (Continued)
   hydralazine
      correct substance properly administered 695.4
      overdose or wrong substance given or taken 972.6
   miliaris disseminatus faciei 017.0●
   nephritis 710.0 [583.81]
      acute 710.0 [580.81]
      chronic 710.0 [582.81]
   nontuberculous, not disseminated 695.4
   pernio (Besnier) 135
   tuberculous (see also Tuberculosis) 017.0●
      eyelid (see also Tuberculosis) 017.0● [373.4]
   vulgaris 017.0●
Luschka's joint disease 721.90
Luteinoma (M8610/0) 220
Lutembacher's disease or syndrome (atrial septal defect with mitral stenosis) 745.5
Luteoma (M8610/0) 220
Lutz-Miescher disease (elastosis perforans serpiginosa) 701.1
Lutz-Splendore-de Almeida disease (Brazilian blastomycosis) 116.1
Luxatio
   bulbi due to birth injury 767.8
   coxae congenita (see also Dislocation, hip, congenital) 754.30
   erecta - see Dislocation, shoulder
   imperfecta - see Sprain, by site
   perinealis - see Dislocation, hip
Luxation - see also Dislocation, by site
   eyeball 360.81
      due to birth injury 767.8
      lateral 376.36
   genital organs (external) NEC - see Wound, open, genital organs
   globe (eye) 360.81
      lateral 376.36
   lacrimal gland (postinfectional) 375.16
   lens (old) (partial) 379.32
      congenital 743.37
         syphilitic 090.49 [379.32]
         Marfan's disease 090.49
      spontaneous 379.32
   penis - see Wound, open, penis
   scrotum - see Wound, open, scrotum
   testis - see Wound, open, testis
L-xyloketosuria 271.8
Lycanthropy (see also Psychosis) 298.9
Lyell's disease or syndrome (toxic epidermal necrolysis) 695.15
   due to drug
      correct substance properly administered 695.15
      overdose or wrong substance given or taken 977.9
         specified drug - see Table of Drugs and Chemicals
Lyme disease 088.81
Lymph
   gland or node - see condition
   scrotum (see also Infestation, filarial) 125.9
Lymphadenitis 289.3
   with
      abortion - see Abortion, by type, with sepsis
      ectopic pregnancy (see also categories 633.0–633.9) 639.0
      molar pregnancy (see also categories 630–632) 639.0
   acute 683
      mesenteric 289.2
   any site, except mesenteric 289.3
      acute 683
      chronic 289.1
      mesenteric (acute) (chronic) (nonspecific) (subacute) 289.2
      subacute 289.1
         mesenteric 289.2
   breast, puerperal, postpartum 675.2●

Lymphadenitis (Continued)
   chancroidal (congenital) 099.0
   chronic 289.1
      mesenteric 289.2
   dermatopathic 695.89
   due to
      anthracosis (occupational) 500
      Brugia (Wuchereria) malayi 125.1
      diphtheria (toxin) 032.89
      lymphogranuloma venereum 099.1
      Wuchereria bancrofti 125.0
   following
      abortion 639.0
      ectopic or molar pregnancy 639.0
   generalized 289.3
   gonorrheal 098.89
   granulomatous 289.1
   infectional 683
   mesenteric (acute) (chronic) (nonspecific) (subacute) 289.2
      due to Bacillus typhi 002.0
      tuberculous (see also Tuberculosis) 014.8●
   mycobacterial 031.8
   purulent 683
   pyogenic 683
   regional 078.3
   septic 683
   streptococcal 683
   subacute, unspecified site 289.1
   suppurative 683
   syphilitic (early) (secondary) 091.4
      late 095.8
   tuberculous - see Tuberculosis, lymph gland
   venereal 099.1
Lymphadenoid goiter 245.2
Lymphadenopathy (general) 785.6
   due to toxoplasmosis (acquired) 130.7
      congenital (active) 771.2
Lymphadenopathy-associated virus (disease) (illness) (infection) - see Human immunodeficiency virus (disease) (illness) (infection)
Lymphadenosis 785.6
   acute 075
Lymphangiectasis 457.1
   conjunctiva 372.89
   postinfectional 457.1
   scrotum 457.1
Lymphangiectatic elephantiasis, nonfilarial 457.1
Lymphangioendothelioma (M9170/0) 228.1
   malignant (M9170/3) - see Neoplasm, connective tissue, malignant
Lymphangioleiomyomatosis 516.4
Lymphangioma (M9170/0) 228.1
   capillary (M9171/0) 228.1
   cavernous (M9172/0) 228.1
   cystic (M9173/0) 228.1
   malignant (M9170/3) - see Neoplasm, connective tissue, malignant
Lymphangiomyoma (M9174/0) 228.1
Lymphangiomyomatosis 516.4
Lymphangiosarcoma (M9170/3) - see Neoplasm, connective tissue, malignant
Lymphangitis 457.2
   with
      abortion - see Abortion, by type, with sepsis
      abscess - see Abscess, by site
      cellulitis - see Abscess, by site
      ectopic pregnancy (see also categories 633.0–633.9) 639.0
      molar pregnancy (see also categories 630–632) 639.0
   acute (with abscess or cellulitis) 682.9
      specified site - see Abscess, by site
   breast, puerperal, postpartum 675.2●
   chancroidal 099.0
   chronic (any site) 457.2
   due to
      Brugia (Wuchereria) malayi 125.1
      Wuchereria bancrofti 125.0

Lymphangitis (Continued)
   following
      abortion 639.0
      ectopic or molar pregnancy 639.0
   gangrenous 457.2
   penis
      acute 607.2
      gonococcal (acute) 098.0
         chronic or duration of 2 months or more 098.2
   puerperal, postpartum, childbirth 670.8●
   strumous, tuberculous (see also Tuberculosis) 017.2●
   subacute (any site) 457.2
   tuberculous - see Tuberculosis, lymph gland
Lymphatic (vessel) - see condition
Lymphatism 254.8
   scrofulous (see also Tuberculosis) 017.2●
Lymphectasia 457.1
Lymphedema (see also Elephantiasis) 457.1
   acquired (chronic) 457.1
   chronic hereditary 757.0
   congenital 757.0
   idiopathic hereditary 757.0
   praecox 457.1
   secondary 457.1
   surgical NEC 997.99
      postmastectomy (syndrome) 457.0
Lymph-hemangioma (M9120/0) - see Hemangioma, by site
Lymphoblastic - see condition
Lymphoblastoma (diffuse) (M9630/3) 200.1●
   giant follicular (M9690/3) 202.0●
   macrofollicular (M9690/3) 202.0●
Lymphoblastosis, acute benign 075
Lymphocele 457.8
Lymphocythemia 288.51
Lymphocytic - see also condition
   chorioencephalitis (acute) (serous) 049.0
   choriomeningitis (acute) (serous) 049.0
Lymphocytoma (diffuse) (malignant) (M9620/3) 200.1●
Lymphocytomatosis (M9620/3) 200.1●
Lymphocytopenia 288.51
Lymphocytosis (symptomatic) 288.61
   infectious (acute) 078.89
Lymphoepithelioma (M8082/3) - see Neoplasm, by site, malignant
Lymphogranuloma (malignant) (M9650/3) 201.9●
   inguinale 099.1
   venereal (any site) 099.1
      with stricture of rectum 099.1
   venereum 099.1
Lymphogranulomatosis (malignant) (M9650/3) 201.9●
   benign (Boeck's sarcoid) (Schaumann's) 135
   Hodgkin's (M9650/3) 201.9●
Lymphohistiocytosis, familial hemophagocytic 288.4
Lymphoid - see condition
Lympholeukoblastoma (M9850/3) 207.8●
Lympholeukosarcoma (M9850/3) 207.8●
Lymphoma (malignant) (M9590/3) 202.8●

Note: Use the following fifth-digit subclassification with categories 200–202:

0 unspecified site, extranodal and solid organ sites
1 lymph nodes of head, face, and neck
2 intrathoracic lymph nodes
3 intra-abdominal lymph nodes
4 lymph nodes of axilla and upper limb
5 lymph nodes of inguinal region and lower limb
6 intrapelvic lymph nodes
7 spleen
8 lymph nodes of multiple sites

Lymphoma (Continued)
- benign (M9590/0) - see Neoplasm, by site, benign
- Burkitt's type (lymphoblastic) (undifferentiated) (M9750/3) 200.2
- Castleman's (mediastinal lymph node hyperplasia) 785.6
- centroblastic-centrocytic
  - diffuse (M9614/3) 202.8
  - follicular (M9692/3) 202.0
- centroblastic type (diffuse) (M9632/3) 202.8
  - follicular (M9697/3) 202.0
- centrocytic (M9622/3) 202.8
- compound (M9613/3) 200.8
- convoluted cell type (lymphoblastic) (M9602/3) 202.8
- diffuse NEC (M9590/3) 202.8
  - large B cell 202.8
- follicular (giant) (M9690/3) 202.0
  - center cell (diffuse) (M9615/3) 202.8
    - cleaved (diffuse) (M9623/3) 202.8
      - follicular (M9695/3) 202.0
    - non-cleaved (diffuse) (M9633/3) 202.8
      - follicular (M9698/3) 202.0
  - centroblastic-centrocytic (M9692/3) 202.0
  - centroblastic type (M9697/3) 202.0
  - large cell 202.0
  - lymphocytic
    - intermediate differentiation (M9694/3) 202.0
    - poorly differentiated (M9696/3) 202.0
  - mixed (cell type) (lymphocytic-histiocytic) (small cell and large cell) (M9691/3) 202.0
- germinocytic (M9622/3) 202.8
- giant, follicular or follicle (M9690/3) 202.0
- histiocytic (diffuse) (M9640/3) 200.0
  - nodular (M9642/3) 200.0
  - pleomorphic cell type (M9641/3) 200.0
- Hodgkin's (M9650/3) (see also Disease, Hodgkin's) 201.9
- immunoblastic (type) (M9612/3) 200.8
- large cell (M9640/3) 200.7
  - anaplastic 200.6
  - nodular (M9642/3) 202.0
  - pleomorphic cell type (M9641/3) 200.0
- lymphoblastic (diffuse) (M9630/3) 200.1
  - Burkitt's type (M9750/3) 200.2
  - convoluted cell type (M9602/3) 202.8

Lymphoma (Continued)
- lymphocytic (cell type) (diffuse) (M9620/3) 200.1
  - with plasmacytoid differentiation, diffuse (M9611/3) 200.8
  - intermediate differentiation (diffuse) (M9621/3) 200.1
    - follicular (M9694/3) 202.0
    - nodular (M9694/3) 202.0
  - nodular (M9690/3) 202.0
  - poorly differentiated (diffuse) (M9630/3) 200.1
    - follicular (M9696/3) 202.0
    - nodular (M9696/3) 202.0
  - well differentiated (diffuse) (M9620/3) 200.1
    - follicular (M9693/3) 202.0
    - nodular (M9693/3) 202.0
- lymphocytic-histiocytic, mixed (diffuse) (M9613/3) 200.8
  - follicular (M9691/3) 202.0
  - nodular (M9691/3) 202.0
- lymphoplasmacytoid type (M9611/3) 200.8
- lymphosarcoma type (M9610/3) 200.1
- macrofollicular (M9690/3) 202.0
- mantle cell 200.4
- marginal zone 200.3
  - extranodal B-cell 200.3
  - nodal B-cell 200.3
  - splenic B-cell 200.3
- mixed cell type (diffuse) (M9613/3) 200.8
  - follicular (M9691/3) 202.0
  - nodular (M9691/3) 202.0
- nodular (M9690/3) 202.0
  - histiocytic (M9642/3) 200.0
  - lymphocytic (M9690/3) 202.0
    - intermediate differentiation (M9694/3) 202.0
    - poorly differentiated (M9696/3) 202.0
  - mixed (cell type) (lymphocytic-histiocytic) (small cell and large cell) (M9691/3) 202.0
- non-Hodgkin's type NEC (M9591/3) 202.8
- peripheral T-cell 202.7
- primary central nervous system 200.5
- reticulum cell (type) (M9640/3) 200.0
- small cell and large cell, mixed (diffuse) (M9613/3) 200.8
  - follicular (M9691/3) 202.0
  - nodular (M9691/3) 202.0
- stem cell (type) (M9601/3) 202.8

Lymphoma (Continued)
- T-cell 202.1
  - peripheral 202.7
  - undifferentiated (cell type) (non-Burkitt's) (M9600/3) 202.8
  - Burkitt's type (M9750/3) 200.2

Lymphomatosis (M9590/3) - see also Lymphoma
- granulomatous 099.1

Lymphopathia
- venereum 099.1
- veneris 099.1

Lymphopenia 288.51
- familial 279.2

Lymphoreticulosis, benign (of inoculation) 078.3

Lymphorrhea 457.8

Lymphosarcoma (M9610/3) 200.1
- diffuse (M9610/3) 200.1
  - with plasmacytoid differentiation (M9611/3) 200.8
  - lymphoplasmacytic (M9611/3) 200.8
- follicular (giant) (M9690/3) 202.0
  - lymphoblastic (M9696/3) 202.0
  - lymphocytic, intermediate differentiation (M9694/3) 202.0
  - mixed cell type (M9691/3) 202.0
- giant follicular (M9690/3) 202.0
- Hodgkin's (M9650/3) 201.9
- immunoblastic (M9612/3) 200.8
- lymphoblastic (diffuse) (M9630/3) 200.1
  - follicular (M9696/3) 202.0
  - nodular (M9696/3) 202.0
- lymphocytic (diffuse) (M9620/3) 200.1
  - intermediate differentiation (diffuse) (M9621/3) 200.1
    - follicular (M9694/3) 202.0
    - nodular (M9694/3) 202.0
  - mixed cell type (diffuse) (M9613/3) 200.8
    - follicular (M9691/3) 202.0
    - nodular (M9691/3) 202.0
- nodular (M9690/3) 202.0
  - lymphoblastic (M9696/3) 202.0
  - lymphocytic, intermediate differentiation (M9694/3) 202.0
  - mixed cell type (M9691/3) 202.0
- prolymphocytic (M9631/3) 200.1
- reticulum cell (M9640/3) 200.0

Lymphostasis 457.8

Lypemania (see also Melancholia) 296.2

Lyssa 071

M

Macacus ear 744.29
Maceration
    fetus (cause not stated) 779.9
    wet feet, tropical (syndrome) 991.4
Machado-Joseph disease 334.8
Machupo virus hemorrhagic fever 078.7
Macleod's syndrome (abnormal transradiancy, one lung) 492.8
Macrocephalia, macrocephaly 756.0
Macrocheilia (congenital) 744.81
Macrochilia (congenital) 744.81
Macrocolon (congenital) 751.3
Macrocornea 743.41
    associated with buphthalmos 743.22
Macrocytic - *see* condition
Macrocytosis 289.89
Macrodactylia, macrodactylism (fingers) (thumbs) 755.57
    toes 755.65
Macrodontia 520.2
Macroencephaly 742.4
Macrogenia 524.05
Macrogenitosomia (female) (male) (praecox) 255.2
Macrogingivae 523.8
Macroglobulinemia (essential) (idiopathic) (monoclonal) (primary) (syndrome) (Waldenström's) 273.3
Macroglossia (congenital) 750.15
    acquired 529.8
Macrognathia, macrognathism (congenital) 524.00
    mandibular 524.02
        alveolar 524.72
    maxillary 524.01
        alveolar 524.71
Macrogyria (congenital) 742.4
Macrohydrocephalus (*see also* Hydrocephalus) 331.4
Macromastia (*see also* Hypertrophy, breast) 611.1
Macrophage activation syndrome 288.4
Macropsia 368.14
Macrosigmoid 564.7
    congenital 751.3
Macrospondylitis, acromegalic 253.0
Macrostomia (congenital) 744.83
Macrotia (external ear) (congenital) 744.22
Macula
    cornea, corneal
        congenital 743.43
            interfering with vision 743.42
        interfering with central vision 371.03
        not interfering with central vision 371.02
        degeneration (*see also* Degeneration, macula) 362.50
        hereditary (*see also* Dystrophy, retina) 362.70
    edema, cystoid 362.53
Maculae ceruleae 132.1
Macules and papules 709.8
Maculopathy, toxic 362.55
Madarosis 374.55
Madelung's
    deformity (radius) 755.54
    disease (lipomatosis) 272.8
    lipomatosis 272.8
Madness (*see also* Psychosis) 298.9
    myxedema (acute) 293.0
        subacute 293.1
Madura
    disease (actinomycotic) 039.9
        mycotic 117.4
    foot (actinomycotic) 039.4
        mycotic 117.4
Maduromycosis (actinomycotic) 039.9
    mycotic 117.4
Maffucci's syndrome (dyschondroplasia with hemangiomas) 756.4

Magenblase syndrome 306.4
Main en griffe (acquired) 736.06
    congenital 755.59
Maintenance
    chemotherapy regimen or treatment V58.11
    dialysis regimen or treatment
        extracorporeal (renal) V56.0
        peritoneal V56.8
        renal V56.0
    drug therapy or regimen
        chemotherapy, antineoplastic V58.11
        immunotherapy, antineoplastic V58.12
    external fixation NEC V54.89
    methadone 304.00
    radiotherapy V58.0
    traction NEC V54.89
Majocchi's
    disease (purpura annularis telangiectodes) 709.1
    granuloma 110.6
Major - *see* condition
Mal
    cerebral (idiopathic) (*see also* Epilepsy) 345.9●
    comital (*see also* Epilepsy) 345.9●
    de los pintos (*see also* Pinta) 103.9
    de Meleda 757.39
    de mer 994.6
    lie - *see* Presentation, fetal
    perforant (*see also* Ulcer, lower extremity) 707.15
Malabar itch 110.9
    beard 110.0
    foot 110.4
    scalp 110.0
Malabsorption 579.9
    calcium 579.8
    carbohydrate 579.8
    disaccharide 271.3
    drug-induced 579.8
    due to bacterial overgrowth 579.8
    fat 579.8
    folate, congenital 281.2
    galactose 271.1
    glucose-galactose (congenital) 271.3
    intestinal 579.9
    isomaltose 271.3
    lactose (hereditary) 271.3
    methionine 270.4
    monosaccharide 271.8
    postgastrectomy 579.3
    postsurgical 579.3
    protein 579.8
    sucrose (-isomaltose) (congenital) 271.3
    syndrome 579.9
        postgastrectomy 579.3
        postsurgical 579.3
Malacia, bone 268.2
    juvenile (*see also* Rickets) 268.0
    Kienböck's (juvenile) (lunate) (wrist) 732.3
        adult 732.8
Malacoplakia
    bladder 596.89
    colon 569.89
    pelvis (kidney) 593.89
    ureter 593.89
    urethra 599.84
Malacosteon 268.2
    juvenile (*see also* Rickets) 268.0
Maladaptation - *see* Maladjustment
Maladie de Roger 745.4
Maladjustment
    conjugal V61.10
        involving
            divorce V61.03
            estrangement V61.09
    educational V62.3
    family V61.9
        specified circumstance NEC V61.8

Maladjustment (*Continued*)
    marital V61.10
        involving
            divorce V61.03
            estrangement V61.09
    occupational V62.29
        current military deployment status V62.21
    simple, adult (*see also* Reaction, adjustment) 309.9
    situational acute (*see also* Reaction, adjustment) 309.9
    social V62.4
Malaise 780.79
Malakoplakia - *see* Malacoplakia
Malaria, malarial (fever) 084.6
    algid 084.9
    any type, with
        algid malaria 084.9
        blackwater fever 084.8
        fever
            blackwater 084.8
            hemoglobinuric (bilious) 084.8
        hemoglobinuria, malarial 084.8
        hepatitis 084.9 [573.2]
        nephrosis 084.9 [581.81]
        pernicious complication NEC 084.9
            cardiac 084.9
            cerebral 084.9
    cardiac 084.9
    carrier (suspected) of V02.9
    cerebral 084.9
    complicating pregnancy, childbirth, or puerperium 647.4●
    congenital 771.2
    congestion, congestive 084.6
        brain 084.9
    continued 084.0
    estivo-autumnal 084.0
    falciparum (malignant tertian) 084.0
    hematinuria 084.8
    hematuria 084.8
    hemoglobinuria 084.8
    hemorrhagic 084.6
    induced (therapeutically) 084.7
        accidental - *see* Malaria, by type
    liver 084.9 [573.2]
    malariae (quartan) 084.2
    malignant (tertian) 084.0
    mixed infections 084.5
    monkey 084.4
    ovale 084.3
    pernicious, acute 084.0
    Plasmodium, P.
        falciparum 084.0
        malariae 084.2
        ovale 084.3
        vivax 084.1
    quartan 084.2
    quotidian 084.0
    recurrent 084.6
        induced (therapeutically) 084.7
            accidental - *see* Malaria, by type
    remittent 084.6
    specified types NEC 084.4
    spleen 084.6
    subtertian 084.0
    tertian (benign) 084.1
        malignant 084.0
    tropical 084.0
    typhoid 084.6
    vivax (benign tertian) 084.1
Malassez's disease (testicular cyst) 608.89
Malassimilation 579.9
Maldescent, testis 752.51
Maldevelopment - *see also* Anomaly, by site
    brain 742.9
    colon 751.5
    hip (joint) 755.63
        congenital dislocation (*see also* Dislocation, hip, congenital) 754.30
    mastoid process 756.0

SECTION I INDEX TO DISEASES AND INJURIES / Malposition

Maldevelopment *(Continued)*
  middle ear, except ossicles 744.03
    ossicles 744.04
  newborn (not malformation) 764.9 ●
  ossicles, ear 744.04
  spine 756.10
  toe 755.66
Male type pelvis 755.69
  with disproportion (fetopelvic) 653.2 ●
    affecting fetus or newborn 763.1
    causing obstructed labor 660.1 ●
      affecting fetus or newborn 763.1
Malformation (congenital) - *see also* Anomaly
  arteriovenous
    pulmonary 747.32
  bone 756.9
  bursa 756.9
  Chiari
    type I 348.4
    type II (*see also* Spina bifida) 741.0 ●
    type III 742.0
    type IV 742.2
  circulatory system NEC 747.9
    specified type NEC 747.89
  cochlea 744.05
  digestive system NEC 751.9
    lower 751.5
    specified type NEC 751.8
    upper 750.9
  eye 743.9
  gum 750.9
  heart NEC 746.9
    specified type NEC 746.89
    valve 746.9
  internal ear 744.05
  joint NEC 755.9
    specified type NEC 755.8
  Mondini's (congenital) (malformation, cochlea) 744.05
  muscle 756.9
  nervous system (central) 742.9
  pelvic organs or tissues
    in pregnancy or childbirth 654.9 ●
      affecting fetus or newborn 763.89
      causing obstructed labor 660.2 ●
        affecting fetus or newborn 763.1
  placenta (*see also* Placenta, abnormal) 656.7 ●
  respiratory organs 748.9
    specified type NEC 748.8
  Rieger's 743.44
  sense organs NEC 742.9
    specified type NEC 742.8
  skin 757.9
    specified type NEC 757.8
  spinal cord 742.9
  teeth, tooth NEC 520.9
  tendon 756.9
  throat 750.9
  umbilical cord (complicating delivery) 663.9 ●
    affecting fetus or newborn 762.6
  umbilicus 759.9
  urinary system NEC 753.9
    specified type NEC 753.8
  venous - *see* Anomaly, vein
Malfunction - *see also* Dysfunction
  arterial graft 996.1
  cardiac pacemaker 996.01
  catheter device - *see* Complications, mechanical, catheter
  colostomy 569.62
    valve 569.62
  cystostomy 596.82
    infection 596.81
    mechanical 596.82
    specified complication NEC 596.83
  device, implant, or graft NEC - *see* Complications, mechanical
  enteric stoma 569.62
  enterostomy 569.62
  esophagostomy 530.87

Malfunction *(Continued)*
  gastroenteric 536.8
  gastrostomy 536.42
  ileostomy
    valve 569.62
  nephrostomy 997.5
  pacemaker - *see* Complications, mechanical, pacemaker
  prosthetic device, internal - *see* Complications, mechanical
  tracheostomy 519.02
  valve
    colostomy 569.62
    ileostomy 569.62
  vascular graft or shunt 996.1
Malgaigne's fracture (closed) 808.43
  open 808.53
Malherbe's
  calcifying epithelioma (M8110/0) - *see* Neoplasm, skin, benign
  tumor (M8110/0) - *see* Neoplasm, skin, benign
Malibu disease 919.8
  infected 919.9
Malignancy (M8000/3) - *see* Neoplasm, by site, malignant
Malignant - *see* condition
Malingerer, malingering V65.2
Mallet, finger (acquired) 736.1
  congenital 755.59
  late effect of rickets 268.1
Malleus 024
Mallory's bodies 034.1
Mallory-Weiss syndrome 530.7
Malnutrition (calorie) 263.9
  complicating pregnancy 648.9 ●
  degree
    first 263.1
    second 263.0
    third 262
    mild (protein) 263.1
    moderate (protein) 263.0
    severe 261
      protein-calorie 262
  fetus 764.2 ●
    "light-for-dates" 764.1 ●
  following gastrointestinal surgery 579.3
  intrauterine or fetal 764.2 ●
    fetus or infant "light-for-dates" 764.1 ●
  lack of care, or neglect (child) (infant) 995.52
    adult 995.84
  malignant 260
  mild (protein) 263.1
  moderate (protein) 263.0
  protein 260
  protein-calorie 263.9
    mild 263.1
    moderate 263.0
    severe 262
    specified type NEC 263.8
  severe 261
    protein-calorie NEC 262
Malocclusion (teeth) 524.4
  angle's class I 524.21
  angle's class II 524.22
  angle's class III 524.23
  due to
    abnormal swallowing 524.59
    accessory teeth (causing crowding) 524.31
    dentofacial abnormality NEC 524.89
    impacted teeth (causing crowding) 520.6
    missing teeth 524.30
    mouth breathing 524.59
    sleep postures 524.59
    supernumerary teeth (causing crowding) 524.31
    thumb sucking 524.59
    tongue, lip, or finger habits 524.59
  temporomandibular (joint) 524.69

Malposition
  cardiac apex (congenital) 746.87
  cervix - *see* Malposition, uterus
  congenital
    adrenal (gland) 759.1
    alimentary tract 751.8
      lower 751.5
      upper 750.8
    aorta 747.21
    appendix 751.5
    arterial trunk 747.29
    artery (peripheral) NEC (*see also* Malposition, congenital, peripheral vascular system) 747.60
      coronary 746.85
      pulmonary 747.39
    auditory canal 744.29
      causing impairment of hearing 744.02
    auricle (ear) 744.29
      causing impairment of hearing 744.02
      cervical 744.43
    biliary duct or passage 751.69
    bladder (mucosa) 753.8
      exteriorized or extroverted 753.5
    brachial plexus 742.8
    brain tissue 742.4
    breast 757.6
    bronchus 748.3
    cardiac apex 746.87
    cecum 751.5
    clavicle 755.51
    colon 751.5
    digestive organ or tract NEC 751.8
      lower 751.5
      upper 750.8
    ear (auricle) (external) 744.29
      ossicles 744.04
    endocrine (gland) NEC 759.2
    epiglottis 748.3
    Eustachian tube 744.24
    eye 743.8
    facial features 744.89
    fallopian tube 752.19
    finger(s) 755.59
      supernumerary 755.01
    foot 755.67
    gallbladder 751.69
    gastrointestinal tract 751.8
    genitalia, genital organ(s) or tract
      female 752.89
        external 752.49
        internal NEC 752.89
      male 752.89
        penis 752.69
        scrotal transposition 752.81
    glottis 748.3
    hand 755.59
    heart 746.87
      dextrocardia 746.87
        with complete transposition of viscera 759.3
    hepatic duct 751.69
    hip (joint) (*see also* Dislocation, hip, congenital) 754.30
    intestine (large) (small) 751.5
      with anomalous adhesions, fixation, or malrotation 751.4
    joint NEC 755.8
    kidney 753.3
    larynx 748.3
    limb 755.8
      lower 755.69
      upper 755.59
    liver 751.69
    lung (lobe) 748.69
    nail(s) 757.5
    nerve 742.8
    nervous system NEC 742.8
    nose, nasal (septum) 748.1
    organ or site NEC - *see* Anomaly, specified type NEC, by site

303

Malposition (Continued)
- congenital (Continued)
  - ovary 752.0
  - pancreas 751.7
  - parathyroid (gland) 759.2
  - patella 755.64
  - peripheral vascular system 747.60
    - gastrointestinal 747.61
    - lower limb 747.64
    - renal 747.62
    - specified NEC 747.69
    - spinal 747.82
    - upper limb 747.63
  - pituitary (gland) 759.2
  - respiratory organ or system NEC 748.9
  - rib (cage) 756.3
    - supernumerary in cervical region 756.2
  - scapula 755.59
  - shoulder 755.59
  - spinal cord 742.59
  - spine 756.19
  - spleen 759.0
  - sternum 756.3
  - stomach 750.7
  - symphysis pubis 755.69
  - testis (undescended) 752.51
  - thymus (gland) 759.2
  - thyroid (gland) (tissue) 759.2
    - cartilage 748.3
  - toe(s) 755.66
    - supernumerary 755.02
  - tongue 750.19
  - trachea 748.3
  - uterus 752.39
  - vein(s) (peripheral) NEC (see also Malposition, congenital, peripheral vascular system) 747.60
    - great 747.49
    - portal 747.49
    - pulmonary 747.49
  - vena cava (inferior) (superior) 747.49
- device, implant, or graft - see Complications, mechanical
- fetus NEC (see also Presentation, fetal) 652.9●
  - with successful version 652.1●
  - affecting fetus or newborn 763.1
  - before labor, affecting fetus or newborn 761.7
  - causing obstructed labor 660.0●
  - in multiple gestation (one fetus or more) 652.6●
  - with locking 660.5●
  - causing obstructed labor 660.0●
- gallbladder (see also Disease, gallbladder) 575.8
- gastrointestinal tract 569.89
  - congenital 751.8
- heart (see also Malposition, congenital, heart) 746.87
- intestine 569.89
  - congenital 751.5
- pelvic organs or tissues
  - in pregnancy or childbirth 654.4●
    - affecting fetus or newborn 763.89
    - causing obstructed labor 660.2●
      - affecting fetus or newborn 763.1
- placenta - see Placenta, previa
- stomach 537.89
  - congenital 750.7
- tooth, teeth 524.30
  - with impaction 520.6
- uterus (acquired) (acute) (adherent) (any degree) (asymptomatic) (postinfectional) (postpartal, old) 621.6
  - anteflexion or anteversion (see also Anteversion, uterus) 621.6
  - congenital 752.39
  - flexion 621.6
    - lateral (see also Lateroversion, uterus) 621.6

Malposition (Continued)
- uterus (Continued)
  - in pregnancy or childbirth 654.4●
    - affecting fetus or newborn 763.89
    - causing obstructed labor 660.2●
      - affecting fetus or newborn 763.1
  - inversion 621.6
  - lateral (flexion) (version) (see also Lateroversion, uterus) 621.6
  - lateroflexion (see also Lateroversion, uterus) 621.6
  - lateroversion (see also Lateroversion, uterus) 621.6
  - retroflexion or retroversion (see also Retroversion, uterus) 621.6

Malposture 729.90
Malpresentation, fetus (see also Presentation, fetal) 652.9●
Malrotation
- cecum 751.4
- colon 751.4
- intestine 751.4
- kidney 753.3

MALT (mucosa associated lymphoid tissue) 200.3●
Malt workers' lung 495.4
Malta fever (see also Brucellosis) 023.9
Maltosuria 271.3
Maltreatment (of)
- adult 995.80
  - emotional 995.82
  - multiple forms 995.85
  - neglect (nutritional) 995.84
  - physical 995.81
  - psychological 995.82
  - sexual 995.83
- child 995.50
  - emotional 995.51
  - multiple forms 995.59
  - neglect (nutritional) 995.52
  - physical 995.54
  - shaken infant syndrome 995.55
  - psychological 995.51
  - sexual 995.53
- spouse (see also Maltreatment, adult) 995.80

Malum coxae senilis 715.25
Malunion, fracture 733.81
Mammillitis (see also Mastitis) 611.0
- puerperal, postpartum 675.2●
Mammitis (see also Mastitis) 611.0
- puerperal, postpartum 675.2●
Mammographic
- calcification 793.89
- calculus 793.89
- microcalcification 793.81
Mammoplasia 611.1
Management
- contraceptive V25.9
  - specified type NEC V25.8
- procreative V26.9
  - specified type NEC V26.89
Mangled NEC (see also nature and site of injury) 959.9
Mania (monopolar) (see also Psychosis, affective) 296.0●
- alcoholic (acute) (chronic) 291.9
- Bell's - see Mania, chronic
- chronic 296.0●
  - recurrent episode 296.1●
  - single episode 296.0●
- compulsive 300.3
- delirious (acute) 296.0●
  - recurrent episode 296.1●
  - single episode 296.0●
- epileptic (see also Epilepsy) 345.4●
- hysterical 300.10
- inhibited 296.89
- puerperal (after delivery) 296.0●
  - recurrent episode 296.1●
  - single episode 296.0●
- recurrent episode 296.1●

Mania (Continued)
- senile 290.8
- single episode 296.0●
- stupor 296.89
- stuporous 296.89
- unproductive 296.89

Manic-depressive insanity, psychosis, reaction, or syndrome (see also Psychosis, affective) 296.80
- circular (alternating) 296.7
  - currently
    - depressed 296.5●
    - episode unspecified 296.7
    - hypomanic, previously depressed 296.4●
    - manic 296.4●
    - mixed 296.6●
- depressed (type), depressive 296.2●
  - atypical 296.82
  - recurrent episode 296.3●
  - single episode 296.2●
- hypomanic 296.0●
  - recurrent episode 296.1●
  - single episode 296.0●
- manic 296.0●
  - atypical 296.81
  - recurrent episode 296.1●
  - single episode 296.0●
- mixed NEC 296.89
- perplexed 296.89
- stuporous 296.89

Manifestations, rheumatoid
- lungs 714.81
- pannus - see Arthritis, rheumatoid
- subcutaneous nodules - see Arthritis, rheumatoid

Mankowsky's syndrome (familial dysplastic osteopathy) 731.2
Mannoheptulosuria 271.8
Mannosidosis 271.8
Manson's
- disease (schistosomiasis) 120.1
- pyosis (pemphigus contagiosus) 684
- schistosomiasis 120.1
Mansonellosis 125.5
Manual - see condition
Maple bark disease 495.6
Maple bark-strippers' lung 495.6
Maple syrup (urine) disease or syndrome 270.3
Marable's syndrome (celiac artery compression) 447.4
Marasmus 261
- brain 331.9
- due to malnutrition 261
- intestinal 569.89
- nutritional 261
- senile 797
- tuberculous NEC (see also Tuberculosis) 011.9●
Marble
- bones 756.52
- skin 782.61
Marburg disease (virus) 078.89
March
- foot 733.94
- hemoglobinuria 283.2
Marchand multiple nodular hyperplasia (liver) 571.5
Marchesani (-Weill) **syndrome** (brachymorphism and ectopia lentis) 759.89
Marchiafava (-Bignami) **disease or syndrome** 341.8
Marchiafava-Micheli syndrome (paroxysmal nocturnal hemoglobinuria) 283.2
Marcus Gunn's syndrome (jaw-winking syndrome) 742.8
Marfan's
- congenital syphilis 090.49
- disease 090.49

Marfan's (Continued)
 syndrome (arachnodactyly) 759.82
  meaning congenital syphilis 090.49
   with luxation of lens 090.49 [379.32]
Marginal
 implantation, placenta - see Placenta, previa
 placenta - see Placenta, previa
 sinus (hemorrhage) (rupture) 641.2●
  affecting fetus or newborn 762.1
Marie's
 cerebellar ataxia 334.2
 syndrome (acromegaly) 253.0
Marie-Bamberger disease or syndrome
  (hypertrophic) (pulmonary) (secondary) 731.2
 idiopathic (acropachyderma) 757.39
 primary (acropachyderma) 757.39
Marie-Charcôt-Tooth neuropathic atrophy, muscle 356.1
Marie-Strümpell arthritis or disease
  (ankylosing spondylitis) 720.0
Marihuana, marijuana
 abuse (see also Abuse, drugs, nondependent) 305.2●
 dependence (see also Dependence) 304.3●
Marion's disease (bladder neck obstruction) 596.0
Marital conflict V61.10
Mark
 port wine 757.32
 raspberry 757.32
 strawberry 757.32
 stretch 701.3
 tattoo 709.09
Maroteaux-Lamy syndrome
  (mucopolysaccharidosis VI) 277.5
Marriage license examination V70.3
Marrow (bone)
 arrest 284.9
 megakaryocytic 287.30
 poor function 289.9
Marseilles fever 082.1
Marsh's disease (exophthalmic goiter) 242.0●
Marshall's (hidrotic) ectodermal dysplasia 757.31
Marsh fever (see also Malaria) 084.6
Martin's disease 715.27
Martin-Albright syndrome
  (pseudohypoparathyroidism) 275.49
Martorell-Fabre syndrome (pulseless disease) 446.7
Masculinization, female, with adrenal hyperplasia 255.2
Masculinovoblastoma (M8670/0) 220
Masochism 302.83
Masons' lung 502
Mass
 abdominal 789.3●
 anus 787.99
 bone 733.90
 breast 611.72
 cheek 784.2
 chest 786.6
 cystic - see Cyst
 ear 388.8
 epigastric 789.3●
 eye 379.92
 female genital organ 625.8
 gum 784.2
 head 784.2
 intracranial 784.2
 joint 719.60
  ankle 719.67
  elbow 719.62
  foot 719.67
  hand 719.64
  hip 719.65
  knee 719.66
  multiple sites 719.69
  pelvic region 719.65
  shoulder (region) 719.61

Mass (Continued)
 joint (Continued)
  specified site NEC 719.68
  wrist 719.63
 kidney (see also Disease, kidney) 593.9
 lung 786.6
 lymph node 785.6
 malignant (M8000/3) - see Neoplasm, by site, malignant
 mediastinal 786.6
 mouth 784.2
 muscle (limb) 729.89
 neck 784.2
 nose or sinus 784.2
 palate 784.2
 pelvis, pelvic 789.3●
 penis 607.89
 perineum 625.8
 rectum 787.99
 scrotum 608.89
 skin 782.2
 specified organ NEC - see Disease of specified organ or site
 splenic 789.2
 substernal 786.6
  thyroid (see also Goiter) 240.9
 superficial (localized) 782.2
 testes 608.89
 throat 784.2
 tongue 784.2
 umbilicus 789.3●
 uterus 625.8
 vagina 625.8
 vulva 625.8
Massive - see condition
Mastalgia 611.71
 psychogenic 307.89
Mast cell
 disease 757.33
  systemic (M9741/3) 202.6●
 leukemia (M9900/3) 207.8●
 sarcoma (M9740/3) 202.6●
 tumor (M9740/1) 238.5
  malignant (M9740/3) 202.6●
Masters-Allen syndrome 620.6
Mastitis (acute) (adolescent) (diffuse) (interstitial) (lobular) (nonpuerperal) (nonsuppurative) (parenchymatous) (phlegmonous) (simple) (subacute) (suppurative) 611.0
 chronic (cystic) (fibrocystic) 610.1
 cystic 610.1
  Schimmelbusch's type 610.1
 fibrocystic 610.1
 infective 611.0
 lactational 675.2●
 lymphangitis 611.0
 neonatal (noninfective) 778.7
  infective 771.5
 periductal 610.4
 plasma cell 610.4
 puerperal, postpartum, (interstitial) (nonpurulent) (parenchymatous) 675.2●
  purulent 675.1●
  stagnation 676.2●
 puerperalis 675.2●
 retromammary 611.0
  puerperal, postpartum 675.1●
 submammary 611.0
  puerperal, postpartum 675.1●
Mastocytoma (M9740/1) 238.5
 malignant (M9740/3) 202.6●
Mastocytosis 757.33
 malignant (M9741/3) 202.6●
 systemic (M9741/3) 202.6●
Mastodynia 611.71
 psychogenic 307.89
Mastoid - see condition
Mastoidalgia (see also Otalgia) 388.70

Mastoiditis (coalescent) (hemorrhagic) (pneumococcal) (streptococcal) (suppurative) 383.9
 acute or subacute 383.00
  with
   Gradenigo's syndrome 383.02
   petrositis 383.02
   specified complication NEC 383.02
   subperiosteal abscess 383.01
 chronic (necrotic) (recurrent) 383.1
 tuberculous (see also Tuberculosis) 015.6●
Mastopathy, mastopathia 611.9
 chronica cystica 610.1
 diffuse cystic 610.1
 estrogenic 611.89
 ovarian origin 611.89
Mastoplasia 611.1
Masturbation 307.9
Maternal condition, affecting fetus or newborn
 acute yellow atrophy of liver 760.8
 albuminuria 760.1
 anesthesia or analgesia 763.5
 blood loss 762.1
 chorioamnionitis 762.7
 circulatory disease, chronic (conditions classifiable to 390–459, 745–747) 760.3
 congenital heart disease (conditions classifiable to 745–746) 760.3
 cortical necrosis of kidney 760.1
 death 761.6
 diabetes mellitus 775.0
  manifest diabetes in the infant 775.1
 disease NEC 760.9
  circulatory system, chronic (conditions classifiable to 390–459, 745–747) 760.3
  genitourinary system (conditions classifiable to 580–599) 760.1
  respiratory (conditions classifiable to 490–519, 748) 760.3
 eclampsia 760.0
 hemorrhage NEC 762.1
 hepatitis acute, malignant, or subacute 760.8
 hyperemesis (gravidarum) 761.8
 hypertension (arising during pregnancy) (conditions classifiable to 642) 760.0
 infection
  disease classifiable to 001–136 760.2
  genital tract NEC 760.8
  urinary tract 760.1
 influenza 760.2
  manifest influenza in the infant 771.2
 injury (conditions classifiable to 800–996) 760.5
 malaria 760.2
  manifest malaria in infant or fetus 771.2
 malnutrition 760.4
 necrosis of liver 760.8
 nephritis (conditions classifiable to 580–583) 760.1
 nephrosis (conditions classifiable to 581) 760.1
 noxious substance transmitted via breast milk or placenta 760.70
  alcohol 760.71
  anticonvulsants 760.77
  antifungals 760.74
  anti-infective agents 760.74
  antimetabolics 760.78
  cocaine 760.75
  "crack" 760.75
  diethylstilbestrol [DES] 760.76
  hallucinogenic agents 760.73
  medicinal agents NEC 760.79
  narcotics 760.72
  obstetric anesthetic or analgesic drug 760.72
  specified agent NEC 760.79
 nutritional disorder (conditions classifiable to 260–269) 760.4

New   Revised   deleted Deleted   ● Use Additional Digit(s)   Omit code

SECTION I INDEX TO DISEASES AND INJURIES / Maternal condition, affecting fetus or newborn

Maternal condition, affecting fetus or newborn *(Continued)*
    operation unrelated to current delivery *(see also* Newborn, affected by) 760.64
    pre-eclampsia 760.0
    pyelitis or pyelonephritis, arising during pregnancy (conditions classifiable to 590) 760.1
    renal disease or failure 760.1
    respiratory disease, chronic (conditions classifiable to 490–519, 748) 760.3
    rheumatic heart disease (chronic) (conditions classifiable to 393–398) 760.3
    rubella (conditions classifiable to 056) 760.2
        manifest rubella in the infant or fetus 771.0
    surgery unrelated to current delivery *(see also* Newborn, affected by) 760.64
        to uterus or pelvic organs 760.64
    syphilis (conditions classifiable to 090–097) 760.2
        manifest syphilis in the infant or fetus 090.0
    thrombophlebitis 760.3
    toxemia (of pregnancy) 760.0
        pre-eclamptic 760.0
    toxoplasmosis (conditions classifiable to 130) 760.2
        manifest toxoplasmosis in the infant or fetus 771.2
    transmission of chemical substance through the placenta 760.70
        alcohol 760.71
        anticonvulsants 760.77
        antifungals 760.74
        anti-infective 760.74
        antimetabolics 760.78
        cocaine 760.75
        "crack" 760.75
        diethylstilbestrol [DES] 760.76
        hallucinogenic agents 760.73
        narcotics 760.72
        specified substance NEC 760.79
    uremia 760.1
    urinary tract conditions (conditions classifiable to 580–599) 760.1
    vomiting (pernicious) (persistent) (vicious) 761.8
Maternity - *see* Delivery
Matheiu's disease (leptospiral jaundice) 100.0
Mauclaire's disease or osteochondrosis 732.3
Maxcy's disease 081.0
Maxilla, maxillary - *see* condition
May (-Hegglin) anomaly or syndrome 288.2
Mayaro fever 066.3
Mazoplasia 610.8
MBD (minimal brain dysfunction), child *(see also* Hyperkinesia) 314.9
MCAD (medium chain acyl CoA dehydrogenase deficiency) 277.85
McArdle (-Schmid-Pearson) disease or syndrome (glycogenosis V) 271.0
McCune-Albright syndrome (osteitis fibrosa disseminata) 756.59
MCLS (mucocutaneous lymph node syndrome) 446.1
McQuarrie's syndrome (idiopathic familial hypoglycemia) 251.2
Measles (black) (hemorrhagic) (suppressed) 055.9
    with
        encephalitis 055.0
        keratitis 055.71
        keratoconjunctivitis 055.71
        otitis media 055.2
        pneumonia 055.1
        complication 055.8
            specified type NEC 055.79
    encephalitis 055.0
    French 056.9
    German 056.9

Measles *(Continued)*
    keratitis 055.71
    keratoconjunctivitis 055.71
    liberty 056.9
    otitis media 055.2
    pneumonia 055.1
    specified complications NEC 055.79
    vaccination, prophylactic (against) V04.2
Meatitis, urethral *(see also* Urethritis) 597.89
Meat poisoning - *see* Poisoning, food
Meatus, meatal - *see* condition
Meat-wrappers' asthma 506.9
Meckel's
    diverticulitis 751.0
    diverticulum (displaced) (hypertrophic) 751.0
Meconium
    aspiration 770.11
        with
            pneumonia 770.12
            pneumonitis 770.12
            respiratory symptoms 770.12
        below vocal cords 770.11
            with respiratory symptoms 770.12
        syndrome 770.12
    delayed passage in newborn 777.1
    ileus 777.1
        due to cystic fibrosis 277.01
    in liquor 792.3
        noted during delivery - 656.8 ●
    insufflation 770.11
        with respiratory symptoms 770.12
    obstruction
        fetus or newborn 777.1
            in mucoviscidosis 277.01
    passage of 792.3
        noted during delivery 763.84
    peritonitis 777.6
    plug syndrome (newborn) NEC 777.1
    staining 779.84
Median - *see also* condition
    arcuate ligament syndrome 447.4
    bar (prostate) 600.90
        with
            other lower urinary tract symptoms (LUTS) 600.91
            urinary
                obstruction 600.91
                retention 600.91
    rhomboid glossitis 529.2
    vesical orifice 600.90
        with
            other lower urinary tract symptoms (LUTS) 600.91
            urinary
                obstruction 600.91
                retention 600.91
Mediastinal shift 793.2
Mediastinitis (acute) (chronic) 519.2
    actinomycotic 039.8
    syphilitic 095.8
    tuberculous *(see also* Tuberculosis) 012.8 ●
Mediastinopericarditis *(see also* Pericarditis) 423.9
    acute 420.90
    chronic 423.8
        rheumatic 393
    rheumatic, chronic 393
Mediastinum, mediastinal - *see* condition
Medical services provided for - *see* Health, services provided because (of)
Medicine poisoning (by overdose) (wrong substance given or taken in error) 977.9
    specified drug or substance - *see* Table of Drugs and Chemicals
Medin's disease (poliomyelitis) 045.9 ●
Mediterranean
    anemia 282.40
        with other hemoglobinopathy 282.49
    disease or syndrome (hemopathic) 282.40
        with other hemoglobinopathy 282.49

Mediterranean *(Continued)*
    fever *(see also* Brucellosis) 023.9
        familial 277.31
    kala-azar 085.0
    leishmaniasis 085.0
    tick fever 082.1
Medulla - *see* condition
Medullary
    cystic kidney 753.16
    sponge kidney 753.17
Medullated fibers
    optic (nerve) 743.57
    retina 362.85
Medulloblastoma (M9470/3)
    desmoplastic (M9471/3) 191.6
    specified site - *see* Neoplasm, by site, malignant
    unspecified site 191.6
Medulloepithelioma (M9501/3) - *see also* Neoplasm, by site, malignant
    teratoid (M9502/3) - *see* Neoplasm, by site, malignant
Medullomyoblastoma (M9472/3)
    specified site - *see* Neoplasm, by site, malignant
    unspecified site 191.6
Meekeren-Ehlers-Danlos syndrome 756.83
Megacaryocytic - *see* condition
Megacolon (acquired) (functional) (not Hirschsprung's disease) 564.7
    aganglionic 751.3
    congenital, congenitum 751.3
    Hirschsprung's (disease) 751.3
    psychogenic 306.4
    toxic *(see also* Colitis, ulcerative) 556.9
Megaduodenum 537.3
Megaesophagus (functional) 530.0
    congenital 750.4
Megakaryocytic - *see* condition
Megalencephaly 742.4
Megalerythema (epidermicum) (infectiosum) 057.0
Megalia, cutis et ossium 757.39
Megaloappendix 751.5
Megalocephalus, megalocephaly NEC 756.0
Megalocornea 743.41
    associated with buphthalmos 743.22
Megalocytic anemia 281.9
Megalodactylia (fingers) (thumbs) 755.57
    toes 755.65
Megaloduodenum 751.5
Megaloesophagus (functional) 530.0
    congenital 750.4
Megalogastria (congenital) 750.7
Megalomania 307.9
Megalophthalmos 743.8
Megalopsia 368.14
Megalosplenia *(see also* Splenomegaly) 789.2
Megaloureter 593.89
    congenital 753.22
Megarectum 569.49
Megasigmoid 564.7
    congenital 751.3
Megaureter 593.89
    congenital 753.22
Megrim 346.9 ●
Meibomian
    cyst 373.2
        infected 373.12
    gland - *see* condition
    infarct (eyelid) 374.85
    stye 373.11
Meibomitis 373.12
Meige
    -Milroy disease (chronic hereditary edema) 757.0
    syndrome (blepharospasm-oromandibular dystonia) 333.82
Melalgia, nutritional 266.2

Melancholia (see also Psychosis, affective) 296.90
- climacteric 296.2 ●
  - recurrent episode 296.3 ●
  - single episode 296.2 ●
- hypochondriac 300.7
- intermittent 296.2 ●
  - recurrent episode 296.3 ●
  - single episode 296.2 ●
- involutional 296.2 ●
  - recurrent episode 296.3 ●
  - single episode 296.2 ●
- menopausal 296.2 ●
  - recurrent episode 296.3 ●
  - single episode 296.2 ●
- puerperal 296.2 ●
- reactive (from emotional stress, psychological trauma) 298.0
- recurrent 296.3 ●
- senile 290.21
- stuporous 296.2 ●
  - recurrent episode 296.3 ●
  - single episode 296.2 ●

Melanemia 275.09
Melanoameloblastoma (M9363/0) - see Neoplasm, bone, benign
Melanoblastoma (M8720/3) - see Melanoma
Melanoblastosis
- Block-Sulzberger 757.33
- cutis linearis sive systematisata 757.33

Melanocarcinoma (M8720/3) - see Melanoma
Melanocytoma, eyeball (M8726/0) 224.0
Melanocytosis, neurocutaneous 757.33
Melanoderma, melanodermia 709.09
- Addison's (primary adrenal insufficiency) 255.41

Melanodontia, infantile 521.05
Melanodontoclasia 521.05
Melanoepithelioma (M8720/3) - see Melanoma
Melanoma (malignant) (M8720/3) 172.9

> Note: Except where otherwise indicated, the morphological varieties of melanoma in the list below should be coded by site as for "Melanoma (malignant)." Internal sites should be coded to malignant neoplasm of those sites.

- abdominal wall 172.5
- ala nasi 172.3
- amelanotic (M8730/3) - see Melanoma, by site
- ankle 172.7
- anus, anal 154.3
  - canal 154.2
- arm 172.6
- auditory canal (external) 172.2
- auricle (ear) 172.2
- auricular canal (external) 172.2
- axilla 172.5
- axillary fold 172.5
- back 172.5
- balloon cell (M8722/3) - see Melanoma, by site
- benign (M8720/0) - see Neoplasm, skin, benign
- breast (female) (male) 172.5
- brow 172.3
- buttock 172.5
- canthus (eye) 172.1
- cheek (external) 172.3
- chest wall 172.5
- chin 172.3
- choroid 190.6
- conjunctiva 190.3
- ear (external) 172.2
- epithelioid cell (M8771/3) - see also Melanoma, by site
  - and spindle cell, mixed (M8775/3) - see Melanoma, by site
- external meatus (ear) 172.2

Melanoma (Continued)
- eye 190.9
- eyebrow 172.3
- eyelid (lower) (upper) 172.1
- face NEC 172.3
- female genital organ (external) NEC 184.4
- finger 172.6
- flank 172.5
- foot 172.7
- forearm 172.6
- forehead 172.3
- foreskin 187.1
- gluteal region 172.5
- groin 172.5
- hand 172.6
- heel 172.7
- helix 172.2
- hip 172.7
- in
  - giant pigmented nevus (M8761/3) - see Melanoma, by site
  - Hutchinson's melanotic freckle (M8742/3) - see Melanoma, by site
  - junctional nevus (M8740/3) - see Melanoma, by site
  - precancerous melanosis (M8741/3) - see Melanoma, by site
- in situ - see Melanoma, by site
  - skin 172.9
- interscapular region 172.5
- iris 190.0
- jaw 172.3
- juvenile (M8770/0) - see Neoplasm, skin, benign
- knee 172.7
- labium
  - majus 184.1
  - minus 184.2
- lacrimal gland 190.2
- leg 172.7
- lip (lower) (upper) 172.0
- liver 197.7
- lower limb NEC 172.7
- male genital organ (external) NEC 187.9
- meatus, acoustic (external) 172.2
- meibomian gland 172.1
- metastatic
  - of or from specified site - see Melanoma, by site
  - site not of skin - see Neoplasm, by site, malignant, secondary
  - to specified site - see Neoplasm, by site, malignant, secondary
  - unspecified site 172.9
- nail 172.9
  - finger 172.6
  - toe 172.7
- neck 172.4
- nodular (M8721/3) - see Melanoma, by site
- nose, external 172.3
- orbit 190.1
- penis 187.4
- perianal skin 172.5
- perineum 172.5
- pinna 172.2
- popliteal (fossa) (space) 172.7
- prepuce 187.1
- pubes 172.5
- pudendum 184.4
- retina 190.5
- scalp 172.4
- scrotum 187.7
- septum nasal (skin) 172.3
- shoulder 172.6
- skin NEC 172.8
  - in situ 172.9
- spindle cell (M8772/3) - see also Melanoma, by site
  - type A (M8773/3) 190.0
  - type B (M8774/3) 190.0
- submammary fold 172.5

Melanoma (Continued)
- superficial spreading (M8743/3) - see Melanoma, by site
- temple 172.3
- thigh 172.7
- toe 172.7
- trunk NEC 172.5
- umbilicus 172.5
- upper limb NEC 172.6
- vagina vault 184.0
- vulva 184.4

Melanoplakia 528.9
Melanosarcoma (M8720/3) - see also Melanoma
- epithelioid cell (M8771/3) - see Melanoma

Melanosis 709.09
- addisonian (primary adrenal insufficiency) 255.41
  - tuberculous (see also Tuberculosis) 017.6 ●
- adrenal 255.41
- colon 569.89
- conjunctiva 372.55
  - congenital 743.49
- corii degenerativa 757.33
- cornea (presenile) (senile) 371.12
  - congenital 743.43
    - interfering with vision 743.42
  - prenatal 743.43
    - interfering with vision 743.42
- eye 372.55
  - congenital 743.49
- jute spinners' 709.09
- lenticularis progressiva 757.33
- liver 573.8
- precancerous (M8741/2) - see also Neoplasm, skin, in situ
  - malignant melanoma in (M8741/3) - see Melanoma
- Riehl's 709.09
- sclera 379.19
  - congenital 743.47
- suprarenal 255.41
- tar 709.09
- toxic 709.09

Melanuria 791.9
MELAS syndrome (mitochondrial encephalopathy, lactic acidosis and stroke-like episodes) 277.87
Melasma 709.09
- adrenal (gland) 255.41
- suprarenal (gland) 255.41

Melena 578.1
- due to
  - swallowed maternal blood 777.3
  - ulcer - see Ulcer, by site, with hemorrhage
- newborn 772.4
  - due to swallowed maternal blood 777.3

Meleney's
- gangrene (cutaneous) 686.09
- ulcer (chronic undermining) 686.09

Melioidosis 025
Melitensis, febris 023.0
Melitococcosis 023.0
Melkersson (-Rosenthal) syndrome 351.8
Mellitus, diabetes - see Diabetes
Melorheostosis (bone) (leri) 733.99
Meloschisis 744.83
Melotia 744.29
Membrana
- capsularis lentis posterior 743.39
- epipapillaris 743.57

Membranacea placenta - see Placenta, abnormal
Membranaceous uterus 621.8
Membrane, membranous - see also condition
- folds, congenital - see Web
- Jackson's 751.4
- over face (causing asphyxia), fetus or newborn 768.9
- premature rupture - see Rupture, membranes, premature
- pupillary 364.74
  - persistent 743.46

SECTION 1 INDEX TO DISEASES AND INJURIES / Membrane, membranous

Membrane, membranous (Continued)
  retained (complicating delivery) (with hemorrhage) 666.2●
    without hemorrhage 667.1●
  secondary (eye) 366.50
  unruptured (causing asphyxia) 768.9
  vitreous humor 379.25
Membranitis, fetal 658.4●
  affecting fetus or newborn 762.7
Memory disturbance, loss or lack (see also Amnesia) 780.93
  mild, following organic brain damage 310.89
MEN (multiple endocrine neoplasia) syndromes
  type I 258.01
  type IIA 258.02
  type IIB 258.03
Menadione (vitamin K) deficiency 269.0
Menarche, precocious 259.1
Mendacity, pathologic 301.7
Mende's syndrome (ptosis-epicanthus) 270.2
Mendelson's syndrome (resulting from a procedure) 997.32
  obstetric 668.0●
Ménétrier's disease or syndrome (hypertrophic gastritis) 535.2●
Ménière's disease, syndrome, or vertigo 386.00
  cochlear 386.02
  cochleovestibular 386.01
  inactive 386.04
  in remission 386.04
  vestibular 386.03
Meninges, meningeal - see condition
Meningioma (M9530/0) - see also Neoplasm, meninges, benign
  angioblastic (M9535/0) - see Neoplasm, meninges, benign
  angiomatous (M9534/0) - see Neoplasm, meninges, benign
  endotheliomatous (M9531/0) - see Neoplasm, meninges, benign
  fibroblastic (M9532/0) - see Neoplasm, meninges, benign
  fibrous (M9532/0) - see Neoplasm, meninges, benign
  hemangioblastic (M9535/0) - see Neoplasm, meninges, benign
  hemangiopericytic (M9536/0) - see Neoplasm, meninges, benign
  malignant (M9530/3) - see Neoplasm, meninges, malignant
  meningiothelial (M9531/0) - see Neoplasm, meninges, benign
  meningotheliomatous (M9531/0) - see Neoplasm, meninges, benign
  mixed (M9537/0) - see Neoplasm, meninges, benign
  multiple (M9530/1) 237.6
  papillary (M9538/1) 237.6
  psammomatous (M9533/0) - see Neoplasm, meninges, benign
  syncytial (M9531/0) - see Neoplasm, meninges, benign
  transitional (M9537/0) - see Neoplasm, meninges, benign
Meningiomatosis (diffuse) (M9530/1) 237.6
Meningism (see also Meningismus) 781.6
Meningismus (infectional) (pneumococcal) 781.6
  due to serum or vaccine 997.09 [321.8]
  influenzal NEC (see also Influenza) 487.8
Meningitis (basal) (basic) (basilar) (brain) (cerebral) (cervical) (congestive) (diffuse) (hemorrhagic) (infantile) (membranous) (metastatic) (nonspecific) (pontine) (progressive) (simple) (spinal) (subacute) (sympathetica) (toxic) 322.9
  abacterial NEC (see also Meningitis, aseptic) 047.9
  actinomycotic 039.8 [320.7]
  adenoviral 049.1
  aerobacter aerogenes 320.82

Meningitis (Continued)
  anaerobes (cocci) (gram-negative) (gram-positive) (mixed) (NEC) 320.81
  arbovirus NEC 066.9 [321.2]
    specified type NEC 066.8 [321.2]
  aseptic (acute) NEC 047.9
    adenovirus 049.1
    Coxsackie virus 047.0
    due to
      adenovirus 049.1
      Coxsackie virus 047.0
      ECHO virus 047.1
      enterovirus 047.9
      mumps 072.1
      poliovirus (see also Poliomyelitis) 045.2● [321.2]
    ECHO virus 047.1
    herpes (simplex) virus 054.72
    zoster 053.0
    leptospiral 100.81
    lymphocytic choriomeningitis 049.0
    noninfective 322.0
  Bacillus pyocyaneus 320.89
  bacterial NEC 320.9
    anaerobic 320.81
    gram-negative 320.82
      anaerobic 320.81
  Bacteroides (fragilis) (oralis) (melaninogenicus) 320.81
  cancerous (M8000/6) 198.4
  candidal 112.83
  carcinomatous (M8010/6) 198.4
  caseous (see also Tuberculosis, meninges) 013.0●
  cerebrospinal (acute) (chronic) (diplococcal) (endemic) (epidemic) (fulminant) (infectious) (malignant) (meningococcal) (sporadic) 036.0
    carrier (suspected) of V02.59
  chronic NEC 322.2
  clear cerebrospinal fluid NEC 322.0
  Clostridium (haemolyticum) (novyi) NEC 320.81
  coccidioidomycosis 114.2
  Coxsackie virus 047.0
  cryptococcal 117.5 [321.0]
  diplococcal 036.0
    gram-negative 036.0
    gram-positive 320.1
  Diplococcus pneumoniae 320.1
  due to
    actinomycosis 039.8 [320.7]
    adenovirus 049.1
    coccidiomycosis 114.2
    enterovirus 047.9
      specified NEC 047.8
    histoplasmosis (see also Histoplasmosis) 115.91
    Listerosis 027.0 [320.7]
    Lyme disease 088.81 [320.7]
    moniliasis 112.83
    mumps 072.1
    neurosyphilis 094.2
    nonbacterial organisms NEC 321.8
    oidiomycosis 112.83
    poliovirus (see also Poliomyelitis) 045.2● [321.2]
    preventive immunization, inoculation, or vaccination 997.09 [321.8]
    sarcoidosis 135 [321.4]
    sporotrichosis 117.1 [321.1]
    syphilis 094.2
      acute 091.81
      congenital 090.42
      secondary 091.81
    trypanosomiasis (see also Trypanosomiasis) 086.9 [321.3]
    whooping cough 033.9 [320.7]
  E. coli 320.82
  ECHO virus 047.1

Meningitis (Continued)
  endothelial-leukocytic, benign, recurrent 047.9
  Enterobacter aerogenes 320.82
  enteroviral 047.9
    specified type NEC 047.8
  enterovirus 047.9
    specified NEC 047.8
  eosinophilic 322.1
  epidemic NEC 036.0
  Escherichia coli (E. coli) 320.82
  Eubacterium 320.81
  fibrinopurulent NEC 320.9
    specified type NEC 320.89
  Friedländer (bacillus) 320.82
  fungal NEC 117.9 [321.1]
  Fusobacterium 320.81
  gonococcal 098.82
  gram-negative bacteria NEC 320.82
    anaerobic 320.81
    cocci 036.0
      specified NEC 320.82
  gram-negative cocci NEC 036.0
    specified NEC 320.82
  gram-positive cocci NEC 320.9
  H. influenzae 320.0
  herpes (simplex) virus 054.72
    zoster 053.0
  infectious NEC 320.9
  influenzal 320.0
  Klebsiella pneumoniae 320.82
  late effect - see Late, effect, meningitis
  leptospiral (aseptic) 100.81
  Listerella (monocytogenes) 027.0 [320.7]
  Listeria monocytogenes 027.0 [320.7]
  lymphocytic (acute) (benign) (serous) 049.0
    choriomeningitis virus 049.0
  meningococcal (chronic) 036.0
  Mima polymorpha 320.82
  Mollaret's 047.9
  monilial 112.83
  mumps (virus) 072.1
  mycotic NEC 117.9 [321.1]
  Neisseria 036.0
  neurosyphilis 094.2
  nonbacterial NEC (see also Meningitis, aseptic) 047.9
  nonpyogenic NEC 322.0
  oidiomycosis 112.83
  ossificans 349.2
  Peptococcus 320.81
  PeptoStreptococcus 320.81
  pneumococcal 320.1
  poliovirus (see also Poliomyelitis) 045.2● [321.2]
  Proprionibacterium 320.81
  Proteus morganii 320.82
  Pseudomonas (aeruginosa) (pyocyaneus) 320.82
  purulent NEC 320.9
    specified organism NEC 320.89
  pyogenic NEC 320.9
    specified organism NEC 320.89
  Salmonella 003.21
  septic NEC 320.9
    specified organism NEC 320.89
  serosa circumscripta NEC 322.0
  serous NEC (see also Meningitis, aseptic) 047.9
    lymphocytic 049.0
    syndrome 348.2
  Serratia (marcescens) 320.82
  specified organism NEC 320.89
  sporadic cerebrospinal 036.0
  sporotrichosis 117.1 [321.1]
  staphylococcal 320.3
  sterile 997.09
  streptococcal (acute) 320.2
  suppurative 320.9
    specified organism NEC 320.89

Meningitis (Continued)
 syphilitic 094.2
  acute 091.81
  congenital 090.42
  secondary 091.81
 torula 117.5 [321.0]
 traumatic (complication of injury) 958.8
 Treponema (denticola) (macrodenticum) 320.81
 trypanosomiasis 086.1 [321.3]
 tuberculous (see also Tuberculosis, meninges) 013.0●
 typhoid 002.0 [320.7]
 Veillonella 320.81
 Vibrio vulnificus 320.82
 viral, virus NEC (see also Meningitis, aseptic) 047.9
 Wallgren's (see also Meningitis, aseptic) 047.9
Meningocele (congenital) (spinal) (see also Spina bifida) 741.9●
 acquired (traumatic) 349.2
 cerebral 742.0
 cranial 742.0
Meningocerebritis - see Meningoencephalitis
Meningococcemia (acute) (chronic) 036.2
Meningococcus, meningococcal (see also condition) 036.9
 adrenalitis, hemorrhagic 036.3
 carditis 036.40
 carrier (suspected) of V02.59
 cerebrospinal fever 036.0
 encephalitis 036.1
 endocarditis 036.42
 exposure to V01.84
 infection NEC 036.9
 meningitis (cerebrospinal) 036.0
 myocarditis 036.43
 optic neuritis 036.81
 pericarditis 036.41
 septicemia (chronic) 036.2
Meningoencephalitis (see also Encephalitis) 323.9
 acute NEC 048
 bacterial, purulent, pyogenic, or septic - see Meningitis
 chronic NEC 094.1
 diffuse NEC 094.1
 diphasic 063.2
 due to
  actinomycosis 039.8 [320.7]
  blastomycosis NEC (see also Blastomycosis) 116.0 [323.41]
  free-living amebae 136.29
  Listeria monocytogenes 027.0 [320.7]
  Lyme disease 088.81 [320.7]
  mumps 072.2
  Naegleria (amebae) (gruberi) (organisms) 136.29
  rubella 056.01
  sporotrichosis 117.1 [321.1]
  toxoplasmosis (acquired) 130.0
   congenital (active) 771.2 [323.41]
  Trypanosoma 086.1 [323.2]
 epidemic 036.0
 herpes 054.3
 herpetic 054.3
 H. influenzae 320.0
 infectious (acute) 048
 influenzal 320.0
 late effect - see category 326
 Listeria monocytogenes 027.0 [320.7]
 lymphocytic (serous) 049.0
 mumps 072.2
 parasitic NEC 123.9 [323.41]
 pneumococcal 320.1
 primary amebic 136.29
 rubella 056.01
 serous 048
  lymphocytic 049.0
 specific 094.2
 staphylococcal 320.3

Meningoencephalitis (Continued)
 streptococcal 320.2
 syphilitic 094.2
 toxic NEC 989.9 [323.71]
  due to
   carbon tetrachloride (vapor) 987.8 [323.71]
   hydroxyquinoline derivatives poisoning 961.3 [323.71]
   lead 984.9 [323.71]
   mercury 985.0 [323.71]
   thallium 985.8 [323.71]
 toxoplasmosis (acquired) 130.0
 trypanosomic 086.1 [323.2]
 tuberculous (see also Tuberculosis, meninges) 013.0●
 virus NEC 048
Meningoencephalocele 742.0
 syphilitic 094.89
  congenital 090.49
Meningoencephalomyelitis (see also Meningoencephalitis) 323.9
 acute NEC 048
  disseminated (postinfectious) 136.9 [323.61]
   postimmunization or postvaccination 323.51
 due to
  actinomycosis 039.8 [320.7]
  torula 117.5 [323.41]
  toxoplasma or toxoplasmosis (acquired) 130.0
   congenital (active) 771.2 [323.41]
 late effect - see category 326
Meningoencephalomyelopathy (see also Meningoencephalomyelitis) 349.9
Meningoencephalopathy (see also Meningoencephalitis) 348.39
Meningoencephalopoliomyelitis (see also Poliomyelitis, bulbar) 045.0●
 late effect 138
Meningomyelitis (see also Meningoencephalitis) 323.9
 blastomycotic NEC (see also Blastomycosis) 116.0 [323.41]
 due to
  actinomycosis 039.8 [320.7]
  blastomycosis (see also Blastomycosis) 116.0 [323.41]
  Meningococcus 036.0
  sporotrichosis 117.1 [323.41]
  torula 117.5 [323.41]
 late effect - see category 326
 lethargic 049.8
 meningococcal 036.0
 syphilitic 094.2
 tuberculous (see also Tuberculosis, meninges) 013.0●
Meningomyelocele (see also Spina bifida) 741.9●
 syphilitic 094.89
Meningomyeloneuritis - see Meningoencephalitis
Meningoradiculitis - see Meningitis
Meningovascular - see condition
Meniscocytosis 282.60
Menkes' syndrome - see Syndrome, Menkes'
Menolipsis 626.0
Menometrorrhagia 626.2
Menopause, menopausal (symptoms) (syndrome) 627.2
 arthritis (any site) NEC 716.3●
 artificial 627.4
 bleeding 627.0
 crisis 627.2
 depression (see also Psychosis, affective) 296.2●
  agitated 296.2●
   recurrent episode 296.3●
   single episode 296.2●

Menopause, menopausal (Continued)
 depression (Continued)
  psychotic 296.2●
   recurrent episode 296.3●
   single episode 296.2●
  recurrent episode 296.3●
  single episode 296.2●
 melancholia (see also Psychosis, affective) 296.2●
  recurrent episode 296.3●
  single episode 296.2●
 paranoid state 297.2
 paraphrenia 297.2
 postsurgical 627.4
 premature 256.31
  postirradiation 256.2
  postsurgical 256.2
 psychoneurosis 627.2
 psychosis NEC 298.8
 surgical 627.4
 toxic polyarthritis NEC 716.39
Menorrhagia (primary) 626.2
 climacteric 627.0
 menopausal 627.0
 postclimacteric 627.1
 postmenopausal 627.1
 preclimacteric 627.0
 premenopausal 627.0
 puberty (menses retained) 626.3
Menorrhalgia 625.3
Menoschesis 626.8
Menostaxis 626.2
Menses, retention 626.8
Menstrual - see also Menstruation
 cycle, irregular 626.4
 disorders NEC 626.9
 extraction V25.3
 fluid, retained 626.8
 molimen 625.4
 period, normal V65.5
 regulation V25.3
Menstruation
 absent 626.0
 anovulatory 628.0
 delayed 626.8
 difficult 625.3
 disorder 626.9
  psychogenic 306.52
  specified NEC 626.8
 during pregnancy 640.8●
 excessive 626.2
 frequent 626.2
 infrequent 626.1
 irregular 626.4
 latent 626.8
 membranous 626.8
 painful (primary) (secondary) 625.3
  psychogenic 306.52
 passage of clots 626.2
 precocious 259.1
 protracted 626.8
 retained 626.8
 retrograde 626.8
 scanty 626.1
 suppression 626.8
 vicarious (nasal) 625.8
Mentagra (see also Sycosis) 704.8
Mental - see also condition
 deficiency (see also Disability, intellectual) 319
 deterioration (see also Psychosis) 298.9
 disorder (see also Disorder, mental) 300.9
 exhaustion 300.5
 insufficiency (congenital) (see also Disability, intellectual) 319
 observation without need for further medical care NEC V71.09
 retardation - see Disability, intellectual
 subnormality (see also Disability, intellectual) 319
  mild 317
  moderate 318.0

SECTION 1 INDEX TO DISEASES AND INJURIES / Mental

Mental (Continued)
  subnormality (Continued)
    profound 318.2
    severe 318.1
  upset (see also Disorder, mental) 300.9
Meralgia paresthetica 355.1
Mercurial - see condition
Mercurialism NEC 985.0
Merergasia 300.9
Merkel cell tumor - see Carcinoma, Merkel cell
Merocele (see also Hernia, femoral) 553.00
Meromelia 755.4
  lower limb 755.30
    intercalary 755.32
      femur 755.34
        tibiofibular (complete) (incomplete) 755.33
      fibula 755.37
      metatarsal(s) 755.38
      tarsal(s) 755.38
      tibia 755.36
      tibiofibular 755.35
    terminal (complete) (partial) (transverse) 755.31
      longitudinal 755.32
        metatarsal(s) 755.38
        phalange(s) 755.39
        tarsal(s) 755.38
    transverse 755.31
  upper limb 755.20
    intercalary 755.22
      carpal(s) 755.28
      humeral 755.24
      radioulnar (complete) (incomplete) 755.23
      metacarpal(s) 755.28
      phalange(s) 755.29
      radial 755.26
      radioulnar 755.25
      ulnar 755.27
    terminal (complete) (partial) (transverse) 755.21
      longitudinal 755.22
        carpal(s) 755.28
        metacarpal(s) 755.28
        phalange(s) 755.29
    transverse 755.21
Merosmia 781.1
MERRF syndrome (myoclonus with epilepsy and with ragged red fibers) 277.87
Merycism - see also Vomiting
  psychogenic 307.53
Merzbacher-Pelizaeus disease 330.0
Mesaortitis - see Aortitis
Mesarteritis - see Arteritis
Mesencephalitis (see also Encephalitis) 323.9
  late effect - see category 326
Mesenchymoma (M8990/1) - see also Neoplasm, connective tissue, uncertain behavior
  benign (M8990/0) - see Neoplasm, connective tissue, benign
  malignant (M8990/3) - see Neoplasm, connective tissue, malignant
Mesenteritis
  retractile 567.82
  sclerosing 567.82
Mesentery, mesenteric - see condition
Mesiodens, mesiodentes 520.1
  causing crowding 524.31
Mesio-occlusion 524.23
Mesocardia (with asplenia) 746.87
Mesocolon - see condition
Mesonephroma (malignant) (M9110/3) - see also Neoplasm, by site, malignant
  benign (M9110/0) - see Neoplasm, by site, benign
Mesophlebitis - see Phlebitis
Mesostromal dysgenesis 743.51

Mesothelioma (malignant) (M9050/3) - see also Neoplasm, by site, malignant
  benign (M9050/0) - see Neoplasm, by site, benign
  biphasic type (M9053/3) - see also Neoplasm, by site, malignant
    benign (M9053/0) - see Neoplasm, by site, benign
  epithelioid (M9052/3) - see also Neoplasm, by site, malignant
    benign (M9052/0) - see Neoplasm, by site, benign
  fibrous (M9051/3) - see also Neoplasm, by site, malignant
    benign (M9051/0) - see Neoplasm, by site, benign
Metabolic syndrome 277.7
Metabolism disorder 277.9
  specified type NEC 277.89
Metagonimiasis 121.5
Metagonimus infestation (small intestine) 121.5
Metal
  pigmentation (skin) 709.00
  polishers' disease 502
Metalliferous miners' lung 503
Metamorphopsia 368.14
Metaplasia
  bone, in skin 709.3
  breast 611.89
  cervix - omit code
  endometrium (squamous) 621.8
  esophagus 530.85
  intestinal, of gastric mucosa 537.89
  kidney (pelvis) (squamous) (see also Disease, renal) 593.89
  myelogenous 289.89
  myeloid 289.89
    agnogenic 238.76
    megakaryocytic 238.76
  spleen 289.59
  squamous cell
    amnion 658.8
    bladder 596.89
    cervix - see condition
    trachea 519.19
    tracheobronchial tree 519.19
    uterus 621.8
      cervix - see condition
Metastasis, metastatic
  abscess - see Abscess
  calcification 275.40
  cancer, neoplasm, or disease
    from specified site (M8000/3) - see Neoplasm, by site, malignant
    to specified site (M8000/6) - see Neoplasm, by site, secondary
  deposits (in) (M8000/6) - see Neoplasm, by site, secondary
  mesentery, of neuroendocrine tumor 209.74
  pneumonia 038.8 [484.8]
  spread (to) (M8000/6) - see Neoplasm, by site, secondary
Metatarsalgia 726.70
  anterior 355.6
  due to Freiberg's disease 732.5
  Morton's 355.6
Metatarsus, metatarsal - see also condition
  abductus valgus (congenital) 754.60
  adductus varus (congenital) 754.53
  primus varus 754.52
  valgus (adductus) (congenital) 754.60
  varus (abductus) (congenital) 754.53
    primus 754.52
Methadone use 304.00
Methemoglobinemia 289.7
  acquired (with sulfhemoglobinemia) 289.7
  congenital 289.7
  enzymatic 289.7
  Hb-M disease 289.7
  hereditary 289.7
  toxic 289.7

Methemoglobinuria (see also Hemoglobinuria) 791.2
Methicillin
  resistant staphylococcus aureus (MRSA) 041.12
    colonization V02.54
    personal history of V12.04
  susceptible staphylococcus aureus (MSSA) 041.11
    colonization V02.53
Methioninemia 270.4
Metritis (catarrhal) (septic) (suppurative) (see also Endometritis) 615.9
  blennorrhagic 098.16
    chronic or duration of 2 months or over 098.36
  cervical (see also Cervicitis) 616.0
  gonococcal 098.16
    chronic or duration of 2 months or over 098.36
  hemorrhagic 626.8
  puerperal, postpartum, childbirth 670.1
  septic 670.2
  tuberculous (see also Tuberculosis) 016.7
Metropathia hemorrhagica 626.8
Metroperitonitis (see also Peritonitis, pelvic, female) 614.5
Metrorrhagia 626.6
  arising during pregnancy - see Hemorrhage, pregnancy
  postpartum NEC 666.2
  primary 626.6
  psychogenic 306.59
  puerperal 666.2
Metrorrhexis - see Rupture, uterus
Metrosalpingitis (see also Salpingo-oophoritis) 614.2
Metrostaxis 626.6
Metrovaginitis (see also Endometritis) 615.9
  gonococcal (acute) 098.16
    chronic or duration of 2 months or over 098.36
Mexican fever - see Typhus, Mexican
Meyenburg-Altherr-Uehlinger syndrome 733.99
Meyer-Schwickerath and Weyers syndrome (dysplasia oculodentodigitalis) 759.89
Meynert's amentia (nonalcoholic) 294.0
  alcoholic 291.1
Mibelli's disease 757.39
Mice, joint (see also Loose, body, joint) 718.1
  knee 717.6
Micheli-Rietti syndrome (thalassemia minor) 282.46
Michotte's syndrome 721.5
Micrencephalon, micrencephaly 742.1
Microalbuminuria 791.0
Microaneurysm, retina 362.14
  diabetic 250.5 [362.01]
    due to secondary diabetes 249.5 [362.01]
Microangiopathy 443.9
  diabetic (peripheral) 250.7 [443.81]
    due to secondary diabetes 249.7 [443.81]
    retinal 250.5 [362.01]
      due to secondary diabetes 249.5 [362.01]
  peripheral 443.9
    diabetic 250.7 [443.81]
      due to secondary diabetes 249.7 [443.81]
  retinal 362.18
    diabetic 250.5 [362.01]
      due to secondary diabetes 249.5 [362.01]
  thrombotic 446.6
    Moschcowitz's (thrombotic thrombocytopenic purpura) 446.6

Microcalcification, mammographic 793.81
Microcephalus, microcephalic, microcephaly 742.1
    due to toxoplasmosis (congenital) 771.2
Microcheilia 744.82
Microcolon (congenital) 751.5
Microcornea (congenital) 743.41
Microcytic - see condition
Microdeletions NEC 758.33
Microdontia 520.2
Microdrepanocytosis (thalassemia-Hb-S disease) 282.41
    with sickle cell crisis 282.42
Microembolism
    atherothrombotic - see Atheroembolism
    retina 362.33
Microencephalon 742.1
Microfilaria streptocerca infestation 125.3
Microgastria (congenital) 750.7
Microgenia 524.06
Microgenitalia (congenital) 752.89
    penis 752.64
Microglioma (M9710/3)
    specified site - see Neoplasm, by site, malignant
    unspecified site 191.9
Microglossia (congenital) 750.16
Micrognathia, micrognathism (congenital) 524.00
    mandibular 524.04
        alveolar 524.74
    maxillary 524.03
        alveolar 524.73
Microgyria (congenital) 742.2
Microinfarct, heart (see also Insufficiency, coronary) 411.89
Microlithiasis, alveolar, pulmonary 516.2
Micromastia 611.82
Micromyelia (congenital) 742.59
Micropenis 752.64
Microphakia (congenital) 743.36
Microphthalmia (congenital) (see also Microphthalmos) 743.10
Microphthalmos (congenital) 743.10
    associated with eye and adnexal anomalies NEC 743.12
    due to toxoplasmosis (congenital) 771.2
    isolated 743.11
    simple 743.11
    syndrome 759.89
Micropsia 368.14
Microsporidiosis 136.8
Microsporosis (see also Dermatophytosis) 110.9
    nigra 111.1
Microsporum furfur infestation 111.0
Microstomia (congenital) 744.84
Microthelia 757.6
Microthromboembolism - see Embolism
Microtia (congenital) (external ear) 744.23
Microtropia 378.34
Microvillus inclusion disease (MVD) 751.5
Micturition
    disorder NEC 788.69
        psychogenic 306.53
    frequency 788.41
        psychogenic 306.53
    nocturnal 788.43
    painful 788.1
        psychogenic 306.53
Middle
    ear - see condition
    lobe (right) syndrome 518.0
Midplane - see condition
Miescher's disease 709.3
    cheilitis 351.8
    granulomatosis disciformi0s 709.3
Miescher-Leder syndrome or granulomatosis 709.3
Mieten's syndrome 759.89

Migraine (idiopathic) 346.9●

Note: The following fifth digit subclassification is for use with category 346:
0   without mention of intractable migraine without mention of status migrainosus
    without mention of refractory migraine without mention of status migrainosus
1   with intractable migraine, so stated, without mention of status migrainosus
    with refractory migraine, so stated, without mention of status migrainosus
2   without mention of intractable migraine with status migrainosus
    without mention of refractory migraine with status migrainosus
3   with intractable migraine, so stated, with status migrainosus
    with refractory migraine, so stated, with status migrainosus

    with aura (acute-onset) (without headache) (prolonged) (typical) 346.0●
    without aura 346.1●
        chronic 346.7●
        transformed 346.7●
    abdominal (syndrome) 346.2●
    allergic (histamine) 346.2●
    atypical 346.8●
    basilar 346.0●
    chronic without aura 346.7●
    classic(al) 346.0●
    common 346.1●
    complicated 346.0●
    hemiplegic 346.3●
        familial 346.3●
        sporadic 346.3●
    lower-half 339.00
    menstrual 346.4●
    menstrually related 346.4●
    ophthalmic 346.8●
    ophthalmoplegic 346.2●
    premenstrual 346.4●
    pure menstrual 346.4●
    retinal 346.0●
    specified form NEC 346.8●
    transformed without aura 346.7●
    variant 346.2●
Migrant, social V60.0
Migratory, migrating - see also condition
    person V60.0
    testis, congenital 752.52
Mikulicz's disease or syndrome (dryness of mouth, absent or decreased lacrimation) 527.1
Milian atrophia blanche 701.3
Miliaria (crystallina) (rubra) (tropicalis) 705.1
    apocrine 705.82
Miliary - see condition
Milium (see also Cyst, sebaceous) 706.2
    colloid 709.3
    eyelid 374.84
Milk
    crust 690.11
    excess secretion 676.6●
    fever, female 672
    poisoning 988.8
    retention 676.2●
    sickness 988.8
    spots 423.1
Milkers' nodes 051.1
Milk-leg (deep vessels) 671.4●
    complicating pregnancy 671.3●
    nonpuerperal 451.19
    puerperal, postpartum, childbirth 671.4●

Milkman (-Looser) disease or syndrome (osteomalacia with pseudofractures) 268.2
Milky urine (see also Chyluria) 791.1
Millar's asthma (laryngismus stridulus) 478.75
Millard-Gubler paralysis or syndrome 344.89
Millard-Gubler-Foville paralysis 344.89
Miller-Dieker syndrome 758.33
Miller's disease (osteomalacia) 268.2
Miller Fisher's syndrome 357.0
Milles' syndrome (encephalocutaneous angiomatosis) 759.6
Mills' disease 335.29
Millstone makers' asthma or lung 502
Milroy's disease (chronic hereditary edema) 757.0
Miners' - see also condition
    asthma 500
    elbow 727.2
    knee 727.2
    lung 500
    nystagmus 300.89
    phthisis (see also Tuberculosis) 011.4●
    tuberculosis (see also Tuberculosis) 011.4●
Minkowski-Chauffard syndrome (see also Spherocytosis) 282.0
Minor - see condition
Minor's disease 336.1
Minot's disease (hemorrhagic disease, newborn) 776.0
Minot-von Willebrand (-Jürgens) disease or syndrome (angiohemophilia) 286.4
Minus (and plus) hand (intrinsic) 736.09
Miosis (persistent) (pupil) 379.42
Mirizzi's syndrome (hepatic duct stenosis) (see also Obstruction, biliary) 576.2
    with calculus, cholelithiasis, or stones - see Choledocholithiasis
Mirror writing 315.09
    secondary to organic lesion 784.69
Misadventure (prophylactic) (therapeutic) (see also Complications) 999.9
    administration of insulin 962.3
    infusion - see Complications, infusion
    local applications (of fomentations, plasters, etc.) 999.9
        burn or scald - see Burn, by site
    medical care (early) (late) NEC 999.9
        adverse effect of drugs or chemicals - see Table of Drugs and Chemicals
        burn or scald - see Burn, by site
    radiation NEC 990
    radiotherapy NEC 990
    surgical procedure (early) (late) - see Complications, surgical procedure
    transfusion - see Complications, transfusion
    vaccination or other immunological procedure - see Complications, vaccination
Misanthropy 301.7
Miscarriage - see Abortion, spontaneous
Mischief, malicious, child (see also Disturbance, conduct) 312.0●
Misdirection
    aqueous 365.83
Mismanagement, feeding 783.3
Misplaced, misplacement
    kidney (see also Disease, renal) 593.0
        congenital 753.3
    organ or site, congenital NEC - see Malposition, congenital
Missed
    abortion 632
    delivery (at or near term) 656.4●
    labor (at or near term) 656.4●
Misshapen reconstructed breast 612.0
Missing - see also Absence
    teeth (acquired) 525.10
        congenital (see also Anodontia) 520.0
        due to
            caries 525.13
            extraction 525.10

Missing (Continued)
   teeth (Continued)
      due to (Continued)
         periodontal disease 525.12
         specified NEC 525.19
         trauma 525.11
   vertebrae (congenital) 756.13
Misuse of drugs NEC (*see also* Abuse, drug, nondependent) 305.9●
Mitchell's disease (erythromelalgia) 443.82
Mite(s)
   diarrhea 133.8
   grain (itch) 133.8
   hair follicle (itch) 133.8
   in sputum 133.8
Mitochondrial encephalopathy, lactic acidosis and stroke-like episodes (MELAS syndrome) 277.87
Mitochondrial neurogastrointestinal encephalopathy syndrome (MNGIE) 277.87
Mitral - *see* condition
Mittelschmerz 625.2
Mixed - *see* condition
Mljet disease (mal de Meleda) 757.39
Mobile, mobility
   cecum 751.4
   coccyx 733.99
   excessive - *see* Hypermobility
   gallbladder 751.69
   kidney 593.0
      congenital 753.3
   organ or site, congenital NEC - *see* Malposition, congenital
   spleen 289.59
Mobitz heart block (atrioventricular) 426.10
   type I (Wenckebach's) 426.13
   type II 426.12
Möbius'
   disease 346.2●
   syndrome
      congenital oculofacial paralysis 352.6
      ophthalmoplegic migraine 346.2●
Moeller (-Barlow) disease (infantile scurvy) 267
   glossitis 529.4
Mohr's syndrome (types I and II) 759.89
Mola destruens (M9100/1) 236.1
Molarization, premolars 520.2
Molar pregnancy 631.8
   hydatidiform (delivered) (undelivered) 630
Mold(s) in vitreous 117.9
Molding, head (during birth) - *omit code*
Mole (pigmented) (M8720/0) - *see also* Neoplasm, skin, benign
   blood 631.8
   Breus' 631.8
   cancerous (M8720/3) - *see* Melanoma
   carneous 631.8
   destructive (M9100/1) 236.1
   ectopic - *see* Pregnancy, ectopic
   fleshy 631.8
   hemorrhagic 631.8
   hydatid, hydatidiform (benign) (complicating pregnancy) (delivered) (undelivered) (*see also* Hydatidiform mole) 630
   invasive (M9100/1) 236.1
   malignant (M9100/1) 236.1
   previous, affecting management of pregnancy V23.1
   invasive (hydatidiform) (M9100/1) 236.1
   malignant
      meaning
         malignant hydatidiform mole (M9100/1) 236.1
         melanoma (M8720/3) - *see* Melanoma
   nonpigmented (M8730/0) - *see* Neoplasm, skin, benign
   pregnancy NEC 631.8
   skin (M8720/0) - *see* Neoplasm, skin, benign
   stone 631.8

Mole (Continued)
   tubal - *see* Pregnancy, tubal
   vesicular (*see also* Hydatidiform mole) 630
Molimen, molimina (menstrual) 625.4
Mollaret's meningitis 047.9
Mollities (cerebellar) (cerebral) 437.8
   ossium 268.2
Molluscum
   contagiosum 078.0
   epitheliale 078.0
   fibrosum (M8851/0) - *see* Lipoma, by site
   pendulum (M8851/0) - *see* Lipoma, by site
Mönckeberg's arteriosclerosis, degeneration, disease, or sclerosis (*see also* Arteriosclerosis, extremities) 440.20
Monday fever 504
Monday morning dyspnea or asthma 504
Mondini's malformation (cochlea) 744.05
Mondor's disease (thrombophlebitis of breast) 451.89
Mongolian, mongolianism, mongolism, mongoloid 758.0
   spot 757.33
Monilethrix (congenital) 757.4
Monilia infestation - *see* Candidiasis
Moniliasis - *see also* Candidiasis
   neonatal 771.7
   vulvovaginitis 112.1
Monkeypox 059.01
Monoarthritis 716.60
   ankle 716.67
   arm 716.62
      lower (and wrist) 716.63
      upper (and elbow) 716.62
   foot (and ankle) 716.67
   forearm (and wrist) 716.63
   hand 716.64
   leg 716.66
      lower 716.66
      upper 716.65
   pelvic region (hip) (thigh) 716.65
   shoulder (region) 716.61
   specified site NEC 716.68
Monoblastic - *see* condition
Monochromatism (cone) (rod) 368.54
Monocytic - *see* condition
Monocytopenia 288.59
Monocytosis (symptomatic) 288.63
Monofixation syndrome 378.34
Monomania (*see also* Psychosis) 298.9
Mononeuritis 355.9
   cranial nerve - *see* Disorder, nerve, cranial
   femoral nerve 355.2
   lateral
      cutaneous nerve of thigh 355.1
      popliteal nerve 355.3
   lower limb 355.8
      specified nerve NEC 355.79
   medial popliteal nerve 355.4
   median nerve 354.1
   multiplex 354.5
   plantar nerve 355.6
   posterior tibial nerve 355.5
   radial nerve 354.3
   sciatic nerve 355.0
   ulnar nerve 354.2
   upper limb 354.9
      specified nerve NEC 354.8
   vestibular 388.5
Mononeuropathy (*see also* Mononeuritis) 355.9
   diabetic NEC 250.6● [355.9]
      due to secondary diabetes 249.6● [355.9]
      lower limb 250.6● [355.8]
         due to secondary diabetes 249.6● [355.8]
      upper limb 250.6● [354.9]
         due to secondary diabetes 249.6● [354.9]
   iliohypogastric nerve 355.79
   ilioinguinal nerve 355.79

Mononeuropathy (Continued)
   obturator nerve 355.79
   saphenous nerve 355.79
Mononucleosis, infectious 075
   with hepatitis 075 [573.1]
Monoplegia 344.5
   brain (current episode) (*see also* Paralysis, brain) 437.8
      fetus or newborn 767.8
   cerebral (current episode) (*see also* Paralysis, brain) 437.8
   congenital or infantile (cerebral) (spastic) (spinal) 343.3
   embolic (current) (*see also* Embolism, brain) 434.1●
      late effect - *see* Late effect(s) (of) cerebrovascular disease
   infantile (cerebral) (spastic) (spinal) 343.3
   lower limb 344.30
      affecting
         dominant side 344.31
         nondominant side 344.32
      due to late effect of cerebrovascular accident - *see* Late effect(s) (of) cerebrovascular accident
   newborn 767.8
   psychogenic 306.0
      specified as conversion reaction 300.11
   thrombotic (current) (*see also* Thrombosis, brain) 434.0●
      late effect - *see* Late effect(s) (of) cerebrovascular disease
   transient 781.4
   upper limb 344.40
      affecting
         dominant side 344.41
         nondominant side 344.42
      due to late effect of cerebrovascular accident - *see* Late effect(s) (of) cerebrovascular accident
Monorchism, monorchidism 752.89
Monteggia's fracture (closed) 813.03
   open 813.13
Mood swings
   brief compensatory 296.99
   rebound 296.99
Moore's syndrome (*see also* Epilepsy) 345.5●
Mooren's ulcer (cornea) 370.07
Mooser-Neill reaction 081.0
Mooser bodies 081.0
Moral
   deficiency 301.7
   imbecility 301.7
Morax-Axenfeld conjunctivitis 372.03
Morbilli (*see also* Measles) 055.9
Morbus
   anglicus, anglorum 268.0
   Beigel 111.2
   caducus (*see also* Epilepsy) 345.9●
   caeruleus 746.89
   celiacus 579.0
   comitialis (*see also* Epilepsy) 345.9●
   cordis - *see also* Disease, heart
      valvulorum - *see* Endocarditis
   coxae 719.95
      tuberculous (*see also* Tuberculosis) 015.1●
   hemorrhagicus neonatorum 776.0
   maculosus neonatorum 772.6
   renum 593.0
   senilis (*see also* Osteoarthrosis) 715.9●
Morel-Kraepelin disease (*see also* Schizophrenia) 295.9●
Morel-Moore syndrome (hyperostosis frontalis interna) 733.3
Morel-Morgagni syndrome (hyperostosis frontalis interna) 733.3
Morgagni
   cyst, organ, hydatid, or appendage 752.89
      fallopian tube 752.11
   disease or syndrome (hyperostosis frontalis interna) 733.3

Morgagni-Adams-Stokes syndrome (syncope with heart block) 426.9
Morgagni-Stewart-Morel syndrome (hyperostosis frontalis interna) 733.3
Moria (see also Psychosis) 298.9
Morning sickness 643.0●
Moron 317
Morphea (guttate) (linear) 701.0
Morphine dependence (see also Dependence) 304.0●
Morphinism (see also Dependence) 304.0●
Morphinomania (see also Dependence) 304.0●
Morphoea 701.0
Morquio (-Brailsford) (-Ullrich) disease or syndrome (mucopolysaccharidosis IV) 277.5
  kyphosis 277.5
Morris syndrome (testicular feminization) 259.51
Morsus humanus (open wound) - see also Wound, open, by site
  skin surface intact - see Contusion
Mortification (dry) (moist) (see also Gangrene) 785.4
Morton's
  disease 355.6
  foot 355.6
  metatarsalgia (syndrome) 355.6
  neuralgia 355.6
  neuroma 355.6
  syndrome (metatarsalgia) (neuralgia) 355.6
  toe 355.6
Morvan's disease 336.0
Mosaicism, mosaic (chromosomal) 758.9
  autosomal 758.5
  sex 758.81
Moschcowitz's syndrome (thrombotic thrombocytopenic purpura) 446.6
Mother yaw 102.0
Motion sickness (from travel, any vehicle) (from roundabouts or swings) 994.6
Mottled teeth (enamel) (endemic) (nonendemic) 520.3
Mottling enamel (endemic) (nonendemic) (teeth) 520.3
Mouchet's disease 732.5
Mould(s) (in vitreous) 117.9
Moulders'
  bronchitis 502
  tuberculosis (see also Tuberculosis) 011.4●
Mounier-Kuhn syndrome 748.3
  with
    acute exacerbation 494.1
    bronchiectasis 494.0
      with (acute) exacerbation 494.1
    acquired 519.19
      with bronchiectasis 494.0
        with (acute) exacerbation 494.1
Mountain
  fever - see Fever, mountain
  sickness 993.2
    with polycythemia, acquired 289.0
    acute 289.0
  tick fever 066.1
Mouse, joint (see also Loose, body, joint) 718.1●
  knee 717.6
Mouth - see condition
Movable
  coccyx 724.71
  kidney (see also Disease, renal) 593.0
    congenital 753.3
  organ or site, congenital NEC - see Malposition, congenital
  spleen 289.59
Movement
  abnormal (dystonic) (involuntary) 781.0
  decreased fetal 655.7●
  paradoxical facial 374.43
Moya Moya disease 437.5
Mozart's ear 744.29

MRSA (methicillin resistant staphylococcus aureus) 041.12
  colonization V02.54
  personal history of V12.04
MSSA (methicillin susceptible staphylococcus aureus) 041.11
  colonization V02.53
Mucha's disease (acute parapsoriasis varioliformis) 696.2
Mucha-Haberman syndrome (acute parapsoriasis varioliformis) 696.2
Mu-chain disease 273.2
Mucinosis (cutaneous) (papular) 701.8
Mucocele
  appendix 543.9
  buccal cavity 528.9
  gallbladder (see also Disease, gallbladder) 575.3
  lacrimal sac 375.43
  orbit (eye) 376.81
  salivary gland (any) 527.6
  sinus (accessory) (nasal) 478.19
  turbinate (bone) (middle) (nasal) 478.19
  uterus 621.8
Mucocutaneous lymph node syndrome (acute) (febrile) (infantile) 446.1
Mucoenteritis 564.9
Mucolipidosis I, II, III 272.7
Mucopolysaccharidosis (types 1–6) 277.5
  cardiopathy 277.5 [425.7]
Mucormycosis (lung) 117.7
Mucosa associated lymphoid tissue (MALT) 200.3●
Mucositis - see also Inflammation, by site 528.00
  cervix (ulcerative) 616.81
  due to
    antineoplastic therapy (ulcerative) 528.01
    other drugs (ulcerative) 528.02
    specified NEC 528.09
  gastrointestinal (ulcerative) 538
  nasal (ulcerative) 478.11
  necroticans agranulocytica (see also Agranulocytosis) 288.09
  ulcerative 528.00
  vagina (ulcerative) 616.81
  vulva (ulcerative) 616.81
Mucous - see also condition
  patches (syphilitic) 091.3
    congenital 090.0
Mucoviscidosis 277.00
  with meconium obstruction 277.01
Mucus
  asphyxia or suffocation (see also Asphyxia, mucus) 933.1
    newborn 770.18
  in stool 792.1
  plug (see also Asphyxia, mucus) 933.1
    aspiration, of newborn 770.17
    tracheobronchial 519.19
      newborn 770.18
Muguet 112.0
Mulberry molars 090.5
Müllerian mixed tumor (M8950/3) - see Neoplasm, by site, malignant
Multicystic kidney 753.19
Multilobed placenta - see Placenta, abnormal
Multinodular prostate 600.10
  with
    urinary
      obstruction 600.11
      retention 600.11
Multiparity V61.5
  affecting
    fetus or newborn 763.89
  management of
    labor and delivery 659.4●
    pregnancy V23.3
  requiring contraceptive management (see also Contraception) V25.9
Multipartita placenta - see Placenta, abnormal

Multiple, multiplex - see also condition
  birth
    affecting fetus or newborn 761.5
    healthy liveborn - see Newborn, multiple
  digits (congenital) 755.00
    fingers 755.01
    toes 755.02
  organ or site NEC - see Accessory
  personality 300.14
  renal arteries 747.62
Mumps 072.9
  with complication 072.8
    specified type NEC 072.79
  encephalitis 072.2
  hepatitis 072.71
  meningitis (aseptic) 072.1
  meningoencephalitis 072.2
  oophoritis 072.79
  orchitis 072.0
  pancreatitis 072.3
  polyneuropathy 072.72
  vaccination, prophylactic (against) V04.6
Mumu (see also Infestation, filarial) 125.9
Münchausen syndrome 301.51
Münchmeyer's disease or syndrome (exostosis luxurians) 728.11
Mural - see condition
Murmur (cardiac) (heart) (nonorganic) (organic) 785.2
  abdominal 787.5
  aortic (valve) (see also Endocarditis, aortic) 424.1
  benign - omit code
  cardiorespiratory 785.2
  diastolic - see condition
  Flint (see also Endocarditis, aortic) 424.1
  functional - omit code
  Graham Steell (pulmonic regurgitation) (see also Endocarditis, pulmonary) 424.3
  innocent - omit code
  insignificant - omit code
  midsystolic 785.2
  mitral (valve) - see Stenosis
  physiologic - see condition
  presystolic, mitral - see Insufficiency, mitral
  pulmonic (valve) (see also Endocarditis, pulmonary) 424.3
  Still's (vibratory) - omit code
  systolic (valvular) - see condition
  tricuspid (valve) - see Endocarditis, tricuspid
  undiagnosed 785.2
  valvular - see condition
  vibratory - omit code
Murri's disease (intermittent hemoglobinuria) 283.2
Muscae volitantes 379.24
Muscle, muscular - see condition
Musculoneuralgia 729.1
Mushrooming hip 718.95
Mushroom workers' (pickers') lung 495.5
Mutation(s)
  factor V Leiden 289.81
  prothrombin gene 289.81
  surfactant, of lung 516.63
Mutism (see also Aphasia) 784.3
  akinetic 784.3
  deaf (acquired) (congenital) 389.7
  hysterical 300.11
  selective (elective) 313.23
    adjustment reaction 309.83
MVD (microvillus inclusion disease) 751.5
MVID (microvillus inclusion disease) 751.5
Myà's disease (congenital dilation, colon) 751.3
Myalgia (intercostal) 729.1
  eosinophilia syndrome 710.5
  epidemic 074.1
    cervical 078.89
  psychogenic 307.89
  traumatic NEC 959.9

 New   Revised   deleted Deleted   ● Use Additional Digit(s)   Omit code

Myasthenia 358.00
  cordis - see Failure, heart
  gravis 358.00
    with exacerbation (acute) 358.01
    in crisis 358.01
    neonatal 775.2
    pseudoparalytica 358.00
  stomach 536.8
    psychogenic 306.4
  syndrome
    in
      botulism 005.1 [358.1]
      diabetes mellitus 250.6● [358.1]
        due to secondary diabetes 249.6●
          [358.1]
      hypothyroidism (see also
          Hypothyroidism) 244.9 [358.1]
      malignant neoplasm NEC 199.1
          [358.1]
      pernicious anemia 281.0 [358.1]
      thyrotoxicosis (see also Thyrotoxicosis)
          242.9● [358.1]
Myasthenic 728.87
Mycelium infection NEC 117.9
Mycetismus 988.1
Mycetoma (actinomycotic) 039.9
  bone 039.8
    mycotic 117.4
  foot 039.4
    mycotic 117.4
  madurae 039.9
    mycotic 117.4
  maduromycotic 039.9
    mycotic 117.4
  mycotic 117.4
  nocardial 039.9
Mycobacteriosis - see Mycobacterium
Mycobacterium, mycobacterial (infection) 031.9
  acid-fast (bacilli) 031.9
  anonymous (see also Mycobacterium,
      atypical) 031.9
  atypical (acid-fast bacilli) 031.9
    cutaneous 031.1
    pulmonary 031.0
      tuberculous (see also Tuberculosis,
          pulmonary) 011.9●
    specified site NEC 031.8
  avium 031.0
    intracellulare complex bacteremia (MAC)
        031.2
  balnei 031.1
  Battey 031.0
  cutaneous 031.1
  disseminated 031.2
    avium-intracellulare complex (DMAC)
        031.2
  fortuitum 031.0
  intracellulare (battey bacillus) 031.0
  kakerifu 031.8
  kansasii 031.0
  kasongo 031.8
  leprae - see Leprosy
  luciflavum 031.0
  marinum 031.1
  pulmonary 031.0
    tuberculous (see also Tuberculosis,
        pulmonary) 011.9●
  scrofulaceum 031.1
  tuberculosis (human, bovine) - see also
      Tuberculosis
    avian type 031.0
  ulcerans 031.1
  xenopi 031.0
Mycosis, mycotic 117.9
  cutaneous NEC 111.9
  ear 111.8 [380.15]
  fungoides (M9700/3) 202.1●
  mouth 112.0
  pharynx 117.9
  skin NEC 111.9
  stomatitis 112.0

Mycosis, mycotic (Continued)
  systemic NEC 117.9
  tonsil 117.9
  vagina, vaginitis 112.1
Mydriasis (persistent) (pupil) 379.43
Myelatelia 742.59
Myelinoclasis, perivascular, acute
    (postinfectious) NEC 136.9 [323.61]
  postimmunization or postvaccinal 323.51
Myelinosis, central pontine 341.8
Myelitis (ascending) (cerebellar) (childhood)
    (chronic) (descending) (diffuse)
    (disseminated) (pressure) (progressive)
    (spinal cord) (subacute) (see also
    Encephalitis) 323.9
  acute (transverse) 341.20
    idiopathic 341.22
    in conditions classified elsewhere 341.21
  due to
    other infection classified elsewhere 136.9
        [323.42]
    specified cause NEC 323.82
    vaccination (any) 323.52
    viral diseases classified elsewhere
        323.02
  herpes simplex 054.74
  herpes zoster 053.14
  late effect - see category 326
  optic neuritis in 341.0
  postchickenpox 052.2
  postimmunization 323.52
  postinfectious 136.9 [323.63]
  postvaccinal 323.52
  postvaricella 052.2
  syphilitic (transverse) 094.89
  toxic 989.9 [323.72]
  transverse 323.82
    acute 341.20
      idiopathic 341.22
      in conditions classified elsewhere
          341.21
    idiopathic 341.22
  tuberculous (see also Tuberculosis) 013.6●
  virus 049.9
Myeloblastic - see condition
Myelocele (see also Spina bifida) 741.9●
  with hydrocephalus 741.0●
Myelocystocele (see also Spina bifida) 741.9●
Myelocytic - see condition
Myelocytoma 205.1●
Myelodysplasia (spinal cord) 742.59
  meaning myelodysplastic syndrome - see
      Syndrome, myelodysplastic
Myeloencephalitis - see Encephalitis
Myelofibrosis 289.83
  with myeloid metaplasia 238.76
  idiopathic (chronic) 238.76
  megakaryocytic 238.79
  primary 238.76
  secondary 289.83
Myelogenous - see condition
Myeloid - see condition
Myelokathexis 288.09
Myeloleukodystrophy 330.0
Myelolipoma (M8870/0) - see Neoplasm, by
    site, benign
Myeloma (multiple) (plasma cell) (plasmacytic)
    (M9730/3) 203.0●
  monostotic (M9731/1) 238.6
  solitary (M9731/1) 238.6
Myelomalacia 336.8
Myelomata, multiple (M9730/3) 203.0●
Myelomatosis (M9730/3) 203.0●
Myelomeningitis - see Meningoencephalitis
Myelomeningocele (spinal cord) (see also Spina
    bifida) 741.9●
  fetal, causing fetopelvic disproportion
      653.7●
Myelo-osteo-musculodysplasia hereditaria
    756.89
Myelopathic - see condition

Myelopathy (spinal cord) 336.9
  cervical 721.1
  diabetic 250.6● [336.3]
    due to secondary diabetes 249.6●
      [336.3]
  drug-induced 336.8
  due to or with
    carbon tetrachloride 987.8 [323.72]
    degeneration or displacement,
        intervertebral disc 722.70
      cervical, cervicothoracic 722.71
      lumbar, lumbosacral 722.73
      thoracic, thoracolumbar 722.72
    hydroxyquinoline derivatives 961.3
      [323.72]
    infection - see Encephalitis
    intervertebral disc disorder 722.70
      cervical, cervicothoracic 722.71
      lumbar, lumbosacral 722.73
      thoracic, thoracolumbar 722.72
    lead 984.9 [323.72]
    mercury 985.0 [323.72]
    neoplastic disease (see also Neoplasm, by
        site) 239.9 [336.3]
    pernicious anemia 281.0 [336.3]
    spondylosis 721.91
      cervical 721.1
      lumbar, lumbosacral 721.42
      thoracic 721.41
    thallium 985.8 [323.72]
  lumbar, lumbosacral 721.42
  necrotic (subacute) 336.1
  radiation-induced 336.8
  spondylogenic NEC 721.91
    cervical 721.1
    lumbar, lumbosacral 721.42
    thoracic 721.41
  thoracic 721.41
  toxic NEC 989.9 [323.72]
  transverse (see also Myelitis) 323.82
  vascular 336.1
Myelophthisis 284.2
Myeloproliferative disease (M9960/1)
    238.79
Myeloradiculitis (see also Polyneuropathy)
    357.0
Myeloradiculodysplasia (spinal) 742.59
Myelosarcoma (M9930/3) 205.3●
Myelosclerosis 289.89
  with myeloid metaplasia (M9961/1)
      238.76
  disseminated, of nervous system 340
  megakaryocytic (M9961/1) 238.79
Myelosis (M9860/3) (see also Leukemia,
    myeloid) 205.9●
  acute (M9861/3) 205.0●
  aleukemic (M9864/3) 205.8●
  chronic (M9863/3) 205.1●
  erythremic (M9840/3) 207.0●
    acute (M9841/3) 207.0●
  megakaryocytic (M9920/3) 207.2●
  nonleukemic (chronic) 288.8
  subacute (M9862/3) 205.2●
Myesthenia - see Myasthenia
Myiasis (cavernous) 134.0
  orbit 134.0 [376.13]
Myoadenoma, prostate 600.20
  with
    other lower urinary tract symptoms
        (LUTS) 600.21
    urinary
      obstruction 600.21
      retention 600.21
Myoblastoma
  granular cell (M9580/0) - see also
      Neoplasm, connective tissue,
      benign
    malignant (M9580/3) - see Neoplasm,
        connective tissue, malignant
  tongue (M9580/0) 210.1
Myocardial - see condition

Myocardiopathy (congestive) (constrictive) (familial) (idiopathic) (infiltrative) (obstructive) (primary) (restrictive) (sporadic) 425.4
  alcoholic 425.5
  amyloid 277.39 [425.7]
  beriberi 265.0 [425.7]
  cobalt-beer 425.5
  due to
    amyloidosis 277.39 [425.7]
    beriberi 265.0 [425.7]
    cardiac glycogenosis 271.0 [425.7]
    Chagas' disease 086.0
    Friedreich's ataxia 334.0 [425.8]
    influenza (see also Influenza) 487.8 [425.8]
    mucopolysaccharidosis 277.5 [425.7]
    myotonia atrophica 359.21 [425.8]
    progressive muscular dystrophy 359.1 [425.8]
    sarcoidosis 135 [425.8]
  glycogen storage 271.0 [425.7]
  hypertrophic 425.18
    nonobstructive 425.18
    obstructive 425.11
  metabolic NEC 277.9 [425.7]
  nutritional 269.9 [425.7]
  obscure (African) 425.2
  peripartum 674.5●
  postpartum 674.5●
  secondary 425.9
  thyrotoxic (see also Thyrotoxicosis) 242.9● [425.7]
  toxic NEC 425.9
Myocarditis (fibroid) (interstitial) (old) (progressive) (senile) (with arteriosclerosis) 429.0
  with
    rheumatic fever (conditions classifiable to 390) 398.0
      active (see also Myocarditis, acute, rheumatic) 391.2
      inactive or quiescent (with chorea) 398.0
  active (nonrheumatic) 422.90
    rheumatic 391.2
      with chorea (acute) (rheumatic) (Sydenham's) 392.0
  acute or subacute (interstitial) 422.90
    due to Streptococcus (beta-hemolytic) 391.2
    idiopathic 422.91
    rheumatic 391.2
      with chorea (acute) (rheumatic) (Sydenham's) 392.0
    specified type NEC 422.99
  aseptic of newborn 074.23
  bacterial (acute) 422.92
  chagasic 086.0
  chronic (interstitial) 429.0
  congenital 746.89
  constrictive 425.4
  Coxsackie (virus) 074.23
  diphtheritic 032.82
  due to or in
    Coxsackie (virus) 074.23
    diphtheria 032.82
    epidemic louse-borne typhus 080 [422.0]
    influenza (see also Influenza) 487.8 [422.0]
    Lyme disease 088.81 [422.0]
    scarlet fever 034.1 [422.0]
    toxoplasmosis (acquired) 130.3
    tuberculosis (see also Tuberculosis) 017.9● [422.0]
    typhoid 002.0 [422.0]
    typhus NEC 081.9 [422.0]
  eosinophilic 422.91
  epidemic of newborn 074.23
  Fiedler's (acute) (isolated) (subacute) 422.91
  giant cell (acute) (subacute) 422.91
  gonococcal 098.85

Myocarditis (Continued)
  granulomatous (idiopathic) (isolated) (nonspecific) 422.91
  hypertensive (see also Hypertension, heart) 402.90
  idiopathic 422.91
    granulomatous 422.91
  infective 422.92
  influenzal (see also Influenza) 487.8 [422.0]
  isolated (diffuse) (granulomatous) 422.91
  malignant 422.99
  meningococcal 036.43
  nonrheumatic, active 422.90
  parenchymatous 422.90
  pneumococcal (acute) (subacute) 422.92
  rheumatic (chronic) (inactive) (with chorea) 398.0
    active or acute 391.2
      with chorea (acute) (rheumatic) (Sydenham's) 392.0
  septic 422.92
  specific (giant cell) (productive) 422.91
  staphylococcal (acute) (subacute) 422.92
  suppurative 422.92
  syphilitic (chronic) 093.82
  toxic 422.93
    rheumatic (see also Myocarditis, acute rheumatic) 391.2
  tuberculous (see also Tuberculosis) 017.9● [422.0]
  typhoid 002.0 [422.0]
  valvular - see Endocarditis
  viral, except Coxsackie 422.91
    Coxsackie 074.23
    of newborn (Coxsackie) 074.23
Myocardium, myocardial - see condition
Myocardosis (see also Cardiomyopathy) 425.4
Myoclonia (essential) 333.2
  epileptica 345.1●
  Friedrich's 333.2
  massive 333.2
Myoclonic
  epilepsy, familial (progressive) 345.1●
  jerks 333.2
Myoclonus (familial essential) (multifocal) (simplex) 333.2
  with epilepsy and with ragged red fibers (MERRF syndrome) 277.87
  facial 351.8
  massive (infantile) 333.2
  palatal 333.2
  pharyngeal 333.2
Myocytolysis 429.1
Myodiastasis 728.84
Myoendocarditis - see also Endocarditis
  acute or subacute 421.9
Myoepithelioma (M8982/0) - see Neoplasm, by site, benign
Myofascitis (acute) 729.1
  low back 724.2
Myofibroma (M8890/0) - see also Neoplasm, connective tissue, benign
  uterus (cervix) (corpus) (see also Leiomyoma) 218.9
Myofibromatosis
  infantile 759.89
Myofibrosis 728.2
  heart (see also Myocarditis) 429.0
  humeroscapular region 726.2
  scapulohumeral 726.2
Myofibrositis (see also Myositis) 729.1
  scapulohumeral 726.2
Myogelosis (occupational) 728.89
Myoglobinuria 791.3
Myoglobulinuria, primary 791.3
Myokymia - see also Myoclonus
  facial 351.8
Myolipoma (M8860/0)
  specified site - see Neoplasm, connective tissue, benign
  unspecified site 223.0

Myoma (M8895/0) - see also Neoplasm, connective tissue, benign
  cervix (stump) (uterus) (see also Leiomyoma) 218.9
  malignant (M8895/3) - see Neoplasm, connective tissue, malignant
  prostate 600.20
    with
      other lower urinary tract symptoms (LUTS) 600.21
      urinary
        obstruction 600.21
        retention 600.21
  uterus (cervix) (corpus) (see also Leiomyoma) 218.9
    in pregnancy or childbirth 654.1●
      affecting fetus or newborn 763.89
      causing obstructed labor 660.2●
        affecting fetus or newborn 763.1
Myomalacia 728.9
  cordis, heart (see also Degeneration, myocardial) 429.1
Myometritis (see also Endometritis) 615.9
Myometrium - see condition
Myonecrosis, clostridial 040.0
Myopathy 359.9
  alcoholic 359.4
  amyloid 277.39 [359.6]
  benign, congenital 359.0
  central core 359.0
  centronuclear 359.0
  congenital (benign) 359.0
  critical illness 359.81
  distal 359.1
  due to drugs 359.4
  endocrine 259.9 [359.5]
    specified type NEC 259.8 [359.5]
  extraocular muscles 376.82
  facioscapulohumeral 359.1
  in
    Addison's disease 255.41 [359.5]
    amyloidosis 277.39 [359.6]
    cretinism 243 [359.5]
    Cushing's syndrome 255.0 [359.5]
    disseminated lupus erythematosus 710.0 [359.6]
    giant cell arteritis 446.5 [359.6]
    hyperadrenocorticism NEC 255.3 [359.5]
    hyperparathyroidism 252.01 [359.5]
    hypopituitarism 253.2 [359.5]
    hypothyroidism (see also Hypothyroidism) 244.9 [359.5]
    malignant neoplasm NEC (M8000/3) 199.1 [359.6]
    myxedema (see also Myxedema) 244.9 [359.5]
    polyarteritis nodosa 446.0 [359.6]
    rheumatoid arthritis 714.0 [359.6]
    sarcoidosis 135 [359.6]
    scleroderma 710.1 [359.6]
    Sjögren's disease 710.2 [359.6]
    thyrotoxicosis (see also Thyrotoxicosis) 242.9● [359.5]
  inflammatory 359.79
    immune NEC 359.79
    specified NEC 359.79
  intensive care (ICU) 359.81
  limb-girdle 359.1
  myotubular 359.0
  necrotizing, acute 359.81
  nemaline 359.0
  ocular 359.1
  oculopharyngeal 359.1
  of critical illness 359.81
  primary 359.89
  progressive NEC 359.89
  proximal myotonic (PROMM) 359.21
  quadriplegic, acute 359.81
  rod body 359.0
  scapulohumeral 359.1

Myopathy (Continued)
  specified type NEC 359.89
  toxic 359.4
Myopericarditis (see also Pericarditis) 423.9
Myopia (axial) (congenital) (increased curvature or refraction, nucleus of lens) 367.1
  degenerative, malignant 360.21
  malignant 360.21
  progressive high (degenerative) 360.21
Myosarcoma (M8895/3) - see Neoplasm, connective tissue, malignant
Myosis (persistent) 379.42
  stromal (endolymphatic) (M8931/1) 236.0
Myositis 729.1
  clostridial 040.0
  due to posture 729.1
  epidemic 074.1
  fibrosa or fibrous (chronic) 728.2
    Volkmann's (complicating trauma) 958.6
  inclusion body (IBM) 359.71
  infective 728.0
  interstitial 728.81
  multiple - see Polymyositis
  occupational 729.1
  orbital, chronic 376.12
  ossificans 728.12
    circumscribed 728.12
    progressive 728.11
    traumatic 728.12

Myositis (Continued)
  progressive fibrosing 728.11
  purulent 728.0
  rheumatic 729.1
  rheumatoid 729.1
  suppurative 728.0
  syphilitic 095.6
  traumatic (old) 729.1
Myospasia impulsiva 307.23
Myotonia (acquisita) (intermittens) 728.85
  atrophica 359.21
  congenita 359.22
    acetazolamide responsive 359.22
    dominant form 359.22
    recessive form 359.22
  drug-induced 359.24
  dystrophica 359.21
  fluctuans 359.29
  levior 359.22
  permanens 359.29
Myotonic pupil 379.46
Myriapodiasis 134.1
Myringitis
  with otitis media - see Otitis media
  acute 384.00
    specified type NEC 384.09
  bullosa hemorrhagica 384.01
  bullous 384.01
  chronic 384.1
Mysophobia 300.29
Mytilotoxism 988.0
Myxadenitis labialis 528.5

Myxedema (adult) (idiocy) (infantile) (juvenile) (thyroid gland) (see also Hypothyroidism) 244.9
  circumscribed 242.9
  congenital 243
  cutis 701.8
  localized (pretibial) 242.9
  madness (acute) 293.0
    subacute 293.1
  papular 701.8
  pituitary 244.8
  postpartum 674.8
  pretibial 242.9
  primary 244.9
Myxochondrosarcoma (M9220/3) - see Neoplasm, cartilage, malignant
Myxofibroma (M8811/0) - see also Neoplasm, connective tissue, benign
  odontogenic (M9320/0) 213.1
  upper jaw (bone) 213.0
Myxofibrosarcoma (M8811/3) - see Neoplasm, connective tissue, malignant
Myxolipoma (M8852/0) (see also Lipoma, by site) 214.9
Myxoliposarcoma (M8852/3) - see Neoplasm, connective tissue, malignant
Myxoma (M8840/0) - see also Neoplasm, connective tissue, benign
  odontogenic (M9320/0) 213.1
  upper jaw (bone) 213.0
Myxosarcoma (M8840/3) - see Neoplasm, connective tissue, malignant

SECTION I INDEX TO DISEASES AND INJURIES / Necrosis, necrotic

N

Naegeli's
  disease (hereditary hemorrhagic thrombasthenia) 287.1
  leukemia, monocytic (M9863/3) 205.1 ●
  syndrome (incontinentia pigmenti) 757.33
Naffziger's syndrome 353.0
Naga sore (see also Ulcer, skin) 707.9
Nägele's pelvis 738.6
  with disproportion (fetopelvic) 653.0 ●
    affecting fetus or newborn 763.1
    causing obstructed labor 660.1 ●
      affecting fetus or newborn 763.1
Nager-de Reynier syndrome (dysostosis mandibularis) 756.0
Nail - see also condition
  biting 307.9
  patella syndrome (hereditary osteoonychodysplasia) 756.89
Nanism, nanosomia (see also Dwarfism) 259.4
  hypophyseal 253.3
  pituitary 253.3
  renis, renalis 588.0
Nanukayami 100.89
Napkin rash 691.0
Narcissism 301.81
Narcolepsy 347.00
  with cataplexy 347.01
  in conditions classified elsewhere 347.10
    with cataplexy 347.11
Narcosis
  carbon dioxide (respiratory) 786.09
  due to drug
    correct substance properly administered 780.09
    overdose or wrong substance given or taken 977.9
      specified drug - see Table of Drugs and Chemicals
Narcotism (chronic) (see also Dependence) 304.9 ●
  acute
    correct substance properly administered 349.82
    overdose or wrong substance given or taken 967.8
      specified drug - see Table of Drugs and Chemicals
NARP (ataxia and retinitis pigmentosa syndrome) 277.87
Narrow
  anterior chamber angle 365.02
  pelvis (inlet) (outlet) - see Contraction, pelvis
Narrowing
  artery NEC 447.1
    auditory, internal 433.8 ●
    basilar 433.0 ●
      with other precerebral artery 433.3 ●
        bilateral 433.3 ●
    carotid 433.1 ●
      with other precerebral artery 433.3 ●
        bilateral 433.3 ●
    cerebellar 433.8 ●
    choroidal 433.8 ●
    communicating posterior 433.8 ●
    coronary - see also Arteriosclerosis, coronary
      congenital 746.85
        due to syphilis 090.5
    hypophyseal 433.8 ●
    pontine 433.8 ●
    precerebral NEC 433.9 ●
      multiple or bilateral 433.3 ●
      specified NEC 433.8 ●
    vertebral 433.2 ●
      with other precerebral artery 433.3 ●
        bilateral 433.3 ●
  auditory canal (external) (see also Stricture, ear canal, acquired) 380.50
  cerebral arteries 437.0

Narrowing (Continued)
  cicatricial - see Cicatrix
  congenital - see Anomaly, congenital
  coronary artery - see Narrowing, artery, coronary
  ear, middle 385.22
  Eustachian tube (see also Obstruction, Eustachian tube) 381.60
  eyelid 374.46
    congenital 743.62
  intervertebral disc or space NEC - see Degeneration, intervertebral disc
  joint space, hip 719.85
  larynx 478.74
  lids 374.46
    congenital 743.62
  mesenteric artery (with gangrene) 557.0
  palate 524.89
  palpebral fissure 374.46
  retinal artery 362.13
  ureter 593.3
  urethra (see also Stricture, urethra) 598.9
Narrowness, abnormal, eyelid 743.62
Nasal - see condition
Nasolacrimal - see condition
Nasopharyngeal - see also condition
  bursa 478.29
  pituitary gland 759.2
  torticollis 723.5
Nasopharyngitis (acute) (infective) (subacute) 460
  chronic 472.2
    due to external agent - see Condition, respiratory, chronic, due to
  due to external agent - see Condition, respiratory, due to
  septic 034.0
  streptococcal 034.0
  suppurative (chronic) 472.2
  ulcerative (chronic) 472.2
Nasopharynx, nasopharyngeal - see condition
Natal tooth, teeth 520.6
Nausea (see also Vomiting) 787.02
  with vomiting 787.01
  epidemic 078.82
  gravidarum - see Hyperemesis, gravidarum
  marina 994.6
Naval - see condition
Neapolitan fever (see also Brucellosis) 023.9
Near drowning 994.1
Nearsightedness 367.1
Near-syncope 780.2
Nebécourt's syndrome 253.3
Nebula, cornea (eye) 371.01
  congenital 743.62
    interfering with vision 743.42
Necator americanus infestation 126.1
Necatoriasis 126.1
Neck - see condition
Necrencephalus (see also Softening, brain) 437.8
Necrobacillosis 040.3
Necrobiosis 799.89
  brain or cerebral (see also Softening, brain) 437.8
  lipoidica 709.3
    diabeticorum 250.8 ● [709.3]
      due to secondary diabetes 249.8 ● [709.3]
Necrodermolysis 695.15
Necrolysis, toxic epidermal 695.15
  due to drug
    correct substance properly administered 695.15
    overdose or wrong substance given or taken 977.9
      specified drug - see Table of Drugs and Chemicals
  Stevens-Johnson syndrome overlap (SJS-TEN overlap syndrome) 695.14

Necrophilia 302.89
Necrosis, necrotic
  adrenal (capsule) (gland) 255.8
  antrum, nasal sinus 478.19
  aorta (hyaline) (see also Aneurysm, aorta) 441.9
    cystic medial 441.00
      abdominal 441.02
      thoracic 441.01
      thoracoabdominal 441.03
    ruptured 441.5
  arteritis 446.0
  artery 447.5
  aseptic, bone 733.40
    femur (head) (neck) 733.42
      medial condyle 733.43
    humoral head 733.41
    jaw 733.45
    medial femoral condyle 733.43
    specific site NEC 733.49
    talus 733.44
  avascular, bone NEC (see also Necrosis, aseptic, bone) 733.40
  bladder (aseptic) (sphincter) 596.89
  bone (see also Osteomyelitis) 730.1 ●
    acute 730.0 ●
    aseptic or avascular 733.40
      femur (head) (neck) 733.42
        medial condyle 733.43
      humoral head 733.41
      jaw 733.45
      medial femoral condyle 733.43
      specified site NEC 733.49
      talus 733.44
    ethmoid 478.19
    ischemic 733.40
    jaw 526.4
      aseptic 733.45
    marrow 289.89
    Paget's (osteitis deformans) 731.0
    tuberculous - see Tuberculosis, bone
  brain (softening) (see also Softening, brain) 437.8
  breast (aseptic) (fat) (segmental) 611.3
  bronchus, bronchi 519.19
  central nervous system NEC (see also Softening, brain) 437.8
  cerebellar (see also Softening, brain) 437.8
  cerebral (softening) (see also Softening, brain) 437.8
  cerebrospinal (softening) (see also Softening, brain) 437.8
  colon 557.0
  cornea (see also Keratitis) 371.40
  cortical, kidney 583.6
  cystic medial (aorta) 441.00
    abdominal 441.02
    thoracic 441.01
    thoracoabdominal 441.03
  dental 521.09
    pulp 522.1
  due to swallowing corrosive substance - see Burn, by site
  ear (ossicle) 385.24
  esophagus 530.89
  ethmoid (bone) 478.19
  eyelid 374.50
  fat, fatty (generalized) (see also Degeneration, fatty) 272.8
    abdominal wall 567.82
    breast (aseptic) (segmental) 611.3
    intestine 569.89
    localized - see Degeneration, by site, fatty
    mesentery 567.82
    omentum 567.82
    pancreas 577.8
    peritoneum 567.82
    skin (subcutaneous) 709.3
      newborn 778.1

◂ New   ◂▥ Revised   ~~deleted~~ Deleted   ● Use Additional Digit(s)   ▨ Omit code   317

Necrosis, necrotic (Continued)
  femur (aseptic) (avascular) 733.42
    head 733.42
    medial condyle 733.43
    neck 733.42
  gallbladder (see also Cholecystitis, acute) 575.0
  gangrenous 785.4
  gastric 537.89
  glottis 478.79
  heart (myocardium) - see Infarct, myocardium
  hepatic (see also Necrosis, liver) 570
  hip (aseptic) (avascular) 733.42
  intestine (acute) (hemorrhagic) (massive) 557.0
  ischemic 785.4
  jaw 526.4
    aseptic 733.45
  kidney (bilateral) 583.9
    acute 584.9
    cortical 583.6
      acute 584.6
        with
          abortion - see Abortion, by type, with renal failure
          ectopic pregnancy (see also categories 633.0–633.9) 639.3
          molar pregnancy (see also categories 630–632) 639.3
        complicating pregnancy 646.2●
          affecting fetus or newborn 760.1
          following labor and delivery 669.3●
    medullary (papillary) (see also Pyelitis) 590.80
      in
        acute renal failure 584.7
        nephritis, nephropathy 583.7
    papillary (see also Pyelitis) 590.80
      in
        acute renal failure 584.7
        nephritis, nephropathy 583.7
    tubular 584.5
      with
        abortion - see Abortion, by type, with renal failure
        ectopic pregnancy (see also categories 633.0–633.9) 639.3
        molar pregnancy (see also categories 630–632) 639.3
        complicating
          abortion 639.3
          ectopic or molar pregnancy 639.3
          pregnancy 646.2●
            affecting fetus or newborn 760.1
          following labor and delivery 669.3●
        traumatic 958.5
  larynx 478.79
  liver (acute) (congenital) (diffuse) (massive) (subacute) 570
    with
      abortion - see Abortion, by type, with specified complication NEC
      ectopic pregnancy (see also categories 633.0–633.9) 639.8

Necrosis, necrotic (Continued)
  liver (Continued)
    with (Continued)
      molar pregnancy (see also categories 630–632) 639.8
      complicating pregnancy 646.7●
        affecting fetus or newborn 760.8
      following
        abortion 639.8
        ectopic or molar pregnancy 639.8
      obstetrical 646.7●
      postabortal 639.8
      puerperal, postpartum 674.8●
      toxic 573.3
  lung 513.0
  lymphatic gland 683
  mammary gland 611.3
  mastoid (chronic) 383.1
  mesentery 557.0
    fat 567.82
  mitral valve - see Insufficiency, mitral
  myocardium, myocardial - see Infarct, myocardium
  nose (septum) 478.19
  omentum 557.0
    with mesenteric infarction 557.0
    fat 567.82
  orbit, orbital 376.10
  ossicles, ear (aseptic) 385.24
  ovary (see also Salpingo-oophoritis) 614.2
  pancreas (aseptic) (duct) (fat) 577.8
    acute 577.0
    infective 577.0
  papillary, kidney (see also Pyelitis) 590.80
  perineum 624.8
  peritoneum 557.0
    with mesenteric infarction 557.0
    fat 567.82
  pharynx 462
    in granulocytopenia 288.09
  phosphorus 983.9
  pituitary (gland) (postpartum) (Sheehan) 253.2
  placenta (see also Placenta, abnormal) 656.7●
  pneumonia 513.0
  pulmonary 513.0
  pulp (dental) 522.1
  pylorus 537.89
  radiation - see Necrosis, by site
  radium - see Necrosis, by site
  renal - see Necrosis, kidney
  sclera 379.19
  scrotum 608.89
  skin or subcutaneous tissue 709.8
    due to burn - see Burn, by site
    gangrenous 785.4
  spine, spinal (column) 730.18
    acute 730.18
    cord 336.1
  spleen 289.59
  stomach 537.89
  stomatitis 528.1

Necrosis, necrotic (Continued)
  subcutaneous fat 709.3
    fetus or newborn 778.1
  subendocardial - see Infarct, myocardium
  suprarenal (capsule) (gland) 255.8
  teeth, tooth 521.09
  testis 608.89
  thymus (gland) 254.8
  tonsil 474.8
  trachea 519.19
  tuberculous NEC - see Tuberculosis
  tubular (acute) (anoxic) (toxic) 584.5
    due to a procedure 997.5
  umbilical cord, affecting fetus or newborn 762.6
  vagina 623.8
  vertebra (lumbar) 730.18
    acute 730.18
    tuberculous (see also Tuberculosis) 015.0● [730.8]
  vesical (aseptic) (bladder) 596.89
  vulva 624.8
  x-ray - see Necrosis, by site
Necrospermia 606.0
Necrotizing angiitis 446.0
Negativism 301.7
Neglect (child) (newborn) NEC 995.52
  adult 995.84
  after or at birth 995.52
  hemispatial 781.8
  left-sided 781.8
  sensory 781.8
  visuospatial 781.8
Negri bodies 071
  Neill-Dingwall syndrome (microcephaly and dwarfism) 759.89
Neisserian infection NEC - see Gonococcus
Nematodiasis NEC (see also Infestation, Nematode) 127.9
  ancylostoma (see also Ancylostomiasis) 126.9
Neoformans cryptococcus infection 117.5
Neonatal - see also condition
  abstinence syndrome 779.5
  adrenoleukodystrophy 277.86
  teeth, tooth 520.6
Neonatorum - see condition
Neoplasia
  anal intraepithelial I (AIN I) (histologically confirmed) 569.44
  anal intraepithelial II (AIN II) (histologically confirmed) 569.44
  anal intraepithelial III (AIN III) 230.6
    anal canal 230.5
  endometrial intraepithelial [EIN] 621.35
  multiple endocrine (MEN)
    type I 258.01
    type IIA 258.02
    type IIB 258.03
  vaginal intraepithelial I (VAIN I) 623.0
  vaginal intraepithelial II (VAIN II) 623.0
  vaginal intraepithelial III (VAIN III) 233.31
  vulvar intraepithelial I (VIN I) 624.01
  vulvar intraepithelial II (VIN II) 624.02
  vulvar intraepithelial III (VIN III) 233.32
Neoplasm, neoplastic - see pages 319–365

SECTION I INDEX TO DISEASES AND INJURIES / Neoplasm, alveolar

	Malignant			Benign	Uncertain Behavior	Unspecified
	Primary	Secondary	Ca in situ			
Neoplasm, neoplastic	199.1	199.1	234.9	229.9	238.9	239.9

Notes — 1. The list below gives the code numbers for neoplasms by anatomical site. For each site there are six possible code numbers according to whether the neoplasm in question is malignant, benign, in situ, of uncertain behavior, or of unspecified nature. The description of the neoplasm will often indicate which of the six columns is appropriate; e.g., malignant melanoma of skin, benign fibroadenoma of breast, carcinoma in situ of cervix uteri.

Where such descriptors are not present, the remainder of the Index should be consulted where guidance is given to the appropriate column for each morphological (histological) variety listed; e.g., Mesonephroma — see Neoplasm, malignant; Embryoma — see also Neoplasm, uncertain behavior; Disease, Bowen's — see Neoplasm, skin, in situ. However, the guidance in the Index can be overridden if one of the descriptors mentioned above is present; e.g., malignant adenoma of colon is coded to 153.9 and not to 211.3 as the adjective "malignant" overrides the Index entry "Adenoma - see also Neoplasm, benign."

2. Sites marked with the sign * (e.g., face NEC*) should be classified to malignant neoplasm of skin of these sites if the variety of neoplasm is a squamous cell carcinoma or an epidermoid carcinoma and to benign neoplasm of skin of these sites if the variety of neoplasm is a papilloma (any type).

	Primary	Secondary	Ca in situ	Benign	Uncertain Behavior	Unspecified
abdomen, abdominal	195.2	198.89	234.8	229.8	238.8	239.89
cavity	195.2	198.89	234.8	229.8	238.8	239.89
organ	195.2	198.89	234.8	229.8	238.8	239.89
viscera	195.2	198.89	234.8	229.8	238.8	239.89
wall	173.50	198.2	232.5	216.5	238.2	239.2
basal cell carcinoma	173.51	—	—	—	—	—
specified type NEC	173.59	—	—	—	—	—
squamous cell carcinoma	173.52	—	—	—	—	—
connective tissue	171.5	198.89	—	215.5	238.1	239.2
abdominopelvic	195.8	198.89	234.8	229.8	238.8	239.89
accessory sinus - see Neoplasm, sinus						
acoustic nerve	192.0	198.4	—	225.1	237.9	239.7
acromion (process)	170.4	198.5	—	213.4	238.0	239.2
adenoid (pharynx) (tissue)	147.1	198.89	230.0	210.7	235.1	239.0
adipose tissue (*see also* Neoplasm, connective tissue)	171.9	198.89	—	215.9	238.1	239.2
adnexa (uterine)	183.9	198.82	233.39	221.8	236.3	239.5
adrenal (cortex) (gland) (medulla)	194.0	198.7	234.8	227.0	237.2	239.7
ala nasi (external)	173.30	198.2	232.3	216.3	238.2	239.2
alimentary canal or tract NEC	159.9	197.8	230.9	211.9	235.5	239.0
alveolar	143.9	198.89	230.0	210.4	235.1	239.0
mucosa	143.9	198.89	230.0	210.4	235.1	239.0
lower	143.1	198.89	230.0	210.4	235.1	239.0
upper	143.0	198.89	230.0	210.4	235.1	239.0
ridge or process	170.1	198.5	—	213.1	238.0	239.2
carcinoma	143.9	—	—	—	—	—
lower	143.1	—	—	—	—	—
upper	143.0	—	—	—	—	—
lower	170.1	198.5	—	213.1	238.0	239.2
mucosa	143.9	198.89	230.0	210.4	235.1	239.0
lower	143.1	198.89	230.0	210.4	235.1	239.0
upper	143.0	198.89	230.0	210.4	235.1	239.0
upper	170.0	198.5	—	213.0	238.0	239.2

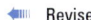 New   Revised   ~~deleted~~ Deleted   ● Use Additional Digit(s)   Omit code

SECTION I INDEX TO DISEASES AND INJURIES / Neoplasm, alveolar

	Malignant			Benign	Uncertain Behavior	Unspecified
	Primary	Secondary	Ca in situ			
Neoplasm (Continued)						
alveolar (Continued)						
sulcus	145.1	198.89	230.0	210.4	235.1	239.0
alveolus	143.9	198.89	230.0	210.4	235.1	239.0
lower	143.1	198.89	230.0	210.4	235.1	239.0
upper	143.0	198.89	230.0	210.4	235.1	239.0
ampulla of Vater	156.2	197.8	230.8	211.5	235.3	239.0
ankle NEC*	195.5	198.89	232.7	229.8	238.8	239.89
anorectum, anorectal (junction)	154.8	197.5	230.7	211.4	235.2	239.0
antecubital fossa or space*	195.4	198.89	232.6	229.8	238.8	239.89
antrum (Highmore) (maxillary)	160.2	197.3	231.8	212.0	235.9	239.1
pyloric	151.2	197.8	230.2	211.1	235.2	239.0
tympanicum	160.1	197.3	231.8	212.0	235.9	239.1
anus, anal	154.3	197.5	230.6	211.4	235.5	239.0
canal	154.2	197.5	230.5	211.4	235.5	239.0
contiguous sites with rectosigmoid junction or rectum	154.8	—	—	—	—	—
margin (see also Neoplasm, anus, skin)	173.50	198.2	232.5	216.5	238.2	239.2
skin	173.50	198.2	232.5	216.5	238.2	239.2
basal cell carcinoma	173.51	—	—	—	—	—
specified type NEC	173.59	—	—	—	—	—
squamous cell carcinoma	173.52	—	—	—	—	—
sphincter	154.2	197.5	230.5	211.4	235.5	239.0
aorta (thoracic)	171.4	198.89	—	215.4	238.1	239.2
abdominal	171.5	198.89	—	215.5	238.1	239.2
aortic body	194.6	198.89	—	227.6	237.3	239.7
aponeurosis	171.9	198.89	—	215.9	238.1	239.2
palmar	171.2	198.89	—	215.2	238.1	239.2
plantar	171.3	198.89	—	215.3	238.1	239.2
appendix	153.5	197.5	230.3	211.3	235.2	239.0
arachnoid (cerebral)	192.1	198.4	—	225.2	237.6	239.7
spinal	192.3	198.4	—	225.4	237.6	239.7
areola (female)	174.0	198.81	233.0	217	238.3	239.3
male	175.0	198.81	233.0	217	238.3	239.3
arm NEC*	195.4	198.89	232.6	229.8	238.8	239.89
artery - see Neoplasm, connective tissue						
aryepiglottic fold	148.2	198.89	230.0	210.8	235.1	239.0
hypopharyngeal aspect	148.2	198.89	230.0	210.8	235.1	239.0
laryngeal aspect	161.1	197.3	231.0	212.1	235.6	239.1
marginal zone	148.2	198.89	230.0	210.8	235.1	239.0
arytenoid (cartilage)	161.3	197.3	231.0	212.1	235.6	239.1
fold - see Neoplasm, aryepiglottic						

◀ New ◁ Revised ~~deleted~~ Deleted ● Use Additional Digit(s) ▨ Omit code

SECTION I INDEX TO DISEASES AND INJURIES / Neoplasm, bladder

	Malignant			Benign	Uncertain Behavior	Unspecified
	Primary	Secondary	Ca in situ			
Neoplasm (Continued)						
associated with transplated organ	199.2	—	—	—	—	—
atlas	170.2	198.5	—	213.2	238.0	239.2
atrium, cardiac	164.1	198.89	—	212.7	238.8	239.89
auditory						
canal (external) (skin) (see also Neoplasm, skin, ear)	173.20	198.2	232.2	216.2	238.2	239.2
internal	160.1	197.3	231.8	212.0	235.9	239.1
nerve	192.0	198.4	—	225.1	237.9	239.7
tube	160.1	197.3	231.8	212.0	235.9	239.1
opening	147.2	198.89	230.0	210.7	235.1	239.0
auricle, ear (see also Neoplasm, skin, ear)	173.20	198.2	232.2	216.2	238.2	239.2
cartilage	171.0	198.89	—	215.0	238.1	239.2
auricular canal (external) (see also Neoplasm, skin, ear)	173.20	198.2	232.2	216.2	238.2	239.2
internal	160.1	197.3	231.8	212.0	235.9	239.1
autonomic nerve or nervous system NEC	171.9	198.89	—	215.9	238.1	239.2
axilla, axillary	195.1	198.89	234.8	229.8	238.8	239.89
fold (see also Neoplasm, skin, trunk)	173.50	198.2	232.5	216.5	238.2	239.2
back NEC*	195.8	198.89	232.5	229.8	238.8	239.89
Bartholin's gland	184.1	198.82	233.39	221.2	236.3	239.5
basal ganglia	191.0	198.3	—	225.0	237.5	239.6
basis pedunculi	191.7	198.3	—	225.0	237.5	239.6
bile or biliary (tract)	156.9	197.8	230.8	211.5	235.3	239.0
canaliculi (biliferi) (intrahepatic)	155.1	197.8	230.8	211.5	235.3	239.0
canals, interlobular	155.1	197.8	230.8	211.5	235.3	239.0
contiguous sites	156.8	—	—	—	—	—
duct or passage (common) (cystic) (extrahepatic)	156.1	197.8	230.8	211.5	235.3	239.0
contiguous sites						
with gallbladder	156.8	—	—	—	—	—
interlobular	155.1	197.8	230.8	211.5	235.3	239.0
intrahepatic	155.1	197.8	230.8	211.5	235.3	239.0
and extrahepatic	156.9	197.8	230.8	211.5	235.3	239.0
bladder (urinary)	188.9	198.1	233.7	223.3	236.7	239.4
contiguous sites	188.8	—	—	—	—	—
dome	188.1	198.1	233.7	223.3	236.7	239.4
neck	188.5	198.1	233.7	223.3	236.7	239.4
orifice	188.9	198.1	233.7	223.3	236.7	239.4
ureteric	188.6	198.1	233.7	223.3	236.7	239.4
urethral	188.5	198.1	233.7	223.3	236.7	239.4
sphincter	188.8	198.1	233.7	223.3	236.7	239.4
trigone	188.0	198.1	233.7	223.3	236.7	239.4
urachus	188.7	—	233.7	223.3	236.7	239.4

◄ New   ◄|||| Revised   ~~deleted~~ Deleted   ● Use Additional Digit(s)   Omit code

SECTION I INDEX TO DISEASES AND INJURIES / Neoplasm, bladder

	Malignant			Benign	Uncertain Behavior	Unspecified
	Primary	Secondary	Ca in situ			
Neoplasm *(Continued)*						
bladder (urinary) *(Continued)*						
wall	188.9	198.1	233.7	223.3	236.7	239.4
anterior	188.3	198.1	233.7	223.3	236.7	239.4
lateral	188.2	198.1	233.7	223.3	236.7	239.4
posterior	188.4	198.1	233.7	223.3	236.7	239.4
blood vessel - *see* Neoplasm, connective tissue						
bone (periosteum)	170.9	198.5	—	213.9	238.0	239.2
Note — Carcinomas and adenocarcinomas, of any type other than intraosseous or odontogenic, of the sites listed under "Neoplasm, bone" should be considered as constituting metastatic spread from an unspecified primary site and coded to 198.5 for morbidity coding.						
acetabulum	170.6	198.5	—	213.6	238.0	239.2
acromion (process)	170.4	198.5	—	213.4	238.0	239.2
ankle	170.8	198.5	—	213.8	238.0	239.2
arm NEC	170.4	198.5	—	213.4	238.0	239.2
astragalus	170.8	198.5	—	213.8	238.0	239.2
atlas	170.2	198.5	—	213.2	238.0	239.2
axis	170.2	198.5	—	213.2	238.0	239.2
back NEC	170.2	198.5	—	213.2	238.0	239.2
calcaneus	170.8	198.5	—	213.8	238.0	239.2
calvarium	170.0	198.5	—	213.0	238.0	239.2
carpus (any)	170.5	198.5	—	213.5	238.0	239.2
cartilage NEC	170.9	198.5	—	213.9	238.0	239.2
clavicle	170.3	198.5	—	213.3	238.0	239.2
clivus	170.0	198.5	—	213.0	238.0	239.2
coccygeal vertebra	170.6	198.5	—	213.6	238.0	239.2
coccyx	170.6	198.5	—	213.6	238.0	239.2
costal cartilage	170.3	198.5	—	213.3	238.0	239.2
costovertebral joint	170.3	198.5	—	213.3	238.0	239.2
cranial	170.0	198.5	—	213.0	238.0	239.2
cuboid	170.8	198.5	—	213.8	238.0	239.2
cuneiform	170.9	198.5	—	213.9	238.0	239.2
ankle	170.8	198.5	—	213.8	238.0	239.2
wrist	170.5	198.5	—	213.5	238.0	239.2
digital	170.9	198.5	—	213.9	238.0	239.2
finger	170.5	198.5	—	213.5	238.0	239.2
toe	170.8	198.5	—	213.8	238.0	239.2
elbow	170.4	198.5	—	213.4	238.0	239.2
ethmoid (labyrinth)	170.0	198.5	—	213.0	238.0	239.2
face	170.0	198.5	—	213.0	238.0	239.2
lower jaw	170.1	198.5	—	213.1	238.0	239.2
femur (any part)	170.7	198.5	—	213.7	238.0	239.2

SECTION I INDEX TO DISEASES AND INJURIES / Neoplasm, bone

	Malignant			Benign	Uncertain Behavior	Unspecified
	Primary	Secondary	Ca in situ			
Neoplasm *(Continued)*						
bone *(Continued)*						
fibula (any part)	170.7	198.5	—	213.7	238.0	239.2
finger (any)	170.5	198.5	—	213.5	238.0	239.2
foot	170.8	198.5	—	213.8	238.0	239.2
forearm	170.4	198.5	—	213.4	238.0	239.2
frontal	170.0	198.5	—	213.0	238.0	239.2
hand	170.5	198.5	—	213.5	238.0	239.2
heel	170.8	198.5	—	213.8	238.0	239.2
hip	170.6	198.5	—	213.6	238.0	239.2
humerus (any part)	170.4	198.5	—	213.4	238.0	239.2
hyoid	170.0	198.5	—	213.0	238.0	239.2
ilium	170.6	198.5	—	213.6	238.0	239.2
innominate	170.6	198.5	—	213.6	238.0	239.2
intervertebral cartilage or disc	170.2	198.5	—	213.2	238.0	239.2
ischium	170.6	198.5	—	213.6	238.0	239.2
jaw (lower)	170.1	198.5	—	213.1	238.0	239.2
upper	170.0	198.5	—	213.0	238.0	239.2
knee	170.7	198.5	—	213.7	238.0	239.2
leg NEC	170.7	198.5	—	213.7	238.0	239.2
limb NEC	170.9	198.5	—	213.9	238.0	239.2
lower (long bones)	170.7	198.5	—	213.7	238.0	239.2
short bones	170.8	198.5	—	213.8	238.0	239.2
upper (long bones)	170.4	198.5	—	213.4	238.0	239.2
short bones	170.5	198.5	—	213.5	238.0	239.2
long	170.9	198.5	—	213.9	238.0	239.2
lower limbs NEC	170.7	198.5	—	213.7	238.0	239.2
upper limbs NEC	170.4	198.5	—	213.4	238.0	239.2
malar	170.0	198.5	—	213.0	238.0	239.2
mandible	170.1	198.5	—	213.1	238.0	239.2
marrow NEC	202.9●	198.5	—	—	—	238.79
mastoid	170.0	198.5	—	213.0	238.0	239.2
maxilla, maxillary (superior)	170.0	198.5	—	213.0	238.0	239.2
inferior	170.1	198.5	—	213.1	238.0	239.2
metacarpus (any)	170.5	198.5	—	213.5	238.0	239.2
metatarsus (any)	170.8	198.5	—	213.8	238.0	239.2
navicular (ankle)	170.8	198.5	—	213.8	238.0	239.2
hand	170.5	198.5	—	213.5	238.0	239.2
nose, nasal	170.0	198.5	—	213.0	238.0	239.2
occipital	170.0	198.5	—	213.0	238.0	239.2
orbit	170.0	198.5	—	213.0	238.0	239.2

SECTION I INDEX TO DISEASES AND INJURIES / Neoplasm, bone

	Malignant			Benign	Uncertain Behavior	Unspecified
	Primary	Secondary	Ca in situ			
Neoplasm *(Continued)*						
bone *(Continued)*						
parietal	170.0	198.5	—	213.0	238.0	239.2
patella	170.8	198.5	—	213.8	238.0	239.2
pelvic	170.6	198.5	—	213.6	238.0	239.2
phalanges	170.9	198.5	—	213.9	238.0	239.2
foot	170.8	198.5	—	213.8	238.0	239.2
hand	170.5	198.5	—	213.5	238.0	239.2
pubic	170.6	198.5	—	213.6	238.0	239.2
radius (any part)	170.4	198.5	—	213.4	238.0	239.2
rib	170.3	198.5	—	213.3	238.0	239.2
sacral vertebra	170.6	198.5	—	213.6	238.0	239.2
sacrum	170.6	198.5	—	213.6	238.0	239.2
scaphoid (of hand)	170.5	198.5	—	213.5	238.0	239.2
of ankle	170.8	198.5	—	213.8	238.0	239.2
scapula (any part)	170.4	198.5	—	213.4	238.0	239.2
sella turcica	170.0	198.5	—	213.0	238.0	239.2
short	170.9	198.5	—	213.9	238.0	239.2
lower limb	170.8	198.5	—	213.8	238.0	239.2
upper limb	170.5	198.5	—	213.5	238.0	239.2
shoulder	170.4	198.5	—	213.4	238.0	239.2
skeleton, skeletal NEC	170.9	198.5	—	213.9	238.0	239.2
skull	170.0	198.5	—	213.0	238.0	239.2
sphenoid	170.0	198.5	—	213.0	238.0	239.2
spine, spinal (column)	170.2	198.5	—	213.2	238.0	239.2
coccyx	170.6	198.5	—	213.6	238.0	239.2
sacrum	170.6	198.5	—	213.6	238.0	239.2
sternum	170.3	198.5	—	213.3	238.0	239.2
tarsus (any)	170.8	198.5	—	213.8	238.0	239.2
temporal	170.0	198.5	—	213.0	238.0	239.2
thumb	170.5	198.5	—	213.5	238.0	239.2
tibia (any part)	170.7	198.5	—	213.7	238.0	239.2
toe (any)	170.8	198.5	—	213.8	238.0	239.2
trapezium	170.5	198.5	—	213.5	238.0	239.2
trapezoid	170.5	198.5	—	213.5	238.0	239.2
turbinate	170.0	198.5	—	213.0	238.0	239.2
ulna (any part)	170.4	198.5	—	213.4	238.0	239.2
unciform	170.5	198.5	—	213.5	238.0	239.2
vertebra (column)	170.2	198.5	—	213.2	238.0	239.2
coccyx	170.6	198.5	—	213.6	238.0	239.2
sacrum	170.6	198.5	—	213.6	238.0	239.2
vomer	170.0	198.5	—	213.0	238.0	239.2

SECTION I INDEX TO DISEASES AND INJURIES / Neoplasm, breast

	Malignant			Benign	Uncertain Behavior	Unspecified
	Primary	Secondary	Ca in situ			
Neoplasm *(Continued)*						
bone *(Continued)*						
wrist	170.5	198.5	—	213.5	238.0	239.2
xiphoid process	170.3	198.5	—	213.3	238.0	239.2
zygomatic	170.0	198.5	—	213.0	238.0	239.2
book-leaf (mouth)	145.8	198.89	230.0	210.4	235.1	239.0
bowel - *see* Neoplasm, intestine						
brachial plexus	171.2	198.89	—	215.2	238.1	239.2
brain NEC	191.9	198.3	—	225.0	237.5	239.6
basal ganglia	191.0	198.3	—	225.0	237.5	239.6
cerebellopontine angle	191.6	198.3	—	225.0	237.5	239.6
cerebellum NOS	191.6	198.3	—	225.0	237.5	239.6
cerebrum	191.0	198.3	—	225.0	237.5	239.6
choroid plexus	191.5	198.3	—	225.0	237.5	239.6
contiguous sites	191.8	—	—	—	—	—
corpus callosum	191.8	198.3	—	225.0	237.5	239.6
corpus striatum	191.0	198.3	—	225.0	237.5	239.6
cortex (cerebral)	191.0	198.3	—	225.0	237.5	239.6
frontal lobe	191.1	198.3	—	225.0	237.5	239.6
globus pallidus	191.0	198.3	—	225.0	237.5	239.6
hippocampus	191.2	198.3	—	225.0	237.5	239.6
hypothalamus	191.0	198.3	—	225.0	237.5	239.6
internal capsule	191.0	198.3	—	225.0	237.5	239.6
medulla oblongata	191.7	198.3	—	225.0	237.5	239.6
meninges	192.1	198.4	—	225.2	237.6	239.7
midbrain	191.7	198.3	—	225.0	237.5	239.6
occipital lobe	191.4	198.3	—	225.0	237.5	239.6
parietal lobe	191.3	198.3	—	225.0	237.5	239.6
peduncle	191.7	198.3	—	225.0	237.5	239.6
pons	191.7	198.3	—	225.0	237.5	239.6
stem	191.7	198.3	—	225.0	237.5	239.6
tapetum	191.8	198.3	—	225.0	237.5	239.6
temporal lobe	191.2	198.3	—	225.0	237.5	239.6
thalamus	191.0	198.3	—	225.0	237.5	239.6
uncus	191.2	198.3	—	225.0	237.5	239.6
ventricle (floor)	191.5	198.3	—	225.0	237.5	239.6
branchial (cleft) (vestiges)	146.8	198.89	230.0	210.6	235.1	239.0
breast (connective tissue) (female) (glandular tissue) (soft parts)	174.9	198.81	233.0	217	238.3	239.3
areola	174.0	198.81	233.0	217	238.3	239.3
male	175.0	198.81	233.0	217	238.3	239.3
axillary tail	174.6	198.81	233.0	217	238.3	239.3
central portion	174.1	198.81	233.0	217	238.3	239.3

SECTION I INDEX TO DISEASES AND INJURIES / Neoplasm, breast

	Malignant			Benign	Uncertain Behavior	Unspecified
	Primary	Secondary	Ca in situ			
Neoplasm *(Continued)*						
breast *(Continued)*						
contiguous sites	174.8	—	—	—	—	—
ectopic sites	174.8	198.81	233.0	217	238.3	239.3
inner	174.8	198.81	233.0	217	238.3	239.3
lower	174.8	198.81	233.0	217	238.3	239.3
lower-inner quadrant	174.3	198.81	233.0	217	238.3	239.3
lower-outer quadrant	174.5	198.81	233.0	217	238.3	239.3
male	175.9	198.81	233.0	217	238.3	239.3
areola	175.0	198.81	233.0	217	238.3	239.3
ectopic tissue	175.9	198.81	233.0	217	238.3	239.3
nipple	175.0	198.81	233.0	217	238.3	239.3
mastectomy site (skin) (*see also* Neoplasm, mastectomy site)	173.50	198.2	—	—	—	—
specified as breast tissue	174.8	198.81	—	—	—	—
midline	174.8	198.81	233.0	217	238.3	239.3
nipple	174.0	198.81	233.0	217	238.3	239.3
male	175.0	198.81	233.0	217	238.3	239.3
outer	174.8	198.81	233.0	217	238.3	239.3
skin (*see also* Neoplasm, mastectomy site)	173.50	198.2	232.5	216.5	238.2	239.2
tail (axillary)	174.6	198.81	233.0	217	238.3	239.3
upper	174.8	198.81	233.0	217	238.3	239.3
upper-inner quadrant	174.2	198.81	233.0	217	238.3	239.3
upper-outer quadrant	174.4	198.81	233.0	217	238.3	239.3
broad ligament	183.3	198.82	233.39	221.0	236.3	239.5
bronchiogenic, bronchogenic (lung)	162.9	197.0	231.2	212.3	235.7	239.1
bronchiole	162.9	197.0	231.2	212.3	235.7	239.1
bronchus	162.9	197.0	231.2	212.3	235.7	239.1
carina	162.2	197.0	231.2	212.3	235.7	239.1
contiguous sites with lung or trachea	162.8	—	—	—	—	—
lower lobe of lung	162.5	197.0	231.2	212.3	235.7	239.1
main	162.2	197.0	231.2	212.3	235.7	239.1
middle lobe of lung	162.4	197.0	231.2	212.3	235.7	239.1
upper lobe of lung	162.3	197.0	231.2	212.3	235.7	239.1
brow	173.30	198.2	232.3	216.3	238.2	239.2
basal cell carcinoma	173.31	—	—	—	—	—
specified type NEC	173.39	—	—	—	—	—
squamous cell carcinoma	173.32	—	—	—	—	—
buccal (cavity)	145.9	198.89	230.0	210.4	235.1	239.0
commissure	145.0	198.89	230.0	210.4	235.1	239.0
groove (lower) (upper)	145.1	198.89	230.0	210.4	235.1	239.0
mucosa	145.0	198.89	230.0	210.4	235.1	239.0
sulcus (lower) (upper)	145.1	198.89	230.0	210.4	235.1	239.0

◄ New ◄▌ Revised ~~deleted~~ Deleted ● Use Additional Digit(s) ▓ Omit code

SECTION I INDEX TO DISEASES AND INJURIES / Neoplasm, cartilage NEC

	Malignant			Benign	Uncertain Behavior	Unspecified
	Primary	Secondary	Ca in situ			
Neoplasm *(Continued)*						
bulbourethral gland	189.3	198.1	233.9	223.81	236.99	239.5
bursa - *see* Neoplasm, connective tissue						
buttock NEC*	195.3	198.89	232.5	229.8	238.8	239.89
calf*	195.5	198.89	232.7	229.8	238.8	239.89
calvarium	170.0	198.5	—	213.0	238.0	239.2
calyx, renal	189.1	198.0	233.9	223.1	236.91	239.5
canal						
anal	154.2	197.5	230.5	211.4	235.5	239.0
auditory (external) (*see also* Neoplasm, skin, ear)	173.20	198.2	232.2	216.2	238.2	239.2
auricular (external) (*see also* Neoplasm, skin, ear)	173.20	198.2	232.2	216.2	238.2	239.2
canaliculi, biliary (biliferi) (intrahepatic)	155.1	197.8	230.8	211.5	235.3	239.0
canthus (eye) (inner) (outer)	173.10	198.2	232.1	216.1	238.2	239.2
basal cell carcinoma	173.11	—	—	—	—	—
specified type NEC	173.19	—	—	—	—	—
squamous cell carcinoma	173.12	—	—	—	—	—
capillary - *see* Neoplasm, connective tissue						
caput coli	153.4	197.5	230.3	211.3	235.2	239.0
cardia (gastric)	151.0	197.8	230.2	211.1	235.2	239.0
cardiac orifice (stomach)	151.0	197.8	230.2	211.1	235.2	239.0
cardio-esophageal junction	151.0	197.8	230.2	211.1	235.2	239.0
cardio-esophagus	151.0	197.8	230.2	211.1	235.2	239.0
carina (bronchus) (trachea)	162.2	197.0	231.2	212.3	235.7	239.1
carotid (artery)	171.0	198.89	—	215.0	238.1	239.2
body	194.5	198.89	—	227.5	237.3	239.7
carpus (any bone)	170.5	198.5	—	213.5	238.0	239.2
cartilage (articular) (joint) NEC - *see also* Neoplasm, bone	170.9	198.5	—	213.9	238.0	239.2
arytenoid	161.3	197.3	231.0	212.1	235.6	239.1
auricular	171.0	198.89	—	215.0	238.1	239.2
bronchi	162.2	197.3	—	212.3	235.7	239.1
connective tissue - *see* Neoplasm, connective tissue						
costal	170.3	198.5	—	213.3	238.0	239.2
cricoid	161.3	197.3	231.0	212.1	235.6	239.1
cuneiform	161.3	197.3	231.0	212.1	235.6	239.1
ear (external)	171.0	198.89	—	215.0	238.1	239.2
ensiform	170.3	198.5	—	213.3	238.0	239.2
epiglottis	161.1	197.3	231.0	212.1	235.6	239.1
anterior surface	146.4	198.89	230.0	210.6	235.1	239.0
eyelid	171.0	198.89	—	215.0	238.1	239.2
intervertebral	170.2	198.5	—	213.2	238.0	239.2
larynx, laryngeal	161.3	197.3	231.0	212.1	235.6	239.1
nose, nasal	160.0	197.3	231.8	212.0	235.9	239.1

SECTION I INDEX TO DISEASES AND INJURIES / Neoplasm, cartilage NEC

	Malignant			Benign	Uncertain Behavior	Unspecified
	Primary	Secondary	Ca in situ			
Neoplasm *(Continued)*						
cartilage NEC *(Continued)*						
pinna	171.0	198.89	—	215.0	238.1	239.2
rib	170.3	198.5	—	213.3	238.0	239.2
semilunar (knee)	170.7	198.5	—	213.7	238.0	239.2
thyroid	161.3	197.3	231.0	212.1	235.6	239.1
trachea	162.0	197.3	231.1	212.2	235.7	239.1
cauda equina	192.2	198.3	—	225.3	237.5	239.7
cavity						
buccal	145.9	198.89	230.0	210.4	235.1	239.0
nasal	160.0	197.3	231.8	212.0	235.9	239.1
oral	145.9	198.89	230.0	210.4	235.1	239.0
peritoneal	158.9	197.6	—	211.8	235.4	239.0
tympanic	160.1	197.3	231.8	212.0	235.9	239.1
cecum	153.4	197.5	230.3	211.3	235.2	239.0
central						
nervous system - *see* Neoplasm, nervous system						
white matter	191.0	198.3	—	225.0	237.5	239.6
cerebellopontine (angle)	191.6	198.3	—	225.0	237.5	239.6
cerebellum, cerebellar	191.6	198.3	—	225.0	237.5	239.6
cerebrum, cerebral (cortex) (hemisphere) (white matter)	191.0	198.3	—	225.0	237.5	239.6
meninges	192.1	198.4	—	225.2	237.6	239.7
peduncle	191.7	198.3	—	225.0	237.5	239.6
ventricle (any)	191.5	198.3	—	225.0	237.5	239.6
cervical region	195.0	198.89	234.8	229.8	238.8	239.89
cervix (cervical) (uteri) (uterus)	180.9	198.82	233.1	219.0	236.0	239.5
canal	180.0	198.82	233.1	219.0	236.0	239.5
contiguous sites	180.8	—	—	—	—	—
endocervix (canal) (gland)	180.0	198.82	233.1	219.0	236.0	239.5
exocervix	180.1	198.82	233.1	219.0	236.0	239.5
external os	180.1	198.82	233.1	219.0	236.0	239.5
nabothian gland	180.0	198.82	233.1	219.0	236.0	239.5
squamocolumnar junction	180.8	198.82	233.1	219.0	236.0	239.5
stump	180.8	198.82	233.1	219.0	236.0	239.5
cheek	195.0	198.89	234.8	229.8	238.8	239.89
external	173.30	198.2	232.3	216.3	238.2	239.2
basal cell carcinoma	173.31	—	—	—	—	—
specified type NEC	173.39	—	—	—	—	—
squamous cell carcinoma	173.32	—	—	—	—	—
inner aspect	145.0	198.89	230.0	210.4	235.1	239.0
internal	145.0	198.89	230.0	210.4	235.1	239.0
mucosa	145.0	198.89	230.0	210.4	235.1	239.0

SECTION I INDEX TO DISEASES AND INJURIES / Neoplasm, connective tissue NEC

	Malignant			Benign	Uncertain Behavior	Unspecified
	Primary	Secondary	Ca in situ			
Neoplasm (Continued)						
chest (wall) NEC	195.1	198.89	234.8	229.8	238.8	239.89
chiasma opticum	192.0	198.4	—	225.1	237.9	239.7
chin	173.30	198.2	232.3	216.3	238.2	239.2
basal cell carcinoma	173.31	—	—	—	—	—
specified type NEC	173.39	—	—	—	—	—
squamous cell carcinoma	173.32	—	—	—	—	—
choana	147.3	198.89	230.0	210.7	235.1	239.0
cholangiole	155.1	197.8	230.8	211.5	235.3	239.0
choledochal duct	156.1	197.8	230.8	211.5	235.3	239.0
choroid	190.6	198.4	234.0	224.6	238.8	239.81
plexus	191.5	198.3	—	225.0	237.5	239.6
ciliary body	190.0	198.4	234.0	224.0	238.8	239.89
clavicle	170.3	198.5	—	213.3	238.0	239.2
clitoris	184.3	198.82	233.32	221.2	236.3	239.5
clivus	170.0	198.5	—	213.0	238.0	239.2
cloacogenic zone	154.8	197.5	230.7	211.4	235.5	239.0
coccygeal						
body or glomus	194.6	198.89	—	227.6	237.3	239.7
vertebra	170.6	198.5	—	213.6	238.0	239.2
coccyx	170.6	198.5	—	213.6	238.0	239.2
colon - see also Neoplasm, intestine, large	153.9	197.5	230.3	211.3	235.2	239.0
with rectum	154.0	197.5	230.4	211.4	235.2	239.0
column, spinal - see Neoplasm, spine						
columnella (see also Neoplasm, skin, face)	173.30	198.2	232.3	216.3	238.2	239.2
commissure						
labial, lip	140.6	198.89	230.0	210.4	235.1	239.0
laryngeal	161.0	197.3	231.0	212.1	235.6	239.1
common (bile) duct	156.1	197.8	230.8	211.5	235.3	239.0
concha (see also Neoplasm, skin, ear)	173.20	198.2	232.2	216.2	238.2	239.2
nose	160.0	197.3	231.8	212.0	235.9	239.1
conjunctiva	190.3	198.4	234.0	224.3	238.8	239.89
connective tissue NEC	171.9	198.89	—	215.9	238.1	239.2

Note — For neoplasms of connective tissue (blood vessel, bursa, fascia, ligament, muscle, peripheral nerves, sympathetic and parasympathetic nerves and ganglia, synovia, tendon, etc.) or of morphological types that indicate connective tissue, code according to the list under "Neoplasm, connective tissue;" for sites that do not appear in this list, code to neoplasm of that site; e.g.,

    liposarcoma, shoulder 171.2
    leiomyosarcoma, stomach 151.9
    neurofibroma, chest wall 215.4

Morphological types that indicate connective tissue appear in their proper place in the alphabetic index with the instruction "see Neoplasm, connective tissue ...."

abdomen	171.5	198.89	—	215.5	238.1	239.2
abdominal wall	171.5	198.89	—	215.5	238.1	239.2

	Malignant			Benign	Uncertain Behavior	Unspecified
	Primary	Secondary	Ca in situ			
Neoplasm *(Continued)*						
connective tissue NEC *(Continued)*						
ankle	171.3	198.89	—	215.3	238.1	239.2
antecubital fossa or space	171.2	198.89	—	215.2	238.1	239.2
arm	171.2	198.89	—	215.2	238.1	239.2
auricle (ear)	171.0	198.89	—	215.0	238.1	239.2
axilla	171.4	198.89	—	215.4	238.1	239.2
back	171.7	198.89	—	215.7	238.1	239.2
breast (female) *(see also* Neoplasm, breast)	174.9	198.81	233.0	217	238.3	239.3
male	175.9	198.81	233.0	217	238.3	239.3
buttock	171.6	198.89	—	215.6	238.1	239.2
calf	171.3	198.89	—	215.3	238.1	239.2
cervical region	171.0	198.89	—	215.0	238.1	239.2
cheek	171.0	198.89	—	215.0	238.1	239.2
chest (wall)	171.4	198.89	—	215.4	238.1	239.2
chin	171.0	198.89	—	215.0	238.1	239.2
contiguous sites	171.8	—	—	—	—	—
diaphragm	171.4	198.89	—	215.4	238.1	239.2
ear (external)	171.0	198.89	—	215.0	238.1	239.2
elbow	171.2	198.89	—	215.2	238.1	239.2
extrarectal	171.6	198.89	—	215.6	238.1	239.2
extremity	171.8	198.89	—	215.8	238.1	239.2
lower	171.3	198.89	—	215.3	238.1	239.2
upper	171.2	198.89	—	215.2	238.1	239.2
eyelid	171.0	198.89	—	215.0	238.1	239.2
face	171.0	198.89	—	215.0	238.1	239.2
finger	171.2	198.89	—	215.2	238.1	239.2
flank	171.7	198.89	—	215.7	238.1	239.2
foot	171.3	198.89	—	215.3	238.1	239.2
forearm	171.2	198.89	—	215.2	238.1	239.2
forehead	171.0	198.89	—	215.0	238.1	239.2
gastric	171.5	198.89	—	215.5	238.1	—
gastrointestinal	171.5	198.89	—	215.5	238.1	—
gluteal region	171.6	198.89	—	215.6	238.1	239.2
great vessels NEC	171.4	198.89	—	215.4	238.1	239.2
groin	171.6	198.89	—	215.6	238.1	239.2
hand	171.2	198.89	—	215.2	238.1	239.2
head	171.0	198.89	—	215.0	238.1	239.2
heel	171.3	198.89	—	215.3	238.1	239.2
hip	171.3	198.89	—	215.3	238.1	239.2
hypochondrium	171.5	198.89	—	215.5	238.1	239.2
iliopsoas muscle	171.6	198.89	—	215.5	238.1	239.2

SECTION I INDEX TO DISEASES AND INJURIES / Neoplasm, connective tissue NEC

	Malignant			Benign	Uncertain Behavior	Unspecified
	Primary	Secondary	Ca in situ			
Neoplasm *(Continued)*						
connective tissue NEC *(Continued)*						
infraclavicular region	171.4	198.89	—	215.4	238.1	239.2
inguinal (canal) (region)	171.6	198.89	—	215.6	238.1	239.2
intestine	171.5	198.89	—	215.5	238.1	—
intrathoracic	171.4	198.89	—	215.4	238.1	239.2
ischorectal fossa	171.6	198.89	—	215.6	238.1	239.2
jaw	143.9	198.89	230.0	210.4	235.1	239.0
knee	171.3	198.89	—	215.3	238.1	239.2
leg	171.3	198.89	—	215.3	238.1	239.2
limb NEC	171.9	198.89	—	215.8	238.1	239.2
lower	171.3	198.89	—	215.3	238.1	239.2
upper	171.2	198.89	—	215.2	238.1	239.2
nates	171.6	198.89	—	215.6	238.1	239.2
neck	171.0	198.89	—	215.0	238.1	239.2
orbit	190.1	198.4	234.0	224.1	238.8	239.89
pararectal	171.6	198.89	—	215.6	238.1	239.2
para-urethral	171.6	198.89	—	215.6	238.1	239.2
paravaginal	171.6	198.89	—	215.6	238.1	239.2
pelvis (floor)	171.6	198.89	—	215.6	238.1	239.2
pelvo-abdominal	171.8	198.89	—	215.8	238.1	239.2
perineum	171.6	198.89	—	215.6	238.1	239.2
perirectal (tissue)	171.6	198.89	—	215.6	238.1	239.2
periurethral (tissue)	171.6	198.89	—	215.6	238.1	239.2
popliteal fossa or space	171.3	198.89	—	215.3	238.1	239.2
presacral	171.6	198.89	—	215.6	238.1	239.2
psoas muscle	171.5	198.89	—	215.5	238.1	239.2
pterygoid fossa	171.0	198.89	—	215.0	238.1	239.2
rectovaginal septum or wall	171.6	198.89	—	215.6	238.1	239.2
rectovesical	171.6	198.89	—	215.6	238.1	239.2
retroperitoneum	158.0	197.6	—	211.8	235.4	239.0
sacrococcygeal region	171.6	198.89	—	215.6	238.1	239.2
scalp	171.0	198.89	—	215.0	238.1	239.2
scapular region	171.4	198.89	—	215.4	238.1	239.2
shoulder	171.2	198.89	—	215.2	238.1	239.2
skin (dermis) NEC	173.90	198.2	232.9	216.9	238.2	239.2
stomach	171.5	198.89	—	215.5	238.1	—
submental	171.0	198.89	—	215.0	238.1	239.2
supraclavicular region	171.0	198.89	—	215.0	238.1	239.2
temple	171.0	198.89	—	215.0	238.1	239.2
temporal region	171.0	198.89	—	215.0	238.1	239.2
thigh	171.3	198.89	—	215.3	238.1	239.2

◀ New ◀◀◀ Revised ~~deleted~~ Deleted ● Use Additional Digit(s) Omit code

SECTION I INDEX TO DISEASES AND INJURIES / Neoplasm, connective tissue NEC

	Malignant			Benign	Uncertain Behavior	Unspecified
	Primary	Secondary	Ca in situ			
Neoplasm *(Continued)*						
connective tissue NEC *(Continued)*						
thoracic (duct) (wall)	171.4	198.89	—	215.4	238.1	239.2
thorax	171.4	198.89	—	215.4	238.1	239.2
thumb	171.2	198.89	—	215.2	238.1	239.2
toe	171.3	198.89	—	215.3	238.1	239.2
trunk	171.7	198.89	—	215.7	238.1	239.2
umbilicus	171.5	198.89	—	215.5	238.1	239.2
vesicorectal	171.6	198.89	—	215.6	238.1	239.2
wrist	171.2	198.89	—	215.2	238.1	239.2
conus medullaris	192.2	198.3	—	225.3	237.5	239.7
cord (true) (vocal)	161.0	197.3	231.0	212.1	235.6	239.1
false	161.1	197.3	231.0	212.1	235.6	239.1
spermatic	187.6	198.82	233.6	222.8	236.6	239.5
spinal (cervical) (lumbar) (thoracic)	192.2	198.3	—	225.3	237.5	239.7
cornea (limbus)	190.4	198.4	234.0	224.4	238.8	239.89
corpus						
albicans	183.0	198.6	233.39	220	236.2	239.5
callosum, brain	191.8	198.3	—	225.0	237.5	239.6
cavernosum	187.3	198.82	233.5	222.1	236.6	239.5
gastric	151.4	197.8	230.2	211.1	235.2	239.0
penis	187.3	198.82	233.5	222.1	236.6	239.5
striatum, cerebrum	191.0	198.3	—	225.0	237.5	239.6
uteri	182.0	198.82	233.2	219.1	236.0	239.5
isthmus	182.1	198.82	233.2	219.1	236.0	239.5
cortex						
adrenal	194.0	198.7	234.8	227.0	237.2	239.7
cerebral	191.0	198.3	—	225.0	237.5	239.6
costal cartilage	170.3	198.5	—	213.3	238.0	239.2
costovertebral joint	170.3	198.5	—	213.3	238.0	239.2
Cowper's gland	189.3	198.1	233.9	223.81	236.99	239.5
cranial (fossa, any)	191.9	198.3	—	225.0	237.5	239.6
meninges	192.1	198.4	—	225.2	237.6	239.7
nerve (any)	192.0	198.4	—	225.1	237.9	239.7
craniobuccal pouch	194.3	198.89	234.8	227.3	237.0	239.7
craniopharyngeal (duct) (pouch)	194.3	198.89	234.8	227.3	237.0	239.7
cricoid	148.0	198.89	230.0	210.8	235.1	239.0
cartilage	161.3	197.3	231.0	212.1	235.6	239.1
cricopharynx	148.0	198.89	230.0	210.8	235.1	239.0
crypt of Morgagni	154.8	197.5	230.7	211.4	235.2	239.0
crystalline lens	190.0	198.4	234.0	224.0	238.8	239.89
cul-de-sac (Douglas')	158.8	197.6	—	211.8	235.4	239.0

	Malignant			Benign	Uncertain Behavior	Unspecified
	Primary	Secondary	Ca in situ			
Neoplasm (Continued)						
cuneiform cartilage	161.3	197.3	231.0	212.1	235.6	239.1
cutaneous - see Neoplasm, skin						
cutis - see Neoplasm, skin						
cystic (bile) duct (common)	156.1	197.8	230.8	211.5	235.3	239.0
dermis - see Neoplasm, skin						
diaphragm	171.4	198.89	—	215.4	238.1	239.2
digestive organs, system, tube, or tract NEC	159.9	197.8	230.9	211.9	235.5	239.0
contiguous sites with peritoneum	159.8	—	—	—	—	—
disc, intervertebral	170.2	198.5	—	213.2	238.0	239.2
disease, generalized	199.0	199.0	234.9	229.9	238.9	199.0
disseminated	199.0	199.0	234.9	229.9	238.9	199.0
Douglas' cul-de-sac or pouch	158.8	197.6	—	211.8	235.4	239.0
duodenojejunal junction	152.8	197.4	230.7	211.2	235.2	239.0
duodenum	152.0	197.4	230.7	211.2	235.2	239.0
dura (cranial) (mater)	192.1	198.4	—	225.2	237.6	239.7
cerebral	192.1	198.4	—	225.2	237.6	239.7
spinal	192.3	198.4	—	225.4	237.6	239.7
ear (external) (see also Neoplasm, ear, skin)	173.20	198.2	232.2	216.2	238.2	239.2
auricle or auris (see also Neoplasm, ear, skin)	173.20	198.2	232.2	216.2	238.2	239.2
canal, external (see also Neoplasm, ear, skin)	173.20	198.2	232.2	216.2	238.2	239.2
cartilage	171.0	198.89	—	215.0	238.1	239.2
external meatus (see also Neoplasm, ear, skin)	173.20	198.2	232.2	216.2	238.2	239.2
inner	160.1	197.3	231.8	212.0	235.9	239.89
lobule (see also Neoplasm, ear, skin)	173.20	198.2	232.2	216.2	238.2	239.2
middle	160.1	197.3	231.8	212.0	235.9	239.89
contiguous sites with accessory sinuses or nasal cavities	160.8	—	—	—	—	—
skin	173.20	198.2	232.2	216.2	238.2	239.2
basal cell carcinoma	173.21	—	—	—	—	—
specified type NEC	173.29	—	—	—	—	—
squamous cell carcinoma	173.22	—	—	—	—	—
earlobe	173.20	198.2	232.2	216.2	238.2	239.2
basal cell carcinoma	173.21	—	—	—	—	—
specified type NEC	173.29	—	—	—	—	—
squamous cell carcinoma	173.22	—	—	—	—	—
ejaculatory duct	187.8	198.82	233.6	222.8	236.6	239.5
elbow NEC*	195.4	198.89	232.6	229.8	238.8	239.89
endocardium	164.1	198.89	—	212.7	238.8	239.89
endocervix (canal) (gland)	180.0	198.82	233.1	219.0	236.0	239.5
endocrine gland NEC	194.9	198.89	—	227.9	237.4	239.7
pluriglandular NEC	194.8	198.89	234.8	227.8	237.4	239.7
endometrium (gland) (stroma)	182.0	198.82	233.2	219.1	236.0	239.5

SECTION I INDEX TO DISEASES AND INJURIES / Neoplasm, ensiform cartilage

	Malignant			Benign	Uncertain Behavior	Unspecified
	Primary	Secondary	Ca in situ			
Neoplasm (Continued)						
ensiform cartilage	170.3	198.5	—	213.3	238.0	239.2
enteric - see Neoplasm, intestine						
ependyma (brain)	191.5	198.3	—	225.0	237.5	239.6
epicardium	164.1	198.89	—	212.7	238.8	239.89
epididymis	187.5	198.82	233.6	222.3	236.6	239.5
epidural	192.9	198.4	—	225.9	237.9	239.7
epiglottis	161.1	197.3	231.0	212.1	235.6	239.1
anterior aspect or surface	146.4	198.89	230.0	210.6	235.1	239.0
cartilage	161.3	197.3	231.0	212.1	235.6	239.1
free border (margin)	146.4	198.89	230.0	210.6	235.1	239.0
junctional region	146.5	198.89	230.0	210.6	235.1	239.0
posterior (laryngeal) surface	161.1	197.3	231.0	212.1	235.6	239.1
suprahyoid portion	161.1	197.3	231.0	212.1	235.6	239.1
esophagogastric junction	151.0	197.8	230.2	211.1	235.2	239.0
esophagus	150.9	197.8	230.1	211.0	235.5	239.0
abdominal	150.2	197.8	230.1	211.0	235.5	239.0
cervical	150.0	197.8	230.1	211.0	235.5	239.0
contiguous sites	150.8	—	—	—	—	—
distal (third)	150.5	197.8	230.1	211.0	235.5	239.0
lower (third)	150.5	197.8	230.1	211.0	235.5	239.0
middle (third)	150.4	197.8	230.1	211.0	235.5	239.0
proximal (third)	150.3	197.8	230.1	211.0	235.5	239.0
specified part NEC	150.8	197.8	230.1	211.0	235.5	239.0
thoracic	150.1	197.8	230.1	211.0	235.5	239.0
upper (third)	150.3	197.8	230.1	211.0	235.5	239.0
ethmoid (sinus)	160.3	197.3	231.8	212.0	235.9	239.1
bone or labyrinth	170.0	198.5	—	213.0	238.0	239.2
Eustachian tube	160.1	197.3	231.8	212.0	235.9	239.1
exocervix	180.1	198.82	233.1	219.0	236.0	239.5
external						
meatus (ear) (see also Neoplasm, skin, ear)	173.20	198.2	232.2	216.2	238.2	239.2
os, cervix uteri	180.1	198.82	233.1	219.0	236.0	239.5
extradural	192.9	198.4	—	225.9	237.9	239.7
extrahepatic (bile) duct	156.1	197.8	230.8	211.5	235.3	239.0
contiguous sites with gallbladder	156.8	—	—	—	—	—
extraocular muscle	190.1	198.4	234.0	224.1	238.8	239.89
extrarectal	195.3	198.89	234.8	229.8	238.8	239.89
extremity*	195.8	198.89	232.8	229.8	238.8	239.89
lower*	195.5	198.89	232.7	229.8	238.8	239.89
upper*	195.4	198.89	232.6	229.8	238.8	239.89

SECTION I INDEX TO DISEASES AND INJURIES / Neoplasm, fornix

	Malignant			Benign	Uncertain Behavior	Unspecified
	Primary	Secondary	Ca in situ			
Neoplasm (Continued)						
eye NEC	190.9	198.4	234.0	224.9	238.8	239.89
contiguous sites	190.8	—	—	—	—	—
specified sites NEC	190.8	198.4	234.0	224.8	238.8	239.89
eyeball	190.0	198.4	234.0	224.0	238.8	239.89
eyebrow	173.30	198.2	232.3	216.3	238.2	239.2
basal cell carcinoma	173.31	—	—	—	—	—
specified type NEC	173.39	—	—	—	—	—
squamous cell carcinoma	173.32	—	—	—	—	—
eyelid (lower) (skin) (upper)	173.10	198.2	232.1	216.1	238.2	239.2
basal cell carcinoma	173.11	—	—	—	—	—
cartilage	171.0	198.89	—	215.0	238.1	239.2
specified type NEC	173.19	—	—	—	—	—
squamous cell carcinoma	173.12	—	—	—	—	—
face NEC*	195.0	198.89	232.3	229.8	238.8	239.89
Fallopian tube (accessory)	183.2	198.82	233.39	221.0	236.3	239.5
falx (cerebella) (cerebri)	192.1	198.4	—	225.2	237.6	239.7
fascia - *see also* Neoplasm, connective tissue						
palmar	171.2	198.89	—	215.2	238.1	239.2
plantar	171.3	198.89	—	215.3	238.1	239.2
fatty tissue - *see* Neoplasm, connective tissue						
fauces, faucial NEC	146.9	198.89	230.0	210.6	235.1	239.0
pillars	146.2	198.89	230.0	210.6	235.1	239.0
tonsil	146.0	198.89	230.0	210.5	235.1	239.0
femur (any part)	170.7	198.5	—	213.7	238.0	239.2
fetal membrane	181	198.82	233.2	219.8	236.1	239.5
fibrous tissue - *see* Neoplasm, connective tissue						
fibula (any part)	170.7	198.5	—	213.7	238.0	239.2
filum terminale	192.2	198.3	—	225.3	237.5	239.7
finger NEC*	195.4	198.89	232.6	229.8	238.8	239.89
flank NEC*	195.8	198.89	232.5	229.8	238.8	239.89
follicle, nabothian	180.0	198.82	233.1	219.0	236.0	239.5
foot NEC*	195.5	198.89	232.7	229.8	238.8	239.89
forearm NEC*	195.4	198.89	232.6	229.8	238.8	239.89
forehead (skin)	173.30	198.2	232.3	216.3	238.2	239.2
basal cell carcinoma	173.31	—	—	—	—	—
specified type NEC	173.39	—	—	—	—	—
squamous cell carcinoma	173.32	—	—	—	—	—
foreskin	187.1	198.82	233.5	222.1	236.6	239.5
fornix						
pharyngeal	147.3	198.89	230.0	210.7	235.1	239.0
vagina	184.0	198.82	233.31	221.1	236.3	239.5

SECTION I INDEX TO DISEASES AND INJURIES / Neoplasm, fossa

	Malignant			Benign	Uncertain Behavior	Unspecified
	Primary	Secondary	Ca in situ			
Neoplasm *(Continued)*						
fossa (of)						
anterior (cranial)	191.9	198.3	—	225.0	237.5	239.6
cranial	191.9	198.3	—	225.0	237.5	239.6
ischiorectal	195.3	198.89	234.8	229.8	238.8	239.89
middle (cranial)	191.9	198.3	—	225.0	237.5	239.6
pituitary	194.3	198.89	234.8	227.3	237.0	239.7
posterior (cranial)	191.9	198.3	—	225.0	237.5	239.6
pterygoid	171.0	198.89	—	215.0	238.1	239.2
pyriform	148.1	198.89	230.0	210.8	235.1	239.0
Rosenmüller	147.2	198.89	230.0	210.7	235.1	239.0
tonsillar	146.1	198.89	230.0	210.6	235.1	239.0
fourchette	184.4	198.82	233.32	221.2	236.3	239.5
frenulum						
labii - *see* Neoplasm, lip, internal						
linguae	141.3	198.89	230.0	210.1	235.1	239.0
frontal						
bone	170.0	198.5	—	213.0	238.0	239.2
lobe, brain	191.1	198.3	—	225.0	237.5	239.6
meninges	192.1	198.4	—	225.2	237.6	239.7
pole	191.1	198.3	—	225.0	237.5	239.6
sinus	160.4	197.3	231.8	212.0	235.9	239.1
fundus						
stomach	151.3	197.8	230.2	211.1	235.2	239.0
uterus	182.0	198.82	233.2	219.1	236.0	239.5
gall duct (extrahepatic)	156.1	197.8	230.8	211.5	235.3	239.0
intrahepatic	155.1	197.8	230.8	211.5	235.3	239.0
gallbladder	156.0	197.8	230.8	211.5	235.3	239.0
contiguous sites with extrahepatic bile ducts	156.8	—	—	—	—	—
ganglia (*see also* Neoplasm, connective tissue)	171.9	198.89	—	215.9	238.1	239.2
basal	191.0	198.3	—	225.0	237.5	239.6
ganglion (*see also* Neoplasm, connective tissue)	171.9	198.89	—	215.9	238.1	239.2
cranial nerve	192.0	198.4	—	225.1	237.9	239.7
Gartner's duct	184.0	198.82	233.31	221.1	236.3	239.5
gastric - *see* Neoplasm, stomach						
gastrocolic	159.8	197.8	230.9	211.9	235.5	239.0
gastroesophageal junction	151.0	197.8	230.2	211.1	235.2	239.0
gastrointestinal (tract) NEC	159.9	197.8	230.9	211.9	235.5	239.0
generalized	199.0	199.0	234.9	229.9	238.9	199.0

SECTION I INDEX TO DISEASES AND INJURIES / Neoplasm, heart

	Malignant			Benign	Uncertain Behavior	Unspecified
	Primary	Secondary	Ca in situ			
Neoplasm (Continued)						
genital organ or tract						
female NEC	184.9	198.82	233.39	221.9	236.3	239.5
contiguous sites	184.8					
specified site NEC	184.8	198.82	233.39	221.8	236.3	239.5
male NEC	187.9	198.82	233.6	222.9	236.6	239.5
contiguous sites	187.8	—	—	—	—	—
specified site NEC	187.8	198.82	233.6	222.8	236.6	239.5
genitourinary tract						
female	184.9	198.82	233.39	221.9	236.3	239.5
male	187.9	198.82	233.6	222.9	236.6	239.5
gingiva (alveolar) (marginal)	143.9	198.89	230.0	210.4	235.1	239.0
lower	143.1	198.89	230.0	210.4	235.1	239.0
mandibular	143.1	198.89	230.0	210.4	235.1	239.0
maxillary	143.0	198.89	230.0	210.4	235.1	239.0
upper	143.0	198.89	230.0	210.4	235.1	239.0
gland, glandular (lymphatic) (system) - see also Neoplasm, lymph gland						
endocrine NEC	194.9	198.89	—	227.9	237.4	239.7
salivary - see Neoplasm, salivary, gland						
glans penis	187.2	198.82	233.5	222.1	236.6	239.5
globus pallidus	191.0	198.3	—	225.0	237.5	239.6
glomus						
coccygeal	194.6	198.89	—	227.6	237.3	239.7
jugularis	194.6	198.89	—	227.6	237.3	239.7
glosso-epiglottic fold(s)	146.4	198.89	230.0	210.6	235.1	239.0
glossopalatine fold	146.2	198.89	230.0	210.6	235.1	239.0
glossopharyngeal sulcus	146.1	198.89	230.0	210.6	235.1	239.0
glottis	161.0	197.3	231.0	212.1	235.6	239.1
gluteal region*	195.3	198.89	232.5	229.8	238.8	239.89
great vessels NEC	171.4	198.89	—	215.4	238.1	239.2
groin NEC	195.3	198.89	232.5	229.8	238.8	239.89
gum	143.9	198.89	230.0	210.4	235.1	239.0
contiguous sites	143.8	—	—	—	—	—
lower	143.1	198.89	230.0	210.4	235.1	239.0
upper	143.0	198.89	230.0	210.4	235.1	239.0
hand NEC*	195.4	198.89	232.6	229.8	238.8	239.89
head NEC*	195.0	198.89	232.4	229.8	238.8	239.89
heart	164.1	198.89	—	212.7	238.8	239.89
contiguous sites with mediastinum or thymus	164.8	—	—	—	—	—

New   Revised   deleted Deleted   Use Additional Digit(s)   Omit code

SECTION I INDEX TO DISEASES AND INJURIES / Neoplasm, heel NEC*

	Malignant			Benign	Uncertain Behavior	Unspecified
	Primary	Secondary	Ca in situ			
Neoplasm (Continued)						
heel NEC*	195.5	198.89	232.7	229.8	238.8	239.89
helix (see also Neoplasm, skin, ear)	173.20	198.2	232.2	216.2	238.2	239.2
hematopoietic, hemopoietic tissue NEC	202.8●	198.89	—	—	—	238.79
hemisphere, cerebral	191.0	198.3	—	225.0	237.5	239.6
hemorrhoidal zone	154.2	197.5	230.5	211.4	235.5	239.0
hepatic	155.2	197.7	230.8	211.5	235.3	239.0
duct (bile)	156.1	197.8	230.8	211.5	235.3	239.0
flexure (colon)	153.0	197.5	230.3	211.3	235.2	239.0
primary	155.0	—	—	—	—	—
hilus of lung	162.2	197.0	231.2	212.3	235.7	239.1
hip NEC*	195.5	198.89	232.7	229.8	238.8	239.89
hippocampus, brain	191.2	198.3	—	225.0	237.5	239.6
humerus (any part)	170.4	198.5	—	213.4	238.0	239.2
hymen	184.0	198.82	233.31	221.1	236.3	239.5
hypopharynx, hypopharyngeal NEC	148.9	198.89	230.0	210.8	235.1	239.0
contiguous sites	148.8	—	—	—	—	—
postcricoid region	148.0	198.89	230.0	210.8	235.1	239.0
posterior wall	148.3	198.89	230.0	210.8	235.1	239.0
pyriform fossa (sinus)	148.1	198.89	230.0	210.8	235.1	239.0
specified site NEC	148.8	198.89	230.0	210.8	235.1	239.0
wall	148.9	198.89	230.0	210.8	235.1	239.0
posterior	148.3	198.89	230.0	210.8	235.1	239.0
hypophysis	194.3	198.89	234.8	227.3	237.0	239.7
hypothalamus	191.0	198.3	—	225.0	237.5	239.6
ileocecum, ileocecal (coil) (junction) (valve)	153.4	197.5	230.3	211.3	235.2	239.0
ileum	152.2	197.4	230.7	211.2	235.2	239.0
ilium	170.6	198.5	—	213.6	238.0	239.2
immunoproliferative NEC	203.8●	—	—	—	—	—
infraclavicular (region)*	195.1	198.89	232.5	229.8	238.8	239.89
inguinal (region)*	195.3	198.89	232.5	229.8	238.8	239.89
insula	191.0	198.3	—	225.0	237.5	239.6
insular tissue (pancreas)	157.4	197.8	230.9	211.7	235.5	239.0
brain	191.0	198.3	—	225.0	237.5	239.6
interarytenoid fold	148.2	198.89	230.0	210.8	235.1	239.0
hypopharyngeal aspect	148.2	198.89	230.0	210.8	235.1	239.0
laryngeal aspect	161.1	197.3	231.0	212.1	235.6	239.1
marginal zone	148.2	198.89	230.0	210.8	235.1	239.0
interdental papillae	143.9	198.89	230.0	210.4	235.1	239.0
lower	143.1	198.89	230.0	210.4	235.1	239.0
upper	143.0	198.89	230.0	210.4	235.1	239.0

	Malignant			Benign	Uncertain Behavior	Unspecified
	Primary	Secondary	Ca in situ			
Neoplasm *(Continued)*						
internal						
capsule	191.0	198.3	—	225.0	237.5	239.6
os (cervix)	180.0	198.82	233.1	219.0	236.0	239.5
intervertebral cartilage or disc	170.2	198.5	—	213.2	238.0	239.2
intestine, intestinal	159.0	197.8	230.7	211.9	235.2	239.0
large	153.9	197.5	230.3	211.3	235.2	239.0
appendix	153.5	197.5	230.3	211.3	235.2	239.0
caput coli	153.4	197.5	230.3	211.3	235.2	239.0
cecum	153.4	197.5	230.3	211.3	235.2	239.0
colon	153.9	197.5	230.3	211.3	235.2	239.0
and rectum	154.0	197.5	230.4	211.4	235.2	239.0
ascending	153.6	197.5	230.3	211.3	235.2	239.0
caput	153.4	197.5	230.3	211.3	235.2	239.0
contiguous sites	153.8	—	—	—	—	—
descending	153.2	197.5	230.3	211.3	235.2	239.0
distal	153.2	197.5	230.3	211.3	235.2	239.0
left	153.2	197.5	230.3	211.3	235.2	239.0
pelvic	153.3	197.5	230.3	211.3	235.2	239.0
right	153.6	197.5	230.3	211.3	235.2	239.0
sigmoid (flexure)	153.3	197.5	230.3	211.3	235.2	239.0
transverse	153.1	197.5	230.3	211.3	235.2	239.0
contiguous sites	153.8	—	—	—	—	—
hepatic flexure	153.0	197.5	230.3	211.3	235.2	239.0
ileocecum, ileocecal (coil) (valve)	153.4	197.5	230.3	211.3	235.2	239.0
sigmoid flexure (lower) (upper)	153.3	197.5	230.3	211.3	235.2	239.0
splenic flexure	153.7	197.5	230.3	211.3	235.2	239.0
small	152.9	197.4	230.7	211.2	235.2	239.0
contiguous sites	152.8	—	—	—	—	—
duodenum	152.0	197.4	230.7	211.2	235.2	239.0
ileum	152.2	197.4	230.7	211.2	235.2	239.0
jejunum	152.1	197.4	230.7	211.2	235.2	239.0
tract NEC	159.0	197.8	230.7	211.9	235.2	239.0
intra-abdominal	195.2	198.89	234.8	229.8	238.8	239.89
intracranial NEC	191.9	198.3	—	225.0	237.5	239.6
intrahepatic (bile) duct	155.1	197.8	230.8	211.5	235.3	239.0
intraocular	190.0	198.4	234.0	224.0	238.8	239.89
intraorbital	190.1	198.4	234.0	224.1	238.8	239.89
intrasellar	194.3	198.89	234.8	227.3	237.0	239.7
intrathoracic (cavity) (organs NEC)	195.1	198.89	234.8	229.8	238.8	239.89
contiguous sites with respiratory organs	165.8	—	—	—	—	—

SECTION I INDEX TO DISEASES AND INJURIES / Neoplasm, iris

	Malignant			Benign	Uncertain Behavior	Unspecified
	Primary	Secondary	Ca in situ			
Neoplasm (Continued)						
iris	190.0	198.4	234.0	224.0	238.8	239.89
ischiorectal (fossa)	195.3	198.89	234.8	229.8	238.8	239.89
ischium	170.6	198.5	—	213.6	238.0	239.2
island of Reil	191.0	198.3	—	225.0	237.5	239.6
islands or islets of Langerhans	157.4	197.8	230.9	211.7	235.5	239.0
isthmus uteri	182.1	198.82	233.2	219.1	236.0	239.5
jaw	195.0	198.89	234.8	229.8	238.8	239.89
bone	170.1	198.5	—	213.1	238.0	239.2
carcinoma	143.9	—	—	—	—	—
lower	143.1	—	—	—	—	—
upper	143.0	—	—	—	—	—
lower	170.1	198.5	—	213.1	238.0	239.2
upper	170.0	198.5	—	213.0	238.0	239.2
carcinoma (any type) (lower) (upper)	195.0	—	—	—	—	—
skin (*see also* Neoplasm, skin, face)	173.30	198.2	232.3	216.3	238.2	239.2
soft tissues	143.9	198.89	230.0	210.4	235.1	239.0
lower	143.1	198.89	230.0	210.4	235.1	239.0
upper	143.0	198.89	230.0	210.4	235.1	239.0
jejunum	152.1	197.4	230.7	211.2	235.2	239.0
joint NEC (*see also* Neoplasm, bone)	170.9	198.5	—	213.9	238.0	239.2
acromioclavicular	170.4	198.5	—	213.4	238.0	239.2
bursa or synovial membrane - *see* Neoplasm, connective tissue						
costovertebral	170.3	198.5	—	213.3	238.0	239.2
sternocostal	170.3	198.5	—	213.3	238.0	239.2
temporomandibular	170.1	198.5	—	213.1	238.0	239.2
junction						
anorectal	154.8	197.5	230.7	211.4	235.5	239.0
cardioesophageal	151.0	197.8	230.2	211.1	235.2	239.0
esophagogastric	151.0	197.8	230.2	211.1	235.2	239.0
gastroesophageal	151.0	197.8	230.2	211.1	235.2	239.0
hard and soft palate	145.5	198.89	230.0	210.4	235.1	239.0
ileocecal	153.4	197.5	230.3	211.3	235.2	239.0
pelvirectal	154.0	197.5	230.4	211.4	235.2	239.0
pelviureteric	189.1	198.0	233.9	223.1	236.91	239.5
rectosigmoid	154.0	197.5	230.4	211.4	235.2	239.0
squamocolumnar, of cervix	180.8	198.82	233.1	219.0	236.0	239.5
kidney (parenchymal)	189.0	198.0	233.9	223.0	236.91	239.5
calyx	189.1	198.0	233.9	223.1	236.91	239.5
hilus	189.1	198.0	233.9	223.1	236.91	239.5
pelvis	189.1	198.0	233.9	223.1	236.91	239.5
knee NEC*	195.5	198.89	232.7	229.8	238.8	239.89

◀ New ◀ Revised ~~deleted~~ Deleted ● Use Additional Digit(s) ▨ Omit code

SECTION I INDEX TO DISEASES AND INJURIES / Neoplasm, ligament

	Malignant			Benign	Uncertain Behavior	Unspecified
	Primary	Secondary	Ca in situ			
Neoplasm (Continued)						
labia (skin)	184.4	198.82	233.32	221.2	236.3	239.5
majora	184.1	198.82	233.32	221.2	236.3	239.5
minora	184.2	198.82	233.32	221.2	236.3	239.5
labial - see also Neoplasm, lip sulcus (lower) (upper)	145.1	198.89	230.0	210.4	235.1	239.0
labium (skin)	184.4	198.82	233.32	221.2	236.3	239.5
majus	184.1	198.82	233.32	221.2	236.3	239.5
minus	184.2	198.82	233.32	221.2	236.3	239.5
lacrimal						
canaliculi	190.7	198.4	234.0	224.7	238.8	239.89
duct (nasal)	190.7	198.4	234.0	224.7	238.8	239.89
gland	190.2	198.4	234.0	224.2	238.8	239.89
punctum	190.7	198.4	234.0	224.7	238.8	239.89
sac	190.7	198.4	234.0	224.7	238.8	239.89
Langerhans, islands or islets	157.4	197.8	230.9	211.7	235.5	239.0
laryngopharynx	148.9	198.89	230.0	210.8	235.1	239.0
larynx, laryngeal NEC	161.9	197.3	231.0	212.1	235.6	239.1
aryepiglottic fold	161.1	197.3	231.0	212.1	235.6	239.1
cartilage (arytenoid) (cricoid) (cuneiform) (thyroid)	161.3	197.3	231.0	212.1	235.6	239.1
commissure (anterior) (posterior)	161.0	197.3	231.0	212.1	235.6	239.1
contiguous sites	161.8	—	—	—	—	—
extrinsic NEC	161.1	197.3	231.0	212.1	235.6	239.1
meaning hypopharynx	148.9	198.89	230.0	210.8	235.1	239.0
interarytenoid fold	161.1	197.3	231.0	212.1	235.6	239.1
intrinsic	161.0	197.3	231.0	212.1	235.6	239.1
ventricular band	161.1	197.3	231.0	212.1	235.6	239.1
leg NEC*	195.5	198.89	232.7	229.8	238.8	239.89
lens, crystalline	190.0	198.4	234.0	224.0	238.8	239.89
lid (lower) (upper)	173.10	198.2	232.1	216.1	238.2	239.2
basal cell carcinoma	173.11	—	—	—	—	—
specified type NEC	173.19	—	—	—	—	—
squamous cell carcinoma	173.12	—	—	—	—	—
ligament - see also Neoplasm, connective tissue						
broad	183.3	198.82	233.39	221.0	236.3	239.5
Mackenrodt's	183.8	198.82	233.39	221.8	236.3	239.5
non-uterine - see Neoplasm, connective tissue						
round	183.5	198.82	—	221.0	236.3	239.5
sacro-uterine	183.4	198.82	—	221.0	236.3	239.5
uterine	183.4	198.82	—	221.0	236.3	239.5
utero-ovarian	183.8	198.82	233.39	221.8	236.3	239.5
uterosacral	183.4	198.82	—	221.0	236.3	239.5

SECTION I INDEX TO DISEASES AND INJURIES / Neoplasm, limb*

	Malignant			Benign	Uncertain Behavior	Unspecified
	Primary	Secondary	Ca in situ			
Neoplasm (Continued)						
limb*	195.8	198.89	232.8	229.8	238.8	239.89
lower*	195.5	198.89	232.7	229.8	238.8	239.89
upper*	195.4	198.89	232.6	229.8	238.8	239.89
limbus of cornea	190.4	198.4	234.0	224.4	238.8	239.89
lingual NEC (see also Neoplasm, tongue)	141.9	198.89	230.0	210.1	235.1	239.0
lingula, lung	162.3	197.0	231.2	212.3	235.7	239.1
lip (external) (lipstick area) (vermillion border)	140.9	198.89	230.0	210.0	235.1	239.0
buccal aspect - see Neoplasm, lip, internal						
commissure	140.6	198.89	230.0	210.4	235.1	239.0
contiguous sites	140.8	—	—	—	—	—
with oral cavity or pharynx	149.8	—	—	—	—	—
frenulum - see Neoplasm, lip, internal						
inner aspect - see Neoplasm, lip, internal						
internal (buccal) (frenulum) (mucosa) (oral)	140.5	198.89	230.0	210.0	235.1	239.0
lower	140.4	198.89	230.0	210.0	235.1	239.0
upper	140.3	198.89	230.0	210.0	235.1	239.0
lower	140.1	198.89	230.0	210.0	235.1	239.0
internal (buccal) (frenulum) (mucosa) (oral)	140.4	198.89	230.0	210.0	235.1	239.0
mucosa - see Neoplasm, lip, internal						
oral aspect - see Neoplasm, lip, internal						
skin (commissure) (lower) (upper)	173.00	198.2	232.0	216.0	238.2	239.2
basal cell carcinoma	173.01	—	—	—	—	—
specified type NEC	173.09	—	—	—	—	—
squamous cell carcinoma	173.02	—	—	—	—	—
upper	140.0	198.89	230.0	210.0	235.1	239.0
internal (buccal) (frenulum) (mucosa) (oral)	140.3	198.89	230.0	210.0	235.1	239.0
liver	155.2	197.7	230.8	211.5	235.3	239.0
primary	155.0	—	—	—	—	—
lobe						
azygos	162.3	197.0	231.2	212.3	235.7	239.1
frontal	191.1	198.3	—	225.0	237.5	239.6
lower	162.5	197.0	231.2	212.3	235.7	239.1
middle	162.4	197.0	231.2	212.3	235.7	239.1
occipital	191.4	198.3	—	225.0	237.5	239.6
parietal	191.3	198.3	—	225.0	237.5	239.6
temporal	191.2	198.3	—	225.0	237.5	239.6
upper	162.3	197.0	231.2	212.3	235.7	239.1
lumbosacral plexus	171.6	198.4	—	215.6	238.1	239.2

SECTION I INDEX TO DISEASES AND INJURIES / Neoplasm, lymph, lymphatic

	Malignant			Benign	Uncertain Behavior	Unspecified
	Primary	Secondary	Ca in situ			
Neoplasm *(Continued)*						
lung	162.9	197.0	231.2	212.3	235.7	239.1
azygos lobe	162.3	197.0	231.2	212.3	235.7	239.1
carina	162.2	197.0	231.2	212.3	235.7	239.1
contiguous sites with bronchus or trachea	162.8	—	—	—	—	—
hilus	162.2	197.0	231.2	212.3	235.7	239.1
lingula	162.3	197.0	231.2	212.3	235.7	239.1
lobe NEC	162.9	197.0	231.2	212.3	235.7	239.1
lower lobe	162.5	197.0	231.2	212.3	235.7	239.1
main bronchus	162.2	197.0	231.2	212.3	235.7	239.1
middle lobe	162.4	197.0	231.2	212.3	235.7	239.1
upper lobe	162.3	197.0	231.2	212.3	235.7	239.1
lymph, lymphatic						
channel NEC (*see also* Neoplasm, connective tissue)	171.9	198.89	—	215.9	238.1	239.2
gland (secondary)	—	196.9	—	229.0	238.8	239.89
abdominal	—	196.2	—	229.0	238.8	239.89
aortic	—	196.2	—	229.0	238.8	239.89
arm	—	196.3	—	229.0	238.8	239.89
auricular (anterior) (posterior)	—	196.0	—	229.0	238.8	239.89
axilla, axillary	—	196.3	—	229.0	238.8	239.89
brachial	—	196.3	—	229.0	238.8	239.89
bronchial	—	196.1	—	229.0	238.8	239.89
bronchopulmonary	—	196.1	—	229.0	238.8	239.89
celiac	—	196.2	—	229.0	238.8	239.89
cervical	—	196.0	—	229.0	238.8	239.89
cervicofacial	—	196.0	—	229.0	238.8	239.89
Cloquet	—	196.5	—	229.0	238.8	239.89
colic	—	196.2	—	229.0	238.8	239.89
common duct	—	196.2	—	229.0	238.8	239.89
cubital	—	196.3	—	229.0	238.8	239.89
diaphragmatic	—	196.1	—	229.0	238.8	239.89
epigastric, inferior	—	196.6	—	229.0	238.8	239.89
epitrochlear	—	196.3	—	229.0	238.8	239.89
esophageal	—	196.1	—	229.0	238.8	239.89
face	—	196.0	—	229.0	238.8	239.89
femoral	—	196.5	—	229.0	238.8	239.89
gastric	—	196.2	—	229.0	238.8	239.89
groin	—	196.5	—	229.0	238.8	239.89
head	—	196.0	—	229.0	238.8	239.89
hepatic	—	196.2	—	229.0	238.8	239.89
hilar (pulmonary)	—	196.1	—	229.0	238.8	239.89
splenic	—	196.2	—	229.0	238.8	239.89

◀ New ◀◀◀ Revised ~~deleted~~ Deleted ● Use Additional Digit(s) ▨ Omit code

SECTION I INDEX TO DISEASES AND INJURIES / Neoplasm, lymph, lymphatic

	Malignant			Benign	Uncertain Behavior	Unspecified
	Primary	Secondary	Ca in situ			
Neoplasm *(Continued)*						
lymph, lymphatic *(Continued)*						
gland *(Continued)*						
hypogastric	—	196.6	—	229.0	238.8	239.89
ileocolic	—	196.2	—	229.0	238.8	239.89
iliac	—	196.6	—	229.0	238.8	239.89
infraclavicular	—	196.3	—	229.0	238.8	239.89
inguina, inguinal	—	196.5	—	229.0	238.8	239.89
innominate	—	196.1	—	229.0	238.8	239.89
intercostal	—	196.1	—	229.0	238.8	239.89
intestinal	—	196.2	—	229.0	238.8	239.89
intrabdominal	—	196.2	—	229.0	238.8	239.89
intrapelvic	—	196.6	—	229.0	238.8	239.89
intrathoracic	—	196.1	—	229.0	238.8	239.9
jugular	—	196.0	—	229.0	238.8	239.89
leg	—	196.5	—	229.0	238.8	239.89
limb						
lower	—	196.5	—	229.0	238.8	239.89
upper	—	196.3	—	229.0	238.8	239.89
lower limb	—	196.5	—	229.0	238.8	239.9
lumbar	—	196.2	—	229.0	238.8	239.89
mandibular	—	196.0	—	229.0	238.8	239.89
mediastinal	—	196.1	—	229.0	238.8	239.89
mesenteric (inferior) (superior)	—	196.2	—	229.0	238.8	239.89
midcolic	—	196.2	—	229.0	238.8	239.89
multiple sites in categories 196.0–196.6	—	196.8	—	229.0	238.8	239.89
neck	—	196.0	—	229.0	238.8	239.89
obturator	—	196.6	—	229.0	238.8	239.89
occipital	—	196.0	—	229.0	238.8	239.89
pancreatic	—	196.2	—	229.0	238.8	239.89
para-aortic	—	196.2	—	229.0	238.8	239.89
paracervical	—	196.6	—	229.0	238.8	239.89
parametrial	—	196.6	—	229.0	238.8	239.89
parasternal	—	196.1	—	229.0	238.8	239.89
parotid	—	196.0	—	229.0	238.8	239.89
pectoral	—	196.3	—	229.0	238.8	239.89
pelvic	—	196.6	—	229.0	238.8	239.89
peri-aortic	—	196.2	—	229.0	238.8	239.89
peripancreatic	—	196.2	—	229.0	238.8	239.89
popliteal	—	196.5	—	229.0	238.8	239.89
porta hepatis	—	196.2	—	229.0	238.8	239.89
portal	—	196.2	—	229.0	238.8	239.89

◄ New   ◄▥ Revised   ~~deleted~~ Deleted   ● Use Additional Digit(s)   Omit code

SECTION I INDEX TO DISEASES AND INJURIES / Neoplasm, mandible

	Malignant			Benign	Uncertain Behavior	Unspecified
	Primary	Secondary	Ca in situ			
Neoplasm *(Continued)*						
lymph, lymphatic *(Continued)*						
gland *(Continued)*						
preauricular	—	196.0	—	229.0	238.8	239.89
prelaryngeal	—	196.0	—	229.0	238.8	239.89
presymphysial	—	196.6	—	229.0	238.8	239.89
pretracheal	—	196.0	—	229.0	238.8	239.89
primary (any site) NEC	202.9●	—	—	—	—	—
pulmonary (hiler)	—	196.1	—	229.0	238.8	239.89
pyloric	—	196.2	—	229.0	238.8	239.89
retroperitoneal	—	196.2	—	229.0	238.8	239.89
retropharyngeal	—	196.0	—	229.0	238.8	239.89
Rosenmüller's	—	196.5	—	229.0	238.8	239.89
sacral	—	196.6	—	229.0	238.8	239.89
scalene	—	196.0	—	229.0	238.8	239.89
site NEC	—	196.9	—	229.0	238.8	239.89
splenic (hilar)	—	196.2	—	229.0	238.8	239.89
subclavicular	—	196.3	—	229.0	238.8	239.89
subinguinal	—	196.5	—	229.0	238.8	239.89
sublingual	—	196.0	—	229.0	238.8	239.89
submandibular	—	196.0	—	229.0	238.8	239.89
submaxillary	—	196.0	—	229.0	238.8	239.89
submental	—	196.0	—	229.0	238.8	239.89
subscapular	—	196.3	—	229.0	238.8	239.89
supraclavicular	—	196.0	—	229.0	238.8	239.89
thoracic	—	196.1	—	229.0	238.8	239.89
tibial	—	196.5	—	229.0	238.8	239.89
tracheal		196.1	—	229.0	238.8	239.89
tracheobronchial	—	196.1	—	229.0	238.8	239.89
upper limb	—	196.3	—	229.0	238.8	239.89
Virchow's	—	196.0	—	229.0	238.8	239.89
node - *see also* Neoplasm, lymph gland	202.9●	—	—	—	—	—
primary NEC						
vessel (*see also* Neoplasm, connective tissue)	171.9	198.89	—	215.9	238.1	239.2
Mackenrodt's ligament	183.8	198.82	233.39	221.8	236.3	239.5
malar region - *see* Neoplasm, cheek	170.0	198.5	—	213.0	238.0	239.2
mammary gland - *see* Neoplasm, breast						
mandible	170.1	198.5	—	213.1	238.0	239.2
alveolar						
mucosa	143.1	198.89	230.0	210.4	235.1	239.0
ridge or process	170.1	198.5	—	213.1	238.0	239.2
carcinoma	143.1	—	—	—	—	—

SECTION I INDEX TO DISEASES AND INJURIES / Neoplasm, mandible

	Malignant			Benign	Uncertain Behavior	Unspecified
	Primary	Secondary	Ca in situ			
Neoplasm *(Continued)*						
mandible *(Continued)*						
carcinoma	143.1	—	—	—	—	—
marrow (bone) NEC	202.9●	198.5	—	—	—	238.79
mastectomy site (skin)	173.50	198.2	—	—	—	—
basal cell carcinoma	173.51	—	—	—	—	—
specified as breast tissue	174.8	198.81	—	—	—	—
specified type NEC	173.59	—	—	—	—	—
squamous cell carcinoma	173.52	—	—	—	—	—
mastoid (air cells) (antrum) (cavity)	160.1	197.3	231.8	212.0	235.9	239.1
bone or process	170.0	198.5	—	213.0	238.0	239.2
maxilla, maxillary (superior)	170.0	198.5	—	213.0	238.0	239.2
alveolar						
mucosa	143.0	198.89	230.0	210.4	235.1	239.0
ridge or process	170.0	198.5	—	213.0	238.0	239.2
carcinoma	143.0	—	—	—	—	—
antrum	160.2	197.3	231.8	212.0	235.9	239.1
carcinoma	143.0	—	—	—	—	—
inferior - *see* Neoplasm, mandible						
sinus	160.2	197.3	231.8	212.0	235.9	239.1
meatus						
external (ear) (*see also* Neoplasm, skin, ear)	173.20	198.2	232.2	216.2	238.2	239.2
Meckel's diverticulum	152.3	197.4	230.7	211.2	235.2	239.0
mediastinum, mediastinal	164.9	197.1	—	212.5	235.8	239.89
anterior	164.2	197.1	—	212.5	235.8	239.89
contiguous sites with heart and thymus	164.8	—	—	—	—	—
posterior	164.3	197.1	—	212.5	235.8	239.89
medulla						
adrenal	194.0	198.7	234.8	227.0	237.2	239.7
oblongata	191.7	198.3	—	225.0	237.5	239.6
meibomian gland	173.10	198.2	232.1	216.1	238.2	239.2
basal cell carcinoma	173.11	—	—	—	—	—
specified type NEC	173.19	—	—	—	—	—
squamous cell carcinoma	173.12	—	—	—	—	—
melanoma - *see* Melanoma						
meninges (brain) (cerebral) (cranial) (intracranial)	192.1	198.4	—	225.2	237.6	239.7
spinal (cord)	192.3	198.4	—	225.4	237.6	239.7
meniscus, knee joint (lateral) (medial)	170.7	198.5	—	213.7	238.0	239.2
mesentery, mesenteric	158.8	197.6	—	211.8	235.4	239.0
mesoappendix	158.8	197.6	—	211.8	235.4	239.0
mesocolon	158.8	197.6	—	211.8	235.4	239.0
mesopharynx - *see* Neoplasm, oropharynx						

SECTION I INDEX TO DISEASES AND INJURIES / Neoplasm, nabothian gland

	Malignant			Benign	Uncertain Behavior	Unspecified
	Primary	Secondary	Ca in situ			
Neoplasm (Continued)						
mesosalpinx	183.3	198.82	233.39	221.0	236.3	239.5
mesovarium	183.3	198.82	233.39	221.0	236.3	239.5
metacarpus (any bone)	170.5	198.5	—	213.5	238.0	239.2
metastatic NEC - see also Neoplasm, by site, secondary	—	199.1	—	—	—	—
metatarsus (any bone)	170.8	198.5	—	213.8	238.0	239.2
midbrain	191.7	198.3	—	225.0	237.5	239.6
milk duct - see Neoplasm, breast						
mons						
pubis	184.4	198.82	233.32	221.2	236.3	239.5
veneris	184.4	198.82	233.32	221.2	236.3	239.5
motor tract	192.9	198.4	—	225.9	237.9	239.7
brain	191.9	198.3	—	225.0	237.5	239.6
spinal	192.2	198.3	—	225.3	237.5	239.7
mouth	145.9	198.89	230.0	210.4	235.1	239.0
contiguous sites	145.8	—	—	—	—	—
floor	144.9	198.89	230.0	210.3	235.1	239.0
anterior portion	144.0	198.89	230.0	210.3	235.1	239.0
contiguous sites	144.8	—	—	—	—	—
lateral portion	144.1	198.89	230.0	210.3	235.1	239.0
roof	145.5	198.89	230.0	210.4	235.1	239.0
specified part NEC	145.8	198.89	230.0	210.4	235.1	239.0
vestibule	145.1	198.89	230.0	210.4	235.1	239.0
mucosa						
alveolar (ridge or process)	143.9	198.89	230.0	210.4	235.1	239.0
lower	143.1	198.89	230.0	210.4	235.1	239.0
upper	143.0	198.89	230.0	210.4	235.1	239.0
buccal	145.0	198.89	230.0	210.4	235.1	239.0
cheek	145.0	198.89	230.0	210.4	235.1	239.0
lip - see Neoplasm, lip, internal						
nasal	160.0	197.3	231.8	212.0	235.9	239.1
oral	145.0	198.89	230.0	210.4	235.1	239.0
Müllerian duct						
female	184.8	198.82	233.39	221.8	236.3	239.5
male	187.8	198.82	233.6	222.8	236.6	239.5
multiple sites NEC	199.0	199.0	234.9	229.9	238.9	199.0
muscle - see also Neoplasm, connective tissue extraocular	190.1	198.4	234.0	224.1	238.8	239.89
myocardium	164.1	198.89	—	212.7	238.8	239.89
myometrium	182.0	198.82	233.2	219.1	236.0	239.5
myopericardium	164.1	198.89	—	212.7	238.8	239.89
nabothian gland (follicle)	180.0	198.82	233.1	219.0	236.0	239.5

 Revised

SECTION 1 INDEX TO DISEASES AND INJURIES / Neoplasm, nail

	Malignant			Benign	Uncertain Behavior	Unspecified
	Primary	Secondary	Ca in situ			
Neoplasm *(Continued)*						
nail	173.90	198.2	232.9	216.9	238.2	239.2
finger *(see also* Neoplasm, skin, limb, upper)	173.60	198.2	232.6	216.6	238.2	239.2
toe *(see also* Neoplasm, skin, limb, lower)	173.70	198.2	232.7	216.7	238.2	239.2
nares, naris (anterior) (posterior)	160.0	197.3	231.8	212.0	235.9	239.1
nasal - *see* Neoplasm, nose						
nasolabial groove *(see also* Neoplasm, skin, face)	173.30	198.2	232.3	216.3	238.2	239.2
nasolacrimal duct	190.7	198.4	234.0	224.7	238.8	239.89
nasopharynx, nasopharyngeal	147.9	198.89	230.0	210.7	235.1	239.0
contiguous sites	147.8	—	—	—	—	—
floor	147.3	198.89	230.0	210.7	235.1	239.0
roof	147.0	198.89	230.0	210.7	235.1	239.0
specified site NEC	147.8	198.89	230.0	210.7	235.1	239.0
wall	147.9	198.89	230.0	210.7	235.1	239.0
anterior	147.3	198.89	230.0	210.7	235.1	239.0
lateral	147.2	198.89	230.0	210.7	235.1	239.0
posterior	147.1	198.89	230.0	210.7	235.1	239.0
superior	147.0	198.89	230.0	210.7	235.1	239.0
nates *(see also* Neoplasm, skin, trunk)	173.50	198.2	232.5	216.5	238.2	239.2
neck NEC*	195.0	198.89	234.8	229.8	238.8	239.89
skin	173.40	198.2	232.4	216.4	238.2	239.2
basal cell carcinoma	173.41	—	—	—	—	—
specified type NEC	173.49	—	—	—	—	—
squamous cell carcinoma	173.42	—	—	—	—	—
nerve (autonomic) (ganglion) (parasympathetic) (peripheral) (sympathetic) - *see also* Neoplasm, connective tissue						
abducens	192.0	198.4	—	225.1	237.9	239.7
accessory (spinal)	192.0	198.4	—	225.1	237.9	239.7
acoustic	192.0	198.4	—	225.1	237.9	239.7
auditory	192.0	198.4	—	225.1	237.9	239.7
brachial	171.2	198.89	—	215.2	238.1	239.2
cranial (any)	192.0	198.4	—	225.1	237.9	239.7
facial	192.0	198.4	—	225.1	237.9	239.7
femoral	171.3	198.89	—	215.3	238.1	239.2
glossopharyngeal	192.0	198.4	—	225.1	237.9	239.7
hypoglossal	192.0	198.4	—	225.1	237.9	239.7
intercostal	171.4	198.89	—	215.4	238.1	239.2
lumbar	171.7	198.89	—	215.7	238.1	239.2
median	171.2	198.89	—	215.2	238.1	239.2
obturator	171.3	198.89	—	215.3	238.1	239.2
oculomotor	192.0	198.4	—	225.1	237.9	239.7
olfactory	192.0	198.4	—	225.1	237.9	239.7

◀ New ⬅ Revised ~~deleted~~ Deleted ● Use Additional Digit(s) ▨ Omit code

SECTION I INDEX TO DISEASES AND INJURIES / Neoplasm, nostril

	Malignant			Benign	Uncertain Behavior	Unspecified
	Primary	Secondary	Ca in situ			
Neoplasm (Continued)						
nerve (Continued)						
optic	192.0	198.4	—	225.1	237.9	239.7
peripheral NEC	171.9	198.89	—	215.9	238.1	239.2
radial	171.2	198.89	—	215.2	238.1	239.2
sacral	171.6	198.89	—	215.6	238.1	239.2
sciatic	171.3	198.89	—	215.3	238.1	239.2
spinal NEC	171.9	198.89	—	215.9	238.1	239.2
trigeminal	192.0	198.4	—	225.1	237.9	239.7
trochlear	192.0	198.4	—	225.1	237.9	239.7
ulnar	171.2	198.89	—	215.2	238.1	239.2
vagus	192.0	198.4	—	225.1	237.9	239.7
nervous system (central) NEC	192.9	198.4	—	225.9	237.9	239.7
autonomic NEC	171.9	198.89	—	215.9	238.1	239.2
brain - see also Neoplasm, brain membrane or meninges	192.1	198.4	—	225.2	237.6	239.7
contiguous sites	192.8	—	—	—	—	—
parasympathetic NEC	171.9	198.89	—	215.9	238.1	239.2
sympathetic NEC	171.9	198.89	—	215.9	238.1	239.2
nipple (female)	174.0	198.81	233.0	217	238.3	239.3
male	175.0	198.81	233.0	217	238.3	239.3
nose, nasal	195.0	198.89	234.8	229.8	238.8	239.89
ala (external) (see also Neoplasm, nose, skin)	173.30	198.2	232.3	216.3	238.2	239.2
bone	170.0	198.5	—	213.0	238.0	239.2
cartilage	160.0	197.3	231.8	212.0	235.9	239.1
cavity	160.0	197.3	231.8	212.0	235.9	239.1
contiguous sites with accessory sinuses or middle ear	160.8	—	—	—	—	—
choana	147.3	198.89	230.0	210.7	235.1	239.0
external (skin) (see also Neoplasm, nose, skin)	173.30	198.2	232.3	216.3	238.2	239.2
fossa	160.0	197.3	231.8	212.0	235.9	239.1
internal	160.0	197.3	231.8	212.0	235.9	239.1
mucosa	160.0	197.3	231.8	212.0	235.9	239.1
septum	160.0	197.3	231.8	212.0	235.9	239.1
posterior margin	147.3	198.89	230.0	210.7	235.1	239.0
sinus - see Neoplasm, sinus						
skin	173.30	198.2	232.3	216.3	238.2	239.2
basal cell carcinoma	173.31	—	—	—	—	—
specified type NEC	173.39	—	—	—	—	—
squamous cell carcinoma	173.32	—	—	—	—	—
turbinate (mucosa)	160.0	197.3	231.8	212.0	235.9	239.1
bone	170.0	198.5	—	213.0	238.0	239.2
vestibule	160.0	197.3	231.8	212.0	235.9	239.1
nostril	160.0	197.3	231.8	212.0	235.9	239.1

SECTION I INDEX TO DISEASES AND INJURIES / Neoplasm, nucleus pulposus

	Malignant			Benign	Uncertain Behavior	Unspecified
	Primary	Secondary	Ca in situ			
Neoplasm (Continued)						
nucleus pulposus	170.2	198.5	—	213.2	238.0	230.2
occipital						
bone	170.0	198.5	—	213.0	238.0	239.2
lobe or pole, brain	191.4	198.3	—	225.0	237.5	239.6
odontogenic - see Neoplasm, jaw bone						
oesophagus - see Neoplasm, esophagus						
olfactory nerve or bulb	192.0	198.4	—	225.1	237.9	239.7
olive (brain)	191.7	198.3	—	225.0	237.5	239.6
omentum	158.8	197.6	—	211.8	235.4	239.0
operculum (brain)	191.0	198.3	—	225.0	237.5	239.6
optic nerve, chiasm, or tract	192.0	198.4	—	225.1	237.9	239.7
oral (cavity)	145.9	198.89	230.0	210.4	235.1	239.0
contiguous sites with lip or pharynx	149.8	—	—	—	—	—
ill-defined	149.9	198.89	230.0	210.4	235.1	239.0
mucosa	145.9	198.89	230.0	210.4	235.1	239.0
orbit	190.1	198.4	234.0	224.1	238.8	239.89
bone	170.0	198.5	—	213.0	238.0	239.2
eye	190.1	198.4	234.0	224.1	238.8	239.89
soft parts	190.1	198.4	234.0	224.1	238.8	239.89
organ of Zuckerkandl	194.6	198.89	—	227.6	237.3	239.7
oropharynx	146.9	198.89	230.0	210.6	235.1	239.0
branchial cleft (vestige)	146.8	198.89	230.0	210.6	235.1	239.0
contiguous sites	146.8	—	—	—	—	—
junctional region	146.5	198.89	230.0	210.6	235.1	239.0
lateral wall	146.6	198.89	230.0	210.6	235.1	239.0
pillars of fauces	146.2	198.89	230.0	210.6	235.1	239.0
posterior wall	146.7	198.89	230.0	210.6	235.1	239.0
specified part NEC	146.8	198.89	230.0	210.6	235.1	239.0
vallecula	146.3	198.89	230.0	210.6	235.1	239.0
os						
external	180.1	198.82	233.1	219.0	236.0	239.5
internal	180.0	198.82	233.1	219.0	236.0	239.5
ovary	183.0	198.6	233.39	220	236.2	239.5
oviduct	183.2	198.82	233.39	221.0	236.3	239.5
palate	145.5	198.89	230.0	210.4	235.1	239.0
hard	145.2	198.89	230.0	210.4	235.1	239.0
junction of hard and soft palate	145.5	198.89	230.0	210.4	235.1	239.0
soft	145.3	198.89	230.0	210.4	235.1	239.0
nasopharyngeal surface	147.3	198.89	230.0	210.7	235.1	239.0
posterior surface	147.3	198.89	230.0	210.7	235.1	239.0
superior surface	147.3	198.89	230.0	210.7	235.1	239.0

SECTION I INDEX TO DISEASES AND INJURIES / Neoplasm, pelvis, pelvic

	Malignant			Benign	Uncertain Behavior	Unspecified
	Primary	Secondary	Ca in situ			
Neoplasm (Continued)						
palatoglossal arch	146.2	198.89	230.0	210.6	235.1	239.0
palatopharyngeal arch	146.2	198.89	230.0	210.6	235.1	239.0
pallium	191.0	198.3	—	225.0	237.5	239.6
palpebra	173.10	198.2	232.1	216.1	238.2	239.2
basal cell carcinoma	173.11	—	—	—	—	—
specified type NEC	173.19	—	—	—	—	—
squamous cell carcinoma	173.12	—	—	—	—	—
pancreas	157.9	197.8	230.9	211.6	235.5	239.0
body	157.1	197.8	230.9	211.6	235.5	239.0
contiguous sites	157.8	—	—	—	—	—
duct (of Santorini) (of Wirsung)	157.3	197.8	230.9	211.6	235.5	239.0
ectopic tissue	157.8	197.8				
head	157.0	197.8	230.9	211.6	235.5	239.0
islet cells	157.4	197.8	230.9	211.7	235.5	239.0
neck	157.8	197.8	230.9	211.6	235.5	239.0
tail	157.2	197.8	230.9	211.6	235.5	239.0
para-aortic body	194.6	198.89	—	227.6	237.3	239.7
paraganglion NEC	194.6	198.89	—	227.6	237.3	239.7
parametrium	183.4	198.82	—	221.0	236.3	239.5
paranephric	158.0	197.6	—	211.8	235.4	239.0
pararectal	195.3	198.89	—	229.8	238.8	239.89
parasagittal (region)	195.0	198.89	234.8	229.8	238.8	239.89
parasellar	192.9	198.4	—	225.9	237.9	239.7
parathyroid (gland)	194.1	198.89	234.8	227.1	237.4	239.7
paraurethral	195.3	198.89	—	229.8	238.8	239.89
gland	189.4	198.1	233.9	223.89	236.99	239.5
paravaginal	195.3	198.89	—	229.8	238.8	239.89
parenchyma, kidney	189.0	198.0	233.9	223.0	236.91	239.5
parietal						
bone	170.0	198.5	—	213.0	238.0	239.2
lobe, brain	191.3	198.3	—	225.0	237.5	239.6
paroophoron	183.3	198.82	233.39	221.0	236.3	239.5
parotid (duct) (gland)	142.0	198.89	230.0	210.2	235.0	239.0
parovarium	183.3	198.82	233.39	221.0	236.3	239.5
patella	170.8	198.5	—	213.8	238.0	239.2
peduncle, cerebral	191.7	198.3	—	225.0	237.5	239.6
pelvirectal junction	154.0	197.5	230.4	211.4	235.2	239.0
pelvis, pelvic	195.3	198.89	234.8	229.8	238.8	239.89
bone	170.6	198.5	—	213.6	238.0	239.2
floor	195.3	198.89	234.8	229.8	238.8	239.89
renal	189.1	198.0	233.9	223.1	236.91	239.5

SECTION I INDEX TO DISEASES AND INJURIES / Neoplasm, pelvis, pelvic

	Malignant			Benign	Uncertain Behavior	Unspecified
	Primary	Secondary	Ca in situ			
Neoplasm *(Continued)*						
pelvis, pelvic *(Continued)*						
viscera	195.3	198.89	234.8	229.8	238.8	239.89
wall	195.3	198.89	234.8	229.8	238.8	239.89
pelvo-abdominal	195.8	198.89	234.8	229.8	238.8	239.89
penis	187.4	198.82	233.5	222.1	236.6	239.5
body	187.3	198.82	233.5	222.1	236.6	239.5
corpus (cavernosum)	187.3	198.82	233.5	222.1	236.6	239.5
glans	187.2	198.82	233.5	222.1	236.6	239.5
skin NEC	187.4	198.82	233.5	222.1	236.6	239.5
periadrenal (tissue)	158.0	197.6	—	211.8	235.4	239.0
perianal (skin) (*see also* Neoplasm, skin, anus)	173.50	198.2	232.5	216.5	238.2	239.2
pericardium	164.1	198.89	—	212.7	238.8	239.89
perinephric	158.0	197.6	—	211.8	235.4	239.0
perineum	195.3	198.89	234.8	229.8	238.8	239.89
periodontal tissue NEC	143.9	198.89	230.0	210.4	235.1	239.0
periosteum - *see* Neoplasm, bone						
peripancreatic	158.0	197.6	—	211.8	235.4	239.0
peripheral nerve NEC	171.9	198.89	—	215.9	238.1	239.2
perirectal (tissue)	195.3	198.89	—	229.8	238.8	239.89
perirenal (tissue)	158.0	197.6	—	211.8	235.4	239.0
peritoneum, peritoneal (cavity)	158.9	197.6	—	211.8	235.4	239.0
contiguous sites	158.8	—	—	—	—	—
with digestive organs	159.8	—	—	—	—	—
parietal	158.8	197.6	—	211.8	235.4	239.0
pelvic	158.8	197.6	—	211.8	235.4	239.0
specified part NEC	158.8	197.6	—	211.8	235.4	239.0
peritonsillar (tissue)	195.0	198.89	234.8	229.8	238.8	239.89
periurethral tissue	195.3	198.89	—	229.8	238.8	239.89
phalanges	170.9	198.5	—	213.9	238.0	239.2
foot	170.8	198.5	—	213.8	238.0	239.2
hand	170.5	198.5	—	213.5	238.0	239.2
pharynx, pharyngeal	149.0	198.89	230.0	210.9	235.1	239.0
bursa	147.1	198.89	230.0	210.7	235.1	239.0
fornix	147.3	198.89	230.0	210.7	235.1	239.0
recess	147.2	198.89	230.0	210.7	235.1	239.0
region	149.0	198.89	230.0	210.9	235.1	239.0
tonsil	147.1	198.89	230.0	210.7	235.1	239.0
wall (lateral) (posterior)	149.0	198.89	230.0	210.9	235.1	239.0
pia mater (cerebral) (cranial)	192.1	198.4	—	225.2	237.6	239.7
spinal	192.3	198.4	—	225.4	237.6	239.7

SECTION I INDEX TO DISEASES AND INJURIES / Neoplasm, pylorus

	Malignant			Benign	Uncertain Behavior	Unspecified
	Primary	Secondary	Ca in situ			
Neoplasm *(Continued)*						
pillars of fauces	146.2	198.89	230.0	210.6	235.1	239.0
pineal (body) (gland)	194.4	198.89	234.8	227.4	237.1	239.7
pinna (ear) NEC (*see also* Neoplasm, skin, ear)	173.20	198.2	232.2	216.2	238.2	239.2
cartilage	171.0	198.89	—	215.0	238.1	239.2
piriform fossa or sinus	148.1	198.89	230.0	210.8	235.1	239.0
pituitary (body) (fossa) (gland) (lobe)	194.3	198.89	234.8	227.3	237.0	239.7
placenta	181	198.82	233.2	219.8	236.1	239.5
pleura, pleural (cavity)	163.9	197.2	—	212.4	235.8	239.1
contiguous sites	163.8	—	—	—	—	—
parietal	163.0	197.2	—	212.4	235.8	239.1
visceral	163.1	197.2	—	212.4	235.8	239.1
plexus						
brachial	171.2	198.89	—	215.2	238.1	239.2
cervical	171.0	198.89	—	215.0	238.1	239.2
choroid	191.5	198.3	—	225.0	237.5	239.6
lumbosacral	171.6	198.89	—	215.6	238.1	239.2
sacral	171.6	198.89	—	215.6	238.1	239.2
pluri-endocrine	194.8	198.89	234.8	227.8	237.4	239.7
pole						
frontal	191.1	198.3	—	225.0	237.5	239.6
occipital	191.4	198.3	—	225.0	237.5	239.6
pons (varolii)	191.7	198.3	—	225.0	237.5	239.6
popliteal fossa or space*	195.5	198.89	234.8	229.8	238.8	239.89
postcricoid (region)	148.0	198.89	230.0	210.8	235.1	239.0
posterior fossa (cranial)	191.9	198.3	—	225.0	237.5	239.6
postnasal space	147.9	198.89	230.0	210.7	235.1	239.0
prepuce	187.1	198.82	233.5	222.1	236.6	239.5
prepylorus	151.1	197.8	230.2	211.1	235.2	239.0
presacral (region)	195.3	198.89	—	229.8	238.8	239.89
prostate (gland)	185	198.82	233.4	222.2	236.5	239.5
utricle	189.3	198.1	233.9	223.81	236.99	239.5
pterygoid fossa	171.0	198.89	—	215.0	238.1	239.2
pubic bone	170.6	198.5	—	213.6	238.0	239.2
pudenda, pudendum (female)	184.4	198.82	233.32	221.2	236.3	239.5
pulmonary	162.9	197.0	231.2	212.3	235.7	239.1
putamen	191.0	198.3	—	225.0	237.5	239.6
pyloric						
antrum	151.2	197.8	230.2	211.1	235.2	239.0
canal	151.1	197.8	230.2	211.1	235.2	239.0
pylorus	151.1	197.8	230.2	211.1	235.2	239.0

   New   Revised   deleted Deleted   ● Use Additional Digit(s)   Omit code

SECTION 1 INDEX TO DISEASES AND INJURIES / Neoplasm, pyramid

	Malignant			Benign	Uncertain Behavior	Unspecified
	Primary	Secondary	Ca in situ			
Neoplasm (Continued)						
pyramid (brain)	191.7	198.3	—	225.0	237.5	239.6
pyriform fossa or sinus	148.1	198.89	230.0	210.8	235.1	239.0
radius (any part)	170.4	198.5	—	213.4	238.0	239.2
Rathke's pouch	194.3	198.89	234.8	227.3	237.0	239.7
rectosigmoid (colon) (junction)	154.0	197.5	230.4	211.4	235.2	239.0
contiguous sites with anus or rectum	154.8	—	—	—	—	—
rectouterine pouch	158.8	197.6	—	211.8	235.4	239.0
rectovaginal septum or wall	195.3	198.89	234.8	229.8	238.8	239.89
rectovesical septum	195.3	198.89	234.8	229.8	238.8	239.89
rectum (ampulla)	154.1	197.5	230.4	211.4	235.2	239.0
and colon	154.0	197.5	230.4	211.4	235.2	239.0
contiguous sites with anus or rectosigmoid junction	154.8	—	—	—	—	—
renal	189.0	198.0	233.9	223.0	236.91	239.5
calyx	189.1	198.0	233.9	223.1	236.91	239.5
hilus	189.1	198.0	233.9	223.1	236.91	239.5
parenchyma	189.0	198.0	233.9	223.0	236.91	239.5
pelvis	189.1	198.0	233.9	223.1	236.91	239.5
respiratory						
organs or system NEC	165.9	197.3	231.9	212.9	235.9	239.1
contiguous sites with intrathoracic organs	165.8	—	—	—	—	—
specified sites NEC	165.8	197.3	231.8	212.8	235.9	239.1
tract NEC	165.9	197.3	231.9	212.9	235.9	239.1
upper	165.0	197.3	231.9	212.9	235.9	239.1
retina	190.5	198.4	234.0	224.5	238.8	239.81
retrobulbar	190.1	198.4	—	224.1	238.8	239.89
retrocecal	158.0	197.6	—	211.8	235.4	239.0
retromolar (area) (triangle) (trigone)	145.6	198.89	230.0	210.4	235.1	239.0
retro-orbital	195.0	198.89	234.8	229.8	238.8	239.89
retroperitoneal (space) (tissue)	158.0	197.6	—	211.8	235.4	239.0
contiguous sites	158.8	—	—	—	—	—
retroperitoneum	158.0	197.6	—	211.8	235.4	239.0
contiguous sites	158.8	—	—	—	—	—
retropharyngeal	149.0	198.89	230.0	210.9	235.1	239.0
retrovesical (septum)	195.3	198.89	234.8	229.8	238.8	239.89
rhinencephalon	191.0	198.3	—	225.0	237.5	239.6
rib	170.3	198.5	—	213.3	238.0	239.2
Rosenmüller's fossa	147.2	198.89	230.0	210.7	235.1	239.0
round ligament	183.5	198.82	—	221.0	236.3	239.5
sacrococcyx, sacrococcygeal	170.6	198.5	—	213.6	238.0	239.2
region	195.3	198.89	234.8	229.8	238.8	239.89

SECTION I INDEX TO DISEASES AND INJURIES / Neoplasm, sinus

	Malignant			Benign	Uncertain Behavior	Unspecified
	Primary	Secondary	Ca in situ			
Neoplasm *(Continued)*						
sacrouterine ligament	183.4	198.82	—	221.0	236.3	239.5
sacrum, sacral (vertebra)	170.6	198.5	—	213.6	238.0	239.2
salivary gland or duct (major)	142.9	198.89	230.0	210.2	235.0	239.0
contiguous sites	142.8	—	—	—	—	—
minor NEC	145.9	198.89	230.0	210.4	235.1	239.0
parotid	142.0	198.89	230.0	210.2	235.0	239.0
pluriglandular	142.8	198.89	230.0	210.2	235.0	239.0
sublingual	142.2	198.89	230.0	210.2	235.0	239.0
submandibular	142.1	198.89	230.0	210.2	235.0	239.0
submaxillary	142.1	198.89	230.0	210.2	235.0	239.0
salpinx (uterine)	183.2	198.82	233.39	221.0	236.3	239.5
Santorini's duct	157.3	197.8	230.9	211.6	235.5	239.0
scalp	173.40	198.2	232.4	216.4	238.2	239.2
basal cell carcinoma	173.41	—	—	—	—	—
specified type NEC	173.49	—	—	—	—	—
squamous cell carcinoma	173.42	—	—	—	—	—
scapula (any part)	170.4	198.5	—	213.4	238.0	239.2
scapular region	195.1	198.89	234.8	229.8	238.8	239.89
scar NEC *(see also* Neoplasm, skin*)*	173.90	198.2	232.9	216.9	238.2	239.2
sciatic nerve	171.3	198.89	—	215.3	238.1	239.2
sclera	190.0	198.4	234.0	224.0	238.8	239.89
scrotum (skin)	187.7	198.82	233.6	222.4	236.6	239.5
sebaceous gland - *see* Neoplasm, skin						
sella turcica	194.3	198.89	234.8	227.3	237.0	239.7
bone	170.0	198.5	—	213.0	238.0	239.2
semilunar cartilage (knee)	170.7	198.5	—	213.7	238.0	239.2
seminal vesicle	187.8	198.82	233.6	222.8	236.6	239.5
septum						
nasal	160.0	197.3	231.8	212.0	235.9	239.1
posterior margin	147.3	198.89	230.0	210.7	235.1	239.0
rectovaginal	195.3	198.89	234.8	229.8	238.8	239.89
rectovesical	195.3	198.89	234.8	229.8	238.8	239.89
urethrovaginal	184.9	198.82	233.39	221.9	236.3	239.5
vesicovaginal	184.9	198.82	233.39	221.9	236.3	239.5
shoulder NEC*	195.4	198.89	232.6	229.8	238.8	239.89
sigmoid flexure (lower) (upper)	153.3	197.5	230.3	211.3	235.2	239.0
sinus (accessory)	160.9	197.3	231.8	212.0	235.9	239.1
bone (any)	170.0	198.5	—	213.0	238.0	239.2
contiguous sites with middle ear or nasal cavities	160.8	—	—	—	—	—
ethmoidal	160.3	197.3	231.8	212.0	235.9	239.1

SECTION 1 INDEX TO DISEASES AND INJURIES / Neoplasm, sinus

	Malignant			Benign	Uncertain Behavior	Unspecified
	Primary	Secondary	Ca in situ			
Neoplasm *(Continued)*						
sinus *(Continued)*						
frontal	160.4	197.3	231.8	212.0	235.9	239.1
maxillary	160.2	197.3	231.8	212.0	235.9	239.1
nasal, paranasal NEC	160.9	197.3	231.8	212.0	235.9	239.1
pyriform	148.1	198.89	230.0	210.8	235.1	239.0
sphenoidal	160.5	197.3	231.8	212.0	235.9	239.1
skeleton, skeletal NEC	170.9	198.5	—	213.9	238.0	239.2
Skene's gland	189.4	198.1	233.9	223.89	236.99	239.5
skin NOS	173.90	198.2	232.9	216.9	238.2	239.2
abdominal wall	173.50	198.2	232.5	216.5	238.2	239.2
basal cell carcinoma	173.51	—	—	—	—	—
specified type NEC	173.59	—	—	—	—	—
squamous cell carcinoma	173.52	—	—	—	—	—
ala nasi *(see also* Neoplasm, skin, face*)*	173.30	198.2	232.3	216.3	238.2	239.2
ankle *(see also* Neoplasm, skin, limb, lower*)*	173.70	198.2	232.7	216.7	238.2	239.2
antecubital space *(see also* Neoplasm, skin, limb, upper*)*	173.60	198.2	232.6	216.6	238.2	239.2
anus	173.50	198.2	232.5	216.5	238.2	239.2
basal cell carcinoma	173.51	—	—	—	—	—
specified type NEC	173.59	—	—	—	—	—
squamous cell carcinoma	173.52	—	—	—	—	—
arm *(see also* Neoplasm, skin, limb, upper*)*	173.60	198.2	232.6	216.6	238.2	239.2
auditory canal (external) *(see also* Neoplasm, skin, ear*)*	173.20	198.2	232.2	216.2	238.2	239.2
auricle (ear) *(see also* Neoplasm, skin, ear*)*	173.20	198.2	232.2	216.2	238.2	239.2
auricular canal (external) *(see also* Neoplasm, skin, ear*)*	173.20	198.2	232.2	216.2	238.2	239.2
axilla, axillary fold *(see also* Neoplasm, skin, trunk*)*	173.50	198.2	232.5	216.5	238.2	239.2
back	173.50	198.2	232.5	216.5	238.2	239.2
basal cell carcinoma	173.51	—	—	—	—	—
specified type NEC	173.59	—	—	—	—	—
squamous cell carcinoma	173.52	—	—	—	—	—
basal cell carcinoma, unspecified site	173.91	—	—	—	—	—
breast *(see also* Neoplasm, skin, trunk*)*	173.50	198.2	232.5	216.5	238.2	239.2
brow *(see also* Neoplasm, skin, face*)*	173.30	198.2	232.3	216.3	238.2	239.2
buttock *(see also* Neoplasm, skin, trunk*)*	173.50	198.2	232.5	216.5	238.2	239.2
calf *(see also* Neoplasm, skin, limb, lower*)*	173.70	198.2	232.7	216.7	238.2	239.2
canthus (eye) (inner) (outer)	173.10	198.2	232.1	216.1	238.2	239.2
basal cell carcinoma	173.11	—	—	—	—	—
specified type NEC	173.19	—	—	—	—	—
squamous cell carcinoma	173.12	—	—	—	—	—
cervical region *(see also* Neoplasm, skin, neck*)*	173.40	198.2	232.4	216.4	238.2	239.2
cheek (external) *(see also* Neoplasm, skin, face*)*	173.30	198.2	232.3	216.3	238.2	239.2
chest (wall) *(see also* Neoplasm, skin, trunk*)*	173.50	198.2	232.5	216.5	238.2	239.2

SECTION I INDEX TO DISEASES AND INJURIES / Neoplasm, skin NOS

	Malignant			Benign	Uncertain Behavior	Unspecified
	Primary	Secondary	Ca in situ			
Neoplasm *(Continued)*						
skin NOS *(Continued)*						
chin *(see also Neoplasm, skin, face)*	173.30	198.2	232.3	216.3	238.2	239.2
clavicular area *(see also Neoplasm, skin, trunk)*	173.50	198.2	232.5	216.5	238.2	239.2
clitoris	184.3	198.82	233.32	221.2	236.3	239.5
columnella *(see also Neoplasm, skin, face)*	173.30	198.2	232.3	216.3	238.2	239.2
concha *(see also Neoplasm, skin, ear)*	173.20	198.2	232.2	216.2	238.2	239.2
contiguous sites	173.80	—	—	—	—	—
basal cell carcinoma	173.81	—	—	—	—	—
specified type NEC	173.89	—	—	—	—	—
squamous cell carcinoma	173.82	—	—	—	—	—
ear (external)	173.20	198.2	232.2	216.2	238.2	239.2
basal cell carcinoma	173.21	—	—	—	—	—
specified type NEC	173.29	—	—	—	—	—
squamous cell carcinoma	173.22	—	—	—	—	—
elbow *(see also Neoplasm, skin, limb, upper)*	173.60	198.2	232.6	216.6	238.2	239.2
eyebrow *(see also Neoplasm, skin, face)*	173.30	198.2	232.3	216.3	238.2	239.2
eyelid	173.10	198.2	232.1	216.1	238.2	239.2
basal cell carcinoma	173.11	—	—	—	—	—
specified type NEC	173.19	—	—	—	—	—
squamous cell carcinoma	173.12	—	—	—	—	—
face NEC	173.30	198.2	232.3	216.3	238.2	239.2
basal cell carcinoma	173.31	—	—	—	—	—
specified type NEC	173.39	—	—	—	—	—
squamous cell carcinoma	173.32	—	—	—	—	—
female genital organs (external)	184.4	198.82	233.30	221.2	236.3	239.5
clitoris	184.3	198.82	233.32	221.2	236.3	239.5
labium NEC	184.4	198.82	233.32	221.2	236.3	239.5
majus	184.1	198.82	233.32	221.2	236.3	239.5
minus	184.2	198.82	233.32	221.2	236.3	239.5
pudendum	184.4	198.82	233.32	221.2	236.3	239.5
vulva	184.4	198.82	233.32	221.2	236.3	239.5
finger *(see also Neoplasm, skin, limb, upper)*	173.60	198.2	232.6	216.6	238.2	239.2
flank *(see also Neoplasm, skin, trunk)*	173.50	198.2	232.5	216.5	238.2	239.2
foot *(see also Neoplasm, skin, limb, lower)*	173.70	198.2	232.7	216.7	238.2	239.2
forearm *(see also Neoplasm, skin, limb, upper)*	173.60	198.2	232.6	216.6	238.2	239.2
forehead *(see also Neoplasm, skin, face)*	173.30	198.2	232.3	216.3	238.2	239.2
glabella *(see also Neoplasm, skin, face)*	173.30	198.2	232.3	216.3	238.2	239.2
gluteal region *(see also Neoplasm, skin, trunk)*	173.50	198.2	232.5	216.5	238.2	239.2
groin *(see also Neoplasm, skin, trunk)*	173.50	198.2	232.5	216.5	238.2	239.2
hand *(see also Neoplasm, skin, limb, upper)*	173.60	198.2	232.6	216.6	238.2	239.2
head NEC *(see also Neoplasm, skin, scalp)*	173.40	198.2	232.4	216.4	238.2	239.2

SECTION I INDEX TO DISEASES AND INJURIES / Neoplasm, skin NOS

	Malignant			Benign	Uncertain Behavior	Unspecified
	Primary	Secondary	Ca in situ			
Neoplasm *(Continued)*						
skin NOS *(Continued)*						
heel *(see also* Neoplasm, skin, limb, lower)	173.70	198.2	232.7	216.7	238.2	239.2
helix *(see also* Neoplasm, skin, ear)	173.20	198.2	232.2	216.2	238.2	239.2
hip	173.70	198.2	232.7	216.7	238.2	239.2
basal cell carcinoma	173.71	—	—	—	—	—
specified type NEC	173.79	—	—	—	—	—
squamous cell carcinoma	173.72	—	—	—	—	—
infraclavicular region *(see also* Neoplasm, skin, trunk)	173.50	198.2	232.5	216.5	238.2	239.2
inguinal region *(see also* Neoplasm, skin, trunk)	173.50	198.2	232.5	216.5	238.2	239.2
jaw *(see also* Neoplasm, skin, face)	173.30	198.2	232.3	216.3	238.2	239.2
knee *(see also* Neoplasm, skin, limb, lower)	173.70	198.2	232.7	216.7	238.2	239.2
labia						
majora	184.1	198.82	233.32	221.2	236.3	239.5
minora	184.2	198.82	233.32	221.2	236.3	239.5
leg *(see also* Neoplasm, skin, limb, lower)	173.70	198.2	232.7	216.7	238.2	239.2
lid (lower) (upper)	173.10	198.2	232.1	216.1	238.2	239.2
basal cell carcinoma	173.11	—	—	—	—	—
specified type NEC	173.19	—	—	—	—	—
squamous cell carcinoma	173.12	—	—	—	—	—
limb NEC	173.90	198.2	232.9	216.9	238.2	239.5
lower	173.70	198.2	232.7	216.7	238.2	239.2
basal cell carcinoma	173.71	—	—	—	—	—
specified type NEC	173.79	—	—	—	—	—
squamous cell carcinoma	173.72	—	—	—	—	—
upper	173.60	198.2	232.6	216.6	238.2	239.2
basal cell carcinoma	173.61	—	—	—	—	—
specified type NEC	173.69	—	—	—	—	—
squamous cell carcinoma	173.62	—	—	—	—	—
lip (lower) (upper)	173.00	198.2	232.0	216.0	238.2	239.2
basal cell carcinoma	173.01	—	—	—	—	—
specified type NEC	173.09	—	—	—	—	—
squamous cell carcinoma	173.02	—	—	—	—	—
male genital organs	187.9	198.82	233.6	222.9	236.6	239.5
penis	187.4	198.82	233.5	222.1	236.6	239.5
prepuce	187.1	198.82	233.5	222.1	236.6	239.5
scrotum	187.7	198.82	233.6	222.4	236.6	239.5
mastectomy site *(see also* Neoplasm, skin, trunk)	173.50	198.2	—	—	—	—
specified as breast tissue	174.8	198.81	—	—	—	—
meatus, acoustic (external) *(see also* Neoplasm, skin, ear)	173.20	198.2	232.2	216.2	238.2	239.2
nates *(see also* Neoplasm, skin, trunk)	173.50	198.2	232.5	216.5	238.2	239.2

	Malignant			Benign	Uncertain Behavior	Unspecified
	Primary	Secondary	Ca in situ			
Neoplasm *(Continued)*						
skin NOS *(Continued)*						
neck	173.40	198.2	232.4	216.4	238.2	239.2
basal cell carcinoma	173.41	—	—	—	—	—
specified type NEC	173.49	—	—	—	—	—
squamous cell carcinoma	173.42	—	—	—	—	—
nose (external) (*see also* Neoplasm, skin, face)	173.30	198.2	232.3	216.3	238.2	239.2
palm (*see also* Neoplasm, skin, limb, upper)	173.60	198.2	232.6	216.6	238.2	239.2
palpebra	173.10	198.2	232.1	216.1	238.2	239.2
basal cell carcinoma	173.11	—	—	—	—	—
specified type NEC	173.19	—	—	—	—	—
squamous cell carcinoma	173.12	—	—	—	—	—
penis NEC	187.4	198.82	233.5	222.1	236.6	239.5
perianal (*see also* Neoplasm, skin, anus)	173.50	198.2	232.5	216.5	238.2	239.2
perineum (*see also* Neoplasm, skin, anus)	173.50	198.2	232.5	216.5	238.2	239.2
pinna (*see also* Neoplasm, skin, ear)	173.20	198.2	232.2	216.2	238.2	239.2
plantar (*see also* Neoplasm, skin, limb, lower)	173.70	198.2	232.7	216.7	238.2	239.2
popliteal fossa or space (*see also* Neoplasm, skin, limb, lower)	173.70	198.2	232.7	216.7	238.2	239.2
prepuce	187.1	198.82	233.5	222.1	236.6	239.5
pubes (*see also* Neoplasm, skin, trunk)	173.50	198.2	232.5	216.5	238.2	239.2
sacrococcygeal region (*see also* Neoplasm, skin, trunk)	173.50	198.2	232.5	216.5	238.2	239.2
scalp	173.40	198.2	232.4	216.4	238.2	239.2
basal cell carcinoma	173.41	—	—	—	—	—
specified type NEC	173.49	—	—	—	—	—
squamous cell carcinoma	173.42	—	—	—	—	—
scapular region (*see also* Neoplasm, skin, trunk)	173.50	198.2	232.5	216.5	238.2	239.2
scrotum	187.7	198.82	233.6	222.4	236.6	239.5
shoulder	173.60	198.2	232.6	216.6	238.2	239.2
basal cell carcinoma	173.61	—	—	—	—	—
specified type NEC	173.69	—	—	—	—	—
squamous cell carcinoma	173.62	—	—	—	—	—
sole (foot) (*see also* Neoplasm, skin, limb, lower)	173.70	198.2	232.7	216.7	238.2	239.2
specified sites NEC	173.80	198.2	232.8	216.8	232.8	239.2
basal cell carcinoma	173.81	—	—	—	—	—
specified type NEC	173.89	—	—	—	—	—
squamous cell carcinoma	173.82	—	—	—	—	—
specified type NEC, unspecified site	173.99	—	—	—	—	—
squamous cell carcinoma, unspecified site	173.92	—	—	—	—	—
submammary fold (*see also* Neoplasm, skin, trunk)	173.50	198.2	232.5	216.5	238.2	239.2
supraclavicular region (*see also* Neoplasm, skin, neck)	173.40	198.2	232.4	216.4	238.2	239.2
temple (*see also* Neoplasm, skin, face)	173.30	198.2	232.3	216.3	238.2	239.2
thigh (*see also* Neoplasm, skin, limb, lower)	173.70	198.2	232.7	216.7	238.2	239.2

SECTION I INDEX TO DISEASES AND INJURIES / Neoplasm, skin NOS

	Malignant			Benign	Uncertain Behavior	Unspecified
	Primary	Secondary	Ca in situ			
Neoplasm *(Continued)*						
skin NOS *(Continued)*						
thoracic wall *(see also* Neoplasm, skin, trunk*)*	173.50	198.2	232.5	216.5	238.2	239.2
thumb *(see also* Neoplasm, skin, limb, upper*)*	173.60	198.2	232.6	216.6	238.2	239.2
toe *(see also* Neoplasm, skin, limb, lower*)*	173.70	198.2	232.7	216.7	238.2	239.2
tragus *(see also* Neoplasm, skin, ear*)*	173.20	198.2	232.2	216.2	238.2	239.2
trunk	173.50	198.2	232.5	216.5	238.2	239.2
basal cell carcinoma	173.51	—	—	—	—	—
specified type NEC	173.59	—	—	—	—	—
squamous cell carcinoma	173.52	—	—	—	—	—
umbilicus *(see also* Neoplasm, skin, trunk*)*	173.50	198.2	232.5	216.5	238.2	239.2
vulva	184.4	198.82	233.32	221.2	236.3	239.5
wrist *(see also* Neoplasm, skin, limb, upper*)*	173.60	198.2	232.6	216.6	238.2	239.2
skull	170.0	198.5	—	213.0	238.0	239.2
soft parts or tissues - *see* Neoplasm, connective tissue						
specified site NEC	195.8	198.89	234.8	229.8	238.8	239.89
spermatic cord	187.6	198.82	233.6	222.8	236.6	239.5
sphenoid	160.5	197.3	231.8	212.0	235.9	239.1
bone	170.0	198.5	—	213.0	238.0	239.2
sinus	160.5	197.3	231.8	212.0	235.9	239.1
sphincter						
anal	154.2	197.5	230.5	211.4	235.5	239.0
of Oddi	156.1	197.8	230.8	211.5	235.3	239.0
spine, spinal (column)	170.2	198.5	—	213.2	238.0	239.2
bulb	191.7	198.3	—	225.0	237.5	239.6
coccyx	170.6	198.5	—	213.6	238.0	239.2
cord (cervical) (lumbar) (sacral) (thoracic)	192.2	198.3	—	225.3	237.5	239.7
dura mater	192.3	198.4	—	225.4	237.6	239.7
lumbosacral	170.2	198.5	—	213.2	238.0	239.2
membrane	192.3	198.4	—	225.4	237.6	239.7
meninges	192.3	198.4	—	225.4	237.6	239.7
nerve (root)	171.9	198.89	—	215.9	238.1	239.2
pia mater	192.3	198.4	—	225.4	237.6	239.7
root	171.9	198.89	—	215.9	238.1	239.2
sacrum	170.6	198.5	—	213.6	238.0	239.2
spleen, splenic NEC	159.1	197.8	230.9	211.9	235.5	239.0
flexure (colon)	153.7	197.5	230.3	211.3	235.2	239.0
stem, brain	191.7	198.3	—	225.0	237.5	239.6
Stensen's duct	142.0	198.89	230.0	210.2	235.0	239.0
sternum	170.3	198.5	—	213.3	238.0	239.2

	Malignant			Benign	Uncertain Behavior	Unspecified
	Primary	Secondary	Ca in situ			
Neoplasm *(Continued)*						
stomach	151.9	197.8	230.2	211.1	235.2	239.0
antrum (pyloric)	151.2	197.8	230.2	211.1	235.2	239.0
body	151.4	197.8	230.2	211.1	235.2	239.0
cardia	151.0	197.8	230.2	211.1	235.2	239.0
cardiac orifice	151.0	197.8	230.2	211.1	235.2	239.0
contiguous sites	151.8	—	—	—	—	—
corpus	151.4	197.8	230.2	211.1	235.2	239.0
fundus	151.3	197.8	230.2	211.1	235.2	239.0
greater curvature NEC	151.6	197.8	230.2	211.1	235.2	239.0
lesser curvature NEC	151.5	197.8	230.2	211.1	235.2	239.0
prepylorus	151.1	197.8	230.2	211.1	235.2	239.0
pylorus	151.1	197.8	230.2	211.1	235.2	239.0
wall NEC	151.9	197.8	230.2	211.1	235.2	239.0
anterior NEC	151.8	197.8	230.2	211.1	235.2	239.0
posterior NEC	151.8	197.8	230.2	211.1	235.2	239.0
stroma, endometrial	182.0	198.82	233.2	219.1	236.0	239.5
stump, cervical	180.8	198.82	233.1	219.0	236.0	239.5
subcutaneous (nodule) (tissue) NEC - *see* Neoplasm, connective tissue						
subdural	192.1	198.4	—	225.2	237.6	239.7
subglottis, subglottic	161.2	197.3	231.0	212.1	235.6	239.1
sublingual	144.9	198.89	230.0	210.3	235.1	239.0
gland or duct	142.2	198.89	230.0	210.2	235.0	239.0
submandibular gland	142.1	198.89	230.0	210.2	235.0	239.0
submaxillary gland or duct	142.1	198.89	230.0	210.2	235.0	239.0
submental	195.0	198.89	234.8	229.8	238.8	239.89
subpleural	162.9	197.0	—	212.3	235.7	239.1
substernal	164.2	197.1	—	212.5	235.8	239.89
sudoriferous, sudoriparous gland, site unspecified	173.90	198.2	232.9	216.9	238.2	239.2
specified site - *see* Neoplasm, skin						
supraclavicular region	195.0	198.89	234.8	229.8	238.8	239.89
supraglottis	161.1	197.3	231.0	212.1	235.6	239.1
suprarenal (capsule) (cortex) (gland) (medulla)	194.0	198.7	234.8	227.0	237.2	239.7
suprasellar (region)	191.9	198.3	—	225.0	237.5	239.6
sweat gland (apocrine) (eccrine), site unspecified	173.90	198.2	232.9	216.9	238.2	239.2
specified site - *see* Neoplasm, skin						
sympathetic nerve or nervous system NEC	171.9	198.89	—	215.9	238.1	239.2
symphysis pubis	170.6	198.5	—	213.6	238.0	239.2
synovial membrane - *see* Neoplasm, connective tissue						
tapetum, brain	191.8	198.3	—	225.0	237.5	239.6
tarsus (any bone)	170.8	198.5	—	213.8	238.0	239.2
temple (skin) (*see also* Neoplasm, skin, face)	173.30	198.2	232.3	216.3	238.2	239.2

SECTION 1 INDEX TO DISEASES AND INJURIES / Neoplasm, temporal

	Malignant			Benign	Uncertain Behavior	Unspecified
	Primary	Secondary	Ca in situ			
Neoplasm (Continued)						
temporal						
bone	170.0	198.5	—	213.0	238.0	239.2
lobe or pole	191.2	198.3	—	225.0	237.5	239.6
region	195.0	198.89	234.8	229.8	238.8	239.89
skin (see also Neoplasm, skin, face)	173.30	198.2	232.3	216.3	238.2	239.2
tendon (sheath) - see Neoplasm, connective tissue						
tentorium (cerebelli)	192.1	198.4	—	225.2	237.6	239.7
testis, testes (descended) (scrotal)	186.9	198.82	233.6	222.0	236.4	239.5
ectopic	186.0	198.82	233.6	222.0	236.4	239.5
retained	186.0	198.82	233.6	222.0	236.4	239.5
undescended	186.0	198.82	233.6	222.0	236.4	239.5
thalamus	191.0	198.3	—	225.0	237.5	239.6
thigh NEC*	195.5	198.89	234.8	229.8	238.8	239.89
thorax, thoracic (cavity) (organs NEC)	195.1	198.89	234.8	229.8	238.8	239.89
duct	171.4	198.89	—	215.4	238.1	239.2
wall NEC	195.1	198.89	234.8	229.8	238.8	239.89
throat	149.0	198.89	230.0	210.9	235.1	239.0
thumb NEC*	195.4	198.89	232.6	229.8	238.8	239.89
thymus (gland)	164.0	198.89	—	212.6	235.8	239.89
contiguous sites with heart and mediastinum	164.8	—	—	—	—	—
thyroglossal duct	193	198.89	234.8	226	237.4	239.7
thyroid (gland)	193	198.89	234.8	226	237.4	239.7
cartilage	161.3	197.3	231.0	212.1	235.6	239.1
tibia (any part)	170.7	198.5	—	213.7	238.0	239.2
toe NEC*	195.5	198.89	232.7	229.8	238.8	239.89
tongue	141.9	198.89	230.0	210.1	235.1	239.0
anterior (two-thirds) NEC	141.4	198.89	230.0	210.1	235.1	239.0
dorsal surface	141.1	198.89	230.0	210.1	235.1	239.0
ventral surface	141.3	198.89	230.0	210.1	235.1	239.0
base (dorsal surface)	141.0	198.89	230.0	210.1	235.1	239.0
border (lateral)	141.2	198.89	230.0	210.1	235.1	239.0
contiguous sites	141.8	—	—	—	—	—
dorsal surface NEC	141.1	198.89	230.0	210.1	235.1	239.0
fixed part NEC	141.0	198.89	230.0	210.1	235.1	239.0
foramen cecum	141.1	198.89	230.0	210.1	235.1	239.0
frenulum linguae	141.3	198.89	230.0	210.1	235.1	239.0
junctional zone	141.5	198.89	230.0	210.1	235.1	239.0
margin (lateral)	141.2	198.89	230.0	210.1	235.1	239.0
midline NEC	141.1	198.89	230.0	210.1	235.1	239.0
mobile part NEC	141.4	198.89	230.0	210.1	235.1	239.0
posterior (third)	141.0	198.89	230.0	210.1	235.1	239.0

SECTION I INDEX TO DISEASES AND INJURIES / Neoplasm, urinary organ or system NEC

	Malignant			Benign	Uncertain Behavior	Unspecified
	Primary	Secondary	Ca in situ			
Neoplasm (Continued)						
tongue (Continued)						
root	141.0	198.89	230.0	210.1	235.1	239.0
surface (dorsal)	141.1	198.89	230.0	210.1	235.1	239.0
base	141.0	198.89	230.0	210.1	235.1	239.0
ventral	141.3	198.89	230.0	210.1	235.1	239.0
tip	141.2	198.89	230.0	210.1	235.1	239.0
tonsil	141.6	198.89	230.0	210.1	235.1	239.0
tonsil	146.0	198.89	230.0	210.5	235.1	239.0
fauces, faucial	146.0	198.89	230.0	210.5	235.1	239.0
lingual	141.6	198.89	230.0	210.1	235.1	239.0
palatine	146.0	198.89	230.0	210.5	235.1	239.0
pharyngeal	147.1	198.89	230.0	210.7	235.1	239.0
pillar (anterior) (posterior)	146.2	198.89	230.0	210.6	235.1	239.0
tonsillar fossa	146.1	198.89	230.0	210.6	235.1	239.0
tooth socket NEC	143.9	198.89	230.0	210.4	235.1	239.0
trachea (cartilage) (mucosa)	162.0	197.3	231.1	212.2	235.7	239.1
contiguous sites with bronchus or lung	162.8	—	—	—	—	—
tracheobronchial	162.8	197.3	231.1	212.2	235.7	239.1
contiguous sites with lung	162.8	—	—	—	—	—
tragus (see also Neoplasm, skin, ear)	173.20	198.2	232.2	216.2	238.2	239.2
trunk NEC*	195.8	198.89	232.5	229.8	238.8	239.89
tubo-ovarian	183.8	198.82	233.39	221.8	236.3	239.5
tunica vaginalis	187.8	198.82	233.6	222.8	236.6	239.5
turbinate (bone)	170.0	198.5	—	213.0	238.0	239.2
nasal	160.0	197.3	231.8	212.0	235.9	239.1
tympanic cavity	160.1	197.3	231.8	212.0	235.9	239.1
ulna (any part)	170.4	198.5	—	213.4	238.0	239.2
umbilicus, umbilical (see also Neoplasm, skin, trunk)	173.50	198.2	232.5	216.5	238.2	239.2
uncus, brain	191.2	198.3	—	225.0	237.5	239.6
unknown site or unspecified	199.1	199.1	234.9	229.9	238.9	239.9
urachus	188.7	198.1	233.7	223.3	236.7	239.4
ureter, ureteral	189.2	198.1	233.9	223.2	236.91	239.5
orifice (bladder)	188.6	198.1	233.7	223.3	236.7	239.4
ureter-bladder (junction)	188.6	198.1	233.7	223.3	236.7	239.4
urethra, urethral (gland)	189.3	198.1	233.9	223.81	236.99	239.5
orifice, internal	188.5	198.1	233.7	223.3	236.7	239.4
urethrovaginal (septum)	184.9	198.82	233.39	221.9	236.3	239.5
urinary organ or system NEC	189.9	198.1	233.9	223.9	236.99	239.5
bladder - see Neoplasm, bladder						
contiguous sites	189.8	—	—	—	—	—
specified sites NEC	189.8	198.1	233.9	223.89	236.99	239.5

SECTION 1 INDEX TO DISEASES AND INJURIES / Neoplasm, utero-ovarian

	Malignant			Benign	Uncertain Behavior	Unspecified
	Primary	Secondary	Ca in situ			
Neoplasm (Continued)						
utero-ovarian	183.8	198.82	233.39	221.8	236.3	239.5
ligament	183.3	198.82	—	221.0	236.3	239.5
uterosacral ligament	183.4	198.82	—	221.0	236.3	239.5
uterus, uteri, uterine	179	198.82	233.2	219.9	236.0	239.5
adnexa NEC	183.9	198.82	233.39	221.8	236.3	239.5
contiguous sites	183.8	—	—	—	—	—
body	182.0	198.82	233.2	219.1	236.0	239.5
contiguous sites	182.8	—	—	—	—	—
cervix	180.9	198.82	233.1	219.0	236.0	239.5
cornu	182.0	198.82	233.2	219.1	236.0	239.5
corpus	182.0	198.82	233.2	219.1	236.0	239.5
endocervix (canal) (gland)	180.0	198.82	233.1	219.0	236.0	239.5
endometrium	182.0	198.82	233.2	219.1	236.0	239.5
exocervix	180.1	198.82	233.1	219.0	236.0	239.5
external os	180.1	198.82	233.1	219.0	236.0	239.5
fundus	182.0	198.82	233.2	219.1	236.0	239.5
internal os	180.0	198.82	233.1	219.0	236.0	239.5
isthmus	182.1	198.82	233.2	219.1	236.0	239.5
ligament	183.4	198.82	—	221.0	236.3	239.5
broad	183.3	198.82	233.39	221.0	236.3	239.5
round	183.5	198.82	—	221.0	236.3	239.5
lower segment	182.1	198.82	233.2	219.1	236.0	239.5
myometrium	182.0	198.82	233.2	219.1	236.0	239.5
squamocolumnar junction	180.8	198.82	233.1	219.0	236.0	239.5
tube	183.2	198.82	233.39	221.0	236.3	239.5
utricle, prostatic	189.3	198.1	233.9	223.81	236.99	239.5
uveal tract	190.0	198.4	234.0	224.0	238.8	239.89
uvula	145.4	198.89	230.0	210.4	235.1	239.0
vagina, vaginal (fornix) (vault) (wall)	184.0	198.82	233.31	221.1	236.3	239.5
vaginovesical	184.9	198.82	233.39	221.9	236.3	239.5
septum	184.9	198.82	233.39	221.9	236.3	239.5
vallecula (epiglottis)	146.3	198.89	230.0	210.6	235.1	239.0
vascular - *see* Neoplasm, connective tissue						
vas deferens	187.6	198.82	233.6	222.8	236.6	239.5
Vater's ampulla	156.2	197.8	230.8	211.5	235.3	239.0
vein, venous - *see* Neoplasm, connective tissue						
vena cava (abdominal) (inferior)	171.5	198.89	—	215.5	238.1	239.2
superior	171.4	198.89	—	215.4	238.1	239.2
ventricle (cerebral) (floor) (fourth) (lateral) (third)	191.5	198.3	—	225.0	237.5	239.6
cardiac (left) (right)	164.1	198.89	—	212.7	238.8	239.89

◀ New ◀ Revised ~~deleted~~ Deleted ● Use Additional Digit(s) ▨ Omit code

	Malignant			Benign	Uncertain Behavior	Unspecified
	Primary	Secondary	Ca in situ			
Neoplasm *(Continued)*						
ventricular band of larynx	161.1	197.3	231.0	212.1	235.6	239.1
ventriculus - *see* Neoplasm, stomach						
vermillion border - *see* Neoplasm, lip						
vermis, cerebellum	191.6	198.3	—	225.0	237.5	239.6
vertebra (column)	170.2	198.5	—	213.2	238.0	239.2
coccyx	170.6	198.5	—	213.6	238.0	239.2
sacrum	170.6	198.5	—	213.6	238.0	239.2
vesical - *see* Neoplasm, bladder						
vesicle, seminal	187.8	198.82	233.6	222.8	236.6	239.5
vesicocervical tissue	184.9	198.82	233.39	221.9	236.3	239.5
vesicorectal	195.3	198.89	234.8	229.8	238.8	239.89
vesicovaginal	184.9	198.82	233.39	221.9	236.3	239.5
septum	184.9	198.82	233.39	221.9	236.3	239.5
vessel (blood) - *see* Neoplasm, connective tissue						
vestibular gland, greater	184.1	198.82	233.32	221.2	236.3	239.5
vestibule						
mouth	145.1	198.89	230.0	210.4	235.1	239.0
nose	160.0	197.3	231.8	212.0	235.9	239.1
Virchow's gland	—	196.0	—	229.0	238.8	239.89
viscera NEC	195.8	198.89	234.8	229.8	238.8	239.89
vocal cords (true)	161.0	197.3	231.0	212.1	235.6	239.1
false	161.1	197.3	231.0	212.1	235.6	239.1
vomer	170.0	198.5	—	213.0	238.0	239.2
vulva	184.4	198.82	233.32	221.2	236.3	239.5
vulvovaginal gland	184.4	198.82	233.32	221.2	236.3	239.5
Waldeyer's ring	149.1	198.89	230.0	210.9	235.1	239.0
Wharton's duct	142.1	198.89	230.0	210.2	235.0	239.0
white matter (central) (cerebral)	191.0	198.3	—	225.0	237.5	239.6
windpipe	162.0	197.3	231.1	212.2	235.7	239.1
Wirsung's duct	157.3	197.8	230.9	211.6	235.5	239.0
wolffian (body) (duct)						
female	184.8	198.82	233.39	221.8	236.3	239.5
male	187.8	198.82	233.6	222.8	236.6	239.5
womb - *see* Neoplasm, uterus						
wrist NEC*	195.4	198.89	232.6	229.8	238.8	239.89
xiphoid process	170.3	198.5	—	213.3	238.0	239.2
Zuckerkandl's organ	194.6	198.89	—	227.6	237.3	239.7

SECTION I INDEX TO DISEASES AND INJURIES / Neovascularization

Neovascularization
    choroid 362.16
    ciliary body 364.42
    cornea 370.60
        deep 370.63
        localized 370.61
    iris 364.42
    retina 362.16
    subretinal 362.16
Nephralgia 788.0
Nephritis, nephritic (albuminuric) (azotemic) (congenital) (degenerative) (diffuse) (disseminated) (epithelial) (familial) (focal) (granulomatous) (hemorrhagic) (infantile) (nonsuppurative, excretory) (uremic) 583.9
    with
        edema - see Nephrosis
        lesion of
            glomerulonephritis
                hypocomplementemic persistent 583.2
                      with nephrotic syndrome 581.2
                      chronic 582.2
                lobular 583.2
                    with nephrotic syndrome 581.2
                    chronic 582.2
                membranoproliferative 583.2
                    with nephrotic syndrome 581.2
                    chronic 582.2
                membranous 583.1
                    with nephrotic syndrome 581.1
                    chronic 582.1
                mesangiocapillary 583.2
                    with nephrotic syndrome 581.2
                    chronic 582.2
                mixed membranous and proliferative 583.2
                    with nephrotic syndrome 581.2
                    chronic 582.2
                proliferative (diffuse) 583.0
                    with nephrotic syndrome 581.0
                    acute 580.0
                    chronic 582.0
                rapidly progressive 583.4
                    acute 580.4
                    chronic 582.4
            interstitial nephritis (diffuse) (focal) 583.89
                with nephrotic syndrome 581.89
                acute 580.89
                chronic 582.89
            necrotizing glomerulitis 583.4
                acute 580.4
                chronic 582.4
            renal necrosis 583.9
                cortical 583.6
                medullary 583.7
            specified pathology NEC 583.89
                with nephrotic syndrome 581.89
                acute 580.89
                chronic 582.89
        necrosis, renal 583.9
            cortical 583.6
            medullary (papillary) 583.7
        nephrotic syndrome (see also Nephrosis) 581.9
        papillary necrosis 583.7
        specified pathology NEC 583.89
    acute 580.9
        extracapillary with epithelial crescents 580.4
        hypertensive (see also Hypertension, kidney) 403.90
        necrotizing 580.4
        poststreptococcal 580.0
        proliferative (diffuse) 580.0
        rapidly progressive 580.4
        specified pathology NEC 580.89
    amyloid 277.39 [583.81]
        chronic 277.39 [582.81]

Nephritis, nephritic (Continued)
    arteriolar (see also Hypertension, kidney) 403.90
    arteriosclerotic (see also Hypertension, kidney) 403.90
    ascending (see also Pyelitis) 590.80
    atrophic 582.9
    basement membrane NEC 583.89
        with pulmonary hemorrhage (Goodpasture's syndrome) 446.21 [583.81]
    calculous, calculus 592.0
    cardiac (see also Hypertension, kidney) 403.90
    cardiovascular (see also Hypertension, kidney) 403.90
    chronic 582.9
        arteriosclerotic (see also Hypertension, kidney) 403.90
        hypertensive (see also Hypertension, kidney) 403.90
    cirrhotic (see also Sclerosis, renal) 587
    complicating pregnancy, childbirth, or puerperium 646.2
        with hypertension 642.1
            affecting fetus or newborn 760.0
        affecting fetus or newborn 760.1
    croupous 580.9
    desquamative - see Nephrosis
    due to
        amyloidosis 277.39 [583.81]
            chronic 277.39 [582.81]
        arteriosclerosis (see also Hypertension, kidney) 403.90
        diabetes mellitus 250.4 [583.81]
            due to secondary diabetes 249.4 [583.81]
            with nephrotic syndrome 250.4 [581.81]
                due to secondary diabetes 249.4 [581.81]
        diphtheria 032.89 [580.81]
        gonococcal infection (acute) 098.19 [583.81]
            chronic or duration of 2 months or over 098.39 [583.81]
        gout 274.10
        infectious hepatitis 070.9 [580.81]
        mumps 072.79 [580.81]
        specified kidney pathology NEC 583.89
            acute 580.89
            chronic 582.89
        streptotrichosis 039.8 [583.81]
        subacute bacterial endocarditis 421.0 [580.81]
        systemic lupus erythematosus 710.0 [583.81]
            chronic 710.0 [582.81]
        typhoid fever 002.0 [580.81]
    endothelial 582.2
    end state (chronic) (terminal) NEC 585.6
    epimembranous 581.1
    exudative 583.89
        with nephrotic syndrome 581.89
        acute 580.89
        chronic 582.89
    gonococcal (acute) 098.19 [583.81]
        chronic or duration of 2 months or over 098.39 [583.81]
    gouty 274.10
    hereditary (Alport's syndrome) 759.89
    hydremic - see Nephrosis
    hypertensive (see also Hypertension, kidney) 403.90
    hypocomplementemic persistent 583.2
        with nephrotic syndrome 581.2
        chronic 582.2
    immune complex NEC 583.89
    infective (see also Pyelitis) 590.80

Nephritis, nephritic (Continued)
    interstitial (diffuse) (focal) 583.89
        with nephrotic syndrome 581.89
        acute 580.89
        chronic 582.89
    latent or quiescent - see Nephritis, chronic
    lead 984.9
        specified type of lead - see Table of Drugs and Chemicals
    lobular 583.2
        with nephrotic syndrome 581.2
        chronic 582.2
    lupus 710.0 [583.81]
        acute 710.0 [580.81]
        chronic 710.0 [582.81]
    membranoproliferative 583.2
        with nephrotic syndrome 581.2
        chronic 582.2
    membranous 583.1
        with nephrotic syndrome 581.1
        chronic 582.1
    mesangiocapillary 583.2
        with nephrotic syndrome 581.2
        chronic 582.2
    minimal change 581.3
    mixed membranous and proliferative 583.2
        with nephrotic syndrome 581.2
        chronic 582.2
    necrotic, necrotizing 583.4
        acute 580.4
        chronic 582.4
    nephrotic - see Nephrosis
    old - see Nephritis, chronic
    parenchymatous 581.89
    polycystic 753.12
        adult type (APKD) 753.13
        autosomal dominant 753.13
        autosomal recessive 753.14
        childhood type (CPKD) 753.14
        infantile type 753.14
    poststreptococcal 580.0
    pregnancy - see Nephritis, complicating pregnancy
    proliferative 583.0
        with nephrotic syndrome 581.0
        acute 580.0
        chronic 582.0
    purulent (see also Pyelitis) 590.80
    rapidly progressive 583.4
        acute 580.4
        chronic 582.4
    salt-losing or salt-wasting (see also Disease, renal) 593.9
    saturnine 584.9
        specified type of lead - see Table of Drugs and Chemicals
    septic (see also Pyelitis) 590.80
    specified pathology NEC 583.89
        acute 580.89
        chronic 582.89
    staphylococcal (see also Pyelitis) 590.80
    streptotrichosis 039.8 [583.81]
    subacute (see also Nephrosis) 581.9
    suppurative (see also Pyelitis) 590.80
    syphilitic (late) 095.4
        congenital 090.5 [583.81]
        early 091.69 [583.81]
    terminal (chronic) (end-stage) NEC 585.6
    toxic - see Nephritis, acute
    tubal, tubular - see Nephrosis, tubular
    tuberculous (see also Tuberculosis) 016.0 [583.81]
    type II (Ellis) - see Nephrosis
    vascular - see also Hypertension, kidney
    war 580.9
Nephroblastoma (M8960/3) 189.0
    epithelial (M8961/3) 189.0
    mesenchymal (M8962/3) 189.0
Nephrocalcinosis 275.49
Nephrocystitis, pustular (see also Pyelitis) 590.80

Nephrolithiasis (congenital) (pelvis) (recurrent) 592.0
  uric acid 274.11
Nephroma (M8960/3) 189.0
  mesoblastic (M8960/1) 236.9
Nephronephritis (*see also* Nephrosis) 581.9
Nephronopthisis 753.16
Nephropathy (*see also* Nephritis) 583.9
  with
      exudative nephritis 583.89
      interstitial nephritis (diffuse) (focal) 583.89
      medullary necrosis 583.7
      necrosis 583.9
          cortical 583.6
          medullary or papillary 583.7
      papillary necrosis 583.7
      specified lesion or cause NEC 583.89
  analgesic 583.89
      with medullary necrosis, acute 584.7
  arteriolar (*see also* Hypertension, kidney) 403.90
  arteriosclerotic (*see also* Hypertension, kidney) 403.90
  complicating pregnancy 646.2 ●
  diabetic 250.4 ● [583.81]
      due to secondary diabetes 249.4 ● [583.81]
  gouty 274.10
      specified type NEC 274.19
  hereditary amyloid 277.31
  hypercalcemic 588.89
  hypertensive (*see also* Hypertension, kidney) 403.90
  hypokalemic (vacuolar) 588.89
  IgA 583.9
  obstructive 593.89
      congenital 753.20
  phenacetin 584.7
  phosphate-losing 588.0
  potassium depletion 588.89
  proliferative (*see also* Nephritis, proliferative) 583.0
  protein-losing 588.89
  salt-losing or salt-wasting (*see also* Disease, renal) 593.9
  sickle-cell (*see also* Disease, sickle-cell) 282.60 [583.81]
  toxic 584.5
  vasomotor 584.5
  water-losing 588.89
Nephroptosis (*see also* Disease, renal) 593.0
  congenital (displaced) 753.3
Nephropyosis (*see also* Abscess, kidney) 590.2
Nephrorrhagia 593.81
Nephrosclerosis (arteriolar) (arteriosclerotic) (chronic) (hyaline) (*see also* Hypertension, kidney) 403.90
  gouty 274.10
  hyperplastic (arteriolar) (*see also* Hypertension, kidney) 403.90
  senile (*see also* Sclerosis, renal) 587
Nephrosis, nephrotic (Epstein's) (syndrome) 581.9
  with
      lesion of
          focal glomerulosclerosis 581.1
          glomerulonephritis
              endothelial 581.2
              hypocomplementemic persistent 581.2
              lobular 581.2
              membranoproliferative 581.2
              membranous 581.1
              mesangiocapillary 581.2
              minimal change 581.3
              mixed membranous and proliferative 581.2
              proliferative 581.0
          segmental hyalinosis 581.1
          specified pathology NEC 581.89
  acute - *see* Nephrosis, tubular

Nephrosis, nephrotic (*Continued*)
  anoxic - *see* Nephrosis, tubular
  arteriosclerotic (*see also* Hypertension, kidney) 403.90
  chemical - *see* Nephrosis, tubular
  cholemic 572.4
  complicating pregnancy, childbirth, or puerperium - *see* Nephritis, complicating pregnancy
  diabetic 250.4 ● [581.81]
      due to secondary diabetes 249.4 ● [581.81]
  Finnish type (congenital) 759.89
  hemoglobinuric - *see* Nephrosis, tubular
  in
      amyloidosis 277.39 [581.81]
      diabetes mellitus 250.4 ● [581.81]
          due to secondary diabetes 249.4 ● [581.81]
      epidemic hemorrhagic fever 078.6
      malaria 084.9 [581.81]
      polyarteritis 446.0 [581.81]
      systemic lupus erythematosus 710.0 [581.81]
  ischemic - *see* Nephrosis, tubular
  lipoid 581.3
  lower nephron - *see* Nephrosis, tubular
  lupoid 710.0 [581.81]
  lupus 710.0 [581.81]
  malarial 084.9 [581.81]
  minimal change 581.3
  necrotizing - *see* Nephrosis, tubular
  osmotic (sucrose) 588.89
  polyarteritic 446.0 [581.81]
  radiation 581.9
  specified lesion or cause NEC 581.89
  syphilitic 095.4
  toxic - *see* Nephrosis, tubular
  tubular (acute) 584.5
      due to a procedure 997.5
      radiation 581.9
Nephrosonephritis hemorrhagic (endemic) 078.6
Nephrostomy status V44.6
  with complication 997.5
Nerve - *see* condition
Nerves 799.21
Nervous (*see also* condition) 799.21
  breakdown 300.9
  heart 306.2
  stomach 306.4
  tension 799.21
Nervousness 799.21
Nesidioblastoma (M8150/0)
  pancreas 211.7
  specified site NEC - *see* Neoplasm, by site, benign
  unspecified site 211.7
Netherton's syndrome (ichthyosiform erythroderma) 757.1
Nettle rash 708.8
Nettleship's disease (urticaria pigmentosa) 757.33
Neumann's disease (pemphigus vegetans) 694.4
Neuralgia, neuralgic (acute) (*see also* Neuritis) 729.2
  accessory (nerve) 352.4
  acoustic (nerve) 388.5
  ankle 355.8
  anterior crural 355.8
  anus 787.99
  arm 723.4
  auditory (nerve) 388.5
  axilla 353.0
  bladder 788.1
  brachial 723.4
  brain - *see* Disorder, nerve, cranial
  broad ligament 625.9
  cerebral - *see* Disorder, nerve, cranial
  ciliary 339.00

Neuralgia, neuralgic (*Continued*)
  cranial nerve - *see also* Disorder, nerve, cranial
      fifth or trigeminal (*see also* Neuralgia, trigeminal) 350.1
  ear 388.71
      middle 352.1
  facial 351.8
  finger 354.9
  flank 355.8
  foot 355.8
  forearm 354.9
  Fothergill's (*see also* Neuralgia, trigeminal) 350.1
      postherpetic 053.12
  glossopharyngeal (nerve) 352.1
  groin 355.8
  hand 354.9
  heel 355.8
  Horton's 339.00
  Hunt's 053.11
  hypoglossal (nerve) 352.5
  iliac region 355.8
  infraorbital (*see also* Neuralgia, trigeminal) 350.1
  inguinal 355.8
  intercostal (nerve) 353.8
      postherpetic 053.19
  jaw 352.1
  kidney 788.0
  knee 355.8
  loin 355.8
  malarial (*see also* Malaria) 084.6
  mastoid 385.89
  maxilla 352.1
  median thenar 354.1
  metatarsal 355.6
  middle ear 352.1
  migrainous 339.00
  Morton's 355.6
  nerve, cranial - *see* Disorder, nerve, cranial
  nose 352.0
  occipital 723.8
  olfactory (nerve) 352.0
  ophthalmic 377.30
      postherpetic 053.19
  optic (nerve) 377.30
  penis 607.9
  perineum 355.8
  pleura 511.0
  postherpetic NEC 053.19
      geniculate ganglion 053.11
      ophthalmic 053.19
      trifacial 053.12
      trigeminal 053.12
  pubic region 355.8
  radial (nerve) 723.4
  rectum 787.99
  sacroiliac joint 724.3
  sciatic (nerve) 724.3
  scrotum 608.9
  seminal vesicle 608.9
  shoulder 354.9
  sluder's 337.09
  specified nerve NEC - *see* Disorder, nerve
  spermatic cord 608.9
  sphenopalatine (ganglion) 337.09
  subscapular (nerve) 723.4
  suprascapular (nerve) 723.4
  testis 608.89
  thenar (median) 354.1
  thigh 355.8
  tongue 352.5
  trifacial (nerve) (*see also* Neuralgia, trigeminal) 350.1
  trigeminal (nerve) 350.1
      postherpetic 053.12
  tympanic plexus 388.71
  ulnar (nerve) 723.4
  vagus (nerve) 352.3

SECTION I INDEX TO DISEASES AND INJURIES / Neuralgia, neuralgic

Neuralgia, neuralgic (Continued)
- wrist 354.9
- writers' 300.89
  - organic 333.84

Neurapraxia - see Injury, nerve, by site

Neurasthenia 300.5
- cardiac 306.2
- gastric 306.4
- heart 306.2
- postfebrile 780.79
- postviral 780.79

Neurilemmoma (M9560/0) - see also Neoplasm, connective tissue, benign
- acoustic (nerve) 225.1
- malignant (M9560/3) - see also Neoplasm, connective tissue, malignant
  - acoustic (nerve) 192.0

Neurilemmosarcoma (M9560/3) - see Neoplasm, connective tissue, malignant

Neurilemoma - see Neurilemmoma

Neurinoma (M9560/0) - see Neurilemmoma

Neurinomatosis (M9560/1) - see also Neoplasm, connective tissue, uncertain behavior
- centralis 759.5

Neuritis (see also Neuralgia) 729.2
- abducens (nerve) 378.54
- accessory (nerve) 352.4
- acoustic (nerve) 388.5
  - syphilitic 094.86
- alcoholic 357.5
  - with psychosis 291.1
- amyloid, any site 277.39 [357.4]
- anterior crural 355.8
- arising during pregnancy 646.4●
- arm 723.4
- ascending 355.2
- auditory (nerve) 388.5
- brachial (nerve) NEC 723.4
  - due to displacement, intervertebral disc 722.0
- cervical 723.4
- chest (wall) 353.8
- costal region 353.8
- cranial nerve - see also Disorder, nerve, cranial
  - first or olfactory 352.0
  - second or optic 377.30
  - third or oculomotor 378.52
  - fourth or trochlear 378.53
  - fifth or trigeminal (see also Neuralgia, trigeminal) 350.1
  - sixth or abducens 378.54
  - seventh or facial 351.8
    - newborn 767.5
  - eighth or acoustic 388.5
  - ninth or glossopharyngeal 352.1
  - tenth or vagus 352.3
  - eleventh or accessory 352.4
  - twelfth or hypoglossal 352.5
- Déjérine-Sottas 356.0
- diabetic 250.6● [357.2]
  - due to secondary diabetes 249.6● [357.2]
- diphtheritic 032.89 [357.4]
- due to
  - beriberi 265.0 [357.4]
  - displacement, prolapse, protrusion, or rupture of intervertebral disc 722.2
    - cervical 722.0
    - lumbar, lumbosacral 722.10
    - thoracic, thoracolumbar 722.11
  - herniation, nucleus pulposus 722.2
    - cervical 722.0
    - lumbar, lumbosacral 722.10
    - thoracic, thoracolumbar 722.11
- endemic 265.0 [357.4]
- facial (nerve) 351.8
  - newborn 767.5
- general - see Polyneuropathy
- geniculate ganglion 351.1
  - due to herpes 053.11
- glossopharyngeal (nerve) 352.1

Neuritis (Continued)
- gouty 274.89 [357.4]
- hypoglossal (nerve) 352.5
- ilioinguinal (nerve) 355.8
- in diseases classified elsewhere - see Polyneuropathy, in
- infectious (multiple) 357.0
- intercostal (nerve) 353.8
- interstitial hypertrophic progressive NEC 356.9
- leg 355.8
- lumbosacral NEC 724.4
- median (nerve) 354.1
  - thenar 354.1
- multiple (acute) (infective) 356.9
  - endemic 265.0 [357.4]
- multiplex endemica 265.0 [357.4]
- nerve root (see also Radiculitis) 729.2
- oculomotor (nerve) 378.52
- olfactory (nerve) 352.0
- optic (nerve) 377.30
  - in myelitis 341.0
  - meningococcal 036.81
- pelvic 355.8
- peripheral (nerve) - see also Neuropathy, peripheral
  - complicating pregnancy or puerperium 646.4●
  - specified nerve NEC - see Mononeuritis
- pneumogastric (nerve) 352.3
- postchickenpox 052.7
- postherpetic 053.19
- progressive hypertrophic interstitial NEC 356.9
- puerperal, postpartum 646.4●
- radial (nerve) 723.4
- retrobulbar 377.32
  - syphilitic 094.85
- rheumatic (chronic) 729.2
- sacral region 355.8
- sciatic (nerve) 724.3
  - due to displacement of intervertebral disc 722.10
- serum 999.59
- specified nerve NEC - see Disorder, nerve
- spinal (nerve) 355.9
  - root (see also Radiculitis) 729.2
- subscapular (nerve) 723.4
- suprascapular (nerve) 723.4
- syphilitic 095.8
- thenar (median) 354.1
- thoracic NEC 724.4
- toxic NEC 357.7
- trochlear (nerve) 378.53
- ulnar (nerve) 723.4
- vagus (nerve) 352.3

Neuroangiomatosis, encephalofacial 759.6

Neuroastrocytoma (M9505/1) - see Neoplasm, by site, uncertain behavior

Neuro-avitaminosis 269.2

Neuroblastoma (M9500/3)
- olfactory (M9522/3) 160.0
- specified site - see Neoplasm, by site, malignant
- unspecified site 194.0

Neurochorioretinitis (see also Chorioretinitis) 363.20

Neurocirculatory asthenia 306.2

Neurocytoma (M9506/0) - see Neoplasm, by site, benign

Neurodermatitis (circumscribed) (circumscripta) (local) 698.3
- atopic 691.8
- diffuse (Brocq) 691.8
- disseminated 691.8
- nodulosa 698.3

Neuroencephalomyelopathy, optic 341.0

Neuroendocrine tumor - see Tumor, neuroendocrine

Neuroepithelioma (M9503/3) - see also Neoplasm, by site, malignant
- olfactory (M9521/3) 160.0

Neurofibroma (M9540/0) - see also Neoplasm, connective tissue, benign
- melanotic (M9541/0) - see Neoplasm, connective tissue, benign
- multiple (M9540/1) 237.70
  - type 1 237.71
  - type 2 237.72
- plexiform (M9550/0) - see Neoplasm, connective tissue, benign

Neurofibromatosis (multiple) (M9540/1) 237.70
- acoustic 237.72
- malignant (M9540/3) - see also Neoplasm, connective tissue, malignant
- Schwannomatosis 237.73
- specified type NEC 237.79
- type 1 237.71
- type 2 237.72
- von Recklinghausen's 237.71

Neurofibrosarcoma (M9540/3) - see Neoplasm, connective tissue, malignant

Neurogenic - see also condition
- bladder (atonic) (automatic) (autonomic) (flaccid) (hypertonic) (hypotonic) (inertia) (infranuclear) (irritable) (motor) (nonreflex) (nuclear) (paralysis) (reflex) (sensory) (spastic) (supranuclear) (uninhibited) 596.54
  - with cauda equina syndrome 344.61
- bowel 564.81
- heart 306.2

Neuroglioma (M9505/1) - see Neoplasm, by site, uncertain behavior

Neurolabyrinthitis (of Dix and Hallpike) 386.12

Neurolathyrism 988.2

Neuroleprosy 030.1

Neuroleptic malignant syndrome 333.92

Neurolipomatosis 272.8

Neuroma (M9570/0) - see also Neoplasm, connective tissue, benign
- acoustic (nerve) (M9560/0) 225.1
- amputation (traumatic) - see also Injury, nerve, by site
  - surgical complication (late) 997.61
- appendix 211.3
- auditory nerve 225.1
- digital 355.6
  - toe 355.6
- interdigital (toe) 355.6
- intermetatarsal 355.6
- Morton's 355.6
- multiple 237.70
  - type 1 237.71
  - type 2 237.72
- nonneoplastic 355.9
  - arm NEC 354.9
  - leg NEC 355.8
  - lower extremity NEC 355.8
  - specified site NEC - see Mononeuritis, by site
  - upper extremity NEC 354.9
- optic (nerve) 225.1
- plantar 355.6
- plexiform (M9550/0) - see Neoplasm, connective tissue, benign
- surgical (nonneoplastic) 355.9
  - arm NEC 354.9
  - leg NEC 355.8
  - lower extremity NEC 355.8
  - upper extremity NEC 354.9
- traumatic - see also Injury, nerve, by site
  - old - see Neuroma, nonneoplastic

Neuromyalgia 729.1

Neuromyasthenia (epidemic) 049.8

Neuromyelitis 341.8
- ascending 357.0
- optica 341.0

Neuromyopathy NEC 358.9

Neuromyositis 729.1

Neuronevus (M8725/0) - see Neoplasm, skin, benign
Neuronitis 357.0
　ascending (acute) 355.2
　vestibular 386.12
Neuroparalytic - see condition
Neuropathy, neuropathic (see also Disorder, nerve) 355.9
　acute motor 357.82
　alcoholic 357.5
　　with psychosis 291.1
　arm NEC 354.9
　ataxia and retinitis pigmentosa (NARP syndrome) 277.87
　autonomic (peripheral) - see Neuropathy, peripheral, autonomic
　axillary nerve 353.0
　brachial plexus 353.0
　cervical plexus 353.2
　chronic
　　progressive segmentally demyelinating 357.89
　　relapsing demyelinating 357.89
　congenital sensory 356.2
　Déjérine-Sottas 356.0
　diabetic 250.6● [357.2]
　　autonomic (peripheral) 250.6 [337.1]
　　due to secondary diabetes 249.6● [357.2]
　　　autonomic (peripheral) 249.6 [337.1]
　entrapment 355.9
　　iliohypogastric nerve 355.79
　　ilioinguinal nerve 355.79
　　lateral cutaneous nerve of thigh 355.1
　　median nerve 354.0
　　obturator nerve 355.79
　　peroneal nerve 355.3
　　posterior tibial nerve 355.5
　　saphenous nerve 355.79
　　ulnar nerve 354.2
　facial nerve 351.9
　hereditary 356.9
　　peripheral 356.0
　　sensory (radicular) 356.2
　hypertrophic
　　Charcôt-Marie-Tooth 356.1
　　Déjérine-Sottas 356.0
　　interstitial 356.9
　　Refsum 356.3
　intercostal nerve 354.8
　ischemic - see Disorder, nerve
　Jamaican (ginger) 357.7
　leg NEC 355.8
　lower extremity NEC 355.8
　lumbar plexus 353.1
　median nerve 354.1
　motor
　　acute 357.82
　multiple (acute) (chronic) (see also Polyneuropathy) 356.9
　optic 377.39
　　ischemic 377.41
　　nutritional 377.33
　　toxic 377.34
　peripheral (nerve) (see also Polyneuropathy) 356.9
　　arm NEC 354.9
　　autonomic 337.9
　　　amyloid 277.39 [337.1]
　　　idiopathic 337.00
　　　in
　　　　amyloidosis 277.39 [337.1]
　　　　diabetes (mellitus) 250.6● [337.1]
　　　　　due to secondary diabetes 249.6● [337.1]
　　　　diseases classified elsewhere 337.1
　　　　gout 274.89 [337.1]
　　　　hyperthyroidism 242.9● [337.1]
　　　due to
　　　　antitetanus serum 357.6
　　　　arsenic 357.7
　　　　drugs 357.6

Neuropathy, neuropathic (Continued)
　peripheral (Continued)
　　due to (Continued)
　　　lead 357.7
　　　organophosphate compounds 357.7
　　　toxic agent NEC 357.7
　　hereditary 356.0
　　idiopathic 356.9
　　　progressive 356.4
　　　specified type NEC 356.8
　　in diseases classified elsewhere - see Polyneuropathy, in
　　leg NEC 355.8
　　lower extremity NEC 355.8
　　upper extremity NEC 354.9
　plantar nerves 355.6
　progressive
　　hypertrophic interstitial 356.9
　　inflammatory 357.89
　radicular NEC 729.2
　　brachial 723.4
　　cervical NEC 723.4
　　hereditary sensory 356.2
　　lumbar 724.4
　　lumbosacral 724.4
　　thoracic NEC 724.4
　sacral plexus 353.1
　sciatic 355.0
　spinal nerve NEC 355.9
　　root (see also Radiculitis) 729.2
　toxic 357.7
　trigeminal sensory 350.8
　ulnar nerve 354.2
　upper extremity NEC 354.9
　uremic 585.9 [357.4]
　vitamin B$_{12}$ 266.2 [357.4]
　　with anemia (pernicious) 281.0 [357.4]
　　due to dietary deficiency 281.1 [357.4]
Neurophthisis - see also Disorder, nerve
　peripheral 356.9
　diabetic 250.6● [357.2]
　　due to secondary diabetes 249.6● [357.2]
Neuropraxia - see Injury, nerve
Neuroretinitis 363.05
　syphilitic 094.85
Neurosarcoma (M9540/3) - see Neoplasm, connective tissue, malignant
Neurosclerosis - see Disorder, nerve
Neurosis, neurotic 300.9
　accident 300.16
　anancastic, anankastic 300.3
　anxiety (state) 300.00
　　generalized 300.02
　　panic type 300.01
　asthenic 300.5
　bladder 306.53
　cardiac (reflex) 306.2
　cardiovascular 306.2
　climacteric, unspecified type 627.2
　colon 306.4
　compensation 300.16
　compulsive, compulsion 300.3
　conversion 300.11
　craft 300.89
　cutaneous 306.3
　depersonalization 300.6
　depressive (reaction) (type) 300.4
　endocrine 306.6
　environmental 300.89
　fatigue 300.5
　functional (see also Disorder, psychosomatic) 306.9
　gastric 306.4
　gastrointestinal 306.4
　genitourinary 306.50
　heart 306.2
　hypochondriacal 300.7
　hysterical 300.10
　　conversion type 300.11
　　dissociative type 300.15
　impulsive 300.3

Neurosis, neurotic (Continued)
　incoordination 306.0
　　larynx 306.1
　　vocal cord 306.1
　intestine 306.4
　larynx 306.1
　　hysterical 300.11
　　sensory 306.1
　menopause, unspecified type 627.2
　mixed NEC 300.89
　musculoskeletal 306.0
　obsessional 300.3
　　phobia 300.3
　obsessive-compulsive 300.3
　occupational 300.89
　ocular 306.7
　oral (see also Disorder, fluency) 315.35
　organ (see also Disorder, psychosomatic) 306.9
　pharynx 306.1
　phobic 300.20
　posttraumatic (acute) (situational) 309.81
　　chronic 309.81
　psychasthenic (type) 300.89
　railroad 300.16
　rectum 306.4
　respiratory 306.1
　rumination 306.4
　senile 300.89
　sexual 302.70
　situational 300.89
　specified type NEC 300.89
　state 300.9
　　with depersonalization episode 300.6
　stomach 306.4
　vasomotor 306.2
　visceral 306.4
　war 300.16
Neurospongioblastosis diffusa 759.5
Neurosyphilis (arrested) (early) (inactive) (late) (latent) (recurrent) 094.9
　with ataxia (cerebellar) (locomotor) (spastic) (spinal) 094.0
　acute meningitis 094.2
　aneurysm 094.89
　arachnoid (adhesive) 094.2
　arteritis (any artery) 094.89
　asymptomatic 094.3
　congenital 090.40
　dura (mater) 094.89
　general paresis 094.1
　gumma 094.9
　hemorrhagic 094.9
　juvenile (asymptomatic) (meningeal) 090.40
　leptomeninges (aseptic) 094.2
　meningeal 094.2
　meninges (adhesive) 094.2
　meningovascular (diffuse) 094.2
　optic atrophy 094.84
　parenchymatous (degenerative) 094.1
　paresis (see also Paresis, general) 094.1
　paretic (see also Paresis, general) 094.1
　relapse 094.9
　remission in (sustained) 094.9
　serological 094.3
　specified nature or site NEC 094.89
　tabes (dorsalis) 094.0
　　juvenile 090.40
　tabetic 094.0
　　juvenile 090.40
　taboparesis 094.1
　　juvenile 090.40
　thrombosis 094.89
　vascular 094.89
Neurotic (see also Neurosis) 300.9
　excoriation 698.4
　　psychogenic 306.3
Neurotmesis - see Injury, nerve, by site
Neurotoxemia - see Toxemia
Neuro-occlusion 524.21

Neutropenia, neutropenic (idiopathic) (pernicious) (primary) 288.00
  chronic 288.09
    hypoplastic 288.09
  congenital (nontransient) 288.01
  cyclic 288.02
  drug induced 288.03
  due to infection 288.04
  fever 288.00
  genetic 288.01
  immune 288.09
  infantile 288.01
  malignant 288.09
  neonatal, transitory (isoimmune) (maternal transfer) 776.7
  periodic 288.02
  splenic 289.53
  splenomegaly 289.53
  toxic 288.09
Neutrophilia, hereditary giant 288.2
Nevocarcinoma (M8720/3) - *see* Melanoma
Nevus (M8720/0) - *see also* Neoplasm, skin, benign

> Note: Except where otherwise indicated, varieties of nevus in the list below that are followed by a morphology code number (M----/0) should be coded by site as for "Neoplasm, skin, benign."

  acanthotic 702.8
  achromic (M8730/0)
  amelanotic (M8730/0)
  anemic, anemicus 709.09
  angiomatous (M9120/0) (*see also* Hemangioma) 228.00
  araneus 448.1
  avasculosus 709.09
  balloon cell (M8722/0)
  bathing trunk (M8761/1) 238.2
  blue (M8780/0)
    cellular (M8790/0)
    giant (M8790/0)
    Jadassohn's (M8780/0)
    malignant (M8780/3) - *see* Melanoma
  capillary (M9131/0) (*see also* Hemangioma) 228.00
  cavernous (M9121/0) (*see also* Hemangioma) 228.00
  cellular (M8720/0)
    blue (M8790/0)
  comedonicus 757.33
  compound (M8760/0)
  conjunctiva (M8720/0) 224.3
  dermal (M8750/0)
    and epidermal (M8760/0)
  epithelioid cell (and spindle cell) (M8770/0)
  flammeus 757.32
    osteohypertrophic 759.89
  hairy (M8720/0)
  halo (M8723/0)
  hemangiomatous (M9120/0) (*see also* Hemangioma) 228.00
  intradermal (M8750/0)
  intraepidermal (M8740/0)
  involuting (M8724/0)
  Jadassohn's (blue) (M8780/0)
  junction, junctional (M8740/0)
    malignant melanoma in (M8740/3) - *see* Melanoma
  juvenile (M8770/0)
  lymphatic (M9170/0) 228.1
  magnocellular (M8726/0)
    specified site - *see* Neoplasm, by site, benign
    unspecified site 224.0
  malignant (M8720/3) - *see* Melanoma
  meaning hemangioma (M9120/0) (*see also* Hemangioma) 228.00
  melanotic (pigmented) (M8720/0)
  multiplex 759.5

Nevus (*Continued*)
  nonneoplastic 448.1
  nonpigmented (M8730/0)
  nonvascular (M8720/0)
  oral mucosa, white sponge 750.26
  osteohypertrophic, flammeus 759.89
  papillaris (M8720/0)
  papillomatosus (M8720/0)
  pigmented (M8720/0)
    giant (M8761/1) - *see also* Neoplasm, skin, uncertain behavior
      malignant melanoma in (M8761/3) - *see* Melanoma
    systematicus 757.33
  pilosus (M8720/0)
  port wine 757.32
  sanguineous 757.32
  sebaceous (senile) 702.8
  senile 448.1
  spider 448.1
  spindle cell (and epithelioid cell) (M8770/0)
  stellar 448.1
  strawberry 757.32
  syringocystadenomatous papilliferous (M8406/0)
  unius lateris 757.33
  Unna's 757.32
  vascular 757.32
  verrucous 757.33
  white sponge (oral mucosa) 750.26
Newborn (infant) (liveborn)
  abstinence syndrome 779.5
  affected by
    amniocentesis 760.61
    maternal abuse of drugs (gestational) (via placenta) (via breast milk) (*see also* Noxious, substances transmitted through placenta or breast milk (affecting fetus or newborn)) 760.70
      methamphetamine(s) 760.72
    procedure
      amniocentesis 760.61
      in utero NEC 760.62
      surgical on mother
        during pregnancy NEC 760.63
        previous not associated with pregnancy 760.64
  apnea 770.81
    obstructive 770.82
    specified NEC 770.82
  breast buds 779.89
  cardiomyopathy 425.4
    congenital 425.3
  convulsion 779.0
  electrolyte imbalance NEC (transitory) 775.5
  fever (environmentally-induced) 778.4
  gestation
    24 completed weeks 765.22
    25–26 completed weeks 765.23
    27–28 completed weeks 765.24
    29–30 completed weeks 765.25
    31–32 completed weeks 765.26
    33–34 completed weeks 765.27
    35–36 completed weeks 765.28
    37 or more completed weeks 765.29
    less than 24 completed weeks 765.21
    unspecified completed weeks 765.20
  infection 771.89
    candida 771.7
    mastitis 771.5
    specified NEC 771.89
    urinary tract 771.82
  mastitis 771.5
  multiple NEC
    born in hospital (without mention of cesarean delivery or section) V37.00
    with cesarean delivery or section V37.01
    born outside hospital
      hospitalized V37.1 ●
      not hospitalized V37.2 ●

Newborn (*Continued*)
  multiple NEC (*Continued*)
    mates all liveborn
      born in hospital (without mention of cesarean delivery or section) V34.00
        with cesarean delivery or section V34.01
      born outside hospital
        hospitalized V34.1 ●
        not hospitalized V34.2 ●
    mates all stillborn
      born in hospital (without mention of cesarean delivery or section) V35.00
        with cesarean delivery or section V35.01
      born outside hospital
        hospitalized V35.1 ●
        not hospitalized V35.2 ●
    mates liveborn and stillborn
      born in hospital (without mention of cesarean delivery or section) V36.00
        with cesarean delivery or section V36.01
      born outside hospital
        hospitalized V36.1 ●
        not hospitalized V36.2 ●
  omphalitis 771.4
  seizure 779.0
  sepsis 771.81
  single
    born in hospital (without mention of cesarean delivery or section) V30.00
      with cesarean delivery or section V30.01
    born outside hospital
      hospitalized V30.1 ●
      not hospitalized V30.2 ●
  specified condition NEC 779.89
  twin NEC
    born in hospital (without mention of cesarean delivery or section) V33.00
      with cesarean delivery or section V33.01
    born outside hospital
      hospitalized V33.1 ●
      not hospitalized V33.2 ●
    mate liveborn
      born in hospital V31.0 ●
      born outside hospital
        hospitalized V31.1 ●
        not hospitalized V31.2 ●
    mate stillborn
      born in hospital V32.0 ●
      born outside hospital
        hospitalized V32.1 ●
        not hospitalized V32.2 ●
  unspecified as to single or multiple birth
    born in hospital (without mention of cesarean delivery or section) V39.00
      with cesarean delivery or section V39.01
    born outside hospital
      hospitalized V39.1 ●
      not hospitalized V39.2 ●
  weight check V20.32
Newcastle's conjunctivitis or disease 077.8
Nezelof's syndrome (pure alymphocytosis) 279.13
Niacin (amide) deficiency 265.2
Nicolas-Durand-Favre disease (climatic bubo) 099.1
Nicolas-Favre disease (climatic bubo) 099.1
Nicotinic acid (amide) deficiency 265.2
Niemann-Pick disease (lipid histiocytosis) (splenomegaly) 272.7

Night
- blindness (*see also* Blindness, night) 368.60
  - congenital 368.61
    - vitamin A deficiency 264.5
- cramps 729.82
- sweats 780.8
- terrors, child 307.46

Nightmare 307.47
- REM-sleep type 307.47

Nipple - *see* condition
Nisbet's chancre 099.0
Nishimoto (-Takeuchi) disease 437.5
Nitritoid crisis or reaction - *see* Crisis, nitritoid
Nitrogen retention, extrarenal 788.99
Nitrosohemoglobinemia 289.89
Njovera 104.0
No
- diagnosis 799.9
- disease (found) V71.9
- room at the inn V65.0

Nocardiasis - *see* Nocardiosis
Nocardiosis 039.9
- with pneumonia 039.1
- lung 039.1
- specified type NEC 039.8

Nocturia 788.43
- psychogenic 306.53

Nocturnal - *see also* condition
- dyspnea (paroxysmal) 786.09
- emissions 608.89
- enuresis 788.36
  - psychogenic 307.6
- frequency (micturition) 788.43
  - psychogenic 306.53

Nodal rhythm disorder 427.89
Nodding of head 781.0
Node(s) - *see also* Nodules
- Heberden's 715.04
- larynx 478.79
- lymph - *see* condition
- milkers' 051.1
- Osler's 421.0
- rheumatic 729.89
- Schmorl's 722.30
  - lumbar, lumbosacral 722.32
  - specified region NEC 722.39
  - thoracic, thoracolumbar 722.31
- singers' 478.5
- skin NEC 782.2
- tuberculous - *see* Tuberculosis, lymph gland
- vocal cords 478.5

Nodosities, Haygarth's 715.04
Nodule(s), nodular
- actinomycotic (*see also* Actinomycosis) 039.9
- arthritic - *see* Arthritis, nodosa
- breast 793.89
- cutaneous 782.2
- Haygarth's 715.04
- inflammatory - *see* Inflammation
- juxta-articular 102.7
  - syphilitic 095.7
  - yaws 102.7
- larynx 478.79
- lung
  - emphysematous 492.8
  - solitary 793.11
- milkers' 051.1
- prostate 600.10
  - with
    - urinary
      - obstruction 600.11
      - retention 600.11
- pulmonary, solitary (subsegmental branch of the bronchial tree) 793.11
  - multiple 793.19
- retrocardiac 785.9
- rheumatic 729.89
- rheumatoid - *see* Arthritis rheumatoid
- scrotum (inflammatory) 608.4
- singers' 478.5
- skin NEC 782.2

Nodule(s), nodular (*Continued*)
- solitary, lung 518.89
  - emphysematous 492.8
- subcutaneous 782.2
- thyroid (gland) (nontoxic) (uninodular) 241.0
  - with
    - hyperthyroidism 242.1●
    - thyrotoxicosis 242.1●
  - toxic or with hyperthyroidism 242.1●
- vocal cords 478.5

Noma (gangrenous) (hospital) (infective) 528.1
- auricle (*see also* Gangrene) 785.4
- mouth 528.1
- pudendi (*see also* Vulvitis) 616.10
- vulvae (*see also* Vulvitis) 616.10

Nomadism V60.0
Non-adherence
- artificial skin graft 996.55
- decellularized allodermis graft 996.55

Non-autoimmune hemolytic anemia NEC 283.10
Nonclosure - *see also* Imperfect, closure
- ductus
  - arteriosus 747.0
  - Botalli 747.0
- Eustachian valve 746.89
- foramen
  - Botalli 745.5
  - ovale 745.5

Noncompliance with medical treatment V15.81
- renal dialysis V45.12

Nondescent (congenital) - *see also* Malposition, congenital
- cecum 751.4
- colon 751.4
- testis 752.51

Nondevelopment
- brain 742.1
  - specified part 742.2
- heart 746.89
- organ or site, congenital NEC - *see* Hypoplasia

Nonengagement
- head NEC 652.5●
  - in labor 660.1●
    - affecting fetus or newborn 763.1

Nonexanthematous tick fever 066.1
Nonexpansion, lung (newborn) NEC 770.4
Nonfunctioning
- cystic duct (*see also* Disease, gallbladder) 575.8
- gallbladder (*see also* Disease, gallbladder) 575.8
- kidney (*see also* Disease, renal) 593.9
- labyrinth 386.58

Nonhealing
- stump (surgical) 997.69
- wound, surgical 998.83

Nonimplantation of ovum, causing infertility 628.3
Noninsufflation, fallopian tube 628.2
Nonne-Milroy-Meige syndrome (chronic hereditary edema) 757.0
Nonovulation 628.0
Nonpatent fallopian tube 628.2
Nonpneumatization, lung NEC 770.4
Nonreflex bladder 596.54
- with cauda equina 344.61

Nonretention of food - *see* Vomiting
Nonrotation - *see* Malrotation
Nonsecretion, urine (*see also* Anuria) 788.5
- newborn 753.3

Nonunion
- fracture 733.82
- organ or site, congenital NEC - *see* Imperfect, closure
- symphysis pubis, congenital 755.69
- top sacrum, congenital 756.19

Nonviability 765.0●
Nonvisualization, gallbladder 793.3
Nonvitalized tooth 522.9

Non-working side interference 524.56
Normal
- delivery - *see* category 650
- menses V65.5
- state (feared complaint unfounded) V65.5

Normoblastosis 289.89
Normocytic anemia (infectional) 285.9
- due to blood loss (chronic) 280.0
  - acute 285.1

Norrie's disease (congenital) (progressive oculoacousticocerebral degeneration) 743.8
North American blastomycosis 116.0
Norwegian itch 133.0
Nose, nasal - *see* condition
Nosebleed 784.7
Nosomania 298.9
Nosophobia 300.29
Nostalgia 309.89
Notch of iris 743.46
Notched lip, congenital (*see also* Cleft, lip) 749.10
Notching nose, congenital (tip) 748.1
Nothnagel's
- syndrome 378.52
- vasomotor acroparesthesia 443.89

Novy's relapsing fever (American) 087.1
Noxious
- foodstuffs, poisoning by
  - fish 988.0
  - fungi 988.1
  - mushrooms 988.1
  - plants (food) 988.2
  - shellfish 988.0
  - specified type NEC 988.8
  - toadstool 988.1
- substances transmitted through placenta or breast milk (affecting fetus or newborn) 760.70
  - acetretin 760.78
  - alcohol 760.71
  - aminopterin 760.78
  - antiandrogens 760.79
  - anticonvulsant 760.77
  - antifungal 760.74
  - anti-infective agents 760.74
  - antimetabolic 760.78
  - atorvastatin 760.78
  - carbamazepine 760.77
  - cocaine 760.75
  - "crack" 760.75
  - diethylstilbestrol (DES) 760.76
  - divalproex sodium 760.77
  - endocrine disrupting chemicals 760.79
  - estrogens 760.79
  - etretinate 760.78
  - fluconazole 760.74
  - fluvastatin 760.78
  - hallucinogenic agents NEC 760.73
  - hormones 760.79
  - lithium 760.79
  - lovastatin 760.78
  - medicinal agents NEC 760.79
  - methotrexate 760.78
  - misoprostil 760.79
  - narcotics 760.72
  - obstetric anesthetic or analgesic 763.5
  - phenobarbital 760.77
  - phenytoin 760.77
  - pravastatin 760.78
  - progestins 760.79
  - retinoic acid 760.78
  - simvastatin 760.78
  - solvents 760.79
  - specified agent NEC 760.79
  - statins 760.79
  - suspected, affecting management of pregnancy 655.5●
  - tetracycline 760.74
  - thalidomide 760.79
  - trimethadione 760.77

Noxious (Continued)
  substances transmitted through placenta or breast milk (Continued)
    valproate 760.77
    valproic acid 760.77
    vitamin A 760.78
NPDH (new persistent daily headache) 339.42
Nuchal hitch (arm) 652.8
Nucleus pulposus - *see* condition
Numbness 782.0
Nuns' knee 727.2
Nursemaid's
  elbow 832.2
  shoulder 831.0
Nutmeg liver 573.8

Nutrition, deficient or insufficient (particular kind of food) 269.9
  due to
    insufficient food 994.2
    lack of
      care (child) (infant) 995.52
        adult 995.84
      food 994.2
Nyctalopia (*see also* Blindness, night) 368.60
  vitamin A deficiency 264.5
Nycturia 788.43
  psychogenic 306.53
Nymphomania 302.89
Nystagmus 379.50
  associated with vestibular system disorders 379.54

Nystagmus (Continued)
  benign paroxysmal positional 386.11
  central positional 386.2
  congenital 379.51
  deprivation 379.53
  dissociated 379.55
  latent 379.52
  miners' 300.89
  positional
    benign paroxysmal 386.11
    central 386.2
  specified NEC 379.56
  vestibular 379.54
  visual deprivation 379.53

SECTION I INDEX TO DISEASES AND INJURIES / Obstruction, obstructed, obstructive

O

Oasthouse urine disease 270.2
Obermeyer's relapsing fever (European) 087.0
Obesity (constitutional) (exogenous) (familial) (nutritional) (simple) 278.00
  adrenal 255.8
  complicating pregnancy, childbirth, or puerperium 649.1 •
  due to hyperalimentation 278.00
  endocrine NEC 259.9
  endogenous 259.9
  Fröhlich's (adiposogenital dystrophy) 253.8
  glandular NEC 259.9
  hypothyroid (see also Hypothyroidism) 244.9
  hypoventilation syndrome 278.03
  morbid 278.01
  of pregnancy 649.1 •
  pituitary 253.8
  severe 278.01
  thyroid (see also Hypothyroidism) 244.9
Oblique - see also condition
  lie before labor, affecting fetus or newborn 761.7
Obliquity, pelvis 738.6
Obliteration
  abdominal aorta 446.7
  appendix (lumen) 543.9
  artery 447.1
  ascending aorta 446.7
  bile ducts 576.8
    with calculus, choledocholithiasis, or stones - see Choledocholithiasis
    congenital 751.61
      jaundice from 751.61 [774.5]
  common duct 576.8
    with calculus, choledocholithiasis, or stones - see Choledocholithiasis
    congenital 751.61
  cystic duct 575.8
    with calculus, choledocholithiasis, or stones - see Choledocholithiasis
  disease, arteriolar 447.1
  endometrium 621.8
  eye, anterior chamber 360.34
  fallopian tube 628.2
  lymphatic vessel 457.1
    postmastectomy 457.0
  organ or site, congenital NEC - see Atresia
  placental blood vessels   see Placenta, abnormal
  supra-aortic branches 446.7
  ureter 593.89
  urethra 599.84
  vein 459.9
  vestibule (oral) 525.8
Observation (for) V71.9
  without need for further medical care V71.9
  accident NEC V71.4
    at work V71.3
  criminal assault V71.6
  deleterious agent ingestion V71.89
  disease V71.9
    cardiovascular V71.7
    heart V71.7
    mental V71.09
    specified condition NEC V71.89
  foreign body ingestion V71.89
  growth and development variations V21.8
  injuries (accidental) V71.4
    inflicted NEC V71.6
      during alleged rape or seduction V71.5
  malignant neoplasm, suspected V71.1
  postpartum
    immediately after delivery V24.0
    routine follow-up V24.2
  pregnancy
    high-risk V23.9
      inconclusive fetal viability V23.87
      specified problem NEC V23.89

Observation (Continued)
  pregnancy (Continued)
    normal (without complication) V22.1
      with nonobstetric complication V22.2
      first V22.0
  rape or seduction, alleged V71.5
    injury during V71.5
  suicide attempt, alleged V71.89
  suspected (undiagnosed) (unproven)
    abuse V71.81
    cardiovascular disease V71.7
    child or wife battering victim V71.6
    concussion (cerebral) V71.6
    condition NEC V71.89
      infant - see Observation, suspected, condition, newborn
      maternal and fetal
        amniotic cavity and membrane problem V89.01
        cervical shortening V89.05
        fetal anomaly V89.03
        fetal growth problem V89.04
        oligohydramnios V89.01
        other specified problem NEC V89.09
        placental problem V89.02
        polyhydramnios V89.01
      newborn V29.9
        cardiovascular disease V29.8
        congenital anomaly V29.8
        genetic V29.3
        infectious V29.0
        ingestion foreign object V29.8
        injury V29.8
        metabolic V29.3
        neoplasm V29.8
        neurological V29.1
        poison, poisoning V29.8
        respiratory V29.2
        specified NEC V29.8
    exposure
      anthrax V71.82
      biologic agent NEC V71.83
      SARS V71.83
    infectious disease not requiring isolation V71.89
    malignant neoplasm V71.1
    mental disorder V71.09
    neglect V71.81
    neoplasm
      benign V71.89
      malignant V71.1
    specified condition NEC V71.89
    tuberculosis V71.2
  tuberculosis, suspected V71.2
Obsession, obsessional 300.3
  ideas and mental images 300.3
  impulses 300.3
  neurosis 300.3
  phobia 300.3
  psychasthenia 300.3
  ruminations 300.3
  state 300.3
  syndrome 300.3
Obsessive-compulsive 300.3
  neurosis 300.3
  personality 301.4
  reaction 300.3
Obstetrical trauma NEC (complicating delivery) 665.9 •
  with
    abortion - see Abortion, by type, with damage to pelvic organs
    ectopic pregnancy (see also categories 633.0-633.9) 639.2
    molar pregnancy (see also categories 630-632) 639.2
  affecting fetus or newborn 763.89
  following
    abortion 639.2
    ectopic or molar pregnancy 639.2

Obstipation (see also Constipation) 564.00
  psychogenic 306.4
Obstruction, obstructed, obstructive
  airway NEC 519.8
    with
      allergic alveolitis NEC 495.9
      asthma NEC (see also Asthma) 493.9 •
      bronchiectasis 494.0
        with acute exacerbation 494.1
      bronchitis (see also Bronchitis, with, obstruction) 491.20
      emphysema NEC 492.8
    chronic 496
      with
        allergic alveolitis NEC 495.5
        asthma NEC (see also Asthma) 493.2 •
        bronchiectasis 494.0
          with acute exacerbation 494.1
        bronchitis (chronic) (see also Bronchitis, chronic, obstructive) 491.20
        emphysema NEC 492.8
    due to
      bronchospasm 519.11
      foreign body 934.9
      inhalation of fumes or vapors 506.9
      laryngospasm 478.75
  alimentary canal (see also Obstruction, intestine) 560.9
  ampulla of Vater 576.2
    with calculus, cholelithiasis, or stones - see Choledocholithiasis
  aortic (heart) (valve) (see also Stenosis, aortic) 424.1
    rheumatic (see also Stenosis, aortic, rheumatic) 395.0
  aortoiliac 444.09
  aqueduct of Sylvius 331.4
    congenital 742.3
      with spina bifida (see also Spina bifida) 741.0 •
  Arnold-Chiari (see also Spina bifida) 741.0 •
  artery (see also Embolism, artery) 444.9
    basilar (complete) (partial) (see also Occlusion, artery, basilar) 433.0 •
    carotid (complete) (partial) (see also Occlusion, artery, carotid) 433.1 •
    precerebral - see Occlusion, artery, precerebral NEC
    retinal (central) (see also Occlusion, retina) 362.30
    vertebral (complete) (partial) (see also Occlusion, artery, vertebral) 433.2 •
  asthma (chronic) (with obstructive pulmonary disease) 493.2 •
  band (intestinal) 560.81
  bile duct or passage (see also Obstruction, biliary) 576.2
    congenital 751.61
      jaundice from 751.61 [774.5]
  biliary (duct) (tract) 576.2
    with calculus 574.51
      with cholecystitis (chronic) 574.41
        acute 574.31
    congenital 751.61
      jaundice from 751.61 [774.5]
    gallbladder 575.2
      with calculus 574.21
        with cholecystitis (chronic) 574.11
          acute 574.01
  bladder neck (acquired) 596.0
    congenital 753.6
  bowel (see also Obstruction, intestine) 560.9
  bronchus 519.19
  canal, ear (see also Stricture, ear canal, acquired) 380.50
  cardia 537.89
  caval veins (inferior) (superior) 459.2
  cecum (see also Obstruction, intestine) 560.9
  circulatory 459.9

373

Obstruction, obstructed, obstructive
(Continued)
- colon (*see also* Obstruction, intestine) 560.9
  - sympathicotonic 560.89
- common duct (*see also* Obstruction, biliary) 576.2
  - congenital 751.61
- coronary (artery) (heart) - *see also* Arteriosclerosis, coronary)
  - acute (*see also* Infarct, myocardium) 410.9●
    - without myocardial infarction 411.81
- cystic duct (*see also* Obstruction, gallbladder) 575.2
  - congenital 751.61
- device, implant, or graft - *see* Complications, due to (presence of) any device, implant, or graft classified to 996.0–996.5 NEC
- due to foreign body accidentally left in operation wound 998.4
- duodenum 537.3
  - congenital 751.1
  - due to
    - compression NEC 537.3
    - cyst 537.3
    - intrinsic lesion or disease NEC 537.3
    - scarring 537.3
    - torsion 537.3
    - ulcer 532.91
    - volvulus 537.3
- ejaculatory duct 608.89
- endocardium 424.90
  - arteriosclerotic 424.99
  - specified cause, except rheumatic 424.99
- esophagus 530.3
- Eustachian tube (complete) (partial) 381.60
  - cartilaginous
    - extrinsic 381.63
    - intrinsic 381.62
  - due to
    - cholesteatoma 381.61
    - osseous lesion NEC 381.61
    - polyp 381.61
  - osseous 381.61
- fallopian tube (bilateral) 628.2
- fecal 560.32
  - with hernia - *see also* Hernia, by site, with obstruction
    - gangrenous - *see* Hernia, by site, with gangrene
- foramen of Monro (congenital) 742.3
  - with spina bifida (*see also* Spina bifida) 741.0●
- foreign body - *see* Foreign body
- gallbladder 575.2
  - with calculus, cholelithiasis, or stones 574.21
    - with cholecystitis (chronic) 574.11
      - acute 574.01
  - congenital 751.69
    - jaundice from 751.69 [774.5]
- gastric outlet 537.0
- gastrointestinal (*see also* Obstruction, intestine) 560.9
- glottis 478.79
- hepatic 573.8
  - duct (*see also* Obstruction, biliary) 576.2
    - congenital 751.61
- icterus (*see also* Obstruction, biliary) 576.8
  - congenital 751.61
- ileocecal coil (*see also* Obstruction, intestine) 560.9
- ileum (*see also* Obstruction, intestine) 560.9
- iliofemoral (artery) 444.81
- internal anastomosis - *see* Complications, mechanical, graft

Obstruction, obstructed, obstructive
(Continued)
- intestine (mechanical) (neurogenic) (paroxysmal) (postinfectional) (reflex) 560.9
  - with
    - adhesions (intestinal) (peritoneal) 560.81
    - hernia - *see also* Hernia, by site, with obstruction
      - gangrenous - *see* Hernia, by site, with gangrene
  - adynamic (*see also* Ileus) 560.1
  - by gallstone 560.31
  - congenital or infantile (small) 751.1
    - large 751.2
  - due to
    - Ascaris lumbricoides 127.0
    - mural thickening 560.89
    - procedure 997.49
      - involving urinary tract 997.5
  - impaction 560.32
  - infantile - *see* Obstruction, intestine, congenital
  - newborn
    - due to
      - fecaliths 777.1
      - inspissated milk 777.2
      - meconium (plug) 777.1
        - in mucoviscidosis 277.01
      - transitory 777.4
  - specified cause NEC 560.89
  - transitory, newborn 777.4
  - volvulus 560.2
- intracardiac ball valve prosthesis 996.02
- jaundice (*see also* Obstruction, biliary) 576.8
  - congenital 751.61
- jejunum (*see also* Obstruction, intestine) 560.9
- kidney 593.89
- labor 660.9●
  - affecting fetus or newborn 763.1
  - by
    - bony pelvis (conditions classifiable to 653.0–653.9) 660.1●
    - deep transverse arrest 660.3●
    - impacted shoulder 660.4●
    - locked twins 660.5●
    - malposition (fetus) (conditions classifiable to 652.0–652.9) 660.0●
    - head during labor 660.3●
    - persistent occipitoposterior position 660.3●
    - soft tissue, pelvic (conditions classifiable to 654.0–654.9) 660.2●
- lacrimal
  - canaliculi 375.53
  - congenital 743.65
  - punctum 375.52
  - sac 375.54
- lacrimonasal duct 375.56
  - congenital 743.65
  - neonatal 375.55
- lacteal, with steatorrhea 579.2
- laryngitis (*see also* Laryngitis) 464.01
- larynx 478.79
  - congenital 748.3
- liver 573.8
  - cirrhotic (*see also* Cirrhosis, liver) 571.5
- lung 518.89
  - with
    - asthma - *see* Asthma
    - bronchitis (chronic) 491.20
    - emphysema NEC 492.8
  - airway, chronic 496
  - chronic NEC 496
    - with
      - asthma (chronic) (obstructive) 493.2●

Obstruction, obstructed, obstructive
(Continued)
- lung *(Continued)*
  - disease, chronic 496
    - with
      - asthma (chronic) (obstructive) 493.2●
  - emphysematous 492.8
- lymphatic 457.1
- meconium
  - fetus or newborn 777.1
    - in mucoviscidosis 277.01
  - newborn due to fecaliths 777.1
- mediastinum 519.3
- mitral (rheumatic) - *see* Stenosis, mitral
- nasal 478.19
  - duct 375.56
    - neonatal 375.55
  - sinus - *see* Sinusitis
- nasolacrimal duct 375.56
  - congenital 743.65
  - neonatal 375.55
- nasopharynx 478.29
- nose 478.19
- organ or site, congenital NEC - *see* Atresia
- pancreatic duct 577.8
- parotid gland 527.8
- pelviureteral junction (*see also* Obstruction, ureter) 593.4
- pharynx 478.29
- portal (circulation) (vein) 452
- prostate 600.90
  - with
    - other lower urinary tract symptoms (LUTS) 600.91
    - urinary
      - obstruction 600.91
      - retention 600.91
  - valve (urinary) 596.0
- pulmonary
  - valve (heart) (*see also* Endocarditis, pulmonary) 424.3
  - vein, isolated 747.49
- pyemic - *see* Septicemia
- pylorus (acquired) 537.0
  - congenital 750.5
  - infantile 750.5
- rectosigmoid (*see also* Obstruction, intestine) 560.9
- rectum 569.49
- renal 593.89
- respiratory 519.8
  - chronic 496
- retinal (artery) (vein) (central) (*see also* Occlusion, retina) 362.30
- salivary duct (any) 527.8
  - with calculus 527.5
- sigmoid (*see also* Obstruction, intestine) 560.9
- sinus (accessory) (nasal) (*see also* Sinusitis) 473.9
- Stensen's duct 527.8
- stomach 537.89
  - acute 536.1
  - congenital 750.7
- submaxillary gland 527.8
  - with calculus 527.5
- thoracic duct 457.1
- thrombotic - *see* Thrombosis
- tooth eruption 520.6
- trachea 519.19
- tracheostomy airway 519.09
- tricuspid - *see* Endocarditis, tricuspid
- upper respiratory, congenital 748.8
- ureter (functional) 593.4
  - congenital 753.20
  - due to calculus 592.1
- ureteropelvic junction, congenital 753.21
- ureterovesical junction, congenital 753.22
- urethra 599.60
  - congenital 753.6

Obstruction, obstructed, obstructive
(Continued)
   urinary (moderate) 599.60
      organ or tract (lower) 599.60
         due to
            benign prostatic hypertrophy
               (BPH) - *see* category 600
         specified NEC 599.69
            due to
               benign prostatic hypertrophy
                  (BPH) - *see* category 600
      prostatic valve 596.0
      specified NEC 599.69
         due to
            benign prostatic hypertrophy
               (BPH) - *see* category 600
   uropathy 599.60
   uterus 621.8
   vagina 623.2
   valvular - *see* Endocarditis
   vascular graft or shunt 996.1
      atherosclerosis - *see* Arteriosclerosis, coronary
      embolism 996.74
      occlusion NEC 996.74
      thrombus 996.74
   vein, venous 459.2
      caval (inferior) (superior) 459.2
      thrombotic - *see* Thrombosis
   vena cava (inferior) (superior) 459.2
   ventricular shunt 996.2
   vesical 596.0
   vesicourethral orifice 596.0
   vessel NEC 459.9
Obturator - *see* condition
Occlusal
   plane deviation 524.76
   wear, teeth 521.10
Occlusion
   anus 569.49
      congenital 751.2
      infantile 751.2
   aortoiliac (chronic) 444.09
   aqueduct of Sylvius 331.4
      congenital 742.3
         with spina bifida (*see also* Spina bifida) 741.0●
   arteries of extremities, lower 444.22
      without thrombus or embolus (*see also* Arteriosclerosis, extremities) 440.20
      due to stricture or stenosis 447.1
      upper 444.21
         without thrombus or embolus (*see also* Arteriosclerosis, extremities) 440.20
         due to stricture or stenosis 447.1
   artery NEC (*see also* Embolism, artery) 444.9
      auditory, internal 433.8●
      basilar 433.0●
         with other precerebral artery 433.3●
         bilateral 433.3●
      brain or cerebral (*see also* Infarct, brain) 434.9●
      carotid 433.1●
         with other precerebral artery 433.3●
         bilateral 433.3●
      cerebellar (anterior inferior) (posterior inferior) (superior) 433.8●
      cerebral (*see also* Infarct, brain) 434.9●
      choroidal (anterior) 433.8●
      chronic total
         coronary 414.2
         extremity(ies) 440.4
      communicating posterior 433.8●
      complete
         coronary 414.2
         extremity(ies) 440.4

Occlusion *(Continued)*
   artery NEC *(Continued)*
      coronary (thrombotic) (*see also* Infarct, myocardium) 410.9●
         acute 410.9●
            without myocardial infarction 411.81
         chronic total 414.2
         complete 414.2
         healed or old 412
         total 414.2
      extremity(ies)
         chronic total 440.4
         complete 440.4
         total 440.4
      hypophyseal 433.8●
      iliac 444.81
      mesenteric (embolic) (thrombotic) (with gangrene) 557.0
      pontine 433.8●
      precerebral NEC 433.9●
         late effect - *see* Late effect(s) (of) cerebrovascular disease
         multiple or bilateral 433.3●
         puerperal, postpartum, childbirth 674.0●
         specified NEC 433.8●
      renal 593.81
      retinal - *see* Occlusion, retina, artery
      spinal 433.8●
      vertebral 433.2●
         with other precerebral artery 433.3●
         bilateral 433.3●
   basilar (artery) - *see* Occlusion, artery, basilar
   bile duct (any) (*see also* Obstruction, biliary) 576.2
   bowel (*see also* Obstruction, intestine) 560.9
   brain (artery) (vascular) (*see also* Infarct, brain) 434.9●
   breast (duct) 611.89
   carotid (artery) (common) (internal) - *see* Occlusion, artery, carotid
   cerebellar (anterior inferior) (artery) (posterior inferior) (superior) 433.8●
   cerebral (artery) (*see also* Infarct, brain) 434.9●
   cerebrovascular (*see also* Infarct, brain) 434.9●
      diffuse 437.0
   cervical canal (*see also* Stricture, cervix) 622.4
      by falciparum malaria 084.0
   cervix (uteri) (*see also* Stricture, cervix) 622.4
   choanal 748.0
   choroidal (artery) 433.8●
   colon (*see also* Obstruction, intestine) 560.9
   communicating posterior artery 433.8●
   coronary (artery) (thrombotic) (*see also* Infarct, myocardium) 410.9●
      acute 410.9●
         without myocardial infarction 411.81
      healed or old 412
   cystic duct (*see also* Obstruction, gallbladder) 575.2
      congenital 751.69
   disto
      division I 524.22
      division II 524.22
   embolic - *see* Embolism
   fallopian tube 628.2
      congenital 752.19
   gallbladder (*see also* Obstruction, gallbladder) 575.2
      congenital 751.69
         jaundice from 751.69 [744.5]
   gingiva, traumatic 523.8
   hymen 623.3
      congenital 752.42
   hypophyseal (artery) 433.8●
   iliac (artery) 444.81
   intestine (*see also* Obstruction, intestine) 560.9
   kidney 593.89

Occlusion *(Continued)*
   lacrimal apparatus - *see* Stenosis, lacrimal
   lung 518.89
   lymph or lymphatic channel 457.1
   mammary duct 611.89
   mesenteric artery (embolic) (thrombotic) (with gangrene) 557.0
   nose 478.19
      congenital 748.0
   organ or site, congenital NEC - *see* Atresia
   oviduct 628.2
      congenital 752.19
   periodontal, traumatic 523.8
   peripheral arteries (lower extremity) 444.22
      without thrombus or embolus (*see also* Arteriosclerosis, extremities) 440.20
      due to stricture or stenosis 447.1
      upper extremity 444.21
         without thrombus or embolus (*see also* Arteriosclerosis, extremities) 440.20
         due to stricture or stenosis 447.1
   pontine (artery) 433.8●
   posterior lingual, of mandibular teeth 524.29
   precerebral artery - *see* Occlusion, artery, precerebral NEC
   puncta lacrimalia 375.52
   pupil 364.74
   pylorus (*see also* Stricture, pylorus) 537.0
   renal artery 593.81
   retina, retinal (vascular) 362.30
      artery, arterial 362.30
         branch 362.32
         central (total) 362.31
         partial 362.33
         transient 362.34
         tributary 362.32
      vein 362.30
         branch 362.36
         central (total) 362.35
         incipient 362.37
         partial 362.37
         tributary 362.36
   spinal artery 433.8●
   stent
      coronary 996.72
   teeth (mandibular) (posterior lingual) 524.29
   thoracic duct 457.1
   tubal 628.2
   ureter (complete) (partial) 593.4
      congenital 753.29
   urethra (*see also* Stricture, urethra) 598.9
      congenital 753.6
   uterus 621.8
   vagina 623.2
   vascular NEC 459.9
   vein - *see* Thrombosis
   vena cava
      inferior 453.2
      superior (acute) 453.87
         chronic 453.77
   ventricle (brain) NEC 331.4
   vertebral (artery) - *see* Occlusion, artery, vertebral
   vessel (blood) NEC 459.9
   vulva 624.8
Occlusio pupillae 364.74
Occupational
   problems NEC V62.29
   therapy V57.21
Ochlophobia 300.29
Ochronosis (alkaptonuric) (congenital) (endogenous) 270.2
   with chloasma of eyelid 270.2
Ocular muscle - *see also* condition
   myopathy 359.1
   torticollis 781.93
Oculoauriculovertebral dysplasia 756.0
Oculogyric
   crisis or disturbance 378.87
      psychogenic 306.7

Oculomotor syndrome 378.81
Oddi's sphincter spasm 576.5
Odelberg's disease (juvenile osteochondrosis) 732.1
Odontalgia 525.9
Odontoameloblastoma (M9311/0) 213.1
    upper jaw (bone) 213.0
Odontoclasia 521.05
Odontoclasis 873.63
    complicated 873.73
Odontodysplasia, regional 520.4
Odontogenesis imperfecta 520.5
Odontoma (M9280/0) 213.1
    ameloblastic (M9311/0) 213.1
        upper jaw (bone) 213.0
    calcified (M9280/0) 213.1
        upper jaw (bone) 213.0
    complex (M9282/0) 213.1
        upper jaw (bone) 213.0
    compound (M9281/0) 213.1
        upper jaw (bone) 213.0
    fibroameloblastic (M9290/0) 213.1
        upper jaw (bone) 213.0
    follicular 526.0
        upper jaw (bone) 213.0
Odontomyelitis (closed) (open) 522.0
Odontonecrosis 521.09
Odontorrhagia 525.8
Odontosarcoma, ameloblastic (M9290/3) 170.1
    upper jaw (bone) 170.0
Odynophagia 787.20
Oesophagostomiasis 127.7
Oesophagostomum infestation 127.7
Oestriasis 134.0
Ogilvie's syndrome (sympathicotonic colon obstruction) 560.89
Oguchi's disease (retina) 368.61
Ohara's disease (see also Tularemia) 021.9
Oidiomycosis (see also Candidiasis) 112.9
Oidiomycotic meningitis 112.83
Oidium albicans infection (see also Candidiasis) 112.9
Old age 797
    dementia (of) 290.0
Olfactory - see condition
Oligemia 285.9
Oligergasia (see also Disability, intellectual) 319
Oligoamnios 658.0●
    affecting fetus or newborn 761.2
Oligoastrocytoma, mixed (M9382/3)
    specified site - see Neoplasm, by site, malignant
    unspecified site 191.9
Oligocythemia 285.9
Oligodendroblastoma (M9460/3)
    specified site - see Neoplasm, by site, malignant
    unspecified site 191.9
Oligodendroglioma (M9450/3)
    anaplastic type (M9451/3)
        specified site - see Neoplasm, by site, malignant
        unspecified site 191.9
    specified site - see Neoplasm, by site, malignant
    unspecified site 191.9
Oligodendroma - see Oligodendroglioma
Oligodontia (see also Anodontia) 520.0
Oligoencephalon 742.1
Oligohydramnios 658.0●
    affecting fetus or newborn 761.2
    due to premature rupture of membranes 658.1●
        affecting fetus or newborn 761.2
Oligohydrosis 705.0
Oligomenorrhea 626.1
Oligophrenia (see also Disability, intellectual) 319
    phenylpyruvic 270.1
Oligospermia 606.1

Oligotrichia 704.09
    congenita 757.4
Oliguria 788.5
    with
        abortion - see Abortion, by type, with renal failure
        ectopic pregnancy (see also categories 633.0–633.9) 639.3
        molar pregnancy (see also categories 630–632) 639.3
    complicating
        abortion 639.3
        ectopic or molar pregnancy 639.3
        pregnancy 646.2●
            with hypertension - see Toxemia, of pregnancy
    due to a procedure 997.5
    following labor and delivery 669.3●
    heart or cardiac - see Failure, heart
    puerperal, postpartum 669.3●
    specified due to a procedure 997.5
Ollier's disease (chondrodysplasia) 756.4
Omentitis (see also Peritonitis) 567.9
Omentocele (see also Hernia, omental) 553.8
Omentum, omental - see condition
Omphalitis (congenital) (newborn) 771.4
    not of newborn 686.9
    tetanus 771.3
Omphalocele 756.72
Omphalomesenteric duct, persistent 751.0
Omphalorrhagia, newborn 772.3
Omsk hemorrhagic fever 065.1
Onanism 307.9
Onchocerciasis 125.3
    eye 125.3 [360.13]
Onchocercosis 125.3
Oncocytoma (M8290/0) - see Neoplasm, by site, benign
Ondine's curse 348.89
Oneirophrenia (see also Schizophrenia) 295.4●
Onychauxis 703.8
    congenital 757.5
Onychia (with lymphangitis) 681.9
    dermatophytic 110.1
    finger 681.02
    toe 681.11
Onychitis (with lymphangitis) 681.9
    finger 681.02
    toe 681.11
Onychocryptosis 703.0
Onychodystrophy 703.8
    congenital 757.5
Onychogryphosis 703.8
Onychogryposis 703.8
Onycholysis 703.8
Onychomadesis 703.8
Onychomalacia 703.8
Onychomycosis 110.1
    finger 110.1
    toe 110.1
Onycho-osteodysplasia 756.89
Onychophagy 307.9
Onychoptosis 703.8
Onychorrhexis 703.8
    congenital 757.5
Onychoschizia 703.8
Onychotrophia (see also Atrophy, nail) 703.8
O'Nyong Nyong fever 066.3
Onyxis (finger) (toe) 703.0
Onyxitis (with lymphangitis) 681.9
    finger 681.02
    toe 681.11
Oocyte (egg) (ovum)
    donor V59.70
        over age 35 V59.73
            anonymous recipient V59.73
            designated recipient V59.74
        under age 35 V59.71
            anonymous recipient V59.71
            designated recipient V59.72

Oophoritis (cystic) (infectional) (interstitial) (see also Salpingo-oophoritis) 614.2
    complicating pregnancy 646.6●
    fetal (acute) 752.0
    gonococcal (acute) 098.19
        chronic or duration of 2 months or over 098.39
    tuberculous (see also Tuberculosis) 016.6●
Opacity, opacities
    cornea 371.00
        central 371.03
        congenital 743.43
            interfering with vision 743.42
        degenerative (see also Degeneration, cornea) 371.40
        hereditary (see also Dystrophy, cornea) 371.50
        inflammatory (see also Keratitis) 370.9
        late effect of trachoma (healed) 139.1
        minor 371.01
        peripheral 371.02
    enamel (fluoride) (nonfluoride) (teeth) 520.3
    lens (see also Cataract) 366.9
    snowball 379.22
    vitreous (humor) 379.24
        congenital 743.51
Opalescent dentin (hereditary) 520.5
Open, opening
    abnormal, organ or site, congenital - see Imperfect, closure
    angle
        with
            borderline findings
                high risk 365.05
                intraocular pressure 365.01
                low risk 365.01
                cupping of discs 365.01
            high risk 365.05
            low risk 365.01
    bite
        anterior 524.24
        posterior 524.25
    false - see Imperfect, closure
    margin on tooth restoration 525.61
    restoration margins 525.61
    wound - see Wound, open, by site
Operation
    causing mutilation of fetus 763.89
    destructive, on live fetus, to facilitate birth 763.89
    for delivery, fetus or newborn 763.89
    maternal, unrelated to current delivery, affecting fetus or newborn (see also Newborn, affected by) 760.64
Operational fatigue 300.89
Operative - see condition
Operculitis (chronic) 523.40
    acute 523.30
Operculum, retina 361.32
    with detachment 361.01
Ophiasis 704.01
Ophthalmia (see also Conjunctivitis) 372.30
    actinic rays 370.24
    allergic (acute) 372.05
        chronic 372.14
    blennorrhagic (neonatorum) 098.40
    catarrhal 372.03
    diphtheritic 032.81
    Egyptian 076.1
    electric, electrica 370.24
    gonococcal (neonatorum) 098.40
    metastatic 360.11
    migraine 346.8●
    neonatorum, newborn 771.6
        gonococcal 098.40
    nodosa 360.14
    phlyctenular 370.31
        with ulcer (see also Ulcer, cornea) 370.00
    sympathetic 360.11
Ophthalmitis - see Ophthalmia
Ophthalmocele (congenital) 743.66

SECTION I INDEX TO DISEASES AND INJURIES / Osteochondrosis

Ophthalmoneuromyelitis 341.0
Ophthalmopathy, infiltrative with thyrotoxicosis 242.0●
Ophthalmoplegia (see also Strabismus) 378.9
   anterior internuclear 378.86
   ataxia-areflexia syndrome 357.0
   bilateral 378.9
   diabetic 250.5● [378.86]
      due to secondary diabetes 249.5● [378.86]
   exophthalmic 242.0● [376.22]
   external 378.55
      progressive 378.72
      total 378.56
   internal (complete) (total) 367.52
   internuclear 378.86
   migraine 346.2●
   painful 378.55
   Parinaud's 378.81
   progressive external 378.72
   supranuclear, progressive 333.0
   total (external) 378.56
      internal 367.52
   unilateral 378.9
Opisthognathism 524.00
Opisthorchiasis (felineus) (tenuicollis) (viverrini) 121.0
Opisthotonos, opisthotonus 781.0
Opitz's disease (congestive splenomegaly) 289.51
Opiumism (see also Dependence) 304.0●
Oppenheim's disease 358.8
Oppenheim-Urbach disease or syndrome (necrobiosis lipoidica diabeticorum) 250.8● [709.3]
   due to secondary diabetes 249.8● [709.3]
Opsoclonia 379.59
Optic nerve - see condition
Orbit - see condition
Orchioblastoma (M9071/3) 186.9
Orchitis (nonspecific) (septic) 604.90
   with abscess 604.0
   blennorrhagic (acute) 098.13
      chronic or duration of 2 months or over 098.33
   diphtheritic 032.89 [604.91]
   filarial 125.9 [604.91]
   gangrenous 604.99
   gonococcal (acute) 098.13
      chronic or duration of 2 months or over 098.33
   mumps 072.0
   parotidea 072.0
   suppurative 604.99
   syphilitic 095.8 [604.91]
   tuberculous (see also Tuberculosis) 016.5● [608.81]
Orf 051.2
Organic - see also condition
   heart - see Disease, heart
   insufficiency 799.89
Oriental
   bilharziasis 120.2
   schistosomiasis 120.2
   sore 085.1
Orientation
   ego-dystonic sexual 302.0
Orifice - see condition
Origin, both great vessels from right ventricle 745.11
Ormond's disease or syndrome 593.4
Ornithosis 073.9
   with
      complication 073.8
         specified NEC 073.7
      pneumonia 073.0
      pneumonitis (lobular) 073.0
Orodigitofacial dysostosis 759.89
Oropouche fever 066.3
Orotaciduria, oroticaciduria (congenital) (hereditary) (pyrimidine deficiency) 281.4
Oroya fever 088.0

Orthodontics V58.5
   adjustment V53.4
   aftercare V58.5
   fitting V53.4
Orthopnea 786.02
Os, uterus - see condition
Osgood-Schlatter
   disease 732.4
   osteochondrosis 732.4
Osler's
   disease (M9950/1) (polycythemia vera) 238.4
   nodes 421.0
Osler-Rendu disease (familial hemorrhagic telangiectasia) 448.0
Osler-Vaquez disease (M9950/1) (polycythemia vera) 238.4
Osler-Weber-Rendu syndrome (familial hemorrhagic telangiectasia) 448.0
Osmidrosis 705.89
Osseous - see condition
Ossification
   artery - see Arteriosclerosis
   auricle (ear) 380.39
   bronchus 519.19
   cardiac (see also Degeneration, myocardial) 429.1
   cartilage (senile) 733.99
   coronary - see Arteriosclerosis, coronary
   diaphragm 728.10
   ear 380.39
      middle (see also Otosclerosis) 387.9
   falx cerebri 349.2
   fascia 728.10
   fontanel
      defective or delayed 756.0
      premature 756.0
   heart (see also Degeneration, myocardial) 429.1
      valve - see Endocarditis
   larynx 478.79
   ligament
      posterior longitudinal 724.8
         cervical 723.7
   meninges (cerebral) 349.2
      spinal 336.8
   multiple, eccentric centers 733.99
   muscle 728.10
      heterotopic, postoperative 728.13
   myocardium, myocardial (see also Degeneration, myocardial) 429.1
   penis 607.81
   periarticular 728.89
   sclera 379.16
   tendon 727.82
   trachea 519.19
   tympanic membrane (see also Tympanosclerosis) 385.00
   vitreous (humor) 360.44
Osteitis (see also Osteomyelitis) 730.2●
   acute 730.0●
   alveolar 526.5
   chronic 730.1●
   condensans (ilii) 733.5
   deformans (Paget's) 731.0
      due to or associated with malignant neoplasm (see also Neoplasm, bone, malignant) 170.9 [731.1]
   due to yaws 102.6
   fibrosa NEC 733.29
      cystica (generalisata) 252.01
      disseminata 756.59
      osteoplastica 252.01
   fragilitans 756.51
   Garré's (sclerosing) 730.1●
   infectious (acute) (subacute) 730.0●
      chronic or old 730.1●
   jaw (acute) (chronic) (lower) (neonatal) (suppurative) (upper) 526.4
   parathyroid 252.01
   petrous bone (see also Petrositis) 383.20
   pubis 733.5

Osteitis (Continued)
   sclerotic, nonsuppurative 730.1●
   syphilitic 095.5
   tuberculosa
      cystica (of Jüngling) 135
      multiplex cystoides 135
Osteoarthritica spondylitis (spine) (see also Spondylosis) 721.90
Osteoarthritis (see also Osteoarthrosis) 715.9●
   distal interphalangeal 715.9●
   hyperplastic 731.2
   interspinalis (see also Spondylosis) 721.90
   spine, spinal NEC (see also Spondylosis) 721.90
Osteoarthropathy (see also Osteoarthrosis) 715.9●
   chronic idiopathic hypertrophic 757.39
   familial idiopathic 757.39
   hypertrophic pulmonary 731.2
      secondary 731.2
   idiopathic hypertrophic 757.39
   primary hypertrophic 731.2
   pulmonary hypertrophic 731.2
   secondary hypertrophic 731.2
Osteoarthrosis (degenerative) (hypertrophic) (rheumatoid) 715.9●

> Note: Use the following fifth-digit subclassification with category 715:
> 0   site unspecified
> 1   shoulder region
> 2   upper arm
> 3   forearm
> 4   hand
> 5   pelvic region and thigh
> 6   lower leg
> 7   ankle and foot
> 8   other specified sites except spine
> 9   multiple sites

   Deformans alkaptonurica 270.2
   generalized 715.09
   juvenilis (Köhler's) 732.5
   localized 715.3●
      idiopathic 715.1●
      primary 715.1●
      secondary 715.2●
   multiple sites, not specified as generalized 715.89
   polyarticular 715.09
   spine (see also Spondylosis) 721.90
   temporomandibular joint 524.69
Osteoblastoma (M9200/0) - see Neoplasm, bone, benign
Osteochondritis (see also Osteochondrosis) 732.9
   dissecans 732.7
      hip 732.7
   ischiopubica 732.1
   multiple 756.59
   syphilitic (congenital) 090.0
Osteochondrodermodysplasia 756.59
Osteochondrodystrophy 277.5
   deformans 277.5
   familial 277.5
   fetalis 756.4
Osteochondrolysis 732.7
Osteochondroma (M9210/0) - see also Neoplasm, bone, benign
   multiple, congenital 756.4
Osteochondromatosis (M9210/1) 238.0
   synovial 727.82
Osteochondromyxosarcoma (M9180/3) - see Neoplasm, bone, malignant
Osteochondropathy NEC 732.9
Osteochondrosarcoma (M9180/3) - see Neoplasm, bone, malignant
Osteochondrosis 732.9
   acetabulum 732.1
   adult spine 732.8
   astragalus 732.5
   Blount's 732.4

Osteochondrosis (Continued)
  Buchanan's (juvenile osteochondrosis of iliac crest) 732.1
  Buchman's (juvenile osteochondrosis) 732.1
  Burns' 732.3
  calcaneus 732.5
  capitular epiphysis (femur) 732.1
  carpal
    lunate (wrist) 732.3
    scaphoid 732.3
  coxae juvenilis 732.1
  deformans juvenilis (coxae) (hip) 732.1
    Scheuermann's 732.0
    spine 732.0
    tibia 732.4
    vertebra 732.0
  Diaz's (astragalus) 732.5
  dissecans (knee) (shoulder) 732.7
  femoral capital epiphysis 732.1
  femur (head) (juvenile) 732.1
  foot (juvenile) 732.5
  Freiberg's (disease) (second metatarsal) 732.5
  Haas' 732.3
  Haglund's (os tibiale externum) 732.5
  hand (juvenile) 732.3
  head of
    femur 732.1
    humerus (juvenile) 732.3
  hip (juvenile) 732.1
  humerus (juvenile) 732.3
  iliac crest (juvenile) 732.1
  ilium (juvenile) 732.1
  ischiopubic synchondrosis 732.1
  Iselin's (osteochondrosis fifth metatarsal) 732.5
  juvenile, juvenilis 732.6
    arm 732.3
    capital femoral epiphysis 732.1
    capitellum humeri 732.3
    capitular epiphysis 732.1
    carpal scaphoid 732.3
    clavicle, sternal epiphysis 732.6
    coxae 732.1
    deformans 732.1
    foot 732.5
    hand 732.3
    hip and pelvis 732.1
    lower extremity, except foot 732.4
    lunate, wrist 732.3
    medial cuneiform bone 732.5
    metatarsal (head) 732.5
    metatarsophalangeal 732.5
    navicular, ankle 732.5
    patella 732.4
    primary patellar center (of Köhler) 732.4
    specified site NEC 732.6
    spine 732.0
    tarsal scaphoid 732.5
    tibia (epiphysis) (tuberosity) 732.4
    upper extremity 732.3
    vertebra (body) (Calvé) 732.0
      epiphyseal plates (of Scheuermann) 732.0
  Kienböck's (disease) 732.3
  Köhler's (disease) (navicular, ankle) 732.5
    patellar 732.4
    tarsal navicular 732.5
  Legg-Calvé-Perthes (disease) 732.1
  lower extremity (juvenile) 732.4
  lunate bone 732.3
  Mauclaire's 732.3
  metacarpal heads (of Mauclaire) 732.3
  metatarsal (fifth) (head) (second) 732.5
  navicular, ankle 732.5
  os calcis 732.5
  Osgood-Schlatter 732.4
  os tibiale externum 732.5
  Panner's 732.3
  patella (juvenile) 732.4

Osteochondrosis (Continued)
  patellar center
    primary (of Köhler) 732.4
    secondary (of Sinding-Larsen) 732.4
  pelvis (juvenile) 732.1
  Pierson's 732.1
  radial head (juvenile) 732.3
  Scheuermann's 732.0
  Sever's (calcaneum) 732.5
  Sinding-Larsen (secondary patellar center) 732.4
  spine (juvenile) 732.0
    adult 732.8
  symphysis pubis (of Pierson) (juvenile) 732.1
  syphilitic (congenital) 090.0
  tarsal (navicular) (scaphoid) 732.5
  tibia (proximal) (tubercle) 732.4
  tuberculous - see Tuberculosis, bone
  ulna 732.3
  upper extremity (juvenile) 732.3
  van Neck's (juvenile osteochondrosis) 732.1
  vertebral (juvenile) 732.0
    adult 732.8
Osteoclastoma (M9250/1) 238.0
  malignant (M9250/3) - see Neoplasm, bone, malignant
Osteocopic pain 733.90
Osteodynia 733.90
Osteodystrophy
  azotemic 588.0
  chronica deformans hypertrophica 731.0
  congenital 756.50
    specified type NEC 756.59
  deformans 731.0
  fibrosa localisata 731.0
  parathyroid 252.01
  renal 588.0
Osteofibroma (M9262/0) - see Neoplasm, bone, benign
Osteofibrosarcoma (M9182/3) - see Neoplasm, bone, malignant
Osteogenesis imperfecta 756.51
Osteogenic - see condition
Osteoma (M9180/0) - see also Neoplasm, bone, benign
  osteoid (M9191/0) - see also Neoplasm, bone, benign
    giant (M9200/0) - see Neoplasm, bone, benign
Osteomalacia 268.2
  chronica deformans hypertrophica 731.0
  due to vitamin D deficiency 268.2
  infantile (see also Rickets) 268.0
  juvenile (see also Rickets) 268.0
  oncogenic 275.8
  pelvis 268.2
  vitamin D-resistant 275.3
Osteomalacic bone 268.2
Osteomalacosis 268.2
Osteomyelitis (general) (infective) (localized) (neonatal) (purulent) (pyogenic) (septic) (staphylococcal) (streptococcal) (suppurative) (with periostitis) 730.2●

Note: Use the following fifth-digit subclassification with category 730:

  0 site unspecified
  1 shoulder region
  2 upper arm
  3 forearm
  4 hand
  5 pelvic region and thigh
  6 lower leg
  7 ankle and foot
  8 other specified sites
  9 multiple sites

  acute or subacute 730.0●
  chronic or old 730.1●

Osteomyelitis (Continued)
  due to or associated with
    diabetes mellitus 250.8● [731.8]
      due to secondary diabetes 249.8● [731.8]
    tuberculosis (see also Tuberculosis, bone) 015.9● [730.8]●
      limb bones 015.5● [730.8]●
      specified bones NEC 015.7● [730.8]●
      spine 015.0● [730.8]●
    typhoid 002.0 [730.8]●
  Garré's 730.1●
  jaw (acute) (chronic) (lower) (neonatal) (suppurative) (upper) 526.4
  nonsuppurating 730.1●
  orbital 376.03
  petrous bone (see also Petrositis) 383.20
  Salmonella 003.24
  sclerosing, nonsuppurative 730.1●
  sicca 730.1●
  syphilitic 095.5
    congenital 090.0 [730.8]●
  tuberculous - see Tuberculosis, bone
  typhoid 002.0 [730.8]●
Osteomyelofibrosis 289.89
Osteomyelosclerosis 289.89
Osteonecrosis 733.40
  meaning osteomyelitis 730.1●
Osteo-onycho-arthro dysplasia 756.89
Osteo-onychodysplasia, hereditary 756.89
Osteopathia
  condensans disseminata 756.53
  hyperostotica multiplex infantilis 756.59
  hypertrophica toxica 731.2
  striata 756.4
Osteopathy resulting from poliomyelitis (see also Poliomyelitis) 045.9● [730.7]
  familial dysplastic 731.2
Osteopecilia 756.53
Osteopenia 733.90
  borderline 733.90
Osteoperiostitis (see also Osteomyelitis) 730.2●
  ossificans toxica 731.2
  toxica ossificans 731.2
Osteopetrosis (familial) 756.52
Osteophyte - see Exostosis
Osteophytosis - see Exostosis
Osteopoikilosis 756.53
Osteoporosis (generalized) 733.00
  circumscripta 731.0
  disuse 733.03
  drug-induced 733.09
  idiopathic 733.02
  postmenopausal 733.01
  posttraumatic 733.7
  screening V82.81
  senile 733.01
  specified type NEC 733.09
Osteoporosis-osteomalacia syndrome 268.2
Osteopsathyrosis 756.51
Osteoradionecrosis, jaw 526.89
Osteosarcoma (M9180/3) - see also Neoplasm, bone, malignant
  chondroblastic (M9181/3) - see Neoplasm, bone, malignant
  fibroblastic (M9182/3) - see Neoplasm, bone, malignant
  in Paget's disease of bone (M9184/3) - see Neoplasm, bone, malignant
  juxtacortical (M9190/3) - see Neoplasm, bone, malignant
  parosteal (M9190/3) - see Neoplasm, bone, malignant
  telangiectatic (M9183/3) - see Neoplasm, bone, malignant
Osteosclerosis 756.52
  fragilis (generalisata) 756.52
Osteosclerotic anemia 289.89
Osteosis
  acromegaloid 757.39
  cutis 709.3

Osteosis (Continued)
  parathyroid 252.01
  renal fibrocystic 588.0
Österreicher-Turner syndrome 756.89
Ostium
  atrioventriculare commune 745.69
  primum (arteriosum) (defect) (persistent) 745.61
  secundum (arteriosum) (defect) (patent) (persistent) 745.5
Ostrum-Furst syndrome 756.59
Otalgia 388.70
  otogenic 388.71
  referred 388.72
Othematoma 380.31
Otitic hydrocephalus 348.2
Otitis 382.9
  with effusion 381.4
    purulent 382.4
    secretory 381.4
    serous 381.4
    suppurative 382.4
  acute 382.9
  adhesive (see also Adhesions, middle ear) 385.10
  chronic 382.9
    with effusion 381.3
    mucoid, mucous (simple) 381.20
    purulent 382.3
    secretory 381.3
    serous 381.10
    suppurative 382.3
  diffuse parasitic 136.8
  externa (acute) (diffuse) (hemorrhagica) 380.10
    actinic 380.22
    candidal 112.82
    chemical 380.22
    chronic 380.23
      mycotic - see Otitis, externa, mycotic
      specified type NEC 380.23
    circumscribed 380.10
    contact 380.22
    due to
      erysipelas 035 [380.13]
      impetigo 684 [380.13]
      seborrheic dermatitis 690.10 [380.13]
    eczematoid 380.22
    furuncular 680.0 [380.13]
    infective 380.10
      chronic 380.16
    malignant 380.14
    mycotic (chronic) 380.15
      due to
        aspergillosis 117.3 [380.15]
        moniliasis 112.82
        otomycosis 111.8 [380.15]
    reactive 380.22
    specified type NEC 380.22
    tropical 111.8 [380.15]
  insidiosa (see also Otosclerosis) 387.9
  interna (see also Labyrinthitis) 386.30
  media (hemorrhagic) (staphylococcal) (streptococcal) 382.9
    acute 382.9
      with effusion 381.00
        allergic 381.04
          mucoid 381.05
          sanguineous 381.06
          serous 381.04
        catarrhal 381.00
        exudative 381.00
        mucoid 381.02
          allergic 381.05
        necrotizing 382.00
          with spontaneous rupture of ear drum 382.01
        in
          influenza (see also Influenza) 487.8 [382.02]
          measles 055.2
          scarlet fever 034.1 [382.02]

Otitis (Continued)
  media (Continued)
    acute (Continued)
      nonsuppurative 381.00
      purulent 382.00
        with spontaneous rupture of ear drum 382.01
      sanguineous 381.03
        allergic 381.06
      secretory 381.01
      seromucinous 381.02
      serous 381.01
        allergic 381.04
      suppurative 382.00
        with spontaneous rupture of ear drum 382.01
        due to
          influenza (see also Influenza) 487.8 [382.02]
          scarlet fever 034.1 [382.02]
      transudative 381.00
    adhesive (see also Adhesions, middle ear) 385.10
    allergic 381.4
      acute 381.04
        mucoid 381.05
        sanguineous 381.06
        serous 381.04
      chronic 381.3
    catarrhal 381.4
      acute 381.00
      chronic (simple) 381.10
    chronic 382.9
      with effusion 381.3
      adhesive (see also Adhesions, middle ear) 385.10
      allergic 381.3
      atticoantral, suppurative (with posterior or superior marginal perforation of ear drum) 382.2
      benign suppurative (with anterior perforation of ear drum) 382.1
      catarrhal 381.10
      exudative 381.3
      mucinous 381.20
      mucoid, mucous (simple) 381.20
      mucosanguineous 381.29
      nonsuppurative 381.3
      purulent 382.3
      secretory 381.3
      seromucinous 381.3
      serosanguineous 381.19
      serous (simple) 381.10
      suppurative 382.3
        atticoantral (with posterior or superior marginal perforation of ear drum) 382.2
        benign (with anterior perforation of ear drum) 382.1
        tuberculous (see also Tuberculosis) 017.4●
        tubotympanic 382.1
      transudative 381.3
    exudative 381.4
      acute 381.00
      chronic 381.3
    fibrotic (see also Adhesions, middle ear) 385.10
    mucoid, mucous 381.4
      acute 381.02
      chronic (simple) 381.20
    mucosanguineous, chronic 381.29
    nonsuppurative 381.4
      acute 381.00
      chronic 381.3
    postmeasles 055.2
    purulent 382.4
      acute 382.00
        with spontaneous rupture of ear drum 382.01
      chronic 382.3

Otitis (Continued)
  media (Continued)
    sanguineous, acute 381.03
      allergic 381.06
    secretory 381.4
      acute or subacute 381.01
      chronic 381.3
    seromucinous 381.4
      acute or subacute 381.02
      chronic 381.3
    serosanguineous, chronic 381.19
    serous 381.4
      acute or subacute 381.01
      chronic (simple) 381.10
    subacute - see Otitis, media, acute
    suppurative 382.4
      acute 382.00
        with spontaneous rupture of ear drum 382.01
      chronic 382.3
        atticoantral 382.2
        benign 382.1
        tuberculous (see also Tuberculosis) 017.4●
        tubotympanic 382.1
    transudative 381.4
      acute 381.00
      chronic 381.3
    tuberculous (see also Tuberculosis) 017.4●
    postmeasles 055.2
Otoconia 386.8
Otolith syndrome 386.19
Otomycosis 111.8 [380.15]
  in
    aspergillosis 117.3 [380.15]
    moniliasis 112.82
Otopathy 388.9
Otoporosis (see also Otosclerosis) 387.9
Otorrhagia 388.69
  traumatic - see nature of injury
Otorrhea 388.60
  blood 388.69
  cerebrospinal (fluid) 388.61
Otosclerosis (general) 387.9
  cochlear (endosteal) 387.2
  involving
    otic capsule 387.2
    oval window
      nonobliterative 387.0
      obliterative 387.1
    round window 387.2
  nonobliterative 387.0
  obliterative 387.1
  specified type NEC 387.8
Otospongiosis (see also Otosclerosis) 387.9
Otto's disease or pelvis 715.35
Outburst, aggressive (see also Disturbance, conduct) 312.0●
  in children or adolescents 313.9
Outcome of delivery
  multiple birth NEC V27.9
    all liveborn V27.5
    all stillborn V27.7
    some liveborn V27.6
    unspecified V27.9
  single V27.9
    liveborn V27.0
    stillborn V27.1
  twins V27.9
    both liveborn V27.2
    both stillborn V27.4
    one liveborn, one stillborn V27.3
Outlet - see also condition
  syndrome (thoracic) 353.0
Outstanding ears (bilateral) 744.29
Ovalocytosis (congenital) (hereditary) (see also Elliptocytosis) 282.1
Ovarian - see also condition
  pregnancy - see Pregnancy, ovarian
  remnant syndrome 620.8
  vein syndrome 593.4

SECTION I INDEX TO DISEASES AND INJURIES / Ovaritis

Ovaritis (cystic) (*see also* Salpingo-oophoritis) 614.2
Ovary, ovarian - *see* condition
Overactive - *see also* Hyperfunction
    bladder 596.51
    eye muscle (*see also* Strabismus) 378.9
    hypothalamus 253.8
    thyroid (*see also* Thyrotoxicosis) 242.9●
Overactivity, child 314.01
Overbite (deep) (excessive) (horizontal) (vertical) 524.29
Overbreathing (*see also* Hyperventilation) 786.01
Overconscientious personality 301.4
Overdevelopment - *see also* Hypertrophy
    breast (female) (male) 611.1
    nasal bones 738.0
    prostate, congenital 752.89
Overdistention - *see* Distention
Overdose, overdosage (drug) 977.9
    specified drug or substance - *see* Table of Drugs and Chemicals
Overeating 783.6
    nonorganic origin 307.51
Overexertion (effects) (exhaustion) 994.5
Overexposure (effects) 994.9
    exhaustion 994.4
Overfeeding (*see also* Overeating) 783.6
Overfill, endodontic 526.62
Overgrowth, bone NEC 733.99
Overhanging
    tooth restoration 525.62
    unrepairable, dental restorative materials 525.62
Overheated (effects) (places) - *see* Heat
Overinhibited child 313.0

Overjet 524.29
    excessive horizontal 524.26
Overlaid, overlying (suffocation) 994.7
Overlap
    excessive horizontal 524.26
Overlapping toe (acquired) 735.8
    congenital (fifth toe) 755.66
Overload
    fluid 276.69
        due to transfusion (blood) (blood components) 276.61
    iron, due to repeated red blood cell transfusions 275.02
    potassium (K) 276.7
    sodium (Na) 276.0
    transfusion associated circulatory (TACO) 276.61
Overnutrition (*see also* Hyperalimentation) 783.6
Overproduction - *see also* Hypersecretion
    ACTH 255.3
    cortisol 255.0
    growth hormone 253.0
    thyroid-stimulating hormone (TSH) 242.8●
Overriding
    aorta 747.21
    finger (acquired) 736.29
        congenital 755.59
    toe (acquired) 735.8
        congenital 755.66
Oversize
    fetus (weight of 4500 grams or more) 766.0
        affecting management of pregnancy 656.6●

Oversize (*Continued*)
    fetus (*Continued*)
        causing disproportion 653.5●
            with obstructed labor 660.1●
        affecting fetus or newborn 763.1
Overstimulation, ovarian 256.1
Overstrained 780.79
    heart - *see* Hypertrophy, cardiac
Overweight (*see also* Obesity) 278.02
Overwork 780.79
Oviduct - *see* condition
Ovotestis 752.7
Ovulation (cycle)
    failure or lack of 628.0
    pain 625.2
Ovum
    blighted 631.8
    donor V59.70
        over age 35 V59.73
            anonymous recipient V59.73
            designated recipient V59.74
        under age 35 V59.71
            anonymous recipient V59.71
            designated recipient V59.72
    dropsical 631.8
    pathologic 631.8
Owren's disease or syndrome (parahemophilia) (*see also* Defect, coagulation) 286.3
Oxalosis 271.8
Oxaluria 271.8
Ox heart - *see* Hypertrophy, cardiac
OX syndrome 758.6
Oxycephaly, oxycephalic 756.0
    syphilitic, congenital 090.0
Oxyuriasis 127.4
Oxyuris vermicularis (infestation) 127.4
Ozena 472.0

P

Pacemaker syndrome 429.4
Pachyderma, pachydermia 701.8
   laryngis 478.5
   laryngitis 478.79
   larynx (verrucosa) 478.79
Pachydermatitis 701.8
Pachydermatocele (congenital) 757.39
   acquired 701.8
Pachydermatosis 701.8
Pachydermoperiostitis
   secondary 731.2
Pachydermoperiostosis
   primary idiopathic 757.39
   secondary 731.2
Pachymeningitis (adhesive) (basal) (brain) (cerebral) (cervical) (chronic) (circumscribed) (external) (fibrous) (hemorrhagic) (hypertrophic) (internal) (purulent) (spinal) (suppurative) (see also Meningitis) 322.9
   gonococcal 098.82
Pachyonychia (congenital) 757.5
   acquired 703.8
Pachyperiosteodermia
   primary or idiopathic 757.39
   secondary 731.2
Pachyperiostosis
   primary or idiopathic 757.39
   secondary 731.2
Pacinian tumor (M9507/0) - see Neoplasm, skin, benign
Pads, knuckle or Garrod's 728.79
Paget's disease (osteitis deformans) 731.0
   with infiltrating duct carcinoma of the breast (M8541/3) - see Neoplasm, breast, malignant
   bone 731.0
      osteosarcoma in (M9184/3) - see Neoplasm, bone, malignant
   breast (M8540/3) 174.0
   extramammary (M8542/3) - see also Neoplasm, skin, malignant
      anus 154.3
      skin 173.59
   malignant (M8540/3)
      breast 174.0
      specified site NEC (M8542/3) - see Neoplasm, skin, malignant
      unspecified site 174.0
   mammary (M8540/3) 174.0
   necrosis of bone 731.0
   nipple (M8540/3) 174.0
   osteitis deformans 731.0
Paget-Schroetter syndrome (intermittent venous claudication) 453.89
Pain(s) (see also Painful) 780.96
   abdominal 789.0
   acute 338.19
      due to trauma 338.11
      postoperative 338.18
         post-thoracotomy 338.12
   adnexa (uteri) 625.9
   alimentary, due to vascular insufficiency 557.9
   anginoid (see also Pain, precordial) 786.51
   anus 569.42
   arch 729.5
   arm 729.5
   axillary 729.5
   back (postural) 724.5
      low 724.2
      psychogenic 307.89
   bile duct 576.9
   bladder 788.99
   bone 733.90
   breast 611.71
      psychogenic 307.89
   broad ligament 625.9
   cancer associated 338.3

Pain(s) (Continued)
   cartilage NEC 733.90
   cecum 789.0
   cervicobrachial 723.3
   chest (central) 786.50
      atypical 786.59
      midsternal 786.51
      musculoskeletal 786.59
      noncardiac 786.59
      substernal 786.51
      wall (anterior) 786.52
   chronic 338.29
      associated with significant psychosocial dysfunction 338.4
      due to trauma 338.21
      postoperative 338.28
         post-thoracotomy 338.22
      syndrome 338.4
   coccyx 724.79
   colon 789.0
   common duct 576.9
   coronary - see Angina
   costochondral 786.52
   diaphragm 786.52
   due to (presence of) any device, implant, or graft classifiable to 996.0–996.5 - see Complications, due to (presence of) any device, implant, or graft classified to 996.0–996.5 NEC
   malignancy (primary) (secondary) 338.3
   ear (see also Otalgia) 388.70
   epigastric, epigastrium 789.06
   extremity (lower) (upper) 729.5
   eye 379.91
   face, facial 784.0
      atypical 350.2
      nerve 351.8
   false (labor) 644.1
   female genital organ NEC 625.9
      psychogenic 307.89
   finger 729.5
   flank 789.0
   foot 729.5
   gallbladder 575.9
   gas (intestinal) 787.3
   gastric 536.8
   generalized 780.96
   genital organ
      female 625.9
      male 608.9
      psychogenic 307.89
   groin 789.0
   growing 781.99
   hand 729.5
   head (see also Headache) 784.0
   heart (see also Pain, precordial) 786.51
   infraorbital (see also Neuralgia, trigeminal) 350.1
   intermenstrual 625.2
   jaw 784.92
   joint 719.40
      ankle 719.47
      elbow 719.42
      foot 719.47
      hand 719.44
      hip 719.45
      knee 719.46
      multiple sites 719.49
      pelvic region 719.45
      psychogenic 307.89
      shoulder (region) 719.41
      specified site NEC 719.48
      wrist 719.43
   kidney 788.0
   labor, false or spurious 644.1
   laryngeal 784.1
   leg 729.5
   limb 729.5
   low back 724.2
   lumbar region 724.2
   mandible, mandibular 784.92

Pain(s) (Continued)
   mastoid (see also Otalgia) 388.70
   maxilla 784.92
   menstrual 625.3
   metacarpophalangeal (joint) 719.44
   metatarsophalangeal (joint) 719.47
   mouth 528.9
   muscle 729.1
      intercostal 786.59
   musculoskeletal (see also Pain, by site) 729.1
   nasal 478.19
   nasopharynx 478.29
   neck NEC 723.1
      psychogenic 307.89
   neoplasm related (acute) (chronic) 338.3
   nerve NEC 729.2
   neuromuscular 729.1
   nose 478.19
   ocular 379.91
   ophthalmic 379.91
   orbital region 379.91
   osteocopic 733.90
   ovary 625.9
      psychogenic 307.89
   over heart (see also Pain, precordial) 786.51
   ovulation 625.2
   pelvic (female) 625.9
      male NEC 789.0
         psychogenic 307.89
      psychogenic 307.89
   penis 607.9
      psychogenic 307.89
   pericardial (see also Pain, precordial) 786.51
   perineum
      female 625.9
      male 608.9
   pharynx 478.29
   pleura, pleural, pleuritic 786.52
   postoperative 338.18
      acute 338.18
      chronic 338.28
   post-thoracotomy 338.12
      acute 338.12
      chronic 338.22
   preauricular 388.70
   precordial (region) 786.51
      psychogenic 307.89
   premenstrual 625.4
   psychogenic 307.80
      cardiovascular system 307.89
      gastrointestinal system 307.89
      genitourinary system 307.89
      heart 307.89
      musculoskeletal system 307.89
      respiratory system 307.89
      skin 306.3
   radicular (spinal) (see also Radiculitis) 729.2
   rectum 569.42
   respiration 786.52
   retrosternal 786.51
   rheumatic NEC 729.0
      muscular 729.1
   rib 786.50
   root (spinal) (see also Radiculitis) 729.2
   round ligament (stretch) 625.9
   sacroiliac 724.6
   sciatic 724.3
   scrotum 608.9
      psychogenic 307.89
   seminal vesicle 608.9
   sinus 478.19
   skin 782.0
   spermatic cord 608.9
   spinal root (see also Radiculitis) 729.2
   stomach 536.8
      psychogenic 307.89
   substernal 786.51
   temporomandibular (joint) 524.62
   testis 608.9
      psychogenic 307.89

SECTION 1 INDEX TO DISEASES AND INJURIES / Pain(s)

Pain(s) *(Continued)*
  thoracic spine 724.1
    with radicular and visceral pain 724.4
  throat 784.1
  tibia 733.90
  toe 729.5
  tongue 529.6
  tooth 525.9
  trigeminal (*see also* Neuralgia, trigeminal) 350.1
  tumor associated 338.3
  umbilicus 789.05
  ureter 788.0
  urinary (organ) (system) 788.0
  uterus 625.9
    psychogenic 307.89
  vagina 625.9
  vertebrogenic (syndrome) 724.5
  vesical 788.99
  vulva 625.9
  xiphoid 733.90
Painful - *see also* Pain
  arc syndrome 726.19
  coitus
    female 625.0
    male 608.89
    psychogenic 302.76
  ejaculation (semen) 608.89
    psychogenic 302.79
  erection 607.3
  feet syndrome 266.2
  menstruation 625.3
    psychogenic 306.52
  micturition 788.1
  ophthalmoplegia 378.55
  respiration 786.52
  scar NEC 709.2
  total hip replacement 996.77
  total knee replacement 996.77
  urination 788.1
  wire sutures 998.89
Painters' colic 984.9
  specified type of lead - *see* Table of Drugs and Chemicals
Palate - *see* condition
Palatoplegia 528.9
Palatoschisis (*see also* Cleft, palate) 749.00
Palilalia 784.69
Palindromic arthritis (*see also* Rheumatism, palindromic) 719.3●
Palliative care V66.7
Pallor 782.61
  temporal, optic disc 377.15
Palmar - *see also* condition
  fascia - *see* condition
Palpable
  cecum 569.89
  kidney 593.89
  liver 573.9
  lymph nodes 785.6
  ovary 620.8
  prostate 602.9
  spleen (*see also* Splenomegaly) 789.2
  uterus 625.8
Palpitation (heart) 785.1
  psychogenic 306.2
Palsy (*see also* Paralysis) 344.9
  atrophic diffuse 335.20
  Bell's 351.0
    newborn 767.5
  birth 767.7
  brachial plexus 353.0
    fetus or newborn 767.6
  brain - *see also* Palsy, cerebral
    noncongenital or noninfantile 344.89
      late effect - *see* Late effect(s) (of) cerebrovascular disease
    syphilitic 094.89
      congenital 090.49

Palsy *(Continued)*
  bulbar (chronic) (progressive) 335.22
    pseudo NEC 335.23
    supranuclear NEC 344.89
  cerebral (congenital) (infantile) (spastic) 343.9
    athetoid 333.71
    diplegic 343.0
      late effect - *see* Late effect(s) (of) cerebrovascular disease
    hemiplegic 343.1
    monoplegic 343.3
    noncongenital or noninfantile 437.8
      late effect - *see* Late effect(s) (of) cerebrovascular disease
    paraplegic 343.0
    quadriplegic 343.2
    spastic, not congenital or infantile 344.89
    syphilitic 094.89
      congenital 090.49
    tetraplegic 343.2
  cranial nerve - *see also* Disorder, nerve, cranial
    multiple 352.6
  creeping 335.21
  divers' 993.3
  Erb's (birth injury) 767.6
  facial 351.0
    newborn 767.5
  glossopharyngeal 352.2
  Klumpke (-Déjérine) 767.6
  lead 984.9
    specified type of lead - *see* Table of Drugs and Chemicals
  median nerve (tardy) 354.0
  peroneal nerve (acute) (tardy) 355.3
  progressive supranuclear 333.0
  pseudobulbar NEC 335.23
  radial nerve (acute) 354.3
  seventh nerve 351.0
    newborn 767.5
  shaking (*see also* Parkinsonism) 332.0
  spastic (cerebral) (spinal) 343.9
    hemiplegic 343.1
  specified nerve NEC - *see* Disorder, nerve
  supranuclear NEC 356.8
    progressive 333.0
  ulnar nerve (tardy) 354.2
  wasting 335.21
Paltauf-Sternberg disease 201.9●
Paludism - *see* Malaria
Panama fever 084.0
Panaris (with lymphangitis) 681.9
  finger 681.02
  toe 681.11
Panaritium (with lymphangitis) 681.9
  finger 681.02
  toe 681.11
Panarteritis (nodosa) 446.0
  brain or cerebral 437.4
Pancake heart 793.2
  with cor pulmonale (chronic) 416.9
Pancarditis (acute) (chronic) 429.89
  with
    rheumatic
      fever (active) (acute) (chronic) (subacute) 391.8
      inactive or quiescent 398.99
    rheumatic, acute 391.8
    chronic or inactive 398.99
Pancoast's syndrome or tumor (carcinoma, pulmonary apex) (M8010/3) 162.3
Pancoast-Tobias syndrome (M8010/3) (carcinoma, pulmonary apex) 162.3
Pancolitis 556.6
Pancreas, pancreatic - *see* condition
Pancreatitis 577.0
  acute (edematous) (hemorrhagic) (recurrent) 577.0
  annular 577.0
  apoplectic 577.0

Pancreatitis *(Continued)*
  calcereous 577.0
  chronic (infectious) 577.1
    recurrent 577.1
  cystic 577.2
  fibrous 577.8
  gangrenous 577.0
  hemorrhagic (acute) 577.0
  interstitial (chronic) 577.1
    acute 577.0
  malignant 577.0
  mumps 072.3
  painless 577.1
  recurrent 577.1
  relapsing 577.1
  subacute 577.0
  suppurative 577.0
  syphilitic 095.8
Pancreatolithiasis 577.8
Pancytolysis 289.9
Pancytopenia (acquired) 284.19
  with
    malformations 284.09
    myelodysplastic syndrome - *see* Syndrome, myelodysplastic
  congenital 284.09
  due to
    antineoplastic chemotherapy 284.11
    drug, specified NEC 284.12
  specified NEC 284.19
Panencephalitis - *see also* Encephalitis
  subacute, sclerosing 046.2
Panhematopenia 284.81
  congenital 284.09
  constitutional 284.09
  splenic, primary 289.4
Panhemocytopenia 284.81
  congenital 284.09
  constitutional 284.09
Panhypogonadism 257.2
Panhypopituitarism 253.2
  prepubertal 253.3
Panic (attack) (state) 300.01
  reaction to exceptional stress (transient) 308.0
Panmyelopathy, familial constitutional 284.09
Panmyelophthisis 284.2
  acquired (secondary) 284.81
  congenital 284.2
  idiopathic 284.9
Panmyelosis (acute) (M9951/1) 238.79
Panner's disease 732.3
  capitellum humeri 732.3
  head of humerus 732.3
  tarsal navicular (bone) (osteochondrosis) 732.5
Panneuritis endemica 265.0 [357.4]
Panniculitis 729.30
  back 724.8
  knee 729.31
  mesenteric 567.82
  neck 723.6
  nodular, nonsuppurative 729.30
  sacral 724.8
  specified site NEC 729.39
Panniculus adiposus (abdominal) 278.1
Pannus (corneal) 370.62
  abdominal (symptomatic) 278.1
  allergic eczematous 370.62
  degenerativus 370.62
  keratic 370.62
  rheumatoid - *see* Arthritis, rheumatoid
  trachomatosus, trachomatous (active) 076.1 [370.62]
  late effect 139.1
Panophthalmitis 360.02
Panotitis - *see* Otitis media
Pansinusitis (chronic) (hyperplastic) (nonpurulent) (purulent) 473.8
  acute 461.8
  due to fungus NEC 117.9
  tuberculous (*see also* Tuberculosis) 012.8●

Panuveitis 360.12
    sympathetic 360.11
Panvalvular disease - *see* Endocarditis, mitral
Papageienkrankheit 073.9
Papanicolaou smear
    anus 796.70
        with
            atypical squamous cells
                cannot exclude high grade
                    squamous intraepithelial
                    lesion (ASC-H) 796.72
                of undetermined significance
                    (ASC-US) 796.71
            cytologic evidence of malignancy
                796.76
            high grade squamous intraepithelial
                lesion (HGSIL) 796.74
            low grade squamous intraepithelial
                lesion (LGSIL) 796.73
    glandular 796.70
    specified finding NEC 796.79
    unsatisfactory cytology 796.78
    cervix (screening test) V76.2
        as part of gynecological examination
            V72.31
        for suspected malignant neoplasm V76.2
            no disease found V71.1
        inadequate cytology sample 795.08
        nonspecific abnormal finding 795.00
            with
                atypical squamous cells
                    cannot exclude high grade
                        squamous intraepithelial
                        lesion (ASC-H) 795.02
                    of undetermined significance
                        (ASC-US) 795.01
                cytologic evidence of malignancy
                    795.06
                high grade squamous
                    intraepithelial lesion (HGSIL)
                    795.04
                low grade squamous intraepithelial
                    lesion (LGSIL) 795.03
        nonspecific finding NEC 795.09
        to confirm findings of recent normal
            smear following initial abnormal
            smear V72.32
        satisfactory smear but lacking
            transformation zone 795.07
        unsatisfactory cervical cytology 795.08
    other specified site - *see also* Screening,
        malignant neoplasm
        for suspected malignant neoplasm - *see*
            also Screening, malignant neoplasm
            no disease found V71.1
        nonspecific abnormal finding 796.9
    vagina V76.47
        with
            atypical squamous cells
                cannot exclude high grade
                    squamous intraepithelial
                    lesion (ASC-H) 795.12
                of undetermined significance
                    (ASC-US) 795.11
            cytologic evidence of malignancy
                795.16
            high grade squamous
                intraepithelial lesion (HGSIL)
                795.14
            low grade squamous intraepithelial
                lesion (LGSIL) 795.13
        abnormal NEC 795.19
        following hysterectomy for malignant
            condition V67.01
        inadequate cytology sample 795.18
        unsatisfactory cytology 795.18
Papilledema 377.00
    associated with
        decreased ocular pressure 377.02
        increased intracranial pressure 377.01
        retinal disorder 377.03

Papilledema (*Continued*)
    choked disc 377.00
    infectional 377.00
Papillitis 377.31
    anus 569.49
    chronic lingual 529.4
    necrotizing, kidney 584.7
    optic 377.31
    rectum 569.49
    renal, necrotizing 584.7
    tongue 529.0
Papilloma (M8050/0) - *see also* Neoplasm, by
    site, benign

> Note: Except where otherwise indicated, the morphological varieties of papilloma in the list below should be coded by site as for "Neoplasm, benign".

    acuminatum (female) (male) 078.11
    bladder (urinary) (transitional cell)
        (M8120/1) 236.7
        benign (M8120/0) 223.3
    choroid plexus (M9390/0) 225.0
        anaplastic type (M9390/3) 191.5
        malignant (M9390/3) 191.5
    ductal (M8503/0)
    dyskeratotic (M8052/0)
    epidermoid (M8052/0)
    hyperkeratotic (M8052/0)
    intracystic (M8504/0)
    intraductal (M8503/0)
    inverted (M8053/0)
    keratotic (M8052/0)
    parakeratotic (M8052/0)
    pinta (primary) 103.0
    renal pelvis (transitional cell) (M8120/1)
        236.99
        benign (M8120/0) 223.1
    Schneiderian (M8121/0)
        specified site - *see* Neoplasm, by site,
            benign
        unspecified site 212.0
    serous surface (M8461/0)
        borderline malignancy (M8461/1)
            specified site - *see* Neoplasm, by site,
                uncertain behavior
            unspecified site 236.2
        specified site - *see* Neoplasm, by site,
            benign
        unspecified site 220
    squamous (cell) (M8052/0)
    transitional (cell) (M8120/0)
        bladder (urinary) (M8120/1) 236.7
        inverted type (M8121/1) - *see* Neoplasm,
            by site, uncertain behavior
        renal pelvis (M8120/1) 236.91
        ureter (M8120/1) 236.91
    ureter (transitional cell) (M8120/1)
        236.91
        benign (M8120/0) 223.2
    urothelial (M8120/1) - *see* Neoplasm, by site,
        uncertain behavior
    verrucous (M8051/0)
    villous (M8261/1) - *see* Neoplasm, by site,
        uncertain behavior
    yaws, plantar or palmar 102.1
Papillomata, multiple, of yaws 102.1
Papillomatosis (M8060/0) - *see also* Neoplasm,
    by site, benign
    confluent and reticulate 701.8
    cutaneous 701.8
    ductal, breast 610.1
    Gougerot-Carteaud (confluent reticulate)
        701.8
    intraductal (diffuse) (M8505/0) - *see*
        Neoplasm, by site, benign
    subareolar duct (M8506/0) 217
Papillon-Léage and Psaume syndrome
    (orodigitofacial dysostosis)
    759.89

Papule 709.8
    carate (primary) 103.0
    fibrous, of nose (M8724/0) 216.3
    pinta (primary) 103.0
Papulosis
    lymphomatoid 709.8
    malignant 447.8
Papyraceous fetus 779.89
    complicating pregnancy 646.0●
Paracephalus 759.7
Parachute mitral valve 746.5
Paracoccidioidomycosis 116.1
    mucocutaneous-lymphangitic 116.1
    pulmonary 116.1
    visceral 116.1
Paracoccidiomycosis - *see*
    Paracoccidioidomycosis
Paracusis 388.40
Paradentosis 523.5
Paradoxical facial movements 374.43
Paraffinoma 999.9
Paraganglioma (M8680/1)
    adrenal (M8700/0) 227.0
        malignant (M8700/3) 194.0
    aortic body (M8691/1) 237.3
        malignant (M8691/3) 194.6
    carotid body (M8692/1) 237.3
        malignant (M8692/3) 194.5
    chromaffin (M8700/0) - *see also* Neoplasm,
        by site, benign
        malignant (M8700/3) - *see* Neoplasm, by
            site, malignant
    extra-adrenal (M8693/1)
        malignant (M8693/3)
            specified site - *see* Neoplasm, by site,
                malignant
            unspecified site 194.6
        specified site - *see* Neoplasm, by site,
            uncertain behavior
        unspecified site 237.3
    glomus jugulare (M8690/1) 237.3
        malignant (M8690/3) 194.6
    jugular (M8690/1) 237.3
    malignant (M8680/3)
        specified site - *see* Neoplasm, by site,
            malignant
        unspecified site 194.6
    nonchromaffin (M8693/1)
        malignant (M8693/3)
            specified site - *see* Neoplasm, by site,
                malignant
            unspecified site 194.6
        specified site - *see* Neoplasm, by site,
            uncertain behavior
        unspecified site 237.3
    parasympathetic (M8682/1)
        specified site - *see* Neoplasm, by site,
            uncertain behavior
        unspecified site 237.3
    specified site - *see* Neoplasm, by site,
        uncertain behavior
    sympathetic (M8681/1)
        specified site - *see* Neoplasm, by site,
            uncertain behavior
        unspecified site 237.3
    unspecified site 237.3
Parageusia 781.1
    psychogenic 306.7
Paragonimiasis 121.2
Paragranuloma, Hodgkin's (M9660/3) 201.0●
Parahemophilia (*see also* Defect, coagulation)
    286.3
Parakeratosis 690.8
    psoriasiformis 696.2
    variegata 696.2
Paralysis, paralytic (complete) (incomplete)
    344.9
    with
        broken
            back - *see* Fracture, vertebra, by site,
                with spinal cord injury

SECTION I INDEX TO DISEASES AND INJURIES / Paralysis, paralytic

Paralysis, paralytic (Continued)
  with (Continued)
    broken (Continued)
      neck - see Fracture, vertebra, cervical, with spinal cord injury
      fracture, vertebra - see Fracture, vertebra, by site, with spinal cord injury
    syphilis 094.89
  abdomen and back muscles 355.9
  abdominal muscles 355.9
  abducens (nerve) 378.54
  abductor 355.9
    lower extremity 355.8
    upper extremity 354.9
  accessory nerve 352.4
  accommodation 367.51
    hysterical 300.11
  acoustic nerve 388.5
  agitans 332.0
    arteriosclerotic 332.0
  alternating 344.89
    oculomotor 344.89
  amyotrophic 335.20
  ankle 355.8
  anterior serratus 355.9
  anus (sphincter) 569.49
  apoplectic (current episode) (see also Disease, cerebrovascular, acute) 436
    late effect - see Late effect(s) (of) cerebrovascular disease
  arm 344.40
    affecting
      dominant side 344.41
      nondominant side 344.42
    both 344.2
    hysterical 300.11
    late effect - see Late effect(s) (of) cerebrovascular disease
    psychogenic 306.0
    transient 781.4
      traumatic NEC (see also Injury, nerve, upper limb) 955.9
  arteriosclerotic (current episode) 437.0
    late effect - see Late effect(s) (of) cerebrovascular disease
  ascending (spinal), acute 357.0
  associated, nuclear 344.89
  asthenic bulbar 358.00
  ataxic NEC 334.9
    general 094.1
  athetoid 333.71
  atrophic 356.9
    infantile, acute (see also Poliomyelitis, with paralysis) 045.1●
    muscle NEC 355.9
    progressive 335.21
    spinal (acute) (see also Poliomyelitis, with paralysis) 045.1●
  attack (see also Disease, cerebrovascular, acute) 436
  axillary 353.0
  Babinski-Nageotte's 344.89
  Bell's 351.0
    newborn 767.5
  Benedikt's 344.89
  birth (injury) 767.7
    brain 767.0
    intracranial 767.0
    spinal cord 767.4
  bladder (sphincter) 596.53
    neurogenic 596.54
      with cauda equina syndrome 344.61
    puerperal, postpartum, childbirth 665.5●
    sensory 596.54
      with cauda equina 344.61
    spastic 596.54
      with cauda equina 344.61
  bowel, colon, or intestine (see also Ileus) 560.1
  brachial plexus 353.0
    due to birth injury 767.6
    newborn 767.6

Paralysis, paralytic (Continued)
  brain
    congenital - see Palsy, cerebral
    current episode 437.8
    diplegia 344.2
      late effect - see Late effect(s) (of) cerebrovascular disease
    hemiplegia 342.9●
      late effect - see Late effect(s) (of) cerebrovascular disease
    infantile - see Palsy, cerebral
    monoplegia - see also Monoplegia
      late effect - see Late effect(s) (of) cerebrovascular disease
    paraplegia 344.1
    quadriplegia - see Quadriplegia
    syphilitic, congenital 090.49
    triplegia 344.89
  bronchi 519.19
  Brown-Séquard's 344.89
  bulbar (chronic) (progressive) 335.22
    infantile (see also Poliomyelitis, bulbar) 045.0●
    poliomyelitic (see also Poliomyelitis, bulbar) 045.0●
    pseudo 335.23
    supranuclear 344.89
  bulbospinal 358.00
  cardiac (see also Failure, heart) 428.9
  cerebral
    current episode 437.8
    spastic, infantile - see Palsy, cerebral
  cerebrocerebellar 437.8
    diplegic infantile 343.0
  cervical
    plexus 353.2
    sympathetic NEC 337.09
  Céstan-Chenais 344.89
  Charcôt-Marie-Tooth type 356.1
  childhood - see Palsy, cerebral
  Clark's 343.9
  colon (see also Ileus) 560.1
  compressed air 993.3
  compression
    arm NEC 354.9
    cerebral - see Paralysis, brain
    leg NEC 355.8
    lower extremity NEC 355.8
    upper extremity NEC 354.9
  congenital (cerebral) (spastic) (spinal) - see Palsy, cerebral
  conjugate movement (of eye) 378.81
  cortical (nuclear) (supranuclear) 378.81
  convergence 378.83
  cordis (see also Failure, heart) 428.9
  cortical (see also Paralysis, brain) 437.8
  cranial or cerebral nerve (see also Disorder, nerve, cranial) 352.9
  creeping 335.21
  crossed leg 344.89
  crutch 953.4
  deglutition 784.99
    hysterical 300.11
  dementia 094.1
  descending (spinal) NEC 335.9
  diaphragm (flaccid) 519.4
    due to accidental section of phrenic nerve during procedure 998.2
  digestive organs NEC 564.89
  diplegic - see Diplegia
  divergence (nuclear) 378.85
  divers' 993.3
  Duchenne's 335.22
  due to intracranial or spinal birth injury - see Palsy, cerebral
  embolic (current episode) (see also Embolism, brain) 434.1●
    late effect - see Late effect(s) (of) cerebrovascular disease

Paralysis, paralytic (Continued)
  enteric (see also Ileus) 560.1
    with hernia - see Hernia, by site, with obstruction
  Erb's syphilitic spastic spinal 094.89
  Erb (-Duchenne) (birth) (newborn) 767.6
  esophagus 530.89
  essential, infancy (see also Poliomyelitis) 045.9●
  extremity
    lower - see Paralysis, leg
    spastic (hereditary) 343.3
      noncongenital or noninfantile 344.1
    transient (cause unknown) 781.4
    upper - see Paralysis, arm
  eye muscle (extrinsic) 378.55
    intrinsic 367.51
  facial (nerve) 351.0
    birth injury 767.5
    congenital 767.5
    following operation NEC 998.2
    newborn 767.5
  familial 359.3
    periodic 359.3
    spastic 334.1
  fauces 478.29
  finger NEC 354.9
  foot NEC 355.8
  gait 781.2
  gastric nerve 352.3
  gaze 378.81
  general 094.1
    ataxic 094.1
    insane 094.1
    juvenile 090.40
    progressive 094.1
    tabetic 094.1
  glossopharyngeal (nerve) 352.2
  glottis (see also Paralysis, vocal cord) 478.30
  gluteal 353.4
  Gubler (-Millard) 344.89
  hand 354.9
    hysterical 300.11
    psychogenic 306.0
  heart (see also Failure, heart) 428.9
  hemifacial, progressive 349.89
  hemiplegic - see Hemiplegia
  hyperkalemic periodic (familial) 359.3
  hypertensive (current episode) 437.8
  hypoglossal (nerve) 352.5
  hypokalemic periodic 359.3
  Hyrtl's sphincter (rectum) 569.49
  hysterical 300.11
  ileus (see also Ileus) 560.1
  infantile (see also Poliomyelitis) 045.9●
    atrophic acute 045.1●
    bulbar 045.0●
    cerebral - see Palsy, cerebral
    paralytic 045.1●
    progressive acute 045.9●
    spastic - see Palsy, cerebral
    spinal 045.9●
  infective (see also Poliomyelitis) 045.9●
  inferior nuclear 344.9
  insane, general or progressive 094.1
  internuclear 378.86
  interosseous 355.9
  intestine (see also Ileus) 560.1
  intracranial (current episode) (see also Paralysis, brain) 437.8
    due to birth injury 767.0
  iris 379.49
    due to diphtheria (toxin) 032.81 [379.49]
  ischemic, Volkmann's (complicating trauma) 958.6
  isolated sleep, recurrent 327.43
  Jackson's 344.89
  jake 357.7
  Jamaica ginger (jake) 357.7
  juvenile general 090.40
  Klumpke (-Déjérine) (birth) (newborn) 767.6

Paralysis, paralytic *(Continued)*
  labioglossal (laryngeal) (pharyngeal) 335.22
  Landry's 357.0
  laryngeal nerve (recurrent) (superior) (*see also* Paralysis, vocal cord) 478.30
  larynx (*see also* Paralysis, vocal cord) 478.30
    due to diphtheria (toxin) 032.3
  late effect
    due to
      birth injury, brain or spinal (cord) - *see* Palsy, cerebral
      edema, brain or cerebral - *see* Paralysis, brain
      lesion
        late effect - *see* Late effect(s) (of) cerebrovascular disease
      spinal (cord) - *see* Paralysis, spinal
  lateral 335.24
  lead 984.9
    specified type of lead - *see* Table of Drugs and Chemicals
  left side - *see* Hemiplegia
  leg 344.30
    affecting
      dominant side 344.31
      nondominant side 344.32
    both (*see also* Paraplegia) 344.1
    crossed 344.89
    hysterical 300.11
    psychogenic 306.0
    transient or transitory 781.4
      traumatic NEC (*see also* Injury, nerve, lower limb) 956.9
  levator palpebrae superioris 374.31
  limb NEC 344.5
    all four - *see* Quadriplegia
    quadriplegia - *see* Quadriplegia
  lip 528.5
  Lissauer's 094.1
  local 355.9
  lower limb - *see also* Paralysis, leg
    both (*see also* Paraplegia) 344.1
  lung 518.89
    newborn 770.89
  median nerve 354.1
  medullary (tegmental) 344.89
  mesencephalic NEC 344.89
    tegmental 344.89
  middle alternating 344.89
  Millard-Gubler-Foville 344.89
  monoplegic - *see* Monoplegia
  motor NEC 344.9
    cerebral - *see* Paralysis, brain
    spinal - *see* Paralysis, spinal
  multiple
    cerebral - *see* Paralysis, brain
    spinal - *see* Paralysis, spinal
  muscle (flaccid) 359.9
    due to nerve lesion NEC 355.9
    eye (extrinsic) 378.55
      intrinsic 367.51
      oblique 378.51
      iris sphincter 364.89
      ischemic (complicating trauma) (Volkmann's) 958.6
    pseudohypertrophic 359.1
  muscular (atrophic) 359.9
    progressive 335.21
  musculocutaneous nerve 354.9
  musculospiral 354.9
  nerve - *see also* Disorder, nerve
    third or oculomotor (partial) 378.51
      total 378.52
    fourth or trochlear 378.53
    sixth or abducens 378.54
    seventh or facial 351.0
      birth injury 767.5
      due to
        injection NEC 999.9
        operation NEC 997.09
      newborn 767.5

Paralysis, paralytic *(Continued)*
  nerve *(Continued)*
    accessory 352.4
    auditory 388.5
    birth injury 767.7
    cranial or cerebral (*see also* Disorder, nerve, cranial) 352.9
    facial 351.0
      birth injury 767.5
      newborn 767.5
    laryngeal (*see also* Paralysis, vocal cord) 478.30
    newborn 767.7
    phrenic 354.8
      newborn 767.7
    radial 354.3
      birth injury 767.6
      newborn 767.6
    syphilitic 094.89
    traumatic NEC (*see also* Injury, nerve, by site) 957.9
    trigeminal 350.9
    ulnar 354.2
  newborn NEC 767.0
  normokalemic periodic 359.3
  obstetrical, newborn 767.7
  ocular 378.9
  oculofacial, congenital 352.6
  oculomotor (nerve) (partial) 378.51
    alternating 344.89
    external bilateral 378.55
    total 378.52
  olfactory nerve 352.0
  palate 528.9
  palatopharyngolaryngeal 352.6
  paratrigeminal 350.9
  periodic (familial) (hyperkalemic) (hypokalemic) (normokalemic) (potassium sensitive) (secondary) 359.3
  peripheral
    autonomic nervous system - *see* Neuropathy, peripheral, autonomic
    nerve NEC 355.9
  peroneal (nerve) 355.3
  pharynx 478.29
  phrenic nerve 354.8
  plantar nerves 355.6
  pneumogastric nerve 352.3
  poliomyelitis (current) (*see also* Poliomyelitis, with paralysis) 045.1 ●
    bulbar 045.0 ●
  popliteal nerve 355.3
  pressure (*see also* Neuropathy, entrapment) 355.9
  progressive 335.21
    atrophic 335.21
    bulbar 335.22
    general 094.1
    hemifacial 349.89
    infantile, acute (*see also* Poliomyelitis) 045.9 ●
    multiple 335.20
  pseudobulbar 335.23
  pseudohypertrophic 359.1
    muscle 359.1
  psychogenic 306.0
  pupil, pupillary 379.49
  quadriceps 355.8
  quadriplegic (*see also* Quadriplegia) 344.0
  radial nerve 354.3
    birth injury 767.6
  rectum (sphincter) 569.49
  rectus muscle (eye) 378.55
  recurrent
    isolated sleep 327.43
    laryngeal nerve (*see also* Paralysis, vocal cord) 478.30

Paralysis, paralytic *(Continued)*
  respiratory (muscle) (system) (tract) 786.09
    center NEC 344.89
      fetus or newborn 770.87
    congenital 768.9
    newborn 768.9
  right side - *see* Hemiplegia
  Saturday night 354.3
  saturnine 984.9
    specified type of lead - *see* Table of Drugs and Chemicals
  sciatic nerve 355.0
  secondary - *see* Paralysis, late effect
  seizure (cerebral) (current episode) (*see also* Disease, cerebrovascular, acute) 436
    late effect - *see* Late effect(s) (of) cerebrovascular disease
  senile NEC 344.9
  serratus magnus 355.9
  shaking (*see also* Parkinsonism) 332.0
  shock (*see also* Disease, cerebrovascular, acute) 436
    late effect - *see* Late effect(s) (of) cerebrovascular disease
  shoulder 354.9
  soft palate 528.9
  spasmodic - *see* Paralysis, spastic
  spastic 344.9
    cerebral infantile - *see* Palsy, cerebral
    congenital (cerebral) - *see* Palsy, cerebral
    familial 334.1
    hereditary 334.1
    infantile 343.9
    noncongenital or noninfantile, cerebral 344.9
    syphilitic 094.0
    spinal 094.89
  sphincter, bladder (*see also* Paralysis, bladder) 596.53
  spinal (cord) NEC 344.1
    accessory nerve 352.4
    acute (*see also* Poliomyelitis) 045.9 ●
    ascending acute 357.0
    atrophic (acute) (*see also* Poliomyelitis, with paralysis) 045.1 ●
      spastic, syphilitic 094.89
    congenital NEC 343.9
    hemiplegic - *see* Hemiplegia
    hereditary 336.8
    infantile (*see also* Poliomyelitis) 045.9 ●
    late effect NEC 344.89
    monoplegic - *see* Monoplegia
    nerve 355.9
    progressive 335.10
    quadriplegic - *see* Quadriplegia
    spastic NEC 343.9
    traumatic - *see* Injury, spinal, by site
  sternomastoid 352.4
  stomach 536.3
    diabetic 250.6 ● [536.3]
      due to secondary diabetes 249.6 ● [536.3]
    nerve (nondiabetic) 352.3
  stroke (current episode) - *see* Infarct, brain
    late effect - *see* Late effect(s) (of) cerebrovascular disease
  subscapularis 354.8
  superior nuclear NEC 334.9
  supranuclear 356.8
  sympathetic
    cervical NEC 337.09
    nerve NEC (*see also* Neuropathy, peripheral, autonomic) 337.9
    nervous system - *see* Neuropathy, peripheral, autonomic
  syndrome 344.9
    specified NEC 344.89
  syphilitic spastic spinal (Erb's) 094.89
  tabetic general 094.1
  thigh 355.8

SECTION 1 INDEX TO DISEASES AND INJURIES / Paralysis, paralytic

Paralysis, paralytic (Continued)
 throat 478.29
  diphtheritic 032.0
  muscle 478.29
 thrombotic (current episode) (see also Thrombosis, brain) 434.0●
  late effect - see Late effect(s) (of) cerebrovascular disease
 thumb NEC 354.9
 tick (-bite) 989.5
 Todd's (postepileptic transitory paralysis) 344.89
 toe 355.6
 tongue 529.8
 transient
  arm or leg NEC 781.4
  traumatic NEC (see also Injury, nerve, by site) 957.9
 trapezius 352.4
 traumatic, transient NEC (see also Injury, nerve, by site) 957.9
 trembling (see also Parkinsonism) 332.0
 triceps brachii 354.9
 trigeminal nerve 350.9
 trochlear nerve 378.53
 ulnar nerve 354.2
 upper limb - see also Paralysis, arm
  both (see also Diplegia) 344.2
 uremic - see Uremia
 uveoparotitic 135
 uvula 528.9
  hysterical 300.11
  postdiphtheritic 032.0
 vagus nerve 352.3
 vasomotor NEC 337.9
 velum palati 528.9
 vesical (see also Paralysis, bladder) 596.53
 vestibular nerve 388.5
 visual field, psychic 368.16
 vocal cord 478.30
  bilateral (partial) 478.33
   complete 478.34
  complete (bilateral) 478.34
  unilateral (partial) 478.31
   complete 478.32
 Volkmann's (complicating trauma) 958.6
 wasting 335.21
 Weber's 344.89
 wrist NEC 354.9
Paramedial orifice, urethrovesical 753.8
Paramenia 626.9
Parametritis (chronic) (see also Disease, pelvis, inflammatory) 614.4
 acute 614.3
 puerperal, postpartum, childbirth 670.8●
Parametrium, parametric - see condition
Paramnesia (see also Amnesia) 780.93
Paramolar 520.1
 causing crowding 524.31
Paramyloidosis 277.30
Paramyoclonus multiplex 333.2
Paramyotonia 359.29
 congenita (of von Eulenburg) 359.29
Paraneoplastic syndrome - see condition
Parangi (see also Yaws) 102.9
Paranoia 297.1
 alcoholic 291.5
 querulans 297.8
 senile 290.20
Paranoid
 dementia (see also Schizophrenia) 295.3●
  praecox (acute) 295.3●
  senile 290.20
 personality 301.0
 psychosis 297.9
  alcoholic 291.5
  climacteric 297.2
  drug-induced 292.11
  involutional 297.2
  menopausal 297.2
  protracted reactive 298.4

Paranoid (Continued)
 psychosis (Continued)
  psychogenic 298.4
   acute 298.3
   senile 290.20
  reaction (chronic) 297.9
   acute 298.3
  schizophrenia (acute) (see also Schizophrenia) 295.3●
  state 297.9
   alcohol-induced 291.5
   climacteric 297.2
   drug-induced 292.11
   due to or associated with
    arteriosclerosis (cerebrovascular) 290.42
    presenile brain disease 290.12
    senile brain disease 290.20
   involutional 297.2
   menopausal 297.2
   senile 290.20
   simple 297.0
   specified type NEC 297.8
  tendencies 301.0
  traits 301.0
  trends 301.0
  type, psychopathic personality 301.0
Paraparesis (see also Paraplegia) 344.1
Paraphasia 784.3
Paraphilia (see also Deviation, sexual) 302.9
Paraphimosis (congenital) 605
 chancroidal 099.0
Paraphrenia, paraphrenic (late) 297.2
 climacteric 297.2
 dementia (see also Schizophrenia) 295.3●
 involutional 297.2
 menopausal 297.2
 schizophrenia (acute) (see also Schizophrenia) 295.3●
Paraplegia 344.1
 with
  broken back - see Fracture, vertebra, by site, with spinal cord injury
  fracture, vertebra - see Fracture, vertebra, by site, with spinal cord injury
 ataxic - see Degeneration, combined, spinal cord
 brain (current episode) (see also Paralysis, brain) 437.8
 cerebral (current episode) (see also Paralysis, brain) 437.8
 congenital or infantile (cerebral) (spastic) (spinal) 343.0
 cortical - see Paralysis, brain
 familial spastic 334.1
 functional (hysterical) 300.11
 hysterical 300.11
 infantile 343.0
 late effect 344.1
 Pott's (see also Tuberculosis) 015.0● [730.88]
 psychogenic 306.0
 spastic
  Erb's spinal 094.89
  hereditary 334.1
  not infantile or congenital 344.1
 spinal (cord)
  traumatic NEC - see Injury, spinal, by site
 syphilitic (spastic) 094.89
 traumatic NEC - see Injury, spinal, by site
Paraproteinemia 273.2
 benign (familial) 273.1
 monoclonal 273.1
 secondary to malignant or inflammatory disease 273.1
Parapsoriasis 696.2
 en plaques 696.2
 guttata 696.2
 lichenoides chronica 696.2
 retiformis 696.2
 varioliformis (acuta) 696.2
Parascarlatina 057.8

Parasitic - see also condition
 disease NEC (see also Infestation, parasitic) 136.9
  contact V01.89
  exposure to V01.89
  intestinal NEC 129
  skin NEC 134.9
 stomatitis 112.0
 sycosis 110.0
  beard 110.0
  scalp 110.0
 twin 759.4
Parasitism NEC 136.9
 intestinal NEC 129
 skin NEC 134.9
 specified - see Infestation
Parasitophobia 300.29
Parasomnia 307.47
 alcohol induced 291.82
 drug induced 292.85
 nonorganic origin 307.47
 organic 327.40
  in conditions classified elsewhere 327.44
  other 327.49
Paraspadias 752.69
Paraspasm facialis 351.8
Parathyroid gland - see condition
Parathyroiditis (autoimmune) 252.1
Parathyroprival tetany 252.1
Paratrachoma 077.0
Paratyphilitis (see also Appendicitis) 541
Paratyphoid (fever) - see Fever, paratyphoid
Paratyphus - see Fever, paratyphoid
Paraurethral duct 753.8
Para-urethritis 597.89
 gonococcal (acute) 098.0
  chronic or duration of 2 months or over 098.2
Paravaccinia NEC 051.9
 milkers' node 051.1
Paravaginitis (see also Vaginitis) 616.10
Parencephalitis (see also Encephalitis) 323.9
 late effect - see category 326
Parergasia 298.9
Paresis (see also Paralysis) 344.9
 accommodation 367.51
 bladder (spastic) (sphincter) (see also Paralysis, bladder) 596.53
  tabetic 094.0
 bowel, colon, or intestine (see also Ileus) 560.1
 brain or cerebral - see Paralysis, brain
 extrinsic muscle, eye 378.55
 general 094.1
  arrested 094.1
  brain 094.1
  cerebral 094.1
  insane 094.1
  juvenile 090.40
   remission 090.49
  progressive 094.1
  remission (sustained) 094.1
  tabetic 094.1
 heart (see also Failure, heart) 428.9
 infantile (see also Poliomyelitis) 045.9●
 insane 094.1
 juvenile 090.40
 late effect - see Paralysis, late effect
 luetic (general) 094.1
 peripheral progressive 356.9
 pseudohypertrophic 359.1
 senile NEC 344.9
 stomach 536.3
  diabetic 250.6● [536.3]
   due to secondary diabetes 249.6● [536.3]
 syphilitic (general) 094.1
  congenital 090.40
 transient, limb 781.4
 vesical (sphincter) NEC 596.53

Paresthesia (see also Disturbance, sensation) 782.0
    Berger's (paresthesia of lower limb) 782.0
    Bernhardt 355.1
    Magnan's 782.0
Paretic - see condition
Parinaud's
    conjunctivitis 372.02
    oculoglandular syndrome 372.02
    ophthalmoplegia 378.81
    syndrome (paralysis of conjugate upward gaze) 378.81
Parkes Weber and Dimitri syndrome (encephalocutaneous angiomatosis) 759.6
Parkinson's disease, syndrome, or tremor - see Parkinsonism
Parkinsonism (arteriosclerotic) (idiopathic) (primary) 332.0
    associated with orthostatic hypotension (idiopathic) (symptomatic) 333.0
    due to drugs 332.1
    neuroleptic-induced 332.1
    secondary 332.1
    syphilitic 094.82
Parodontitis 523.40
Parodontosis 523.5
Paronychia (with lymphangitis) 681.9
    candidal (chronic) 112.3
    chronic 681.9
        candidal 112.3
        finger 681.02
        toe 681.11
    finger 681.02
    toe 681.11
    tuberculous (primary) (see also Tuberculosis) 017.0●
Parorexia NEC 307.52
    hysterical 300.11
Parosmia 781.1
    psychogenic 306.7
Parotid gland - see condition
Parotiditis (see also Parotitis) 527.2
    epidemic 072.9
    infectious 072.9
Parotitis 527.2
    allergic 527.2
    chronic 527.2
    epidemic (see also Mumps) 072.9
    infectious (see also Mumps) 072.9
    noninfectious 527.2
    nonspecific toxic 527.2
    not mumps 527.2
    postoperative 527.2
    purulent 527.2
    septic 527.2
    suppurative (acute) 527.2
    surgical 527.2
    toxic 527.2
Paroxysmal - see also condition
    dyspnea (nocturnal) 786.09
Parrot's disease (syphilitic osteochondritis) 090.0
Parrot fever 073.9
Parry's disease or syndrome (exophthalmic goiter) 242.0●
Parry-Romberg syndrome 349.89
Parson's disease (exophthalmic goiter) 242.0●
Parsonage-Aldren-Turner syndrome 353.5
Parsonage-Turner syndrome 353.5
Pars planitis 363.21
Particolored infant 757.39
Parturition - see Delivery
Parvovirus 079.83
    B19 079.83
    human 079.83
Passage
    false, urethra 599.4
    meconium noted during delivery 763.84
    of sounds or bougies (see also Attention to artificial opening) V55.9

Passive - see condition
Pasteurella septica 027.2
Pasteurellosis (see also Infection, Pasteurella) 027.2
PAT (paroxysmal atrial tachycardia) 427.0
Patau's syndrome (trisomy D1) 758.1
Patch
    herald 696.3
Patches
    mucous (syphilitic) 091.3
        congenital 090.0
    smokers' (mouth) 528.6
Patellar - see condition
Patellofemoral syndrome 719.46
Patent - see also Imperfect closure
    atrioventricular ostium 745.69
    canal of Nuck 752.41
    cervix 622.5
        complicating pregnancy 654.5●
            affecting fetus or newborn 761.0
    ductus arteriosus or Botalli 747.0
    Eustachian
        tube 381.7
        valve 746.89
    foramen
        Botalli 745.5
        ovale 745.5
    interauricular septum 745.5
    interventricular septum 745.4
    omphalomesenteric duct 751.0
    os (uteri) - see Patent, cervix
    ostium secundum 745.5
    urachus 753.7
    vitelline duct 751.0
Paternity testing V70.4
Paterson's syndrome (sideropenic dysphagia) 280.8
Paterson (-Brown) (-Kelly) syndrome (sideropenic dysphagia) 280.8
Paterson-Kelly syndrome or web (sideropenic dysphagia) 280.8
Pathologic, pathological - see also condition
    asphyxia 799.01
    drunkenness 291.4
    emotionality 301.3
    fracture - see Fracture, pathologic
    liar 301.7
    personality 301.9
    resorption, tooth 521.40
        external 521.42
        internal 521.41
        specified NEC 521.49
    sexuality (see also Deviation, sexual) 302.9
Pathology (of) - see also Disease
    periradicular, associated with previous endodontic treatment 526.69
Patterned motor discharge, idiopathic (see also Epilepsy) 345.5●
Patulous - see also Patent
    anus 569.49
    Eustachian tube 381.7
Pause, sinoatrial 427.81
Pavor nocturnus 307.46
Pavy's disease 593.6
Paxton's disease (white piedra) 111.2
Payr's disease or syndrome (splenic flexure syndrome) 569.89
PBA (pseudobulbar affect) 310.81
Pearls
    Elschnig 366.51
    enamel 520.2
Pearl-workers' disease (chronic osteomyelitis) (see also Osteomyelitis) 730.1●
Pectenitis 569.49
Pectenosis 569.49
Pectoral - see condition
Pectus
    carinatum (congenital) 754.82
        acquired 738.3
        rachitic (see also Rickets) 268.0

Pectus (Continued)
    excavatum (congenital) 754.81
        acquired 738.3
        rachitic (see also Rickets) 268.0
    recurvatum (congenital) 754.81
        acquired 738.3
Pedatrophia 261
Pederosis 302.2
Pediculosis (infestation) 132.9
    capitis (head louse) (any site) 132.0
    corporis (body louse) (any site) 132.1
    eyelid 132.0 [373.6]
    mixed (classifiable to more than one category in 132.0–132.2) 132.3
    pubis (pubic louse) (any site) 132.2
    vestimenti 132.1
    vulvae 132.2
Pediculus (infestation) - see Pediculosis
Pedophilia 302.2
Peg-shaped teeth 520.2
Pel's crisis 094.0
Pel-Ebstein disease - see Disease, Hodgkin's
Pelade 704.01
Pelger-Huët anomaly or syndrome (hereditary hyposegmentation) 288.2
Peliosis (rheumatica) 287.0
Pelizaeus-Merzbacher
    disease 330.0
    sclerosis, diffuse cerebral 330.0
Pellagra (alcoholic or with alcoholism) 265.2
    with polyneuropathy 265.2 [357.4]
Pellagra-cerebellar-ataxia-renal aminoaciduria syndrome 270.0
Pellegrini's disease (calcification, knee joint) 726.62
Pellegrini (-Stieda) disease or syndrome (calcification, knee joint) 726.62
Pellizzi's syndrome (pineal) 259.8
Pelvic - see also condition
    congestion-fibrosis syndrome 625.5
    kidney 753.3
Pelvioectasis 591
Pelviolithiasis 592.0
Pelviperitonitis
    female (see also Peritonitis, pelvic, female) 614.5
    male (see also Peritonitis) 567.21
Pelvis, pelvic - see also condition or type
    infantile 738.6
    Nägele's 738.6
    obliquity 738.6
    Robert's 755.69
Pemphigoid 694.5
    benign, mucous membrane 694.60
        with ocular involvement 694.61
    bullous 694.5
    cicatricial 694.60
        with ocular involvement 694.61
    juvenile 694.2
Pemphigus 694.4
    benign 694.5
        chronic familial 757.39
    Brazilian 694.4
    circinatus 694.0
    congenital, traumatic 757.39
    conjunctiva 694.61
    contagiosus 684
    erythematodes 694.4
    erythematosus 694.4
    foliaceus 694.4
    frambesiodes 694.4
    gangrenous (see also Gangrene) 785.4
    malignant 694.4
    neonatorum, newborn 684
    ocular 694.61
    papillaris 694.4
    seborrheic 694.4
    South American 694.4
    syphilitic (congenital) 090.0
    vegetans 694.4

Pemphigus (Continued)
  vulgaris 694.4
  wildfire 694.4
Pendred's syndrome (familial goiter with deaf-mutism) 243
Pendulous
  abdomen 701.9
    in pregnancy or childbirth 654.4●
      affecting fetus or newborn 763.89
  breast 611.89
Penetrating wound - *see also* Wound, open, by site
  with internal injury - *see* Injury, internal, by site, with open wound
  eyeball 871.7
    with foreign body (nonmagnetic) 871.6
      magnetic 871.5
  ocular (*see also* Penetrating wound, eyeball) 871.7
    adnexa 870.3
      with foreign body 870.4
    orbit 870.3
      with foreign body 870.4
Penetration, pregnant uterus by instrument
  with
    abortion - *see* Abortion, by type, with damage to pelvic organs
    ectopic pregnancy (*see also* categories 633.0–633.9) 639.2
    molar pregnancy (*see also* categories 630–632) 639.2
  complication of delivery 665.1●
    affecting fetus or newborn 763.89
  following
    abortion 639.2
    ectopic or molar pregnancy 639.2
Penfield's syndrome (*see also* Epilepsy) 345.5●
Penicilliosis of lung 117.3
Penis - *see* condition
Penitis 607.2
Penta X syndrome 758.81
Pentalogy (of Fallot) 745.2
Pentosuria (benign) (essential) 271.8
Peptic acid disease 536.8
Peregrinating patient V65.2
Perforated - *see* Perforation
Perforation, perforative (nontraumatic)
  antrum (*see also* Sinusitis, maxillary) 473.0
  appendix 540.0
    with peritoneal abscess 540.1
  atrial septum, multiple 745.5
  attic, ear 384.22
    healed 384.81
  bile duct, except cystic (*see also* Disease, biliary) 576.3
    cystic 575.4
  bladder (urinary) 596.6
    with
      abortion - *see* Abortion, by type, with damage to pelvic organs
      ectopic pregnancy (*see also* categories 633.0–633.9) 639.2
      molar pregnancy (*see also* categories 630–632) 639.2
    following
      abortion 639.2
      ectopic or molar pregnancy 639.2
    obstetrical trauma 665.5●
  bowel 569.83
    with
      abortion - *see* Abortion, by type, with damage to pelvic organs
      ectopic pregnancy (*see also* categories 633.0–633.9) 639.2
      molar pregnancy (*see also* categories 630–632) 639.2
    fetus or newborn 777.6
    following
      abortion 639.2
      ectopic or molar pregnancy 639.2
    obstetrical trauma 665.5●

Perforation, perforative (Continued)
  broad ligament
    with
      abortion - *see* Abortion, by type, with damage to pelvic organs
      ectopic pregnancy (*see also* categories 633.0–633.9) 639.2
      molar pregnancy (*see also* categories 630–632) 639.2
    following
      abortion 639.2
      ectopic or molar pregnancy 639.2
    obstetrical trauma 665.6●
  by
    device, implant, or graft - *see* Complications, mechanical
    foreign body left accidentally in operation wound 998.4
    instrument (any) during a procedure, accidental 998.2
  cecum 540.0
    with peritoneal abscess 540.1
  cervix (uteri) - *see also* Injury, internal, cervix
    with
      abortion - *see* Abortion, by type, with damage to pelvic organs
      ectopic pregnancy (*see also* categories 633.0–633.9) 639.2
      molar pregnancy (*see also* categories 630–632) 639.2
    following
      abortion 639.2
      ectopic or molar pregnancy 639.2
    obstetrical trauma 665.3●
  colon 569.83
  common duct (bile) 576.3
  cornea (*see also* Ulcer, cornea) 370.00
    due to ulceration 370.06
  cystic duct 575.4
  diverticulum (*see also* Diverticula) 562.10
    small intestine 562.00
  duodenum, duodenal (ulcer) - *see* Ulcer, duodenum, with perforation
  ear drum - *see* Perforation, tympanum
  enteritis - *see* Enteritis
  esophagus 530.4
  ethmoidal sinus (*see also* Sinusitis, ethmoidal) 473.2
  foreign body (external site) - *see also* Wound, open, by site, complicated
    internal site, by ingested object - *see* Foreign body
  frontal sinus (*see also* Sinusitis, frontal) 473.1
  gallbladder or duct (*see also* Disease, gallbladder) 575.4
  gastric (ulcer) - *see* Ulcer, stomach, with perforation
  heart valve - *see* Endocarditis
  ileum (*see also* Perforation, intestine) 569.83
  instrumental
    external - *see* Wound, open, by site
    pregnant uterus, complicating delivery 665.9●
    surgical (accidental) (blood vessel) (nerve) (organ) 998.2
  intestine 569.83
    with
      abortion - *see* Abortion, by type, with damage to pelvic organs
      ectopic pregnancy (*see also* categories 633.0–633.9) 639.2
      molar pregnancy (*see also* categories 630–632) 639.2
    fetus or newborn 777.6
    obstetrical trauma 665.5●
    ulcerative NEC 569.83
  jejunum, jejunal 569.83
    ulcer - *see* Ulcer, gastrojejunal, with perforation
  mastoid (antrum) (cell) 383.89

Perforation, perforative (Continued)
  maxillary sinus (*see also* Sinusitis, maxillary) 473.0
  membrana tympani - *see* Perforation, tympanum
  nasal
    septum 478.19
      congenital 748.1
      syphilitic 095.8
    sinus (*see also* Sinusitis) 473.9
      congenital 748.1
  palate (hard) 526.89
    soft 528.9
      syphilitic 095.8
    syphilitic 095.8
  palatine vault 526.89
    syphilitic 095.8
      congenital 090.5
  pelvic
    floor
      with
        abortion - *see* Abortion, by type, with damage to pelvic organs
        ectopic pregnancy (*see also* categories 633.0–633.9) 639.2
        molar pregnancy (*see also* categories 630–632) 639.2
      obstetrical trauma 664.1●
    organ
      with
        abortion - *see* Abortion, by type, with damage to pelvic organs
        ectopic pregnancy (*see also* categories 633.0–633.9) 639.2
        molar pregnancy (*see also* categories 630–632) 639.2
      following
        abortion 639.2
        ectopic or molar pregnancy 639.2
      obstetrical trauma 665.5●
  perineum - *see* Laceration, perineum
  periurethral tissue
    with
      abortion - *see* Abortion, by type, with damage to pelvic organs
      ectopic pregnancy (*see also* categories 630–632) 639.2
      molar pregnancy (*see also* categories 630–632) 639.2
  pharynx 478.29
  pylorus, pyloric (ulcer) - *see* Ulcer, stomach, with perforation
  rectum 569.49
  root canal space 526.61
  sigmoid 569.83
  sinus (accessory) (chronic) (nasal) (*see also* Sinusitis) 473.9
  sphenoidal sinus (*see also* Sinusitis, sphenoidal) 473.3
  stomach (due to ulcer) - *see* Ulcer, stomach, with perforation
  surgical (accidental) (by instrument) (blood vessel) (nerve) (organ) 998.2
  traumatic
    external - *see* Wound, open, by site
    eye (*see also* Penetrating wound, ocular) 871.7
    internal organ - *see* Injury, internal, by site
  tympanum (membrane) (persistent posttraumatic) (postinflammatory) 384.20
    with
      otitis media - *see* Otitis media
    attic 384.22
    central 384.21
    healed 384.81
    marginal NEC 384.23
    multiple 384.24
    pars flaccida 384.22
    total 384.25
    traumatic - *see* Wound, open, ear, drum

Perforation, perforative (Continued)
  typhoid, gastrointestinal 002.0
  ulcer - see Ulcer, by site, with perforation
  ureter 593.89
  urethra
    with
      abortion - see Abortion, by type, with damage to pelvic organs
      ectopic pregnancy (see also categories 633.0–633.9) 639.2
      molar pregnancy (see also categories 630–632) 639.2
    following
      abortion 639.2
      ectopic or molar pregnancy 639.2
      obstetrical trauma 665.5●
  uterus - see also Injury, internal, uterus
    with
      abortion - see Abortion, by type, with damage to pelvic organs
      ectopic pregnancy (see also categories 633.0–633.9) 639.2
      molar pregnancy (see also categories 630–632) 639.2
      by intrauterine contraceptive device 996.32
    following
      abortion 639.2
      ectopic or molar pregnancy 639.2
      obstetrical trauma - see Injury, internal, uterus, obstetrical trauma
  uvula 528.9
    syphilitic 095.8
  vagina - see Laceration, vagina
  viscus NEC 799.89
    traumatic 868.00
      with open wound into cavity 868.10
Periadenitis mucosa necrotica recurrens 528.2
Periangiitis 446.0
Periantritis 535.4●
Periappendicitis (acute) (see also Appendicitis) 541
Periarteritis (disseminated) (infectious) (necrotizing) (nodosa) 446.0
Periarthritis (joint) 726.90
  Duplay's 726.2
  gonococcal 098.50
  humeroscapularis 726.2
  scapulohumeral 726.2
  shoulder 726.2
  wrist 726.4
Periarthrosis (angioneural) - see Periarthritis
Peribronchitis 491.9
  tuberculous (see also Tuberculosis) 011.3●
Pericapsulitis, adhesive (shoulder) 726.0
Pericarditis (granular) (with decompensation) (with effusion) 423.9
  with
    rheumatic fever (conditions classifiable to 390)
      active (see also Pericarditis, rheumatic) 391.0
      inactive or quiescent 393
  actinomycotic 039.8 [420.0]
  acute (nonrheumatic) 420.90
    with chorea (acute) (rheumatic) (Sydenham's) 392.0
    bacterial 420.99
    benign 420.91
    hemorrhagic 420.90
    idiopathic 420.91
    infective 420.90
    nonspecific 420.91
    rheumatic 391.0
      with chorea (acute) (rheumatic) (Sydenham's) 392.0
    sicca 420.90
    viral 420.91

Pericarditis (Continued)
  adhesive or adherent (external) (internal) 423.1
    acute - see Pericarditis, acute
    rheumatic (external) (internal) 393
  amebic 006.8 [420.0]
  bacterial (acute) (subacute) (with serous or seropurulent effusion) 420.99
  calcareous 423.2
  cholesterol (chronic) 423.8
    acute 420.90
  chronic (nonrheumatic) 423.8
    rheumatic 393
  constrictive 423.2
  Coxsackie 074.21
  due to
    actinomycosis 039.8 [420.0]
    amebiasis 006.8 [420.0]
    Coxsackie (virus) 074.21
    histoplasmosis (see also Histoplasmosis) 115.93
    nocardiosis 039.8 [420.0]
    tuberculosis (see also Tuberculosis) 017.9● [420.0]
  fibrinocaseous (see also Tuberculosis) 017.9● [420.0]
  fibrinopurulent 420.99
  fibrinous - see Pericarditis, rheumatic
  fibropurulent 420.99
  fibrous 423.1
  gonococcal 098.83
  hemorrhagic 423.0
  idiopathic (acute) 420.91
  infective (acute) 420.90
  meningococcal 036.41
  neoplastic (chronic) 423.8
    acute 420.90
  nonspecific 420.91
  obliterans, obliterating 423.1
  plastic 423.1
  pneumococcal (acute) 420.99
  postinfarction 411.0
  purulent (acute) 420.99
  rheumatic (active) (acute) (with effusion) (with pneumonia) 391.0
    with chorea (acute) (rheumatic) (Sydenham's) 392.0
    chronic or inactive (with chorea) 393
  septic (acute) 420.99
  serofibrinous - see Pericarditis, rheumatic
  staphylococcal (acute) 420.99
  streptococcal (acute) 420.99
  suppurative (acute) 420.99
  syphilitic 093.81
  tuberculous (acute) (chronic) (see also Tuberculosis) 017.9● [420.0]
  uremic 585.9 [420.0]
  viral (acute) 420.91
Pericardium, pericardial - see condition
Pericellulitis (see also Cellulitis) 682.9
Pericementitis 523.40
  acute 523.30
  chronic (suppurative) 523.40
Pericholecystitis (see also Cholecystitis) 575.10
Perichondritis
  auricle 380.00
    acute 380.01
    chronic 380.02
  bronchus 491.9
  ear (external) 380.00
    acute 380.01
    chronic 380.02
  larynx 478.71
    syphilitic 095.8
    typhoid 002.0 [478.71]
  nose 478.19
  pinna 380.00
    acute 380.01
    chronic 380.02
  trachea 478.9

Periclasia 523.5
Pericolitis 569.89
Pericoronitis (chronic) 523.40
  acute 523.33
Pericystitis (see also Cystitis) 595.9
Pericytoma (M9150/1) - see also Neoplasm, connective tissue, uncertain behavior
  benign (M9150/0) - see Neoplasm, connective tissue, benign
  malignant (M9150/3) - see Neoplasm, connective tissue, malignant
Peridacryocystitis, acute 375.32
Peridiverticulitis (see also Diverticulitis) 562.11
Periduodenitis 535.6●
Periendocarditis (see also Endocarditis) 424.90
  acute or subacute 421.9
Periepididymitis (see also Epididymitis) 604.90
Perifolliculitis (abscedens) 704.8
  capitis, abscedens et suffodiens 704.8
  dissecting, scalp 704.8
  scalp 704.8
  superficial pustular 704.8
Perigastritis (acute) 535.0●
Perigastrojejunitis (acute) 535.0●
Perihepatitis (acute) 573.3
  chlamydial 099.56
  gonococcal 098.86
Peri-ileitis (subacute) 569.89
Perilabyrinthitis (acute) - see Labyrinthitis
Perimeningitis - see Meningitis
Perimetritis (see also Endometritis) 615.9
Perimetrosalpingitis (see also Salpingo-oophoritis) 614.2
Perineocele 618.05
Perinephric - see condition
Perinephritic - see condition
Perinephritis (see also Infection, kidney) 590.9
  purulent (see also Abscess, kidney) 590.2
Perineum, perineal - see condition
Perineuritis NEC 729.2
Periodic - see also condition
  disease (familial) 277.31
  edema 995.1
    hereditary 277.6
  fever 277.31
  headache syndromes in child or adolescent 346.2●
  limb movement disorder 327.51
  paralysis (familial) 359.3
  peritonitis 277.31
  polyserositis 277.31
  somnolence (see also Narcolepsy) 347.00
Periodontal
  cyst 522.8
  pocket 523.8
Periodontitis (chronic) (complex) (compound) (simplex) 523.40
  acute 523.33
  aggressive 523.30
    generalized 523.32
    localized 523.31
  apical 522.6
    acute (pulpal origin) 522.4
  generalized 523.42
  localized 523.41
Periodontoclasia 523.5
Periodontosis 523.5
Periods - see also Menstruation
  heavy 626.2
  irregular 626.4
Perionychia (with lymphangitis) 681.9
  finger 681.02
  toe 681.11
Perioophoritis (see also Salpingo-oophoritis) 614.2
Periorchitis (see also Orchitis) 604.90
Periosteum, periosteal - see condition

Periostitis (circumscribed) (diffuse) (infective) 730.3●

> Note: Use the following fifth-digit subclassification with category 730:
>
> 0 site unspecified
> 1 shoulder region
> 2 upper arm
> 3 forearm
> 4 hand
> 5 pelvic region and thigh
> 6 lower leg
> 7 ankle and foot
> 8 other specified sites
> 9 multiple sites

    with osteomyelitis (see also Osteomyelitis) 730.2●
        acute or subacute 730.0●
        chronic or old 730.1●
    albuminosa, albuminosus 730.3●
    alveolar 526.5
    alveolodental 526.5
    dental 526.5
    gonorrheal 098.89
    hyperplastica, generalized 731.2
    jaw (lower) (upper) 526.4
    monomelic 733.99
    orbital 376.02
    syphilitic 095.5
        congenital 090.0 [730.8]●
        secondary 091.61
    tuberculous (see also Tuberculosis, bone) 015.9● [730.8]●
    yaws (early) (hypertrophic) (late) 102.6
Periostosis (see also Periostitis) 730.3●
    with osteomyelitis (see also Osteomyelitis) 730.2●
        acute or subacute 730.0●
        chronic or old 730.1●
    hyperplastic 756.59
Peripartum cardiomyopathy 674.5●
Periphlebitis (see also Phlebitis) 451.9
    lower extremity 451.2
        deep (vessels) 451.19
        superficial (vessels) 451.0
    portal 572.1
    retina 362.18
    superficial (vessels) 451.0
    tuberculous (see also Tuberculosis) 017.9●
        retina 017.3● [362.18]
Peripneumonia - see Pneumonia
Periproctitis 569.49
Periprostatitis (see also Prostatitis) 601.9
Perirectal - see condition
Perirenal - see condition
Perisalpingitis (see also Salpingo-oophoritis) 614.2
Perisigmoiditis 569.89
Perisplenitis (infectional) 289.59
Perispondylitis - see Spondylitis
Peristalsis reversed or visible 787.4
Peritendinitis (see also Tenosynovitis) 726.90
    adhesive (shoulder) 726.0
Perithelioma (M9150/1) - see Pericytoma
Peritoneum, peritoneal - see also condition
    equilibration test V56.32
Peritonitis (acute) (adhesive) (fibrinous) (hemorrhagic) (idiopathic) (localized) (perforative) (primary) (with adhesions) (with effusion) 567.9
    with or following
        abortion - see Abortion, by type, with sepsis
        abscess 567.21
        appendicitis 540.0
            with peritoneal abscess 540.1
        ectopic pregnancy (see also categories 633.0–633.9) 639.0
        molar pregnancy (see also categories 630–632) 639.0

Peritonitis (Continued)
    aseptic 998.7
    bacterial 567.29
        spontaneous 567.23
    bile, biliary 567.81
    chemical 998.7
    chlamydial 099.56
    chronic proliferative 567.89
    congenital NEC 777.6
    diaphragmatic 567.22
    diffuse NEC 567.29
    diphtheritic 032.83
    disseminated NEC 567.29
    due to
        bile 567.81
        foreign
            body or object accidentally left during a procedure (instrument) (sponge) (swab) 998.4
            substance accidentally left during a procedure (chemical) (powder) (talc) 998.7
        talc 998.7
        urine 567.89
    fibrinopurulent 567.29
    fibrinous 567.29
    fibrocaseous (see also Tuberculosis) 014.0●
    fibropurulent 567.29
    general, generalized (acute) 567.21
    gonococcal 098.86
    in infective disease NEC 136.9 [567.0]
    meconium (newborn) 777.6
    pancreatic 577.8
    paroxysmal, benign 277.31
    pelvic
        female (acute) 614.5
            chronic NEC 614.7
                with adhesions 614.6
            puerperal, postpartum, childbirth 670.8●
        male (acute) 567.21
    periodic (familial) 277.31
    phlegmonous 567.29
    pneumococcal 567.1
    postabortal 639.0
    proliferative, chronic 567.89
    puerperal, postpartum, childbirth 670.8●
    purulent 567.29
    septic 567.29
    spontaneous bacterial 567.23
    staphylococcal 567.29
    streptococcal 567.29
    subdiaphragmatic 567.29
    subphrenic 567.29
    suppurative 567.29
    syphilitic 095.2
        congenital 090.0 [567.0]
    talc 998.7
    tuberculous (see also Tuberculosis) 014.0●
    urine 567.89
Peritonsillar - see condition
Peritonsillitis 475
Perityphlitis (see also Appendicitis) 541
Periureteritis 593.89
Periurethral - see condition
Periurethritis (gangrenous) 597.89
Periuterine - see condition
Perivaginitis (see also Vaginitis) 616.10
Perivasculitis, retinal 362.18
Perivasitis (chronic) 608.4
Periventricular leukomalacia 779.7
Perivesiculitis (seminal) (see also Vesiculitis) 608.0
Perlèche 686.8
    due to
        moniliasis 112.0
        riboflavin deficiency 266.0
Pernicious - see condition
Pernio, perniosis 991.5

Persecution
    delusion 297.9
    social V62.4
Perseveration (tonic) 784.69
Persistence, persistent (congenital) 759.89
    anal membrane 751.2
    arteria stapedia 744.04
    atrioventricular canal 745.69
    bloody ejaculate 792.2
    branchial cleft 744.41
    bulbus cordis in left ventricle 745.8
    canal of Cloquet 743.51
    capsule (opaque) 743.51
    cilioretinal artery or vein 743.51
    cloaca 751.5
    communication - see Fistula, congenital
    convolutions
        aortic arch 747.21
        fallopian tube 752.19
        oviduct 752.19
        uterine tube 752.19
    double aortic arch 747.21
    ductus
        arteriosus 747.0
        Botalli 747.0
    fetal
        circulation 747.83
        form of cervix (uteri) 752.49
        hemoglobin (hereditary) ("Swiss variety") 282.7
        pulmonary hypertension 747.83
    foramen
        Botalli 745.5
        ovale 745.5
    Gartner's duct 752.41
    hemoglobin, fetal (hereditary) (HPFH) 282.7
    hyaloid
        artery (generally incomplete) 743.51
        system 743.51
    hymen (tag)
        in pregnancy or childbirth 654.8●
            causing obstructed labor 660.2●
    lanugo 757.4
    left
        posterior cardinal vein 747.49
        root with right arch of aorta 747.21
        superior vena cava 747.49
    Meckel's diverticulum 751.0
    mesonephric duct 752.89
        fallopian tube 752.11
    mucosal disease (middle ear) (with posterior or superior marginal perforation of ear drum) 382.2
    nail(s), anomalous 757.5
    occiput, anterior or posterior 660.3●
        fetus or newborn 763.1
    omphalomesenteric duct 751.0
    organ or site NEC - see Anomaly, specified type NEC
    ostium
        atrioventriculare commune 745.69
        primum 745.61
        secundum 745.5
    ovarian rests in fallopian tube 752.19
    pancreatic tissue in intestinal tract 751.5
    primary (deciduous)
        teeth 520.6
        vitreous hyperplasia 743.51
    pulmonary hypertension 747.83
    pupillary membrane 743.46
        iris 743.46
    Rhesus (Rh) titer (see also Complications, transfusion) 999.70
    right aortic arch 747.21
    sinus
        urogenitalis 752.89
        venosus with imperfect incorporation in right auricle 747.49
    thymus (gland) 254.8
        hyperplasia 254.0
    thyroglossal duct 759.2

Persistence, persistent *(Continued)*
    thyrolingual duct 759.2
    truncus arteriosus or communis 745.0
    tunica vasculosa lentis 743.39
    umbilical sinus 753.7
    urachus 753.7
    vegetative state 780.03
    vitelline duct 751.0
    wolffian duct 752.89
Person (with)
    admitted for clinical research, as participant or control subject V70.7
    affected by
        family member
            currently on deployment (military) V61.01
            returned from deployment (military) (current or past conflict) V61.02
    awaiting admission to adequate facility elsewhere V63.2
    undergoing social agency investigation V63.8
    concern (normal) about sick person in family V61.49
    consulting on behalf of another V65.19
        pediatric
            pre-adoption visit for adoptive parents V65.11
            pre-birth visit for expectant parents V65.11
    currently deployed in theater or in support of military war, peacekeeping and humanitarian operations V62.21
    feared
        complaint in whom no diagnosis was made V65.5
        condition not demonstrated V65.5
    feigning illness V65.2
    healthy, accompanying sick person V65.0
    history of military war, peacekeeping and humanitarian deployment (current or past conflict) V62.22
    living (in)
        alone V60.3
        boarding school V60.6
        residence remote from hospital or medical care facility V63.0
        residential institution V60.6
        without
            adequate
                financial resources V60.2
                housing (heating) (space) V60.1
            housing (permanent) (temporary) V60.0
            material resources V60.2
            person able to render necessary care V60.4
            shelter V60.0
    medical services in home not available V63.1
    on waiting list V63.2
        undergoing social agency investigation V63.8
    sick or handicapped in family V61.49
    "worried well" V65.5
Personality
    affective 301.10
    aggressive 301.3
    amoral 301.7
    anancastic, anankastic 301.4
    antisocial 301.7
    asocial 301.7
    asthenic 301.6
    avoidant 301.82
    borderline 301.83
    change 310.1
    compulsive 301.4
    cycloid 301.13
    cyclothymic 301.13
    dependent 301.6
    depressive (chronic) 301.12

Personality *(Continued)*
    disorder, disturbance NEC 301.9
        with
            antisocial disturbance 301.7
            pattern disturbance NEC 301.9
            sociopathic disturbance 301.7
            trait disturbance 301.9
    dual 300.14
    dyssocial 301.7
    eccentric 301.89
        "haltlose" type 301.89
    emotionally unstable 301.59
    epileptoid 301.3
    explosive 301.3
    fanatic 301.0
    histrionic 301.50
    hyperthymic 301.11
    hypomanic 301.11
    hypothymic 301.12
    hysterical 301.50
    immature 301.89
    inadequate 301.6
    labile 301.59
    masochistic 301.89
    morally defective 301.7
    multiple 300.14
    narcissistic 301.81
    obsessional 301.4
    obsessive-compulsive 301.4
    overconscientious 301.4
    paranoid 301.0
    passive (-dependent) 301.6
    passive-aggressive 301.84
    pathologic NEC 301.9
    pattern defect or disturbance 301.9
    pseudosocial 301.7
    psychoinfantile 301.59
    psychoneurotic NEC 301.89
    psychopathic 301.9
        with
            amoral trend 301.7
            antisocial trend 301.7
            asocial trend 301.7
            pathologic sexuality (*see also* Deviation, sexual) 302.9
        mixed types 301.9
    schizoid 301.20
        introverted 301.21
        schizotypal 301.22
    type A 301.4
    unstable (emotional) 301.59
Perthes' disease (capital femoral osteochondrosis) 732.1
Pertussis (*see also* Whooping cough) 033.9
    vaccination, prophylactic (against) V03.6
Peruvian wart 088.0
Perversion, perverted
    appetite 307.52
        hysterical 300.11
    function
        pineal gland 259.8
        pituitary gland 253.9
            anterior lobe
                deficient 253.2
                excessive 253.1
            posterior lobe 253.6
    placenta - *see* Placenta, abnormal
    sense of smell or taste 781.1
        psychogenic 306.7
    sexual (*see also* Deviation, sexual) 302.9
Pervious, congenital - *see also* Imperfect, closure
    ductus arteriosus 747.0
Pes (congenital) (*see also* Talipes) 754.70
    abductus (congenital) 754.60
        acquired 736.79
    acquired NEC 736.79
        planus 734
    adductus (congenital) 754.79
        acquired 736.79
    cavus 754.71
        acquired 736.73

Pes *(Continued)*
    planovalgus (congenital) 754.69
        acquired 736.79
    planus (acquired) (any degree) 734
        congenital 754.61
        rachitic 268.1
    valgus (congenital) 754.61
        acquired 736.79
    varus (congenital) 754.50
        acquired 736.79
Pest (*see also* Plague) 020.9
Pestis (*see also* Plague) 020.9
    bubonica 020.0
    fulminans 020.0
    minor 020.8
    pneumonica - *see* Plague, pneumonic
Petechia, petechiae 782.7
    fetus or newborn 772.6
Petechial
    fever 036.0
    typhus 081.9
Petges-Cléjat or Petges-Clégat syndrome (poikilodermatomyositis) 710.3
Petit's
    disease (*see also* Hernia, lumbar) 553.8
Petit mal (idiopathic) (*see also* Epilepsy) 345.0 •
    status 345.2
Petrellidosis 117.6
Petrositis 383.20
    acute 383.21
    chronic 383.22
Peutz-Jeghers disease or syndrome 759.6
Peyronie's disease 607.85
Pfeiffer's disease 075
Phacentocele 379.32
    traumatic 921.3
Phacoanaphylaxis 360.19
Phacocele (old) 379.32
    traumatic 921.3
Phaehyphomycosis 117.8
Phagedena (dry) (moist) (*see also* Gangrene) 785.4
    arteriosclerotic 440.24
    geometric 686.09
    penis 607.89
    senile 440.24
    sloughing 785.4
    tropical (*see also* Ulcer, skin) 707.9
    vulva 616.50
Phagedenic - *see also* condition
    abscess - *see also* Abscess
        chancroid 099.0
    bubo NEC 099.8
    chancre 099.0
    ulcer (tropical) (*see also* Ulcer, skin) 707.9
Phagomania 307.52
Phakoma 362.89
Phantom limb (syndrome) 353.6
Pharyngeal - *see also* condition
    arch remnant 744.41
    pouch syndrome 279.11
Pharyngitis (acute) (catarrhal) (gangrenous) (infective) (malignant) (membranous) (phlegmonous) (pneumococcal) (pseudomembranous) (simple) (staphylococcal) (subacute) (suppurative) (ulcerative) (viral) 462
    with influenza, flu, or grippe (*see also* Influenza) 487.1
    aphthous 074.0
    atrophic 472.1
    chlamydial 099.51
    chronic 472.1
    Coxsackie virus 074.0
    diphtheritic (membranous) 032.0
    follicular 472.1
    fusospirochetal 101
    gonococcal 098.6
    granular (chronic) 472.1
    herpetic 054.79
    hypertrophic 472.1

SECTION I INDEX TO DISEASES AND INJURIES / Pharyngitis

Pharyngitis (Continued)
  infectional, chronic 472.1
  influenzal (see also Influenza) 487.1
  lymphonodular, acute 074.8
  septic 034.0
  streptococcal 034.0
  tuberculous (see also Tuberculosis) 012.8●
  vesicular 074.0
Pharyngoconjunctival fever 077.2
Pharyngoconjunctivitis, viral 077.2
Pharyngolaryngitis (acute) 465.0
  chronic 478.9
  septic 034.0
Pharyngoplegia 478.29
Pharyngotonsillitis 465.8
  tuberculous 012.8●
Pharyngotracheitis (acute) 465.8
  chronic 478.9
Pharynx, pharyngeal - see condition
Phase of life problem NEC V62.89
Phenomenon
  Arthus 995.21
  flashback (drug) 292.89
  jaw-winking 742.8
  Jod-Basedow 242.8●
  L. E. cell 710.0
  lupus erythematosus cell 710.0
  Pelger-Huët (hereditary hyposegmentation) 288.2
  Raynaud's (paroxysmal digital cyanosis) (secondary) 443.0
  Reilly's (see also Neuropathy, peripheral, autonomic) 337.9
  vasomotor 780.2
  vasospastic 443.9
  vasovagal 780.2
  Wenckebach's, heart block (second degree) 426.13
Phenylketonuria (PKU) 270.1
Phenylpyruvicaciduria 270.1
Pheochromoblastoma (M8700/3)
  specified site - see Neoplasm, by site, malignant
  unspecified site 194.0
Pheochromocytoma (M8700/0)
  malignant (M8700/3)
    specified site - see Neoplasm, by site, malignant
    unspecified site 194.0
  specified site - see Neoplasm, by site, benign
  unspecified site 227.0
Phimosis (congenital) 605
  chancroidal 099.0
  due to infection 605
Phlebectasia (see also Varicose, vein) 454.9
  congenital NEC 747.60
  esophagus (see also Varix, esophagus) 456.1
    with hemorrhage (see also Varix, esophagus, bleeding) 456.0
Phlebitis (infective) (pyemic) (septic) (suppurative) 451.9
  antecubital vein 451.82
  arm NEC 451.84
    axillary vein 451.89
    basilic vein 451.82
    deep 451.83
    superficial 451.82
  axillary vein 451.89
  basilic vein 451.82
  blue 451.9
  brachial vein 451.83
  breast, superficial 451.89
  cavernous (venous) sinus - see Phlebitis, intracranial sinus
  cephalic vein 451.82
  cerebral (venous) sinus - see Phlebitis, intracranial sinus
  chest wall, superficial 451.89
  complicating pregnancy or puerperium 671.2●
    affecting fetus or newborn 760.3

Phlebitis (Continued)
  cranial (venous) sinus - see Phlebitis, intracranial sinus
  deep (vessels) 451.19
    femoral vein 451.11
    specified vessel NEC 451.19
  due to implanted device - see Complications, due to (presence of) any device, implant, or graft classified to 996.0–996.5 NEC
  during or resulting from a procedure 997.2
  femoral vein (deep) (superficial) 451.11
  femoropopliteal 451.19
  following infusion, perfusion, or transfusion 999.2
  gouty 274.89 [451.9]
  hepatic veins 451.89
  iliac vein 451.81
  iliofemoral 451.11
  intracranial sinus (any) (venous) 325
    late effect - see category 326
    nonpyogenic 437.6
      in pregnancy or puerperium 671.5●
  jugular vein 451.89
  lateral (venous) sinus - see Phlebitis, intracranial sinus
  leg 451.2
    deep (vessels) 451.19
      specified vessel NEC 451.19
    superficial (vessels) 451.0
      femoral vein 451.11
  longitudinal sinus - see Phlebitis, intracranial sinus
  lower extremity 451.2
    deep (vessels) 451.19
      specified vessel NEC 451.19
    superficial (vessels) 451.0
      femoral vein 451.11
  migrans, migrating (superficial) 453.1
  pelvic
    with
      abortion - see Abortion, by type, with sepsis
      ectopic pregnancy (see also categories 633.0–633.9) 639.0
      molar pregnancy (see also categories 630–632) 639.0
    following
      abortion 639.0
      ectopic or molar pregnancy 639.0
    puerperal, postpartum 671.4●
  popliteal vein 451.19
  portal (vein) 572.1
  postoperative 997.2
  pregnancy 671.2●
    deep 671.3●
    specified type NEC 671.5●
  superficial 671.2●
  puerperal, postpartum, childbirth 671.2●
    deep 671.4●
    lower extremities 671.2●
    pelvis 671.4●
    specified site NEC 671.5●
    superficial 671.2●
  radial vein 451.83
  retina 362.18
  saphenous (great) (long) 451.0
    accessory or small 451.0
  sinus (meninges) - see Phlebitis, intracranial sinus
  specified site NEC 451.89
  subclavian vein 451.89
  syphilitic 093.89
  tibial vein 451.19
  ulcer, ulcerative 451.9
    leg 451.2
      deep (vessels) 451.19
        specified vessel NEC 451.19
      superficial (vessels) 451.0
        femoral vein 451.11

Phlebitis (Continued)
  ulcer, ulcerative (Continued)
    lower extremity 451.2
      deep (vessels) 451.19
        femoral vein 451.11
        specified vessel NEC 451.19
      superficial (vessels) 451.0
    ulnar vein 451.83
    umbilicus 451.89
    upper extremity - see Phlebitis, arm
      deep (veins) 451.83
        brachial vein 451.83
        radial vein 451.83
        ulnar vein 451.83
      superficial (veins) 451.82
        antecubital vein 451.82
        basilic vein 451.82
        cephalic vein 451.82
    uterus (septic) (see also Endometritis) 615.9
    varicose (leg) (lower extremity) (see also Varicose, vein) 454.1
Phlebofibrosis 459.89
Pheboliths 459.89
Phlebosclerosis 459.89
Phlebothrombosis - see Thrombosis
Phlebotomus fever 066.0
Phlegm, choked on 933.1
Phlegmasia
  alba dolens (deep vessels) 451.19
    complicating pregnancy 671.3●
    nonpuerperal 451.19
    puerperal, postpartum, childbirth 671.4●
  cerulea dolens 451.19
Phlegmon (see also Abscess) 682.9
  erysipelatous (see also Erysipelas) 035
  iliac 682.2
  fossa 540.1
  throat 478.29
Phlegmonous - see condition
Phlyctenulosis (allergic) (keratoconjunctivitis) (nontuberculous) 370.31
  cornea 370.31
    with ulcer (see also Ulcer, cornea) 370.00
  tuberculous (see also Tuberculosis) 017.3● [370.31]
Phobia, phobic (reaction) 300.20
  animal 300.29
  isolated NEC 300.29
  obsessional 300.3
  simple NEC 300.29
  social 300.23
  specified NEC 300.29
  state 300.20
Phocas' disease 610.1
Phocomelia 755.4
  lower limb 755.32
    complete 755.33
    distal 755.35
    proximal 755.34
  upper limb 755.22
    complete 755.23
    distal 755.25
    proximal 755.24
Phoria (see also Heterophoria) 378.40
Phosphate-losing tubular disorder 588.0
Phosphatemia 275.3
Phosphaturia 275.3
Photoallergic response 692.72
Photocoproporphyria 277.1
Photodermatitis (sun) 692.72
  light other than sun 692.82
Photokeratitis 370.24
Photo-ophthalmia 370.24
Photophobia 368.13
Photopsia 368.15
Photoretinitis 363.31
Photoretinopathy 363.31
Photosensitiveness (sun) 692.72
  light other than sun 692.82

Photosensitization skin (sun) 692.72
    light other than sun 692.82
Phototoxic response 692.72
Phrenitis 323.9
Phrynoderma 264.8
Phthiriasis (pubis) (any site) 132.2
    with any infestation classifiable to 132.0 and 132.1 132.3
Phthirus infestation - see Phthiriasis
Phthisis (see also Tuberculosis) 011.9 ●
    bulbi (infectional) 360.41
    colliers' 011.4 ●
    cornea 371.05
    eyeball (due to infection) 360.41
    millstone makers' 011.4 ●
    miners' 011.4 ●
    potters' 011.4 ●
    sandblasters' 011.4 ●
    stonemasons' 011.4 ●
Phycomycosis 117.7
Physalopteriasis 127.7
Physical therapy NEC V57.1
    breathing exercises V57.0
Physiological cup, optic papilla
    borderline, glaucoma suspect 365.00
    enlarged 377.14
    glaucomatous 377.14
Phytobezoar 938
    intestine 936
    stomach 935.2
Pian (see also Yaws) 102.9
Pianoma 102.1
Piarhemia, piarrhemia (see also Hyperlipemia) 272.4
    bilharziasis 120.9
Pica 307.52
    hysterical 300.11
Pick's
    cerebral atrophy 331.11
        with dementia
            with behavioral disturbance 331.11 [294.11]
            without behavioral disturbance 331.11 [294.10]
    disease
        brain 331.11
            dementia in
                with behavioral disturbance 331.11 [294.11]
                without behavioral disturbance 331.11 [294.10]
        lipid histiocytosis 272.7
        liver (pericardial pseudocirrhosis of liver) 423.2
        pericardium (pericardial pseudocirrhosis of liver) 423.2
        polyserositis (pericardial pseudocirrhosis of liver) 423.2
    syndrome
        heart (pericardial pseudocirrhosis of liver) 423.2
        liver (pericardial pseudocirrhosis of liver) 423.2
    tubular adenoma (M8640/0)
        specified site - see Neoplasm, by site, benign
        unspecified site
            female 220
            male 222.0
Pick-Herxheimer syndrome (diffuse idiopathic cutaneous atrophy) 701.8
Pick-Niemann disease (lipid histiocytosis) 272.7
Pickwickian syndrome (cardiopulmonary obesity) 278.03
Piebaldism, classic 709.09
Piedra 111.2
    beard 111.2
        black 111.3
        white 111.2
    black 111.3

Piedra (Continued)
    scalp 111.3
        black 111.3
        white 111.2
    white 111.2
Pierre Marie's syndrome (pulmonary hypertrophic osteoarthropathy) 731.2
Pierre Marie-Bamberger syndrome (hypertrophic pulmonary osteoarthropathy) 731.2
Pierre Mauriac's syndrome (diabetes-dwarfism-obesity) 258.1
Pierre Robin deformity or syndrome (congenital) 756.0
Pierson's disease or osteochondrosis 732.1
Pigeon
    breast or chest (acquired) 738.3
        congenital 754.82
        rachitic (see also Rickets) 268.0
    breeders' disease or lung 495.2
    fanciers' disease or lung 495.2
    toe 735.8
Pigmentation (abnormal) 709.00
    anomalies NEC 709.00
        congenital 757.33
        specified NEC 709.09
    conjunctiva 372.55
    cornea 371.10
        anterior 371.11
        posterior 371.13
        stromal 371.12
    lids (congenital) 757.33
        acquired 374.52
    limbus corneae 371.10
    metals 709.00
    optic papilla, congenital 743.57
    retina (congenital) (grouped) (nevoid) 743.53
        acquired 362.74
    scrotum, congenital 757.33
Piles - see Hemorrhoids
Pili
    annulati or torti (congenital) 757.4
    incarnati 704.8
Pill roller hand (intrinsic) 736.09
Pilomatrixoma (M8110/0) - see Neoplasm, skin, benign
Pilonidal - see condition
Pimple 709.8
PIN I (prostatic intraepithelial neoplasia I) 602.3
PIN II (prostatic intraepithelial neoplasia II) 602.3
PIN III (prostatic intraepithelial neoplasia III) 233.4
Pinched nerve - see Neuropathy, entrapment
Pineal body or gland - see condition
Pinealoblastoma (M9362/3) 194.4
Pinealoma (M9360/1) 237.1
    malignant (M9360/3) 194.4
Pineoblastoma (M9362/3) 194.4
Pineocytoma (M9361/1) 237.1
Pinguecula 372.51
Pingueculitis 372.34
Pinhole meatus (see also Stricture, urethra) 598.9
Pink
    disease 985.0
    eye 372.03
    puffer 492.8
Pinkus' disease (lichen nitidus) 697.1
Pinpoint
    meatus (see also Stricture, urethra) 598.9
    os (uteri) (see also Stricture, cervix) 622.4
Pinselhaare (congenital) 757.4
Pinta 103.9
    cardiovascular lesions 103.2
    chancre (primary) 103.0
    erythematous plaques 103.1
    hyperchromic lesions 103.1
    hyperkeratosis 103.1

Pinta (Continued)
    lesions 103.9
        cardiovascular 103.2
        hyperchromic 103.1
        intermediate 103.1
        late 103.2
        mixed 103.3
        primary 103.0
        skin (achromic) (cicatricial) (dyschromic) 103.2
            hyperchromic 103.1
            mixed (achromic and hyperchromic) 103.3
    papule (primary) 103.0
    skin lesions (achromic) (cicatricial) (dyschromic) 103.2
        hyperchromic 103.1
        mixed (achromic and hyperchromic) 103.3
    vitiligo 103.2
Pintid 103.0
Pinworms (disease) (infection) (infestation) 127.4
Piry fever 066.8
Pistol wound - see Gunshot wound
Pit, lip (mucus), congenital 750.25
Pitchers' elbow 718.82
Pithecoid pelvis 755.69
    with disproportion (fetopelvic) 653.2 ●
        affecting fetus or newborn 763.1
        causing obstructed labor 660.1 ●
Pithiatism 300.11
Pitted - see also Pitting
    teeth 520.4
Pitting (edema) (see also Edema) 782.3
    lip 782.3
    nail 703.8
    congenital 757.5
Pituitary gland - see condition
Pituitary snuff-takers' disease 495.8
Pityriasis 696.5
    alba 696.5
    capitis 690.11
    circinata (et maculata) 696.3
    Hebra's (exfoliative dermatitis) 695.89
    lichenoides et varioliformis 696.2
    maculata (et circinata) 696.3
    nigra 111.1
    pilaris 757.39
        acquired 701.1
        Hebra's 696.4
    rosea 696.3
    rotunda 696.3
    rubra (Hebra) 695.89
        pilaris 696.4
    sicca 690.18
    simplex 690.18
    specified type NEC 696.5
    streptogenes 696.5
    versicolor 111.0
        scrotal 111.0
Placenta, placental
    ablatio 641.2 ●
        affecting fetus or newborn 762.1
    abnormal, abnormality 656.7 ●
        with hemorrhage 641.8 ●
            affecting fetus or newborn 762.1
        affecting fetus or newborn 762.2
    abruptio 641.2 ●
        affecting fetus or newborn 762.1
    accessory lobe - see Placenta, abnormal
    accreta (without hemorrhage) 667.0 ●
        with hemorrhage 666.0 ●
    adherent (without hemorrhage) 667.0 ●
        with hemorrhage 666.0 ●
    apoplexy - see Placenta, separation
    battledore - see Placenta, abnormal
    bilobate - see Placenta, abnormal
    bipartita - see Placenta, abnormal
    carneous mole 631.8
    centralis - see Placenta, previa
    circumvallata - see Placenta, abnormal

SECTION I INDEX TO DISEASES AND INJURIES / Placenta, placental

Placenta, placental *(Continued)*
   cyst (amniotic) - *see* Placenta, abnormal
   deficiency - *see* Placenta, insufficiency
   degeneration - *see* Placenta, insufficiency
   detachment (partial) (premature) (with hemorrhage) 641.2●
      affecting fetus or newborn 762.1
   dimidiata - *see* Placenta, abnormal
   disease 656.7●
      affecting fetus or newborn 762.2
   duplex - *see* Placenta, abnormal
   dysfunction - *see* Placenta, insufficiency
   fenestrata - *see* Placenta, abnormal
   fibrosis - *see* Placenta, abnormal
   fleshy mole 631.8
   hematoma - *see* Placenta, abnormal
   hemorrhage NEC - *see* Placenta, separation
   hormone disturbance or malfunction - *see* Placenta, abnormal
   hyperplasia - *see* Placenta, abnormal
   increta (without hemorrhage) 667.0●
      with hemorrhage 666.0●
   infarction 656.7●
      affecting fetus or newborn 762.2
   insertion, vicious - *see* Placenta, previa
   insufficiency
      affecting
         fetus or newborn 762.2
         management of pregnancy 656.5●
   lateral - *see* Placenta, previa
   low implantation or insertion - *see* Placenta, previa
   low-lying - *see* Placenta, previa
   malformation - *see* Placenta, abnormal
   malposition - *see* Placenta, previa
   marginalis, marginata - *see* Placenta, previa
   marginal sinus (hemorrhage) (rupture) 641.2●
      affecting fetus or newborn 762.1
   membranacea - *see* Placenta, abnormal
   multilobed - *see* Placenta, abnormal
   multipartita - *see* Placenta, abnormal
   necrosis - *see* Placenta, abnormal
   percreta (without hemorrhage) 667.0●
      with hemorrhage 666.0●
   polyp 674.4●
   previa (central) (centralis) (complete) (lateral) (marginal) (marginalis) (partial) (partialis) (total) (with hemorrhage) 641.1●
      affecting fetus or newborn 762.0
      noted
         before labor, without hemorrhage (with cesarean delivery) 641.0●
         during pregnancy (without hemorrhage) 641.0●
      without hemorrhage (before labor and delivery) (during pregnancy) 641.0●
   retention (with hemorrhage) 666.0●
      fragments, complicating puerperium (delayed hemorrhage) 666.2●
         without hemorrhage 667.1●
      postpartum, puerperal 666.2●
         without hemorrhage 667.0●
   separation (normally implanted) (partial) (premature) (with hemorrhage) 641.2●
      affecting fetus or newborn 762.1
   septuplex - *see* Placenta, abnormal
   small - *see* Placenta, insufficiency
   softening (premature) - *see* Placenta, abnormal
   spuria - *see* Placenta, abnormal
   succenturiata - *see* Placenta, abnormal
   syphilitic 095.8
   transfusion syndromes 762.3
   transmission of chemical substance - *see* Absorption, chemical, through placenta
   trapped (with hemorrhage) 666.0●
      without hemorrhage 667.0●

Placenta, placental *(Continued)*
   trilobate - *see* Placenta, abnormal
   tripartita - *see* Placenta, abnormal
   triplex - *see* Placenta, abnormal
   varicose vessel - *see* Placenta, abnormal
   vicious insertion - *see* Placenta, previa
Placentitis
   affecting fetus or newborn 762.7
   complicating pregnancy 658.4●
Plagiocephaly (skull) 754.0
Plague 020.9
   abortive 020.8
   ambulatory 020.8
   bubonic 020.0
   cellulocutaneous 020.1
   lymphatic gland 020.0
   pneumonic 020.5
      primary 020.3
      secondary 020.4
   pulmonary - *see* Plague, pneumonic
   pulmonic - *see* Plague, pneumonic
   septicemic 020.2
   tonsillar 020.9
      septicemic 020.2
   vaccination, prophylactic (against) V03.3
Planning, family V25.09
   contraception V25.9
   natural
      procreative V26.41
      to avoid pregnancy V25.04
   procreation V26.49
      natural V26.41
Plaque
   artery, arterial - *see* Arteriosclerosis
   calcareous - *see* Calcification
   Hollenhorst's (retinal) 362.33
   tongue 528.6
Plasma cell myeloma 203.0●
Plasmacytoma, plasmocytoma (solitary) (M9731/1) 238.6
   benign (M9731/0) - *see* Neoplasm, by site, benign
   malignant (M9731/3) 203.8●
Plasmacytopenia 288.59
Plasmacytosis 288.64
Plaster ulcer (*see also* Ulcer, pressure) 707.00
Plateau iris syndrome (without glaucoma) 364.82
   with glaucoma 365.23
Platybasia 756.0
Platyonychia (congenital) 757.5
   acquired 703.8
Platypelloid pelvis 738.6
   with disproportion (fetopelvic) 653.2●
      affecting fetus or newborn 763.1
   causing obstructed labor 660.1●
      affecting fetus or newborn 763.1
   congenital 755.69
Platyspondylia 756.19
Plethora 782.62
   newborn 776.4
Pleura, pleural - *see* condition
Pleuralgia 786.52
Pleurisy (acute) (adhesive) (chronic) (costal) (diaphragmatic) (double) (dry) (fetid) (fibrinous) (fibrous) (interlobar) (latent) (lung) (old) (plastic) (primary) (residual) (sicca) (sterile) (subacute) (unresolved) (with adherent pleura) 511.0
   with
      effusion (without mention of cause) 511.9
         bacterial, nontuberculous 511.1
         nontuberculous NEC 511.9
            bacterial 511.1
         pneumococcal 511.1
         specified type NEC 511.89
         staphylococcal 511.1
         streptococcal 511.1
         tuberculous (*see also* Tuberculosis, pleura) 012.0●
            primary, progressive 010.1●

Pleurisy *(Continued)*
   with *(Continued)*
      influenza, flu, or grippe (*see also* Influenza) 487.1
      tuberculosis - *see* Pleurisy, tuberculous
   encysted 511.89
   exudative (*see also* Pleurisy, with effusion) 511.9
      bacterial, nontuberculous 511.1
   fibrinopurulent 510.9
      with fistula 510.0
   fibropurulent 510.9
      with fistula 510.0
   hemorrhagic 511.89
   influenzal (*see also* Influenza) 487.1
   pneumococcal 511.0
      with effusion 511.1
   purulent 510.9
      with fistula 510.0
   septic 510.9
      with fistula 510.0
   serofibrinous (*see also* Pleurisy, with effusion) 511.9
      bacterial, nontuberculous 511.1
   seropurulent 510.9
      with fistula 510.0
   serous (*see also* Pleurisy, with effusion) 511.9
      bacterial, nontuberculous 511.1
   staphylococcal 511.0
      with effusion 511.1
   streptococcal 511.0
      with effusion 511.1
   suppurative 510.9
      with fistula 510.0
   traumatic (post) (current) 862.29
      with open wound into cavity 862.39
   tuberculous (with effusion) (*see also* Tuberculosis, pleura) 012.0●
      primary, progressive 010.1●
Pleuritis sicca - *see* Pleurisy
Pleurobronchopneumonia (*see also* Pneumonia, broncho-) 485
Pleurodynia 786.52
   epidemic 074.1
   viral 074.1
Pleurohepatitis 573.8
Pleuropericarditis (*see also* Pericarditis) 423.9
   acute 420.90
Pleuropneumonia (acute) (bilateral) (double) (septic) (*see also* Pneumonia) 486
   chronic (*see also* Fibrosis, lung) 515
Pleurorrhea (*see also* Hydrothorax) 511.89
Plexitis, brachial 353.0
Plica
   knee 727.83
   polonica 132.0
   tonsil 474.8
Plicae dysphonia ventricularis 784.49
Plicated tongue 529.5
   congenital 750.13
Plug
   bronchus NEC 519.19
   meconium (newborn) NEC 777.1
   mucus - *see* Mucus, plug
Plumbism 984.9
   specified type of lead - *see* Table of Drugs and Chemicals
Plummer's disease (toxic nodular goiter) 242.3●
Plummer-Vinson syndrome (sideropenic dysphagia) 280.8
Pluricarential syndrome of infancy 260
Plurideficiency syndrome of infancy 260
Plus (and minus) hand (intrinsic) 736.09
PMDD (premenstrual dysphoric disorder) 625.4
PMS 625.4
Pneumathemia - *see* Air, embolism, by type
Pneumatic drill or hammer disease 994.9
Pneumatocele (lung) 518.89
   intracranial 348.89
   tension 492.0

Pneumatosis
   cystoides intestinalis 569.89
   peritonei 568.89
   pulmonum 492.8
Pneumaturia 599.84
Pneumoblastoma (M8981/3) - *see* Neoplasm, lung, malignant
Pneumocephalus 348.89
Pneumococcemia 038.2
Pneumococcus, pneumococcal - *see* condition
Pneumoconiosis (due to) (inhalation of) 505
   aluminum 503
   asbestos 501
   bagasse 495.1
   bauxite 503
   beryllium 503
   carbon electrode makers' 503
   coal
      miners' (simple) 500
      workers' (simple) 500
   cotton dust 504
   diatomite fibrosis 502
   dust NEC 504
      inorganic 503
      lime 502
      marble 502
      organic NEC 504
   fumes or vapors (from silo) 506.9
   graphite 503
   hard metal 503
   mica 502
   moldy hay 495.0
   rheumatoid 714.81
   silica NEC 502
      and carbon 500
   silicate NEC 502
   talc 502
Pneumocystis carinii pneumonia 136.3
Pneumocystis jiroveci pneumonia 136.3
Pneumocystosis 136.3
   with pneumonia 136.3
Pneumoenteritis 025
Pneumohemopericardium (*see also* Pericarditis) 423.9
Pneumohemothorax (*see also* Hemothorax) 511.89
   traumatic 860.4
      with open wound into thorax 860.5
Pneumohydropericardium (*see also* Pericarditis) 423.9
Pneumohydrothorax (*see also* Hydrothorax) 511.89
Pneumomediastinum 518.1
   congenital 770.2
   fetus or newborn 770.2
Pneumomycosis 117.9
Pneumonia (acute) (Alpenstich) (benign) (bilateral) (brain) (cerebral) (circumscribed) (congestive) (creeping) (delayed resolution) (double) (epidemic) (fever) (flash) (fulminant) (fungoid) (granulomatous) (hemorrhagic) (incipient) (infantile) (infectious) (infiltration) (insular) (intermittent) (latent) (lobe) (migratory) (newborn) (organized) (overwhelming) (primary) (progressive) (pseudolobar) (purulent) (resolved) (secondary) (senile) (septic) (suppurative) (terminal) (true) (unresolved) (vesicular) 486
   with influenza, flu, or grippe 487.0
      due to
         identified (virus)
            avian 488.01
            (novel) 2009 H1N1 488.11
         novel influenza A 488.81
   adenoviral 480.0
   adynamic 514
   alba 090.0
   allergic 518.3
   alveolar - *see* Pneumonia, lobar

Pneumonia (*Continued*)
   anaerobes 482.81
   anthrax 022.1 [484.5]
   apex, apical - *see* Pneumonia, lobar
   ascaris 127.0 [484.8]
   aspiration 507.0
      due to
         aspiration of microorganisms
            bacterial 482.9
               specified type NEC 482.89
            specified organism NEC 483.8
               bacterial NEC 482.89
            viral 480.9
               specified type NEC 480.8
         food (regurgitated) 507.0
         gastric secretions 507.0
         milk 507.0
         oils, essences 507.1
         solids, liquids NEC 507.8
         vomitus 507.0
      fetal 770.18
         due to
            blood 770.16
            clear amniotic fluid 770.14
            meconium 770.12
            postnatal stomach contents 770.86
      newborn 770.18
         due to
            blood 770.16
            clear amniotic fluid 770.14
            meconium 770.12
            postnatal stomach contents 770.86
   asthenic 514
   atypical (disseminated) (focal) (primary) 486
      with influenza (*see also* Influenza) 487.0
   bacillus 482.9
      specified type NEC 482.89
   bacterial 482.9
      specified type NEC 482.89
   Bacteroides (fragilis) (oralis) (melaninogenicus) 482.81
   basal, basic, basilar - *see* Pneumonia, by type
   bronchiolitis obliterans organized (BOOP) 516.8
   broncho-, bronchial (confluent) (croupous) (diffuse) (disseminated) (hemorrhagic) (involving lobes) (lobar) (terminal) 485
      with influenza 487.0
      due to
         identified (virus)
            avian 488.01
            (novel) 2009 H1N1 488.11
         novel influenza A 488.81
   allergic 518.3
   aspiration (*see also* Pneumonia, aspiration) 507.0
   bacterial 482.9
      specified type NEC 482.89
   capillary 466.19
      with bronchospasm or obstruction 466.19
   chronic (*see also* Fibrosis, lung) 515
   congenital (infective) 770.0
   diplococcal 481
   Eaton's agent 483.0
   Escherichia coli (E. coli) 482.82
   Friedländer's bacillus 482.0
   Hemophilus influenzae 482.2
   hiberno-vernal 083.0 [484.8]
   hypostatic 514
   influenzal (*see also* Influenza) 487.0
   inhalation (*see also* Pneumonia, aspiration) 507.0
      due to fumes or vapors (chemical) 506.0
   Klebsiella 482.0
   lipid 507.1
      endogenous 516.8
   Mycoplasma (pneumoniae) 483.0
   ornithosis 073.0

Pneumonia (*Continued*)
   broncho-, bronchial (*Continued*)
      pleuropneumonia-like organisms (PPLO) 483.0
      pneumococcal 481
      Proteus 482.83
      Pseudomonas 482.1
      specified organism NEC 483.8
         bacterial NEC 482.89
      staphylococcal 482.40
         aureus 482.41
            methicillin
               resistant (MRSA) 482.42
               susceptible (MSSA) 482.41
         specified type NEC 482.49
      streptococcal - *see* Pneumonia, streptococcal
      typhoid 002.0 [484.8]
      viral, virus (*see also* Pneumonia, viral) 480.9
   Butyrivibrio (fibriosolvens) 482.81
   Candida 112.4
   capillary 466.19
      with bronchospasm or obstruction 466.19
   caseous (*see also* Tuberculosis) 011.6 ●
   catarrhal - *see* Pneumonia, broncho-
   central - *see* Pneumonia, lobar
   Chlamydia, chlamydial 483.1
      pneumoniae 483.1
      psittaci 073.0
      specified type NEC 483.1
      trachomatis 483.1
   cholesterol 516.8
   chronic (*see also* Fibrosis, lung) 515
   cirrhotic (chronic) (*see also* Fibrosis, lung) 515
   Clostridium (haemolyticum) (novyi) NEC 482.81
   confluent - *see* Pneumonia, broncho-
   congenital (infective) 770.0
      aspiration 770.18
   croupous - *see* Pneumonia, lobar
   cryptogenic organizing 516.36
   cytomegalic inclusion 078.5 [484.1]
   deglutition (*see also* Pneumonia, aspiration) 507.0
   desquamative interstitial 516.37
   diffuse - *see* Pneumonia, broncho-
   diplococcal, diplococcus (broncho-) (lobar) 481
   disseminated (focal) - *see* Pneumonia, broncho-
   due to
      adenovirus 480.0
      anaerobes 482.81
      Bacterium anitratum 482.83
      Chlamydia, chlamydial 483.1
         pneumoniae 483.1
         psittaci 073.0
         specified type NEC 483.1
         trachomatis 483.1
      coccidioidomycosis 114.0
      Diplococcus (pneumoniae) 481
      Eaton's agent 483.0
      Escherichia coli (E. coli) 482.82
      Friedländer's bacillus 482.0
      fumes or vapors (chemical) (inhalation) 506.0
      fungus NEC 117.9 [484.7]
         coccidioidomycosis 114.0
      Hemophilus influenzae (H. influenzae) 482.2
      Herellea 482.83
      influenza (*see also* Influenza) 487.0
      Klebsiella pneumoniae 482.0
      Mycoplasma (pneumoniae) 483.0
      parainfluenza virus 480.2
      pleuropneumonia-like organism (PPLO) 483.0
      Pneumococcus 481

SECTION I INDEX TO DISEASES AND INJURIES / Pneumonia

Pneumonia (Continued)
  due to (Continued)
    Pneumocystis carinii 136.3
    Pneumocystis jiroveci 136.3
    Proteus 482.83
    Pseudomonas 482.1
    respiratory syncytial virus 480.1
    rickettsia 083.9 [484.8]
    SARS-associated coronavirus 480.3
    specified
      bacteria NEC 482.89
      organism NEC 483.8
      virus NEC 480.8
    Staphylococcus 482.40
      aureus 482.41
        methicillin
          resistant (MRSA) 482.42
          susceptible (MSSA) 482.41
      specified type NEC 482.49
    Streptococcus - *see also* Pneumonia, streptococcal
      pneumoniae 481
    virus (*see also* Pneumonia, viral) 480.9
      SARS-associated coronavirus 480.3
  Eaton's agent 483.0
  embolic, embolism (*see* Embolism, pulmonary)
  eosinophilic 518.3
  Escherichia coli (E. coli) 482.82
  Eubacterium 482.81
  fibrinous - *see* Pneumonia, lobar
  fibroid (chronic) (*see also* Fibrosis, lung) 515
  fibrous (*see also* Fibrosis, lung) 515
  Friedländer's bacillus 482.0
  fusobacterium (nucleatum) 482.81
  gangrenous 513.0
  giant cell (*see also* Pneumonia, viral) 480.9
  gram-negative bacteria NEC 482.83
    anaerobic 482.81
  grippal (*see also* Influenza) 487.0
  Hemophilus influenzae (bronchial) (lobar) 482.2
  hypostatic (broncho-) (lobar) 514
  in
    actinomycosis 039.1
    anthrax 022.1 [484.5]
    aspergillosis 117.3 [484.6]
    candidiasis 112.4
    coccidioidomycosis 114.0
    cytomegalic inclusion disease 078.5 [484.1]
    histoplasmosis (*see also* Histoplasmosis) 115.95
    infectious disease NEC 136.9 [484.8]
    measles 055.1
    mycosis, systemic NEC 117.9 [484.7]
    nocardiasis, nocardiosis 039.1
    ornithosis 073.0
    pneumocystosis 136.3
    psittacosis 073.0
    Q fever 083.0 [484.8]
    salmonellosis 003.22
    toxoplasmosis 130.4
    tularemia 021.2
    typhoid (fever) 002.0 [484.8]
    varicella 052.1
    whooping cough (*see also* Whooping cough) 033.9 [484.3]
  infective, acquired prenatally 770.0
  influenzal (broncho) (lobar) (virus) (*see also* Influenza) 487.0
  inhalation (*see also* Pneumonia, aspiration) 507.0
    fumes or vapors (chemical) 506.0

Pneumonia (Continued)
  interstitial 516.8
    with influenzal (*see also* Influenza) 487.0
    acute
      due to Pneumocystis (carinii) (jiroveci) 136.3
      meaning:
        acute interstitial pneumonitis 516.33
        atypical pneumonia - *see* Pneumonia, atypical
        bacterial pneumonia - *see* Pneumonia, bacterial
    chronic (*see also* Fibrosis, lung) 515
    desquamative 516.37
    hypostatic 514
    idiopathic 516.30
      lymphoid 516.35
    lipoid 507.1
    lymphoid (due to known underlying cause) 516.8
    non-specific (due to known underlying cause) 516.8
    organizing (due to known underlying cause) 516.8
    plasma cell 136.3
    Pseudomonas 482.1
  intrauterine (infective) 770.0
    aspiration 770.18
    blood 770.16
    clear amniotic fluid 770.14
    meconium 770.12
    postnatal stomach contents 770.86
  Klebsiella pneumoniae 482.0
  Legionnaires' 482.84
  lipid, lipoid (exogenous) (interstitial) 507.1
    endogenous 516.8
  lobar (diplococcal) (disseminated) (double) (interstitial) (pneumococcal, any type) 481
    with influenza (*see also* Influenza) 487.0
    bacterial 482.9
      specified type NEC 482.89
    chronic (*see also* Fibrosis, lung) 515
    Escherichia coli (E. coli) 482.82
    Friedländer's bacillus 482.0
    Hemophilus influenzae (H. influenzae) 482.2
    hypostatic 514
    influenzal (*see also* Influenza) 487.0
    Klebsiella 482.0
    ornithosis 073.0
    Proteus 482.83
    Pseudomonas 482.1
    psittacosis 073.0
    specified organism NEC 483.8
      bacterial NEC 482.89
    staphylococcal 482.40
      aureus 482.41
        methicillin
          resistant (MRSA) 482.42
          susceptible (MSSA) 482.41
      specified type NEC 482.49
    streptococcal - *see* Pneumonia, streptococcal
    viral, virus (*see also* Pneumonia, viral) 480.9
  lobular (confluent) - *see* Pneumonia, broncho-
  Löffler's 518.3
  massive - *see* Pneumonia, lobar
  meconium aspiration 770.12
  metastatic NEC 038.8 [484.8]
  methicillin resistant Staphylococcus aureus (MRSA) 482.42
  methicillin susceptible Staphylococcus aureus (MSSA) 482.41
  MRSA (methicillin resistant Staphylococcus aureus) 482.42
  MSSA (methicillin susceptible Staphylococcus aureus) 482.41

Pneumonia (Continued)
  multilobar - *see* Pneumonia, by type
  Mycoplasma (pneumoniae) 483.0
  necrotic 513.0
  nitrogen dioxide 506.9
  orthostatic 514
  parainfluenza virus 480.2
  parenchymatous (*see also* Fibrosis, lung) 515
  passive 514
  patchy - *see* Pneumonia, broncho-
  Peptococcus 482.81
  Peptostreptococcus 482.81
  plasma cell 136.3
  pleurolobar - *see* Pneumonia, lobar
  pleuropneumonia-like organism (PPLO) 483.0
  pneumococcal (broncho) (lobar) 481
  Pneumocystis (carinii) (jiroveci) 136.3
  postinfectional NEC 136.9 [484.8]
  postmeasles 055.1
  postoperative 997.39
    aspiration 997.32
  primary atypical 486
  Proprionibacterium 482.81
  Proteus 482.83
  Pseudomonas 482.1
  psittacosis 073.0
  radiation 508.0
  respiratory syncytial virus 480.1
  resulting from a procedure 997.39
    aspiration 997.32
  rheumatic 390 [517.1]
  Salmonella 003.22
  SARS-associated coronavirus 480.3
  segmented, segmental - *see* Pneumonia, broncho-
  Serratia (marcascens) 482.83
  specified
    bacteria NEC 482.89
    organism NEC 483.8
    virus NEC 480.8
  spirochetal 104.8 [484]
  staphylococcal (broncho) (lobar) 482.40
    aureus 482.41
      methicillin
        resistant (MRSA) 482.42
        susceptible (MSSA) 482.41
    specified type NEC 482.49
  static, stasis 514
  streptococcal (broncho) (lobar) NEC 482.30
    Group
      A 482.31
      B 482.32
      specified NEC 482.39
    pneumoniae 481
    specified type NEC 482.39
  Streptococcus pneumoniae 481
  traumatic (complication) (early) (secondary) 958.8
  tuberculous (any) (*see also* Tuberculosis) 011.6 ●
  tularemic 021.2
  TWAR agent 483.1
  varicella 052.1
  Veillonella 482.81
  ventilator associated 997.31
  viral, virus (broncho) (interstitial) (lobar) 480.9
    with influenza, flu, or grippe (*see also* Influenza) 487.0
    adenoviral 480.0
    parainfluenza 480.2
    respiratory syncytial 480.1
    SARS-associated coronavirus 480.3
    specified type NEC 480.8
  white (congenital) 090.0
Pneumonic - *see* condition
Pneumonitis (acute) (primary) (*see also* Pneumonia) 486
  allergic 495.9
    specified type NEC 495.8

SECTION 1 INDEX TO DISEASES AND INJURIES / Poison ivy, oak, sumac or other plant dermatitis

Pneumonitis (*Continued*)
  aspiration 507.0
    due to fumes or gases 506.0
      fetal 770.18
        due to
          blood 770.16
          clear amniotic fluid 770.14
          meconium 770.12
          postnatal stomach contents 770.86
      newborn 770.18
        due to
          blood 770.16
          clear amniotic fluid 770.14
          meconium 770.12
          postnatal stomach contents 770.86
      obstetric 668.0 ●
  chemical 506.0
    due to fumes or gases 506.0
    resulting from a procedure 997.32
  cholesterol 516.8
  chronic (*see also* Fibrosis, lung) 515
  congenital rubella 771.0
  crack 506.0
  due to
    crack (cocaine) 506.0
    fumes or vapors 506.0
    inhalation
      food (regurgitated), milk, vomitus 507.0
      oils, essences 507.1
      saliva 507.0
      solids, liquids NEC 507.8
    toxoplasmosis (acquired) 130.4
      congenital (active) 771.2 [484.8]
  eosinophilic 518.3
  fetal aspiration 770.18
    due to
      blood 770.16
      clear amniotic fluid 770.14
      meconium 770.12
      postnatal stomach contents 770.86
  hypersensitivity 495.9
  interstitial (chronic) (*see also* Fibrosis, lung) 515
    acute 516.33
    idiopathic
      lymphocytic 516.35
      non-specific 516.32
    lymphoid 516.8
  lymphoid, interstitial 516.8
  meconium aspiration 770.12
  postanesthetic
    correct substance properly administered 507.0
    obstetric 668.0 ●
    overdose or wrong substance given 968.4
      specified anesthetic - *see* Table of Drugs and Chemicals
  postoperative 997.39
    aspiration 997.32
    obstetric 668.0 ●
  radiation 508.0
  rubella, congenital 771.0
  "ventilation" 495.7
  ventilator associated 997.31
  wood-dust 495.8
Pneumonoconiosis - *see* Pneumoconiosis
Pneumoparotid 527.8
Pneumopathy NEC 518.89
  alveolar 516.9
    specified NEC 516.8
    due to dust NEC 504
  parietoalveolar 516.9
    specified condition NEC 516.8
Pneumopericarditis (*see also* Pericarditis) 423.9
  acute 420.90
Pneumopericardium - *see also* Pericarditis
  congenital 770.2
  fetus or newborn 770.2
  traumatic (post) (*see also* Pneumothorax, traumatic) 860.0
    with open wound into thorax 860.1

Pneumoperitoneum 568.89
  fetus or newborn 770.2
Pneumophagia (psychogenic) 306.4
Pneumopleurisy, pneumopleuritis (*see also* Pneumonia) 486
Pneumopyopericardium 420.99
Pneumopyothorax (*see also* Pyopneumothorax) 510.9
  with fistula 510.0
Pneumorrhagia 786.30
  newborn 770.3
  tuberculous (*see also* Tuberculosis, pulmonary) 011.9 ●
Pneumosiderosis (occupational) 503
Pneumothorax 512.89
  acute 512.89
  chronic 512.83
  congenital 770.2
  due to operative injury of chest wall or lung 512.1
    accidental puncture or laceration 512.1
  fetus or newborn 770.2
  iatrogenic 512.1
  postoperative 512.1
  specified type NEC 512.89
  spontaneous 512.89
    fetus or newborn 770.2
    primary 512.81
    secondary 512.82
    tension 512.0
  sucking 512.89
    iatrogenic 512.1
    postoperative 512.1
  tense valvular, infectional 512.0
  tension 512.0
    iatrogenic 512.1
    postoperative 512.1
    spontaneous 512.0
  traumatic 860.0
    with
      hemothorax 860.4
        with open wound into thorax 860.5
      open wound into thorax 860.1
  tuberculous (*see also* Tuberculosis) 011.7 ●
Pocket(s)
  endocardial (*see also* Endocarditis) 424.90
  periodontal 523.8
Podagra 274.01
Podencephalus 759.89
Poikilocytosis 790.09
Poikiloderma 709.09
  Civatte's 709.09
  congenital 757.33
  vasculare atrophicans 696.2
Poikilodermatomyositis 710.3
Pointed ear 744.29
Poise imperfect 729.90
Poisoned - *see* Poisoning
Poisoning (acute) - *see also* Table of Drugs and Chemicals
  Bacillus, B.
    aertrycke (*see also* Infection, Salmonella) 003.9
    botulinus 005.1
    cholerae (suis) (*see also* Infection, Salmonella) 003.9
    paratyphosus (*see also* Infection, Salmonella) 003.9
    suipestifer (*see also* Infection, Salmonella) 003.9
  bacterial toxins NEC 005.9
  berries, noxious 988.2
  blood (general) - *see* Septicemia
  botulism 005.1
  bread, moldy, mouldy - *see* Poisoning, food
  Ciguatera 988.0
  damaged meat - *see* Poisoning, food
  death-cap (Amanita phalloides) (Amanita verna) 988.1
  decomposed food - *see* Poisoning, food
  diseased food - *see* Poisoning, food

Poisoning (*Continued*)
  drug - *see* Table of Drugs and Chemicals
  epidemic, fish, meat, or other food - *see* Poisoning, food
  fava bean 282.2
  fish (bacterial) - *see also* Poisoning, food
    noxious 988.0
  food (acute) (bacterial) (diseased) (infected) NEC 005.9
    due to
      bacillus
        aertrycke (*see also* Poisoning, food, due to Salmonella) 003.9
        botulinus 005.1
        cereus 005.89
        choleraesuis (*see also* Poisoning, food, due to Salmonella) 003.9
        paratyphosus (*see also* Poisoning, food, due to Salmonella) 003.9
        suipestifer (*see also* Poisoning, food, due to Salmonella) 003.9
      Clostridium 005.3
        botulinum 005.1
        perfringens 005.2
        welchii 005.2
      Salmonella (aertrycke) (callinarum) (choleraesuis) (enteritidis) (paratyphi) (suipestifer) 003.9
        with
          gastroenteritis 003.0
          localized infection(s) (*see also* Infection, Salmonella) 003.20
          septicemia 003.1
          specified manifestation NEC 003.8
      specified bacterium NEC 005.89
      Staphylococcus 005.0
      Streptococcus 005.89
      Vibrio parahaemolyticus 005.4
      Vibrio vulnificus 005.81
    noxious or naturally toxic 988.0
      berries 988.2
      fish 988.0
      mushroom 988.1
      plants NEC 988.2
  ice cream - *see* Poisoning, food
  ichthyotoxism (bacterial) 005.9
  kreotoxism, food 005.9
  malarial - *see* Malaria
  meat - *see* Poisoning, food
  mushroom (noxious) 988.1
  mussel - *see also* Poisoning, food
    noxious 988.0
  noxious foodstuffs (*see also* Poisoning, food, noxious) 988.9
    specified type NEC 988.8
  plants, noxious 988.2
  pork - *see also* Poisoning, food
    specified NEC 988.8
    Trichinosis 124
  ptomaine - *see* Poisoning, food
  putrefaction, food - *see* Poisoning, food
  radiation 508.0
  Salmonella (*see also* Infection, Salmonella) 003.9
  sausage - *see also* Poisoning, food
    Trichinosis 124
  saxitoxin 988.0
  shellfish - *see also* Poisoning, food
    noxious (amnesic) (azaspiracid) (diarrheic) (neurotoxic) (paralytic) 988.0
  Staphylococcus, food 005.0
  toxic, from disease NEC 799.89
  truffles - *see* Poisoning, food
  uremic - *see* Uremia
  uric acid 274.9
  water 276.69
Poison ivy, oak, sumac or other plant dermatitis 692.6

Poker spine 720.0
Policeman's disease 729.2
Polioencephalitis (acute) (bulbar) (see also
      Poliomyelitis, bulbar) 045.0●
   inferior 335.22
   influenzal (see also Influenza) 487.8
   superior hemorrhagic (acute) (Wernicke's)
      265.1
   Wernicke's (superior hemorrhagic) 265.1
Polioencephalomyelitis (acute) (anterior)
      (bulbar) (see also Polioencephalitis)
      045.0●
Polioencephalopathy, superior hemorrhagic
      265.1
   with
      beriberi 265.0
      pellagra 265.2
Poliomeningoencephalitis - see
      Meningoencephalitis
Poliomyelitis (acute) (anterior) (epidemic)
      045.9●

Note: Use the following fifth-digit
subclassification with category 045:
   0   poliovirus, unspecified type
   1   poliovirus, type I
   2   poliovirus, type II
   3   poliovirus, type III

   with
      paralysis 045.1●
         bulbar 045.0●
   abortive 045.2●
   ascending 045.9●
      progressive 045.9●
   bulbar 045.0●
   cerebral 045.0●
   chronic 335.21
   congenital 771.2
   contact V01.2
   deformities 138
   exposure to V01.2
   late effect 138
   nonepidemic 045.9●
   nonparalytic 045.2●
   old with deformity 138
   posterior, acute 053.19
   residual 138
   sequelae 138
   spinal, acute 045.9●
   syphilitic (chronic) 094.89
   vaccination, prophylactic (against) V04.0
Poliosis (eyebrow) (eyelashes) 704.3
   circumscripta (congenital) 757.4
      acquired 704.3
   congenital 757.4
Pollakiuria 788.41
   psychogenic 306.53
Pollinosis 477.0
Pollitzer's disease (hidradenitis suppurativa)
      705.83
Polyadenitis (see also Adenitis) 289.3
   malignant 020.0
Polyalgia 729.99
Polyangiitis (essential) 446.0
Polyarteritis (nodosa) (renal) 446.0
Polyarthralgia 719.49
   psychogenic 306.0
Polyarthritis, polyarthropathy NEC 716.59
   due to or associated with other specified
      conditions - see Arthritis, due to or
      associated with
   endemic (see also Disease, Kaschin-Beck)
      716.0●
   inflammatory 714.9
      specified type NEC 714.89
   juvenile (chronic) 714.30
      acute 714.31
   migratory - see Fever, rheumatic
   rheumatic 714.0
      fever (acute) - see Fever, rheumatic

Polycarential syndrome of infancy 260
Polychondritis (atrophic) (chronic) (relapsing)
      733.99
Polycoria 743.46
Polycystic (congenital) (disease) 759.89
   degeneration, kidney - see Polycystic, kidney
   kidney (congenital) 753.12
      adult type (APKD) 753.13
      autosomal dominant 753.13
      autosomal recessive 753.14
      childhood type (CPKD) 753.14
      infantile type 753.14
   liver 751.62
   lung 518.89
      congenital 748.4
   ovary, ovaries 256.4
   spleen 759.0
Polycythemia (primary) (rubra) (vera)
      (M9950/1) 238.4
   acquired 289.0
   benign 289.0
      familial 289.6
   due to
      donor twin 776.4
      fall in plasma volume 289.0
      high altitude 289.0
      maternal-fetal transfusion 776.4
      stress 289.0
   emotional 289.0
   erythropoietin 289.0
   familial (benign) 289.6
   Gaisböck's (hypertonica) 289.0
   high altitude 289.0
   hypertonica 289.0
   hypoxemic 289.0
   neonatorum 776.4
   nephrogenous 289.0
   relative 289.0
   secondary 289.0
   spurious 289.0
   stress 289.0
Polycytosis cryptogenica 289.0
Polydactylism, polydactyly 755.00
   fingers 755.01
   toes 755.02
Polydipsia 783.5
Polydystrophic oligophrenia 277.5
Polyembryoma (M9072/3) - see Neoplasm, by
      site, malignant
Polygalactia 676.6●
Polyglandular
   deficiency 258.9
   dyscrasia 258.9
   dysfunction 258.9
   syndrome 258.8
Polyhydramnios (see also Hydramnios) 657●
Polymastia 757.6
Polymenorrhea 626.2
Polymicrogyria 742.2
Polymyalgia 725
   arteritica 446.5
   rheumatica 725
Polymyositis (acute) (chronic) (hemorrhagic)
      710.4
   with involvement of
      lung 710.4 [517.8]
      skin 710.3
   ossificans (generalisata) (progressiva) 728.19
   Wagner's (dermatomyositis) 710.3
Polyneuritis, polyneuritic (see also
      Polyneuropathy) 356.9
   alcoholic 357.5
      with psychosis 291.1
   cranialis 352.6
   demyelinating, chronic inflammatory (CIDP)
      357.81
   diabetic 250.6● [357.2]
      due to secondary diabetes 249.6● [357.2]
   due to lack of vitamin NEC 269.2 [357.4]
   endemic 265.0 [357.4]
   erythredema 985.0

Polyneuritis, polyneuritic (Continued)
   febrile 357.0
   hereditary ataxic 356.3
   idiopathic, acute 357.0
   infective (acute) 357.0
   nutritional 269.9 [357.4]
   postinfectious 357.0
Polyneuropathy (peripheral) 356.9
   alcoholic 357.5
   amyloid 277.39 [357.4]
   arsenical 357.7
   critical illness 357.82
   demyelinating, chronic inflammatory (CIDP)
      357.81
   diabetic 250.6● [357.2]
      due to secondary diabetes 249.6● [357.2]
   due to
      antitetanus serum 357.6
      arsenic 357.7
      drug or medicinal substance 357.6
         correct substance properly
            administered 357.6
         overdose or wrong substance given or
            taken 977.9
         specified drug - see Table of Drugs
            and Chemicals
      lack of vitamin NEC 269.2 [357.4]
      lead 357.7
      organophosphate compounds 357.7
      pellagra 265.2 [357.4]
      porphyria 277.1 [357.4]
      serum 357.6
      toxic agent NEC 357.7
   hereditary 356.0
   idiopathic 356.9
      progressive 356.4
   in
      amyloidosis 277.39 [357.4]
      avitaminosis 269.2 [357.4]
         specified NEC 269.1 [357.4]
      beriberi 265.0 [357.4]
      collagen vascular disease NEC 710.9
         [357.1]
      deficiency
         B-complex NEC 266.2 [357.4]
         vitamin B 266.9 [357.4]
         vitamin B_6 266.1 [357.4]
      diabetes 250.6● [357.2]
         due to secondary diabetes 249.6●
            [357.2]
      diphtheria (see also Diphtheria) 032.89
         [357.4]
      disseminated lupus erythematosus 710.0
         [357.1]
      herpes zoster 053.13
      hypoglycemia 251.2 [357.4]
      malignant neoplasm (M8000/3) NEC
         199.1 [357.3]
      mumps 072.72
      pellagra 265.2 [357.4]
      polyarteritis nodosa 446.0 [357.1]
      porphyria 277.1 [357.4]
      rheumatoid arthritis 714.0 [357.1]
      sarcoidosis 135 [357.4]
      uremia 585.9 [357.4]
   lead 357.7
   nutritional 269.9 [357.4]
      specified NEC 269.8 [357.4]
   postherpetic 053.13
   progressive 356.4
   sensory (hereditary) 356.2
   specified NEC 356.8
Polyonychia 757.5
Polyopia 368.2
   refractive 368.15
Polyorchism, polyorchidism (three testes)
      752.89
Polyorrhymenitis (peritoneal) (see also
      Polyserositis) 568.82
   pericardial 423.2
Polyostotic fibrous dysplasia 756.54

Polyotia 744.1
Polyp, polypus

> Note: Polyps of organs or sites that do not appear in the list below should be coded to the residual category for diseases of the organ or site concerned.

    accessory sinus 471.8
    adenoid tissue 471.0
    adenomatous (M8210/0) - see also Neoplasm, by site, benign
        adenocarcinoma in (M8210/3) - see Neoplasm, by site, malignant
        carcinoma in (M8210/3) - see Neoplasm, by site, malignant
        multiple (M8221/0) - see Neoplasm, by site, benign
    antrum 471.8
    anus, anal (canal) (nonadenomatous) 569.0
        adenomatous 211.4
    Bartholin's gland 624.6
    bladder (M8120/1) 236.7
    broad ligament 620.8
    cervix (uteri) 622.7
        adenomatous 219.0
        in pregnancy or childbirth 654.6 •
            affecting fetus or newborn 763.89
            causing obstructed labor 660.2 •
        mucous 622.7
        nonneoplastic 622.7
    choanal 471.0
    cholesterol 575.6
    clitoris 624.6
    colon (M8210/0) (see also Polyp, adenomatous) 211.3
    corpus uteri 621.0
    dental 522.0
    ear (middle) 385.30
    endometrium 621.0
    ethmoidal (sinus) 471.8
    fallopian tube 620.8
    female genital organs NEC 624.8
    frontal (sinus) 471.8
    gallbladder 575.6
    gingiva 523.8
    gum 523.8
    labia 624.6
    larynx (mucous) 478.4
    malignant (M8000/3) - see Neoplasm, by site, malignant
    maxillary (sinus) 471.8
    middle ear 385.30
    myometrium 621.0
    nares
        anterior 471.9
        posterior 471.0
    nasal (mucous) 471.9
        cavity 471.0
        septum 471.9
    nasopharyngeal 471.0
    neoplastic (M8210/0) - see Neoplasm, by site, benign
    nose (mucous) 471.9
    oviduct 620.8
    paratubal 620.8
    pharynx 478.29
        congenital 750.29
    placenta, placental 674.4 •
    prostate 600.20
        with
            other lower urinary tract symptoms (LUTS) 600.21
            urinary
                obstruction 600.21
                retention 600.21
    pudenda 624.6
    pulp (dental) 522.0
    rectosigmoid 211.4
    rectum (nonadenomatous) 569.0
        adenomatous 211.4

Polyp, polypus (Continued)
    septum (nasal) 471.9
    sinus (accessory) (ethmoidal) (frontal) (maxillary) (sphenoidal) 471.8
    sphenoidal (sinus) 471.8
    stomach (M8210/0) 211.1
    tube, fallopian 620.8
    turbinate, mucous membrane 471.8
    ureter 593.89
    urethra 599.3
    uterine
        ligament 620.8
        tube 620.8
    uterus (body) (corpus) (mucous) 621.0
        in pregnancy or childbirth 654.1 •
            affecting fetus or newborn 763.89
            causing obstructed labor 660.2 •
    vagina 623.7
    vocal cord (mucous) 478.4
    vulva 624.6
Polyphagia 783.6
Polypoid - see condition
Polyposis - see also Polyp
    coli (adenomatous) (M8220/0) 211.3
        adenocarcinoma in (M8220/3) 153.9
        carcinoma in (M8220/3) 153.9
    familial (M8220/0) 211.3
    intestinal (adenomatous) (M8220/0) 211.3
    multiple (M8221/0) - see Neoplasm, by site, benign
Polyradiculitis (acute) 357.0
Polyradiculoneuropathy (acute) (segmentally demyelinating) 357.0
Polysarcia 278.00
Polyserositis (peritoneal) 568.82
    due to pericarditis 423.2
    paroxysmal (familial) 277.31
    pericardial 423.2
    periodic (familial) 277.31
    pleural - see Pleurisy
    recurrent 277.31
    tuberculous (see also Tuberculosis, polyserositis) 018.9 •
Polysialia 527.7
Polysplenia syndrome 759.0
Polythelia 757.6
Polytrichia (see also Hypertrichosis) 704.1
Polyunguia (congenital) 757.5
    acquired 703.8
Polyuria 788.42
Pompe's disease (glycogenosis II) 271.0
Pompholyx 705.81
Poncet's disease (tuberculous rheumatism) (see also Tuberculosis) 015.9 •
Pond fracture - see Fracture, skull, vault
Ponos 085.0
Pons, pontine - see condition
Poor
    aesthetics of existing restoration of tooth 525.67
    contractions, labor 661.2 •
        affecting fetus or newborn 763.7
    fetal growth NEC 764.9 •
        affecting management of pregnancy 656.5 •
    incorporation
        artificial skin graft 996.55
        decellularized allodermis graft 996.55
    obstetrical history V13.29
        affecting management of current pregnancy V23.49
            ectopic pregnancy V23.42
            pre-term labor V23.41
        pre-term labor V13.21
    sucking reflex (newborn) 796.1
    vision NEC 369.9
Poradenitis, nostras 099.1
Porencephaly (congenital) (developmental) (true) 742.4
    acquired 348.0
    nondevelopmental 348.0
    traumatic (post) 310.2

Porocephaliasis 134.1
Porokeratosis 757.39
    disseminated superficial actinic (DSAP) 692.75
Poroma, eccrine (M8402/0) - see Neoplasm, skin, benign
Porphyria (acute) (congenital) (constitutional) (erythropoietic) (familial) (hepatica) (idiopathic) (idiosyncratic) (intermittent) (latent) (mixed hepatic) (photosensitive) (South African genetic) (Swedish) 277.1
    acquired 277.1
    cutaneatarda
        hereditaria 277.1
        symptomatica 277.1
    due to drugs
        correct substance properly administered 277.1
        overdose or wrong substance given or taken 977.9
            specified drug - see Table of Drugs and Chemicals
    secondary 277.1
    toxic NEC 277.1
    variegata 277.1
Porphyrinuria (acquired) (congenital) (secondary) 277.1
Porphyruria (acquired) (congenital) 277.1
Portal - see condition
Port wine nevus or mark 757.32
Posadas-Wernicke disease 114.9
Position
    fetus, abnormal (see also Presentation, fetal) 652.9 •
    teeth, faulty (see also Anomaly, position tooth) 524.30
Positive
    culture (nonspecific) 795.39
        AIDS virus V08
        blood 790.7
        HIV V08
        human immunodeficiency virus V08
        nose 795.39
            Staphylococcus - see Carrier (suspected) of, Staphylococcus
        skin lesion NEC 795.39
        spinal fluid 792.0
        sputum 795.39
        stool 792.1
        throat 795.39
        urine 791.9
        wound 795.39
    findings, anthrax 795.31
    HIV V08
    human immunodeficiency virus (HIV) V08
    PPD 795.51
    serology
        AIDS virus V08
            inconclusive 795.71
        HIV V08
            inconclusive 795.71
        human immunodeficiency virus V08
            inconclusive 795.71
        syphilis 097.1
            with signs or symptoms - see Syphilis, by site and stage
            false 795.6
    skin test 795.7
        tuberculin (without active tuberculosis) 795.51
    VDRL 097.1
        with signs or symptoms - see Syphilis, by site and stage
        false 795.6
    Wassermann reaction 097.1
        false 795.6
Postcardiotomy syndrome 429.4
Postcaval ureter 753.4
Postcholecystectomy syndrome 576.0
Postclimacteric bleeding 627.1
Postcommissurotomy syndrome 429.4

SECTION I INDEX TO DISEASES AND INJURIES / Postconcussional syndrome

Postconcussional syndrome 310.2
Postcontusional syndrome 310.2
Postcricoid region - *see* condition
Post-dates (pregnancy) - *see* Pregnancy
Postencephalitic - *see also* condition
   syndrome 310.89
Posterior - *see* condition
Posterolateral sclerosis (spinal cord) - *see*
   Degeneration, combined
Postexanthematous - *see* condition
Postfebrile - *see* condition
Postgastrectomy dumping syndrome 564.2
Posthemiplegic chorea 344.89
Posthemorrhagic anemia (chronic) 280.0
   acute 285.1
   newborn 776.5
Posthepatitis syndrome 780.79
Postherpetic neuralgia (intercostal) (syndrome)
   (zoster) 053.19
   geniculate ganglion 053.11
   ophthalmica 053.19
   trigeminal 053.12
Posthitis 607.1
Postimmunization complication or reaction -
   see Complications, vaccination
Postinfectious - *see* condition
Postinfluenzal syndrome 780.79
Postlaminectomy syndrome 722.80
   cervical, cervicothoracic 722.81
   kyphosis 737.12
   lumbar, lumbosacral 722.83
   thoracic, thoracolumbar 722.82
Postleukotomy syndrome 310.0
Postlobectomy syndrome 310.0
Postmastectomy lymphedema (syndrome)
   457.0
Postmaturity, postmature (fetus or newborn)
   (gestation period over 42 completed
   weeks) 766.22
   affecting management of pregnancy
     post-term pregnancy 645.1●
     prolonged pregnancy 645.2●
   syndrome 766.22
Postmeasles - *see also* condition
   complication 055.8
   specified NEC 055.79
Postmenopausal
   endometrium (atrophic) 627.8
     suppurative (*see also* Endometritis) 615.9
   hormone replacement therapy V07.4
   status (age related) (natural) V49.81
Postnasal drip 784.91
Postnatal - *see* condition
Postoperative - *see also* condition
   confusion state 293.9
   psychosis 293.9
   status NEC (*see also* Status (post)) V45.89
Postpancreatectomy hyperglycemia 251.3
Postpartum - *see also* condition
   anemia 648.2●
     cardiomyopathy 674.5●
   observation
     immediately after delivery V24.0
     routine follow-up V24.2
Postperfusion syndrome NEC 999.89
   bone marrow 996.85
Postpoliomyelitic - *see* condition
Postsurgery status NEC (*see also* Status (post))
   V45.89
Post-term (pregnancy) 645.1●
   infant (gestation period over 40 completed
     weeks to 42 completed weeks) 766.21
Post-transplant lymphoproliferative disorder
   (PTLD) 238.77
Posttraumatic - *see* condition
Posttraumatic brain syndrome, nonpsychotic
   310.2
Post-Traumatic Stress Disorder (PTSD)
   309.81
Post-typhoid abscess 002.0
Postures, hysterical 300.11

Postvaccinal reaction or complication - *see*
   Complications, vaccination
Postvagotomy syndrome 564.2
Postvalvulotomy syndrome 429.4
Postvasectomy sperm count V25.8
Potain's disease (pulmonary edema) 514
Potain's syndrome (gastrectasis with
   dyspepsia) 536.1
Pott's
   curvature (spinal) (*see also* Tuberculosis)
     015.0● *[737.43]*
   disease or paraplegia (*see also* Tuberculosis)
     015.0● *[730.88]*
   fracture (closed) 824.4
     open 824.5
   gangrene 440.24
   osteomyelitis (*see also* Tuberculosis) 015.0●
     [730.88]
   spinal curvature (*see also* Tuberculosis)
     015.0● *[737.43]*
   tumor, puffy (*see also* Osteomyelitis) 730.2●
Potter's
   asthma 502
   disease 753.0
   facies 754.0
   lung 502
   syndrome (with renal agenesis) 753.0
Pouch
   bronchus 748.3
   Douglas' - *see* condition
   esophagus, esophageal (congenital) 750.4
     acquired 530.6
   gastric 537.1
   Hartmann's (abnormal sacculation of
     gallbladder neck) 575.8
   of intestine V44.3
     attention to V55.3
   pharynx, pharyngeal (congenital) 750.27
Pouchitis 569.71
Poulet's disease 714.2
Poultrymen's itch 133.8
Poverty V60.2
PPE (palmar plantar erythrodysesthesia)
   693.0
Prader-Labhart-Willi-Fanconi syndrome
   (hypogenital dystrophy with diabetic
   tendency) 759.81
Prader-Willi syndrome (hypogenital dystrophy
   with diabetic tendency) 759.81
Preachers' voice 784.49
Pre-AIDS - *see* Human immunodeficiency virus
   (disease) (illness) (infection)
Preauricular appendage 744.1
Prebetalipoproteinemia (acquired) (essential)
   (familial) (hereditary) (primary)
   (secondary) 272.1
   with chylomicronemia 272.3
Precipitate labor 661.3●
   affecting fetus or newborn 763.6
Preclimacteric bleeding 627.0
   menorrhagia 627.0
Precocious
   adrenarche 259.1
   menarche 259.1
   menstruation 259.1
   pubarche 259.1
   puberty NEC 259.1
   sexual development NEC 259.1
   thelarche 259.1
Precocity, sexual (constitutional) (cryptogenic)
   (female) (idiopathic) (male) NEC 259.1
   with adrenal hyperplasia 255.2
Precordial pain 786.51
   psychogenic 307.89
Predeciduous teeth 520.2
Prediabetes, prediabetic 790.29
   complicating pregnancy, childbirth, or
     puerperium 648.8●
   fetus or newborn 775.89
Predislocation status of hip, at birth (*see also*
   Subluxation, congenital, hip) 754.32

Pre-eclampsia (mild) 642.4●
   with pre-existing hypertension 642.7●
   affecting fetus or newborn 760.0
   severe 642.5●
   superimposed on pre-existing hypertensive
     disease 642.7●
Preeruptive color change, teeth, tooth
   520.8
Preexcitation 426.7
   atrioventricular conduction 426.7
   ventricular 426.7
Preglaucoma 365.00
Pregnancy (single) (uterine) (without sickness)
   V22.2

> Note: Use the following fifth-digit subclassification with categories 640–649, 651–679:
>
> 0   unspecified as to episode of care
> 1   delivered, with or without mention of antepartum condition
> 2   delivered, with mention of postpartum complication
> 3   antepartum condition or complication
> 4   postpartum condition or complication

   abdominal (ectopic) 633.00
     with intrauterine pregnancy 633.01
     affecting fetus or newborn 761.4
   abnormal NEC 646.9●
   ampullar - *see* Pregnancy, tubal
   biochemical 631.0
   broad ligament - *see* Pregnancy, cornual
   cervical - *see* Pregnancy, cornual
   chemical 631.0
   combined (extrauterine and intrauterine) -
     see Pregnancy, cornual
   complicated (by) 646.9●
     abnormal, abnormality NEC 646.9●
       cervix 654.6●
       cord (umbilical) 663.9●
       glucose tolerance (conditions
         classifiable to 790.21–790.29)
         648.8●
       pelvic organs or tissues NEC 654.9●
       pelvis (bony) 653.0●
       perineum or vulva 654.8●
       placenta, placental (vessel) 656.7●
       position
         cervix 654.4●
         placenta 641.1●
           without hemorrhage 641.0●
         uterus 654.4●
       size, fetus 653.5●
       uterus (congenital) 654.0●
     abscess or cellulitis
       bladder 646.6●
       genitourinary tract (conditions
         classifiable to 590, 595, 597, 599.0,
         614.0–614.5, 614.7–614.9, 615)
         646.6●
       kidney 646.6●
       urinary tract NEC 646.6●
     adhesion, pelvic peritoneal 648.9●
     air embolism 673.0●
     albuminuria 646.2●
       with hypertension - *see* Toxemia, of
         pregnancy
     amnionitis 658.4●
     amniotic fluid embolism 673.1●
     anemia (conditions classifiable to
       280–285) 648.2●
     appendicitis 648.9●
     atrophy, yellow (acute) (liver) (subacute)
       646.7●
     bacilluria, asymptomatic 646.5●
     bacteriuria, asymptomatic 646.5●
     bariatric surgery status 649.2●
     bicornis or bicornuate uterus 654.0●
     biliary problems 646.8●

SECTION I INDEX TO DISEASES AND INJURIES / Pregnancy

Pregnancy (Continued)
    complicated (Continued)
        bone and joint disorders (conditions classifiable to 720–724 or conditions affecting lower limbs classifiable to 711–719, 725–738) 648.7●
        breech presentation (buttocks) (complete) (frank) 652.2●
            with successful version 652.1●
        cardiovascular disease (conditions classifiable to 390–398, 410–429) 648.6●
            congenital (conditions classifiable to 745–747) 648.5●
        cerebrovascular disorders (conditions classifiable to 430–434, 436–437) 674.0●
        cervicitis (conditions classifiable to 616.0) 646.6●
        chloasma (gravidarum) 646.8●
        cholelithiasis 646.8●
        cholestasis 646.7●
        chorea (gravidarum) - see Eclampsia, pregnancy
        coagulation defect 649.3●
        conjoined twins 678.1●
        contraction, pelvis (general) 653.1●
            inlet 653.2●
            outlet 653.3●
        convulsions (eclamptic) (uremic) 642.6●
            with pre-existing hypertension 642.7●
        current disease or condition (nonobstetric)
            abnormal glucose tolerance 648.8●
            anemia 648.2●
            biliary tract 646.7●
            bone and joint (lower limb) 648.7●
            cardiovascular 648.6●
                congenital 648.5●
            cerebrovascular 674.0●
            diabetes (conditions classifiable to 249 and 250) 648.0●
            drug dependence 648.3●
            female genital mutilation 648.9●
            genital organ or tract 646.6●
            gonorrheal 647.1●
            hypertensive 642.2●
                chronic kidney 642.2●
                renal 642.1●
            infectious 647.9●
                specified type NEC 647.8●
            liver 646.7●
            malarial 647.4●
            nutritional deficiency 648.9●
            parasitic NEC 647.8●
            periodontal disease 648.9●
            renal 646.2●
                hypertensive 642.1●
            rubella 647.5●
            specified condition NEC 648.9●
            syphilitic 647.0●
            thyroid 648.1●
            tuberculous 647.3●
            urinary 646.6●
            venereal 647.2●
            viral NEC 647.6●
        cystitis 646.6●
        cystocele 654.4●
        death of fetus (near term) 656.4●
            early pregnancy (before 22 completed weeks' gestation) 632
        deciduitis 646.6●
        decreased fetal movements 655.7●
        diabetes (mellitus) (conditions classifiable to 249 and 250) 648.0●
        disorders of liver and biliary tract 646.7●
        displacement, uterus NEC 654.4●
        disproportion - see Disproportion
        double uterus 654.0●
        drug dependence (conditions classifiable to 304) 648.3●

Pregnancy (Continued)
    complicated (Continued)
        dysplasia, cervix 654.6●
        early onset of delivery (spontaneous) 644.2●
        eclampsia, eclamptic (coma) (convulsions) (delirium) (nephritis) (uremia) 642.6●
            with pre-existing hypertension 642.7●
        edema 646.1●
            with hypertension - see Toxemia, of pregnancy
        effusion, amniotic fluid 658.1●
            delayed delivery following 658.2●
        embolism
            air 673.0●
            amniotic fluid 673.1●
            blood-clot 673.2●
            cerebral 674.0●
            pulmonary NEC 673.2●
            pyemic 673.3●
            septic 673.3●
        emesis (gravidarum) - see Pregnancy, complicated, vomiting
        endometritis (conditions classifiable to 615.0–615.9) 670.1●
            decidual 646.6●
        epilepsy 649.4●
        excessive weight gain NEC 646.1●
        face presentation 652.4●
        failure, fetal head to enter pelvic brim 652.5●
        false labor (pains) 644.1●
        fatigue 646.8●
        fatty metamorphosis of liver 646.7●
        female genital mutilation 648.9●
        fetal
            anemia 678.0●
            complications from in utero procedure 679.1●
            conjoined twins 678.1●
            death (near term) 656.4●
                early (before 22 completed weeks' gestation) 632
            deformity 653.7●
            distress 656.8●
            hematologic conditions 678.0●
            reduction of multiple fetuses reduced to single fetus 651.7●
            thrombocytopenia 678.0●
            twin to twin transfusion 678.0●
        fibroid (tumor) (uterus) 654.1●
        footling presentation 652.8●
            with successful version 652.1●
        gallbladder disease 646.8●
        gastric banding status 649.2●
        gastric bypass status for obesity 649.2●
        genital herpes (asymptomatic) (history of) (inactive) 647.6●
        goiter 648.1●
        gonococcal infection (conditions classifiable to 098) 647.1●
        gonorrhea (conditions classifiable to 098) 647.1●
        hemorrhage 641.9●
            accidental 641.2●
            before 22 completed weeks' gestation NEC 640.9●
            cerebrovascular 674.0●
            due to
                afibrinogenemia or other coagulation defect (conditions classifiable to 286.0–286.9) 641.3●
                leiomyoma, uterine 641.8●
                marginal sinus (rupture) 641.2●
                premature separation, placenta 641.2●
                trauma 641.8●

Pregnancy (Continued)
    complicated (Continued)
        hemorrhage (Continued)
            early (before 22 completed weeks' gestation) 640.9●
            threatened abortion 640.0●
            unavoidable 641.1●
        hepatitis (acute) (malignant) (subacute) 646.7●
            viral 647.6●
        herniation of uterus 654.4●
        high head at term 652.5●
        hydatidiform mole (delivered) (undelivered) 630
        hydramnios 657●
        hydrocephalic fetus 653.6●
        hydrops amnii 657●
        hydrorrhea 658.1●
        hyperemesis (gravidarum) - see Hyperemesis, gravidarum
        hypertension - see Hypertension, complicating pregnancy
        hypertensive
            chronic kidney disease 642.2●
            heart and chronic kidney disease 642.2●
            heart and renal disease 642.2●
            heart disease 642.2●
            renal disease 642.2●
        hypertensive heart and chronic kidney disease 642.2●
        hyperthyroidism 648.1●
        hypothyroidism 648.1●
        hysteralgia 646.8●
        icterus gravis 646.7●
        incarceration, uterus 654.3●
        incompetent cervix (os) 654.5●
        infection 647.9●
            amniotic fluid 658.4●
            bladder 646.6●
            genital organ (conditions classifiable to 614.0– 614.5, 614.7–614.9, 615) 646.6●
            kidney (conditions classifiable to 590.0–590.9) 646.6●
            urinary (tract) 646.6●
                asymptomatic 646.5●
        infective and parasitic diseases NEC 647.8●
        inflammation
            bladder 646.6●
            genital organ (conditions classifiable to 614.0) 646.6●
            urinary tract NEC 646.6●
        injury 648.9●
            obstetrical NEC 665.9●
        insufficient weight gain 646.8●
        insulin resistance 648.8●
        intrauterine fetal death (near term) NEC 656.4●
            early (before 22 completed weeks' gestation) 632
        malaria (conditions classifiable to 084) 647.4●
        malformation, uterus (congenital) 654.0●
        malnutrition (conditions classifiable to 260–269) 648.9●
        malposition
            fetus - see Pregnancy, complicated, malpresentation
            uterus or cervix 654.4●
        malpresentation 652.9●
            with successful version 652.1●
            in multiple gestation 652.6●
            specified type NEC 652.8●
        marginal sinus hemorrhage or rupture 641.2●
        maternal complications from in utero procedure 679.0●
        maternal drug abuse 648.4●
        maternal obesity syndrome 646.1●

◀ New ◀|||| Revised deleted Deleted ● Use Additional Digit(s) Omit code 401

Pregnancy (Continued)
    complicated (Continued)
        menstruation 640.8●
        mental disorders (conditions classifiable to 290–303, 305.0, 305.2–305.9, 306–316, 317–319) 648.4●
        mentum presentation 652.4●
        missed
            abortion 632
            delivery (at or near term) 656.4●
            labor (at or near term) 656.4●
        necrosis
            genital organ or tract (conditions classifiable to 614.0–614.5, 614.7–614.9, 615) 646.6●
            liver (conditions classifiable to 570) 646.7●
            renal, cortical 646.2●
        nephritis or nephrosis (conditions classifiable to 580–589) 646.2●
            with hypertension 642.1●
        nephropathy NEC 646.2●
        neuritis (peripheral) 646.4●
        nutritional deficiency (conditions classifiable to 260–269) 648.9●
        obesity 649.1●
            surgery status 649.2●
        oblique lie or presentation 652.3●
            with successful version 652.1●
        obstetrical trauma NEC 665.9●
        oligohydramnios NEC 658.0●
        onset of contractions before 37 weeks 644.0●
        oversize fetus 653.5●
        papyraceous fetus 646.0●
        patent cervix 654.5●
        pelvic inflammatory disease (conditions classifiable to 614.0–614.5, 614.7–614.9, 615) 646.6●
        pelvic peritoneal adhesion 648.9●
        placenta, placental
            abnormality 656.7●
            abruptio or ablatio 641.2●
            detachment 641.2●
            disease 656.7●
            infarct 656.7●
            low implantation 641.1●
                without hemorrhage 641.0●
            malformation 656.7●
            malposition 641.1●
                without hemorrhage 641.0●
            marginal sinus hemorrhage 641.2●
            previa 641.1●
                without hemorrhage 641.0●
            separation (premature) (undelivered) 641.2●
        placentitis 658.4●
        pneumonia 648.9
        polyhydramnios 657●
        postmaturity
            post-term 645.1●
            prolonged 645.2●
        prediabetes 648.8●
        pre-eclampsia (mild) 642.4●
            severe 642.5●
            superimposed on pre-existing hypertensive disease 642.7●
        premature rupture of membranes 658.1●
            with delayed delivery 658.2●
        previous
            ectopic pregnancy V23.42
            infertility V23.0
            in utero procedure during previous pregnancy V23.86
            nonobstetric condition V23.89
            poor obstetrical history V23.49
            premature delivery V23.41
            trophoblastic disease (conditions classifiable to 630) V23.1
        prolapse, uterus 654.4●

Pregnancy (Continued)
    complicated (Continued)
        proteinuria (gestational) 646.2●
            with hypertension - see Toxemia, of pregnancy
        pruritus (neurogenic) 646.8●
        psychosis or psychoneurosis 648.4●
        ptyalism 646.8●
        pyelitis (conditions classifiable to 590.0–590.9) 646.6●
        renal disease or failure NEC 646.2●
            with secondary hypertension 642.1●
            hypertensive 642.2●
        retention, retained dead ovum 631.8
        retroversion, uterus 654.3●
        Rh immunization, incompatibility, or sensitization 656.1●
        rubella (conditions classifiable to 056) 647.5●
        rupture
            amnion (premature) 658.1●
                with delayed delivery 658.2●
            marginal sinus (hemorrhage) 641.2●
            membranes (premature) 658.1●
                with delayed delivery 658.2●
            uterus (before onset of labor) 665.0●
        salivation (excessive) 646.8●
        salpingo-oophoritis (conditions classifiable to 614.0–614.2) 646.6●
        septicemia (conditions classifiable to 038.0–038.9) 647.8●
            postpartum 670.2●
            puerperal 670.2●
            smoking 649.0●
        spasms, uterus (abnormal) 646.8●
        specified condition NEC 646.8●
        spotting 649.5●
        spurious labor pains 644.1●
        status post
            bariatric surgery 649.2●
            gastric banding 649.2●
            gastric bypass for obesity 649.2●
            obesity surgery 649.2●
        superfecundation 651.9●
        superfetation 651.9●
        syphilis (conditions classifiable to 090–097) 647.0●
        threatened
            abortion 640.0●
            premature delivery 644.2●
            premature labor 644.0●
        thrombophlebitis (superficial) 671.2●
            deep 671.3●
            septic 670.3●
        thrombosis 671.2●
            venous (superficial) 671.2●
                deep 671.3●
        thyroid dysfunction (conditions classifiable to 240–246) 648.1●
        thyroiditis 648.1●
        thyrotoxicosis 648.1●
        tobacco use disorder 649.0●
        torsion of uterus 654.4●
        toxemia - see Toxemia, of pregnancy
        transverse lie or presentation 652.3●
            with successful version 652.1●
        trauma 648.9●
            obstetrical 665.9●
        tuberculosis (conditions classifiable to 010–018) 647.3●
        tumor
            cervix 654.6●
            ovary 654.4●
            pelvic organs or tissue NEC 654.4●
            uterus (body) 654.1●
                cervix 654.6●
            vagina 654.7●
            vulva 654.8●
        unstable lie 652.0●

Pregnancy (Continued)
    complicated (Continued)
        uremia - see Pregnancy, complicated, renal disease
        urethritis 646.6●
        vaginitis or vulvitis (conditions classifiable to 616.1) 646.6●
        varicose
            placental vessels 656.7●
            veins (legs) 671.0●
                perineum 671.1●
                vulva 671.1●
        varicosity, labia or vulva 671.1●
        venereal disease NEC (conditions classifiable to 099) 647.2●
        venous complication 671.9●
        viral disease NEC (conditions classifiable to 042, 050–055, 057–079, 795.05, 795.15, 796.75) 647.6●
        vomiting (incoercible) (pernicious) (persistent) (uncontrollable) (vicious) 643.9●
            due to organic disease or other cause 643.8●
            early - see Hyperemesis, gravidarum
            late (after 22 completed weeks gestation) 643.2●
        young maternal age 659.8●
    complications NEC 646.9●
    cornual 633.80
        with intrauterine pregnancy 633.81
        affecting fetus or newborn 761.4
    death, maternal NEC 646.9●
    delivered - see Delivery
    ectopic (ruptured) NEC 633.90
        with intrauterine pregnancy 633.91
        abdominal - see Pregnancy, abdominal
        affecting fetus or newborn 761.4
        combined (extrauterine and intrauterine) - see Pregnancy, cornual
        ovarian - see Pregnancy, ovarian
        specified type NEC 633.80
            with intrauterine pregnancy 633.81
            affecting fetus or newborn 761.4
        tubal - see Pregnancy, tubal
    examination, pregnancy
        negative result V72.41
        not confirmed V72.40
        positive result V72.42
    extrauterine - see Pregnancy, ectopic
    fallopian - see Pregnancy, tubal
    false 300.11
        labor (pains) 644.1●
    fatigue 646.8●
    illegitimate V61.6
    incidental finding V22.2
    in double uterus 654.0●
    interstitial - see Pregnancy, cornual
    intraligamentous - see Pregnancy, cornual
    intramural - see Pregnancy, cornual
    intraperitoneal - see Pregnancy, abdominal
    isthmian - see Pregnancy, tubal
    management affected by
        abnormal, abnormality
            fetus (suspected) 655.9●
                specified NEC 655.8●
            placenta 656.7●
        advanced maternal age NEC 659.6●
            multigravida 659.6●
            primigravida 659.5●
        antibodies (maternal)
            anti-c 656.1●
            anti-d 656.1●
            anti-e 656.1●
            blood group (ABO) 656.2●
                Rh(esus) 656.1●
        appendicitis 648.9●
        bariatric surgery status 649.2●
        coagulation defect 649.3●
        elderly multigravida 659.6●

Pregnancy (Continued)
  management affected by (Continued)
    elderly primigravida 659.5
    epilepsy 649.4
    fetal (suspected)
      abnormality 655.9
        abdominal 655.8
        acid-base balance 656.8
        cardiovascular 655.8
        facial 655.8
        gastrointestinal 655.8
        genitourinary 655.8
        heart rate or rhythm 659.7
        limb 655.8
        specified NEC 655.8
      acidemia 656.3
      anencephaly 655.0
      aneuploidy 655.1
      bradycardia 659.7
      central nervous system malformation 655.0
      chromosomal abnormalities (conditions classifiable to 758.0–758.9) 655.1
      damage from
        drugs 655.5
          obstetric, anesthetic, or sedative 655.5
        environmental toxins 655.8
        intrauterine contraceptive device 655.8
        maternal
          alcohol addiction 655.4
          disease NEC 655.4
          drug use 655.5
          listeriosis 655.4
          rubella 655.3
          toxoplasmosis 655.4
          viral infection 655.3
        radiation 655.6
      death (near term) 656.4
        early (before 22 completed weeks' gestation) 632
      distress 656.8
      excessive growth 656.6
      growth retardation 656.5
      hereditary disease 655.2
      hydrocephalus 655.0
      intrauterine death 656.4
      poor growth 656.5
      spina bifida (with myelomeningocele) 655.0
    fetal-maternal hemorrhage 656.0
    gastric banding status 649.2
    gastric bypass status for obesity 649.2
    hereditary disease in family (possibly) affecting fetus 655.2
    incompatibility, blood groups (ABO) 656.2
      Rh(esus) 656.1
    insufficient prenatal care V23.7
    insulin resistance 648.8
    intrauterine death 656.4
    isoimmunization (ABO) 656.2
      Rh(esus) 656.1
    large-for-dates fetus 656.6
    light-for-dates fetus 656.5
    meconium in liquor 656.8
    mental disorder (conditions classifiable to 290–303, 305.0, 305.2–305.9, 306–316, 317–319) 648.4
    multiparity (grand) 659.4
    obesity 649.1
      surgery status 649.2
    poor obstetric history V23.49
      pre-term labor V23.41
    postmaturity
      post-term 645.1
      prolonged 645.2
    post-term pregnancy 645.1

Pregnancy (Continued)
  management affected by (Continued)
    previous
      abortion V23.2
        habitual 646.3
      cesarean delivery 654.2
      difficult delivery V23.49
      ectopic pregnancy V23.42
      forceps delivery V23.49
      habitual abortions 646.3
      hemorrhage, antepartum or postpartum V23.49
      hydatidiform mole V23.1
      infertility V23.0
      in utero procedure during previous pregnancy V23.86
      malignancy NEC V23.89
      nonobstetrical conditions V23.89
      premature delivery V23.41
      recurrent pregnancy loss 646.3
      trophoblastic disease (conditions in 630) V23.1
      vesicular mole V23.1
    prolonged pregnancy 645.2
    recurrent pregnancy loss 646.3
    small-for-dates fetus 656.5
    smoking 649.0
    spotting 649.5
    suspected conditions not found
      amniotic cavity and membrane problem V89.01
      cervical shortening V89.05
      fetal anomaly V89.03
      fetal growth problem V89.04
      oligohydramnios V89.01
      other specified problem NEC V89.09
      placental problem V89.02
      polyhydramnios V89.01
    tobacco use disorder 649.0
    venous complication 671.9
    young maternal age 659.8
  maternal death NEC 646.9
  mesometric (mural) - see Pregnancy, cornual
  molar 631.8
    hydatidiform (see also Hydatidiform mole) 630
      previous, affecting management of pregnancy V23.1
    previous, affecting management of pregnancy V23.49
  multiple NEC 651.9
    with fetal loss and retention of one or more fetus(es) 651.6
    affecting fetus or newborn 761.5
    following (elective) fetal reduction 651.7
    specified type NEC 651.8
      with fetal loss and retention of one or more fetus(es) 651.6
      following (elective) fetal reduction 651.7
  mural - see Pregnancy, cornual
  observation NEC V22.1
    first pregnancy V22.0
    high-risk V23.9
      inconclusive fetal viability V23.87
      specified problem NEC V23.89
  ovarian 633.20
    with intrauterine pregnancy 633.21
    affecting fetus or newborn 761.4
  possible, not (yet) confirmed V72.40
  postmature
    post-term 645.1
    prolonged 645.2
  post-term 645.1
  prenatal care only V22.1
    first pregnancy V22.0
    high-risk V23.9
      inconclusive fetal viability V23.87
      specified problem NEC V23.89
  prolonged 645.2

Pregnancy (Continued)
  quadruplet NEC 651.2
    with fetal loss and retention of one or more fetus(es) 651.5
    affecting fetus or newborn 761.5
    following (elective) fetal reduction 651.7
  quintuplet NEC 651.8
    with fetal loss and retention of one or more fetus(es) 651.6
    affecting fetus or newborn 761.5
    following (elective) fetal reduction 651.7
  resulting from
    assisted reproductive technology V23.85
    in vitro fertilization V23.85
  sextuplet NEC 651.8
    with fetal loss and retention of one or more fetus(es) 651.6
    affecting fetus or newborn 761.5
    following (elective) fetal reduction 651.7
  spurious 300.11
  superfecundation NEC 651.9
    with fetal loss and retention of one or more fetus(es) 651.6
    following (elective) fetal reduction 651.7
  superfetation NEC 651.9
    with fetal loss and retention of one or more fetus(es) 651.6
    following (elective) fetal reduction 651.7
  supervision (of) (for) - see also Pregnancy, management affected by
    elderly
      multigravida V23.82
      primigravida V23.81
    high-risk V23.9
      inconclusive fetal viability V23.87
      insufficient prenatal care V23.7
      specified problem NEC V23.89
    inconclusive fetal viability V23.87
    multiparity V23.3
    normal NEC V22.1
      first V22.0
    poor
      obstetric history V23.49
        ectopic pregnancy V23.42
        pre-term labor V23.41
      reproductive history V23.5
    previous
      abortion V23.2
      hydatidiform mole V23.1
      infertility V23.0
      neonatal death V23.5
      stillbirth V23.5
      trophoblastic disease V23.1
      vesicular mole V23.1
    specified problem NEC V23.89
    young
      multigravida V23.84
      primigravida V23.83
  triplet NEC 651.1
    with fetal loss and retention of one or more fetus(es) 651.4
    affecting fetus or newborn 761.5
    following (elective) fetal reduction 651.7
  tubal (with rupture) 633.10
    with intrauterine pregnancy 633.11
    affecting fetus or newborn 761.4
  twin NEC 651.0
    with fetal loss and retention of one fetus 651.3
    affecting fetus or newborn 761.5
    conjoined 678.1
    following (elective) fetal reduction 651.7
  unconfirmed V72.40
  undelivered (no other diagnosis) V22.2
    with false labor 644.1
    high-risk V23.9
      specified problem NEC V23.89
  unwanted NEC V61.7
Pregnant uterus - see condition
Preiser's disease (osteoporosis) 733.09
Prekwashiorkor 260

Preleukemia 238.75
Preluxation of hip, congenital (see also
    Subluxation, congenital, hip) 754.32
Premature - see also condition
    beats (nodal) 427.60
        atrial 427.61
        auricular 427.61
        postoperative 997.1
        specified type NEC 427.69
        supraventricular 427.61
        ventricular 427.69
    birth NEC 765.1
    closure
        cranial suture 756.0
        fontanel 756.0
        foramen ovale 745.8
    contractions 427.60
        atrial 427.61
        auricular 427.61
        auriculoventricular 427.61
        heart (extrasystole) 427.60
        junctional 427.60
        nodal 427.60
        postoperative 997.1
        ventricular 427.69
    ejaculation 302.75
    infant NEC 765.1
        excessive 765.0
        light-for-dates - see Light-for-dates
    labor 644.2
        threatened 644.0
    lungs 770.4
    menopause 256.31
    puberty 259.1
    rupture of membranes or amnion
        658.1
        affecting fetus or newborn 761.1
        delayed delivery following 658.2
    senility (syndrome) 259.8
    separation, placenta (partial) - see Placenta,
        separation
    ventricular systole 427.69
Prematurity NEC 765.1
    extreme 765.0
Premenstrual syndrome 625.4
Premenstrual tension 625.4
Premolarization, cuspids 520.2
Premyeloma 273.1
Prenatal
    care, normal pregnancy V22.1
        first V22.0
    death, cause unknown - see Death, fetus
    screening - see Antenatal, screening
    teeth 520.6
Prepartum - see condition
Preponderance, left or right ventricular
    429.3
Prepuce - see condition
PRES (posterior reversible encephalopathy
    syndrome) 348.39
Presbycardia 797
    hypertensive (see also Hypertension, heart)
        402.90
Presbycusis 388.01
Presbyesophagus 530.89
Presbyophrenia 310.1
Presbyopia 367.4
Prescription of contraceptives NEC
    V25.02
    diaphragm V25.02
    oral (pill) V25.01
        emergency V25.03
        postcoital V25.03
        repeat V25.41
    repeat V25.40
        oral (pill) V25.41
Presenile - see also condition
    aging 259.8
    dementia (see also Dementia, presenile)
        290.10
Presenility 259.8

Presentation, fetal
    abnormal 652.9
        with successful version 652.1
        before labor, affecting fetus or newborn
            761.7
        causing obstructed labor 660.0
            affecting fetus or newborn, any, except
                breech 763.1
        in multiple gestation (one or more) 652.6
        specified NEC 652.8
    arm 652.7
        causing obstructed labor 660.0
    breech (buttocks) (complete) (frank) 652.2
        with successful version 652.1
            before labor, affecting fetus or
                newborn 761.7
        before labor, affecting fetus or newborn
            761.7
    brow 652.4
        causing obstructed labor 660.0
    buttocks 652.2
    chin 652.4
    complete 652.2
    compound 652.8
    cord 663.0
    extended head 652.4
    face 652.4
        to pubes 652.8
    footling 652.8
    frank 652.2
    hand, leg, or foot NEC 652.8
    incomplete 652.8
    mentum 652.4
    multiple gestation (one fetus or more) 652.6
    oblique 652.3
        with successful version 652.1
    shoulder 652.8
        affecting fetus or newborn 763.1
    transverse 652.3
        with successful version 652.1
    umbilical cord 663.0
    unstable 652.0
Prespondylolisthesis (congenital)
    (lumbosacral) 756.11
Pressure
    area, skin ulcer (see also Ulcer, pressure)
        707.00
    atrophy, spine 733.99
    birth, fetus or newborn NEC 767.9
    brachial plexus 353.0
    brain 348.4
        injury at birth 767.0
    cerebral - see Pressure, brain
    chest 786.59
    cone, tentorial 348.4
        injury at birth 767.0
    funis - see Compression, umbilical cord
    hyposystolic (see also Hypotension) 458.9
    increased
        intracranial 781.99
            due to
                benign intracranial hypertension
                    348.2
                hydrocephalus - see hydrocephalus
                injury at birth 767.8
        intraocular 365.00
    lumbosacral plexus 353.1
    mediastinum 519.3
    necrosis (chronic) (skin) (see also Decubitus)
        707.00
    nerve - see Compression, nerve
    paralysis (see also Neuropathy, entrapment)
        355.9
    pre-ulcer skin changes limited to persistent
        focal erythema (see also Ulcer, pressure)
        707.21
    sore (chronic) (see also Ulcer, pressure)
        707.00
    spinal cord 336.9
    ulcer (chronic) (see also Ulcer, pressure)
        707.00

Pressure (Continued)
    umbilical cord - see Compression, umbilical
        cord
    venous, increased 459.89
Pre-syncope 780.2
Preterm infant NEC 765.1
    extreme 765.0
Priapism (penis) 607.3
Prickling sensation (see also Disturbance,
    sensation) 782.0
Prickly heat 705.1
Primary - see also condition
    angle closure suspect 365.02
Primigravida, elderly
    affecting
        fetus or newborn 763.89
        management of pregnancy, labor, and
            delivery 659.5
Primipara, old
    affecting
        fetus or newborn 763.89
        management of pregnancy, labor, and
            delivery 659.5
Primula dermatitis 692.6
Primus varus (bilateral) (metatarsus) 754.52
PRIND (prolonged reversible ischemic
    neurologic deficit) 434.91
    history of (personal) V12.54
Pringle's disease (tuberous sclerosis) 759.5
Prinzmetal's angina 413.1
Prinzmetal-Massumi syndrome (anterior chest
    wall) 786.52
Prizefighter ear 738.7
Problem (with) V49.9
    academic V62.3
    acculturation V62.4
    adopted child V61.24
    aged
        in-law V61.3
        parent V61.3
        person NEC V61.8
    alcoholism in family V61.41
    anger reaction (see also Disturbance, conduct)
        312.0
    behavior, child 312.9
    behavioral V40.9
        specified NEC V40.39
    betting V69.3
    biological child V61.23
    cardiorespiratory NEC V47.2
    care of sick or handicapped person in family
        or household V61.49
    career choice V62.29
    communication V40.1
    conscience regarding medical care V62.6
    delinquency (juvenile) 312.9
    diet, inappropriate V69.1
    digestive NEC V47.3
    ear NEC V41.3
    eating habits, inappropriate V69.1
    economic V60.2
        affecting care V60.9
        specified type NEC V60.89
    educational V62.3
    enuresis, child 307.6
    exercise, lack of V69.0
    eye NEC V41.1
    family V61.9
        specified circumstance NEC V61.8
    fear reaction, child 313.0
    feeding (elderly) (infant) 783.3
        newborn 779.31
        nonorganic 307.59
    fetal, affecting management of pregnancy
        656.9
        specified type NEC 656.8
    financial V60.2
    foster child V61.25
    functional V41.9
        specified type NEC V41.8
    gambling V69.3

Problem (Continued)
- genital NEC V47.5
- head V48.9
  - deficiency V48.0
  - disfigurement V48.6
  - mechanical V48.2
  - motor V48.2
  - movement of V48.2
  - sensory V48.4
  - specified condition NEC V48.8
- hearing V41.2
- high-risk sexual behavior V69.2
- identity 313.82
- influencing health status NEC V49.89
- internal organ NEC V47.9
  - deficiency V47.0
  - mechanical or motor V47.1
- interpersonal NEC V62.81
- jealousy, child 313.3
- learning V40.0
- legal V62.5
- life circumstance NEC V62.89
- lifestyle V69.9
  - specified NEC V69.8
- limb V49.9
  - deficiency V49.0
  - disfigurement V49.4
  - mechanical V49.1
  - motor V49.2
  - movement, involving
    - musculoskeletal system V49.1
    - nervous system V49.2
  - sensory V49.3
  - specified condition NEC V49.5
- litigation V62.5
- living alone V60.3
- loneliness NEC V62.89
- marital V61.10
  - involving
    - divorce V61.03
    - estrangement V61.09
    - psychosexual disorder 302.9
    - sexual function V41.7
  - relationship V61.10
- mastication V41.6
- medical care, within family V61.49
- mental V40.9
  - specified NEC V40.2
- mental hygiene, adult V40.9
- multiparity V61.5
- nail biting, child 307.9
- neck V48.9
  - deficiency V48.1
  - disfigurement V48.7
  - mechanical V48.3
  - motor V48.3
  - movement V48.3
  - sensory V48.5
  - specified condition NEC V48.8
- neurological NEC 781.99
- none (feared complaint unfounded) V65.5
- occupational V62.29
- parent-child V61.20
  - adopted child V61.24
  - biological child V61.23
  - foster child V61.25
  - relationship V61.20
- partner V61.10
  - relationship V61.10
- personal NEC V62.89
  - interpersonal conflict NEC V62.81
- personality (see also Disorder, personality) 301.9
- phase of life V62.89
- placenta, affecting management of pregnancy 656.9●
  - specified type NEC 656.8●
- poverty V60.2
- presence of sick or handicapped person in family or household V61.49
- psychiatric 300.9

Problem (Continued)
- psychosocial V62.9
  - specified type NEC V62.89
- relational NEC V62.81
- relationship, childhood 313.3
- religious or spiritual belief
  - other than medical care V62.89
  - regarding medical care V62.6
- self-damaging behavior V69.8
- sexual
  - behavior, high-risk V69.2
  - function NEC V41.7
- sibling
  - relational V61.8
  - relationship V61.8
- sight V41.0
- sleep, lack of V69.4
- sleep disorder, child 307.40
- smell V41.5
- speech V40.1
- spite reaction, child (see also Disturbance, conduct) 312.0●
- spoiled child reaction (see also Disturbance, conduct) 312.1●
- substance abuse in family V61.42
- swallowing V41.6
- tantrum, child (see also Disturbance, conduct) 312.1●
- taste V41.5
- thumb sucking, child 307.9
- tic (child) 307.21
- trunk V48.9
  - deficiency V48.1
  - disfigurement V48.7
  - mechanical V48.3
  - motor V48.3
  - movement V48.3
  - sensory V48.5
  - specified condition NEC V48.8
- unemployment V62.0
- urinary NEC V47.4
- voice production V41.4

Procedure (surgical) not done NEC V64.3
- because of
  - contraindication V64.1
  - patient's decision V64.2
    - for reasons of conscience or religion V62.6
  - specified reason NEC V64.3

Procidentia
- anus (sphincter) 569.1
- rectum (sphincter) 569.1
- stomach 537.89
- uteri 618.1

Proctalgia 569.42
- fugax 564.6
- spasmodic 564.6
  - psychogenic 307.89

Proctitis 569.49
- amebic 006.8
- chlamydial 099.52
- gonococcal 098.7
- granulomatous 555.1
- idiopathic 556.2
  - with ulcerative sigmoiditis 556.3
- tuberculous (see also Tuberculosis) 014.8●
- ulcerative (chronic) (nonspecific) 556.2
  - with ulcerative sigmoiditis 556.3

Proctocele
- female (without uterine prolapse) 618.04
  - with uterine prolapse 618.4
    - complete 618.3
    - incomplete 618.2
- male 569.49

Proctocolitis, idiopathic 556.2
- with ulcerative sigmoiditis 556.3

Proctoptosis 569.1

Proctosigmoiditis 569.89
- ulcerative (chronic) 556.3

Proctospasm 564.6
- psychogenic 306.4

Prodromal-AIDS - see Human immunodeficiency virus (disease) (illness) (infection)

Profichet's disease or syndrome 729.90

Progeria (adultorum) (syndrome) 259.8

Prognathism (mandibular) (maxillary) 524.10

Progonoma (melanotic) (M9363/0) - see Neoplasm, by site, benign

Progressive - see condition

Prolapse, prolapsed
- anus, anal (canal) (sphincter) 569.1
- arm or hand, complicating delivery 652.7●
  - causing obstructed labor 660.0●
    - affecting fetus or newborn 763.1
  - fetus or newborn 763.1
- bladder (acquired) (mucosa) (sphincter)
  - congenital (female) (male) 756.71
  - female (see also Cystocele, female) 618.01
  - male 596.89
- breast implant (prosthetic) 996.54
- cecostomy 569.69
- cecum 569.89
- cervix, cervical (hypertrophied) 618.1
  - anterior lip, obstructing labor 660.2●
    - affecting fetus or newborn 763.1
  - congenital 752.49
  - postpartal (old) 618.1
  - stump 618.84
- ciliary body 871.1
- colon (pedunculated) 569.89
- colostomy 569.69
- conjunctiva 372.73
- cord - see Prolapse, umbilical cord
- cystostomy 596.83
- disc (intervertebral) - see Displacement, intervertebral disc
- duodenum 537.89
- eye implant (orbital) 996.59
  - lens (ocular) 996.53
- fallopian tube 620.4
- fetal extremity, complicating delivery 652.8●
  - causing obstructed labor 660.0●
  - fetus or newborn 763.1
- funis - see Prolapse, umbilical cord
- gastric (mucosa) 537.89
- genital, female 618.9
  - specified NEC 618.89
- globe 360.81
- ileostomy bud 569.69
- intervertebral disc - see Displacement, intervertebral disc
- intestine (small) 569.89
- iris 364.89
  - traumatic 871.1
- kidney (see also Disease, renal) 593.0
  - congenital 753.3
- laryngeal muscles or ventricle 478.79
- leg, complicating delivery 652.8●
  - causing obstructed labor 660.0●
  - fetus or newborn 763.1
- liver 573.8
- meatus urinarius 599.5
- mitral valve 424.0
- ocular lens implant 996.53
- organ or site, congenital NEC - see Malposition, congenital
- ovary 620.4
- pelvic (floor), female 618.89
- perineum, female 618.89
- pregnant uterus 654.4●
- rectum (mucosa) (sphincter) 569.1
  - due to Trichuris trichiuria 127.3
- spleen 289.59
- stomach 537.89
- umbilical cord
  - affecting fetus or newborn 762.4
  - complicating delivery 663.0●
- ureter 593.89
  - with obstruction 593.4
- ureterovesical orifice 593.89

Prolapse, prolapsed (Continued)
urethra (acquired) (infected) (mucosa) 599.5
    congenital 753.8
uterovaginal 618.4
    complete 618.3
    incomplete 618.2
    specified NEC 618.89
uterus (first degree) (second degree) (third degree) (complete) (without vaginal wall prolapse) 618.1
    with mention of vaginal wall prolapse - see Prolapse, uterovaginal
    congenital 752.39
    in pregnancy or childbirth 654.4 ●
        affecting fetus or newborn 763.1
        causing obstructed labor 660.2 ●
            affecting fetus or newborn 763.1
    postpartal (old) 618.1
uveal 871.1
vagina (anterior) (posterior) (vault) (wall) (without uterine prolapse) 618.00
    with uterine prolapse 618.4
        complete 618.3
        incomplete 618.2
    paravaginal 618.02
    posthysterectomy 618.5
    specified NEC 618.09
vitreous (humor) 379.26
    traumatic 871.1
womb - see Prolapse, uterus

Prolapsus, female 618.9
Proliferative - see condition
Prolinemia 270.8
Prolinuria 270.8
Prolonged, prolongation
bleeding time (see also Defect, coagulation) 790.92
"idiopathic" (in von Willebrand's disease) 286.4
coagulation time (see also Defect, coagulation) 790.92
gestation syndrome 766.22
labor 662.1 ●
    affecting fetus or newborn 763.89
    first stage 662.0 ●
    second stage 662.2 ●
PR interval 426.11
pregnancy 645.2 ●
prothrombin time (see also Defect, coagulation) 790.92
QT interval 794.31
    syndrome 426.82
rupture of membranes (24 hours or more prior to onset of labor) 658.2 ●
uterine contractions in labor 661.4 ●
    affecting fetus or newborn 763.7

Prominauris 744.29
Prominence
auricle (ear) (congenital) 744.29
    acquired 380.32
ischial spine or sacral promontory
    with disproportion (fetopelvic) 653.3 ●
        affecting fetus or newborn 763.1
        causing obstructed labor 660.1 ●
            affecting fetus or newborn 763.1
nose (congenital) 748.1
    acquired 738.0

PROMM (proximal myotonic myotonia) 359.21
Pronation
ankle 736.79
foot 736.79
    congenital 755.67

Prophylactic
administration of
    antibiotics, long-term V58.62
        short-term - omit code
    antitoxin, any V07.2
    antivenin V07.2
    chemotherapeutic agent NEC V07.39
        fluoride V07.31

Prophylactic (Continued)
administration of (Continued)
    diphtheria antitoxin V07.2
    drug V07.39
    gamma globulin V07.2
    immune sera (gamma globulin) V07.2
    RhoGAM V07.2
    tetanus antitoxin V07.2
chemotherapy NEC V07.39
    fluoride V07.31
hormone replacement (postmenopausal) V07.4
immunotherapy V07.2
measure V07.9
    specified type NEC V07.8
medication V07.39
postmenopausal hormone replacement V07.4
sterilization V25.2

Proptosis (ocular) (see also Exophthalmos) 376.30
thyroid 242.0 ●
Propulsion
eyeball 360.81
Prosecution, anxiety concerning V62.5
Prosopagnosia 368.16
Prostate, prostatic - see condition
Prostatism 600.90
with
    other lower urinary tract symptoms (LUTS) 600.91
    urinary
        obstruction 600.91
        retention 600.91

Prostatitis (congestive) (suppurative) 601.9
acute 601.0
cavitary 601.8
chlamydial 099.54
chronic 601.1
diverticular 601.8
due to Trichomonas (vaginalis) 131.03
fibrous 600.90
    with
        other lower urinary tract symptoms (LUTS) 600.91
        urinary
            obstruction 600.91
            retention 600.91
gonococcal (acute) 098.12
    chronic or duration of 2 months or over 098.32
granulomatous 601.8
hypertrophic 600.00
    with
        other lower urinary tract symptoms (LUTS) 600.01
        urinary
            obstruction 600.01
            retention 600.01
specified type NEC 601.8
subacute 601.1
trichomonal 131.03
tuberculous (see also Tuberculosis) 016.5 ●
    [601.4]

Prostatocystitis 601.3
Prostatorrhea 602.8
Prostatoseminovesiculitis, trichomonal 131.03
Prostration 780.79
heat 992.5
    anhydrotic 992.3
    due to
        salt (and water) depletion 992.4
        water depletion 992.3
nervous 300.5
newborn 779.89
senile 797

Protanomaly 368.51
Protanopia (anomalous trichromat) (complete) (incomplete) 368.51
Protection (against) (from) - see Prophylactic

Protein
deficiency 260
malnutrition 260
sickness (prophylactic) (therapeutic) 999.59
Proteinemia 790.99
Proteinosis
alveolar, lung or pulmonary 516.0
lipid 272.8
lipoid (of Urbach) 272.8
Proteinuria (see also Albuminuria) 791.0
Bence-Jones NEC 791.0
gestational 646.2 ●
    with hypertension - see Toxemia, of pregnancy
orthostatic 593.6
postural 593.6
Proteolysis, pathologic 286.6
Protocoproporphyria 277.1
Protoporphyria (erythrohepatic) (erythropoietic) 277.1
Protrusio acetabuli 718.65
Protrusion
acetabulum (into pelvis) 718.65
device, implant, or graft - see Complications, mechanical
ear, congenital 744.29
intervertebral disc - see Displacement, intervertebral disc
nucleus pulposus - see Displacement, intervertebral disc
Proud flesh 701.5
Prune belly (syndrome) 756.71
Prurigo (ferox) (gravis) (Hebra's) (hebrae) (mitis) (simplex) 698.2
agria 698.3
asthma syndrome 691.8
Besnier's (atopic dermatitis) (infantile eczema) 691.8
eczematodes allergicum 691.8
estivalis (Hutchinson's) 692.72
Hutchinson's 692.72
nodularis 698.3
psychogenic 306.3
Pruritus, pruritic 698.9
ani 698.0
    psychogenic 306.3
conditions NEC 698.9
    psychogenic 306.3
due to Onchocerca volvulus 125.3
ear 698.9
essential 698.9
genital organ(s) 698.1
    psychogenic 306.3
gravidarum 646.8 ●
hiemalis 698.8
neurogenic (any site) 306.3
perianal 698.0
psychogenic (any site) 306.3
scrotum 698.1
    psychogenic 306.3
senile, senilis 698.8
Trichomonas 131.9
vulva, vulvae 698.1
    psychogenic 306.3
Psammocarcinoma (M8140/3) - see Neoplasm, by site, malignant
Pseudarthrosis, pseudoarthrosis (bone) 733.82
joint following fusion V45.4
Pseudoacanthosis
nigricans 701.8
Pseudoaneurysm - see Aneurysm
Pseudoangina (pectoris) - see Angina
Pseudoangioma 452
Pseudo-Argyll-Robertson pupil 379.45
Pseudoarteriosus 747.89
Pseudoarthrosis - see Pseudarthrosis
Pseudoataxia 799.89
Pseudobulbar affect (PBA) 310.81
Pseudobursa 727.89
Pseudocholera 025
Pseudochromidrosis 705.89

Pseudocirrhosis, liver, pericardial 423.2
Pseudocoarctation 747.21
Pseudocowpox 051.1
Pseudocoxalgia 732.1
Pseudocroup 478.75
Pseudocyesis 300.11
Pseudocyst
    lung 518.89
    pancreas 577.2
    retina 361.19
Pseudodementia 300.16
Pseudoelephantiasis neuroarthritica 757.0
Pseudoemphysema 518.89
Pseudoencephalitis
    superior (acute) hemorrhagic 265.1
Pseudoerosion cervix, congenital 752.49
Pseudoexfoliation, lens capsule 366.11
Pseudofracture (idiopathic) (multiple)
    (spontaneous) (symmetrical) 268.2
Pseudoglanders 025
Pseudoglioma 360.44
Pseudogout - see Chondrocalcinosis
Pseudohallucination 780.1
Pseudohemianesthesia 782.0
Pseudohemophilia (Bernuth's) (hereditary)
    (type B) 286.4
    type A 287.8
    vascular 287.8
Pseudohermaphroditism 752.7
    with chromosomal anomaly - see Anomaly,
        chromosomal
    adrenal 255.2
    female (without adrenocortical disorder)
        752.7
        with adrenocortical disorder 255.2
        adrenal 255.2
    male (without gonadal disorder) 752.7
        with
            adrenocortical disorder 255.2
            cleft scrotum 752.7
            feminizing testis 259.51
            gonadal disorder 257.9
        adrenal 255.2
Pseudohole, macula 362.54
Pseudo-Hurler's disease (mucolipidosis III)
    272.7
Pseudohydrocephalus 348.2
Pseudohypertrophic muscular dystrophy
    (Erb's) 359.1
Pseudohypertrophy, muscle 359.1
Pseudohypoparathyroidism 275.49
Pseudoinfluenza (see also Influenza) 487.1
Pseudoinsomnia 307.49
Pseudoleukemia 288.8
    infantile 285.8
Pseudomembranous - see condition
Pseudomeningocele (cerebral) (infective) 349.2
    postprocedural 997.01
    spinal 349.2
Pseudomenstruation 626.8
Pseudomucinous
    cyst (ovary) (M8470/0) 220
    peritoneum 568.89
Pseudomyeloma 273.1
Pseudomyxoma peritonei (M8480/6) 197.6
Pseudoneuritis optic (nerve) 377.24
    papilla 377.24
        congenital 743.57
Pseudoneuroma - see Injury, nerve, by site
Pseudo-obstruction
    intestine (chronic) (idiopathic) (intermittent
        secondary) (primary) 564.89
        acute 560.89
Pseudopapilledema 377.24
Pseudoparalysis
    arm or leg 781.4
    atonic, congenital 358.8
Pseudopelade 704.09
Pseudophakia V43.1
Pseudopolycythemia 289.0
Pseudopolyposis, colon 556.4

Pseudoporencephaly 348.0
Pseudopseudohypoparathyroidism 275.49
Pseudopsychosis 300.16
Pseudopterygium 372.52
Pseudoptosis (eyelid) 374.34
Pseudorabies 078.89
Pseudoretinitis, pigmentosa 362.65
Pseudorickets 588.0
    senile (Pozzi's) 731.0
Pseudorubella 057.8
Pseudoscarlatina 057.8
Pseudosclerema 778.1
Pseudosclerosis (brain)
    Jakob's 046.19
    of Westphal (-Strümpell) (hepatolenticular
        degeneration) 275.1
    spastic 046.19
        with dementia
            with behavioral disturbance 046.19
                [294.11]
            without behavioral disturbance 046.19
                [294.10]
Pseudoseizure 780.39
    non-psychiatric 780.39
    psychiatric 300.11
Pseudotabes 799.89
    diabetic 250.6● [337.1]
    due to secondary diabetes 249.6● [337.1]
Pseudotetanus (see also Convulsions) 780.39
Pseudotetany 781.7
    hysterical 300.11
Pseudothalassemia 285.0
Pseudotrichinosis 710.3
Pseudotruncus arteriosus 747.29
Pseudotuberculosis, pasteurella (infection)
    027.2
Pseudotumor
    cerebri 348.2
    orbit (inflammatory) 376.11
Pseudo-Turner's syndrome 759.89
Pseudoxanthoma elasticum 757.39
Psilosis (sprue) (tropical) 579.1
    Monilia 112.89
    nontropical 579.0
    not sprue 704.00
Psittacosis 073.9
Psoitis 728.89
Psora NEC 696.1
Psoriasis 696.1
    any type, except arthropathic 696.1
    arthritic, arthropathic 696.0
    buccal 528.6
    flexural 696.1
    follicularis 696.1
    guttate 696.1
    inverse 696.1
    mouth 528.6
    nummularis 696.1
    psychogenic 316 [696.1]
    punctata 696.1
    pustular 696.1
    rupioides 696.1
    vulgaris 696.1
Psorospermiasis 136.4
Psorospermosis 136.4
    follicularis (vegetans) 757.39
Psychalgia 307.80
Psychasthenia 300.89
    compulsive 300.3
    mixed compulsive states 300.3
    obsession 300.3
Psychiatric disorder or problem NEC 300.9
Psychogenic - see also condition
    factors associated with physical conditions
        316
Psychoneurosis, psychoneurotic (see also
    Neurosis) 300.9
    anxiety (state) 300.00
    climacteric 627.2
    compensation 300.16
    compulsion 300.3

Psychoneurosis, psychoneurotic (Continued)
    conversion hysteria 300.11
    depersonalization 300.6
    depressive type 300.4
    dissociative hysteria 300.15
    hypochondriacal 300.7
    hysteria 300.10
        conversion type 300.11
        dissociative type 300.15
    mixed NEC 300.89
    neurasthenic 300.5
    obsessional 300.3
    obsessive-compulsive 300.3
    occupational 300.89
    personality NEC 301.89
    phobia 300.20
    senile NEC 300.89
Psychopathic - see also condition
    constitution, posttraumatic 310.2
        with psychosis 293.9
    personality 301.9
        amoral trends 301.7
        antisocial trends 301.7
        asocial trends 301.7
        mixed types 301.7
    state 301.9
Psychopathy, sexual (see also Deviation, sexual)
    302.9
Psychophysiologic, psychophysiological
    condition - see Reaction,
    psychophysiologic
Psychose passionelle 297.8
Psychosexual identity disorder 302.6
    adult-life 302.85
    childhood 302.6
Psychosis 298.9
    acute hysterical 298.1
    affecting management of pregnancy,
        childbirth, or puerperium 648.4●
    affective (see also Disorder, mood) 296.90

Note:	Use the following fifth-digit subclassification with categories 296.0–296.6:
0	unspecified
1	mild
2	moderate
3	severe, without mention of psychotic behavior
4	severe, specified as with psychotic behavior
5	in partial or unspecified remission
6	in full remission

        drug-induced 292.84
        due to or associated with physical
            condition 293.9
        involutional 293.83
            recurrent episode 296.3●
            single episode 296.2●
        manic-depressive 296.80
            circular (alternating) 296.7
                currently depressed 296.5●
                currently manic 296.4●
            depressed type 296.2●
                atypical 296.82
                recurrent episode 296.3●
                single episode 296.2●
            manic 296.0●
                atypical 296.81
                recurrent episode 296.1●
                single episode 296.0●
            mixed type NEC 296.89
            specified type NEC 296.89
        senile 290.21
        specified type NEC 296.99
    alcoholic 291.9
        with
            anxiety 291.89
            delirium tremens 291.0
            delusions 291.5
            dementia 291.2

 <!-- deleted strikethrough -->

◄ New   ⬅ Revised   ~~deleted~~ Deleted   ● Use Additional Digit(s)   Omit code

SECTION I INDEX TO DISEASES AND INJURIES / Psychosis

Psychosis (Continued)
- alcoholic (Continued)
    - with (Continued)
        - hallucinosis 291.3
        - jealousy 291.5
        - mood disturbance 291.89
        - paranoia 291.5
        - persisting amnesia 291.1
        - sexual dysfunction 291.89
        - sleep disturbance 291.89
    - amnestic confabulatory 291.1
    - delirium tremens 291.0
    - hallucinosis 291.3
    - Korsakoff's, Korsakov's, Korsakow's 291.1
    - paranoid type 291.5
    - pathological intoxication 291.4
    - polyneuritic 291.1
    - specified type NEC 291.89
- alternating (see also Psychosis, manic-depressive, circular) 296.7
- anergastic (see also Psychosis, organic) 294.9
- arteriosclerotic 290.40
    - with
        - acute confusional state 290.41
        - delirium 290.41
        - delusions 290.42
        - depressed mood 290.43
    - depressed type 290.43
    - paranoid type 290.42
    - simple type 290.40
    - uncomplicated 290.40
- atypical 298.9
    - depressive 296.82
    - manic 296.81
- borderline (schizophrenia) (see also Schizophrenia) 295.5
    - of childhood (see also Psychosis, childhood) 299.8
    - prepubertal 299.8
- brief reactive 298.8
- childhood, with origin specific to 299.9

Note: Use the following fifth-digit subclassification with category 299:
0 current or active state
1 residual state

- atypical 299.8
- specified type NEC 299.8
- circular (see also Psychosis, manic-depressive, circular) 296.7
- climacteric (see also Psychosis, involutional) 298.8
- confusional 298.9
    - acute 293.0
    - reactive 298.2
    - subacute 293.1
- depressive (see also Psychosis, affective) 296.2
    - atypical 296.82
    - involutional 296.2
        - with hypomania (bipolar II) 296.89
        - recurrent episode 296.3
        - single episode 296.2
    - psychogenic 298.0
    - reactive (emotional stress) (psychological trauma) 298.0
    - recurrent episode 296.3
        - with hypomania (bipolar II) 296.89
    - single episode 296.2
- disintegrative, childhood (see also Psychosis, childhood) 299.1
- drug 292.9
    - with
        - affective syndrome 292.84
        - amnestic syndrome 292.83
        - anxiety 292.89
        - delirium 292.81
            - withdrawal 292.0
        - delusions 292.11

Psychosis (Continued)
- drug (Continued)
    - with (Continued)
        - dementia 292.82
        - depressive state 292.84
        - hallucinations 292.12
        - hallucinosis 292.12
        - mood disorder 292.84
        - mood disturbance 292.84
        - organic personality syndrome NEC 292.89
        - sexual dysfunction 292.89
        - sleep disturbance 292.89
        - withdrawal syndrome (and delirium) 292.0
    - affective syndrome 292.84
    - delusions 292.11
    - hallucinatory state 292.12
    - hallucinosis 292.12
    - paranoid state 292.11
    - specified type NEC 292.89
    - withdrawal syndrome (and delirium) 292.0
- due to or associated with physical condition (see also Psychosis, organic) 294.9
- epileptic NEC 293.9
- excitation (psychogenic) (reactive) 298.1
- exhaustive (see also Reaction, stress, acute) 308.9
- hypomanic (see also Psychosis, affective) 296.0
    - recurrent episode 296.1
    - single episode 296.0
- hysterical 298.8
    - acute 298.1
- incipient 298.8
    - schizophrenia (see also Schizophrenia) 295.5
- induced 297.3
- infantile (see also Psychosis, childhood) 299.0
- infective 293.9
    - acute 293.0
    - subacute 293.1
- in
    - conditions classified elsewhere
        - with
            - delusions 293.81
            - hallucinations 293.82
    - pregnancy, childbirth, or puerperium 648.4
- interactional (childhood) (see also Psychosis, childhood) 299.1
- involutional 298.8
    - depressive (see also Psychosis, affective) 296.2
        - recurrent episode 296.3
        - single episode 296.2
    - melancholic 296.2
        - recurrent episode 296.3
        - single episode 296.2
    - paranoid state 297.2
    - paraphrenia 297.2
- Korsakoff's, Korakov's, Korsakow's (nonalcoholic) 294.0
    - alcoholic 291.1
- mania (phase) (see also Psychosis, affective) 296.0
    - recurrent episode 296.1
    - single episode 296.0
- manic (see also Psychosis, affective) 296.0
    - atypical 296.81
    - recurrent episode 296.1
    - single episode 296.0
- manic-depressive 296.80
    - circular 296.7
        - currently
            - depressed 296.5
            - manic 296.4
            - mixed 296.6

Psychosis (Continued)
- manic-depressive (Continued)
    - depressive 296.2
        - recurrent episode 296.3
            - with hypomania (bipolar II) 296.89
        - single episode 296.2
    - hypomanic 296.0
        - recurrent episode 296.1
        - single episode 296.0
    - manic 296.0
        - atypical 296.81
        - recurrent episode 296.1
        - single episode 296.0
    - mixed NEC 296.89
    - perplexed 296.89
    - stuporous 296.89
- menopausal (see also Psychosis, involutional) 298.8
- mixed schizophrenic and affective (see also Schizophrenia) 295.7
- multi-infarct (cerebrovascular) (see also Psychosis, arteriosclerotic) 290.40
- organic NEC 294.9
    - due to or associated with
        - addiction
            - alcohol (see also Psychosis, alcoholic) 291.9
            - drug (see also Psychosis, drug) 292.9
        - alcohol intoxication, acute (see also Psychosis, alcoholic) 291.9
        - alcoholism (see also Psychosis, alcoholic) 291.9
        - arteriosclerosis (cerebral) (see also Psychosis, arteriosclerotic) 290.40
        - cerebrovascular disease
            - acute (psychosis) 293.0
            - arteriosclerotic (see also Psychosis, arteriosclerotic) 290.40
        - childbirth - see Psychosis, puerperal
        - dependence
            - alcohol (see also Psychosis, alcoholic) 291.9
            - drug 292.9
        - disease
            - alcoholic liver (see also Psychosis, alcoholic) 291.9
            - brain
                - arteriosclerotic (see also Psychosis, arteriosclerotic) 290.40
            - cerebrovascular
                - acute (psychosis) 293.0
                - arteriosclerotic (see also Psychosis, arteriosclerotic) 290.40
            - endocrine or metabolic 293.9
                - acute (psychosis) 293.0
                - subacute (psychosis) 293.1
            - Jakob-Creutzfeldt 046.19
                - with behavioral disturbance 046.19 [294.11]
                - without behavioral disturbance 046.19 [294.10]
                - familial 046.19
                - iatrogenic 046.19
                - specified NEC 046.19
                - sporadic 046.19
                - variant 046.11
                    - with dementia
                        - with behavioral disturbance 046.11 [294.11]
                        - without behavioral disturbance 046.11 [294.10]
            - liver, alcoholic (see also Psychosis, alcoholic) 291.9

Psychosis (Continued)
   organic NEC (Continued)
      due to or associated with (Continued)
         disorder
            cerebrovascular
               acute (psychosis) 293.0
            endocrine or metabolic 293.9
               acute (psychosis) 293.0
               subacute (psychosis) 293.1
            epilepsy
               with behavioral disturbance 345.9 [294.11]●
               without behavioral disturbance 345.9 [294.10]●
               transient (acute) 293.0
            Huntington's chorea
               with behavioral disturbance 333.4 [294.11]
               without behavioral disturbance 333.4 [294.10]
         infection
            brain 293.9
               acute (psychosis) 293.0
               chronic 294.8
               subacute (psychosis) 293.1
            intracranial NEC 293.9
               acute (psychosis) 293.0
               chronic 294.8
               subacute (psychosis) 293.1
         intoxication
            alcoholic (acute) (see also Psychosis, alcoholic) 291.9
               pathological 291.4
            drug (see also Psychosis, drug) 292.9
         ischemia
            cerebrovascular (generalized) (see also Psychosis, arteriosclerotic) 290.40
         Jakob-Creutzfeldt disease (syndrome) 046.19
            with behavioral disturbance 046.19 [294.11]
            without behavioral disturbance 046.19 [294.10]
            variant 046.11
               with dementia
                  with behavioral disturbance 046.11 [294.11]
                  without behavioral disturbance 046.11 [294.10]
         multiple sclerosis
            with behavioral disturbance 340 [294.11]
            without behavioral disturbance 340 [294.10]
         physical condition NEC 293.9
            with
               delusions 293.81
               hallucinations 293.82
         presenility 290.10
         puerperium - see Psychosis, puerperal
         sclerosis, multiple
            with behavioral disturbance 340 [294.11]
            without behavioral disturbance 340 [294.10]
         senility 290.20
         status epilepticus
            with behavioral disturbance 345.3 [294.11]
            without behavioral disturbance 345.3 [294.10]
         trauma
            brain (birth) (from electrical current) (surgical) 293.9
               acute (psychosis) 293.0
               chronic 294.8
               subacute (psychosis) 293.1

Psychosis (Continued)
   organic NEC (Continued)
      due to or associated with (Continued)
         unspecified physical condition 293.9
            with
               delusions 293.81
               hallucinations 293.82
      infective 293.9
         acute (psychosis) 293.0
         subacute 293.1
      posttraumatic 293.9
         acute 293.0
         subacute 293.1
      specified type NEC 294.8
      transient 293.9
         with
            anxiety 293.84
            delusions 293.81
            depression 293.83
            hallucinations 293.82
         depressive type 293.83
         hallucinatory type 293.82
         paranoid type 293.81
         specified type NEC 293.89
   paranoic 297.1
   paranoid (chronic) 297.9
      alcoholic 291.5
      chronic 297.1
      climacteric 297.2
      involutional 297.2
      menopausal 297.2
      protracted reactive 298.4
      psychogenic 298.4
         acute 298.3
      schizophrenic (see also Schizophrenia) 295.3●
      senile 290.20
   paroxysmal 298.9
      senile 290.20
   polyneuritic, alcoholic 291.1
   postoperative 293.9
   postpartum - see Psychosis, puerperal
   prepsychotic (see also Schizophrenia) 295.5●
   presbyophrenic (type) 290.8
   presenile (see also Dementia, presenile) 290.10
   prison 300.16
   psychogenic 298.8
      depressive 298.0
      paranoid 298.4
         acute 298.3
   puerperal
      specified type - see categories 295–298
      unspecified type 293.89
         acute 293.0
         chronic 293.89
         subacute 293.1
   reactive (emotional stress) (psychological trauma) 298.8
      brief 298.8
      confusion 298.2
      depressive 298.0
      excitation 298.1
   schizo-affective (depressed) (excited) (see also Schizophrenia) 295.7●
   schizophrenia, schizophrenic (see also Schizophrenia) 295.9●
      borderline type 295.5●
         of childhood (see also Psychosis, childhood) 299.8●
      catatonic (excited) (withdrawn) 295.2●
      childhood type (see also Psychosis, childhood) 299.9●
      hebephrenic 295.1●
      incipient 295.5●
      latent 295.5●
      paranoid 295.3●
      prepsychotic 295.5●
      prodromal 295.5●
      pseudoneurotic 295.5●
      pseudopsychopathic 295.5●
      schizophreniform 295.4●

Psychosis (Continued)
   schizophrenia, schizophrenic (Continued)
      simple 295.0●
      undifferentiated type 295.9●
   schizophreniform 295.4●
   senile NEC 290.20
      with
         delusional features 290.20
         depressive features 290.21
      depressed type 290.21
      paranoid type 290.20
      simple deterioration 290.20
      specified type - see categories 295–298
   shared 297.3
   situational (reactive) 298.8
   symbiotic (childhood) (see also Psychosis, childhood) 299.1●
   toxic (acute) 293.9
Psychotic (see also condition) 298.9
   episode 298.9
      due to or associated with physical conditions (see also Psychosis, organic) 293.9
Pterygium (eye) 372.40
   central 372.43
   colli 744.5
   double 372.44
   peripheral (stationary) 372.41
      progressive 372.42
   recurrent 372.45
Ptilosis 374.55
PTLD (post-transplant lymphoproliferative disorder) 238.77
Ptomaine (poisoning) (see also Poisoning, food) 005.9
Ptosis (adiposa) 374.30
   breast 611.81
   cecum 569.89
   colon 569.89
   congenital (eyelid) 743.61
      specified site NEC - see Anomaly, specified type NEC
   epicanthus syndrome 270.2
   eyelid 374.30
      congenital 743.61
      mechanical 374.33
      myogenic 374.32
      paralytic 374.31
   gastric 537.5
   intestine 569.89
   kidney (see also Disease, renal) 593.0
      congenital 753.3
   liver 573.8
   renal (see also Disease, renal) 593.0
      congenital 753.3
   splanchnic 569.89
   spleen 289.59
   stomach 537.5
   viscera 569.89
PTP (posttransfusion purpura) 287.41
PTSD (Post-Traumatic Stress Disorder) 309.81
Ptyalism 527.7
   hysterical 300.11
   periodic 527.2
   pregnancy 646.8●
   psychogenic 306.4
Ptyalolithiasis 527.5
Pubalgia 848.8
Pubarche, precocious 259.1
Pubertas praecox 259.1
Puberty V21.1
   abnormal 259.9
   bleeding 626.3
   delayed 259.0
   precocious (constitutional) (cryptogenic) (idiopathic) NEC 259.1
      due to
         adrenal
            cortical hyperfunction 255.2
            hyperplasia 255.2
            cortical hyperfunction 255.2

Puberty (Continued)
  precocious NEC (Continued)
    due to (Continued)
      ovarian hyperfunction 256.1
        estrogen 256.0
        pineal tumor 259.8
        testicular hyperfunction 257.0
    premature 259.1
      due to
        adrenal cortical hyperfunction 255.2
        pineal tumor 259.8
        pituitary (anterior) hyperfunction 253.1
Puckering, macula 362.56
Pudenda, pudendum - see condition
Puente's disease (simple glandular cheilitis) 528.5
Puerperal
  abscess
    areola 675.1
    Bartholin's gland 646.6
    breast 675.1
    cervix (uteri) 670.8
    fallopian tube 670.8
    genital organ 670.8
    kidney 646.6
    mammary 675.1
    mesosalpinx 670.8
    nabothian 646.6
    nipple 675.0
    ovary, ovarian 670.8
    oviduct 670.8
    parametric 670.8
    para-uterine 670.8
    pelvic 670.8
    perimetric 670.8
    periuterine 670.8
    retro-uterine 670.8
    subareolar 675.1
    suprapelvic 670.8
    tubal (ruptured) 670.8
    tubo-ovarian 670.8
    urinary tract NEC 646.6
    uterine, uterus 670.8
    vagina (wall) 646.6
    vaginorectal 646.6
    vulvovaginal gland 646.6
  accident 674.9
  adnexitis 670.8
  afibrinogenemia, or other coagulation defect 666.3
  albuminuria (acute) (subacute) 646.2
    pre-eclamptic 642.4
  anemia (conditions classifiable to 280–285) 648.2
  anuria 669.3
  apoplexy 674.0
  asymptomatic bacteriuria 646.5
  atrophy, breast 676.3
  blood dyscrasia 666.3
  caked breast 676.2
  cardiomyopathy 674.5
  cellulitis - see Puerperal, abscess
  cerebrovascular disorder (conditions classifiable to 430–434, 436–437) 674.0
  cervicitis (conditions classifiable to 616.0) 646.6
  coagulopathy (any) 666.3
  complications 674.9
    specified type NEC 674.8
  convulsions (eclamptic) (uremic) 642.6
    with pre-existing hypertension 642.7
  cracked nipple 676.1
  cystitis 646.6
  cystopyelitis 646.6
  deciduitis (acute) 670.8
  delirium NEC 293.9
  diabetes (mellitus) (conditions classifiable to 249 and 250) 648.0

Puerperal (Continued)
  disease 674.9
    breast NEC 676.3
    cerebrovascular (acute) 674.0
    nonobstetric NEC (see also Pregnancy, complicated, current disease or condition) 648.9
    pelvis inflammatory 670.8
    renal NEC 646.2
    tubo-ovarian 670.8
    Valsuani's (progressive pernicious anemia) 648.2
  disorder
    lactation 676.9
      specified type NEC 676.8
    nonobstetric NEC (see also Pregnancy, complicated, current disease or condition) 648.9
  disruption
    cesarean wound 674.1
    episiotomy wound 674.2
    perineal laceration wound 674.2
  drug dependence (conditions classifiable to 304) 648.3
  eclampsia 642.6
    with pre-existing hypertension 642.7
  embolism (pulmonary) 673.2
    air 673.0
    amniotic fluid 673.1
    blood clot 673.2
    brain or cerebral 674.0
    cardiac 674.8
    fat 673.8
    intracranial sinus (venous) 671.5
    pyemic 673.3
    septic 673.3
    spinal cord 671.5
  endometritis (conditions classifiable to 615.0–615.9) 670.1
  endophlebitis - see Puerperal, phlebitis
  endotrachelitis 646.6
  engorgement, breasts 676.2
  erysipelas 670.8
  failure
    lactation 676.4
    renal, acute 669.3
  fever 672
    meaning pyrexia (of unknown origin) 672
    meaning sepsis 670.2
  fissure, nipple 676.1
  fistula
    breast 675.1
    mammary gland 675.1
    nipple 675.0
  galactophoritis 675.2
  galactorrhea 676.6
  gangrene
    gas 670.8
      with sepsis 670.2
    uterus 670.8
  gonorrhea (conditions classifiable to 098) 647.1
  hematoma, subdural 674.0
  hematosalpinx, infectional 670.8
  hemiplegia, cerebral 674.0
  hemorrhage 666.1
    brain 674.0
    bulbar 674.0
    cerebellar 674.0
    cerebral 674.0
    cortical 674.0
    delayed (after 24 hours) (uterine) 666.2
    extradural 674.0
    internal capsule 674.0
    intracranial 674.0
    intrapontine 674.0
    meningeal 674.0
    pontine 674.0
    subarachnoid 674.0
    subcortical 674.0

Puerperal (Continued)
  hemorrhage (Continued)
    subdural 674.0
    uterine, delayed 666.2
    ventricular 674.0
  hemorrhoids 671.8
  hepatorenal syndrome 674.8
  hypertrophy
    breast 676.3
    mammary gland 676.3
  induration breast (fibrous) 676.3
  infarction
    lung - see Puerperal, embolism
    pulmonary - see Puerperal, embolism
  infection
    Bartholin's gland 646.6
    breast 675.2
      with nipple 675.9
        specified type NEC 675.8
    cervix 646.6
    endocervix 646.6
    fallopian tube 670.8
    generalized 670.0
    genital tract (major) 670.0
      minor or localized 646.6
    kidney (bacillus coli) 646.6
    mammary gland 675.2
      with nipple 675.9
        specified type NEC 675.8
    nipple 675.0
      with breast 675.9
        specified type NEC 675.8
    ovary 670.8
    pelvic 670.8
    peritoneum 670.8
    renal 646.6
    tubo-ovarian 670.8
    urinary (tract) NEC 646.6
      asymptomatic 646.5
    uterus, uterine 670.8
    vagina 646.6
  inflammation - see also Puerperal, infection
    areola 675.1
    Bartholin's gland 646.6
    breast 675.2
    broad ligament 670.8
    cervix (uteri) 646.6
    fallopian tube 670.8
    genital organs 670.8
      localized 646.6
    mammary gland 675.2
    nipple 675.0
    ovary 670.8
    oviduct 670.8
    pelvis 670.8
    periuterine 670.8
    tubal 670.8
    vagina 646.6
    vein - see Puerperal, phlebitis
  inversion, nipple 676.3
  ischemia, cerebral 674.0
  lymphangitis 670.8
    breast 675.2
  malaria (conditions classifiable to 084) 647.4
  malnutrition 648.9
  mammillitis 675.0
  mammitis 675.2
  mania 296.0
    recurrent episode 296.1
    single episode 296.0
  mastitis 675.2
    purulent 675.1
    retromammary 675.1
    submammary 675.1
  melancholia 296.2
    recurrent episode 296.3
    single episode 296.2
  mental disorder (conditions classifiable to 290–303, 305.0, 305.2–305.9, 306–316, 317–319) 648.4

Puerperal (Continued)
  metritis (suppurative) 670.1●
    septic 670.2●
  metroperitonitis 670.8●
  metrorrhagia 666.2●
  metrosalpingitis 670.8●
  metrovaginitis 670.8●
  milk leg 671.4●
  monoplegia, cerebral 674.0●
  necrosis
    kidney, tubular 669.3●
    liver (acute) (subacute) (conditions classifiable to 570) 674.8●
    ovary 670.8●
    renal cortex 669.3●
  nephritis or nephrosis (conditions classifiable to 580–589) 646.2●
    with hypertension 642.1●
  nutritional deficiency (conditions classifiable to 260–269) 648.9●
  occlusion, precerebral artery 674.0●
  oliguria 669.3●
  oophoritis 670.8●
  ovaritis 670.8●
  paralysis●
    bladder (sphincter) 665.5●
    cerebral 674.0●
  paralytic stroke 674.0●
  parametritis 670.8●
  paravaginitis 646.6●
  pelviperitonitis 670.8●
  perimetritis 670.8●
  perimetrosalpingitis 670.8●
  perinephritis 646.6●
  perioophoritis 670.8●
  periphlebitis - *see* Puerperal, phlebitis
  perisalpingitis 670.8●
  peritoneal infection 670.8●
  peritonitis (pelvic) 670.8●
  perivaginitis 646.6●
  phlebitis 671.2●
    deep 671.4●
    intracranial sinus (venous) 671.5●
    pelvic 671.4●
    specified site NEC 671.5●
    superficial 671.2●
  phlegmasia alba dolens 671.4●
  placental polyp 674.4●
  pneumonia, embolic - *see* Puerperal, embolism
  prediabetes 648.8●
  pre-eclampsia (mild) 642.4●
    with pre-existing hypertension 642.7●
    severe 642.5●
  psychosis, unspecified (*see also* Psychosis, puerperal) 293.89
  pyelitis 646.6●
  pyelocystitis 646.6●
  pyelohydronephrosis 646.6●
  pyelonephritis 646.6●
  pyelonephrosis 646.6●
  pyemia 670.2●
  pyocystitis 646.6●
  pyohemia 670.2●
  pyometra 670.8●
  pyonephritis 646.6●
  pyonephrosis 646.6●
  pyo-oophoritis 670.8●
  pyosalpingitis 670.8●
  pyosalpinx 670.8●
  pyrexia (of unknown origin) 672●
  renal
    disease NEC 646.2●
    failure, acute 669.3●
  retention
    decidua (fragments) (with delayed hemorrhage) 666.2●
      without hemorrhage 667.1●
    placenta (fragments) (with delayed hemorrhage) 666.2●
      without hemorrhage 667.1●

Puerperal (Continued)
  retention (Continued)
    secundines (fragments) (with delayed hemorrhage) 666.2●
      without hemorrhage 667.1●
  retracted nipple 676.0●
  rubella (conditions classifiable to 056) 647.5●
  salpingitis 670.8●
  salpingo-oophoritis 670.8●
  salpingo-ovaritis 670.8●
  salpingoperitonitis 670.8●
  sapremia 670.2●
  secondary perineal tear 674.2●
  sepsis (pelvic) 670.2●
  septicemia 670.2●
  subinvolution (uterus) 674.8●
  sudden death (cause unknown) 674.9●
  suppuration - *see* Puerperal, abscess
  syphilis (conditions classifiable to 090–097) 647.0●
  tetanus 670.8●
  thelitis 675.0●
  thrombocytopenia 666.3●
  thrombophlebitis (superficial) 671.2●
    deep 671.4●
    pelvic 671.4●
    septic 670.3●
    specified site NEC 671.5●
  thrombosis (venous) - *see* Thrombosis, puerperal
  thyroid dysfunction (conditions classifiable to 240–246) 648.1●
  toxemia (*see also* Toxemia, of pregnancy) 642.4●
    eclamptic 642.6●
      with pre-existing hypertension 642.7●
    pre-eclamptic (mild) 642.4●
      with
        convulsions 642.6●
        pre-existing hypertension 642.7●
      severe 642.5●
  tuberculosis (conditions classifiable to 010–018) 647.3●
  uremia 669.3●
  vaginitis (conditions classifiable to 616.1) 646.6●
  varicose veins (legs) 671.0●
    vulva or perineum 671.1●
  venous complication 671.9●
  vulvitis (conditions classifiable to 616.1) 646.6●
  vulvovaginitis (conditions classifiable to 616.1) 646.6●
  white leg 671.4●
Pulled muscle - *see* Sprain, by site
Pulmolithiasis 518.89
Pulmonary - *see* condition
Pulmonitis (unknown etiology) 486
Pulpitis (acute) (anachoretic) (chronic) (hyperplastic) (putrescent) (suppurative) (ulcerative) 522.0
Pulpless tooth 522.9
Pulse
  alternating 427.89
    psychogenic 306.2
  bigeminal 427.89
  fast 785.0
  feeble, rapid, due to shock following injury 958.4
  rapid 785.0
  slow 427.89
  strong 785.9
  trigeminal 427.89
  water-hammer (*see also* Insufficiency, aortic) 424.1
  weak 785.9
Pulseless disease 446.7
Pulsus
  alternans or trigeminy 427.89
    psychogenic 306.2

Punch drunk 310.2
Puncta lacrimalia occlusion 375.52
Punctiform hymen 752.49
Puncture (traumatic) - *see also* Wound, open, by site
  accidental, complicating surgery 998.2
  bladder, nontraumatic 596.6
  by
    device, implant, or graft - *see* Complications, mechanical
    foreign body
      internal organs - *see also* Injury, internal, by site
        by ingested object - *see* Foreign body
      left accidentally in operation wound 998.4
    instrument (any) during a procedure, accidental 998.2
  internal organs, abdomen, chest, or pelvis - *see* Injury, internal, by site
  kidney, nontraumatic 593.89
Pupil - *see* condition
Pupillary membrane 364.74
  persistent 743.46
Pupillotonia 379.46
  pseudotabetic 379.46
Purpura 287.2
  abdominal 287.0
  allergic 287.0
  anaphylactoid 287.0
  annularis telangiectodes 709.1
  arthritic 287.0
  autoerythrocyte sensitization 287.2
  autoimmune 287.0
  bacterial 287.0
  Bateman's (senile) 287.2
  capillary fragility (hereditary) (idiopathic) 287.8
  cryoglobulinemic 273.2
  devil's pinches 287.2
  fibrinolytic (*see also* Fibrinolysis) 286.6
  fulminans, fulminous 286.6
  gangrenous 287.0
  hemorrhagic (*see also* Purpura, thrombocytopenic) 287.39
    nodular 272.7
    nonthrombocytopenic 287.0
    thrombocytopenic 287.39
  Henoch's (purpura nervosa) 287.0
  Henoch-Schönlein (allergic) 287.0
  hypergammaglobulinemic (benign primary) (Waldenström's) 273.0
  idiopathic 287.31
    nonthrombocytopenic 287.0
    thrombocytopenic 287.31
  immune thrombocytopenic 287.31
  infectious 287.0
  malignant 287.0
  neonatorum 772.6
  nervosa 287.0
  newborn NEC 772.6
  nonthrombocytopenic 287.2
    hemorrhagic 287.0
    idiopathic 287.0
  nonthrombopenic 287.2
  peliosis rheumatica 287.0
  pigmentaria, progressiva 709.09
  posttransfusion (PTP) 287.41
    from whole blood (fresh) or blood products 287.41
  primary 287.0
  primitive 287.0
  red cell membrane sensitivity 287.2
  rheumatica 287.0
  Schönlein (-Henoch) (allergic) 287.0
  scorbutic 267
  senile 287.2
  simplex 287.2
  symptomatica 287.0
  telangiectasia annularis 709.1

SECTION I INDEX TO DISEASES AND INJURIES / Purpura

Purpura (Continued)
   thrombocytopenic (*see also* Thrombocytopenia) 287.30
      congenital 287.33
      essential 287.30
      hereditary 287.31
      idiopathic 287.31
      immune 287.31
      neonatal, transitory (*see also* Thrombocytopenia, neonatal transitory) 776.1
      primary 287.30
      puerperal, postpartum 666.3●
      thrombotic 446.6
   thrombohemolytic (*see also* Fibrinolysis) 286.6
   thrombopenic (*see also* Thrombocytopenia) 287.30
      congenital 287.33
      essential 287.30
   thrombotic 446.6
      thrombocytic 446.6
      thrombocytopenic 446.6
   toxic 287.0
   variolosa 050.0
   vascular 287.0
   visceral symptoms 287.0
   Werlhof's (*see also* Purpura, thrombocytopenic) 287.39
Purpuric spots 782.7
Purulent - *see* condition
Pus
   absorption, general - *see* Septicemia
   in
      stool 792.1
      urine 791.9
   tube (rupture) (*see also* Salpingo-oophoritis) 614.2
Pustular rash 782.1
Pustule 686.9
   malignant 022.0
   nonmalignant 686.9
Putnam's disease (subacute combined sclerosis with pernicious anemia) 281.0 *[336.2]*
Putnam-Dana syndrome (subacute combined sclerosis with pernicious anemia) 281.0 *[336.2]*
Putrefaction, intestinal 569.89
Putrescent pulp (dental) 522.1
Pyarthritis - *see* Pyarthrosis
Pyarthrosis (*see also* Arthritis, pyogenic) 711.0●
   tuberculous - *see* Tuberculosis, joint
Pycnoepilepsy, pycnolepsy (idiopathic) (*see also* Epilepsy) 345.0●
Pyelectasia 593.89
Pyelectasis 593.89
Pyelitis (congenital) (uremic) 590.80
   with
      abortion - *see* Abortion, by type, with specified complication NEC
      contracted kidney 590.00
      ectopic pregnancy (*see also* categories 633.0–633.9) 639.8
      molar pregnancy (*see also* categories 630–632) 639.8
   acute 590.10
      with renal medullary necrosis 590.11
   chronic 590.00
      with
         renal medullary necrosis 590.01
   complicating pregnancy, childbirth, or puerperium 646.6●
      affecting fetus or newborn 760.1

Pyelitis (Continued)
   cystica 590.3
   following
      abortion 639.8
      ectopic or molar pregnancy 639.8
   gonococcal 098.19
      chronic or duration of 2 months or over 098.39
   tuberculous (*see also* Tuberculosis) 016.0● *[590.81]*
Pyelocaliectasis 593.89
Pyelocystitis (*see also* Pyelitis) 590.80
Pyelohydronephrosis 591
Pyelonephritis (*see also* Pyelitis) 590.80
   acute 590.10
      with renal medullary necrosis 590.11
   chronic 590.00
   syphilitic (late) 095.4
   tuberculous (*see also* Tuberculosis) 016.0● *[590.81]*
Pyelonephrosis (*see also* Pyelitis) 590.80
   chronic 590.00
Pyelophlebitis 451.89
Pyelo-ureteritis cystica 590.3
Pyemia, pyemic (purulent) (*see also* Septicemia) 038.9
   abscess - *see* Abscess
   arthritis (*see also* Arthritis, pyogenic) 711.0●
   Bacillus coli 038.42
   embolism (*see also* Septicemia) 415.12
   fever 038.9
   infection 038.9
   joint (*see also* Arthritis, pyogenic) 711.0●
   liver 572.1
   meningococcal 036.2
   newborn 771.81
   phlebitis - *see* Phlebitis
   pneumococcal 038.2
   portal 572.1
   postvaccinal 999.39
   puerperal 670.2●
   specified organism NEC 038.8
   staphylococcal 038.10
      aureus 038.11
      methicillin
         resistant 038.12
         susceptible 038.11
      specified organism NEC 038.19
   streptococcal 038.0
   tuberculous - *see* Tuberculosis, miliary
Pygopagus 759.4
Pykno-epilepsy, pyknolepsy (idiopathic) (*see also* Epilepsy) 345.0●
Pyle (-Cohn) disease (craniometaphyseal dysplasia) 756.89
Pylephlebitis (suppurative) 572.1
Pylethrombophlebitis 572.1
Pylethrombosis 572.1
Pyloritis (*see also* Gastritis) 535.5●
Pylorospasm (reflex) 537.81
   congenital or infantile 750.5
   neurotic 306.4
   newborn 750.5
   psychogenic 306.4
Pylorus, pyloric - *see* condition
Pyoarthrosis - *see* Pyarthrosis
Pyocele
   mastoid 383.00
   sinus (accessory) (nasal) (*see also* Sinusitis) 473.9
   turbinate (bone) 473.9
   urethra (*see also* Urethritis) 597.0

Pyococcal dermatitis 686.00
Pyococcide, skin 686.00
Pyocolpos (*see also* Vaginitis) 616.10
Pyocyaneus dermatitis 686.09
Pyocystitis (*see also* Cystitis) 595.9
Pyoderma, pyodermia 686.00
   gangrenosum 686.01
   specified type NEC 686.09
   vegetans 686.8
Pyodermatitis 686.00
   vegetans 686.8
Pyogenic - *see* condition
Pyohemia - *see* Septicemia
Pyohydronephrosis (*see also* Pyelitis) 590.80
Pyometra 615.9
Pyometritis (*see also* Endometritis) 615.9
Pyometrium (*see also* Endometritis) 615.9
Pyomyositis 728.0
   ossificans 728.19
   tropical (bungpagga) 040.81
Pyonephritis (*see also* Pyelitis) 590.80
   chronic 590.00
Pyonephrosis (congenital) (*see also* Pyelitis) 590.80
   acute 590.10
Pyo-oophoritis (*see also* Salpingo-oophoritis) 614.2
Pyo-ovarium (*see also* Salpingo-oophoritis) 614.2
Pyopericarditis 420.99
Pyopericardium 420.99
Pyophlebitis - *see* Phlebitis
Pyopneumopericardium 420.99
Pyopneumothorax (infectional) 510.9
   with fistula 510.0
   subdiaphragmatic (*see also* Peritonitis) 567.29
   subphrenic (*see also* Peritonitis) 567.29
   tuberculous (*see also* Tuberculosis, pleura) 012.0●
Pyorrhea (alveolar) (alveolaris) 523.40
   degenerative 523.5
Pyosalpingitis (*see also* Salpingo-oophoritis) 614.2
Pyosalpinx (*see also* Salpingo-oophoritis) 614.2
Pyosepticemia - *see* Septicemia
Pyosis
   Corlett's (impetigo) 684
   Manson's (pemphigus contagiosus) 684
Pyothorax 510.9
   with fistula 510.0
   tuberculous (*see also* Tuberculosis, pleura) 012.0●
Pyoureter 593.89
   tuberculous (*see also* Tuberculosis) 016.2●
Pyramidopallidonigral syndrome 332.0
Pyrexia (of unknown origin) (P.U.O.) 780.60
   atmospheric 992.0
   during labor 659.2●
   environmentally-induced newborn 778.4
   heat 992.0
   newborn, environmentally-induced 778.4
   puerperal 672●
Pyroglobulinemia 273.8
Pyromania 312.33
Pyrosis 787.1
Pyrroloporphyria 277.1
Pyuria (bacterial) 791.9

Q

Q fever 083.0
- with pneumonia 083.0 [484.8]

Quadricuspid aortic valve 746.89

Quadrilateral fever 083.0

Quadriparesis - see Quadriplegia
- meaning muscle weakness 728.87

Quadriplegia 344.00
- with fracture, vertebra (process) - see Fracture, vertebra, cervical, with spinal cord injury
- brain (current episode) 437.8
- C_1–C_4
  - complete 344.01
  - incomplete 344.02
- C_5–C_7
  - complete 344.03
  - incomplete 344.04
- cerebral (current episode) 437.8
- congenital or infantile (cerebral) (spastic) (spinal) 343.2
- cortical 437.8
- embolic (current episode) (see also Embolism, brain) 434.1●

Quadriplegia (Continued)
- functional 780.72
- infantile (cerebral) (spastic) (spinal) 343.2
- newborn NEC 767.0
- specified NEC 344.09
- thrombotic (current episode) (see also Thrombosis, brain) 434.0●
- traumatic - see Injury, spinal, cervical

Quadruplet
- affected by maternal complications of pregnancy 761.5
- healthy liveborn - see Newborn, multiple
- pregnancy (complicating delivery) NEC 651.8●
  - with fetal loss and retention of one or more fetus(es) 651.5●
  - following (elective) fetal reduction 651.7●

Quarrelsomeness 301.3

Quartan
- fever 084.2
- malaria (fever) 084.2

Queensland fever 083.0
- coastal 083.0
- seven-day 100.89

Quervain's disease 727.04
- thyroid (subacute granulomatous thyroiditis) 245.1

Queyrat's erythroplasia (M8080/2)
- specified site - see Neoplasm, skin, in situ
- unspecified site 233.5

Quincke's disease or edema - see Edema, angioneurotic

Quinquaud's disease (acne decalvans) 704.09

Quinsy (gangrenous) 475

Quintan fever 083.1

Quintuplet
- affected by maternal complications of pregnancy 761.5
- healthy liveborn - see Newborn, multiple
- pregnancy (complicating delivery) NEC 651.2●
  - with fetal loss and retention of one or more fetus(es) 651.6●
  - following (elective) fetal reduction 651.7●

Quotidian
- fever 084.0
- malaria (fever) 084.0

R

Rabbia 071
Rabbit fever (see also Tularemia) 021.9
Rabies 071
   contact V01.5
   exposure to V01.5
   inoculation V04.5
      reaction - see Complications, vaccination
   vaccination, prophylactic (against) V04.5
Rachischisis (see also Spina bifida) 741.9●
Rachitic - see also condition
   deformities of spine 268.1
   pelvis 268.1
      with disproportion (fetopelvic) 653.2●
         affecting fetus or newborn 763.1
         causing obstructed labor 660.1●
            affecting fetus or newborn 763.1
Rachitis, rachitism - see also Rickets
   acute 268.0
   fetalis 756.4
   renalis 588.0
   tarda 268.0
Racket nail 757.5
Radial nerve - see condition
Radiation effects or sickness - see also Effect, adverse, radiation
   cataract 366.46
   dermatitis 692.82
      sunburn (see also Sunburn) 692.71
Radiculitis (pressure) (vertebrogenic) 729.2
   accessory nerve 723.4
   anterior crural 724.4
   arm 723.4
   brachial 723.4
   cervical NEC 723.4
   due to displacement of intervertebral disc - see Neuritis, due to, displacement intervertebral disc
   leg 724.4
   lumbar NEC 724.4
   lumbosacral 724.4
   rheumatic 729.2
   syphilitic 094.89
   thoracic (with visceral pain) 724.4
Radiculomyelitis 357.0
   toxic, due to
      Clostridium tetani 037
      corynebacterium diphtheriae 032.89
Radiculopathy (see also Radiculitis) 729.2
Radioactive substances, adverse effect - see Effect, adverse, radioactive substance
Radiodermal burns (acute) (chronic) (occupational) - see Burn, by site
Radiodermatitis 692.82
Radionecrosis - see Effect, adverse, radiation
Radiotherapy session V58.0
Radium, adverse effect - see Effect, adverse, radioactive substance
Raeder-Harbitz syndrome (pulseless disease) 446.7
Rage (see also Disturbance, conduct) 312.0●
   meaning rabies 071
Rag sorters' disease 022.1
Raillietiniasis 123.8
Railroad neurosis 300.16
Railway spine 300.16
Raised - see Elevation
Raiva 071
Rake teeth, tooth 524.39
Rales 786.7
Ramifying renal pelvis 753.3
Ramsay Hunt syndrome (herpetic geniculate ganglionitis) 053.11
   meaning dyssynergia cerebellaris myoclonica 334.2
Ranke's primary infiltration (see also Tuberculosis) 010.0●
Ranula 527.6
   congenital 750.26

Rape
   adult 995.83
   alleged, observation or examination V71.5
   child 995.53
Rapid
   feeble pulse, due to shock, following injury 958.4
   heart (beat) 785.0
      psychogenic 306.2
   respiration 786.06
      psychogenic 306.1
   second stage (delivery) 661.3●
      affecting fetus or newborn 763.6
   time-zone change syndrome 327.35
Rarefaction, bone 733.99
Rash 782.1
   canker 034.1
   diaper 691.0
   drug (internal use) 693.0
      contact 692.3
   ECHO 9 virus 078.89
   enema 692.89
   food (see also Allergy, food) 693.1
   heat 705.1
   napkin 691.0
   nettle 708.8
   pustular 782.1
   rose 782.1
      epidemic 056.9
      of infants 057.8
   scarlet 034.1
   serum (prophylactic) (therapeutic) 999.59
   toxic 782.1
   wandering tongue 529.1
Rasmussen's aneurysm (see also Tuberculosis) 011.2●
Rat-bite fever 026.9
   due to Streptobacillus moniliformis 026.1
   spirochetal (morsus muris) 026.0
Rathke's pouch tumor (M9350/1) 237.0
Raymond (-Céstan) syndrome 433.8●
Raynaud's
   disease or syndrome (paroxysmal digital cyanosis) 443.0
   gangrene (symmetric) 443.0 [785.4]
   phenomenon (paroxysmal digital cyanosis) (secondary) 443.0
RDS 769
Reaction
   acute situational maladjustment (see also Reaction, adjustment) 309.9
   adaptation (see also Reaction, adjustment) 309.9
   adjustment 309.9
      with
         anxious mood 309.24
            with depressed mood 309.28
         conduct disturbance 309.3
            combined with disturbance of emotions 309.4
         depressed mood 309.0
            brief 309.0
               with anxious mood 309.28
            prolonged 309.1
         elective mutism 309.83
         mixed emotions and conduct 309.4
         mutism, elective 309.83
         physical symptoms 309.82
         predominant disturbance (of)
            conduct 309.3
            emotions NEC 309.29
               mixed 309.28
            mixed, emotions and conduct 309.4
         specified type NEC 309.89
         specific academic or work inhibition 309.23
         withdrawal 309.83

Reaction (Continued)
   adjustment (Continued)
      depressive 309.0
         with conduct disturbance 309.4
         brief 309.0
         prolonged 309.1
      specified type NEC 309.89
   adverse food NEC 995.7
   affective (see also Psychosis, affective) 296.90
      specified type NEC 296.99
   aggressive 301.3
      unsocialized (see also Disturbance, conduct) 312.0●
   allergic (see also Allergy) 995.3
      drug, medicinal substance, and biological - see Allergy, drug
      due to correct medical substance properly administered 995.27
      food - see Allergy, food
      serum 999.59
   anaphylactic - see Anaphylactic reaction
   anesthesia - see Anesthesia, complication
   anger 312.0●
   antisocial 301.7
   antitoxin (prophylactic) (therapeutic) - see Complications, vaccination
   anxiety 300.00
   Arthus 995.21
   asthenic 300.5
   compulsive 300.3
   conversion (anesthetic) (autonomic) (hyperkinetic) (mixed paralytic) (paresthetic) 300.11
   deoxyribonuclease (DNA) (DNase) hypersensitivity NEC 287.2
   depressive 300.4
      acute 309.0
      affective (see also Psychosis, affective) 296.2●
      recurrent episode 296.3●
      single episode 296.2●
      brief 309.0
      manic (see also Psychosis, affective) 296.80
      neurotic 300.4
      psychoneurotic 300.4
      psychotic 298.0
   dissociative 300.15
   drug NEC (see also Table of Drugs and Chemicals) 995.20
      allergic - see also Allergy, drug 995.27
      correct substance properly administered 995.20
      obstetric anesthetic or analgesic NEC 668.9●
         affecting fetus or newborn 763.5
         specified drug - see Table of Drugs and Chemicals
      overdose or poisoning 977.9
         specified drug - see Table of Drugs and Chemicals
      specific to newborn 779.4
      transmitted via placenta or breast milk - see Absorption, drug, through placenta
      withdrawal NEC 292.0
         infant of dependent mother 779.5
      wrong substance given or taken in error 977.9
         specified drug - see Table of Drugs and Chemicals
   dyssocial 301.7
   dystonic, acute, due to drugs 333.72
   erysipeloid 027.1
   fear 300.20
      child 313.0
   fluid loss, cerebrospinal 349.0
   food - see also Allergy, food
      adverse NEC 995.7
      anaphylactic shock - see Anaphylactic reaction or shock, due to, food

Reaction (Continued)
  foreign
    body NEC 728.82
      in operative wound (inadvertently left) 998.4
        due to surgical material intentionally left - see Complications, due to (presence of) any device, implant, or graft classified to 996.0–996.5 NEC
    substance accidentally left during a procedure (chemical) (powder) (talc) 998.7
      body or object (instrument) (sponge) (swab) 998.4
  graft-versus-host (GVH) 279.50
  grief (acute) (brief) 309.0
    prolonged 309.1
  gross stress (see also Reaction, stress, acute) 308.9
  group delinquent (see also Disturbance, conduct) 312.2
  Herxheimer's 995.91
  hyperkinetic (see also Hyperkinesia) 314.9
  hypochondriacal 300.7
  hypoglycemic, due to insulin 251.0
    therapeutic misadventure 962.3
  hypomanic (see also Psychosis, affective) 296.0
    recurrent episode 296.1
    single episode 296.0
  hysterical 300.10
    conversion type 300.11
    dissociative 300.15
  id (bacterial cause) 692.89
  immaturity NEC 301.89
    aggressive 301.3
    emotional instability 301.59
  immunization - see Complications, vaccination
  incompatibility
    blood group (see also Complications, transfusion) 999.80
      ABO (due to transfusion of blood or blood products) (see also Complications, transfusion) 999.60
        minor blood group 999.89
        non-ABO (see also Complications, transfusion) 999.75
      ABO 999.6
      minor blood group 999.89
      Rh antigen (C) (c) (D) (E) (e) (factor) (infusion) (transfusion) (see also Complications, transfusion) 999.70
  inflammatory - see Infection
  infusion - see Complications, infusion
  inoculation (immune serum) - see Complications, vaccination
  insulin 995.23
  involutional
    paranoid 297.2
    psychotic (see also Psychosis, affective, depressive) 296.2
  leukemoid (basophilic) (lymphocytic) (monocytic) (myelocytic) (neutrophilic) 288.62
  LSD (see also Abuse, drugs, nondependent) 305.3
  lumbar puncture 349.0
  manic-depressive (see also Psychosis, affective) 296.80
    depressed 296.2
      recurrent episode 296.3
      single episode 296.2
    hypomanic 296.0
  neurasthenic 300.5
  neurogenic (see also Neurosis) 300.9
  neurotic NEC 300.9
  neurotic-depressive 300.4

Reaction (Continued)
  nitritoid - see Crisis, nitritoid
  nonspecific
    to
      cell mediated immunity measurement of gamma interferon antigen response without active tuberculosis 795.52
      QuantiFERON-TB test (QFT) without active tuberculosis 795.52
      tuberculin test (see also Reaction, tuberculin skin test) 795.51
  obsessive-compulsive 300.3
  organic 293.9
    acute 293.0
    subacute 293.1
  overanxious, child or adolescent 313.0
  paranoid (chronic) 297.9
    acute 298.3
    climacteric 297.2
    involutional 297.2
    menopausal 297.2
    senile 290.20
    simple 297.0
  passive
    aggressive 301.84
    dependency 301.6
  personality (see also Disorder, personality) 301.9
  phobic 300.20
  postradiation - see Effect, adverse, radiation
  psychogenic NEC 300.9
  psychoneurotic (see also Neurosis) 300.9
    anxiety 300.00
    compulsive 300.3
    conversion 300.11
    depersonalization 300.6
    depressive 300.4
    dissociative 300.15
    hypochondriacal 300.7
    hysterical 300.10
      conversion type 300.11
      dissociative type 300.15
    neurasthenic 300.5
    obsessive 300.3
    obsessive-compulsive 300.3
    phobic 300.20
    tension state 300.9
  psychophysiologic NEC (see also Disorder, psychosomatic) 306.9
    cardiovascular 306.2
    digestive 306.4
    endocrine 306.6
    gastrointestinal 306.4
    genitourinary 306.50
    heart 306.2
    hemic 306.8
    intestinal (large) (small) 306.4
    laryngeal 306.1
    lymphatic 306.8
    musculoskeletal 306.0
    pharyngeal 306.1
    respiratory 306.1
    skin 306.3
    special sense organs 306.7
  psychosomatic (see also Disorder, psychosomatic) 306.9
  psychotic (see also Psychosis) 298.9
    depressive 298.0
    due to or associated with physical condition (see also Psychosis, organic) 293.9
    involutional (see also Psychosis, affective) 296.2
      recurrent episode 296.3
      single episode 296.2
  pupillary (myotonic) (tonic) 379.46
  radiation - see Effect, adverse, radiation
  runaway - see also Disturbance, conduct
    socialized 312.2
    undersocialized, unsocialized 312.1

Reaction (Continued)
  scarlet fever toxin - see Complications, vaccination
  schizophrenic (see also Schizophrenia) 295.9
    latent 295.5
  serological for syphilis - see Serology for syphilis
  serum (prophylactic) (therapeutic) 999.59
    anaphylactic 999.49
    due to
      administration of blood and blood products 999.51
        anaphylactic 999.41
      vaccination 999.52
        anaphylactic 999.41
    immediate 999.49
  situational (see also Reaction, adjustment) 309.9
    acute, to stress 308.3
    adjustment (see also Reaction, adjustment) 309.9
  somatization (see also Disorder, psychosomatic) 306.9
  spinal puncture 349.0
  spite, child (see also Disturbance, conduct) 312.0
  stress, acute 308.9
    with predominant disturbance (of)
      consciousness 308.1
      emotions 308.0
      mixed 308.4
      psychomotor 308.2
      specified type NEC 308.3
    bone or cartilage - see Fracture, stress
  surgical procedure - see Complications, surgical procedure
  tetanus antitoxin - see Complications, vaccination
  toxin-antitoxin - see Complications, vaccination
  transfusion (blood) (bone marrow) (lymphocytes) (allergic) (see also Complications, transfusion) 999.80
  tuberculin skin test, nonspecific (without active tuberculosis) 795.51
    positive (without active tuberculosis) 795.51
  ultraviolet - see Effect, adverse, ultraviolet
  undersocialized, unsocialized - see also Disturbance, conduct
    aggressive (type) 312.0
    unaggressive (type) 312.1
  vaccination (any) - see Complications, vaccination
  white graft (skin) 996.52
  withdrawing, child or adolescent 313.22
  x-ray - see Effect, adverse, x-rays
Reactive depression (see also Reaction, depressive) 300.4
  neurotic 300.4
  psychoneurotic 300.4
  psychotic 298.0
Rebound tenderness 789.6
Recalcitrant patient V15.81
Recanalization, thrombus - see Thrombosis
Recession, receding
  chamber angle (eye) 364.77
  chin 524.06
  gingival (postinfective) (postoperative) 523.20
    generalized 523.25
    localized 523.24
    minimal 523.21
    moderate 523.22
    severe 523.23
Recklinghausen's disease (M9540/1) 237.71
  bones (osteitis fibrosa cystica) 252.01
Recklinghausen-Applebaum disease (hemochromatosis) 275.03
Reclus' disease (cystic) 610.1
Recrudescent typhus (fever) 081.1

Recruitment, auditory 388.44
Rectalgia 569.42
Rectitis 569.49
Rectocele
  female (without uterine prolapse) 618.04
    with uterine prolapse 618.4
      complete 618.3
      incomplete 618.2
  in pregnancy or childbirth 654.4●
    causing obstructed labor 660.2●
      affecting fetus or newborn 763.1
  male 569.49
  vagina, vaginal (outlet) 618.04
Rectosigmoiditis 569.89
  ulcerative (chronic) 556.3
Rectosigmoid junction - *see* condition
Rectourethral - *see* condition
Rectovaginal - *see* condition
Rectovesical - *see* condition
Rectum, rectal - *see* condition
Recurrent - *see* condition
  pregnancy loss - *see* Pregnancy, management affected by, abortion, habitual
Red bugs 133.8
Red cedar asthma 495.8
Redness
  conjunctiva 379.93
  eye 379.93
  nose 478.19
Reduced ventilatory or vital capacity 794.2
Reduction
  function
    kidney (*see also* Disease, renal) 593.9
    liver 573.8
  ventilatory capacity 794.2
  vital capacity 794.2
Redundant, redundancy
  abdomen 701.9
  anus 751.5
  cardia 537.89
  clitoris 624.2
  colon (congenital) 751.5
  foreskin (congenital) 605
  intestine 751.5
  labia 624.3
  organ or site, congenital NEC - *see* Accessory
  panniculus (abdominal) 278.1
  prepuce (congenital) 605
  pylorus 537.89
  rectum 751.5
  scrotum 608.89
  sigmoid 751.5
  skin (of face) 701.9
    eyelids 374.30
  stomach 537.89
  uvula 528.9
  vagina 623.8
Reduplication - *see* Duplication
Referral
  adoption (agency) V68.89
  nursing care V63.8
  patient without examination or treatment V68.81
  social services V63.8
Reflex - *see also* condition
  blink, deficient 374.45
  hyperactive gag 478.29
  neurogenic bladder NEC 596.54
    atonic 596.54
      with cauda equina syndrome 344.61
  vasoconstriction 443.9
  vasovagal 780.2
Reflux 530.81
  acid 530.81
  esophageal 530.81
    with esophagitis 530.11
  esophagitis 530.11
  gastroesophageal 530.81
  mitral - *see* Insufficiency, mitral
  ureteral - *see* Reflux, vesicoureteral

Reflux (*Continued*)
  vesicoureteral 593.70
    with
      reflux nephropathy 593.73
        bilateral 593.72
        unilateral 593.71
Reformed gallbladder 576.0
Reforming, artificial openings (*see also* Attention to, artificial, opening) V55.9
Refractive error (*see also* Error, refractive) 367.9
Refsum's disease or syndrome (heredopathia atactica polyneuritiformis) 356.3
Refusal of
  food 307.59
    hysterical 300.11
  treatment because of, due to
    patient's decision NEC V64.2
    reason of conscience or religion V62.6
Regaud
  tumor (M8082/3) - *see* Neoplasm, nasopharynx, malignant
  type carcinoma (M8082/3) - *see* Neoplasm, nasopharynx, malignant
Regional - *see* condition
Regulation feeding (elderly) (infant) 783.3
  newborn 779.31
Regurgitated
  food, choked on 933.1
  stomach contents, choked on 933.1
Regurgitation 787.03
  aortic (valve) (*see also* Insufficiency, aortic) 424.1
    congenital 746.4
    syphilitic 093.22
  food - *see also* Vomiting
    with reswallowing - *see* Rumination
    newborn 779.33
  gastric contents - *see* Vomiting
  heart - *see* Endocarditis
  mitral (valve) - *see also* Insufficiency, mitral
    congenital 746.6
  myocardial - *see* Endocarditis
  pulmonary (heart) (valve) (*see also* Endocarditis, pulmonary) 424.3
  stomach - *see* Vomiting
  tricuspid - *see* Endocarditis, tricuspid
  valve, valvular - *see* Endocarditis
  vesicoureteral - *see* Reflux, vesicoureteral
Rehabilitation V57.9
  multiple types V57.89
  occupational V57.21
  specified type NEC V57.89
  speech (-language) V57.3
  vocational V57.22
Reichmann's disease or syndrome (gastrosuccorrhea) 536.8
Reifenstein's syndrome (hereditary familial hypogonadism, male) 259.52
Reilly's syndrome or phenomenon (*see also* Neuropathy, peripheral, autonomic) 337.9
Reimann's periodic disease 277.31
Reinsertion, contraceptive device V25.42
  intrauterine V25.13
Reiter's disease, syndrome, or urethritis 099.3 [711.1]●
Rejection
  food, hysterical 300.11
  transplant 996.80
    bone marrow 996.85
    corneal 996.51
    organ (immune or nonimmune cause) 996.80
      bone marrow 996.85
      heart 996.83
      intestines 996.87
      kidney 996.81
      liver 996.82
      lung 996.84
      pancreas 996.86
      specified NEC 996.89

Rejection (*Continued*)
  transplant (*Continued*)
    skin 996.52
      artificial 996.55
      decellularized allodermis 996.55
    stem cell(s) 996.88
      from
        peripheral blood 996.88
        umbilical cord 996.88
Relapsing fever 087.9
  Carter's (Asiatic) 087.0
  Dutton's (West African) 087.1
  Koch's 087.9
  louse-borne (epidemic) 087.0
  Novy's (American) 087.1
  Obermeyer's (European) 087.0
  Spirillum 087.9
  tick-borne (endemic) 087.1
Relaxation
  anus (sphincter) 569.49
    due to hysteria 300.11
  arch (foot) 734
    congenital 754.61
  back ligaments 728.4
  bladder (sphincter) 596.59
  cardio-esophageal 530.89
  cervix (*see also* Incompetency, cervix) 622.5
  diaphragm 519.4
  inguinal rings - *see* Hernia, inguinal
  joint (capsule) (ligament) (paralytic) (*see also* Derangement, joint) 718.90
    congenital 755.8
  lumbosacral joint 724.6
  pelvic floor 618.89
  pelvis 618.89
  perineum 618.89
  posture 729.90
  rectum (sphincter) 569.49
  sacroiliac (joint) 724.6
  scrotum 608.89
  urethra (sphincter) 599.84
  uterus (outlet) 618.89
  vagina (outlet) 618.89
  vesical 596.59
Remains
  canal of Cloquet 743.51
  capsule (opaque) 743.51
Remittent fever (malarial) 084.6
Remnant
  canal of Cloquet 743.51
  capsule (opaque) 743.51
  cervix, cervical stump (acquired) (postoperative) 622.8
  cystic duct, postcholecystectomy 576.0
  fingernail 703.8
    congenital 757.5
  meniscus, knee 717.5
  thyroglossal duct 759.2
  tonsil 474.8
    infected 474.00
  urachus 753.7
Remote effect of cancer - *see* condition
Removal (of)
  catheter (urinary) (indwelling) V53.6
    from artificial opening - *see* Attention to, artificial, opening
    non-vascular V58.82
    vascular V58.81
  cerebral ventricle (communicating) shunt V53.01
  device - *see also* Fitting (of)
    contraceptive V25.12
      with reinsertion V25.13
    fixation
      external V54.89
      internal V54.01
    traction V54.89
  drains V58.49

Removal *(Continued)*
- dressing
  - wound V58.30
    - nonsurgical V58.30
    - surgical V58.31
- ileostomy V55.2
- Kirschner wire V54.89
- non-vascular catheter V58.82
- pin V54.01
- plaster cast V54.89
- plate (fracture) V54.01
- rod V54.01
- screw V54.01
- splint, external V54.89
- staples V58.32
- subdermal implantable contraceptive V25.43
- sutures V58.32
- traction device, external V54.89
- vascular catheter V58.81
- wound packing V58.30
  - nonsurgical V58.30
  - surgical V58.31

Ren
- arcuatus 753.3
- mobile, mobilis (*see also* Disease, renal) 593.0
  - congenital 753.3
- unguliformis 753.3

Renal - *see also* condition
- glomerulohyalinosis-diabetic syndrome 250.4● [581.81]
  - due to secondary diabetes 249.4● [581.81]

Rendu-Osler-Weber disease or syndrome (familial hemorrhagic telangiectasia) 448.0

Reninoma (M8361/1) 236.91

Rénon-Delille syndrome 253.8

Repair
- pelvic floor, previous, in pregnancy or childbirth 654.4●
  - affecting fetus or newborn 763.89
- scarred tissue V51.8

Replacement by artificial or mechanical device or prosthesis of (*see also* Fitting (of))
- artificial skin V43.83
- bladder V43.5
- blood vessel V43.4
- breast V43.82
- eye globe V43.0
- heart
  - with
    - assist device V43.21
    - fully implantable artificial heart V43.22
  - valve V43.3
- intestine V43.89
- joint V43.60
  - ankle V43.66
  - elbow V43.62
  - finger V43.69
  - hip (partial) (total) V43.64
  - knee V43.65
  - shoulder V43.61
  - specified NEC V43.69
  - wrist V43.63
- kidney V43.89
- larynx V43.81
- lens V43.1
- limb(s) V43.7
- liver V43.89
- lung V43.89
- organ NEC V43.89
- pancreas V43.89
- skin (artificial) V43.83
- tissue NEC V43.89

Reprogramming
- cardiac pacemaker V53.31

Request for expert evidence V68.2

Reserve, decreased or low
- cardiac - *see* Disease, heart
  - kidney (*see also* Disease, renal) 593.9

Residual - *see also* condition
- bladder 596.89
- foreign body - *see* Retention, foreign body
- state, schizophrenic (*see also* Schizophrenia) 295.6●
- urine 788.69

Resistance, resistant (to)
- activated protein C 289.81

> Note: Use the following subclassification for categories V09.5, V09.7, V09.8, V09.9
>
> 0 without mention of resistance to multiple drugs
> 1 with resistance to multiple drugs
> V09.5 quinolones and fluoro-quinolones
> V09.7 antimycobacterial agents
> V09.8 specified drugs NEC
> V09.9 unspecified drugs

- drugs by microorganisms V09.90
  - amikacin V09.4
  - aminoglycosides V09.4
  - amodiaquine V09.5●
  - amoxicillin V09.0
  - ampicillin V09.0
  - antimycobacterial agents V09.7●
  - azithromycin V09.2
  - azlocillin V09.0
  - aztreonam V09.1
  - B-lactam antibiotics V09.1
  - bacampicillin V09.0
  - bacitracin V09.8●
  - benznidazole V09.8●
  - capreomycin V09.7●
  - carbenicillin V09.0
  - cefaclor V09.1
  - cefadroxil V09.1
  - cefamandole V09.1
  - cefatetan V09.1
  - cefazolin V09.1
  - cefixime V09.1
  - cefonicid V09.1
  - cefoperazone V09.1
  - ceforanide V09.1
  - cefotaxime V09.1
  - cefoxitin V09.1
  - ceftazidine V09.1
  - ceftizoxime V09.1
  - ceftriaxone V09.1
  - cefuroxime V09.1
  - cephalexin V09.1
  - cephaloglycin V09.1
  - cephaloridine V09.1
  - cephalosporins V09.1
  - cephalothin V09.1
  - cephapirin V09.1
  - cephradine V09.1
  - chloramphenicol V09.8●
  - chloraquine V09.5●
  - chlorguanide V09.8●
  - chlorproguanil V09.8●
  - chlortetracycline V09.3
  - cinoxacin V09.5●
  - ciprofloxacin V09.5●
  - clarithromycin V09.2
  - clindamycin V09.8●
  - clioquinol V09.5●
  - clofazimine V09.7●
  - cloxacillin V09.0
  - cyclacillin V09.0
  - cycloserine V09.7●
  - dapsone [Dz] V09.7●
  - demeclocycline V09.3
  - dicloxacillin V09.0
  - doxycycline V09.3
  - enoxacin V09.5●
  - erythromycin V09.2
  - ethambutol [EMB] V09.7●
  - ethionamide [ETA] V09.7●
  - fluoroquinolones NEC V09.5●

Resistance, resistant *(Continued)*
- drugs by microorganisms *(Continued)*
  - gentamicin V09.4
  - halofantrine V09.8●
  - imipenem V09.1
  - iodoquinol V09.5●
  - isoniazid [INH] V09.7●
  - kanamycin V09.4
  - macrolides V09.2
  - mafenide V09.6
  - MDRO (multiple drug resistant organisms) NOS V09.91
  - mefloquine V09.8●
  - melarsoprol V09.8●
  - methicillin - *see* Infection, Methicillin
  - methacycline V09.3
  - methenamine V09.8●
  - metronidazole V09.8●
  - mezlocillin V09.0
  - minocycline V09.3
  - multiple drug resistant organisms NOS V09.91
  - nafcillin V09.0
  - nalidixic acid V09.5●
  - natamycin V09.2
  - neomycin V09.4
  - netilmicin V09.4
  - nimorazole V09.8●
  - nitrofurantoin V09.8●
  - norfloxacin V09.5●
  - nystatin V09.2
  - ofloxacin V09.5●
  - oleandomycin V09.2
  - oxacillin V09.0
  - oxytetracycline V09.3
  - para-amino salicyclic acid [PAS] V09.7●
  - paromomycin V09.4
  - penicillin (G) (V) (Vk) V09.0
  - penicillins V09.0
  - pentamidine V09.8●
  - piperacillin V09.0
  - primaquine V09.5●
  - proguanil V09.8●
  - pyrazinamide [PZA] V09.7●
  - pyrimethamine/sulfalene V09.8●
  - pyrimethamine/sulfodoxine V09.8●
  - quinacrine V09.5●
  - quinidine V09.8●
  - quinine V09.8●
  - quinolones V09.5●
  - rifabutin V09.7●
  - rifampin [Rif] V09.7●
  - rifamycin V09.7●
  - rolitetracycline V09.3
  - specified drugs NEC V09.8●
  - spectinomycin V09.8●
  - spiramycin V09.2
  - streptomycin [Sm] V09.4
  - sulfacetamide V09.6
  - sulfacytine V09.6
  - sulfadiazine V09.6
  - sulfadoxine V09.6
  - sulfamethoxazole V09.6
  - sulfapyridine V09.6
  - sulfasalizine V09.6
  - sulfasoxazone V09.6
  - sulfonamides V09.6
  - sulfoxone V09.7●
  - tetracycline V09.3
  - tetracyclines V09.3
  - thiamphenicol V09.8●
  - ticarcillin V09.0
  - tinidazole V09.8●
  - tobramycin V09.4
  - triamphenicol V09.8●
  - trimethoprim V09.8●
  - vancomycin V09.8●
- insulin 277.7
  - complicating pregnancy 648.8●
- thyroid hormone 246.8

Resorption
- biliary 576.8
  - purulent or putrid (see also Cholecystitis) 576.8
- dental (roots) 521.40
  - alveoli 525.8
  - pathological
    - external 521.42
    - internal 521.41
    - specified NEC 521.49
- septic - see Septicemia
- teeth (roots) 521.40
  - pathological
    - external 521.42
    - internal 521.41
    - specified NEC 521.49

Respiration
- asymmetrical 786.09
- bronchial 786.09
- Cheyne-Stokes (periodic respiration) 786.04
- decreased, due to shock following injury 958.4
- disorder of 786.00
  - psychogenic 306.1
  - specified NEC 786.09
- failure 518.81
  - acute 518.81
    - following trauma and surgery 518.51
  - acute and chronic 518.84
    - following trauma and surgery 518.53
  - chronic 518.83
    - following trauma and surgery 518.51
  - newborn 770.84
- insufficiency 786.09
  - acute 518.82
  - newborn NEC 770.89
- Kussmaul (air hunger) 786.09
- painful 786.52
- periodic 786.09
- high altitude 327.22
- poor 786.09
  - newborn NEC 770.89
- sighing 786.7
  - psychogenic 306.1
- wheezing 786.07

Respiratory - see also condition
- distress 786.09
  - acute 518.82
  - fetus or newborn NEC 770.89
  - syndrome (newborn) 769
    - adult (following trauma and surgery) 518.52
      - specified NEC 518.82
- failure 518.81
  - acute 518.81
    - following trauma and surgery 518.51
  - acute and chronic 518.84
    - following trauma and surgery 518.53
  - chronic 518.83
    - following trauma and surgery 518.51

Respiratory syncytial virus (RSV) 079.6
- bronchiolitis 466.11
- pneumonia 480.1
- vaccination, prophylactic (against) V04.82

Response
- photoallergic 692.72
- phototoxic 692.72

Rest, rests
- mesonephric duct 752.89
  - fallopian tube 752.11
- ovarian, in fallopian tubes 752.19
- wolffian duct 752.89

Restless legs syndrome (RLS) 333.94

Restlessness 799.29

Restoration of organ continuity from previous sterilization (tuboplasty) (vasoplasty) V26.0

Restriction of housing space V60.1

Restzustand, schizophrenic (see also Schizophrenia) 295.6●

Retained - see Retention

Retardation
- development, developmental, specific (see also Disorder, development, specific) 315.9
  - learning, specific 315.2
    - arithmetical 315.1
    - language (skills) 315.31
      - expressive 315.31
      - mixed receptive-expressive 315.32
    - mathematics 315.1
    - reading 315.00
      - phonological 315.39
    - written expression 315.2
  - motor 315.4
- endochondral bone growth 733.91
- growth (physical) in childhood 783.43
  - due to malnutrition 263.2
  - fetal (intrauterine) 764.9●
    - affecting management of pregnancy 656.5●
- intrauterine growth 764.9●
  - affecting management of pregnancy 656.5●
- mental - see Disability, intellectual
- motor, specific 315.4
- physical 783.43
  - child 783.43
  - due to malnutrition 263.2
  - fetus (intrauterine) 764.9●
    - affecting management of pregnancy 656.5●
- psychomotor NEC 307.9
- reading 315.00

Retching - see Vomiting

Retention, retained
- bladder (see also Retention, urine) 788.20
  - psychogenic 306.53
- carbon dioxide 276.2
- cholelithiasis, following cholecystectomy 997.41
- cyst - see Cyst
- dead
  - fetus (after 22 completed weeks' gestation) 656.4●
  - early fetal death (before 22 completed weeks' gestation) 632
  - ovum 631.8
- decidua (following delivery) (fragments) (with hemorrhage) 666.2●
  - without hemorrhage 667.1●
- deciduous tooth 520.6
- dental root 525.3
- fecal (see also Constipation) 564.00
- fluid 276.69
- foreign body - see also Foreign body, retained
  - bone 733.99
  - current trauma - see Foreign body, by site or type
  - middle ear 385.83
  - muscle 729.6
  - soft tissue NEC 729.6
- gallstones, following cholecystectomy 997.41
- gastric 536.8
- membranes (following delivery) (with hemorrhage) 666.2●
  - with abortion - see Abortion, by type
  - without hemorrhage 667.1●
- menses 626.8
- milk (puerperal) 676.2●
- nitrogen, extrarenal 788.99
- placenta (total) (with hemorrhage) 666.0●
  - with abortion - see Abortion, by type
  - portions or fragments 666.2●
    - without hemorrhage 667.1●
  - without hemorrhage 667.0●
- products of conception
  - early pregnancy (fetal death before 22 completed weeks' gestation) 632

Retention, retained (Continued)
- products of conception (Continued)
  - following
    - abortion - see Abortion, by type
    - delivery 666.2●
      - with hemorrhage 666.2●
      - without hemorrhage 667.1●
  - secundines (following delivery) (with hemorrhage) 666.2●
    - with abortion - see Abortion, by type
    - complicating puerperium (delayed hemorrhage) 666.2●
    - without hemorrhage 667.1●
- smegma, clitoris 624.8
- urine NEC 788.20
  - bladder, incomplete emptying 788.21
  - due to
    - benign prostatic hypertrophy (BPH) - see category 600
  - due to
    - benign prostatic hypertrophy (BPH) - see category 600
  - psychogenic 306.53
  - specified NEC 788.29
- water (in tissue) (see also Edema) 782.3

Reticulation, dust (occupational) 504

Reticulocytosis NEC 790.99

Reticuloendotheliosis
- acute infantile (M9722/3) 202.5●
- leukemic (M9940/3) 202.4●
- malignant (M9720/3) 202.3●
- nonlipid (M9722/3) 202.5●

Reticulohistiocytoma (giant cell) 277.89

Reticulohistiocytosis, multicentric 272.8

Reticulolymphosarcoma (diffuse) (M9613/3) 200.8●
- follicular (M9691/3) 202.0●
- nodular (M9691/3) 202.0●

Reticulosarcoma (M9640/3) 200.0●
- nodular (M9642/3) 200.0●
- pleomorphic cell type (M9641/3) 200.0●

Reticulosis (skin)
- acute of infancy (M9722/3) 202.5●
- familial hemophagocytic 288.4
- histiocytic medullary (M9721/3) 202.3●
- lipomelanotic 695.89
- malignant (M9720/3) 202.3●
- Sézary's (M9701/3) 202.2●

Retina, retinal - see condition

Retinitis (see also Chorioretinitis) 363.20
- albuminurica 585.9 [363.10]
- arteriosclerotic 440.8 [362.13]
- central angiospastic 362.41
- Coat's 362.12
- diabetic 250.5● [362.01]
  - due to secondary diabetes 249.5● [362.01]
- disciformis 362.52
- disseminated 363.10
  - metastatic 363.14
  - neurosyphilitic 094.83
  - pigment epitheliopathy 363.15
- exudative 362.12
- focal 363.00
  - in histoplasmosis 115.92
    - capsulatum 115.02
    - duboisii 115.12
  - juxtapapillary 363.05
  - macular 363.06
  - paramacular 363.06
  - peripheral 363.08
  - posterior pole NEC 363.07
- gravidarum 646.8●
- hemorrhagica externa 362.12
- juxtapapillary (Jensen's) 363.05
- luetic - see Retinitis, syphilitic
- metastatic 363.14
- pigmentosa 362.74
- proliferans 362.29
- proliferating 362.29
- punctata albescens 362.76
- renal 585.9 [363.13]

SECTION I INDEX TO DISEASES AND INJURIES / **Rheumatism, rheumatic**

Retinitis (Continued)
  syphilitic (secondary) 091.51
    congenital 090.0 [363.13]
    early 091.51
    late 095.8 [363.13]
  syphilitica, central, recurrent 095.8 [363.13]
  tuberculous (see also Tuberculous) 017.3●
    [363.13]
Retinoblastoma (M9510/3) 190.5
  differentiated type (M9511/3) 190.5
  undifferentiated type (M9512/3) 190.5
Retinochoroiditis (see also Chorioretinitis)
  363.20
  central angiospastic 362.41
  disseminated 363.10
    metastatic 363.14
    neurosyphilitic 094.83
    pigment epitheliopathy 363.15
    syphilitic 094.83
  due to toxoplasmosis (acquired) (focal)
    130.2
  focal 363.00
    in histoplasmosis 115.92
      capsulatum 115.02
      duboisii 115.12
    juxtapapillary (Jensen's) 363.05
    macular 363.06
    paramacular 363.06
    peripheral 363.08
    posterior pole NEC 363.07
  juxtapapillaris 363.05
  syphilitic (disseminated) 094.83
Retinopathy (background) 362.10
  arteriosclerotic 440.8 [362.13]
  atherosclerotic 440.8 [362.13]
  central serous 362.41
  circinate 362.10
  Coat's 362.12
  diabetic 250.5● [362.01]
    due to secondary diabetes 249.5●
      [362.01]
    nonproliferative 250.5● [362.03]
      due to secondary diabetes 249.5●
        [362.03]
      mild 250.5● [362.04]
        due to secondary diabetes 249.5●
          [362.04]
      moderate 250.5● [362.05]
        due to secondary diabetes 249.5●
          [362.05]
      severe 250.5● [362.06]
        due to secondary diabetes 249.5●
          [362.06]
    proliferative 250.5● [362.02]
      due to secondary diabetes 249.5●
        [362.02]
  exudative 362.12
  hypertensive 362.11
  nonproliferative
    diabetic 250.5● [362.03]
      due to secondary diabetes 249.5●
        [362.03]
      mild 250.5● [362.04]
        due to secondary diabetes 249.5●
          [362.04]
      moderate 250.5● [362.05]
        due to secondary diabetes 249.5●
          [362.05]
      severe 250.5● [362.06]
        due to secondary diabetes 249.5●
          [362.06]
  of prematurity 362.20
    cicatricial 362.21
    stage
      0 362.22
      1 362.23
      2 362.24
      3 362.25
      4 362.26
      5 362.27
  pigmentary, congenital 362.74

Retinopathy (Continued)
  proliferative 362.29
    diabetic 250.5● [362.02]
      due to secondary diabetes 249.5●
        [362.02]
    sickle-cell 282.60 [362.29]
  solar 363.31
Retinoschisis 361.10
  bullous 361.12
  congenital 743.56
  flat 361.11
  juvenile 362.73
Retractile testis 752.52
Retraction
  cervix see Retraction, uterus
  drum (membrane) 384.82
  eyelid 374.41
  finger 736.29
  head 781.0
  lid 374.41
  lung 518.89
  mediastinum 519.3
  nipple 611.79
    congenital 757.6
    puerperal, postpartum 676.0●
  palmar fascia 728.6
  pleura (see also Pleurisy) 511.0
  ring, uterus (Bandl's) (pathological) 661.4●
    affecting fetus or newborn 763.7
  sternum (congenital) 756.3
    acquired 738.3
    during respiration 786.9
  substernal 738.3
  supraclavicular 738.8
  syndrome (Duane's) 378.71
  uterus 621.6
  valve (heart) - see Endocarditis
Retrobulbar - see condition
Retrocaval ureter 753.4
Retrocecal - see also condition
  appendix (congenital) 751.5
Retrocession - see Retroversion
Retrodisplacement - see Retroversion
Retroflection, retroflexion - see Retroversion
Retrognathia, retrognathism (mandibular)
  (maxillary) 524.10
Retrograde
  ejaculation 608.87
  menstruation 626.8
Retroiliac ureter 753.4
Retroperineal - see condition
Retroperitoneal - see condition
Retroperitonitis 567.39
Retropharyngeal - see condition
Retroplacental - see condition
Retroposition - see Retroversion
Retroprosthetic membrane 996.51
Retrosternal thyroid (congenital) 759.2
Retroversion, retroverted
  cervix - see Retroversion, uterus
  female NEC (see also Retroversion, uterus)
    621.6
  iris 364.70
  testis (congenital) 752.51
  uterus, uterine (acquired) (acute) (adherent)
    (any degree) (asymptomatic) (cervix)
    (postinfectional) (postpartal, old)
    621.6
    congenital 752.39
    in pregnancy or childbirth 654.3●
      affecting fetus or newborn 763.89
      causing obstructed labor 660.2●
        affecting fetus or newborn 763.1
Retrusion, premaxilla (developmental)
  524.04
Rett's syndrome 330.8
Reverse, reversed
  peristalsis 787.4
Reye's syndrome 331.81
Reye-Sheehan syndrome (postpartum pituitary
  necrosis) 253.2

Rh antigen (C) (c) (D) (E) (e) (factor)
  hemolytic disease 773.0
  incompatibility, immunization, or
    sensitization
    affecting management of pregnancy
      656.1●
    fetus or newborn 773.0
    transfusion reaction (see also
      Complications, transfusion) 999.70
  negative mother, affecting fetus or newborn
    773.0
  titer elevated (see also Complications,
    transfusion) 999.70
  transfusion reaction (see also Complications,
    transfusion) 999.70
Rhabdomyolysis (idiopathic) 728.88
Rhabdomyoma (M8900/0) - see also Neoplasm,
  connective tissue, benign
  adult (M8904/0) - see Neoplasm, connective
    tissue, benign
  fetal (M8903/0) - see Neoplasm, connective
    tissue, benign
  glycogenic (M8904/0) - see Neoplasm,
    connective tissue, benign
Rhabdomyosarcoma (M8900/3) - see also
  Neoplasm, connective tissue, malignant
  alveolar (M8920/3) - see Neoplasm,
    connective tissue, malignant
  embryonal (M8910/3) - see Neoplasm,
    connective tissue, malignant
  mixed type (M8902/3) - see Neoplasm,
    connective tissue, malignant
  pleomorphic (M8901/3) - see Neoplasm,
    connective tissue, malignant
Rhabdosarcoma (M8900/3) - see
  Rhabdomyosarcoma
Rhesus (factor) (Rh) incompatibility - see Rh,
  incompatibility
Rheumaticosis - see Rheumatism
Rheumatism, rheumatic (acute NEC) 729.0
  adherent pericardium 393
  arthritis
    acute or subacute - see Fever, rheumatic
    chronic 714.0
      spine 720.0
  articular (chronic) NEC (see also Arthritis)
    716.9●
    acute or subacute - see Fever, rheumatic
  back 724.9
  blennorrhagic 098.59
  carditis - see Disease, heart, rheumatic
  cerebral - see Fever, rheumatic
  chorea (acute) - see Chorea, rheumatic
  chronic NEC 729.0
  coronary arteritis 391.9
    chronic 398.99
  degeneration, myocardium (see also
    Degeneration, myocardium, with
    rheumatic fever) 398.0
  desert 114.0
  febrile - see Fever, rheumatic
  fever - see Fever, rheumatic
  gonococcal 098.59
  gout 714.0
  heart
    disease (see also Disease, heart, rheumatic)
      398.90
    failure (chronic) (congestive) (inactive)
      398.91
  hemopericardium - see Rheumatic,
    pericarditis
  hydropericardium - see Rheumatic,
    pericarditis
  inflammatory (acute) (chronic) (subacute) -
    see Fever, rheumatic
  intercostal 729.0
    meaning Tietze's disease 733.6
  joint (chronic) NEC (see also Arthritis) 716.9●
    acute - see Fever, rheumatic
  mediastinopericarditis - see Rheumatic,
    pericarditis

SECTION 1 INDEX TO DISEASES AND INJURIES / Rheumatism, rheumatic

Rheumatism, rheumatic (Continued)
- muscular 729.0
- myocardial degeneration (see also
    - Degeneration, myocardium, with rheumatic fever) 398.0
- myocarditis (chronic) (inactive) (with chorea) 398.0
    - active or acute 391.2
        - with chorea (acute) (rheumatic) (Sydenham's) 392.0
- myositis 729.1
- neck 724.9
- neuralgic 729.0
- neuritis (acute) (chronic) 729.2
- neuromuscular 729.0
- nodose - see Arthritis, nodosa
- nonarticular 729.0
- palindromic 719.30
    - ankle 719.37
    - elbow 719.32
    - foot 719.37
    - hand 719.34
    - hip 719.35
    - knee 719.36
    - multiple sites 719.39
    - pelvic region 719.35
    - shoulder (region) 719.31
    - specified site NEC 719.38
    - wrist 719.33
- pancarditis, acute 391.8
    - with chorea (acute) (rheumatic) (Sydenham's) 392.0
    - chronic or inactive 398.99
- pericarditis (active) (acute) (with effusion) (with pneumonia) 391.0
    - with chorea (acute) (rheumatic) (Sydenham's) 392.0
    - chronic or inactive 393
- pericardium - see Rheumatic, pericarditis
- pleuropericarditis - see Rheumatic, pericarditis
- pneumonia 390 [517.1]
- pneumonitis 390 [517.1]
- pneumopericarditis - see Rheumatic, pericarditis
- polyarthritis
    - acute or subacute - see Fever, rheumatic
    - chronic 714.0
- polyarticular NEC (see also Arthritis) 716.9●
- psychogenic 306.0
- radiculitis 729.2
- sciatic 724.3
- septic - see Fever, rheumatic
- spine 724.9
- subacute NEC 729.0
- torticollis 723.5
- tuberculous NEC (see also Tuberculosis) 015.9●
- typhoid fever 002.0

Rheumatoid - see also condition
- lungs 714.81

Rhinitis (atrophic) (catarrhal) (chronic) (croupous) (fibrinous) (hyperplastic) (hypertrophic) (membranous) (purulent) (suppurative) (ulcerative) 472.0
- with
    - hay fever (see also Fever, hay) 477.9
        - with asthma (bronchial) 493.0●
    - sore throat - see Nasopharyngitis
- acute 460
- allergic (nonseasonal) (seasonal) (see also Fever, hay) 477.9
    - with asthma (see also Asthma) 493.0●
    - due to food 477.1
- granulomatous 472.0
- infective 460
- obstructive 472.0
- pneumococcal 460
- syphilitic 095.8
    - congenital 090.0
- tuberculous (see also Tuberculosis) 012.8●
- vasomotor (see also Fever, hay) 477.9

Rhinoantritis (chronic) 473.0
- acute 461.0

Rhinodacryolith 375.57

Rhinolalia (aperta) (clausa) (open) 784.43

Rhinolith 478.19
- nasal sinus (see also Sinusitis) 473.9

Rhinomegaly 478.19

Rhinopharyngitis (acute) (subacute) (see also Nasopharyngitis) 460
- chronic 472.2
- destructive ulcerating 102.5
- mutilans 102.5

Rhinophyma 695.3

Rhinorrhea 478.19
- cerebrospinal (fluid) 349.81
- paroxysmal (see also Fever, hay) 477.9
- spasmodic (see also Fever, hay) 477.9

Rhinosalpingitis 381.50
- acute 381.51
- chronic 381.52

Rhinoscleroma 040.1

Rhinosporidiosis 117.0

Rhinovirus infection 079.3

Rhizomelic chrondrodysplasia punctata 277.86

Rhizomelique, pseudopolyarthritic 446.5

Rhoads and Bomford anemia (refractory) 238.72

Rhus
- diversiloba dermatitis 692.6
- radicans dermatitis 692.6
- toxicodendron dermatitis 692.6
- venenata dermatitis 692.6
- verniciflua dermatitis 692.6

Rhythm
- atrioventricular nodal 427.89
- disorder 427.9
    - coronary sinus 427.89
    - ectopic 427.89
    - nodal 427.89
- escape 427.89
- heart, abnormal 427.9
    - fetus or newborn - see Abnormal, heart rate
- idioventricular 426.89
    - accelerated 427.89
- nodal 427.89
- sleep, inversion 327.39
    - nonorganic origin 307.45

Rhytidosis facialis 701.8

Rib - see also condition
- cervical 756.2

Riboflavin deficiency 266.0

Rice bodies (see also Loose, body, joint) 718.1●
- knee 717.6

Richter's hernia - see Hernia, Richter's

Ricinism 988.2

Rickets (active) (acute) (adolescent) (adult) (chest wall) (congenital) (current) (infantile) (intestinal) 268.0
- celiac 579.0
- fetal 756.4
- hemorrhagic 267
- hypophosphatemic with nephrotic-glycosuric dwarfism 270.0
- kidney 588.0
- late effect 268.1
- renal 588.0
- scurvy 267
- vitamin D-resistant 275.3

Rickettsial disease 083.9
- specified type NEC 083.8

Rickettsialpox 083.2

Rickettsiosis NEC 083.9
- specified type NEC 083.8
- tick-borne 082.9
    - specified type NEC 082.8
- vesicular 083.2

Ricord's chancre 091.0

Riddoch's syndrome (visual disorientation) 368.16

Rider's
- bone 733.99
- chancre 091.0

Ridge, alveolus - see also condition
- edentulous
    - atrophy 525.20
        - mandible 525.20
            - minimal 525.21
            - moderate 525.22
            - severe 525.23
        - maxilla 525.20
            - minimal 525.24
            - moderate 525.25
            - severe 525.26
    - flabby 525.20

Ridged ear 744.29

Riedel's
- disease (ligneous thyroiditis) 245.3
- lobe, liver 751.69
- struma (ligneous thyroiditis) 245.3
- thyroiditis (ligneous) 245.3

Rieger's anomaly or syndrome (mesodermal dysgenesis, anterior ocular segment) 743.44

Riehl's melanosis 709.09

Rietti-Greppi-Micheli anemia or syndrome 282.46

Rieux's hernia - see Hernia, Rieux's

Rift Valley fever 066.3

Riga's disease (cachectic aphthae) 529.0

Riga-Fede disease (cachectic aphthae) 529.0

Riggs' disease (compound periodontitis) 523.40

Right middle lobe syndrome 518.0

Rigid, rigidity - see also condition
- abdominal 789.4●
- articular, multiple congenital 754.89
- back 724.8
- cervix uteri
    - in pregnancy or childbirth 654.6●
        - affecting fetus or newborn 763.89
        - causing obstructed labor 660.2●
            - affecting fetus or newborn 763.1
- hymen (acquired) (congenital) 623.3
- nuchal 781.6
- pelvic floor
    - in pregnancy or childbirth 654.4●
        - affecting fetus or newborn 763.89
        - causing obstructed labor 660.2●
            - affecting fetus or newborn 763.1
- perineum or vulva
    - in pregnancy or childbirth 654.8●
        - affecting fetus or newborn 763.89
        - causing obstructed labor 660.2●
            - affecting fetus or newborn 763.1
- spine 724.8
- vagina
    - in pregnancy or childbirth 654.7●
        - affecting fetus or newborn 763.89
        - causing obstructed labor 660.2●
            - affecting fetus or newborn 763.1

Rigors 780.99

Riley-Day syndrome (familial dysautonomia) 742.8

RIND (reversible ischemic neurological deficit) 434.91
- history of (personal) V12.54

Ring(s)
- aorta 747.21
- Bandl's, complicating delivery 661.4●
    - affecting fetus or newborn 763.7
- contraction, complicating delivery 661.4●
    - affecting fetus or newborn 763.7
- esophageal (congenital) 750.3
- Fleischer (-Kayser) (cornea) 275.1 [371.14]
- hymenal, tight (acquired) (congenital) 623.3
- Kayser-Fleischer (cornea) 275.1 [371.14]
- retraction, uterus, pathological 661.4●
    - affecting fetus or newborn 763.7
- Schatzki's (esophagus) (congenital) (lower) 750.3
    - acquired 530.3

Ring(s) (Continued)
    Soemmering's 366.51
    trachea, abnormal 748.3
    vascular (congenital) 747.21
    Vossius' 921.3
        late effect 366.21
Ringed hair (congenital) 757.4
Ringing in the ear (see also Tinnitus) 388.30
Ringworm 110.9
    beard 110.0
    body 110.5
    Burmese 110.9
    corporeal 110.5
    foot 110.4
    groin 110.3
    hand 110.2
    honeycomb 110.0
    nails 110.1
    perianal (area) 110.3
    scalp 110.0
    specified site NEC 110.8
    Tokelau 110.5
Rise, venous pressure 459.89
Risk
    factor - see Problem
    falling V15.88
    suicidal 300.9
Ritter's disease (dermatitis exfoliativa neonatorum) 695.81
Rivalry, sibling 313.3
Rivalta's disease (cervicofacial actinomycosis) 039.3
River blindness 125.3 [360.13]
Robert's pelvis 755.69
    with disproportion (fetopelvic) 653.0
        affecting fetus or newborn 763.1
        causing obstructed labor 660.1
            affecting fetus or newborn 763.1
Robin's syndrome 756.0
Robinson's (hidrotic) ectodermal dysplasia 757.31
Robles' disease (onchocerciasis) 125.3 [360.13]
Rochalimea - see Rickettsial disease
Rocky Mountain fever (spotted) 082.0
Rodent ulcer (M8090/3) - see also Neoplasm, skin, malignant
    cornea 370.07
Roentgen ray, adverse effect - see Effect, adverse, x-ray
Roetheln 056.9
Roger's disease (congenital interventricular septal defect) 745.4
Rokitansky's
    disease (see also Necrosis, liver) 570
    tumor 620.2
Rokitansky-Aschoff sinuses (mucosal outpouching of gallbladder) (see also Disease, gallbladder) 575.8
Rokitansky-Kuster-Hauser syndrome (congenital absence vagina) 752.45
Rollet's chancre (syphilitic) 091.0
Rolling of head 781.0
Romano-Ward syndrome (prolonged QT interval syndrome) 426.82
Romanus lesion 720.1
Romberg's disease or syndrome 349.89
Roof, mouth - see condition
Rosacea 695.3
    acne 695.3
    keratitis 695.3 [370.49]
Rosary, rachitic 268.0
Rose
    cold 477.0
    fever 477.0
    rash 782.1
        epidemic 056.9
        of infants 057.8
Rosen-Castleman-Liebow syndrome (pulmonary proteinosis) 516.0
Rosenbach's erysipelatoid or erysipeloid 027.1
Rosenthal's disease (factor XI deficiency) 286.2

Roseola 057.8
    infantum, infantilis (see also Exanthem subitum) 058.10
Rossbach's disease (hyperchlorhydria) 536.8
    psychogenic 306.4
Rossle-Urbach-Wiethe lipoproteinosis 272.8
Ross river fever 066.3
Rostan's asthma (cardiac) (see also Failure, ventricular, left) 428.1
Rot
    Barcoo (see also Ulcer, skin) 707.9
    knife-grinders' (see also Tuberculosis) 011.4
Rot-Bernhardt disease 355.1
Rotation
    anomalous, incomplete or insufficient - see Malrotation
    cecum (congenital) 751.4
    colon (congenital) 751.4
    manual, affecting fetus or newborn 763.89
    spine, incomplete or insufficient 737.8
    tooth, teeth 524.35
    vertebra, incomplete or insufficient 737.8
Röteln 056.9
Roth's disease or meralgia 355.1
Roth-Bernhardt disease or syndrome 355.1
Rothmund (-Thomson) syndrome 757.33
Rotor's disease or syndrome (idiopathic hyperbilirubinemia) 277.4
Rotundum ulcus - see Ulcer, stomach
Round
    back (with wedging of vertebrae) 737.10
        late effect of rickets 268.1
    hole, retina 361.31
        with detachment 361.01
    ulcer (stomach) - see Ulcer, stomach
    worms (infestation) (large) NEC 127.0
Roussy-Lévy syndrome 334.3
Routine postpartum follow-up V24.2
Roy (-Jutras) syndrome (acropachyderma) 757.39
Rubella (German measles) 056.9
    complicating pregnancy, childbirth, or puerperium 647.5
    complication 056.8
        neurological 056.00
            encephalomyelitis 056.01
            specified type NEC 056.09
        specified type NEC 056.79
    congenital 771.0
    contact V01.4
    exposure to V01.4
    maternal
        with suspected fetal damage affecting management of pregnancy 655.3
        affecting fetus or newborn 760.2
            manifest rubella in infant 771.0
    specified complications NEC 056.79
    vaccination, prophylactic (against) V04.3
Rubeola (measles) (see also Measles) 055.9
    complicated 055.8
    meaning rubella (see also Rubella) 056.9
    scarlatinosis 057.8
Rubeosis iridis 364.42
    diabetica 250.5 [364.42]
        due to secondary diabetes 249.5 [364.42]
Rubinstein-Taybi's syndrome (brachydactylia, short stature and intellectual disabilities) 759.89
Rud's syndrome (mental deficiency, epilepsy, and infantilism) 759.89
Rudimentary (congenital) - see also Agenesis
    arm 755.22
    bone 756.9
    cervix uteri 752.43
    eye (see also Microphthalmos) 743.10
    fallopian tube 752.19
    leg 755.32
    lobule of ear 744.21
    patella 755.64
    respiratory organs in thoracopagus 759.4
    tracheal bronchus 748.3
    uterine horn 752.39

Rudimentary (Continued)
    uterus 752.39
        in male 752.7
        solid or with cavity 752.39
    vagina 752.45
Ruiter-Pompen (-Wyers) syndrome (angiokeratoma corporis diffusum) 272.7
Ruled out condition (see also Observation, suspected) V71.9
Rumination - see also Vomiting
    disorder 307.53
    neurotic 300.3
    obsessional 300.3
    psychogenic 307.53
Runaway reaction - see also Disturbance, conduct
    socialized 312.2
    undersocialized, unsocialized 312.1
Runeberg's disease (progressive pernicious anemia) 281.0
Runge's syndrome (postmaturity) 766.22
Runny nose 784.99
Rupia 091.3
    congenital 090.0
    tertiary 095.9
Rupture, ruptured 553.9
    abdominal viscera NEC 799.89
        obstetrical trauma 665.5
    abscess (spontaneous) - see Abscess, by site
    amnion - see Rupture, membranes
    aneurysm - see Aneurysm
    anus (sphincter) - see Laceration, anus
    aorta, aortic 441.5
        abdominal 441.3
        arch 441.1
        ascending 441.1
        descending 441.5
            abdominal 441.3
            thoracic 441.1
        syphilitic 093.0
        thoracoabdominal 441.6
        thorax, thoracic 441.1
        transverse 441.1
        traumatic (thoracic) 901.0
            abdominal 902.0
        valve or cusp (see also Endocarditis, aortic) 424.1
    appendix (with peritonitis) 540.0
        with peritoneal abscess 540.1
        traumatic - see Injury, internal, gastrointestinal tract
    arteriovenous fistula, brain (congenital) 430
    artery 447.2
        brain (see also Hemorrhage, brain) 431
        coronary (see also Infarct, myocardium) 410.9
        heart (see also Infarct, myocardium) 410.9
        pulmonary 417.8
        traumatic (complication) (see also Injury, blood vessel, by site) 904.9
    bile duct, except cystic (see also Disease, biliary) 576.3
        cystic 575.4
        traumatic - see Injury, internal, intra-abdominal
    bladder (sphincter) 596.6
        with
            abortion - see Abortion, by type, with damage to pelvic organs
            ectopic pregnancy (see also categories 633.0–633.9) 639.2
            molar pregnancy (see also categories 630–632) 639.2
        following
            abortion 639.2
            ectopic or molar pregnancy 639.2
        nontraumatic 596.6
        obstetrical trauma 665.5
        spontaneous 596.6
        traumatic - see Injury, internal, bladder

 New | Revised | deleted Deleted | Use Additional Digit(s) | Omit code

SECTION 1 INDEX TO DISEASES AND INJURIES / Rupture, ruptured

Rupture, ruptured *(Continued)*
- blood vessel *(see also* Hemorrhage) 459.0
  - brain *(see also* Hemorrhage, brain) 431
  - heart *(see also* Infarct, myocardium) 410.9●
  - traumatic (complication) *(see also* Injury, blood vessel, by site) 904.9
- bone - *see* Fracture, by site
- bowel 569.89
  - traumatic - *see* Injury, internal, intestine
- Bowman's membrane 371.31
- brain
  - aneurysm (congenital) *(see also* Hemorrhage, subarachnoid) 430
    - late effect - *see* Late effect(s) (of) cerebrovascular disease
    - syphilitic 094.87
  - hemorrhagic *(see also* Hemorrhage, brain) 431
  - injury at birth 767.0
  - syphilitic 094.89
- capillaries 448.9
- cardiac *(see also* Infarct, myocardium) 410.9●
- cartilage (articular) (current) - *see also* Sprain, by site
  - knee - *see* Tear, meniscus
  - semilunar - *see* Tear, meniscus
- cecum (with peritonitis) 540.0
  - with peritoneal abscess 540.1
  - traumatic 863.89
    - with open wound into cavity 863.99
- cerebral aneurysm (congenital) *(see also* Hemorrhage, subarachnoid) 430
  - late effect - *see* Late effect(s) (of) cerebrovascular disease
- cervix (uteri)
  - with
    - abortion - *see* Abortion, by type, with damage to pelvic organs
    - ectopic pregnancy *(see also* categories 633.0–633.9) 639.2
    - molar pregnancy *(see also* categories 630–632) 639.2
  - following
    - abortion 639.2
    - ectopic or molar pregnancy 639.2
  - obstetrical trauma 665.3●
  - traumatic - *see* Injury, internal, cervix
- chordae tendineae 429.5
- choroid (direct) (indirect) (traumatic) 363.63
- circle of Willis *(see also* Hemorrhage, subarachnoid) 430
  - late effect - *see* Late effect(s) (of) cerebrovascular disease
- colon 569.89
  - traumatic - *see* Injury, internal, colon
- cornea (traumatic) - *see also* Rupture, eye
  - due to ulcer 370.00
- coronary (artery) (thrombotic) *(see also* Infarct, myocardium) 410.9●
- corpus luteum (infected) (ovary) 620.1
- cyst - *see* Cyst
- cystic duct *(see also* Disease, gallbladder) 575.4
- Descemet's membrane 371.33
  - traumatic - *see* Rupture, eye
- diaphragm - *see also* Hernia, diaphragm
  - traumatic - *see* Injury, internal, diaphragm
- diverticulum
  - bladder 596.3
  - intestine (large) *(see also* Diverticula) 562.10
    - small 562.00
- duodenal stump 537.89
- duodenum (ulcer) - *see* Ulcer, duodenum, with perforation
- ear drum *(see also* Perforation, tympanum) 384.20
  - with otitis media - *see* Otitis media
  - traumatic - *see* Wound, open, ear

Rupture, ruptured *(Continued)*
- esophagus 530.4
  - traumatic 862.22
    - with open wound into cavity 862.32
    - cervical region - *see* Wound, open, esophagus
- eye (without prolapse of intraocular tissue) 871.0
  - with
    - exposure of intraocular tissue 871.1
    - partial loss of intraocular tissue 871.2
    - prolapse of intraocular tissue 871.1
  - due to burn 940.5
- fallopian tube 620.8
  - due to pregnancy - *see* Pregnancy, tubal
  - traumatic - *see* Injury, internal, fallopian tube
- fontanel 767.3
- free wall (ventricle) *(see also* Infarct, myocardium) 410.9●
- gallbladder or duct *(see also* Disease, gallbladder) 575.4
  - traumatic - *see* Injury, internal, gallbladder
- gastric *(see also* Rupture, stomach) 537.89
  - vessel 459.0
- globe (eye) (traumatic) - *see* Rupture, eye
- graafian follicle (hematoma) 620.0
- heart (auricle) (ventricle) *(see also* Infarct, myocardium) 410.9●
  - infectional 422.90
  - traumatic - *see* Rupture, myocardium, traumatic
- hymen 623.8
- internal
  - organ, traumatic - *see also* Injury, internal, by site
    - heart - *see* Rupture, myocardium, traumatic
    - kidney - *see* Rupture, kidney
    - liver - *see* Rupture, liver
    - spleen - *see* Rupture, spleen, traumatic
    - semilunar cartilage - *see* Tear, meniscus
  - intervertebral disc - *see* Displacement, intervertebral disc
    - traumatic (current) - *see* Dislocation, vertebra
- intestine 569.89
  - traumatic - *see* Injury, internal, intestine
- intracranial, birth injury 767.0
- iris 364.76
  - traumatic - *see* Rupture, eye
- joint capsule - *see* Sprain, by site
- kidney (traumatic) 866.03
  - with open wound into cavity 866.13
  - due to birth injury 767.8
  - nontraumatic 593.89
- lacrimal apparatus (traumatic) 870.2
- lens (traumatic) 366.20
- ligament - *see also* Sprain, by site
  - with open wound - *see* Wound, open, by site
  - old *(see also* Disorder, cartilage, articular) 718.0●
- liver (traumatic) 864.04
  - with open wound into cavity 864.14
  - due to birth injury 767.8
  - nontraumatic 573.8
- lymphatic (node) (vessel) 457.8
- marginal sinus (placental) (with hemorrhage) 641.2●
  - affecting fetus or newborn 762.1
- meaning hernia - *see* Hernia
- membrana tympani *(see also* Perforation, tympanum) 384.20
  - with otitis media - *see* Otitis media
  - traumatic - *see* Wound, open, ear
- membranes (spontaneous)
  - artificial
    - delayed delivery following 658.3●
      - affecting fetus or newborn 761.1
      - fetus or newborn 761.1

Rupture, ruptured *(Continued)*
- membranes *(Continued)*
  - delayed delivery following 658.2●
    - affecting fetus or newborn 761.1
  - premature (less than 24 hours prior to onset of labor) 658.1●
    - affecting fetus or newborn 761.1
    - delayed delivery following 658.2●
      - affecting fetus or newborn 761.1
- meningeal artery *(see also* Hemorrhage, subarachnoid) 430
  - late effect - *see* Late effect(s) (of) cerebrovascular disease
- meniscus (knee) - *see also* Tear, meniscus
  - old *(see also* Derangement, meniscus) 717.5
    - site other than knee - *see* Disorder, cartilage, articular
    - site other than knee - *see* Sprain, by site
- mesentery 568.89
  - traumatic - *see* Injury, internal, mesentery
- mitral - *see* Insufficiency, mitral
- muscle (traumatic) NEC - *see also* Sprain, by site
  - with open wound - *see* Wound, open, by site
  - nontraumatic 728.83
- musculotendinous cuff (nontraumatic) (shoulder) 840.4
- mycotic aneurysm, causing cerebral hemorrhage *(see also* Hemorrhage, subarachnoid) 430
  - late effect - *see* Late effect(s) (of) cerebrovascular disease
- myocardium, myocardial *(see also* Infarct, myocardium) 410.9●
  - traumatic 861.03
    - with open wound into thorax 861.13
- nontraumatic (meaning hernia) *(see also* Hernia, by site) 553.9
- obstructed *(see also* Hernia, by site, with obstruction) 552.9
  - gangrenous *(see also* Hernia, by site, with gangrene) 551.9
- operation wound *(see also* Dehiscence) 998.32
  - internal 998.31
- ovary, ovarian 620.8
  - corpus luteum 620.1
  - follicle (graafian) 620.0
- oviduct 620.8
  - due to pregnancy - *see* Pregnancy, tubal
- pancreas 577.8
  - traumatic - *see* Injury, internal, pancreas
- papillary muscle (ventricular) 429.6
- pelvic
  - floor, complicating delivery 664.1●
  - organ NEC - *see* Injury, pelvic, organs
- penis (traumatic) - *see* Wound, open, penis
- perineum 624.8
  - during delivery *(see also* Laceration, perineum, complicating delivery) 664.4●
- pharynx (nontraumatic) (spontaneous) 478.29
- pregnant uterus (before onset of labor) 665.0●
- prostate (traumatic) - *see* Injury, internal, prostate
- pulmonary
  - artery 417.8
  - valve (heart) *(see also* Endocarditis, pulmonary) 424.3
  - vein 417.8
  - vessel 417.8
- pupil, sphincter 364.75
- pus tube *(see also* Salpingo-oophoritis) 614.2
- pyosalpinx *(see also* Salpingo-oophoritis) 614.2
- rectum 569.49
  - traumatic - *see* Injury, internal, rectum

SECTION I INDEX TO DISEASES AND INJURIES / Rytand-Lipsitch syndrome

Rupture, ruptured (Continued)
- retina, retinal (traumatic) (without detachment) 361.30
  - with detachment (see also Detachment, retina, with retinal defect) 361.00
- rotator cuff (capsule) (traumatic) 840.4
  - nontraumatic (complete) 727.61
  - partial 726.13
- sclera 871.0
- semilunar cartilage, knee (see also Tear, meniscus) 836.2
  - old (see also Derangement, meniscus) 717.5
- septum (cardiac) 410.8 ●
- sigmoid 569.89
  - traumatic - see Injury, internal, colon, sigmoid
- sinus of Valsalva 747.29
- spinal cord - see also Injury, spinal, by site
  - due to injury at birth 767.4
  - fetus or newborn 767.4
  - syphilitic 094.89
  - traumatic - see also Injury, spinal, by site
    - with fracture - see Fracture, vertebra, by site, with spinal cord injury
- spleen 289.59
  - congenital 767.8
  - due to injury at birth 767.8
  - malarial 084.9
  - nontraumatic 289.59
  - spontaneous 289.59
  - traumatic 865.04
    - with open wound into cavity 865.14
- splenic vein 459.0
- stomach 537.89
  - due to injury at birth 767.8
  - traumatic - see Injury, internal, stomach
  - ulcer - see Ulcer, stomach, with perforation
- synovium 727.50
  - specified site NEC 727.59
- tendon (traumatic) - see also Sprain, by site
  - with open wound - see Wound, open, by site
  - Achilles 845.09
    - nontraumatic 727.67
  - ankle 845.09
    - nontraumatic 727.68
  - biceps (long head) 840.8
    - nontraumatic 727.62
  - foot 845.10
    - interphalangeal (joint) 845.13
    - metatarsophalangeal (joint) 845.12
    - nontraumatic 727.68
    - specified site NEC 845.19
    - tarsometatarsal (joint) 845.11
  - hand 842.10
    - carpometacarpal (joint) 842.11
    - interphalangeal (joint) 842.13
    - metacarpophalangeal (joint) 842.12

Rupture, ruptured (Continued)
- tendon (Continued)
  - hand (Continued)
    - nontraumatic 727.63
      - extensors 727.63
      - flexors 727.64
    - specified site NEC 842.19
  - nontraumatic 727.60
    - specified site NEC 727.69
  - patellar 844.8
    - nontraumatic 727.66
  - quadriceps 844.8
    - nontraumatic 727.65
  - rotator cuff (capsule) 840.4
    - nontraumatic (complete) 727.61
    - partial 726.13
  - wrist 842.00
    - carpal (joint) 842.01
    - nontraumatic 727.63
      - extensors 727.63
      - flexors 727.64
    - radiocarpal (joint) (ligament) 842.02
    - radioulnar (joint), distal 842.09
    - specified site NEC 842.09
- testis (traumatic) 878.2
  - complicated 878.3
  - due to syphilis 095.8
- thoracic duct 457.8
- tonsil 474.8
- traumatic
  - with open wound - see Wound, open, by site
  - aorta - see Rupture, aorta, traumatic
  - ear drum - see Wound, open, ear, drum
  - external site - see Wound, open, by site
  - eye 871.2
  - globe (eye) - see Wound, open, eyeball
  - internal organ (abdomen, chest, or pelvis) - see also Injury, internal, by site
    - heart - see Rupture, myocardium, traumatic
    - kidney - see Rupture, kidney
    - liver - see Rupture, liver
    - spleen - see Rupture, spleen, traumatic
  - ligament, muscle, or tendon - see also Sprain, by site
    - with open wound - see Wound, open, by site
  - meaning hernia - see Hernia
- tricuspid (heart) (valve) - see Endocarditis, tricuspid
- tube, tubal 620.8
  - abscess (see also Salpingo-oophoritis) 614.2
  - due to pregnancy - see Pregnancy, tubal
- tympanum, tympanic (membrane) (see also Perforation, tympanum) 384.20
  - with otitis media - see Otitis media
  - traumatic - see Wound, open, ear, drum

Rupture, ruptured (Continued)
- umbilical cord 663.8 ●
  - fetus or newborn 772.0
- ureter (traumatic) (see also Injury, internal, ureter) 867.2
  - nontraumatic 593.89
- urethra 599.84
  - with
    - abortion - see Abortion, by type, with damage to pelvic organs
    - ectopic pregnancy (see also categories 633.0–633.9) 639.2
    - molar pregnancy (see also categories 630–632) 639.2
  - following
    - abortion 639.2
    - ectopic or molar pregnancy 639.2
  - obstetrical trauma 665.5 ●
  - traumatic - see Injury, internal urethra
- uterosacral ligament 620.8
- uterus (traumatic) - see also Injury, internal uterus
  - affecting fetus or newborn 763.89
  - during labor 665.1 ●
  - nonpuerperal, nontraumatic 621.8
  - nontraumatic 621.8
  - pregnant (during labor) 665.1 ●
    - before labor 665.0 ●
- vagina 878.6
  - complicated 878.7
  - complicating delivery - see Laceration, vagina, complicating delivery
- valve, valvular (heart) - see Endocarditis
- varicose vein - see Varicose, vein
- varix - see Varix
- vena cava 459.0
- ventricle (free wall) (left) (see also Infarct, myocardium) 410.9 ●
- vesical (urinary) 596.6
  - traumatic - see Injury, internal, bladder
- vessel (blood) 459.0
  - pulmonary 417.8
- viscus 799.89
- vulva 878.4
  - complicated 878.5
  - complicating delivery 664.0 ●

Russell's dwarf (uterine dwarfism and craniofacial dysostosis) 759.89
Russell's dysentery 004.8
Russell (-Silver) syndrome (congenital hemihypertrophy and short stature) 759.89
Russian spring-summer type encephalitis 063.0
Rust's disease (tuberculous spondylitis) 015.0 ● [720.81]
Rustitskii's disease (multiple myeloma) (M9730/3) 203.0 ●
Ruysch's disease (Hirschsprung's disease) 751.3
Rytand-Lipsitch syndrome (complete atrioventricular block) 426.0

S

Saber
  shin 090.5
  tibia 090.5
Sac, lacrimal - *see* condition
Saccharomyces infection (*see also* Candidiasis) 112.9
Saccharopinuria 270.7
Saccular - *see* condition
Sacculation
  aorta (nonsyphilitic) (*see also* Aneurysm, aorta) 441.9
    ruptured 441.5
    syphilitic 093.0
  bladder 596.3
  colon 569.89
  intralaryngeal (congenital) (ventricular) 748.3
  larynx (congenital) (ventricular) 748.3
  organ or site, congenital - *see* Distortion
  pregnant uterus, complicating delivery 654.4●
    affecting fetus or newborn 763.1
      causing obstructed labor 660.2●
        affecting fetus or newborn 763.1
  rectosigmoid 569.89
  sigmoid 569.89
  ureter 593.89
  urethra 599.2
  vesical 596.3
Sachs (-Tay) disease (amaurotic familial idiocy) 330.1
Sacks-Libman disease 710.0 [424.91]
Sacralgia 724.6
Sacralization
  fifth lumbar vertebra 756.15
  incomplete (vertebra) 756.15
Sacrodynia 724.6
Sacroiliac joint - *see* condition
Sacroiliitis NEC 720.2
Sacrum - *see* condition
Saddle
  back 737.8
  embolus
    abdominal aorta 444.01
    pulmonary artery 415.13
  injury - code to condition
  nose 738.0
    congenital 754.0
    due to syphilis 090.5
Sadism (sexual) 302.84
Saemisch's ulcer 370.04
Saenger's syndrome 379.46
Sago spleen 277.39
Sailors' skin 692.74
Saint
  Anthony's fire (*see also* Erysipelas) 035
  Guy's dance - *see* Chorea
  Louis-type encephalitis 062.3
  triad (*see also* Hernia, diaphragm) 553.3
  Vitus' dance - *see* Chorea
Salicylism
  correct substance properly administered 535.4●
  overdose or wrong substance given or taken 965.1
Salivary duct or gland - *see also* condition
  virus disease 078.5
Salivation (excessive) (*see also* Ptyalism) 527.7
Salmonella (aertrycke) (choleraesuis) (enteritidis) (gallinarum) (suipestifer) (typhimurium) (*see also* Infection, Salmonella) 003.9
  arthritis 003.23
  carrier (suspected) of V02.3
  meningitis 003.21
  osteomyelitis 003.24
  pneumonia 003.22
  septicemia 003.1

Salmonella (*Continued*)
  typhosa 002.0
    carrier (suspected) of V02.1
Salmonellosis 003.0
  with pneumonia 003.22
Salpingitis (catarrhal) (fallopian tube) (nodular) (pseudofollicular) (purulent) (septic) (*see also* Salpingo-oophoritis) 614.2
  ear 381.50
    acute 381.51
    chronic 381.52
  Eustachian (tube) 381.50
    acute 381.51
    chronic 381.52
  follicularis 614.1
  gonococcal (chronic) 098.37
    acute 098.17
  interstitial, chronic 614.1
  isthmica nodosa 614.1
  old - *see* Salpingo-oophoritis, chronic
  puerperal, postpartum, childbirth 670.8●
  specific (chronic) 098.37
    acute 098.17
  tuberculous (acute) (chronic) (*see also* Tuberculosis) 016.6●
  venereal (chronic) 098.37
    acute 098.17
Salpingocele 620.4
Salpingo-oophoritis (catarrhal) (purulent) (ruptured) (septic) (suppurative) 614.2
  acute 614.0
    with
      abortion - *see* Abortion, by type, with sepsis
      ectopic pregnancy (*see also* categories 633.0–633.9) 639.0
      molar pregnancy (*see also* categories 630–632) 639.0
    following
      abortion 639.0
      ectopic or molar pregnancy 639.0
    gonococcal 098.17
    puerperal, postpartum, childbirth 670.8●
    tuberculous (*see also* Tuberculosis) 016.6●
  chronic 614.1
    gonococcal 098.37
    tuberculous (*see also* Tuberculosis) 016.6●
  complicating pregnancy 646.6●
    affecting fetus or newborn 760.8
  gonococcal (chronic) 098.37
    acute 098.17
  old - *see* Salpingo-oophoritis, chronic
  puerperal 670.8●
  specific - *see* Salpingo-oophoritis, gonococcal
  subacute (*see also* Salpingo-oophoritis, acute) 614.0
  tuberculous (acute) (chronic) (*see also* Tuberculosis) 016.6●
  venereal - *see* Salpingo-oophoritis, gonococcal
Salpingo-ovaritis (*see also* Salpingo-oophoritis) 614.2
Salpingoperitonitis (*see also* Salpingo-oophoritis) 614.2
Salt-losing
  nephritis (*see also* Disease, renal) 593.9
  syndrome (*see also* Disease, renal) 593.9
Salt-rheum (*see also* Eczema) 692.9
Salzmann's nodular dystrophy 371.46
Sampling
  chorionic villus V28.89
Sampson's cyst or tumor 617.1
Sandblasters'
  asthma 502
  lung 502
Sander's disease (paranoia) 297.1
Sandfly fever 066.0
Sandhoff's disease 330.1
Sanfilippo's syndrome (mucopolysaccharidosis III) 277.5
Sanger-Brown's ataxia 334.2

San Joaquin Valley fever 114.0
Sao Paulo fever or typhus 082.0
Saponification, mesenteric 567.89
Sapremia - *see* Septicemia
Sarcocele (benign)
  syphilitic 095.8
    congenital 090.5
Sarcoepiplocele (*see also* Hernia) 553.9
Sarcoepiplomphalocele (*see also* Hernia, umbilicus) 553.1
Sarcoid (any site) 135
  with lung involvement 135 [517.8]
  Boeck's 135
  Darier-Roussy 135
  Spiegler-Fendt 686.8
Sarcoidosis 135
  cardiac 135 [425.8]
  lung 135 [517.8]
Sarcoma (M8800/3) - *see also* Neoplasm, connective tissue, malignant
  alveolar soft part (M9581/3) - *see* Neoplasm, connective tissue, malignant
  ameloblastic (M9330/3) 170.1
    upper jaw (bone) 170.0
  botryoid (M8910/3) - *see* Neoplasm, connective tissue, malignant
  botryoides (M8910/3) - *see* Neoplasm, connective tissue, malignant
  cerebellar (M9480/3) 191.6
    circumscribed (arachnoidal) (M9471/3) 191.6
  circumscribed (arachnoidal) cerebellar (M9471/3) 191.6
  clear cell, of tendons and aponeuroses (M9044/3) - *see* Neoplasm, connective tissue, malignant
  embryonal (M8991/3) - *see* Neoplasm, connective tissue, malignant
  endometrial (stromal) (M8930/3) 182.0
    isthmus 182.1
  endothelial (M9130/3) - *see also* Neoplasm, connective tissue, malignant
    bone (M9260/3) - *see* Neoplasm, bone, malignant
  epithelioid cell (M8804/3) - *see* Neoplasm, connective tissue, malignant
  Ewing's (M9260/3) - *see* Neoplasm, bone, malignant
  follicular dendritic cell 202.9●
  germinoblastic (diffuse) (M9632/3) 202.8●
    follicular (M9697/3) 202.0●
  giant cell (M8802/3) - *see also* Neoplasm, connective tissue, malignant
    bone (M9250/3) - *see* Neoplasm, bone, malignant
  glomoid (M8710/3) - *see* Neoplasm, connective tissue, malignant
  granulocytic (M9930/3) 205.3●
  hemangioendothelial (M9130/3) - *see* Neoplasm, connective tissue, malignant
  hemorrhagic, multiple (M9140/3) - *see* Kaposi's, sarcoma
  Hodgkin's (M9662/3) 201.2●
  immunoblastic (M9612/3) 200.8●
  interdigitating dendritic cell 202.9●
  Kaposi's (M9140/3) - *see* Kaposi's, sarcoma
  Kupffer cell (M9124/3) 155.0
  Langerhans cell 202.9●
  leptomeningeal (M9530/3) - *see* Neoplasm, meninges, malignant
  lymphangioendothelial (M9170/3) - *see* Neoplasm, connective tissue, malignant
  lymphoblastic (M9630/3) 200.1●
  lymphocytic (M9620/3) 200.1●
  mast cell (M9740/3) 202.6●
  melanotic (M8720/3) - *see* Melanoma
  meningeal (M9530/3) - *see* Neoplasm, meninges, malignant

Sarcoma (Continued)
 meningothelial (M9530/3) - see Neoplasm, meninges, malignant
 mesenchymal (M8800/3) - see also Neoplasm, connective tissue, malignant
  mixed (M8990/3) - see Neoplasm, connective tissue, malignant
 mesothelial (M9050/3) - see Neoplasm, by site, malignant
 monstrocellular (M9481/3)
  specified site - see Neoplasm, by site, malignant
  unspecified site 191.9
 myeloid (M9930/3) 205.3 ●
 neurogenic (M9540/3) - see Neoplasm, connective tissue, malignant
 odontogenic (M9270/3) 170.1
  upper jaw (bone) 170.0
 osteoblastic (M9180/3) - see Neoplasm, bone, malignant
 osteogenic (M9180/3) - see also Neoplasm, bone, malignant
  juxtacortical (M9190/3) - see Neoplasm, bone, malignant
  periosteal (M9190/3) - see Neoplasm, bone, malignant
 periosteal (M8812/3) - see also Neoplasm, bone, malignant
  osteogenic (M9190/3) - see Neoplasm, bone, malignant
 plasma cell (M9731/3) 203.8 ●
 pleomorphic cell (M8802/3) - see Neoplasm, connective tissue, malignant
 reticuloendothelial (M9720/3) 202.3 ●
 reticulum cell (M9640/3) 200.0 ●
  nodular (M9642/3) 200.0 ●
   pleomorphic cell type (M9641/3) 200.0 ●
 round cell (M8803/3) - see Neoplasm, connective tissue, malignant
 small cell (M8803/3) - see Neoplasm, connective tissue, malignant
 spindle cell (M8801/3) - see Neoplasm, connective tissue, malignant
 stromal (endometrial) (M8930/3) 182.0
  isthmus 182.1
 synovial (M9040/3) - see also Neoplasm, connective tissue, malignant
  biphasic type (M9043/3) - see Neoplasm, connective tissue, malignant
  epithelioid cell type (M9042/3) - see Neoplasm, connective tissue, malignant
  spindle cell type (M9041/3) - see Neoplasm, connective tissue, malignant

Sarcomatosis
 meningeal (M9539/3) - see Neoplasm, meninges, malignant
 specified site NEC (M8800/3) - see Neoplasm, connective tissue, malignant
 unspecified site (M8800/6) 171.9

Sarcosinemia 270.8
Sarcosporidiosis 136.5
Satiety, early 780.94
Satisfactory smear but lacking transformation zone
 anal 796.77
 cervical 795.07
Saturnine - see condition
Saturnism 984.9
 specified type of lead - see Table of Drugs and Chemicals
Satyriasis 302.89
Sauriasis - see Ichthyosis
Sauriderma 757.39
Sauriosis - see Ichthyosis
Savill's disease (epidemic exfoliative dermatitis) 695.89
SBE (subacute bacterial endocarditis) 421.0

Scabies (any site) 133.0
Scabs 782.8
Scaglietti-Dagnini syndrome (acromegalic macrospondylitis) 253.0
Scald, scalded - see also Burn, by site
 skin syndrome 695.81
Scalenus anticus (anterior) syndrome 353.0
Scales 782.8
Scalp - see condition
Scaphocephaly 756.0
Scaphoiditis, tarsal 732.5
Scapulalgia 733.90
Scapulohumeral myopathy 359.1
Scar, scarring (see also Cicatrix) 709.2
 adherent 709.2
 atrophic 709.2
 cervix
  in pregnancy or childbirth 654.6 ●
   affecting fetus or newborn 763.89
   causing obstructed labor 660.2 ●
    affecting fetus or newborn 763.1
 cheloid 701.4
 chorioretinal 363.30
  disseminated 363.35
  macular 363.32
  peripheral 363.34
  posterior pole NEC 363.33
 choroid (see also Scar, chorioretinal) 363.30
 compression, pericardial 423.9
 congenital 757.39
 conjunctiva 372.64
 cornea 371.00
  xerophthalmic 264.6
 due to previous cesarean delivery, complicating pregnancy or childbirth 654.2 ●
  affecting fetus or newborn 763.89
 duodenal (bulb) (cap) 537.3
 hypertrophic 701.4
 keloid 701.4
 labia 624.4
 lung (base) 518.89
 macula 363.32
  disseminated 363.35
  peripheral 363.34
 muscle 728.89
 myocardium, myocardial 412
 painful 709.2
 papillary muscle 429.81
 posterior pole NEC 363.33
  macular - see Scar, macula
 postnecrotic (hepatic) (liver) 571.9
 psychic V15.49
 retina (see also Scar, chorioretinal) 363.30
 trachea 478.9
 uterus 621.8
  in pregnancy or childbirth NEC 654.9 ●
   affecting fetus or newborn 763.89
   from previous cesarean delivery 654.2 ●
 vulva 624.4
Scarabiasis 134.1
Scarlatina 034.1
 anginosa 034.1
 maligna 034.1
 myocarditis, acute 034.1 [422.0]
  old (see also Myocarditis) 429.0
 otitis media 034.1 [382.02]
 ulcerosa 034.1
Scarlatinella 057.8
Scarlet fever (albuminuria) (angina) (convulsions) (lesions of lid) (rash) 034.1
Schamberg's disease, dermatitis, or dermatosis (progressive pigmentary dermatosis) 709.09
Schatzki's ring (esophagus) (lower) (congenital) 750.3
 acquired 530.3
Schaufenster krankheit 413.9

Schaumann's
 benign lymphogranulomatosis 135
 disease (sarcoidosis) 135
 syndrome (sarcoidosis) 135
Scheie's syndrome (mucopolysaccharidosis IS) 277.5
Schenck's disease (sporotrichosis) 117.1
Scheuermann's disease or osteochondrosis 732.0
Scheuthauer-Marie-Sainton syndrome (cleidocranialis dysostosis) 755.59
Schilder (-Flatau) disease 341.1
Schilling-type monocytic leukemia (M9890/3) 206.9 ●
Schimmelbusch's disease, cystic mastitis, or hyperplasia 610.1
Schirmer's syndrome (encephalocutaneous angiomatosis) 759.6
Schistocelia 756.79
Schistoglossia 750.13
Schistosoma infestation - see Infestation, Schistosoma
Schistosomiasis 120.9
 Asiatic 120.2
 bladder 120.0
 chestermani 120.8
 colon 120.1
 cutaneous 120.3
 due to
  S. hematobium 120.0
  S. japonicum 120.2
  S. mansoni 120.1
  S. mattheii 120.8
 eastern 120.2
 genitourinary tract 120.0
 intestinal 120.1
 lung 120.2
 Manson's (intestinal) 120.1
 Oriental 120.2
 pulmonary 120.2
 specified type NEC 120.8
 vesical 120.0
Schizencephaly 742.4
Schizo-affective psychosis (see also Schizophrenia) 295.7 ●
Schizodontia 520.2
Schizoid personality 301.20
 introverted 301.21
 schizotypal 301.22
Schizophrenia, schizophrenic (reaction) 295.9 ●

> Note: Use the following fifth-digit subclassification with category 295:
>
> 0 unspecified
> 1 subchronic
> 2 chronic
> 3 subchronic with acute exacerbation
> 4 chronic with acute exacerbation
> 5 in remission

 acute (attack) NEC 295.8 ●
  episode 295.4 ●
 atypical form 295.8 ●
 borderline 295.5 ●
 catalepsy 295.2 ●
 catatonic (type) (acute) (excited) (withdrawn) 295.2 ●
 childhood (type) (see also Psychosis, childhood) 299.9 ●
 chronic NEC 295.6 ●
 coenesthesiopathic 295.8 ●
 cyclic (type) 295.7 ●
 disorganized (type) 295.1 ●
 flexibilitas cerea 295.2 ●
 hebephrenic (type) (acute) 295.1 ●
 incipient 295.5 ●
 latent 295.5 ●
 paranoid (type) (acute) 295.3 ●
 paraphrenic (acute) 295.3 ●
 prepsychotic 295.5 ●
 primary (acute) 295.0 ●

SECTION I INDEX TO DISEASES AND INJURIES / Schizophrenia, schizophrenic

Schizophrenia, schizophrenic (Continued)
- prodromal 295.5●
- pseudoneurotic 295.5●
- pseudopsychopathic 295.5●
- reaction 295.9●
- residual type (state) 295.6●
- restzustand 295.6●
- schizo-affective (type) (depressed) (excited) 295.7●
- schizophreniform type 295.4●
- simple (type) (acute) 295.0●
- simplex (acute) 295.0●
- specified type NEC 295.8●
- syndrome of childhood NEC (see also Psychosis, childhood) 299.9●
- undifferentiated type 295.9●
    - acute 295.8●
    - chronic 295.6●

Schizothymia 301.20
- introverted 301.21
- schizotypal 301.22

Schlafkrankheit 086.5

Schlatter's tibia (osteochondrosis) 732.4

Schlatter-Osgood disease (osteochondrosis, tibial tubercle) 732.4

Schloffer's tumor (see also Peritonitis) 567.29

Schmidt's syndrome
- sphallo-pharyngo-laryngeal hemiplegia 352.6
- thyroid-adrenocortical insufficiency 258.1
- vagoaccessory 352.6

Schmincke
- carcinoma (M8082/3) - see Neoplasm, nasopharynx, malignant
- tumor (M8082/3) - see Neoplasm, nasopharynx, malignant

Schmitz (-Stutzer) dysentery 004.0

Schmorl's disease or nodes 722.30
- lumbar, lumbosacral 722.32
- specified region NEC 722.39
- thoracic, thoracolumbar 722.31

Schneider's syndrome 047.9

Schneiderian
- carcinoma (M8121/3)
    - specified site - see Neoplasm, by site, malignant
    - unspecified site 160.0
- papilloma (M8121/0)
    - specified site - see Neoplasm, by site, benign
    - unspecified site 212.0

Schnitzler syndrome 273.1

Schoffer's tumor (see also Peritonitis) 567.29

Scholte's syndrome (malignant carcinoid) 259.2

Scholz's disease 330.0

Scholz (-Bielschowsky-Henneberg) syndrome 330.0

Schönlein (-Henoch) disease (primary) (purpura) (rheumatic) 287.0

School examination V70.3
- following surgery V67.09

Schottmüller's disease (see also Fever, paratyphoid) 002.9

Schroeder's syndrome (endocrine-hypertensive) 255.3

Schüller-Christian disease or syndrome (chronic histiocytosis X) 277.89

Schultz's disease or syndrome (agranulocytosis) 288.09

Schultze's acroparesthesia, simple 443.89

Schwalbe-Ziehen-Oppenheimer disease 333.6

Schwannoma (M9560/0) - see also Neoplasm, connective tissues, benign
- malignant (M9560/3) - see Neoplasm, connective tissue, malignant

Schwannomatosis 237.73

Schwartz (-Jampel) syndrome 359.23

Schwartz-Bartter syndrome (inappropriate secretion of antidiuretic hormone) 253.6

Schweninger-Buzzi disease (macular atrophy) 701.3

Sciatic - see condition

Sciatica (infectional) 724.3
- due to
    - displacement of intervertebral disc 722.10
    - herniation, nucleus pulposus 722.10
- wallet 724.3

Scimitar syndrome (anomalous venous drainage, right lung to inferior vena cava) 747.49

Sclera - see condition

Sclerectasia 379.11

Scleredema
- adultorum 710.1
- Buschke's 710.1
- newborn 778.1

Sclerema
- adiposum (newborn) 778.1
- adultorum 710.1
- edematosum (newborn) 778.1
- neonatorum 778.1
- newborn 778.1

Scleriasis - see Scleroderma

Scleritis 379.00
- with corneal involvement 379.05
- anterior (annular) (localized) 379.03
- brawny 379.06
- granulomatous 379.09
- posterior 379.07
- specified NEC 379.09
- suppurative 379.09
- syphilitic 095.0
- tuberculous (nodular) (see also Tuberculosis) 017.3● [379.09]

Sclerochoroiditis (see also Scleritis) 379.00

Scleroconjunctivitis (see also Scleritis) 379.00

Sclerocystic ovary (syndrome) 256.4

Sclerodactylia 701.0

Scleroderma, sclerodermia (acrosclerotic) (diffuse) (generalized) (progressive) (pulmonary) 710.1
- circumscribed 701.0
- linear 701.0
- localized (linear) 701.0
- newborn 778.1

Sclerokeratitis 379.05
- meaning sclerosing keratitis 370.54
- tuberculous (see also Tuberculosis) 017.3● [379.09]

Scleroma, trachea 040.1

Scleromalacia
- multiple 731.0
- perforans 379.04

Scleromyxedema 701.8

Scleroperikeratitis 379.05

Sclerose en plaques 340

Sclerosis, sclerotic
- adrenal (gland) 255.8
- Alzheimer's 331.0
    - with dementia - see Alzheimer's, dementia
- amyotrophic (lateral) 335.20
- annularis fibrosi
    - aortic 424.1
    - mitral 424.0
- aorta, aortic 440.0
    - valve (see also Endocarditis, aortic) 424.1
- artery, arterial, arteriolar, arteriovascular - see Arteriosclerosis
- ascending multiple 340
- Baló's (concentric) 341.1
- basilar - see Sclerosis, brain
- bone (localized) NEC 733.99
- brain (general) (lobular) 348.89
    - Alzheimer's - see Alzheimer's, dementia
    - artery, arterial 437.0
    - atrophic lobar 331.0
        - with dementia
            - with behavioral disturbance 331.0 [294.11]
            - without behavioral disturbance 331.0 [294.10]

Sclerosis, sclerotic (Continued)
- brain (Continued)
    - diffuse 341.1
        - familial (chronic) (infantile) 330.0
        - infantile (chronic) (familial) 330.0
        - Pelizaeus-Merzbacher type 330.0
    - disseminated 340
    - hereditary 334.2
    - hippocampal 348.81
    - infantile (degenerative) (diffuse) 330.0
    - insular 340
    - Krabbe's 330.0
    - mesial temporal 348.81
    - miliary 340
    - multiple 340
    - Pelizaeus-Merzbacher 330.0
    - progressive familial 330.0
    - senile 437.0
    - temporal 348.81
        - mesial 348.81
    - tuberous 759.5
- bulbar, progressive 340
- bundle of His 426.50
    - left 426.3
    - right 426.4
- cardiac - see Arteriosclerosis, coronary
- cardiorenal (see also Hypertension, cardiorenal) 404.90
- cardiovascular (see also Disease, cardiovascular) 429.2
    - renal (see also Hypertension, cardiorenal) 404.90
- centrolobar, familial 330.0
- cerebellar - see Sclerosis, brain
- cerebral - see Sclerosis, brain
- cerebrospinal 340
    - disseminated 340
    - multiple 340
- cerebrovascular 437.0
- choroid 363.40
    - diffuse 363.56
- combined (spinal cord) - see also Degeneration, combined
    - multiple 340
- concentric, Baló's 341.1
- cornea 370.54
- coronary (artery) - see Arteriosclerosis, coronary
- corpus cavernosum
    - female 624.8
    - male 607.89
- Dewitzky's
    - aortic 424.1
    - mitral 424.0
- diffuse NEC 341.1
- disease, heart - see Arteriosclerosis, coronary
- disseminated 340
- dorsal 340
- dorsolateral (spinal cord) - see Degeneration, combined
- endometrium 621.8
- extrapyramidal 333.90
- eye, nuclear (senile) 366.16
- Friedreich's (spinal cord) 334.0
- funicular (spermatic cord) 608.89
- gastritis 535.4●
- general (vascular) - see Arteriosclerosis
- gland (lymphatic) 457.8
- hepatic 571.9
- hereditary
    - cerebellar 334.2
    - spinal 334.0
- hippocampal 348.81
- idiopathic cortical (Garre's) (see also Osteomyelitis) 730.1●
- ilium, piriform 733.5
- insular 340
    - pancreas 251.8
- Islands of Langerhans 251.8
- kidney - see Sclerosis, renal
- larynx 478.79

Sclerosis, sclerotic (Continued)
  lateral 335.24
    amyotrophic 335.20
    descending 335.24
    primary 335.24
    spinal 335.24
  liver 571.9
  lobar, atrophic (of brain) 331.0
    with dementia
      with behavioral disturbance 331.0 [294.11]
      without behavioral disturbance 331.0 [294.10]
  lung (see also Fibrosis, lung) 515
  mastoid 383.1
  mesial temporal 348.81
  mitral - see Endocarditis, mitral
  Mönckeberg's (medial) (see also Arteriosclerosis, extremities) 440.20
  multiple (brain stem) (cerebral) (generalized) (spinal cord) 340
  myocardium, myocardial - see Arteriosclerosis, coronary
  nuclear (senile), eye 366.16
  ovary 620.8
  pancreas 577.8
  penis 607.89
  peripheral arteries (see also Arteriosclerosis, extremities) 440.20
  plaques 340
  pluriglandular 258.8
  polyglandular 258.8
  posterior (spinal cord) (syphilitic) 094.0
  posterolateral (spinal cord) - see Degeneration, combined
  prepuce 607.89
  primary lateral 335.24
  progressive systemic 710.1
  pulmonary (see also Fibrosis, lung) 515
    artery 416.0
    valve (heart) (see also Endocarditis, pulmonary) 424.3
  renal 587
    with
      cystine storage disease 270.0
      hypertension (see also Hypertension, kidney) 403.90
      hypertensive heart disease (conditions classifiable to 402) (see also Hypertension, cardiorenal) 404.90
    arteriolar (hyaline) (see also Hypertension, kidney) 403.90
    hyperplastic (see also Hypertension, kidney) 403.90
  retina (senile) (vascular) 362.17
  rheumatic
    aortic valve 395.9
    mitral valve 394.9
  Schilder's 341.1
  senile - see Arteriosclerosis
  spinal (cord) (general) (progressive) (transverse) 336.8
    ascending 357.0
    combined - see also Degeneration, combined
      multiple 340
      syphilitic 094.89
    disseminated 340
    dorsolateral - see Degeneration, combined
    hereditary (Friedreich's) (mixed form) 334.0
    lateral (amyotrophic) 335.24
    multiple 340
    posterior (syphilitic) 094.0
  stomach 537.89
  subendocardial, congenital 425.3
  systemic (progressive) 710.1
    with lung involvement 710.1 [517.2]
  temporal 348.81
    mesial 348.81

Sclerosis, sclerotic (Continued)
  tricuspid (heart) (valve) - see Endocarditis, tricuspid
  tuberous (brain) 759.5
  tympanic membrane (see also Tympanosclerosis) 385.00
  valve, valvular (heart) - see Endocarditis
  vascular - see Arteriosclerosis
  vein 459.89
Sclerotenonitis 379.07
Sclerotitis (see also Scleritis) 379.00
  syphilitic 095.0
  tuberculous (see also Tuberculosis) 017.3 ● [379.09]
Scoliosis (acquired) (postural) 737.30
  congenital 754.2
  due to or associated with
    Charcôt-Marie-Tooth disease 356.1 [737.43]
    mucopolysaccharidosis 277.5 [737.43]
    neurofibromatosis 237.71 [737.43]
    osteitis
      deformans 731.0 [737.43]
      fibrosa cystica 252.01 [737.43]
    osteoporosis (see also Osteoporosis) 733.00 [737.43]
    poliomyelitis 138 [737.43]
    radiation 737.33
    tuberculosis (see also Tuberculosis) 015.0 ● [737.43]
  idiopathic 737.30
  infantile
    progressive 737.32
    resolving 737.31
  paralytic 737.39
  rachitic 268.1
  sciatic 724.3
  specified NEC 737.39
  thoracogenic 737.34
  tuberculous (see also Tuberculosis) 015.0 ● [737.43]
Scoliotic pelvis 738.6
  with disproportion (fetopelvic) 653.0 ●
    affecting fetus or newborn 763.1
    causing obstructed labor 660.1 ●
      affecting fetus or newborn 763.1
Scorbutus, scorbutic 267
  anemia 281.8
Scotoma (ring) 368.44
  arcuate 368.43
  Bjerrum 368.43
  blind spot area 368.42
  central 368.41
  centrocecal 368.41
  paracecal 368.42
  paracentral 368.41
  scintillating 368.12
  Seidel 368.43
Scratch - see Injury, superficial, by site
Scratchy throat 784.99
Screening (for) V82.9
  alcoholism V79.1
  anemia, deficiency NEC V78.1
    iron V78.0
  anomaly, congenital V82.89
  antenatal, of mother V28.9
    alphafetoprotein levels, raised V28.1
    based on amniocentesis V28.2
      chromosomal anomalies V28.0
      raised alphafetoprotein levels V28.1
    fetal growth retardation using ultrasonics V28.4
    genomic V28.89
    isoimmunization V28.5
    malformations using ultrasonics V28.3
    proteomic V28.89
    raised alphafetoprotein levels V28.1
    risk
      pre-term labor V28.82
    specified condition NEC V28.89
    Streptococcus B V28.6

Screening (Continued)
  arterial hypertension V81.1
  arthropod-borne viral disease NEC V73.5
  asymptomatic bacteriuria V81.5
  bacterial
    and spirochetal sexually transmitted diseases V74.5
    conjunctivitis V74.4
    disease V74.9
      sexually transmitted V74.5
      specified condition NEC V74.8
  bacteriuria, asymptomatic V81.5
  blood disorder NEC V78.9
    specified type NEC V78.8
  bronchitis, chronic V81.3
  brucellosis V74.8
  cancer - see Screening, malignant neoplasm
  cardiovascular disease NEC V81.2
  cataract V80.2
  Chagas' disease V75.3
  chemical poisoning V82.5
  cholera V74.0
  cholesterol level V77.91
  chromosomal
    anomalies
      by amniocentesis, antenatal V28.0
      maternal postnatal V82.4
    athletes V70.3
  colonoscopy V76.51
  condition
    cardiovascular NEC V81.2
    eye NEC V80.2
    genitourinary NEC V81.6
    neurological NEC V80.09
    respiratory NEC V81.4
    skin V82.0
    specified NEC V82.89
  congenital
    anomaly V82.89
      eye V80.2
    dislocation of hip V82.3
    eye condition or disease V80.2
  conjunctivitis, bacterial V74.4
  contamination NEC (see also Poisoning) V82.5
  coronary artery disease V81.0
  cystic fibrosis V77.6
  deficiency anemia NEC V78.1
    iron V78.0
  dengue fever V73.5
  depression V79.0
  developmental handicap V79.9
    in early childhood V79.3
    specified type NEC V79.8
  diabetes mellitus V77.1
  diphtheria V74.3
  disease or disorder V82.9
    bacterial V74.9
      specified NEC V74.8
    blood V78.9
      specified type NEC V78.8
    blood-forming organ V78.9
      specified type NEC V78.8
    cardiovascular NEC V81.2
      hypertensive V81.1
      ischemic V81.0
  Chagas' V75.3
  chlamydial V73.98
    specified NEC V73.88
  ear NEC V80.3
  endocrine NEC V77.99
  eye NEC V80.2
  genitourinary NEC V81.6
  heart NEC V81.2
    hypertensive V81.1
    ischemic V81.0
  HPV (human papillomavirus) V73.81
  human papillomavirus (HPV) V73.81
  immunity NEC V77.99
  infectious NEC V75.9
  lipoid NEC V77.91

SECTION I INDEX TO DISEASES AND INJURIES / Screening

Screening (Continued)
- disease or disorder (Continued)
  - mental V79.9
    - specified type NEC V79.8
  - metabolic NEC V77.99
    - inborn NEC V77.7
  - neurological NEC V80.09
  - nutritional NEC V77.99
  - rheumatic NEC V82.2
  - rickettsial V75.0
  - sexually transmitted V74.5
    - bacterial V74.5
    - spirochetal V74.5
  - sickle-cell V78.2
    - trait V78.2
  - specified type NEC V82.89
  - thyroid V77.0
  - vascular NEC V81.2
    - ischemic V81.0
  - venereal V74.5
  - viral V73.99
    - arthropod-borne NEC V73.5
    - specified type NEC V73.89
- dislocation of hip, congenital V82.3
- drugs in athletes V70.3
- elevated titer V82.9
- emphysema (chronic) V81.3
- encephalitis, viral (mosquito or tick borne) V73.5
- endocrine disorder NEC V77.99
- eye disorder NEC V80.2
  - congenital V80.2
- fever
  - dengue V73.5
  - hemorrhagic V73.5
  - yellow V73.4
- filariasis V75.6
- galactosemia V77.4
- genetic V82.79
  - disease carrier status V82.71
- genitourinary condition NEC V81.6
- glaucoma V80.1
- gonorrhea V74.5
- gout V77.5
- Hansen's disease V74.2
- heart disease NEC V81.2
  - hypertensive V81.1
  - ischemic V81.0
- heavy metal poisoning V82.5
- helminthiasis, intestinal V75.7
- hematopoietic malignancy V76.89
- hemoglobinopathies NEC V78.3
- hemorrhagic fever V73.5
- Hodgkin's disease V76.89
- hormones in athletes V70.3
- HPV (human papillomavirus) V73.81
- human papillomavirus (HPV) V73.81
- hypercholesterolemia V77.91
- hyperlipidemia V77.91
- hypertension V81.1
- immunity disorder NEC V77.99
- inborn errors of metabolism NEC V77.7
- infection
  - bacterial V74.9
    - specified type NEC V74.8
  - mycotic V75.4
  - parasitic NEC V75.8
- infectious disease V75.9
  - specified type NEC V75.8
- ingestion of radioactive substance V82.5
- intellectual disabilities V79.2
- intestinal helminthiasis V75.7
- iron deficiency anemia V78.0
- ischemic heart disease V81.0
- lead poisoning V82.5
- leishmaniasis V75.2
- leprosy V74.2
- leptospirosis V74.8
- leukemia V76.89
- lipoid disorder NEC V77.91
- lymphoma V76.89

Screening (Continued)
- malaria V75.1
- malignant neoplasm (of) V76.9
  - bladder V76.3
  - blood V76.89
  - breast V76.10
    - mammogram NEC V76.12
      - for high-risk patient V76.11
    - specified type NEC V76.19
  - cervix V76.2
  - colon V76.51
  - colorectal V76.51
  - hematopoietic system V76.89
  - intestine V76.50
    - colon V76.51
    - small V76.52
  - lung V76.0
  - lymph (glands) V76.89
  - nervous system V76.81
  - oral cavity V76.42
  - other specified neoplasm NEC V76.89
  - ovary V76.46
  - prostate V76.44
  - rectum V76.41
  - respiratory organs V76.0
  - skin V76.43
  - specified sites NEC V76.49
  - testis V76.45
  - vagina V76.47
    - following hysterectomy for malignant condition V67.01
- malnutrition V77.2
- mammogram NEC V76.12
  - for high-risk patient V76.11
- maternal postnatal chromosomal anomalies V82.4
- measles V73.2
- mental
  - disorder V79.9
    - specified type NEC V79.8
  - retardation - see Screening, intellectual disabilities
- metabolic disorder NEC V77.99
- metabolic errors, inborn V77.7
- mucoviscidosis V77.6
- multiphasic V82.6
- mycosis V75.4
- mycotic infection V75.4
- nephropathy V81.5
- neurological condition NEC V80.09
- nutritional disorder NEC V77.99
- obesity V77.8
- osteoporosis V82.81
- parasitic infection NEC V75.8
- phenylketonuria V77.3
- plague V74.8
- poisoning
  - chemical NEC V82.5
  - contaminated water supply V82.5
  - heavy metal V82.5
- poliomyelitis V73.0
- postnatal chromosomal anomalies, maternal V82.4
- prenatal - see Screening, antenatal
- pulmonary tuberculosis V74.1
- radiation exposure V82.5
- renal disease V81.5
- respiratory condition NEC V81.4
- rheumatic disorder NEC V82.2
- rheumatoid arthritis V82.1
- rickettsial disease V75.0
- rubella V73.3
- schistosomiasis V75.5
- senile macular lesions of eye V80.2
- sexually transmitted diseases V74.5
  - bacterial V74.5
  - spirochetal V74.5
- sickle-cell anemia, disease, or trait V78.2
- skin condition V82.0
- sleeping sickness V75.3
- smallpox V73.1

Screening (Continued)
- special V82.9
  - specified condition NEC V82.89
- specified type NEC V82.89
- spirochetal disease V74.9
  - sexually transmitted V74.5
  - specified type NEC V74.8
- stimulants in athletes V70.3
- syphilis V74.5
- tetanus V74.8
- thyroid disorder V77.0
- trachoma V73.6
- traumatic brain injury V80.01
- trypanosomiasis V75.3
- tuberculosis, pulmonary V74.1
- venereal disease V74.5
- viral encephalitis
  - mosquito-borne V73.5
  - tick-borne V73.5
- whooping cough V74.8
- worms, intestinal V75.7
- yaws V74.6
- yellow fever V73.4

Scrofula (see also Tuberculosis) 017.2●
Scrofulide (primary) (see also Tuberculosis) 017.0●
Scrofuloderma, scrofulodermia (any site) (primary) (see also Tuberculosis) 017.0●
Scrofulosis (universal) (see also Tuberculosis) 017.2●
Scrofulosis lichen (primary) (see also Tuberculosis) 017.0●
Scrofulous - see condition
Scrotal tongue 529.5
- congenital 750.13
Scrotum - see condition
Scurvy (gum) (infantile) (rickets) (scorbutic) 267
Sea-blue histiocyte syndrome 272.7
Seabright-Bantam syndrome (pseudohypoparathyroidism) 275.49
Sealpox 059.12
Seasickness 994.6
Seatworm 127.4
Sebaceous
- cyst (see also Cyst, sebaceous) 706.2
- gland disease NEC 706.9
Sebocystomatosis 706.2
Seborrhea, seborrheic 706.3
- adiposa 706.3
- capitis 690.11
- congestiva 695.4
- corporis 706.3
- dermatitis 690.10
  - infantile 690.12
- diathesis in infants 695.89
- eczema 690.18
  - infantile 690.12
- keratosis 702.19
  - inflamed 702.11
- nigricans 759.89
- sicca 690.18
- wart 702.19
  - inflamed 702.11
Seckel's syndrome 759.89
Seclusion pupil 364.74
Seclusiveness, child 313.22
Secondary - see also condition
- neoplasm - see Neoplasm, by site, malignant, secondary
Secretan's disease or syndrome (posttraumatic edema) 782.3
Secretion
- antidiuretic hormone, inappropriate (syndrome) 253.6
- catecholamine, by pheochromocytoma 255.6
- hormone
  - antidiuretic, inappropriate (syndrome) 253.6

Secretion *(Continued)*
  hormone *(Continued)*
    by
      carcinoid tumor 259.2
      pheochromocytoma 255.6
    ectopic NEC 259.3
  urinary
    excessive 788.42
    suppression 788.5
Section
  cesarean
    affecting fetus or newborn 763.4
      post mortem, affecting fetus or newborn 761.6
    previous, in pregnancy or childbirth 654.2 ●
      affecting fetus or newborn 763.89
  nerve, traumatic - *see* Injury, nerve, by site
Seeligmann's syndrome (ichthyosis congenita) 757.1
Segmentation, incomplete (congenital) - *see also* Fusion
  bone NEC 756.9
  lumbosacral (joint) 756.15
  vertebra 756.15
    lumbosacral 756.15
Seizure(s) 780.39
  akinetic (idiopathic) (*see also* Epilepsy) 345.0 ●
    psychomotor 345.4 ●
  apoplexy, apoplectic (*see also* Disease, cerebrovascular, acute) 436
  atonic (*see also* Epilepsy) 345.0 ●
  autonomic 300.11
  brain or cerebral (*see also* Disease, cerebrovascular, acute) 436
  convulsive (*see also* Convulsions) 780.39
  cortical (focal) (motor) (*see also* Epilepsy) 345.5 ●
  disorder (*see also* Epilepsy) 345.9
  due to stroke 438.89
  epilepsy, epileptic (cryptogenic) (*see also* Epilepsy) 345.9 ●
  epileptiform, epileptoid 780.39
    focal (*see also* Epilepsy) 345.5 ●
  febrile (simple) 780.31
    with status epilepticus 345.3
    atypical 780.32
    complex 780.32
    complicated 780.32
  heart - *see* Disease, heart
  hysterical 300.11
  Jacksonian (focal) (*see also* Epilepsy) 345.5 ●
    motor type 345.5 ●
    sensory type 345.5 ●
  migraine triggered 346.0 ●
  newborn 779.0
  paralysis (*see also* Disease, cerebrovascular, acute) 436
  post traumatic 780.33
  recurrent 345.8 ●
    epileptic - *see* Epilepsy
  repetitive 780.39
    epileptic - *see* Epilepsy
  salaam (*see also* Epilepsy) 345.6 ●
  uncinate (*see also* Epilepsy) 345.4 ●
Self-mutilation 300.9
Semicoma 780.09
Semiconsciousness 780.09
Seminal
  vesicle - *see* condition
  vesiculitis (*see also* Vesiculitis) 608.0
Seminoma (M9061/3)
  anaplastic type (M9062/3)
    specified site - *see* Neoplasm, by site, malignant
    unspecified site 186.9
  specified site - *see* Neoplasm, by site, malignant

Seminoma *(Continued)*
  spermatocytic (M9063/3)
    specified site - *see* Neoplasm, by site, malignant
    unspecified site 186.9
  unspecified site 186.9
Semliki Forest encephalitis 062.8
Senear-Usher disease or syndrome (pemphigus erythematosus) 694.4
Senecio jacobae dermatitis 692.6
Senectus 797
Senescence 797
Senile (*see also* condition) 797
  cervix (atrophic) 622.8
  degenerative atrophy, skin 701.3
  endometrium (atrophic) 621.8
  fallopian tube (atrophic) 620.3
  heart (failure) 797
  lung 492.8
  ovary (atrophic) 620.3
  syndrome 259.8
  vagina, vaginitis (atrophic) 627.3
  wart 702.0
Senility 797
  with
    acute confusional state 290.3
    delirium 290.3
    mental changes 290.9
    psychosis NEC (*see also* Psychosis, senile) 290.20
  premature (syndrome) 259.8
Sensation
  burning (*see also* Disturbance, sensation) 782.0
    tongue 529.6
  choking 784.99
  loss of (*see also* Disturbance, sensation) 782.0
  prickling (*see also* Disturbance, sensation) 782.0
  tingling (*see also* Disturbance, sensation) 782.0
Sense loss (touch) (*see also* Disturbance, sensation) 782.0
  smell 781.1
  taste 781.1
Sensibility disturbance NEC (cortical) (deep) (vibratory) (*see also* Disturbance, sensation) 782.0
Sensitive dentine 521.89
Sensitiver Beziehungswahn 297.8
Sensitivity, sensitization - *see also* Allergy
  autoerythrocyte 287.2
  carotid sinus 337.01
  child (excessive) 313.21
  cold, autoimmune 283.0
  methemoglobin 289.7
  suxamethonium 289.89
  tuberculin, without clinical or radiological symptoms 795.51
Sensory
  extinction 781.8
  neglect 781.8
Separation
  acromioclavicular - *see* Dislocation, acromioclavicular
  anxiety, abnormal 309.21
  apophysis, traumatic - *see* Fracture, by site
  choroid 363.70
    hemorrhagic 363.72
    serous 363.71
  costochondral (simple) (traumatic) - *see* Dislocation, costochondral
  delayed
    umbilical cord 779.83
  epiphysis, epiphyseal
    nontraumatic 732.9
      upper femoral 732.2
    traumatic - *see* Fracture, by site
  fracture - *see* Fracture, by site
  infundibulum cardiac from right ventricle by a partition 746.83

Separation *(Continued)*
  joint (current) (traumatic) - *see* Dislocation, by site
  placenta (normally implanted) - *see* Placenta, separation
  pubic bone, obstetrical trauma 665.6 ●
  retina, retinal (*see also* Detachment, retina) 361.9
    layers 362.40
      sensory (*see also* Retinoschisis) 361.10
      pigment epithelium (exudative) 362.42
        hemorrhagic 362.43
  sternoclavicular (traumatic) - *see* Dislocation, sternoclavicular
  symphysis pubis, obstetrical trauma 665.6 ●
  tracheal ring, incomplete (congenital) 748.3
Sepsis (generalized) 995.91
  with
    abortion - *see* Abortion, by type, with sepsis
    acute organ dysfunction 995.92
    ectopic pregnancy (*see also* categories 633.0–633.9) 639.0
    molar pregnancy (*see also* categories 630–632) 639.0
    multiple organ dysfunction (MOD) 995.92
  buccal 528.3
  complicating labor 659.3 ●
  dental (pulpal origin) 522.4
  female genital organ NEC 614.9
  fetus (intrauterine) 771.81
  following
    abortion 639.0
    ectopic or molar pregnancy 639.0
    infusion, perfusion, or transfusion 999.39
  Friedländer's 038.49
  intra-abdominal 567.22
  intraocular 360.00
  localized - code to specific localized infection
    in operation wound 998.59
    skin (*see also* Abscess) 682.9
  malleus 024
  nadir 038.9
  newborn (organism unspecified) NEC 771.81
  oral 528.3
  puerperal, postpartum, childbirth (pelvic) 670.2 ●
  resulting from infusion, injection, transfusion, or vaccination 999.39
  severe 995.92
  skin, localized (*see also* Abscess) 682.9
  umbilical (newborn) (organism unspecified) 771.89
    tetanus 771.3
  urinary 599.0
    meaning sepsis 995.91
    meaning urinary tract infection 599.0
Septate - *see also* Septum
Septic - *see also* condition
  adenoids 474.01
    and tonsils 474.02
  arm (with lymphangitis) 682.3
  embolus - *see* Embolism
  finger (with lymphangitis) 681.00
  foot (with lymphangitis) 682.7
  gallbladder (*see also* Cholecystitis) 575.8
  hand (with lymphangitis) 682.4
  joint (*see also* Arthritis, septic) 711.0 ●
  kidney (*see also* Infection, kidney) 590.9
  leg (with lymphangitis) 682.6
  mouth 528.3
  nail 681.9
    finger 681.02
    toe 681.11
  shock (endotoxic) 785.52
  postoperative 998.02
  sore (*see also* Abscess) 682.9
  throat 034.0
    milk-borne 034.0
    streptococcal 034.0
  spleen (acute) 289.59

SECTION 1 INDEX TO DISEASES AND INJURIES / Septic

Septic (Continued)
   teeth (pulpal origin) 522.4
   throat 034.0
   thrombus - see Thrombosis
   toe (with lymphangitis) 681.10
   tonsils 474.00
     and adenoids 474.02
   umbilical cord (newborn) (organism unspecified) 771.89
   uterus (see also Endometritis) 615.9
Septicemia, septicemic (generalized) (suppurative) 038.9
   with
     abortion - see Abortion, by type, with sepsis
     ectopic pregnancy (see also categories 633.0–633.9) 639.0
     molar pregnancy (see also categories 630–632) 639.0
   Aerobacter aerogenes 038.49
   anaerobic 038.3
   anthrax 022.3
   Bacillus coli 038.42
   Bacteroides 038.3
   Clostridium 038.3
   complicating labor 659.3●
   cryptogenic 038.9
   enteric gram-negative bacilli 038.40
   Enterobacter aerogenes 038.49
   Erysipelothrix (insidiosa) (rhusiopathiae) 027.1
   Escherichia coli 038.42
   following
     abortion 639.0
     ectopic or molar pregnancy 639.0
     infusion, injection, transfusion, or vaccination 999.39
   Friedländer's (bacillus) 038.49
   gangrenous 038.9
   gonococcal 098.89
   gram-negative (organism) 038.40
     anaerobic 038.3
   Hemophilus influenzae 038.41
   herpes (simplex) 054.5
   herpetic 054.5
   Listeria monocytogenes 027.0
   meningeal - see Meningitis
   meningococcal (chronic) (fulminating) 036.2
   methicillin
     resistant Staphylococcus aureus (MRSA) 038.12
     susceptible Staphylococcus aureus (MSSA) 038.11
   MRSA (methicillin resistant Staphylococcus aureus) 038.12
   MSSA (methicillin susceptible Staphylococcus aureus) 038.11
   navel, newborn (organism unspecified) 771.89
   newborn (organism unspecified) 771.81
   plague 020.2
   pneumococcal 038.2
   postabortal 639.0
   postoperative 998.59
   Proteus vulgaris 038.49
   Pseudomonas (aeruginosa) 038.43
   puerperal, postpartum 670.2●
   Salmonella (aertrycke) (callinarum) (choleraesuis) (enteritidis) (suipestifer) 003.1
   Serratia 038.44
   Shigella (see also Dysentery, bacillary) 004.9
   specified organism NEC 038.8
   staphylococcal 038.10
     aureus 038.11
     methicillin
       resistant (MRSA) 038.12
       susceptible (MSSA) 038.11
     specified organism NEC 038.19
   streptococcal (anaerobic) 038.0
   Streptococcus pneumoniae 038.2

Septicemia, septicemic (Continued)
   suipestifer 003.1
   umbilicus, newborn (organism unspecified) 771.89
   viral 079.99
   Yersinia enterocolitica 038.49
Septum, septate (congenital) - see also Anomaly, specified type NEC
   anal 751.2
   aqueduct of Sylvius 742.3
     with spina bifida (see also Spina bifida) 741.0●
   hymen 752.49
   uterus (complete) (partial) 752.35
   vagina
     in pregnancy or childbirth 654.7●
       affecting fetus or newborn 763.89
       causing obstructed labor 660.2●
         affecting fetus or newborn 763.1
     longitudinal (with or without obstruction) 752.47
     transverse 752.46
Sequestration
   lung (congenital) (extralobar) (intralobar) 748.5
   orbit 376.10
   pulmonary artery (congenital) 747.39
   splenic 289.52
Sequestrum
   bone (see also Osteomyelitis) 730.1●
     jaw 526.4
   dental 525.8
   jaw bone 526.4
   sinus (accessory) (nasal) (see also Sinusitis) 473.9
     maxillary 473.0
Sequoiosis asthma 495.8
Serology for syphilis
   doubtful
     with signs or symptoms - see Syphilis, by site and stage
     follow-up of latent syphilis - see Syphilis, latent
   false positive 795.6
   negative, with signs or symptoms - see Syphilis, by site and stage
   positive 097.1
     with signs or symptoms - see Syphilis, by site and stage
     false 795.6
     follow-up of latent syphilis - see Syphilis, latent
     only finding - see Syphilis, latent
   reactivated 097.1
Seroma - (postoperative) (non-infected) 998.13
   infected 998.51
   post-traumatic 729.91
Seropurulent - see condition
Serositis, multiple 569.89
   pericardial 423.2
   peritoneal 568.82
   pleural - see Pleurisy
Serotonin syndrome 333.99
Serous - see condition
Sertoli cell
   adenoma (M8640/0)
     specified site - see Neoplasm, by site, benign
     unspecified site
       female 220
       male 222.0
   carcinoma (M8640/3)
     specified site - see Neoplasm, by site, malignant
     unspecified site 186.9
   syndrome (germinal aplasia) 606.0
   tumor (M8640/0)
     with lipid storage (M8641/0)
       specified site - see Neoplasm, by site, benign

Sertoli cell (Continued)
   tumor (Continued)
     with lipid storage (Continued)
       unspecified site
         female 220
         male 222.0
     specified site - see Neoplasm, by site, benign
     unspecified site
       female 220
       male 222.0
Sertoli-Leydig cell tumor (M8631/0)
   specified site - see Neoplasm, by site, benign
   unspecified site
     female 220
     male 222.0
Serum
   allergy, allergic reaction 999.59
     shock 999.49
   arthritis 999.59 [713.6]
   complication or reaction NEC 999.59
   disease NEC 999.59
   hepatitis 070.3●
   intoxication 999.59
   jaundice (homologous) - see Hepatitis, viral, type B
   neuritis 999.59
   poisoning NEC 999.59
   rash NEC 999.59
   reaction NEC 999.59
   sickness NEC 999.59
Sesamoiditis 733.99
Seven-day fever 061
   of
     Japan 100.89
     Queensland 100.89
Sever's disease or osteochondrosis (calcaneum) 732.5
Sex chromosome mosaics 758.81
Sex reassignment surgery status (see also Trans-sexualism) 302.50
Sextuplet
   affected by maternal complication of pregnancy 761.5
   healthy liveborn - see Newborn, multiple
   pregnancy (complicating delivery) NEC 651.8●
     with fetal loss and retention of one or more fetus(es) 651.6●
     following (elective) fetal reduction 651.7●
Sexual
   anesthesia 302.72
   deviation (see also Deviation, sexual) 302.9
   disorder (see also Deviation, sexual) 302.9
   frigidity (female) 302.72
   function, disorder of (psychogenic) 302.70
     specified type NEC 302.79
   immaturity (female) (male) 259.0
   impotence 607.84
     organic origin NEC 607.84
     psychogenic 302.72
   precocity (constitutional) (cryptogenic) (female) (idiopathic) (male) NEC 259.1
     with adrenal hyperplasia 255.2
   sadism 302.84
Sexuality, pathological (see also Deviation, sexual) 302.9
Sézary's disease, reticulosis, or syndrome (M9701/3) 202.2●
Shadow, lung 793.19
Shaken infant syndrome 995.55
Shaking
   head (tremor) 781.0
   palsy or paralysis (see also Parkinsonism) 332.0
Shallowness, acetabulum 736.39
Shaver's disease or syndrome (bauxite pneumoconiosis) 503
Shearing
   artificial skin graft 996.55
   decellularized allodermis graft 996.55

SECTION I INDEX TO DISEASES AND INJURIES / Shunt

Sheath (tendon) - see condition
Shedding
- nail 703.8
- teeth, premature, primary (deciduous) 520.6

Sheehan's disease or syndrome (postpartum pituitary necrosis) 253.2
Shelf, rectal 569.49
Shell
- shock (current) (see also Reaction, stress, acute) 308.9
  - lasting state 300.16
- teeth 520.5

Shield kidney 753.3
Shift, mediastinal 793.2
Shifting
- pacemaker 427.89
- sleep-work schedule (affecting sleep) 327.36

Shiga's
- bacillus 004.0
- dysentery 004.0

Shigella (dysentery) (see also Dysentery, bacillary) 004.9
- carrier (suspected) of V02.3

Shigellosis (see also Dysentery, bacillary) 004.9
Shingles (see also Herpes, zoster) 053.9
- eye NEC 053.29

Shin splints 844.9
Shipyard eye or disease 077.1
Shirodkar suture, in pregnancy 654.5 ●
Shock 785.50
- with
  - abortion - see Abortion, by type, with shock
  - ectopic pregnancy (see also categories 633.0–633.9) 639.5
  - molar pregnancy (see also categories 630–632) 639.5
- allergic - see Anaphylactic reaction or shock
- anaclitic 309.21
- anaphylactic see also Anaphylactic reaction or shock
  - due to administration of blood and blood products 999.41
- anaphylactoid - see Anaphylactic reaction or shock
- anesthetic
  - correct substance properly administered 995.4
  - overdose or wrong substance given 968.4
    - specified anesthetic - see Table of Drugs and Chemicals
- birth, fetus or newborn NEC 779.89
- cardiogenic 785.51
- chemical substance - see Table of Drugs and Chemicals
- circulatory 785.59
- complicating
  - abortion - see Abortion, by type, with shock
  - ectopic pregnancy - (see also categories 633.0–633.9) 639.5
  - labor and delivery 669.1 ●
  - molar pregnancy (see also categories 630–632) 639.5
- culture 309.29
- due to
  - drug 995.0
    - correct substance properly administered 995.0
    - overdose or wrong substance given or taken 977.9
    - specified drug - see Table of Drugs and Chemicals
  - food - see Anaphylactic shock, due to, food
- during labor and delivery 669.1 ●
- electric 994.8
  - from electroshock gun (taser) 994.8
- endotoxic 785.52
  - due to surgical procedure 998.02
  - postoperative 998.02

Shock (Continued)
- following
  - abortion 639.5
  - ectopic or molar pregnancy 639.5
  - injury (immediate) (delayed) 958.4
  - labor and delivery 669.1 ●
- gram-negative 785.52
  - postoperative 998.02
- hematogenic 785.59
- hemorrhagic
  - due to
    - disease 785.59
    - surgery (intraoperative) (postoperative) 998.09
    - trauma 958.4
- hypovolemic NEC 785.59
  - surgical 998.09
  - traumatic 958.4
- insulin 251.0
  - therapeutic misadventure 962.3
- kidney 584.5
  - traumatic (following crushing) 958.5
- lightning 994.0
- lung 518.82
  - related to trauma and surgery 518.52
- nervous (see also Reaction, stress, acute) 308.9
- obstetric 669.1 ●
  - with
    - abortion - see Abortion, by type, with shock
    - ectopic pregnancy (see also categories 633.0–633.9) 639.5
    - molar pregnancy (see also categories 630–632) 639.5
  - following
    - abortion 639.5
    - ectopic or molar pregnancy 639.5
- paralysis, paralytic (see also Disease, cerebrovascular, acute) 436
  - late effect - see Late effect(s) (of) cerebrovascular disease
- pleural (surgical) 998.09
  - due to trauma 958.4
- postoperative 998.00
  - with
    - abortion - see Abortion, by type, with shock
    - ectopic pregnancy (see also categories 633.0–633.9) 639.5
    - molar pregnancy (see also categories 630–632) 639.5
  - cardiogenic 998.01
  - following
    - abortion 639.5
    - ectopic or molar pregnancy 639.5
  - hypovolemic 998.09
  - specified NEC 998.09
  - septic (endotoxic) (gram-negative) 998.02
- psychic (see also Reaction, stress, acute) 308.9
  - past history (of) V15.49
- psychogenic (see also Reaction, stress, acute) 308.9
- septic 785.52
  - with
    - abortion - see Abortion, by type, with shock
    - ectopic pregnancy (see also categories 633.0–633.9) 639.5
    - molar pregnancy (see also categories 630–632) 639.5
  - due to
    - surgical procedure 998.02
    - transfusion NEC 999.89
      - bone marrow 996.85
  - following
    - abortion 639.5
    - ectopic or molar pregnancy 639.5
    - surgical procedure 998.02
    - transfusion NEC 999.89
      - bone marrow 996.85
  - postoperative 998.02

Shock (Continued)
- spinal - see also Injury, spinal, by site
  - with spinal bone injury - see Fracture, vertebra, by site, with spinal cord injury
- surgical 998.00
- therapeutic misadventure NEC (see also Complications) 998.89
- thyroxin 962.7
- toxic 040.82
- transfusion - see Complications, transfusion
- traumatic (immediate) (delayed) 958.4

Shoemakers' chest 738.3
Short, shortening, shortness
- Achilles tendon (acquired) 727.81
- arm 736.89
  - congenital 755.20
- back 737.9
- bowel syndrome 579.3
- breath 786.05
- cervical, cervix 649.7 ●
  - gravid uterus 649.7 ●
  - non-gravid uterus 622.5
    - acquired 622.5
    - congenital 752.49
- chain acyl CoA dehydrogenase deficiency (SCAD) 277.85
- common bile duct, congenital 751.69
- cord (umbilical) 663.4 ●
  - affecting fetus or newborn 762.6
- cystic duct, congenital 751.69
- esophagus (congenital) 750.4
- femur (acquired) 736.81
  - congenital 755.34
- frenulum linguae 750.0
- frenum, lingual 750.0
- hamstrings 727.81
- hip (acquired) 736.39
  - congenital 755.63
- leg (acquired) 736.81
  - congenital 755.30
- metatarsus (congenital) 754.79
  - acquired 736.79
- organ or site, congenital NEC - see Distortion
- palate (congenital) 750.26
- P-R interval syndrome 426.81
- radius (acquired) 736.09
  - congenital 755.26
- round ligament 629.89
- sleeper 307.49
- stature, constitutional (hereditary) (idiopathic) 783.43
- tendon 727.81
  - Achilles (acquired) 727.81
  - congenital 754.79
  - congenital 756.89
- thigh (acquired) 736.81
  - congenital 755.34
- tibialis anticus 727.81
- umbilical cord 663.4 ●
  - affecting fetus or newborn 762.6
- urethra 599.84
- uvula (congenital) 750.26
- vagina 623.8

Shortsightedness 367.1
Shoshin (acute fulminating beriberi) 265.0
Shoulder - see condition
Shovel-shaped incisors 520.2
Shower, thromboembolic - see Embolism
Shunt (status)
- aortocoronary bypass V45.81
- arterial-venous (dialysis) V45.11
- arteriovenous, pulmonary (acquired) 417.0
  - congenital 747.39
  - traumatic (complication) 901.40
- cerebral ventricle (communicating) in situ V45.2
- coronary artery bypass V45.81
- surgical, prosthetic, with complications - see Complications, shunt
- vascular NEC V45.89

 New · Revised · deleted Deleted · ● Use Additional Digit(s) · Omit code

Shutdown
  renal 586
    with
      abortion - *see* Abortion, by type, with renal failure
      ectopic pregnancy (*see also* categories 633.0–633.9) 639.3
      molar pregnancy (*see also* categories 630–632) 639.3
    complicating
      abortion 639.3
      ectopic or molar pregnancy 639.3
    following labor and delivery 669.3●
Shwachman's syndrome 288.02
Shy-Drager syndrome (orthostatic hypotension with multisystem degeneration) 333.0
Sialadenitis (any gland) (chronic) (supportive) 527.2
  epidemic - *see* Mumps
Sialadenosis, periodic 527.2
Sialaporia 527.7
Sialectasia 527.8
Sialitis 527.2
Sialoadenitis (*see also* Sialadenitis) 527.2
Sialoangitis 527.2
Sialodochitis (fibrinosa) 527.2
Sialodocholithiasis 527.5
Sialolithiasis 527.5
Sialorrhea (*see also* Ptyalism) 527.7
  periodic 527.2
Sialosis 527.8
  rheumatic 710.2
Siamese twin 759.4
  complicating pregnancy 678.1●
Sicard's syndrome 352.6
Sicca syndrome (keratoconjunctivitis) 710.2
Sick 799.9
  cilia syndrome 759.89
  or handicapped person in family V61.49
Sickle-cell
  anemia (*see also* Disease, sickle-cell) 282.60
  disease (*see also* Disease, sickle-cell) 282.60
  hemoglobin
    C disease (without crisis) 282.63
      with
        crisis 282.64
          vaso-occlusive pain 282.64
    D disease (without crisis) 282.68
      with crisis 282.69
    E disease (without crisis) 282.68
      with crisis 282.69
  thalassemia (without crisis) 282.41
    with
      crisis 282.42
        vaso-occlusive pain 282.42
  trait 282.5
Sicklemia (*see also* Disease, sickle-cell) 282.60
  trait 282.5
Sickness
  air (travel) 994.6
  airplane 994.6
  alpine 993.2
  altitude 993.2
  Andes 993.2
  aviators' 993.2
  balloon 993.2
  car 994.6
  compressed air 993.3
  decompression 993.3
  green 280.9
  harvest 100.89
  milk 988.8
  morning 643.0●
  motion 994.6
  mountain 993.2
    acute 289.0
  protein (*see also* Complications, vaccination) 999.59
  radiation NEC 990
  roundabout (motion) 994.6
  sea 994.6

Sickness (*Continued*)
  serum NEC 999.59
  sleeping (African) 086.5
    by Trypanosoma 086.5
      gambiense 086.3
      rhodesiense 086.4
    Gambian 086.3
    late effect 139.8
    Rhodesian 086.4
  sweating 078.2
  swing (motion) 994.6
  train (railway) (travel) 994.6
  travel (any vehicle) 994.6
Sick sinus syndrome 427.81
Sideropenia (*see also* Anemia, iron deficiency) 280.9
Siderosis (lung) (occupational) 503
  central nervous system (CNS) 437.8
  cornea 371.15
  eye (bulbi) (vitreous) 360.23
  lens 360.23
Siegal-Cattan-Mamou disease (periodic) 277.31
Siemens' syndrome
  ectodermal dysplasia 757.31
  keratosis follicularis spinulosa (decalvans) 757.39
Sighing respiration 786.7
Sigmoid
  flexure - *see* condition
  kidney 753.3
Sigmoiditis - *see* Enteritis
Silfverskiöld's syndrome 756.50
Silicosis, silicotic (complicated) (occupational) (simple) 502
  fibrosis, lung (confluent) (massive) (occupational) 502
  non-nodular 503
  pulmonum 502
Silicotuberculosis (*see also* Tuberculosis) 011.4●
Silo fillers' disease 506.9
Silver's syndrome (congenital hemihypertrophy and short stature) 759.89
Silver wire arteries, retina 362.13
Silvestroni-Bianco syndrome (thalassemia minima) 282.49
Simian crease 757.2
Simmonds' cachexia or disease (pituitary cachexia) 253.2
Simons' disease or syndrome (progressive lipodystrophy) 272.6
Simple, simplex - *see* condition
Sinding-Larsen disease (juvenile osteopathia patellae) 732.4
Singapore hemorrhagic fever 065.4
Singers' node or nodule 478.5
Single
  atrium 745.69
  coronary artery 746.85
  umbilical artery 747.5
  ventricle 745.3
Singultus 786.8
  epidemicus 078.89
Sinus - *see also* Fistula
  abdominal 569.81
  arrest 426.6
  arrhythmia 427.89
  bradycardia 427.89
    chronic 427.81
  branchial cleft (external) (internal) 744.41
  coccygeal (infected) 685.1
    with abscess 685.0
  dental 522.7
  dermal (congenital) 685.1
    with abscess 685.0
  draining - *see* Fistula
  infected, skin NEC 686.9
  marginal, rupture or bleeding 641.2●
    affecting fetus or newborn 762.1
  pause 426.6
  pericranii 742.0

Sinus (*Continued*)
  pilonidal (infected) (rectum) 685.1
    with abscess 685.0
  preauricular 744.46
  rectovaginal 619.1
  sacrococcygeal (dermoid) (infected) 685.1
    with abscess 685.0
  skin
    infected NEC 686.9
    noninfected- *see* Ulcer, skin
  tachycardia 427.89
  tarsi syndrome 726.79
  testis 608.89
  tract (postinfectional) - *see* Fistula
  urachus 753.7
Sinuses, Rokitansky-Aschoff (*see also* Disease, gallbladder) 575.8
Sinusitis (accessory) (chronic) (hyperplastic) (nasal) (nonpurulent) (purulent) 473.9
  with influenza, flu, or grippe (*see also* Influenza) 487.1
  acute 461.9
    ethmoidal 461.2
    frontal 461.1
    maxillary 461.0
    specified type NEC 461.8
    sphenoidal 461.3
  allergic (*see also* Fever, hay) 477.9
  antrum - *see* Sinusitis, maxillary
  due to
    fungus, any sinus 117.9
    high altitude 993.1
  ethmoidal 473.2
    acute 461.2
  frontal 473.1
    acute 461.1
  influenzal (*see also* Influenza) 487.1
  maxillary 473.0
    acute 461.0
  specified site NEC 473.8
  sphenoidal 473.3
    acute 461.3
  syphilitic, any sinus 095.8
  tuberculous, any sinus (*see also* Tuberculosis) 012.8●
Sinusitis-bronchiectasis-situs inversus (syndrome) (triad) 759.3
Sipple's syndrome (medullary thyroid carcinoma-pheochromocytoma) 258.02
Sirenomelia 759.89
Siriasis 992.0
Sirkari's disease 085.0
SIRS (systemic inflammatory response syndrome) 995.90
  due to
    infectious process 995.91
      with acute organ dysfunction 995.92
    non-infectious process 995.93
      with acute organ dysfunction 995.94
Siti 104.0
Sitophobia 300.29
Situation, psychiatric 300.9
Situational
  disturbance (transient) (*see also* Reaction, adjustment) 309.9
    acute 308.3
  maladjustment, acute (*see also* Reaction, adjustment) 309.9
  reaction (*see also* Reaction, adjustment) 309.9
    acute 308.3
Situs inversus or transversus 759.3
  abdominalis 759.3
  thoracis 759.3
Sixth disease
  due to
    human herpesvirus 6 058.11
    human herpesvirus 7 058.12
Sjögren (-Gougerot) **syndrome or disease** (keratoconjunctivitis sicca) 710.2
  with lung involvement 710.2 [517.8]

Sjögren-Larsson syndrome (ichthyosis congenita) 757.1
SJS-TEN (Stevens-Johnson syndrome-toxic epidermal necrolysis overlap syndrome) 695.14
Skeletal - see condition
Skene's gland - see condition
Skenitis (see also Urethritis) 597.89
   gonorrheal (acute) 098.0
      chronic or duration of 2 months or over 098.2
Skerljevo 104.0
Skevas-Zerfus disease 989.5
Skin - see also condition
   donor V59.1
   hidebound 710.9
SLAP lesion (superior glenoid labrum) 840.7
Slate-dressers' lung 502
Slate-miners' lung 502
Sleep
   deprivation V69.4
   disorder 780.50
      with apnea - see Apnea, sleep
      child 307.40
      movement, unspecified 780.58
      nonorganic origin 307.40
         specified type NEC 307.49
   disturbance 780.50
      with apnea - see Apnea, sleep
      nonorganic origin 307.40
         specified type NEC 307.49
   drunkenness 307.47
   movement disorder, unspecified 780.58
   paroxysmal (see also Narcolepsy) 347.00
   related movement disorder, unspecified 780.58
   rhythm inversion 327.39
      nonorganic origin 307.45
   walking 307.46
      hysterical 300.13
Sleeping sickness 086.5
   late effect 139.8
Sleeplessness (see also Insomnia) 780.52
   menopausal 627.2
   nonorganic origin 307.41
Slipped, slipping
   epiphysis (postinfectional) 732.9
      traumatic (old) 732.9
         current - see Fracture, by site
      upper femoral (nontraumatic) 732.2
   intervertebral disc - see Displacement, intervertebral disc
   ligature, umbilical 772.3
   patella 717.89
   rib 733.99
   sacroiliac joint 724.6
   tendon 727.9
   ulnar nerve, nontraumatic 354.2
   vertebra NEC (see also Spondylolisthesis) 756.12
Slocumb's syndrome 255.3
Sloughing (multiple) (skin) 686.9
   abscess - see Abscess, by site
   appendix 543.9
   bladder 596.89
   fascia 728.9
   graft - see Complications, graft
   phagedena (see also Gangrene) 785.4
   reattached extremity (see also Complications, reattached extremity) 996.90
   rectum 569.49
   scrotum 608.89
   tendon 727.9
   transplanted organ (see also Rejection, transplant, organ, by site) 996.80
   ulcer (see also Ulcer, skin) 707.9
Slow
   feeding newborn 779.31
   fetal, growth NEC 764.9●
      affecting management of pregnancy 656.5●

Slowing
   heart 427.89
   urinary stream 788.62
Sluder's neuralgia or syndrome 337.09
Slurred, slurring, speech 784.59
Small, smallness
   cardia reserve - see Disease, heart
   for dates
      fetus or newborn 764.0●
         with malnutrition 764.1●
         affecting management of pregnancy 656.5●
      infant, term 764.0●
         with malnutrition 764.1●
         affecting management of pregnancy 656.5●
   introitus, vagina 623.3
   kidney, unknown cause 589.9
      bilateral 589.1
      unilateral 589.0
   ovary 620.8
   pelvis
      with disproportion (fetopelvic) 653.1●
         affecting fetus or newborn 763.1
      causing obstructed labor 660.1●
         affecting fetus or newborn 763.1
   placenta - see Placenta, insufficiency
   uterus 621.8
   white kidney 582.9
Small-for-dates (see also Light-for-dates) 764.0●
   affecting management of pregnancy 656.5●
Smallpox 050.9
   contact V01.3
   exposure to V01.3
   hemorrhagic (pustular) 050.0
   malignant 050.0
   modified 050.2
   vaccination
      complications - see Complications, vaccination
      prophylactic (against) V04.1
Smearing, fecal 787.62
Smith's fracture (separation) (closed) 813.41
   open 813.51
Smith-Lemli-Opitz syndrome (cerebrohepatorenal syndrome) 759.89
Smith-Magenis syndrome 758.33
Smith-Strang disease (oasthouse urine) 270.2
Smokers'
   bronchitis 491.0
   cough 491.0
   syndrome (see also Abuse, drugs, nondependent) 305.1
   throat 472.1
   tongue 528.6
Smoking complicating pregnancy, childbirth, or the puerperium 649.0●
Smothering spells 786.09
Snaggle teeth, tooth 524.39
Snapping
   finger 727.05
   hip 719.65
   jaw 524.69
      temporomandibular joint sounds on opening or closing 524.64
   knee 717.9
   thumb 727.05
Sneddon-Wilkinson disease or syndrome (subcorneal pustular dermatosis) 694.1
Sneezing 784.99
   intractable 478.19
Sniffing
   cocaine (see also Dependence) 304.2●
   either (see also Dependence) 304.6●
   glue (airplane) (see also Dependence) 304.6●
Snoring 786.09
Snow blindness 370.24
Snuffles (nonsyphilitic) 460
   syphilitic (infant) 090.0
Social migrant V60.0
Sodoku 026.0

Soemmering's ring 366.51
Soft - see also condition
   enlarged prostate 600.00
      with
         other lower urinary tract symptoms (LUTS) 600.01
         urinary
            obstruction 600.01
            retention 600.01
   nails 703.8
Softening
   bone 268.2
   brain (necrotic) (progressive) 348.89
      arteriosclerotic 437.0
      congenital 742.4
      due to cerebrovascular accident 438.89
      embolic (see also Embolism, brain) 434.1●
      hemorrhagic (see also Hemorrhage, brain) 431
      occlusive 434.9●
      thrombotic (see also Thrombosis, brain) 434.0●
   cartilage 733.92
   cerebellar - see Softening, brain
   cerebral - see Softening, brain
   cerebrospinal - see Softening, brain
   myocardial, heart (see also Degeneration, myocardial) 429.1
   nails 703.8
   spinal cord 336.8
   stomach 537.89
Soiling, fecal 787.62
Solar fever 061
Soldier's
   heart 306.2
   patches 423.1
Solitary
   cyst
      bone 733.21
      kidney 593.2
   kidney (congenital) 753.0
   tubercle, brain (see also Tuberculosis, brain) 013.2●
   ulcer, bladder 596.89
Somatization reaction, somatic reaction (see also Disorder, psychosomatic) 306.9
   disorder 300.81
Somatoform disorder 300.82
   atypical 300.82
   severe 300.81
   undifferentiated 300.82
Somnambulism 307.46
   hysterical 300.13
Somnolence 780.09
   nonorganic origin 307.43
   periodic 349.89
Sonne dysentery 004.3
Soor 112.0
Sore
   Delhi 085.1
   desert (see also Ulcer, skin) 707.9
   eye 379.99
   Lahore 085.1
   mouth 528.9
      canker 528.2
      due to dentures 528.9
   muscle 729.1
   naga (see also Ulcer, skin) 707.9
   oriental 085.1
   pressure (see also Ulcer, pressure) 707.00
      with gangrene (see also Ulcer, pressure) 707.00 [785.4]
   skin NEC 709.9
   soft 099.0
   throat 462
      with influenza, flu, or grippe (see also Influenza) 487.1
      acute 462
      chronic 472.1
      clergyman's 784.49
      Coxsackie (virus) 074.0

SECTION I INDEX TO DISEASES AND INJURIES / Sore

Sore (Continued)
  throat (Continued)
    diphtheritic 032.0
    epidemic 034.0
    gangrenous 462
    herpetic 054.79
    influenzal (see also Influenza) 487.1
    malignant 462
    purulent 462
    putrid 462
    septic 034.0
    streptococcal (ulcerative) 034.0
    ulcerated 462
    viral NEC 462
      Coxsackie 074.0
  tropical (see also Ulcer, skin) 707.9
  veldt (see also Ulcer, skin) 707.9
Sotos' syndrome (cerebral gigantism) 253.0
Sounds
  friction, pleural 786.7
  succussion, chest 786.7
  temporomandibular joint
    on opening or closing 524.64
South African cardiomyopathy syndrome 425.2
South American
  blastomycosis 116.1
  trypanosomiasis - see Trypanosomiasis
Southeast Asian hemorrhagic fever 065.4
Spacing, teeth, abnormal 524.30
  excessive 524.32
Spade-like hand (congenital) 754.89
Spading nail 703.8
  congenital 757.5
Spanemia 285.9
Spanish collar 605
Sparganosis 123.5
Spasm, spastic, spasticity (see also condition) 781.0
  accommodation 367.53
  ampulla of Vater (see also Disease, gallbladder) 576.8
  anus, ani (sphincter) (reflex) 564.6
    psychogenic 306.4
  artery NEC 443.9
    basilar 435.0
    carotid 435.8
    cerebral 435.9
      specified artery NEC 435.8
    retinal (see also Occlusion, retinal, artery) 362.30
    vertebral 435.1
    vertebrobasilar 435.3
  Bell's 351.0
  bladder (sphincter, external or internal) 596.89
  bowel 564.9
    psychogenic 306.4
  bronchus, bronchiole 519.11
  cardia 530.0
  cardiac - see Angina
  carpopedal (see also Tetany) 781.7
  cecum 564.9
    psychogenic 306.4
  cerebral (arteries) (vascular) 435.9
    specified artery NEC 435.8
  cerebrovascular 435.9
  cervix, complicating delivery 661.4●
    affecting fetus or newborn 763.7
  ciliary body (of accommodation) 367.53
  colon 564.1
    psychogenic 306.4
  common duct (see also Disease, biliary) 576.8
  compulsive 307.22
  conjugate 378.82
  convergence 378.84
  coronary (artery) - see Angina
  diaphragm (reflex) 786.8
    psychogenic 306.1
  duodenum, duodenal (bulb) 564.89

Spasm, spastic, spasticity (Continued)
  esophagus (diffuse) 530.5
    psychogenic 306.4
  facial 351.8
  fallopian tube 620.8
  gait 781.2
  gastrointestinal (tract) 536.8
    psychogenic 306.4
  glottis 478.75
    hysterical 300.11
    psychogenic 306.1
      specified as conversion reaction 300.11
    reflex through recurrent laryngeal nerve 478.75
  habit 307.20
    chronic 307.22
    transient (of childhood) 307.21
  heart - see Angina
  hourglass - see Contraction, hourglass
  hysterical 300.11
  infantile (see also Epilepsy) 345.6●
  internal oblique, eye 378.51
  intestinal 564.9
    psychogenic 306.4
  larynx, laryngeal 478.75
    hysterical 300.11
    psychogenic 306.1
      specified as conversion reaction 300.11
  levator palpebrae superioris 333.81
  lightning (see also Epilepsy) 345.6●
  mobile 781.0
  muscle 728.85
    back 724.8
    psychogenic 306.0
  nerve, trigeminal 350.1
  nervous 306.0
  nodding 307.3
    infantile (see also Epilepsy) 345.6●
  occupational 300.89
  oculogyric 378.87
  ophthalmic artery 362.30
  orbicularis 781.0
  perineal 625.8
  peroneo-extensor (see also Flat, foot) 734
  pharynx (reflex) 478.29
    hysterical 300.11
    psychogenic 306.1
      specified as conversion reaction 300.11
  pregnant uterus, complicating delivery 661.4●
  psychogenic 306.0
  pylorus 537.81
    adult hypertrophic 537.0
    congenital or infantile 750.5
    psychogenic 306.4
  rectum (sphincter) 564.6
    psychogenic 306.4
  retinal artery NEC (see also Occlusion, retina, artery) 362.30
  sacroiliac 724.6
  salaam (infantile) (see also Epilepsy) 345.6●
  saltatory 781.0
  sigmoid 564.9
    psychogenic 306.4
  sphincter of Oddi (see also Disease, gallbladder) 576.5
  stomach 536.8
    neurotic 306.4
  throat 478.29
    hysterical 300.11
    psychogenic 306.1
      specified as conversion reaction 300.11
  tic 307.20
    chronic 307.22
    transient (of childhood) 307.21
  tongue 529.8
  torsion 333.6
  trigeminal nerve 350.1
    postherpetic 053.12
  ureter 593.89
  urethra (sphincter) 599.84

Spasm, spastic, spasticity (Continued)
  uterus 625.8
    complicating labor 661.4●
      affecting fetus or newborn 763.7
  vagina 625.1
    psychogenic 306.51
  vascular NEC 443.9
  vasomotor NEC 443.9
  vein NEC 459.89
  vesical (sphincter, external or internal) 596.89
  viscera 789.0●
Spasmodic - see condition
Spasmophilia (see also Tetany) 781.7
Spasmus nutans 307.3
Spastic - see also Spasm
  child 343.9
Spasticity - see also Spasm
  cerebral, child 343.9
Speakers' throat 784.49
Specific, specified - see condition
Speech
  defect, disorder, disturbance, impediment NEC 784.59
    psychogenic 307.9
  (language) therapy V57.3
Spells 780.39
  breath-holding 786.9
Spencer's disease (epidemic vomiting) 078.82
Spens' syndrome (syncope with heart block) 426.9
Spermatic cord - see condition
Spermatocele 608.1
  congenital 752.89
Spermatocystitis 608.4
Spermatocytoma (M9063/3)
  specified site - see Neoplasm, by site, malignant
  unspecified site 186.9
Spermatorrhea 608.89
Sperm counts
  fertility testing V26.21
  following sterilization reversal V26.22
  postvasectomy V25.8
Sphacelus (see also Gangrene) 785.4
Sphenoidal - see condition
Sphenoiditis (chronic) (see also Sinusitis, sphenoidal) 473.3
Sphenopalatine ganglion neuralgia 337.09
Sphericity, increased, lens 743.36
Spherocytosis (congenital) (familial) (hereditary) 282.0
  hemoglobin disease 282.7
  sickle-cell (disease) 282.60
Spherophakia 743.36
Sphincter - see condition
Sphincteritis, sphincter of Oddi (see also Cholecystitis) 576.8
Sphingolipidosis 272.7
Sphingolipodystrophy 272.7
Sphingomyelinosis 272.7
Spicule tooth 520.2
Spider
  finger 755.59
  nevus 448.1
  vascular 448.1
Spiegler-Fendt sarcoid 686.8
Spielmeyer-Stock disease 330.1
Spielmeyer-Vogt disease 330.1
Spina bifida (aperta) 741.9●

> Note: Use the following fifth-digit subclassification with category 741:
>
> 0 unspecified region
> 1 cervical region
> 2 dorsal [thoracic] region
> 3 lumbar region

  with hydrocephalus 741.0●
    fetal (suspected), affecting management of pregnancy 655.0●
  occulta 756.17

Spindle, Krukenberg's 371.13
Spine, spinal - see condition
Spiradenoma (eccrine) (M8403/0) - see
    Neoplasm, skin, benign
Spirillosis NEC (see also Fever, relapsing) 087.9
Spirillum minus 026.0
Spirillum obermeieri infection 087.0
Spirochetal - see condition
Spirochetosis 104.9
    arthritic, arthritica 104.9 [711.8]●
    bronchopulmonary 104.8
    icterohemorrhagica 100.0
    lung 104.8
Spitting blood (see also Hemoptysis) 786.30
Splanchnomegaly 569.89
Splanchnoptosis 569.89
Spleen, splenic - see also condition
    agenesis 759.0
    flexure syndrome 569.89
    neutropenia syndrome 289.53
    sequestration syndrome 289.52
Splenectasis (see also Splenomegaly) 789.2
Splenitis (interstitial) (malignant) (nonspecific)
        289.59
    malarial (see also Malaria) 084.6
    tuberculous (see also Tuberculosis) 017.7●
Splenocele 289.59
Splenomegalia - see Splenomegaly
Splenomegalic - see condition
Splenomegaly 789.2
    Bengal 789.2
    cirrhotic 289.51
    congenital 759.0
    congestive, chronic 289.51
    cryptogenic 789.2
    Egyptian 120.1
    Gaucher's (cerebroside lipidosis) 272.7
    idiopathic 789.2
    malarial (see also Malaria) 084.6
    neutropenic 289.53
    Niemann-Pick (lipid histiocytosis) 272.7
    siderotic 289.51
    syphilitic 095.8
        congenital 090.0
    tropical (Bengal) (idiopathic) 789.2
Splenopathy 289.50
Splenopneumonia - see Pneumonia
Splenoptosis 289.59
Splinter - see Injury, superficial, by site
Split, splitting
    heart sounds 427.89
    lip, congenital (see also Cleft, lip) 749.10
    nails 703.8
    urinary stream 788.61
Spoiled child reaction (see also Disturbance,
        conduct) 312.1●
Spondylarthritis (see also Spondylosis) 721.90
Spondylarthrosis (see also Spondylosis) 721.90
Spondylitis 720.9
    ankylopoietica 720.0
    ankylosing (chronic) 720.0
    atrophic 720.9
        ligamentous 720.9
    chronic (traumatic) (see also Spondylosis)
        721.90
    deformans (chronic) (see also Spondylosis)
        721.90
    gonococcal 098.53
    gouty 274.00
    hypertrophic (see also Spondylosis) 721.90
    infectious NEC 720.9
    juvenile (adolescent) 720.0
    Kummell's 721.7
    Marie-Strümpell (ankylosing) 720.0
    muscularis 720.9
    ossificans ligamentosa 721.6
    osteoarthritica (see also Spondylosis) 721.90
    posttraumatic 721.7
    proliferative 720.0
    rheumatoid 720.0
    rhizomelica 720.0

Spondylitis (Continued)
    sacroiliac NEC 720.2
    senescent (see also Spondylosis) 721.90
    senile (see also Spondylosis) 721.90
    static (see also Spondylosis) 721.90
    traumatic (chronic) (see also Spondylosis)
        721.90
    tuberculous (see also Tuberculosis) 015.0●
        [720.81]
    typhosa 002.0 [720.81]
Spondyloarthrosis (see also Spondylosis) 721.90
Spondylolisthesis (congenital) (lumbosacral)
        756.12
    with disproportion (fetopelvic) 653.3●
        affecting fetus or newborn 763.1
        causing obstructed labor 660.1●
            affecting fetus or newborn 763.1
    acquired 738.4
    degenerative 738.4
    traumatic 738.4
        acute (lumbar) - see Fracture, vertebra,
            lumbar
        site other than lumbosacral - see
            Fracture, vertebra, by site
Spondylolysis (congenital) 756.11
    acquired 738.4
    cervical 756.19
    lumbosacral region 756.11
        with disproportion (fetopelvic) 653.3●
            affecting fetus or newborn 763.1
            causing obstructed labor 660.1●
                affecting fetus or newborn 763.1
Spondylopathy
    inflammatory 720.9
        specified type NEC 720.89
    traumatic 721.7
Spondylose rhizomelique 720.0
Spondylosis 721.90
    with
        disproportion 653.3●
            affecting fetus or newborn 763.1
            causing obstructed labor 660.1●
                affecting fetus or newborn 763.1
        myelopathy NEC 721.91
    cervical, cervicodorsal 721.0
        with myelopathy 721.1
    inflammatory 720.9
    lumbar, lumbosacral 721.3
        with myelopathy 721.42
    sacral 721.3
        with myelopathy 721.42
    thoracic 721.2
        with myelopathy 721.41
    traumatic 721.7
Sponge
    divers' disease 989.5
    inadvertently left in operation wound
        998.4
    kidney (medullary) 753.17
Spongioblastoma (M9422/3)
    multiforme (M9440/3)
        specified site - see Neoplasm, by site,
            malignant
        unspecified site 191.9
    polare (M9423/3)
        specified site - see Neoplasm, by site,
            malignant
        unspecified site 191.9
    primitive polar (M9443/3)
        specified site - see Neoplasm, by site,
            malignant
        unspecified site 191.9
    specified site - see Neoplasm, by site,
        malignant
    unspecified site 191.9
Spongiocytoma (M9400/3)
    specified site - see Neoplasm, by site,
        malignant
    unspecified site 191.9
Spongioneuroblastoma (M9504/3) - see
    Neoplasm, by site, malignant

Spontaneous - see also condition
    fracture - see Fracture, pathologic
Spoon nail 703.8
    congenital 757.5
Sporadic - see condition
Sporotrichosis (bones) (cutaneous)
        (disseminated) (epidermal) (lymphatic)
        (lymphocutaneous) (mucous membranes)
        (pulmonary) (skeletal) (visceral) 117.1
Sporotrichum schenckii infection 117.1
Spots, spotting
    atrophic (skin) 701.3
    Bitôt's (in the young child) 264.1
    café au lait 709.09
    cayenne pepper 448.1
    complicating pregnancy 649.5●
    cotton wool (retina) 362.83
    de Morgan's (senile angiomas) 448.1
    Fúchs' black (myopic) 360.21
    intermenstrual
        irregular 626.6
        regular 626.5
    interpalpebral 372.53
    Koplik's 055.9
    liver 709.09
    Mongolian (pigmented) 757.33
    of pregnancy 649.5●
    purpuric 782.7
    ruby 448.1
Spotted fever - see Fever, spotted
Sprain, strain (joint) (ligament) (muscle)
        (tendon) 848.9
    abdominal wall (muscle) 848.8
    Achilles tendon 845.09
    acromioclavicular 840.0
    ankle 845.00
        and foot 845.00
    anterior longitudinal, cervical 847.0
    arm 840.9
        upper 840.9
            and shoulder 840.9
    astragalus 845.00
    atlanto-axial 847.0
    atlanto-occipital 847.0
    atlas 847.0
    axis 847.0
    back (see also Sprain, spine) 847.9
    breast bone 848.40
    broad ligaments - see Injury, internal, broad
        ligament
    calcaneofibular 845.02
    carpal 842.01
    carpometacarpal 842.11
    cartilage
        costal, without mention of injury to
            sternum 848.3
            involving sternum 848.42
        ear 848.8
        knee 844.9
            with current tear (see also Tear,
                meniscus) 836.2
            semilunar (knee) 844.8
                with current tear (see also Tear,
                    meniscus) 836.2
        septal, nose 848.0
        thyroid region 848.2
        xiphoid 848.49
    cervical, cervicodorsal, cervicothoracic 847.0
    chondrocostal, without mention of injury to
        sternum 848.3
        involving sternum 848.42
    chondrosternal 848.42
    chronic (joint) - see Derangement, joint
    clavicle 840.9
    coccyx 847.4
    collar bone 840.9
    collateral, knee (medial) (tibial) 844.1
        lateral (fibular) 844.0
        recurrent or old 717.89
            lateral 717.81
            medial 717.82

SECTION I INDEX TO DISEASES AND INJURIES / Sprain, strain

Sprain, strain (Continued)
   coracoacromial 840.8
   coracoclavicular 840.1
   coracohumeral 840.2
   coracoid (process) 840.9
   coronary, knee 844.8
   costal cartilage, without mention of injury to sternum 848.3
      involving sternum 848.42
   cricoarytenoid articulation 848.2
   cricothyroid articulation 848.2
   cruciate
      knee 844.2
      old 717.89
         anterior 717.83
         posterior 717.84
   deltoid
      ankle 845.01
      shoulder 840.8
   dorsal (spine) 847.1
   ear cartilage 848.8
   elbow 841.9
      and forearm 841.9
      specified site NEC 841.8
   femur (proximal end) 843.9
      distal end 844.9
   fibula (proximal end) 844.9
      distal end 845.00
   fibulocalcaneal 845.02
   finger(s) 842.10
   foot 845.10
      and ankle 845.00
   forearm 841.9
      and elbow 841.9
      specified site NEC 841.8
   glenoid (shoulder) - (see also SLAP lesion) 840.8
   hand 842.10
   hip 843.9
      and thigh 843.9
   humerus (proximal end) 840.9
      distal end 841.9
   iliofemoral 843.0
   infraspinatus 840.3
   innominate
      acetabulum 843.9
      pubic junction 848.5
      sacral junction 846.1
   internal
      collateral, ankle 845.01
      semilunar cartilage 844.8
         with current tear (see also Tear, meniscus) 836.2
         old 717.5
   interphalangeal
      finger 842.13
      toe 845.13
   ischiocapsular 843.1
   jaw (cartilage) (meniscus) 848.1
      old 524.69
   knee 844.9
      and leg 844.9
      old 717.5
         collateral
            lateral 717.81
            medial 717.82
         cruciate
            anterior 717.83
            posterior 717.84
   late effect - see Late, effects (of), sprain
   lateral collateral, knee 844.0
      old 717.81
   leg 844.9
      and knee 844.9
   ligamentum teres femoris 843.8
   low back 846.9
   lumbar (spine) 847.2
   lumbosacral 846.0
      chronic or old 724.6
   mandible 848.1
      old 524.69

Sprain, strain (Continued)
   maxilla 848.1
   medial collateral, knee 844.1
      old 717.82
   meniscus
      jaw 848.1
         old 524.69
      knee 844.8
         with current tear (see also Tear, meniscus) 836.2
         old 717.5
      mandible 848.1
         old 524.69
      specified site NEC 848.8
   metacarpal 842.10
      distal 842.12
      proximal 842.11
   metacarpophalangeal 842.12
   metatarsal 845.10
   metatarsophalangeal 845.12
   midcarpal 842.19
   midtarsal 845.19
   multiple sites, except fingers alone or toes alone 848.8
   neck 847.0
   nose (septal cartilage) 848.0
   occiput from atlas 847.0
   old - see Derangement, joint
   orbicular, hip 843.8
   patella(r) 844.8
      old 717.89
   pelvis 848.5
   phalanx
      finger 842.10
      toe 845.10
   radiocarpal 842.02
   radiohumeral 841.2
   radioulnar 841.9
      distal 842.09
   radius, radial (proximal end) 841.9
      and ulna 841.9
         distal 842.09
      collateral 841.0
      distal end 842.00
   recurrent - see Sprain, by site
   rib (cage), without mention of injury to sternum 848.3
      involving sternum 848.42
   rotator cuff (capsule) 840.4
   round ligament - see also Injury, internal, round ligament
      femur 843.8
   sacral (spine) 847.3
   sacrococcygeal 847.3
   sacroiliac (region) 846.9
      chronic or old 724.6
      ligament 846.1
      specified site NEC 846.8
   sacrospinatus 846.2
   sacrospinous 846.2
   sacrotuberous 846.3
   scaphoid bone, ankle 845.00
   scapula(r) 840.9
   semilunar cartilage (knee) 844.8
      with current tear (see also Tear, meniscus) 836.2
      old 717.5
   septal cartilage (nose) 848.0
   shoulder 840.9
      and arm, upper 840.9
      blade 840.9
   specified site NEC 848.8
   spine 847.9
      cervical 847.0
      coccyx 847.4
      dorsal 847.1
      lumbar 847.2
      lumbosacral 846.0
         chronic or old 724.6
      sacral 847.3

Sprain, strain (Continued)
   spine (Continued)
      sacroiliac (see also Sprain, sacroiliac) 846.9
         chronic or old 724.6
      thoracic 847.1
   sternoclavicular 848.41
   sternum 848.40
   subglenoid - (see also SLAP lesion) 840.8
   subscapularis 840.5
   supraspinatus 840.6
   symphysis
      jaw 848.1
         old 524.69
      mandibular 848.1
         old 524.69
      pubis 848.5
   talofibular 845.09
   tarsal 845.10
   tarsometatarsal 845.11
   temporomandibular 848.1
      old 524.69
   teres
      ligamentum femoris 843.8
      major or minor 840.8
   thigh (proximal end) 843.9
      and hip 843.9
      distal end 844.9
   thoracic (spine) 847.1
   thorax 848.8
   thumb 842.10
   thyroid cartilage or region 848.2
   tibia (proximal end) 844.9
      distal end 845.00
   tibiofibular
      distal 845.03
      superior 844.3
   toe(s) 845.10
   trachea 848.8
   trapezoid 840.8
   ulna, ulnar (proximal end) 841.9
      collateral 841.1
      distal end 842.00
   ulnohumeral 841.3
   vertebrae (see also Sprain, spine) 847.9
      cervical, cervicodorsal, cervicothoracic 847.0
   wrist (cuneiform) (scaphoid) (semilunar) 842.00
   xiphoid cartilage 848.49

Sprengel's deformity (congenital) 755.52
Spring fever 309.23
Sprue 579.1
   celiac 579.0
   idiopathic 579.0
   meaning thrush 112.0
   nontropical 579.0
   tropical 579.1
Spur - see also Exostosis
   bone 726.91
      calcaneal 726.73
   calcaneal 726.73
   iliac crest 726.5
   nose (septum) 478.19
      bone 726.91
   septal 478.19
Spuria placenta - see Placenta, abnormal
Spurway's syndrome (brittle bones and blue sclera) 756.51
Sputum, abnormal (amount) (color) (excessive) (odor) (purulent) 786.4
   bloody 786.30
Squamous - see also condition
   cell metaplasia
      bladder 596.89
      cervix - see condition
   epithelium in
      cervical canal (congenital) 752.49
      uterine mucosa (congenital) 752.39
   metaplasia
      bladder 596.89
      cervix - see condition

SECTION I INDEX TO DISEASES AND INJURIES / Status

Squashed nose 738.0
  congenital 754.0
Squeeze, divers' 993.3
Squint (see also Strabismus) 378.9
  accommodative (see also Esotropia) 378.00
  concomitant (see also Heterotropia) 378.30
Stab - see also Wound, open, by site
  internal organs - see Injury, internal, by site, with open wound
Staggering gait 781.2
  hysterical 300.11
Staghorn calculus 592.0
Stähli's
  ear 744.29
  pigment line (cornea) 371.11
Stähli's pigment lines (cornea) 371.11
Stain, staining
  meconium 779.84
  port wine 757.32
  tooth, teeth (hard tissues) 521.7
    due to
      accretions 523.6
      deposits (betel) (black) (green) (materia alba) (orange) (tobacco) 523.6
      metals (copper) (silver) 521.7
      nicotine 523.6
      pulpal bleeding 521.7
      tobacco 523.6
Stammering (see also Disorder, fluency) 315.35
Standstill
  atrial 426.6
  auricular 426.6
  cardiac (see also Arrest, cardiac) 427.5
  sinoatrial 426.6
  sinus 426.6
  ventricular (see also Arrest, cardiac) 427.5
Stannosis 503
Stanton's disease (melioidosis) 025
Staphylitis (acute) (catarrhal) (chronic) (gangrenous) (membranous) (suppurative) (ulcerative) 528.3
Staphylococcemia 038.10
  aureus 038.11
  specified organism NEC 038.19
Staphylococcus, staphylococcal - see condition
Staphyloderma (skin) 686.00
Staphyloma 379.11
  anterior, localized 379.14
  ciliary 379.11
  cornea 371.73
  equatorial 379.13
  posterior 379.12
  posticum 379.12
  ring 379.15
  sclera NEC 379.11
Starch eating 307.52
Stargardt's disease 362.75
Starvation (inanition) (due to lack of food) 994.2
  edema 262
  voluntary NEC 307.1
Stasis
  bile (duct) (see also Disease, biliary) 576.8
  bronchus (see also Bronchitis) 490
  cardiac (see also Failure, heart) 428.0
  cecum 564.89
  colon 564.89
  dermatitis (see also Varix, with stasis dermatitis) 454.1
  duodenal 536.8
  eczema (see also Varix, with stasis dermatitis) 454.1
  edema (see also Hypertension, venous) 459.30
  foot 991.4
  gastric 536.3
  ileocecal coil 564.89
  ileum 564.89
  intestinal 564.89
  jejunum 564.89
  kidney 586
  liver 571.9
    cirrhotic - see Cirrhosis, liver

Stasis (Continued)
  lymphatic 457.8
  pneumonia 514
  portal 571.9
  pulmonary 514
  rectal 564.89
  renal 586
    tubular 584.5
  stomach 536.3
  ulcer
    with varicose veins 454.0
    without varicose veins 459.81
  urine NEC (see also Retention, urine) 788.20
  venous 459.81
State
  affective and paranoid, mixed, organic psychotic 294.8
  agitated 307.9
    acute reaction to stress 308.2
  anxiety (neurotic) (see also Anxiety) 300.00
    specified type NEC 300.09
  apprehension (see also Anxiety) 300.00
    specified type NEC 300.09
  climacteric, female 627.2
    following induced menopause 627.4
  clouded
    epileptic (see also Epilepsy) 345.9●
    paroxysmal (idiopathic) (see also Epilepsy) 345.9●
  compulsive (mixed) (with obsession) 300.3
  confusional 298.9
    acute 293.0
      with
        arteriosclerotic dementia 290.41
        presenile brain disease 290.11
        senility 290.3
    alcoholic 291.0
    drug-induced 292.81
    epileptic 293.0
    postoperative 293.9
    reactive (emotional stress) (psychological trauma) 298.2
    subacute 293.1
  constitutional psychopathic 301.9
  convulsive (see also Convulsions) 780.39
  depressive NEC 311
    induced by drug 292.84
    neurotic 300.4
  dissociative 300.15
  hallucinatory 780.1
    induced by drug 292.12
  hypercoagulable (primary) 289.81
    secondary 289.82
  hyperdynamic beta-adrenergic circulatory 429.82
  locked-in 344.81
  menopausal 627.2
    artificial 627.4
    following induced menopause 627.4
  neurotic NEC 300.9
    with depersonalization episode 300.6
  obsessional 300.3
  oneiroid (see also Schizophrenia) 295.4●
  panic 300.01
  paranoid 297.9
    alcohol-induced 291.5
    arteriosclerotic 290.42
    climacteric 297.2
    drug-induced 292.11
    in
      presenile brain disease 290.12
      senile brain disease 290.20
    involutional 297.2
    menopausal 297.2
    senile 290.20
    simple 297.0
  postleukotomy 310.0
  pregnant (see also Pregnancy) V22.2
  psychogenic, twilight 298.2

State (Continued)
  psychotic, organic (see also Psychosis, organic) 294.9
    mixed paranoid and affective 294.8
    senile or presenile NEC 290.9
    transient NEC 293.9
      with
        anxiety 293.84
        delusions 293.81
        depression 293.83
        hallucinations 293.82
  residual schizophrenic (see also Schizophrenia) 295.6●
  tension (see also Anxiety) 300.9
  transient organic psychotic 293.9
    anxiety type 293.84
    depressive type 293.83
    hallucinatory type 293.83
    paranoid type 293.81
    specified type NEC 293.89
  twilight
    epileptic 293.0
    psychogenic 298.2
  vegetative (persistent) 780.03
Status (post)
  absence
    epileptic (see also Epilepsy) 345.2
    of organ, acquired (postsurgical) - see Absence, by site, acquired
  administration of tPA (rtPA) in a different institution within the last 24 hours prior to admission to facility V45.88
  anastomosis of intestine (for bypass) V45.3
  anginosus 413.9
  angioplasty, percutaneous transluminal coronary V45.82
  ankle prosthesis V43.66
  aortocoronary bypass or shunt V45.81
  arthrodesis V45.4
  artificially induced condition NEC V45.89
  artificial opening (of) V44.9
    gastrointestinal tract NEC V44.4
    specified site NEC V44.8
    urinary tract NEC V44.6
    vagina V44.7
  aspirator V46.0
  asthmaticus (see also Asthma) 493.9●
  awaiting organ transplant V49.83
  bariatric surgery V45.86
    complicating pregnancy, childbirth, or the puerperium 649.2●
  bed confinement V49.84
  breast
    correction V43.82
    implant removal V45.83
    reconstruction V43.82
  cardiac
    device (in situ) V45.00
      carotid sinus V45.09
        fitting or adjustment V53.39
      defibrillator, automatic implantable (with synchronous cardiac pacemaker) V45.02
      pacemaker V45.01
        fitting or adjustment V53.31
  carotid sinus stimulator V45.09
  cataract extraction V45.61
  chemotherapy V66.2
    current V58.69
  circumcision, female 629.20
  clitorectomy (female genital mutilation type I) 629.21
    with excision of labia minora (female genital mutilation type II) 629.22
  colonization - see Carrier (suspected) of
  colostomy V44.3
  contraceptive device V45.59
    intrauterine V45.51
    subdermal V45.52
  convulsivus idiopathicus (see also Epilepsy) 345.3

SECTION I INDEX TO DISEASES AND INJURIES / Status

Status (Continued)
- coronary artery bypass or shunt V45.81
- cutting
  - female genital 629.20
    - specified NEC 629.29
    - type I 629.21
    - type II 629.22
    - type III 629.23
    - type IV 629.29
- cystostomy V44.50
  - appendico-vesicostomy V44.52
  - cutaneous-vesicostomy V44.51
  - specifed type NEC V44.59
- defibrillator, automatic implantable cardiac (with synchronous cardiac pacemaker) V45.02
- delinquent immunization V15.83
- dental crowns V45.84
- dental fillings V45.84
- dental restoration V45.84
- dental sealant V49.82
- dialysis (hemo) (peritoneal) V45.11
- donor V59.9
- do not resuscitate V49.86
- drug therapy or regimen V67.59
  - high-risk medication NEC V67.51
- elbow prosthesis V43.62
- embedded
  - fragment - see Foreign body, retained
  - splinter - see Foreign body, retained
- enterostomy V44.4
- epileptic, epilepticus (absence) (grand mal) (see also Epilepsy) 345.3
  - focal motor 345.7 ●
  - partial 345.7 ●
  - petit mal 345.2
  - psychomotor 345.7 ●
  - temporal lobe 345.7 ●
- estrogen receptor
  - negative [ER-] V86.1
  - positive [ER+] V86.0
- explantation of joint prosthesis NEC V88.29
  - hip V88.21
  - knee V88.22
- eye (adnexa) surgery V45.69
- female genital
  - cutting 629.20
    - specified NEC 629.29
    - type I 629.21
    - type II 629.22
    - type III 629.23
    - type IV 629.29
  - mutilation 629.20
    - type I 629.21
    - type II 629.22
    - type III 629.23
    - type IV 629.29
- filtering bleb (eye) (postglaucoma) V45.69
  - with rupture or complication 997.99
  - postcataract extraction (complication) 997.99
- finger joint prosthesis V43.69
- foster care V60.81
- gastric
  - banding V45.86
    - complicating pregnancy, childbirth, or the puerperium 649.2 ●
  - bypass for obesity V45.86
    - complicating pregnancy, childbirth, or the puerperium 649.2 ●
- gastrostomy V44.1
- grand mal 345.3
- heart valve prosthesis V43.3
- hemodialysis V45.11
- hip prosthesis (joint) (partial) (total) V43.64
  - explantation V88.21
- hysterectomy V88.01
  - partial with remaining cervical stump V88.02
  - total V88.01
- ileostomy V44.2

Status (Continued)
- infibulation (female genital mutilation type III) 629.23
- insulin pump V45.85
- intestinal bypass V45.3
- intrauterine contraceptive device V45.51
- jejunostomy V44.4
- joint prosthesis NEC V43.69
  - explantation V88.29
- knee joint prosthesis V43.65
  - explantation V88.22
- lacunaris 437.8
- lacunosis 437.8
- lapsed immunization schedule V15.83
- low birth weight V21.30
  - less than 500 grams V21.31
  - 500–999 grams V21.32
  - 1000–1499 grams V21.33
  - 1500–1999 grams V21.34
  - 2000–2500 grams V21.35
- lymphaticus 254.8
- malignant neoplasm, ablated or excised - see History, malignant neoplasm
- marmoratus 333.79
- military deployment V62.22
- mutilation, female 629.20
  - type I 629.21
  - type II 629.22
  - type III 629.23
  - type IV 629.29
- nephrostomy V44.6
- neuropacemaker NEC V45.89
  - brain V45.89
  - carotid sinus V45.09
  - neurologic NEC V45.89
- obesity surgery V45.86
  - complicating pregnancy, childbirth, or the puerperium 649.2 ●
- organ replacement
  - by artificial or mechanical device or prosthesis of
    - artery V43.4
    - artificial skin V43.83
    - bladder V43.5
    - blood vessel V43.4
    - breast V43.82
    - eye globe V43.0
    - heart
      - assist device V43.21
      - fully implantable artificial heart V43.22
      - valve V43.3
    - intestine V43.89
    - joint V43.60
      - ankle V43.66
      - elbow V43.62
      - finger V43.69
      - hip (partial) (total) V43.64
      - knee V43.65
      - shoulder V43.61
      - specified NEC V43.69
      - wrist V43.63
    - kidney V43.89
    - larynx V43.81
    - lens V43.1
    - limb(s) V43.7
    - liver V43.89
    - lung V43.89
    - organ NEC V43.89
    - pancreas V43.89
    - skin (artificial) V43.83
    - tissue NEC V43.89
    - vein V43.4
  - by organ transplant (heterologous) (homologous) - see Status, transplant
- pacemaker
  - brain V45.89
  - cardiac V45.01
  - carotid sinus V45.09

Status (Continued)
- pacemaker (Continued)
  - neurologic NEC V45.89
  - specified site NEC V45.89
- percutaneous transluminal coronary angioplasty V45.82
- peritoneal dialysis V45.11
- petit mal 345.2
- physical restraints V49.87
- postcommotio cerebri 310.2
- postmenopausal (age related) (natural) V49.81
- postoperative NEC V45.89
- postpartum NEC V24.2
  - care immediately following delivery V24.0
  - routine follow-up V24.2
- postsurgical NEC V45.89
- renal dialysis V45.11
  - noncompliance V45.12
- respirator [ventilator] V46.11
  - encounter
    - during
      - mechanical failure V46.14
      - power failure V46.12
    - for weaning V46.13
- retained foreign body - see Foreign body, retained
- reversed jejunal transposition (for bypass) V45.3
- sex reassignment surgery (see also Transsexualism) 302.50
- shoulder prosthesis V43.61
- shunt
  - aortocoronary bypass V45.81
  - arteriovenous (for dialysis) V45.11
  - cerebrospinal fluid V45.2
  - vascular NEC V45.89
    - aortocoronary (bypass) V45.81
  - ventricular (communicating) (for drainage) V45.2
- sterilization
  - tubal ligation V26.51
  - vasectomy V26.52
- subdermal contraceptive device V45.52
- thymicolymphaticus 254.8
- thymicus 254.8
- thymolymphaticus 254.8
- tooth extraction 525.10
- tracheostomy V44.0
- transplant
  - blood vessel V42.89
  - bone V42.4
    - marrow V42.81
  - cornea V42.5
  - heart V42.1
    - valve V42.2
  - intestine V42.84
  - kidney V42.0
  - liver V42.7
  - lung V42.6
  - organ V42.9
    - removal (due to complication, failure, rejection or infection) V45.87
    - specified site NEC V42.89
  - pancreas V42.83
  - peripheral stem cells V42.82
  - skin V42.3
  - stem cells, peripheral V42.82
  - tissue V42.9
    - specified type NEC V42.89
  - vessel, blood V42.89
- tubal ligation V26.51
- underimmunization V15.83
- ureterostomy V44.6
- urethrostomy V44.6
- vagina, artificial V44.7
- vascular shunt NEC V45.89
  - aortocoronary (bypass) V45.81
- vasectomy V26.52

Status (Continued)
　　ventilator [respirator] V46.11
　　　encounter
　　　　during
　　　　　mechanical failure V46.14
　　　　　power failure V46.12
　　　　for weaning V46.13
　　wheelchair confinement V46.3
　　wrist prosthesis V43.63
Stave fracture - see Fracture, metacarpus, metacarpal bone(s)
Steal
　　subclavian artery 435.2
　　vertebral artery 435.1
Stealing, solitary, child problem (see also Disturbance, conduct) 312.1●
Steam burn - see Burn, by site
Steatocystoma multiplex 706.2
Steatoma (infected) 706.2
　　eyelid (cystic) 374.84
　　　infected 373.13
Steatorrhea (chronic) 579.8
　　with lacteal obstruction 579.2
　　idiopathic 579.0
　　　adult 579.0
　　　infantile 579.0
　　pancreatic 579.4
　　primary 579.0
　　secondary 579.8
　　specified cause NEC 579.8
　　tropical 579.1
Steatosis 272.8
　　heart (see also Degeneration, myocardial) 429.1
　　kidney 593.89
　　liver 571.8
Steele-Richardson (-Olszewski) syndrome 333.0
Stein's syndrome (polycystic ovary) 256.4
Stein-Leventhal syndrome (polycystic ovary) 256.4
Steinbrocker's syndrome (see also Neuropathy, peripheral, autonomic) 337.9
Steinert's disease 359.21
STEMI (ST elevation myocardial infarction) (see also - Infarct, myocardium, ST elevation) 410.9●
Stenocardia (see also Angina) 413.9
Stenocephaly 756.0
Stenosis (cicatricial) - see also Stricture
　　ampulla of Vater 576.2
　　　with calculus, cholelithiasis, or stones - see Choledocholithiasis
　　anus, anal (canal) (sphincter) 569.2
　　　congenital 751.2
　　aorta (ascending) 747.22
　　　arch 747.10
　　　arteriosclerotic 440.0
　　　calcified 440.0
　　aortic (valve) 424.1
　　　with
　　　　mitral (valve)
　　　　　insufficiency or incompetence 396.2
　　　　　stenosis or obstruction 396.0
　　　atypical 396.0
　　　congenital 746.3
　　　rheumatic 395.0
　　　　with
　　　　　insufficiency, incompetency or regurgitation 395.2
　　　　　　with mitral (valve) disease 396.8
　　　　　mitral (valve)
　　　　　　disease (stenosis) 396.0
　　　　　　insufficiency or incompetence 396.2
　　　　　　stenosis or obstruction 396.0
　　　specified cause, except rheumatic 424.1
　　　syphilitic 093.22
　　aqueduct of Sylvius (congenital) 742.3
　　　with spina bifida (see also Spina bifida) 741.0●
　　　acquired 331.4

Stenosis (Continued)
　　artery NEC (see also Arteriosclerosis) 447.1
　　　basilar - see Narrowing, artery, basilar
　　　carotid (common) (internal) - see Narrowing, artery, carotid
　　　celiac 447.4
　　　cerebral 437.0
　　　　due to
　　　　　embolism (see also Embolism, brain) 434.1●
　　　　　thrombus (see also Thrombosis, brain) 434.0●
　　　extremities 440.20
　　　precerebral - see Narrowing, artery, precerebral
　　　pulmonary (congenital) 747.31
　　　　acquired 417.8
　　　renal 440.1
　　　vertebral - see Narrowing, artery, vertebral
　　bile duct or biliary passage (see also Obstruction, biliary) 576.2
　　　congenital 751.61
　　bladder neck (acquired) 596.0
　　　congenital 753.6
　　brain 348.89
　　bronchus 519.19
　　　syphilitic 095.8
　　cardia (stomach) 537.89
　　　congenital 750.7
　　cardiovascular (see also Disease, cardiovascular) 429.2
　　carotid artery - see Narrowing, artery, carotid
　　cervix, cervical (canal) 622.4
　　　congenital 752.49
　　　in pregnancy or childbirth 654.6●
　　　　affecting fetus or newborn 763.89
　　　　causing obstructed labor 660.2●
　　　　　affecting fetus or newborn 763.1
　　colon (see also Obstruction, intestine) 560.9
　　　congenital 751.2
　　colostomy 569.62
　　common bile duct (see also Obstruction, biliary) 576.2
　　　congenital 751.61
　　coronary (artery) - see Arteriosclerosis, coronary
　　cystic duct (see also Obstruction, gallbladder) 575.2
　　　congenital 751.61
　　due to (presence of) any device, implant, or graft classifiable to 996.0–996.5 - see Complications, due to (presence of) any device, implant, or graft classified to 996.0–996.5 NEC
　　duodenum 537.3
　　　congenital 751.1
　　ejaculatory duct NEC 608.89
　　endocervical os - see Stenosis, cervix
　　enterostomy 569.62
　　esophagostomy 530.87
　　esophagus 530.3
　　　congenital 750.3
　　　syphilitic 095.8
　　　　congenital 090.5
　　external ear canal 380.50
　　　secondary to
　　　　inflammation 380.53
　　　　surgery 380.52
　　　　trauma 380.51
　　gallbladder (see also Obstruction, gallbladder) 575.2
　　glottis 478.74
　　heart valve (acquired) - see also Endocarditis
　　　congenital NEC 746.89
　　　　aortic 746.3
　　　　mitral 746.5
　　　　pulmonary 746.02
　　　　tricuspid 746.1
　　hepatic duct (see also Obstruction, biliary) 576.2
　　hymen 623.3

Stenosis (Continued)
　　hypertrophic subaortic (idiopathic) 425.11
　　infundibulum cardiac 746.83
　　intestine (see also Obstruction, intestine) 560.9
　　　congenital (small) 751.1
　　　　large 751.2
　　lacrimal
　　　canaliculi 375.53
　　　duct 375.56
　　　　congenital 743.65
　　　punctum 375.52
　　　　congenital 743.65
　　　sac 375.54
　　　　congenital 743.65
　　lacrimonasal duct 375.56
　　　congenital 743.65
　　　neonatal 375.55
　　larynx 478.74
　　　congenital 748.3
　　　syphilitic 095.8
　　　　congenital 090.5
　　mitral (valve) (chronic) (inactive) 394.0
　　　with
　　　　aortic (valve)
　　　　　disease (insufficiency) 396.1
　　　　　insufficiency or incompetence 396.1
　　　　　stenosis or obstruction 396.0
　　　　incompetency, insufficiency or regurgitation 394.2
　　　　　with aortic valve disease 396.8
　　　active or acute 391.1
　　　　with chorea (acute) (rheumatic) (Sydenham's) 392.0
　　　congenital 746.5
　　　specified cause, except rheumatic 424.0
　　　syphilitic 093.21
　　myocardium, myocardial (see also Degeneration, myocardial) 429.1
　　　hypertrophic subaortic (idiopathic) 425.11
　　nares (anterior) (posterior) 478.19
　　　congenital 748.0
　　nasal duct 375.56
　　　congenital 743.65
　　nasolacrimal duct 375.56
　　　congenital 743.65
　　　neonatal 375.55
　　organ or site, congenital NEC - see Atresia
　　papilla of Vater 576.2
　　　with calculus, cholelithiasis, or stones - see Choledocholithiasis
　　pulmonary (artery) (congenital) 747.31
　　　with ventricular septal defect, dextraposition of aorta and hypertrophy of right ventricle 745.2
　　　acquired 417.8
　　　infundibular 746.83
　　　in tetralogy of Fallot 745.2
　　　subvalvular 746.83
　　　valve (see also Endocarditis, pulmonary) 424.3
　　　　congenital 746.02
　　　vein 747.49
　　　　acquired 417.8
　　　vessel NEC 417.8
　　pulmonic (congenital) 746.02
　　　infundibular 746.83
　　　subvalvular 746.83
　　pylorus (hypertrophic) 537.0
　　　adult 537.0
　　　congenital 750.5
　　　infantile 750.5
　　rectum (sphincter) (see also Stricture, rectum) 569.2
　　renal artery 440.1
　　salivary duct (any) 527.8
　　sphincter of Oddi (see also Obstruction, biliary) 576.2

SECTION 1 INDEX TO DISEASES AND INJURIES / Stenosis

Stenosis (Continued)
  spinal 724.00
    cervical 723.0
    lumbar, lumbosacral (without neurogenic claudication) 724.02
      with neurogenic claudication 724.03
    nerve (root) NEC 724.9
    specified region NEC 724.09
    thoracic, thoracolumbar 724.01
  stomach, hourglass 537.6
  subaortic 746.81
    hypertrophic (idiopathic) 425.11
  supra (valvular)-aortic 747.22
  trachea 519.19
    congenital 748.3
    syphilitic 095.8
    tuberculous (see also Tuberculosis) 012.8●
  tracheostomy 519.02
  tricuspid (valve) (see also Endocarditis, tricuspid) 397.0
    congenital 746.1
    nonrheumatic 424.2
  tubal 628.2
  ureter (see also Stricture, ureter) 593.3
    congenital 753.29
  urethra (see also Stricture, urethra) 598.9
  vagina 623.2
    congenital 752.49
    in pregnancy or childbirth 654.7●
      affecting fetus or newborn 763.89
      causing obstructed labor 660.2●
        affecting fetus or newborn 763.1
  valve (cardiac) (heart) (see also Endocarditis) 424.90
    congenital NEC 746.89
      aortic 746.3
      mitral 746.5
      pulmonary 746.02
      tricuspid 746.1
      urethra 753.6
  valvular (see also Endocarditis) 424.90
    congenital NEC 746.89
      urethra 753.6
  vascular graft or shunt 996.1
    atherosclerosis - see Arteriosclerosis, extremities
    embolism 996.74
    occlusion NEC 996.74
    thrombus 996.74
  vena cava (inferior) (superior) 459.2
    congenital 747.49
  ventricular shunt 996.2
  vulva 624.8
Stent jail 996.72
Stercolith (see also Fecalith) 560.32
  appendix 543.9
Stercoraceous, stercoral ulcer 569.82
  anus or rectum 569.41
Stereopsis, defective
  with fusion 368.33
  without fusion 368.32
Stereotypies NEC 307.3
Sterility
  female - see Infertility, female
  male (see also Infertility, male) 606.9
Sterilization, admission for V25.2
  status
    tubal ligation V26.51
    vasectomy V26.52
Sternalgia (see also Angina) 413.9
Sternopagus 759.4
Sternum bifidum 756.3
Sternutation 784.99
Steroid
  effects (adverse) (iatrogenic)
    cushingoid
      correct substance properly administered 255.0
      overdose or wrong substance given or taken 962.0

Steroid (Continued)
  effects (Continued)
    diabetes - see Diabetes, secondary
      correct substance properly administered 251.8
      overdose or wrong substance given or taken 962.0
    due to
      correct substance properly administered 255.8
      overdose or wrong substance given or taken 962.0
    fever
      correct substance properly administered 780.60
      overdose or wrong substance given or taken 962.0
    withdrawal
      correct substance properly administered 255.41
      overdose or wrong substance given or taken 962.0
  responder 365.03
Stevens-Johnson disease or syndrome (erythema multiforme exudativum) 695.13
  toxic epidermal necrolysis overlap (SJS-TEN overlap syndrome) 695.14
Stewart-Morel syndrome (hyperostosis frontalis interna) 733.3
Sticker's disease (erythema infectiosum) 057.0
Stickler syndrome 759.89
Sticky eye 372.03
Stieda's disease (calcification, knee joint) 726.62
Stiff
  back 724.8
  neck (see also Torticollis) 723.5
Stiff-baby 759.89
Stiff-man syndrome 333.91
Stiffness, joint NEC 719.50
  ankle 719.57
  back 724.8
  elbow 719.52
  finger 719.54
  hip 719.55
  knee 719.56
  multiple sites 719.59
  sacroiliac 724.6
  shoulder 719.51
  specified site NEC 719.58
  spine 724.9
  surgical fusion V45.4
  wrist 719.53
Stigmata, congenital syphilis 090.5
Still's disease or syndrome 714.30
  adult onset 714.2
Still-Felty syndrome (rheumatoid arthritis with splenomegaly and leukopenia) 714.1
Stillbirth, stillborn NEC 779.9
Stiller's disease (asthenia) 780.79
Stilling-Türk-Duane syndrome (ocular retraction syndrome) 378.71
Stimulation, ovary 256.1
Sting (animal) (bee) (fish) (insect) (jellyfish) (Portuguese man-o-war) (wasp) (venomous) 989.5
  anaphylactic shock or reaction 989.5
  plant 692.6
Stippled epiphyses 756.59
Stitch
  abscess 998.59
  burst (in external operation wound) (see also Dehiscence) 998.32
    internal 998.31
  in back 724.5
Stojano's (subcostal) syndrome 098.86
Stokes' disease (exophthalmic goiter) 242.0●
Stokes-Adams syndrome (syncope with heart block) 426.9
Stokvis' (-Talma) disease (enterogenous cyanosis) 289.7

Stomach - see condition
Stoma malfunction
  colostomy 569.62
  cystostomy 596.82
    infection 596.81
    mechanical 596.82
    specified complication NEC 596.83
  enterostomy 569.62
  esophagostomy 530.87
  gastrostomy 536.42
  ileostomy 569.62
  nephrostomy 997.5
  tracheostomy 519.02
  ureterostomy 997.5
Stomatitis 528.00
  angular 528.5
    due to dietary or vitamin deficiency 266.0
  aphthous 528.2
  bovine 059.11
  candidal 112.0
  catarrhal 528.00
  denture 528.9
  diphtheritic (membranous) 032.0
  due to
    dietary deficiency 266.0
    thrush 112.0
    vitamin deficiency 266.0
  epidemic 078.4
  epizootic 078.4
  follicular 528.00
  gangrenous 528.1
  herpetic 054.2
  herpetiformis 528.2
  malignant 528.00
  membranous acute 528.00
  monilial 112.0
  mycotic 112.0
  necrotic 528.1
    ulcerative 101
  necrotizing ulcerative 101
  parasitic 112.0
  septic 528.00
  specified NEC 528.09
  spirochetal 101
  suppurative (acute) 528.00
  ulcerative 528.00
    necrotizing 101
  ulceromembranous 101
  vesicular 528.00
    with exanthem 074.3
  Vincent's 101
Stomatocytosis 282.8
Stomatomycosis 112.0
Stomatorrhagia 528.9
Stone(s) - see also Calculus
  bladder 594.1
    diverticulum 594.0
  cystine 270.0
  heart syndrome (see also Failure, ventricular, left) 428.1
  kidney 592.0
  prostate 602.0
  pulp (dental) 522.2
  renal 592.0
  salivary duct or gland (any) 527.5
  ureter 592.1
  urethra (impacted) 594.2
  urinary (duct) (impacted) (passage) 592.9
    bladder 594.1
      diverticulum 594.0
    lower tract NEC 594.9
    specified site 594.8
  xanthine 277.2
Stonecutters' lung 502
  tuberculous (see also Tuberculosis) 011.4●
Stonemasons'
  asthma, disease, or lung 502
    tuberculous (see also Tuberculosis) 011.4●
  phthisis (see also Tuberculosis) 011.4●

Stoppage
  bowel (*see also* Obstruction, intestine) 560.9
  heart (*see also* Arrest, cardiac) 427.5
  intestine (*see also* Obstruction, intestine) 560.9
  urine NEC (*see also* Retention, urine) 788.20
Storm, thyroid (apathetic) (*see also* Thyrotoxicosis) 242.9●
Strabismus (alternating) (congenital) (nonparalytic) 378.9
  concomitant (*see also* Heterotropia) 378.30
    convergent (*see also* Esotropia) 378.00
    divergent (*see also* Exotropia) 378.10
  convergent (*see also* Esotropia) 378.00
  divergent (*see also* Exotropia) 378.10
  due to adhesions, scars - *see* Strabismus, mechanical
  in neuromuscular disorder NEC 378.73
    intermittent 378.20
      vertical 378.31
  latent 378.40
    convergent (esophoria) 378.41
    divergent (exophoria) 378.42
    vertical 378.43
  mechanical 378.60
    due to
      Brown's tendon sheath syndrome 378.61
      specified musculofascial disorder NEC 378.62
  paralytic 378.50
    third or oculomotor nerve (partial) 378.51
      total 378.52
    fourth or trochlear nerve 378.53
    sixth or abducens nerve 378.54
  specified type NEC 378.73
  vertical (hypertropia) 378.31
Strain - *see also* Sprain, by site
  eye NEC 368.13
  heart - *see* Disease, heart
  meaning gonorrhea - *see* Gonorrhea
  on urination 788.65
  physical NEC V62.89
  postural 729.90
  psychological NEC V62.89
Strands
  conjunctiva 372.62
  vitreous humor 379.25
Strangulation, strangulated 994.7
  appendix 543.9
  asphyxiation or suffocation by 994.7
  bladder neck 596.0
  bowel - *see* Strangulation, intestine
  colon - *see* Strangulation, intestine
  cord (umbilical) - *see* Compression, umbilical cord
  due to birth injury 767.8
  food or foreign body (*see also* Asphyxia, food) 933.1
  hemorrhoids 455.8
    external 455.5
    internal 455.2
  hernia - *see also* Hernia, by site, with obstruction
    gangrenous - *see* Hernia, by site, with gangrene
  intestine (large) (small) 560.2
    with hernia - *see also* Hernia, by site, with obstruction
      gangrenous - *see* Hernia, by site, with gangrene
    congenital (small) 751.1
      large 751.2
  mesentery 560.2
  mucus (*see also* Asphyxia, mucus) 933.1
    newborn 770.18
  omentum 560.2
  organ or site, congenital NEC - *see* Atresia
  ovary 620.8
    due to hernia 620.4
  penis 607.89
    foreign body 939.3

Strangulation, strangulated (*Continued*)
  rupture (*see also* Hernia, by site, with obstruction) 552.9
    gangrenous (*see also* Hernia, by site, with gangrene) 551.9
  stomach, due to hernia (*see also* Hernia, by site, with obstruction) 552.9
    with gangrene (*see also* Hernia, by site, with gangrene) 551.9
  umbilical cord - *see* Compression, umbilical cord
  vesicourethral orifice 596.0
Strangury 788.1
Strawberry
  gallbladder (*see also* Disease, gallbladder) 575.6
  mark 757.32
  tongue (red) (white) 529.3
Straw itch 133.8
Streak, ovarian 752.0
Strephosymbolia 315.01
  secondary to organic lesion 784.69
Streptobacillary fever 026.1
Streptobacillus moniliformis 026.1
Streptococcemia 038.0
Streptococcicosis - *see* Infection, streptococcal
Streptococcus, streptococcal - *see* condition
Streptoderma 686.00
Streptomycosis - *see* Actinomycosis
Streptothricosis - *see* Actinomycosis
Streptothrix - *see* Actinomycosis
Streptotrichosis - *see* Actinomycosis
Stress 308.9
  fracture - *see* Fracture, stress
  polycythemia 289.0
  reaction (gross) (*see also* Reaction, stress, acute) 308.9
Stretching, nerve - *see* Injury, nerve, by site
Striae (albicantes) (atrophicae) (cutis distensae) (distensae) 701.3
Striations of nails 703.8
Stricture (*see also* Stenosis) 799.89
  ampulla of Vater 576.2
    with calculus, cholelithiasis, or stones - *see* Choledocholithiasis
  anus (sphincter) 569.2
    congenital 751.2
    infantile 751.2
  aorta (ascending) 747.22
    arch 747.10
    arteriosclerotic 440.0
    calcified 440.0
  aortic (valve) (*see also* Stenosis, aortic) 424.1
    congenital 746.3
  aqueduct of Sylvius (congenital) 742.3
    with spina bifida (*see also* Spina bifida) 741.0●
    acquired 331.4
  artery 447.1
    basilar - *see* Narrowing, artery, basilar
    carotid (common) (internal) - *see* Narrowing, artery, carotid
    celiac 447.4
    cerebral 437.0
      congenital 747.81
      due to
        embolism (*see also* Embolism, brain) 434.1●
        thrombus (*see also* Thrombosis, brain) 434.0●
    congenital (peripheral) 747.60
      cerebral 747.81
      coronary 746.85
      gastrointestinal 747.61
      lower limb 747.64
      renal 747.62
      retinal 743.58
      specified NEC 747.69
      spinal 747.82
      umbilical 747.5
      upper limb 747.63

Stricture (*Continued*)
  artery (*Continued*)
    coronary - *see* Arteriosclerosis, coronary
      congenital 746.85
    precerebral - *see* Narrowing, artery, precerebral NEC
    pulmonary (congenital) 747.31
      acquired 417.8
    renal 440.1
    vertebral - *see* Narrowing, artery, vertebral
  auditory canal (congenital) (external) 744.02
    acquired (*see also* Stricture, ear canal, acquired) 380.50
  bile duct or passage (any) (postoperative) (*see also* Obstruction, biliary) 576.2
    congenital 751.61
  bladder 596.89
    congenital 753.6
    neck 596.0
      congenital 753.6
  bowel (*see also* Obstruction, intestine) 560.9
  brain 348.89
  bronchus 519.19
    syphilitic 095.8
  cardia (stomach) 537.89
    congenital 750.7
  cardiac - *see also* Disease, heart orifice (stomach) 537.89
  cardiovascular (*see also* Disease, cardiovascular) 429.2
  carotid artery - *see* Narrowing, artery, carotid
  cecum (*see also* Obstruction, intestine) 560.9
  cervix, cervical (canal) 622.4
    congenital 752.49
    in pregnancy or childbirth 654.6●
      affecting fetus or newborn 763.89
      causing obstructed labor 660.2●
        affecting fetus or newborn 763.1
  colon (*see also* Obstruction, intestine) 560.9
    congenital 751.2
  colostomy 569.62
  common bile duct (*see also* Obstruction, biliary) 576.2
    congenital 751.61
  coronary (artery) - *see* Arteriosclerosis, coronary
    congenital 746.85
  cystic duct (*see also* Obstruction, gallbladder) 575.2
    congenital 751.61
  cystostomy 596.83
  digestive organs NEC, congenital 751.8
  duodenum 537.3
    congenital 751.1
  ear canal (external) (congenital) 744.02
    acquired 380.50
      secondary to
        inflammation 380.53
        surgery 380.52
        trauma 380.51
  ejaculatory duct 608.85
  enterostomy 569.62
  esophagostomy 530.87
  esophagus (corrosive) (peptic) 530.3
    congenital 750.3
    syphilitic 095.8
      congenital 090.5
  Eustachian tube (*see also* Obstruction, Eustachian tube) 381.60
    congenital 744.24
  fallopian tube 628.2
    gonococcal (chronic) 098.37
      acute 098.17
    tuberculous (*see also* Tuberculosis) 016.6●
  gallbladder (*see also* Obstruction, gallbladder) 575.2
    congenital 751.69
  glottis 478.74

 New   Revised   ~~deleted~~ Deleted   ● Use Additional Digit(s)   Omit code

Stricture (Continued)
  heart - see also Disease, heart
    congenital NEC 746.89
    valve - see also Endocarditis
      congenital NEC 746.89
        aortic 746.3
        mitral 746.5
        pulmonary 746.02
        tricuspid 746.1
  hepatic duct (see also Obstruction, biliary) 576.2
  hourglass, of stomach 537.6
  hymen 623.3
  hypopharynx 478.29
  intestine (see also Obstruction, intestine) 560.9
    congenital (small) 751.1
      large 751.2
    ischemic 557.1
  lacrimal
    canaliculi 375.53
      congenital 743.65
    punctum 375.52
      congenital 743.65
    sac 375.54
      congenital 743.65
  lacrimonasal duct 375.56
    congenital 743.65
    neonatal 375.55
  larynx 478.79
    congenital 748.3
    syphilitic 095.8
      congenital 090.5
  lung 518.89
  meatus
    ear (congenital) 744.02
      acquired (see also Stricture, ear canal, acquired) 380.50
    osseous (congenital) (ear) 744.03
      acquired (see also Stricture, ear canal, acquired) 380.50
    urinarius (see also Stricture, urethra) 598.9
      congenital 753.6
  mitral (valve) (see also Stenosis, mitral) 394.0
    congenital 746.5
    specified cause, except rheumatic 424.0
  myocardium, myocardial (see also Degeneration, myocardial) 429.1
    hypertrophic subaortic (idiopathic) 425.11
  nares (anterior) (posterior) 478.19
    congenital 748.0
  nasal duct 375.56
    congenital 743.65
    neonatal 375.55
  nasolacrimal duct 375.56
    congenital 743.65
    neonatal 375.55
  nasopharynx 478.29
    syphilitic 095.8
  nephrostomy 997.5
  nose 478.19
    congenital 748.0
  nostril (anterior) (posterior) 478.19
    congenital 748.0
  organ or site, congenital NEC - see Atresia
  osseous meatus (congenital) (ear) 744.03
    acquired (see also Stricture, ear canal, acquired) 380.50
  os uteri (see also Stricture, cervix) 622.4
  oviduct - see Stricture, fallopian tube
  pelviureteric junction 593.3
  pharynx (dilation) 478.29
  prostate 602.8
  pulmonary, pulmonic
    artery (congenital) 747.31
      acquired 417.8
      noncongenital 417.8
    infundibulum (congenital) 746.83
    valve (see also Endocarditis, pulmonary) 424.3
      congenital 746.02

Stricture (Continued)
  pulmonary, pulmonic (Continued)
    vein (congenital) 747.49
      acquired 417.8
    vessel NEC 417.8
  punctum lacrimale 375.52
    congenital 743.65
  pylorus (hypertrophic) 537.0
    adult 537.0
    congenital 750.5
    infantile 750.5
  rectosigmoid 569.89
  rectum (sphincter) 569.2
    congenital 751.2
    due to
      chemical burn 947.3
      irradiation 569.2
      lymphogranuloma venereum 099.1
    gonococcal 098.7
    inflammatory 099.1
    syphilitic 095.8
    tuberculous (see also Tuberculosis) 014.8 ●
  renal artery 440.1
  salivary duct or gland (any) 527.8
  sigmoid (flexure) (see also Obstruction, intestine) 560.9
  spermatic cord 608.85
  stoma (following) (of)
    colostomy 569.62
    cystostomy 596.83
    enterostomy 569.62
    esophagostomy 530.87
    gastrostomy 536.42
    ileostomy 569.62
    nephrostomy 997.5
    tracheostomy 519.02
    ureterostomy 997.5
  stomach 537.89
    congenital 750.7
    hourglass 537.6
  subaortic 746.81
    hypertrophic (acquired) (idiopathic) 425.11
  subglottic 478.74
  syphilitic NEC 095.8
  tendon (sheath) 727.81
  trachea 519.19
    congenital 748.3
    syphilitic 095.8
    tuberculous (see also Tuberculosis) 012.8 ●
  tracheostomy 519.02
  tricuspid (valve) (see also Endocarditis, tricuspid) 397.0
    congenital 746.1
    nonrheumatic 424.2
  tunica vaginalis 608.85
  ureter (postoperative) 593.3
    congenital 753.29
    tuberculous (see also Tuberculosis) 016.2 ●
  ureteropelvic junction 593.3
    congenital 753.21
  ureterovesical orifice 593.3
    congenital 753.22
  urethra (anterior) (meatal) (organic) (posterior) (spasmodic) 598.9
    associated with schistosomiasis (see also Schistosomiasis) 120.9 [598.01]
    congenital (valvular) 753.6
    due to
      infection 598.00
        syphilis 095.8 [598.01]
      trauma 598.1
    gonococcal 098.2 [598.01]
    gonorrheal 098.2 [598.01]
    infective 598.00
    late effect of injury 598.1
    postcatheterization 598.2
    postobstetric 598.1
    postoperative 598.2
    specified cause NEC 598.8
    syphilitic 095.8 [598.01]

Stricture (Continued)
  urethra (Continued)
    traumatic 598.1
    valvular, congenital 753.6
  urinary meatus (see also Stricture, urethra) 598.9
    congenital 753.6
  uterus, uterine 621.5
    os (external) (internal) - see Stricture, cervix
  vagina (outlet) 623.2
    congenital 752.49
  valve (cardiac) (heart) (see also Endocarditis) 424.90
    congenital (cardiac) (heart) NEC 746.89
      aortic 746.3
      mitral 746.5
      pulmonary 746.02
      tricuspid 746.1
      urethra 753.6
  valvular (see also Endocarditis) 424.90
  vascular graft or shunt 996.1
    atherosclerosis - see Arteriosclerosis, extremities
    embolism 996.74
    occlusion NEC 996.74
    thrombus 996.74
  vas deferens 608.85
    congenital 752.89
  vein 459.2
  vena cava (inferior) (superior) NEC 459.2
    congenital 747.49
  ventricular shunt 996.2
  vesicourethral orifice 596.0
    congenital 753.6
  vulva (acquired) 624.8
Stridor 786.1
  congenital (larynx) 748.3
Stridulous - see condition
Strippling of nails 703.8
Stroke 434.91
  apoplectic (see also Disease, cerebrovascular, acute) 436
  brain - see Infarct, brain
  embolic 434.11
  epileptic - see Epilepsy
  healed or old V12.54
  heart - see Disease, heart
  heat 992.0
  hemorrhagic - see Hemorrhage, brain
  iatrogenic 997.02
  in evolution 434.91
  ischemic 434.91
  late effect - see Late effect(s) (of) cerebrovascular disease
  lightning 994.0
  paralytic - see Infarct, brain
  postoperative 997.02
  progressive 435.9
  thrombotic 434.01
Stromatosis, endometrial (M8931/1) 236.0
Strong pulse 785.9
Strongyloides stercoralis infestation 127.2
Strongyloidiasis 127.2
Strongyloidosis 127.2
Strongylus (gibsoni) infestation 127.7
Strophulus (newborn) 779.89
  pruriginosus 698.2
Struck by lighting 994.0
Struma (see also Goiter) 240.9
  fibrosa 245.3
  Hashimoto (struma lymphomatosa) 245.2
  lymphomatosa 245.2
  nodosa (simplex) 241.9
    endemic 241.9
    multinodular 241.1
    sporadic 241.9
    toxic or with hyperthyroidism 242.3 ●
      multinodular 242.2 ●
      uninodular 242.1 ●

Struma (Continued)
   nodosa (Continued)
      toxicosa 242.3●
         multinodular 242.2●
         uninodular 242.1●
      uninodular 241.0
   ovarii (M9090/0) 220
      and carcinoid (M9091/1) 236.2
      malignant (M9090/3) 183.0
   Riedel's (ligneous thyroiditis) 245.3
   scrofulous (see also Tuberculosis) 017.2●
   tuberculous (see also Tuberculosis) 017.2●
      abscess 017.2●
      adenitis 017.2●
      lymphangitis 017.2●
      ulcer 017.2●
Strumipriva cachexia (see also Hypothyroidism) 244.9
Strümpell-Marie disease or spine (ankylosing spondylitis) 720.0
Strümpell-Westphal pseudosclerosis (hepatolenticular degeneration) 275.1
Stuart's disease (congenital factor X deficiency) (see also Defect, coagulation) 286.3
Stuart-Prower factor deficiency (congenital factor X deficiency) (see also Defect, coagulation) 286.3
Students' elbow 727.2
Stuffy nose 478.19
Stump - see also Amputation
   cervix, cervical (healed) 622.8
Stupor 780.09
   catatonic (see also Schizophrenia) 295.2●
   circular (see also Psychosis, manic-depressive, circular) 296.7
   manic 296.89
   manic-depressive (see also Psychosis, affective) 296.89
   mental (anergic) (delusional) 298.9
   psychogenic 298.8
   reaction to exceptional stress (transient) 308.2
   traumatic NEC - see also Injury, intracranial
      with spinal (cord)
         lesion - see Injury, spinal, by site
         shock - see Injury, spinal, by site
Sturge (-Weber) (-Dimitri) disease or syndrome (encephalocutaneous angiomatosis) 759.6
Sturge-Kalischer-Weber syndrome (encephalocutaneous angiomatosis) 759.6
Stuttering 315.35
   adult onset 307.0
   childhood onset 315.35
   due to late effect of cerebrovascular disease (see also Late effect(s) (of) cerebrovascular disease) 438.14
   in conditions classified elsewhere 784.52
Sty, stye 373.11
   external 373.11
   internal 373.12
   meibomian 373.12
Subacidity, gastric 536.8
   psychogenic 306.4
Subacute - see condition
Subarachnoid - see condition
Subclavian steal syndrome 435.2
Subcortical - see condition
Subcostal syndrome 098.86
   nerve compression 354.8
Subcutaneous, subcuticular - see condition
Subdelirium 293.1
Subdural - see condition
Subendocardium - see condition
Subependymoma (M9383/1) 237.5
Suberosis 495.3
Subglossitis - see Glossitis
Subhemophilia 286.0
Subinvolution (uterus) 621.1
   breast (postlactational) (postpartum) 611.89
   chronic 621.1
   puerperal, postpartum 674.8●

Sublingual - see condition
Sublinguitis 527.2
Subluxation - see also Dislocation, by site
   congenital NEC - see also Malposition, congenital
      hip (unilateral) 754.32
         with dislocation of other hip 754.35
         bilateral 754.33
      joint
         lower limb 755.69
         shoulder 755.59
         upper limb 755.59
   lower limb (joint) 755.69
   shoulder (joint) 755.59
   upper limb (joint) 755.59
   lens 379.32
      anterior 379.33
      posterior 379.34
   radial head 832.2
   rotary, cervical region of spine - see Fracture, vertebra, cervical
Submaxillary - see condition
Submersion (fatal) (nonfatal) 994.1
Submissiveness (undue), in child 313.0
Submucous - see condition
Subnormal, subnormality
   accommodation (see also Disorder, accommodation) 367.9
   mental (see also Disability, intellectual) 319
      mild 317
      moderate 318.0
      profound 318.2
      severe 318.1
   temperature (accidental) 991.6
      not associated with low environmental temperature 780.99
Subphrenic - see condition
Subscapular nerve - see condition
Subseptus uterus 752.35
Subsiding appendicitis 542
Substance abuse in family V61.42
Substernal thyroid (see also Goiter) 240.9
   congenital 759.2
Substitution disorder 300.11
Subtentorial - see condition
Subtertian
   fever 084.0
   malaria (fever) 084.0
Subthyroidism (acquired) (see also Hypothyroidism) 244.9
   congenital 243
Succenturiata placenta - see Placenta, abnormal
Succussion sounds, chest 786.7
Sucking thumb, child 307.9
Sudamen 705.1
Sudamina 705.1
Sudanese kala-azar 085.0
Sudden
   death, cause unknown (less than 24 hours) 798.1
      cardiac (SCD)
         family history of V17.41
         personal history of, successfully resuscitated V12.53
      during childbirth 669.9●
      infant 798.0
      puerperal, postpartum 674.9●
   hearing loss NEC 388.2
   heart failure (see also Failure, heart) 428.9
   infant death syndrome 798.0
Sudeck's atrophy, disease, or syndrome 733.7
SUDS (Sudden unexplained death) 798.2
Suffocation (see also Asphyxia) 799.01
   by
      bed clothes 994.7
      bunny bag 994.7
      cave-in 994.7
      constriction 994.7
      drowning 994.1

Suffocation (Continued)
   by (Continued)
      inhalation
         food or foreign body (see also Asphyxia, food or foreign body) 933.1
         oil or gasoline (see also Asphyxia, food or foreign body) 933.1
      overlying 994.7
      plastic bag 994.7
      pressure 994.7
      strangulation 994.7
   during birth 768.1
   mechanical 994.7
Sugar
   blood
      high 790.29
      low 251.2
   in urine 791.5
Suicide, suicidal (attempted)
   by poisoning - see Table of Drugs and Chemicals
   ideation V62.84
   risk 300.9
   tendencies 300.9
   trauma NEC (see also nature and site of injury) 959.9
Suipestifer infection (see also Infection, Salmonella) 003.9
Sulfatidosis 330.0
Sulfhemoglobinemia, sulphemoglobinemia (acquired) (congenital) 289.7
Sumatran mite fever 081.2
Summer - see condition
Sunburn 692.71
   dermatitis 692.71
   due to
      other ultraviolet radiation 692.82
      tanning bed 692.82
   first degree 692.71
   second degree 692.76
   third degree 692.77
SUNCT (short lasting unilateral neuralgiform headache with conjunctival injection and tearing) 339.05
Sunken
   acetabulum 718.85
   fontanels 756.0
Sunstroke 992.0
Superfecundation 651.9●
   with fetal loss and retention of one or more fetus(es) 651.6●
   following (elective) fetal reduction 651.7●
Superfetation 651.9●
   with fetal loss and retention of one or more fetus(es) 651.6●
   following (elective) fetal reduction 651.7●
Superinvolution uterus 621.8
Supernumerary (congenital)
   aortic cusps 746.89
   auditory ossicles 744.04
   bone 756.9
   breast 757.6
   carpal bones 755.56
   cusps, heart valve NEC 746.89
      mitral 746.5
      pulmonary 746.09
   digit(s) 755.00
      finger 755.01
      toe 755.02
   ear (lobule) 744.1
   fallopian tube 752.19
   finger 755.01
   hymen 752.49
   kidney 753.3
   lacrimal glands 743.64
   lacrimonasal duct 743.65
   lobule (ear) 744.1
   mitral cusps 746.5
   muscle 756.82
   nipples 757.6

SECTION I INDEX TO DISEASES AND INJURIES / Supernumerary

Supernumerary (Continued)
  organ or site NEC - see Accessory
  ossicles, auditory 744.04
  ovary 752.0
  oviduct 752.19
  pulmonic cusps 746.09
  rib 756.3
    cervical or first 756.2
      syndrome 756.2
  roots (of teeth) 520.2
  spinal vertebra 756.19
  spleen 759.0
  tarsal bones 755.67
  teeth 520.1
    causing crowding 524.31
  testis 752.89
  thumb 755.01
  toe 755.02
  uterus 752.2
  vagina 752.49
  vertebra 756.19
Supervision (of)
  contraceptive method previously prescribed V25.40
    intrauterine device V25.42
    oral contraceptive (pill) V25.41
    specified type NEC V25.49
    subdermal implantable contraceptive V25.43
  dietary (for) V65.3
    allergy (food) V65.3
    colitis V65.3
    diabetes mellitus V65.3
    food allergy intolerance V65.3
    gastritis V65.3
    hypercholesterolemia V65.3
    hypoglycemia V65.3
    intolerance (food) V65.3
    obesity V65.3
    specified NEC V65.3
  lactation V24.1
  newborn health
    8 to 28 days old V20.32
    under 8 days old V20.31
  pregnancy - see Pregnancy, supervision of
Supplemental teeth 520.1
  causing crowding 524.31
Suppression
  binocular vision 368.31
  lactation 676.5 ●
  menstruation 626.8
  ovarian secretion 256.39
  renal 586
  urinary secretion 788.5
  urine 788.5
Suppuration, suppurative - see also condition
  accessory sinus (chronic) (see also Sinusitis) 473.9
  adrenal gland 255.8
  antrum (chronic) (see also Sinusitis, maxillary) 473.0
  bladder (see also Cystitis) 595.89
  bowel 569.89
  brain 324.0
    late effect 326
  breast 611.0
    puerperal, postpartum 675.1 ●
  dental periosteum 526.5
  diffuse (skin) 686.00
  ear (middle) (see also Otitis media) 382.4
    external (see also Otitis, externa) 380.10
    internal 386.33
  ethmoidal (sinus) (chronic) (see also Sinusitis, ethmoidal) 473.2
  fallopian tube (see also Salpingo-oophoritis) 614.2
  frontal (sinus) (chronic) (see also Sinusitis, frontal) 473.1
  gallbladder (see also Cholecystitis, acute) 575.0
  gum 523.30

Suppuration, suppurative (Continued)
  hernial sac - see Hernia, by site
  intestine 569.89
  joint (see also Arthritis, suppurative) 711.0 ●
  labyrinthine 386.33
  lung 513.0
  mammary gland 611.0
    puerperal, postpartum 675.1 ●
  maxilla, maxillary 526.4
    sinus (chronic) (see also Sinusitis, maxillary) 473.0
  muscle 728.0
  nasal sinus (chronic) (see also Sinusitis) 473.9
  pancreas 577.0
  parotid gland 527.2
  pelvis, pelvic
    female (see also Disease, pelvis, inflammatory) 614.4
      acute 614.3
    male (see also Peritonitis) 567.21
  pericranial (see also Osteomyelitis) 730.2 ●
  salivary duct or gland (any) 527.2
  sinus (nasal) (see also Sinusitis) 473.9
  sphenoidal (sinus) (chronic) (see also Sinusitis, sphenoidal) 473.3
  thymus (gland) 254.1
  thyroid (gland) 245.0
  tonsil 474.8
  uterus (see also Endometritis) 615.9
  vagina 616.10
  wound - see also Wound, open, by site, complicated
    dislocation - see Dislocation, by site, compound
    fracture - see Fracture, by site, open
    scratch or other superficial injury - see Injury, superficial, by site
Supraeruption, teeth 524.34
Supraglottitis 464.50
  with obstruction 464.51
Suprapubic drainage 596.89
Suprarenal (gland) - see condition
Suprascapular nerve - see condition
Suprasellar - see condition
Supraspinatus syndrome 726.10
Surfer knots 919.8
  infected 919.9
Surgery
  cosmetic NEC V50.1
    breast reconstruction following mastectomy V51.0
    following healed injury or operation V51.8
    hair transplant V50.0
  elective V50.9
    breast
      augmentation or reduction V50.1
      reconstruction following mastectomy V51.0
    circumcision, ritual or routine (in absence of medical indication) V50.2
    cosmetic NEC V50.1
    ear piercing V50.3
    face-lift V50.1
    following healed injury or operation V51.8
    hair transplant V50.0
  not done because of
    contraindication V64.1
    patient's decision V64.2
    specified reason NEC V64.3
  plastic
    breast
      augmentation or reduction V50.1
      reconstruction following mastectomy V51.0
    cosmetic V50.1
    face-lift V50.1
    following healed injury or operation V51.8

Surgery (Continued)
  plastic (Continued)
    repair of scarred tissue (following healed injury or operation) V51.8
    specified type NEC V50.8
  previous, in pregnancy or childbirth
    cervix 654.6 ●
      affecting fetus or newborn (see also Newborn, affected by) 760.63
      causing obstructed labor 660.2 ●
        affecting fetus or newborn 763.1
    pelvic soft tissues NEC 654.9 ●
      affecting fetus or newborn (see also Newborn, affected by) 760.63
      causing obstructed labor 660.2 ●
        affecting fetus or newborn 763.1
    perineum or vulva 654.8 ●
    uterus NEC 654.9 ●
      affecting fetus or newborn (see also Newborn, affected by) 760.63
      causing obstructed labor 660.2 ●
        affecting fetus or newborn 763.1
      from previous cesarean delivery 654.2 ●
    vagina 654.7 ●
Surgical
  abortion - see Abortion, legal
  emphysema 998.81
  kidney (see also Pyelitis) 590.80
  operation NEC 799.9
  procedures, complication or misadventure - see Complications, surgical procedure
  shock 998.00
Survey
  fetal anatomic V28.81
Susceptibility
  genetic
    to
      MEN (multiple endocrine neoplasia) V84.81
      neoplasia
        multiple endocrine (MEN) V84.81
      neoplasm
        malignant, of
          breast V84.01
          endometrium V84.04
          other V84.09
          ovary V84.02
          prostate V84.03
        specified disease NEC V84.89
Suspected condition, ruled out (see also Observation, suspected) V71.9
  specified condition NEC V71.89
Suspended uterus, in pregnancy or childbirth 654.4 ●
  affecting fetus or newborn 763.89
  causing obstructed labor 660.2 ●
    affecting fetus or newborn 763.1
Sutton's disease 709.09
Sutton and Gull's disease (arteriolar nephrosclerosis) (see also Hypertension, kidney) 403.90
Suture
  burst (in external operation wound) (see also Dehiscence) 998.32
    internal 998.31
  inadvertently left in operation wound 998.4
  removal V58.32
  Shirodkar, in pregnancy (with or without cervical incompetence) 654.5 ●
Swab inadvertently left in operation wound 998.4
Swallowed, swallowing
  difficulty (see also Dysphagia) 787.20
  foreign body NEC (see also Foreign body) 938
Swamp fever 100.89
Swan neck hand (intrinsic) 736.09
Sweat(s), sweating
  disease or sickness 078.2
  excessive (see also Hyperhidrosis) 780.8

444 ◀ New ⬅ Revised ~~deleted~~ Deleted ● Use Additional Digit(s) ▮ Omit code

Sweat(s), sweating (Continued)
- fetid 705.89
- fever 078.2
- gland disease 705.9
  - specified type NEC 705.89
- miliary 078.2
- night 780.8

Sweeley-Klionsky disease (angiokeratoma corporis diffusum) 272.7

Sweet's syndrome (acute febrile neutrophilic dermatosis) 695.89

Swelling 782.3
- abdominal (not referable to specific organ) 789.3●
- adrenal gland, cloudy 255.8
- ankle 719.07
- anus 787.99
- arm 729.81
- breast 611.72
- Calabar 125.2
- cervical gland 785.6
- cheek 784.2
- chest 786.6
- ear 388.8
- epigastric 789.3●
- extremity (lower) (upper) 729.81
- eye 379.92
- female genital organ 625.8
- finger 729.81
- foot 729.81
- glands 785.6
- gum 784.2
- hand 729.81
- head 784.2
- inflammatory - *see* Inflammation
- joint (*see also* Effusion, joint) 719.0●
  - tuberculous - *see* Tuberculosis, joint
- kidney, cloudy 593.89
- leg 729.81
- limb 729.81
- liver 573.8
- lung 786.6
- lymph nodes 785.6
- mediastinal 786.6
- mouth 784.2
- muscle (limb) 729.81
- neck 784.2
- nose or sinus 784.2
- palate 784.2
- pelvis 789.3●
- penis 607.83
- perineum 625.8
- rectum 787.99
- scrotum 608.86
- skin 782.2
- splenic (*see also* Splenomegaly) 789.2
- substernal 786.6
- superficial, localized (skin) 782.2
- testicle 608.86
- throat 784.2
- toe 729.81
- tongue 784.2
- tubular (*see also* Disease, renal) 593.9
- umbilicus 789.3●
- uterus 625.8
- vagina 625.8
- vulva 625.8
- wandering, due to Gnathostoma (spinigerum) 128.1
- white - *see* Tuberculosis, arthritis

Swift's disease 985.0

Swimmers'
- ear (acute) 380.12
- itch 120.3

Swimming in the head 780.4

Swollen - *see also* Swelling
- glands 785.6

Swyer-James syndrome (unilateral hyperlucent lung) 492.8

Swyer's syndrome (XY pure gonadal dysgenesis) 752.7

Sycosis 704.8
- barbae (not parasitic) 704.8
- contagiosa 110.0
- lupoid 704.8
- mycotic 110.0
- parasitic 110.0
- vulgaris 704.8

Sydenham's chorea - *see* Chorea, Sydenham's

Sylvatic yellow fever 060.0

Sylvest's disease (epidemic pleurodynia) 074.1

Symblepharon 372.63
- congenital 743.62

Symonds' syndrome 348.2

Sympathetic - *see* condition

Sympatheticotonia (*see also* Neuropathy, peripheral, autonomic) 337.9

Sympathicoblastoma (M9500/3)
- specified site - *see* Neoplasm, by site, malignant
- unspecified site 194.0

Sympathicogonioma (M9500/3) - *see* Sympathicoblastoma

Sympathoblastoma (M9500/3) - *see* Sympathicoblastoma

Sympathogonioma (M9500/3) - *see* Sympathicoblastoma

Symphalangy (*see also* Syndactylism) 755.10

Symptoms, specified (general) NEC 780.99
- abdomen NEC 789.9
- bone NEC 733.90
- breast NEC 611.79
- cardiac NEC 785.9
- cardiovascular NEC 785.9
- chest NEC 786.9
- cognition 799.59
- development NEC 783.9
- digestive system NEC 787.99
- emotional state NEC 799.29
- eye NEC 379.99
- gastrointestinal tract NEC 787.99
- genital organs NEC
  - female 625.9
  - male 608.9
- head and neck NEC 784.99
- heart NEC 785.9
- jaw 784.92
- joint NEC 719.60
  - ankle 719.67
  - elbow 719.62
  - foot 719.67
  - hand 719.64
  - hip 719.65
  - knee 719.66
  - multiple sites 719.69
  - pelvic region 719.65
  - shoulder (region) 719.61
  - specified site NEC 719.68
  - temporomandibular 524.69
  - wrist 719.63
- larynx NEC 784.99
- limbs NEC 729.89
- lymphatic system NEC 785.9
- maxilla 784.92
- menopausal 627.2
- metabolism NEC 783.9
- mouth NEC 528.9
- muscle NEC 728.9
- musculoskeletal NEC 781.99
  - limbs NEC 729.89
- nervous system NEC 781.99
- neurotic NEC 300.9
- nutrition, metabolism, and development NEC 783.9
- pelvis NEC 789.9
  - female 625.9
- peritoneum NEC 789.9
- respiratory system NEC 786.9
- skin and integument NEC 782.9
- subcutaneous tissue NEC 782.9
- throat NEC 784.99
- tonsil NEC 784.99

Symptoms, specified (Continued)
- urinary system NEC 788.99
- vascular NEC 785.9

Sympus 759.89

Synarthrosis 719.80
- ankle 719.87
- elbow 719.82
- foot 719.87
- hand 719.84
- hip 719.85
- knee 719.86
- multiple sites 719.89
- pelvic region 719.85
- shoulder (region) 719.81
- specified site NEC 719.88
- wrist 719.83

Syncephalus 759.4

Synchondrosis 756.9
- abnormal (congenital) 756.9
- ischiopubic (van Neck's) 732.1

Synchysis (senile) (vitreous humor) 379.21
- scintillans 379.22

Syncope (near) (pre-) 780.2
- anginosa 413.9
- bradycardia 427.89
- cardiac 780.2
- carotid sinus 337.01
- complicating delivery 669.2●
- due to lumbar puncture 349.0
- fatal 798.1
- heart 780.2
- heat 992.1
- laryngeal 786.2
- tussive 786.2
- vasoconstriction 780.2
- vasodepressor 780.2
- vasomotor 780.2
- vasovagal 780.2

Syncytial infarct - *see* Placenta, abnormal

Syndactylism, syndactyly (multiple sites) 755.10
- fingers (without fusion of bone) 755.11
  - with fusion of bone 755.12
- toes (without fusion of bone) 755.13
  - with fusion of bone 755.14

Syndrome - *see also* Disease
- 5q minus 238.74
- abdominal
  - acute 789.0●
  - migraine 346.2●
  - muscle deficiency 756.79
- Abercrombie's (amyloid degeneration) 277.39
- abnormal innervation 374.43
- abstinence
  - alcohol 291.81
  - drug 292.0
  - neonatal 779.5
- Abt-Letterer-Siwe (acute histiocytosis X) (M9722/3) 202.5●
- Achard-Thiers (adrenogenital) 255.2
- acid pulmonary aspiration 997.39
  - obstetric (Mendelson's) 668.0●
- acquired immune deficiency 042
- acquired immunodeficiency 042
- acrocephalosyndactylism 755.55
- acute abdominal 789.0●
- acute chest 517.3
- acute coronary 411.1
- Adair-Dighton (brittle bones and blue sclera, deafness) 756.51
- Adams-Stokes (-Morgagni) (syncope with heart block) 426.9
- Addisonian 255.41
- Adie (-Holmes) (pupil) 379.46
- adiposogenital 253.8
- adrenal
  - hemorrhage 036.3
  - meningococcic 036.3
- adrenocortical 255.3

SECTION 1 INDEX TO DISEASES AND INJURIES / Syndrome

Syndrome (Continued)
- adrenogenital (acquired) (congenital) 255.2
  - feminizing 255.2
  - iatrogenic 760.79
  - virilism (acquired) (congenital) 255.2
- affective organic NEC 293.89
  - drug-induced 292.84
- afferent loop NEC 537.89
- African macroglobulinemia 273.3
- Ahumada-Del Castillo (nonpuerperal galactorrhea and amenorrhea) 253.1
- air blast concussion - see Injury, internal, by site
- Alagille 759.89
- Albright (-Martin) (pseudohypoparathyroidism) 275.49
- Albright-McCune-Sternberg (osteitis fibrosa disseminata) 756.59
- alcohol withdrawal 291.81
- Alder's (leukocyte granulation anomaly) 288.2
- Aldrich (-Wiskott) (eczema-thrombocytopenia) 279.12
- Alibert-Bazin (mycosis fungoides) (M9700/3) 202.1●
- Alice in Wonderland 293.89
- alien hand 781.8
- Allen-Masters 620.6
- Alligator baby (ichthyosis congenita) 757.1
- Alport's (hereditary hematuria-nephropathy-deafness) 759.89
- Alvarez (transient cerebral ischemia) 435.9
- alveolar capillary block 516.8
- Alzheimer's 331.0
  - with dementia - see Alzheimer's, dementia
- amnestic (confabulatory) 294.0
  - alcohol-induced persisting 291.1
  - drug-induced 292.83
  - posttraumatic 294.0
- amotivational 292.89
- amyostatic 275.1
- amyotrophic lateral sclerosis 335.20
- androgen insensitivity 259.51
  - partial 259.52
- Angelman 759.89
- angina (see also Angina) 413.9
- ankyloglossia superior 750.0
- anterior
  - chest wall 786.52
  - compartment (tibial) 958.8
  - spinal artery 433.8●
    - compression 721.1
  - tibial (compartment) 958.8
- antibody deficiency 279.00
  - agammaglobulinemic 279.00
  - congenital 279.04
  - hypogammaglobulinemic 279.00
- anticardiolipin antibody 289.81
- antimongolism 758.39
- antiphospholipid antibody 289.81
- Anton (-Babinski) (hemiasomatognosia) 307.9
- anxiety (see also Anxiety) 300.00
  - organic 293.84
- aortic
  - arch 446.7
  - bifurcation (occlusion) 444.09
  - ring 747.21
- Apert's (acrocephalosyndactyly) 755.55
- Apert-Gallais (adrenogenital) 255.2
- aphasia-apraxia-alexia 784.69
- apical ballooning 429.83
- "approximate answers" 300.16
- arcuate ligament (-celiac axis) 447.4
- arcus aortae 446.7
- arc welders' 370.24
- argentaffin, argentaffinoma 259.2
- Argonz-Del Castillo (nonpuerperal galactorrhea and amenorrhea) 253.1

Syndrome (Continued)
- Argyll Robertson's (syphilitic) 094.89
  - nonsyphilitic 379.45
- Armenian 277.31
- arm-shoulder (see also Neuropathy, peripheral, autonomic) 337.9
- Arnold-Chiari (see also Spina bifida) 741.0●
  - type I 348.4
  - type II 741.0●
  - type III 742.0
  - type IV 742.2
- Arrillaga-Ayerza (pulmonary artery sclerosis with pulmonary hypertension) 416.0
- arteriomesenteric duodenum occlusion 537.89
- arteriovenous steal 996.73
- arteritis, young female (obliterative brachiocephalic) 446.7
- aseptic meningitis - see Meningitis, aseptic
- Asherman's 621.5
- Asperger's 299.8●
- asphyctic (see also Anxiety) 300.00
- aspiration, of newborn (massive 770.18)
  - meconium 770.12
- ataxia-telangiectasia 334.8
- Audry's (acropachyderma) 757.39
- auriculotemporal 350.8
- autoimmune lymphoproliferative (ALPS) 279.41
- autosomal - see also Abnormal, autosomes NEC
  - deletion 758.39
    - 5p 758.31
    - 22q11.2 758.32
- Avellis' 344.89
- Axenfeld's 743.44
- Ayerza (-Arrillaga) (pulmonary artery sclerosis with pulmonary hypertension) 416.0
- Baader's (erythema multiforme exudativum) 695.19
- Baastrup's 721.5
- Babinski (-Vaquez) (cardiovascular syphilis) 093.89
- Babinski-Fröhlich (adiposogenital dystrophy) 253.8
- Babinski-Nageotte 344.89
- Bagratuni's (temporal arteritis) 446.5
- Bakwin-Krida (craniometaphyseal dysplasia) 756.89
- Balint's (psychic paralysis of visual disorientation) 368.16
- Ballantyne (-Runge) (postmaturity) 766.22
- ballooning posterior leaflet 424.0
- Banti's - see Cirrhosis, liver
- Bard-Pic's (carcinoma, head of pancreas) 157.0
- Bardet-Biedl (obesity, polydactyly, and intellectual disabilities) 759.89
- Barlow's (mitral valve prolapse) 424.0
- Barlow (-Möller) (infantile scurvy) 267
- Baron Munchausen's 301.51
- Barré-Guillain 357.0
- Barré-Liéou (posterior cervical sympathetic) 723.2
- Barrett's (chronic peptic ulcer of esophagus) 530.85
- Bársony-Polgár (corkscrew esophagus) 530.5
- Bársony-Teschendorf (corkscrew esophagus) 530.5
- Barth 759.89
- Bartter's (secondary hyperaldosteronism with juxtaglomerular hyperplasia) 255.13
- basal cell nevus 759.89
- Basedow's (exophthalmic goiter) 242.0●
- basilar artery 435.0
- basofrontal 377.04
- Bassen-Kornzweig (abetalipoproteinemia) 272.5
- Batten-Steinert 359.21

Syndrome (Continued)
- battered
  - adult 995.81
  - baby or child 995.54
  - spouse 995.81
- Baumgarten-Cruveilhier (cirrhosis of liver) 571.5
- Beals 759.82
- Bearn-Kunkel (-Slater) (lupoid hepatitis) 571.49
- Beau's (see also Degeneration, myocardial) 429.1
- Bechterew-Strümpell-Marie (ankylosing spondylitis) 720.0
- Beck's (anterior spinal artery occlusion) 433.8●
- Beckwith (-Wiedemann) 759.89
- Behçet's 136.1
- Bekhterev-Strümpell-Marie (ankylosing spondylitis) 720.0
- Benedikt's 344.89
- Béquez César (-Steinbrinck-Chédiak-Higashi) (congenital gigantism of peroxidase granules) 288.2
- Bernard-Horner (see also Neuropathy, peripheral, autonomic) 337.9
- Bernard-Sergent (acute adrenocortical insufficiency) 255.41
- Bernhardt-Roth 355.1
- Bernheim's (see also Failure, heart) 428.0
- Bertolotti's (sacralization of fifth lumbar vertebra) 756.15
- Besnier-Boeck-Schaumann (sarcoidosis) 135
- Bianchi's (aphasia-apraxia-alexia syndrome) 784.69
- Biedl-Bardet (obesity, polydactyly, and intellectual disabilities) 759.89
- Biemond's (obesity, polydactyly, and intellectual disabilities) 759.89
- big spleen 289.4
- bilateral polycystic ovarian 256.4
- Bing-Horton's 339.00
- Biörck (-Thorson) (malignant carcinoid) 259.2
- Birt-Hogg-Dube 759.89
- Blackfan-Diamond (congenital hypoplastic anemia) 284.01
- black lung 500
- black widow spider bite 989.5
- bladder neck (see also Incontinence, urine) 788.30
- blast (concussion) - see Blast, injury
- blind loop (postoperative) 579.2
- Block-Siemens (incontinentia pigmenti) 757.33
- Bloch-Sulzberger (incontinentia pigmenti) 757.33
- Bloom (-Machacek) (-Torre) 757.39
- Blount-Barber (tibia vara) 732.4
- blue
  - bloater 491.20
    - with
      - acute bronchitis 491.22
      - exacerbation (acute) 491.21
  - diaper 270.0
  - drum 381.02
  - sclera 756.51
  - toe 445.02
- Boder-Sedgwick (ataxia-telangiectasia) 334.8
- Boerhaave's (spontaneous esophageal rupture) 530.4
- Bonnevie-Ullrich 758.6
- Bonnier's 386.19
- Borjeson-Forssman-Lehmann 759.89
- Bouillaud's (rheumatic heart disease) 391.9
- Bourneville (-Pringle) (tuberous sclerosis) 759.5
- Bouveret (-Hoffmann) (paroxysmal tachycardia) 427.2
- brachial plexus 353.0

SECTION I INDEX TO DISEASES AND INJURIES / Syndrome

Syndrome (Continued)
- Brachman-de Lange (Amsterdam dwarf, intellectual disabilities, and brachycephaly) 759.89
- bradycardia-tachycardia 427.81
- Brailsford-Morquio (dystrophy) (mucopolysaccharidosis IV) 277.5
- brain (acute) (chronic) (nonpsychotic) (organic) (with behavioral reaction) (with neurotic reaction) 310.9
  - with
    - presenile brain disease (see also Dementia, presenile) 290.10
    - psychosis, psychotic reaction (see also Psychosis, organic) 294.9
  - chronic alcoholic 291.2
  - congenital (see also Disability, intellectual) 319
  - postcontusional 310.2
  - posttraumatic
    - nonpsychotic 310.2
    - psychotic 293.9
      - acute 293.0
      - chronic (see also Psychosis, organic) 294.8
      - subacute 293.1
  - psycho-organic (see also Syndrome, psycho-organic) 310.9
  - psychotic (see also Psychosis, organic) 294.9
  - senile (see also Dementia, senile) 290.0
- branchial arch 744.41
- Brandt's (acrodermatitis enteropathica) 686.8
- Brennemann's 289.2
- Briquet's 300.81
- Brissaud-Meige (infantile myxedema) 244.9
- broad ligament laceration 620.6
- Brock's (atelectasis due to enlarged lymph nodes) 518.0
- broken heart 429.83
- Brown's tendon sheath 378.61
- Brown-Séquard 344.89
- brown spot 756.59
- Brugada 746.89
- Brugsch's (acropachyderma) 757.39
- bubbly lung 770.7
- Buchem's (hyperostosis corticalis) 733.3
- Budd-Chiari (hepatic vein thrombosis) 453.0
- Büdinger-Ludloff-Läwen 717.89
- bulbar 335.22
  - lateral (see also Disease, cerebrovascular, acute) 436
- Bullis fever 082.8
- bundle of Kent (anomalous atrioventricular excitation) 426.7
- Bürger-Grutz (essential familial hyperlipemia) 272.3
- Burke's (pancreatic insufficiency and chronic neutropenia) 577.8
- Burnett's (milk-alkali) 275.42
- Burnier's (hypophyseal dwarfism) 253.3
- burning feet 266.2
- Bywaters' 958.5
- Caffey's (infantile cortical hyperostosis) 756.59
- Calvé-Legg-Perthes (osteochrondrosis, femoral capital) 732.1
- Caplan (-Colinet) syndrome 714.81
- capsular thrombosis (see also Thrombosis, brain) 434.0●
- carbohydrate-deficient glycoprotein (CDGS) 271.8
- carcinogenic thrombophlebitis 453.1
- carcinoid 259.2
- cardiac asthma (see also Failure, ventricular, left) 428.1
- cardiacos negros 416.0
- cardiofaciocutaneous 759.89
- cardiopulmonary obesity 278.03
- cardiorenal (see also Hypertension, cardiorenal) 404.90

Syndrome (Continued)
- cardiorespiratory distress (idiopathic), newborn 769
- cardiovascular renal (see also Hypertension, cardiorenal) 404.90
- cardiovasorenal 272.7
- Carini's (ichthyosis congenita) 757.1
- carotid
  - artery (internal) 435.8
  - body or sinus 337.01
- carpal tunnel 354.0
- Carpenter's 759.89
- Cassidy (-Scholte) (malignant carcinoid) 259.2
- cat-cry 758.31
- cauda equina 344.60
- causalgia 355.9
  - lower limb 355.71
  - upper limb 354.4
- cavernous sinus 437.6
- celiac 579.0
  - artery compression 447.4
  - axis 447.4
- central pain 338.0
- cerebellomedullary malformation (see also Spina bifida) 741.0●
- cerebral gigantism 253.0
- cerebrohepatorenal 759.89
- cervical (root) (spine) NEC 723.8
  - disc 722.71
  - posterior, sympathetic 723.2
  - rib 353.0
  - sympathetic paralysis 337.09
  - traumatic (acute) NEC 847.0
- cervicobrachial (diffuse) 723.3
- cervicocranial 723.2
- cervicodorsal outlet 353.2
- Céstan's 344.89
- Céstan (-Raymond) 433.8●
- Céstan-Chenais 344.89
- chancriform 114.1
- Charcôt's (intermittent claudication) 443.9
  - angina cruris 443.9
  - due to atherosclerosis 440.21
- Charcôt-Marie-Tooth 356.1
- Charcôt-Weiss-Baker 337.01
- CHARGE association 759.89
- Cheadle (-Möller) (-Barlow) (infantile scurvy) 267
- Chédiak-Higashi (-Steinbrinck) (congenital gigantism of peroxidase granules) 288.2
- chest wall 786.52
- Chiari's (hepatic vein thrombosis) 453.0
- Chiari-Frommel 676.6●
- chiasmatic 368.41
- Chilaiditi's (subphrenic displacement, colon) 751.4
- chondroectodermal dysplasia 756.55
- chorea-athetosis-agitans 275.1
- Christian's (chronic histiocytosis X) 277.89
- chromosome 4 short arm deletion 758.39
- chronic pain 338.4
- Churg-Strauss 446.4
- Clarke-Hadfield (pancreatic infantilism) 577.8
- Claude's 352.6
- Claude Bernard-Horner (see also Neuropathy, peripheral, autonomic) 337.9
- Clérambault's
  - automatism 348.89
  - erotomania 297.8
- Clifford's (postmaturity) 766.22
- climacteric 627.2
- Clouston's (hidrotic ectodermal dysplasia) 757.31
- clumsiness 315.4
- Cockayne's (microencephaly and dwarfism) 759.89
- Cockayne-Weber (epidermolysis bullosa) 757.39

Syndrome (Continued)
- Coffin-Lowry 759.89
- Cogan's (nonsyphilitic interstitial keratitis) 370.52
- cold injury (newborn) 778.2
- Collet (-Sicard) 352.6
- combined immunity deficiency 279.2
- compartment(al) (anterior) (deep) (posterior) 958.8
  - nontraumatic
    - abdomen 729.73
    - arm 729.71
    - buttock 729.72
    - fingers 729.71
    - foot 729.72
    - forearm 729.71
    - hand 729.71
    - hip 729.72
    - leg 729.72
    - lower extremity 729.72
    - shoulder 729.71
    - specified site NEC 729.79
    - thigh 729.72
    - toes 729.72
    - upper extremity 729.71
    - wrist 729.71
  - post-surgical (see also Syndrome, compartment, non-traumatic) 998.89
  - traumatic 958.90
    - abdomen 958.93
    - arm 958.91
    - buttock 958.92
    - fingers 958.91
    - foot 958.92
    - forearm 958.91
    - hand 958.91
    - hip 958.92
    - leg 958.92
    - lower extremity 958.92
    - shoulder 958.91
    - specified site NEC 958.99
    - thigh 958.92
    - tibial 958.92
    - toes 958.92
    - upper extremity 958.91
    - wrist 958.91
- complex regional pain - see also Dystrophy, sympathetic
  - type I - see Dystrophy, sympathetic (posttraumatic) (reflex)
  - type II - see Causalgia
- compression 958.5
  - cauda equina 344.60
    - with neurogenic bladder 344.61
- concussion 310.2
- congenital
  - affecting more than one system 759.7
    - specified type NEC 759.89
  - congenital central alveolar hypoventilation 327.25
  - facial diplegia 352.6
  - muscular hypertrophy-cerebral 759.89
- congestion-fibrosis (pelvic) 625.5
- conjunctivourethrosynovial 099.3
- Conn (-Louis) (primary aldosteronism) 255.12
- Conradi (-Hünermann) (chondrodysplasia calcificans congenita) 756.59
- conus medullaris 336.8
- Cooke-Apert-Gallais (adrenogenital) 255.2
- Cornelia de Lange's (Amsterdam dwarf, intellectual disabilities, and brachycephaly) 759.8
- coronary insufficiency or intermediate 411.1
- cor pulmonale 416.9
- corticosexual 255.2
- Costen's (complex) 524.60
- costochondral junction 733.6
- costoclavicular 353.0
- costovertebral 253.0

◀ New ⬅ Revised ~~deleted~~ Deleted Use Additional Digit(s) ▭ Omit code

SECTION 1 INDEX TO DISEASES AND INJURIES / Syndrome

Syndrome (Continued)
- Cotard's (paranoia) 297.1
- Cowden 759.6
- craniovertebral 723.2
- Creutzfeldt-Jakob 046.19
  - with dementia
    - with behavioral disturbance 046.19 [294.11]
    - without behavioral disturbance 046.19 [294.10]
  - variant 046.11
    - with dementia
      - with behavioral disturbance 046.11 [294.11]
      - without behavioral disturbance 046.11 [294.10]
- crib death 798.0
- cricopharyngeal 787.20
- cri-du-chat 758.31
- Crigler-Najjar (congenital hyperbilirubinemia) 277.4
- crocodile tears 351.8
- Cronkhite-Canada 211.3
- croup 464.4
- CRST (cutaneous systemic sclerosis) 710.1
- crush 958.5
- crushed lung (see also Injury, internal, lung) 861.20
- Cruveilhier-Baumgarten (cirrhosis of liver) 571.5
- cubital tunnel 354.2
- Cuiffini-Pancoast (M8010/3) (carcinoma, pulmonary apex) 162.3
- Curschmann (-Batten) (-Steinert) 359.21
- Cushing's (iatrogenic) (idiopathic) (pituitary basophilism) (pituitary-dependent) 255.0
  - overdose or wrong substance given or taken 962.0
- Cyriax's (slipping rib) 733.99
- cystic duct stump 576.0
- Da Costa's (neurocirculatory asthenia) 306.2
- Dameshek's (erythroblastic anemia) 282.49
- Dana-Putnam (subacute combined sclerosis with pernicious anemia) 281.0 [336.2]
- Danbolt (-Closs) (acrodermatitis enteropathica) 686.8
- Dandy-Walker (atresia, foramen of Magendie) 742.3
  - with spina bifida (see also Spina bifida) 741.0●
- Danlos' 756.83
- Davies-Colley (slipping rib) 733.99
- dead fetus 641.3●
- defeminization 255.2
- defibrination (see also Fibrinolysis) 286.6
- Degos' 447.8
- Deiters' nucleus 386.19
- Déjérine-Roussy 338.0
- Déjérine-Thomas 333.0
- de Lange's (Amsterdam dwarf, intellectual disabilities, and brachycephaly) (Cornelia) 759.89
- Del Castillo's (germinal aplasia) 606.0
- deletion chromosomes 758.39
- delusional
  - induced by drug 292.11
- dementia-aphonia, of childhood (see also Psychosis, childhood) 299.1●
- demyelinating NEC 341.9
- denial visual hallucination 307.9
- depersonalization 300.6
- de Quervain's 259.51
- Dercum's (adiposis dolorosa) 272.8
- de Toni-Fanconi (-Debre) (cystinosis) 270.0
- diabetes-dwarfism-obesity (juvenile) 258.1
- diabetes mellitus-hypertension-nephrosis 250.4● [581.81]
  - due to secondary diabetes 249.4● [581.81]
- diabetes mellitus in newborn infant 775.1

Syndrome (Continued)
- diabetes-nephrosis 250.4● [581.81]
  - due to secondary diabetes 249.4● [581.81]
- diabetic amyotrophy 250.6● [353.5]
  - due to secondary diabetes 249.6● [353.5]
- Diamond-Blackfan (congenital hypoplastic anemia) 284.01
- Diamond-Gardner (autoerythrocyte sensitization) 287.2
- DIC (diffuse or disseminated intravascular coagulopathy) (see also Fibrinolysis) 286.6
- diencephalohypophyseal NEC 253.8
- diffuse cervicobrachial 723.3
- diffuse obstructive pulmonary 496
- DiGeorge's (thymic hypoplasia) 279.11
- Dighton's 756.51
- Di Guglielmo's (erythremic myelosis) (M9841/3) 207.0●
- disequilibrium 276.9
- disseminated platelet thrombosis 446.6
- Ditthomska 307.81
- Doan-Wiseman (primary splenic neutropenia) 289.53
- Döhle body-panmyelopathic 288.2
- Donohue's (leprechaunism) 259.8
- dorsolateral medullary (see also Disease, cerebrovascular, acute) 436
- double athetosis 333.71
- double whammy 360.81
- Down's (mongolism) 758.0
- Dresbach's (elliptocytosis) 282.1
- Dressler's (postmyocardial infarction) 411.0
  - hemoglobinuria 283.2
  - postcardiotomy 429.4
- drug withdrawal, infant, of dependent mother 779.5
- dry skin 701.1
  - eye 375.15
- DSAP (disseminated superficial actinic porokeratosis) 692.75
- Duane's (retraction) 378.71
- Duane-Stilling-Türk (ocular retraction syndrome) 378.71
- Dubin-Johnson (constitutional hyperbilirubinemia) 277.4
- Dubin-Sprinz (constitutional hyperbilirubinemia) 277.4
- Duchenne's 335.22
- due to abnormality
  - autosomal NEC (see also Abnormal, autosomes NEC) 758.5
    - 13 758.1
    - 18 758.2
    - 21 or 22 758.0
    - D_1 758.1
    - E_3 758.2
    - G 758.0
  - chromosomal 758.89
  - sex 758.81
- dumping 564.2
  - nonsurgical 536.8
- Duplay's 726.2
- Dupré's (meningism) 781.6
- Dyke-Young (acquired macrocytic hemolytic anemia) 283.9
- dyspraxia 315.4
- dystocia, dystrophia 654.9●
- Eagle-Barret 756.71
- Eales' 362.18
- Eaton-Lambert (see also Syndrome, Lambert-Eaton) 358.30
- Ebstein's (downward displacement, tricuspid valve into right ventricle) 746.2
- ectopic ACTH secretion 255.0
- eczema-thrombocytopenia 279.12
- Eddowes' (brittle bones and blue sclera) 756.51
- Edwards' 758.2
- efferent loop 537.89

Syndrome (Continued)
- effort (aviators') (psychogenic) 306.2
- Ehlers-Danlos 756.83
- Eisenmenger's (ventricular septal defect) 745.4
- Ekbom's (restless legs) 333.94
- Ekman's (brittle bones and blue sclera) 756.51
- electric feet 266.2
- Elephant man 237.71
- Ellison-Zollinger (gastric hypersecretion with pancreatic islet cell tumor) 251.5
- Ellis-van Creveld (chondroectodermal dysplasia) 756.55
- embryonic fixation 270.2
- empty sella (turcica) 253.8
- endocrine-hypertensive 255.3
- Engel-von Recklinghausen (osteitis fibrosa cystica) 252.01
- enteroarticular 099.3
- entrapment - see Neuropathy, entrapment
- eosinophilia myalgia 710.5
- epidemic vomiting 078.82
- Epstein's - see Nephrosis
- Erb (-Oppenheim)-Goldflam 358.00
- Erdheim-Chester 277.89
- Erdheim's (acromegalic macrospondylitis) 253.0
- Erlacher-Blount (tibia vara) 732.4
- erythrocyte fragmentation 283.19
- euthyroid sick 790.94
- Evans' (thrombocytopenic purpura) 287.32
- excess cortisol, iatrogenic 255.0
- exhaustion 300.5
- extrapyramidal 333.90
- eyelid-malar-mandible 756.0
- eye retraction 378.71
- Faber's (achlorhydric anemia) 280.9
- Fabry (-Anderson) (angiokeratoma corporis diffusum) 272.7
- facet 724.8
- Fallot's 745.2
- falx (see also Hemorrhage, brain) 431
- familial eczema-thrombocytopenia 279.12
- Fanconi's (anemia) (congenital pancytopenia) 284.09
- Fanconi (-de Toni) (-Debré) (cystinosis) 270.0
- Farber (-Uzman) (disseminated lipogranulomatosis) 272.8
- fatigue NEC 300.5
  - chronic 780.71
- faulty bowel habit (idiopathic megacolon) 564.7
- FDH (focal dermal hypoplasia) 757.39
- fecal reservoir 560.39
- Feil-Klippel (brevicollis) 756.16
- Felty's (rheumatoid arthritis with splenomegaly and leukopenia) 714.1
- fertile eunuch 257.2
- fetal alcohol 760.71
  - late effect 760.71
- fibrillation-flutter 427.32
- fibrositis (periarticular) 729.0
- Fiedler's (acute isolated myocarditis) 422.91
- Fiessinger-Leroy (-Reiter) 099.3
- Fiessinger-Rendu (erythema multiforme exudativum) 695.19
- first arch 756.0
- Fisher's 357.0
- fish odor 270.8
- Fitz's (acute hemorrhagic pancreatitis) 577.0
- Fitz-Hugh and Curtis 098.86
  - due to
    - Chlamydia trachomatis 099.56
    - Neisseria gonorrhoeae (gonococcal peritonitis) 098.86
- Flajani (-Basedow) (exophthalmic goiter) 242.0●
- flat back
  - acquired 737.29
  - postprocedural 738.5

Syndrome (Continued)
- floppy
  - infant 781.99
  - iris 364.81
  - valve (mitral) 424.0
- flush 259.2
- Foix-Alajouanine 336.1
- Fong's (hereditary osteo-onychodysplasia) 756.89
- foramen magnum 348.4
- Forbes-Albright (nonpuerperal amenorrhea and lactation associated with pituitary tumor) 253.1
- Foster-Kennedy 377.04
- Foville's (peduncular) 344.89
- fragile X 759.83
- Franceschetti's (mandibulofacial dysostosis) 756.0
- Fraser's 759.89
- Freeman-Sheldon 759.89
- Frey's (auriculotemporal) 705.22
- Friderichsen-Waterhouse 036.3
- Friedrich-Erb-Arnold (acropachyderma) 757.39
- Fröhlich's (adiposogenital dystrophy) 253.8
- Froin's 336.8
- Frommel-Chiari 676.6 ●
- frontal lobe 310.0
- Fukuhara 277.87
- Fuller Albright's (osteitis fibrosa disseminata) 756.59
- functional
  - bowel 564.9
  - prepubertal castrate 752.89
- Gaisböck's (polycythemia hypertonica) 289.0
- ganglion (basal, brain) 333.90
  - geniculi 351.1
- Ganser's, hysterical 300.16
- Gardner-Diamond (autoerythrocyte sensitization) 287.2
- gastroesophageal junction 530.0
- gastroesophageal laceration-hemorrhage 530.7
- gastrojejunal loop obstruction 537.89
- Gayet-Wernicke's (superior hemorrhagic polioencephalitis) 265.1
- Gee-Herter-Heubner (nontropical sprue) 579.0
- Gélineau's (*see also* Narcolepsy) 347.00
- genito-anorectal 099.1
- Gerhardt's (vocal cord paralysis) 478.30
- Gerstmann's (finger agnosia) 784.69
- Gerstmann-Sträussler-Scheinker (GSS) 046.71
- Gianotti Crosti 057.8
  - due to known virus - *see* Infection, virus
  - due to unknown virus 057.8
- Gilbert's 277.4
- Gilford (-Hutchinson) (progeria) 259.8
- Gilles de la Tourette's 307.23
- Gillespie's (dysplasia oculodentodigitalis) 759.89
- Glénard's (enteroptosis) 569.89
- Glinski-Simmonds (pituitary cachexia) 253.2
- glucuronyl transferase 277.4
- glue ear 381.20
- Goldberg (-Maxwell) (-Morris) (testicular feminization) 259.51
- Goldenhar's (oculoauriculovertebral dysplasia) 756.0
- Goldflam-Erb 358.00
- Goltz-Gorlin (dermal hypoplasia) 757.39
- Goodpasture's (pneumorenal) 446.21
- Good's 279.06
- Gopalan's (burning feet) 266.2
- Gorlin-Chaudhry-Moss 759.89
- Gorlin's 759.89
- Gougerot (-Houwer)-Sjögren (keratoconjunctivitis sicca) 710.2
- Gougerot-Blum (pigmented purpuric lichenoid dermatitis) 709.1

Syndrome (Continued)
- Gougerot-Carteaud (confluent reticulate papillomatosis) 701.8
- Gouley's (constrictive pericarditis) 423.2
- Gowers' (vasovagal attack) 780.2
- Gowers-Paton-Kennedy 377.04
- Gradenigo's 383.02
- Gray or grey (chloramphenicol) (newborn) 779.4
- Greig's (hypertelorism) 756.0
- GSS (Gerstmann-Sträussler-Scheinker) 046.71
- Gubler-Millard 344.89
- Guérin-Stern (arthrogryposis multiplex congenita) 754.89
- Guillain-Barré (-Strohl) 357.0
- Gunn's (jaw-winking syndrome) 742.8
- Günther's (congenital erythropoietic porphyria) 277.1
- gustatory sweating 350.8
- H$_3$O 759.81
- Hadfield-Clarke (pancreatic infantilism) 577.8
- Haglund-Läwen-Fründ 717.89
- hair tourniquet - *see also* Injury, superficial, by site
  - finger 915.8
    - infected 915.9
  - penis 911.8
    - infected 911.9
  - toe 917.8
    - infected 917.9
- hairless women 257.8
- Hallermann-Strieff 756.0
- Hallervorden-Spatz 333.0
- Hamman's (spontaneous mediastinal emphysema) 518.1
- Hamman-Rich (diffuse interstitial pulmonary fibrosis) 516.33
- Hand-Schüller-Christian (chronic histiocytosis X) 277.89
- hand-foot 693.0
- Hanot-Chauffard (-Troisier) (bronze diabetes) 275.01
- Harada's 363.22
- Hare's (M8010/3) (carcinoma, pulmonary apex) 162.3
- Harkavy's 446.0
- harlequin color change 779.89
- Harris' (organic hyperinsulinism) 251.1
- Hart's (pellagra-cerebellar ataxia-renal aminoaciduria) 270.0
- Hayem-Faber (achlorhydric anemia) 280.9
- Hayem-Widal (acquired hemolytic jaundice) 283.9
- headache - *see* Headache, syndrome
- Heberden's (angina pectoris) 413.9
- Hedinger's (malignant carcinoid) 259.2
- Hegglin's 288.2
- Heller's (infantile psychosis) (*see also* Psychosis, childhood) 299.1 ●
- H.E.L.L.P. 642.5 ●
- hemolytic-uremic (adult) (child) 283.11
- hemophagocytic 288.4
  - infection-associated 288.4
- Hench-Rosenberg (palindromic arthritis) (*see also* Rheumatism, palindromic) 719.3 ●
- Henoch-Schönlein (allergic purpura) 287.0
- hepatic flexure 569.89
- hepatopulmonary 573.5
- hepatorenal 572.4
  - due to a procedure 997.49
  - following delivery 674.8 ●
- hepatourologic 572.4
- Herrick's (hemoglobin S disease) 282.61
- Herter (-Gee) (nontropical sprue) 579.0
- Heubner-Herter (nontropical sprue) 579.0
- Heyd's (hepatorenal) 572.4
- HHHO 759.81
- high grade myelodysplastic 238.73
  - with 5q deletion 238.73
- Hilger's 337.09

Syndrome (Continued)
- histiocytic 288.4
- Hoffa (-Kastert) (liposynovitis prepatellaris) 272.8
- Hoffmann's 244.9 [359.5]
- Hoffmann-Bouveret (paroxysmal tachycardia) 427.2
- Hoffmann-Werdnig 335.0
- Holländer-Simons (progressive lipodystrophy) 272.6
- Holmes' (visual disorientation) 368.16
- Holmes-Adie 379.46
- Hoppe-Goldflam 358.00
- Horner's (*see also* Neuropathy, peripheral, autonomic) 337.9
  - traumatic - *see* Injury, nerve, cervical sympathetic
- hospital addiction 301.51
- hungry bone 275.5
- Hunt's (herpetic geniculate ganglionitis) 053.11
  - dyssynergia cerebellaris myoclonica 334.2
- Hunter (-Hurler) (mucopolysaccharidosis II) 277.5
- hunterian glossitis 529.4
- Hurler (-Hunter) (mucopolysaccharidosis II) 277.5
- Hutchinson's incisors or teeth 090.5
- Hutchinson-Boeck (sarcoidosis) 135
- Hutchinson-Gilford (progeria) 259.8
- hydralazine
  - correct substance properly administered 695.4
  - overdose or wrong substance given or taken 972.6
- hydraulic concussion (abdomen) (*see also* Injury, internal, abdomen) 868.00
- hyperabduction 447.8
- hyperactive bowel 564.9
- hyperaldosteronism with hypokalemic alkalosis (Bartter's) 255.13
- hypercalcemic 275.42
- hypercoagulation NEC 289.89
- hypereosinophilic (idiopathic) 288.3
- hyperkalemic 276.7
- hyperkinetic - *see also* Hyperkinesia, heart 429.82
- hyperlipemia-hemolytic anemia-icterus 571.1
- hypermobility 728.5
- hypernatremia 276.0
- hyperosmolarity 276.0
- hyperperfusion 997.01
- hypersomnia-bulimia 349.89
- hypersplenic 289.4
- hypersympathetic (*see also* Neuropathy, peripheral, autonomic) 337.9
- hypertransfusion, newborn 776.4
- hyperventilation, psychogenic 306.1
- hyperviscosity (of serum) NEC 273.3
  - polycythemic 289.0
  - sclerothymic 282.8
- hypoglycemic (familial) (neonatal) 251.2
  - functional 251.1
- hypokalemic 276.8
- hypophyseal 253.8
- hypophyseothalamic 253.8
- hypopituitarism 253.2
- hypoplastic left heart 746.7
- hypopotassemia 276.8
- hyposmolality 276.1
- hypotension, maternal 669.2 ●
- hypothenar hammer 443.89
- hypotonia-hypomentia-hypogonadism-obesity 759.81
- ICF (intravascular coagulation-fibrinolysis) (*see also* Fibrinolysis) 286.6
- idiopathic cardiorespiratory distress, newborn 769
- idiopathic nephrotic (infantile) 581.9
- iliotibial band 728.89

SECTION 1 INDEX TO DISEASES AND INJURIES / Syndrome

Syndrome (Continued)
- Imerslund (-Gräsbeck) (anemia due to familial selective vitamin B_{12} malabsorption) 281.1
- immobility (paraplegic) 728.3
- immune reconstitution inflammatory (IRIS) 995.90
- immunity deficiency, combined 279.2
- impending coronary 411.1
- impingement
  - shoulder 726.2
  - vertebral bodies 724.4
- inappropriate secretion of antidiuretic hormone (ADH) 253.6
- incomplete
  - mandibulofacial 756.0
- infant
  - death, sudden (SIDS) 798.0
  - Hercules 255.2
  - of diabetic mother 775.0
  - shaken 995.55
- infantilism 253.3
- inferior vena cava 459.2
- influenza-like (see also Influenza) 487.1
- inspissated bile, newborn 774.4
- insufficient sleep 307.44
- intermediate coronary (artery) 411.1
- internal carotid artery (see also Occlusion, artery, carotid) 433.1●
- interspinous ligament 724.8
- intestinal
  - carcinoid 259.2
  - gas 787.3
  - knot 560.2
- intraoperative floppy iris (IFIS) 364.81
- intravascular
  - coagulation-fibrinolysis (ICF) (see also Fibrinolysis) 286.6
  - coagulopathy (see also Fibrinolysis) 286.6
- inverted Marfan's 759.89
- IRDS (idiopathic respiratory distress, newborn) 769
- irritable
  - bowel 564.1
  - heart 306.2
  - weakness 300.5
- ischemic bowel (transient) 557.9
  - chronic 557.1
  - due to mesenteric artery insufficiency 557.1
- Itsenko-Cushing (pituitary basophilism) 255.0
- IVC (intravascular coagulopathy) (see also Fibrinolysis) 286.6
- Ivemark's (asplenia with congenital heart disease) 759.0
- Jaccoud's 714.4
- Jackson's 344.89
- Jadassohn-Lewandowski (pachyonchia congenita) 757.5
- Jaffe-Lichtenstein (-Uehlinger) 252.01
- Jahnke's (encephalocutaneous angiomatosis) 759.6
- Jakob-Creutzfeldt 046.19
  - with dementia
    - with behavioral disturbance 046.19 [294.11]
    - without behavioral disturbance 046.19 [294.10]
  - variant 046.11
    - with dementia
      - with behavioral disturbance 046.11 [294.11]
      - without behavioral disturbance 046.11 [294.10]
- Jaksch's (pseudoleukemia infantum) 285.8
- Jaksch-Hayem (-Luzet) (pseudoleukemia infantum) 285.8
- jaw-winking 742.8
- jejunal 564.2
- Jervell-Lange-Nielsen 426.82

Syndrome (Continued)
- jet lag 327.35
- Jeune's (asphyxiating thoracic dystrophy of newborn) 756.4
- Job's (chronic granulomatous disease) 288.1
- Jordan's 288.2
- Joseph-Diamond-Blackfan (congenital hypoplastic anemia) 284.01
- Joubert 759.89
- jugular foramen 352.6
- Kabuki 759.89
- Kahler's (multiple myeloma) (M9730/3) 203.0●
- Kalischer's (encephalocutaneous angiomatosis) 759.6
- Kallmann's (hypogonadotropic hypogonadism with anosmia) 253.4
- Kanner's (autism) (see also Psychosis, childhood) 299.0●
- Kartagener's (sinusitis, bronchiectasis, situs inversus) 759.3
- Kasabach-Merritt (capillary hemangioma associated with thrombocytopenic purpura) 287.39
- Kast's (dyschondroplasia with hemangiomas) 756.4
- Kaznelson's (congenital hypoplastic anemia) 284.01
- Kearns-Sayre 277.87
- Kelly's (sideropenic dysphagia) 280.8
- Kimmelstiel-Wilson (intercapillary glomerulosclerosis) 250.4● [581.81]
  - due to secondary diabetes 249.4● [581.81]
- Klauder's (erythema multiforme exudativum) 695.19
- Klein-Waardenburg (ptosis-epicanthus) 270.2
- Kleine-Levin 327.13
- Klinefelter's 758.7
- Klippel-Feil (brevicollis) 756.16
- Klippel-Trenaunay 759.89
- Klumpke (-Déjérine) (injury to brachial plexus at birth) 767.6
- Klüver-Bucy (-Terzian) 310.0
- Köhler-Pelligrini-Stieda (calcification, knee joint) 726.62
- König's 564.89
- Korsakoff's (nonalcoholic) 294.0
  - alcoholic 291.1
- Korsakoff (-Wernicke) (nonalcoholic) 294.0
  - alcoholic 291.1
- Kostmann's (infantile genetic agranulocytosis) 288.01
- Krabbe's
  - congenital muscle hypoplasia 756.89
  - cutaneocerebral angioma 759.6
- Kunkel (lupoid hepatitis) 571.49
- labyrinthine 386.50
- laceration, broad ligament 620.6
- Lambert-Eaton 358.30
  - in
    - diseases classified elsewhere 358.39
    - neoplastic disease 358.31
- Landau-Kleffner 345.8●
- Langdon Down (mongolism) 758.0
- Larsen's (flattened facies and multiple congenital dislocations) 755.8
- lateral
  - cutaneous nerve of thigh 355.1
  - medullary (see also Disease, cerebrovascular, acute) 436
- Launois' (pituitary gigantism) 253.0
- Launois-Cléret (adiposogenital dystrophy) 253.8
- Laurence-Moon (-Bardet)-Biedl (obesity, polydactyly, and intellectual disabilities) 759.89
- Lawford's (encephalocutaneous angiomatosis) 759.6
- lazy
  - leukocyte 288.09
  - posture 728.3

Syndrome (Continued)
- Lederer-Brill (acquired infectious hemolytic anemia) 283.19
- Legg-Calvé-Perthes (osteochondrosis capital femoral) 732.1
- Lemiere 451.89
- Lennox-Gastaut syndrome 345.0●
  - with tonic seizures 345.1●
- Lennox's (see also Epilepsy) 345.0●
- lenticular 275.1
- Léopold-Lévi's (paroxysmal thyroid instability) 242.9●
- Lepore hemoglobin 282.45
- Léri-Weill 756.59
- Leriche's (aortic bifurcation occlusion) 444.09
- Lermoyez's (see also Disease, Ménière's) 386.00
- Lesch-Nyhan (hypoxanthine-guanine-phosphoribosyltransferase deficiency) 277.2
- leukoencephalopathy, reversible, posterior 348.5
- Lev's (acquired complete heart block) 426.0
- Levi's (pituitary dwarfism) 253.3
- Lévy-Roussy 334.3
- Lichtheim's (subacute combined sclerosis with pernicious anemia) 281.0 [336.2]
- Li-Fraumeni V84.01
- Lightwood's (renal tubular acidosis) 588.89
- Lignac (-de Toni) (-Fanconi) (-Debré) (cystinosis) 270.0
- Likoff's (angina in menopausal women) 413.9
- liver-kidney 572.4
- Lloyd's 258.1
- lobotomy 310.0
- Löffler's (eosinophilic pneumonitis) 518.3
- Löfgren's (sarcoidosis) 135
- long arm 18 or 21 deletion 758.39
- Looser (-Debray)-Milkman (osteomalacia with pseudofractures) 268.2
- Lorain-Levi (pituitary dwarfism) 253.3
- Louis-Bar (ataxia-telangiectasia) 334.8
- low
  - atmospheric pressure 993.2
  - back 724.2
    - psychogenic 306.0
  - output (cardiac) (see also Failure, heart) 428.9
- Lowe's (oculocerebrorenal dystrophy) 270.8
- Lowe-Terrey-MacLachlan (oculocerebrorenal dystrophy) 270.8
- lower radicular, newborn 767.4
- Lown (-Ganong)-Levine (short P-R internal, normal QRS complex, and supraventricular tachycardia) 426.81
- Lucey-Driscoll (jaundice due to delayed conjugation) 774.30
- Luetscher's (dehydration) 276.51
- lumbar vertebral 724.4
- Lutembacher's (atrial septal defect with mitral stenosis) 745.5
- Lyell's (toxic epidermal necrolysis) 695.15
  - due to drug
    - correct substance properly administered 695.15
    - overdose or wrong substance given or taken 977.9
    - specified drug - see Table of Drugs and Chemicals
- MacLeod's 492.8
- macrogenitosomia praecox 259.8
- macroglobulinemia 273.3
- macrophage activation 288.4
- Maffucci's (dyschondroplasia with hemangiomas) 756.4
- Magenblase 306.4
- magnesium-deficiency 781.7

SECTION I INDEX TO DISEASES AND INJURIES / Syndrome

Syndrome (Continued)
- malabsorption 579.9
    - postsurgical 579.3
    - spinal fluid 331.3
- Mal de Debarquement 780.4
- malignant carcinoid 259.2
- Mallory-Weiss 530.7
- mandibulofacial dysostosis 756.0
- manic-depressive (see also Psychosis, affective) 296.80
- Mankowsky's (familial dysplastic osteopathy) 731.2
- maple syrup (urine) 270.3
- Marable's (celiac artery compression) 447.4
- Marchesani (-Weill) (brachymorphism and ectopia lentis) 759.89
- Marchiafava-Bignami 341.8
- Marchiafava-Micheli (paroxysmal nocturnal hemoglobinuria) 283.2
- Marcus Gunn's (jaw-winking syndrome) 742.8
- Marfan's (arachnodactyly) 759.82
    - meaning congenital syphilis 090.49
        - with luxation of lens 090.49 [379.32]
- Marie's (acromegaly) 253.0
    - primary or idiopathic (acropachyderma) 757.39
    - secondary (hypertrophic pulmonary osteoarthropathy) 731.2
- Markus-Adie 379.46
- Maroteaux-Lamy (mucopolysaccharidosis VI) 277.5
- Martin's 715.27
- Martin-Albright (pseudohypoparathyroidism) 275.49
- Martorell-Fabré (pulseless disease) 446.7
- massive aspiration of newborn 770.18
- Masters-Allen 620.6
- mastocytosis 757.33
- maternal hypotension 669.2●
- maternal obesity 646.1●
- May (-Hegglin) 288.2
- McArdle (-Schmid) (-Pearson) (glycogenosis V) 271.0
- McCune-Albright (osteitis fibrosa disseminata) 756.59
- McQuarrie's (idiopathic familial hypoglycemia) 251.2
- meconium
    - aspiration 770.12
    - plug (newborn) NEC 777.1
- median arcuate ligament 447.4
- mediastinal fibrosis 519.3
- Meekeren-Ehlers-Danlos 756.83
- Meige (blepharospasm-oromandibular dystonia) 333.82
    - -Milroy (chronic hereditary edema) 757.0
- MELAS (mitochondrial encephalopathy, lactic acidosis and stroke-like episodes) 277.87
- Melkersson (-Rosenthal) 351.8
- MEN (multiple endocrine neoplasia)
    - type I 258.01
    - type IIA 258.02
    - type IIB 258.03
- Mende's (ptosis-epicanthus) 270.2
- Mendelson's (resulting from a procedure) 997.32
    - during labor 668.0●
    - obstetric 668.0●
- Ménétrier's (hypertrophic gastritis) 535.2●
- Ménière's (see also Disease, Ménière's) 386.00
- meningo-eruptive 047.1
- Menkes' 759.89
    - glutamic acid 759.89
    - maple syrup (urine) disease 270.3
- menopause 627.2
    - postartificial 627.4
- menstruation 625.4
- MERRF (myoclonus with epilepsy and with ragged red fibers) 277.87

Syndrome (Continued)
- mesenteric
    - artery, superior 557.1
    - vascular insufficiency (with gangrene) 557.1
- metabolic 277.7
- metastatic carcinoid 259.2
- Meyenburg-Altherr-Uehlinger 733.99
- Meyer-Schwickerath and Weyers (dysplasia oculodentodigitalis) 759.89
- Micheli-Rietti (thalassemia minor) 282.46
- Michotte's 721.5
- micrognathia-glossoptosis 756.0
- microphthalmos (congenital) 759.89
- midbrain 348.89
- middle
    - lobe (lung) (right) 518.0
    - radicular 353.0
- Miescher's
    - familial acanthosis nigricans 701.2
    - granulomatosis disciformis 709.3
- Mieten's 759.89
- migraine 346.0●
- Mikity-Wilson (pulmonary dysmaturity) 770.7
- Mikulicz's (dryness of mouth, absent or decreased lacrimation) 527.1
- milk alkali (milk drinkers') 275.42
- Milkman (-Looser) (osteomalacia with pseudofractures) 268.2
- Millard-Gubler 344.89
- Miller-Dieker 758.33
- Miller Fisher's 357.0
- Milles' (encephalocutaneous angiomatosis) 759.6
- Minkowski-Chauffard (see also Spherocytosis) 282.0
- Mirizzi's (hepatic duct stenosis) 576.2
    - with calculus, cholelithiasis, or stones - see Choledocholithiasis
- mitochondrial neurogastrointestinal encephalopathy (MNGIE) 277.87
- mitral
    - click (-murmur) 785.2
    - valve prolapse 424.0
- MNGIE (mitochondrial neurogastrointestinal encephalopathy) 277.87
- Möbius'
    - congenital oculofacial paralysis 352.6
    - ophthalmoplegic migraine 346.2●
- Mohr's (types I and II) 759.89
- monofixation 378.34
- Moore's (see also Epilepsy) 345.5●
- Morel-Moore (hyperostosis frontalis interna) 733.3
- Morel-Morgagni (hyperostosis frontalis interna) 733.3
- Morgagni (-Stewart-Morel) (hyperostosis frontalis interna) 733.3
- Morgagni-Adams-Stokes (syncope with heart block) 426.9
- Morquio (-Brailsford) (-Ullrich) (mucopolysaccharidosis IV) 277.5
- Morris (testicular feminization) 259.51
- Morton's (foot) (metatarsalgia) (metatarsal neuralgia) (neuralgia) (neuroma) (toe) 355.6
- Moschcowitz (-Singer-Symmers) (thrombotic thrombocytopenic purpura) 446.6
- Mounier-Kuhn 748.3
    - with
        - acute exacerbation 494.1
        - bronchiectasis 494.0
            - with (acute) exacerbation 494.1
        - acquired 519.19
            - with bronchiectasis 494.0
                - with (acute) exacerbation 494.1
- Mucha-Haberman (acute parapsoriasis varioliformis) 696.2
- mucocutaneous lymph node (acute) (febrile) (infantile) (MCLS) 446.1

Syndrome (Continued)
- multiple
    - deficiency 260
    - endocrine neoplasia (MEN)
        - type I 258.01
        - type IIA 258.02
        - type IIB 258.03
    - operations 301.51
- Munchausen's 301.51
- Munchmeyer's (exostosis luxurians) 728.11
- Murchison-Sanderson - see Disease, Hodgkin's
- myasthenic - see Myasthenia, syndrome
- myelodysplastic 238.75
    - with 5q deletion 238.74
    - high grade with 5q deletion 238.73
    - lesions, low grade 238.72
    - therapy-related 289.83
- myeloproliferative (chronic) (M9960/1) 238.79
- myofascial pain NEC 729.1
- Naffziger's 353.0
- Nager-de Reynier (dysostosis mandibularis) 756.0
- nail-patella (hereditary osteo-onychodysplasia) 756.89
- NARP (neuropathy, ataxia and retinitis pigmentosa) 277.87
- Nebécourt's 253.3
- Neill Dingwall (microencephaly and dwarfism) 759.89
- nephrotic (see also Nephrosis) 581.9
    - diabetic 250.4● [581.81]
    - due to secondary diabetes 249.4● [581.81]
- Netherton's (ichthyosiform erythroderma) 757.1
- neurocutaneous 759.6
- neuroleptic malignant 333.92
- Nezelof's (pure alymphocytosis) 279.13
- Niemann-Pick (lipid histiocytosis) 272.7
- Nonne-Milroy-Meige (chronic hereditary edema) 757.0
- nonsense 300.16
- Noonan's 759.89
- Nothnagel's
    - ophthalmoplegia-cerebellar ataxia 378.52
    - vasomotor acroparesthesia 443.89
- nucleus ambiguous-hypoglossal 352.6
- OAV (oculoauriculovertebral dysplasia) 756.0
- obesity hypoventilation 278.03
- obsessional 300.3
- oculocutaneous 364.24
- oculomotor 378.81
- oculourethroarticular 099.3
- Ogilvie's (sympathicotonic colon obstruction) 560.89
- ophthalmoplegia-cerebellar ataxia 378.52
- Oppenheim-Urbach (necrobiosis lipoidica diabeticorum) 250.8● [709.3]
    - due to secondary diabetes 249.8● [709.3]
- oral-facial-digital 759.89
- organic
    - affective NEC 293.83
        - drug-induced 292.84
    - anxiety 293.84
    - delusional 293.81
        - alcohol-induced 291.5
        - drug-induced 292.11
        - due to or associated with
            - arteriosclerosis 290.42
            - presenile brain disease 290.12
            - senility 290.20
    - depressive 293.83
        - drug-induced 292.84
        - due to or associated with
            - arteriosclerosis 290.43
            - presenile brain disease 290.13
            - senile brain disease 290.21

SECTION I INDEX TO DISEASES AND INJURIES / Syndrome

Syndrome (Continued)
- organic (Continued)
  - hallucinosis 293.82
    - drug-induced 292.84
  - organic affective 293.83
    - induced by drug 292.84
  - organic personality 310.1
    - induced by drug 292.89
- Ormond's 593.4
- orodigitofacial 759.89
- orthostatic hypotensive-dysautonomic-dyskinetic 333.0
- Osler-Weber-Rendu (familial hemmorrhagic telangiectasia) 448.0
- osteodermopathic hyperostosis 757.39
- osteoporosis-osteomalacia 268.2
- Österreicher-Turner (hereditary osteo-onychodysplasia) 756.89
- os trigonum 755.69
- Ostrum-Furst 756.59
- otolith 386.19
- otopalatodigital 759.89
- outlet (thoracic) 353.0
- ovarian remnant 620.8
- Owren's (see also Defect, coagulation) 286.3
- OX 758.6
- pacemaker 429.4
- Paget-Schroetter (intermittent venous claudication) 453.89
- pain - see also Pain
  - central 338.0
  - chronic 338.4
  - complex regional 355.9
    - type I 337.20
      - lower limb 337.22
      - specified site NEC 337.29
      - upper limb 337.21
    - type II
      - lower limb 355.71
      - upper limb 354.4
  - myelopathic 338.0
  - thalamic (hyperesthetic) 338.0
- painful
  - apicocostal vertebral (M8010/3) 162.3
  - arc 726.19
  - bruising 287.2
  - feet 266.2
- Pancoast's (carcinoma, pulmonary apex) (M8010/3) 162.3
- panhypopituitary (postpartum) 253.2
- papillary muscle 429.81
  - with myocardial infarction 410.8●
- Papillon-Léage and Psaume (orodigitofacial dysostosis) 759.89
- parabiotic (transfusion)
  - donor (twin) 772.0
  - recipient (twin) 776.4
- paralysis agitans 332.0
- paralytic 344.9
  - specified type NEC 344.89
- paraneoplastic - see Condition
- Parinaud's (paralysis of conjugate upward gaze) 378.81
  - oculoglandular 372.02
- Parkes Weber and Dimitri (encephalocutaneous angiomatosis) 759.6
- Parkinson's (see also Parkinsonism) 332.0
- parkinsonian (see also Parkinsonism) 332.0
- Parry's (exophthalmic goiter) 242.0●
- Parry-Romberg 349.82
- Parsonage-Aldren-Turner 353.5
- Parsonage-Turner 353.5
- Patau's (trisomy D_1) 758.1
- patella clunk 719.66
- patellofemoral 719.46
- Paterson (-Brown) (-Kelly) (sideropenic dysphagia) 280.8
- Payr's (splenic flexure syndrome) 569.89
- pectoral girdle 447.8
- pectoralis minor 447.8

Syndrome (Continued)
- Pelger-Huët (hereditary hyposegmentation) 288.2
- pellagra-cerebellar ataxia-renal aminoaciduria 270.0
- Pellegrini-Stieda 726.62
- pellagroid 265.2
- Pellizzi's (pineal) 259.8
- pelvic congestion (-fibrosis) 625.5
- Pendred's (familial goiter with deaf-mutism) 243
- Penfield's (see also Epilepsy) 345.5●
- Penta X 758.81
- peptic ulcer - see Ulcer, peptic 533.9
- perabduction 447.8
- periodic 277.31
- periurethral fibrosis 593.4
- persistent fetal circulation 747.83
- Petges-Cléjat (poikilodermatomyositis) 710.3
- Peutz-Jeghers 759.6
- Pfeiffer (acrocephalosyndactyly) 755.55
- phantom limb 353.6
- pharyngeal pouch 279.11
- Pick's (pericardial pseudocirrhosis of liver) 423.2
  - heart 423.2
  - liver 423.2
- Pick-Herxheimer (diffuse idiopathic cutaneous atrophy) 701.8
- Pickwickian (cardiopulmonary obesity) 278.03
- PIE (pulmonary infiltration with eosinophilia) 518.3
- Pierre Marie-Bamberger (hypertrophic pulmonary osteoarthropathy) 731.2
- Pierre Mauriac's (diabetes-dwarfism-obesity) 258.1
- Pierre Robin 756.0
- pigment dispersion, iris 364.53
- pineal 259.8
- pink puffer 492.8
- pituitary 253.0
- placental
  - dysfunction 762.2
  - insufficiency 762.2
  - transfusion 762.3
- plantar fascia 728.71
- plateau iris (without glaucoma) 364.82
  - with glaucoma 365.23
- plica knee 727.83
- Plummer-Vinson (sideropenic dysphagia) 280.8
- pluricarential of infancy 260
- plurideficiency of infancy 260
- pluriglandular (compensatory) 258.8
- Poland 756.81
- polycarential of infancy 260
- polyglandular 258.8
- polysplenia 759.0
- pontine 433.8●
- popliteal
  - artery entrapment 447.8
  - web 756.89
- post chemoembolization - code to associated conditions
- postartificial menopause 627.4
- postcardiac injury
  - postcardiotomy 429.4
  - postmyocardial infarction 411.0
- postcardiotomy 429.4
- postcholecystectomy 576.0
- postcommissurotomy 429.4
- postconcussional 310.2
- postcontusional 310.2
- postencephalitic 310.89
- posterior
  - cervical sympathetic 723.2
  - fossa compression 348.4
  - inferior cerebellar artery (see also Disease, cerebrovascular, acute) 436
  - reversible encephalopathy (PRES) 348.39

Syndrome (Continued)
- postgastrectomy (dumping) 564.2
- post-gastric surgery 564.2
- posthepatitis 780.79
- postherpetic (neuralgia) (zoster) 053.19
  - geniculate ganglion 053.11
  - ophthalmica 053.19
- postimmunization - see Complications, vaccination
- postinfarction 411.0
- postinfluenza (asthenia) 780.79
- postirradiation 990
- postlaminectomy 722.80
  - cervical, cervicothoracic 722.81
  - lumbar, lumbosacral 722.83
  - thoracic, thoracolumbar 722.82
- postleukotomy 310.0
- postlobotomy 310.0
- postmastectomy lymphedema 457.0
- postmature (of newborn) 766.22
- postmyocardial infarction 411.0
- postoperative NEC 998.9
  - blind loop 579.2
- postpartum panhypopituitary 253.2
- postperfusion NEC 999.89
  - bone marrow 996.85
- postpericardiotomy 429.4
- postphlebitic (asymptomatic) 459.10
  - with
    - complications NEC 459.19
    - inflammation 459.12
      - and ulcer 459.13
    - stasis dermatitis 459.12
      - with ulcer 459.13
    - ulcer 459.11
      - with inflammation 459.13
- postpolio (myelitis) 138
- postvagotomy 564.2
- postvalvulotomy 429.4
- postviral (asthenia) NEC 780.79
- Potain's (gastrectasis with dyspepsia) 536.1
- potassium intoxication 276.7
- Potter's 753.0
- Prader (-Labhart)-Willi (-Fanconi) 759.81
- preinfarction 411.1
- preleukemic 238.75
- premature senility 259.8
- premenstrual 625.4
- premenstrual tension 625.4
- pre ulcer 536.9
- Prinzmetal-Massumi (anterior chest wall syndrome) 786.52
- Profichet's 729.90
- progeria 259.8
- progressive pallidal degeneration 333.0
- prolonged gestation 766.22
- Proteus (dermal hypoplasia) 757.39
- prune belly 756.71
- prurigo-asthma 691.8
- pseudocarpal tunnel (sublimis) 354.0
- pseudohermaphroditism-virilism hirsutism 255.2
- pseudoparalytica 358.00
- pseudo-Turner's 759.89
- psycho-organic 293.9
  - acute 293.0
  - anxiety type 293.84
  - depressive type 293.83
  - hallucinatory type 293.82
  - nonpsychotic severity 310.1
    - specified focal (partial) NEC 310.89
  - paranoid type 293.81
  - specified type NEC 293.89
  - subacute 293.1
- pterygolymphangiectasia 758.6
- ptosis-epicanthus 270.2
- pulmonary
  - arteriosclerosis 416.0
  - hypoperfusion (idiopathic) 769
  - renal (hemorrhagic) 446.21
- pulseless 446.7

SECTION I INDEX TO DISEASES AND INJURIES / Syndrome

Syndrome (Continued)
- Putnam-Dana (subacute combined sclerosis with pernicious anemia) 281.0 [336.2]
- pyloroduodenal 537.89
- pyramidopallidonigral 332.0
- pyriformis 355.0
- QT interval prolongation 426.82
- radicular NEC 729.2
  - lower limbs 724.4
  - upper limbs 723.4
  - newborn 767.4
- Raeder-Harbitz (pulseless disease) 446.7
- Ramsay Hunt's
  - dyssynergia cerebellaris myoclonica 334.2
  - herpetic geniculate ganglionitis 053.11
- rapid time-zone change 327.35
- Raymond (-Céstan) 433.8 ●
- Raynaud's (paroxysmal digital cyanosis) 443.0
- RDS (respiratory distress syndrome, newborn) 769
- Refsum's (heredopathia atactica polyneuritiformis) 356.3
- Reichmann's (gastrosuccorrhea) 536.8
- Reifenstein's (hereditary familial hypogonadism, male) 259.52
- Reilly's (see also Neuropathy, peripheral, autonomic 337.9
- Reiter's 099.3
- renal glomerulohyalinosis-diabetic 250.4 ● [581.81]
  - due to secondary diabetes 249.4 ● [581.81]
- Rendu-Osler-Weber (familial hemorrhagic telangiectasia) 448.0
- renofacial (congenital biliary fibroangiomatosis) 753.0
- Rénon-Delille 253.8
- respiratory distress (idiopathic) (newborn) 769
  - adult (following trauma and surgery) 518.52
  - specified NEC 518.82
  - type II 770.6
- restless legs (RLS) 333.94
- retinoblastoma (familial) 190.5
- retraction (Duane's) 378.71
- retroperitoneal fibrosis 593.4
- retroviral seroconversion (acute) V08
- Rett's 330.8
- Reye's 331.81
- Reye-Sheehan (postpartum pituitary necrosis) 253.2
- Riddoch's (visual disorientation) 368.16
- Ridley's (see also Failure, ventricular, left) 428.1
- Rieger's (mesodermal dysgenesis, anterior ocular segment) 743.44
- Rietti-Greppi-Micheli (thalassemia minor) 282.46
- right ventricular obstruction - see Failure, heart
- Riley-Day (familial dysautonomia) 742.8
- Robin's 756.0
- Rokitansky-Kuster-Hauser (congenital absence, vagina) 752.45
- Romano-Ward (prolonged QT interval syndrome) 426.82
- Romberg's 349.89
- Rosen-Castleman-Liebow (pulmonary proteinosis) 516.0
- rotator cuff, shoulder 726.10
- Roth's 355.1
- Rothmund's (congenital poikiloderma) 757.33
- Rotor's (idiopathic hyperbilirubinemia) 277.4
- Roussy-Lévy 334.3
- Roy (-Jutras) (acropachyderma) 757.39
- rubella (congenital) 771.0
- Rubinstein-Taybi's (brachydactylia, short stature, and intellectual disabilities) 759.89

Syndrome (Continued)
- Rud's (mental deficiency, epilepsy, and infantilism) 759.89
- Ruiter-Pompen (-Wyers) (angiokeratoma corporis diffusum) 272.7
- Runge's (postmaturity) 766.22
- Russell (-Silver) (congenital hemihypertrophy and short stature) 759.89
- Rytand-Lipsitch (complete atrioventricular block) 426.0
- sacralization-scoliosis-sciatica 756.15
- sacroiliac 724.6
- Saenger's 379.46
- salt
  - depletion (see also Disease, renal) 593.9
    - due to heat NEC 992.8
      - causing heat exhaustion or prostration 992.4
  - low (see also Disease, renal) 593.9
- salt-losing (see also Disease, renal) 593.9
- Sanfilippo's (mucopolysaccharidosis III) 277.5
- Scaglietti-Dagnini (acromegalic macrospondylitis) 253.0
- scalded skin 695.81
- scalenus anticus (anterior) 353.0
- scapulocostal 354.8
- scapuloperoneal 359.1
- scapulovertebral 723.4
- Schaumann's (sarcoidosis) 135
- Scheie's (mucopolysaccharidosis IS) 277.5
- Scheuthauer-Marie-Sainton (cleidocranialis dysostosis) 755.59
- Schirmer's (encephalocutaneous angiomatosis) 759.6
- schizophrenic, of childhood NEC (see also Psychosis, childhood) 299.9 ●
- Schmidt's
  - sphallo-pharyngo-laryngeal hemiplegia 352.6
  - thyroid-adrenocortical insufficiency 258.1
  - vagoaccessory 352.6
- Schneider's 047.9
- Schnitzler 273.1
- Scholte's (malignant carcinoid) 259.2
- Scholz (-Bielschowsky-Henneberg) 330.0
- Schroeder's (endocrine-hypertensive) 255.3
- Schüller-Christian (chronic histiocytosis X) 277.89
- Schultz's (agranulocytosis) 288.09
- Schwachman's - see Syndrome, Shwachman's
- Schwartz (-Jampel) 359.23
- Schwartz-Bartter (inappropriate secretion of antidiuretic hormone) 253.6
- Scimitar (anomalous venous drainage, right lung to inferior vena cava) 747.49
- sclerocystic ovary 256.4
- sea-blue histiocyte 272.7
- Seabright-Bantam (pseudohypoparathyroidism) 275.49
- Seckel's 759.89
- Secretan's (posttraumatic edema) 782.3
- secretoinhibitor (keratoconjunctivitis sicca) 710.2
- Seeligmann's (ichthyosis congenita) 757.1
- Senear-Usher (pemphigus erythematosus) 694.4
- senilism 259.8
- seroconversion, retroviral (acute) V08
- serotonin 333.99
- serous meningitis 348.2
- Sertoli cell (germinal aplasia) 606.0
- sex chromosome mosaic 758.81
- Sézary's (reticulosis) (M9701/3) 202.2 ●
- shaken infant 995.55
- Shaver's (bauxite pneumoconiosis) 503
- Sheehan's (postpartum pituitary necrosis) 253.2

Syndrome (Continued)
- shock (traumatic) 958.4
  - kidney 584.5
    - following crush injury 958.5
  - lung 518.82
    - related to trauma and surgery 518.52
  - neurogenic 308.9
  - psychic 308.9
- Shone's 746.84
- short
  - bowel 579.3
  - P-R interval 426.81
- shoulder-arm (see also Neuropathy, peripheral, autonomic) 337.9
- shoulder-girdle 723.4
- shoulder-hand (see also Neuropathy, peripheral, autonomic) 337.9
- Shwachman's 288.02
- Shy-Drager (orthostatic hypotension with multisystem degeneration) 333.0
- Sicard's 352.6
- sicca (keratoconjunctivitis) 710.2
- sick
  - cell 276.1
  - cilia 759.89
  - sinus 427.81
- sideropenic 280.8
- Siemens'
  - ectodermal dysplasia 757.31
  - keratosis follicularis spinulosa (decalvans) 757.39
- Silfverskiöld's (osteochondrodystrophy, extremities) 756.50
- Silver's (congenital hemihypertrophy and short stature) 759.89
- Silvestroni-Bianco (thalassemia minima) 282.46
- Simons' (progressive lipodystrophy) 272.6
- sinus tarsi 726.79
- sinusitis-bronchiectasis-situs inversus 759.3
- Sipple's (medullary thyroid carcinoma-pheochromocytoma) 258.02
- Sjögren (-Gougerot) (keratoconjunctivitis sicca) 710.2
  - with lung involvement 710.2 [517.8]
- Sjögren-Larsson (ichthyosis congenita) 757.1
- SJS-TEN (Stevens-Johnson syndrome-toxic epidermal necrolysis overlap) 695.14
- Slocumb's 255.3
- Sluder's 337.09
- Smith-Lemli-Opitz (cerebrohepatorenal syndrome) 759.89
- Smith-Magenis 758.33
- smokers' 305.1
- Sneddon-Wilkinson (subcorneal pustular dermatosis) 694.1
- Sotos' (cerebral gigantism) 253.0
- South African cardiomyopathy 425.2
- spasmodic
  - upward movement, eye(s) 378.82
  - winking 307.20
- Spens' (syncope with heart block) 426.9
- spherophakia-brachymorphia 759.89
- spinal cord injury - see also Injury, spinal, by site
  - with fracture, vertebra - see Fracture, vertebra, by site, with spinal cord injury
  - cervical - see Injury, spinal, cervical
  - fluid malabsorption (acquired) 331.3
- splenic
  - agenesis 759.0
  - flexure 569.89
  - neutropenia 289.53
  - sequestration 289.52
- Spurway's (brittle bones and blue sclera) 756.51
- staphylococcal scalded skin 695.81
- Stein's (polycystic ovary) 256.4
- Stein-Leventhal (polycystic ovary) 256.4

◀ New   Revised   ~~deleted~~ Deleted   Use Additional Digit(s)   Omit code

SECTION I INDEX TO DISEASES AND INJURIES / Syndrome

Syndrome (Continued)
- Steinbrocker's (see also Neuropathy, peripheral, autonomic) 337.9
- Stevens-Johnson (erythema multiforme exudativum) 695.13
  - toxic epidermal necrolysis overlap (SJS-TEN overlap syndrome) 695.14
- Stewart-Morel (hyperostosis frontalis interna) 733.3
- Stickler 759.89
- stiff-baby 759.89
- stiff-man 333.91
- Still's (juvenile rheumatoid arthritis) 714.30
- Still-Felty (rheumatoid arthritis with splenomegaly and leukopenia) 714.1
- Stilling-Türk-Duane (ocular retraction syndrome) 378.71
- Stojano's (subcostal) 098.86
- Stokes (-Adams) (syncope with heart block) 426.9
- Stokvis-Talma (enterogenous cyanosis) 289.7
- stone heart (see also Failure, ventricular, left) 428.1
- straight-back 756.19
- stroke (see also Disease, cerebrovascular, acute) 436
  - little 435.9
- Sturge-Kalischer-Weber (encephalotrigeminal angiomatosis) 759.6
- Sturge-Weber (-Dimitri) (encephalocutaneous angiomatosis) 759.6
- subclavian-carotid obstruction (chronic) 446.7
- subclavian steal 435.2
- subcoracoid-pectoralis minor 447.8
- subcostal 098.86
  - nerve compression 354.8
- subperiosteal hematoma 267
- subphrenic interposition 751.4
- sudden infant death (SIDS) 798.0
- Sudeck's 733.7
- Sudeck-Leriche 733.7
- superior
  - cerebellar artery (see also Disease, cerebrovascular, acute) 436
  - mesenteric artery 557.1
  - pulmonary sulcus (tumor) (M8010/3) 162.3
  - semi-circular canal dehiscence 386.8
  - vena cava 459.2
- suprarenal cortical 255.3
- supraspinatus 726.10
- Susac 348.39
- swallowed blood 777.3
- sweat retention 705.1
- Sweet's (acute febrile neutrophilic dermatosis) 695.89
- Swyer-James (unilateral hyperlucent lung) 492.8
- Swyer's (XY pure gonadal dysgenesis) 752.7
- Symonds' 348.2
- sympathetic
  - cervical paralysis 337.09
  - pelvic 625.5
- syndactylic oxycephaly 755.55
- syphilitic-cardiovascular 093.89
- systemic
  - fibrosclerosing 710.8
  - inflammatory response (SIRS) 995.90
    - due to
      - infectious process 995.91
        - with acute organ dysfunction 995.92
      - non-infectious process 995.93
        - with acute organ dysfunction 995.94
- systolic click (-murmur) 785.2
- Tabagism 305.1
- tachycardia-bradycardia 427.81

Syndrome (Continued)
- Takayasu (-Onishi) (pulseless disease) 446.7
- Takotsubo 429.83
- Tapia's 352.6
- tarsal tunnel 355.5
- Taussig-Bing (transposition, aorta and overriding pulmonary artery) 745.11
- Taybi's (otopalatodigital) 759.89
- Taylor's 625.5
- teething 520.7
- tegmental 344.89
- telangiectasis-pigmentation-cataract 757.33
- temporal 383.02
  - lobectomy behavior 310.0
- temporomandibular joint-pain-dysfunction [TMJ] NEC 524.60
  - specified NEC 524.69
- Terry's (see also Retinopathy of prematurity) 362.21
- testicular feminization 259.51
- testis, nonvirilizing 257.8
- tethered (spinal) cord 742.59
- thalamic 338.0
- Thibierge-Weissenbach (cutaneous systemic sclerosis) 710.1
- Thiele 724.6
- thoracic outlet (compression) 353.0
- thoracogenous rheumatic (hypertrophic pulmonary osteoarthropathy) 731.2
- Thorn's (see also Disease, renal) 593.9
- Thorson-Biörck (malignant carcinoid) 259.2
- thrombopenia-hemangioma 287.39
- thyroid-adrenocortical insufficiency 258.1
- Tietze's 733.6
- time-zone (rapid) 327.35
- Tobias' (carcinoma, pulmonary apex) (M8010/3) 162.3
- toilet seat 926.0
- Tolosa-Hunt 378.55
- Toni-Fanconi (cystinosis) 270.0
- Touraine's (hereditary osteo-onychodysplasia) 756.89
- Touraine-Solente-Golé (acropachyderma) 757.39
- toxic
  - oil 710.5
  - shock 040.82
- transfusion
  - fetal-maternal 772.0
  - twin
    - donor (infant) 772.0
    - recipient (infant) 776.4
- transient left ventricular apical ballooning 429.83
- Treacher Collins' (incomplete mandibulofacial dysostosis) 756.0
- trigeminal plate 259.8
- triplex X female 758.81
- trisomy NEC 758.5
  - 13 or D_1 758.1
  - 16–18 or E 758.2
  - 18 or E_3 758.2
  - 20 758.5
  - 21 or G (mongolism) 758.0
  - 22 or G (mongolism) 758.0
  - G 758.0
- Troisier-Hanot-Chauffard (bronze diabetes) 275.01
- tropical wet feet 991.4
- Trousseau's (thrombophlebitis migrans visceral cancer) 453.1
- tumor lysis (following antineoplastic drug therapy) (spontaneous) 277.88
- Türk's (ocular retraction syndrome) 378.71
- Turner's 758.6
- Turner-Varny 758.6
- Twiddler's (due to)
  - automatic implantable defibrillator 996.04
  - pacemaker 996.01
- twin-to-twin transfusion 762.3
  - recipient twin 776.4

Syndrome (Continued)
- Uehlinger's (acropachyderma) 757.39
- Ullrich (-Bonnevie) (-Turner) 758.6
- Ullrich-Feichtiger 759.89
- underwater blast injury (abdominal) (see also Injury, internal, abdomen) 868.00
- universal joint, cervix 620.6
- Unverricht (-Lundborg) 345.1●
- Unverricht-Wagner (dermatomyositis) 710.3
- upward gaze 378.81
- Urbach-Oppenheim (necrobiosis lipoidica diabeticorum) 250.8● [709.3]
  - due to secondary diabetes 249.8● [709.3]
- Urbach-Wiethe (lipoid proteinosis) 272.8
- uremia, chronic 585.9
- urethral 597.81
- urethro-oculoarticular 099.3
- urethro-oculosynovial 099.3
- urohepatic 572.4
- uveocutaneous 364.24
- uveomeningeal, uveomeningitis 363.22
- vagohypoglossal 352.6
- vagovagal 780.2
- van Buchem's (hyperostosis corticalis) 733.3
- van der Hoeve's (brittle bones and blue sclera, deafness) 756.51
- van der Hoeve-Halbertsma-Waardenburg (ptosis-epicanthus) 270.2
- van der Hoeve-Waarderburg-Gualdi (ptosis-epicanthus) 270.2
- vanishing twin 651.33
- van Neck-Odelberg (juvenile osteochondrosis) 732.1
- vascular splanchnic 557.0
- vasomotor 443.9
- vasovagal 780.2
- VATER 759.89
- Velo-cardio-facial 758.32
- vena cava (inferior) (superior) (obstruction) 459.2
- Verbiest's (claudicatio intermittens spinalis) 435.1
- Vernet's 352.6
- vertebral
  - artery 435.1
    - compression 721.1
  - lumbar 724.4
  - steal 435.1
- vertebrogenic (pain) 724.5
- vertiginous NEC 386.9
- video display tube 723.8
- Villaret's 352.6
- Vinson-Plummer (sideropenic dysphagia) 280.8
- virilizing adrenocortical hyperplasia, congenital 255.2
- virus, viral 079.99
- visceral larval migrans 128.0
- visual disorientation 368.16
- vitamin B_6 deficiency 266.1
- vitreous touch 997.99
- Vogt's (corpus striatum) 333.71
- Vogt-Koyanagi 364.24
- Volkmann's 958.6
- von Bechterew-Stumpell (ankylosing spondylitis) 720.0
- von Graefe's 378.72
- von Hippel-Lindau (angiomatosis retinocerebellosa) 759.6
- von Schroetter's (intermittent venous claudication) 453.89
- von Willebrand (-Jürgens) (angiohemophilia) 286.4
- Waardenburg-Klein (ptosis epicanthus) 270.2
- Wagner (-Unverricht) (dermatomyositis) 710.3
- Waldenström's (macroglobulinemia) 273.3
- Waldenström-Kjellberg (sideropenic dysphagia) 280.8

SECTION 1 INDEX TO DISEASES AND INJURIES / Syphilis, syphilitic

Syndrome (Continued)
  Wallenberg's (posterior inferior cerebellar artery) (see also Disease, cerebrovascular, acute) 436
  Waterhouse (-Friderichsen) 036.3
  water retention 276.69
  Weber's 344.89
  Weber-Christian (nodular nonsuppurative panniculitis) 729.30
  Weber-Cockayne (epidermolysis bullosa) 757.39
  Weber-Dimitri (encephalocutaneous angiomatosis) 759.6
  Weber-Gubler 344.89
  Weber-Leyden 344.89
  Weber-Osler (familial hemorrhagic telangiectasia) 448.0
  Wegener's (necrotizing respiratory granulomatosis) 446.4
  Weill-Marchesani (brachymorphism and ectopia lentis) 759.89
  Weingarten's (tropical eosinophilia) 518.3
  Weiss-Baker (carotid sinus syncope) 337.01
  Weissenbach-Thibierge (cutaneous systemic sclerosis) 710.1
  Werdnig-Hoffmann 335.0
  Werlhof-Wichmann (see also Purpura, thrombocytopenic) 287.39
  Wermer's (polyendocrine adenomatosis) 258.01
  Werner's (progeria adultorum) 259.8
  Wernicke's (nonalcoholic) (superior hemorrhagic polioencephalitis) 265.1
  Wernicke-Korsakoff (nonalcoholic) 294.0
    alcoholic 291.1
  Westphal-Strümpell (hepatolenticular degeneration) 275.1
  wet
    brain (alcoholic) 303.9 ●
    feet (maceration) (tropical) 991.4
    lung
      adult 518.52
      newborn 770.6
  whiplash 847.0
  Whipple's (intestinal lipodystrophy) 040.2
  "whistling face" (craniocarpotarsal dystrophy) 759.89
  Widal (-Abrami) (acquired hemolytic jaundice) 283.9
  Wilkie's 557.1
  Wilkinson-Sneddon (subcorneal pustular dermatosis) 694.1
  Willan-Plumbe (psoriasis) 696.1
  Willebrand (-Jürgens) (angiohemophilia) 286.4
  Willi-Prader (hypogenital dystrophy with diabetic tendency) 759.81
  Wilson's (hepatolenticular degeneration) 275.1
  Wilson-Mikity 770.7
  Wiskott-Aldrich (eczema-thrombocytopenia) 279.12
  withdrawal
    alcohol 291.81
    drug 292.0
    infant of dependent mother 779.5
  Woakes' (ethmoiditis) 471.1
  Wolff-Parkinson-White (anomalous atrioventricular excitation) 426.7
  Wright's (hyperabduction) 447.8
  X
    cardiac 413.9
    dysmetabolic 277.7
  xiphoidalgia 733.99
  XO 758.6
  XXX 758.81
  XXXXY 758.81
  XXY 758.7
  yellow vernix (placental dysfunction) 762.2
  Zahorsky's 074.0
  Zellweger 277.86

Syndrome (Continued)
  Zieve's (jaundice, hyperlipemia and hemolytic anemia) 571.1
  Zollinger-Ellison (gastric hypersecretion with pancreatic islet cell tumor) 251.5
  Zuelzer-Ogden (nutritional megaloblastic anemia) 281.2
Synechia (iris) (pupil) 364.70
  anterior 364.72
    peripheral 364.73
  intrauterine (traumatic) 621.5
  posterior 364.71
  vulvae, congenital 752.49
Synesthesia (see also Disturbance, sensation) 782.0
Synodontia 520.2
Synophthalmus 759.89
Synorchidism 752.89
Synorchism 752.89
Synostosis (congenital) 756.59
  astragaloscaphoid 755.67
  radioulnar 755.53
  talonavicular (bar) 755.67
  tarsal 755.67
Synovial - see condition
Synovioma (M9040/3) - see also Neoplasm, connective tissue, malignant
  benign (M9040/0) - see Neoplasm, connective tissue, benign
Synoviosarcoma (M9040/3) - see Neoplasm, connective tissue, malignant
Synovitis (see also Tenosynovitis) 727.00
  chronic crepitant, wrist 727.2
  due to crystals - see Arthritis, due to crystals
  gonococcal 098.51
  gouty 274.00
  specified NEC 727.09
  syphilitic 095.7
    congenital 090.0
  traumatic, current - see Sprain, by site
  tuberculous - see Tuberculosis, synovitis
  villonodular 719.20
    ankle 719.27
    elbow 719.22
    foot 719.27
    hand 719.24
    hip 719.25
    knee 719.26
    multiple sites 719.29
    pelvic region 719.25
    shoulder (region) 719.21
    specified site NEC 719.28
    wrist 719.23
Syphilide 091.3
  congenital 090.0
  newborn 090.0
  tubercular 095.8
    congenital 090.0
Syphilis, syphilitic (acquired) 097.9
  with lung involvement 095.1
  abdomen (late) 095.2
  acoustic nerve 094.86
  adenopathy (secondary) 091.4
  adrenal (gland) 095.8
    with cortical hypofunction 095.8
  age under 2 years NEC (see also Syphilis, congenital) 090.9
    acquired 097.9
  alopecia (secondary) 091.82
  anemia 095.8
  aneurysm (artery) (ruptured) 093.89
    aorta 093.0
    central nervous system 094.89
    congenital 090.5
  anus 095.8
    primary 091.1
    secondary 091.3
  aorta, aortic (arch) (abdominal) (insufficiency) (pulmonary) (regurgitation) (stenosis) (thoracic) 093.89
    aneurysm 093.0

Syphilis, syphilitic (Continued)
  arachnoid (adhesive) 094.2
  artery 093.89
    cerebral 094.89
    spinal 094.89
  arthropathy (neurogenic) (tabetic) 094.0 [713.5]
  asymptomatic - see Syphilis, latent
  ataxia, locomotor (progressive) 094.0
  atrophoderma maculatum 091.3
  auricular fibrillation 093.89
  Bell's palsy 094.89
  bladder 095.8
  bone 095.5
    secondary 091.61
  brain 094.89
  breast 095.8
  bronchus 095.8
  bubo 091.0
  bulbar palsy 094.89
  bursa (late) 095.7
  cardiac decompensation 093.89
  cardiovascular (early) (late) (primary) (secondary) (tertiary) 093.9
    specified type and site NEC 093.89
  causing death under 2 years of age (see also Syphilis, congenital) 090.9
    stated to be acquired NEC 097.9
  central nervous system (any site) (early) (late) (latent) (primary) (recurrent) (relapse) (secondary) (tertiary) 094.9
    with
      ataxia 094.0
      paralysis, general 094.1
        juvenile 090.40
      paresis (general) 094.1
        juvenile 090.40
      tabes (dorsalis) 094.0
        juvenile 090.40
      taboparesis 094.1
        juvenile 090.40
    aneurysm (ruptured) 094.87
    congenital 090.40
    juvenile 090.40
    remission in (sustained) 094.9
    serology doubtful, negative, or positive 094.9
    specified nature or site NEC 094.89
    vascular 094.89
  cerebral 094.89
    meningovascular 094.2
    nerves 094.89
    sclerosis 094.89
    thrombosis 094.89
  cerebrospinal 094.89
    tabetic 094.0
  cerebrovascular 094.89
  cervix 095.8
  chancre (multiple) 091.0
    extragenital 091.2
    Rollet's 091.2
  Charcôt's joint 094.0 [713.5]
  choked disc 094.89 [377.00]
  chorioretinitis 091.51
    congenital 090.0 [363.13]
    late 094.83
  choroiditis 091.51
    congenital 090.0 [363.13]
    late 094.83
    prenatal 090.0 [363.13]
  choroidoretinitis (secondary) 091.51
    congenital 090.0 [363.13]
    late 094.83
  ciliary body (secondary) 091.52
    late 095.8 [364.11]
  colon (late) 095.8
  combined sclerosis 094.89
  complicating pregnancy, childbirth, or puerperium 647.0 ●
    affecting fetus or newborn 760.2
  condyloma (latum) 091.3

 New   Revised   ~~deleted~~ Deleted   ● Use Additional Digit(s)   Omit code

455

Syphilis, syphilitic (Continued)
 congenital 090.9
  with
   encephalitis 090.41
   paresis (general) 090.40
   tabes (dorsalis) 090.40
   taborparesis 090.40
  chorioretinitis, choroiditis 090.0 [363.13]
  early or less than 2 years after birth NEC 090.2
   with manifestations 090.0
   latent (without manifestations) 090.1
    negative spinal fluid test 090.1
    serology, positive 090.1
   symptomatic 090.0
  interstitial keratitis 090.3
  juvenile neurosyphilis 090.40
  late or 2 years or more after birth NEC 090.7
   chorioretinitis, choroiditis 090.5 [363.13]
   interstitial keratitis 090.3
   juvenile neurosyphilis NEC 090.40
   latent (without manifestations) 090.6
    negative spinal fluid test 090.6
    serology, positive 090.6
   symptomatic or with manifestations NEC 090.5
   interstitial keratitis 090.3
 conjugal 097.9
  tabes 094.0
 conjunctiva 095.8 [372.10]
 contact V01.6
 cord, bladder 094.0
 cornea, late 095.8 [370.59]
 coronary (artery) 093.89
  sclerosis 093.89
 coryza 095.8
  congenital 090.0
 cranial nerve 094.89
 cutaneous - see Syphilis, skin
 dacryocystitis 095.8
 degeneration, spinal cord 094.89
 d'emblée 095.8
 dementia 094.1
  paralytica 094.1
   juvenilis 090.40
 destruction of bone 095.5
 dilatation, aorta 093.0
 due to blood transfusion 097.9
 dura mater 094.89
 ear 095.8
  inner 095.8
   nerve (eighth) 094.86
   neurorecurrence 094.86
 early NEC 091.0
  cardiovascular 093.9
  central nervous system 094.9
   paresis 094.1
   tabes 094.0
  latent (without manifestations) (less than 2 years after infection) 092.9
   negative spinal fluid test 092.9
   serological relapse following treatment 092.0
   serology positive 092.9
  paresis 094.1
  relapse (treated, untreated) 091.7
  skin 091.3
  symptomatic NEC 091.89
   extragenital chancre 091.2
   primary, except extragenital chancre 091.0
   secondary (see also Syphilis, secondary) 091.3
    relapse (treated, untreated) 091.7
  tabes 094.0
  ulcer 091.3
 eighth nerve 094.86
 endemic, nonveneral 104.0

Syphilis, syphilitic (Continued)
 endocarditis 093.20
  aortic 093.22
  mitral 093.21
  pulmonary 093.24
  tricuspid 093.23
 epididymis (late) 095.8
 epiglottis 095.8
 epiphysitis (congenital) 090.0
 esophagus 095.8
 Eustachian tube 095.8
 exposure to V01.6
 eye 095.8 [363.13]
  neuromuscular mechanism 094.85
 eyelid 095.8 [373.5]
  with gumma 095.8 [373.5]
  ptosis 094.89
 fallopian tube 095.8
 fracture 095.5
 gallbladder (late) 095.8
 gastric 095.8
  crisis 094.0
  polyposis 095.8
 general 097.9
  paralysis 094.1
   juvenile 090.40
 genital (primary) 091.0
 glaucoma 095.8
 gumma (late) NEC 095.9
  cardiovascular system 093.9
  central nervous system 094.9
  congenital 090.5
  heart or artery 093.89
 heart 093.89
  block 093.89
  decompensation 093.89
  disease 093.89
  failure 093.89
  valve (see also Syphilis, endocarditis) 093.20
 hemianesthesia 094.89
 hemianopsia 095.8
 hemiparesis 094.89
 hemiplegia 094.89
 hepatic artery 093.89
 hepatitis 095.3
 hepatomegaly 095.3
  congenital 090.0
 hereditaria tarda (see also Syphilis, congenital, late) 090.7
 hereditary (see also Syphilis, congenital) 090.9
  interstitial keratitis 090.3
 Hutchinson's teeth 090.5
 hyalitis 095.8
 inactive - see Syphilis, latent
 infantum NEC (see also Syphilis, congenital) 090.9
 inherited - see Syphilis, congenital
 internal ear 095.8
 intestine (late) 095.8
 iris, iritis (secondary) 091.52
  late 095.8 [364.11]
 joint (late) 095.8
 keratitis (congenital) (early) (interstitial) (late) (parenchymatous) (punctata profunda) 090.3
 kidney 095.4
 lacrimal apparatus 095.8
 laryngeal paralysis 095.8
 larynx 095.8
 late 097.0
  cardiovascular 093.9
  central nervous system 094.9
  latent or 2 years or more after infection (without manifestation) 096
   negative spinal fluid test 096
   serology positive 096
  paresis 094.1
  specified site NEC 095.8
  symptomatic or with symptoms 095.9
  tabes 094.0

Syphilis, syphilitic (Continued)
 latent 097.1
  central nervous system 094.9
  date of infection unspecified 097.1
  early or less than 2 years after infection 092.9
  late or 2 years or more after infection 096
  serology
   doubtful
    follow-up of latent syphilis 097.1
     central nervous system 094.9
     date of infection unspecified 097.1
     early or less than 2 years after infection 092.9
     late or 2 years or more after infection 096
   positive, only finding 097.1
    date of infection unspecified 097.1
    early or less than 2 years after infection 097.1
    late or 2 years or more after infection 097.1
 lens 095.8
 leukoderma 091.3
  late 095.8
 lienis 095.8
 lip 091.3
  chancre 091.2
  late 095.8
  primary 091.2
 Lissauer's paralysis 094.1
 liver 095.3
  secondary 091.62
 locomotor ataxia 094.0
 lung 095.1
 lymphadenitis (secondary) 091.4
 lymph gland (early) (secondary) 091.4
  late 095.8
 macular atrophy of skin 091.3
  striated 095.8
 maternal, affecting fetus or newborn 760.2
  manifest syphilis in newborn - see Syphilis, congenital
 mediastinum (late) 095.8
 meninges (adhesive) (basilar) (brain) (spinal cord) 094.2
 meningitis 094.2
  acute 091.81
  congenital 090.42
 meningoencephalitis 094.2
 meningovascular 094.2
  congenital 090.49
 mesarteritis 093.89
  brain 094.89
  spine 094.89
 middle ear 095.8
 mitral stenosis 093.21
 monoplegia 094.89
 mouth (secondary) 091.3
  late 095.8
 mucocutaneous 091.3
  late 095.8
 mucous
  membrane 091.3
   late 095.8
  patches 091.3
   congenital 090.0
 mulberry molars 090.5
 muscle 095.6
 myocardium 093.82
 myositis 095.6
 nasal sinus 095.8
 neonatorum NEC (see also Syphilis, congenital) 090.9
 nerve palsy (any cranial nerve) 094.89
 nervous system, central 094.9
 neuritis 095.8
  acoustic nerve 094.86
 neurorecidive of retina 094.83
 neuroretinitis 094.85

Syphilis, syphilitic *(Continued)*
    newborn (*see also* Syphilis, congenital) 090.9
    nodular superficial 095.8
    nonvenereal, endemic 104.0
    nose 095.8
        saddle back deformity 090.5
        septum 095.8
            perforated 095.8
    occlusive arterial disease 093.89
    ophthalmic 095.8 [363.13]
    ophthalmoplegia 094.89
    optic nerve (atrophy) (neuritis) (papilla) 094.84
    orbit (late) 095.8
    orchitis 095.8
    organic 097.9
    osseous (late) 095.5
    osteochondritis (congenital) 090.0
    osteoporosis 095.5
    ovary 095.8
    oviduct 095.8
    palate 095.8
        gumma 095.8
        perforated 090.5
    pancreas (late) 095.8
    pancreatitis 095.8
    paralysis 094.89
        general 094.1
        juvenile 090.40
    paraplegia 094.89
    paresis (general) 094.1
        juvenile 090.40
    paresthesia 094.89
    Parkinson's disease or syndrome 094.82
    paroxysmal tachycardia 093.89
    pemphigus (congenital) 090.0
    penis 091.0
        chancre 091.0
        late 095.8
    pericardium 093.81
    perichondritis, larynx 095.8
    periosteum 095.5
        congenital 090.0
        early 091.61
        secondary 091.61
    peripheral nerve 095.8
    petrous bone (late) 095.5
    pharynx 095.8
        secondary 091.3
    pituitary (gland) 095.8
    placenta 095.8
    pleura (late) 095.8
    pneumonia, white 090.0
    pontine (lesion) 094.89
    portal vein 093.89
    primary NEC 091.2
        anal 091.1
        and secondary (*see also* Syphilis, secondary) 091.9
        cardiovascular 093.9
        central nervous system 094.9
        extragenital chancre NEC 091.2
        fingers 091.2
        genital 091.0
        lip 091.2
        specified site NEC 091.2
        tonsils 091.2
    prostate 095.8
    psychosis (intracranial gumma) 094.89
    ptosis (eyelid) 094.89
    pulmonary (late) 095.1
        artery 093.89
    pulmonum 095.1
    pyelonephritis 095.4
    recently acquired, symptomatic NEC 091.89
    rectum 095.8
    respiratory tract 095.8
    retina
        late 094.83
        neurorecidive 094.83
    retrobulbar neuritis 094.85

Syphilis, syphilitic *(Continued)*
    salpingitis 095.8
    sclera (late) 095.0
    sclerosis
        cerebral 094.89
        coronary 093.89
        multiple 094.89
        subacute 094.89
    scotoma (central) 095.8
    scrotum 095.8
    secondary (and primary) 091.9
        adenopathy 091.4
        anus 091.3
        bone 091.61
        cardiovascular 093.9
        central nervous system 094.9
        chorioretinitis, choroiditis 091.51
        hepatitis 091.62
        liver 091.62
        lymphadenitis 091.4
        meningitis, acute 091.81
        mouth 091.3
        mucous membranes 091.3
        periosteum 091.61
        periostitis 091.61
        pharynx 091.3
        relapse (treated) (untreated) 091.7
        skin 091.3
        specified form NEC 091.89
        tonsil 091.3
        ulcer 091.3
        viscera 091.69
        vulva 091.3
    seminal vesicle (late) 095.8
    seronegative
        with signs or symptoms - *see* Syphilis, by site and stage
    seropositive
        with signs or symptoms - *see* Syphilis, by site or stage
        follow-up of latent syphilis - *see* Syphilis, latent
        only finding - *see* Syphilis, latent
    seventh nerve (paralysis) 094.89
    sinus 095.8
    sinusitis 095.8
    skeletal system 095.5
    skin (early) (secondary) (with ulceration) 091.3
        late or tertiary 095.8
    small intestine 095.8
    spastic spinal paralysis 094.0
    spermatic cord (late) 095.8
    spinal (cord) 094.89
        with
            paresis 094.1
            tabes 094.0
    spleen 095.8
    splenomegaly 095.8
    spondylitis 095.5
    staphyloma 095.8
    stigmata (congenital) 090.5
    stomach 095.8
    synovium (late) 095.7
    tabes dorsalis (early) (late) 094.0
        juvenile 090.40
    tabetic type 094.0
        juvenile 090.40
    taboparesis 094.1
        juvenile 090.40
    tachycardia 093.89
    tendon (late) 095.7
    tertiary 097.0
        with symptoms 095.8
        cardiovascular 093.9
        central nervous system 094.9
        multiple NEC 095.8
        specified site NEC 095.8
    testis 095.8
    thorax 095.8
    throat 095.8

Syphilis, syphilitic *(Continued)*
    thymus (gland) 095.8
    thyroid (late) 095.8
    tongue 095.8
    tonsil (lingual) 095.8
        primary 091.2
        secondary 091.3
    trachea 095.8
    tricuspid valve 093.23
    tumor, brain 094.89
    tunica vaginalis (late) 095.8
    ulcer (any site) (early) (secondary) 091.3
        late 095.9
        perforating 095.9
            foot 094.0
    urethra (stricture) 095.8
    urogenital 095.8
    uterus 095.8
    uveal tract (secondary) 091.50
        late 095.8 [363.13]
    uveitis (secondary) 091.50
        late 095.8 [363.13]
    uvula (late) 095.8
        perforated 095.8
    vagina 091.0
        late 095.8
    valvulitis NEC 093.20
    vascular 093.89
        brain or cerebral 094.89
    vein 093.89
        cerebral 094.89
    ventriculi 095.8
    vesicae urinariae 095.8
    viscera (abdominal) 095.2
        secondary 091.69
    vitreous (hemorrhage) (opacities) 095.8
    vulva 091.0
        late 095.8
        secondary 091.3
Syphiloma 095.9
    cardiovascular system 093.9
    central nervous system 094.9
    circulatory system 093.9
    congenital 090.5
Syphilophobia 300.29
Syringadenoma (M8400/0) - *see also* Neoplasm, skin, benign
    papillary (M8406/0) - *see* Neoplasm, skin, benign
Syringobulbia 336.0
Syringocarcinoma (M8400/3) - *see* Neoplasm, skin, malignant
Syringocystadenoma (M8400/0) - *see also* Neoplasm, skin, benign
    papillary (M8406/0) - *see* Neoplasm, skin, benign
Syringocystoma (M8407/0) - *see* Neoplasm, skin, benign
Syringoma (M8407/0) - *see also* Neoplasm, skin, benign
    chondroid (M8940/0) - *see* Neoplasm, by site, benign
Syringomyelia 336.0
Syringomyelitis 323.9
    late effect - *see* category 326
Syringomyelocele (*see also* Spina bifida) 741.9 ●
Syringopontia 336.0
System, systemic - *see also* condition
    disease, combined - *see* Degeneration, combined
    fibrosclerosing syndrome 710.8
    inflammatory response syndrome (SIRS) 995.90
        due to
            infectious process 995.91
                with acute organ dysfunction 995.92
            non-infectious process 995.93
                with acute organ dysfunction 995.94
    lupus erythematosus 710.0
        inhibitor 795.79

T

Tab - see Tag
Tabacism 989.84
Tabacosis 989.84
Tabardillo 080
- flea-borne 081.0
- louse-borne 080

Tabes, tabetic
- with
  - central nervous system syphilis 094.0
  - Charcôt's joint 094.0 [713.5]
  - cord bladder 094.0
  - crisis, viscera (any) 094.0
  - paralysis, general 094.1
  - paresis (general) 094.1
  - perforating ulcer 094.0
- arthropathy 094.0 [713.5]
- bladder 094.0
- bone 094.0
- cerebrospinal 094.0
- congenital 090.40
- conjugal 094.0
- dorsalis 094.0
  - neurosyphilis 094.0
- early 094.0
- juvenile 090.40
- latent 094.0
- mesenterica (see also Tuberculosis) 014.8●
- paralysis insane, general 094.1
- peripheral (nonsyphilitic) 799.89
- spasmodic 094.0
  - not dorsal or dorsalis 343.9
- syphilis (cerebrospinal) 094.0

Taboparalysis 094.1
Taboparesis (remission) 094.1
- with
  - Charcôt's joint 094.1 [713.5]
  - cord bladder 094.1
  - perforating ulcer 094.1
- juvenile 090.40

Tache noir 923.20
Tachyalimentation 579.3
Tachyarrhythmia, tachyrhythmia - see also Tachycardia
- paroxysmal with sinus bradycardia 427.81

Tachycardia 785.0
- atrial 427.89
- auricular 427.89
- AV nodal re-entry (re-entrant) 427.89
- junctional ectopic 427.0
- newborn 779.82
- nodal 427.89
  - nonparoxysmal atrioventricular 426.89
  - nonparoxysmal atrioventricular (nodal) 426.89
- nonsustained 427.2
- paroxysmal 427.2
  - with sinus bradycardia 427.81
  - atrial (PAT) 427.0
    - psychogenic 316 [427.0]
  - atrioventricular (AV) 427.0
    - psychogenic 316 [427.0]
  - essential 427.2
  - junctional 427.0
  - nodal 427.0
  - psychogenic 316 [427.2]
    - atrial 316 [427.0]
      - supraventricular 316 [427.0]
      - ventricular 316 [427.1]
  - supraventricular 427.0
    - psychogenic 316 [427.0]
  - ventricular 427.1
    - psychogenic 316 [427.1]
- postoperative 997.1
- psychogenic 306.2
- sick sinus 427.81
- sinoauricular 427.89
- sinus 427.89
- supraventricular 427.89

Tachycardia (Continued)
- sustained 427.2
  - supraventricular 427.0
  - ventricular 427.1
- ventricular (paroxysmal) 427.1
  - psychogenic 316 [427.1]

Tachygastria 536.8
Tachypnea 786.06
- hysterical 300.11
- newborn (idiopathic) (transitory) 770.6
- psychogenic 306.1
- transitory, of newborn 770.6

TACO (transfusion associated circulatory overload) 276.61
Taenia (infection) (infestation) (see also Infestation, taenia) 123.3
- diminuta 123.6
- echinococcal infestation (see also Echinococcus) 122.9
- nana 123.6
- saginata infestation 123.2
- solium (intestinal form) 123.0
  - larval form 123.1

Taeniasis (intestine) (see also Infestation, taenia) 123.3
- saginata 123.2
- solium 123.0

Taenzer's disease 757.4
Tag (hypertrophied skin) (infected) 701.9
- adenoid 474.8
- anus 455.9
- endocardial (see also Endocarditis) 424.90
- hemorrhoidal 455.9
- hymen 623.8
- perineal 624.8
- preauricular 744.1
- rectum 455.9
- sentinel 455.9
- skin 701.9
  - accessory 757.39
  - anus 455.9
  - congenital 757.39
  - preauricular 744.1
  - rectum 455.9
- tonsil 474.8
- urethra, urethral 599.84
- vulva 624.8

Tahyna fever 062.5
Takayasu (-Onishi) disease or syndrome (pulseless disease) 446.7
Takotsubo syndrome 429.83
Talc granuloma 728.82
- in operation wound 998.7

Talcosis 502
Talipes (congenital) 754.70
- acquired NEC 736.79
  - planus 734
- asymmetric 754.79
  - acquired 736.79
- calcaneovalgus 754.62
  - acquired 736.76
- calcaneovarus 754.59
  - acquired 736.76
- calcaneus 754.79
  - acquired 736.76
- cavovarus 754.59
  - acquired 736.75
- cavus 754.71
  - acquired 736.73
- equinovalgus 754.69
  - acquired 736.72
- equinovarus 754.51
  - acquired 736.71
- equinus 754.79
  - acquired, NEC 736.72
- percavus 754.71
  - acquired 736.73
- planovalgus 754.69
  - acquired 736.79

Talipes (Continued)
- planus (acquired) (any degree) 734
  - congenital 754.61
  - due to rickets 268.1
- valgus 754.60
  - acquired 736.79
- varus 754.50
  - acquired 736.79

Talma's disease 728.85
Talon noir 924.20
- hand 923.20
- heel 924.20
- toe 924.3

Tamponade heart (Rose's) (see also Pericarditis) 423.3
Tanapox 059.21
Tangier disease (familial high-density lipoprotein deficiency) 272.5
Tank ear 380.12
Tantrum (childhood) (see also Disturbance, conduct) 312.1●
Tapeworm (infection) (infestation) (see also Infestation, tapeworm) 123.9
Tapia's syndrome 352.6
Tarantism 297.8
Target-oval cell anemia 285.8
- with thalassemia - see Thalassemia

Tarlov's cyst 355.9
Tarral-Besnier disease (pityriasis rubra pilaris) 696.4
Tarsalgia 729.2
Tarsal tunnel syndrome 355.5
Tarsitis (eyelid) 373.00
- syphilitic 095.8 [373.00]
- tuberculous (see also Tuberculosis) 017.0● [373.4]

Tartar (teeth) 523.6
Tattoo (mark) 709.09
Taurodontism 520.2
Taussig-Bing defect, heart, or syndrome (transposition, aorta and overriding pulmonary artery) 745.11
Tay's choroiditis 363.41
Tay-Sachs
- amaurotic familial idiocy 330.1
- disease 330.1

Taybi's syndrome (otopalatodigital) 759.89
Taylor's
- disease (diffuse idiopathic cutaneous atrophy) 701.8
- syndrome 625.5

TBI (traumatic brain injury) (see also Injury, intracranial) 854.0●
- with skull fracture - see Fracture, skull, by site

Tear, torn (traumatic) - see also Wound, open, by site
- annular fibrosis 722.51
- anus, anal (sphincter) 863.89
  - with open wound in cavity 863.99
  - complicating delivery (healed) (old) 654.8●
    - with mucosa 664.3●
    - not associated with third-degree perineal laceration 664.6●
  - nontraumatic, nonpuerperal (healed) (old) 569.43
- articular cartilage, old (see also Disorder, cartilage, articular) 718.0●
- bladder
  - with
    - abortion - see Abortion, by type, with damage to pelvic organs
    - ectopic pregnancy (see also categories 633.0–633.9) 639.2
    - molar pregnancy (see also categories 630–632) 639.2
  - following
    - abortion 639.2
    - ectopic or molar pregnancy 639.2
  - obstetrical trauma 665.5●

Tear, torn (Continued)
  bowel
    with
      abortion - see Abortion, by type, with damage to pelvic organs
      ectopic pregnancy (see also categories 633.0–633.9) 639.2
      molar pregnancy (see also categories 630–632) 639.2
    following
      abortion 639.2
      ectopic or molar pregnancy 639.2
    obstetrical trauma 665.5 ●
  broad ligament
    with
      abortion - see Abortion, by type, with damage to pelvic organs
      ectopic pregnancy (see also categories 633.0–633.9) 639.2
      molar pregnancy (see also categories 630–632) 639.2
    following
      abortion 639.2
      ectopic or molar pregnancy 639.2
    obstetrical trauma 665.6 ●
  bucket handle (knee) (meniscus) - see Tear, meniscus
  capsule
    joint - see Sprain, by site
    spleen - see Laceration, spleen, capsule
  cartilage - see also Sprain, by site
    articular, old (see also Disorder, cartilage, articular) 718.0 ●
    knee - see Tear, meniscus
    semilunar (knee) (current injury) - see Tear, meniscus
  cervix
    with
      abortion - see Abortion, by type, with damage to pelvic organs
      ectopic pregnancy (see also categories 633.0–633.9) 639.2
      molar pregnancy (see also categories 630–632) 639.2
    following
      abortion 639.2
      ectopic or molar pregnancy 639.2
    obstetrical trauma (current) 665.3 ●
    old 622.3
  dural 349.31
    accidental puncture or laceration during a procedure 349.31
    incidental (inadvertent) 349.31
    nontraumatic NEC 349.39
  internal organ (abdomen, chest, or pelvis) - see Injury, internal, by site
  ligament - see also Sprain, by site
    with open wound - see Wound, open, by site
  meniscus (knee) (current injury) 836.2
    bucket handle 836.0
      old 717.0
    lateral 836.1
      anterior horn 836.1
        old 717.42
      bucket handle 836.1
        old 717.41
      old 717.40
      posterior horn 836.1
        old 717.43
      specified site NEC 836.1
        old 717.49
    medial 836.0
      anterior horn 836.0
        old 717.1
      bucket handle 836.0
        old 717.0
      old 717.3
      posterior horn 836.0
        old 717.2

Tear, torn (Continued)
  meniscus (Continued)
    old NEC 717.5
    site other than knee - see Sprain, by site
  muscle - see also Sprain, by site
    with open wound - see Wound, open, by site
  pelvic
    floor, complicating delivery 664.1 ●
    organ NEC
      with
        abortion - see Abortion, by type, with damage to pelvic organs
        ectopic pregnancy (see also categories 633.0–633.9) 639.2
        molar pregnancy (see also categories 630–632) 639.2
      following
        abortion 639.2
        ectopic or molar pregnancy 639.2
      obstetrical trauma 665.5 ●
  perineum - see also Laceration, perineum
    obstetrical trauma 665.5 ●
  periurethral tissue
    with
      abortion - see Abortion, by type, with damage to pelvic organs
      ectopic pregnancy (see also categories 633.0–633.9) 639.2
      molar pregnancy (see also categories 630–632) 639.2
    following
      abortion 639.2
      ectopic or molar pregnancy 639.2
    obstetrical trauma 664.8 ●
  rectovaginal septum - see Laceration, rectovaginal septum
  retina, retinal (recent) (with detachment) 361.00
    without detachment 361.30
    dialysis (juvenile) (with detachment) 361.04
    giant (with detachment) 361.03
    horseshoe (without detachment) 361.32
    multiple (with detachment) 361.02
      without detachment 361.33
    old
      delimited (partial) 361.06
      partial 361.06
      total or subtotal 361.07
    partial (without detachment)
      giant 361.03
      multiple defects 361.02
      old (delimited) 361.06
      single defect 361.01
    round hole (without detachment) 361.31
    single defect (with detachment) 361.01
    total or subtotal (recent) 361.05
      old 361.07
  rotator cuff (traumatic) 840.4
    current injury 840.4
    degenerative 726.10
    nontraumatic (complete) 727.61
      partial 726.13
  semilunar cartilage, knee (see also Tear, meniscus) 836.2
    old 717.5
  tendon - see also Sprain, by site
    with open wound - see Wound, open, by site
  tentorial, at birth 767.0
  umbilical cord
    affecting fetus or newborn 772.0
    complicating delivery 663.8 ●
  urethra
    with
      abortion - see Abortion, by type, with damage to pelvic organs
      ectopic pregnancy (see also categories 633.0–633.9) 639.2
      molar pregnancy (see also categories 630–632) 639.2

Tear, torn (Continued)
  urethra (Continued)
    following
      abortion 639.2
      ectopic or molar pregnancy 639.2
      obstetrical trauma 665.5 ●
  uterus - see Injury, internal, uterus
  vagina - see Laceration, vagina
  vessel, from catheter 998.2
  vulva, complicating delivery 664.0 ●
Tear stone 375.57
Teeth, tooth - see also condition
  grinding 306.8
  prenatal 520.6
Teething 520.7
  syndrome 520.7
Tegmental syndrome 344.89
Telangiectasia, telangiectasis (verrucous) 448.9
  ataxic (cerebellar) 334.8
  familial 448.0
  hemorrhagic, hereditary (congenital) (senile) 448.0
  hereditary hemorrhagic 448.0
  retina 362.15
  spider 448.1
Telecanthus (congenital) 743.63
Telescoped bowel or intestine (see also Intussusception) 560.0
Teletherapy, adverse effect NEC 990
Telogen effluvium 704.02
Temperature
  body, high (of unknown origin) (see also Pyrexia) 780.60
  cold, trauma from 991.9
    newborn 778.2
    specified effect NEC 991.8
  high
    body (of unknown origin) (see also Pyrexia) 780.60
    trauma from - see Heat
Temper tantrum (childhood) (see also Disturbance, conduct) 312.1 ●
Temple - see condition
Temporal - see also condition
  lobe syndrome 310.0
Temporomandibular joint-pain-dysfunction syndrome 524.60
Temporosphenoidal - see condition
Tendency
  bleeding (see also Defect, coagulation) 286.9
  homosexual, ego-dystonic 302.0
  paranoid 301.0
  suicide 300.9
Tenderness
  abdominal (generalized) (localized) 789.6 ●
  rebound 789.6 ●
  skin 782.0
Tendinitis, tendonitis (see also Tenosynovitis) 726.90
  Achilles 726.71
  adhesive 726.90
    shoulder 726.0
  calcific 727.82
    shoulder 726.11
  gluteal 726.5
  patellar 726.64
  peroneal 726.79
  pes anserinus 726.61
  psoas 726.5
  tibialis (anterior) (posterior) 726.72
  trochanteric 726.5
Tendon - see condition
Tendosynovitis - see Tenosynovitis
Tendovaginitis - see Tenosynovitis
Tenesmus 787.99
  rectal 787.99
  vesical 788.99
Tenia - see Taenia
Teniasis - see Taeniasis
Tennis elbow 726.32

Tenonitis - *see also* Tenosynovitis
    eye (capsule) 376.04
Tenontosynovitis - *see* Tenosynovitis
Tenontothecitis - *see* Tenosynovitis
Tenophyte 727.9
Tenosynovitis (*see also* Synovitis) 727.00
    adhesive 726.90
        shoulder 726.0
    ankle 727.06
    bicipital (calcifying) 726.12
    buttock 727.09
    due to crystals - *see* Arthritis, due to crystals
    elbow 727.09
    finger 727.05
    foot 727.06
    gonococcal 098.51
    hand 727.05
    hip 727.09
    knee 727.09
    radial styloid 727.04
    shoulder 726.10
        adhesive 726.0
    specified NEC 727.09
    spine 720.1
    supraspinatus 726.10
    toe 727.06
    tuberculous - *see* Tuberculosis, tenosynovitis
    wrist 727.05
Tenovaginitis - *see* Tenosynovitis
Tension
    arterial, high (*see also* Hypertension) 401.9
        without diagnosis of hypertension 796.2
    headache 307.81
    intraocular (elevated) 365.00
    nervous 799.21
    ocular (elevated) 365.00
    pneumothorax 512.0
        iatrogenic 512.1
        postoperative 512.1
        spontaneous 512.0
    premenstrual 625.4
    state 300.9
Tentorium - *see* condition
Teratencephalus 759.89
Teratism 759.7
Teratoblastoma (malignant) (M9080/3) - *see* Neoplasm, by site, malignant
Teratocarcinoma (M9081/3) - *see also* Neoplasm, by site, malignant
    liver 155.0
Teratoma (solid) (M9080/1) - *see also* Neoplasm, by site, uncertain behavior
    adult (cystic) (M9080/0) - *see* Neoplasm, by site, benign
    and embryonal carcinoma, mixed (M9081/3) - *see* Neoplasm, by site, malignant
    benign (M9080/0) - *see* Neoplasm, by site, benign
    combined with choriocarcinoma (M9101/3) - *see* Neoplasm, by site, malignant
    cystic (adult) (M9080/0) - *see* Neoplasm, by site, benign
    differentiated type (M9080/0) - *see* Neoplasm, by site, benign
    embryonal (M9080/3) - *see also* Neoplasm, by site, malignant
        liver 155.0
    fetal
        sacral, causing fetopelvic disproportion 653.7●
    immature (M9080/3) - *see* Neoplasm, by site, malignant
    liver (M9080/3) 155.0
        adult, benign, cystic, differentiated type, or mature (M9080/0) 211.5
    malignant (M9080/3) - *see also* Neoplasm, by site, malignant
        anaplastic type (M9082/3) - *see* Neoplasm, by site, malignant

Teratoma (Continued)
    malignant (Continued)
        intermediate type (M9083/3) - *see* Neoplasm, by site, malignant
        liver (M9080/3) 155.0
        trophoblastic (M9102/3)
            specified site - *see* Neoplasm, by site, malignant
            unspecified site 186.9
        undifferentiated type (M9082/3) - *see* Neoplasm, by site, malignant
    mature (M9080/0) - *see* Neoplasm, by site, benign
        malignant (M9080/3) - *see* Neoplasm, by site, malignant
    ovary (M9080/0) 220
        embryonal, immature, or malignant (M9080/3) 183.0
    suprasellar (M9080/3) - *see* Neoplasm, by site, malignant
    testis (M9080/3) 186.9
        adult, benign, cystic, differentiated type or mature (M9080/0) 222.0
        undescended 186.0
Terminal care V66.7
Termination
    anomalous - *see also* Malposition, congenital
        portal vein 747.49
        right pulmonary vein 747.42
    pregnancy (legal) (therapeutic) (*see* Abortion, legal) 635.9●
        fetus NEC 779.6
        illegal (*see also* Abortion, illegal) 636.9●
Ternidens diminutus infestation 127.7
Terrors, night (child) 307.46
Terry's syndrome (*see also* Retinopathy of prematurity) 362.21
Tertiary - *see* condition
Tessellated fundus, retina (tigroid) 362.89
Test(s)
    adequacy
        hemodialysis V56.31
        peritoneal dialysis V56.32
    AIDS virus V72.69
    allergen V72.7
    bacterial disease NEC (*see also* Screening, by name of disease) V74.9
    basal metabolic rate V72.69
    blood
        alcohol V70.4
        drug V70.4
            for therapeutic drug monitoring V58.83
            for routine general physical examination V72.62
        prior to treatment or procedure V72.63
        typing V72.86
            Rh typing V72.86
    developmental, infant or child V20.2
    Dick V74.8
    fertility V26.21
    genetic
        female V26.32
        for genetic disease carrier status
            female V26.31
            male V26.34
        male V26.39
    hearing V72.19
        following failed hearing screening V72.11
        routine, for infant and child V20.2
    HIV V72.69
    human immunodeficiency virus V72.69
    immunity status V72.61
    Kveim V82.89
    laboratory V72.60
        for medicolegal reason V70.4
        ordered as part of a routine general medical examination V72.62
    pre-operative V72.63
    pre-procedural V72.63
    specified NEC V72.69

Test(s) (Continued)
    male partner of female with recurrent pregnancy loss V26.35
    Mantoux (for tuberculosis) V74.1
    mycotic organism V75.4
    nuchal translucency V28.89
    parasitic agent NEC V75.8
    paternity V70.4
    peritoneal equilibration V56.32
    pregnancy
        negative result V72.41
        positive result V72.42
            first pregnancy V72.42
        unconfirmed V72.40
    preoperative V72.84
        cardiovascular V72.81
        respiratory V72.82
        specified NEC V72.83
    procreative management NEC V26.29
        genetic disease carrier status
            female V26.31
            male V26.34
    Rh typing V72.86
    sarcoidosis V82.89
    Schick V74.3
    Schultz-Charlton V74.8
    skin, diagnostic
        allergy V72.7
        bacterial agent NEC (*see also* Screening, by name of disease) V74.9
        Dick V74.8
        hypersensitivity V72.7
        Kveim V82.89
        Mantoux V74.1
        mycotic organism V75.4
        parasitic agent NEC V75.8
        sarcoidosis V82.89
        Schick V74.3
        Schultz-Charlton V74.8
        tuberculin V74.1
    specified type NEC V72.85
    tuberculin V74.1
    vision V72.0
        routine, for infant and child V20.2
    Wassermann
        positive (*see also* Serology for syphilis, positive) 097.1
        false 795.6
Testicle, testicular, testis - *see also* condition
    feminization (syndrome) 259.51
Tetanus, tetanic (cephalic) (convulsions) 037
    with
        abortion - *see* Abortion, by type, with sepsis
        ectopic pregnancy (*see also* categories 633.0–633.9) 639.0
        molar pregnancy (*see* categories 630–632) 639.0
    following
        abortion 639.0
        ectopic or molar pregnancy 639.0
    inoculation V03.7
        reaction (due to serum) - *see* Complications, vaccination
    neonatorum 771.3
    puerperal, postpartum, childbirth 670.8●
Tetany, tetanic 781.7
    alkalosis 276.3
    associated with rickets 268.0
    convulsions 781.7
        hysterical 300.11
    functional (hysterical) 300.11
    hyperkinetic 781.7
        hysterical 300.11
    hyperpnea 786.01
        hysterical 300.11
        psychogenic 306.1
    hyperventilation 786.01
        hysterical 300.11
        psychogenic 306.1
    hypocalcemic, neonatal 775.4

SECTION I INDEX TO DISEASES AND INJURIES / Thrombophlebitis

Tetany, tetanic *(Continued)*
- hysterical 300.11
- neonatal 775.4
- parathyroid (gland) 252.1
- parathyroprival 252.1
- postoperative 252.1
- postthyroidectomy 252.1
- pseudotetany 781.7
  - hysterical 300.11
- psychogenic 306.1
  - specified as conversion reaction 300.11

Tetralogy of Fallot 745.2
Tetraplegia - *see* Quadriplegia
Thailand hemorrhagic fever 065.4
Thalassanemia 282.40
Thalassemia (disease) 282.40
- with other hemoglobinopathy 282.49
- alpha (major) (severe) (triple gene defect) 282.43
  - silent carrier 282.46
- beta (homozygous) (major) (severe) 282.44
- delta-beta (homozygous) 282.45
- dominant 282.49
- Hb-S (without crisis) 282.41
  - with
    - crisis 282.42
      - vaso-occlusive pain 282.42
  - hemoglobin
    - C (Hb-C) 282.49
    - D (Hb-D) 282.49
    - E (Hb-E) 282.49
    - E-beta 282.47
    - H (Hb-H) 282.49
    - I (Hb-I) 282.49
- high fetal gene (*see also* Thalassemia) 282.40
- high fetal hemoglobin (*see also* Thalassemia) 282.40
- intermedia 282.44
- major 282.44
- minor (alpha) (beta) 282.46
- mixed 282.49
- sickle-cell (without crisis) 282.41
  - with
    - crisis 282.42
      - vaso-occlusive pain 282.42
- specified NEC 282.49
- trait (alpha) (beta) (delta-beta) 282.46

Thalassemic variants 282.49
Thaysen-Gee disease (nontropical sprue) 579.0
Thecoma (M8600/0) 220
- malignant (M8600/3) 183.0

Thelarche, precocious 259.1
Thelitis 611.0
- puerperal, postpartum 675.0●

Therapeutic - *see* condition
Therapy V57.9
- blood transfusion, without reported diagnosis V58.2
- breathing V57.0
- chemotherapy, antineoplastic V58.11
  - fluoride V07.31
  - prophylactic NEC V07.39
- dialysis (intermittent) (treatment)
  - extracorporeal V56.0
  - peritoneal V56.8
  - renal V56.0
  - specified type NEC V56.8
- exercise NEC V57.1
  - breathing V57.0
- extracorporeal dialysis (renal) V56.0
- fluoride prophylaxis V07.31
- hemodialysis V56.0
- hormone replacement (postmenopausal) V07.4
- immunotherapy antineoplastic V58.12
- long term oxygen therapy V46.2
- occupational V57.21
- orthoptic V57.4
- orthotic V57.81
- peritoneal dialysis V56.8
- physical NEC V57.1

Therapy *(Continued)*
- postmenopausal hormone replacement V07.4
- radiation V58.0
- speech (-language) V57.3
- vocational V57.22

Thermalgesia 782.0
Thermalgia 782.0
Thermanalgesia 782.0
Thermanesthesia 782.0
Thermic - *see* condition
Thermography (abnormal) 793.99
- breast 793.89

Thermoplegia 992.0
Thesaurismosis
- amyloid 277.39
- bilirubin 277.4
- calcium 275.40
- cystine 270.0
- glycogen (*see also* Disease, glycogen storage) 271.0
- kerasin 272.7
- lipoid 272.7
- melanin 255.41
- phosphatide 272.7
- urate 274.9

Thiaminic deficiency 265.1
- with beriberi 265.0

Thibierge-Weissenbach syndrome (cutaneous systemic sclerosis) 710.1
Thickened endometrium 793.5
Thickening
- bone 733.99
  - extremity 733.99
- breast 611.79
- hymen 623.3
- larynx 478.79
- nail 703.8
  - congenital 757.5
- periosteal 733.99
- pleura (*see also* Pleurisy) 511.0
- skin 782.8
- subepiglottic 478.79
- tongue 529.8
- valve, heart - *see* Endocarditis

Thiele syndrome 724.6
Thigh - *see* condition
Thinning vertebra (*see also* Osteoporosis) 733.00
Thirst, excessive 783.5
- due to deprivation of water 994.3

Thomsen's disease 359.22
Thomson's disease (congenital poikiloderma) 757.33
Thoracic - *see also* condition
- kidney 753.3
- outlet syndrome 353.0
- stomach - *see* Hernia, diaphragm

Thoracogastroschisis (congenital) 759.89
Thoracopagus 759.4
Thoracoschisis 756.3
Thoracoscopic surgical procedure converted to open procedure V64.42
Thorax - *see* condition
Thorn's syndrome (*see also* Disease, renal) 593.9
Thornwaldt's, Tornwaldt's
- bursitis (pharyngeal) 478.29
- cyst 478.26
- disease (pharyngeal bursitis) 478.29

Thorson-Biörck syndrome (malignant carcinoid) 259.2
Threadworm (infection) (infestation) 127.4
Threatened
- abortion or miscarriage 640.0●
  - with subsequent abortion (*see also* Abortion, spontaneous) 634.9●
  - affecting fetus 762.1
- labor 644.1●
  - affecting fetus or newborn 761.8
  - premature 644.0●
- miscarriage 640.0●
  - affecting fetus 762.1

Threatened *(Continued)*
- premature
  - delivery 644.2●
    - affecting fetus or newborn 761.8
  - labor 644.0●
    - before 22 completed weeks gestation 640.0●

Three-day fever 066.0
Threshers' lung 495.0
Thrix annulata (congenital) 757.4
Throat - *see* condition
Thrombasthenia (Glanzmann's) (hemorrhagic) (hereditary) 287.1
Thromboangiitis 443.1
- obliterans (general) 443.1
  - cerebral 437.1
  - vessels
    - brain 437.1
    - spinal cord 437.1

Thromboarteritis - *see* Arteritis
Thromboasthenia (Glanzmann's) (hemorrhagic) (hereditary) 287.1
Thrombocytasthenia (Glanzmann's) 287.1
Thrombocythemia (primary) (M9962/1) 238.71
- essential 238.71
- hemorrhagic 238.71
- idiopathic (hemorrhagic) (M9962/1) 238.71

Thrombocytopathy (dystrophic) (granulopenic) 287.1
Thrombocytopenia, thrombocytopenic 287.5
- with
  - absent radii (TAR) syndrome 287.33
  - giant hemangioma 287.39
- amegakaryocytic, congenital 287.33
- congenital 287.33
- cyclic 287.39
- dilutional 287.49
- due to
  - drugs 287.49
  - extracorporeal circulation of blood 287.49
  - massive blood transfusion 287.49
  - platelet alloimmunization 287.49
- essential 287.30
- fetal 678.0●
- heparin-induced (HIT) 289.84
- hereditary 287.33
- Kasabach-Merritt 287.39
- neonatal, transitory 776.1
  - due to
    - exchange transfusion 776.1
    - idiopathic maternal thrombocytopenia 776.1
    - isoimmunization 776.1
- primary 287.30
- puerperal, postpartum 666.3●
- purpura (*see also* Purpura, thrombocytopenic) 287.30
  - thrombotic 446.6
- secondary NEC 287.49
- sex-linked 287.39

Thrombocytosis 238.71
- essential 238.71
- primary 238.71

Thromboembolism - *see* Embolism
Thrombopathy (Bernard-Soulier) 287.1
- constitutional 286.4
- Willebrand-Jürgens (angiohemophilia) 286.4

Thrombopenia (*see also* Thrombocytopenia) 287.5
Thrombophlebitis 451.9
- antecubital vein 451.82
- antepartum (superficial) 671.2●
  - affecting fetus or newborn 760.3
  - deep 671.3●
- arm 451.89
  - deep 451.83
  - superficial 451.82
- breast, superficial 451.89
- cavernous (venous) sinus - *see* Thrombophlebitis, intracranial venous sinus

◀ New ◀ Revised ~~deleted~~ Deleted ● Use Additional Digit(s) ▓ Omit code

461

Thrombophlebitis (Continued)
cephalic vein 451.82
cerebral (sinus) (vein) 325
  late effect - see category 326
  nonpyogenic 437.6
    in pregnancy or puerperium 671.5●
    late effect - see Late effect(s) (of) cerebrovascular disease
  due to implanted device - see Complications, due to (presence of) any device, implant, or graft classified to 996.0–996.5 NEC
  during or resulting from a procedure NEC 997.2
femoral 451.11
femoropopliteal 451.19
following infusion, perfusion, or transfusion 999.2
hepatic (vein) 451.89
idiopathic, recurrent 453.1
iliac vein 451.81
iliofemoral 451.11
intracranial venous sinus (any) 325
  late effect - see category 326
  nonpyogenic 437.6
    in pregnancy or puerperium 671.5●
    late effect - see Late effect(s) (of) cerebrovascular disease
jugular vein 451.89
lateral (venous) sinus - see Thrombophlebitis, intracranial venous sinus
leg 451.2
  deep (vessels) 451.19
    femoral vein 451.11
    specified vessel NEC 451.19
  superficial (vessels) 451.0
    femoral vein 451.11
longitudinal (venous) sinus - see Thrombophlebitis, intracranial venous sinus
lower extremity 451.2
  deep (vessels) 451.19
    femoral vein 451.11
    specified vessel NEC 451.19
  superficial (vessels) 451.0
migrans, migrating 453.1
pelvic
  with
    abortion - see Abortion, by type, with sepsis
    ectopic pregnancy (see also categories 633.0–633.9) 639.0
    molar pregnancy (see also categories 630–632) 639.0
  following
    abortion 639.0
    ectopic or molar pregnancy 639.0
  puerperal 671.4●
popliteal vein 451.19
portal (vein) 572.1
postoperative 997.2
pregnancy (superficial) 671.2●
  affecting fetus or newborn 760.3
  deep 671.3●
puerperal, postpartum, childbirth (extremities) (superficial) 671.2●
  deep 671.4●
  pelvic 671.4●
  septic 670.3●
  specified site NEC 671.5●
radial vein 451.82
saphenous (greater) (lesser) 451.0
sinus (intracranial) - see Thrombophlebitis, intracranial venous sinus
specified site NEC 451.89
tibial vein 451.19

Thrombosis, thrombotic (marantic) (multiple) (progressive) (vein) (vessel) 453.9
with childbirth or during the puerperium - see Thrombosis, puerperal, postpartum
antepartum - see Thrombosis, pregnancy

Thrombosis, thrombotic (Continued)
aorta, aortic 444.1
  abdominal 444.09
    saddle 444.01
  bifurcation 444.09
    saddle 444.01
  terminal 444.09
  thoracic 444.1
  valve - see Endocarditis, aortic
apoplexy (see also Thrombosis, brain) 434.0●
  late effect - see Late effect(s) (of) cerebrovascular disease
appendix, septic - see Appendicitis, acute
arteriolar-capillary platelet, disseminated 446.6
artery, arteries (postinfectional) 444.9
  auditory, internal 433.8●
  basilar (see also Occlusion, artery, basilar) 433.0●
  carotid (common) (internal) (see also Occlusion, artery, carotid) 433.1●
    with other precerebral artery 433.3●
  cerebellar (anterior inferior) (posterior inferior) (superior) 433.8●
  cerebral (see also Thrombosis, brain) 434.0●
  choroidal (anterior) 433.8●
  communicating posterior 433.8●
  coronary (see also Infarct, myocardium) 410.9●
    without myocardial infarction 411.81
    due to syphilis 093.89
    healed or specified as old 412
  extremities 444.22
    lower 444.22
    upper 444.21
  femoral 444.22
  hepatic 444.89
  hypophyseal 433.8●
  meningeal, anterior or posterior 433.8●
  mesenteric (with gangrene) 557.0
  ophthalmic (see also Occlusion, retina) 362.30
  pontine 433.8●
  popliteal 444.22
  precerebral - see Occlusion, artery, precerebral NEC
  pulmonary 415.19
    iatrogenic 415.11
    personal history of V12.55
    postoperative 415.11
    septic 415.12
  renal 593.81
  retinal (see also Occlusion, retina) 362.30
  specified site NEC 444.89
  spinal, anterior or posterior 433.8●
  traumatic (complication) (early) (see also Injury, blood vessel, by site) 904.9
  vertebral (see also Occlusion, artery, vertebral) 433.2●
    with other precerebral artery 433.3●
atrial (endocardial) 424.90
  without endocarditis 429.89
  due to syphilis 093.89
auricular (see also Infarct, myocardium) 410.9●
axillary (acute) (vein) 453.84
  chronic 453.74
  personal history of V12.51
basilar (artery) (see also Occlusion, artery, basilar) 433.0●
bland NEC 453.9
brain (artery) (stem) 434.0●
  due to syphilis 094.89
  iatrogenic 997.02
  late effect - see Late effect(s) (of) cerebrovascular disease
  postoperative 997.02
  puerperal, postpartum, childbirth 674.0●
  sinus (see also Thrombosis, intracranial venous sinus) 325

Thrombosis, thrombotic (Continued)
capillary 448.9
  arteriolar, generalized 446.6
cardiac (see also Infarct, myocardium) 410.9●
  due to syphilis 093.89
  healed or specified as old 412
  valve - see Endocarditis
carotid (artery) (common) (internal) (see also Occlusion, artery, carotid) 433.1●
  with other precerebral artery 433.3●
cavernous sinus (venous) - see Thrombosis, intracranial venous sinus
cerebellar artery (anterior inferior) (posterior inferior) (superior) 433.8●
  late effect - see Late effect(s) (of) cerebrovascular disease
cerebral (arteries) (see also Thrombosis, brain) 434.0●
  late effect - see Late effect(s) (of) cerebrovascular disease
coronary (artery) (see also Infarct, myocardium) 410.9●
  without myocardial infarction 411.81
  due to syphilis 093.89
  healed or specified as old 412
corpus cavernosum 607.82
cortical (see also Thrombosis, brain) 434.0●
due to (presence of) any device, implant, or graft classifiable to 996.0–996.5 - see Complications, due to (presence of) any device, implant, or graft classified to 996.0–996.5 NEC
effort 453.89
endocardial - see Infarct, myocardium
eye (see also Occlusion, retina) 362.30
femoral (vein) 453.6
  with inflammation or phlebitis 451.11
  artery 444.22
  deep 453.41
  personal history of V12.51
genital organ, male 608.83
heart (chamber) (see also Infarct, myocardium) 410.9●
hepatic (vein) 453.0
  artery 444.89
  infectional or septic 572.1
iliac (acute) (vein) 453.41
  with inflammation or phlebitis 451.81
  artery (common) (external) (internal) 444.81
  chronic 453.51
  personal history of V12.51
inflammation, vein - see Thrombophlebitis
internal carotid artery (see also Occlusion, artery, carotid) 433.1●
  with other precerebral artery 433.3●
intestine (with gangrene) 557.0
intracranial (see also Thrombosis, brain) 434.0●
  venous sinus (any) 325
    nonpyogenic origin 437.6
      in pregnancy or puerperium 671.5●
intramural (see also Infarct, myocardium) 410.9●
  without
    cardiac condition 429.89
    coronary artery disease 429.89
    myocardial infarction 429.89
  healed or specified as old 412
jugular (bulb)
  external (acute) 453.89
    chronic 453.79
  internal (acute) 453.86
    chronic 453.76
kidney 593.81
  artery 593.81
lateral sinus (venous) - see Thrombosis, intracranial venous sinus

SECTION I INDEX TO DISEASES AND INJURIES / Thyroiditis

Thrombosis, thrombotic (Continued)
  leg (see also Thrombosis, lower extremity) 453.6
    with inflammation or phlebitis - see Thrombophlebitis
    deep (vessels) 453.40
      acute 453.40
        lower (distal) 453.42
        upper (proximal) 453.41
      chronic 453.50
        lower (distal) 453.52
        upper (proximal) 453.51
      lower (distal) 453.42
      upper (proximal) 453.41
    personal history of V12.51
    superficial (vessels) 453.6
  liver (venous) 453.0
    artery 444.89
    infectional or septic 572.1
    portal vein 452
  longitudinal sinus (venous) - see Thrombosis, intracranial venous sinus
  lower extremity (superficial) 453.6
    deep vessels 453.40
      acute 453.40
        calf 453.42
        distal (lower leg) 453.42
        femoral 453.41
        iliac 453.41
        lower leg 453.42
        peroneal 453.42
        popliteal 453.41
        proximal (upper leg) 453.41
        thigh 453.41
        tibial 453.42
      chronic 453.50
        calf 453.52
        distal (lower leg) 453.52
        femoral 453.51
        iliac 453.51
        lower leg 453.52
        peroneal 453.52
        popliteal 453.51
        proximal (upper leg) 453.51
        thigh 453.51
        tibial 453.52
    personal history of V12.51
    saphenous (greater) (lesser) 453.6
    superficial 453.6
  lung 415.19
    iatrogenic 415.11
    personal history of V12.55
    postoperative 415.11
    septic 415.12
  marantic, dural sinus 437.6
  meninges (brain) (see also Thrombosis, brain) 434.0●
  mesenteric (artery) (with gangrene) 557.0
    vein (inferior) (superior) 557.0
  mitral - see Insufficiency, mitral
  mural (heart chamber) (see also Infarct, myocardium) 410.9●
    without
      cardiac condition 429.89
      coronary artery disease 429.89
      myocardial infarction 429.89
    due to syphilis 093.89
    following myocardial infarction 429.79
    healed or specified as old 412
  omentum (with gangrene) 557.0
  ophthalmic (artery) (see also Occlusion, retina) 362.30
  pampiniform plexus (male) 608.83
    female 620.8
  parietal (see also Infarct, myocardium) 410.9●
  penis, penile 607.82
  peripheral arteries 444.22
    lower 444.22
    upper 444.21
  platelet 446.6

Thrombosis, thrombotic (Continued)
  portal 452
    due to syphilis 093.89
    infectional or septic 572.1
  precerebral artery - see also Occlusion, artery, precerebral NEC
  pregnancy 671.2●
    deep (vein) 671.3●
    superficial (vein) 671.2●
  puerperal, postpartum, childbirth 671.2●
    brain (artery) 674.0●
      venous 671.5●
    cardiac 674.8●
    cerebral (artery) 674.0●
      venous 671.5●
    deep (vein) 671.4●
    intracranial sinus (nonpyogenic) (venous) 671.5●
    pelvic 671.4●
    pulmonary (artery) 673.2●
    specified site NEC 671.5●
    superficial 671.2●
  pulmonary (artery) (vein) 415.19
    iatrogenic 415.11
    personal history of V12.55
    postoperative 415.11
    septic 415.12
  renal (artery) 593.81
    vein 453.3
  resulting from presence of shunt or other internal prosthetic device - see Complications, due to (presence of) any device, implant, or graft classifiable to 996.0–996.5 NEC
  retina, retinal (artery) 362.30
    arterial branch 362.32
    central 362.31
    partial 362.33
    vein
      central 362.35
      tributary (branch) 362.36
  saphenous vein (greater) (lesser) 453.6
  scrotum 608.83
  seminal vesicle 608.83
  sigmoid (venous) sinus (see Thrombosis, intracranial venous sinus) 325
  silent NEC 453.9
  sinus, intracranial (venous) (any) (see also Thrombosis, intracranial venous sinus) 325
  softening, brain (see also Thrombosis, brain) 434.0●
  specified site NEC (acute) 453.89
    chronic 453.79
  spermatic cord 608.83
  spinal cord 336.1
    due to syphilis 094.89
    in pregnancy or puerperium 671.5●
    pyogenic origin 324.1
      late effect - see category 326
  spleen, splenic 289.59
    artery 444.89
  testis 608.83
  traumatic (complication) (early) (see also Injury, blood vessel, by site) 904.9
  tricuspid - see Endocarditis, tricuspid
  tumor - see Neoplasm, by site
  tunica vaginalis 608.83
  umbilical cord (vessels) 663.6●
    affecting fetus or newborn 762.6
  upper extremity (acute) 453.83
    deep 453.82
    superficial 453.81
    chronic 453.73
      deep 453.72
      superficial 453.71
  vas deferens 608.83
  vein
    antecubital (acute) 453.81
    chronic 453.71

Thrombosis, thrombotic (Continued)
  vein (Continued)
    axillary (acute) 453.84
      chronic 453.74
    basilic (acute) 453.81
      chronic 453.71
    brachial (acute) 453.82
      chronic 453.72
    brachiocephalic (innominate) (acute) 453.87
      chronic 453.77
    cephalic (acute) 453.81
      chronic 453.71
    deep 453.40
      personal history of V12.51
    internal jugular (acute) 453.86
      chronic 453.76
    lower extremity - see Thrombosis, lower extremity
    personal history of V12.51
    radial (acute) 453.82
      chronic 453.72
    saphenous (greater) (lesser) 453.6
    specified site NEC (acute) 453.89
      chronic 453.79
    subclavian (acute) 453.85
      chronic 453.75
    superior vena cava (acute) 453.87
      chronic 453.77
    thoracic (acute) 453.87
      chronic 453.77
    ulnar (acute) 453.82
      chronic 453.72
    upper extremity - see Thrombosis, upper extremity
  vena cava
    inferior 453.2
    personal history of V12.51
    superior (acute) 453.87
      chronic 453.77

Thrombus - see Thrombosis
Thrush 112.0
  newborn 771.7
Thumb - see also condition
  gamekeeper's 842.12
  sucking (child problem) 307.9
Thygeson's superficial punctate keratitis 370.21
Thymergasia (see also Psychosis, affective) 296.80
Thymitis 254.8
Thymoma (benign) (M8580/0) 212.6
  malignant (M8580/3) 164.0
Thymus, thymic (gland) - see condition
Thyrocele (see also Goiter) 240.9
Thyroglossal - see also condition
  cyst 759.2
  duct, persistent 759.2
Thyroid (body) (gland) - see also condition
  hormone resistance 246.8
  lingual 759.2
Thyroiditis 245.9
  acute (pyogenic) (suppurative) 245.0
    nonsuppurative 245.0
  autoimmune 245.2
  chronic (nonspecific) (sclerosing) 245.8
    fibrous 245.3
    lymphadenoid 245.2
    lymphocytic 245.2
    lymphoid 245.2
  complicating pregnancy, childbirth, or puerperium 648.1●
  de Quervain's (subacute granulomatous) 245.1
  fibrous (chronic) 245.3
  giant (cell) (follicular) 245.1
  granulomatous (de Quervain's) (subacute) 245.1
  Hashimoto's (struma lymphomatosa) 245.2
  iatrogenic 245.4
  invasive (fibrous) 245.3

SECTION I INDEX TO DISEASES AND INJURIES / Thyroiditis

Thyroiditis (Continued)
- ligneous 245.3
- lymphocytic (chronic) 245.2
- lymphoid 245.2
- lymphomatous 245.2
- pseudotuberculous 245.1
- pyogenic 245.0
- radiation 245.4
- Riedel's (ligneous) 245.3
- subacute 245.1
- suppurative 245.0
- tuberculous (see also Tuberculosis) 017.5●
- viral 245.1
- woody 245.3

Thyrolingual duct, persistent 759.2

Thyromegaly 240.9

Thyrotoxic
- crisis or storm (see also Thyrotoxicosis) 242.9●
- heart failure (see also Thyrotoxicosis) 242.9● [425.7]

Thyrotoxicosis 242.9●

Note: Use the following fifth-digit subclassification with category 242:
- 0 without mention of thyrotoxic crisis or storm
- 1 with mention of thyrotoxic crisis or storm

with
- goiter (diffuse) 242.0●
  - adenomatous 242.3●
    - multinodular 242.2●
    - uninodular 242.1●
  - nodular 242.3●
    - multinodular 242.2●
    - uninodular 242.1●
  - infiltrative
    - dermopathy 242.0●
    - ophthalmopathy 242.0●
    - thyroid acropachy 242.0●
- complicating pregnancy, childbirth, or puerperium 648.1●
- due to
  - ectopic thyroid nodule 242.4●
  - ingestion of (excessive) thyroid material 242.8●
  - specified cause NEC 242.8●
- factitia 242.8●
- heart 242.9● [425.7]
- neonatal (transient) 775.3

TIA (transient ischemic attack) 435.9
- with transient neurologic deficit 435.9
- late effect - see Late effect(s) (of) cerebrovascular disease

Tibia vara 732.4

Tic 307.20
- breathing 307.20
- child problem 307.21
- compulsive 307.22
- convulsive 307.20
- degenerative (generalized) (localized) 333.3
  - facial 351.8
- douloureux (see also Neuralgia, trigeminal) 350.1
  - atypical 350.2
- habit 307.20
  - chronic (motor or vocal) 307.22
  - transient (of childhood) 307.21
- lid 307.20
  - transient (of childhood) 307.21
- motor-verbal 307.23
- occupational 300.89
- orbicularis 307.20
  - transient (of childhood) 307.21
- organic origin 333.3
- postchoreic - see Chorea
- psychogenic 307.20
  - compulsive 307.22

Tic (Continued)
- salaam 781.0
- spasm 307.20
  - chronic (motor or vocal) 307.22
  - transient (of childhood) 307.21

Tick (-borne) fever NEC 066.1
- American mountain 066.1
- Colorado 066.1
- hemorrhagic NEC 065.3
  - Crimean 065.0
  - Kyasanur Forest 065.2
  - Omsk 065.1
- mountain 066.1
- nonexanthematous 066.1

Tick-bite fever NEC 066.1
- African 087.1
- Colorado (virus) 066.1
- Rocky Mountain 082.0

Tick paralysis 989.5

Tics and spasms, compulsive 307.22

Tietze's disease or syndrome 733.6

Tight, tightness
- anus 564.89
- chest 786.59
- fascia (lata) 728.9
- foreskin (congenital) 605
- hymen 623.3
- introitus (acquired) (congenital) 623.3
- rectal sphincter 564.89
- tendon 727.81
  - Achilles (heel) 727.81
- urethral sphincter 598.9

Tilting vertebra 737.9

Timidity, child 313.21

Tinea (intersecta) (tarsi) 110.9
- amiantacea 110.0
- asbestina 110.0
- barbae 110.0
- beard 110.0
- black dot 110.0
- blanca 111.2
- capitis 110.0
- corporis 110.5
- cruris 110.3
- decalvans 704.09
- flava 111.0
- foot 110.4
- furfuracea 111.0
- imbricata (Tokelau) 110.5
- lepothrix 039.0
- manuum 110.2
- microsporic (see also Dermatophytosis) 110.9
- nigra 111.1
- nodosa 111.2
- pedis 110.4
- scalp 110.0
- specified site NEC 110.8
- sycosis 110.0
- tonsurans 110.0
- trichophytic (see also Dermatophytosis) 110.9
- unguium 110.1
- versicolor 111.0

Tingling sensation (see also Disturbance, sensation) 782.0

Tin-miners' lung 503

Tinnitus (aurium) 388.30
- audible 388.32
- objective 388.32
- subjective 388.31

Tipped, teeth 524.33

Tipping
- pelvis 738.6
  - with disproportion (fetopelvic) 653.0●
    - affecting fetus or newborn 763.1
    - causing obstructed labor 660.1●
      - affecting fetus or newborn 763.1
- teeth 524.33

Tiredness 780.79

Tissue - see condition

Tobacco
- abuse (affecting health) NEC (see also Abuse, drugs, nondependent) 305.1
- heart 989.84
- use disorder complicating pregnancy, childbirth, or the puerperium 649.0●

Tobias' syndrome (carcinoma, pulmonary apex) (M8010/3) 162.3

Tocopherol deficiency 269.1

Todd's
- cirrhosis - see Cirrhosis, biliary
- paralysis (postepileptic transitory paralysis) 344.89

Toe - see condition

Toilet, artificial opening (see also Attention to, artificial, opening) V55.9

Tokelau ringworm 110.5

Tollwut 071

Tolosa-Hunt syndrome 378.55

Tommaselli's disease
- correct substance properly administered 599.70
- overdose or wrong substance given or taken 961.4

Tongue - see also condition
- worms 134.1

Tongue tie 750.0

Toni-Fanconi syndrome (cystinosis) 270.0

Tonic pupil 379.46

Tonsil - see condition

Tonsillitis (acute) (catarrhal) (croupous) (follicular) (gangrenous) (infective) (lacunar) (lingual) (malignant) (membranous) (phlegmonous) (pneumococcal) (pseudomembranous) (purulent) (septic) (staphylococcal) (subacute) (suppurative) (toxic) (ulcerative) (vesicular) (viral) 463
- with influenza, flu, or grippe (see also Influenza) 487.1
- chronic 474.00
- diphtheritic (membranous) 032.0
- hypertrophic 474.00
- influenzal (see also Influenza) 487.1
- parenchymatous 475
- streptococcal 034.0
- tuberculous (see also Tuberculosis) 012.8●
- Vincent's 101

Tonsillopharyngitis 465.8

Tooth, teeth - see condition

Toothache 525.9

Topagnosis 782.0

Tophi (gouty) 274.03
- ear 274.81
- heart 274.82
- specified site NEC 274.82

TORCH infection - (see also Infection, congenital) 760.2

Torn - see Tear, torn

Tornwaldt's bursitis (disease) (pharyngeal bursitis) 478.29
- cyst 478.26

Torpid liver 573.9

Torsion
- accessory tube 620.5
- adnexa (female) 620.5
- aorta (congenital) 747.29
  - acquired 447.1
- appendix
  - epididymis 608.24
  - testis 608.23
- bile duct 576.8
  - with calculus, choledocholithiasis or stones - see Choledocholithiasis
  - congenital 751.69
- bowel, colon, or intestine 560.2
- cervix - see Malposition, uterus
- duodenum 537.3
- dystonia - see Dystonia, torsion
- epididymis 608.24
  - appendix 608.24

Torsion (Continued)
- fallopian tube 620.5
- gallbladder (see also Disease, gallbladder) 575.8
  - congenital 751.69
- gastric 537.89
- hydatid of Morgagni (female) 620.5
- kidney (pedicle) 593.89
- Meckel's diverticulum (congenital) 751.0
- mesentery 560.2
- omentum 560.2
- organ or site, congenital NEC - see Anomaly, specified type NEC
- ovary (pedicle) 620.5
  - congenital 752.0
- oviduct 620.5
- penis 607.89
  - congenital 752.69
- renal 593.89
- spasm - see Dystonia, torsion
- spermatic cord 608.22
  - extravaginal 608.21
  - intravaginal 608.22
- spleen 289.59
- testicle, testis 608.20
  - appendix 608.23
- tibia 736.89
- umbilical cord - see Compression, umbilical cord
- uterus (see also Malposition, uterus) 621.6

Torticollis (intermittent) (spastic) 723.5
- congenital 754.1
  - sternomastoid 754.1
- due to birth injury 767.8
- hysterical 300.11
- ocular 781.93
- psychogenic 306.0
  - specified as conversion reaction 300.11
- rheumatic 723.5
- rheumatoid 714.0
- spasmodic 333.83
- traumatic, current NEC 847.0

Tortuous
- artery 447.1
- fallopian tube 752.19
- organ or site, congenital NEC - see Distortion
- renal vessel (congenital) 747.62
- retina vessel (congenital) 743.58
  - acquired 362.17
- ureter 593.4
- urethra 599.84
- vein - see Varicose, vein

Torula, torular (infection) 117.5
- histolytica 117.5
- lung 117.5

Torulosis 117.5

Torus
- fracture
  - fibula 823.41
    - with tibia 823.42
  - humerus 812.49
  - radius (alone) 813.45
    - with ulna 813.47
  - tibia 823.40
    - with fibula 823.42
  - ulna (alone) 813.46
    - with radius 813.47
- mandibularis 526.81
- palatinus 526.81

Touch, vitreous 997.99
Touraine's syndrome (hereditary osteo-onychodysplasia) 756.89
Touraine-Solente-Golé syndrome (acropachyderma) 757.39
Tourette's disease (motor-verbal tic) 307.23
Tower skull 756.0
- with exophthalmos 756.0

Toxemia 799.89
- with
  - abortion - see Abortion, by type, with toxemia

Toxemia (Continued)
- bacterial - see Septicemia
- biliary (see also Disease, biliary) 576.8
- burn - see Burn, by site
- congenital NEC 779.89
- eclamptic 642.6●
  - with pre-existing hypertension 642.7●
- erysipelatous (see also Erysipelas) 035
- fatigue 799.89
- fetus or newborn NEC 779.89
- food (see also Poisoning, food) 005.9
- gastric 537.89
- gastrointestinal 558.2
- intestinal 558.2
- kidney (see also Disease, renal) 593.9
- lung 518.89
- malarial NEC (see also Malaria) 084.6
- maternal (of pregnancy), affecting fetus or newborn 760.0
- myocardial - see Myocarditis, toxic
- of pregnancy (mild) (pre-eclamptic) 642.4●
  - with
    - convulsions 642.6●
    - pre-existing hypertension 642.7●
  - affecting fetus or newborn 760.0
  - severe 642.5●
- pre-eclamptic - see Toxemia, of pregnancy
- puerperal, postpartum - see Toxemia, of pregnancy
- pulmonary 518.89
- renal (see also Disease, renal) 593.9
- septic (see also Septicemia) 038.9
- small intestine 558.2
- staphylococcal 038.10
  - aureus 038.11
  - due to food 005.0
  - specified organism NEC 038.19
- stasis 799.89
- stomach 537.89
- uremic (see also Uremia) 586
- urinary 586

Toxemica cerebropathia psychica (nonalcoholic) 294.0
- alcoholic 291.1

Toxic (poisoning) - see also condition
- from drug or poison - see Table of Drugs and Chemicals
- oil syndrome 710.5
- shock syndrome 040.82
- thyroid (gland) (see also Thyrotoxicosis) 242.9●

Toxicemia - see Toxemia

Toxicity
- dilantin
  - asymptomatic 796.0
  - symptomatic - see Table of Drugs and Chemicals
- drug
  - asymptomatic 796.0
  - symptomatic - see Table of Drugs and Chemicals
- fava bean 282.2
- from drug or poison
  - asymptomatic 796.0
  - symptomatic - see Table of Drugs and Chemicals

Toxicosis (see also Toxemia) 799.89
- capillary, hemorrhagic 287.0

Toxinfection 799.89
- gastrointestinal 558.2

Toxocariasis 128.0
Toxoplasma infection, generalized 130.9
Toxoplasmosis (acquired) 130.9
- with pneumonia 130.4
- congenital, active 771.2
- disseminated (multisystemic) 130.8
- maternal
  - with suspected damage to fetus affecting management of pregnancy 655.4●

Toxoplasmosis (Continued)
- maternal (Continued)
  - affecting fetus or newborn 760.2
    - manifest toxoplasmosis in fetus or newborn 771.2
- multiple sites 130.8
- multisystemic disseminated 130.8
- specified site NEC 130.7

Trabeculation, bladder 596.89
Trachea - see condition
Tracheitis (acute) (catarrhal) (infantile) (membranous) (plastic) (pneumococcal) (septic) (suppurative) (viral) 464.10
- with
  - bronchitis 490
    - acute or subacute 466.0
    - chronic 491.8
    - tuberculosis - see Tuberculosis, pulmonary
  - laryngitis (acute) 464.20
    - with obstruction 464.21
    - chronic 476.1
    - tuberculous (see also Tuberculosis, larynx) 012.3●
  - obstruction 464.11
- chronic 491.8
  - with
    - bronchitis (chronic) 491.8
    - laryngitis (chronic) 476.1
  - due to external agent - see Condition, respiratory, chronic, due to
- diphtheritic (membranous) 032.3
  - due to external agent - see Inflammation, respiratory, upper, due to
- edematous 464.11
- influenzal (see also Influenza) 487.1
- streptococcal 034.0
- syphilitic 095.8
- tuberculous (see also Tuberculosis) 012.8●

Trachelitis (nonvenereal) (see also Cervicitis) 616.0
- trichomonal 131.09

Tracheobronchial - see condition
Tracheobronchitis (see also Bronchitis) 490
- acute or subacute 466.0
  - with bronchospasm or obstruction 466.0
- chronic 491.8
- influenzal (see also Influenza) 487.1
- senile 491.8

Tracheobronchomegaly (congenital) 748.3
- with bronchiectasis 494.0
  - with (acute) exacerbation 494.1
- acquired 519.19
  - with bronchiectasis 494.0
    - with (acute) exacerbation 494.1

Tracheobronchopneumonitis - see Pneumonia, broncho
Tracheocele (external) (internal) 519.19
- congenital 748.3

Tracheomalacia 519.19
- congenital 748.3

Tracheopharyngitis (acute) 465.8
- chronic 478.9
  - due to external agent - see Condition, respiratory, chronic, due to
- due to external agent - see Inflammation, respiratory, upper, due to

Tracheostenosis 519.19
- congenital 748.3

Tracheostomy
- attention to V55.0
- complication 519.00
- granuloma 519.09
- hemorrhage 519.09
- infection 519.01
- malfunctioning 519.02
- obstruction 519.09
- sepsis 519.01
- status V44.0
- stenosis 519.02

SECTION I INDEX TO DISEASES AND INJURIES / Trachoma, trachomatous

Trachoma, trachomatous 076.9
   active (stage) 076.1
   contraction of conjunctiva 076.1
   dubium 076.0
   healed or late effect 139.1
   initial (stage) 076.0
   Türck's (chronic catarrhal laryngitis) 476.0
Trachyphonia 784.49
Traction, vitreomacular 379.27
Training
   insulin pump V65.46
   orthoptic V57.4
   orthotic V57.81
Train sickness 994.6
Trait
   hemoglobin
     abnormal NEC 282.7
       with thalassemia 282.46
     C (see also Disease, hemoglobin, C) 282.7
       with elliptocytosis 282.7
     S (Hb-S) 282.5
     Lepore 282.49
       with other abnormal hemoglobin NEC 282.49
   paranoid 301.0
   sickle-cell 282.5
     with
       elliptocytosis 282.5
       spherocytosis 282.5
   thalassemia (alpha) (beta) (delta-beta) 282.46
Traits, paranoid 301.0
Tramp V60.0
Trance 780.09
   hysterical 300.13
Transaminasemia 790.4
Transfusion, blood
   donor V59.01
     stem cells V59.02
   fetal twin to twin 678.0 •
   incompatible (see also Complications, transfusion) 999.80
     ABO (see also Complications, transfusion) 999.60
     minor blood group 999.89
     non-ABO (see also Complications, transfusion) 999.75
     Rh (antigen) (C) (c) (D) (E) (e) (see also Complications, transfusion) 999.70
   reaction or complication - see Complications, transfusion
   related acute lung injury (TRALI) 518.7
   syndrome
     fetomaternal 772.0
     twin-to-twin
       blood loss (donor twin) 772.0
       recipient twin 776.4
   twin to twin fetal 678.0 •
   without reported diagnosis V58.2
Transient - see also condition
   alteration of awareness 780.02
   blindness 368.12
   deafness (ischemic) 388.02
   global amnesia 437.7
   hyperglycemia (post-procedural) 790.29
   hypoglycemia (post-procedural) 251.2
   person (homeless) NEC V60.0
Transitional, lumbosacral joint of vertebra 756.19
Translocation
   autosomes NEC 758.5
     13–15 758.1
     16–18 758.2
     21 or 22 758.0
     balanced in normal individual 758.4
     D_1 758.1
     E_3 758.2
     G 758.0
   balanced autosomal in normal individual 758.4
   chromosomes NEC 758.89
   Down's syndrome 758.0

Translucency, iris 364.53
Transmission of chemical substances through the placenta (affecting fetus or newborn) 760.70
   alcohol 760.71
   anticonvulsants 760.77
   antifungals 760.74
   anti-infective agents 760.74
   antimetabolics 760.78
   cocaine 760.75
   "crack" 760.75
   diethylstilbestrol [DES] 760.76
   hallucinogenic agents 760.73
   medicinal agents NEC 760.79
   narcotics 760.72
   obstetric anesthetic or analgesic drug 763.5
   specified agent NEC 760.79
   suspected, affecting management of pregnancy 655.5 •
Transplant (ed)
   bone V42.4
     marrow V42.81
   complication - see also Complications, due to (presence of) any device, implant, or graft classified to 996.0–996.5 NEC
     bone marrow 996.85
     corneal graft NEC 996.79
       infection or inflammation 996.69
       reaction 996.51
       rejection 996.51
     organ (failure) (immune or nonimmune cause) (infection) (rejection) 996.80
       bone marrow 996.85
       heart 996.83
       intestines 996.87
       kidney 996.81
       liver 996.82
       lung 996.84
       pancreas 996.86
       specified NEC 996.89
     previously removed due to complication, failure, rejection or infection V45.87
     removal status V45.87
     skin NEC 996.79
       infection or inflammation 996.69
       rejection 996.52
       artificial 996.55
         decellularized allodermis 996.55
     stem cell(s) 996.88
       from
         peripheral blood 996.88
         umbilical cord 996.88
   cornea V42.5
   hair V50.0
   heart V42.1
     valve V42.2
   intestine V42.84
   kidney V42.0
   liver V42.7
   lung V42.6
   organ V42.9
     specified NEC V42.89
   pancreas V42.83
   peripheral stem cells V42.82
   skin V42.3
   stem cells, peripheral V42.82
   tissue V42.9
     specified NEC V42.89
Transplants, ovarian, endometrial 617.1
Transposed - see Transposition
Transposition (congenital) - see also Malposition, congenital
   abdominal viscera 759.3
   aorta (dextra) 745.11
   appendix 751.5
   arterial trunk 745.10
   colon 751.5
   great vessels (complete) 745.10
     both originating from right ventricle 745.11
     corrected 745.12

Transposition (Continued)
   great vessels (Continued)
     double outlet right ventricle 745.11
     incomplete 745.11
     partial 745.11
     specified type NEC 745.19
   heart 746.87
     with complete transposition of viscera 759.3
   intestine (large) (small) 751.5
   pulmonary veins 747.49
   reversed jejunal (for bypass) (status) V45.3
   scrotal 752.81
   stomach 750.7
     with general transposition of viscera 759.3
   teeth, tooth 524.30
   vessels (complete) 745.10
     partial 745.11
   viscera (abdominal) (thoracic) 759.3
Trans-sexualism 302.50
   with
     asexual history 302.51
     heterosexual history 302.53
     homosexual history 302.52
Transverse - see also condition
   arrest (deep), in labor 660.3 •
     affecting fetus or newborn 763.1
   lie 652.3 •
     before labor, affecting fetus or newborn 761.7
     causing obstructed labor 660.0 •
       affecting fetus or newborn 763.1
     during labor, affecting fetus or newborn 763.1
Transvestism, transvestitism (transvestic fetishism) 302.3
Trapped placenta (with hemorrhage) 666.0 •
   without hemorrhage 667.0 •
Trauma, traumatism (see also Injury, by site) 959.9
   birth - see Birth, injury NEC
   causing hemorrhage of pregnancy or delivery 641.8 •
   complicating
     abortion - see Abortion, by type, with damage to pelvic organs
     ectopic pregnancy (see also categories 633.0–633.9) 639.2
     molar pregnancy (see also categories 630–632) 639.2
   during delivery NEC 665.9 •
   following
     abortion 639.2
     ectopic or molar pregnancy 639.2
   maternal, during pregnancy, affecting fetus or newborn 760.5
   neuroma - see Injury, nerve, by site
   previous major, affecting management of pregnancy, childbirth, or puerperium V23.89
   psychic (current) - see also Reaction, adjustment
     previous (history) V15.49
   psychologic, previous (affecting health) V15.49
   transient paralysis - see Injury, nerve, by site
Traumatic - see also condition
   brain injury (TBI) (see also Injury, intracranial) 854.0 •
     with skull fracture - see Fracture, skull, by site
Treacher Collins' syndrome (incomplete facial dysostosis) 756.0
Treitz's hernia - see Hernia, Treitz's
Trematode infestation NEC 121.9
Trematodiasis NEC 121.9
Trembles 988.8
Trembling paralysis (see also Parkinsonism) 332.0

Tremor 781.0
　essential (benign) 333.1
　familial 333.1
　flapping (liver) 572.8
　hereditary 333.1
　hysterical 300.11
　intention 333.1
　medication-induced postural 333.1
　mercurial 985.0
　muscle 728.85
　Parkinson's (see also Parkinsonism) 332.0
　psychogenic 306.0
　　specified as conversion reaction 300.11
　senilis 797
　specified type NEC 333.1
Trench
　fever 083.1
　foot 991.4
　mouth 101
　nephritis - see Nephritis, acute
Treponema pallidum infection (see also Syphilis) 097.9
Treponematosis 102.9
　due to
　　T. pallidum - see Syphilis
　　T. pertenue (yaws) (see also Yaws) 102.9
Triad
　Kartagener's 759.3
　Reiter's (complete) (incomplete) 099.3
　Saint's (see also Hernia, diaphragm) 553.3
Trichiasis 704.2
　cicatricial 704.2
　eyelid 374.05
　　with entropion (see also Entropion) 374.00
Trichinella spiralis (infection) (infestation) 124
Trichinelliasis 124
Trichinellosis 124
Trichiniasis 124
Trichinosis 124
Trichobezoar 938
　intestine 936
　stomach 935.2
Trichocephaliasis 127.3
Trichocephalosis 127.3
Trichocephalus infestation 127.3
Trichoclasis 704.2
Trichoepithelioma (M8100/0) - see also Neoplasm, skin, benign
　breast 217
　genital organ NEC - see Neoplasm, by site, benign
　malignant (M8100/3) - see Neoplasm, skin, malignant
Trichofolliculoma (M8101/0) - see Neoplasm, skin, benign
Tricholemmoma (M8102/0) - see Neoplasm, skin, benign
Trichomatosis 704.2
Trichomoniasis 131.9
　bladder 131.09
　cervix 131.09
　intestinal 007.3
　prostate 131.03
　seminal vesicle 131.09
　specified site NEC 131.8
　urethra 131.02
　urogenitalis 131.00
　vagina 131.01
　vulva 131.01
　vulvovaginal 131.01
Trichomycosis 039.0
　axillaris 039.0
　nodosa 111.2
　nodularis 111.2
　rubra 039.0

Trichonocardiosis (axillaris) (palmellina) 039.0
Trichonodosis 704.2
Trichophytid, trichophyton infection (see also Dermatophytosis) 110.9
Trichophytide - see Dermatophytosis
Trichophytobezoar 938
　intestine 936
　stomach 935.2
Trichophytosis - see Dermatophytosis
Trichoptilosis 704.2
Trichorrhexis (nodosa) 704.2
Trichosporosis nodosa 111.2
Trichostasis spinulosa (congenital) 757.4
Trichostrongyliasis (small intestine) 127.6
Trichostrongylosis 127.6
Trichostrongylus (instabilis) infection 127.6
Trichotillomania 312.39
Trichromat, anomalous (congenital) 368.59
Trichromatopsia, anomalous (congenital) 368.59
Trichuriasis 127.3
Trichuris trichiuria (any site) (infection) (infestation) 127.3
Tricuspid (valve) - see condition
Trifid - see also Accessory
　kidney (pelvis) 753.3
　tongue 750.13
Trigeminal neuralgia (see also Neuralgia, trigeminal) 350.1
Trigeminoencephaloangiomatosis 759.6
Trigeminy 427.89
　postoperative 997.1
Trigger finger (acquired) 727.03
　congenital 756.89
Trigonitis (bladder) (chronic) (pseudomembranous) 595.3
　tuberculous (see also Tuberculosis) 016.1 ●
Trigonocephaly 756.0
Trihexosidosis 272.7
Trilobate placenta - see Placenta, abnormal
Trilocular heart 745.8
Trimethylaminuria 270.8
Tripartita placenta - see Placenta, abnormal
Triple - see also Accessory
　kidneys 753.3
　uteri 752.2
　X female 758.81
Triplegia 344.89
　congenital or infantile 343.8
Triplet
　affected by maternal complications of pregnancy 761.5
　healthy liveborn - see Newborn, multiple
　pregnancy (complicating delivery) NEC 651.1 ●
　　with fetal loss and retention of one or more fetus(es) 651.4 ●
　　following (elective) fetal reduction 651.7 ●
Triplex placenta - see Placenta, abnormal
Triplication - see Accessory
Trismus 781.0
　neonatorum 771.3
　newborn 771.3
Trisomy (syndrome) NEC 758.5
　13 (partial) 758.1
　16–18 758.2
　18 (partial) 758.2
　21 (partial) 758.0
　22 758.0
　autosomes NEC 758.5
　D$_1$ 758.1
　E$_3$ 758.2
　G (group) 758.0
　group D$_1$ 758.1
　group E 758.2
　group G 758.0
Tritanomaly 368.53
Tritanopia 368.53

Troisier-Hanot-Chauffard syndrome (bronze diabetes) 275.01
Trombidiosis 133.8
Trophedema (hereditary) 757.0
　congenital 757.0
Trophoblastic disease (see also Hydatidiform mole) 630
　previous, affecting management of pregnancy V23.1
Tropholymphedema 757.0
Trophoneurosis NEC 356.9
　arm NEC 354.9
　disseminated 710.1
　facial 349.89
　leg NEC 355.8
　lower extremity NEC 355.8
　upper extremity NEC 354.9
Tropical - see also condition
　maceration feet (syndrome) 991.4
　wet foot (syndrome) 991.4
Trouble - see also Disease
　bowel 569.9
　heart - see Disease, heart
　intestine 569.9
　kidney (see also Disease, renal) 593.9
　nervous 799.21
　sinus (see also Sinusitis) 473.9
Trousseau's syndrome (thrombophlebitis migrans) 453.1
Truancy, childhood - see also Disturbance, conduct
　socialized 312.2 ●
　undersocialized, unsocialized 312.1 ●
Truncus
　arteriosus (persistent) 745.0
　common 745.0
　communis 745.0
Trunk - see condition
Trychophytide - see Dermatophytosis
Trypanosoma infestation - see Trypanosomiasis
Trypanosomiasis 086.9
　with meningoencephalitis 086.9 [323.2]
　African 086.5
　　due to Trypanosoma 086.5
　　　gambiense 086.3
　　　rhodesiense 086.4
　American 086.2
　　with
　　　heart involvement 086.0
　　　other organ involvement 086.1
　　without mention of organ involvement 086.2
　Brazilian - see Trypanosomiasis, American
　Chagas' - see Trypanosomiasis, American
　due to Trypanosoma
　　cruzi - see Trypanosomiasis, American
　　gambiense 086.3
　　rhodesiense 086.4
　gambiensis, Gambian 086.3
　North American - see Trypanosomiasis, American
　rhodesiensis, Rhodesian 086.4
　South American - see Trypanosomiasis, American
T-shaped incisors 520.2
Tsutsugamushi fever 081.2
Tube, tubal, tubular - see also condition
　ligation, admission for V25.2
Tubercle - see also Tuberculosis
　brain, solitary 013.2 ●
　Darwin's 744.29
　epithelioid noncaseating 135
　Ghon, primary infection 010.0 ●
Tuberculid, tuberculide (indurating) (lichenoid) (miliary) (papulonecrotic) (primary) (skin) (subcutaneous) (see also Tuberculosis) 017.0 ●
Tuberculoma - see also Tuberculosis
　brain (any part) 013.2 ●
　meninges (cerebral) (spinal) 013.1 ●
　spinal cord 013.4 ●

SECTION I INDEX TO DISEASES AND INJURIES / Tuberculosis, tubercular, tuberculous

Tuberculosis, tubercular, tuberculous
(calcification) (calcified) (caseous)
(chromogenic acid-fast bacilli)
(congenital) (degeneration) (disease)
(fibrocaseous) (fistula) (gangrene)
(interstitial) (isolated circumscribed
lesions) (necrosis) (parenchymatous)
(ulcerative) 011.9●

> Note: Use the following fifth-digit subclassification with categories 010–018:
> 0 unspecified
> 1 bacteriological or histological examination not done
> 2 bacteriological or histological examination unknown (at present)
> 3 tubercle bacilli found (in sputum) by microscopy
> 4 tubercle bacilli not found (in sputum) by microscopy, but found by bacterial culture
> 5 tubercle bacilli not found by bacteriological examination, but tuberculosis confirmed histologically
> 6 tubercle bacilli not found by bacteriological or histological examination, but tuberculosis confirmed by other methods [inoculation of animals]
>
> For tuberculous conditions specified as late effects or sequelae, see category 137.

    abdomen 014.8●
        lymph gland 014.8●
    abscess 011.9●
        arm 017.9
        bone (see also Osteomyelitis, due to, tuberculosis) 015.9● [730.8]●
            hip 015.1● [730.85]
            knee 015.2● [730.86]
            sacrum 015.0● [730.88]
            specified site NEC 015.7● [730.88]
            spinal 015.0● [730.88]
            vertebra 015.0● [730.88]
        brain 013.3●
        breast 017.9●
        Cowper's gland 016.5●
        dura (mater) 013.8●
            brain 013.3●
            spinal cord 013.5●
        epidural 013.8●
            brain 013.3●
            spinal cord 013.5●
        frontal sinus - see Tuberculosis, sinus
        genital organs NEC 016.9●
            female 016.7●
            male 016.5●
        genitourinary NEC 016.9●
        gland (lymphatic) - see Tuberculosis, lymph gland
        hip 015.1●
        iliopsoas 015.0● [730.88]
        intestine 014.8●
        ischiorectal 014.8●
        joint 015.9●
            hip 015.1●
            knee 015.2●
            specified joint NEC 015.8●
            vertebral 015.0● [730.88]
        kidney 016.0● [590.81]
        knee 015.2●
        lumbar 015.0● [730.88]
        lung 011.2●
            primary, progressive 010.8●
        meninges (cerebral) (spinal) 013.0●
        pelvic 016.9●
            female 016.7●
            male 016.5●

Tuberculosis, tubercular, tuberculous (Continued)
    abscess (Continued)
        perianal 014.8●
            fistula 014.8●
        perinephritic 016.0● [590.81]
        perineum 017.9●
        perirectal 014.8●
        psoas 015.0● [730.88]
        rectum 014.8●
        retropharyngeal 012.8●
        sacrum 015.0● [730.88]
        scrofulous 017.2●
        scrotum 016.5●
        skin 017.0●
            primary 017.0●
        spinal cord 013.5●
        spine or vertebra (column) 015.0● [730.88]
        strumous 017.2●
        subdiaphragmatic 014.8●
        testis 016.5●
        thigh 017.9●
        urinary 016.3●
            kidney 016.0● [590.81]
        uterus 016.7●
    accessory sinus - see Tuberculosis, sinus
    Addison's disease 017.6●
    adenitis (see also Tuberculosis, lymph gland) 017.2●
    adenoids 012.8●
    adenopathy (see also Tuberculosis, lymph gland) 017.2●
        tracheobronchial 012.1●
            primary progressive 010.8●
    adherent pericardium 017.9● [420.0]
    adnexa (uteri) 016.7●
    adrenal (capsule) (gland) 017.6●
    air passage NEC 012.8●
    alimentary canal 014.8●
    anemia 017.9●
    ankle (joint) 015.8●
        bone 015.5● [730.87]
    anus 014.8●
    apex (see also Tuberculosis, pulmonary) 011.9●
    apical (see also Tuberculosis, pulmonary) 011.9●
    appendicitis 014.8●
    appendix 014.8●
    arachnoid 013.0●
    artery 017.9●
    arthritis (chronic) (synovial) 015.9● [711.40]
        ankle 015.8● [730.87]
        hip 015.1● [711.45]
        knee 015.2● [711.46]
        specified site NEC 015.8● [711.48]
        spine or vertebra (column) 015.0● [720.81]
        wrist 015.8● [730.83]
    articular - see Tuberculosis, joint
    ascites 014.0●
    asthma (see also Tuberculosis, pulmonary) 011.9●
    axilla, axillary 017.2●
        gland 017.2●
    bilateral (see also Tuberculosis, pulmonary) 011.9●
    bladder 016.1●
    bone (see also Osteomyelitis, due to, tuberculosis) 015.9● [730.8]
        hip 015.1● [730.85]
        knee 015.2● [730.86]
        limb NEC 015.5● [730.88]
        sacrum 015.0● [730.88]
        specified site NEC 015.7● [730.88]
        spinal or vertebral column 015.0● [730.88]
    bowel 014.8●
        miliary 018.9●
    brain 013.2●
    breast 017.9●

Tuberculosis, tubercular, tuberculous (Continued)
    broad ligament 016.7●
    bronchi, bronchial, bronchus 011.3●
        ectasia, ectasis 011.5●
        fistula 011.3●
            primary, progressive 010.8●
        gland 012.1●
            primary, progressive 010.8●
        isolated 012.2●
        lymph gland or node 012.1●
            primary, progressive 010.8●
    bronchiectasis 011.5●
    bronchitis 011.3●
    bronchopleural 012.0●
    bronchopneumonia, bronchopneumonic 011.6●
    bronchorrhagia 011.3●
    bronchotracheal 011.3●
        isolated 012.2●
    bronchus - see Tuberculosis, bronchi
    bronze disease (Addison's) 017.6●
    buccal cavity 017.9●
    bulbourethral gland 016.5●
    bursa (see also Tuberculosis, joint) 015.9●
    cachexia NEC (see also Tuberculosis, pulmonary) 011.9●
    cardiomyopathy 017.9● [425.8]
    caries (see also Tuberculosis, bone) 015.9● [730.8]●
    cartilage (see also Tuberculosis, bone) 015.9● [730.8]●
        intervertebral 015.0● [730.88]
    catarrhal (see also Tuberculosis, pulmonary) 011.9●
    cecum 014.8●
    cellular tissue (primary) 017.0●
    cellulitis (primary) 017.0●
    central nervous system 013.9●
        specified site NEC 013.8●
    cerebellum (current) 013.2●
    cerebral (current) 013.2●
        meninges 013.0●
    cerebrospinal 013.6●
        meninges 013.0●
    cerebrum (current) 013.2●
    cervical 017.2●
        gland 017.2●
        lymph nodes 017.2●
    cervicitis (uteri) 016.7●
    cervix 016.7●
    chest (see also Tuberculosis, pulmonary) 011.9●
    childhood type or first infection 010.0●
    choroid 017.3● [363.13]
    choroiditis 017.3● [363.13]
    ciliary body 017.3● [364.11]
    colitis 014.8●
    colliers' 011.4●
    colliquativa (primary) 017.0●
    colon 014.8●
        ulceration 014.8●
    complex, primary 010.0●
    complicating pregnancy, childbirth, or puerperium 647.3●
        affecting fetus or newborn 760.2
    congenital 771.2
    conjunctiva 017.3● [370.31]
    connective tissue 017.9●
        bone - see Tuberculosis, bone
    contact V01.1
    converter (tuberculin skin test) (without disease) 795.51
    cornea (ulcer) 017.3● [370.31]
    Cowper's gland 016.5●
    coxae 015.1● [730.85]
    coxalgia 015.1● [730.85]
    cul-de-sac of Douglas 014.8●
    curvature, spine 015.0● [737.40]
    cutis (colliquativa) (primary) 017.0●
    cyst, ovary 016.6●

Tuberculosis, tubercular, tuberculous
(Continued)
cystitis 016.1
dacryocystitis 017.3 [375.32]
dactylitis 015.5
diarrhea 014.8
diffuse (see also Tuberculosis, miliary) 018.9
    lung - see Tuberculosis, pulmonary
    meninges 013.0
digestive tract 014.8
disseminated (see also Tuberculosis, miliary) 018.9
    meninges 013.0
duodenum 014.8
dura (mater) 013.9
    abscess 013.8
        cerebral 013.3
        spinal 013.5
dysentery 014.8
ear (inner) (middle) 017.4
    bone 015.6
    external (primary) 017.0
    skin (primary) 017.0
elbow 015.8
emphysema - see Tuberculosis, pulmonary
empyema 012.0
encephalitis 013.6
endarteritis 017.9
endocarditis (any valve) 017.9 [424.91]
endocardium (any valve) 017.9 [424.91]
endocrine glands NEC 017.9
endometrium 016.7
enteric, enterica 014.8
enteritis 014.8
enterocolitis 014.8
epididymis 016.4
epididymitis 016.4
epidural abscess 013.8
    brain 013.3
    spinal cord 013.5
epiglottis 012.3
episcleritis 017.3 [379.00]
erythema (induratum) (nodosum) (primary) 017.1
esophagus 017.8
Eustachian tube 017.4
exposure to V01.1
exudative 012.0
    primary, progressive 010.1
eye 017.3
eyelid (primary) 017.0
    lupus 017.0 [373.4]
fallopian tube 016.6
fascia 017.9
fauces 012.8
finger 017.9
first infection 010.0
fistula, perirectal 014.8
Florida 011.6
foot 017.9
funnel pelvis 137.3
gallbladder 017.9
galloping (see also Tuberculosis, pulmonary) 011.9
ganglionic 015.9
gastritis 017.9
gastrocolic fistula 014.8
gastroenteritis 014.8
gastrointestinal tract 014.8
general, generalized 018.9
    acute 018.0
    chronic 018.8
genital organs NEC 016.9
    female 016.7
    male 016.5
genitourinary NEC 016.9
genu 015.2
glandulae suprarenalis 017.6
glandular, general 017.2
glottis 012.3
grinders' 011.4

Tuberculosis, tubercular, tuberculous
(Continued)
groin 017.2
gum 017.9
hand 017.9
heart 017.9 [425.8]
hematogenous - see Tuberculosis, miliary
hemoptysis (see also Tuberculosis, pulmonary) 011.9
hemorrhage NEC (see also Tuberculosis, pulmonary) 011.9
hemothorax 012.0
hepatitis 017.9
hilar lymph nodes 012.1
    primary, progressive 010.8
hip (disease) (joint) 015.1
    bone 015.1 [730.85]
hydrocephalus 013.8
hydropneumothorax 012.0
hydrothorax 012.0
hypoadrenalism 017.6
hypopharynx 012.8
ileocecal (hyperplastic) 014.8
ileocolitis 014.8
ileum 014.8
iliac spine (superior) 015.0 [730.88]
incipient NEC (see also Tuberculosis, pulmonary) 011.9
indurativa (primary) 017.1
infantile 010.0
infection NEC 011.9
    without clinical manifestation 010.0
infraclavicular gland 017.2
inguinal gland 017.2
inguinalis 017.2
intestine (any part) 014.8
iris 017.3 [364.11]
iritis 017.3 [364.11]
ischiorectal 014.8
jaw 015.7 [730.88]
jejunum 014.8
joint 015.9
    hip 015.1
    knee 015.2
    specified site NEC 015.8
    vertebral 015.0 [730.88]
keratitis 017.3 [370.31]
    interstitial 017.3 [370.59]
keratoconjunctivitis 017.3 [370.31]
kidney 016.0
knee (joint) 015.2
kyphoscoliosis 015.0 [737.43]
kyphosis 015.0 [737.41]
lacrimal apparatus, gland 017.3
laryngitis 012.3
larynx 012.3
latent 795.51
leptomeninges, leptomeningitis (cerebral) (spinal) 013.0
lichenoides (primary) 017.0
linguae 017.9
lip 017.9
liver 017.9
lordosis 015.0 [737.42]
lung - see Tuberculosis, pulmonary
luposa 017.0
    eyelid 017.0 [373.4]
lymphadenitis - see Tuberculosis, lymph gland
lymphangitis - see Tuberculosis, lymph gland
lymphatic (gland) (vessel) - see Tuberculosis, lymph gland
lymph gland or node (peripheral) 017.2
    abdomen 014.8
    bronchial 012.1
        primary, progressive 010.8
    cervical 017.2
    hilar 012.1
        primary, progressive 010.8
    intrathoracic 012.1
        primary, progressive 010.8

Tuberculosis, tubercular, tuberculous
(Continued)
lymph gland or node *(Continued)*
    mediastinal 012.1
        primary, progressive 010.8
    mesenteric 014.8
    peripheral 017.2
    retroperitoneal 014.8
    tracheobronchial 012.1
        primary, progressive 010.8
malignant NEC (see also Tuberculosis, pulmonary) 011.9
mammary gland 017.9
marasmus NEC (see also Tuberculosis, pulmonary) 011.9
mastoiditis 015.6
maternal, affecting fetus or newborn 760.2
mediastinal (lymph) gland or node 012.1
    primary, progressive 010.8
mediastinitis 012.8
    primary, progressive 010.8
mediastinopericarditis 017.9 [420.0]
mediastinum 012.8
    primary, progressive 010.8
medulla 013.9
    brain 013.2
    spinal cord 013.4
melanosis, Addisonian 017.6
membrane, brain 013.0
meninges (cerebral) (spinal) 013.0
meningitis (basilar) (brain) (cerebral) (cerebrospinal) (spinal) 013.0
meningoencephalitis 013.0
mesentery, mesenteric 014.8
    lymph gland or node 014.8
miliary (any site) 018.9
    acute 018.0
    chronic 018.8
    specified type NEC 018.8
millstone makers' 011.4
miners' 011.4
moulders' 011.4
mouth 017.9
multiple 018.9
    acute 018.0
    chronic 018.8
muscle 017.9
myelitis 013.6
myocarditis 017.9 [422.0]
myocardium 017.9 [422.0]
nasal (passage) (sinus) 012.8
nasopharynx 012.8
neck gland 017.2
nephritis 016.0 [583.81]
nerve 017.9
nose (septum) 012.8
ocular 017.3
old NEC 137.0
    without residuals V12.01
omentum 014.8
oophoritis (acute) (chronic) 016.6
optic 017.3 [377.39]
    nerve trunk 017.3 [377.39]
    papilla, papillae 017.3 [377.39]
orbit 017.3
orchitis 016.5 [608.81]
organ, specified NEC 017.9
orificialis (primary) 017.0
osseous (see also Tuberculosis, bone) 015.9 [730.8]
osteitis (see also Tuberculosis, bone) 015.9 [730.8]
osteomyelitis (see also Tuberculosis, bone) 015.9 [730.8]
otitis (media) 017.4
ovaritis (acute) (chronic) 016.6
ovary (acute) (chronic) 016.6
oviducts (acute) (chronic) 016.6
pachymeningitis 013.0
palate (soft) 017.9
pancreas 017.9

SECTION I INDEX TO DISEASES AND INJURIES / Tuberculosis, tubercular, tuberculous

Tuberculosis, tubercular, tuberculous (Continued)
- papulonecrotic (primary) 017.0 ●
- parathyroid glands 017.9 ●
- paronychia (primary) 017.0 ●
- parotid gland or region 017.9 ●
- pelvic organ NEC 016.9 ●
  - female 016.7 ●
  - male 016.5 ●
- pelvis (bony) 015.7 ● [730.85]
- penis 016.5 ●
- peribronchitis 011.3 ●
- pericarditis 017.9 ● [420.0]
- pericardium 017.9 ● [420.0]
- perichondritis, larynx 012.3 ●
- perineum 017.9 ●
- periostitis (see also Tuberculosis, bone) 015.9 ● [730.8]
- periphlebitis 017.9 ●
  - eye vessel 017.3 ● [362.18]
  - retina 017.3 ● [362.18]
- perirectal fistula 014.8 ●
- peritoneal gland 014.8 ●
- peritoneum 014.0 ●
- peritonitis 014.0 ●
- pernicious NEC (see also Tuberculosis, pulmonary) 011.9 ●
- pharyngitis 012.8 ●
- pharynx 012.8 ●
- phlyctenulosis (conjunctiva) 017.3 ● [370.31]
- phthisis NEC (see also Tuberculosis, pulmonary) 011.9 ●
- pituitary gland 017.9 ●
- placenta 016.7 ●
- pleura, pleural, pleurisy, pleuritis (fibrinous) (obliterative) (purulent) (simple plastic) (with effusion) 012.0 ●
  - primary, progressive 010.1 ●
- pneumonia, pneumonic 011.6 ●
- pneumothorax 011.7 ●
- polyserositis 018.9 ●
  - acute 018.0 ●
  - chronic 018.8 ●
- potters' 011.4 ●
- prepuce 016.5 ●
- primary 010.9 ●
  - complex 010.0 ●
  - complicated 010.8 ●
    - with pleurisy or effusion 010.1 ●
  - progressive 010.8 ●
    - with pleurisy or effusion 010.1 ●
  - skin 017.0 ●
- proctitis 014.8 ●
- prostate 016.5 ● [601.4]
- prostatitis 016.5 ● [601.4]
- pulmonaris (see also Tuberculosis, pulmonary) 011.9 ●
- pulmonary (artery) (incipient) (malignant) (multiple round foci) (pernicious) (reinfection stage) 011.9 ●
  - cavitated or with cavitation 011.2 ●
    - primary, progressive 010.8 ●
  - childhood type or first infection 010.0 ●
  - chromogenic acid-fast bacilli 795.39
  - fibrosis or fibrotic 011.4 ●
  - infiltrative 011.0 ●
    - primary, progressive 010.9 ●
  - nodular 011.1 ●
  - specified NEC 011.8 ●
  - sputum positive only 795.39
  - status following surgical collapse of lung NEC 011.9 ●
- pyelitis 016.0 ● [590.81]
- pyelonephritis 016.0 ● [590.81]
- pyemia - see Tuberculosis, miliary
- pyonephrosis 016.0 ●
- pyopneumothorax 012.0 ●
- pyothorax 012.0 ●
- rectum (with abscess) 014.8 ●
  - fistula 014.8 ●

Tuberculosis, tubercular, tuberculous (Continued)
- reinfection stage (see also Tuberculosis, pulmonary) 011.9 ●
- renal 016.0 ●
- renis 016.0 ●
- reproductive organ 016.7 ●
- respiratory NEC (see also Tuberculosis, pulmonary) 011.9 ●
  - specified site NEC 012.8 ●
- retina 017.3 ● [363.13]
- retroperitoneal (lymph gland or node) 014.8 ●
  - gland 014.8 ●
- retropharyngeal abscess 012.8 ●
- rheumatism 015.9 ●
- rhinitis 012.8 ●
- sacroiliac (joint) 015.8 ●
- sacrum 015.0 ● [730.88]
- salivary gland 017.9 ●
- salpingitis (acute) (chronic) 016.6 ●
- sandblasters' 011.4 ●
- sclera 017.3 ● [379.09]
- scoliosis 015.0 ● [737.43]
- scrofulous 017.2 ●
- scrotum 016.5 ●
- seminal tract or vesicle 016.5 ● [608.81]
- senile NEC (see also Tuberculosis, pulmonary) 011.9 ●
- septic NEC (see also Tuberculosis, miliary) 018.9 ●
- shoulder 015.8 ●
  - blade 015.7 ● [730.8]
- sigmoid 014.8 ●
- sinus (accessory) (nasal) 012.8 ●
  - bone 015.7 ● [730.88]
  - epididymis 016.4 ●
- skeletal NEC (see also Osteomyelitis, due to tuberculosis) 015.9 ● [730.8]
- skin (any site) (primary) 017.0 ●
- small intestine 014.8 ●
- soft palate 017.9 ●
- spermatic cord 016.5 ●
- spinal
  - column 015.0 ● [730.88]
  - cord 013.4 ●
  - disease 015.0 ● [730.88]
  - medulla 013.4 ●
  - membrane 013.0 ●
  - meninges 013.0 ●
- spine 015.0 ● [730.88]
- spleen 017.7 ●
- splenitis 017.7 ●
- spondylitis 015.0 ● [720.81]
- spontaneous pneumothorax - see Tuberculosis, pulmonary
- sternoclavicular joint 015.8 ●
- stomach 017.9 ●
- stonemasons' 011.4 ●
- struma 017.2 ●
- subcutaneous tissue (cellular) (primary) 017.0 ●
- subcutis (primary) 017.0 ●
- subdeltoid bursa 017.9 ●
- submaxillary 017.9 ●
  - region 017.9 ●
- supraclavicular gland 017.2 ●
- suprarenal (capsule) (gland) 017.6 ●
- swelling, joint (see also Tuberculosis, joint) 015.9 ●
- symphysis pubis 015.7 ● [730.88]
- synovitis 015.9 ● [727.01]
  - hip 015.1 ● [727.01]
  - knee 015.2 ● [727.01]
  - specified site NEC 015.8 ● [727.01]
  - spine or vertebra 015.0 ● [727.01]
- systemic - see Tuberculosis, miliary
- tarsitis (eyelid) 017.0 ● [373.4]
  - ankle (bone) 015.5 ● [730.87]
- tendon (sheath) - see Tuberculosis, tenosynovitis

Tuberculosis, tubercular, tuberculous (Continued)
- tenosynovitis 015.9 ● [727.01]
  - hip 015.1 ● [727.01]
  - knee 015.2 ● [727.01]
  - specified site NEC 015.8 ● [727.01]
  - spine or vertebra 015.0 ● [727.01]
- testis 016.5 ● [608.81]
- throat 012.8 ●
- thymus gland 017.9 ●
- thyroid gland 017.5 ●
- toe 017.9 ●
- tongue 017.9 ●
- tonsil (lingual) 012.8 ●
- tonsillitis 012.8 ●
- trachea, tracheal 012.8 ●
  - gland 012.1 ●
    - primary, progressive 010.8 ●
  - isolated 012.2 ●
- tracheobronchial 011.3 ●
  - glandular 012.1 ●
    - primary, progressive 010.8 ●
  - isolated 012.2 ●
  - lymph gland or node 012.1 ●
    - primary, progressive 010.8 ●
- tubal 016.6 ●
- tunica vaginalis 016.5 ●
- typhlitis 014.8 ●
- ulcer (primary) (skin) 017.0 ●
  - bowel or intestine 014.8 ●
  - specified site NEC - see Tuberculosis, by site
  - unspecified site - see Tuberculosis, pulmonary
- ureter 016.2 ●
- urethra, urethral 016.3 ●
- urinary organ or tract 016.3 ●
  - kidney 016.0 ●
- uterus 016.7 ●
- uveal tract 017.3 ● [363.13]
- uvula 017.9 ●
- vaccination, prophylactic (against) V03.2
- vagina 016.7 ●
- vas deferens 016.5 ●
- vein 017.9 ●
- verruca (primary) 017.0 ●
- verrucosa (cutis) (primary) 017.0 ●
- vertebra (column) 015.0 ● [730.88]
- vesiculitis 016.5 ● [608.81]
- viscera NEC 014.8 ●
- vulva 016.7 ● [616.51]
- wrist (joint) 015.8 ●
  - bone 015.5 ● [730.83]

Tuberculum
- auriculae 744.29
- occlusal 520.2
- paramolare 520.2

Tuberosity
- jaw, excessive 524.07
- maxillary, entire 524.07

Tuberous sclerosis (brain) 759.5

Tubo-ovarian - see condition

Tuboplasty, after previous sterilization V26.0

Tubotympanitis 381.10

Tularemia 021.9
- with
  - conjunctivitis 021.3
  - pneumonia 021.2
- bronchopneumonic 021.2
- conjunctivitis 021.3
- cryptogenic 021.1
- disseminated 021.8
- enteric 021.1
- generalized 021.8
- glandular 021.8
- intestinal 021.1
- oculoglandular 021.3
- ophthalmic 021.3
- pneumonia 021.2
- pulmonary 021.2
- specified NEC 021.8

SECTION 1 INDEX TO DISEASES AND INJURIES / Tumor

Tularemia *(Continued)*
 typhoidal 021.1
 ulceroglandular 021.0
 vaccination, prophylactic (against) V03.4
Tularensis conjunctivitis 021.3
Tumefaction - *see also* Swelling
 liver *(see also* Hypertrophy, liver) 789.1
Tumor (M8000/1) - *see also* Neoplasm, by site, unspecified nature
 Abrikossov's (M9580/0) - *see also* Neoplasm, connective tissue, benign
  malignant (M9580/3) - *see* Neoplasm, connective tissue, malignant
 acinar cell (M8550/1) - *see* Neoplasm, by site, uncertain behavior
 acinic cell (M8550/1) - *see* Neoplasm, by site, uncertain behavior
 adenomatoid (M9054/0) - *see also* Neoplasm, by site, benign
  odontogenic (M9300/0) 213.1
   upper jaw (bone) 213.0
 adnexal (skin) (M8390/0) - *see* Neoplasm, skin, benign
 adrenal
  cortical (benign) (M8370/0) 227.0
   malignant (M8370/3) 194.0
  rest (M8671/0) - *see* Neoplasm, by site, benign
 alpha cell (M8152/0)
  malignant (M8152/3)
   pancreas 157.4
   specified site NEC - *see* Neoplasm, by site, malignant
   unspecified site 157.4
  pancreas 211.7
  specified site NEC - *see* Neoplasm, by site, benign
  unspecified site 211.7
 aneurysmal *(see also* Aneurysm) 442.9
 aortic body (M8691/1) 237.3
  malignant (M8691/3) 194.6
 argentaffin (M8241/1) - *see* Neoplasm, by site, uncertain behavior
 basal cell (M8090/1) - *see also* Neoplasm, skin, uncertain behavior
 benign (M8000/0) - *see* Neoplasm, by site, benign
 beta cell (M8151/0)
  malignant (M8151/3)
   pancreas 157.4
   specified site - *see* Neoplasm, by site, malignant
   unspecified site 157.4
  pancreas 211.7
  specified site NEC - *see* Neoplasm, by site, benign
  unspecified site 211.7
 blood - *see* Hematoma
 brenner (M9000/0) 220
  borderline malignancy (M9000/1) 236.2
  malignant (M9000/3) 183.0
  proliferating (M9000/1) 236.2
 Brooke's (M8100/0) - *see* Neoplasm, skin, benign
 brown fat (M8880/0) - *see* Lipoma, by site
 Burkitt's (M9750/3) 200.2●
 calcifying epithelial odontogenic (M9340/0) 213.1
  upper jaw (bone) 213.0
 carcinoid (M8240/1) 209.60
  benign 209.60
   appendix 209.51
   ascending colon 209.53
   bronchus 209.61
   cecum 209.52
   colon 209.50
   descending colon 209.55
   duodenum 209.41
   foregut 209.65
   hindgut 209.67
   ileum 209.43

Tumor *(Continued)*
 carcinoid *(Continued)*
  benign *(Continued)*
   jejunum 209.42
   kidney 209.64
   large intestine 209.50
   lung 209.61
   midgut 209.66
   rectum 209.57
   sigmoid colon 209.56
   small intestine 209.40
   specified NEC 209.69
   stomach 209.63
   thymus 209.62
   transverse colon 209.54
  malignant (of) 209.20
   appendix 209.11
   ascending colon 209.13
   bronchus 209.21
   cecum 209.12
   colon 209.10
   descending colon 209.15
   duodenum 209.01
   foregut 209.25
   hindgut 209.27
   ileum 209.03
   jejunum 209.02
   kidney 209.24
   large intestine 209.10
   lung 209.21
   midgut 209.26
   rectum 209.17
   sigmoid colon 209.16
   small intestine 209.00
   specified NEC 209.29
   stomach 209.23
   thymus 209.22
   transverse colon 209.14
  secondary - *see* Tumor, neuroendocrine, secondary
 carotid body (M8692/1) 237.3
  malignant (M8692/3) 194.5
 Castleman's (mediastinal lymph node hyperplasia) 785.6
 cells (M8001/1) - *see also* Neoplasm, by site, unspecified nature
  benign (M8001/0) - *see* Neoplasm, by site, benign
  malignant (M8001/3) - *see* Neoplasm, by site, malignant
  uncertain whether benign or malignant (M8001/1) - *see* Neoplasm, by site, uncertain nature
 cervix
  in pregnancy or childbirth 654.6●
   affecting fetus or newborn 763.89
   causing obstructed labor 660.2●
    affecting fetus or newborn 763.1
 chondromatous giant cell (M9230/0) - *see* Neoplasm, bone, benign
 chromaffin (M8700/0) - *see also* Neoplasm, by site, benign
  malignant (M8700/3) - *see* Neoplasm, by site, malignant
 Cock's peculiar 706.2
 Codman's (benign chondroblastoma) (M9230/0) - *see* Neoplasm, bone, benign
 dentigerous, mixed (M9282/0) 213.1
  upper jaw (bone) 213.0
 dermoid (M9084/0) - *see* Neoplasm, by site, benign
  with malignant transformation (M9084/3) 183.0
 desmoid (extra-abdominal) (M8821/1) - *see also* Neoplasm, connective tissue, uncertain behavior
  abdominal (M8822/1) - *see* Neoplasm, connective tissue, uncertain behavior

Tumor *(Continued)*
 embryonal (mixed) (M9080/1) - *see also* Neoplasm, by site, uncertain behavior
  liver (M9080/3) 155.0
 endodermal sinus (M9071/3)
  specified site - *see* Neoplasm, by site, malignant
  unspecified site
   female 183.0
   male 186.9
 epithelial
  benign (M8010/0) - *see* Neoplasm, by site, benign
  malignant (M8010/3) - *see* Neoplasm, by site, malignant
 Ewing's (M9260/3) - *see* Neoplasm, bone, malignant
 fatty - *see* Lipoma
 fetal, causing disproportion 653.7●
  causing obstructed labor 660.1●
 fibroid (M8890/0) - *see* Leiomyoma
 G cell (M8153/1)
  malignant (M8153/3)
   pancreas 157.4
   specified site NEC - *see* Neoplasm, by site, malignant
   unspecified site 157.4
  specified site - *see* Neoplasm, by site, uncertain behavior
  unspecified site 235.5
 giant cell (type) (M8003/1) - *see also* Neoplasm, by site, unspecified nature
  bone (M9250/1) 238.0
   malignant (M9250/3) - *see* Neoplasm, bone, malignant
  chondromatous (M9230/0) - *see* Neoplasm, bone, benign
  malignant (M8003/3) - *see* Neoplasm, by site, malignant
  peripheral (gingiva) 523.8
  soft parts (M9251/1) - *see also* Neoplasm, connective tissue, uncertain behavior
   malignant (M9251/3) - *see* Neoplasm, connective tissue, malignant
  tendon sheath 727.02
 glomus (M8711/0) - *see also* Hemangioma, by site
  jugulare (M8690/1) 237.3
   malignant (M8690/3) 194.6
 gonadal stromal (M8590/1) - *see* Neoplasm, by site, uncertain behavior
 granular cell (M9580/0) - *see also* Neoplasm, connective tissue, benign
  malignant (M9580/3) - *see* Neoplasm, connective tissue, malignant
 granulosa cell (M8620/1) 236.2
  malignant (M8620/3) 183.0
 granulosa cell-theca cell (M8621/1) 236.2
  malignant (M8621/3) 183.0
 Grawitz's (hypernephroma) (M8312/3) 189.0
 hazard-crile (M8350/3) 193
 hemorrhoidal - *see* Hemorrhoids
 hilar cell (M8660/0) 220
 Hürthle cell (benign) (M8290/0) 226
  malignant (M8290/3) 193
 hydatid *(see also* Echinococcus) 122.9
 hypernephroid (M8311/1) - *see also* Neoplasm, by site, uncertain behavior
 interstitial cell (M8650/1) - *see also* Neoplasm, by site, uncertain behavior
  benign (M8650/0) - *see* Neoplasm, by site, benign
  malignant (M8650/3) - *see* Neoplasm, by site, malignant
 islet cell (M8150/0)
  malignant (M8150/3)
   pancreas 157.4
   specified site - *see* Neoplasm, by site, malignant
   unspecified site 157.4

Tumor (Continued)
  islet cell (Continued)
    pancreas 211.7
    specified site NEC - see Neoplasm, by site, benign
    unspecified site 211.7
  juxtaglomerular (M8361/1) 236.91
  Krukenberg's (M8490/6) 198.6
  Leydig cell (M8650/1)
    benign (M8650/0)
      specified site - see Neoplasm, by site, benign
      unspecified site
        female 220
        male 222.0
    malignant (M8650/3)
      specified site - see Neoplasm, by site, malignant
      unspecified site
        female 183.0
        male 186.9
    specified site - see Neoplasm, by site, uncertain behavior
    unspecified site
      female 236.2
      male 236.4
  lipid cell, ovary (M8670/0) 220
  lipoid cell, ovary (M8670/0) 220
  lymphomatous, benign (M9590/0) - see also Neoplasm, by site, benign
  lysis syndrome (following antineoplastic drug therapy) (spontaneous) 277.88
  Malherbe's (M8110/0) - see Neoplasm, skin, benign
  malignant (M8000/3) - see also Neoplasm, by site, malignant
    fusiform cell (type) (M8004/3) - see Neoplasm, by site, malignant
    giant cell (type) (M8003/3) - see Neoplasm, by site, malignant
    mixed NEC (M8940/3) - see Neoplasm, by site, malignant
    small cell (type) (M8002/3) - see Neoplasm, by site, malignant
    spindle cell (type) (M8004/3) - see Neoplasm, by site, malignant
  mast cell (M9740/1) 238.5
    malignant (M9740/3) 202.6 ●
  melanotic, neuroectodermal (M9363/0) - see Neoplasm, by site, benign
  Merkel cell - see Carcinoma, Merkel cell
  mesenchymal
    malignant (M8800/3) - see Neoplasm, connective tissue, malignant
    mixed (M8990/1) - see Neoplasm, connective tissue, uncertain behavior
  mesodermal, mixed (M8951/3) - see also Neoplasm, by site, malignant
    liver 155.0
  mesonephric (M9110/1) - see also Neoplasm, by site, uncertain behavior
    malignant (M9110/3) - see Neoplasm, by site, malignant
  metastatic
    from specified site (M8000/3) - see Neoplasm, by site, malignant
    to specified site (M8000/6) - see Neoplasm, by site, malignant, secondary
  mixed NEC (M8940/0) - see also Neoplasm, by site, benign
    malignant (M8940/3) - see Neoplasm, by site, malignant
  mucocarcinoid, malignant (M8243/3) - see Neoplasm, by site, malignant
  mucoepidermoid (M8430/1) - see Neoplasm, by site, uncertain behavior
  Müllerian, mixed (M8950/3) - see Neoplasm, by site, malignant

Tumor (Continued)
  myoepithelial (M8982/0) - see Neoplasm, by site, benign
  neuroendocrine 209.60
    malignant poorly differentiated 209.30
    secondary 209.70
      bone 209.73
      distant lymph nodes 209.71
      liver 209.72
      peritoneum 209.74
      site specified NEC 209.79
  neurogenic olfactory (M9520/3) 160.0
  nonencapsulated sclerosing (M8350/3) 193
  odontogenic (M9270/1) 238.0
    adenomatoid (M9300/0) 213.1
      upper jaw (bone) 213.0
    benign (M9270/0) 213.1
      upper jaw (bone) 213.0
    calcifying epithelial (M9340/0) 213.1
      upper jaw (bone) 213.0
    malignant (M9270/3) 170.1
      upper jaw (bone) 170.0
    squamous (M9312/0) 213.1
      upper jaw (bone) 213.0
  ovarian stromal (M8590/1) 236.2
  ovary
    in pregnancy or childbirth 654.4 ●
      affecting fetus or newborn 763.89
      causing obstructed labor 660.2 ●
        affecting fetus or newborn 763.1
  pacinian (M9507/0) - see Neoplasm, skin, benign
  Pancoast's (M8010/3) 162.3
  papillary - see Papilloma
  pelvic, in pregnancy or childbirth 654.9 ●
    affecting fetus or newborn 763.89
    causing obstructed labor 660.2 ●
      affecting fetus or newborn 763.1
  phantom 300.11
  plasma cell (M9731/1) 238.6
    benign (M9731/0) - see Neoplasm, by site, benign
    malignant (M9731/3) 203.8 ●
  polyvesicular vitelline (M9071/3)
    specified site - see Neoplasm, by site, malignant
    unspecified site
      female 183.0
      male 186.9
  Pott's puffy (see also Osteomyelitis) 730.2 ●
  Rathke's pouch (M9350/1) 237.0
  regaud's (M8082/3) - see Neoplasm, nasopharynx, malignant
  rete cell (M8140/0) 222.0
  retinal anlage (M9363/0) - see Neoplasm, by site, benign
  Rokitansky's 620.2
  salivary gland type, mixed (M8940/0) - see also Neoplasm, by site, benign
    malignant (M8940/3) - see Neoplasm, by site, malignant
  Sampson's 617.1
  Schloffer's (see also Peritonitis) 567.29
  Schmincke (M8082/3) - see Neoplasm, nasopharynx, malignant
  sebaceous (see also Cyst, sebaceous) 706.2
  secondary (M8000/6) - see Neoplasm, by site, secondary
    carcinoid - see Tumor, neuroendocrine, secondary
    neuroendocrine - see Tumor, neuroendocrine, secondary
  Sertoli cell (M8640/0)
    with lipid storage (M8641/0)
      specified site, - see Neoplasm, by site, benign
      unspecified site
        female 220
        male 222.0
    specified site - see Neoplasm, by site, benign

Tumor (Continued)
  Sertoli cell (Continued)
    unspecified site
      female 220
      male 222.0
  Sertoli-Leydig cell (M8631/0)
    specified site - see Neoplasm, by site, benign
    unspecified site
      female 220
      male 222.0
  sex cord (-stromal) (M8590/1) - see Neoplasm, by site, uncertain behavior
  skin appendage (M8390/0) - see Neoplasm, skin, benign
  soft tissue
    benign (M8800/0) - see Neoplasm, connective tissue, benign
    malignant (M8800/3) - see Neoplasm, connective tissue, malignant
  sternomastoid 754.1
  stromal
    abdomen
      benign 215.5
      malignant NEC 171.5
      uncertain behavior 238.1
    digestive system 238.1
      benign 215.5
      malignant NEC 171.5
      uncertain behavior 238.1
    endometrium (endometrial) 236.0
    gastric 238.1
      benign 215.5
      malignant 151.9
      uncertain behavior 238.1
    gastrointestinal 238.1
      benign 215.5
      malignant NEC 171.5
      uncertain behavior 238.1
    intestine (small) 238.1
      benign 215.5
      malignant 152.9
      uncertain behavior 238.1
    stomach 238.1
      benign 215.5
      malignant 151.9
      uncertain behavior 238.1
  superior sulcus (lung) (pulmonary) (syndrome) (M8010/3) 162.3
  suprasulcus (M8010/3) 162.3
  sweat gland (M8400/1) - see also Neoplasm, skin, uncertain behavior
    benign (M8400/0) - see Neoplasm, skin, benign
    malignant (M8400/3) - see Neoplasm, skin, malignant
  syphilitic brain 094.89
    congenital 090.49
  testicular stromal (M8590/1) 236.4
  theca cell (M8600/0) 220
  theca cell-granulosa cell (M8621/1) 236.2
  theca-lutein (M8610/0) 220
  turban (M8200/0) 216.4
  uterus
    in pregnancy or childbirth 654.1 ●
      affecting fetus or newborn 763.89
      causing obstructed labor 660.2 ●
        affecting fetus or newborn 763.1
  vagina
    in pregnancy or childbirth 654.7 ●
      affecting fetus or newborn 763.89
      causing obstructed labor 660.2 ●
        affecting fetus or newborn 763.1
  varicose (see also Varicose, vein) 454.9
  von Recklinghausen's (M9540/1) 237.71
  vulva
    in pregnancy or childbirth 654.8 ●
      affecting fetus or newborn 763.89
      causing obstructed labor 660.2 ●
        affecting fetus or newborn 763.1
  Warthin's (salivary gland) (M8561/0) 210.2

Tumor (Continued)
  white - *see also* Tuberculosis, arthritis
  White-Darier 757.39
  Wilms' (nephroblastoma) (M8960/3) 189.0
  yolk sac (M9071/3)
    specified site - *see* Neoplasm, by site, malignant
    unspecified site
      female 183.0
      male 186.9
Tumorlet (M8040/1) - *see* Neoplasm, by site, uncertain behavior
Tungiasis 134.1
Tunica vasculosa lentis 743.39
Tunnel vision 368.45
Turban tumor (M8200/0) 216.4
Türck's trachoma (chronic catarrhal laryngitis) 476.0
Türk's syndrome (ocular retraction syndrome) 378.71
Turner's
  hypoplasia (tooth) 520.4
  syndrome 758.6
  tooth 520.4
Turner-Kieser syndrome (hereditary osteo-onychodysplasia) 756.89
Turner-Varny syndrome 758.6
Turricephaly 756.0
Tussis convulsiva (*see also* Whooping cough) 033.9
Twiddler's syndrome (due to)
  automatic implantable defibrillator 996.04
  pacemaker 996.01
Twin
  affected by maternal complications of pregnancy 761.5
  conjoined 759.4
    fetal 678.1●
  healthy liveborn - *see* Newborn, twin
  pregnancy (complicating delivery) NEC 651.0●
    with fetal loss and retention of one fetus 651.3●
    conjoined 678.1●
    following (elective) fetal reduction 651.7●
Twinning, teeth 520.2
Twist, twisted
  bowel, colon, or intestine 560.2
  hair (congenital) 757.4
  mesentery 560.2
  omentum 560.2

Twist, twisted (Continued)
  organ or site, congenital NEC - *see* Anomaly, specified type NEC
  ovarian pedicle 620.5
    congenital 752.0
  umbilical cord - *see* Compression, umbilical cord
Twitch 781.0
Tylosis 700
  buccalis 528.6
  gingiva 523.8
  linguae 528.6
  palmaris et plantaris 757.39
Tympanism 787.3
Tympanites (abdominal) (intestine) 787.3
Tympanitis - *see* Myringitis
Tympanosclerosis 385.00
  involving
    combined sites NEC 385.09
      with tympanic membrane 385.03
    tympanic membrane 385.01
      with ossicles 385.02
        and middle ear 385.03
Tympanum - *see* condition
Tympany
  abdomen 787.3
  chest 786.7
Typhlitis (*see also* Appendicitis) 541
Typhoenteritis 002.0
Typhogastric fever 002.0
Typhoid (abortive) (ambulant) (any site) (fever) (hemorrhagic) (infection) (intermittent) (malignant) (rheumatic) 002.0
  with pneumonia 002.0 [484.8]
  abdominal 002.0
  carrier (suspected) of V02.1
  cholecystitis (current) 002.0
  clinical (Widal and blood test negative) 002.0
  endocarditis 002.0 [421.1]
  inoculation reaction - *see* Complications, vaccination
  meningitis 002.0 [320.7]
  mesenteric lymph nodes 002.0
  myocarditis 002.0 [422.0]
  osteomyelitis (*see also* Osteomyelitis, due to, typhoid) 002.0 [730.8]●
  perichondritis, larynx 002.0 [478.71]
  pneumonia 002.0 [484.8]
  spine 002.0 [720.81]
  ulcer (perforating) 002.0

Typhoid (Continued)
  vaccination, prophylactic (against) V03.1
  Widal negative 002.0
Typhomalaria (fever) (*see also* Malaria) 084.6
Typhomania 002.0
Typhoperitonitis 002.0
Typhus (fever) 081.9
  abdominal, abdominalis 002.0
  African tick 082.1
  amarillic (*see also* Fever, Yellow) 060.9
  brain 081.9
  cerebral 081.9
  classical 080
  endemic (flea-borne) 081.0
  epidemic (louse-borne) 080
  exanthematic NEC 080
  exanthematicus SAI 080
    brillii SAI 081.1
    Mexicanus SAI 081.0
    pediculo vestimenti causa 080
    typhus murinus 081.0
  flea-borne 081.0
  Indian tick 082.1
  Kenya tick 082.1
  louse-borne 080
  Mexican 081.0
    flea-borne 081.0
    louse-borne 080
    tabardillo 080
  mite-borne 081.2
  murine 081.0
  North Asian tick-borne 082.2
  petechial 081.9
  Queensland tick 082.3
  rat 081.0
  recrudescent 081.1
  recurrent (*see also* Fever, relapsing) 087.9
  Saõ Paulo 082.0
  scrub (China) (India) (Malaya) (New Guinea) 081.2
  shop (of Malaya) 081.0
  Siberian tick 082.2
  tick-borne NEC 082.9
  tropical 081.2
  vaccination, prophylactic (against) V05.8
Tyrosinemia 270.2
  neonatal 775.89
Tyrosinosis (Medes) (Sakai) 270.2
Tyrosinuria 270.2
Tyrosyluria 270.2

SECTION 1 INDEX TO DISEASES AND INJURIES / Uehlinger's syndrome

U

Uehlinger's syndrome (acropachyderma) 757.39
Uhl's anomaly or disease (hypoplasia of myocardium, right ventricle) 746.84
Ulcer, ulcerated, ulcerating, ulceration, ulcerative 707.9
- with gangrene 707.9 [785.4]
- abdomen (wall) (see also Ulcer, skin) 707.8
- ala, nose 478.19
- alveolar process 526.5
- amebic (intestine) 006.9
  - skin 006.6
- anastomotic - see Ulcer, gastrojejunal
- anorectal 569.41
- antral - see Ulcer, stomach
- anus (sphincter) (solitary) 569.41
  - varicose - see Varicose, ulcer, anus
- aorta - see Aneurysm
- aphthous (oral) (recurrent) 528.2
  - genital organ(s)
    - female 616.50
    - male 608.89
  - mouth 528.2
- arm (see also Ulcer, skin) 707.8
- arteriosclerotic plaque - see Arteriosclerosis, by site
- artery NEC 447.2
  - without rupture 447.8
- atrophic NEC - see Ulcer, skin
- Barrett's (chronic peptic ulcer of esophagus) 530.85
- bile duct 576.8
- bladder (solitary) (sphincter) 596.89
  - bilharzial (see also Schistosomiasis) 120.9 [595.4]
  - submucosal (see also Cystitis) 595.1
  - tuberculous (see also Tuberculosis) 016.1●
- bleeding NEC - see Ulcer, peptic, with hemorrhage
- bone 730.9●
- bowel (see also Ulcer, intestine) 569.82
- breast 611.0
- bronchitis 491.8
- bronchus 519.19
- buccal (cavity) (traumatic) 528.9
- burn (acute) - see Ulcer, duodenum
- Buruli 031.1
- buttock (see also Ulcer, skin) 707.8
  - decubitus (see also Ulcer, pressure) 707.00
- cancerous (M8000/3) - see Neoplasm, by site, malignant
- cardia - see Ulcer, stomach
- cardio-esophageal (peptic) 530.20
  - with bleeding 530.21
- cecum (see also Ulcer, intestine) 569.82
- cervix (uteri) (trophic) 622.0
  - with mention of cervicitis 616.0
- chancroidal 099.0
- chest (wall) (see also Ulcer, skin) 707.8
- Chiclero 085.4
- chin (pyogenic) (see also Ulcer, skin) 707.8
- chronic (cause unknown) - see also Ulcer, skin
  - penis 607.89
- Cochin-China 085.1
- colitis - see Colitis, ulcerative
- colon (see also Ulcer, intestine) 569.82
- conjunctiva (acute) (postinfectional) 372.00
- cornea (infectional) 370.00
  - with perforation 370.06
  - annular 370.02
  - catarrhal 370.01
  - central 370.03
  - dendritic 054.42
  - marginal 370.01
  - mycotic 370.05
  - phlyctenular, tuberculous (see also Tuberculosis) 017.3● [370.31]
  - ring 370.02
  - rodent 370.07

Ulcer, ulcerated, ulcerating, ulceration, ulcerative (Continued)
- cornea (Continued)
  - serpent, serpiginous 370.04
  - superficial marginal 370.01
  - tuberculous (see also Tuberculosis) 017.3● [370.31]
- corpus cavernosum (chronic) 607.89
- crural - see Ulcer, lower extremity
- Curling's - see Ulcer, duodenum
- Cushing's - see Ulcer, peptic
- cystitis (interstitial) 595.1
- decubitus (unspecified site) (see also Ulcer, pressure) 707.00
  - with gangrene 707.00 [785.4]
  - ankle 707.06
  - back
    - lower 707.03
    - upper 707.02
  - buttock 707.05
  - coccyx 707.03
  - elbow 707.01
  - head 707.09
  - heel 707.07
  - hip 707.04
  - other site 707.09
  - sacrum 707.03
  - shoulder blades 707.02
- dendritic 054.42
- diabetes, diabetic (mellitus) 250.8● [707.9]
  - due to secondary diabetes 249.8● [707.9]
  - lower limb 250.8● [707.10]
    - due to secondary diabetes 249.8● [707.10]
    - ankle 250.8● [707.13]
      - due to secondary diabetes 249.8● [707.13]
    - calf 250.8● [707.12]
      - due to secondary diabetes 249.8● [707.12]
    - foot 250.8● [707.15]
      - due to secondary diabetes 249.8● [707.15]
    - heel 250.8● [707.14]
      - due to secondary diabetes 249.8● [707.14]
    - knee 250.8● [707.19]
      - due to secondary diabetes 249.8● [707.19]
    - specified site NEC 250.8● [707.19]
      - due to secondary diabetes 249.8● [707.19]
    - thigh 250.8● [707.11]
      - due to secondary diabetes 249.8● [707.11]
    - toes 250.8● [707.15]
      - due to secondary diabetes 249.8● [707.15]
  - specified site NEC 250.8● [707.8]
    - due to secondary diabetes 249.8● [707.8]
- Dieulafoy - see Lesion, Dieulafoy
- due to
  - infection NEC - see Ulcer, skin
  - radiation, radium - see Ulcer, by site
  - trophic disturbance (any region) - see Ulcer, skin
  - x-ray - see Ulcer, by site
- duodenum, duodenal (eroded) (peptic) 532.9●

> Note: Use the following fifth-digit subclassification with categories 531–534:
> 0 without mention of obstruction
> 1 with obstruction

- with
  - hemorrhage (chronic) 532.4●
    - and perforation 532.6●
  - perforation (chronic) 532.5●
    - and hemorrhage 532.6●

Ulcer, ulcerated, ulcerating, ulceration, ulcerative (Continued)
- duodenum, duodenal (Continued)
  - acute 532.3●
    - with
      - hemorrhage 532.0●
        - and perforation 532.2●
      - perforation 532.1●
        - and hemorrhage 532.2●
  - bleeding (recurrent) - see Ulcer, duodenum, with hemorrhage
  - chronic 532.7●
    - with
      - hemorrhage 532.4●
        - and perforation 532.6●
      - perforation 532.5●
        - and hemorrhage 532.6●
  - penetrating - see Ulcer, duodenum, with perforation
  - perforating - see Ulcer, duodenum, with perforation
- dysenteric NEC 009.0
- elusive 595.1
- endocarditis (any valve) (acute) (chronic) (subacute) 421.0
- enteritis - see Colitis, ulcerative
- enterocolitis 556.0
- epiglottis 478.79
- esophagus (peptic) 530.20
  - with bleeding 530.21
  - due to ingestion
    - aspirin 530.20
    - chemicals 530.20
    - medicinal agents 530.20
  - fungal 530.20
  - infectional 530.20
  - varicose (see also Varix, esophagus) 456.1
    - bleeding (see also Varix, esophagus, bleeding) 456.0
- eye NEC 360.00
  - dendritic 054.42
- eyelid (region) 373.01
- face (see also Ulcer, skin) 707.8
- fauces 478.29
- Fenwick (-Hunner) (solitary) (see also Cystitis) 595.1
- fistulous NEC - see Ulcer, skin
- foot (indolent) (see also Ulcer, lower extremity) 707.15
  - perforating 707.15
    - leprous 030.1
    - syphilitic 094.0
  - trophic 707.15
  - varicose 454.0
    - inflamed or infected 454.2
- frambesial, initial or primary 102.0
- gallbladder or duct 575.8
- gall duct 576.8
- gangrenous (see also Gangrene) 785.4
- gastric - see Ulcer, stomach
- gastrocolic - see Ulcer, gastrojejunal
- gastroduodenal - see Ulcer, peptic
- gastroesophageal - see Ulcer, stomach
- gastrohepatic - see Ulcer, stomach
- gastrointestinal - see Ulcer, gastrojejunal
- gastrojejunal (eroded) (peptic) 534.9●

> Note: Use the following fifth-digit subclassification with categories 531–534:
> 0 without mention of obstruction
> 1 with obstruction

- with
  - hemorrhage (chronic) 534.4●
    - and perforation 534.6●
  - perforation 534.5●
    - and hemorrhage 534.6●

474 ◀ New ⬅ Revised ~~deleted~~ Deleted ● Use Additional Digit(s) ▮ Omit code

SECTION I INDEX TO DISEASES AND INJURIES / Ulcer, ulcerated, ulcerating, ulceration, ulcerative

Ulcer, ulcerated, ulcerating, ulceration, ulcerative (Continued)
gastrojejunal (Continued)
  acute 534.3●
    with
      hemorrhage 534.0●
        and perforation 534.2●
      perforation 534.1●
        and hemorrhage 534.2●
    bleeding (recurrent) - see Ulcer, gastrojejunal, with hemorrhage
    chronic 534.7●
      with
        hemorrhage 534.4●
          and perforation 534.6●
        perforation 534.5●
          and hemorrhage 534.6●
    penetrating - see Ulcer, gastrojejunal, with perforation
    perforating - see Ulcer, gastrojejunal, with perforation
  gastrojejunocolic - see Ulcer, gastrojejunal
  genital organ
    female 629.89
    male 608.89
  gingiva 523.8
  gingivitis 523.10
  glottis 478.79
  granuloma of pudenda 099.2
  groin (see also Ulcer, skin) 707.8
  gum 523.8
  gumma, due to yaws 102.4
  hand (see also Ulcer, skin) 707.8
  hard palate 528.9
  heel (see also Ulcer, lower extremity) 707.14
    decubitus (see also Ulcer, pressure) 707.07
  hemorrhoids 455.8
    external 455.5
    internal 455.2
  hip (see also Ulcer, skin) 707.8
    decubitus (see also Ulcer, pressure) 707.04
  Hunner's 595.1
  hypopharynx 478.29
  hypopyon (chronic) (subacute) 370.04
  hypostaticum - see Ulcer, varicose
  ileocolitis 556.1
  ileum (see also Ulcer, intestine) 569.82
  intestine, intestinal 569.82
    with perforation 569.83
    amebic 006.9
    duodenal - see Ulcer, duodenum
    granulocytopenic (with hemorrhage) 288.09
    marginal 569.82
    perforating 569.83
    small, primary 569.82
    stercoraceous 569.82
    stercoral 569.82
    tuberculous (see also Tuberculosis) 014.8●
    typhoid (fever) 002.0
    varicose 456.8
  ischemic 707.9
    lower extremity (see also Ulcer, lower extremity) 707.10
      ankle 707.13
      calf 707.12
      foot 707.15
      heel 707.14
      knee 707.19
      specified site NEC 707.19
      thigh 707.11
      toes 707.15
  jejunum, jejunal - see Ulcer, gastrojejunal
  keratitis (see also Ulcer, cornea) 370.00
  knee - see Ulcer, lower extremity
  labium (majus) (minus) 616.50
  laryngitis (see also Laryngitis) 464.00
    with obstruction 464.01
  larynx (aphthous) (contact) 478.79
    diphtheritic 032.3
  leg - see Ulcer, lower extremity

Ulcer, ulcerated, ulcerating, ulceration, ulcerative (Continued)
  lip 528.5
  Lipschütz's 616.50
  lower extremity (atrophic) (chronic) (neurogenic) (perforating) (pyogenic) (trophic) (tropical) 707.10
    with gangrene (see also Ulcer, lower extremity) 707.10 [785.4]
      arteriosclerotic 440.24
    ankle 707.13
    arteriosclerotic 440.23
      with gangrene 440.24
    calf 707.12
    decubitus (see also Ulcer, pressure) 707.00
      with gangrene 707.00 [785.4]
      ankle 707.06
      buttock 707.05
      heel 707.07
      hip 707.04
    foot 707.15
    heel 707.14
    knee 707.19
    specified site NEC 707.19
    thigh 707.11
    toes 707.15
    varicose 454.0
      inflamed or infected 454.2
  luetic - see Ulcer, syphilitic
  lung 518.89
    tuberculous (see also Tuberculosis) 011.2●
  malignant (M8000/3) - see Neoplasm, by site, malignant
  marginal NEC - see Ulcer, gastrojejunal
  meatus (urinarius) 597.89
  Meckel's diverticulum 751.0
  Meleney's (chronic undermining) 686.09
  Mooren's (cornea) 370.07
  mouth (traumatic) 528.9
  mycobacterial (skin) 031.1
  nasopharynx 478.29
  navel cord (newborn) 771.4
  neck (see also Ulcer, skin) 707.8
    uterus 622.0
  neurogenic NEC - see Ulcer, skin
  nose, nasal (infectional) (passage) 478.19
    septum 478.19
    varicose 456.8
    skin - see Ulcer, skin
    spirochetal NEC 104.8
  oral mucosa (traumatic) 528.9
  palate (soft) 528.9
  penetrating NEC - see Ulcer, peptic, with perforation
  penis (chronic) 607.89
  peptic (site unspecified) 533.9

> Note: Use the following fifth-digit subclassification with categories 531–534:
> 0 without mention of obstruction
> 1 with obstruction

    with
      hemorrhage 533.4●
        and perforation 533.6●
      perforation (chronic) 533.5●
        and hemorrhage 533.6●
    acute 533.3●
      with
        hemorrhage 533.0●
          and perforation 533.2●
        perforation 533.1●
          and hemorrhage 533.2●
    bleeding (recurrent) - see Ulcer, peptic, with hemorrhage
    chronic 533.7●
      with
        hemorrhage 533.4●
          and perforation 533.6●
        perforation 533.5●
          and hemorrhage 533.6●

Ulcer, ulcerated, ulcerating, ulceration, ulcerative (Continued)
  peptic (Continued)
    penetrating - see Ulcer, peptic, with perforation
    perforating NEC (see also Ulcer, peptic, with perforation) 533.5●
    skin 707.9
  perineum (see also Ulcer, skin) 707.8
  peritonsillar 474.8
  phagedenic (tropical) NEC - see Ulcer, skin
  pharynx 478.29
  phlebitis - see Phlebitis
  plaster (see also Ulcer, pressure) 707.00
  popliteal space - see Ulcer, lower extremity
  postpyloric - see Ulcer, duodenum
  prepuce 607.89
  prepyloric - see Ulcer, stomach
  pressure 707.00
    with
      abrasion, blister, partial thickness skin loss involving epidermis and/or dermis 707.22
      full thickness skin loss involving damage or necrosis of subcutaneous tissue 707.23
      gangrene 707.00 [785.4]
      necrosis of soft tissues through to underlying muscle, tendon, or bone 707.24
    ankle 707.06
    back
      lower 707.03
      upper 707.02
    buttock 707.05
    coccyx 707.03
    elbow 707.01
    head 707.09
    healed - omit code
    healing - code to Ulcer, pressure, by stage
    heel 707.07
    hip 707.04
    other site 707.09
    sacrum 707.03
    shoulder blades 707.02
    stage
      I (healing) 707.21
      II (healing) 707.22
      III (healing) 707.23
      IV (healing) 707.24
      unspecified (healing) 707.20
    unstageable 707.25
  primary of intestine 569.82
    with perforation 569.83
  proctitis 556.2
    with ulcerative sigmoiditis 556.3
  prostate 601.8
  pseudopeptic - see Ulcer, peptic
  pyloric - see Ulcer, stomach
  rectosigmoid 569.82
    with perforation 569.83
  rectum (sphincter) (solitary) 569.41
    stercoraceous, stercoral 569.41
    varicose - see Varicose, ulcer, anus
  retina (see also Chorioretinitis) 363.20
  rodent (M8090/3) - see Neoplasm, skin, malignant
    cornea 370.07
  round - see Ulcer, stomach
  sacrum (region) (see also Ulcer, skin) 707.8
  Saemisch's 370.04
  scalp (see also Ulcer, skin) 707.8
  sclera 379.09
  scrofulous (see also Tuberculosis) 017.2●
  scrotum 608.89
    tuberculous (see also Tuberculosis) 016.5●
    varicose 456.4
  seminal vesicle 608.89
  sigmoid 569.82
    with perforation 569.83

◄ New   ◄··· Revised   ~~deleted~~ Deleted   ● Use Additional Digit(s)   Omit code

475

SECTION I INDEX TO DISEASES AND INJURIES / Ulcer, ulcerated, ulcerating, ulceration, ulcerative

Ulcer, ulcerated, ulcerating, ulceration, ulcerative *(Continued)*
  skin (atrophic) (chronic) (neurogenic) (non-healing) (perforating) (pyogenic) (trophic) 707.9
    with gangrene 707.9 *[785.4]*
    amebic 006.6
    decubitus *(see also* Ulcer, pressure*)* 707.00
      with gangrene 707.00 *[785.4]*
      in granulocytopenia 288.09
    lower extremity *(see also* Ulcer, lower extremity*)* 707.10
      with gangrene 707.10 *[785.4]*
        arteriosclerotic 440.24
      ankle 707.13
      arteriosclerotic 440.23
        with gangrene 440.24
      calf 707.12
      foot 707.15
      heel 707.14
      knee 707.19
      specified site NEC 707.19
      thigh 707.11
      toes 707.15
    mycobacterial 031.1
    syphilitic (early) (secondary) 091.3
    tuberculous (primary) *(see also* Tuberculosis*)* 017.0●
    varicose - *see* Ulcer, varicose
  sloughing NEC - *see* Ulcer, skin
  soft palate 528.9
  solitary, anus or rectum (sphincter) 569.41
  sore throat 462
    streptococcal 034.0
  spermatic cord 608.89
  spine (tuberculous) 015.0● *[730.88]*
  stasis (leg) (venous) 454.0
    with varicose veins 454.0
    without varicose veins 459.81
    inflamed or infected 454.2
  stercoral, stercoraceous 569.82
    with perforation 569.83
    anus or rectum 569.41
  stoma, stomal - *see* Ulcer, gastrojejunal
  stomach (eroded) (peptic) (round) 531.9●

> Note: Use the following fifth-digit subclassification with categories 531–534:
> 0 without mention of obstruction
> 1 with obstruction

    with
      hemorrhage 531.4●
        and perforation 531.6●
      perforation (chronic) 531.5●
        and hemorrhage 531.6●
      acute 531.3●
        with
          hemorrhage 531.0●
            and perforation 531.2●
          perforation 531.1●
            and hemorrhage 531.2●
      bleeding (recurrent) - *see* Ulcer, stomach, with hemorrhage
      chronic 531.7●
        with
          hemorrhage 531.4●
            and perforation 531.6●
          perforation 531.5●
            and hemorrhage 531.6●
      penetrating - *see* Ulcer, stomach, with perforation
      perforating - *see* Ulcer, stomach, with perforation
  stomatitis 528.00
  stress - *see* Ulcer, peptic
  strumous (tuberculous) *(see also* Tuberculosis*)* 017.2●
  submental *(see also* Ulcer, skin*)* 707.8
  submucosal, bladder 595.1

Ulcer, ulcerated, ulcerating, ulceration, ulcerative *(Continued)*
  syphilitic (any site) (early) (secondary) 091.3
    late 095.9
    perforating 095.9
      foot 094.0
  testis 608.89
  thigh - *see* Ulcer, lower extremity
  throat 478.29
    diphtheritic 032.0
  toe - *see* Ulcer, lower extremity
  tongue (traumatic) 529.0
  tonsil 474.8
    diphtheritic 032.0
  trachea 519.19
  trophic - *see* Ulcer, skin
  tropical NEC *(see also* Ulcer, skin*)* 707.9
  tuberculous - *see* Tuberculosis, ulcer
  tunica vaginalis 608.89
  turbinate 730.9●
  typhoid (fever) 002.0
    perforating 002.0
  umbilicus (newborn) 771.4
  unspecified site NEC - *see* Ulcer, skin
  urethra (meatus) *(see also* Urethritis*)* 597.89
  uterus 621.8
    cervix 622.0
      with mention of cervicitis 616.0
    neck 622.0
      with mention of cervicitis 616.0
  vagina 616.89
  valve, heart 421.0
  varicose (lower extremity, any part) 454.0
    anus - *see* Varicose, ulcer, anus
    broad ligament 456.5
    esophagus *(see also* Varix, esophagus*)* 456.1
      bleeding *(see also* Varix, esophagus, bleeding*)* 456.0
    inflamed or infected 454.2
    nasal septum 456.8
    perineum 456.6
    rectum - *see* Varicose, ulcer, anus
    scrotum 456.4
    specified site NEC 456.8
    sublingual 456.3
    vulva 456.6
  vas deferens 608.89
  vesical *(see also* Ulcer, bladder*)* 596.89
  vulva (acute) (infectional) 616.50
    Behçet's syndrome 136.1 *[616.51]*
    herpetic 054.12
    tuberculous 016.7● *[616.51]*
  vulvobuccal, recurring 616.50
  x-ray - *see* Ulcer, by site
  yaws 102.4
Ulcerosa scarlatina 034.1
Ulcus - *see also* Ulcer
  cutis tuberculosum *(see also* Tuberculosis*)* 017.0●
  duodeni - *see* Ulcer, duodenum
  durum 091.0
    extragenital 091.2
  gastrojejunale - *see* Ulcer, gastrojejunal
  hypostaticum - *see* Ulcer, varicose
  molle (cutis) (skin) 099.0
  serpens corneae (pneumococcal) 370.04
  ventriculi - *see* Ulcer, stomach
Ulegyria 742.4
Ulerythema
  acneiforma 701.8
  centrifugum 695.4
  ophryogenes 757.4
Ullrich (-Bonnevie) (-Turner) **syndrome** 758.6
Ullrich-Feichtiger syndrome 759.89
Ulnar - *see* condition
Ulorrhagia 523.8
Ulorrhea 523.8
Umbilicus, umbilical - *see also* condition
  cord necrosis, affecting fetus or newborn 762.6

Unacceptable
  existing dental restoration
    contours 525.65
    morphology 525.65
Unavailability of medical facilities (at) V63.9
  due to
    investigation by social service agency V63.8
    lack of services at home V63.1
    remoteness from facility V63.0
    waiting list V63.2
  home V63.1
  outpatient clinic V63.0
  specified reason NEC V63.8
Uncinaria americana infestation 126.1
Uncinariasis *(see also* Ancylostomiasis*)* 126.9
Unconscious, unconsciousness 780.09
Underdevelopment - *see also* Undeveloped
  sexual 259.0
Underfill, endodontic 526.63
Undernourishment 269.9
Undernutrition 269.9
Under observation - *see* Observation
Underweight 783.22
  for gestational age - *see* Light-for-dates
Underwood's disease (sclerema neonatorum) 778.1
Undescended - *see also* Malposition, congenital
  cecum 751.4
  colon 751.4
  testis 752.51
Undetermined diagnosis or cause 799.9
Undeveloped, undevelopment - *see also* Hypoplasia
  brain (congenital) 742.1
  cerebral (congenital) 742.1
  fetus or newborn 764.9●
  heart 746.89
  lung 748.5
  testis 257.2
  uterus 259.0
Undiagnosed (disease) 799.9
Undulant fever *(see also* Brucellosis*)* 023.9
Unemployment, anxiety concerning V62.0
Unequal leg (acquired) (length) 736.81
  congenital 755.30
Unerupted teeth, tooth 520.6
Unextracted dental root 525.3
Unguis incarnatus 703.0
Unicornis uterus 752.33
Unicornuate uterus (with or without a separate uterine horn) 752.33
Unicorporeus uterus 752.39
Uniformis uterus 752.39
Unilateral - *see also* condition
  development, breast 611.89
  organ or site, congenital NEC - *see* Agenesis
  vagina 752.49
Unilateralis uterus 752.39
Unilocular heart 745.8
Uninhibited bladder 596.54
  with cauda equina syndrome 344.61
  neurogenic *(see also* Neurogenic, bladder*)* 596.54
Union, abnormal - *see also* Fusion
  divided tendon 727.89
  larynx and trachea 748.3
Universal
  joint, cervix 620.6
  mesentery 751.4
Unknown
  cause of death 799.9
  diagnosis 799.9
Unna's disease (seborrheic dermatitis) 690.10
Unresponsiveness, adrenocorticotropin (ACTH) 255.41
Unsatisfactory
  cytology smear
    anal 796.78
    cervical 795.08
    vaginal 795.18

SECTION I INDEX TO DISEASES AND INJURIES / Urticaria

Unsatisfactory (Continued)
  restoration, tooth (existing) 525.60
    specified NEC 525.69
Unsoundness of mind (see also Psychosis) 298.9
Unspecified cause of death 799.9
Unstable
  back NEC 724.9
  colon 569.89
  joint - see Instability, joint
  lie 652.0●
    affecting fetus or newborn (before labor) 761.7
    causing obstructed labor 660.0●
      affecting fetus or newborn 763.1
  lumbosacral joint (congenital) 756.19
    acquired 724.6
  sacroiliac 724.6
  spine NEC 724.9
Untruthfulness, child problem (see also Disturbance, conduct) 312.0●
Unverricht (-Lundborg) disease, syndrome, or epilepsy 345.1●
Unverricht-Wagner syndrome (dermatomyositis) 710.3
Upper respiratory - see condition
Upset
  gastric 536.8
    psychogenic 306.4
  gastrointestinal 536.8
    psychogenic 306.4
    virus (see also Enteritis, viral) 008.8
  intestinal (large) (small) 564.9
    psychogenic 306.4
  menstruation 626.9
  mental 300.9
  stomach 536.8
    psychogenic 306.4
Urachus - see also condition
  patent 753.7
  persistent 753.7
Uratic arthritis 274.00
Urbach's lipoid proteinosis 272.8
Urbach-Oppenheim disease or syndrome (necrobiosis lipoidica diabeticorum) 250.8● [709.3]
  due to secondary diabetes 249.8● [709.3]
Urbach-Wiethe disease or syndrome (lipoid proteinosis) 272.8
Urban yellow fever 060.1
Urea, blood, high - see Uremia
Uremia, uremic (absorption) (amaurosis) (amblyopia) (aphasia) (apoplexy) (coma) (delirium) (dementia) (dropsy) (dyspnea) (fever) (intoxication) (mania) (paralysis) (poisoning) (toxemia) (vomiting) 586
  with
    abortion - see Abortion, by type, with renal failure
    ectopic pregnancy (see also categories 633.0–633.9) 639.3
    hypertension (see also Hypertension, kidney) 403.91
    molar pregnancy (see also categories 630–632) 639.3
  chronic 585.9
  complicating
    abortion 639.3
    ectopic or molar pregnancy 639.3
    hypertension (see also Hypertension, kidney) 403.91
    labor and delivery 669.3●
  congenital 779.89
  extrarenal 788.99
  hypertensive (chronic) (see also Hypertension, kidney) 403.91
  maternal NEC, affecting fetus or newborn 760.1
  neuropathy 585.9 [357.4]
  pericarditis 585.9 [420.0]
  prerenal 788.99
  pyelitic (see also Pyelitis) 590.80

Ureter, ureteral - see condition
Ureteralgia 788.0
Ureterectasis 593.89
Ureteritis 593.89
  cystica 590.3
  due to calculus 592.1
  gonococcal (acute) 098.19
    chronic or duration of 2 months or over 098.39
  nonspecific 593.89
Ureterocele (acquired) 593.89
  congenital 753.23
Ureterolith 592.1
Ureterolithiasis 592.1
Ureterostomy status V44.6
  with complication 997.5
Urethra, urethral - see condition
Urethralgia 788.99
Urethritis (abacterial) (acute) (allergic) (anterior) (chronic) (nonvenereal) (posterior) (recurrent) (simple) (subacute) (ulcerative) (undifferentiated) 597.80
  diplococcal (acute) 098.0
    chronic or duration of 2 months or over 098.2
  due to Trichomonas (vaginalis) 131.02
  gonococcal (acute) 098.0
    chronic or duration of 2 months or over 098.2
  nongonococcal (sexually transmitted) 099.40
    Chlamydia trachomatis 099.41
    Reiter's 099.3
    specified organism NEC 099.49
  nonspecific (sexually transmitted) (see also Urethritis, nongonococcal) 099.40
  not sexually transmitted 597.80
  Reiter's 099.3
  trichomonal or due to Trichomonas (vaginalis) 131.02
  tuberculous (see also Tuberculosis) 016.3●
  venereal NEC (see also Urethritis, nongonococcal) 099.40
Urethrocele
  female 618.03
    with uterine prolapse 618.4
      complete 618.3
      incomplete 618.2
  male 599.5
Urethrolithiasis 594.2
Urethro-oculoarticular syndrome 099.3
Urethro-oculosynovial syndrome 099.3
Urethrorectal - see condition
Urethrorrhagia 599.84
Urethrorrhea 788.7
Urethrostomy status V44.6
  with complication 997.5
Urethrotrigonitis 595.3
Urethrovaginal - see condition
Urgency
  fecal 787.63
  hypertensive - see Hypertension
Urhidrosis, uridrosis 705.89
Uric acid
  diathesis 274.9
  in blood 790.6
Uricacidemia 790.6
Uricemia 790.6
Uricosuria 791.9
Urination
  frequent 788.41
  painful 788.1
  urgency 788.63
Urine, urinary - see also condition
  abnormality NEC 788.69
  blood in (see also Hematuria) 599.70
  discharge, excessive 788.42
  enuresis 788.30
    nonorganic origin 307.6
  extravasation 788.8
  frequency 788.41
  hesitancy 788.64

Urine, urinary (Continued)
  incontinence 788.30
    active 788.30
    female 788.30
      stress 625.6
      and urge 788.33
    male 788.30
      stress 788.32
      and urge 788.33
    mixed (stress and urge) 788.33
    neurogenic 788.39
    nonorganic origin 307.6
    overflow 788.38
    stress (female) 625.6
      male NEC 788.32
  intermittent stream 788.61
  pus in 791.9
  retention or stasis NEC 788.20
    bladder, incomplete emptying 788.21
    psychogenic 306.53
    specified NEC 788.29
  secretion
    deficient 788.5
    excessive 788.42
    frequency 788.41
  strain 788.65
  stream
    intermittent 788.61
    slowing 788.62
    splitting 788.61
    weak 788.62
  urgency 788.63
Urinemia - see Uremia
Urinoma NEC 599.9
  bladder 596.89
  kidney 593.89
  renal 593.89
  ureter 593.89
  urethra 599.84
Uroarthritis, infectious 099.3
Urodialysis 788.5
Urolithiasis 592.9
Uronephrosis 593.89
Uropathy 599.9
  obstructive 599.60
Urosepsis 599.0
  meaning sepsis 995.91
  meaning urinary tract infection 599.0
Urticaria 708.9
  with angioneurotic edema 995.1
    hereditary 277.6
  allergic 708.0
  cholinergic 708.5
  chronic 708.8
  cold, familial 708.2
  dermatographic 708.3
  due to
    cold or heat 708.2
    drugs 708.0
    food 708.0
    inhalants 708.0
    plants 708.8
    serum 999.59
  factitial 708.3
  giant 995.1
    hereditary 277.6
  gigantea 995.1
    hereditary 277.6
  idiopathic 708.1
  larynx 995.1
    hereditary 277.6
  neonatorum 778.8
  nonallergic 708.1
  papulosa (Hebra) 698.2
  perstans hemorrhagica 757.39
  pigmentosa 757.33
  recurrent periodic 708.8
  serum 999.59
  solare 692.72
  specified type NEC 708.8

SECTION I INDEX TO DISEASES AND INJURIES / Urticaria

Urticaria (Continued)
    thermal (cold) (heat) 708.2
    vibratory 708.4
Urticarioides acarodermatitis 133.9
Use of
    agents affecting estrogen receptors and estrogen levels NEC V07.59
    anastrozole (Arimidex) V07.52
    aromatase inhibitors V07.52
    estrogen receptor downregulators V07.59
    exemestane (Aromasin) V07.52
    fulvestrant (Faslodex) V07.59
    gonadotropin-releasing hormone (GnRH) agonist V07.59
    goserelin acetate (Zoladex) V07.59
    letrozole (Femara) V07.52
    leuprolide acetate (leuprorelin) (Lupron) V07.59
    megestrol acetate (Megace) V07.59
    methadone 304.00
    nonprescribed drugs (see also Abuse, drugs, nondependent) 305.9●
    patent medicines (see also Abuse, drugs, nondependent) 305.9●
    raloxifene (Evista) V07.51
    selective estrogen receptor modulators (SERMs) V07.51
    tamoxifen (Nolvadex) V07.51
    toremifene (Fareston) V07.51

Usher-Senear disease (pemphigus erythematosus) 694.4
Uta 085.5
Uterine size-date discrepancy 649.6●
Uteromegaly 621.2
Uterovaginal - see condition
Uterovesical - see condition
Uterus - see also condition
    with only one functioning horn 752.33
Utriculitis (utriculus prostaticus) 597.89
Uveal - see condition
Uveitis (anterior) (see also Iridocyclitis) 364.3
    acute or subacute 364.00
        due to or associated with
            gonococcal infection 098.41
            herpes (simplex) 054.44
            zoster 053.22
        primary 364.01
        recurrent 364.02
        secondary (noninfectious) 364.04
            infectious 364.03
    allergic 360.11
    chronic 364.10
        due to or associated with
            sarcoidosis 135 [364.11]
            tuberculosis (see also Tuberculosis) 017.3● [364.11]

Uveitis (Continued)
    due to
        operation 360.11
        toxoplasmosis (acquired) 130.2
            congenital (active) 771.2
    granulomatous 364.10
    heterochromic 364.21
    lens-induced 364.23
    nongranulomatous 364.00
    posterior 363.20
        disseminated - see Chorioretinitis, disseminated
        focal - see Chorioretinitis, focal
    recurrent 364.02
    sympathetic 360.11
    syphilitic (secondary) 091.50
        congenital 090.0 [363.13]
        late 095.8 [363.13]
    tuberculous (see also Tuberculosis) 017.3● [364.11]
Uveoencephalitis 363.22
Uveokeratitis (see also Iridocyclitis) 364.3
Uveoparotid fever 135
Uveoparotitis 135
Uvula - see condition
Uvulitis (acute) (catarrhal) (chronic) (gangrenous) (membranous) (suppurative) (ulcerative) 528.3

V

Vaccination
  complication or reaction - *see* Complications, vaccination
  delayed V64.00
  not carried out V64.00
    because of
      acute illness V64.01
      allergy to vaccine or component V64.04
      caregiver refusal V64.05
      chronic illness V64.02
      guardian refusal V64.05
      immune compromised state V64.03
      parent refusal V64.05
      patient had disease being vaccinated against V64.08
      patient refusal V64.06
      reason NEC V64.09
      religious reasons V64.07
  prophylactic (against) V05.9
    arthropod-borne viral
      disease NEC V05.1
      encephalitis V05.0
    chicken pox V05.4
    cholera (alone) V03.0
      with typhoid-paratyphoid (cholera + TAB) V06.0
    common cold V04.7
    diphtheria (alone) V03.5
      with
        poliomyelitis (DTP + polio) V06.3
        tetanus V06.5
          pertussis combined [DTP] (DTaP) V06.1
        typhoid-paratyphoid (DTP + TAB) V06.2
    disease (single) NEC V05.9
      bacterial NEC V03.9
        specified type NEC V03.89
      combination NEC V06.9
        specified type NEC V06.8
      specified type NEC V05.8
    encephalitis, viral, arthropod-borne V05.0
    Hemophilus influenzae, type B [Hib] V03.81
    hepatitis, viral V05.3
    influenza V04.81
      with
        Streptococcus pneumoniae [pneumococcus] V06.6
    leishmaniasis V05.2
    measles (alone) V04.2
      with mumps-rubella (MMR) V06.4
    mumps (alone) V04.6
      with measles and rubella (MMR) V06.4
    pertussis alone V03.6
    plague V03.3
    poliomyelitis V04.0
      with diphtheria-tetanus-pertussis (DTP polio) V06.3
    rabies V04.5
    respiratory syncytial virus (RSV) V04.82
    rubella (alone) V04.3
      with measles and mumps (MMR) V06.4
    smallpox V04.1
    Streptococcus pneumoniae [pneumococcus] V03.82
      with
        influenza V06.6
    tetanus toxoid (alone) V03.7
      with diphtheria [Td] [DT] V06.5
        with
          pertussis (DTP) (DTaP) V06.1
            with poliomyelitis (DTP + polio) V06.3
    tuberculosis (BCG) V03.2
    tularemia V03.4

Vaccination *(Continued)*
  prophylactic *(Continued)*
    typhoid-paratyphoid (TAB) (alone) V03.1
      with diphtheria-tetanus-pertussis (TAB + DTP) V06.2
    varicella V05.4
    viral
      disease NEC V04.89
      encephalitis, arthropod-borne V05.0
      hepatitis V05.3
    yellow fever V04.4
Vaccinia (generalized) 999.0
  congenital 771.2
  conjunctiva 999.39
  eyelids 999.0 *[373.5]*
  localized 999.39
  nose 999.39
  not from vaccination 051.02
    eyelid 051.02 *[373.5]*
  sine vaccinatione 051.02
  without vaccination 051.02
Vacuum
  extraction of fetus or newborn 763.3
  in sinus (accessory) (nasal) (*see also* Sinusitis) 473.9
Vagabond V60.0
Vagabondage V60.0
Vagabonds' disease 132.1
Vagina, vaginal - *see also* condition
  high risk human papillomavirus (HPV) DNA test positive 795.15
  low risk human papillomavirus (HPV) DNA test positive 795.19
Vaginalitis (tunica) 608.4
Vaginismus (reflex) 625.1
  functional 306.51
  hysterical 300.11
  psychogenic 306.51
Vaginitis (acute) (chronic) (circumscribed) (diffuse) (emphysematous) (Hemophilus vaginalis) (nonspecific) (nonvenereal) (ulcerative) 616.10
  with
    abortion - *see* Abortion, by type, with sepsis
    ectopic pregnancy (*see also* categories 633.0–633.9) 639.0
    molar pregnancy (*see also* categories 630–632) 639.0
  adhesive, congenital 752.49
  atrophic, postmenopausal 627.3
  bacterial 616.10
  blennorrhagic (acute) 098.0
    chronic or duration of 2 months or over 098.2
  candidal 112.1
  chlamydial 099.53
  complicating pregnancy or puerperium 646.6 ●
    affecting fetus or newborn 760.8
  congenital (adhesive) 752.49
  due to
    C. albicans 112.1
    Trichomonas (vaginalis) 131.01
  following
    abortion 639.0
    ectopic or molar pregnancy 639.0
  gonococcal (acute) 098.0
    chronic or duration of 2 months or over 098.2
  granuloma 099.2
  Monilia 112.1
  mycotic 112.1
  pinworm 127.4 *[616.11]*
  postirradiation 616.10
  postmenopausal atrophic 627.3
  senile (atrophic) 627.3
  syphilitic (early) 091.0
    late 095.8
  trichomonal 131.01

Vaginitis *(Continued)*
  tuberculous (*see also* Tuberculosis) 016.7 ●
  venereal NEC 099.8
Vaginosis - *see* Vaginitis
Vagotonia 352.3
Vagrancy V60.0
VAIN I (vaginal intraepithelial neoplasia I) 623.0
VAIN II (vaginal intraepithelial neoplasia II) 623.0
VAIN III (vaginal intraepithelial neoplasia III) 233.31
Vallecula - *see* condition
Valley fever 114.0
Valsuani's disease (progressive pernicious anemia, puerperal) 648.2 ●
Valve, valvular (formation) - *see also* condition
  cerebral ventricle (communicating) in situ V45.2
  cervix, internal os 752.49
  colon 751.5
  congenital NEC - *see* Atresia
  formation congenital NEC - *see* Atresia
  heart defect - *see* Anomaly, heart, valve
  ureter 753.29
    pelvic junction 753.21
    vesical orifice 753.22
  urethra 753.6
Valvulitis (chronic) (*see also* Endocarditis) 424.90
  rheumatic (chronic) (inactive) (with chorea) 397.9
    active or acute (aortic) (mitral) (pulmonary) (tricuspid) 391.1
  syphilitic NEC 093.20
    aortic 093.22
    mitral 093.21
    pulmonary 093.24
    tricuspid 093.23
Valvulopathy - *see* Endocarditis
van Bogaert's leukoencephalitis (sclerosing) (subacute) 046.2
van Bogaert-Nijssen (-Peiffer) **disease** 330.0
van Buchem's syndrome (hyperostosis corticalis) 733.3
Vancomycin (glycopeptide)
  intermediate staphylococcus aureus (VISA/GISA) V09.8
  resistant
    enterococcus (VRE) V09.8
    staphylococcus aureus (VRSA/GRSA) V09.8
van Creveld-von Gierke disease (glycogenosis I) 271.0
van den Bergh's disease (enterogenous cyanosis) 289.7
van der Hoeve's syndrome (brittle bones and blue sclera, deafness) 756.51
van der Hoeve-Halbertsma-Waardenburg syndrome (ptosis-epicanthus) 270.2
van der Hoeve-Waardenburg-Gualdi syndrome (ptosis-epicanthus) 270.2
Vanillism 692.89
Vanishing lung 492.0
Vanishing twin 651.33
van Neck (-Odelberg) **disease or syndrome** (juvenile osteochondrosis) 732.1
Vapor asphyxia or suffocation NEC 987.9
  specified agent - *see* Table of Drugs and Chemicals
Vaquez's disease (M9950/1) 238.4
Vaquez-Osler disease (polycythemia vera) (M9950/1) 238.4
Variance, lethal ball, prosthetic heart valve 996.02
Variants, thalassemic 282.49
Variations in hair color 704.3

Varicella 052.9
- with
    - complication 052.8
        - specified NEC 052.7
    - pneumonia 052.1
- exposure to V01.71
- vaccination and inoculation (against) (prophylactic) V05.4

Varices - see Varix

Varicocele (scrotum) (thrombosed) 456.4
- ovary 456.5
- perineum 456.6
- spermatic cord (ulcerated) 456.4

Varicose
- aneurysm (ruptured) (see also Aneurysm) 442.9
- dermatitis (lower extremity) - see Varicose, vein, inflamed or infected
- eczema - see Varicose, vein
- phlebitis - see Varicose, vein, inflamed or infected
- placental vessel - see Placenta, abnormal
- tumor - see Varicose, vein
- ulcer (lower extremity, any part) 454.0
    - anus 455.8
        - external 455.5
        - internal 455.2
    - esophagus (see also Varix, esophagus) 456.1
        - bleeding (see also Varix, esophagus, bleeding) 456.0
    - inflamed or infected 454.2
    - nasal septum 456.8
    - perineum 456.6
    - rectum - see Varicose, ulcer, anus
    - scrotum 456.4
    - specified site NEC 456.8
- vein (lower extremity) (ruptured) (see also Varix) 454.9
    - with
        - complications NEC 454.8
        - edema 454.8
        - inflammation or infection 454.1
            - ulcerated 454.2
        - pain 454.8
        - stasis dermatitis 454.1
            - with ulcer 454.2
        - swelling 454.8
        - ulcer 454.0
            - inflamed or infected 454.2
    - anus - see Hemorrhoids
    - broad ligament 456.5
    - congenital (peripheral) 747.60
        - gastrointestinal 747.61
        - lower limb 747.64
        - renal 747.62
        - specified NEC 747.69
        - upper limb 747.63
    - esophagus (ulcerated) (see also Varix, esophagus) 456.1
        - bleeding (see also Varix, esophagus, bleeding) 456.0
    - inflamed or infected 454.1
        - with ulcer 454.2
    - in pregnancy or puerperium 671.0●
        - vulva or perineum 671.1●
    - nasal septum (with ulcer) 456.8
    - pelvis 456.5
    - perineum 456.6
        - in pregnancy, childbirth, or puerperium 671.1●
    - rectum - see Hemorrhoids
    - scrotum (ulcerated) 456.4
    - specified site NEC 456.8
    - sublingual 456.3
    - ulcerated 454.0
        - inflamed or infected 454.2
    - umbilical cord, affecting fetus or newborn 762.6
    - urethra 456.8

Varicose (Continued)
- vein (Continued)
    - vulva 456.6
        - in pregnancy, childbirth, or puerperium 671.1●
    - vessel - see also Varix
    - placenta - see Placenta, abnormal

Varicosis, varicosities, varicosity (see also Varix) 454.9

Variola 050.9
- hemorrhagic (pustular) 050.0
- major 050.0
- minor 050.1
- modified 050.2

Varioloid 050.2

Variolosa, purpura 050.0

Varix (lower extremity) (ruptured) 454.9
- with
    - complications NEC 454.8
    - edema 454.8
    - inflammation or infection 454.1
        - with ulcer 454.2
    - pain 454.8
    - stasis dermatitis 454.1
        - with ulcer 454.2
    - swelling 454.8
    - ulcer 454.0
        - with inflammation or infection 454.2
- aneurysmal (see also Aneurysm) 442.9
- anus - see Hemorrhoids
- arteriovenous (congenital) (peripheral) NEC 747.60
    - gastrointestinal 747.61
    - lower limb 747.64
    - renal 747.62
    - specified NEC 747.69
    - spinal 747.82
    - upper limb 747.63
- bladder 456.5
- broad ligament 456.5
- congenital (peripheral) 747.60
- esophagus (ulcerated) 456.1
    - bleeding 456.0
        - in
            - cirrhosis of liver 571.5 [456.20]
            - portal hypertension 572.3 [456.20]
    - congenital 747.69
    - in
        - cirrhosis of liver 571.5 [456.21]
            - with bleeding 571.5 [456.20]
        - portal hypertension 572.3 [456.21]
            - with bleeding 572.3 [456.20]
- gastric 456.8
- inflamed or infected 454.1
    - ulcerated 454.2
- in pregnancy or puerperium 671.0●
    - perineum 671.1●
    - vulva 671.1●
- labia (majora) 456.6
- orbit 456.8
    - congenital 747.69
- ovary 456.5
- papillary 448.1
- pelvis 456.5
- perineum 456.6
    - in pregnancy or puerperium 671.1●
- pharynx 456.8
- placenta - see Placenta, abnormal
- prostate 456.8
- rectum - see Hemorrhoids
- renal papilla 456.8
- retina 362.17
- scrotum (ulcerated) 456.4
- sigmoid colon 456.8
- specified site NEC 456.8
- spinal (cord) (vessels) 456.8
- spleen, splenic (vein) (with phlebolith) 456.8
- sublingual 456.3
- ulcerated 454.0
    - inflamed or infected 454.2

Varix (Continued)
- umbilical cord, affecting fetus or newborn 762.6
- uterine ligament 456.5
- vocal cord 456.8
- vulva 456.6
    - in pregnancy, childbirth, or puerperium 671.1●

Vasa previa 663.5●
- affecting fetus or newborn 762.6
- hemorrhage from, affecting fetus or newborn 772.0

Vascular - see also condition
- loop on papilla (optic) 743.57
- sheathing, retina 362.13
- spasm 443.9
- spider 448.1

Vascularity, pulmonary, congenital 747.39

Vascularization
- choroid 362.16
- cornea 370.60
    - deep 370.63
    - localized 370.61
- retina 362.16
- subretinal 362.16

Vasculitis 447.6
- allergic 287.0
- cryoglobulinemic 273.2
- disseminated 447.6
- kidney 447.8
- leukocytoclastic 446.29
- nodular 695.2
- retinal 362.18
- rheumatic - see Fever, rheumatic

Vasculopathy
- cardiac allograft 996.83

Vas deferens - see condition

Vas deferentitis 608.4

Vasectomy, admission for V25.2

Vasitis 608.4
- nodosa 608.4
- scrotum 608.4
- spermatic cord 608.4
- testis 608.4
- tuberculous (see also Tuberculosis) 016.5●
- tunica vaginalis 608.4
- vas deferens 608.4

Vasodilation 443.9

Vasomotor - see condition

Vasoplasty, after previous sterilization V26.0

Vasoplegia, splanchnic (see also Neuropathy, peripheral, autonomic) 337.9

Vasospasm 443.9
- cerebral (artery) 435.9
    - with transient neurologic deficit 435.9
- coronary 413.1
- nerve
    - arm NEC 354.9
    - autonomic 337.9
    - brachial plexus 353.0
    - cervical plexus 353.2
    - leg NEC 355.8
    - lower extremity NEC 355.8
    - peripheral NEC 335.9
    - spinal NEC 355.9
    - sympathetic 337.9
    - upper extremity NEC 354.9
- peripheral NEC 443.9
- retina (artery) (see also Occlusion, retinal, artery) 362.30

Vasospastic - see condition

Vasovagal attack (paroxysmal) 780.2
- psychogenic 306.2

Vater's ampulla - see condition

VATER syndrome 759.89

vCJD (variant Creutzfeldt-Jakob disease) 046.11

Vegetation, vegetative
- adenoid (nasal fossa) 474.2
- consciousness (persistent) 780.03
- endocarditis (acute) (any valve) (chronic) (subacute) 421.0

Vegetation, vegetative (Continued)
  heart (mycotic) (valve) 421.0
  state (persistent) 780.03
Veil
  Jackson's 751.4
  over face (causing asphyxia) 768.9
Vein, venous - *see* condition
Veldt sore (*see also* Ulcer, skin) 707.9
Velo-cardio-facial syndrome 758.32
Velpeau's hernia - *see* Hernia, femoral
Venereal
  balanitis NEC 099.8
  bubo 099.1
  disease 099.9
    specified nature or type NEC 099.8
  granuloma inguinale 099.2
  lymphogranuloma (Durand-Nicolas-Favre),
    any site 099.1
  salpingitis 098.37
  urethritis (*see also* Urethritis, nongonococcal)
    099.40
  vaginitis NEC 099.8
  warts 078.11
Vengefulness, in child (*see also* Disturbance,
    conduct) 312.0●
Venofibrosis 459.89
Venom, venomous
  bite or sting (animal or insect) 989.5
  poisoning 989.5
Venous - *see* condition
Ventouse delivery NEC 669.5●
  affecting fetus or newborn 763.3
Ventral - *see* condition
Ventricle, ventricular - *see also* condition
  escape 427.69
  standstill (*see also* Arrest, cardiac) 427.5
Ventriculitis, cerebral (*see also* Meningitis)
    322.9
Ventriculostomy status V45.2
Verbiest's syndrome (claudicatio intermittens
    spinalis) 435.1
Vernet's syndrome 352.6
Verneuil's disease (syphilitic bursitis) 095.7
Verruca (filiformis) 078.10
  acuminata (any site) 078.11
  necrogenica (primary) (*see also* Tuberculosis)
    017.0●
  peruana 088.0
  peruviana 088.0
  plana (juvenilis) 078.19
  plantaris 078.12
  seborrheica 702.19
    inflamed 702.11
  senilis 702.0
  tuberculosa (primary) (*see also* Tuberculosis)
    017.0●
  venereal 078.11
  viral 078.10
    specified NEC 078.19
  vulgaris 078.10
Verrucosities (*see also* Verruca) 078.10
Verrucous endocarditis (acute) (any valve)
    (chronic) (subacute) 710.0 *[424.91]*
  nonbacterial 710.0 *[424.91]*
Verruga
  peruana 088.0
  peruviana 088.0
Verse's disease (calcinosis intervertebralis)
    275.49 *[722.90]*
Version
  before labor, affecting fetus or newborn
    761.7
  cephalic (correcting previous malposition)
    652.1●
    affecting fetus or newborn 763.1
  cervix - *see* Version, uterus
  uterus (postinfectional) (postpartal, old) (*see
    also* Malposition, uterus) 621.6
    forward - *see* Anteversion, uterus
    lateral - *see* Lateroversion, uterus
Vertebra, vertebral - *see* condition

Vertigo 780.4
  auditory 386.19
  aural 386.19
  benign paroxysmal positional 386.11
  central origin 386.2
  cerebral 386.2
  Dix and Hallpike (epidemic) 386.12
  endemic paralytic 078.81
  epidemic 078.81
    Dix and Hallpike 386.12
    Gerlier's 078.81
    Pedersen's 386.12
    vestibular neuronitis 386.12
  epileptic - *see* Epilepsy
  Gerlier's (epidemic) 078.81
  hysterical 300.11
  labyrinthine 386.10
  laryngeal 786.2
  malignant positional 386.2
  Ménière's (*see also* Disease, Ménière's) 386.00
  menopausal 627.2
  otogenic 386.19
  paralytic 078.81
  paroxysmal positional, benign 386.11
  Pedersen's (epidemic) 386.12
  peripheral 386.10
    specified type NEC 386.19
  positional
    benign paroxysmal 386.11
    malignant 386.2
Verumontanitis (chronic) (*see also* Urethritis)
    597.89
Vesania (*see also* Psychosis) 298.9
Vesical - *see* condition
Vesicle
  cutaneous 709.8
  seminal - *see* condition
  skin 709.8
Vesicocolic - *see* condition
Vesicoperineal - *see* condition
Vesicorectal - *see* condition
Vesicourethrorectal - *see* condition
Vesicovaginal - *see* condition
Vesicular - *see* condition
Vesiculitis (seminal) 608.0
  amebic 006.8
  gonorrheal (acute) 098.14
    chronic or duration of 2 months or over
      098.34
  trichomonal 131.09
  tuberculous (*see also* Tuberculosis) 016.5●
    [608.81]
Vestibulitis (ear) (*see also* Labyrinthitis) 386.30
  nose (external) 478.19
  vulvar 625.71
Vestibulopathy, acute peripheral (recurrent)
    386.12
Vestige, vestigial - *see also* Persistence
  branchial 744.41
  structures in vitreous 743.51
Vibriosis NEC 027.9
Vidal's disease (lichen simplex chronicus) 698.3
Video display tube syndrome 723.8
Vienna-type encephalitis 049.8
Villaret's syndrome 352.6
Villous - *see* condition
VIN I (vulvar intraepithelial neoplasia I)
    624.01
VIN II (vulvar intraepithelial neoplasia II)
    624.02
VIN III (vulvar intraepithelial neoplasia III)
    233.32
Vincent's
  angina 101
  bronchitis 101
  disease 101
  gingivitis 101
  infection (any site) 101
  laryngitis 101
  stomatitis 101
  tonsillitis 101

Vinson-Plummer syndrome (sideropenic
    dysphagia) 280.8
Viosterol deficiency (*see also* Deficiency,
    calciferol) 268.9
Virchow's disease 733.99
Viremia 790.8
Virilism (adrenal) (female) NEC 255.2
  with
    3-beta-hydroxysteroid dehydrogenase
      defect 255.2
    11-hydroxylase defect 255.2
    21-hydroxylase defect 255.2
    adrenal
      hyperplasia 255.2
      insufficiency (congenital) 255.2
    cortical hyperfunction 255.2
Virilization (female) (suprarenal) (*see also*
    Virilism) 255.2
  isosexual 256.4
Virulent bubo 099.0
Virus, viral - *see also* condition
  infection NEC (*see also* Infection, viral) 079.99
  septicemia 079.99
  yaba monkey tumor 059.22
**VISA (vancomycin intermediate
    staphylococcus aureus)** V09.8
Viscera, visceral - *see* condition
Visceroptosis 569.89
Visible peristalsis 787.4
Vision, visual
  binocular, suppression 368.31
  blurred, blurring 368.8
    hysterical 300.11
  defect, defective (*see also* Impaired, vision)
    369.9
  disorientation (syndrome) 368.16
  disturbance NEC (*see also* Disturbance,
    vision) 368.9
    hysterical 300.11
  examination V72.0
  field, limitation 368.40
  fusion, with defective steropsis 368.33
  hallucinations 368.16
  halos 368.16
  loss 369.9
    both eyes (*see also* Blindness, both eyes)
      369.3
    complete (*see also* Blindness, both eyes)
      369.00
    one eye 369.8
    sudden 368.16
  low (both eyes) 369.20
    one eye (other eye normal) (*see also*
      Impaired, vision) 369.70
    blindness, other eye 369.10
  perception, simultaneous without fusion
    368.32
  tunnel 368.45
Vitality, lack or want of 780.79
  newborn 779.89
Vitamin deficiency NEC (*see also* Deficiency,
    vitamin) 269.2
Vitelline duct, persistent 751.0
Vitiligo 709.01
  due to pinta (carate) 103.2
  eyelid 374.53
  vulva 624.8
Vitium cordis - *see* Disease, heart
Vitreous - *see also* condition
  touch syndrome 997.99
VLCAD (long chain/very long chain acyl CoA
    dehydrogenase deficiency, LCAD) 277.85
Vocal cord - *see* condition
Vocational rehabilitation V57.22
Vogt's (Cecile) disease or syndrome 333.7
Vogt-Koyanagi syndrome 364.24
Vogt-Spielmeyer disease (amaurotic familial
    idiocy) 330.1
Voice
  change (*see also* Dysphonia) 784.49
  loss (*see also* Aphonia) 784.41

Volhard-Fahr disease (malignant nephrosclerosis) 403.00
Volhynian fever 083.1
Volkmann's ischemic contracture or paralysis (complicating trauma) 958.6
Voluntary starvation 307.1
Volvulus (bowel) (colon) (intestine) 560.2
- with
    - hernia - *see also* Hernia, by site, with obstruction
        - gangrenous - *see* Hernia, by site, with gangrene
    - perforation 560.2
- congenital 751.5
- duodenum 537.3
- fallopian tube 620.5
- oviduct 620.5
- stomach (due to absence of gastrocolic ligament) 537.89

Vomiting 787.03
- with nausea 787.01
- allergic 535.4●
- asphyxia 933.1
- bilious (cause unknown) 787.04
    - following gastrointestinal surgery 564.3
    - newborn 779.32
- blood (*see also* Hematemesis) 578.0
- causing asphyxia, choking, or suffocation (*see also* Asphyxia, food) 933.1
- cyclical 536.2
    - associated with migraine 346.2●
    - psychogenic 306.4
- epidemic 078.82
- fecal matter 569.87
- following gastrointestinal surgery 564.3
- functional 536.8
    - psychogenic 306.4
- habit 536.2
- hysterical 300.11
- nervous 306.4
- neurotic 306.4
- newborn 779.33
    - bilious 779.32
- of or complicating pregnancy 643.9●
    - due to
        - organic disease 643.8●
        - specific cause NEC 643.8●
    - early - *see* Hyperemesis, gravidarum
    - late (after 22 completed weeks of gestation) 643.2●

Vomiting (*Continued*)
- pernicious or persistent 536.2
    - complicating pregnancy - *see* Hyperemesis, gravidarum
    - psychogenic 306.4
- physiological 787.03
    - bilious 787.04
- psychic 306.4
- psychogenic 307.54
- stercoral 569.89
- uncontrollable 536.2
    - psychogenic 306.4
- uremic - *see* Uremia
- winter 078.82

von Bechterew (-Strümpell) disease or syndrome (ankylosing spondylitis) 720.0
von Bezold's abscess 383.01
von Economo's disease (encephalitis lethargica) 049.8
von Eulenburg's disease (congenital paramyotonia) 359.29
von Gierke's disease (glycogenosis I) 271.0
von Gies' joint 095.8
von Graefe's disease or syndrome 378.72
von Hippel (-Lindau) disease or syndrome (retinocerebral angiomatosis) 759.6
von Jaksch's anemia or disease (pseudoleukemia infantum) 285.8
von Recklinghausen's
- disease or syndrome (nerves) (skin) (M9540/1) 237.71
    - bones (osteitis fibrosa cystica) 252.01
- tumor (M9540/1) 237.71

von Recklinghausen-Applebaum disease (hemochromatosis) (*see also* Hemochromatosis) 275.03
von Schroetter's syndrome (intermittent venous claudication) 453.89
von Willebrand (-Jürgens) (-Minot) disease or syndrome (angiohemophilia) 286.4
von Zambusch's disease (lichen sclerosus et atrophicus) 701.0
Voorhoeve's disease or dyschondroplasia 756.4
Vossius' ring 921.3
- late effect 366.21
Voyeurism 302.82
VRE (vancomycin resistant enterococcus) V09.8

Vrolik's disease (osteogenesis imperfecta) 756.51
VRSA (vancomycin resistant staphylococcus aureus) V09.8
Vulva - *see* condition
Vulvismus 625.1
Vulvitis (acute) (allergic) (chronic) (gangrenous) (hypertrophic) (intertriginous) 616.10
- with
    - abortion - *see* Abortion, by type, with sepsis
    - ectopic pregnancy (*see also* categories 633.0–633.9) 639.0
    - molar pregnancy (*see also* categories 630–632) 639.0
- adhesive, congenital 752.49
- blennorrhagic (acute) 098.0
    - chronic or duration of 2 months or over 098.2
- chlamydial 099.53
- complicating pregnancy or puerperium 646.6●
- due to Ducrey's bacillus 099.0
- following
    - abortion 639.0
    - ectopic or molar pregnancy 639.0
- gonococcal (acute) 098.0
    - chronic or duration of 2 months or over 098.2
- herpetic 054.11
- leukoplakic 624.09
- monilial 112.1
- puerperal, postpartum, childbirth 646.6●
- syphilitic (early) 091.0
    - late 095.8
- trichomonal 131.01

Vulvodynia 625.70
- specified NEC 625.79
Vulvorectal - *see* condition
Vulvovaginitis (*see also* Vulvitis) 616.10
- amebic 006.8
- chlamydial 099.53
- gonococcal (acute) 098.0
    - chronic or duration of 2 months or over 098.2
- herpetic 054.11
- monilial 112.1
- trichomonal (Trichomonas vaginalis) 131.01

W

Waardenburg's syndrome 756.89
  meaning ptosis-epicanthus 270.2
Waardenburg-Klein syndrome (ptosis-epicanthus) 270.2
Wagner's disease (colloid milium) 709.3
Wagner (-Unverricht) **syndrome** (dermatomyositis) 710.3
Waiting list, person on V63.2
  undergoing social agency investigation V63.8
Wakefulness disorder (see also Hypersomnia) 780.54
  nonorganic origin 307.43
Waldenström's
  disease (osteochondrosis, capital femoral) 732.1
  hepatitis (lupoid hepatitis) 571.49
  hypergammaglobulinemia 273.0
  macroglobulinemia 273.3
  purpura, hypergammaglobulinemic 273.0
  syndrome (macroglobulinemia) 273.3
Waldenström-Kjellberg syndrome (sideropenic dysphagia) 280.8
Walking
  difficulty 719.7
    psychogenic 307.9
  sleep 307.46
    hysterical 300.13
Wall, abdominal - see condition
Wallenberg's syndrome (posterior inferior cerebellar artery) (see also Disease, cerebrovascular, acute) 436
Wallgren's
  disease (obstruction of splenic vein with collateral circulation) 459.89
  meningitis (see also Meningitis, aseptic) 047.9
Wandering
  acetabulum 736.39
  gallbladder 751.69
  in diseases classified elsewhere V40.31
  kidney, congenital 753.3
  organ or site, congenital NEC - see Malposition, congenital
  pacemaker (atrial) (heart) 427.89
  spleen 289.59
Wardrop's disease (with lymphangitis) 681.9
  finger 681.02
  toe 681.11
War neurosis 300.16
Wart (digitate) (filiform) (infectious) (viral) 078.10
  common 078.19
  external genital organs (venereal) 078.11
  fig 078.19
  flat 078.19
  genital 078.11
  Hassall-Henle's (of cornea) 371.41
  Henle's (of cornea) 371.41
  juvenile 078.19
  moist 078.10
  Peruvian 088.0
  plantar 078.12
  prosector (see also Tuberculosis) 017.0 ●
  seborrheic 702.19
    inflamed 702.11
  senile 702.0
  specified NEC 078.19
  syphilitic 091.3
  tuberculous (see also Tuberculosis) 017.0 ●
  venereal (female) (male) 078.11
Warthin's tumor (salivary gland) (M8561/0) 210.2
Washerwoman's itch 692.4
Wassilieff's disease (leptospiral jaundice) 100.0
Wasting
  disease 799.4
    due to malnutrition 261
    extreme (due to malnutrition) 261
  muscular NEC 728.2

Wasting (Continued)
  palsy, paralysis 335.21
  pelvic muscle 618.83
Water
  clefts 366.12
  deprivation of 994.3
  in joint (see also Effusion, joint) 719.0 ●
  intoxication 276.69
  itch 120.3
  lack of 994.3
  loading 276.69
  on
    brain - see Hydrocephalus
    chest 511.89
  poisoning 276.69
Waterbrash 787.1
Water-hammer pulse (see also Insufficiency, aortic) 424.1
Waterhouse (-Friderichsen) **disease or syndrome** 036.3
Water-losing nephritis 588.89
Watermelon stomach 537.82
  with hemorrhage 537.83
  without hemorrhage 537.82
Wax in ear 380.4
Waxy
  degeneration, any site 277.39
  disease 277.39
  kidney 277.39 [583.81]
  liver (large) 277.39
  spleen 277.39
Weak, weakness (generalized) 780.79
  arches (acquired) 734
    congenital 754.61
  bladder sphincter 596.59
  congenital 779.89
  eye muscle - see Strabismus
  facial 781.94
  foot (double) - see Weak, arches
  heart, cardiac (see also Failure, heart) 428.9
    congenital 746.9
  mind 317
  muscle (generalized) 728.87
  myocardium (see also Failure, heart) 428.9
  newborn 779.89
  pelvic fundus
    pubocervical tissue 618.81
    rectovaginal tissue 618.82
  pulse 785.9
  senile 797
  urinary stream 788.62
  valvular - see Endocarditis
Wear, worn, tooth, teeth (approximal) (hard tissues) (interproximal) (occlusal) - see also Attrition, teeth 521.10
Weather, weathered
  effects of
    cold NEC 991.9
      specified effect NEC 991.8
    hot (see also Heat) 992.9
  skin 692.74
Web, webbed (congenital) - see also Anomaly, specified type NEC
  canthus 743.63
  digits (see also Syndactylism) 755.10
  duodenal 751.5
  esophagus 750.3
  fingers (see also Syndactylism, fingers) 755.11
  larynx (glottic) (subglottic) 748.2
  neck (pterygium colli) 744.5
  Paterson-Kelly (sideropenic dysphagia) 280.8
  popliteal syndrome 756.89
  toes (see also Syndactylism, toes) 755.13
Weber's paralysis or syndrome 344.89
Weber-Christian disease or syndrome (nodular nonsuppurative panniculitis) 729.30
Weber-Cockayne syndrome (epidermolysis bullosa) 757.39
Weber-Dimitri syndrome 759.6
Weber-Gubler syndrome 344.89
Weber-Leyden syndrome 344.89

Weber-Osler syndrome (familial hemorrhagic telangiectasia) 448.0
Wedge-shaped or wedging vertebra (see also Osteoporosis) 733.00
Wegener's granulomatosis or syndrome 446.4
Wegner's disease (syphilitic osteochondritis) 090.0
Weight
  gain (abnormal) (excessive) 783.1
    during pregnancy 646.1 ●
      insufficient 646.8 ●
  less than 1000 grams at birth 765.0 ●
  loss (cause unknown) 783.21
Weightlessness 994.9
Weil's disease (leptospiral jaundice) 100.0
Weill-Marchesani syndrome (brachymorphism and ectopia lentis) 759.89
Weingarten's syndrome (tropical eosinophilia) 518.3
Weir Mitchell's disease (erythromelalgia) 443.82
Weiss-Baker syndrome (carotid sinus syncope) 337.01
Weissenbach-Thibierge syndrome (cutaneous systemic sclerosis) 710.1
Wen (see also Cyst, sebaceous) 706.2
Wenckebach's phenomenon, heart block (second degree) 426.13
Werdnig-Hoffmann syndrome (muscular atrophy) 335.0
Werlhof's disease (see also Purpura, thrombocytopenic) 287.39
Werlhof-Wichmann syndrome (see also Purpura, thrombocytopenic) 287.39
Wermer's syndrome or disease (polyendocrine adenomatosis) 258.01
Werner's disease or syndrome (progeria adultorum) 259.8
Werner-His disease (trench fever) 083.1
Werner-Schultz disease (agranulocytosis) 288.09
Wernicke's encephalopathy, disease, or syndrome (superior hemorrhagic polioencephalitis) 265.1
Wernicke-Korsakoff syndrome or psychosis (nonalcoholic) 294.0
  alcoholic 291.1
Wernicke-Posadas disease (see also Coccidioidomycosis) 114.9
Wesselsbron fever 066.3
West African fever 084.8
West Nile
  encephalitis 066.41
  encephalomyelitis 066.41
  fever 066.40
    with
      cranial nerve disorders 066.42
      encephalitis 066.41
      optic neuritis 066.42
      other complications 066.49
      other neurologic manifestations 066.42
      polyradiculitis 066.42
  virus 066.40
Westphal-Strümpell syndrome (hepatolenticular degeneration) 275.1
Wet
  brain (alcoholic) (see also Alcoholism) 303.9 ●
  feet, tropical (syndrome) (maceration) 991.4
  lung (syndrome)
    adult 518.52
    newborn 770.6
Wharton's duct - see condition
Wheal 709.8
Wheelchair confinement status V46.3
Wheezing 786.07
Whiplash injury or syndrome 847.0
Whipple's disease or syndrome (intestinal lipodystrophy) 040.2
Whipworm 127.3
"Whistling face" syndrome (craniocarpotarsal dystrophy) 759.89

SECTION 1 INDEX TO DISEASES AND INJURIES / White

White - see also condition
   kidney
      large - see Nephrosis
      small 582.9
   leg, puerperal, postpartum, childbirth 671.4●
      nonpuerperal 451.19
   mouth 112.0
   patches of mouth 528.6
   sponge nevus of oral mucosa 750.26
   spot lesions, teeth 521.01
White's disease (congenital) (keratosis follicularis) 757.39
Whitehead 706.2
Whitlow (with lymphangitis) 681.01
   herpetic 054.6
Whitmore's disease or fever (melioidosis) 025
Whooping cough 033.9
   with pneumonia 033.9 [484.3]
   due to
      Bordetella
         bronchoseptica 033.8
            with pneumonia 033.8 [484.3]
         parapertussis 033.1
            with pneumonia 033.1 [484.3]
         pertussis 033.0
            with pneumonia 033.0 [484.3]
      specified organism NEC 033.8
         with pneumonia 033.8 [484.3]
   vaccination, prophylactic (against) V03.6
Wichmann's asthma (laryngismus stridulus) 478.75
Widal (-Abrami) syndrome (acquired hemolytic jaundice) 283.9
Widening aorta (see also Ectasia, aortic) 447.70
   with aneurysm 441.9
   ruptured 441.5
Wilkie's disease or syndrome 557.1
Wilkinson-Sneddon disease or syndrome (subcorneal pustular dermatosis) 694.1
Willan's lepra 696.1
Willan-Plumbe syndrome (psoriasis) 696.1
Willebrand (-Jürgens) syndrome or thrombopathy (angiohemophilia) 286.4
Willi-Prader syndrome (hypogenital dystrophy with diabetic tendency) 759.81
Willis' disease (diabetes mellitus) (see also Diabetes) 250.0●
   due to secondary diabetes 249.0●
Wilms' tumor or neoplasm (nephroblastoma) (M8960/3) 189.0
Wilson's
   disease or syndrome (hepatolenticular degeneration) 275.1
   hepatolenticular degeneration 275.1
   lichen ruber 697.0
Wilson-Brocq disease (dermatitis exfoliativa) 695.89
Wilson-Mikity syndrome 770.7
Window - see also Imperfect, closure
   aorticopulmonary 745.0
Winged scapula 736.89
Winter - see also condition
   vomiting disease 078.82
Wise's disease 696.2
Wiskott-Aldrich syndrome (eczema-thrombocytopenia) 279.12
Withdrawal symptoms, syndrome
   alcohol 291.81
      delirium (acute) 291.0
         chronic 291.1
         newborn 760.71
   drug or narcotic 292.0
   newborn, infant of dependent mother 779.5
   steroid NEC
      correct substance properly administered 255.41
      overdose or wrong substance given or taken 962.0
Withdrawing reaction, child or adolescent 313.22
Witts' anemia (achlorhydric anemia) 280.9

Witzelsucht 301.9
Woakes' syndrome (ethmoiditis) 471.1
Wohlfart-Kugelberg-Welander disease 335.11
Woillez's disease (acute idiopathic pulmonary congestion) 518.52
Wolff-Parkinson-White syndrome (anomalous atrioventricular excitation) 426.7
Wolhynian fever 083.1
Wolman's disease (primary familial xanthomatosis) 272.7
Wood asthma 495.8
Woolly, wooly hair (congenital) (nevus) 757.4
Wool-sorters' disease 022.1
Word
   blindness (congenital) (developmental) 315.01
      secondary to organic lesion 784.61
   deafness (secondary to organic lesion) 784.69
      developmental 315.31
Worm(s) (colic) (fever) (infection) (infestation) (see also Infestation) 128.9
   guinea 125.7
   in intestine NEC 127.9
Worm-eaten soles 102.3
Worn out (see also Exhaustion) 780.79
   artificial heart valve 996.02
   cardiac defibrillator (with synchronous cardiac pacemaker) V53.32
   cardiac pacemaker lead or battery V53.31
   joint prosthesis (see also Complications, mechanical, device NEC, prosthetic NEC, joint) 996.46
"Worried well" V65.5
Wound, open (by cutting or piercing instrument) (by firearms) (cut) (dissection) (incised) (laceration) (penetration) (perforating) (puncture) (with initial hemorrhage, not internal) 879.8

> Note: For fracture with open wound, see Fracture.
>
> For laceration, traumatic rupture, tear, or penetrating wound of internal organs, such as heart, lung, liver, kidney, pelvic organs, etc., whether or not accompanied by open wound or fracture in the same region, see Injury, internal. For contused wound, see Contusion. For crush injury, see Crush. For abrasion, insect bite (nonvenomous), blister, or scratch, see Injury, superficial.
>
> Complicated includes wounds with:
>   delayed healing
>   delayed treatment
>   foreign body
>   primary infection
>
> For late effect of open wound, see Late, effect, wound, open, by site.

   abdomen, abdominal (external) (muscle) 879.2
      complicated 879.3
      wall (anterior) 879.2
         complicated 879.3
         lateral 879.4
            complicated 879.5
   alveolar (process) 873.62
      complicated 873.72
   ankle 891.0
      with tendon involvement 891.2
      complicated 891.1
   anterior chamber, eye (see also Wound, open, intraocular) 871.9
   anus 863.89
   arm 884.0
      with tendon involvement 884.2
      complicated 884.1

Wound, open (Continued)
   arm (Continued)
      forearm 881.00
         with tendon involvement 881.20
         complicated 881.10
      multiple sites - see Wound, open, multiple, upper limb
      upper 880.03
         with tendon involvement 880.23
         complicated 880.13
         multiple sites (with axillary or shoulder regions) 880.09
            with tendon involvement 880.29
            complicated 880.19
   artery - see Injury, blood vessel, by site
   auditory
      canal (external) (meatus) 872.02
         complicated 872.12
      ossicles (incus) (malleus) (stapes) 872.62
         complicated 872.72
   auricle, ear 872.01
      complicated 872.11
   axilla 880.02
      with tendon involvement 880.22
      complicated 880.12
         with tendon involvement 880.29
      involving other sites of upper arm 880.09
         complicated 880.19
   back 876.0
      complicated 876.1
   bladder - see Injury, internal, bladder
   blood vessel - see Injury, blood vessel, by site
   brain - see Injury, intracranial, with open intracranial wound
   breast 879.0
      complicated 879.1
   brow 873.42
      complicated 873.52
   buccal mucosa 873.61
      complicated 873.71
   buttock 877.0
      complicated 877.1
   calf 891.0
      with tendon involvement 891.2
      complicated 891.1
   canaliculus lacrimalis 870.8
      with laceration of eyelid 870.2
   canthus, eye 870.8
      laceration - see Laceration, eyelid
   cavernous sinus - see Injury, intracranial
   cerebellum - see Injury, intracranial
   cervical esophagus 874.4
      complicated 874.5
   cervix - see Injury, internal, cervix
   cheek(s) (external) 873.41
      complicated 873.51
      internal 873.61
         complicated 873.71
   chest (wall) (external) 875.0
      complicated 875.1
   chin 873.44
      complicated 873.54
   choroid 363.63
   ciliary body (eye) (see also Wound, open, intraocular) 871.9
   clitoris 878.8
      complicated 878.9
   cochlea 872.64
      complicated 872.74
   complicated 879.9
   conjunctiva - see Wound, open, intraocular
   cornea (nonpenetrating) (see also Wound, open, intraocular) 871.9
   costal region 875.0
      complicated 875.1
   Descemet's membrane (see also Wound, open, intraocular) 871.9
   digit(s)
      foot 893.0
         with tendon involvement 893.2
         complicated 893.1

SECTION I INDEX TO DISEASES AND INJURIES / Wound, open

Wound, open *(Continued)*
  digit(s) *(Continued)*
    hand 883.0
      with tendon involvement 883.2
      complicated 883.1
  drumhead, ear 872.61
    complicated 872.71
  ear 872.8
    canal 872.02
      complicated 872.12
    complicated 872.9
    drum 872.61
      complicated 872.71
    external 872.00
      complicated 872.10
    multiple sites 872.69
      complicated 872.79
    ossicles (incus) (malleus) (stapes) 872.62
      complicated 872.72
    specified part NEC 872.69
      complicated 872.79
  elbow 881.01
    with tendon involvement 881.21
    complicated 881.11
  epididymis 878.2
    complicated 878.3
  epigastric region 879.2
    complicated 879.3
  epiglottis 874.01
    complicated 874.11
  esophagus (cervical) 874.4
    complicated 874.5
    thoracic - *see* Injury, internal, esophagus
  Eustachian tube 872.63
    complicated 872.73
  extremity
    lower (multiple) NEC 894.0
      with tendon involvement 894.2
      complicated 894.1
    upper (multiple) NEC 884.0
      with tendon involvement 884.2
      complicated 884.1
  eye(s) (globe) - *see* Wound, open, intraocular
  eyeball NEC 871.9
    laceration (*see also* Laceration, eyeball) 871.4
    penetrating (*see also* Penetrating wound, eyeball) 871.7
  eyebrow 873.42
    complicated 873.52
  eyelid NEC 870.8
    laceration - *see* Laceration, eyelid
  face 873.40
    complicated 873.50
    multiple sites 873.49
      complicated 873.59
    specified part NEC 873.49
      complicated 873.59
  fallopian tube - *see* Injury, internal, fallopian tube
  finger(s) (nail) (subungual) 883.0
    with tendon involvement 883.2
    complicated 883.1
  flank 879.4
    complicated 879.5
  foot (any part, except toe(s) alone) 892.0
    with tendon involvement 892.2
    complicated 892.1
  forearm 881.00
    with tendon involvement 881.20
    complicated 881.10
  forehead 873.42
    complicated 873.52
  genital organs (external) NEC 878.8
    complicated 878.9
    internal - *see* Injury, internal, by site
  globe (eye) (*see also* Wound, open, eyeball) 871.9
  groin 879.4
    complicated 879.5

Wound, open *(Continued)*
  gum(s) 873.62
    complicated 873.72
  hand (except finger(s) alone) 882.0
    with tendon involvement 882.2
    complicated 882.1
  head NEC 873.8
    with intracranial injury - *see* Injury, intracranial
    due to or associated with skull fracture - *see* Fracture, skull
    complicated 873.9
    scalp - *see* Wound, open, scalp
  heel 892.0
    with tendon involvement 892.2
    complicated 892.1
  high-velocity (grease gun) - *see* Wound, open, complicated, by site
  hip 890.0
    with tendon involvement 890.2
    complicated 890.1
  hymen 878.6
    complicated 878.7
  hypochondrium 879.4
    complicated 879.5
  hypogastric region 879.2
    complicated 879.3
  iliac (region) 879.4
    complicated 879.5
  incidental to
    dislocation - *see* Dislocation, open, by site
    fracture - *see* Fracture, open, by site
    intracranial injury - *see* Injury, intracranial, with open intracranial wound
    nerve injury - *see* Injury, nerve, by site
  inguinal region 879.4
    complicated 879.5
  instep 892.0
    with tendon involvement 892.2
    complicated 892.1
  interscapular region 876.0
    complicated 876.1
  intracranial - *see* Injury, intracranial, with open intracranial wound
  intraocular 871.9
    with
      partial loss (of intraocular tissue) 871.2
      prolapse or exposure (of intraocular tissue) 871.1
    laceration (*see also* Laceration, eyeball) 871.4
    penetrating 871.7
      with foreign body (nonmagnetic) 871.6
        magnetic 871.5
      without prolapse (of intraocular tissue) 871.0
  iris (*see also* Wound, open, eyeball) 871.9
  jaw (fracture not involved) 873.44
    with fracture - *see* Fracture, jaw
    complicated 873.54
  knee 891.0
    with tendon involvement 891.2
    complicated 891.1
  labium (majus) (minus) 878.4
    complicated 878.5
  lacrimal apparatus, gland, or sac 870.8
    with laceration of eyelid 870.2
  larynx 874.01
    with trachea 874.00
      complicated 874.10
    complicated 874.11
  leg (multiple) 891.0
    with tendon involvement 891.2
    complicated 891.1
    lower 891.0
      with tendon involvement 891.2
      complicated 891.1
    thigh 890.0
      with tendon involvement 890.2
      complicated 890.1

Wound, open *(Continued)*
  leg *(Continued)*
    upper 890.0
      with tendon involvement 890.2
      complicated 890.1
  lens (eye) (alone) (*see also* Cataract, traumatic) 366.20
    with involvement of other eye structures - *see* Wound, open, eyeball
  limb
    lower (multiple) NEC 894.0
      with tendon involvement 894.2
      complicated 894.1
    upper (multiple) NEC 884.0
      with tendon involvement 884.2
      complicated 884.1
  lip 873.43
    complicated 873.53
  loin 876.0
    complicated 876.1
  lumbar region 876.0
    complicated 876.1
  malar region 873.41
    complicated 873.51
  mastoid region 873.49
    complicated 873.59
  mediastinum - *see* Injury, internal, mediastinum
  midthoracic region 875.0
    complicated 875.1
  mouth 873.60
    complicated 873.70
    floor 873.64
      complicated 873.74
    multiple sites 873.69
      complicated 873.79
    specified site NEC 873.69
      complicated 873.79
  multiple, unspecified site(s) 879.8

> Note: Multiple open wounds of sites classifiable to the same four-digit category should be classified to that category unless they are in different limbs.
>
> Multiple open wounds of sites classifiable to different four-digit categories, or to different limbs, should be coded separately.

    complicated 879.9
    lower limb(s) (one or both) (sites classifiable to more than one three-digit category in 890–893) 894.0
      with tendon involvement 894.2
      complicated 894.1
    upper limb(s) (one or both) (sites classifiable to more than one three-digit category in 880–883) 884.0
      with tendon involvement 884.2
      complicated 884.1
  muscle - *see* Sprain, by site
  nail
    finger(s) 883.0
      complicated 883.1
    thumb 883.0
      complicated 883.1
    toe(s) 893.0
      complicated 893.1
  nape (neck) 874.8
    complicated 874.9
    specified part NEC 874.8
      complicated 874.9
  nasal - *see also* Wound, open, nose
    cavity 873.22
      complicated 873.32
    septum 873.21
      complicated 873.31
    sinuses 873.23
      complicated 873.33

SECTION I INDEX TO DISEASES AND INJURIES / Wound, open

Wound, open (Continued)
   nasopharynx 873.22
      complicated 873.32
   neck 874.8
      complicated 874.9
      nape 874.8
         complicated 874.9
      specified part NEC 874.8
         complicated 874.9
   nerve - *see* Injury, nerve, by site
   non-healing surgical 998.83
   nose 873.20
      complicated 873.30
      multiple sites 873.29
         complicated 873.39
      septum 873.21
         complicated 873.31
      sinuses 873.23
         complicated 873.33
   occipital region - *see* Wound, open, scalp
   ocular NEC 871.9
      adnexa 870.9
         specified region NEC 870.8
      laceration (*see also* Laceration, ocular) 871.4
      muscle (extraocular) 870.3
         with foreign body 870.4
         eyelid 870.1
         intraocular - *see* Wound, open, eyeball
      penetrating (*see also* Penetrating wound, ocular) 871.7
   orbit 870.8
      penetrating 870.3
         with foreign body 870.4
   orbital region 870.9
   ovary - *see* Injury, internal, pelvic organs
   palate 873.65
      complicated 873.75
   palm 882.0
      with tendon involvement 882.2
      complicated 882.1
   parathyroid (gland) 874.2
      complicated 874.3
   parietal region - *see* Wound, open, scalp
   pelvic floor or region 879.6
      complicated 879.7
   penis 878.0
      complicated 878.1
   perineum 879.6
      complicated 879.7
   periocular area 870.8
      laceration of skin 870.0
   pharynx 874.4
      complicated 874.5
   pinna 872.01
      complicated 872.11
   popliteal space 891.0
      with tendon involvement 891.2
      complicated 891.1
   prepuce 878.0
      complicated 878.1
   pubic region 879.2
      complicated 879.3
   pudenda 878.8
      complicated 878.9
   rectovaginal septum 878.8
      complicated 878.9

Wound, open (Continued)
   sacral region 877.0
      complicated 877.1
   sacroiliac region 877.0
      complicated 877.1
   salivary (ducts) (glands) 873.69
      complicated 873.79
   scalp 873.0
      complicated 873.1
   scalpel, fetus or newborn 767.8
   scapular region 880.01
      with tendon involvement 880.21
      complicated 880.11
      involving other sites of upper arm 880.09
         with tendon involvement 880.29
         complicated 880.19
   sclera (*see also* Wound, open, intraocular) 871.9
   scrotum 878.2
      complicated 878.3
   seminal vesicle - *see* Injury, internal, pelvic organs
   shin 891.0
      with tendon involvement 891.2
      complicated 891.1
   shoulder 880.00
      with tendon involvement 880.20
      complicated 880.10
      involving other sites of upper arm 880.09
         with tendon involvement 880.29
         complicated 880.19
   skin NEC 879.8
      complicated 879.9
   skull - *see also* Injury, intracranial, with open intracranial wound
      with skull fracture - *see* Fracture, skull
   spermatic cord (scrotal) 878.2
      complicated 878.3
      pelvic region - *see* Injury, internal, spermatic cord
   spinal cord - *see* Injury, spinal
   sternal region 875.0
      complicated 875.1
   subconjunctival - *see* Wound, open, intraocular
   subcutaneous NEC 879.8
      complicated 879.9
   submaxillary region 873.44
      complicated 873.54
   submental region 873.44
      complicated 873.54
   subungual
      finger(s) (thumb) - *see* Wound, open, finger
      toe(s) - *see* Wound, open, toe
   supraclavicular region 874.8
      complicated 874.9
   supraorbital 873.42
      complicated 873.52
   surgical, non-healing 998.83
   temple 873.49
      complicated 873.59
   temporal region 873.49
      complicated 873.59
   testis 878.2
      complicated 878.3
   thigh 890.0
      with tendon involvement 890.2
      complicated 890.1

Wound, open (Continued)
   thorax, thoracic (external) 875.0
      complicated 875.1
   throat 874.8
      complicated 874.9
   thumb (nail) (subungual) 883.0
      with tendon involvement 883.2
      complicated 883.1
   thyroid (gland) 874.2
      complicated 874.3
   toe(s) (nail) (subungual) 893.0
      with tendon involvement 893.2
      complicated 893.1
   tongue 873.64
      complicated 873.74
   tonsil - *see* Wound, open, neck
   trachea (cervical region) 874.02
      with larynx 874.00
         complicated 874.10
      complicated 874.12
      intrathoracic - *see* Injury, internal, trachea
   trunk (multiple) NEC 879.6
      complicated 879.7
      specified site NEC 879.6
         complicated 879.7
   tunica vaginalis 878.2
      complicated 878.3
   tympanic membrane 872.61
      complicated 872.71
   tympanum 872.61
      complicated 872.71
   umbilical region 879.2
      complicated 879.3
   ureter - *see* Injury, internal, ureter
   urethra - *see* Injury, internal, urethra
   uterus - *see* Injury, internal, uterus
   uvula 873.69
      complicated 873.79
   vagina 878.6
      complicated 878.7
   vas deferens - *see* Injury, internal, vas deferens
   vitreous (humor) 871.2
   vulva 878.4
      complicated 878.5
   wrist 881.02
      with tendon involvement 881.22
      complicated 881.12

Wright's syndrome (hyperabduction) 447.8
   pneumonia 390 [517.1]

Wringer injury - *see* Crush injury, by site

Wrinkling of skin 701.8

Wrist - *see also* condition
   drop (acquired) 736.05

Wrong drug (given in error) NEC 977.9
   specified drug or substance - *see* Table of Drugs and Chemicals

Wry neck - *see also* Torticollis
   congenital 754.1

Wuchereria infestation 125.0
   bancrofti 125.0
   Brugia malayi 125.1
   malayi 125.1

Wuchereriasis 125.0

Wuchereriosis 125.0

Wuchernde struma langhans (M8332/3) 193

X

Xanthelasma 272.2
- eyelid 272.2 *[374.51]*
- palpebrarum 272.2 *[374.51]*

Xanthelasmatosis (essential) 272.2

Xanthelasmoidea 757.33

Xanthine stones 277.2

Xanthinuria 277.2

Xanthofibroma (M8831/0) - *see* Neoplasm, connective tissue, benign

Xanthoma(s), xanthomatosis 272.2
- with
  - hyperlipoproteinemia
    - type I 272.3
    - type III 272.2
    - type IV 272.1
    - type V 272.3
- bone 272.7
- craniohypophyseal 277.89
- cutaneotendinous 272.7
- diabeticorum 250.8 ● *[272.2]*
  - due to secondary diabetes 249.8 ● *[272.2]*
- disseminatum 272.7
- eruptive 272.2
- eyelid 272.2 *[374.51]*
- familial 272.7
- hereditary 272.7
- hypercholesterinemic 272.0

Xanthoma(s) *(Continued)*
- hypercholesterolemic 272.0
- hyperlipemic 272.4
- hyperlipidemic 272.4
- infantile 272.7
- joint 272.7
- juvenile 272.7
- multiple 272.7
- multiplex 272.7
- primary familial 272.7
- tendon (sheath) 272.7
- tuberosum 272.2
- tuberous 272.2
- tubo-eruptive 272.2

Xanthosis 709.09
- surgical 998.81

Xenophobia 300.29

Xeroderma (congenital) 757.39
- acquired 701.1
- eyelid 373.33
- pigmentosum 757.33
- vitamin A deficiency 264.8

Xerophthalmia 372.53
- vitamin A deficiency 264.7

Xerosis
- conjunctiva 372.53
  - with Bitôt's spot 372.53
    - vitamin A deficiency 264.1
  - vitamin A deficiency 264.0

Xerosis *(Continued)*
- cornea 371.40
  - with corneal ulceration 370.00
    - vitamin A deficiency 264.3
  - vitamin A deficiency 264.2
- cutis 706.8
- skin 706.8

Xerostomia 527.7

Xiphodynia 733.90

Xiphoidalgia 733.90

Xiphoiditis 733.99

Xiphopagus 759.4

XO syndrome 758.6

X-ray
- effects, adverse, NEC 990
- of chest
  - for suspected tuberculosis V71.2
  - routine V72.5

XXX syndrome 758.81

XXXXY syndrome 758.81

XXY syndrome 758.7

Xyloketosuria 271.8

Xylosuria 271.8

Xylulosuria 271.8

XYY syndrome 758.81

Y

Yaba monkey tumor virus 059.22
Yawning 786.09
    psychogenic 306.1
Yaws 102.9
    bone or joint lesions 102.6
    butter 102.1
    chancre 102.0
    cutaneous, less than five years after infection 102.2
    early (cutaneous) (macular) (maculopapular) (micropapular) (papular) 102.2
        frambeside 102.2
        skin lesions NEC 102.2
    eyelid 102.9 [373.4]
    ganglion 102.6
    gangosis, gangosa 102.5
    gumma, gummata 102.4
        bone 102.6

Yaws (Continued)
    gummatous
        frambeside 102.4
        osteitis 102.6
        periostitis 102.6
    hydrarthrosis 102.6
    hyperkeratosis (early) (late) (palmar) (plantar) 102.3
    initial lesions 102.0
    joint lesions 102.6
    juxta-articular nodules 102.7
    late nodular (ulcerated) 102.4
    latent (without clinical manifestations) (with positive serology) 102.8
    mother 102.0
    mucosal 102.7
    multiple papillomata 102.1
    nodular, late (ulcerated) 102.4
    osteitis 102.6

Yaws (Continued)
    papilloma, papillomata (palmar) (plantar) 102.1
    periostitis (hypertrophic) 102.6
    ulcers 102.4
    wet crab 102.1
Yeast infection (see also Candidiasis) 112.9
Yellow
    atrophy (liver) 570
        chronic 571.8
        resulting from administration of blood, plasma, serum, or other biological substance (within 8 months of administration) - see Hepatitis, viral
    fever - see Fever, yellow
    jack (see also Fever, yellow) 060.9
    jaundice (see also Jaundice) 782.4
Yersinia septica 027.8

Z

Zagari's disease (xerostomia) 527.7
Zahorsky's disease (exanthema subitum) (*see also* Exanthem subitum) 058.10
— syndrome (herpangina) 074.0
Zellweger syndrome 277.86
Zenker's diverticulum (esophagus) 530.6
Ziehen-Oppenheim disease 333.6

Zieve's syndrome (jaundice, hyperlipemia, and hemolytic anemia) 571.1
Zika fever 066.3
Zollinger-Ellison syndrome (gastric hypersecretion with pancreatic islet cell tumor) 251.5
Zona (*see also* Herpes, zoster) 053.9
Zoophilia (erotica) 302.1
Zoophobia 300.29

Zoster (herpes) (*see also* Herpes, zoster) 053.9
Zuelzer (-Ogden) anemia or syndrome (nutritional megaloblastic anemia) 281.2
Zygodactyly (*see also* Syndactylism) 755.10
Zygomycosis 117.7
Zymotic - *see* condition

SECTION II TABLE OF DRUGS AND CHEMICALS

ALPHABETIC INDEX TO POISONING AND EXTERNAL CAUSES OF ADVERSE EFFECTS OF DRUGS AND OTHER CHEMICAL SUBSTANCES

This table contains a classification of drugs and other chemical substances to identify poisoning states and external causes of adverse effects.

Each of the listed substances in the table is assigned a code according to the poisoning classification (960–989). These codes are used when there is a statement of poisoning, overdose, wrong substance given or taken, or intoxication.

The table also contains a listing of external causes of adverse effects. An adverse effect is a pathologic manifestation due to ingestion or exposure to drugs or other chemical substances (e.g., dermatitis, hypersensitivity reaction, aspirin gastritis). The adverse effect is to be identified by the appropriate code found in Section I, Index to Diseases and Injuries. An external cause code can then be used to identify the circumstances involved. The table headings pertaining to external causes are defined below:

Accidental poisoning (E850–E869)-accidental overdose of drug, wrong substance given or taken, drug taken inadvertently, accidents in the usage of drugs and biologicals in medical and surgical procedures, and to show external causes of poisonings classifiable to 980–989.

Therapeutic use (E930–E949)-a correct substance properly administered in therapeutic or prophylactic dosage as the external cause of adverse effects.

Suicide attempt (E950–E952)-instances in which self-inflicted injuries or poisonings are involved.

Assault (E961–E962)-injury or poisoning inflicted by another person with the intent to injure or kill.

Undetermined (E980–E982)-to be used when the intent of the poisoning or injury cannot be determined whether it was intentional or accidental.

The American Hospital Formulary Service (AHFS) list numbers are included in the table to help classify new drugs not identified in the table by name. The AHFS list numbers are keyed to the continually revised AHFS (American Hospital Formulary Service, 2 vol. Washington, D.C.: American Society of Hospital Pharmacists, 1959-). These listings are found in the table under the main term **Drug.**

Excluded from the table are radium and other radioactive substances. The classification of adverse effects and complications pertaining to these substances will be found in Index to Diseases and Injuries, and Index to External Causes of Injuries.

Although certain substances are indexed with one or more subentries, the majority are listed according to one use or state. It is recognized that many substances may be used in various ways, in medicine and in industry, and may cause adverse effects whatever the state of the agent (solid, liquid, or fumes arising from a liquid). In cases in which the reported data indicate a use or state not in the table, or which is clearly different from the one listed, an attempt should be made to classify the substance in the form which most nearly expresses the reported facts.

TABLE OF DRUGS AND CHEMICALS / Acetylcarbromal

| Substance | Poisoning | External Cause (E Code) |||||
		Accident	Therapeutic Use	Suicide Attempt	Assault	Undetermined
1-propanol	980.3	E860.4	—	E950.9	E962.1	E980.9
2-propanol	980.2	E860.3	—	E950.9	E962.1	E980.9
2,4-D (dichlorophenoxyacetic acid)	989.4	E863.5	—	E950.6	E962.1	E980.7
2,4-toluene diisocyanate	983.0	E864.0	—	E950.7	E962.1	E980.6
2,4,5-T (trichlorophenoxyacetic acid)	989.2	E863.5	—	E950.6	E962.1	E980.7
14-hydroxydihydromorphinone	965.09	E850.2	E935.2	E950.0	E962.0	E980.0
ABOB	961.7	E857	E931.7	E950.4	E962.0	E980.4
Abrus (seed)	988.2	E865.3	—	E950.9	E962.1	E980.9
Absinthe	980.0	E860.1	—	E950.9	E962.1	E980.9
beverage	980.0	E860.0	—	E950.9	E962.1	E980.9
Acenocoumarin, acenocoumarol	964.2	E858.2	E934.2	E950.4	E962.0	E980.4
Acepromazine	969.1	E853.0	E939.1	E950.3	E962.0	E980.3
Acetal	982.8	E862.4	—	E950.9	E962.1	E980.9
Acetaldehyde (vapor)	987.8	E869.8	—	E952.8	E962.2	E982.8
liquid	989.89	E866.8	—	E950.9	E962.1	E980.9
Acetaminophen	965.4	E850.4	E935.4	E950.0	E962.0	E980.0
Acetaminosalol	965.1	E850.3	E935.3	E950.0	E962.0	E980.0
Acetanilid(e)	965.4	E850.4	E935.4	E950.0	E962.0	E980.0
Acetarsol, acetarsone	961.1	E857	E931.1	E950.4	E962.0	E980.4
Acetazolamide	974.2	E858.5	E944.2	E950.4	E962.0	E980.4
Acetic	—	—	—	—	—	—
acid	983.1	E864.1	—	E950.7	E962.1	E980.6
with sodium acetate (ointment)	976.3	E858.7	E946.3	E950.4	E962.0	E980.4
irrigating solution	974.5	E858.5	E944.5	E950.4	E962.0	E980.4
lotion	976.2	E858.7	E946.2	E950.4	E962.0	E980.4
anhydride	983.1	E864.1	—	E950.7	E962.1	E980.6
ether (vapor)	982.8	E862.4	—	E950.9	E962.1	E980.9
Acetohexamide	962.3	E858.0	E932.3	E950.4	E962.0	E980.4
Acetomenaphthone	964.3	E858.2	E934.3	E950.4	E962.0	E980.4
Acetomorphine	965.01	E850.0	E935.0	E950.0	E962.0	E980.0
Acetone (oils) (vapor)	982.8	E862.4	—	E950.9	E962.1	E980.9
Acetophenazine (maleate)	969.1	E853.0	E939.1	E950.3	E962.0	E980.3
Acetophenetidin	965.4	E850.4	E935.4	E950.0	E962.0	E980.0
Acetophenone	982.0	E862.4	—	E950.9	E962.1	E980.9
Acetorphine	965.09	E850.2	E935.2	E950.0	E962.0	E980.0
Acetosulfone (sodium)	961.8	E857	E931.8	E950.4	E962.0	E980.4
Acetrizoate (sodium)	977.8	E858.8	E947.8	E950.4	E962.0	E980.4
Acetylcarbromal	967.3	E852.2	E937.3	E950.2	E962.0	E980.2

TABLE OF DRUGS AND CHEMICALS / Acetylcholine

Substance	Poisoning	External Cause (E Code) Accident	Therapeutic Use	Suicide Attempt	Assault	Undetermined
Acetylcholine (chloride)	971.0	E855.3	E941.0	E950.4	E962.0	E980.4
Acetylcysteine	975.5	E858.6	E945.5	E950.4	E962.0	E980.4
Acetyldigitoxin	972.1	E858.3	E942.1	E950.4	E962.0	E980.4
Acetyldihydrocodeine	965.09	E850.2	E935.2	E950.0	E962.0	E980.0
Acetyldihydrocodeinone	965.09	E850.2	E935.2	E950.0	E962.0	E980.0
Acetylene (gas) (industrial)	987.1	E868.1	—	E951.8	E962.2	E981.8
incomplete combustion of - see Carbon monoxide, fuel, utility	—	—	—	—	—	—
tetrachloride (vapor)	982.3	E862.4	—	E950.9	E962.1	E980.9
Acetyliodosalicylic acid	965.1	E850.3	E935.3	E950.0	E962.0	E980.0
Acetylphenylhydrazine	965.8	E850.8	E935.8	E950.0	E962.0	E980.0
Acetylsalicylic acid	965.1	E850.3	E935.3	E950.0	E962.0	E980.0
Achromycin	960.4	E856	E930.4	E950.4	E962.0	E980.4
ophthalmic preparation	976.5	E858.7	E946.5	E950.4	E962.0	E980.4
topical NEC	976.0	E858.7	E946.0	E950.4	E962.0	E980.4
Acidifying agents	963.2	E858.1	E933.2	E950.4	E962.0	E980.4
Acids (corrosive) NEC	983.1	E864.1	—	E950.7	E962.1	E980.6
Aconite (wild)	988.2	E865.4	—	E950.9	E962.1	E980.9
Aconitine (liniment)	976.8	E858.7	E946.8	E950.4	E962.0	E980.4
Aconitum ferox	988.2	E865.4	—	E950.9	E962.1	E980.9
Acridine	983.0	E864.0	—	E950.7	E962.1	E980.6
vapor	987.8	E869.8	—	E952.8	E962.2	E982.8
Acriflavine	961.9	E857	E931.9	E950.4	E962.0	E980.4
Acrisorcin	976.0	E858.7	E946.0	E950.4	E962.0	E980.4
Acrolein (gas)	987.8	E869.8	—	E952.8	E962.2	E982.8
liquid	989.89	E866.8	—	E950.9	E962.1	E980.9
Actaea spicata	988.2	E865.4	—	E950.9	E962.1	E980.9
Acterol	961.5	E857	E931.5	E950.4	E962.0	E980.4
ACTH	962.4	E858.0	E932.4	E950.4	E962.0	E980.4
Acthar	962.4	E858.0	E932.4	E950.4	E962.0	E980.4
Actinomycin (C) (D)	960.7	E856	E930.7	E950.4	E962.0	E980.4
Adalin (acetyl)	967.3	E852.2	E937.3	E950.2	E962.0	E980.2
Adenosine (phosphate)	977.8	E858.8	E947.8	E950.4	E962.0	E980.4
Adhesives	989.89	E866.6	—	E950.9	E962.1	E980.9
ADH	962.5	E858.0	E932.5	E950.4	E962.0	E980.4
Adicillin	960.0	E856	E930.0	E950.4	E962.0	E980.4
Adiphenine	975.1	E855.6	E945.1	E950.4	E962.0	E980.4
Adjunct, pharmaceutical	977.4	E858.8	E947.4	E950.4	E962.0	E980.4

TABLE OF DRUGS AND CHEMICALS / Alcohol

Substance	Poisoning	External Cause (E Code) Accident	Therapeutic Use	Suicide Attempt	Assault	Undetermined
Adrenal (extract, cortex or medulla) (glucocorticoids) (hormones) (mineralocorticoids)	962.0	E858.0	E932.0	E950.4	E962.0	E980.4
ENT agent	976.6	E858.7	E946.6	E950.4	E962.0	E980.4
ophthalmic preparation	976.5	E858.7	E946.5	E950.4	E962.0	E980.4
topical NEC	976.0	E858.7	E946.0	E950.4	E962.0	E980.4
Adrenalin	971.2	E855.5	E941.2	E950.4	E962.0	E980.4
Adrenergic blocking agents	971.3	E855.6	E941.3	E950.4	E962.0	E980.4
Adrenergics	971.2	E855.5	E941.2	E950.4	E962.0	E980.4
Adrenochrome (derivatives)	972.8	E858.3	E942.8	E950.4	E962.0	E980.4
Adrenocorticotropic hormone	962.4	E858.0	E932.4	E950.4	E962.0	E980.4
Adrenocorticotropin	962.4	E858.0	E932.4	E950.4	E962.0	E980.4
Adriamycin	960.7	E856	E930.7	E950.4	E962.0	E980.4
Aerosol spray - see Sprays	—	—	—	—	—	—
Aerosporin	960.8	E856	E930.8	E950.4	E962.0	E980.4
ENT agent	976.6	E858.7	E946.6	E950.4	E962.0	E980.4
ophthalmic preparation	976.5	E858.7	E946.5	E950.4	E962.0	E980.4
topical NEC	976.0	E858.7	E946.0	E950.4	E962.0	E980.4
Aethusa cynapium	988.2	E865.4	—	E950.9	E962.1	E980.9
Afghanistan black	969.6	E854.1	E939.6	E950.3	E962.0	E980.3
Aflatoxin	989.7	E865.9	—	E950.9	E962.1	E980.9
African boxwood	988.2	E865.4	—	E950.9	E962.1	E980.9
Agar (-agar)	973.3	E858.4	E943.3	E950.4	E962.0	E980.4
Agricultural agent NEC	989.89	E863.9	—	E950.6	E962.1	E980.7
Agrypnal	967.0	E851	E937.0	E950.1	E962.0	E980.1
Air contaminant(s), source or type not specified	—	—	—	—	—	—
specified type - see specific substance	987.9	E869.9	—	E952.9	E962.2	E982.9
Akee	988.2	E865.4	—	E950.9	E962.1	E980.9
Akrinol	976.0	E858.7	E946.0	E950.4	E962.0	E980.4
Alantolactone	961.6	E857	E931.6	E950.4	E962.0	E980.4
Albamycin	960.8	E856	E930.8	E950.4	E962.0	E980.4
Albumin (normal human serum)	964.7	E858.2	E934.7	E950.4	E962.0	E980.4
Albuterol	975.7	E858.6	E945.7	E950.4	E962.0	E980.4
Alcohol	980.9	E860.9	—	E950.9	E962.1	E980.9
absolute	980.0	E860.1	—	E950.9	E962.1	E980.9
beverage	980.0	E860.0	E947.8	E950.9	E962.1	E980.9
amyl	980.3	E860.4	—	E950.9	E962.1	E980.9
antifreeze	980.1	E860.2	—	E950.9	E962.1	E980.9
butyl	980.3	E860.4	—	E950.9	E962.1	E980.9

TABLE OF DRUGS AND CHEMICALS / Alcohol

Substance	Poisoning	External Cause (E Code) Accident	Therapeutic Use	Suicide Attempt	Assault	Undetermined
Alcohol *(Continued)*						
dehydrated	980.0	E860.1	—	E950.9	E862.1	E980.9
beverage	980.0	E860.0	E947.8	E950.9	E962.1	E980.9
denatured	980.0	E860.1	—	E950.9	E962.1	E980.9
deterrents	977.3	E858.8	E947.3	E950.4	E962.0	E980.4
diagnostic (gastric function)	977.8	E858.8	E947.8	E950.4	E962.0	E980.4
ethyl	980.0	E860.1	—	E950.9	E962.1	E980.9
beverage	980.0	E860.0	E947.8	E950.9	E962.1	E980.9
grain	980.0	E860.1	—	E950.9	E962.1	E980.9
beverage	980.0	E860.0	E947.8	E950.9	E962.1	E980.9
industrial	980.9	E860.9	—	E950.9	E962.1	E980.9
isopropyl	980.2	E860.3	—	E950.9	E962.1	E980.9
methyl	980.1	E860.2	—	E950.9	E962.1	E980.9
preparation for consumption	980.0	E860.0	E947.8	E950.9	E962.1	E980.9
propyl	980.3	E860.4	—	E950.9	E962.1	E980.9
secondary	980.2	E860.3	—	E950.9	E962.1	E980.9
radiator	980.1	E860.2	—	E950.9	E962.1	E980.9
rubbing	980.2	E860.3	—	E950.9	E962.1	E980.9
specified type NEC	980.8	E860.8	—	E950.9	E962.1	E980.9
surgical	980.9	E860.9	—	E950.9	E962.1	E980.9
vapor (from any type of alcohol)	987.8	E869.8	—	E952.8	E962.2	E982.8
wood	980.1	E860.2	—	E950.9	E962.1	E980.9
Alcuronium chloride	975.2	E858.6	E945.2	E950.4	E962.0	E980.4
Aldactone	974.4	E858.5	E944.4	E950.4	E962.0	E980.4
Aldicarb	989.3	E863.2	—	E950.6	E962.1	E980.7
Aldomet	972.6	E858.3	E942.6	E950.4	E962.0	E980.4
Aldosterone	962.0	E858.0	E932.0	E950.4	E962.0	E980.4
Aldrin (dust)	989.2	E863.0	—	E950.6	E962.1	E980.7
Aleve - *see* Naproxen	—	—	—	—	—	—
Algeldrate	973.0	E858.4	E943.0	E950.4	E962.0	E980.4
Alidase	963.4	E858.1	E933.4	E950.4	E962.0	E980.4
Aliphatic thiocyanates	989.0	E866.8	—	E950.9	E962.1	E980.9
Alkaline antiseptic solution (aromatic)	976.6	E858.7	E946.6	E950.4	E962.0	E980.4
Alkalinizing agents (medicinal)	963.3	E858.1	E933.3	E950.4	E962.0	E980.4
Alkalis, caustic	983.2	E864.2	—	E950.7	E962.1	E980.6
Alkalizing agents (medicinal)	963.3	E858.1	E933.3	E950.4	E962.0	E980.4
Alka-seltzer	965.1	E850.3	E935.3	E950.0	E962.0	E980.0
Alkavervir	972.6	E858.3	E942.6	E950.4	E962.0	E980.4

TABLE OF DRUGS AND CHEMICALS / Amethocaine

Substance	Poisoning	External Cause (E Code)				
		Accident	Therapeutic Use	Suicide Attempt	Assault	Undetermined
Allegron	969.05	E854.0	E939.0	E950.3	E962.0	E980.3
Allobarbital, allobarbitone	967.0	E851	E937.0	E950.1	E962.0	E980.1
Allopurinol	974.7	E858.5	E944.7	E950.4	E962.0	E980.4
Allylestrenol	962.2	E858.0	E932.2	E950.4	E962.0	E980.4
Allylisopropylacetylurea	967.8	E852.8	E937.8	E950.2	E962.0	E980.2
Allylisopropylmalonylurea	967.0	E851	E937.0	E950.1	E962.0	E980.1
Allyltribromide	967.3	E852.2	E937.3	E950.2	E962.0	E980.2
Aloe, aloes, aloin	973.1	E858.4	E943.1	E950.4	E962.0	E980.4
Alosetron	973.8	E858.4	E943.8	E950.4	E962.0	E980.4
Aloxidone	966.0	E855.0	E936.0	E950.4	E962.0	E980.4
Aloxiprin	965.1	E850.3	E935.3	E950.0	E962.0	E980.0
Alpha amylase	963.4	E858.1	E933.4	E950.4	E962.0	E980.4
Alpha-1 blockers	971.3	E855.6	E941.3	E950.4	E962.0	E980.4
Alphaprodine (hydrochloride)	965.09	E850.2	E935.2	E950.0	E962.0	E980.0
Alpha tocopherol	963.5	E858.1	E933.5	E950.4	E962.0	E980.4
Alseroxylon	972.6	E858.3	E942.6	E950.4	E962.0	E980.4
Alum (ammonium) (potassium)	983.2	E864.2	—	E950.7	E962.1	E980.6
medicinal (astringent) NEC	976.2	E858.7	E946.2	E950.4	E962.0	E980.4
Aluminium, aluminum (gel) (hydroxide)	973.0	E858.4	E943.0	E950.4	E962.0	E980.4
acetate solution	976.2	E858.7	E946.2	E950.4	E962.0	E980.4
aspirin	965.1	E850.3	E935.3	E950.0	E962.0	E980.0
carbonate	973.0	E858.4	E943.0	E950.4	E962.0	E980.4
glycinate	973.0	E858.4	E943.0	E950.4	E962.0	E980.4
nicotinate	972.2	E858.3	E942.2	E950.4	E962.0	E980.4
ointment (surgical) (topical)	976.3	E858.7	E946.3	E950.4	E962.0	E980.4
phosphate	973.0	E858.4	E943.0	E950.4	E962.0	E980.4
subacetate	976.2	E858.7	E946.2	E950.4	E962.0	E980.4
topical NEC	976.3	E858.7	E946.3	E950.4	E962.0	E980.4
Alurate	967.0	E851	E937.0	E950.1	E962.0	E980.1
Alverine (citrate)	975.1	E858.6	E945.1	E950.4	E962.0	E980.4
Alvodine	965.09	E850.2	E935.2	E950.0	E962.0	E980.0
Amanita phalloides	988.1	E865.5	—	E950.9	E962.1	E980.9
Amantadine (hydrochloride)	966.4	E855.0	E936.4	E950.4	E962.0	E980.4
Ambazone	961.9	E857	E931.9	E950.4	E962.0	E980.4
Ambenonium	971.0	E855.3	E941.0	E950.4	E962.0	E980.4
Ambutonium bromide	971.1	E855.4	E941.1	E950.4	E962.0	E980.4
Ametazole	977.8	E858.8	E947.8	E950.4	E962.0	E980.4
Amethocaine (infiltration) (topical)	968.5	E855.2	E938.5	E950.4	E962.0	E980.4
nerve block (peripheral) (plexus)	968.6	E855.2	E938.6	E950.4	E962.0	E980.4
spinal	968.7	E855.2	E938.7	E950.4	E962.0	E980.4

◀ New   ⬅ Revised   ~~deleted~~ Deleted   ● Use Additional Digit(s)

TABLE OF DRUGS AND CHEMICALS / Amethopterin

Substance	Poisoning	External Cause (E Code)				
		Accident	Therapeutic Use	Suicide Attempt	Assault	Undetermined
Amethopterin	963.1	E858.1	E933.1	E950.4	E962.0	E980.4
Amfepramone	977.0	E858.8	E947.0	E950.4	E962.0	E980.4
Amidone	965.02	E850.1	E935.1	E950.0	E962.0	E980.0
Amidopyrine	965.5	E850.5	E935.5	E950.0	E962.0	E980.0
Aminacrine	976.0	E858.7	E946.0	E950.4	E962.0	E980.4
Aminitrozole	961.5	E857	E931.5	E950.4	E962.0	E980.4
Aminoacetic acid	974.5	E858.5	E944.5	E950.4	E962.0	E980.4
Amino acids	974.5	E858.5	E944.5	E950.4	E962.0	E980.4
Aminocaproic acid	964.4	E858.2	E934.4	E950.4	E962.0	E980.4
Aminoethylisothiourium	963.8	E858.1	E933.8	E950.4	E962.0	E980.4
Aminoglutethimide	966.3	E855.0	E936.3	E950.4	E962.0	E980.4
Aminometradine	974.3	E858.5	E944.3	E950.4	E962.0	E980.4
Aminopentamide	971.1	E855.4	E941.1	E950.4	E962.0	E980.4
Aminophenazone	965.5	E850.5	E935.5	E950.0	E962.0	E980.0
Aminophenol	983.0	E864.0	—	E950.7	E962.1	E980.6
Aminophenylpyridone	969.5	E853.8	E939.5	E950.3	E962.0	E980.3
Aminophylline	975.7	E858.6	E945.7	E950.4	E962.0	E980.4
Aminopterin	963.1	E858.1	E933.1	E950.4	E962.0	E980.4
Aminopyrine	965.5	E850.5	E935.5	E950.0	E962.0	E980.0
Aminosalicylic acid	961.8	E857	E931.8	E950.4	E962.0	E980.4
Amiphenazole	970.1	E854.3	E940.1	E950.4	E962.0	E980.4
Amiquinsin	972.6	E858.3	E942.6	E950.4	E962.0	E980.4
Amisometradine	974.3	E858.5	E944.3	E950.4	E962.0	E980.4
Amitriptyline	969.05	E854.0	E939.0	E950.3	E962.0	E980.3
Ammonia (fumes) (gas) (vapor)	987.8	E869.8	—	E952.8	E962.2	E982.8
liquid (household) NEC	983.2	E861.4	—	E950.7	E962.1	E980.6
spirit, aromatic	970.89	E854.3	E940.8	E950.4	E962.0	E980.4
Ammoniated mercury	976.0	E858.7	E946.0	E950.4	E962.0	E980.4
Ammonium	—	—	—	—	—	—
carbonate	983.2	E864.2	—	E950.7	E962.1	E980.6
chloride (acidifying agent)	963.2	E858.1	E933.2	E950.4	E962.0	E980.4
expectorant	975.5	E858.6	E945.5	E950.4	E962.0	E980.4
compounds (household) NEC	983.2	E861.4	—	E950.7	E962.1	E980.6
fumes (any usage)	987.8	E869.8	—	E952.8	E962.2	E982.8
industrial	983.2	E864.2	—	E950.7	E962.1	E980.6
ichthosulfonate	976.4	E858.7	E946.4	E950.4	E962.0	E980.4
mandelate	961.9	E857	E931.9	E950.4	E962.0	E980.4
Amobarbital	967.0	E851	E937.0	E950.1	E962.0	E980.1
Amodiaquin(e)	961.4	E857	E931.4	E950.4	E962.0	E980.4
Amopyroquin(e)	961.4	E857	E931.4	E950.4	E962.0	E980.4

◀ New ◀▥ Revised ~~deleted~~ Deleted ● Use Additional Digit(s)

TABLE OF DRUGS AND CHEMICALS / Anesthesia, anesthetic NEC

Substance	Poisoning	External Cause (E Code)				
		Accident	Therapeutic Use	Suicide Attempt	Assault	Undetermined
Amphenidone	969.5	E853.8	E939.5	E950.3	E962.0	E980.3
Amphetamine	969.72	E854.2	E939.7	E950.3	E962.0	E980.3
Amphomycin	960.8	E856	E930.8	E950.4	E962.0	E980.4
Amphotericin B	960.1	E856	E930.1	E950.4	E962.0	E980.4
topical	976.0	E858.7	E946.0	E950.4	E962.0	E980.4
Ampicillin	960.0	E856	E930.0	E950.4	E962.0	E980.4
Amprotropine	971.1	E855.4	E941.1	E950.4	E962.0	E980.4
Amygdalin	977.8	E858.8	E947.8	E950.4	E962.0	E980.4
Amyl	—	—	—	—	—	—
acetate (vapor)	982.8	E862.4	—	E950.9	E962.1	E980.9
alcohol	980.3	E860.4	—	E950.9	E962.1	E980.9
nitrite (medicinal)	972.4	E858.3	E942.4	E950.4	E962.0	E980.4
Amylase (alpha)	963.4	E858.1	E933.4	E950.4	E962.0	E980.4
Amylene hydrate	980.8	E860.8	—	E950.9	E962.1	E980.9
Amylobarbitone	967.0	E851	E937.0	E950.1	E962.0	E980.1
Amylocaine	968.9	E855.2	E938.9	E950.4	E962.0	E980.4
infiltration (subcutaneous)	968.5	E855.2	E938.5	E950.4	E962.0	E980.4
nerve block (peripheral) (plexus)	968.6	E855.2	E938.6	E950.4	E962.0	E980.4
spinal	968.7	E855.2	E938.7	E950.4	E962.0	E980.4
topical (surface)	968.5	E855.2	E938.5	E950.4	E962.0	E980.4
Amytal (sodium)	967.0	E851	E937.0	E950.1	E962.0	E980.1
Analeptics	970.0	E854.3	E940.0	E950.4	E962.0	E980.4
Analgesics	965.9	E850.9	E935.9	E950.0	E962.0	E980.0
aromatic NEC	965.4	E850.4	E935.4	E950.0	E962.0	E980.0
non-narcotic NEC	965.7	E850.7	E935.7	E950.0	E962.0	E980.0
specified NEC	965.8	E850.8	E935.8	E950.0	E962.0	E980.0
Anamirta cocculus	988.2	E865.3	—	E950.9	E962.1	E980.9
Ancillin	960.0	E856	E930.0	E950.4	E962.0	E980.4
Androgens (anabolic congeners)	962.1	E858.0	E932.1	E950.4	E962.0	E980.4
Androstalone	962.1	E858.0	E932.1	E950.4	E962.0	E980.4
Androsterone	962.1	E858.0	E932.1	E950.4	E962.0	E980.4
Anemone pulsatilia	988.2	E865.4	—	E950.9	E962.1	E980.9
Anesthesia, anesthetic (general) NEC	968.4	E855.1	E938.4	E950.4	E962.0	E980.4
block (nerve) (plexus)	968.6	E855.2	E938.6	E950.4	E962.0	E980.4
gaseous NEC	968.2	E855.1	E938.2	E950.4	E962.0	E980.4
halogenated hydrocarbon derivatives NEC	968.2	E855.1	E938.2	E950.4	E962.0	E980.4
infiltration (intradermal) (subcutaneous) (submucosal)	968.5	E855.2	E938.5	E950.4	E962.0	E980.4
intravenous	968.3	E855.1	E938.3	E950.4	E962.0	E980.4
local NEC	968.9	E855.2	E938.9	E950.4	E962.0	E980.4

◂ New   ◂▥ Revised   ~~deleted~~ Deleted   ● Use Additional Digit(s)

TABLE OF DRUGS AND CHEMICALS / Anesthesia, anesthetic NEC

Substance	Poisoning	External Cause (E Code)				
		Accident	Therapeutic Use	Suicide Attempt	Assault	Undetermined
Anesthesia, anesthetic NEC *(Continued)*						
nerve blocking (peripheral) (plexus)	968.6	E855.2	E938.6	E950.4	E962.0	E980.4
rectal NEC	968.3	E855.1	E938.3	E950.4	E962.0	E980.4
spinal	968.7	E855.2	E938.7	E950.4	E962.0	E980.4
surface	968.5	E855.2	E938.5	E950.4	E962.0	E980.4
topical	968.5	E855.2	E938.5	E950.4	E962.0	E980.4
Aneurine	963.5	E858.1	E933.5	E950.4	E962.0	E980.4
Anginine - *see* Glyceryl trinitrate	971.2	E855.5	E941.2	E950.4	E962.0	E980.4
Angio-Conray	977.8	E858.8	E947.8	E950.4	E962.0	E980.4
Angiotensin	971.2	E855.5	E941.2	E950.4	E962.0	E980.4
Anhydrohydroxyprogesterone	962.2	E858.0	E932.2	E950.4	E962.0	E980.4
Anhydron	974.3	E858.5	E944.3	E950.4	E962.0	E980.4
Anileridine	965.09	E850.2	E935.2	E950.0	E962.0	E980.0
Aniline (dye) (liquid)	983.0	E864.0	—	E950.7	E962.1	E980.6
analgesic	965.4	E850.4	E935.4	E950.0	E962.0	E980.0
derivatives, therapeutic NEC	965.4	E850.4	E935.4	E950.0	E962.0	E980.0
vapor	987.8	E869.8	—	E952.8	E962.2	E982.8
Aniscoropine	971.1	E855.4	E941.1	E950.4	E962.0	E980.4
Anisindione	964.2	E858.2	E934.2	E950.4	E962.0	E980.4
Anorexic agents	977.0	E858.8	E947.0	E950.4	E962.0	E980.4
Ant (bite) (sting)	989.5	E905.5	—	E950.9	E962.1	E980.9
Antabuse	977.3	E858.8	E947.3	E950.4	E962.0	E980.4
Antacids	973.0	E858.4	E943.0	E950.4	E962.0	E980.4
Antazoline	963.0	E858.1	E933.0	E950.4	E962.0	E980.4
Anthelmintics	961.6	E857	E931.6	E950.4	E962.0	E980.4
Anthralin	976.4	E858.7	E946.4	E950.4	E962.0	E980.4
Anthramycin	960.7	E856	E930.7	E950.4	E962.0	E980.4
Antiadrenergics	971.3	E855.6	E941.3	E950.4	E962.0	E980.4
Antiallergic agents	963.0	E858.1	E933.0	E950.4	E962.0	E980.4
Antianemic agents NEC	964.1	E858.2	E934.1	E950.4	E962.0	E980.4
Antiaris toxicaria	988.2	E865.4	—	E950.9	E962.1	E980.9
Antiarteriosclerotic agents	972.2	E858.3	E942.2	E950.4	E962.0	E980.4
Antiasthmatics	975.7	E858.6	E945.7	E950.4	E962.0	E980.4
Antibiotics	960.9	E856	E930.9	E950.4	E962.0	E980.4
antifungal	960.1	E856	E930.1	E950.4	E962.0	E980.4
antimycobacterial	960.6	E856	E930.6	E950.4	E962.0	E980.4
antineoplastic	960.7	E856	E930.7	E950.4	E962.0	E980.4
cephalosporin (group)	960.5	E856	E930.5	E950.4	E962.0	E980.4
chloramphenicol (group)	960.2	E856	E930.2	E950.4	E962.0	E980.4
macrolides	960.3	E856	E930.3	E950.4	E962.0	E980.4

TABLE OF DRUGS AND CHEMICALS / Antihypertensive agents NEC

Substance	Poisoning	External Cause (E Code)				
		Accident	Therapeutic Use	Suicide Attempt	Assault	Undetermined
Antibiotics *(Continued)*						
specified NEC	960.8	E856	E930.8	E950.4	E962.0	E980.4
tetracycline (group)	960.4	E856	E930.4	E950.4	E962.0	E980.4
Anticancer agents NEC	963.1	E858.1	E933.1	E950.4	E962.0	E980.4
antibiotics	960.7	E856	E930.7	E950.4	E962.0	E980.4
Anticholinergics	971.1	E855.4	E941.1	E950.4	E962.0	E980.4
Anticholinesterase (organophosphorus) (reversible)	971.0	E855.3	E941.0	E950.4	E962.0	E980.4
Anticoagulants	964.2	E858.2	E934.2	E950.4	E962.0	E980.4
antagonists	964.5	E858.2	E934.5	E950.4	E962.0	E980.4
Anti-common cold agents NEC	975.6	E858.6	E945.6	E950.4	E962.0	E980.4
Anticonvulsants NEC	966.3	E855.0	E936.3	E950.4	E962.0	E980.4
Antidepressants	969.00	E854.0	E939.0	E950.3	E962.0	E980.3
monoamine oxidase inhibitors (MAOI)	969.01	E854.0	E939.0	E950.3	E962.0	E980.3
specified type NEC	969.09	E854.0	E939.0	E950.3	E962.0	E980.3
SSNRI (selective serotonin and norepinephrine reuptake inhibitors)	969.02	E854.0	E939.0	E950.3	E962.0	E980.3
SSRI (selective serotonin reuptake inhibitors)	969.03	E854.0	E939.0	E950.3	E962.0	E980.3
tetracyclic	969.04	E854.0	E939.0	E950.3	E962.0	E980.3
tricyclic	969.05	E854.0	E939.0	E950.3	E962.0	E980.3
Antidiabetic agents	962.3	E858.0	E932.3	E950.4	E962.0	E980.4
Antidiarrheal agents	973.5	E858.4	E943.5	E950.4	E962.0	E980.4
Antidiuretic hormone	962.5	E858.0	E932.5	E950.4	E962.0	E980.4
Antidotes NEC	977.2	E858.8	E947.2	E950.4	E962.0	E980.4
Antiemetic agents	963.0	E858.1	E933.0	E950.4	E962.0	E980.4
Antiepilepsy agent NEC	966.3	E855.0	E936.3	E950.4	E962.0	E980.4
Antifertility pills	962.2	E858.0	E932.2	E950.4	E962.0	E980.4
Antiflatulents	973.8	E858.4	E943.8	E950.4	E962.0	E980.4
Antifreeze	989.89	E866.8	—	E950.9	E962.1	E980.9
alcohol	980.1	E860.2	—	E950.9	E962.1	E980.9
ethylene glycol	982.8	E862.4	—	E950.9	E962.1	E980.9
Antifungals (nonmedicinal) (sprays)	989.4	E863.6	—	E950.6	E962.1	E980.7
medicinal NEC	961.9	E857	E931.9	E950.4	E962.0	E980.4
antibiotic	960.1	E856	E930.1	E950.4	E962.0	E980.4
topical	976.0	E858.7	E946.0	E950.4	E962.0	E980.4
Antigastric secretion agents	973.0	E858.4	E943.0	E950.4	E962.0	E980.4
Antihelmintics	961.6	E857	E931.6	E950.4	E962.0	E980.4
Antihemophilic factor (human)	964.7	E858.2	E934.7	E950.4	E962.0	E980.4
Antihistamine	963.0	E858.1	E933.0	E950.4	E962.0	E980.4
Antihypertensive agents NEC	972.6	E858.3	E942.6	E950.4	E962.0	E980.4

TABLE OF DRUGS AND CHEMICALS / Anti-infectives NEC

		External Cause (E Code)				
Substance	Poisoning	Accident	Therapeutic Use	Suicide Attempt	Assault	Undetermined
Anti-infectives NEC	961.9	E857	E931.9	E950.4	E962.0	E980.4
antibiotics	960.9	E856	E930.9	E950.4	E962.0	E980.4
specified NEC	960.8	E856	E930.8	E950.4	E962.0	E980.4
anthelmintic	961.6	E857	E931.6	E950.4	E962.0	E980.4
antimalarial	961.4	E857	E931.4	E950.4	E962.0	E980.4
antimycobacterial NEC	961.8	E857	E931.8	E950.4	E962.0	E980.4
antibiotics	960.6	E856	E930.6	E950.4	E962.0	E980.4
antiprotozoal NEC	961.5	E857	E931.5	E950.4	E962.0	E980.4
blood	961.4	E857	E931.4	E950.4	E962.0	E980.4
antiviral	961.7	E857	E931.7	E950.4	E962.0	E980.4
arsenical	961.1	E857	E931.1	E950.4	E962.0	E980.4
ENT agents	976.6	E858.7	E946.6	E950.4	E962.0	E980.4
heavy metals NEC	961.2	E857	E931.2	E950.4	E962.0	E980.4
local	976.0	E858.7	E946.0	E950.4	E962.0	E980.4
ophthalmic preparation	976.5	E858.7	E946.5	E950.4	E962.0	E980.4
topical NEC	976.0	E858.7	E946.0	E950.4	E962.0	E980.4
Anti-inflammatory agents (topical)	976.0	E858.7	E946.0	E950.4	E962.0	E980.4
Antiknock (tetraethyl lead)	984.1	E862.1	—	E950.9	E962.1	E980.9
Antilipemics	972.2	E858.3	E942.2	E950.4	E962.0	E980.4
Antimalarials	961.4	E857	E931.4	E950.4	E962.0	E980.4
Antimony (compounds) (vapor) NEC	985.4	E866.2	—	E950.9	E962.1	E980.9
anti-infectives	961.2	E857	E931.2	E950.4	E962.0	E980.4
pesticides (vapor)	985.4	E863.4	—	E950.6	E962.2	E980.7
potassium tartrate	961.2	E857	E931.2	E950.4	E962.0	E980.4
tartrated	961.2	E857	E931.2	E950.4	E962.0	E980.4
Antimuscarinic agents	971.1	E855.4	E941.1	E950.4	E962.0	E980.4
Antimycobacterials NEC	961.8	E857	E931.8	E950.4	E962.0	E980.4
antibiotics	960.6	E856	E930.6	E950.4	E962.0	E980.4
Antineoplastic agents	963.1	E858.1	E933.1	E950.4	E962.0	E980.4
antibiotics	960.7	E856	E930.7	E950.4	E962.0	E980.4
Anti-Parkinsonism agents	966.4	E855.0	E936.4	E950.4	E962.0	E980.4
Antiphlogistics	965.69	E850.6	E935.6	E950.0	E962.0	E980.0
Antiprotozoals NEC	961.5	E857	E931.5	E950.4	E962.0	E980.4
blood	961.4	E857	E931.4	E950.4	E962.0	E980.4
Antipruritics (local)	976.1	E858.7	E946.1	E950.4	E962.0	E980.4
Antipsychotic agents NEC	969.3	E853.8	E939.3	E950.3	E962.0	E980.3
Antipyretics	965.9	E850.9	E935.9	E950.0	E962.0	E980.0
specified NEC	965.8	E850.8	E935.8	E950.0	E962.0	E980.0
Antipyrine	965.5	E850.5	E935.5	E950.0	E962.0	E980.0
Antirabies serum (equine)	979.9	E858.8	E949.9	E950.4	E962.0	E980.4

TABLE OF DRUGS AND CHEMICALS / Arsenic, arsenicals NEC

Substance	Poisoning	External Cause (E Code)				
		Accident	Therapeutic Use	Suicide Attempt	Assault	Undetermined
Antirheumatics	965.69	E850.6	E935.6	E950.0	E962.0	E980.0
Antiseborrheics	976.4	E858.7	E946.4	E950.4	E962.0	E980.4
Antiseptics (external) (medicinal)	976.0	E858.7	E946.0	E950.4	E962.0	E980.4
Antistine	963.0	E858.1	E933.0	E950.4	E962.0	E980.4
Antithyroid agents	962.8	E858.0	E932.8	E950.4	E962.0	E980.4
Antitoxin, any	979.9	E858.8	E949.9	E950.4	E962.0	E980.4
Antituberculars	961.8	E857	E931.8	E950.4	E962.0	E980.4
antibiotics	960.6	E856	E930.6	E950.4	E962.0	E980.4
Antitussives	975.4	E858.6	E945.4	E950.4	E962.0	E980.4
Antivaricose agents (sclerosing)	972.7	E858.3	E942.7	E950.4	E962.0	E980.4
Antivenin (crotaline) (spider-bite)	979.9	E858.8	E949.9	E950.4	E962.0	E980.4
Antivert	963.0	E858.1	E933.0	E950.4	E962.0	E980.4
Antivirals NEC	961.7	E857	E931.7	E950.4	E962.0	E980.4
Ant poisons - *see* Pesticides	—	—	—	—	—	—
Antrol	989.4	E863.4	—	E950.6	E962.1	E980.7
fungicide	989.4	E863.6	—	E950.6	E962.1	E980.7
Apomorphine hydrochloride (emetic)	973.6	E858.4	E943.6	E950.4	E962.0	E980.4
Appetite depressants, central	977.0	E858.8	E947.0	E950.4	E962.0	E980.4
Apresoline	972.6	E858.3	E942.6	E950.4	E962.0	E980.4
Aprobarbital, aprobarbitone	967.0	E851	E937.0	E950.1	E962.0	E980.1
Apronalide	967.8	E852.8	E937.8	E950.2	E962.0	E980.2
Aqua fortis	983.1	E864.1	—	E950.7	E962.1	E980.6
Arachis oil (topical)	976.3	E858.7	E946.3	E950.4	E962.0	E980.4
cathartic	973.2	E858.4	E943.2	E950.4	E962.0	E980.4
Aralen	961.4	E857	E931.4	E950.4	E962.0	E980.4
Arginine salts	974.5	E858.5	E944.5	E950.4	E962.0	E980.4
Argyrol	976.0	E858.7	E946.0	E950.4	E962.0	E980.4
ENT agent	976.6	E858.7	E946.6	E950.4	E962.0	E980.4
ophthalmic preparation	976.5	E858.7	E946.5	E950.4	E962.0	E980.4
Aristocort	962.0	E858.0	E932.0	E950.4	E962.0	E980.4
ENT agent	976.6	E858.7	E946.6	E950.4	E962.0	E980.4
ophthalmic preparation	976.5	E858.7	E946.5	E950.4	E962.0	E980.4
topical NEC	976.0	E858.7	E946.0	E950.4	E962.0	E980.4
Aromatics, corrosive	983.0	E864.0	—	E950.7	E962.1	E980.6
disinfectants	983.0	E861.4	—	E950.7	E962.1	E980.6
Arsenate of lead (insecticide)	985.1	E863.4	—	E950.8	E962.1	E980.8
herbicide	985.1	E863.5	—	E950.8	E962.1	E980.8
Arsenic, arsenicals (compounds) (dust) (fumes) (vapor) NEC	985.1	E866.3	—	E950.8	E962.1	E980.8
anti-infectives	961.1	E857	E931.1	E950.4	E962.0	E980.4
pesticide (dust) (fumes)	985.1	E863.4	—	E950.8	E962.1	E980.8

TABLE OF DRUGS AND CHEMICALS / Arsine

Substance	Poisoning	External Cause (E Code) Accident	Therapeutic Use	Suicide Attempt	Assault	Undetermined
Arsine (gas)	985.1	E866.3	—	E950.8	E962.1	E980.8
Arsphenamine (silver)	961.1	E857	E931.1	E950.4	E962.0	E980.4
Arsthinol	961.1	E857	E931.1	E950.4	E962.0	E980.4
Artane	971.1	E855.4	E941.1	E950.4	E962.0	E980.4
Arthropod (venomous) NEC	989.5	E905.5	—	E950.9	E962.1	E980.9
Asbestos	989.81	E866.8	—	E950.9	E962.1	E980.9
Ascaridole	961.6	E857	E931.6	E950.4	E962.0	E980.4
Ascorbic acid	963.5	E858.1	E933.5	E950.4	E962.0	E980.4
Asiaticoside	976.0	E858.7	E946.0	E950.4	E962.0	E980.4
Aspidium (oleoresin)	961.6	E857	E931.6	E950.4	E962.0	E980.4
Aspirin	965.1	E850.3	E935.3	E950.0	E962.0	E980.0
Astringents (local)	976.2	E858.7	E946.2	E950.4	E962.0	E980.4
Atabrine	961.3	E857	E931.3	E950.4	E962.0	E980.4
Ataractics	969.5	E853.8	E939.5	E950.3	E962.0	E980.3
Atonia drug, intestinal	973.3	E858.4	E943.3	E950.4	E962.0	E980.4
Atophan	974.7	E858.5	E944.7	E950.4	E962.0	E980.4
Atropine	971.1	E855.4	E941.1	E950.4	E962.0	E980.4
Attapulgite	973.5	E858.4	E943.5	E950.4	E962.0	E980.4
Attenuvax	979.4	E858.8	E949.4	E950.4	E962.0	E980.4
Aureomycin	960.4	E856	E930.4	E950.4	E962.0	E980.4
ophthalmic preparation	976.5	E858.7	E946.5	E950.4	E962.0	E980.4
topical NEC	976.0	E858.7	E946.0	E950.4	E962.0	E980.4
Aurothioglucose	965.69	E850.6	E935.6	E950.0	E962.0	E980.0
Aurothioglycanide	965.69	E850.6	E935.6	E950.0	E962.0	E980.0
Aurothiomalate	965.69	E850.6	E935.6	E950.0	E962.0	E980.0
Automobile fuel	981	E862.1	—	E950.9	E962.1	E980.9
Autonomic nervous system agents NEC	971.9	E855.9	E941.9	E950.4	E962.0	E980.4
Avlosulfon	961.8	E857	E931.8	E950.4	E962.0	E980.4
Avomine	967.8	E852.8	E937.8	E950.2	E962.0	E980.2
Azacyclonol	969.5	E853.8	E939.5	E950.3	E962.0	E980.3
Azapetine	971.3	E855.6	E941.3	E950.4	E962.0	E980.4
Azaribine	963.1	E858.1	E933.1	E950.4	E962.0	E980.4
Azaserine	960.7	E856	E930.7	E950.4	E962.0	E980.4
Azathioprine	963.1	E858.1	E933.1	E950.4	E962.0	E980.4
Azosulfamide	961.0	E857	E931.0	E950.4	E962.0	E980.4
Azulfidine	961.0	E857	E931.0	E950.4	E962.0	E980.4
Azuresin	977.8	E858.8	E947.8	E950.4	E962.0	E980.4
Bacimycin	976.0	E858.7	E946.0	E950.4	E962.0	E980.4
ophthalmic preparation	976.5	E858.7	E946.5	E950.4	E962.0	E980.4

TABLE OF DRUGS AND CHEMICALS / Benzamidosalicylate

Substance	Poisoning	External Cause (E Code)				
		Accident	Therapeutic Use	Suicide Attempt	Assault	Undetermined
Bacitracin	960.8	E856	E930.8	E950.4	E962.0	E980.4
ENT agent	976.6	E858.7	E946.6	E950.4	E962.0	E980.4
ophthalmic preparation	976.5	E858.7	E946.5	E950.4	E962.0	E980.4
topical NEC	976.0	E858.7	E946.0	E950.4	E962.0	E980.4
Baking soda	963.3	E858.1	E933.3	E950.4	E962.0	E980.4
BAL	963.8	E858.1	E933.8	E950.4	E962.0	E980.4
Bamethan (sulfate)	972.5	E858.3	E942.5	E950.4	E962.0	E980.4
Bamipine	963.0	E858.1	E933.0	E950.4	E962.0	E980.4
Baneberry	988.2	E865.4	—	E950.9	E962.1	E980.9
Banewort	988.2	E865.4	—	E950.9	E962.1	E980.9
Barbenyl	967.0	E851	E937.0	E950.1	E962.0	E980.1
Barbital, barbitone	967.0	E851	E937.0	E950.1	E962.0	E980.1
Barbiturates, barbituric acid	967.0	E851	E937.0	E950.1	E962.0	E980.1
anesthetic (intravenous)	968.3	E855.1	E938.3	E950.4	E962.0	E980.4
Barium (carbonate) (chloride) (sulfate)	985.8	E866.4	—	E950.9	E962.1	E980.9
diagnostic agent	977.8	E858.8	E947.8	E950.4	E962.0	E980.4
pesticide	985.8	E863.4	—	E950.6	E962.1	E980.7
rodenticide	985.8	E863.7	—	E950.6	E962.1	E980.7
Barrier cream	976.3	E858.7	E946.3	E950.4	E962.0	E980.4
Battery acid or fluid	983.1	E864.1	—	E950.7	E962.1	E980.6
Bay rum	980.8	E860.8	—	E950.9	E962.1	E980.9
BCG vaccine	978.0	E858.8	E948.0	E950.4	E962.0	E980.4
Bearsfoot	988.2	E865.4	—	E950.9	E962.1	E980.9
Beclamide	966.3	E855.0	E936.3	E950.4	E962.0	E980.4
Bee (sting) (venom)	989.5	E905.3	—	E950.9	E962.1	E980.9
Belladonna (alkaloids)	971.1	E855.4	E941.1	E950.4	E962.0	E980.4
Bemegride	970.0	E854.3	E940.0	E950.4	E962.0	E980.4
Benactyzine	969.8	E855.8	E939.8	E950.3	E962.0	E980.3
Benadryl	963.0	E858.1	E933.0	E950.4	E962.0	E980.4
Bendrofluazide	974.3	E858.5	E944.3	E950.4	E962.0	E980.4
Bendroflumethiazide	974.3	E858.5	E944.3	E950.4	E962.0	E980.4
Benemid	974.7	E858.5	E944.7	E950.4	E962.0	E980.4
Benethamine penicillin G	960.0	E856	E930.0	E950.4	E962.0	E980.4
Benisone	976.0	E858.7	E946.0	E950.4	E962.0	E980.4
Benoquin	976.8	E858.7	E946.8	E950.4	E962.0	E980.4
Benoxinate	968.5	E855.2	E938.5	E950.4	E962.0	E980.4
Bentonite	976.3	E858.7	E946.3	E950.4	E962.0	E980.4
Benzalkonium (chloride)	976.0	E858.7	E946.0	E950.4	E962.0	E980.4
ophthalmic preparation	976.5	E858.7	E946.5	E950.4	E962.0	E980.4
Benzamidosalicylate (calcium)	961.8	E857	E931.8	E950.4	E962.0	E980.4

◀ New ⬅ Revised ~~deleted~~ Deleted ● Use Additional Digit(s)

TABLE OF DRUGS AND CHEMICALS / Benzathine penicillin

		External Cause (E Code)				
Substance	**Poisoning**	**Accident**	**Therapeutic Use**	**Suicide Attempt**	**Assault**	**Undetermined**
Benzathine penicillin	960.0	E856	E930.0	E950.4	E962.0	E980.4
Benzcarbimine	963.1	E858.1	E933.1	E950.4	E962.0	E980.4
Benzedrex	971.2	E855.5	E941.2	E950.4	E962.0	E980.4
Benzedrine (amphetamine)	969.72	E854.2	E939.7	E950.3	E962.0	E980.3
Benzene (acetyl) (dimethyl) (methyl) (solvent) (vapor)	982.0	E862.4	—	E950.9	E962.1	E980.9
hexachloride (gamma) (insecticide) (vapor)	989.2	E863.0	—	E950.6	E962.1	E980.7
Benzethonium	976.0	E858.7	E946.0	E950.4	E962.0	E980.4
Benzhexol (chloride)	966.4	E855.0	E936.4	E950.4	E962.0	E980.4
Benzilonium	971.1	E855.4	E941.1	E950.4	E962.0	E980.4
Benzin(e) - *see* Ligroin	—	—	—	—	—	—
Benziodarone	972.4	E858.3	E942.4	E950.4	E962.0	E980.4
Benzocaine	968.5	E855.2	E938.5	E950.4	E962.0	E980.4
Benzodiapin	969.4	E853.2	E939.4	E950.3	E962.0	E980.3
Benzodiazepines (tranquilizers) NEC	969.4	E853.2	E939.4	E950.3	E962.0	E980.3
Benzoic acid (with salicylic acid) (anti-infective)	976.0	E858.7	E946.0	E950.4	E962.0	E980.4
Benzoin	976.3	E858.7	E946.3	E950.4	E962.0	E980.4
Benzol (vapor)	982.0	E862.4	—	E950.9	E962.1	E980.9
Benzomorphan	965.09	E850.2	E935.2	E950.0	E962.0	E980.0
Benzonatate	975.4	E858.6	E945.4	E950.4	E962.0	E980.4
Benzothiadiazides	974.3	E858.5	E944.3	E950.4	E962.0	E980.4
Benzoylpas	961.8	E857	E931.8	E950.4	E962.0	E980.4
Benzperidol	969.5	E853.8	E939.5	E950.3	E962.0	E980.3
Benzphetamine	977.0	E858.8	E947.0	E950.4	E962.0	E980.4
Benzpyrinium	971.0	E855.3	E941.0	E950.4	E962.0	E980.4
Benzquinamide	963.0	E858.1	E933.0	E950.4	E962.0	E980.4
Benzthiazide	974.3	E858.5	E944.3	E950.4	E962.0	E980.4
Benztropine	971.1	E855.4	E941.1	E950.4	E962.0	E980.4
Benzyl	—	—	—	—	—	—
acetate	982.8	E862.4	—	E950.9	E962.1	E980.9
benzoate (anti-infective)	976.0	E858.7	E946.0	E950.4	E962.0	E980.4
morphine	965.09	E850.2	E935.2	E950.0	E962.0	E980.0
penicillin	960.0	E856	E930.0	E950.4	E962.0	E980.4
Bephenium	—	—	—	—	—	—
hydroxynapthoate	961.6	E857	E931.6	E950.4	E962.0	E980.4
Bergamot oil	989.89	E866.8	—	E950.9	E962.1	E980.9
Berries, poisonous	988.2	E865.3	—	E950.9	E962.1	E980.9
Beryllium (compounds) (fumes)	985.3	E866.4	—	E950.9	E962.1	E980.9
Beta-carotene	976.3	E858.7	E946.3	E950.4	E962.0	E980.4
Beta-Chlor	967.1	E852.0	E937.1	E950.2	E962.0	E980.2

TABLE OF DRUGS AND CHEMICALS / Bleomycin

Substance	Poisoning	External Cause (E Code) Accident	Therapeutic Use	Suicide Attempt	Assault	Undetermined
Betamethasone	962.0	E858.0	E932.0	E950.4	E962.0	E980.4
topical	976.0	E858.7	E946.0	E950.4	E962.0	E980.4
Betazole	977.8	E858.8	E947.8	E950.4	E962.0	E980.4
Bethanechol	971.0	E855.3	E941.0	E950.4	E962.0	E980.4
Bethanidine	972.6	E858.3	E942.6	E950.4	E962.0	E980.4
Betula oil	976.3	E858.7	E946.3	E950.4	E962.0	E980.4
Bhang	969.6	E854.1	E939.6	E950.3	E962.0	E980.3
Bialamicol	961.5	E857	E931.5	E950.4	E962.0	E980.4
Bichloride of mercury - see Mercury, chloride	—	—	—	—	—	—
Bichromates (calcium) (crystals) (potassium) (sodium)	983.9	E864.3	—	E950.7	E962.1	E980.6
fumes	987.8	E869.8	—	E952.8	E962.2	E982.8
Biguanide derivatives, oral	962.3	E858.0	E932.3	E950.4	E962.0	E980.4
Biligrafin	977.8	E858.8	E947.8	E950.4	E962.0	E980.4
Bilopaque	977.8	E858.8	E947.8	E950.4	E962.0	E980.4
Bioflavonoids	972.8	E858.3	E942.8	E950.4	E962.0	E980.4
Biological substance NEC	979.9	E858.8	E949.9	E950.4	E962.0	E980.4
Biperiden	966.4	E855.0	E936.4	E950.4	E962.0	E980.4
Bisacodyl	973.1	E858.4	E943.1	E950.4	E962.0	E980.4
Bishydroxycoumarin	964.2	E858.2	E934.2	E950.4	E962.0	E980.4
Bismarsen	961.1	E857	E931.1	E950.4	E962.0	E980.4
Bismuth (compounds) NEC	985.8	E866.4	—	E950.9	E962.1	E980.9
anti-infectives	961.2	E857	E931.2	E950.4	E962.0	E980.4
subcarbonate	973.5	E858.4	E943.5	E950.4	E962.0	E980.4
sulfarsphenamine	961.1	E857	E931.1	E950.4	E962.0	E980.4
Bisphosphonates	—	—	—	—	—	—
intravenous	963.1	E858.1	E933.7	E950.4	E962.0	E980.4
oral	963.1	E858.1	E933.6	E950.4	E962.0	E980.4
Bithionol	961.6	E857	E931.6	E950.4	E962.0	E980.4
Bitter almond oil	989.0	E866.8	—	E950.9	E962.1	E980.9
Bittersweet	988.2	E865.4	—	E950.9	E962.1	E930.9
Black	—	—	—	—	—	—
flag	989.4	E863.4	—	E950.6	E962.1	E980.7
henbane	988.2	E865.4	—	E950.9	E962.1	E980.9
leaf (40)	989.4	E863.4	—	E950.6	E962.1	E980.7
widow spider (bite)	989.5	E905.1	—	E950.9	E962.1	E980.9
antivenin	979.9	E858.8	E949.9	E950.4	E962.0	E980.4
Blast furnace gas (carbon monoxide from)	986	E868.8	—	E952.1	E962.2	E982.1
Bleach NEC	983.9	E864.3	—	E950.7	E962.1	E980.6
Bleaching solutions	983.9	E864.3	—	E950.7	E962.1	E980.6
Bleomycin (sulfate)	960.7	E856	E930.7	E950.4	E962.0	E980.4

TABLE OF DRUGS AND CHEMICALS / Blockain

Substance	Poisoning	Accident	Therapeutic Use	Suicide Attempt	Assault	Undetermined
Blockain	968.9	E855.2	E938.9	E950.4	E962.0	E980.4
infiltration (subcutaneous)	968.5	E855.2	E938.5	E950.4	E962.0	E980.4
nerve block (peripheral) (plexus)	968.6	E855.2	E938.6	E950.4	E962.0	E980.4
topical (surface)	968.5	E855.2	E938.5	E950.4	E962.0	E980.4
Blood (derivatives) (natural) (plasma) (whole)	964.7	E858.2	E934.7	E950.4	E962.0	E980.4
affecting agent	964.9	E858.2	E934.9	E950.4	E962.0	E980.4
specified NEC	964.8	E858.2	E934.8	E950.4	E962.0	E980.4
substitute (macromolecular)	964.8	E858.2	E934.8	E950.4	E962.0	E980.4
Blue velvet	965.09	E850.2	E935.2	E950.0	E962.0	E980.0
Bone meal	989.89	E866.5	—	E950.9	E962.1	E980.9
Bonine	963.0	E858.1	E933.0	E950.4	E962.0	E980.4
Boracic acid	976.0	E858.7	E946.0	E950.4	E962.0	E980.4
ENT agent	976.6	E858.7	E946.6	E950.4	E962.0	E980.4
ophthalmic preparation	976.5	E858.7	E946.5	E950.4	E962.0	E980.4
Borate (cleanser) (sodium)	989.6	E861.3	—	E950.9	E962.1	E980.9
Borax (cleanser)	989.6	E861.3	—	E950.9	E962.1	E980.9
Boric acid	976.0	E858.7	E946.0	E950.4	E962.0	E980.4
ENT agent	976.6	E858.7	E946.6	E950.4	E962.0	E980.4
ophthalmic preparation	976.5	E858.7	E946.5	E950.4	E962.0	E980.4
Boron hydride NEC	989.89	E866.8	—	E950.9	E962.1	E980.9
fumes or gas	987.8	E869.8	—	E952.8	E962.2	E982.8
Botox	975.3	E858.6	E945.3	E950.4	E962.0	E980.4
Brake fluid vapor	987.8	E869.8	—	E952.8	E962.2	E982.8
Brass (compounds) (fumes)	985.8	E866.4	—	E950.9	E962.1	E980.9
Brasso	981	E861.3	—	E950.9	E962.1	E980.9
Bretylium (tosylate)	972.6	E858.3	E942.6	E950.4	E962.0	E980.4
Brevital (sodium)	968.3	E855.1	E938.3	E950.4	E962.0	E980.4
British antilewisite	963.8	E858.1	E933.8	E950.4	E962.0	E980.4
Bromal (hydrate)	967.3	E852.2	E937.3	E950.2	E962.0	E980.2
Bromelains	963.4	E858.1	E933.4	E950.4	E962.0	E980.4
Bromides NEC	967.3	E852.2	E937.3	E950.2	E962.0	E980.2
Bromine (vapor)	987.8	E869.8	—	E952.8	E962.2	E982.8
compounds (medicinal)	967.3	E852.2	E937.3	E950.2	E962.0	E980.2
Bromisovalum	967.3	E852.2	E937.3	E950.2	E962.0	E980.2
Bromobenzyl cyanide	987.5	E869.3	—	E952.8	E962.2	E982.8
Bromodiphenhydramine	963.0	E858.1	E933.0	E950.4	E962.0	E980.4
Bromoform	967.3	E852.2	E937.3	E950.2	E962.0	E980.2
Bromophenol blue reagent	977.8	E858.8	E947.8	E950.4	E962.0	E980.4
Bromosalicylhydroxamic acid	961.8	E857	E931.8	E950.4	E962.0	E980.4
Bromo-seltzer	965.4	E850.4	E935.4	E950.0	E962.0	E980.0

TABLE OF DRUGS AND CHEMICALS / Butyl

Substance	Poisoning	External Cause (E Code)				
		Accident	Therapeutic Use	Suicide Attempt	Assault	Undetermined
Brompheniramine	963.0	E858.1	E933.0	E950.4	E962.0	E980.4
Bromural	967.3	E852.2	E937.3	E950.2	E962.0	E980.2
Brown spider (bite) (venom)	989.5	E905.1	—	E950.9	E962.1	E980.9
Brucia	988.2	E865.3	—	E950.9	E962.1	E980.9
Brucine	989.1	E863.7	—	E950.6	E962.1	E980.7
Brunswick green - see Copper	—	—	—	—	—	—
Bruten - see Ibuprofen	—	—	—	—	—	—
Bryonia (alba) (dioica)	988.2	E865.4	—	E950.9	E962.1	E980.9
Buclizine	969.5	E853.8	E939.5	E950.3	E962.0	E980.3
Bufferin	965.1	E850.3	E935.3	E950.0	E962.0	E980.0
Bufotenine	969.6	E854.1	E939.6	E950.3	E962.0	E980.3
Buphenine	971.2	E855.5	E941.2	E950.4	E962.0	E980.4
Bupivacaine	968.9	E855.2	E938.9	E950.4	E962.0	E980.4
infiltration (subcutaneous)	968.5	E855.2	E938.5	E950.4	E962.0	E980.4
nerve block (peripheral) (plexus)	968.6	E855.2	E938.6	E950.4	E962.0	E980.4
Busulfan	963.1	E858.1	E933.1	E950.4	E962.0	E980.4
Butabarbital (sodium)	967.0	E851	E937.0	E950.1	E962.0	E980.1
Butabarbitone	967.0	E851	E937.0	E950.1	E962.0	E980.1
Butabarpal	967.0	E851	E937.0	E950.1	E962.0	E980.1
Butacaine	968.5	E855.2	E938.5	E950.4	E962.0	E980.4
Butallylonal	967.0	E851	E937.0	E950.1	E962.0	E980.1
Butane (distributed in mobile container)	987.0	E868.0	—	E951.1	E962.2	E981.1
distributed through pipes	987.0	E867	—	E951.0	E962.2	E981.0
incomplete combustion of - see Carbon monoxide, butane	—	—	—	—	—	—
Butanol	980.3	E860.4	—	E950.9	E962.1	E980.9
Butanone	982.8	E862.4	—	E950.9	E962.1	E980.9
Butaperazine	969.1	E853.0	E939.1	E950.3	E962.0	E980.3
Butazolidin	965.5	E850.5	E935.5	E950.0	E962.0	E980.0
Butethal	967.0	E851	E937.0	E950.1	E962.0	E980.1
Butethamate	971.1	E855.4	E941.1	E950.4	E962.0	E980.4
Buthalitone (sodium)	968.3	E855.1	E938.3	E950.4	E962.0	E980.4
Butisol (sodium)	967.0	E851	E937.0	E950.1	E962.0	E980.1
Butobarbital, butobarbitone	967.0	E851	E937.0	E950.1	E962.0	E980.1
Butriptyline	969.05	E854.0	E939.0	E950.3	E962.0	E980.3
Buttercups	988.2	E865.4	—	E950.9	E962.1	E980.9
Butter of antimony - see Antimony	—	—	—	—	—	—
Butyl	—	—	—	—	—	—
acetate (secondary)	982.8	E862.4	—	E950.9	E962.1	E980.9
alcohol	980.3	E860.4	—	E950.9	E962.1	E980.9

◀ New   ⬅ Revised   ~~deleted~~ Deleted   ● Use Additional Digit(s)

TABLE OF DRUGS AND CHEMICALS / Butyl

Substance	Poisoning	External Cause (E Code) Accident	Therapeutic Use	Suicide Attempt	Assault	Undetermined
Butyl (Continued)						
carbinol	980.8	E860.8	—	E950.9	E962.1	E980.9
carbitol	982.8	E862.4	—	E950.9	E962.1	E980.9
cellosolve	982.8	E862.4	—	E950.9	E962.1	E980.9
chloral (hydrate)	967.1	E852.0	E937.1	E950.2	E962.0	E980.2
formate	982.8	E862.4	—	E950.9	E962.1	E980.9
scopolammonium bromide	971.1	E855.4	E941.1	E950.4	E962.0	E980.4
Butyn	968.5	E855.2	E938.5	E950.4	E962.0	E980.4
Butyrophenone (-based tranquilizers)	969.2	E853.1	E939.2	E950.3	E962.0	E980.3
Cacodyl, cacodylic acid - see Arsenic	—	—	—	—	—	—
Cactinomycin	960.7	E856	E930.7	E950.4	E962.0	E980.4
Cade oil	976.4	E858.7	E946.4	E950.4	E962.0	E980.4
Cadmium (chloride) (compounds) (dust) (fumes) (oxide)	985.5	E866.4	—	E950.9	E962.1	E980.9
sulfide (medicinal) NEC	976.4	E858.7	E946.4	E950.4	E962.0	E980.4
Caffeine	969.71	E854.2	E939.7	E950.3	E962.0	E980.3
Calabar bean	988.2	E865.4	—	E950.9	E962.1	E980.9
Caladium seguinium	988.2	E865.4	—	E950.9	E962.1	E980.9
Calamine (liniment) (lotion)	976.3	E858.7	E946.3	E950.4	E962.0	E980.4
Calciferol	963.5	E858.1	E933.5	E950.4	E962.0	E980.4
Calcium (salts) NEC	974.5	E858.5	E944.5	E950.4	E962.0	E980.4
acetylsalicylate	965.1	E850.3	E935.3	E950.0	E962.0	E980.0
benzamidosalicylate	961.8	E857	E931.8	E950.4	E962.0	E980.4
carbaspirin	965.1	E850.3	E935.3	E950.0	E962.0	E980.0
carbimide (citrated)	977.3	E858.8	E947.3	E950.4	E962.0	E980.4
carbonate (antacid)	973.0	E858.4	E943.0	E950.4	E962.0	E980.4
cyanide (citrated)	977.3	E858.8	E947.3	E950.4	E962.0	E980.4
dioctyl sulfosuccinate	973.2	E858.4	E943.2	E950.4	E962.0	E980.4
disodium edathamil	963.8	E858.1	E933.8	E950.4	E962.0	E980.4
disodium edetate	963.8	E858.1	E933.8	E950.4	E962.0	E980.4
EDTA	963.8	E858.1	E933.8	E950.4	E962.0	E980.4
hydrate, hydroxide	983.2	E864.2	—	E950.7	E962.1	E980.6
mandelate	961.9	E857	E931.9	E950.4	E962.0	E980.4
oxide	983.2	E864.2	—	E950.7	E962.1	E980.6
Calomel - see Mercury, chloride	—	—	—	—	—	—
Caloric agents NEC	974.5	E858.5	E944.5	E950.4	E962.0	E980.4
Calusterone	963.1	E858.1	E933.1	E950.4	E962.0	E980.4
Camoquin	961.4	E857	E931.4	E950.4	E962.0	E980.4
Camphor (oil)	976.1	E858.7	E946.1	E950.4	E962.0	E980.4
Candeptin	976.0	E858.7	E946.0	E950.4	E962.0	E980.4

TABLE OF DRUGS AND CHEMICALS / Carbon

Substance	Poisoning	External Cause (E Code) Accident	Therapeutic Use	Suicide Attempt	Assault	Undetermined
Candicidin	976.0	E858.7	E946.0	E950.4	E962.0	E980.4
Cannabinols	969.6	E854.1	E939.6	E950.3	E962.0	E980.3
Cannabis (derivatives) (indica) (sativa)	969.6	E854.1	E939.6	E950.3	E962.0	E980.3
Canned heat	980.1	E860.2	—	E950.9	E962.1	E980.9
Cantharides, cantharidin, cantharis	976.8	E858.7	E946.8	E950.4	E962.0	E980.4
Capillary agents	972.8	E858.3	E942.8	E950.4	E962.0	E980.4
Capreomycin	960.6	E856	E930.6	E950.4	E962.0	E980.4
Captodiame, captodiamine	969.5	E853.8	E939.5	E950.3	E962.0	E980.3
Caramiphen (hydrochloride)	971.1	E855.4	E941.1	E950.4	E962.0	E980.4
Carbachol	971.0	E855.3	E941.0	E950.4	E962.0	E980.4
Carbacrylamine resins	974.5	E858.5	E944.5	E950.4	E962.0	E980.4
Carbamate (sedative)	967.8	E852.8	E937.8	E950.2	E962.0	E980.2
herbicide	989.3	E863.5	—	E950.6	E962.1	E980.7
insecticide	989.3	E863.2	—	E950.6	E962.1	E980.7
Carbamazepine	966.3	E855.0	E936.3	E950.4	E962.0	E980.4
Carbamic esters	967.8	E852.8	E937.8	E950.2	E962.0	E980.2
Carbamide	974.4	E858.5	E944.4	E950.4	E962.0	E980.4
topical	976.8	E858.7	E946.8	E950.4	E962.0	E980.4
Carbamylcholine chloride	971.0	E855.3	E941.0	E950.4	E962.0	E980.4
Carbarsone	961.1	E857	E931.1	E950.4	E962.0	E980.4
Carbaryl	989.3	E863.2	—	E950.6	E962.1	E980.7
Carbaspirin	965.1	E850.3	E935.3	E950.0	E962.0	E980.0
Carbazochrome	972.8	E858.3	E942.8	E950.4	E962.0	E980.4
Carbenicillin	960.0	E856	E930.0	E950.4	E962.0	E980.4
Carbenoxolone	973.8	E858.4	E943.8	E950.4	E962.0	E980.4
Carbetapentane	975.4	E858.6	E945.4	E950.4	E962.0	E980.4
Carbimazole	962.8	E858.0	E932.8	E950.4	E962.0	E980.4
Carbinol	980.1	E860.2	—	E950.9	E962.1	E980.9
Carbinoxamine	963.0	E858.1	E933.0	E950.4	E962.0	E980.4
Carbitol	982.8	E862.4	—	E950.9	E962.1	E980.9
Carbocaine	968.9	E855.2	E938.9	E950.4	E962.0	E980.4
infiltration (subcutaneous)	968.5	E855.2	E938.5	E950.4	E962.0	E980.4
nerve block (peripheral) (plexus)	968.6	E855.2	E938.6	E950.4	E962.0	E980.4
topical (surface)	968.5	E855.2	E938.5	E950.4	E962.0	E980.4
Carbol-fuchsin solution	976.0	E858.7	E946.0	E950.4	E962.0	E980.4
Carbolic acid (see also Phenol)	983.0	E864.0	—	E950.7	E962.1	E980.6
Carbomycin	960.8	E856	E930.8	E950.4	E962.0	E980.4
Carbon	—	—	—	—	—	—
bisulfide (liquid) (vapor)	982.2	E862.4	—	E950.9	E962.1	E980.9

TABLE OF DRUGS AND CHEMICALS / Carbon

		External Cause (E Code)				
Substance	Poisoning	Accident	Therapeutic Use	Suicide Attempt	Assault	Undetermined
Carbon *(Continued)*						
dioxide (gas)	987.8	E869.8	—	E952.8	E962.2	E982.8
disulfide (liquid) (vapor)	982.2	E862.4	—	E950.9	E962.1	E980.9
monoxide (from incomplete combustion of) (in) NEC	986	E868.9	—	E952.1	E962.2	E982.1
blast furnace gas	986	E868.8	—	E952.1	E962.2	E982.1
butane (distributed in mobile container)	986	E868.0	—	E951.1	E962.2	E981.1
distributed through pipes	986	E867	—	E951.0	E962.2	E981.0
charcoal fumes	986	E868.3	—	E952.1	E962.2	E982.1
coal						
gas (piped)	986	E867	—	E951.0	E962.2	E981.0
solid (in domestic stoves, fireplaces)	986	E868.3	—	E952.1	E962.2	E982.1
coke (in domestic stoves, fireplaces)	986	E868.3	—	E952.1	E962.2	E982.1
exhaust gas (motor) not in transit	986	E868.2	—	E952.0	E962.2	E982.0
combustion engine, any not in watercraft	986	E868.2	—	E952.0	E962.2	E982.0
farm tractor, not in transit	986	E868.2	—	E952.0	E962.2	E982.0
gas engine	986	E868.2	—	E952.0	E962.2	E982.0
motor pump	986	E868.2	—	E952.0	E962.2	E982.0
motor vehicle, not in transit	986	E868.2	—	E952.0	E962.2	E982.0
fuel (in domestic use)	986	E868.3	—	E952.1	E962.2	E982.1
gas (piped)	986	E867	—	E951.0	E962.2	E981.0
in mobile container	986	E868.0	—	E951.1	E962.2	E981.1
utility	986	E868.1	—	E951.8	E962.2	E981.1
in mobile container	986	E868.0	—	E951.1	E962.2	E981.1
piped (natural)	986	E867	—	E951.0	E962.2	E981.0
illuminating gas	986	E868.1	—	E951.8	E962.2	E981.8
industrial fuels or gases, any	986	E868.8	—	E952.1	E962.2	E982.1
kerosene (in domestic stoves, fireplaces)	986	E868.3	—	E952.1	E962.2	E982.1
kiln gas or vapor	986	E868.8	—	E952.1	E962.2	E982.1
motor exhaust gas, not in transit	986	E868.2	—	E952.0	E962.2	E982.0
piped gas (manufactured) (natural)	986	E867	—	E951.0	E962.2	E981.0
producer gas	986	E868.8	—	E952.1	E962.2	E982.1
propane (distributed in mobile container)	986	E868.0	—	E951.1	E962.2	E981.1
distributed through pipes	986	E867	—	E951.0	E962.2	E981.0
specified source NEC	986	E868.8	—	E952.1	E962.2	E982.1
stove gas	986	E868.1	—	E951.8	E962.2	E981.8
piped	986	E867	—	E951.0	E962.2	E981.0
utility gas	986	E868.1	—	E951.8	E962.2	E981.8
piped	986	E867	—	E951.0	E962.2	E981.0

TABLE OF DRUGS AND CHEMICALS / Cathomycin

Substance	Poisoning	External Cause (E Code)				
		Accident	Therapeutic Use	Suicide Attempt	Assault	Undetermined
Carbon *(Continued)*						
monoxide (from incomplete combustion of) (in) NEC *(Continued)*						
water gas	986	E868.1	—	E951.8	E962.2	E981.8
wood (in domestic stoves, fireplaces)	986	E868.3	—	E952.1	E962.2	E982.1
tetrachloride (vapor) NEC	987.8	E869.8	—	E952.8	E962.2	E982.8
liquid (cleansing agent) NEC	982.1	E861.3	—	E950.9	E962.1	E980.9
solvent	982.1	E862.4	—	E950.9	E962.1	E980.9
Carbonic acid (gas)	987.8	E869.8	—	E952.8	E962.2	E982.8
anhydrase inhibitors	974.2	E858.5	E944.2	E950.4	E962.0	E980.4
Carbowax	976.3	E858.7	E946.3	E950.4	E962.0	E980.4
Carbrital	967.0	E851	E937.0	E950.1	E962.0	E980.1
Carbromal (derivatives)	967.3	E852.2	E937.3	E950.2	E962.0	E980.2
Cardiac	—	—	—	—	—	—
depressants	972.0	E858.3	E942.0	E950.4	E962.0	E980.4
rhythm regulators	972.0	E858.3	E942.0	E950.4	E962.0	E980.4
Cardiografin	977.8	E858.8	E947.8	E950.4	E962.0	E980.4
Cardio-green	977.8	E858.8	E947.8	E950.4	E962.0	E980.4
Cardiotonic glycosides	972.1	E858.3	E942.1	E950.4	E962.0	E980.4
Cardiovascular agents NEC	972.9	E858.3	E942.9	E950.4	E962.0	E980.4
Cardrase	974.2	E858.5	E944.2	E950.4	E962.0	E980.4
Carfusin	976.0	E858.7	E946.0	E950.4	E962.0	E980.4
Carisoprodol	968.0	E855.1	E938.0	E950.4	E962.0	E980.4
Carmustine	963.1	E858.1	E933.1	E950.4	E962.0	E980.4
Carotene	963.5	E858.1	E933.5	E950.4	E962.0	E980.4
Carphenazine (maleate)	969.1	E853.0	E939.1	E950.3	E962.0	E980.3
Carter's Little Pills	973.1	E858.4	E943.1	E950.4	E962.0	E980.4
Cascara (sagrada)	973.1	E858.4	E943.1	E950.4	E962.0	E980.4
Cassava	988.2	E865.4	—	E950.9	E962.1	E980.9
Castellani's paint	976.0	E858.7	E946.0	E950.4	E962.0	E980.4
Castor	—	—	—	—	—	—
bean	988.2	E865.3	—	E950.9	E962.1	E980.9
oil	973.1	E858.4	E943.1	E950.4	E962.0	E980.4
Caterpillar (sting)	989.5	E905.5	—	E950.9	E962.1	E980.9
Catha (edulis)	970.89	E854.3	E940.8	E950.4	E962.0	E980.4
Cathartics NEC	973.3	E858.4	E943.3	E950.4	E962.0	E980.4
contact	973.1	E858.4	E943.1	E950.4	E962.0	E980.4
emollient	973.2	E858.4	E943.2	E950.4	E962.0	E980.4
intestinal irritants	973.1	E858.4	E943.1	E950.4	E962.0	E980.4
saline	973.3	E858.4	E943.3	E950.4	E962.0	E980.4
Cathomycin	960.8	E856	E930.8	E950.4	E962.0	E980.4

TABLE OF DRUGS AND CHEMICALS / Caustic(s)

Substance	Poisoning	External Cause (E Code)				
		Accident	Therapeutic Use	Suicide Attempt	Assault	Undetermined
Caustic(s)	983.9	E864.4	—	E950.7	E962.1	E980.6
alkali	983.2	E864.2	—	E950.7	E962.1	E980.6
hydroxide	983.2	E864.2	—	E950.7	E962.1	E980.6
potash	983.2	E864.2	—	E950.7	E962.1	E980.6
soda	983.2	E864.2	—	E950.7	E962.1	E980.6
specified NEC	983.9	E864.3	—	E950.7	E962.1	E980.6
Ceepryn	976.0	E858.7	E946.0	E950.4	E962.0	E980.4
ENT agent	976.6	E858.7	E946.6	E950.4	E962.0	E980.4
lozenges	976.6	E858.7	E946.6	E950.4	E962.0	E980.4
Celestone	962.0	E858.0	E932.0	E950.4	E962.0	E980.4
topical	976.0	E858.7	E946.0	E950.4	E962.0	E980.4
Cellosolve	982.8	E862.4	—	E950.9	E962.1	E980.9
Cell stimulants and proliferants	976.8	E858.7	E946.8	E950.4	E962.0	E980.4
Cellulose derivatives, cathartic	973.3	E858.4	E943.3	E950.4	E962.0	E980.4
nitrates (topical)	976.3	E858.7	E946.3	E950.4	E962.0	E980.4
Centipede (bite)	989.5	E905.4	—	E950.9	E962.1	E980.9
Central nervous system	—	—	—	—	—	—
depressants	968.4	E855.1	E938.4	E950.4	E962.0	E980.4
anesthetic (general) NEC	968.4	E855.1	E938.4	E950.4	E962.0	E980.4
gases NEC	968.2	E855.1	E938.2	E950.4	E962.0	E980.4
intravenous	968.3	E855.1	E938.3	E950.4	E962.0	E980.4
barbiturates	967.0	E851	E937.0	E950.1	E962.0	E980.1
bromides	967.3	E852.2	E937.3	E950.2	E962.0	E980.2
cannabis sativa	969.6	E854.1	E939.6	E950.3	E962.0	E980.3
chloral hydrate	967.1	E852.0	E937.1	E950.2	E962.0	E980.2
hallucinogenics	969.6	E854.1	E939.6	E950.3	E962.0	E980.3
hypnotics	967.9	E852.9	E937.9	E950.2	E962.0	E980.2
specified NEC	967.8	E852.8	E937.8	E950.2	E962.0	E980.2
muscle relaxants	968.0	E855.1	E938.0	E950.4	E962.0	E980.4
paraldehyde	967.2	E852.1	E937.2	E950.2	E962.0	E980.2
sedatives	967.9	E852.9	E937.9	E950.2	E962.0	E980.2
mixed NEC	967.6	E852.5	E937.6	E950.2	E962.0	E980.2
specified NEC	967.8	E852.8	E937.8	E950.2	E962.0	E980.2
muscle-tone depressants	968.0	E855.1	E938.0	E950.4	E962.0	E980.4
stimulants	970.9	E854.3	E940.9	E950.4	E962.0	E980.4
amphetamines	969.72	E854.2	E939.7	E950.3	E962.0	E980.3
analeptics	970.0	E854.3	E940.0	E950.4	E962.0	E980.4
antidepressants	969.00	E854.0	E939.0	E950.3	E962.0	E980.3
opiate antagonists	970.1	E854.3	E940.0	E950.4	E962.0	E980.4
specified NEC	970.89	E854.3	E940.8	E950.4	E962.0	E980.4

◀ New ◀|||| Revised ~~deleted~~ Deleted ● Use Additional Digit(s)

TABLE OF DRUGS AND CHEMICALS / Chloramphenicol

Substance	Poisoning	External Cause (E Code)				
		Accident	Therapeutic Use	Suicide Attempt	Assault	Undetermined
Cephalexin	960.5	E856	E930.5	E950.4	E962.0	E980.4
Cephaloglycin	960.5	E856	E930.5	E950.4	E962.0	E980.4
Cephaloridine	960.5	E856	E930.5	E950.4	E962.0	E980.4
Cephalosporins NEC	960.5	E856	E930.5	E950.4	E962.0	E980.4
N (adicillin)	960.0	E856	E930.0	E950.4	E962.0	E980.4
Cephalothin (sodium)	960.5	E856	E930.5	E950.4	E962.0	E980.4
Cerbera (odallam)	988.2	E865.4	—	E950.9	E962.1	E980.9
Cerberin	972.1	E858.3	E942.1	E950.4	E962.0	E980.4
Cerebral stimulants	970.9	E854.3	E940.9	E950.4	E962.0	E980.4
psychotherapeutic	969.79	E854.2	E939.7	E950.3	E962.0	E980.3
specified NEC	970.89	E854.3	E940.8	E950.4	E962.0	E980.4
Cetalkonium (chloride)	976.0	E858.7	E946.0	E950.4	E962.0	E980.4
Cetoxime	963.0	E858.1	E933.0	E950.4	E962.0	E980.4
Cetrimide	976.2	E858.7	E946.2	E950.4	E962.0	E980.4
Cetylpyridinium	976.0	E858.7	E946.0	E950.4	E962.0	E980.4
ENT agent	976.6	E858.7	E946.6	E950.4	E962.0	E980.4
lozenges	976.6	E858.7	E946.6	E950.4	E962.0	E980.4
Cevadilla - see Sabadilla	—	—	—	—	—	—
Cevitamic acid	963.5	E858.1	E933.5	E950.4	E962.0	E980.4
Chalk, precipitated	973.0	E858.4	E943.0	E950.4	E962.0	E980.4
Charcoal	—	—	—	—	—	—
fumes (carbon monoxide)	986	E868.3	—	E952.1	E962.2	E982.1
industrial	986	E868.8	—	E952.1	E962.2	E982.1
medicinal (activated)	973.0	E858.4	E943.0	E950.4	E962.0	E980.4
Chelating agents NEC	977.2	E858.8	E947.2	E950.4	E962.0	E980.4
Chelidonium majus	988.2	E865.4	—	E950.9	E962.1	E980.9
Chemical substance	989.9	E866.9	—	E950.9	E962.1	E980.9
specified NEC	989.89	E866.8	—	E950.9	E962.1	E980.9
Chemotherapy, antineoplastic	963.1	E858.1	E933.1	E950.4	E962.0	E980.4
Chenopodium (oil)	961.6	E857	E931.6	E950.4	E962.0	E980.4
Cherry laurel	988.2	E865.4	—	E950.9	E962.1	E980.9
Chiniofon	961.3	E857	E931.3	E950.4	E962.0	E980.4
Chlophedianol	975.4	E858.6	E945.4	E950.4	E962.0	E980.4
Chloral (betaine) (formamide) (hydrate)	967.1	E852.0	E937.1	E950.2	E962.0	E980.2
Chloralamide	967.1	E852.0	E937.1	E950.2	E962.0	E980.2
Chlorambucil	963.1	E858.1	E933.1	E950.4	E962.0	E980.4
Chloramphenicol	960.2	E856	E930.2	E950.4	E962.0	E980.4
ENT agent	976.6	E858.7	E946.6	E950.4	E962.0	E980.4
ophthalmic preparation	976.5	E858.7	E946.5	E950.4	E962.0	E980.4
topical NEC	976.0	E858.7	E946.0	E950.4	E962.0	E980.4

TABLE OF DRUGS AND CHEMICALS / Chlorate(s) NEC

		External Cause (E Code)				
Substance	**Poisoning**	**Accident**	**Therapeutic Use**	**Suicide Attempt**	**Assault**	**Undetermined**
Chlorate(s) (potassium) (sodium) NEC	983.9	E864.3	—	E950.7	E962.1	E980.6
herbicides	989.4	E863.5	—	E950.6	E962.1	E980.7
Chlorcyclizine	963.0	E858.1	E933.0	E950.4	E962.0	E980.4
Chlordan(e) (dust)	989.2	E863.0	—	E950.6	E962.1	E980.7
Chlordantoin	976.0	E858.7	E946.0	E950.4	E962.0	E980.4
Chlordiazepoxide	969.4	E853.2	E939.4	E950.3	E962.0	E980.3
Chloresium	976.8	E858.7	E946.8	E950.4	E962.0	E980.4
Chlorethiazol	967.1	E852.0	E937.1	E950.2	E962.0	E980.2
Chlorethyl - see Ethyl, chloride	—	—	—	—	—	—
Chloretone	967.1	E852.0	E937.1	E950.2	E962.0	E980.2
Chlorex	982.3	E862.4	—	E950.9	E962.1	E980.9
Chlorhexadol	967.1	E852.0	E937.1	E950.2	E962.0	E980.2
Chlorhexidine (hydrochloride)	976.0	E858.7	E946.0	E950.4	E962.0	E980.4
Chlorhydroxyquinolin	976.0	E858.7	E946.0	E950.4	E962.0	E980.4
Chloride of lime (bleach)	983.9	E864.3	—	E950.7	E962.1	E980.6
Chlorinated	—	—	—	—	—	—
camphene	989.2	E863.0	—	E950.6	E962.1	E980.7
diphenyl	989.89	E866.8	—	E950.9	E962.1	E980.9
hydrocarbons NEC	989.2	E863.0	—	E950.6	E962.1	E980.7
solvent	982.3	E862.4	—	E950.9	E962.1	E980.9
lime (bleach)	983.9	E864.3	—	E950.7	E962.1	E980.6
naphthalene - see Naphthalene	—	—	—	—	—	—
pesticides NEC	989.2	E863.0	—	E950.6	E962.1	E980.7
soda - see Sodium, hypochlorite	—	—	—	—	—	—
Chlorine (fumes) (gas)	987.6	E869.8	—	E952.8	E962.2	E982.8
bleach	983.9	E864.3	—	E950.7	E962.1	E980.6
compounds NEC	983.9	E864.3	—	E950.7	E962.1	E980.6
disinfectant	983.9	E861.4	—	E950.7	E962.1	E980.6
releasing agents NEC	983.9	E864.3	—	E950.7	E962.1	E980.6
Chlorisondamine	972.3	E858.3	E942.3	E950.4	E962.0	E980.4
Chlormadinone	962.2	E858.0	E932.2	E950.4	E962.0	E980.4
Chlormerodrin	974.0	E858.5	E944.0	E950.4	E962.0	E980.4
Chlormethiazole	967.1	E852.0	E937.1	E950.2	E962.0	E980.2
Chlormethylenecycline	960.4	E856	E930.4	E950.4	E962.0	E980.4
Chlormezanone	969.5	E853.8	E939.5	E950.3	E962.0	E980.3
Chloroacetophenone	987.5	E869.3	—	E952.8	E962.2	E982.8
Chloroaniline	983.0	E864.0	—	E950.7	E962.1	E980.6
Chlorobenzene, chlorobenzol	982.0	E862.4	—	E950.9	E962.1	E980.9
Chlorobutanol	967.1	E852.0	E937.1	E950.2	E962.0	E980.2

TABLE OF DRUGS AND CHEMICALS / Chlorproguanil

Substance	Poisoning	External Cause (E Code) Accident	Therapeutic Use	Suicide Attempt	Assault	Undetermined
Chlorodinitrobenzene	983.0	E864.0	—	E950.7	E962.1	E980.6
dust or vapor	987.8	E869.8	—	E952.8	E962.2	E982.8
Chloroethane - see Ethyl, chloride	—	—	—	—	—	—
Chloroform (fumes) (vapor)	987.8	E869.8	—	E952.8	E962.2	E982.8
anesthetic (gas)	968.2	E855.1	E938.2	E950.4	E962.0	E980.4
liquid NEC	968.4	E855.1	E938.4	E950.4	E962.0	E980.4
solvent	982.3	E862.4	—	E950.9	E962.1	E980.9
Chloroguanide	961.4	E857	E931.4	E950.4	E962.0	E980.4
Chloromycetin	960.2	E856	E930.2	E950.4	E962.0	E980.4
ENT agent	976.6	E858.7	E946.6	E950.4	E962.0	E980.4
ophthalmic preparation	976.5	E858.7	E946.5	E950.4	E962.0	E980.4
otic solution	976.6	E858.7	E946.6	E950.4	E962.0	E980.4
topical NEC	976.0	E858.7	E946.0	E950.4	E962.0	E980.4
Chloronitrobenzene	983.0	E864.0	—	E950.7	E962.1	E980.6
dust or vapor	987.8	E869.8	—	E952.8	E962.2	E982.8
Chlorophenol	983.0	E864.0	—	E950.7	E962.1	E980.6
Chlorophenothane	989.2	E863.0	—	E950.6	E962.1	E980.7
Chlorophyll (derivatives)	976.8	E858.7	E946.8	E950.4	E962.0	E980.4
Chloropicrin (fumes)	987.8	E869.8	—	E952.8	E962.2	E982.8
fumigant	989.4	E863.8	—	E950.6	E962.1	E980.7
fungicide	989.4	E863.6	—	E950.6	E962.1	E980.7
pesticide (fumes)	989.4	E863.4	—	E950.6	E962.1	E980.7
Chloroprocaine	968.9	E855.2	E938.9	E950.4	E962.0	E980.4
infiltration (subcutaneous)	968.5	E855.2	E938.5	E950.4	E962.0	E980.4
nerve block (peripheral) (plexus)	968.6	E855.2	E938.6	E950.4	E962.0	E980.4
Chloroptic	976.5	E858.7	E946.5	E950.4	E962.0	E980.4
Chloropurine	963.1	E858.1	E933.1	E950.4	E962.0	E980.4
Chloroquine (hydrochloride) (phosphate)	961.4	E857	E931.4	E950.4	E962.0	E980.4
Chlorothen	963.0	E858.1	E933.0	E950.4	E962.0	E980.4
Chlorothiazide	974.3	E858.5	E944.3	E950.4	E962.0	E980.4
Chlorotrianisene	962.2	E858.0	E932.2	E950.4	E962.0	E980.4
Chlorovinyldichloroarsine	985.1	E866.3	—	E950.8	E962.1	E980.8
Chloroxylenol	976.0	E858.7	E946.0	E950.4	E962.0	E980.4
Chlorphenesin (carbamate)	968.0	E855.1	E938.0	E950.4	E962.0	E980.4
topical (antifungal)	976.0	E858.7	E946.0	E950.4	E962.0	E980.4
Chlorpheniramine	963.0	E858.1	E933.0	E950.4	E962.0	E980.4
Chlorphenoxamine	966.4	E855.0	E936.4	E950.4	E962.0	E980.4
Chlorphentermine	977.0	E858.8	E947.0	E950.4	E962.0	E980.4
Chlorproguanil	961.4	E857	E931.4	E950.4	E962.0	E980.4

◀ New   ◀▥ Revised   ~~deleted~~ Deleted   ● Use Additional Digit(s)

TABLE OF DRUGS AND CHEMICALS / Chlorpromazine

Substance	Poisoning	External Cause (E Code) Accident	Therapeutic Use	Suicide Attempt	Assault	Undetermined
Chlorpromazine	969.1	E853.0	E939.1	E950.3	E962.0	E980.3
Chlorpropamide	962.3	E858.0	E932.3	E950.4	E962.0	E980.4
Chlorprothixene	969.3	E853.8	E939.3	E950.3	E962.0	E980.3
Chlorquinaldol	976.0	E858.7	E946.0	E950.4	E962.0	E980.4
Chlortetracycline	960.4	E856	E930.4	E950.4	E962.0	E980.4
Chlorthalidone	974.4	E858.5	E944.4	E950.4	E962.0	E980.4
Chlortrianisene	962.2	E858.0	E932.2	E950.4	E962.0	E980.4
Chlor-Trimeton	963.0	E858.1	E933.0	E950.4	E962.0	E980.4
Chlorzoxazone	968.0	E855.1	E938.0	E950.4	E962.0	E980.4
Choke damp	987.8	E869.8	—	E952.8	E962.2	E982.8
Cholebrine	977.8	E858.8	E947.8	E950.4	E962.0	E980.4
Cholera vaccine	978.2	E858.8	E948.2	E950.4	E962.0	E980.4
Cholesterol-lowering agents	972.2	E858.3	E942.2	E950.4	E962.0	E980.4
Cholestyramine (resin)	972.2	E858.3	E942.2	E950.4	E962.0	E980.4
Cholic acid	973.4	E858.4	E943.4	E950.4	E962.0	E980.4
Choline	—	—	—	—	—	—
dihydrogen citrate	977.1	E858.8	E947.1	E950.4	E962.0	E980.4
salicylate	965.1	E850.3	E935.3	E950.0	E962.0	E980.0
theophyllinate	974.1	E858.5	E944.1	E950.4	E962.0	E980.4
Cholinergics	971.0	E855.3	E941.0	E950.4	E962.0	E980.4
Cholografin	977.8	E858.8	E947.8	E950.4	E962.0	E980.4
Chorionic gonadotropin	962.4	E858.0	E932.4	E950.4	E962.0	E980.4
Chromates	983.9	E864.3	—	E950.7	E962.1	E980.6
dust or mist	987.8	E869.8	—	E952.8	E962.2	E982.8
lead	984.0	E866.0	—	E950.9	E962.1	E980.9
paint	984.0	E861.5	—	E950.9	E962.1	E980.9
Chromic acid	983.9	E864.3	—	E950.7	E962.1	E980.6
dust or mist	987.8	E869.8	—	E952.8	E962.2	E982.8
Chromium	985.6	E866.4	—	E950.9	E962.1	E980.9
compounds - see Chromates	—	—	—	—	—	—
Chromonar	972.4	E858.3	E942.4	E950.4	E962.0	E980.4
Chromyl chloride	983.9	E864.3	—	E950.7	E962.1	E980.6
Chrysarobin (ointment)	976.4	E858.7	E946.4	E950.4	E962.0	E980.4
Chrysazin	973.1	E858.4	E943.1	E950.4	E962.0	E980.4
Chymar	963.4	E858.1	E933.4	E950.4	E962.0	E980.4
ophthalmic preparation	976.5	E858.7	E946.5	E950.4	E962.0	E980.4
Chymotrypsin	963.4	E858.1	E933.4	E950.4	E962.0	E980.4
ophthalmic preparation	976.5	E858.7	E946.5	E950.4	E962.0	E980.4
Cicuta maculata or virosa	988.2	E865.4	—	E950.9	E962.1	E980.9

◀ New ⬅ Revised ~~deleted~~ Deleted ● Use Additional Digit(s)

TABLE OF DRUGS AND CHEMICALS / Coal

Substance	Poisoning	External Cause (E Code)				
		Accident	Therapeutic Use	Suicide Attempt	Assault	Undetermined
Cigarette lighter fluid	981	E862.1	—	E950.9	E962.1	E980.9
Cinchocaine (spinal)	968.7	E855.2	E938.7	E950.4	E962.0	E980.4
topical (surface)	968.5	E855.2	E938.5	E950.4	E962.0	E980.4
Cinchona	961.4	E857	E931.4	E950.4	E962.0	E980.4
Cinchonine alkaloids	961.4	E857	E931.4	E950.4	E962.0	E980.4
Cinchophen	974.7	E858.5	E944.7	E950.4	E962.0	E980.4
Cinnarizine	963.0	E858.1	E933.0	E950.4	E962.0	E980.4
Citanest	968.9	E855.2	E938.9	E950.4	E962.0	E980.4
infiltration (subcutaneous)	968.5	E855.2	E938.5	E950.4	E962.0	E980.4
nerve block (peripheral) (plexus)	968.6	E855.2	E938.6	E950.4	E962.0	E980.4
Citric acid	989.89	E866.8	—	E950.9	E962.1	E980.9
Citrovorum factor	964.1	E858.2	E934.1	E950.4	E962.0	E980.4
Claviceps purpurea	988.2	E865.4	—	E950.9	E962.1	E980.9
Cleaner, cleansing agent, type not specified	989.89	E861.9	—	E950.9	E962.1	E980.9
of paint or varnish	982.8	E862.9	—	E950.9	E962.1	E980.9
specified type NEC	989.89	E861.3	—	E950.9	E962.1	E980.9
Clematis vitalba	988.2	E865.4	—	E950.9	E962.1	E980.9
Clemizole	963.0	E858.1	E933.0	E950.4	E962.0	E980.4
penicillin	960.0	E856	E930.0	E950.4	E962.0	E980.4
Clidinium	971.1	E855.4	E941.1	E950.4	E962.0	E980.4
Clindamycin	960.8	E856	E930.8	E950.4	E962.0	E980.4
Cliradon	965.09	E850.2	E935.2	E950.0	E962.0	E980.0
Clocortolone	962.0	E858.0	E932.0	E950.4	E962.0	E980.4
Clofedanol	975.4	E858.6	E945.4	E950.4	E962.0	E980.4
Clofibrate	972.2	E858.3	E942.2	E950.4	E962.0	E980.4
Clomethiazole	967.1	E852.0	E937.1	E950.2	E962.0	E980.2
Clomiphene	977.8	E858.8	E947.8	E950.4	E962.0	E980.4
Clonazepam	969.4	E853.2	E939.4	E950.3	E962.0	E980.3
Clonidine	972.6	E858.3	E942.6	E950.4	E962.0	E980.4
Clopamide	974.3	E858.5	E944.3	E950.4	E962.0	E980.4
Clorazepate	969.4	E853.2	E939.4	E950.3	E962.0	E980.3
Clorexolone	974.4	E858.5	E944.4	E950.4	E962.0	E980.4
Clorox (bleach)	983.9	E864.3	—	E950.7	E962.1	E980.6
Clortermine	977.0	E858.8	E947.0	E950.4	E962.0	E980.4
Clotrimazole	976.0	E858.7	E946.0	E950.4	E962.0	E980.4
Cloxacillin	960.0	E856	E930.0	E950.4	E962.0	E980.4
Coagulants NEC	964.5	E858.2	E934.5	E950.4	E962.0	E980.4
Coal (carbon monoxide from) - see also Carbon, monoxide, coal	—	—	—	—	—	—
oil - see Kerosene	—	—	—	—	—	—

TABLE OF DRUGS AND CHEMICALS / Coal

Substance	Poisoning	External Cause (E Code)				
		Accident	Therapeutic Use	Suicide Attempt	Assault	Undetermined
Coal (carbon monoxide from) *(Continued)*						
tar NEC	983.0	E864.0	—	E950.7	E962.1	E980.6
fumes	987.8	E869.8	—	E952.8	E962.2	E982.8
medicinal (ointment)	976.4	E858.7	E946.4	E950.4	E962.0	E980.4
analgesics NEC	965.5	E850.5	E935.5	E950.0	E962.0	E980.0
naphtha (solvent)	981	E862.0	—	E950.9	E962.1	E980.9
Cobalt (fumes) (industrial)	985.8	E866.4	—	E950.9	E962.1	E980.9
Cobra (venom)	989.5	E905.0	—	E950.9	E962.1	E980.9
Coca (leaf)	970.81	E854.3	E940.8	E950.4	E962.0	E980.4
Cocaine (hydrochloride) (salt)	970.81	E854.3	E940.8	E950.4	E962.0	E980.4
topical anesthetic	968.5	E855.2	E938.5	E950.4	E962.0	E980.4
Coccidioidin	977.8	E858.8	E947.8	E950.4	E962.0	E980.4
Cocculus indicus	988.2	E865.3	—	E950.9	E962.1	E980.9
Cochineal	989.89	E866.8	—	E950.9	E962.1	E980.9
medicinal products	977.4	E858.8	E947.4	E950.4	E962.0	E980.4
Codeine	965.09	E850.2	E935.2	E950.0	E962.0	E980.0
Coffee	989.89	E866.8	—	E950.9	E962.1	E980.9
Cogentin	971.1	E855.4	E941.1	E950.4	E962.0	E980.4
Coke fumes or gas (carbon monoxide)	986	E868.3	—	E952.1	E962.2	E982.1
industrial use	986	E868.8	—	E952.1	E962.2	E982.1
Colace	973.2	E858.4	E943.2	E950.4	E962.0	E980.4
Colchicine	974.7	E858.5	E944.7	E950.4	E962.0	E980.4
Colchicum	988.2	E865.3	—	E950.9	E962.1	E980.9
Cold cream	976.3	E858.7	E946.3	E950.4	E962.0	E980.4
Colestipol	972.2	E858.3	E942.2	E950.4	E962.0	E980.4
Colistimethate	960.8	E856	E930.8	E950.4	E962.0	E980.4
Colistin	960.8	E856	E930.8	E950.4	E962.0	E980.4
Collagen	977.8	E866.8	E947.8	E950.9	E962.1	E980.9
Collagenase	976.8	E858.7	E946.8	E950.4	E962.0	E980.4
Collodion (flexible)	976.3	E858.7	E946.3	E950.4	E962.0	E980.4
Colocynth	973.1	E858.4	E943.1	E950.4	E962.0	E980.4
Coloring matter - *see* Dye(s)	—	—	—	—	—	—
Combustion gas - *see* Carbon, monoxide	—	—	—	—	—	—
Compazine	969.1	E853.0	E939.1	E950.3	E962.0	E980.3
Compound	—	—	—	—	—	—
42 (warfarin)	989.4	E863.7	—	E950.6	E962.1	E980.7
269 (endrin)	989.2	E863.0	—	E950.6	E962.1	E980.7
497 (dieldrin)	989.2	E863.0	—	E950.6	E962.1	E980.7

TABLE OF DRUGS AND CHEMICALS / Corrosive

Substance	Poisoning	Accident	Therapeutic Use	Suicide Attempt	Assault	Undetermined
Compound *(Continued)*						
1080 (sodium fluoroacetate)	989.4	E863.7	—	E950.6	E962.1	E980.7
3422 (parathion)	989.3	E863.1	—	E950.6	E962.1	E980.7
3911 (phorate)	989.3	E863.1	—	E950.6	E962.1	E980.7
3956 (toxaphene)	989.2	E863.0	—	E950.6	E962.1	E980.7
4049 (malathion)	989.3	E863.1	—	E950.6	E962.1	E980.7
4124 (dicapthon)	989.4	E863.4	—	E950.6	E962.1	E980.7
E (cortisone)	962.0	E858.0	E932.0	E950.4	E962.0	E980.4
F (hydrocortisone)	962.0	E858.0	E932.0	E950.4	E962.0	E980.4
Congo red	977.8	E858.8	E947.8	E950.4	E962.0	E980.4
Coniine, conine	965.7	E850.7	E935.7	E950.0	E962.0	E980.0
Conium (maculatum)	988.2	E865.4	—	E950.9	E962.1	E980.9
Conjugated estrogens (equine)	962.2	E858.0	E932.2	E950.4	E962.0	E980.4
Contac	975.6	E858.6	E945.6	E950.4	E962.0	E980.4
Contact lens solution	976.5	E858.7	E946.5	E950.4	E962.0	E980.4
Contraceptives (oral)	962.2	E858.0	E932.2	E950.4	E962.0	E980.4
vaginal	976.8	E858.7	E946.8	E950.4	E962.0	E980.4
Contrast media (roentgenographic)	977.8	E858.8	E947.8	E950.4	E962.0	E980.4
Convallaria majalis	988.2	E865.4	—	E950.9	E962.1	E980.9
Copper (dust) (fumes) (salts) NEC	985.8	E866.4	—	E950.9	E962.1	E980.9
arsenate, arsenite	985.1	E866.3	—	E950.8	E962.1	E980.8
insecticide	985.1	E863.4	—	E950.8	E962.1	E980.8
emetic	973.6	E858.4	E943.6	E950.4	E962.0	E980.4
fungicide	985.8	E863.6	—	E950.6	E962.1	E980.7
insecticide	985.8	E863.4	—	E950.6	E962.1	E980.7
oleate	976.0	E858.7	E946.0	E950.4	E962.0	E980.4
sulfate	983.9	E864.3	—	E950.7	E962.1	E980.6
fungicide	983.9	E863.6	—	E950.7	E962.1	E980.6
cupric	973.6	E858.4	E943.6	E950.4	E962.0	E980.4
cuprous	983.9	E864.3	—	E950.7	E962.1	E980.6
Copperhead snake (bite) (venom)	989.5	E905.0	—	E950.9	E962.1	E980.9
Coral (sting)	989.5	E905.6	—	E950.9	E962.1	E980.9
snake (bite) (venom)	989.5	E905.0	—	E950.9	E962.1	E980.9
Cordran	976.0	E858.7	E946.0	E950.4	E962.0	E980.4
Corn cures	976.4	E858.7	E946.4	E950.4	E962.0	E980.4
Cornhusker's lotion	976.3	E858.7	E946.3	E950.4	E962.0	E980.4
Corn starch	976.3	E858.7	E946.3	E950.4	E962.0	E980.4
Corrosive	983.9	E864.4	—	E950.7	E962.1	E980.6
acids NEC	983.1	E864.1	—	E950.7	E962.1	E980.6

◀ New ◀ Revised ~~deleted~~ Deleted ● Use Additional Digit(s)

TABLE OF DRUGS AND CHEMICALS / Corrosive

Substance	Poisoning	External Cause (E Code)				
		Accident	Therapeutic Use	Suicide Attempt	Assault	Undetermined
Corrosive *(Continued)*						
aromatics	983.0	E864.0	—	E950.7	E962.1	E980.6
disinfectant	983.0	E861.4	—	E950.7	E962.1	E980.6
fumes NEC	987.9	E869.9	—	E952.9	E962.2	E982.9
specified NEC	983.9	E864.3	—	E950.7	E962.1	E980.6
sublimate - *see* Mercury, chloride	—	—	—	—	—	—
Cortate	962.0	E858.0	E932.0	E950.4	E962.0	E980.4
Cort-Dome	962.0	E858.0	E932.0	E950.4	E962.0	E980.4
ENT agent	976.6	E858.7	E946.6	E950.4	E962.0	E980.4
ophthalmic preparation	976.5	E858.7	E946.5	E950.4	E962.0	E980.4
topical NEC	976.0	E858.7	E946.0	E950.4	E962.0	E980.4
Cortef	962.0	E858.0	E932.0	E950.4	E962.0	E980.4
ENT agent	976.6	E858.7	E946.6	E950.4	E962.0	E980.4
ophthalmic preparation	976.5	E858.7	E946.5	E950.4	E962.0	E980.4
topical NEC	976.0	E858.7	E946.0	E950.4	E962.0	E980.4
Corticosteroids (fluorinated)	962.0	E858.0	E932.0	E950.4	E962.0	E980.4
ENT agent	976.6	E858.7	E946.6	E950.4	E962.0	E980.4
ophthalmic preparation	976.5	E858.7	E946.5	E950.4	E962.0	E980.4
topical NEC	976.0	E858.7	E946.0	E950.4	E962.0	E980.4
Corticotropin	962.4	E858.0	E932.4	E950.4	E962.0	E980.4
Cortisol	962.0	E858.0	E932.0	E950.4	E962.0	E980.4
ENT agent	976.6	E858.7	E946.6	E950.4	E962.0	E980.4
ophthalmic preparation	976.5	E858.7	E946.5	E950.4	E962.0	E980.4
topical NEC	976.0	E858.7	E946.0	E950.4	E962.0	E980.4
Cortisone derivatives (acetate)	962.0	E858.0	E932.0	E950.4	E962.0	E980.4
ENT agent	976.6	E858.7	E946.6	E950.4	E962.0	E980.4
ophthalmic preparation	976.5	E858.7	E946.5	E950.4	E962.0	E980.4
topical NEC	976.0	E858.7	E946.0	E950.4	E962.0	E980.4
Cortogen	962.0	E858.0	E932.0	E950.4	E962.0	E980.4
ENT agent	976.6	E858.7	E946.6	E950.4	E962.0	E980.4
ophthalmic preparation	976.5	E858.7	E946.5	E950.4	E962.0	E980.4
Cortone	962.0	E858.0	E932.0	E950.4	E962.0	E980.4
ENT agent	976.6	E858.7	E946.6	E950.4	E962.0	E980.4
ophthalmic preparation	976.5	E858.7	E946.5	E950.4	E962.0	E980.4
Cortril	962.0	E858.0	E932.0	E950.4	E962.0	E980.4
ENT agent	976.6	E858.7	E946.6	E950.4	E962.0	E980.4
ophthalmic preparation	976.5	E858.7	E946.5	E950.4	E962.0	E980.4
topical NEC	976.0	E858.7	E946.0	E950.4	E962.0	E980.4
Cosmetics	989.89	E866.7	—	E950.9	E962.1	E980.9

TABLE OF DRUGS AND CHEMICALS / Curare, curarine

Substance	Poisoning	External Cause (E Code)				
		Accident	Therapeutic Use	Suicide Attempt	Assault	Undetermined
Cosyntropin	977.8	E858.8	E947.8	E950.4	E962.0	E980.4
Cotarnine	964.5	E858.2	E934.5	E950.4	E962.0	E980.4
Cottonseed oil	976.3	E858.7	E946.3	E950.4	E962.0	E980.4
Cough mixtures (antitussives)	975.4	E858.6	E945.4	E950.4	E962.0	E980.4
containing opiates	965.09	E850.2	E935.2	E950.0	E962.0	E980.0
expectorants	975.5	E858.6	E945.5	E950.4	E962.0	E980.4
Coumadin	964.2	E858.2	E934.2	E950.4	E962.0	E980.4
rodenticide	989.4	E863.7	—	E950.6	E962.1	E980.7
Coumarin	964.2	E858.2	E934.2	E950.4	E962.0	E980.4
Coumetarol	964.2	E858.2	E934.2	E950.4	E962.0	E980.4
Cowbane	988.2	E865.4	—	E950.9	E962.1	E980.9
Cozyme	963.5	E858.1	E933.5	E950.4	E962.0	E980.4
Crack	970.81	E854.3	E940.8	E950.4	E962.0	E980.4
Creolin	983.0	E864.0	—	E950.7	E962.1	E980.6
disinfectant	983.0	E861.4	—	E950.7	E962.1	E980.6
Creosol (compound)	983.0	E864.0	—	E950.7	E962.1	E980.6
Creosote (beechwood) (coal tar)	983.0	E864.0	—	E950.7	E962.1	E980.6
medicinal (expectorant)	975.5	E858.6	E945.5	E950.4	E962.0	E980.4
syrup	975.5	E858.6	E945.5	E950.4	E962.0	E980.4
Cresol	983.0	E864.0	—	E950.7	E962.1	E980.6
disinfectant	983.0	E861.4	—	E950.7	E962.1	E980.6
Cresylic acid	983.0	E864.0	—	E950.7	E962.1	E980.6
Cropropamide	965.7	E850.7	E935.7	E950.0	E962.0	E980.0
with crotethamide	970.0	E854.3	E940.0	E950.4	E962.0	E980.4
Crotamiton	976.0	E858.7	E946.0	E950.4	E962.0	E980.4
Crotethamide	965.7	E850.7	E935.7	E950.0	E962.0	E980.0
with cropropamide	970.0	E854.3	E940.0	E950.4	E962.0	E980.4
Croton (oil)	973.1	E858.4	E943.1	E950.4	E962.0	E980.4
chloral	967.1	E852.0	E937.1	E950.2	E962.0	E980.2
Crude oil	981	E862.1	—	E950.9	E962.1	E980.9
Cryogenine	965.8	E850.8	E935.8	E950.0	E962.0	E980.0
Cryolite (pesticide)	989.4	E863.4	—	E950.6	E962.1	E980.7
Cryptenamine	972.6	E858.3	E942.6	E950.4	E962.0	E980.4
Crystal violet	976.0	E858.7	E946.0	E950.4	E962.0	E980.4
Cuckoopint	988.2	E865.4	—	E950.9	E962.1	E980.9
Cumetharol	964.2	E858.2	E934.2	E950.4	E962.0	E980.4
Cupric sulfate	973.6	E858.4	E943.6	E950.4	E962.0	E980.4
Cuprous sulfate	983.9	E864.3	—	E950.7	E962.1	E980.6
Curare, curarine	975.2	E858.6	E945.2	E950.4	E962.0	E980.4

◀ New   ◀▦ Revised   ~~deleted~~ Deleted   ● Use Additional Digit(s)

TABLE OF DRUGS AND CHEMICALS / Cyanic acid

Substance	Poisoning	External Cause (E Code) Accident	Therapeutic Use	Suicide Attempt	Assault	Undetermined
Cyanic acid - *see* Cyanide(s)	—	—	—	—	—	—
Cyanide(s) (compounds) (hydrogen) (potassium) (sodium) NEC	989.0	E866.8	—	E950.9	E962.1	E980.9
dust or gas (inhalation) NEC	987.7	E869.8	—	E952.8	E962.2	E982.8
fumigant	989.0	E863.8	—	E950.6	E962.1	E980.7
mercuric - *see* Mercury	—	—	—	—	—	—
pesticide (dust) (fumes)	989.0	E863.4	—	E950.6	E962.1	E980.7
Cyanocobalamin	964.1	E858.2	E934.1	E950.4	E962.0	E980.4
Cyanogen (chloride) (gas)	—	—	—	—	—	—
NEC	987.8	E869.8	—	E952.8	E962.2	E982.8
Cyclaine	968.5	E855.2	E938.5	E950.4	E962.0	E980.4
Cyclamen europaeum	988.2	E865.4	—	E950.9	E962.1	E980.9
Cyclandelate	972.5	E858.3	E942.5	E950.4	E962.0	E980.4
Cyclazocine	965.09	E850.2	E935.2	E950.0	E962.0	E980.0
Cyclizine	963.0	E858.1	E933.0	E950.4	E962.0	E980.4
Cyclobarbital, cyclobarbitone	967.0	E851	E937.0	E950.1	E962.0	E980.1
Cycloguanil	961.4	E857	E931.4	E950.4	E962.0	E980.4
Cyclohexane	982.0	E862.4	—	E950.9	E962.1	E980.9
Cyclohexanol	980.8	E860.8	—	E950.9	E962.1	E980.9
Cyclohexanone	982.8	E862.4	—	E950.9	E962.1	E980.9
Cyclomethycaine	968.5	E855.2	E938.5	E950.4	E962.0	E980.4
Cyclopentamine	971.2	E855.5	E941.2	E950.4	E962.0	E980.4
Cyclopenthiazide	974.3	E858.5	E944.3	E950.4	E962.0	E980.4
Cyclopentolate	971.1	E855.4	E941.1	E950.4	E962.0	E980.4
Cyclophosphamide	963.1	E858.1	E933.1	E950.4	E962.0	E980.4
Cyclopropane	968.2	E855.1	E938.2	E950.4	E962.0	E980.4
Cycloserine	960.6	E856	E930.6	E950.4	E962.0	E980.4
Cyclothiazide	974.3	E858.5	E944.3	E950.4	E962.0	E980.4
Cycrimine	966.4	E855.0	E936.4	E950.4	E962.0	E980.4
Cymarin	972.1	E858.3	E942.1	E950.4	E962.0	E980.4
Cyproheptadine	963.0	E858.1	E933.0	E950.4	E962.0	E980.4
Cyprolidol	969.09	E854.0	E939.0	E950.3	E962.0	E980.3
Cytarabine	963.1	E858.1	E933.1	E950.4	E962.0	E980.4
Cytisus	—	—	—	—	—	—
laburnum	988.2	E865.4	—	E950.9	E962.1	E980.9
scoparius	988.2	E865.4	—	E950.9	E962.1	E980.9
Cytomel	962.7	E858.0	E932.7	E950.4	E962.0	E980.4
Cytosine (antineoplastic)	963.1	E858.1	E933.1	E950.4	E962.0	E980.4
Cytoxan	963.1	E858.1	E933.1	E950.4	E962.0	E980.4
Dacarbazine	963.1	E858.1	E933.1	E950.4	E962.0	E980.4

TABLE OF DRUGS AND CHEMICALS / Delalutin

| Substance | Poisoning | External Cause (E Code) |||||
		Accident	Therapeutic Use	Suicide Attempt	Assault	Undetermined
Dactinomycin	960.7	E856	E930.7	E950.4	E962.0	E980.4
DADPS	961.8	E857	E931.8	E950.4	E962.0	E980.4
Dakin's solution (external)	976.0	E858.7	E946.0	E950.4	E962.0	E980.4
Dalmane	969.4	E853.2	E939.4	E950.3	E962.0	E980.3
DAM	977.2	E858.8	E947.2	E950.4	E962.0	E980.4
Danilone	964.2	E858.2	E934.2	E950.4	E962.0	E980.4
Danthron	973.1	E858.4	E943.1	E950.4	E962.0	E980.4
Dantrolene	975.2	E858.6	E945.2	E950.4	E962.0	E980.4
Daphne (gnidium) (mezereum)	988.2	E865.4	—	E950.9	E962.1	E980.9
berry	988.2	E865.3	—	E950.9	E962.1	E980.9
Dapsone	961.8	E857	E931.8	E950.4	E962.0	E980.4
Daraprim	961.4	E857	E931.4	E950.4	E962.0	E980.4
Darnel	988.2	E865.3	—	E950.9	E962.1	E980.9
Darvon	965.8	E850.8	E935.8	E950.0	E962.0	E980.0
Daunorubicin	960.7	E856	E930.7	E950.4	E962.0	E980.4
DBI	962.3	E858.0	E932.3	E950.4	E962.0	E980.4
D-Con (rodenticide)	989.4	E863.7	—	E950.6	E962.1	E980.7
DDS	961.8	E857	E931.8	E950.4	E962.0	E980.4
DDT	989.2	E863.0	—	E950.6	E962.1	E980.7
Deadly nightshade	988.2	E865.4	—	E950.9	E962.1	E980.9
berry	988.2	E865.3	—	E950.9	E962.1	E980.9
Deanol	969.79	E854.2	E939.7	E950.3	E962.0	E980.3
Debrisoquine	972.6	E858.3	E942.6	E950.4	E962.0	E980.4
Decaborane	989.89	E866.8	—	E950.9	E962.1	E980.9
fumes	987.8	E869.8	—	E952.8	E962.2	E982.8
Decadron	962.0	E858.0	E932.0	E950.4	E962.0	E980.4
ENT agent	976.6	E858.7	E946.6	E950.4	E962.0	E980.4
ophthalmic preparation	976.5	E858.7	E946.5	E950.4	E962.0	E980.4
topical NEC	976.0	E858.7	E946.0	E950.4	E962.0	E980.4
Decahydronaphthalene	982.0	E862.4	—	E950.9	E962.1	E980.9
Decalin	982.0	E862.4	—	E950.9	E962.1	E980.9
Decamethonium	975.2	E858.6	E945.2	E950.4	E962.0	E980.4
Decholin	973.4	E858.4	E943.4	E950.4	E962.0	E980.4
sodium (diagnostic)	977.8	E858.8	E947.8	E950.4	E962.0	E980.4
Declomycin	960.4	E856	E930.4	E950.4	E962.0	E980.4
Deferoxamine	963.8	E858.1	E933.8	E950.4	E962.0	E980.4
Dehydrocholic acid	973.4	E858.4	E943.4	E950.4	E962.0	E980.4
Dekalin	982.0	E862.4	—	E950.9	E962.1	E980.9
Delalutin	962.2	E858.0	E932.2	E950.4	E962.0	E980.4

TABLE OF DRUGS AND CHEMICALS / Delphinium

Substance	Poisoning	External Cause (E Code)				
		Accident	Therapeutic Use	Suicide Attempt	Assault	Undetermined
Delphinium	988.2	E865.3	—	E950.9	E962.1	E980.9
Deltasone	962.0	E858.0	E932.0	E950.4	E962.0	E980.4
Deltra	962.0	E858.0	E932.0	E950.4	E962.0	E980.4
Delvinal	967.0	E851	E937.0	E950.1	E962.0	E980.1
Demecarium (bromide)	971.0	E855.3	E941.0	E950.4	E962.0	E980.4
Demeclocycline	960.4	E856	E930.4	E950.4	E962.0	E980.4
Demecolcine	963.1	E858.1	E933.1	E950.4	E962.0	E980.4
Demelanizing agents	976.8	E858.7	E946.8	E950.4	E962.0	E980.4
Demerol	965.09	E850.2	E935.2	E950.0	E962.0	E980.0
Demethylchlortetracycline	960.4	E856	E930.4	E950.4	E962.0	E980.4
Demethyltetracycline	960.4	E856	E930.4	E950.4	E962.0	E980.4
Demeton	989.3	E863.1	—	E950.6	E962.1	E980.7
Demulcents	976.3	E858.7	E946.3	E950.4	E962.0	E980.4
Demulen	962.2	E858.0	E932.2	E950.4	E962.0	E980.4
Denatured alcohol	980.0	E860.1	—	E950.9	E962.1	E980.9
Dendrid	976.5	E858.7	E946.5	E950.4	E962.0	E980.4
Dental agents, topical	976.7	E858.7	E946.7	E950.4	E962.0	E980.4
Deodorant spray (feminine hygiene)	976.8	E858.7	E946.8	E950.4	E962.0	E980.4
Deoxyribonuclease	963.4	E858.1	E933.4	E950.4	E962.0	E980.4
Depressants	—	—	—	—	—	—
appetite, central	977.0	E858.8	E947.0	E950.4	E962.0	E980.4
cardiac	972.0	E858.3	E942.0	E950.4	E962.0	E980.4
central nervous system (anesthetic)	968.4	E855.1	E938.4	E950.4	E962.0	E980.4
psychotherapeutic	969.5	E853.9	E939.5	E950.3	E962.0	E980.3
Dequalinium	976.0	E858.7	E946.0	E950.4	E962.0	E980.4
Dermolate	976.2	E858.7	E946.2	E950.4	E962.0	E980.4
DES	962.2	E858.0	E932.2	E950.4	E962.0	E980.4
Desenex	976.0	E858.7	E946.0	E950.4	E962.0	E980.4
Deserpidine	972.6	E858.3	E942.6	E950.4	E962.0	E980.4
Desipramine	969.05	E854.0	E939.0	E950.3	E962.0	E980.3
Deslanoside	972.1	E858.3	E942.1	E950.4	E962.0	E980.4
Desocodeine	965.09	E850.2	E935.2	E950.0	E962.0	E980.0
Desomorphine	965.09	E850.2	E935.2	E950.0	E962.0	E980.0
Desonide	976.0	E858.7	E946.0	E950.4	E962.0	E980.4
Desoxycorticosterone derivatives	962.0	E858.0	E932.0	E950.4	E962.0	E980.4
Desoxyephedrine	969.72	E854.2	E939.7	E950.3	E962.0	E980.3
DET	969.6	E854.1	E939.6	E950.3	E962.0	E980.3
Detergents (ingested) (synthetic)	989.6	E861.0	—	E950.9	E962.1	E980.9
external medication	976.2	E858.7	E946.2	E950.4	E962.0	E980.4

TABLE OF DRUGS AND CHEMICALS / Diazinon

Substance	Poisoning	External Cause (E Code)				
		Accident	Therapeutic Use	Suicide Attempt	Assault	Undetermined
Deterrent, alcohol	977.3	E858.8	E947.3	E950.4	E962.0	E980.4
Detrothyronine	962.7	E858.0	E932.7	E950.4	E962.0	E980.4
Dettol (external medication)	976.0	E858.7	E946.0	E950.4	E962.0	E980.4
Dexamethasone	962.0	E858.0	E932.0	E950.4	E962.0	E980.4
ENT agent	976.6	E858.7	E946.6	E950.4	E962.0	E980.4
ophthalmic preparation	976.5	E858.7	E946.5	E950.4	E962.0	E980.4
topical NEC	976.0	E858.7	E946.0	E950.4	E962.0	E980.4
Dexamphetamine	969.72	E854.2	E939.7	E950.3	E962.0	E980.3
Dexedrine	969.72	E854.2	E939.7	E950.3	E962.0	E980.3
Dexpanthenol	963.5	E858.1	E933.5	E950.4	E962.0	E980.4
Dextran	964.8	E858.2	E934.8	E950.4	E962.0	E980.4
Dextriferron	964.0	E858.2	E934.0	E950.4	E962.0	E980.4
Dextroamphetamine	969.72	E854.2	E939.7	E950.3	E962.0	E980.3
Dextro calcium pantothenate	963.5	E858.1	E933.5	E950.4	E962.0	E980.4
Dextromethorphan	975.4	E858.6	E945.4	E950.4	E962.0	E980.4
Dextromoramide	965.09	E850.2	E935.2	E950.0	E962.0	E980.0
Dextro pantothenyl alcohol	963.5	E858.1	E933.5	E950.4	E962.0	E980.4
topical	976.8	E858.7	E946.8	E950.4	E962.0	E980.4
Dextropropoxyphene (hydrochloride)	965.8	E850.8	E935.8	E950.0	E962.0	E980.0
Dextrorphan	965.09	E850.2	E935.2	E950.0	E962.0	E980.0
Dextrose NEC	974.5	E858.5	E944.5	E950.4	E962.0	E980.4
Dextrothyroxine	962.7	E858.0	E932.7	E950.4	E962.0	E980.4
DFP	971.0	E855.3	E941.0	E950.4	E962.0	E980.4
DHE-45	972.9	E858.3	E942.9	E950.4	E962.0	E980.4
Diabinese	962.3	E858.0	E932.3	E950.4	E962.0	E980.4
Diacetyl monoxime	977.2	E858.8	E947.2	E950.4	E962.0	E980.4
Diacetylmorphine	965.01	E850.0	E935.0	E950.0	E962.0	E980.0
Diagnostic agents	977.8	E858.8	E947.8	E950.4	E962.0	E980.4
Dial (soap)	976.2	E858.7	E946.2	E950.4	E962.0	E980.4
sedative	967.0	E851	E937.0	E950.1	E962.0	E980.1
Diallylbarbituric acid	967.0	E851	E937.0	E950.1	E962.0	E980.1
Diaminodiphenyisulfone	961.8	E857	E931.8	E950.4	E962.0	E980.4
Diamorphine	965.01	E850.0	E935.0	E950.0	E962.0	E980.0
Diamox	974.2	E858.5	E944.2	E950.4	E962.0	E980.4
Diamthazole	976.0	E858.7	E946.0	E950.4	E962.0	E980.4
Diaphenyisulfone	961.8	E857	E931.8	E950.4	E962.0	E980.4
Diasone (sodium)	961.8	E857	E931.8	E950.4	E962.0	E980.4
Diazepam	969.4	E853.2	E939.4	E950.3	E962.0	E980.3
Diazinon	989.3	E863.1	—	E950.6	E962.1	E980.7

◀ New   ⬅ Revised   ~~deleted~~ Deleted   ● Use Additional Digit(s)

TABLE OF DRUGS AND CHEMICALS / Diazomethane

Substance	Poisoning	External Cause (E Code) Accident	Therapeutic Use	Suicide Attempt	Assault	Undetermined
Diazomethane (gas)	987.8	E869.8	—	E952.8	E962.2	E982.8
Diazoxide	972.5	E858.3	E942.5	E950.4	E962.0	E980.4
Dibenamine	971.3	E855.6	E941.3	E950.4	E962.0	E980.4
Dibenzheptropine	963.0	E858.1	E933.0	E950.4	E962.0	E980.4
Dibenzyline	971.3	E855.6	E941.3	E950.4	E962.0	E980.4
Diborane (gas)	987.8	E869.8	—	E952.8	E962.2	E982.8
Dibromomannitol	963.1	E858.1	E933.1	E950.4	E962.0	E980.4
Dibucaine (spinal)	968.7	E855.2	E938.7	E950.4	E962.0	E980.4
topical (surface)	968.5	E855.2	E938.5	E950.4	E962.0	E980.4
Dibunate sodium	975.4	E858.6	E945.4	E950.4	E962.0	E980.4
Dibutoline	971.1	E855.4	E941.1	E950.4	E962.0	E980.4
Dicapthon	989.4	E863.4	—	E950.6	E962.1	E980.7
Dichloralphenazone	967.1	E852.0	E937.1	E950.2	E962.0	E980.2
Dichlorodifluoromethane	987.4	E869.2	—	E952.8	E962.2	E982.8
Dichloroethane	982.3	E862.4	—	E950.9	E962.1	E980.9
Dichloroethylene	982.3	E862.4	—	E950.9	E962.1	E980.9
Dichloroethyl sulfide	987.8	E869.8	—	E952.8	E962.2	E982.8
Dichlorohydrin	982.3	E862.4	—	E950.9	E962.1	E980.9
Dichloromethane (solvent) (vapor)	982.3	E862.4	—	E950.9	E962.1	E980.9
Dichlorophen(e)	961.6	E857	E931.6	E950.4	E962.0	E980.4
Dichlorphenamide	974.2	E858.5	E944.2	E950.4	E962.0	E980.4
Dichlorvos	989.3	E863.1	—	E950.6	E962.1	E980.7
Diclofenac sodium	965.69	E850.6	E935.6	E950.0	E962.0	E980.0
Dicoumarin, dicumarol	964.2	E858.2	E934.2	E950.4	E962.0	E980.4
Dicyanogen (gas)	987.8	E869.8	—	E952.8	E962.2	E982.8
Dicyclomine	971.1	E855.4	E941.1	E950.4	E962.0	E980.4
Dieldrin (vapor)	989.2	E863.0	—	E950.6	E962.1	E980.7
Dienestrol	962.2	E858.0	E932.2	E950.4	E962.0	E980.4
Dietetics	977.0	E858.8	E947.0	E950.4	E962.0	E980.4
Diethazine	966.4	E855.0	E936.4	E950.4	E962.0	E980.4
Diethyl	—	—	—	—	—	—
barbituric acid	967.0	E851	E937.0	E950.1	E962.0	E980.1
carbamazine	961.6	E857	E931.6	E950.4	E962.0	E980.4
carbinol	980.8	E860.8	—	E950.9	E962.1	E980.9
carbonate	982.8	E862.4	—	E950.9	E962.1	E980.9
ether (vapor) - see Ether(s)	—	—	—	—	—	—
propion	977.0	E858.8	E947.0	E950.4	E962.0	E980.4
stilbestrol	962.2	E858.0	E932.2	E950.4	E962.0	E980.4

TABLE OF DRUGS AND CHEMICALS / Dimethindene

Substance	Poisoning	External Cause (E Code)				
		Accident	Therapeutic Use	Suicide Attempt	Assault	Undetermined
Diethylene	—	—	—	—	—	—
dioxide	982.8	E862.4	—	E950.9	E962.1	E980.9
glycol (monoacetate) (monoethyl ether)	982.8	E862.4	—	E950.9	E962.1	E980.9
Diethylsulfone-diethylmethane	967.8	E852.8	E937.8	E950.2	E962.0	E980.2
Difencloxazine	965.09	E850.2	E935.2	E950.0	E962.0	E980.0
Diffusin	963.4	E858.1	E933.4	E950.4	E962.0	E980.4
Diflos	971.0	E855.3	E941.0	E950.4	E962.0	E980.4
Digestants	973.4	E858.4	E943.4	E950.4	E962.0	E980.4
Digitalin(e)	972.1	E858.3	E942.1	E950.4	E962.0	E980.4
Digitalis glycosides	972.1	E858.3	E942.1	E950.4	E962.0	E980.4
Digitoxin	972.1	E858.3	E942.1	E950.4	E962.0	E980.4
Digoxin	972.1	E858.3	E942.1	E950.4	E962.0	E980.4
Dihydrocodeine	965.09	E850.2	E935.2	E950.0	E962.0	E980.0
Dihydrocodeinone	965.09	E850.2	E935.2	E950.0	E962.0	E980.0
Dihydroergocristine	972.9	E858.3	E942.9	E950.4	E962.0	E980.4
Dihydroergotamine	972.9	E858.3	E942.9	E950.4	E962.0	E980.4
Dihydroergotoxine	972.9	E858.3	E942.9	E950.4	E962.0	E980.4
Dihydrohydroxycodeinone	965.09	E850.2	E935.2	E950.0	E962.0	E980.0
Dihydrohydroxymorphinone	965.09	E850.2	E935.2	E950.0	E962.0	E980.0
Dihydroisocodeine	965.09	E850.2	E935.2	E950.0	E962.0	E980.0
Dihydromorphine	965.09	E850.2	E935.2	E950.0	E962.0	E980.0
Dihydromorphinone	965.09	E850.2	E935.2	E950.0	E962.0	E980.0
Dihydrostreptomycin	960.6	E856	E930.6	E950.4	E962.0	E980.4
Dihydrotachysterol	962.6	E858.0	E932.6	E950.4	E962.0	E980.4
Dihydroxyanthraquinone	973.1	E858.4	E943.1	E950.4	E962.0	E980.4
Dihydroxycodeinone	965.09	E850.2	E935.2	E950.0	E962.0	E980.0
Diiodohydroxyquin	961.3	E857	E931.3	E950.4	E962.0	E980.4
topical	976.0	E858.7	E946.0	E950.4	E962.0	E980.4
Diiodohydroxyquinoline	961.3	E857	E931.3	E950.4	E962.0	E980.4
Dilantin	966.1	E855.0	E936.1	E950.4	E962.0	E980.4
Dilaudid	965.09	E850.2	E935.2	E950.0	E962.0	E980.0
Diloxanide	961.5	E857	E931.5	E950.4	E962.0	E980.4
Dimefline	970.0	E854.3	E940.0	E950.4	E962.0	E980.4
Dimenhydrinate	963.0	E858.1	E933.0	E950.4	E962.0	E980.4
Dimercaprol	963.8	E858.1	E933.8	E950.4	E962.0	E980.4
Dimercaptopropanol	963.8	E858.1	E933.8	E950.4	E962.0	E980.4
Dimetane	963.0	E858.1	E933.0	E950.4	E962.0	E980.4
Dimethicone	976.3	E858.7	E946.3	E950.4	E962.0	E980.4
Dimethindene	963.0	E858.1	E933.0	E950.4	E962.0	E980.4

◀ New ◀◀ Revised ~~deleted~~ Deleted ● Use Additional Digit(s)

TABLE OF DRUGS AND CHEMICALS / Dimethisoquin

		External Cause (E Code)				
Substance	Poisoning	Accident	Therapeutic Use	Suicide Attempt	Assault	Undetermined
Dimethisoquin	968.5	E855.2	E938.5	E950.4	E962.0	E980.4
Dimethisterone	962.2	E858.0	E932.2	E950.4	E962.0	E980.4
Dimethoxanate	975.4	E858.6	E945.4	E950.4	E962.0	E980.4
Dimethyl	—	—	—	—	—	—
arsine, arsinic acid - see Arsenic	—	—	—	—	—	—
carbinol	980.2	E860.3	—	E950.9	E962.1	E980.9
diguanide	962.3	E858.0	E932.3	E950.4	E962.0	E980.4
ketone	982.8	E862.4	—	E950.9	E962.1	E980.9
vapor	987.8	E869.8	—	E952.8	E962.2	E982.8
meperidine	965.09	E850.2	E935.2	E950.0	E962.0	E980.0
parathion	989.3	E863.1	—	E950.6	E962.1	E980.7
polysiloxane	973.8	E858.4	E943.8	E950.4	E962.0	E980.4
sulfate (fumes)	987.8	E869.8	—	E952.8	E962.2	E982.8
liquid	983.9	E864.3	—	E950.7	E962.1	E980.6
sulfoxide NEC	982.8	E862.4	—	E950.9	E962.1	E980.9
medicinal	976.4	E858.7	E946.4	E950.4	E962.0	E980.4
triptamine	969.6	E854.1	E939.6	E950.3	E962.0	E980.3
tubocurarine	975.2	E858.6	E945.2	E950.4	E962.0	E980.4
Dindevan	964.2	E858.2	E934.2	E950.4	E962.0	E980.4
Dinitro (-ortho-) cresol (herbicide) (spray)	989.4	E863.5	—	E950.6	E962.1	E980.7
insecticide	989.4	E863.4	—	E950.6	E962.1	E980.7
Dinitrobenzene	983.0	E864.0	—	E950.7	E962.1	E980.6
vapor	987.8	E869.8	—	E952.8	E962.2	E982.8
Dinitro-orthocresol (herbicide)	989.4	E863.5	—	E950.6	E962.1	E980.7
insecticide	989.4	E863.4	—	E950.6	E962.1	E980.7
Dinitrophenol (herbicide) (spray)	989.4	E863.5	—	E950.6	E962.1	E980.7
insecticide	989.4	E863.4	—	E950.6	E962.1	E980.7
Dinoprost	975.0	E858.6	E945.0	E950.4	E962.0	E980.4
Dioctyl sulfosuccinate (calcium) (sodium)	973.2	E858.4	E943.2	E950.4	E962.0	E980.4
Diodoquin	961.3	E857	E931.3	E950.4	E962.0	E980.4
Dione derivatives NEC	966.3	E855.0	E936.3	E950.4	E962.0	E980.4
Dionin	965.09	E850.2	E935.2	E950.0	E962.0	E980.0
Dioxane	982.8	E862.4	—	E950.9	E962.1	E980.9
Dioxin - see herbicide	—	—	—	—	—	—
Dioxyline	972.5	E858.3	E942.5	E950.4	E962.0	E980.4
Dipentene	982.8	E862.4	—	E950.9	E962.1	E980.9
Diphemanil	971.1	E855.4	E941.1	E950.4	E962.0	E980.4
Diphenadione	964.2	E858.2	E934.2	E950.4	E962.0	E980.4
Diphenhydramine	963.0	E858.1	E933.0	E950.4	E962.0	E980.4

TABLE OF DRUGS AND CHEMICALS / D-lysergic acid diethylamide

		External Cause (E Code)				
Substance	Poisoning	Accident	Therapeutic Use	Suicide Attempt	Assault	Undetermined
Diphenidol	963.0	E858.1	E933.0	E950.4	E962.0	E980.4
Diphenoxylate	973.5	E858.4	E943.5	E950.4	E962.0	E980.4
Diphenylchlorarsine	985.1	E866.3	—	E950.8	E962.1	E980.8
Diphenylhydantoin (sodium)	966.1	E855.0	E936.1	E950.4	E962.0	E980.4
Diphenylpyraline	963.0	E858.1	E933.0	E950.4	E962.0	E980.4
Diphtheria	—	—	—	—	—	—
antitoxin	979.9	E858.8	E949.9	E950.4	E962.0	E980.4
toxoid	978.5	E858.8	E948.5	E950.4	E962.0	E980.4
with tetanus toxoid	978.9	E858.8	E948.9	E950.4	E962.0	E980.4
with pertussis component	978.6	E858.8	E948.6	E950.4	E962.0	E980.4
vaccine	978.5	E858.8	E948.5	E950.4	E962.0	E980.4
Dipipanone	965.09	E850.2	E935.2	E950.0	E962.0	E980.0
Diplovax	979.5	E858.8	E949.5	E950.4	E962.0	E980.4
Diprophylline	975.1	E858.6	E945.1	E950.4	E962.0	E980.4
Dipyridamole	972.4	E858.3	E942.4	E950.4	E962.0	E980.4
Dipyrone	965.5	E850.5	E935.5	E950.0	E962.0	E980.0
Diquat	989.4	E863.5	—	E950.6	E962.1	E980.7
Disinfectant NEC	983.9	E861.4	—	E950.7	E962.1	E980.6
alkaline	983.2	E861.4	—	E950.7	E962.1	E980.6
aromatic	983.0	E861.4	—	E950.7	E962.1	E980.6
Disipal	966.4	E855.0	E936.4	E950.4	E962.0	E980.4
Disodium edetate	963.8	E858.1	E933.8	E950.4	E962.0	E980.4
Disulfamide	974.4	E858.5	E944.4	E950.4	E962.0	E980.4
Disulfanilamide	961.0	E857	E931.0	E950.4	E962.0	E980.4
Disulfiram	977.3	E858.8	E947.3	E950.4	E962.0	E980.4
Dithiazanine	961.6	E857	E931.6	E950.4	E962.0	E980.4
Dithioglycerol	963.8	E858.1	E933.8	E950.4	E962.0	E980.4
Dithranol	976.4	E858.7	E946.4	E950.4	E962.0	E980.4
Diucardin	974.3	E858.5	E944.3	E950.4	E962.0	E980.4
Diupres	974.3	E858.5	E944.3	E950.4	E962.0	E980.4
Diuretics NEC	974.4	E858.5	E944.4	E950.4	E962.0	E980.4
carbonic acid anhydrase inhibitors	974.2	E858.5	E944.2	E950.4	E962.0	E980.4
mercurial	974.0	E858.5	E944.0	E950.4	E962.0	E980.4
osmotic	974.4	E858.5	E944.4	E950.4	E962.0	E980.4
purine derivatives	974.1	E858.5	E944.1	E950.4	E962.0	E980.4
saluretic	974.3	E858.5	E944.3	E950.4	E962.0	E980.4
Diuril	974.3	E858.5	E944.3	E950.4	E962.0	E980.4
Divinyl ether	968.2	E855.1	E938.2	E950.4	E962.0	E980.4
D-lysergic acid diethylamide	969.6	E854.1	E939.6	E950.3	E962.0	E980.3

TABLE OF DRUGS AND CHEMICALS / DMCT

Substance	Poisoning	External Cause (E Code) Accident	Therapeutic Use	Suicide Attempt	Assault	Undetermined
DMCT	960.4	E856	E930.4	E950.4	E962.0	E980.4
DMSO	982.8	E862.4	—	E950.9	E962.1	E980.9
DMT	969.6	E854.1	E939.6	E950.3	E962.0	E980.3
DNOC	989.4	E863.5	—	E950.6	E962.1	E980.7
DOCA	962.0	E858.0	E932.0	E950.4	E962.0	E980.4
Dolophine	965.02	E850.1	E935.1	E950.0	E962.0	E980.0
Doloxene	965.8	E850.8	E935.8	E950.0	E962.0	E980.0
DOM	969.6	E854.1	E939.6	E950.3	E962.0	E980.3
Domestic gas - see Gas, utility	—	—	—	—	—	—
Domiphen (bromide) (lozenges)	976.6	E858.7	E946.6	E950.4	E962.0	E980.4
Dopa (levo)	966.4	E855.0	E936.4	E950.4	E962.0	E980.4
Dopamine	971.2	E855.5	E941.2	E950.4	E962.0	E980.4
Doriden	967.5	E852.4	E937.5	E950.2	E962.0	E980.2
Dormiral	967.0	E851	E937.0	E950.1	E962.0	E980.1
Dormison	967.8	E852.8	E937.8	E950.2	E962.0	E980.2
Dornase	963.4	E858.1	E933.4	E950.4	E962.0	E980.4
Dorsacaine	968.5	E855.2	E938.5	E950.4	E962.0	E980.4
Dothiepin hydrochloride	969.05	E854.0	E939.0	E950.3	E962.0	E980.3
Doxapram	970.0	E854.3	E940.0	E950.4	E962.0	E980.4
Doxepin	969.05	E854.0	E939.0	E950.3	E962.0	E980.3
Doxorubicin	960.7	E856	E930.7	E950.4	E962.0	E980.4
Doxycycline	960.4	E856	E930.4	E950.4	E962.0	E980.4
Doxylamine	963.0	E858.1	E933.0	E950.4	E962.0	E980.4
Dramamine	963.0	E858.1	E933.0	E950.4	E962.0	E980.4
Drano (drain cleaner)	983.2	E864.2	—	E950.7	E962.1	E980.6
Dromoran	965.09	E850.2	E935.2	E950.0	E962.0	E980.0
Dromostanolone	962.1	E858.0	E932.1	E950.4	E962.0	E980.4
Droperidol	969.2	E853.1	E939.2	E950.3	E962.0	E980.3
Drotrecogin alfa	964.2	E858.2	E934.2	E950.4	E962.0	E980.4
Drug	977.9	E858.9	E947.9	E950.5	E962.0	E980.5
specified NEC	977.8	E858.8	E947.8	E950.4	E962.0	E980.4
AHFS List	—	—	—	—	—	—
4:00 antihistamine drugs	963.0	E858.1	E933.0	E950.4	E962.0	E980.4
8:04 amebacides	961.5	E857	E931.5	E950.4	E962.0	E980.4
arsenical anti-infectives	961.1	E857	E931.1	E950.4	E962.0	E980.4
quinoline derivatives	961.3	E857	E931.3	E950.4	E962.0	E980.4
8:08 anthelmintics	961.6	E857	E931.6	E950.4	E962.0	E980.4
quinoline derivatives	961.3	E857	E931.3	E950.4	E962.0	E980.4
8:12.04 antifungal antibiotics	960.1	E856	E930.1	E950.4	E962.0	E980.4

TABLE OF DRUGS AND CHEMICALS / Drug

Substance	Poisoning	External Cause (E Code)				
		Accident	Therapeutic Use	Suicide Attempt	Assault	Undetermined
Drug *(Continued)*						
8:12.06 cephalosporins	960.5	E856	E930.5	E950.4	E962.0	E980.4
8:12.08 chloramphenicol	960.2	E856	E930.2	E950.4	E962.0	E980.4
8:12.12 erythromycins	960.3	E856	E930.3	E950.4	E962.0	E980.4
8:12.16 penicillins	960.0	E856	E930.0	E950.4	E962.0	E980.4
8:12.20 streptomycins	960.6	E856	E930.6	E950.4	E962.0	E980.4
8:12.24 tetracyclines	960.4	E856	E930.4	E950.4	E962.0	E980.4
8:12.28 other antibiotics	960.8	E856	E930.8	E950.4	E962.0	E980.4
antimycobacterial	960.6	E856	E930.6	E950.4	E962.0	E980.4
macrolides	960.3	E856	E930.3	E950.4	E962.0	E980.4
8:16 antituberculars	961.8	E857	E931.8	E950.4	E962.0	E980.4
antibiotics	960.6	E856	E930.6	E950.4	E962.0	E980.4
8:18 antivirals	961.7	E857	E931.7	E950.4	E962.0	E980.4
8:20 plasmodicides (antimalarials)	961.4	E857	E931.4	E950.4	E962.0	E980.4
8:24 sulfonamides	961.0	E857	E931.0	E950.4	E962.0	E980.4
8:26 sulfones	961.8	E857	E931.8	E950.4	E962.0	E980.4
8:28 treponemicides	961.2	E857	E931.2	E950.4	E962.0	E980.4
8:32 trichomonacides	961.5	E857	E931.5	E950.4	E962.0	E980.4
quinoline derivatives	961.3	E857	E931.3	E950.4	E962.0	E980.4
nitrofuran derivatives	961.9	E857	E931.9	E950.4	E962.0	E980.4
8:36 urinary germicides	961.9	E857	E931.9	E950.4	E962.0	E980.4
quinoline derivatives	961.3	E857	E931.3	E950.4	E962.0	E980.4
8:40 other anti-infectives	961.9	E857	E931.9	E950.4	E962.0	E980.4
10:00 antineoplastic agents	963.1	E858.1	E933.1	E950.4	E962.0	E980.4
antibiotics	960.7	E856	E930.7	E950.4	E962.0	E980.4
progestogens	962.2	E858.0	E932.2	E950.4	E962.0	E980.4
12:04 parasympathomimetic (cholinergic) agents	971.0	E855.3	E941.0	E950.4	E962.0	E980.4
12:08 parasympatholytic (cholinergic-blocking) agents	971.1	E855.4	E941.1	E950.4	E962.0	E980.4
12:12 sympathomimetic (adrenergic) agents	971.2	E855.5	E941.2	E950.4	E962.0	E980.4
12:16 sympatholytic (adrenergic-blocking) agents	971.3	E855.6	E941.3	E950.4	E962.0	E980.4
12:20 skeletal muscle relaxants	—	—	—	—	—	—
central nervous system muscle-tone depressants	968.0	E855.1	E938.0	E950.4	E962.0	E980.4
myoneural blocking agents	975.2	E858.6	E945.2	E950.4	E962.0	E980.4
16:00 blood derivatives	964.7	E858.2	E934.7	E950.4	E962.0	E980.4
20:04 antianemia drugs	964.1	E858.2	E934.1	E950.4	E962.0	E980.4
20:04.04 iron preparations	964.0	E858.2	E934.0	E950.4	E962.0	E980.4
20:04.08 liver and stomach preparations	964.1	E858.2	E934.1	E950.4	E962.0	E980.4
20:12.04 anticoagulants	964.2	E858.2	E934.2	E950.4	E962.0	E980.4
20:12.08 antiheparin agents	964.5	E858.2	E934.5	E950.4	E962.0	E980.4

TABLE OF DRUGS AND CHEMICALS / Drug

Substance	Poisoning	External Cause (E Code)				
		Accident	Therapeutic Use	Suicide Attempt	Assault	Undetermined
Drug *(Continued)*						
20:12.12 coagulants	964.5	E858.2	E934.5	E950.4	E962.0	E980.4
20:12.16 hemostatics NEC	964.5	E858.2	E934.5	E950.4	E962.0	E980.4
capillary active drugs	972.8	E858.3	E942.8	E950.4	E962.0	E980.4
24:04 cardiac drugs	972.9	E858.3	E942.9	E950.4	E962.0	E980.4
cardiotonic agents	972.1	E858.3	E942.1	E950.4	E962.0	E980.4
rhythm regulators	972.0	E858.3	E942.0	E950.4	E962.0	E980.4
24:06 antilipemic agents	972.2	E858.3	E942.2	E950.4	E962.0	E980.4
thyroid derivatives	962.7	E858.0	E932.7	E950.4	E962.0	E980.4
24:08 hypotensive agents	972.6	E858.3	E942.6	E950.4	E962.0	E980.4
adrenergic blocking agents	971.3	E855.6	E941.3	E950.4	E962.0	E980.4
ganglion blocking agents	972.3	E858.3	E942.3	E950.4	E962.0	E980.4
vasodilators	972.5	E858.3	E942.5	E950.4	E962.0	E980.4
24:12 vasodilating agents NEC	972.5	E858.3	E942.5	E950.4	E962.0	E980.4
coronary	972.4	E858.3	E942.4	E950.4	E962.0	E980.4
nicotinic acid derivatives	972.2	E858.3	E942.2	E950.4	E962.0	E980.4
24:16 sclerosing agents	972.7	E858.3	E942.7	E950.4	E962.0	E980.4
28:04 general anesthetics	968.4	E855.1	E938.4	E950.4	E962.0	E980.4
gaseous anesthetics	968.2	E855.1	E938.2	E950.4	E962.0	E980.4
halothane	968.1	E855.1	E938.1	E950.4	E962.0	E980.4
intravenous anesthetics	968.3	E855.1	E938.3	E950.4	E962.0	E980.4
28:08 analgesics and antipyretics	965.9	E850.9	E935.9	E950.0	E962.0	E980.0
antirheumatics	965.69	E850.6	E935.6	E950.0	E962.0	E980.0
aromatic analgesics	965.4	E850.4	E935.4	E950.0	E962.0	E980.0
non-narcotic NEC	965.7	E850.7	E935.7	E950.0	E962.0	E980.0
opium alkaloids	965.00	E850.2	E935.2	E950.0	E962.0	E980.0
heroin	965.01	E850.0	E935.0	E950.0	E962.0	E980.0
methadone	965.02	E850.1	E935.1	E950.0	E962.0	E980.0
specified type NEC	965.09	E850.2	E935.2	E950.0	E962.0	E980.0
pyrazole derivatives	965.5	E850.5	E935.5	E950.0	E962.0	E980.0
salicylates	965.1	E850.3	E935.3	E950.0	E962.0	E980.0
specified NEC	965.8	E850.8	E935.8	E950.0	E962.0	E980.0
28:10 narcotic antagonists	970.1	E854.3	E940.1	E950.4	E962.0	E980.4
28:12 anticonvulsants	966.3	E855.0	E936.3	E950.4	E962.0	E980.4
barbiturates	967.0	E851	E937.0	E950.1	E962.0	E980.1
benzodiazepine-based tranquilizers	969.4	E853.2	E939.4	E950.3	E962.0	E980.3
bromides	967.3	E852.2	E937.3	E950.2	E962.0	E980.2
hydantoin derivatives	966.1	E855.0	E936.1	E950.4	E962.0	E980.4
oxazolidine (derivatives)	966.0	E855.0	E936.0	E950.4	E962.0	E980.4
succinimides	966.2	E855.0	E936.2	E950.4	E962.0	E980.4

◀ New   ◀◀◀◀ Revised   ~~deleted~~ Deleted   ● Use Additional Digit(s)

TABLE OF DRUGS AND CHEMICALS / Drug

Substance	Poisoning	External Cause (E Code)				
		Accident	Therapeutic Use	Suicide Attempt	Assault	Undetermined
Drug *(Continued)*						
28:16.04 antidepressants	969.00	E854.0	E939.0	E950.3	E962.0	E980.3
28:16.08 tranquilizers	969.5	E853.9	E939.5	E950.3	E962.0	E980.3
benzodiazepine-based	969.4	E853.2	E939.4	E950.3	E962.0	E980.3
butyrophenone-based	969.2	E853.1	E939.2	E950.3	E962.0	E980.3
major NEC	969.3	E853.8	E939.3	E950.3	E962.0	E980.3
phenothiazine-based	969.1	E853.0	E939.1	E950.3	E962.0	E980.3
28:16.12 other psychotherapeutic agents	969.8	E855.8	E939.8	E950.3	E962.0	E980.3
28:20 respiratory and cerebral stimulants	970.9	E854.3	E940.9	E950.4	E962.0	E980.4
analeptics	970.0	E854.3	E940.0	E950.4	E962.0	E980.4
anorexigenic agents	977.0	E858.8	E947.0	E950.4	E962.0	E980.4
psychostimulants	969.70	E854.2	E939.7	E950.3	E962.0	E980.3
specified NEC	970.89	E854.3	E940.8	E950.4	E962.0	E980.4
28:24 sedatives and hypnotics	967.9	E852.9	E937.9	E950.2	E962.0	E980.2
barbiturates	967.0	E851	E937.0	E950.1	E962.0	E980.1
benzodiazepine-based tranquilizers	969.4	E853.2	E939.4	E950.3	E962.0	E980.3
chloral hydrate (group)	967.1	E852.0	E937.1	E950.2	E962.0	E980.2
glutethimide group	967.5	E852.4	E937.5	E950.2	E962.0	E980.2
intravenous anesthetics	968.3	E855.1	E938.3	E950.4	E962.0	E980.4
methaqualone (compounds)	967.4	E852.3	E937.4	E950.2	E962.0	E980.2
paraldehyde	967.2	E852.1	E937.2	E950.2	E962.0	E980.2
phenothiazine-based tranquilizers	969.1	E853.0	E939.1	E950.3	E962.0	E980.3
specified NEC	967.8	E852.8	E937.8	E950.2	E962.0	E980.2
thiobarbiturates	968.3	E855.1	E938.3	E950.4	E962.0	E980.4
tranquilizer NEC	969.5	E853.9	E939.5	E950.3	E962.0	E980.3
36:04 to 36:88 diagnostic agents	977.8	E858.8	E947.8	E950.4	E962.0	E980.4
40:00 electrolyte, caloric, and water balance agents NEC	974.5	E858.5	E944.5	E950.4	E962.0	E980.4
40:04 acidifying agents	963.2	E858.1	E933.2	E950.4	E962.0	E980.4
40:08 alkalinizing agents	963.3	E858.1	E933.3	E950.4	E962.0	E980.4
40:10 ammonia detoxicants	974.5	E858.5	E944.5	E950.4	E962.0	E980.4
40:12 replacement solutions	974.5	E858.5	E944.5	E950.4	E962.0	E980.4
plasma expanders	964.8	E858.2	E934.8	E950.4	E962.0	E980.4
40:16 sodium-removing resins	974.5	E858.5	E944.5	E950.4	E962.0	E980.4
40:18 potassium-removing resins	974.5	E858.5	E944.5	E950.4	E962.0	E980.4
40:20 caloric agents	974.5	E858.5	E944.5	E950.4	E962.0	E980.4
40:24 salt and sugar substitutes	974.5	E858.5	E944.5	E950.4	E962.0	E980.4
40:28 diuretics NEC	974.4	E858.5	E944.4	E950.4	E962.0	E980.4
carbonic acid anhydrase inhibitors	974.2	E858.5	E944.2	E950.4	E962.0	E980.4

◀ New   ◀◀◀ Revised   ~~deleted~~ Deleted   Use Additional Digit(s)

TABLE OF DRUGS AND CHEMICALS / Drug

Substance	Poisoning	External Cause (E Code)				
		Accident	Therapeutic Use	Suicide Attempt	Assault	Undetermined
Drug *(Continued)*						
40:28 diuretics NEC *(Continued)*						
mercurials	974.0	E858.5	E944.0	E950.4	E962.0	E980.4
purine derivatives	974.1	E858.5	E944.1	E950.4	E962.0	E980.4
saluretics	974.3	E858.5	E944.3	E950.4	E962.0	E980.4
thiazides	974.3	E858.5	E944.3	E950.4	E962.0	E980.4
40:36 irrigating solutions	974.5	E858.5	E944.5	E950.4	E962.0	E980.4
40:40 uricosuric agents	974.7	E858.5	E944.7	E950.4	E962.0	E980.4
44:00 enzymes	963.4	E858.1	E933.4	E950.4	E962.0	E980.4
fibrinolysis-affecting agents	964.4	E858.2	E934.4	E950.4	E962.0	E980.4
gastric agents	973.4	E858.4	E943.4	E950.4	E962.0	E980.4
48:00 expectorants and cough preparations	—	—	—	—	—	—
antihistamine agents	963.0	E858.1	E933.0	E950.4	E962.0	E980.4
antitussives	975.4	E858.6	E945.4	E950.4	E962.0	E980.4
codeine derivatives	965.09	E850.2	E935.2	E950.0	E962.0	E980.0
expectorants	975.5	E858.6	E945.5	E950.4	E962.0	E980.4
narcotic agents NEC	965.09	E850.2	E935.2	E950.0	E962.0	E980.0
52:04 anti-infectives (EENT)	—	—	—	—	—	—
ENT agent	976.6	E858.7	E946.6	E950.4	E962.0	E980.4
ophthalmic preparation	976.5	E858.7	E946.5	E950.4	E962.0	E980.4
52:04.04 antibiotics (EENT)	—	—	—	—	—	—
ENT agent	976.6	E858.7	E946.6	E950.4	E962.0	E980.4
ophthalmic preparation	976.5	E858.7	E946.5	E950.4	E962.0	E980.4
52:04.06 antivirals (EENT)	—	—	—	—	—	—
ENT agent	976.6	E858.7	E946.6	E950.4	E962.0	E980.4
ophthalmic preparation	976.5	E858.7	E946.5	E950.4	E962.0	E980.4
52:04.08 sulfonamides (EENT)	—	—	—	—	—	—
ENT agent	976.6	E858.7	E946.6	E950.4	E962.0	E980.4
ophthalmic preparation	976.5	E858.7	E946.5	E950.4	E962.0	E980.4
52:04.12 miscellaneous anti-infectives (EENT)	—	—	—	—	—	—
ENT agent	976.6	E858.7	E946.6	E950.4	E962.0	E980.4
ophthalmic preparation	976.5	E858.7	E946.5	E950.4	E962.0	E980.4
52:08 anti-inflammatory agents (EENT)	—	—	—	—	—	—
ENT agent	976.6	E858.7	E946.6	E950.4	E962.0	E980.4
ophthalmic preparation	976.5	E858.7	E946.5	E950.4	E962.0	E980.4
52:10 carbonic anhydrase inhibitors	974.2	E858.5	E944.2	E950.4	E962.0	E980.4
52:12 contact lens solutions	976.5	E858.7	E946.5	E950.4	E962.0	E980.4
52:16 local anesthetics (EENT)	968.5	E855.2	E938.5	E950.4	E962.0	E980.4

TABLE OF DRUGS AND CHEMICALS / Drug

Substance	Poisoning	External Cause (E Code)				
		Accident	Therapeutic Use	Suicide Attempt	Assault	Undetermined
Drug *(Continued)*						
52:20 miotics	971.0	E855.3	E941.0	E950.4	E962.0	E980.4
52:24 mydriatics	—	—	—	—	—	—
adrenergics	971.2	E855.5	E941.2	E950.4	E962.0	E980.4
anticholinergics	971.1	E855.4	E941.1	E950.4	E962.0	E980.4
antimuscarinics	971.1	E855.4	E941.1	E950.4	E962.0	E980.4
parasympatholytics	971.1	E855.4	E941.1	E950.4	E962.0	E980.4
spasmolytics	971.1	E855.4	E941.1	E950.4	E962.0	E980.4
sympathomimetics	971.2	E855.5	E941.2	E950.4	E962.0	E980.4
52:28 mouth washes and gargles	976.6	E858.7	E946.6	E950.4	E962.0	E980.4
52:32 vasoconstrictors (EENT)	971.2	E855.5	E941.2	E950.4	E962.0	E980.4
52:36 unclassified agents (EENT)	—	—	—	—	—	—
ENT agent	976.6	E858.7	E946.6	E950.4	E962.0	E980.4
ophthalmic preparation	976.5	E858.7	E946.5	E950.4	E962.0	E980.4
56:04 antacids and adsorbents	973.0	E858.4	E943.0	E950.4	E962.0	E980.4
56:08 antidiarrhea agents	973.5	E858.4	E943.5	E950.4	E962.0	E980.4
56:10 antiflatulents	973.8	E858.4	E943.8	E950.4	E962.0	E980.4
56:12 cathartics NEC	973.3	E858.4	E943.3	E950.4	E962.0	E980.4
emollients	973.2	E858.4	E943.2	E950.4	E962.0	E980.4
irritants	973.1	E858.4	E943.1	E950.4	E962.0	E980.4
56:16 digestants	973.4	E858.4	E943.4	E950.4	E962.0	E980.4
56:20 emetics and antiemetics	—	—	—	—	—	—
antiemetics	963.0	E858.1	E933.0	E950.4	E962.0	E980.4
emetics	973.6	E858.4	E943.6	E950.4	E962.0	E980.4
56:24 lipotropic agents	977.1	E858.8	E947.1	E950.4	E962.0	E980.4
56:40 miscellaneous G.I. drugs	973.8	E858.4	E943.8	E950.4	E962.0	E980.4
60:00 gold compounds	965.69	E850.6	E935.6	E950.0	E962.0	E980.0
64:00 heavy metal antagonists	963.8	E858.1	E933.8	E950.4	E962.0	E980.4
68:04 adrenals	962.0	E858.0	E932.0	E950.4	E962.0	E980.4
68:08 androgens	962.1	E858.0	E932.1	E950.4	E962.0	E980.4
68:12 contraceptives, oral	962.2	E858.0	E932.2	E950.4	E962.0	E980.4
68:16 estrogens	962.2	E858.0	E932.2	E950.4	E962.0	E980.4
68:18 gonadotropins	962.4	E858.0	E932.4	E950.4	E962.0	E980.4
68:20 insulins and antidiabetic agents	962.3	E858.0	E932.3	E950.4	E962.0	E980.4
68:20.08 insulins	962.3	E858.0	E932.3	E950.4	E962.0	E980.4
68:24 parathyroid	962.6	E858.0	E932.6	E950.4	E962.0	E980.4
68:28 pituitary (posterior)	962.5	E858.0	E932.5	E950.4	E962.0	E980.4
anterior	962.4	E858.0	E932.4	E950.4	E962.0	E980.4
68:32 progestogens	962.2	E858.0	E932.2	E950.4	E962.0	E980.4

◂ New ◂◂◂ Revised ~~deleted~~ Deleted ● Use Additional Digit(s)

TABLE OF DRUGS AND CHEMICALS / Drug

Substance	Poisoning	External Cause (E Code)				
		Accident	Therapeutic Use	Suicide Attempt	Assault	Undetermined
Drug *(Continued)*						
68:34 other corpus luteum hormones NEC	962.2	E858.0	E932.2	E950.4	E962.0	E980.4
68:36 thyroid and antithyroid	—	—	—	—	—	—
antithyroid	962.8	E858.0	E932.8	E950.4	E962.0	E980.4
thyroid (derivatives)	962.7	E858.0	E932.7	E950.4	E962.0	E980.4
72:00 local anesthetics NEC	968.9	E855.2	E938.9	E950.4	E962.0	E980.4
topical (surface)	968.5	E855.2	E938.5	E950.4	E962.0	E980.4
infiltration (intradermal) (subcutaneous) (submucosal)	968.5	E855.2	E938.5	E950.4	E962.0	E980.4
nerve blocking (peripheral) (plexus) (regional)	968.6	E855.2	E938.6	E950.4	E962.0	E980.4
spinal	968.7	E855.2	E938.7	E950.4	E962.0	E980.4
76:00 oxytocics	975.0	E858.6	E945.0	E950.4	E962.0	E980.4
78:00 radioactive agents	990	—	—	—	—	—
80:04 serums NEC	979.9	E858.8	E949.9	E950.4	E962.0	E980.4
immune gamma globulin (human)	964.6	E858.2	E934.6	E950.4	E962.0	E980.4
80:08 toxoids NEC	978.8	E858.8	E948.8	E950.4	E962.0	E980.4
diphtheria	978.5	E858.8	E948.5	E950.4	E962.0	E980.4
and tetanus	978.9	E858.8	E948.9	E950.4	E962.0	E980.4
with pertussis component	978.6	E858.8	E948.6	E950.4	E962.0	E980.4
tetanus	978.4	E858.8	E948.4	E950.4	E962.0	E980.4
and diphtheria	978.9	E858.8	E948.9	E950.4	E962.0	E980.4
with pertussis component	978.6	E858.8	E948.6	E950.4	E962.0	E980.4
80:12 vaccines	979.9	E858.8	E949.9	E950.4	E962.0	E980.4
bacterial NEC	978.8	E858.8	E948.8	E950.4	E962.0	E980.4
with	—	—	—	—	—	—
other bacterial components	978.9	E858.8	E948.9	E950.4	E962.0	E980.4
pertussis component	978.6	E858.8	E948.6	E950.4	E962.0	E980.4
viral and rickettsial components	979.7	E858.8	E949.7	E950.4	E962.0	E980.4
rickettsial NEC	979.6	E858.8	E949.6	E950.4	E962.0	E980.4
with	—	—	—	—	—	—
bacterial component	979.7	E858.8	E949.7	E950.4	E962.0	E980.4
pertussis component	978.6	E858.8	E948.6	E950.4	E962.0	E980.4
viral component	979.7	E858.8	E949.7	E950.4	E962.0	E980.4
viral NEC	979.6	E858.8	E949.6	E950.4	E962.0	E980.4
with	—	—	—	—	—	—
bacterial component	979.7	E858.8	E949.7	E950.4	E962.0	E980.4
pertussis component	978.6	E858.8	E948.6	E950.4	E962.0	E980.4
rickettsial component	979.7	E858.8	E949.7	E950.4	E962.0	E980.4
84:04.04 antibiotics (skin and mucous membrane)	976.0	E858.7	E946.0	E950.4	E962.0	E980.4
84:04.08 fungicides (skin and mucous membrane)	976.0	E858.7	E946.0	E950.4	E962.0	E980.4

◀ New ◀▥ Revised ~~deleted~~ Deleted ● Use Additional Digit(s)

TABLE OF DRUGS AND CHEMICALS / Dyflos

| Substance | Poisoning | External Cause (E Code) |||||
		Accident	Therapeutic Use	Suicide Attempt	Assault	Undetermined
Drug *(Continued)*						
84:04.12 scabicides and pediculicides (skin and mucous membrane)	976.0	E858.7	E946.0	E950.4	E962.0	E980.4
84:04.16 miscellaneous local anti-infectives (skin and mucous membrane)	976.0	E858.7	E946.0	E950.4	E962.0	E980.4
84:06 anti-inflammatory agents (skin and mucous membrane)	976.0	E858.7	E946.0	E950.4	E962.0	E980.4
84:08 antipruritics and local anesthetics	—	—	—	—	—	—
antipruritics	976.1	E858.7	E946.1	E950.4	E962.0	E980.4
local anesthetics	968.5	E855.2	E938.5	E950.4	E962.0	E980.4
84:12 astringents	976.2	E858.7	E946.2	E950.4	E962.0	E980.4
84:16 cell stimulants and proliferants	976.8	E858.7	E946.8	E950.4	E962.0	E980.4
84:20 detergents	976.2	E858.7	E946.2	E950.4	E962.0	E980.4
84:24 emollients, demulcents, and protectants	976.3	E858.7	E946.3	E950.4	E962.0	E980.4
84:28 keratolytic agents	976.4	E858.7	E946.4	E950.4	E962.0	E980.4
84:32 keratoplastic agents	976.4	E858.7	E946.4	E950.4	E962.0	E980.4
84:36 miscellaneous agents (skin and mucous membrane)	976.8	E858.7	E946.8	E950.4	E962.0	E980.4
86:00 spasmolytic agents	975.1	E858.6	E945.1	E950.4	E962.0	E980.4
antiasthmatics	975.7	E858.6	E945.7	E950.4	E962.0	E980.4
papaverine	972.5	E858.3	E942.5	E950.4	E962.0	E980.4
theophylline	974.1	E858.5	E944.1	E950.4	E962.0	E980.4
88:04 vitamin A	963.5	E858.1	E933.5	E950.4	E962.0	E980.4
88:08 vitamin B complex	963.5	E858.1	E933.5	E950.4	E962.0	E980.4
hematopoietic vitamin	964.1	E858.2	E934.1	E950.4	E962.0	E980.4
nicotinic acid derivatives	972.2	E858.3	E942.2	E950.4	E962.0	E980.4
88:12 vitamin C	963.5	E858.1	E933.5	E950.4	E962.0	E980.4
88:16 vitamin D	963.5	E858.1	E933.5	E950.4	E962.0	E980.4
88:20 vitamin E	963.5	E858.1	E933.5	E950.4	E962.0	E980.4
88:24 vitamin K activity	964.3	E858.2	E934.3	E950.4	E962.0	E980.4
88:28 multivitamin preparations	963.5	E858.1	E933.5	E950.4	E962.0	E980.4
92:00 unclassified therapeutic agents	977.8	E858.8	E947.8	E950.4	E962.0	E980.4
Duboisine	971.1	E855.4	E941.1	E950.4	E962.0	E980.4
Dulcolax	973.1	E858.4	E943.1	E950.4	E962.0	E980.4
Duponol (C) (EP)	976.2	E858.7	E946.2	E950.4	E962.0	E980.4
Durabolin	962.1	E858.0	E932.1	E950.4	E962.0	E980.4
Dyclone	968.5	E855.2	E938.5	E950.4	E962.0	E980.4
Dyclonine	968.5	E855.2	E938.5	E950.4	E962.0	E980.4
Dydrogesterone	962.2	E858.0	E932.2	E950.4	E962.0	E980.4
Dyes NEC	989.89	E866.8	—	E950.9	E962.1	E980.9
diagnostic agents	977.8	E858.8	E947.8	E950.4	E962.0	E980.4
pharmaceutical NEC	977.4	E858.8	E947.4	E950.4	E962.0	E980.4
Dyflos	971.0	E855.3	E941.0	E950.4	E962.0	E980.4

TABLE OF DRUGS AND CHEMICALS / Dymelor

Substance	Poisoning	Accident	Therapeutic Use	Suicide Attempt	Assault	Undetermined
Dymelor	962.3	E858.0	E932.3	E950.4	E962.0	E980.4
Dynamite	989.89	E866.8	—	E950.9	E962.1	E980.9
fumes	987.8	E869.8	—	E952.8	E962.2	E982.8
Dyphylline	975.1	E858.6	E945.1	E950.4	E962.0	E980.4
Ear preparations	976.6	E858.7	E946.6	E950.4	E962.0	E980.4
Echothiopate, ecothiopate	971.0	E855.3	E941.0	E950.4	E962.0	E980.4
Ecstasy	969.72	E854.2	E939.7	E950.3	E962.0	E980.3
Ectylurea	967.8	E852.8	E937.8	E950.2	E962.0	E980.2
Edathamil disodium	963.8	E858.1	E933.8	E950.4	E962.0	E980.4
Edecrin	974.4	E858.5	E944.4	E950.4	E962.0	E980.4
Edetate, disodium (calcium)	963.8	E858.1	E933.8	E950.4	E962.0	E980.4
Edrophonium	971.0	E855.3	E941.0	E950.4	E962.0	E980.4
Elase	976.8	E858.7	E946.8	E950.4	E962.0	E980.4
Elaterium	973.1	E858.4	E943.1	E950.4	E962.0	E980.4
Elder	988.2	E865.4	—	E950.9	E962.1	E980.9
berry (unripe)	988.2	E865.3	—	E950.9	E962.1	E980.9
Electrolytes NEC	974.5	E858.5	E944.5	E950.4	E962.0	E980.4
Electrolytic agent NEC	974.5	E858.5	E944.5	E950.4	E962.0	E980.4
Embramine	963.0	E858.1	E933.0	E950.4	E962.0	E980.4
Emetics	973.6	E858.4	E943.6	E950.4	E962.0	E980.4
Emetine (hydrochloride)	961.5	E857	E931.5	E950.4	E962.0	E980.4
Emollients	976.3	E858.7	E946.3	E950.4	E962.0	E980.4
Emylcamate	969.5	E853.8	E939.5	E950.3	E962.0	E980.3
Encyprate	969.09	E854.0	E939.0	E950.3	E962.0	E980.3
Endocaine	968.5	E855.2	E938.5	E950.4	E962.0	E980.4
Endrin	989.2	E863.0	—	E950.6	E962.1	E980.7
Enflurane	968.2	E855.1	E938.2	E950.4	E962.0	E980.4
Enovid	962.2	E858.0	E932.2	E950.4	E962.0	E980.4
ENT preparations (anti-infectives)	976.6	E858.7	E946.6	E950.4	E962.0	E980.4
Enzodase	963.4	E858.1	E933.4	E950.4	E962.0	E980.4
Enzymes NEC	963.4	E858.1	E933.4	E950.4	E962.0	E980.4
Epanutin	966.1	E855.0	E936.1	E950.4	E962.0	E980.4
Ephedra (tincture)	971.2	E855.5	E941.2	E950.4	E962.0	E980.4
Ephedrine	971.2	E855.5	E941.2	E950.4	E962.0	E980.4
Epiestriol	962.2	E858.0	E932.2	E950.4	E962.0	E980.4
Epilim - see Sodium valproate	—	—	—	—	—	—
Epinephrine	971.2	E855.5	E941.2	E950.4	E962.0	E980.4
Epsom salt	973.3	E858.4	E943.3	E950.4	E962.0	E980.4
Equanil	969.5	E853.8	E939.5	E950.3	E962.0	E980.3

TABLE OF DRUGS AND CHEMICALS / Ethisterone

Substance	Poisoning	External Cause (E Code)				
		Accident	Therapeutic Use	Suicide Attempt	Assault	Undetermined
Equisetum (diuretic)	974.4	E858.5	E944.4	E950.4	E962.0	E980.4
Ergometrine	975.0	E858.6	E945.0	E950.4	E962.0	E980.4
Ergonovine	975.0	E858.6	E945.0	E950.4	E962.0	E980.4
Ergot NEC	988.2	E865.4	—	E950.9	E962.1	E980.9
medicinal (alkaloids)	975.0	E858.6	E945.0	E950.4	E962.0	E980.4
Ergotamine (tartrate) (for migraine) NEC	972.9	E858.3	E942.9	E950.4	E962.0	E980.4
Ergotrate	975.0	E858.6	E945.0	E950.4	E962.0	E980.4
Erythrityl tetranitrate	972.4	E858.3	E942.4	E950.4	E962.0	E980.4
Erythrol tetranitrate	972.4	E858.3	E942.4	E950.4	E962.0	E980.4
Erythromycin	960.3	E856	E930.3	E950.4	E962.0	E980.4
ophthalmic preparation	976.5	E858.7	E946.5	E950.4	E962.0	E980.4
topical NEC	976.0	E858.7	E946.0	E950.4	E962.0	E980.4
Eserine	971.0	E855.3	E941.0	E950.4	E962.0	E980.4
Eskabarb	967.0	E851	E937.0	E950.1	E962.0	E980.1
Eskalith	969.8	E855.8	E939.8	E950.3	E962.0	E980.3
Estradiol (cypionate) (dipropionate) (valerate)	962.2	E858.0	E932.2	E950.4	E962.0	E980.4
Estriol	962.2	E858.0	E932.2	E950.4	E962.0	E980.4
Estrogens (with progestogens)	962.2	E858.0	E932.2	E950.4	E962.0	E980.4
Estrone	962.2	E858.0	E932.2	E950.4	E962.0	E980.4
Etafedrine	971.2	E855.5	E941.2	E950.4	E962.0	E980.4
Ethacrynate sodium	974.4	E858.5	E944.4	E950.4	E962.0	E980.4
Ethacrynic acid	974.4	E858.5	E944.4	E950.4	E962.0	E980.4
Ethambutol	961.8	E857	E931.8	E950.4	E962.0	E980.4
Ethamide	974.2	E858.5	E944.2	E950.4	E962.0	E980.4
Ethamivan	970.0	E854.3	E940.0	E950.4	E962.0	E980.4
Ethamsylate	964.5	E858.2	E934.5	E950.4	E962.0	E980.4
Ethanol	980.0	E860.1	—	E950.9	E962.1	E980.9
beverage	980.0	E860.0	—	E950.9	E962.1	E980.9
Ethchlorvynol	967.8	E852.8	E937.8	E950.2	E962.0	E980.2
Ethebenecid	974.7	E858.5	E944.7	E950.4	E962.0	E980.4
Ether(s) (diethyl) (ethyl) (vapor)	987.8	E869.8	—	E952.8	E962.2	E982.8
anesthetic	968.2	E855.1	E938.2	E950.4	E962.0	E980.4
petroleum - see Ligroin solvent	982.8	E862.4	—	E950.9	E962.1	E980.9
Ethidine chloride (vapor)	987.8	E869.8	—	E952.8	E962.2	E982.8
liquid (solvent)	982.3	E862.4	—	E950.9	E962.1	E980.9
Ethinamate	967.8	E852.8	E937.8	E950.2	E962.0	E980.2
Ethinylestradiol	962.2	E858.0	E932.2	E950.4	E962.0	E980.4
Ethionamide	961.8	E857	E931.8	E950.4	E962.0	E980.4
Ethisterone	962.2	E858.0	E932.2	E950.4	E962.0	E980.4

◀ New   ◀▥ Revised   ~~deleted~~ Deleted   ● Use Additional Digit(s)

TABLE OF DRUGS AND CHEMICALS / Ethobral

Substance	Poisoning	External Cause (E Code)				
		Accident	Therapeutic Use	Suicide Attempt	Assault	Undetermined
Ethobral	967.0	E851	E937.0	E950.1	E962.0	E980.1
Ethocaine (infiltration) (topical)	968.5	E855.2	E938.5	E950.4	E962.0	E980.4
nerve block (peripheral) (plexus)	968.6	E855.2	E938.6	E950.4	E962.0	E980.4
spinal	968.7	E855.2	E938.7	E950.4	E962.0	E980.4
Ethoheptazine (citrate)	965.7	E850.7	E935.7	E950.0	E962.0	E980.0
Ethopropazine	966.4	E855.0	E936.4	E950.4	E962.0	E980.4
Ethosuximide	966.2	E855.0	E936.2	E950.4	E962.0	E980.4
Ethotoin	966.1	E855.0	E936.1	E950.4	E962.0	E980.4
Ethoxazene	961.9	E857	E931.9	E950.4	E962.0	E980.4
Ethoxzolamide	974.2	E858.5	E944.2	E950.4	E962.0	E980.4
Ethyl	—	—	—	—	—	—
acetate (vapor)	982.8	E862.4	—	E950.9	E962.1	E980.9
alcohol	980.0	E860.1	—	E950.9	E962.1	E980.9
beverage	980.0	E860.0	—	E950.9	E962.1	E980.9
aldehyde (vapor)	987.8	E869.8	—	E952.8	E962.2	E982.8
liquid	989.89	E866.8	—	E950.9	E962.1	E980.9
aminobenzoate	968.5	E855.2	E938.5	E950.4	E962.0	E980.4
biscoumacetate	964.2	E858.2	E934.2	E950.4	E962.0	E980.4
bromide (anesthetic)	968.2	E855.1	E938.2	E950.4	E962.0	E980.4
carbamate (antineoplastic)	963.1	E858.1	E933.1	E950.4	E962.0	E980.4
carbinol	980.3	E860.4	—	E950.9	E962.1	E980.9
chaulmoograte	961.8	E857	E931.8	E950.4	E962.0	E980.4
chloride (vapor)	987.8	E869.8	—	E952.8	E962.2	E982.8
anesthetic (local)	968.5	E855.2	E938.5	E950.4	E962.0	E980.4
inhaled	968.2	E855.1	E938.2	E950.4	E962.0	E980.4
solvent	982.3	E862.4	—	E950.9	E962.1	E980.9
estranol	962.1	E858.0	E932.1	E950.4	E962.0	E980.4
ether - *see* Ether(s)	—	—	—	—	—	—
formate (solvent) NEC	982.8	E862.4	—	E950.9	E962.1	E980.9
iodoacetate	987.5	E869.3	—	E952.8	E962.2	E982.8
lactate (solvent) NEC	982.8	E862.4	—	E950.9	E962.1	E980.9
methylcarbinol	980.8	E860.8	—	E950.9	E962.1	E980.9
morphine	965.09	E850.2	E935.2	E950.0	E962.0	E980.0
Ethylene (gas)	987.1	E869.8	—	E952.8	E962.2	E982.8
anesthetic (general)	968.2	E855.1	E938.2	E950.4	E962.0	E980.4
chlorohydrin (vapor)	982.3	E862.4	—	E950.9	E962.1	E980.9
dichloride (vapor)	982.3	E862.4	—	E950.9	E962.1	E980.9
glycol(s) (any) (vapor)	982.8	E862.4	—	E950.9	E962.1	E980.9

TABLE OF DRUGS AND CHEMICALS / Fecal softeners

Substance	Poisoning	External Cause (E Code)				
		Accident	Therapeutic Use	Suicide Attempt	Assault	Undetermined
Ethylidene	—	—	—	—	—	—
chloride NEC	982.3	E862.4	—	E950.9	E962.1	E980.9
diethyl ether	982.8	—	E862.4	E950.9	E962.1	E980.9
Ethynodiol	962.2	E858.0	E932.2	E950.4	E962.0	E980.4
Etidocaine	968.9	E855.2	E938.9	E950.4	E962.0	E980.4
infiltration (subcutaneous)	968.5	E855.2	E938.5	E950.4	E962.0	E980.4
nerve (peripheral) (plexus)	968.6	E855.2	E938.6	E950.4	E962.0	E980.4
Etilfen	967.0	E851	E937.0	E950.1	E962.0	E980.1
Etomide	965.7	E850.7	E935.7	E950.0	E962.0	E980.0
Etorphine	965.09	E850.2	E935.2	E950.0	E962.0	E980.0
Etoval	967.0	E851	E937.0	E950.1	E962.0	E980.1
Etryptamine	969.01	E854.0	E939.0	E950.3	E962.0	E980.3
Eucaine	968.5	E855.2	E938.5	E950.4	E962.0	E980.4
Eucalyptus (oil) NEC	975.5	E858.6	E945.5	E950.4	E962.0	E980.4
Eucatropine	971.1	E855.4	E941.1	E950.4	E962.0	E980.4
Eucodal	965.09	E850.2	E935.2	E950.0	E962.0	E980.0
Euneryl	967.0	E851	E937.0	E950.1	E962.0	E980.1
Euphthalmine	971.1	E855.4	E941.1	E950.4	E962.0	E980.4
Eurax	976.0	E858.7	E946.0	E950.4	E962.0	E980.4
Euresol	976.4	E858.7	E946.4	E950.4	E962.0	E980.4
Euthroid	962.7	E858.0	E932.7	E950.4	E962.0	E980.4
Evans blue	977.8	E858.8	E947.8	E950.4	E962.0	E980.4
Evipal	967.0	E851	E937.0	E950.1	E962.0	E980.1
sodium	968.3	E855.1	E938.3	E950.4	E962.0	E980.4
Evipan	967.0	E851	E937.0	E950.1	E962.0	E980.1
sodium	968.3	E855.1	E938.3	E950.4	E962.0	E980.4
Exalgin	965.4	E850.4	E935.4	E950.0	E962.0	E980.0
Excipients, pharmaceutical	977.4	E858.8	E947.4	E950.4	E962.0	E980.4
Exhaust gas - *see* Carbon, monoxide	—	—	—	—	—	—
Ex-Lax (phenolphthalein)	973.1	E858.4	E943.1	E950.4	E962.0	E980.4
Expectorants	975.5	E858.6	E945.5	E950.4	E962.0	E980.4
External medications (skin) (mucous membrane)	976.9	E858.7	E946.9	E950.4	E962.0	E980.4
dental agent	976.7	E858.7	E946.7	E950.4	E962.0	E980.4
ENT agent	976.6	E858.7	E946.6	E950.4	E962.0	E980.4
ophthalmic preparation	976.5	E858.7	E946.5	E950.4	E962.0	E980.4
specified NEC	976.8	E858.7	E946.8	E950.4	E962.0	E980.4
Eye agents (anti-infective)	976.5	E858.7	E946.5	E950.4	E962.0	E980.4
Factor IX complex (human)	964.5	E858.2	E934.5	E950.4	E962.0	E980.4
Fecal softeners	973.2	E858.4	E943.2	E950.4	E962.0	E980.4

◀ New ◀▥ Revised ~~deleted~~ Deleted ● Use Additional Digit(s)

TABLE OF DRUGS AND CHEMICALS / Fenbutrazate

Substance	Poisoning	External Cause (E Code)			
		Accident	Therapeutic Use	Suicide Attempt	Assault	Undetermined
Fenbutrazate	977.0	E858.8	E947.0	E950.4	E962.0	E980.4
Fencamfamin	970.89	E854.3	E940.8	E950.4	E962.0	E980.4
Fenfluramine	977.0	E858.8	E947.0	E950.4	E962.0	E980.4
Fenoprofen	965.61	E850.6	E935.6	E950.0	E962.0	E980.0
Fentanyl	965.09	E850.2	E935.2	E950.0	E962.0	E980.0
Fentazin	969.1	E853.0	E939.1	E930.3	E962.0	E980.3
Fenticlor, fentichlor	976.0	E858.7	E946.0	E950.4	E962.0	E980.4
Fer de lance (bite) (venom)	989.5	E905.0	—	E950.9	E962.1	E980.9
Ferric - see Iron	—	—	—	—	—	—
Ferrocholinate	964.0	E858.2	E934.0	E950.4	E962.0	E980.4
Ferrous fumerate, gluconate, lactate, salt NEC, sulfate (medicinal)	964.0	E858.2	E934.0	E950.4	E962.0	E980.4
Ferrum - see Iron	—	—	—	—	—	—
Fertilizers NEC	989.89	E866.5	—	E950.9	E962.1	E980.4
with herbicide mixture	989.4	E863.5	—	E950.6	E962.1	E980.7
Fibrinogen (human)	964.7	E858.2	E934.7	E950.4	E962.0	E980.4
Fibrinolysin	964.4	E858.2	E934.4	E950.4	E962.0	E980.4
Fibrinolysis-affecting agents	964.4	E858.2	E934.4	E950.4	E962.0	E980.4
Filix mas	961.6	E857	E931.6	E950.4	E962.0	E980.4
Fiorinal	965.1	E850.3	E935.3	E950.0	E962.0	E980.0
Fire damp	987.1	E869.8	—	E952.8	E962.2	E982.8
Fish, nonbacterial or noxious	988.0	E865.2	—	E950.9	E962.1	E980.9
shell	988.0	E865.1	—	E950.9	E962.1	E980.9
Flagyl	961.5	E857	E931.5	E950.4	E962.0	E980.4
Flavoxate	975.1	E858.6	E945.1	E950.4	E962.0	E980.4
Flaxedil	975.2	E858.6	E945.2	E950.4	E962.0	E980.4
Flaxseed (medicinal)	976.3	E858.7	E946.3	E950.4	E962.0	E980.4
Flomax	971.3	E855.6	E941.3	E950.4	E962.0	E980.4
Florantyrone	973.4	E858.4	E943.4	E950.4	E962.0	E980.4
Floraquin	961.3	E857	E931.3	E950.4	E962.0	E980.4
Florinef	962.0	E858.0	E932.0	E950.4	E962.0	E980.4
ENT agent	976.6	E858.7	E946.6	E950.4	E962.0	E980.4
ophthalmic preparation	976.5	E858.7	E946.5	E950.4	E962.0	E980.4
topical NEC	976.0	E858.7	E946.0	E950.4	E962.0	E980.4
Flowers of sulfur	976.4	E858.7	E946.4	E950.4	E962.0	E980.4
Floxuridine	963.1	E858.1	E933.1	E950.4	E962.0	E980.4
Flucytosine	961.9	E857	E931.9	E950.4	E962.0	E980.4
Fludrocortisone	962.0	E858.0	E932.0	E950.4	E962.0	E980.4
ENT agent	976.6	E858.7	E946.6	E950.4	E962.0	E980.4
ophthalmic preparation	976.5	E858.7	E946.5	E950.4	E962.0	E980.4

TABLE OF DRUGS AND CHEMICALS / Flurbiprofen

Substance	Poisoning	External Cause (E Code)				
		Accident	Therapeutic Use	Suicide Attempt	Assault	Undetermined
Fludrocortisone *(Continued)*						
topical NEC	976.0	E858.7	E946.0	E950.4	E962.0	E980.4
Flumethasone	976.0	E858.7	E946.0	E950.4	E962.0	E980.4
Flumethiazide	974.3	E858.5	E944.3	E950.4	E962.0	E980.4
Flumidin	961.7	E857	E931.7	E950.4	E962.0	E980.4
Flunitrazepam	969.4	E853.2	E939.4	E950.3	E962.0	E980.3
Fluocinolone	976.0	E858.7	E946.0	E950.4	E962.0	E980.4
Fluocortolone	962.0	E858.0	E932.0	E950.4	E962.0	E980.4
Fluohydrocortisone	962.0	E858.0	E932.0	E950.4	E962.0	E980.4
ENT agent	976.6	E858.7	E946.6	E950.4	E962.0	E980.4
ophthalmic preparation	976.5	E858.7	E946.5	E950.4	E962.0	E980.4
topical NEC	976.0	E858.7	E946.0	E950.4	E962.0	E980.4
Fluonid	976.0	E858.7	E946.0	E950.4	E962.0	E980.4
Fluopromazine	969.1	E853.0	E939.1	E950.3	E962.0	E980.3
Fluoracetate	989.4	E863.7	—	E950.6	E962.1	E980.7
Fluorescein (sodium)	977.8	E858.8	E947.8	E950.4	E962.0	E980.4
Fluoride(s) (pesticides) (sodium) NEC	989.4	E863.4	—	E950.6	E962.1	E980.7
hydrogen - *see* Hydrofluoric acid	—	—	—	—	—	—
medicinal	976.7	E858.7	E946.7	E950.4	E962.0	E980.4
not pesticide NEC	983.9	E864.4	—	E950.7	E962.1	E980.6
stannous	976.7	E858.7	E946.7	E950.4	E962.0	E980.4
Fluorinated corticosteroids	962.0	E858.0	E932.0	E950.4	E962.0	E980.4
Fluorine (compounds) (gas)	987.8	E869.8	—	E952.8	E962.2	E982.8
salt - *see* Fluoride(s)	—	—	—	—	—	—
Fluoristan	976.7	E858.7	E946.7	E950.4	E962.0	E980.4
Fluoroacetate	989.4	E863.7	—	E950.6	E962.1	E980.7
Fluorodeoxyuridine	963.1	E858.1	E933.1	E950.4	E962.0	E980.4
Fluorometholone (topical) NEC	976.0	E858.7	E946.0	E950.4	E962.0	E980.4
ophthalmic preparation	976.5	E858.7	E946.5	E950.4	E962.0	E980.4
Fluorouracil	963.1	E858.1	E933.1	E950.4	E962.0	E980.4
Fluothane	968.1	E855.1	E938.1	E950.4	E962.0	E980.4
Fluoxetine hydrochloride	969.03	E854.0	E939.0	E950.3	E962.0	E980.3
Fluoxymesterone	962.1	E858.0	E932.1	E950.4	E962.0	E980.4
Fluphenazine	969.1	E853.0	E939.1	E950.3	E962.0	E980.3
Fluprednisolone	962.0	E858.0	E932.0	E950.4	E962.0	E980.4
Flurandrenolide	976.0	E858.7	E946.0	E950.4	E962.0	E980.4
Flurazepam (hydrochloride)	969.4	E853.2	E939.4	E950.3	E962.0	E980.3
Flurbiprofen	965.61	E850.6	E935.6	E950.0	E962.0	E980.0

 New   Revised   ~~deleted~~ Deleted   ● Use Additional Digit(s)

TABLE OF DRUGS AND CHEMICALS / Flurobate

Substance	Poisoning	External Cause (E Code)				
		Accident	Therapeutic Use	Suicide Attempt	Assault	Undetermined
Flurobate	976.0	E858.7	E946.0	E950.4	E962.0	E980.4
Flurothyl	969.8	E855.8	E939.8	E950.3	E962.0	E980.3
Fluroxene	968.2	E855.1	E938.2	E950.4	E962.0	E980.4
Folacin	964.1	E858.2	E934.1	E950.4	E962.0	E980.4
Folic acid	964.1	E858.2	E934.1	E950.4	E962.0	E980.4
Follicle stimulating hormone	962.4	E858.0	E932.4	E950.4	E962.0	E980.4
Food, foodstuffs, nonbacterial or noxious	988.9	E865.9	—	E950.9	E962.1	E980.9
berries, seeds	988.2	E865.3	—	E950.9	E962.1	E980.9
fish	988.0	E865.2	—	E950.9	E962.1	E980.9
mushrooms	988.1	E865.5	—	E950.9	E962.1	E980.9
plants	988.2	E865.9	—	E950.9	E962.1	E980.9
specified type NEC	988.2	E865.4	—	E950.9	E962.1	E980.9
shellfish	988.0	E865.1	—	E950.9	E962.1	E980.9
specified NEC	988.8	E865.8	—	E950.9	E962.1	E980.9
Fool's parsley	988.2	E865.4	—	E950.9	E962.1	E980.9
Formaldehyde (solution)	989.89	E861.4	—	E950.9	E962.1	E980.9
fungicide	989.4	E863.6	—	E950.6	E962.1	E980.7
gas or vapor	987.8	E869.8	—	E952.8	E962.2	E982.8
Formalin	989.89	E861.4	—	E950.9	E962.1	E980.9
fungicide	989.4	E863.6	—	E950.6	E962.1	E980.7
vapor	987.8	E869.8	—	E952.8	E962.2	E982.8
Formic acid	983.1	E864.1	—	E950.7	E962.1	E980.6
vapor	987.8	E869.8	—	E952.8	E962.2	E982.8
Fowler's solution	985.1	E866.3	—	E950.8	E962.1	E980.8
Foxglove	988.2	E865.4	—	E950.9	E962.1	E980.9
Fox green	977.8	E858.8	E947.8	E950.4	E962.0	E980.4
Framycetin	960.8	E856	E930.8	E950.4	E962.0	E980.4
Frangula (extract)	973.1	E858.4	E943.1	E950.4	E962.0	E980.4
Frei antigen	977.8	E858.8	E947.8	E950.4	E962.0	E980.4
Freons	987.4	E869.2	—	E952.8	E962.2	E982.8
Fructose	974.5	E858.5	E944.5	E950.4	E962.0	E980.4
Frusemide	974.4	E858.5	E944.4	E950.4	E962.0	E980.4
FSH	962.4	E858.0	E932.4	E950.4	E962.0	E980.4
Fuel	—	—	—	—	—	—
automobile	981	E862.1	—	E950.9	E962.1	E980.9
exhaust gas, not in transit	986	E868.2	—	E952.0	E962.2	E982.0
vapor NEC	987.1	E869.8	—	E952.8	E962.2	E982.8

TABLE OF DRUGS AND CHEMICALS / Furacin

Substance	Poisoning	Accident	Therapeutic Use	Suicide Attempt	Assault	Undetermined
Fuel *(Continued)*						
gas (domestic use) - *see also* Carbon, monoxide, fuel	—	—	—	—	—	—
utility	987.1	E868.1	—	E951.8	E962.2	E981.8
incomplete combustion of - *see* Carbon, monoxide, fuel, utility	—	—	—	—	—	—
in mobile container	987.0	E868.0	—	E951.1	E962.2	E981.1
piped (natural)	987.1	E867	—	E951.0	E962.2	E981.0
industrial, incomplete combustion	986	E868.3	—	E952.1	E962.2	E982.1
Fugillin	960.8	E856	E930.8	E950.4	E962.0	E980.4
Fulminate of mercury	985.0	E866.1	—	E950.9	E962.1	E980.9
Fulvicin	960.1	E856	E930.1	E950.4	E962.0	E980.4
Fumadil	960.8	E856	E930.8	E950.4	E962.0	E980.4
Fumagillin	960.8	E856	E930.8	E950.4	E962.0	E980.4
Fumes (from)	987.9	E869.9	—	E952.9	E962.2	E982.9
carbon monoxide - *see* Carbon, monoxide	—	—	—	—	—	—
charcoal (domestic use)	986	E868.3	—	E952.1	E962.2	E982.1
chloroform - *see* Chloroform						
coke (in domestic stoves, fireplaces)	986	E868.3	—	E952.1	E962.2	E982.1
corrosive NEC	987.8	E869.8	—	E952.8	E962.2	E982.8
ether - *see* Ether(s)						
freons	987.4	E869.2	—	E952.8	E962.2	E982.8
hydrocarbons	987.1	E869.8	—	E952.8	E962.2	E982.8
petroleum (liquefied)	987.0	E868.0	—	E951.1	E962.2	E981.1
distributed through pipes (pure or mixed with air)	987.0	E867	—	E951.0	E962.2	E981.0
lead - *see* Lead	—	—	—	—	—	—
metals - *see* specified metal	—	—	—	—	—	—
nitrogen dioxide	987.2	E869.0	—	E952.8	E962.2	E982.8
pesticides - *see* Pesticides	—	—	—	—	—	—
petroleum (liquefied)	987.0	E868.0	—	E951.1	E962.2	E981.1
distributed through pipes (pure or mixed with air)	987.0	E867	—	E951.0	E962.2	E981.0
polyester	987.8	E869.8	—	E952.8	E962.2	E982.8
specified source, other (*see also* substance specified)	987.8	E869.8	—	E952.8	E962.2	E982.8
sulfur dioxide	987.3	E869.1	—	E952.8	E962.2	E982.8
Fumigants	989.4	E863.8	—	E950.6	E962.1	E980.7
Fungi, noxious, used as food	988.1	E865.5	—	E950.9	E962.1	E980.9
Fungicides (*see also* Antifungals)	989.4	E863.6	—	E950.6	E962.1	E980.7
Fungizone	960.1	E856	E930.1	E950.4	E962.0	E980.4
topical	976.0	E858.7	E946.0	E950.4	E962.0	E980.4
Furacin	976.0	E858.7	E946.0	E950.4	E962.0	E980.4

 Use Additional Digit(s)

TABLE OF DRUGS AND CHEMICALS / Furadantin

Substance	Poisoning	Accident	Therapeutic Use	Suicide Attempt	Assault	Undetermined
Furadantin	961.9	E857	E931.9	E950.4	E962.0	E980.4
Furazolidone	961.9	E857	E931.9	E950.4	E962.0	E980.4
Furnace (coal burning) (domestic), gas from	986	E868.3	—	E952.1	E962.2	E982.1
industrial	986	E868.8	—	E952.1	E962.2	E982.1
Furniture polish	989.89	E861.2	—	E950.9	E962.1	E980.9
Furosemide	974.4	E858.5	E944.4	E950.4	E962.0	E980.4
Furoxone	961.9	E857	E931.9	E950.4	E962.0	E980.4
Fusel oil (amyl) (butyl) (propyl)	980.3	E860.4	—	E950.9	E962.1	E980.9
Fusidic acid	960.8	E856	E930.8	E950.4	E962.0	E980.4
Gallamine	975.2	E858.6	E945.2	E950.4	E962.0	E980.4
Gallotannic acid	976.2	E858.7	E946.2	E950.4	E962.0	E980.4
Gamboge	973.1	E858.4	E943.1	E950.4	E962.0	E980.4
Gamimune	964.6	E858.2	E934.6	E950.4	E962.0	E980.4
Gamma-benzene hexachloride (vapor)	989.2	E863.0	—	E950.6	E962.1	E980.7
Gamma globulin	964.6	E858.2	E934.6	E950.4	E962.0	E980.4
Gamma hydroxy butyrate (GHB)	968.4	E855.1	E938.4	E950.4	E962.0	E980.4
Gamulin	964.6	E858.2	E934.6	E950.4	E962.0	E980.4
Ganglionic blocking agents	972.3	E858.3	E942.3	E950.4	E962.0	E980.4
Ganja	969.6	E854.1	E939.6	E950.3	E962.0	E980.3
Garamycin	960.8	E856	E930.8	E950.4	E962.0	E980.4
ophthalmic preparation	976.5	E858.7	E946.5	E950.4	E962.0	E980.4
topical NEC	976.0	E858.7	E946.0	E950.4	E962.0	E980.4
Gardenal	967.0	E851	E937.0	E950.1	E962.0	E980.1
Gardepanyl	967.0	E851	E937.0	E950.1	E962.0	E980.1
Gas	987.9	E869.9	—	E952.9	E962.2	E982.9
acetylene	987.1	E868.1	—	E951.8	E962.2	E981.8
incomplete combustion of - see Carbon, monoxide, fuel, utility	—	—	—	—	—	—
air contaminants, source or type not specified	987.9	E869.9	—	E952.9	E962.2	E982.9
anesthetic (general) NEC	968.2	E855.1	E938.2	E950.4	E962.0	E980.4
blast furnace	986	E868.8	—	E952.1	E962.2	E982.1
butane - see Butane	—	—	—	—	—	—
carbon monoxide - see Carbon, monoxide, chlorine	987.6	E869.8	—	E952.8	E962.2	E982.8
coal - see Carbon, monoxide, coal	—	—	—	—	—	—
cyanide	987.7	E869.8	—	E952.8	E962.2	E982.8
dicyanogen	987.8	E869.8	—	E952.8	E962.2	E982.8
domestic - see Gas, utility	—	—	—	—	—	—
exhaust - see Carbon, monoxide, exhaust gas	—	—	—	—	—	—
from wood- or coal-burning stove or fireplace	986	E868.3	—	E952.1	E962.2	E982.1

TABLE OF DRUGS AND CHEMICALS / Gas

Substance	Poisoning	Accident	Therapeutic Use	Suicide Attempt	Assault	Undetermined
Gas *(Continued)*						
fuel (domestic use) - *see also* Carbon, monoxide, fuel	—	—	—	—	—	—
industrial use	986	E868.8	—	E952.1	E962.2	E982.1
utility	987.1	E868.1	—	E951.8	E962.2	E981.8
incomplete combustion of - *see* Carbon, monoxide, fuel, utility	—	—	—	—	—	—
in mobile container	987.0	E868.0	—	E951.1	E962.2	E981.1
piped (natural)	987.1	E867	—	E951.0	E962.2	E981.0
garage	986	E868.2	—	E952.0	E962.2	E982.0
hydrocarbon NEC	987.1	E869.8	—	E952.8	E962.2	E982.8
incomplete combustion of - *see* Carbon, monoxide, fuel, utility	—	—	—	—	—	—
liquefied (mobile container)	987.0	E868.0	—	E951.1	E962.2	E981.1
piped	987.0	E867	—	E951.0	E962.2	E981.0
hydrocyanic acid	987.7	E869.8	—	E952.8	E962.2	E982.8
illuminating - *see* Gas, utility	—	—	—	—	—	—
incomplete combustion, any - *see* Carbon, monoxide	—	—	—	—	—	—
kiln	986	E868.8	—	E952.1	E962.2	E982.1
lacrimogenic	987.5	E869.3	—	E952.8	E962.2	E982.8
marsh	987.1	E869.8	—	E952.8	E962.2	E982.8
motor exhaust, not in transit	986	E868.8	—	E952.1	E962.2	E982.1
mustard - *see* Mustard, gas	—	—	—	—	—	—
natural	987.1	E867	—	E951.0	E962.2	E981.0
nerve (war)	987.9	E869.9	—	E952.9	E962.2	E982.9
oils	981	E862.1	—	E950.9	E962.1	E980.9
petroleum (liquefied) (distributed in mobile containers)	987.0	E868.0	—	E951.1	E962.2	E981.1
piped (pure or mixed with air)	987.0	E867	—	E951.1	E962.2	E981.1
piped (manufactured) (natural) NEC	987.1	E867	—	E951.0	E962.2	E981.0
producer	986	E868.8	—	E952.1	E962.2	E982.1
propane - *see* Propane	—	—	—	—	—	—
refrigerant (freon)	987.4	E869.2	—	E952.8	E962.2	E982.8
not freon	987.9	E869.9	—	E952.9	E962.2	E982.9
sewer	987.8	E869.8	—	E952.8	E962.2	E982.8
specified source NEC (*see also* substance specified)	987.8	E869.8	—	E952.8	E962.2	E982.8
stove - *see* Gas, utility	—	—	—	—	—	—
tear	987.5	E869.3	—	E952.8	E962.2	E982.8
utility (for cooking, heating, or lighting) (piped) NEC	987.1	E868.1	—	E951.8	E962.2	E981.8
incomplete combustion of - *see* Carbon, monoxide, fuel, utility	—	—	—	—	—	—
in mobile container	987.0	E868.0	—	E951.1	E962.2	E981.1
piped (natural)	987.1	E867	—	E951.0	E962.2	E981.0
water	987.1	E868.1	—	E951.8	E962.2	E981.8
incomplete combustion of - *see* Carbon, monoxide, fuel, utility	—	—	—	—	—	—

TABLE OF DRUGS AND CHEMICALS / Gaseous substance

Substance	Poisoning	Accident	Therapeutic Use	Suicide Attempt	Assault	Undetermined
Gaseous substance - see Gas	—	—	—	—	—	—
Gasoline, gasolene	981	E862.1	—	E950.9	E962.1	E980.9
vapor	987.1	E869.8	—	E952.8	E962.2	E982.8
Gastric enzymes	973.4	E858.4	E943.4	E950.4	E962.0	E980.4
Gastrografin	977.8	E858.8	E947.8	E950.4	E962.0	E980.4
Gastrointestinal agents	973.9	E858.4	E943.9	E950.4	E962.0	E980.4
specified NEC	973.8	E858.4	E943.8	E950.4	E962.0	E980.4
Gaultheria procumbens	988.2	E865.4	—	E950.9	E962.1	E980.9
Gelatin (intravenous)	964.8	E858.2	E934.8	E950.4	E962.0	E980.4
absorbable (sponge)	964.5	E858.2	E934.5	E950.4	E962.0	E980.4
Gelfilm	976.8	E858.7	E946.8	E950.4	E962.0	E980.4
Gelfoam	964.5	E858.2	E934.5	E950.4	E962.0	E980.4
Gelsemine	970.89	E854.3	E940.8	E950.4	E962.0	E980.4
Gelsemium (sempervirens)	988.2	E865.4	—	E950.9	E962.1	E980.9
Gemonil	967.0	E851	E937.0	E950.1	E962.0	E980.1
Gentamicin	960.8	E856	E930.8	E950.4	E962.0	E980.4
ophthalmic preparation	976.5	E858.7	E946.5	E950.4	E962.0	E980.4
topical NEC	976.0	E858.7	E946.0	E950.4	E962.0	E980.4
Gentian violet	976.0	E858.7	E946.0	E950.4	E962.0	E980.4
Gexane	976.0	E858.7	E946.0	E950.4	E962.0	E980.4
Gila monster (venom)	989.5	E905.0	—	E950.9	E962.1	E980.9
Ginger, Jamaica	989.89	E866.8	—	E950.9	E962.1	E980.9
Gitalin	972.1	E858.3	E942.1	E950.4	E962.0	E980.4
Gitoxin	972.1	E858.3	E942.1	E950.4	E962.0	E980.4
Glandular extract (medicinal) NEC	977.9	E858.9	E947.9	E950.5	E962.0	E980.5
Glaucarubin	961.5	E857	E931.5	E950.4	E962.0	E980.4
Globin zinc insulin	962.3	E858.0	E932.3	E950.4	E962.0	E980.4
Glucagon	962.3	E858.0	E932.3	E950.4	E962.0	E980.4
Glucochloral	967.1	E852.0	E937.1	E950.2	E962.0	E980.2
Glucocorticoids	962.0	E858.0	E932.0	E950.4	E962.0	E980.4
Glucose	974.5	E858.5	E944.5	E950.4	E962.0	E980.4
oxidase reagent	977.8	E858.8	E947.8	E950.4	E962.0	E980.4
Glucosulfone sodium	961.8	E857	E931.8	E950.4	E962.0	E980.4
Glue(s)	989.89	E866.6	—	E950.9	E962.1	E980.9
Glutamic acid (hydrochloride)	973.4	E858.4	E943.4	E950.4	E962.0	E980.4
Glutaraldehyde	989.89	E861.4	—	E950.9	E962.1	E980.9
Glutathione	963.8	E858.1	E933.8	E950.4	E962.0	E980.4
Glutethimide (group)	967.5	E852.4	E937.5	E950.2	E962.0	E980.2
Glycerin (lotion)	976.3	E858.7	E946.3	E950.4	E962.0	E980.4
Glycerol (topical)	976.3	E858.7	E946.3	E950.4	E962.0	E980.4

TABLE OF DRUGS AND CHEMICALS / Halethazole

Substance	Poisoning	External Cause (E Code) Accident	Therapeutic Use	Suicide Attempt	Assault	Undetermined
Glyceryl	—	—	—	—	—	—
guaiacolate	975.5	E858.6	E945.5	E950.4	E962.0	E980.4
triacetate (topical)	976.0	E858.7	E946.0	E950.4	E962.0	E980.4
trinitrate	972.4	E858.3	E942.4	E950.4	E962.0	E980.4
Glycine	974.5	E858.5	E944.5	E950.4	E962.0	E980.4
Glycobiarsol	961.1	E857	E931.1	E950.4	E962.0	E980.4
Glycols (ether)	982.8	E862.4	—	E950.9	E962.1	E980.9
Glycopyrrolate	971.1	E855.4	E941.1	E950.4	E962.0	E980.4
Glymidine	962.3	E858.0	E932.3	E950.4	E962.0	E980.4
Gold (compounds) (salts)	965.69	E850.6	E935.6	E950.0	E962.0	E980.0
Golden sulfide of antimony	985.4	E866.2	—	E950.9	E962.1	E980.9
Goldylocks	988.2	E865.4	—	E950.9	E962.1	E980.9
Gonadal tissue extract	962.9	E858.0	E932.9	E950.4	E962.0	E980.4
female	962.2	E858.0	E932.2	E950.4	E962.0	E980.4
male	962.1	E858.0	E932.1	E950.4	E962.0	E980.4
Gonadotropin	962.4	E858.0	E932.4	E950.4	E962.0	E980.4
Grain alcohol	980.0	E860.1	—	E950.9	E962.1	E980.9
beverage	980.0	E860.0	—	E950.9	E962.1	E980.9
Gramicidin	960.8	E856	E930.8	E950.4	E962.0	E980.4
Gratiola officinalis	988.2	E865.4	—	E950.9	E962.1	E980.9
Grease	989.89	E866.8	—	E950.9	E962.1	E980.9
Green hellebore	988.2	E865.4	—	E950.9	E962.1	E980.9
Green soap	976.2	E858.7	E946.2	E950.4	E962.0	E980.4
Grifulvin	960.1	E856	E930.1	E950.4	E962.0	E980.4
Griseofulvin	960.1	E856	E930.1	E950.4	E962.0	E980.4
Growth hormone	962.4	E858.0	E932.4	E950.4	E962.0	E980.4
Guaiacol	975.5	E858.6	E945.5	E950.4	E962.0	E980.4
Givaiac reagent	977.8	E858.8	E947.8	E950.4	E962.0	E980.4
Guaifenesin	975.5	E858.6	E945.5	E950.4	E962.0	E980.4
Guaiphenesin	975.5	E858.6	E945.5	E950.4	E962.0	E980.4
Guanatol	961.4	E857	E931.4	E950.4	E962.0	E980.4
Guanethidine	972.6	E858.3	E942.6	E950.4	E962.0	E980.4
Guano	989.89	E866.5	—	E950.9	E962.1	E980.9
Guanochlor	972.6	E858.3	E942.6	E950.4	E962.0	E980.4
Guanoctine	972.6	E858.3	E942.6	E950.4	E962.0	E980.4
Guanoxan	972.6	E858.3	E942.6	E950.4	E962.0	E980.4
Hair treatment agent NEC	976.4	E858.7	E946.4	E950.4	E962.0	E980.4
Halcinonide	976.0	E858.7	E946.0	E950.4	E962.0	E980.4
Halethazole	976.0	E858.7	E946.0	E950.4	E962.0	E980.4

◀ New   ◀▥ Revised   ~~deleted~~ Deleted   ● Use Additional Digit(s)

TABLE OF DRUGS AND CHEMICALS / Hallucinogens

Substance	Poisoning	External Cause (E Code) Accident	Therapeutic Use	Suicide Attempt	Assault	Undetermined
Hallucinogens	969.6	E854.1	E939.6	E950.3	E962.0	E980.3
Haloperidol	969.2	E853.1	E939.2	E950.3	E962.0	E980.3
Haloprogin	976.0	E858.7	E946.0	E950.4	E962.0	E980.4
Halotex	976.0	E858.7	E946.0	E950.4	E962.0	E980.4
Halothane	968.1	E855.1	E938.1	E950.4	E962.0	E980.4
Halquinols	976.0	E858.7	E946.0	E950.4	E962.0	E980.4
Hand sanitizer	976.0	E858.7	E946.0	E950.4	E962.0	E980.4
Harmonyl	972.6	E858.3	E942.6	E950.4	E962.0	E980.4
Hartmann's solution	974.5	E858.5	E944.5	E950.4	E962.0	E980.4
Hashish	969.6	E854.1	E939.6	E950.3	E962.0	E980.3
Hawaiian wood rose seeds	969.6	E854.1	E939.6	E950.3	E962.0	E980.3
Headache cures, drugs, powders NEC	977.9	E858.9	E947.9	E950.5	E962.0	E980.9
Heavenly Blue (morning glory)	969.6	E854.1	E939.6	E950.3	E962.0	E980.3
Heavy metal antagonists	963.8	E858.1	E933.8	E950.4	E962.0	E980.4
anti-infectives	961.2	E857	E931.2	E950.4	E962.0	E980.4
Hedaquinium	976.0	E858.7	E946.0	E950.4	E962.0	E980.4
Hedge hyssop	988.2	E865.4	—	E950.9	E962.1	E980.9
Heet	976.8	E858.7	E946.8	E950.4	E962.0	E980.4
Helenin	961.6	E857	E931.6	E950.4	E962.0	E980.4
Hellebore (black) (green) (white)	988.2	E865.4	—	E950.9	E962.1	E980.9
Hemlock	988.2	E865.4	—	E950.9	E962.1	E980.9
Hemostatics	964.5	E858.2	E934.5	E950.4	E962.0	E980.4
capillary active drugs	972.8	E858.3	E942.8	E950.4	E962.0	E980.4
Henbane	988.2	E865.4	—	E950.9	E962.1	E980.9
Heparin (sodium)	964.2	E858.2	E934.2	E950.4	E962.0	E980.4
Heptabarbital, heptabarbitone	967.0	E851	E937.0	E950.1	E962.0	E980.1
Heptachlor	989.2	E863.0	—	E950.6	E962.1	E980.7
Heptalgin	965.09	E850.2	E935.2	E950.0	E962.0	E980.0
Herbicides	989.4	E863.5	—	E950.6	E962.1	E980.7
Heroin	965.01	E850.0	E935.0	E950.0	E962.0	E980.0
Herplex	976.5	E858.7	E946.5	E950.4	E962.0	E980.4
HES	964.8	E858.2	E934.8	E950.4	E962.0	E980.4
Hetastarch	964.8	E858.2	E934.8	E950.4	E962.0	E980.7
Hexachlorocyclohexane	989.2	E863.0	—	E950.6	E962.1	E980.7
Hexachlorophene	976.2	E858.7	E946.2	E950.4	E962.0	E980.4
Hexadimethrine (bromide)	964.5	E858.2	E934.5	E950.4	E962.0	E980.4
Hexafluorenium	975.2	E858.6	E945.2	E950.4	E962.0	E980.4
Hexa-germ	976.2	E858.7	E946.2	E950.4	E962.0	E980.4
Hexahydrophenol	980.8	E860.8	—	E950.9	E962.1	E980.9

TABLE OF DRUGS AND CHEMICALS / Hyazyme

| Substance | Poisoning | External Cause (E Code) |||||
		Accident	Therapeutic Use	Suicide Attempt	Assault	Undetermined
Hexalen	980.8	E860.8	—	E950.9	E962.1	E980.9
Hexamethonium	972.3	E858.3	E942.3	E950.4	E962.0	E980.4
Hexamethylenamine	961.9	E857	E931.9	E950.4	E962.0	E980.4
Hexamine	961.9	E857	E931.9	E950.4	E962.0	E980.4
Hexanone	982.8	E862.4	—	E950.9	E962.1	E980.9
Hexapropymate	967.8	E852.8	E937.8	E950.2	E962.0	E980.2
Hexestrol	962.2	E858.0	E932.2	E950.4	E962.0	E980.4
Hexethal (sodium)	967.0	E851	E937.0	E950.1	E962.0	E980.1
Hexetidine	976.0	E858.7	E946.0	E950.4	E962.0	E980.4
Hexobarbital, hexobarbitone	967.0	E851	E937.0	E950.1	E962.0	E980.1
sodium (anesthetic)	968.3	E855.1	E938.3	E950.4	E962.0	E980.4
soluble	968.3	E855.1	E938.3	E950.4	E962.0	E980.4
Hexocyclium	971.1	E855.4	E941.1	E950.4	E962.0	E980.4
Hexoestrol	962.2	E858.0	E932.2	E950.4	E962.0	E980.4
Hexone	982.8	E862.4	—	E950.9	E962.1	E980.9
Hexylcaine	968.5	E855.2	E938.5	E950.4	E962.0	E980.4
Hexylresorcinol	961.6	E857	E931.6	E950.4	E962.0	E980.4
Hinkle's pills	973.1	E858.4	E943.1	E950.4	E962.0	E980.4
Histalog	977.8	E858.8	E947.8	E950.4	E962.0	E980.4
Histamine (phosphate)	972.5	E858.3	E942.5	E950.4	E962.0	E980.4
Histoplasmin	977.8	E858.8	E947.8	E950.4	E962.0	E980.4
Holly berries	988.2	E865.3	—	E950.9	E962.1	E980.9
Homatropine	971.1	E855.4	E941.1	E950.4	E962.0	E980.4
Homo-tet	964.6	E858.2	E934.6	E950.4	E962.0	E980.4
Hormones (synthetic substitute) NEC	962.9	E858.0	E932.9	E950.4	E962.0	E980.4
adrenal cortical steroids	962.0	E858.0	E932.0	E950.4	E962.0	E980.4
antidiabetic agents	962.3	E858.0	E932.3	E950.4	E962.0	E980.4
follicle stimulating	962.4	E858.0	E932.4	E950.4	E962.0	E980.4
gonadotropic	962.4	E858.0	E932.4	E950.4	E962.0	E980.4
growth	962.4	E858.0	E932.4	E950.4	E962.0	E980.4
ovarian (substitutes)	962.2	E858.0	E932.2	E950.4	E962.0	E980.4
parathyroid (derivatives)	962.6	E858.0	E932.6	E950.4	E962.0	E980.4
pituitary (posterior)	962.5	E858.0	E932.5	E950.4	E962.0	E980.4
anterior	962.4	E858.0	E932.4	E950.4	E962.0	E980.4
thyroid (derivative)	962.7	E858.0	E932.7	E950.4	E962.0	E980.4
Hornet (sting)	989.5	E905.3	—	E950.9	E962.1	E980.9
Horticulture agent NEC	989.4	E863.9	—	E950.6	E962.1	E980.7
Hyaluronidase	963.4	E858.1	E933.4	E950.4	E962.0	E980.4
Hyazyme	963.4	E858.1	E933.4	E950.4	E962.0	E980.4

TABLE OF DRUGS AND CHEMICALS / Hycodan

Substance	Poisoning	External Cause (E Code) Accident	Therapeutic Use	Suicide Attempt	Assault	Undetermined
Hycodan	965.09	E850.2	E935.2	E950.0	E962.0	E980.0
Hydantoin derivatives	966.1	E855.0	E936.1	E950.4	E962.0	E980.4
Hydeltra	962.0	E858.0	E932.0	E950.4	E962.0	E980.4
Hydergine	971.3	E855.6	E941.3	E950.4	E962.0	E980.4
Hydrabamine penicillin	960.0	E856	E930.0	E950.4	E962.0	E980.4
Hydralazine, hydrallazine	972.6	E858.3	E942.6	E950.4	E962.0	E980.4
Hydrargaphen	976.0	E858.7	E946.0	E950.4	E962.0	E980.4
Hydrazine	983.9	E864.3	—	E950.7	E962.1	E980.6
Hydriodic acid	975.5	E858.6	E945.5	E950.4	E962.0	E980.4
Hydrocarbon gas	987.1	E869.8	—	E952.8	E962.2	E982.8
incomplete combustion of - see Carbon, monoxide, fuel, utility	—	—	—	—	—	—
liquefied (mobile container)	987.0	E868.0	—	E951.1	E962.2	E981.1
piped (natural)	987.0	E867	—	E951.0	E962.2	E981.0
Hydrochloric acid (liquid)	983.1	E864.1	—	E950.7	E962.1	E980.6
medicinal	973.4	E858.4	E943.4	E950.4	E962.0	E980.4
vapor	987.8	E869.8	—	E952.8	E962.2	E982.8
Hydrochlorothiazide	974.3	E858.5	E944.3	E950.4	E962.0	E980.4
Hydrocodone	965.09	E850.2	E935.2	E950.0	E962.0	E980.0
Hydrocortisone	962.0	E858.0	E932.0	E950.4	E962.0	E980.4
ENT agent	976.6	E858.7	E946.6	E950.4	E962.0	E980.4
ophthalmic preparation	976.5	E858.7	E946.5	E950.4	E962.0	E980.4
topical NEC	976.0	E858.7	E946.0	E950.4	E962.0	E980.4
Hydrocortone	962.0	E858.0	E932.0	E950.4	E962.0	E980.4
ENT agent	976.6	E858.7	E946.6	E950.4	E962.0	E980.4
ophthalmic preparation	976.5	E858.7	E946.5	E950.4	E962.0	E980.4
topical NEC	976.0	E858.7	E946.0	E950.4	E962.0	E980.4
Hydrocyanic acid - see Cyanide(s)	—	—	—	—	—	—
Hydroflumethiazide	974.3	E858.5	E944.3	E950.4	E962.0	E980.4
Hydrofluoric acid (liquid)	983.1	E864.1	—	E950.7	E962.1	E980.6
vapor	987.8	E869.8	—	E952.8	E962.2	E982.8
Hydrogen	987.8	E869.8	—	E952.8	E962.2	E982.8
arsenide	985.1	E866.3	—	E950.8	E962.1	E980.8
arseniurated	985.1	E866.3	—	E950.8	E962.1	E980.8
cyanide (salts)	989.0	E866.8	—	E950.9	E962.1	E980.9
gas	987.7	E869.8	—	E952.8	E962.2	E982.8
fluoride (liquid)	983.1	E864.1	—	E950.7	E962.1	E980.6
vapor	987.8	E869.8	—	E952.8	E962.2	E982.8
peroxide (solution)	976.6	E858.7	E946.6	E950.4	E962.0	E980.4
phosphorated	987.8	E869.8	—	E952.8	E962.2	E982.8

TABLE OF DRUGS AND CHEMICALS / Ichthammol

Substance	Poisoning	External Cause (E Code) Accident	Therapeutic Use	Suicide Attempt	Assault	Undetermined
Hydrogen *(Continued)*						
sulfide (gas)	987.8	E869.8	—	E952.8	E962.2	E982.8
arseniurated	985.1	E866.3	—	E950.8	E962.1	E980.8
sulfureted	987.8	E869.8	—	E952.8	E962.2	E982.8
Hydromorphinol	965.09	E850.2	E935.2	E950.0	E962.0	E980.0
Hydromorphinone	965.09	E850.2	E935.2	E950.0	E962.0	E980.0
Hydromorphone	965.09	E850.2	E935.2	E950.0	E962.0	E980.0
Hydromox	974.3	E858.5	E944.3	E950.4	E962.0	E980.4
Hydrophilic lotion	976.3	E858.7	E946.3	E950.4	E962.0	E980.4
Hydroquinone	983.0	E864.0	—	E950.7	E962.1	E980.6
vapor	987.8	E869.8	—	E952.8	E962.2	E982.8
Hydrosulfuric acid (gas)	987.8	E869.8	—	E952.8	E962.2	E982.8
Hydrous wool fat (lotion)	976.3	E858.7	E946.3	E950.4	E962.0	E980.4
Hydroxide, caustic	983.2	E864.2	—	E950.7	E962.1	E980.6
Hydroxocobalamin	964.1	E858.2	E934.1	E950.4	E962.0	E980.4
Hydroxyamphetamine	971.2	E858.5	E941.2	E950.4	E962.0	E980.4
Hydroxychloroquine	961.4	E857	E931.4	E950.4	E962.0	E980.4
Hydroxydihydrocodeinone	965.09	E850.2	E935.2	E950.0	E962.0	E980.0
Hydroxyethyl starch	964.8	E858.2	E934.8	E950.4	E962.0	E980.4
Hydroxyphenamate	969.5	E853.8	E939.5	E950.3	E962.0	E980.3
Hydroxyphenylbutazone	965.5	E850.5	E935.5	E950.0	E962.0	E980.0
Hydroxyprogesterone	962.2	E858.0	E932.2	E950.4	E962.0	E980.4
Hydroxyquinoline derivatives	961.3	E857	E931.3	E950.4	E962.0	E980.4
Hydroxystilbamidine	961.5	E857	E931.5	E950.4	E962.0	E980.4
Hydroxyurea	963.1	E858.1	E933.1	E950.4	E962.0	E980.4
Hydroxyzine	969.5	E853.8	E939.5	E950.3	E962.0	E980.3
Hyoscine (hydrobromide)	971.1	E855.4	E941.1	E950.4	E962.0	E980.4
Hyoscyamine	971.1	E855.4	E941.1	E950.4	E962.0	E980.4
Hyoscyamus (albus) (niger)	988.2	E865.4	—	E950.9	E962.1	E980.9
Hypaque	977.8	E858.8	E947.8	E950.4	E962.0	E980.4
Hypertussis	964.6	E858.2	E934.6	E950.4	E962.0	E980.4
Hypnotics NEC	967.9	E852.9	E937.9	E950.2	E962.0	E980.2
Hypochlorites - *see* Sodium, hypochlorite	—	—	—	—	—	—
Hypotensive agents NEC	972.6	E858.3	E942.6	E950.4	E962.0	E980.4
Ibufenac	965.69	E850.6	E935.6	E950.0	E962.0	E980.0
Ibuprofen	965.61	E850.6	E935.6	E950.0	E962.0	E980.0
ICG	977.8	E858.8	E947.8	E950.4	E962.0	E980.4
Ichthammol	976.4	E858.7	E946.4	E950.4	E962.0	E980.4

 New   Revised   ~~deleted~~ Deleted   ● Use Additional Digit(s)

TABLE OF DRUGS AND CHEMICALS / Ichthyol

Substance	Poisoning	External Cause (E Code) Accident	Therapeutic Use	Suicide Attempt	Assault	Undetermined
Ichthyol	976.4	E858.7	E946.4	E950.4	E962.0	E980.4
Idoxuridine	976.5	E858.7	E946.5	E950.4	E962.0	E980.4
IDU	976.5	E858.7	E946.5	E950.4	E962.0	E980.4
Iletin	962.3	E858.0	E932.3	E950.4	E962.0	E980.4
Ilex	988.2	E865.4	—	E950.9	E962.1	E980.9
Illuminating gas - see Gas, utility	—	—	—	—	—	—
Ilopan	963.5	E858.1	E933.5	E950.4	E962.0	E980.4
Ilotycin	960.3	E856	E930.3	E950.4	E962.0	E980.4
ophthalmic preparation	976.5	E858.7	E946.5	E950.4	E962.0	E980.4
topical NEC	976.0	E858.7	E946.0	E950.4	E962.0	E980.4
Imipramine	969.05	E854.0	E939.0	E950.3	E962.0	E980.3
Immu-G	964.6	E858.2	E934.6	E950.4	E962.0	E980.4
Immuglobin	964.6	E858.2	E934.6	E950.4	E962.0	E980.4
Immune serum globulin	964.6	E858.2	E934.6	E950.4	E962.0	E980.4
Immunosuppressive agents	963.1	E858.1	E933.1	E950.4	E962.0	E980.4
Immu-tetanus	964.6	E858.2	E934.6	E950.4	E962.0	E980.4
Indandione (derivatives)	964.2	E858.2	E934.2	E950.4	E962.0	E980.4
Inderal	972.0	E858.3	E942.0	E950.4	E962.0	E980.4
Indian	—	—	—	—	—	—
hemp	969.6	E854.1	E939.6	E950.3	E962.0	E980.3
tobacco	988.2	E865.4	—	E950.9	E962.1	E980.9
Indigo carmine	977.8	E858.8	E947.8	E950.4	E962.0	E980.4
Indocin	965.69	E850.6	E935.6	E950.0	E962.0	E980.0
Indocyanine green	977.8	E858.8	E947.8	E950.4	E962.0	E980.4
Indomethacin	965.69	E850.6	E935.6	E950.0	E962.0	E980.0
Industrial	—	—	—	—	—	—
alcohol	980.9	E860.9	—	E950.9	E962.1	E980.9
fumes	987.8	E869.8	—	E952.8	E962.2	E982.8
solvents (fumes) (vapors)	982.8	E862.9	—	E950.9	E962.1	E980.9
Influenza vaccine	979.6	E858.8	E949.6	E950.4	E962.0	E982.8
Ingested substances NEC	989.9	E866.9	—	E950.9	E962.1	E980.9
INH (isoniazid)	961.8	E857	E931.8	E950.4	E962.0	E980.4
Inhalation, gas (noxious) - see Gas	—	—	—	—	—	—
Ink	989.89	E866.8	—	E950.9	E962.1	E980.9
Innovar	967.6	E852.5	E937.6	E950.2	E962.0	E980.2
Inositol niacinate	972.2	E858.3	E942.2	E950.4	E962.0	E980.4
Inproquone	963.1	E858.1	E933.1	E950.4	E962.0	E980.4
Insect (sting), venomous	989.5	E905.5	—	E950.9	E962.1	E980.9

TABLE OF DRUGS AND CHEMICALS / Iproniazid

Substance	Poisoning	External Cause (E Code)				
		Accident	Therapeutic Use	Suicide Attempt	Assault	Undetermined
Insecticides (see also Pesticides)	989.4	E863.4	—	E950.6	E962.1	E980.7
chlorinated	989.2	E863.0	—	E950.6	E962.1	E980.7
mixtures	989.4	E863.3	—	E950.6	E962.1	E980.7
organochlorine (compounds)	989.2	E863.0	—	E950.6	E962.1	E980.7
organophosphorus (compounds)	989.3	E863.1	—	E950.6	E962.1	E980.7
Insular tissue extract	962.3	E858.0	E932.3	E950.4	E962.0	E980.4
Insulin (amorphous) (globin) (isophane) (Lente) (NPH) (Protamine) (Semilente) (Ultralente) (zinc)	962.3	E858.0	E932.3	E950.4	E962.0	E980.4
Intranarcon	968.3	E855.1	E938.3	E950.4	E962.0	E980.4
Inulin	977.8	E858.8	E947.8	E950.4	E962.0	E980.4
Invert sugar	974.5	E858.5	E944.5	E950.4	E962.0	E980.4
Inza - see Naproxen	—	—	—	—	—	—
Iodide NEC (see also Iodine)	976.0	E858.7	E946.0	E950.4	E962.0	E980.4
mercury (ointment)	976.0	E858.7	E946.0	E950.4	E962.0	E980.4
methylate	976.0	E858.7	E946.0	E950.4	E962.0	E980.4
potassium (expectorant) NEC	975.5	E858.6	E945.5	E950.4	E962.0	E980.4
Iodinated glycerol	975.5	E858.6	E945.5	E950.4	E962.0	E980.4
Iodine (antiseptic, external) (tincture) NEC	976.0	E858.7	E946.0	E950.4	E962.0	E980.4
diagnostic	977.8	E858.8	E947.8	E950.4	E962.0	E980.4
for thyroid conditions (antithyroid)	962.8	E858.0	E932.8	E950.4	E962.0	E980.4
vapor	987.8	E869.8	—	E952.8	E962.2	E982.8
Iodized oil	977.8	E858.8	E947.8	E950.4	E962.0	E980.4
Iodobismitol	961.2	E857	E931.2	E950.4	E962.0	E980.4
Iodochlorhydroxyquin	961.3	E857	E931.3	E950.4	E962.0	E980.4
topical	976.0	E858.7	E946.0	E950.4	E962.0	E980.4
Iodoform	976.0	E858.7	E946.0	E950.4	E962.0	E980.4
Iodopanoic acid	977.8	E858.8	E947.8	E950.4	E962.0	E980.4
Iodophthalein	977.8	E858.8	E947.8	E950.4	E962.0	E980.4
Ion exchange resins	974.5	E858.5	E944.5	E950.4	E962.0	E980.4
Iopanoic acid	977.8	E858.8	E947.8	E950.4	E962.0	E980.4
Iophendylate	977.8	E858.8	E947.8	E950.4	E962.0	E980.4
Iothiouracil	962.8	E858.0	E932.8	E950.4	E962.0	E980.4
Ipecac	973.6	E858.4	E943.6	E950.4	E962.0	E980.4
Ipecacuanha	973.6	E858.4	E943.6	E950.4	E962.0	E980.4
Ipodate	977.8	E858.8	E947.8	E950.4	E962.0	E980.4
Ipral	967.0	E851	E937.0	E950.1	E962.0	E980.1
Ipratropium	975.1	E858.6	E945.1	E950.4	E962.0	E980.4
Iproniazid	969.01	E854.0	E939.0	E950.3	E962.0	E980.3

New   Revised   ~~deleted~~ Deleted   Use Additional Digit(s)

TABLE OF DRUGS AND CHEMICALS / Iron

		External Cause (E Code)				
Substance	Poisoning	Accident	Therapeutic Use	Suicide Attempt	Assault	Undetermined
Iron (compounds) (medicinal) (preparations)	964.0	E858.2	E934.0	E950.4	E962.0	E980.4
dextran	964.0	E858.2	E934.0	E950.4	E962.0	E980.4
nonmedicinal (dust) (fumes) NEC	985.8	E866.4	—	E950.9	E962.1	E980.9
Irritant drug	977.9	E858.9	E947.9	E950.5	E962.0	E980.5
Ismelin	972.6	E858.3	E942.6	E950.4	E962.0	E980.4
Isoamyl nitrite	972.4	E858.3	E942.4	E950.4	E962.0	E980.4
Isobutyl acetate	982.8	E862.4	—	E950.9	E962.1	E980.9
Isocarboxazid	969.01	E854.0	E939.0	E950.3	E962.0	E980.3
Isoephedrine	971.2	E855.5	E941.2	E950.4	E962.0	E980.4
Isoetharine	971.2	E855.5	E941.2	E950.4	E962.0	E980.4
Isofluorophate	971.0	E855.3	E941.0	E950.4	E962.0	E980.4
Isoniazid (INH)	961.8	E857	E931.8	E950.4	E962.0	E980.4
Isopentaquine	961.4	E857	E931.4	E950.4	E962.0	E980.4
Isophane insulin	962.3	E858.0	E932.3	E950.4	E962.0	E980.4
Isopregnenone	962.2	E858.0	E932.2	E950.4	E962.0	E980.4
Isoprenaline	971.2	E855.5	E941.2	E950.4	E962.0	E980.4
Isopropamide	971.1	E855.4	E941.1	E950.4	E962.0	E980.4
Isopropanol	980.2	E860.3	—	E950.9	E962.1	E980.9
topical (germicide)	976.0	E858.7	E946.0	E950.4	E962.0	E980.4
Isopropyl	—	—	—	—	—	—
acetate	982.8	E862.4	—	E950.9	E962.1	E980.9
alcohol	980.2	E860.3	—	E950.9	E962.1	E980.9
topical (germicide)	976.0	E858.7	E946.0	E950.4	E962.0	E980.4
ether	982.8	E862.4	—	E950.9	E962.1	E980.9
Isoproterenol	971.2	E855.5	E941.2	E950.4	E962.0	E980.4
Isosorbide dinitrate	972.4	E858.3	E942.4	E950.4	E962.0	E980.4
Isothipendyl	963.0	E858.1	E933.0	E950.4	E962.0	E980.4
Isoxazolyl penicillin	960.0	E856	E930.0	E950.4	E962.0	E980.4
Isoxsuprine hydrochloride	972.5	E858.3	E942.5	E950.4	E962.0	E980.4
l-thyroxine sodium	962.7	E858.0	E932.7	E950.4	E962.0	E980.4
Jaborandi (pilocarpus) (extract)	971.0	E855.3	E941.0	E950.4	E962.0	E980.4
Jalap	973.1	E858.4	E943.1	E950.4	E962.0	E980.4
Jamaica	—	—	—	—	—	—
dogwood (bark)	965.7	E850.7	E935.7	E950.0	E962.0	E980.0
ginger	989.89	E866.8	—	E950.9	E962.1	E980.9
Jatropha	988.2	E865.4	—	E950.9	E962.1	E980.9
curcas	988.2	E865.3	—	E950.9	E962.1	E980.9
Jectofer	964.0	E858.2	E934.0	E950.4	E962.0	E980.4

TABLE OF DRUGS AND CHEMICALS / Lanolin

Substance	Poisoning	External Cause (E Code)				
		Accident	Therapeutic Use	Suicide Attempt	Assault	Undetermined
Jellyfish (sting)	989.5	E905.6	—	E950.9	E962.1	E980.9
Jequirity (bean)	988.2	E865.3	—	E950.9	E962.1	E980.9
Jimson weed	988.2	E865.4	—	E950.9	E962.1	E980.9
seeds	988.2	E865.3	—	E950.9	E962.1	E980.9
Juniper tar (oil) (ointment)	976.4	E858.7	E946.4	E950.4	E962.0	E980.4
Kallikrein	972.5	E858.3	E942.5	E950.4	E962.0	E980.4
Kanamycin	960.6	E856	E930.6	E950.4	E962.0	E980.4
Kantrex	960.6	E856	E930.6	E950.4	E962.0	E980.4
Kaolin	973.5	E858.4	E943.5	E950.4	E962.0	E980.4
Karaya (gum)	973.3	E858.4	E943.3	E950.4	E962.0	E980.4
Kemithal	968.3	E855.1	E938.3	E950.4	E962.0	E980.4
Kenacort	962.0	E858.0	E932.0	E950.4	E962.0	E980.4
Keratolytics	976.4	E858.7	E946.4	E950.4	E962.0	E980.4
Keratoplastics	976.4	E858.7	E946.4	E950.4	E962.0	E980.4
Kerosene, kerosine (fuel) (solvent) NEC	981	E862.1	—	E950.9	E962.1	E980.9
insecticide	981	E863.4	—	E950.6	E962.1	E980.7
vapor	987.1	E869.8	—	E952.8	E962.2	E982.8
Ketamine	968.3	E855.1	E938.3	E950.4	E962.0	E980.4
Ketobemidone	965.09	E850.2	E935.2	E950.0	E962.0	E980.0
Ketols	982.8	E862.4	—	E950.9	E962.1	E980.9
Ketone oils	982.8	E862.4	—	E950.9	E962.1	E980.9
Ketoprofen	965.61	E850.6	E935.6	E950.0	E962.0	E980.0
Kiln gas or vapor (carbon monoxide)	986	E868.8	—	E952.1	E962.2	E982.1
Konsyl	973.3	E858.4	E943.3	E950.4	E962.0	E980.4
Kosam seed	988.2	E865.3	—	E950.9	E962.1	E980.9
Krait (venom)	989.5	E905.0	—	E950.9	E962.1	E980.9
Kwell (insecticide)	989.2	E863.0	—	E950.6	E962.1	E980.7
anti-infective (topical)	976.0	E858.7	E946.0	E950.4	E962.0	E980.4
Laburnum (flowers) (seeds)	988.2	E865.3	—	E950.9	E962.1	E980.9
leaves	988.2	E865.4	—	E950.9	E962.1	E980.9
Lacquers	989.89	E861.6	—	E950.9	E962.1	E980.9
Lacrimogenic gas	987.5	E869.3	—	E952.8	E962.2	E982.8
Lactic acid	983.1	E864.1	—	E950.7	E962.1	E980.6
Lactobacillus acidophilus	973.5	E858.4	E943.5	E950.4	E962.0	E980.4
Lactoflavin	963.5	E858.1	E933.5	E950.4	E962.0	E980.4
Lactuca (virosa) (extract)	967.8	E852.8	E937.8	E950.2	E962.0	E980.2
Lactucarium	967.8	E852.8	E937.8	E950.2	E962.0	E980.2
Laevulose	974.5	E858.5	E944.5	E950.4	E962.0	E980.4
Lanatoside (C)	972.1	E858.3	E942.1	E950.4	E962.0	E980.4
Lanolin (lotion)	976.3	E858.7	E946.3	E950.4	E962.0	E980.4

TABLE OF DRUGS AND CHEMICALS / Largactil

Substance	Poisoning	External Cause (E Code)				
		Accident	Therapeutic Use	Suicide Attempt	Assault	Undetermined
Largactil	969.1	E853.0	E939.1	E950.3	E962.0	E980.3
Larkspur	988.2	E865.3	—	E950.9	E962.1	E980.9
Laroxyl	969.05	E854.0	E939.0	E950.3	E962.0	E980.3
Lasix	974.4	E858.5	E944.4	E950.4	E962.0	E980.4
Latex	989.82	E866.8	—	E950.9	E962.1	E980.9
Lathyrus (seed)	988.2	E865.3	—	E950.9	E962.1	E980.9
Laudanum	965.09	E850.2	E935.2	E950.0	E962.0	E980.0
Laudexium	975.2	E858.6	E945.2	E950.4	E962.0	E980.4
Laurel, black or cherry	988.2	E865.4	—	E950.9	E962.1	E980.9
Laurolinium	976.0	E858.7	E946.0	E950.4	E962.0	E980.4
Lauryl sulfoacetate	976.2	E858.7	E946.2	E950.4	E962.0	E980.4
Laxatives NEC	973.3	E858.4	E943.3	E950.4	E962.0	E980.4
emollient	973.2	E858.4	E943.2	E950.4	E962.0	E980.4
L-dopa	966.4	E855.0	E936.4	E950.4	E962.0	E980.4
L-Tryptophan - *see* amino acid	—	—	—	—	—	—
Lead (dust) (fumes) (vapor) NEC	984.9	E866.0	—	E950.9	E962.1	E980.9
acetate (dust)	984.1	E866.0	—	E950.9	E962.1	E980.9
anti-infectives	961.2	E857	E931.2	E950.4	E962.0	E980.4
antiknock compound (tetra-ethyl)	984.1	E862.1	—	E950.9	E962.1	E980.9
arsenate, arsenite (dust) (insecticide) (vapor)	985.1	E863.4	—	E950.8	E962.1	E980.8
herbicide	985.1	E863.5	—	E950.8	E962.1	E980.8
carbonate	984.0	E866.0	—	E950.9	E962.1	E980.9
paint	984.0	E861.5	—	E950.9	E962.1	E980.9
chromate	984.0	E866.0	—	E950.9	E962.1	E980.9
paint	984.0	E861.5	—	E950.9	E962.1	E980.9
dioxide	984.0	E866.0	—	E950.9	E962.1	E980.9
inorganic (compound)	984.0	E866.0	—	E950.9	E962.1	E980.9
paint	984.0	E861.5	—	E950.9	E962.1	E980.9
iodide	984.0	E866.0	—	E950.9	E962.1	E980.9
pigment (paint)	984.0	E861.5	—	E950.9	E962.1	E980.9
monoxide (dust)	984.0	E866.0	—	E950.9	E962.1	E980.9
paint	984.0	E861.5	—	E950.9	E962.1	E980.9
organic	984.1	E866.0	—	E950.9	E962.1	E980.9
oxide	984.0	E866.0	—	E950.9	E962.1	E980.9
paint	984.0	E861.5	—	E950.9	E962.1	E980.9
paint	984.0	E861.5	—	E950.9	E962.1	E980.9
salts	984.0	E866.0	—	E950.9	E962.1	E980.9
specified compound NEC	984.8	E866.0	—	E950.9	E962.1	E980.9
tetra-ethyl	984.1	E862.1	—	E950.9	E962.1	E980.9
Lebanese red	969.6	E854.1	E939.6	E950.3	E962.0	E980.3

TABLE OF DRUGS AND CHEMICALS / Limonene

Substance	Poisoning	External Cause (E Code)				
		Accident	Therapeutic Use	Suicide Attempt	Assault	Undetermined
Lente Iletin (insulin)	962.3	E858.0	E932.3	E950.4	E962.0	E980.4
Leptazol	970.0	E854.3	E940.0	E950.4	E962.0	E980.4
Leritine	965.09	E850.2	E935.2	E950.0	E962.0	E980.0
Letter	962.7	E858.0	E932.7	E950.4	E962.0	E980.4
Lettuce opium	967.8	E852.8	E937.8	E950.2	E962.0	E980.2
Leucovorin (factor)	964.1	E858.2	E934.1	E950.4	E962.0	E980.4
Leukeran	963.1	E858.1	E933.1	E950.4	E962.0	E980.4
Levalbuterol	975.7	E858.6	E945.7	E950.4	E962.0	E980.4
Levallorphan	970.1	E854.3	E940.1	E950.4	E962.0	E980.4
Levanil	967.8	E852.8	E937.8	E950.2	E962.0	E980.2
Levarterenol	971.2	E855.5	E941.2	E950.4	E962.0	E980.4
Levodopa	966.4	E855.0	E936.4	E950.4	E962.0	E980.4
Levo-dromoran	965.09	E850.2	E935.2	E950.0	E962.0	E980.0
Levoid	962.7	E858.0	E932.7	E950.4	E962.0	E980.4
Levo-iso-methadone	965.02	E850.1	E935.1	E950.0	E962.0	E980.0
Levomepromazine	967.8	E852.8	E937.8	E950.2	E962.0	E980.2
Levoprome	967.8	E852.8	E937.8	E950.2	E962.0	E980.2
Levopropoxyphene	975.4	E858.6	E945.4	E950.4	E962.0	E980.4
Levorphan, levophanol	965.09	E850.2	E935.2	E950.0	E962.0	E980.0
Levothyroxine (sodium)	962.7	E858.0	E932.7	E950.4	E962.0	E980.4
Levsin	971.1	E855.4	E941.1	E950.4	E962.0	E980.4
Levulose	974.5	E858.5	E944.5	E950.4	E962.0	E980.4
Lewisite (gas)	985.1	E866.3	—	E950.8	E962.1	E980.8
Librium	969.4	E853.2	E939.4	E950.3	E962.0	E980.3
Lidex	976.0	E858.7	E946.0	E950.4	E962.0	E980.4
Lidocaine (infiltration) (topical)	968.5	E855.2	E938.5	E950.4	E962.0	E980.4
nerve block (peripheral) (plexus)	968.6	E855.2	E938.6	E950.4	E962.0	E980.4
spinal	968.7	E855.2	E938.7	E950.4	E962.0	E980.4
Lighter fluid	981	E862.1	—	E950.9	E962.1	E980.9
Lignocaine (infiltration) (topical)	968.5	E855.2	E938.5	E950.4	E962.0	E980.4
nerve block (peripheral) (plexus)	968.6	E855.2	E938.6	E950.4	E962.0	E980.4
spinal	968.7	E855.2	E938.7	E950.4	E962.0	E980.4
Ligroin(e) (solvent)	981	E862.0	—	E950.9	E962.1	E980.9
vapor	987.1	E869.8	—	E952.8	E962.2	E982.8
Ligustrum vulgare	988.2	E865.3	—	E950.9	E962.1	E980.9
Lily of the valley	988.2	E865.4	—	E950.9	E962.1	E980.9
Lime (chloride)	983.2	E864.2	—	E950.7	E962.1	E980.6
solution, sulferated	976.4	E858.7	E946.4	E950.4	E962.0	E980.4
Limonene	982.8	E862.4	—	E950.9	E962.1	E980.9

TABLE OF DRUGS AND CHEMICALS / Lincomycin

Substance	Poisoning	External Cause (E Code)				
		Accident	Therapeutic Use	Suicide Attempt	Assault	Undetermined
Lincomycin	960.8	E856	E930.8	E950.4	E962.0	E980.4
Lindane (insecticide) (vapor)	989.2	E863.0	—	E950.6	E962.1	E980.7
anti-infective (topical)	976.0	E858.7	E946.0	E950.4	E962.0	E980.4
Liniments NEC	976.9	E858.7	E946.9	E950.4	E962.0	E980.4
Linoleic acid	972.2	E858.3	E942.2	E950.4	E962.0	E980.4
Liothyronine	962.7	E858.0	E932.7	E950.4	E962.0	E980.4
Liotrix	962.7	E858.0	E932.7	E950.4	E962.0	E980.4
Lipancreatin	973.4	E858.4	E943.4	E950.4	E962.0	E980.4
Lipo-Lutin	962.2	E858.0	E932.2	E950.4	E962.0	E980.4
Lipotropic agents	977.1	E858.8	E947.1	E950.4	E962.0	E980.4
Liquefied petroleum gases	987.0	E868.0	—	E951.1	E962.2	E981.1
piped (pure or mixed with air)	987.0	E867	—	E951.0	E962.2	E981.0
Liquid petrolatum	973.2	E858.4	E943.2	E950.4	E962.0	E980.4
substance	989.9	E866.9	—	E950.9	E962.1	E980.9
specified NEC	989.89	E866.8	—	E950.9	E962.1	E980.9
Lirugen	979.4	E858.8	E949.4	E950.4	E962.0	E980.4
Lithane	969.8	E855.8	E939.8	E950.3	E962.0	E980.3
Lithium	985.8	E866.4	—	E950.9	E962.1	E980.9
carbonate	969.8	E855.8	E939.8	E950.3	E962.0	E980.3
Lithonate	969.8	E855.8	E939.8	E950.3	E962.0	E980.3
Liver (extract) (injection) (preparations)	964.1	E858.2	E934.1	E950.4	E962.0	E980.4
Lizard (bite) (venom)	989.5	E905.0	—	E950.9	E962.1	E980.9
LMD	964.8	E858.2	E934.8	E950.4	E962.0	E980.4
Lobelia	988.2	E865.4	—	E950.9	E962.1	E980.9
Lobeline	970.0	E854.3	E940.0	E950.4	E962.0	E980.4
Locorten	976.0	E858.7	E946.0	E950.4	E962.0	E980.4
Lolium temulentum	988.2	E865.3	—	E950.9	E962.1	E980.9
Lomotil	973.5	E858.4	E943.5	E950.4	E962.0	E980.4
Lomustine	963.1	E858.1	E933.1	E950.4	E962.0	E980.4
Lophophora williamsii	969.6	E854.1	E939.6	E950.3	E962.0	E980.3
Lorazepam	969.4	E853.2	E939.4	E950.3	E962.0	E980.3
Lotions NEC	976.9	E858.7	E946.9	E950.4	E962.0	E980.4
Lotronex	973.8	E858.4	E943.8	E950.4	E962.0	E980.4
Lotusate	967.0	E851	E937.0	E950.1	E962.0	E980.1
Lowila	976.2	E858.7	E946.2	E950.4	E962.0	E980.4
Loxapine	969.3	E853.8	E939.3	E950.3	E962.0	E980.3
Lozenges (throat)	976.6	E858.7	E946.6	E950.4	E962.0	E980.4
LSD (25)	969.6	E854.1	E939.6	E950.3	E962.0	E980.3
Lubricating oil NEC	981	E862.2	—	E950.9	E962.1	E980.9

◀ New   ⬅ Revised   ~~deleted~~ Deleted   ● Use Additional Digit(s)

TABLE OF DRUGS AND CHEMICALS / Manganese compounds NEC

Substance	Poisoning	Accident	Therapeutic Use	Suicide Attempt	Assault	Undetermined
Lucanthone	961.6	E857	E931.6	E950.4	E962.0	E980.4
Luminal	967.0	E851	E937.0	E950.1	E962.0	E980.1
Lung irritant (gas) NEC	987.9	E869.9	—	E952.9	E962.2	E982.9
Lutocylol	962.2	E858.0	E932.2	E950.4	E962.0	E980.4
Lutromone	962.2	E858.0	E932.2	E950.4	E962.0	E980.4
Lututrin	975.0	E858.6	E945.0	E950.4	E962.0	E980.4
Lye (concentrated)	983.2	E864.2	—	E950.7	E962.1	E980.6
Lygranum (skin test)	977.8	E858.8	E947.8	E950.4	E962.0	E980.4
Lymecycline	960.4	E856	E930.4	E950.4	E962.0	E980.4
Lymphogranuloma venereum antigen	977.8	E858.8	E947.8	E950.4	E962.0	E980.4
Lynestrenol	962.2	E858.0	E932.2	E950.4	E962.0	E980.4
Lyovac Sodium Edecrin	974.4	E858.5	E944.4	E950.4	E962.0	E980.4
Lypressin	962.5	E858.0	E932.5	E950.4	E962.0	E980.4
Lysergic acid (amide) (diethylamide)	969.6	E854.1	E939.6	E950.3	E962.0	E980.3
Lysergide	969.6	E854.1	E939.6	E950.3	E962.0	E980.3
Lysine vasopressin	962.5	E858.0	E932.5	E950.4	E962.0	E980.4
Lysol	983.0	E864.0	—	E950.7	E962.1	E980.6
Lytta (vitatta)	976.8	E858.7	E946.8	E950.4	E962.0	E980.4
Mace	987.5	E869.3	—	E952.8	E962.2	E982.8
Macrolides (antibiotics)	960.3	E856	E930.3	E950.4	E962.0	E980.4
Mafenide	976.0	E858.7	E946.0	E950.4	E962.0	E980.4
Magaldrate	973.0	E858.4	E943.0	E950.4	E962.0	E980.4
Magic mushroom	969.6	E854.1	E939.6	E950.3	E962.0	E980.3
Magnamycin	960.8	E856	E930.8	E950.4	E962.0	E980.4
Magnesia magma	973.0	E858.4	E943.0	E950.4	E962.0	E980.4
Magnesium (compounds) (fumes) NEC	985.8	E866.4	—	E950.9	E962.1	E980.9
antacid	973.0	E858.4	E943.0	E950.4	E962.0	E980.4
carbonate	973.0	E858.4	E943.0	E950.4	E962.0	E980.4
cathartic	973.3	E858.4	E943.3	E950.4	E962.0	E980.4
citrate	973.3	E858.4	E943.3	E950.4	E962.0	E980.4
hydroxide	973.0	E858.4	E943.0	E950.4	E962.0	E980.4
oxide	973.0	E858.4	E943.0	E950.4	E962.0	E980.4
sulfate (oral)	973.3	E858.4	E943.3	E950.4	E962.0	E980.4
intravenous	966.3	E855.0	E936.3	E950.4	E962.0	E980.4
trisilicate	973.0	E858.4	E943.0	E950.4	E962.0	E980.4
Malathion (insecticide)	989.3	E863.1	—	E950.6	E962.1	E980.7
Male fern (oleoresin)	961.6	E857	E931.6	E950.4	E962.0	E980.4
Mandelic acid	961.9	E857	E931.9	E950.4	E962.0	E980.4
Manganese compounds (fumes) NEC	985.2	E866.4	—	E950.9	E962.1	E980.9

TABLE OF DRUGS AND CHEMICALS / Mannitol NEC

		External Cause (E Code)				
Substance	Poisoning	Accident	Therapeutic Use	Suicide Attempt	Assault	Undetermined
Mannitol (diuretic) (medicinal) NEC	974.4	E858.5	E944.4	E950.4	E962.0	E980.4
hexanitrate	972.4	E858.3	E942.4	E950.4	E962.0	E980.4
mustard	963.1	E858.1	E933.1	E950.4	E962.0	E980.4
Mannomustine	963.1	E858.1	E933.1	E950.4	E962.0	E980.4
MAO inhibitors	969.01	E854.0	E939.0	E950.3	E962.0	E980.3
Mapharsen	961.1	E857	E931.1	E950.4	E962.0	E980.4
Marcaine	968.9	E855.2	E938.9	E950.4	E962.0	E980.4
infiltration (subcutaneous)	968.5	E855.2	E938.5	E950.4	E962.0	E980.4
nerve block (peripheral) (plexus)	968.6	E855.2	E938.6	E950.4	E962.0	E980.4
Marezine	963.0	E858.1	E933.0	E950.4	E962.0	E980.4
Marihuana, marijuana (derivatives)	969.6	E854.1	E939.6	E950.3	E962.0	E980.3
Marine animals or plants (sting)	989.5	E905.6	—	E950.9	E962.1	E980.9
Marplan	969.01	E854.0	E939.0	E950.3	E962.0	E980.3
Marsh gas	987.1	E869.8	—	E952.8	E962.2	E982.8
Marsilid	969.01	E854.0	E939.0	E950.3	E962.0	E980.3
Matulane	963.1	E858.1	E933.1	E950.4	E962.0	E980.4
Mazindol	977.0	E858.8	E947.0	E950.4	E962.0	E980.4
MDMA	969.72	E854.2	E939.7	E950.3	E962.0	E980.3
Meadow saffron	988.2	E865.3	—	E950.9	E962.1	E980.9
Measles vaccine	979.4	E858.8	E949.4	E950.4	E962.0	E980.4
Meat, noxious or nonbacterial	988.8	E865.0	—	E950.9	E962.1	E980.9
Mebanazine	969.01	E854.0	E939.0	E950.3	E962.0	E980.3
Mebaral	967.0	E851	E937.0	E950.1	E962.0	E980.1
Mebendazole	961.6	E857	E931.6	E950.4	E962.0	E980.4
Mebeverine	975.1	E858.6	E945.1	E950.4	E962.0	E980.4
Mebhydroline	963.0	E858.1	E933.0	E950.4	E962.0	E980.4
Mebrophenhydramine	963.0	E858.1	E933.0	E950.4	E962.0	E980.4
Mebutamate	969.5	E853.8	E939.5	E950.3	E962.0	E980.3
Mecamylamine (chloride)	972.3	E858.3	E942.3	E950.4	E962.0	E980.4
Mechlorethamine hydrochloride	963.1	E858.1	E933.1	E950.4	E962.0	E980.4
Meclizene (hydrochloride)	963.0	E858.1	E933.0	E950.4	E962.0	E980.4
Meclofenoxate	970.0	E854.3	E940.0	E950.4	E962.0	E980.4
Meclozine (hydrochloride)	963.0	E858.1	E933.0	E950.4	E962.0	E980.4
Medazepam	969.4	E853.2	E939.4	E950.3	E962.0	E980.3
Medicine, medicinal substance	977.9	E858.9	E947.9	E950.5	E962.0	E980.5
specified NEC	977.8	E858.8	E947.8	E950.4	E962.0	E980.4
Medinal	967.0	E851	E937.0	E950.1	E962.0	E980.1
Medomin	967.0	E851	E937.0	E950.1	E962.0	E980.1
Medroxyprogesterone	962.2	E858.0	E932.2	E950.4	E962.0	E980.4

TABLE OF DRUGS AND CHEMICALS / Meprobamate

Substance	Poisoning	External Cause (E Code)				
		Accident	Therapeutic Use	Suicide Attempt	Assault	Undetermined
Medrysone	976.5	E858.7	E946.5	E950.4	E962.0	E980.4
Mefenamic acid	965.7	E850.7	E935.7	E950.0	E962.0	E980.0
Megahallucinogen	969.6	E854.1	E939.6	E950.3	E962.0	E980.3
Megestrol	962.2	E858.0	E932.2	E950.4	E962.0	E980.4
Meglumine	977.8	E858.8	E947.8	E950.4	E962.0	E980.4
Meladinin	976.3	E858.7	E946.3	E950.4	E962.0	E980.4
Melanizing agents	976.3	E858.7	E946.3	E950.4	E962.0	E980.4
Melarsoprol	961.1	E857	E931.1	E950.4	E962.0	E980.4
Melia azedarach	988.2	E865.3	—	E950.9	E962.1	E980.9
Mellaril	969.1	E853.0	E939.1	E950.3	E962.0	E980.3
Meloxine	976.3	E858.7	E946.3	E950.4	E962.0	E980.4
Melphalan	963.1	E858.1	E933.1	E950.4	E962.0	E980.4
Memantine hydrochloride	969.8	E854.8	E939.8	E950.3	E962.0	E980.3
Menadiol sodium diphosphate	964.3	E858.2	E934.3	E950.4	E962.0	E980.4
Menadione (sodium bisulfite)	964.3	E858.2	E934.3	E950.4	E962.0	E980.4
Menaphthone	964.3	E858.2	E934.3	E950.4	E962.0	E980.4
Meningococcal vaccine	978.8	E858.8	E948.8	E950.4	E962.0	E980.4
Menningovax-C	978.8	E858.8	E948.8	E950.4	E962.0	E980.4
Menotropins	962.4	E858.0	E932.4	E950.4	E962.0	E980.4
Menthol NEC	976.1	E858.7	E946.1	E950.4	E962.0	E980.4
Mepacrine	961.3	E857	E931.3	E950.4	E962.0	E980.4
Meparfynol	967.8	E852.8	E937.8	E950.2	E962.0	E980.2
Mepazine	969.1	E853.0	E939.1	E950.3	E962.0	E980.3
Mepenzolate	971.1	E855.4	E941.1	E950.4	E962.0	E980.4
Meperidine	965.09	E850.2	E935.2	E950.0	E962.0	E980.0
Mephenamin(e)	966.4	E855.0	E936.4	E950.4	E962.0	E980.4
Mephenesin (carbamate)	968.0	E855.1	E938.0	E950.4	E962.0	E980.4
Mephenoxalone	969.5	E853.8	E939.5	E950.3	E962.0	E980.3
Mephentermine	971.2	E855.5	E941.2	E950.4	E962.0	E980.4
Mephenytoin	966.1	E855.0	E936.1	E950.4	E962.0	E980.4
Mephobarbital	967.0	E851	E937.0	E950.1	E962.0	E980.1
Mepiperphenidol	971.1	E855.4	E941.1	E950.4	E962.0	E980.4
Mepivacaine	968.9	E855.2	E938.9	E950.4	E962.0	E980.4
infiltration (subcutaneous)	968.5	E855.2	E938.5	E950.4	E962.0	E980.4
nerve block (peripheral) (plexus)	968.6	E855.2	E938.6	E950.4	E962.0	E980.4
topical (surface)	968.5	E855.2	E938.5	E950.4	E962.0	E980.4
Meprednisone	962.0	E858.0	E932.0	E950.4	E962.0	E980.4
Meprobam	969.5	E853.8	E939.5	E950.3	E962.0	E980.3
Meprobamate	969.5	E853.8	E939.5	E950.3	E962.0	E980.3

TABLE OF DRUGS AND CHEMICALS / Mepyramine

Substance	Poisoning	External Cause (E Code)				
		Accident	Therapeutic Use	Suicide Attempt	Assault	Undetermined
Mepyramine (maleate)	963.0	E858.1	E933.0	E950.4	E962.0	E980.4
Meralluride	974.0	E858.5	E944.0	E950.4	E962.0	E980.4
Merbaphen	974.0	E858.5	E944.0	E950.4	E962.0	E980.4
Merbromin	976.0	E858.7	E946.0	E950.4	E962.0	E980.4
Mercaptomerin	974.0	E858.5	E944.0	E950.4	E962.0	E980.4
Mercaptopurine	963.1	E858.1	E933.1	E950.4	E962.0	E980.4
Mercumatilin	974.0	E858.5	E944.0	E950.4	E962.0	E980.4
Mercuramide	974.0	E858.5	E944.0	E950.4	E962.0	E980.4
Mercuranin	976.0	E858.7	E946.0	E950.4	E962.0	E980.4
Mercurochrome	976.0	E858.7	E946.0	E950.4	E962.0	E980.4
Mercury, mercuric, mercurous (compounds) (cyanide) (fumes) (nonmedicinal) (vapor) NEC	985.0	E866.1	—	E950.9	E962.1	E980.9
ammoniated	976.0	E858.7	E946.0	E950.4	E962.0	E980.4
anti-infective	961.2	E857	E931.2	E950.4	E962.0	E980.4
topical	976.0	E858.7	E946.0	E950.4	E962.0	E980.4
chloride (antiseptic) NEC	976.0	E858.7	E946.0	E950.4	E962.0	E980.4
fungicide	985.0	E863.6	—	E950.6	E962.1	E980.7
diuretic compounds	974.0	E858.5	E944.0	E950.4	E962.0	E980.4
fungicide	985.0	E863.6	—	E950.6	E962.1	E980.7
organic (fungicide)	985.0	E863.6	—	E950.6	E962.1	E980.7
Merethoxylline	974.0	E858.5	E944.0	E950.4	E962.0	E980.4
Mersalyl	974.0	E858.5	E944.0	E950.4	E962.0	E980.4
Merthiolate (topical)	976.0	E858.7	E946.0	E950.4	E962.0	E980.4
ophthalmic preparation	976.5	E858.7	E946.5	E950.4	E962.0	E980.4
Meruvax	979.4	E858.8	E949.4	E950.4	E962.0	E980.4
Mescal buttons	969.6	E854.1	E939.6	E950.3	E962.0	E980.3
Mescaline (salts)	969.6	E854.1	E939.6	E950.3	E962.0	E980.3
Mesoridazine besylate	969.1	E853.0	E939.1	E950.3	E962.0	E980.3
Mestanolone	962.1	E858.0	E932.1	E950.4	E962.0	E980.4
Mestranol	962.2	E858.0	E932.2	E950.4	E962.0	E980.4
Metactesylacetate	976.0	E858.7	E946.0	E950.4	E962.0	E980.4
Metaldehyde (snail killer) NEC	989.4	E863.4	—	E950.6	E962.1	E980.7
Metals (heavy) (nonmedicinal) NEC	985.9	E866.4	—	E950.9	E962.1	E980.9
dust, fumes, or vapor NEC	985.9	E866.4	—	E950.9	E962.1	E980.9
light NEC	985.9	E866.4	—	E950.9	E962.1	E980.9
dust, fumes, or vapor NEC	985.9	E866.4	—	E950.9	E962.1	E980.9
pesticides (dust) (vapor)	985.9	E863.4	—	E950.6	E962.1	E980.7
Metamucil	973.3	E858.4	E943.3	E950.4	E962.0	E980.4
Metaphen	976.0	E858.7	E946.0	E950.4	E962.0	E980.4

TABLE OF DRUGS AND CHEMICALS / Methoserpidine

| Substance | Poisoning | External Cause (E Code) |||||
		Accident	Therapeutic Use	Suicide Attempt	Assault	Undetermined
Metaproterenol	975.1	E858.6	E945.1	E950.4	E962.0	E980.4
Metaraminol	972.8	E858.3	E942.8	E950.4	E962.0	E980.4
Metaxalone	968.0	E855.1	E938.0	E950.4	E962.0	E980.4
Metformin	962.3	E858.0	E932.3	E950.4	E962.0	E980.4
Methacycline	960.4	E856	E930.4	E950.4	E962.0	E980.4
Methadone	965.02	E850.1	E935.1	E950.0	E962.0	E980.0
Methallenestril	962.2	E858.0	E932.2	E950.4	E962.0	E980.4
Methamphetamine	969.72	E854.2	E939.7	E950.3	E962.0	E980.3
Methandienone	962.1	E858.0	E932.1	E950.4	E962.0	E980.4
Methandriol	962.1	E858.0	E932.1	E950.4	E962.0	E980.4
Methandrostenolone	962.1	E858.0	E932.1	E950.4	E962.0	E980.4
Methane gas	987.1	E869.8	—	E952.8	E962.2	E982.8
Methanol	980.1	E860.2	—	E950.9	E962.1	E980.9
vapor	987.8	E869.8	—	E952.8	E962.2	E982.8
Methantheline	971.1	E855.4	E941.1	E950.4	E962.0	E980.4
Methaphenilene	963.0	E858.1	E933.0	E950.4	E962.0	E980.4
Methapyrilene	963.0	E858.1	E933.0	E950.4	E962.0	E980.4
Methaqualone (compounds)	967.4	E852.3	E937.4	E950.2	E962.0	E980.2
Metharbital, metharbitone	967.0	E851	E937.0	E950.1	E962.0	E980.1
Methazolamide	974.2	E858.5	E944.2	E950.4	E962.0	E980.4
Methdilazine	963.0	E858.1	E933.0	E950.4	E962.0	E980.4
Methedrine	969.72	E854.2	E939.7	E950.3	E962.0	E980.3
Methenamine (mandelate)	961.9	E857	E931.9	E950.4	E962.0	E980.4
Methenolone	962.1	E858.0	E932.1	E950.4	E962.0	E980.4
Methergine	975.0	E858.6	E945.0	E950.4	E962.0	E980.4
Methiacil	962.8	E858.0	E932.8	E950.4	E962.0	E980.4
Methicillin (sodium)	960.0	E856	E930.0	E950.4	E962.0	E980.4
Methimazole	962.8	E858.0	E932.8	E950.4	E962.0	E980.4
Methionine	977.1	E858.8	E947.1	E950.4	E962.0	E980.4
Methisazone	961.7	E857	E931.7	E950.4	E962.0	E980.4
Methitural	967.0	E851	E937.0	E950.1	E962.0	E980.1
Methixene	971.1	E855.4	E941.1	E950.4	E962.0	E980.4
Methobarbital, methobarbitone	967.0	E851	E937.0	E950.1	E962.0	E980.1
Methocarbamol	968.0	E855.1	E938.0	E950.4	E962.0	E980.4
Methohexital, methohexitone (sodium)	968.3	E855.1	E938.3	E950.4	E962.0	E980.4
Methoin	966.1	E855.0	E936.1	E950.4	E962.0	E980.4
Methopholine	965.7	E850.7	E935.7	E950.0	E962.0	E980.0
Methorate	975.4	E858.6	E945.4	E950.4	E962.0	E980.4
Methoserpidine	972.6	E858.3	E942.6	E950.4	E962.0	E980.4

TABLE OF DRUGS AND CHEMICALS / Methotrexate

Substance	Poisoning	External Cause (E Code)				
		Accident	Therapeutic Use	Suicide Attempt	Assault	Undetermined
Methotrexate	963.1	E858.1	E933.1	E950.4	E962.0	E980.4
Methotrimeprazine	967.8	E852.8	E937.8	E950.2	E962.0	E980.2
Methoxa-Dome	976.3	E858.7	E946.3	E950.4	E962.0	E980.4
Methoxamine	971.2	E855.5	E941.2	E950.4	E962.0	E980.4
Methoxsalen	976.3	E858.7	E946.3	E950.4	E962.0	E980.4
Methoxybenzyl penicillin	960.0	E856	E930.0	E950.4	E962.0	E980.4
Methoxychlor	989.2	E863.0	—	E950.6	E962.1	E980.7
Methoxyflurane	968.2	E855.1	E938.2	E950.4	E962.0	E980.4
Methoxyphenamine	971.2	E855.5	E941.2	E950.4	E962.0	E980.4
Methoxypromazine	969.1	E853.0	E939.1	E950.3	E962.0	E980.3
Methoxypsoralen	976.3	E858.7	E946.3	E950.4	E962.0	E980.4
Methscopolamine (bromide)	971.1	E855.4	E941.1	E950.4	E962.0	E980.4
Methsuximide	966.2	E855.0	E936.2	E950.4	E962.0	E980.4
Methyclothiazide	974.3	E858.5	E944.3	E950.4	E962.0	E980.4
Methyl	—	—	—	—	—	—
acetate	982.8	E862.4	—	E950.9	E962.1	E980.9
acetone II	982.8	E862.4	—	E950.9	E962.1	E980.9
alcohol	980.1	E860.2	—	E950.9	E962.1	E980.9
amphetamine	969.72	E854.2	E939.7	E950.3	E962.0	E980.3
androstanolone	962.1	E858.0	E932.1	E950.4	E962.0	E980.4
atropine	971.1	E855.4	E941.1	E950.4	E962.0	E980.4
benzene	982.0	E862.4	—	E950.9	E962.1	E980.9
bromide (gas)	987.8	E869.8	—	E952.8	E962.2	E982.8
fumigant	987.8	E863.8	—	E950.6	E962.2	E980.7
butanol	980.8	E860.8	—	E950.9	E962.1	E980.9
carbinol	980.1	E860.2	—	E950.9	E962.1	E980.9
cellosolve	982.8	E862.4	—	E950.9	E962.1	E980.9
cellulose	973.3	E858.4	E943.3	E950.4	E962.0	E980.4
chloride (gas)	987.8	E869.8	—	E952.8	E962.2	E982.8
cyclohexane	982.8	E862.4	—	E950.9	E962.1	E980.9
cyclohexanone	982.8	E862.4	—	E950.9	E962.1	E980.9
dihydromorphinone	965.09	E850.2	E935.2	E950.0	E962.0	E980.0
ergometrine	975.0	E858.6	E945.0	E950.4	E962.0	E980.4
ergonovine	975.0	E858.6	E945.0	E950.4	E962.0	E980.4
ethyl ketone	982.8	E862.4	—	E950.9	E962.1	E980.9
hydrazine	983.9	E864.3	—	E950.7	E962.1	E980.6
isobutyl ketone	982.8	E862.4	—	E950.9	E962.1	E980.9
morphine NEC	965.09	E850.2	E935.2	E950.0	E962.0	E980.0
parafynol	967.8	E852.8	E937.8	E950.2	E962.0	E980.2

TABLE OF DRUGS AND CHEMICALS / Midol

		External Cause (E Code)				
Substance	Poisoning	Accident	Therapeutic Use	Suicide Attempt	Assault	Undetermined
Methyl (Continued)						
parathion	989.3	E863.1	—	E950.6	E962.1	E980.7
pentynol NEC	967.8	E852.8	E937.8	E950.2	E962.0	E980.2
peridol	969.2	E853.1	E939.2	E950.3	E962.0	E980.3
phenidate	969.73	E854.2	E939.7	E950.3	E962.0	E980.3
prednisolone	962.0	E858.0	E932.0	E950.4	E962.0	E980.4
ENT agent	976.6	E858.7	E946.6	E950.4	E962.0	E980.4
ophthalmic preparation	976.5	E858.7	E946.5	E950.4	E962.0	E980.4
topical NEC	976.0	E858.7	E946.0	E950.4	E962.0	E980.4
propylcarbinol	980.8	E860.8	—	E950.9	E962.1	E980.9
rosaniline NEC	976.0	E858.7	E946.0	E950.4	E962.0	E980.4
salicylate NEC	976.3	E858.7	E946.3	E950.4	E962.0	E980.4
sulfate (fumes)	987.8	E869.8	—	E952.8	E962.2	E982.8
liquid	983.9	E864.3	—	E950.7	E962.1	E980.6
sulfonal	967.8	E852.8	E937.8	E950.2	E962.0	E980.2
testosterone	962.1	E858.0	E932.1	E950.4	E962.0	E980.4
thiouracil	962.8	E858.0	E932.8	E950.4	E962.0	E980.4
Methylated spirit	980.0	E860.1	—	E950.9	E962.1	E980.9
Methyldopa	972.6	E858.3	E942.6	E950.4	E962.0	E980.4
Methylene blue	961.9	E857	E931.9	E950.4	E962.0	E980.4
chloride or dichloride (solvent) NEC	982.3	E862.4	—	E950.9	E962.1	E980.9
Methylhexabital	967.0	E851	E937.0	E950.1	E962.0	E980.1
Methylparaben (ophthalmic)	976.5	E858.7	E946.5	E950.4	E962.0	E980.4
Methyprylon	967.5	E852.4	E937.5	E950.2	E962.0	E980.2
Methysergide	971.3	E855.6	E941.3	E950.4	E962.0	E980.4
Metoclopramide	963.0	E858.1	E933.0	E950.4	E962.0	E980.4
Metofoline	965.7	E850.7	E935.7	E950.0	E962.0	E980.0
Metopon	965.09	E850.2	E935.2	E950.0	E962.0	E980.0
Metronidazole	961.5	E857	E931.5	E950.4	E962.0	E980.4
Metycaine	968.9	E855.2	E938.9	E950.4	E962.0	E980.4
infiltration (subcutaneous)	968.5	E855.2	E938.5	E950.4	E962.0	E980.4
nerve block (peripheral) (plexus)	968.6	E855.2	E938.6	E950.4	E962.0	E980.4
topical (surface)	968.5	E855.2	E938.5	E950.4	E962.0	E980.4
Metyrapone	977.8	E858.8	E947.8	E950.4	E962.0	E980.4
Mevinphos	989.3	E863.1	—	E950.6	E962.1	E980.7
Mezereon (berries)	988.2	E865.3	—	E950.9	E962.1	E980.9
Micatin	976.0	E858.7	E946.0	E950.4	E962.0	E980.4
Miconazole	976.0	E858.7	E946.0	E950.4	E962.0	E980.4
Midol	965.1	E850.3	E935.3	E950.0	E962.0	E980.0

TABLE OF DRUGS AND CHEMICALS / Mifepristone

Substance	Poisoning	External Cause (E Code) Accident	Therapeutic Use	Suicide Attempt	Assault	Undetermined
Mifepristone	962.9	E858.0	E932.9	E950.4	E962.0	E980.4
Milk of magnesia	973.0	E858.4	E943.0	E950.4	E962.0	E980.4
Millipede (tropical) (venomous)	989.5	E905.4	—	E950.9	E962.1	E980.9
Miltown	969.5	E853.8	E939.5	E950.3	E962.0	E980.3
Mineral	—	—	—	—	—	—
oil (medicinal)	973.2	E858.4	E943.2	E950.4	E962.0	E980.4
nonmedicinal	981	E862.1	—	E950.9	E962.1	E980.9
topical	976.3	E858.7	E946.3	E950.4	E962.0	E980.4
salts NEC	974.6	E858.5	E944.6	E950.4	E962.0	E980.4
spirits	981	E862.0	—	E950.9	E962.1	E980.9
Minocycline	960.4	E856	E930.4	E950.4	E962.0	E980.4
Mithramycin (antineoplastic)	960.7	E856	E930.7	E950.4	E962.0	E980.4
Mitobronitol	963.1	E858.1	E933.1	E950.4	E962.0	E980.4
Mitomycin (antineoplastic)	960.7	E856	E930.7	E950.4	E962.0	E980.4
Mitotane	963.1	E858.1	E933.1	E950.4	E962.0	E980.4
Moderil	972.6	E858.3	E942.6	E950.4	E962.0	E980.4
Mogadon - see Nitrazepam	—	—	—	—	—	—
Molindone	969.3	E853.8	E939.3	E950.3	E962.0	E980.3
Monistat	976.0	E858.7	E946.0	E950.4	E962.0	E980.4
Monkshood	988.2	E865.4	—	E950.9	E962.1	E980.9
Monoamine oxidase inhibitors	969.01	E854.0	E939.0	E950.3	E962.0	E980.3
Monochlorobenzene	982.0	E862.4	—	E950.9	E962.1	E980.9
Monosodium glutamate	989.89	E866.8	—	E950.9	E962.1	E980.9
Monoxide, carbon - see Carbon, monoxide	—	—	—	—	—	—
Moperone	969.2	E853.1	E939.2	E950.3	E962.0	E980.3
Morning glory seeds	969.6	E854.1	E939.6	E950.3	E962.0	E980.3
Moroxydine (hydrochloride)	961.7	E857	E931.7	E950.4	E962.0	E980.4
Morphazinamide	961.8	E857	E931.8	E950.4	E962.0	E980.4
Morphinans	965.09	E850.2	E935.2	E950.0	E962.0	E980.0
Morphine NEC	965.09	E850.2	E935.2	E950.0	E962.0	E980.0
antagonists	970.1	E854.3	E940.1	E950.4	E962.0	E980.4
Morpholinylethyl morphine	965.09	E850.2	E935.2	E950.0	E962.0	E980.0
Morrhuate sodium	972.7	E858.3	E942.7	E950.4	E962.0	E980.4
Moth balls (see also Pesticides)	989.4	E863.4	—	E950.6	E962.1	E980.7
naphthalene	983.0	E863.4	—	E950.7	E962.1	E980.6
Motor exhaust gas - see Carbon, monoxide, exhaust gas	—	—	—	—	—	—
Mouth wash	976.6	E858.7	E946.6	E950.4	E962.0	E980.4
Mucolytic agent	975.5	E858.6	E945.5	E950.4	E962.0	E980.4
Mucomyst	975.5	E858.6	E945.5	E950.4	E962.0	E980.4

TABLE OF DRUGS AND CHEMICALS / Nalidixic acid

Substance	Poisoning	External Cause (E Code) Accident	Therapeutic Use	Suicide Attempt	Assault	Undetermined
Mucous membrane agents (external)	976.9	E858.7	E946.9	E950.4	E962.0	E980.4
specified NEC	976.8	E858.7	E946.8	E950.4	E962.0	E980.4
Mumps	—	—	—	—	—	—
immune globulin (human)	964.6	E858.2	E934.6	E950.4	E962.0	E980.4
skin test antigen	977.8	E858.8	E947.8	E950.4	E962.0	E980.4
vaccine	979.6	E858.8	E949.6	E950.4	E962.0	E980.4
Mumpsvax	979.6	E858.8	E949.6	E950.4	E962.0	E980.4
Muriatic acid - see Hydrochloric acid	—	—	—	—	—	—
Muscarine	971.0	E855.3	E941.0	E950.4	E962.0	E980.4
Muscle affecting agents NEC	975.3	E858.6	E945.3	E950.4	E962.0	E980.4
oxytocic	975.0	E858.6	E945.0	E950.4	E962.0	E980.4
relaxants	975.3	E858.6	E945.3	E950.4	E962.0	E980.4
central nervous system	968.0	E855.1	E938.0	E950.4	E962.0	E980.4
skeletal	975.2	E858.6	E945.2	E950.4	E962.0	E980.4
smooth	975.1	E858.6	E945.1	E950.4	E962.0	E980.4
Mushrooms, noxious	988.1	E865.5	—	E950.9	E962.1	E980.9
Mussel, noxious	988.0	E865.1	—	E950.9	E962.1	E980.9
Mustard (emetic)	973.6	E858.4	E943.6	E950.4	E962.0	E980.4
gas	987.8	E869.8	—	E952.8	E962.2	E982.8
nitrogen	963.1	E858.1	E933.1	E950.4	E962.0	E980.4
Mustine	963.1	E858.1	E933.1	E950.4	E962.0	E980.4
M-vac	979.4	E858.8	E949.4	E950.4	E962.0	E980.4
Mycifradin	960.8	E856	E930.8	E950.4	E962.0	E980.4
topical	976.0	E858.7	E946.0	E950.4	E962.0	E980.4
Mycitracin	960.8	E856	E930.8	E950.4	E962.0	E980.4
ophthalmic preparation	976.5	E858.7	E946.5	E950.4	E962.0	E980.4
Mycostatin	960.1	E856	E930.1	E950.4	E962.0	E980.4
topical	976.0	E858.7	E946.0	E950.4	E962.0	E980.4
Mydriacyl	971.1	E855.4	E941.1	E950.4	E962.0	E980.4
Myelobromal	963.1	E858.1	E933.1	E950.4	E962.0	E980.4
Myleran	963.1	E858.1	E933.1	E950.4	E962.0	E980.4
Myochrysin(e)	965.69	E850.6	E935.6	E950.0	E962.0	E980.0
Myoneural blocking agents	975.2	E858.6	E945.2	E950.4	E962.0	E980.4
Myristica fragrans	988.2	E865.3	—	E950.9	E962.1	E980.9
Myristicin	988.2	E865.3	—	E950.9	E962.1	E980.9
Mysoline	966.3	E855.0	E936.3	E950.4	E962.0	E980.4
Nafcillin (sodium)	960.0	E856	E930.0	E950.4	E962.0	E980.4
Nail polish remover	982.8	E862.4	—	E950.9	E962.1	E980.9
Nalidixic acid	961.9	E857	E931.9	E950.4	E962.0	E980.4

TABLE OF DRUGS AND CHEMICALS / Nalorphine

		External Cause (E Code)				
Substance	Poisoning	Accident	Therapeutic Use	Suicide Attempt	Assault	Undetermined
Nalorphine	970.1	E854.3	E940.1	E950.4	E962.0	E980.4
Naloxone	970.1	E854.3	E940.1	E950.4	E962.0	E980.4
Namenda	969.8	E854.8	E939.8	E950.3	E962.0	E980.3
Nandrolone (decanoate) (phenpropionate)	962.1	E858.0	E932.1	E950.4	E962.0	E980.4
Naphazoline	971.2	E855.5	E941.2	E950.4	E962.0	E980.4
Naphtha (painter's) (petroleum)	981	E862.0	—	E950.9	E962.1	E980.9
solvent	981	E862.0	—	E950.9	E962.1	E980.9
vapor	987.1	E869.8	—	E952.8	E962.2	E982.8
Naphthalene (chlorinated)	983.0	E864.0	—	E950.7	E962.1	E980.6
insecticide or moth repellent	983.0	E863.4	—	E950.7	E962.1	E980.6
vapor	987.8	E869.8	—	E952.8	E962.2	E982.8
Naphthol	983.0	E864.0	—	E950.7	E962.1	E980.6
Naphthylamine	983.0	E864.0	—	E950.7	E962.1	E980.6
Naprosyn - see Naproxen	—	—	—	—	—	—
Naproxen	965.61	E850.6	E935.6	E950.0	E962.0	E980.0
Narcotic (drug)	967.9	E852.9	E937.9	E950.2	E962.0	E980.2
analgesic NEC	965.8	E850.8	E935.8	E950.0	E962.0	E980.0
antagonist	970.1	E854.3	E940.1	E950.4	E962.0	E980.4
specified NEC	967.8	E852.8	E937.8	E950.2	E962.0	E980.2
Narcotine	975.4	E858.6	E945.4	E950.4	E962.0	E980.4
Nardil	969.01	E854.0	E939.0	E950.3	E962.0	E980.3
Natrium cyanide - see Cyanide(s)	—	—	—	—	—	—
Natural	—	—	—	—	—	—
blood (product)	964.7	E858.2	E934.7	E950.4	E962.0	E980.4
gas (piped)	987.1	E867	—	E951.0	E962.2	E981.0
incomplete combustion	986	E867	—	E951.0	E962.2	E981.0
Nealbarbital, nealbarbitone	967.0	E851	E937.0	E950.1	E962.0	E980.1
Nectadon	975.4	E858.6	E945.4	E950.4	E962.0	E980.4
Nematocyst (sting)	989.5	E905.6	—	E950.9	E962.1	E980.9
Nembutal	967.0	E851	E937.0	E950.1	E962.0	E980.1
Neoarsphenamine	961.1	E857	E931.1	E950.4	E962.0	E980.4
Neocinchophen	974.7	E858.5	E944.7	E950.4	E962.0	E980.4
Neomycin	960.8	E856	E930.8	E950.4	E962.0	E980.4
ENT agent	976.6	E858.7	E946.6	E950.4	E962.0	E980.4
ophthalmic preparation	976.5	E858.7	E946.5	E950.4	E962.0	E980.4
topical NEC	976.0	E858.7	E946.0	E950.4	E962.0	E980.4
Neonal	967.0	E851	E937.0	E950.1	E962.0	E980.1
Neoprontosil	961.0	E857	E931.0	E950.4	E962.0	E980.4
Neosalvarsan	961.1	E857	E931.1	E950.4	E962.0	E980.4

◀ New ◀▬ Revised ~~deleted~~ Deleted ● Use Additional Digit(s)

TABLE OF DRUGS AND CHEMICALS / Nitrates

Substance	Poisoning	External Cause (E Code)				
		Accident	Therapeutic Use	Suicide Attempt	Assault	Undetermined
Neosilversalvarsan	961.1	E857	E931.1	E950.4	E962.0	E980.4
Neosporin	960.8	E856	E930.8	E950.4	E962.0	E980.4
ENT agent	976.6	E858.7	E946.6	E950.4	E962.0	E980.4
ophthalmic preparation	976.5	E858.7	E946.5	E950.4	E962.0	E980.4
topical NEC	976.0	E858.7	E946.0	E950.4	E962.0	E980.4
Neostigmine	971.0	E855.3	E941.0	E950.4	E962.0	E980.4
Neraval	967.0	E851	E937.0	E950.1	E962.0	E980.1
Neravan	967.0	E851	E937.0	E950.1	E962.0	E980.1
Nerium oleander	988.2	E865.4	—	E950.9	E962.1	E980.9
Nerve gases (war)	987.9	E869.9	—	E952.9	E962.2	E982.9
Nesacaine	968.9	E855.2	E938.9	E950.4	E962.0	E980.4
infiltration (subcutaneous)	968.5	E855.2	E938.5	E950.4	E962.0	E980.4
nerve block (peripheral) (plexus)	968.6	E855.2	E938.6	E950.4	E962.0	E980.4
Neurobarb	967.0	E851	E937.0	E950.1	E962.0	E980.1
Neuroleptics NEC	969.3	E853.8	E939.3	E950.3	E962.0	E980.3
Neuroprotective agent	977.8	E858.8	E947.8	E950.4	E962.0	E980.4
Neutral spirits	980.0	E860.1	—	E950.9	E962.1	E980.9
beverage	980.0	E860.0	—	E950.9	E962.1	E980.9
Niacin, niacinamide	972.2	E858.3	E942.2	E950.4	E962.0	E980.4
Nialamide	969.01	E854.0	E939.0	E950.3	E962.0	E980.3
Nickle (carbonyl) (compounds) (fumes) (tetracarbonyl) (vapor)	985.8	E866.4	—	E950.9	E962.1	E980.9
Niclosamide	961.6	E857	E931.6	E950.4	E962.0	E980.4
Nicomorphine	965.09	E850.2	E935.2	E950.0	E962.0	E980.0
Nicotinamide	972.2	E858.3	E942.2	E950.4	E962.0	E980.4
Nicotine (insecticide) (spray) (sulfate) NEC	989.4	E863.4	—	E950.6	E962.1	E980.7
not insecticide	989.89	E866.8	—	E950.9	E962.1	E980.9
Nicotinic acid (derivatives)	972.2	E858.3	E942.2	E950.4	E962.0	E980.4
Nicotinyl alcohol	972.2	E858.3	E942.2	E950.4	E962.0	E980.4
Nicoumalone	964.2	E858.2	E934.2	E950.4	E962.0	E980.4
Nifenazone	965.5	E850.5	E935.5	E950.0	E962.0	E980.0
Nifuraldezone	961.9	E857	E931.9	E950.4	E962.0	E980.4
Nightshade (deadly)	988.2	E865.4	—	E950.9	E962.1	E980.9
Nikethamide	970.0	E854.3	E940.0	E950.4	E962.0	E980.4
Nilstat	960.1	E856	E930.1	E950.4	E962.0	E980.4
topical	976.0	E858.7	E946.0	E950.4	E962.0	E980.4
Nimodipine	977.8	E858.8	E947.8	E950.4	E962.0	E980.4
Niridazole	961.6	E857	E931.6	E950.4	E962.0	E980.4
Nisentil	965.09	E850.2	E935.2	E950.0	E962.0	E980.0
Nitrates	972.4	E858.3	E942.4	E950.4	E962.0	E980.4

TABLE OF DRUGS AND CHEMICALS / Nitrazepam

| Substance | Poisoning | External Cause (E Code) |||||
		Accident	Therapeutic Use	Suicide Attempt	Assault	Undetermined
Nitrazepam	969.4	E853.2	E939.4	E950.3	E962.0	E980.3
Nitric	—	—	—	—	—	—
acid (liquid)	983.1	E864.1	—	E950.7	E962.1	E980.6
vapor	987.8	E869.8	—	E952.8	E962.2	E982.8
oxide (gas)	987.2	E869.0	—	E952.8	E962.2	E982.8
Nitrite, amyl (medicinal) (vapor)	972.4	E858.3	E942.4	E950.4	E962.0	E980.4
Nitroaniline	983.0	E864.0	—	E950.7	E962.1	E980.6
vapor	987.8	E869.8	—	E952.8	E962.2	E982.8
Nitrobenzene, nitrobenzol	983.0	E864.0	—	E950.7	E962.1	E980.6
vapor	987.8	E869.8	—	E952.8	E962.2	E982.8
Nitrocellulose	976.3	E858.7	E946.3	E950.4	E962.0	E980.4
Nitrofuran derivatives	961.9	E857	E931.9	E950.4	E962.0	E980.4
Nitrofurantoin	961.9	E857	E931.9	E950.4	E962.0	E980.4
Nitrofurazone	976.0	E858.7	E946.0	E950.4	E962.0	E980.4
Nitrogen (dioxide) (gas) (oxide)	987.2	E869.0	—	E952.8	E962.2	E982.8
mustard (antineoplastic)	963.1	E858.1	E933.1	E950.4	E962.0	E980.4
Nitroglycerin, nitroglycerol (medicinal)	972.4	E858.3	E942.4	E950.4	E962.0	E980.4
nonmedicinal	989.89	E866.8	—	E950.9	E962.1	E980.9
fumes	987.8	E869.8	—	E952.8	E962.2	E982.8
Nitrohydrochloric acid	983.1	E864.1	—	E950.7	E962.1	E980.6
Nitromersol	976.0	E858.7	E946.0	E950.4	E962.0	E980.4
Nitronaphthalene	983.0	E864.0	—	E950.7	E962.2	E980.6
Nitrophenol	983.0	E864.0	—	E950.7	E962.2	E980.6
Nitrothiazol	961.6	E857	E931.6	E950.4	E962.0	E980.4
Nitrotoluene, nitrotoluol	983.0	E864.0	—	E950.7	E962.1	E980.6
vapor	987.8	E869.8	—	E952.8	E962.2	E982.8
Nitrous	968.2	E855.1	E938.2	E950.4	E962.0	E980.4
acid (liquid)	983.1	E864.1	—	E950.7	E962.1	E980.6
fumes	987.2	E869.0	—	E952.8	E962.2	E982.8
oxide (anesthetic) NEC	968.2	E855.1	E938.2	E950.4	E962.0	E980.4
Nitrozone	976.0	E858.7	E946.0	E950.4	E962.0	E980.4
Noctec	967.1	E852.0	E937.1	E950.2	E962.0	E980.2
Noludar	967.5	E852.4	E937.5	E950.2	E962.0	E980.2
Noptil	967.0	E851	E937.0	E950.1	E962.0	E980.1
Noradrenalin	971.2	E855.5	E941.2	E950.4	E962.0	E980.4
Noramidopyrine	965.5	E850.5	E935.5	E950.0	E962.0	E980.0
Norepinephrine	971.2	E855.5	E941.2	E950.4	E962.0	E980.4
Norethandrolone	962.1	E858.0	E932.1	E950.4	E962.0	E980.4
Norethindrone	962.2	E858.0	E932.2	E950.4	E962.0	E980.4

TABLE OF DRUGS AND CHEMICALS / Oil NEC

Substance	Poisoning	External Cause (E Code)				
		Accident	Therapeutic Use	Suicide Attempt	Assault	Undetermined
Norethisterone	962.2	E858.0	E932.2	E950.4	E962.0	E980.4
Norethynodrel	962.2	E858.0	E932.2	E950.4	E962.0	E980.4
Norlestrin	962.2	E858.0	E932.2	E950.4	E962.0	E980.4
Norlutin	962.2	E858.0	E932.2	E950.4	E962.0	E980.4
Normison - see Benzodiazepines	—	—	—	—	—	—
Normorphine	965.09	E850.2	E935.2	E950.0	E962.0	E980.0
Nortriptyline	969.05	E854.0	E939.0	E950.3	E962.0	E980.3
Noscapine	975.4	E858.6	E945.4	E950.4	E962.0	E980.4
Nose preparations	976.6	E858.7	E946.6	E950.4	E962.0	E980.4
Novobiocin	960.8	E856	E930.8	E950.4	E962.0	E980.4
Novocain (infiltration) (topical)	968.5	E855.2	E938.5	E950.4	E962.0	E980.4
nerve block (peripheral) (plexus)	968.6	E855.2	E938.6	E950.4	E962.0	E980.4
spinal	968.7	E855.2	E938.7	E950.4	E962.0	E980.4
Noxythiolin	961.9	E857	E931.9	E950.4	E962.0	E980.4
NPH Iletin (insulin)	962.3	E858.0	E932.3	E950.4	E962.0	E980.4
Numorphan	965.09	E850.2	E935.2	E950.0	E962.0	E980.0
Nunol	967.0	E851	E937.0	E950.1	E962.0	E980.1
Nupercaine (spinal anesthetic)	968.7	E855.2	E938.7	E950.4	E962.0	E980.4
topical (surface)	968.5	E855.2	E938.5	E950.4	E962.0	E980.4
Nutmeg oil (liniment)	976.3	E858.7	E946.3	E950.4	E962.0	E980.4
Nux vomica	989.1	E863.7	—	E950.6	E962.1	E980.7
Nydrazid	961.8	E857	E931.8	E950.4	E962.0	E980.4
Nylidrin	971.2	E855.5	E941.2	E950.4	E962.0	E980.4
Nystatin	960.1	E856	E930.1	E950.4	E962.0	E980.4
topical	976.0	E858.7	E946.0	E950.4	E962.0	E980.4
Nytol	963.0	E858.1	E933.0	E950.4	E962.0	E980.4
Oblivion	967.8	E852.8	E937.8	E950.2	E962.0	E980.2
Octyl nitrite	972.4	E858.3	E942.4	E950.4	E962.0	E980.4
Oestradiol (cypionate) (dipropionate) (valerate)	962.2	E858.0	E932.2	E950.4	E962.0	E980.4
Oestriol	962.2	E858.0	E932.2	E950.4	E962.0	E980.4
Oestrone	962.2	E858.0	E932.2	E950.4	E962.0	E980.4
Oil (of) NEC	989.89	E866.8	—	E950.9	E962.1	E980.9
bitter almond	989.0	E866.8	—	E950.9	E962.1	E980.9
camphor	976.1	E858.7	E946.1	E950.4	E962.0	E980.4
colors	989.89	E861.6	—	E950.9	E962.1	E980.9
fumes	987.8	E869.8	—	E952.8	E962.2	E982.8
lubricating	981	E862.2	—	E950.9	E962.1	E980.9
specified source, other - see substance specified	—	—	—	—	—	—

TABLE OF DRUGS AND CHEMICALS / Oil NEC

Substance	Poisoning	External Cause (E Code) Accident	Therapeutic Use	Suicide Attempt	Assault	Undetermined
Oil (of) NEC *(Continued)*						
vitriol (liquid)	983.1	E864.1	—	E950.7	E962.1	E980.6
fumes	987.8	E869.8	—	E952.8	E962.2	E982.8
wintergreen (bitter) NEC	976.3	E858.7	E946.3	E950.4	E962.0	E980.4
Ointments NEC	976.9	E858.7	E946.9	E950.4	E962.0	E980.4
Oleander	988.2	E865.4	—	E950.9	E962.1	E980.9
Oleandomycin	960.3	E856	E930.3	E950.4	E962.0	E980.4
Oleovitamin A	963.5	E858.1	E933.5	E950.4	E962.0	E980.4
Oleum ricini	973.1	E858.4	E943.1	E950.4	E962.0	E980.4
Olive oil (medicinal) NEC	973.2	E858.4	E943.2	E950.4	E962.0	E980.4
OMPA	989.3	E863.1	—	E950.6	E962.1	E980.7
Oncovin	963.1	E858.1	E933.1	E950.4	E962.0	E980.4
Ophthaine	968.5	E855.2	E938.5	E950.4	E962.0	E980.4
Ophthetic	968.5	E855.2	E938.5	E950.4	E962.0	E980.4
Opiates, opioids, opium NEC	965.00	E850.2	E935.2	E950.0	E962.0	E980.0
antagonists	970.1	E854.3	E940.1	E950.4	E962.0	E980.4
Oracon	962.2	E858.0	E932.2	E950.4	E962.0	E980.4
Oragrafin	977.8	E858.8	E947.8	E950.4	E962.0	E980.4
Oral contraceptives	962.2	E858.0	E932.2	E950.4	E962.0	E980.4
Orciprenaline	975.1	E858.6	E945.1	E950.4	E962.0	E980.4
Organidin	975.5	E858.6	E945.5	E950.4	E962.0	E980.4
Organophosphates	989.3	E863.1	—	E950.6	E962.1	E980.7
Orimune	979.5	E858.8	E949.5	E950.4	E962.0	E980.4
Orinase	962.3	E858.0	E932.3	E950.4	E962.0	E980.4
Orphenadrine	966.4	E855.0	E936.4	E950.4	E962.0	E980.4
Ortal (sodium)	967.0	E851	E937.0	E950.1	E962.0	E980.1
Orthoboric acid	976.0	E858.7	E946.0	E950.4	E962.0	E980.4
ENT agent	976.6	E858.7	E946.6	E950.4	E962.0	E980.4
ophthalmic preparation	976.5	E858.7	E946.5	E950.4	E962.0	E980.4
Orthocaine	968.5	E855.2	E938.5	E950.4	E962.0	E980.4
Ortho-Novum	962.2	E858.0	E932.2	E950.4	E962.0	E980.4
Orthotolidine (reagent)	977.8	E858.8	E947.8	E950.4	E962.0	E980.4
Osmic acid (liquid)	983.1	E864.1	—	E950.7	E962.1	E980.6
fumes	987.8	E869.8	—	E952.8	E962.2	E982.8
Osmotic diuretics	974.4	E858.5	E944.4	E950.4	E962.0	E980.4
Ouabain	972.1	E858.3	E942.1	E950.4	E962.0	E980.4
Ovarian hormones (synthetic substitutes)	962.2	E858.0	E932.2	E950.4	E962.0	E980.4
Ovral	962.2	E858.0	E932.2	E950.4	E962.0	E980.4

TABLE OF DRUGS AND CHEMICALS / PABA

Substance	Poisoning	External Cause (E Code)				
		Accident	Therapeutic Use	Suicide Attempt	Assault	Undetermined
Ovulation suppressants	962.2	E858.0	E932.2	E950.4	E962.0	E980.4
Ovulen	962.2	E858.0	E932.2	E950.4	E962.0	E980.4
Oxacillin (sodium)	960.0	E856	E930.0	E950.4	E962.0	E980.4
Oxalic acid	983.1	E864.1	—	E950.7	E962.1	E980.6
Oxanamide	969.5	E853.8	E939.5	E950.3	E962.0	E980.3
Oxandrolone	962.1	E858.0	E932.1	E950.4	E962.0	E980.4
Oxaprozin	965.61	E850.6	E935.6	E950.0	E962.0	E980.0
Oxazepam	969.4	E853.2	E939.4	E950.3	E962.0	E980.3
Oxazolidine derivatives	966.0	E855.0	E936.0	E950.4	E962.0	E980.4
Ox bile extract	973.4	E858.4	E943.4	E950.4	E962.0	E980.4
Oxedrine	971.2	E855.5	E941.2	E950.4	E962.0	E980.4
Oxeladin	975.4	E858.6	E945.4	E950.4	E962.0	E980.4
Oxethazaine NEC	968.5	E855.2	E938.5	E950.4	E962.0	E980.4
Oxidizing agents NEC	983.9	E864.3	—	E950.7	E962.1	E980.6
Oxolinic acid	961.3	E857	E931.3	E950.4	E962.0	E980.4
Oxophenarsine	961.1	E857	E931.1	E950.4	E962.0	E980.4
Oxsoralen	976.3	E858.7	E946.3	E950.4	E962.0	E980.4
Oxtriphylline	976.7	E858.6	E945.7	E950.4	E962.0	E980.4
Oxybuprocaine	968.5	E855.2	E938.5	E950.4	E962.0	E980.4
Oxybutynin	975.1	E858.6	E945.1	E950.4	E962.0	E980.4
Oxycodone	965.09	E850.2	E935.2	E950.0	E962.0	E980.0
Oxygen	987.8	E869.8	—	E952.8	E962.2	E982.8
Oxylone	976.0	E858.7	E946.0	E950.4	E962.0	E980.4
ophthalmic preparation	976.5	E858.7	E946.5	E950.4	E962.0	E980.4
Oxymesterone	962.1	E858.0	E932.1	E950.4	E962.0	E980.4
Oxymetazoline	971.2	E855.5	E941.2	E950.4	E962.0	E980.4
Oxymetholone	962.1	E858.0	E932.1	E950.4	E962.0	E980.4
Oxymorphone	965.09	E850.2	E935.2	E950.0	E962.0	E980.0
Oxypertine	969.09	E854.0	E939.0	E950.3	E962.0	E980.3
Oxyphenbutazone	965.5	E850.5	E935.5	E950.0	E962.0	E980.0
Oxyphencyclimine	971.1	E855.4	E941.1	E950.4	E962.0	E980.4
Oxyphenisatin	973.1	E858.4	E943.1	E950.4	E962.0	E980.4
Oxyphenonium	971.1	E855.4	E941.1	E950.4	E962.0	E980.4
Oxyquinoline	961.3	E857	E931.3	E950.4	E962.0	E980.4
Oxytetracycline	960.4	E856	E930.4	E950.4	E962.0	E980.4
Oxytocics	975.0	E858.6	E945.0	E950.4	E962.0	E980.4
Oxytocin	975.0	E858.6	E945.0	E950.4	E962.0	E980.4
Ozone	987.8	E869.8	—	E952.8	E962.2	E982.8
PABA	976.3	E858.7	E946.3	E950.4	E962.0	E980.4

TABLE OF DRUGS AND CHEMICALS / Packed red cells

Substance	Poisoning	External Cause (E Code) Accident	Therapeutic Use	Suicide Attempt	Assault	Undetermined
Packed red cells	964.7	E858.2	E934.7	E950.4	E962.0	E980.4
Paint NEC	989.89	E861.6	—	E950.9	E962.1	E980.9
cleaner	982.8	E862.9	—	E950.9	E962.1	E980.9
fumes NEC	987.8	E869.8	—	E952.8	E962.1	E982.8
lead (fumes)	984.0	E861.5	—	E950.9	E962.1	E980.9
solvent NEC	982.8	E862.9	—	E950.9	E962.1	E980.9
stripper	982.8	E862.9	—	E950.9	E962.1	E980.9
Palfium	965.09	E850.2	E935.2	E950.0	E962.0	E980.0
Palivizumab	979.9	E858.8	E949.6	E950.4	E962.0	E980.4
Paludrine	961.4	E857	E931.4	E950.4	E962.0	E980.4
PAM	977.2	E855.8	E947.2	E950.4	E962.0	E980.4
Pamaquine (napthoate)	961.4	E857	E931.4	E950.4	E962.0	E980.4
Pamprin	965.1	E850.3	E935.3	E950.0	E962.0	E980.0
Panadol	965.4	E850.4	E935.4	E950.0	E962.0	E980.0
Pancreatic dornase (mucolytic)	963.4	E858.1	E933.4	E950.4	E962.0	E980.4
Pancreatin	973.4	E858.4	E943.4	E950.4	E962.0	E980.4
Pancrelipase	973.4	E858.4	E943.4	E950.4	E962.0	E980.4
Pangamic acid	963.5	E858.1	E933.5	E950.4	E962.0	E980.4
Panthenol	963.5	E858.1	E933.5	E950.4	E962.0	E980.4
topical	976.8	E858.7	E946.8	E950.4	E962.0	E980.4
Pantopaque	977.8	E858.8	E947.8	E950.4	E962.0	E980.4
Pantopon	965.00	E850.2	E935.2	E950.0	E962.0	E980.0
Pantothenic acid	963.5	E858.1	E933.5	E950.4	E962.0	E980.4
Panwarfin	964.2	E858.2	E934.2	E950.4	E962.0	E980.4
Papain	973.4	E858.4	E943.4	E950.4	E962.0	E980.4
Papaverine	972.5	E858.3	E942.5	E950.4	E962.0	E980.4
Para-aminobenzoic acid	976.3	E858.7	E946.3	E950.4	E962.0	E980.4
Para-aminophenol derivatives	965.4	E850.4	E935.4	E950.0	E962.0	E980.0
Para-aminosalicylic acid (derivatives)	961.8	E857	E931.8	E950.4	E962.0	E980.4
Paracetaldehyde (medicinal)	967.2	E852.1	E937.2	E950.2	E962.0	E980.2
Paracetamol	965.4	E850.4	E935.4	E950.0	E962.0	E980.0
Paracodin	965.09	E850.2	E935.2	E950.0	E962.0	E980.0
Paradione	966.0	E855.0	E936.0	E950.4	E962.0	E980.4
Paraffin(s) (wax)	981	E862.3	—	E950.9	E962.1	E980.9
liquid (medicinal)	973.2	E858.4	E943.2	E950.4	E962.0	E980.4
nonmedicinal (oil)	981	E962.1	—	E950.9	E962.1	E980.9
Paraldehyde (medicinal)	967.2	E852.1	E937.2	E950.2	E962.0	E980.2
Paramethadione	966.0	E855.0	E936.0	E950.4	E962.0	E980.4
Paramethasone	962.0	E858.0	E932.0	E950.4	E962.0	E980.4

TABLE OF DRUGS AND CHEMICALS / Pentachlorophenol

Substance	Poisoning	External Cause (E Code)				
		Accident	Therapeutic Use	Suicide Attempt	Assault	Undetermined
Paraquat	989.4	E863.5	—	E950.6	E962.1	E980.7
Parasympatholytics	971.1	E855.4	E941.1	E950.4	E962.0	E980.4
Parasympathomimetics	971.0	E855.3	E941.0	E950.4	E962.0	E980.4
Parathion	989.3	E863.1	—	E950.6	E962.1	E980.7
Parathormone	962.6	E858.0	E932.6	E950.4	E962.0	E980.4
Parathyroid (derivatives)	962.6	E858.0	E932.6	E950.4	E962.0	E980.4
Paratyphoid vaccine	978.1	E858.8	E948.1	E950.4	E962.0	E980.4
Paredrine	971.2	E855.5	E941.2	E950.4	E962.0	E980.4
Paregoric	965.00	E850.2	E935.2	E950.0	E962.0	E980.0
Pargyline	972.3	E858.3	E942.3	E950.4	E962.0	E980.4
Paris green	985.1	E866.3	—	E950.8	E962.1	E980.8
insecticide	985.1	E863.4	—	E950.8	E962.1	E980.8
Parnate	969.01	E854.0	E939.0	E950.3	E962.0	E980.3
Paromomycin	960.8	E856	E930.8	E950.4	E962.0	E980.4
Paroxypropione	963.1	E858.1	E933.1	E950.4	E962.0	E980.4
Parzone	965.09	E850.2	E935.2	E950.0	E962.0	E980.0
PAS	961.8	E857	E931.8	E950.4	E962.0	E980.4
PCBs	981	E862.3	—	E950.9	E962.1	E980.9
PCP (pentachlorophenol)	989.4	E863.6	—	E950.6	E962.1	E980.7
herbicide	989.4	E863.5	—	E950.6	E962.1	E980.7
insecticide	989.4	E863.4	—	E950.6	E962.1	E980.7
phencyclidine	968.3	E855.1	E938.3	E950.4	E962.0	E980.4
Peach kernel oil (emulsion)	973.2	E858.4	E943.2	E950.4	E962.0	E980.4
Peanut oil (emulsion) NEC	973.2	E858.4	E943.2	E950.4	E962.0	E980.4
topical	976.3	E858.7	E946.3	E950.4	E962.0	E980.4
Pearly Gates (morning glory seeds)	969.6	E854.1	E939.6	E950.3	E962.0	E980.3
Pecazine	969.1	E853.0	E939.1	E950.3	E962.0	E980.3
Pecilocin	960.1	E856	E930.1	E950.4	E962.0	E980.4
Pectin (with kaolin) NEC	973.5	E858.4	E943.5	E950.4	E962.0	E980.4
Pelletierine tannate	961.6	E857	E931.6	E950.4	E962.0	E980.4
Pemoline	969.79	E854.2	E939.7	E950.3	E962.0	E980.3
Pempidine	972.3	E858.3	E942.3	E950.4	E962.0	E980.4
Penamecillin	960.0	E856	E930.0	E950.4	E962.0	E980.4
Penethamate hydriodide	960.0	E856	E930.0	E950.4	E962.0	E980.4
Penicillamine	963.8	E858.1	E933.8	E950.4	E962.0	E980.4
Penicillin (any type)	960.0	E856	E930.0	E950.4	E962.0	E980.4
Penicillinase	963.4	E858.1	E933.4	E950.4	E962.0	E980.4
Pentachlorophenol (fungicide)	989.4	E863.6	—	E950.6	E962.1	E980.7
herbicide	989.4	E863.5	—	E950.6	E962.1	E980.7
insecticide	989.4	E863.4	—	E950.6	E962.1	E980.7

TABLE OF DRUGS AND CHEMICALS / Pentaerythritol

Substance	Poisoning	External Cause (E Code)				
		Accident	Therapeutic Use	Suicide Attempt	Assault	Undetermined
Pentaerythritol	972.4	E858.3	E942.4	E950.4	E962.0	E980.4
chloral	967.1	E852.0	E937.1	E950.2	E962.0	E980.2
tetranitrate NEC	972.4	E858.3	E942.4	E950.4	E962.0	E980.4
Pentagastrin	977.8	E858.8	E947.8	E950.4	E962.0	E980.4
Pentalin	982.3	E862.4	—	E950.9	E962.1	E980.9
Pentamethonium (bromide)	972.3	E858.3	E942.3	E950.4	E962.0	E980.4
Pentamidine	961.5	E857	E931.5	E950.4	E962.0	E980.4
Pentanol	980.8	E860.8	—	E950.9	E962.1	E980.9
Pentaquine	961.4	E857	E931.4	E950.4	E962.0	E980.4
Pentazocine	965.8	E850.8	E935.8	E950.0	E962.0	E980.0
Penthienate	971.1	E855.4	E941.1	E950.4	E962.0	E980.4
Pentobarbital, pentobarbitone (sodium)	967.0	E851	E937.0	E950.1	E962.0	E980.1
Pentolinium (tartrate)	972.3	E858.3	E942.3	E950.4	E962.0	E980.4
Pentothal	968.3	E855.1	E938.3	E950.4	E962.0	E980.4
Pentylenetetrazol	970.0	E854.3	E940.0	E950.4	E962.0	E980.4
Pentylsalicylamide	961.8	E857	E931.8	E950.4	E962.0	E980.4
Pepsin	973.4	E858.4	E943.4	E950.4	E962.0	E980.4
Peptavlon	977.8	E858.8	E947.8	E950.4	E962.0	E980.4
Percaine (spinal)	968.7	E855.2	E938.7	E950.4	E962.0	E980.4
topical (surface)	968.5	E855.2	E938.5	E950.4	E962.0	E980.4
Perchloroethylene (vapor)	982.3	E862.4	—	E950.9	E962.1	E980.9
medicinal	961.6	E857	E931.6	E950.4	E962.0	E980.4
Percodan	965.09	E850.2	E935.2	E950.0	E962.0	E980.0
Percogesic	965.09	E850.2	E935.2	E950.0	E962.0	E980.0
Percorten	962.0	E858.0	E932.0	E950.4	E962.0	E980.4
Pergonal	962.4	E858.0	E932.4	E950.4	E962.0	E980.4
Perhexiline	972.4	E858.3	E942.4	E950.4	E962.0	E980.4
Periactin	963.0	E858.1	E933.0	E950.4	E962.0	E980.4
Periclor	967.1	E852.0	E937.1	E950.2	E962.0	E980.2
Pericyazine	969.1	E853.0	E939.1	E950.3	E962.0	E980.3
Peritrate	972.4	E858.3	E942.4	E950.4	E962.0	E980.4
Permanganates NEC	983.9	E864.3	—	E950.7	E962.1	E980.6
potassium (topical)	976.0	E858.7	E946.0	E950.4	E962.0	E980.4
Pernocton	967.0	E851	E937.0	E950.1	E962.0	E980.1
Pernoston	967.0	E851	E937.0	E950.1	E962.0	E980.1
Peronin(e)	965.09	E850.2	E935.2	E950.0	E962.0	E980.0
Perphenazine	969.1	E853.0	E939.1	E950.3	E962.0	E980.3
Pertofrane	969.05	E854	E939.0	E950.3	E962.0	E980.3

TABLE OF DRUGS AND CHEMICALS / Pharmaceutical excipient or adjunct

Substance	Poisoning	External Cause (E Code)				
		Accident	Therapeutic Use	Suicide Attempt	Assault	Undetermined
Pertussis	—	—	—	—	—	—
immune serum (human)	964.6	E858.2	E934.6	E950.4	E962.0	E980.4
vaccine (with diphtheria toxoid) (with tetanus toxoid)	978.6	E858.8	E948.6	E950.4	E962.0	E980.4
Peruvian balsam	976.8	E858.7	E946.8	E950.4	E962.0	E980.4
Pesticides (dust) (fumes) (vapor)	989.4	E863.4	—	E950.6	E962.1	E980.7
arsenic	985.1	E863.4	—	E950.8	E962.1	E980.8
chlorinated	989.2	E863.0	—	E950.6	E962.1	E980.7
cyanide	989.0	E863.4	—	E950.6	E962.1	E980.7
kerosene	981	E863.4	—	E950.6	E962.1	E980.7
mixture (of compounds)	989.4	E863.3	—	E950.6	E962.1	E980.7
naphthalene	983.0	E863.4	—	E950.7	E962.1	E980.6
organochlorine (compounds)	989.2	E863.0	—	E950.6	E962.1	E980.7
petroleum (distillate) (products) NEC	981	E863.4	—	E950.6	E962.1	E980.7
specified ingredient NEC	989.4	E863.4	—	E950.6	E962.1	E980.7
strychnine	989.1	E863.4	—	E950.6	E962.1	E980.7
thallium	985.8	E863.7	—	E950.6	E962.1	E980.7
Pethidine (hydrochloride)	965.09	E850.2	E935.2	E950.0	E962.0	E980.0
Petrichloral	967.1	E852.0	E937.1	E950.2	E962.0	E980.2
Petrol	981	E862.1	—	E950.9	E962.1	E980.9
vapor	987.1	E869.8	—	E952.8	E962.2	E982.8
Petrolatum (jelly) (ointment)	976.3	E858.7	E946.3	E950.4	E962.0	E980.4
hydrophilic	976.3	E858.7	E946.3	E950.4	E962.0	E980.4
liquid	973.2	E858.4	E943.2	E950.4	E962.0	E980.4
topical	976.3	E858.7	E946.3	E950.4	E962.0	E980.4
nonmedicinal	981	E862.1	—	E950.9	E962.1	E980.9
Petroleum (cleaners) (fuels) (products) NEC	981	E862.1	—	E950.9	E962.1	E980.9
benzin(e) - see Ligroin	—	—	—	—	—	—
ether - see Ligroin	—	—	—	—	—	—
jelly - see Petrolatum	—	—	—	—	—	—
aphtha - see Ligroin	—	—	—	—	—	—
pesticide	981	E863.4	—	E950.6	E962.1	E980.7
solids	981	E862.3	—	E950.9	E962.1	E980.9
solvents	981	E862.0	—	E950.9	E962.1	E980.9
vapor	987.1	E869.8	—	E952.8	E962.2	E982.8
Peyote	969.6	E854.1	E939.6	E950.3	E962.0	E980.3
Phanodorm, phanodorn	967.0	E851	E937.0	E950.1	E962.0	E980.1
Phanquinone, phanquone	961.5	E857	E931.5	E950.4	E962.0	E980.4
Pharmaceutical excipient or adjunct	977.4	E858.8	E947.4	E950.4	E962.0	E980.4

TABLE OF DRUGS AND CHEMICALS / Phenacemide

		External Cause (E Code)				
Substance	Poisoning	Accident	Therapeutic Use	Suicide Attempt	Assault	Undetermined
Phenacemide	966.3	E855.0	E936.3	E950.4	E962.0	E980.4
Phenacetin	965.4	E850.4	E935.4	E950.0	E962.0	E980.0
Phenadoxone	965.09	E850.2	E935.2	E950.0	E962.0	E980.0
Phenaglycodol	969.5	E853.8	E939.5	E950.3	E962.0	E980.3
Phenantoin	966.1	E855.0	E936.1	E950.4	E962.0	E980.4
Phenaphthazine reagent	977.8	E858.8	E947.8	E950.4	E962.0	E980.4
Phenazocine	965.09	E850.2	E935.2	E950.0	E962.0	E980.0
Phenazone	965.5	E850.5	E935.5	E950.0	E962.0	E980.0
Phenazopyridine	976.1	E858.7	E946.1	E950.4	E962.0	E980.4
Phenbenicillin	960.0	E856	E930.0	E950.4	E962.0	E980.4
Phenbutrazate	977.0	E858.8	E947.0	E950.4	E962.0	E980.4
Phencyclidine	968.3	E855.1	E938.3	E950.4	E962.0	E980.4
Phendimetrazine	977.0	E858.8	E947.0	E950.4	E962.0	E980.4
Phenelzine	969.01	E854.0	E939.0	E950.3	E962.0	E980.3
Phenergan	967.8	E852.8	E937.8	E950.2	E962.0	E980.2
Phenethicillin (potassium)	960.0	E856	E930.0	E950.4	E962.0	E980.4
Phenetsal	965.1	E850.3	E935.3	E950.0	E962.0	E980.0
Pheneturide	966.3	E855.0	E936.3	E950.4	E962.0	E980.4
Phenformin	962.3	E858.0	E932.3	E950.4	E962.0	E980.4
Phenglutarimide	971.1	E855.4	E941.1	E950.4	E962.0	E980.4
Phenicarbazide	965.8	E850.8	E935.8	E950.0	E962.0	E980.0
Phenindamine (tartrate)	963.0	E858.1	E933.0	E950.4	E962.0	E980.4
Phenindione	964.2	E858.2	E934.2	E950.4	E962.0	E980.4
Pheniprazine	969.01	E854.0	E939.0	E950.3	E962.0	E980.3
Pheniramine (maleate)	963.0	E858.1	E933.0	E950.4	E962.0	E980.4
Phenmetrazine	977.0	E858.8	E947.0	E950.4	E962.0	E980.4
Phenobal	967.0	E851	E937.0	E950.1	E962.0	E980.1
Phenobarbital	967.0	E851	E937.0	E950.1	E962.0	E980.1
Phenobarbitone	967.0	E851	E937.0	E950.1	E962.0	E980.1
Phenoctide	976.0	E858.7	E946.0	E950.4	E962.0	E980.4
Phenol (derivatives) NEC	983.0	E864.0	—	E950.7	E962.1	E980.6
disinfectant	983.0	E864.0	—	E950.7	E962.1	E980.6
pesticide	989.4	E863.4	—	E950.6	E962.1	E980.7
red	977.8	E858.8	E947.8	E950.4	E962.0	E980.4
Phenolphthalein	973.1	E858.4	E943.1	E950.4	E962.0	E980.4
Phenolsulfonphthalein	977.8	E858.8	E947.8	E950.4	E962.0	E980.4
Phenomorphan	965.09	E850.2	E935.2	E950.0	E962.0	E980.0
Phenonyl	967.0	E851	E937.0	E950.1	E962.0	E980.1

TABLE OF DRUGS AND CHEMICALS / Phylloquinone

Substance	Poisoning	External Cause (E Code)				
		Accident	Therapeutic Use	Suicide Attempt	Assault	Undetermined
Phenoperidine	965.09	E850.2	E935.2	E950.0	E962.0	E980.0
Phenoquin	974.7	E858.5	E944.7	E950.4	E962.0	E980.4
Phenothiazines (tranquilizers) NEC	969.1	E853.0	E939.1	E950.3	E962.0	E980.3
insecticide	989.3	E863.4	—	E950.6	E962.1	E980.7
Phenoxybenzamine	971.3	E855.6	E941.3	E950.4	E962.0	E980.4
Phenoxymethyl penicillin	960.0	E856	E930.0	E950.4	E962.0	E980.4
Phenprocoumon	964.2	E858.2	E934.2	E950.4	E962.0	E980.4
Phensuximide	966.2	E855.0	E936.2	E950.4	E962.0	E980.4
Phentermine	977.0	E858.8	E947.0	E950.4	E962.0	E980.4
Phentolamine	971.3	E855.6	E941.3	E950.4	E962.0	E980.4
Phenyl	—	—	—	—	—	—
butazone	965.5	E850.5	E935.5	E950.0	E962.0	E980.0
enediamine	983.0	E864.0	—	E950.7	E962.1	E980.6
hydrazine	983.0	E864.0	—	E950.7	E962.1	E980.6
antineoplastic	963.1	E858.1	E933.1	E950.4	E962.0	E980.4
mercuric compounds - *see* Mercury	—	—	—	—	—	—
salicylate	976.3	E858.7	E946.3	E950.4	E962.0	E980.4
Phenylephrine	971.2	E855.5	E941.2	E950.4	E962.0	E980.4
Phenylethylbiguanide	962.3	E858.0	E932.3	E950.4	E962.0	E980.4
Phenylpropanolamine	971.2	E855.5	E941.2	E950.4	E962.0	E980.4
Phenylsulfthion	989.3	E863.1	—	E950.6	E962.1	E980.7
Phenyramidol, phenyramidon	965.7	E850.7	E935.7	E950.0	E962.0	E980.0
Phenytoin	966.1	E855.0	E936.1	E950.4	E962.0	E980.4
pHisoHex	976.2	E858.7	E946.2	E950.4	E962.0	E980.4
Pholcodine	965.09	E850.2	E935.2	E950.0	E962.0	E980.0
Phorate	989.3	E863.1	—	E950.6	E962.1	E980.7
Phosdrin	989.3	E863.1	—	E950.6	E962.1	E980.7
Phosgene (gas)	987.8	E869.8	—	E952.8	E962.2	E982.8
Phosphate (tricresyl)	989.89	E866.8	—	E950.9	E962.1	E980.9
organic	989.3	E863.1	—	E950.6	E962.1	E980.7
solvent	982.8	E862.4	—	E950.9	E962.1	E980.9
Phosphine	987.8	E869.8	—	E952.8	E962.2	E982.8
fumigant	987.8	E863.8	—	E950.6	E962.2	E980.7
Phospholine	971.0	E855.3	E941.0	E950.4	E962.0	E980.4
Phosphoric acid	983.1	E864.1	—	E950.7	E962.1	E980.6
Phosphorus (compounds) NEC	983.9	E864.3	—	E950.7	E962.1	E980.6
rodenticide	983.9	E863.7	—	E950.7	E962.1	E980.6
Phthalimidoglutarimide	967.8	E852.8	E937.8	E950.2	E962.0	E980.2
Phthalylsulfathiazole	961.0	E857	E931.0	E950.4	E962.0	E980.4
Phylloquinone	964.3	E858.2	E934.3	E950.4	E962.0	E980.4

◀ New   ◀ Revised   ~~deleted~~ Deleted   ● Use Additional Digit(s)

TABLE OF DRUGS AND CHEMICALS / Physeptone

Substance	Poisoning	External Cause (E Code) Accident	Therapeutic Use	Suicide Attempt	Assault	Undetermined
Physeptone	965.02	E850.1	E935.1	E950.0	E962.0	E980.0
Physostigma venenosum	988.2	E865.4	—	E950.9	E962.1	E980.9
Physostigmine	971.0	E855.3	E941.0	E950.4	E962.0	E980.4
Phytolacca decandra	988.2	E865.4	—	E950.9	E962.1	E980.9
Phytomenadione	964.3	E858.2	E934.3	E950.4	E962.0	E980.4
Phytonadione	964.3	E858.2	E934.3	E950.4	E962.0	E980.4
Picric (acid)	983.0	E864.0	—	E950.7	E962.1	E980.6
Picrotoxin	970.0	E854.3	E940.0	E950.4	E962.0	E980.4
Pilocarpine	971.0	E855.3	E941.0	E950.4	E962.0	E980.4
Pilocarpus (jaborandi) extract	971.0	E855.3	E941.0	E950.4	E962.0	E980.4
Pimaricin	960.1	E856	E930.1	E950.4	E962.0	E980.4
Piminodine	965.09	E850.2	E935.2	E950.0	E962.0	E980.0
Pine oil, pinesol (disinfectant)	983.9	E861.4	—	E950.7	E962.1	E980.6
Pinkroot	961.6	E857	E931.6	E950.4	E962.0	E980.4
Pipadone	965.09	E850.2	E935.2	E950.0	E962.0	E980.0
Pipamazine	963.0	E858.1	E933.0	E950.4	E962.0	E980.4
Pipazethate	975.4	E858.6	E945.4	E950.4	E962.0	E980.4
Pipenzolate	971.1	E855.4	E941.1	E950.4	E962.0	E980.4
Piperacetazine	969.1	E853.0	E939.1	E950.3	E962.0	E980.3
Piperazine NEC	961.6	E857	E931.6	E950.4	E962.0	E980.4
estrone sulfate	962.2	E858.0	E932.2	E950.4	E962.0	E980.4
Piper cubeba	988.2	E865.4	—	E950.9	E962.1	E980.9
Piperidione	975.4	E858.6	E945.4	E950.4	E962.0	E980.4
Piperidolate	971.1	E855.4	E941.1	E950.4	E962.0	E980.4
Piperocaine	968.9	E855.2	E938.9	E950.4	E962.0	E980.4
infiltration (subcutaneous)	968.5	E855.2	E938.5	E950.4	E962.0	E980.4
nerve block (peripheral) (plexus)	968.6	E855.2	E938.6	E950.4	E962.0	E980.4
topical (surface)	968.5	E855.2	E938.5	E950.4	E962.0	E980.4
Pipobroman	963.1	E858.1	E933.1	E950.4	E962.0	E980.4
Pipradrol	970.89	E854.3	E940.8	E950.4	E962.0	E980.4
Piscidia (bark) (erythrina)	965.7	E850.7	E935.7	E950.0	E962.0	E980.0
Pitch	983.0	E864.0	—	E950.7	E962.1	E980.6
Pitkin's solution	968.7	E855.2	E938.7	E950.4	E962.0	E980.4
Pitocin	975.0	E858.6	E945.0	E950.4	E962.0	E980.4
Pitressin (tannate)	962.5	E858.0	E932.5	E950.4	E962.0	E980.4
Pituitary extracts (posterior)	962.5	E858.0	E932.5	E950.4	E962.0	E980.4
anterior	962.4	E858.0	E932.4	E950.4	E962.0	E980.4
Pituitrin	962.5	E858.0	E932.5	E950.4	E962.0	E980.4
Placental extract	962.9	E858.0	E932.9	E950.4	E962.0	E980.4
Placidyl	967.8	E852.8	E937.8	E950.2	E962.0	E980.2

TABLE OF DRUGS AND CHEMICALS / Polythiazide

Substance	Poisoning	External Cause (E Code)				
		Accident	Therapeutic Use	Suicide Attempt	Assault	Undetermined
Plague vaccine	978.3	E858.8	E948.3	E950.4	E962.0	E980.4
Plant foods or fertilizers NEC	989.89	E866.5	—	E950.9	E962.1	E980.9
mixed with herbicides	989.4	E863.5	—	E950.6	E962.1	E930.7
Plants, noxious, used as food	988.2	E865.9	—	E950.9	E962.1	E980.9
berries and seeds	988.2	E865.3	—	E950.9	E962.1	E980.9
specified type NEC	988.2	E865.4	—	E950.9	E962.1	E980.9
Plasma (blood)	964.7	E858.2	E934.7	E950.4	E962.0	E980.4
expanders	964.8	E858.2	E934.8	E950.4	E962.0	E980.4
Plasmanate	964.7	E858.2	E934.7	E950.4	E962.0	E980.4
Plegicil	969.1	E853.0	E939.1	E950.3	E962.0	E980.3
Podophyllin	976.4	E858.7	E946.4	E950.4	E962.0	E980.4
Podophyllum resin	976.4	E858.7	E946.4	E950.4	E962.0	E980.4
Poison NEC	989.9	E866.9	—	E950.9	E962.1	E980.9
Poisonous berries	988.2	E865.3	—	E950.9	E962.1	E980.9
Pokeweed (any part)	988.2	E865.4	—	E950.9	E962.1	E980.9
Poldine	971.1	E855.4	E941.1	E950.4	E962.0	E980.4
Poliomyelitis vaccine	979.5	E858.8	E949.5	E950.4	E962.0	E980.4
Poliovirus vaccine	979.5	E858.8	E949.5	E950.4	E962.0	E980.4
Polish (car) (floor) (furniture) (metal) (silver)	989.89	E861.2	—	E950.9	E962.1	E980.9
abrasive	989.89	E861.3	—	E950.9	E962.1	E980.9
porcelain	989.89	E861.3	—	E950.9	E962.1	E980.9
Poloxalkol	973.2	E858.4	E943.2	E950.4	E962.0	E980.4
Polyaminostyrene resins	974.5	E858.5	E944.5	E950.4	E962.0	E980.4
Polychlorinated biphenyl - *see* PCBs	—	—	—	—	—	—
Polycycline	960.4	E856	E930.4	E950.4	E962.0	E980.4
Polyester resin hardener	982.8	E862.4	—	E950.9	E962.1	E980.9
fumes	987.8	E869.8	—	E952.8	E962.2	E982.8
Polyestradiol (phosphate)	962.2	E858.0	E932.2	E950.4	E962.0	E980.4
Polyethanolamine alkyl sulfate	976.2	E858.7	E946.2	E950.4	E962.0	E980.4
Polyethylene glycol	976.3	E858.7	E946.3	E950.4	E962.0	E980.4
Polyferose	964.0	E858.2	E934.0	E950.4	E962.0	E980.4
Polymyxin B	960.8	E856	E930.8	E950.4	E962.0	E980.4
ENT agent	976.6	E858.7	E946.6	E950.4	E962.0	E980.4
ophthalmic preparation	976.5	E858.7	E946.5	E950.4	E962.0	E980.4
topical NEC	976.0	E858.7	E946.0	E950.4	E962.0	E980.4
Polynoxylin(e)	976.0	E858.7	E946.0	E950.4	E962.0	E980.4
Polyoxymethyleneurea	976.0	E858.7	E946.0	E950.4	E962.0	E980.4
Polytetrafluoroethylene (inhaled)	987.8	E869.8	—	E952.8	E962.2	E982.8
Polythiazide	974.3	E858.5	E944.3	E950.4	E962.0	E980.4

◀ New   Revised   deleted Deleted   ● Use Additional Digit(s)

TABLE OF DRUGS AND CHEMICALS / Polyvinylpyrrolidone

		External Cause (E Code)				
Substance	Poisoning	Accident	Therapeutic Use	Suicide Attempt	Assault	Undetermined
Polyvinylpyrrolidone	964.8	E858.2	E934.8	E950.4	E962.0	E980.4
Pontocaine (hydrochloride) (infiltration) (topical)	968.5	E855.2	E938.5	E950.4	E962.0	E980.4
nerve block (peripheral) (plexus)	968.6	E855.2	E938.6	E950.4	E962.0	E980.4
spinal	968.7	E855.2	E938.7	E950.4	E962.0	E980.4
Pot	969.6	E854.1	E939.6	E950.3	E962.0	E980.3
Potash (caustic)	983.2	E864.2	—	E950.7	E962.1	E980.6
Potassic saline injection (lactated)	974.5	E858.5	E944.5	E950.4	E962.0	E980.4
Potassium (salts) NEC	974.5	E858.5	E944.5	E950.4	E962.0	E980.4
aminosalicylate	961.8	E857	E931.8	E950.4	E962.0	E980.4
arsenite (solution)	985.1	E866.3	—	E950.8	E962.1	E980.8
bichromate	983.9	E864.3	—	E950.7	E962.1	E980.6
bisulfate	983.9	E864.3	—	E950.7	E962.1	E980.6
bromide (medicinal) NEC	967.3	E852.2	E937.3	E950.2	E962.0	E980.2
carbonate	983.2	E864.2	—	E950.7	E962.1	E980.6
chlorate NEC	983.9	E864.3	—	E950.7	E962.1	E980.6
cyanide - see Cyanide	—	—	—	—	—	—
hydroxide	983.2	E864.2	—	E950.7	E962.1	E980.6
iodide (expectorant) NEC	975.5	E858.6	E945.5	E950.4	E962.0	E980.4
nitrate	989.89	E866.8	—	E950.9	E962.1	E980.9
oxalate	983.9	E864.3	—	E950.7	E962.1	E980.6
perchlorate NEC	977.8	E858.8	E947.8	E950.4	E962.0	E980.4
antithyroid	962.8	E858.0	E932.8	E950.4	E962.0	E980.4
permanganate	976.0	E858.7	E946.0	E950.4	E962.0	E980.4
nonmedicinal	983.9	E864.3	—	E950.7	E962.1	E980.6
Povidone-iodine (anti-infective) NEC	976.0	E858.7	E946.0	E950.4	E962.0	E980.4
Practolol	972.0	E858.3	E942.0	E950.4	E962.0	E980.4
Pralidoxime (chloride)	977.2	E858.8	E947.2	E950.4	E962.0	E980.4
Pramoxine	968.5	E855.2	E938.5	E950.4	E962.0	E980.4
Prazosin	972.6	E858.3	E942.6	E950.4	E962.0	E980.4
Prednisolone	962.0	E858.0	E932.0	E950.4	E962.0	E980.4
ENT agent	976.6	E858.7	E946.6	E950.4	E962.0	E980.4
ophthalmic preparation	976.5	E858.7	E946.5	E950.4	E962.0	E980.4
topical NEC	976.0	E858.7	E946.0	E950.4	E962.0	E980.4
Prednisone	962.0	E858.0	E932.0	E950.4	E962.0	E980.4
Pregnanediol	962.2	E858.0	E932.2	E950.4	E962.0	E980.4
Pregneninolone	962.2	E858.0	E932.2	E950.4	E962.0	E980.4
Preludin	977.0	E858.8	E947.0	E950.4	E962.0	E980.4
Premarin	962.2	E858.0	E932.2	E950.4	E962.0	E980.4
Prenylamine	972.4	E858.3	E942.4	E950.4	E962.0	E980.4

TABLE OF DRUGS AND CHEMICALS / Promedrol

Substance	Poisoning	Accident	Therapeutic Use	Suicide Attempt	Assault	Undetermined
Preparation H	976.8	E858.7	E946.8	E950.4	E962.0	E980.4
Preservatives	989.89	E866.8	—	E950.9	E962.1	E980.9
Pride of China	988.2	E865.3	—	E950.9	E962.1	E980.9
Prilocaine	968.9	E855.2	E938.9	E950.4	E962.0	E980.4
infiltration (subcutaneous)	968.5	E855.2	E938.5	E950.4	E962.0	E980.4
nerve block (peripheral) (plexus)	968.6	E855.2	E938.6	E950.4	E962.0	E980.4
Primaquine	961.4	E857	E931.4	E950.4	E962.0	E980.4
Primidone	966.3	E855.0	E936.3	E950.4	E962.0	E980.4
Primula (veris)	988.2	E865.4	—	E950.9	E962.1	E980.9
Prinodol	965.09	E850.2	E935.2	E950.0	E962.0	E980.0
Priscol, Priscoline	971.3	E855.6	E941.3	E950.4	E962.0	E980.4
Privet	988.2	E865.4	—	E950.9	E962.1	E980.9
Privine	971.2	E855.5	E941.2	E950.4	E962.0	E980.4
Pro-Banthine	971.1	E855.4	E941.1	E950.4	E962.0	E980.4
Probarbital	967.0	E851	E937.0	E950.1	E962.0	E980.1
Probenecid	974.7	E858.5	E944.7	E950.4	E962.0	E980.4
Procainamide (hydrochloride)	972.0	E858.3	E942.0	E950.4	E962.0	E980.4
Procaine (hydrochloride) (infiltration) (topical)	968.5	E855.2	E938.5	E950.4	E962.0	E980.4
nerve block (peripheral) (plexus)	968.6	E855.2	E938.6	E950.4	E962.0	E980.4
penicillin G	960.0	E856	E930.0	E950.4	E962.0	E980.4
spinal	968.7	E855.2	E938.7	E950.4	E962.0	E980.4
Procalmidol	969.5	E853.8	E939.5	E950.3	E962.0	E980.3
Procarbazine	963.1	E858.1	E933.1	E950.4	E962.0	E980.4
Prochlorperazine	969.1	E853.0	E939.1	E950.3	E962.0	E980.3
Procyclidine	966.4	E855.0	E936.4	E950.4	E962.0	E980.4
Producer gas	986	E868.8	—	E952.1	E962.2	E982.1
Profenamine	966.4	E855.0	E936.4	E950.4	E962.0	E980.4
Profenil	975.1	E858.6	E945.1	E950.4	E962.0	E980.4
Progesterones	962.2	E858.0	E932.2	E950.4	E962.0	E980.4
Progestin	962.2	E858.0	E932.2	E950.4	E962.0	E980.4
Progestogens (with estrogens)	962.2	E858.0	E932.2	E950.4	E962.0	E980.4
Progestone	962.2	E858.0	E932.2	E950.4	E962.0	E980.4
Proguanil	961.4	E857	E931.4	E950.4	E962.0	E980.4
Prolactin	962.4	E858.0	E932.4	E950.4	E962.0	E980.4
Proloid	962.7	E858.0	E932.7	E950.4	E962.0	E980.4
Proluton	962.2	E858.0	E932.2	E950.4	E962.0	E980.4
Promacetin	961.8	E857	E931.8	E950.4	E962.0	E980.4
Promazine	969.1	E853.0	E939.1	E950.3	E962.0	E980.3
Promedrol	965.09	E850.2	E935.2	E950.0	E962.0	E980.0

TABLE OF DRUGS AND CHEMICALS / Promethazine

Substance	Poisoning	External Cause (E Code) Accident	Therapeutic Use	Suicide Attempt	Assault	Undetermined
Promethazine	967.8	E852.8	E937.8	E950.2	E962.0	E980.2
Promine	961.8	E857	E931.8	E950.4	E962.0	E980.4
Pronestyl (hydrochloride)	972.0	E858.3	E942.0	E950.4	E962.0	E980.4
Pronetalol, pronethalol	972.0	E858.3	E942.0	E950.4	E962.0	E980.4
Prontosil	961.0	E857	E931.0	E950.4	E962.0	E980.4
Propamidine isethionate	961.5	E857	E931.5	E950.4	E962.0	E980.4
Propanal (medicinal)	967.8	E852.8	E937.8	E950.2	E962.0	E980.2
Propane (gas) (distributed in mobile container)	987.0	E868.0	—	E951.1	E962.2	E981.1
distributed through pipes	987.0	E867	—	E951.0	E962.2	E981.0
incomplete combustion of - see Carbon monoxide, Propane	—	—	—	—	—	—
Propanidid	968.3	E855.1	E938.3	E950.4	E962.0	E980.4
Propanol	980.3	E860.4	—	E950.9	E962.1	E980.9
Propantheline	971.1	E855.4	E941.1	E950.4	E962.0	E980.4
Proparacaine	968.5	E855.2	E938.5	E950.4	E962.0	E980.4
Propatyl nitrate	972.4	E858.3	E942.4	E950.4	E962.0	E980.4
Propicillin	960.0	E856	E930.0	E950.4	E962.0	E980.4
Propiolactone (vapor)	987.8	E869.8	—	E952.8	E962.2	E982.8
Propiomazine	967.8	E852.8	E937.8	E950.2	E962.0	E980.2
Propionaldehyde (medicinal)	967.8	E852.8	E937.8	E950.2	E962.0	E980.2
Propionate compound	976.0	E858.7	E946.0	E950.4	E962.0	E980.4
Propion gel	976.0	E858.7	E946.0	E950.4	E962.0	E980.4
Propitocaine	968.9	E855.2	E938.9	E950.4	E962.0	E980.4
infiltration (subcutaneous)	968.5	E855.2	E938.5	E950.4	E962.0	E980.4
nerve block (peripheral) (plexus)	968.6	E855.2	E938.6	E950.4	E962.0	E980.4
Propoxur	989.3	E863.2	—	E950.6	E962.1	E980.7
Propoxycaine	968.9	E855.2	E938.9	E950.4	E962.0	E980.4
infiltration (subcutaneous)	968.5	E855.2	E938.5	E950.4	E962.0	E980.4
nerve block (peripheral) (plexus)	968.6	E855.2	E938.6	E950.4	E962.0	E980.4
topical (surface)	968.5	E855.2	E938.5	E950.4	E962.0	E980.4
Propoxyphene (hydrochloride)	965.8	E850.8	E935.8	E950.0	E962.0	E980.0
Propranolol	972.0	E858.3	E942.0	E950.4	E962.0	E980.4
Propyl	—	—	—	—	—	—
alcohol	980.3	E860.4	—	E950.9	E962.1	E980.9
carbinol	980.3	E860.4	—	E950.9	E962.1	E980.9
hexadrine	971.2	E855.5	E941.2	E950.4	E962.0	E980.4
iodone	977.8	E858.8	E947.8	E950.4	E962.0	E980.4
thiouracil	962.8	E858.0	E932.8	E950.4	E962.0	E980.4
Propylene	987.1	E869.8	—	E952.8	E962.2	E982.8
Propylparaben (ophthalmic)	976.5	E858.7	E946.5	E950.4	E962.0	E980.4

TABLE OF DRUGS AND CHEMICALS / Psyllium

| Substance | Poisoning | External Cause (E Code) |||||
		Accident	Therapeutic Use	Suicide Attempt	Assault	Undetermined
Proscillaridin	972.1	E858.3	E942.1	E950.4	E962.0	E980.4
Prostaglandins	975.0	E858.6	E945.0	E950.4	E962.0	E980.4
Prostigmin	971.0	E855.3	E941.0	E950.4	E962.0	E980.4
Protamine (sulfate)	964.5	E858.2	E934.5	E950.4	E962.0	E980.4
zinc insulin	962.3	E858.0	E932.3	E950.4	E962.0	E980.4
Protectants (topical)	976.3	E858.7	E946.3	E950.4	E962.0	E980.4
Protein hydrolysate	974.5	E858.5	E944.5	E950.4	E962.0	E980.4
Prothiaden - see Dothiepin hydrochloride	—	—	—	—	—	—
Prothionamide	961.8	E857	E931.8	E950.4	E962.0	E980.4
Prothipendyl	969.5	E853.8	E939.5	E950.3	E962.0	E980.3
Protokylol	971.2	E855.5	E941.2	E950.4	E962.0	E980.4
Protopam	977.2	E858.8	E947.2	E950.4	E962.0	E980.4
Protoveratrine(s) (A) (B)	972.6	E858.3	E942.6	E950.4	E962.0	E980.4
Protriptyline	969.05	E854.0	E939.0	E950.3	E962.0	E980.3
Provera	962.2	E858.0	E932.2	E950.4	E962.0	E980.4
Provitamin A	963.5	E858.1	E933.5	E950.4	E962.0	E980.4
Proxymetacaine	968.5	E855.2	E938.5	E950.4	E962.0	E980.4
Proxyphylline	975.1	E858.6	E945.1	E950.4	E962.0	E980.4
Prozac - see Fluoxetine hydrochloride	—	—	—	—	—	—
Prunus	—	—	—	—	—	—
laurocerasus	988.2	E865.4	—	E950.9	E962.1	E980.9
virginiana	988.2	E865.4	—	E950.9	E962.1	E980.9
Prussic acid	989.0	E866.8	—	E950.9	E962.1	E980.9
vapor	987.7	E869.8	—	E952.8	E962.2	E982.8
Pseudoephedrine	971.2	E855.5	E941.2	E950.4	E962.0	E980.4
Psilocin	969.6	E854.1	E939.6	E950.3	E962.0	E980.3
Psilocybin	969.6	E854.1	E939.6	E950.3	E962.0	E980.3
PSP	977.8	E858.8	E947.8	E950.4	E962.0	E980.4
Psychedelic agents	969.6	E854.1	E939.6	E950.3	E962.0	E980.3
Psychodysleptics	969.6	E854.1	E939.6	E950.3	E962.0	E980.3
Psychostimulants	969.70	E854.2	E939.7	E950.3	E962.0	E980.3
Psychotherapeutic agents	969.9	E855.9	E939.9	E950.3	E962.0	E980.3
antidepressants	969.00	E854.0	E939.0	E950.3	E962.0	E980.3
specified NEC	969.8	E855.8	E939.8	E950.3	E962.0	E980.3
tranquilizers NEC	969.5	E853.9	E939.5	E950.3	E962.0	E980.3
Psychotomimetic agents	969.6	E854.1	E939.6	E950.3	E962.0	E980.3
Psychotropic agents	969.9	E854.8	E939.9	E950.3	E962.0	E980.3
specified NEC	969.8	E854.8	E939.8	E950.3	E962.0	E980.3
Psyllium	973.3	E858.4	E943.3	E950.4	E962.0	E980.4

TABLE OF DRUGS AND CHEMICALS / Pteroylglutamic acid

Substance	Poisoning	External Cause (E Code)				
		Accident	Therapeutic Use	Suicide Attempt	Assault	Undetermined
Pteroylglutamic acid	964.1	E858.2	E934.1	E950.4	E962.0	E980.4
Pteroyltriglutamate	963.1	E858.1	E933.1	E950.4	E962.0	E980.4
PTFE	987.8	E869.8	—	E952.8	E962.2	E982.8
Pulsatilla	988.2	E865.4	—	E950.9	E962.1	E980.9
Purex (bleach)	983.9	E864.3	—	E950.7	E962.1	E980.6
Purine diuretics	974.1	E858.5	E944.1	E950.4	E962.0	E980.4
Purinethol	963.1	E858.1	E933.1	E950.4	E962.0	E980.4
PVP	964.8	E858.2	E934.8	E950.4	E962.0	E980.4
Pyrabital	965.7	E850.7	E935.7	E950.0	E962.0	E980.0
Pyramidon	965.5	E850.5	E935.5	E950.0	E962.0	E980.0
Pyrantel (pamoate)	961.6	E857	E931.6	E950.4	E962.0	E980.4
Pyrathiazine	963.0	E858.1	E933.0	E950.4	E962.0	E980.4
Pyrazinamide	961.8	E857	E931.8	E950.4	E962.0	E980.4
Pyrazinoic acid (amide)	961.8	E857	E931.8	E950.4	E962.0	E980.4
Pyrazole (derivatives)	965.5	E850.5	E935.5	E950.0	E962.0	E980.0
Pyrazolone (analgesics)	965.5	E850.5	E935.5	E950.0	E962.0	E980.0
Pyrethrins, pyrethrum	989.4	E863.4	—	E950.6	E962.1	E980.7
Pyribenzamine	963.0	E858.1	E933.0	E950.4	E962.0	E980.4
Pyridine (liquid) (vapor)	982.0	E862.4	—	E950.9	E962.1	E980.9
aldoxime chloride	977.2	E858.8	E947.2	E950.4	E962.0	E980.4
Pyridium	976.1	E858.7	E946.1	E950.4	E962.0	E980.4
Pyridostigmine	971.0	E855.3	E941.0	E950.4	E962.0	E980.4
Pyridoxine	963.5	E858.1	E933.5	E950.4	E962.0	E980.4
Pyrilamine	963.0	E858.1	E933.0	E950.4	E962.0	E980.4
Pyrimethamine	961.4	E857	E931.4	E950.4	E962.0	E980.4
Pyrogallic acid	983.0	E864.0	—	E950.7	E962.1	E980.6
Pyroxylin	976.3	E858.7	E946.3	E950.4	E962.0	E980.4
Pyrrobutamine	963.0	E858.1	E933.0	E950.4	E962.0	E980.4
Pyrrocitine	968.5	E855.2	E938.5	E950.4	E962.0	E980.4
Pyrvinium (pamoate)	961.6	E857	E931.6	E950.4	E962.0	E980.4
PZI	962.3	E858.0	E932.3	E950.4	E962.0	E980.4
Quaalude	967.4	E852.3	E937.4	E950.2	E962.0	E980.2
Quaternary ammonium derivatives	971.1	E855.4	E941.1	E950.4	E962.0	E980.4
Quicklime	983.2	E864.2	—	E950.7	E962.1	E980.6
Quinacrine	961.3	E857	E931.3	E950.4	E962.0	E980.4
Quinaglute	972.0	E858.3	E942.0	E950.4	E962.0	E980.4
Quinalbarbitone	967.0	E851	E937.0	E950.1	E962.0	E980.1
Quinestradiol	962.2	E858.0	E932.2	E950.4	E962.0	E980.4
Quinethazone	974.3	E858.5	E944.3	E950.4	E962.0	E980.4

TABLE OF DRUGS AND CHEMICALS / Respiratory agents NEC

Substance	Poisoning	External Cause (E Code)				
		Accident	Therapeutic Use	Suicide Attempt	Assault	Undetermined
Quinidine (gluconate) (polygalacturonate) (salts) (sulfate)	972.0	E858.3	E942.0	E950.4	E962.0	E980.4
Quinine	961.4	E857	E931.4	E950.4	E962.0	E980.4
Quiniobine	961.3	E857	E931.3	E950.4	E962.0	E980.4
Quinolines	961.3	E857	E931.3	E950.4	E962.0	E980.4
Quotane	968.5	E855.2	E938.5	E950.4	E962.0	E980.4
Rabies	—	—	—	—	—	—
immune globulin (human)	964.6	E858.2	E934.6	E950.4	E962.0	E980.4
vaccine	979.1	E858.8	E949.1	E950.4	E962.0	E980.4
Racemoramide	965.09	E850.2	E935.2	E950.0	E962.0	E980.0
Racemorphan	965.09	E850.2	E935.2	E950.0	E962.0	E980.0
Radiator alcohol	980.1	E860.2	—	E950.9	E962.1	E980.9
Radio-opaque (drugs) (materials)	977.8	E858.8	E947.8	E950.4	E962.0	E980.4
Ranunculus	988.2	E865.4	—	E950.9	E962.1	E980.9
Rat poison	989.4	E863.7	—	E950.6	E962.1	E980.7
Rattlesnake (venom)	989.5	E905.0	—	E950.9	E962.1	E980.9
Raudixin	972.6	E858.3	E942.6	E950.4	E962.0	E980.4
Rautensin	972.6	E858.3	E942.6	E950.4	E962.0	E980.4
Rautina	972.6	E858.3	E942.6	E950.4	E962.0	E980.4
Rautotal	972.6	E858.3	E942.6	E950.4	E962.0	E980.4
Rauwiloid	972.6	E858.3	E942.6	E950.4	E962.0	E980.4
Rauwoldin	972.6	E858.3	E942.6	E950.4	E962.0	E980.4
Rauwolfia (alkaloids)	972.6	E858.3	E942.6	E950.4	E962.0	E980.4
Realgar	985.1	E866.3	—	E950.8	E962.1	E980.8
Red cells, packed	964.7	E858.2	E934.7	E950.4	E962.0	E980.4
Reducing agents, industrial NEC	983.9	E864.3	—	E950.7	E962.1	E980.6
Refrigerant gas (freon)	987.4	E869.2	—	E952.8	E962.2	E982.8
not freon	987.9	E869.9	—	E952.9	E962.2	E982.9
Regroton	974.4	E858.5	E944.4	E950.4	E962.0	E980.4
Rela	968.0	E855.1	E938.0	E950.4	E962.0	E980.4
Relaxants, skeletal muscle (autonomic)	975.2	E858.6	E945.2	E950.4	E962.0	E980.4
central nervous system	968.0	E855.1	E938.0	E950.4	E962.0	E980.4
Renese	974.3	E858.5	E944.3	E950.4	E962.0	E980.4
Renografin	977.8	E858.8	E947.8	E950.4	E962.0	E980.4
Replacement solutions	974.5	E858.5	E944.5	E950.4	E962.0	E980.4
Rescinnamine	972.6	E858.3	E942.6	E950.4	E962.0	E980.4
Reserpine	972.6	E858.3	E942.6	E950.4	E962.0	E980.4
Resorcin, resorcinol	976.4	E858.7	E946.4	E950.4	E962.0	E980.4
Respaire	975.5	E858.6	E945.5	E950.4	E962.0	E980.4
Respiratory agents NEC	975.8	E858.6	E945.8	E950.4	E962.0	E980.4

◄ New   ◄▬ Revised   ~~deleted~~ Deleted   ● Use Additional Digit(s)

TABLE OF DRUGS AND CHEMICALS / Retinoic acid

Substance	Poisoning	External Cause (E Code)				
		Accident	Therapeutic Use	Suicide Attempt	Assault	Undetermined
Retinoic acid	976.8	E858.7	E946.8	E950.4	E962.0	E980.4
Retinol	963.5	E858.1	E933.5	E950.4	E962.0	E980.4
Rh (D) immune globulin (human)	964.6	E858.2	E934.6	E950.4	E962.0	E980.4
Rhodine	965.1	E850.3	E935.3	E950.0	E962.0	E980.0
RhoGAM	964.6	E858.2	E934.6	E950.4	E962.0	E980.4
Riboflavin	963.5	E858.1	E933.5	E950.4	E962.0	E980.4
Ricin	989.89	E866.8	—	E950.9	E962.1	E980.9
Ricinus communis	988.2	E865.3	—	E950.9	E962.1	E980.9
Rickettsial vaccine NEC	979.6	E858.8	E949.6	E950.4	E962.0	E980.4
with viral and bacterial vaccine	979.7	E858.8	E949.7	E950.4	E962.0	E980.4
Rifampin	960.6	E856	E930.6	E950.4	E962.0	E980.4
Rimifon	961.8	E857	E931.8	E950.4	E962.0	E980.4
Ringer's injection (lactated)	974.5	E858.5	E944.5	E950.4	E962.0	E980.4
Ristocetin	960.8	E856	E930.8	E950.4	E962.0	E980.4
Ritalin	969.73	E854.2	E939.7	E950.3	E962.0	E980.3
Roach killers - see Pesticides	—	—	—	—	—	—
Rocky Mountain spotted fever vaccine	979.6	E858.8	E949.6	E950.4	E962.0	E980.4
Rodenticides	989.4	E863.7	—	E950.6	E962.1	E980.7
Rohypnol	969.4	E853.2	E939.4	E950.3	E962.0	E980.3
Rolaids	973.0	E858.4	E943.0	E950.4	E962.0	E980.4
Rolitetracycline	960.4	E856	E930.4	E950.4	E962.0	E980.4
Romilar	975.4	E858.6	E945.4	E950.4	E962.0	E980.4
Rose water ointment	976.3	E858.7	E946.3	E950.4	E962.0	E980.4
Rotenone	989.4	E863.7	—	E950.6	E962.1	E980.7
Rotoxamine	963.0	E858.1	E933.0	E950.4	E962.0	E980.4
Rough-on-rats	989.4	E863.7	—	E950.6	E962.1	E980.7
RU486	962.9	E858.0	E932.9	E950.4	E962.0	E980.4
Rubbing alcohol	980.2	E860.3	—	E950.9	E962.1	E980.9
Rubella virus vaccine	979.4	E858.8	E949.4	E950.4	E962.0	E980.4
Rubelogen	979.4	E858.8	E949.4	E950.4	E962.0	E980.4
Rubeovax	979.4	E858.8	E949.4	E950.4	E962.0	E980.4
Rubidomycin	960.7	E856	E930.7	E950.4	E962.0	E980.4
Rue	988.2	E865.4	—	E950.9	E962.1	E980.9
Ruta	988.2	E865.4	—	E950.9	E962.1	E980.9
Sabadilla (medicinal)	976.0	E858.7	E946.0	E950.4	E962.0	E980.4
pesticide	989.4	E863.4	—	E950.6	E962.1	E980.7
Sabin oral vaccine	979.5	E858.8	E949.5	E950.4	E962.0	E980.4
Saccharated iron oxide	964.0	E858.2	E934.0	E950.4	E962.0	E980.4
Saccharin	974.5	E858.5	E944.5	E950.4	E962.0	E980.4

TABLE OF DRUGS AND CHEMICALS / Scouring powder

Substance	Poisoning	External Cause (E Code)				
		Accident	Therapeutic Use	Suicide Attempt	Assault	Undetermined
Safflower oil	972.2	E858.3	E942.2	E950.4	E962.0	E980.4
Salbutamol sulfate	975.7	E858.6	E945.7	E950.4	E962.0	E980.4
Salicylamide	965.1	E850.3	E935.3	E950.0	E962.0	E980.0
Salicylate(s)	965.1	E850.3	E935.3	E950.0	E962.0	E980.0
methyl	976.3	E858.7	E946.3	E950.4	E962.0	E980.4
theobromine calcium	974.1	E858.5	E944.1	E950.4	E962.0	E980.4
Salicylazosulfapyridine	961.0	E857	E931.0	E950.4	E962.0	E980.4
Salicylhydroxamic acid	976.0	E858.7	E946.0	E950.4	E962.0	E980.4
Salicylic acid (keratolytic) NEC	976.4	E858.7	E946.4	E950.4	E962.0	E980.4
congeners	965.1	E850.3	E935.3	E950.0	E962.0	E980.0
salts	965.1	E850.3	E935.3	E950.0	E962.0	E980.0
Saliniazid	961.8	E857	E931.8	E950.4	E962.0	E980.4
Salol	976.3	E858.7	E946.3	E950.4	E962.0	E980.4
Salt (substitute) NEC	974.5	E858.5	E944.5	E950.4	E962.0	E980.4
Saluretics	974.3	E858.5	E944.3	E950.4	E962.0	E980.4
Saluron	974.3	E858.5	E944.3	E950.4	E962.0	E980.4
Salvarsan 606 (neosilver) (silver)	961.1	E857	E931.1	E950.4	E962.0	E980.4
Sambucus canadensis	988.2	E865.4	—	E950.9	E962.1	E980.9
berry	988.2	E865.3	—	E950.9	E962.1	E980.9
Sandril	972.6	E858.3	E942.6	E950.4	E962.0	E980.4
Sanguinaria canadensis	988.2	E865.4	—	E950.9	E962.1	E980.9
Saniflush (cleaner)	983.9	E861.3	—	E950.7	E962.1	E980.6
Santonin	961.6	E857	E931.6	E950.4	E962.0	E980.4
Santyl	976.8	E858.7	E946.8	E950.4	E962.0	E980.4
Sarkomycin	960.7	E856	E930.7	E950.4	E962.0	E980.4
Saroten	969.05	E854.0	E939.0	E950.3	E962.0	E980.3
Saturnine - see Lead	—	—	—	—	—	—
Savin (oil)	976.4	E858.7	E946.4	E950.4	E962.0	E980.4
Scammony	973.1	E858.4	E943.1	E950.4	E962.0	E980.4
Scarlet red	976.8	E858.7	E946.8	E950.4	E962.0	E980.4
Scheele's green	985.1	E866.3	—	E950.8	E962.1	E980.8
insecticide	985.1	E863.4	—	E950.8	E962.1	E980.8
Schradan	989.3	E863.1	—	E950.6	E962.1	E980.7
Schweinfurt(h) green	985.1	E866.3	—	E950.8	E962.1	E980.8
insecticide	985.1	E863.4	—	E950.8	E962.1	E980.8
Scilla - see Squill	—	—	—	—	—	—
Sclerosing agents	972.7	E858.3	E942.7	E950.4	E962.0	E980.4
Scopolamine	971.1	E855.4	E941.1	E950.4	E962.0	E980.4
Scouring powder	989.89	E861.3	—	E950.9	E962.1	E980.9

◀ New   ⬅ Revised   ~~deleted~~ Deleted   ● Use Additional Digit(s)

TABLE OF DRUGS AND CHEMICALS / Sea

	External Cause (E Code)					
Substance	Poisoning	Accident	Therapeutic Use	Suicide Attempt	Assault	Undetermined
Sea	—	—	—	—	—	—
anemone (sting)	989.5	E905.6	—	E950.9	E962.1	E980.9
cucumber (sting)	989.5	E905.6	—	E950.9	E962.1	E980.9
snake (bite) (venom)	989.5	E905.0	—	E950.9	E962.1	E980.9
urchin spine (puncture)	989.5	E905.6	—	E950.9	E962.1	E980.9
Secbutabarbital	967.0	E851	E937.0	E950.1	E962.0	E980.1
Secbutabarbitone	967.0	E851	E937.0	E950.1	E962.0	E980.1
Secobarbital	967.0	E851	E937.0	E950.1	E962.0	E980.1
Seconal	967.0	E851	E937.0	E950.1	E962.0	E980.1
Secretin	977.8	E858.8	E947.8	E950.4	E962.0	E980.4
Sedatives, nonbarbiturate	967.9	E852.9	E937.9	E950.2	E962.0	E980.2
specified NEC	967.8	E852.8	E937.8	E950.2	E962.0	E980.2
Sedormid	967.8	E852.8	E937.8	E950.2	E962.0	E980.2
Seed (plant)	988.2	E865.3	—	E950.9	E962.1	E980.9
disinfectant or dressing	989.89	E866.5	—	E950.9	E962.1	E980.9
Selective serotonin and norepinephrine reuptake inhibitors (SSNRI)	969.02	E854.0	E939.0	E950.3	E962.0	E980.3
Selective serotonin reuptake inhibitors (SSRI)	969.03	E854.0	E939.0	E950.3	E962.0	E980.3
Selenium (fumes) NEC	985.8	E866.4	—	E950.9	E962.1	E980.9
disulfide or sulfide	976.4	E858.7	E946.4	E950.4	E962.0	E980.4
Selsun	976.4	E858.7	E946.4	E950.4	E962.0	E980.4
Senna	973.1	E858.4	E943.1	E950.4	E962.0	E980.4
Septisol	976.2	E858.7	E946.2	E950.4	E962.0	E980.4
Serax	969.4	E853.2	E939.4	E950.3	E962.0	E980.3
Serenesil	967.8	E852.8	E937.8	E950.2	E962.0	E980.2
Serenium (hydrochloride)	961.9	E857	E931.9	E950.4	E962.0	E980.4
Serepax - see Oxazepam	—	—	—	—	—	—
Sernyl	968.3	E855.1	E938.3	E950.4	E962.0	E980.4
Serotonin	977.8	E858.8	E947.8	E950.4	E962.0	E980.4
Serpasil	972.6	E858.3	E942.6	E950.4	E962.0	E980.4
Sewer gas	987.8	E869.8	—	E952.8	E962.2	E982.8
Shampoo	989.6	E861.0	—	E950.9	E962.1	E980.9
Shellfish, nonbacterial or noxious	988.0	E865.1	—	E950.9	E962.1	E980.9
Silicones NEC	989.83	E866.8	E947.8	E950.9	E962.1	E980.9
Silvadene	976.0	E858.7	E946.0	E950.4	E962.0	E980.4
Silver (compound) (medicinal) NEC	976.0	E858.7	E946.0	E950.4	E962.0	E980.4
anti-infectives	976.0	E858.7	E946.0	E950.4	E962.0	E980.4
arsphenamine	961.1	E857	E931.1	E950.4	E962.0	E980.4
nitrate	976.0	E858.7	E946.0	E950.4	E962.0	E980.4
ophthalmic preparation	976.5	E858.7	E946.5	E950.4	E962.0	E980.4
toughened (keratolytic)	976.4	E858.7	E946.4	E950.4	E962.0	E980.4

TABLE OF DRUGS AND CHEMICALS / Sodium

Substance	Poisoning	Accident	Therapeutic Use	Suicide Attempt	Assault	Undetermined
Silver (compound) (medicinal) NEC *(Continued)*						
nonmedicinal (dust)	985.8	E866.4	—	E950.9	E962.1	E980.9
protein (mild) (strong)	976.0	E858.7	E946.0	E950.4	E962.0	E980.4
salvarsan	961.1	E857	E931.1	E950.4	E962.0	E980.4
Simethicone	973.8	E858.4	E943.8	E950.4	E962.0	E980.4
Sinequan	969.05	E854.0	E939.0	E950.3	E962.0	E980.3
Singoserp	972.6	E858.3	E942.6	E950.4	E962.0	E980.4
Sintrom	964.2	E858.2	E934.2	E950.4	E962.0	E980.4
Sitosterols	972.2	E858.3	E942.2	E950.4	E962.0	E980.4
Skeletal muscle relaxants	975.2	E858.6	E945.2	E950.4	E962.0	E980.4
Skin	—	—	—	—	—	—
agents (external)	976.9	E858.7	E946.9	E950.4	E962.0	E980.4
specified NEC	976.8	E858.7	E946.8	E950.4	E962.0	E980.4
test antigen	977.8	E858.8	E947.8	E950.4	E962.0	E980.4
Sleep-eze	963.0	E858.1	E933.0	E950.4	E962.0	E980.4
Sleeping draught (drug) (pill) (tablet)	967.9	E852.9	E937.9	E950.2	E962.0	E980.2
Smallpox vaccine	979.0	E858.8	E949.0	E950.4	E962.0	E980.4
Smelter fumes NEC	985.9	E866.4	—	E950.9	E962.1	E980.9
Smog	987.3	E869.1	—	E952.8	E962.2	E982.8
Smoke NEC	987.9	E869.9	—	E952.9	E962.2	E982.9
Smooth muscle relaxant	975.1	E858.6	E945.1	E950.4	E962.0	E980.4
Snail killer	989.4	E863.4	—	E950.6	E962.1	E980.7
Snake (bite) (venom)	989.5	E905.0	—	E950.9	E962.1	E980.9
Snuff	989.89	E866.8	—	E950.9	E962.1	E980.9
Soap (powder) (product)	989.6	E861.1	—	E950.9	E962.1	E980.9
medicinal, soft	976.2	E858.7	E946.2	E950.4	E962.0	E980.4
Soda (caustic)	983.2	E864.2	—	E950.7	E962.1	E980.6
bicarb	963.3	E858.1	E933.3	E950.4	E962.0	E980.4
chlorinated - *see* Sodium, hypochlorite	—	—	—	—	—	—
Sodium	—	—	—	—	—	—
acetosulfone	961.8	E857	E931.8	E950.4	E962.0	E980.4
acetrizoate	977.8	E858.8	E947.8	E950.4	E962.0	E980.4
amytal	967.0	E851	E937.0	E950.1	E962.0	E980.1
arsenate - *see* Arsenic	—	—	—	—	—	—
bicarbonate	963.3	E858.1	E933.3	E950.4	E962.0	E980.4
bichromate	983.9	E864.3	—	E950.7	E962.1	E980.6
biphosphate	963.2	E858.1	E933.2	E950.4	E962.0	E980.4
bisulfate	983.9	E864.3	—	E950.7	E962.1	E980.6
borate (cleanser)	989.6	E861.3	—	E950.9	E962.1	E980.9
bromide NEC	967.3	E852.2	E937.3	E950.2	E962.0	E980.2

◀ New ◀|||| Revised ~~deleted~~ Deleted ● Use Additional Digit(s)

TABLE OF DRUGS AND CHEMICALS / Sodium

Substance	Poisoning	External Cause (E Code)				
		Accident	Therapeutic Use	Suicide Attempt	Assault	Undetermined
Sodium *(Continued)*						
cacodylate (nonmedicinal) NEC	978.8	E858.8	E948.8	E950.4	E962.0	E980.4
anti-infective	961.1	E857	E931.1	E950.4	E962.0	E980.4
herbicide	989.4	E863.5	—	E950.6	E962.1	E980.7
calcium edetate	963.8	E858.1	E933.8	E950.4	E962.0	E980.4
carbonate NEC	983.2	E864.2	—	E950.7	E962.1	E980.6
chlorate NEC	983.9	E864.3	—	E950.7	E962.1	E980.6
herbicide	983.9	E863.5	—	E950.7	E962.1	E980.6
chloride NEC	974.5	E858.5	E944.5	E950.4	E962.0	E980.4
chromate	983.9	E864.3	—	E950.7	E962.1	E980.6
citrate	963.3	E858.1	E933.3	E950.4	E962.0	E980.4
cyanide - *see* Cyanide(s)	—	—	—	—	—	—
cyclamate	974.5	E858.5	E944.5	E950.4	E962.0	E980.4
diatrizoate	977.8	E858.8	E947.8	E950.4	E962.0	E980.4
dibunate	975.4	E858.6	E945.4	E950.4	E962.0	E980.4
dioctyl sulfosuccinate	973.2	E858.4	E943.2	E950.4	E962.0	E980.4
edetate	963.8	E858.1	E933.8	E950.4	E962.0	E980.4
ethacrynate	974.4	E858.5	E944.4	E950.4	E962.0	E980.4
fluoracetate (dust) (rodenticide)	989.4	E863.7	—	E950.6	E962.1	E980.7
fluoride - *see* Fluoride(s)	—	—	—	—	—	—
free salt	974.5	E858.5	E944.5	E950.4	E962.0	E980.4
glucosulfone	961.8	E857	E931.8	E950.4	E962.0	E980.4
hydroxide	983.2	E864.2	—	E950.7	E962.1	E980.6
hypochlorite (bleach) NEC	983.9	E864.3	—	E950.7	E962.1	E980.6
disinfectant	983.9	E861.4	—	E950.7	E962.1	E980.6
medicinal (anti-infective) (external)	976.0	E858.7	E946.0	E950.4	E962.0	E980.4
vapor	987.8	E869.8	—	E952.8	E962.2	E982.8
hyposulfite	976.0	E858.7	E946.0	E950.4	E962.0	E980.4
indigotindisulfonate	977.8	E858.8	E947.8	E950.4	E962.0	E980.4
iodide	977.8	E858.8	E947.8	E950.4	E962.0	E980.4
iothalamate	977.8	E858.8	E947.8	E950.4	E962.0	E980.4
iron edetate	964.0	E858.2	E934.0	E950.4	E962.0	E980.4
lactate	963.3	E858.1	E933.3	E950.4	E962.0	E980.4
lauryl sulfate	976.2	E858.7	E946.2	E950.4	E962.0	E980.4
L-triiodothyronine	962.7	E858.0	E932.7	E950.4	E962.0	E980.4
metrizoate	977.8	E858.8	E947.8	E950.4	E962.0	E980.4
monofluoracetate (dust) (rodenticide)	989.4	E863.7	—	E950.6	E962.1	E980.7
morrhuate	972.7	E858.3	E942.7	E950.4	E962.0	E980.4
nafcillin	960.0	E856	E930.0	E950.4	E962.0	E980.4

◄ New   ⬅ Revised   ~~deleted~~ Deleted   ● Use Additional Digit(s)

TABLE OF DRUGS AND CHEMICALS / Sominex

Substance	Poisoning	External Cause (E Code)				
		Accident	Therapeutic Use	Suicide Attempt	Assault	Undetermined
Sodium *(Continued)*						
nitrate (oxidizing agent)	983.9	E864.3	—	E950.7	E962.1	E980.6
nitrite (medicinal)	972.4	E858.3	E942.4	E950.4	E962.0	E980.4
nitroferricyanide	972.6	E858.3	E942.6	E950.4	E962.0	E980.4
nitroprusside	972.6	E858.3	E942.6	E950.4	E962.0	E980.4
para-aminohippurate	977.8	E858.8	E947.8	E950.4	E962.0	E980.4
perborate (nonmedicinal) NEC	989.89	E866.8	—	E950.9	E962.1	E980.9
medicinal	976.6	E858.7	E946.6	E950.4	E962.0	E980.4
soap	989.6	E861.1	—	E950.9	E962.1	E980.9
percarbonate - *see* Sodium, perborate	—	—	—	—	—	—
phosphate	973.3	E858.4	E943.3	E950.4	E962.0	E980.4
polystyrene sulfonate	974.5	E858.5	E944.5	E950.4	E962.0	E980.4
propionate	976.0	E858.7	E946.0	E950.4	E962.0	E980.4
psylliate	972.7	E858.3	E942.7	E950.4	E962.0	E980.4
removing resins	974.5	E858.5	E944.5	E950.4	E962.0	E980.4
salicylate	965.1	E850.3	E935.3	E950.0	E962.0	E980.0
sulfate	973.3	E858.4	E943.3	E950.4	E962.0	E980.4
sulfoxone	961.8	E857	E931.8	E950.4	E962.0	E980.4
tetradecyl sulfate	972.7	E858.3	E942.7	E950.4	E962.0	E980.4
thiopental	968.3	E855.1	E938.3	E950.4	E962.0	E980.4
thiosalicylate	965.1	E850.3	E935.3	E950.0	E962.0	E980.0
thiosulfate	976.0	E858.7	E946.0	E950.4	E962.0	E980.4
tolbutamide	977.8	E858.8	E947.8	E950.4	E962.0	E980.4
tyropanoate	977.8	E858.8	E947.8	E950.4	E962.0	E980.4
valproate	966.3	E855.0	E936.3	E950.4	E962.0	E980.4
Solanine	977.8	E858.8	E947.8	E950.4	E962.0	E980.4
Solanum dulcamara	988.2	E865.4	—	E950.9	E962.1	E980.9
Solapsone	961.8	E857	E931.8	E950.4	E962.0	E980.4
Solasulfone	961.8	E857	E931.8	E950.4	E962.0	E980.4
Soldering fluid	983.1	E864.1	—	E950.7	E962.1	E980.6
Solid substance	989.9	E866.9	—	E950.9	E962.1	E980.9
specified NEC	989.9	E866.8	—	E950.9	E962.1	E980.9
Solvents, industrial	982.8	E862.9	—	E950.9	E962.1	E980.9
naphtha	981	E862.0	—	E950.9	E962.1	E980.9
petroleum	981	E862.0	—	E950.9	E962.1	E980.9
specified NEC	982.8	E862.4	—	E950.9	E962.1	E980.9
Soma	968.0	E855.1	E938.0	E950.4	E962.0	E980.4
Somatotropin	962.4	E858.0	E932.4	E950.4	E962.0	E980.4
Sominex	963.0	E858.1	E933.0	E950.4	E962.0	E980.4

◀ New   Revised   ~~deleted~~ Deleted   ● Use Additional Digit(s)

TABLE OF DRUGS AND CHEMICALS / Somnos

Substance	Poisoning	External Cause (E Code)				
		Accident	Therapeutic Use	Suicide Attempt	Assault	Undetermined
Somnos	967.1	E852.0	E937.1	E950.2	E962.0	E980.2
Somonal	967.0	E851	E937.0	E950.1	E962.0	E980.1
Soneryl	967.0	E851	E937.0	E950.1	E962.0	E980.1
Soothing syrup	977.9	E858.9	E947.9	E950.5	E962.0	E980.5
Sopor	967.4	E852.3	E937.4	E950.2	E962.0	E980.2
Soporific drug	967.9	E852.9	E937.9	E950.2	E962.0	E980.2
specified type NEC	967.8	E852.8	E937.8	E950.2	E962.0	E980.2
Sorbitol NEC	977.4	E858.8	E947.4	E950.4	E962.0	E980.4
Sotradecol	972.7	E858.3	E942.7	E950.4	E962.0	E980.4
Spacoline	975.1	E858.6	E945.1	E950.4	E962.0	E980.4
Spanish fly	976.8	E858.7	E946.8	E950.4	E962.0	E980.4
Sparine	969.1	E853.0	E939.1	E950.3	E962.0	E980.3
Sparteine	975.0	E858.6	E945.0	E950.4	E962.0	E980.4
Spasmolytics	975.1	E858.6	E945.1	E950.4	E962.0	E980.4
anticholinergics	971.1	E855.4	E941.1	E950.4	E962.0	E980.4
Spectinomycin	960.8	E856	E930.8	E950.4	E962.0	E980.4
Speed	969.72	E854.2	E939.7	E950.3	E962.0	E980.3
Spermicides	976.8	E858.7	E946.8	E950.4	E962.0	E980.4
Spider (bite) (venom)	989.5	E905.1	—	E950.9	E962.1	E980.9
antivenin	979.9	E858.8	E949.9	E950.4	E962.0	E980.4
Spigelia (root)	961.6	E857	E931.6	E950.4	E962.0	E980.4
Spiperone	969.2	E853.1	E939.2	E950.3	E962.0	E980.3
Spiramycin	960.3	E856	E930.3	E950.4	E962.0	E980.4
Spirilene	969.5	E853.8	E939.5	E950.3	E962.0	E980.3
Spirit(s) (neutral) NEC	980.0	E860.1	—	E950.9	E962.1	E980.9
beverage	980.0	E860.0	—	E950.9	E962.1	E980.9
industrial	980.9	E860.9	—	E950.9	E962.1	E980.9
mineral	981	E862.0	—	E950.9	E962.1	E980.9
of salt - *see* Hydrochloric acid	—	—	—	—	—	—
surgical	980.9	E860.9	—	E950.9	E962.1	E980.9
Spironolactone	974.4	E858.5	E944.4	E950.4	E962.0	E980.4
Sponge, absorbable (gelatin)	964.5	E858.2	E934.5	E950.4	E962.0	E980.4
Sporostacin	976.0	E858.7	E946.0	E950.4	E962.0	E980.4
Sprays (aerosol)	989.89	E866.8	—	E950.9	E962.1	E980.9
cosmetic	989.89	E866.7	—	E950.9	E962.1	E980.9
medicinal NEC	977.9	E858.9	E947.9	E950.5	E962.0	E980.5
pesticides - *see* Pesticides	—	—	—	—	—	—
specified content - *see* substance specified	—	—	—	—	—	—
Spurge flax	988.2	E865.4	—	E950.9	E962.1	E980.9

TABLE OF DRUGS AND CHEMICALS / Stramonium NEC

Substance	Poisoning	Accident	Therapeutic Use	Suicide Attempt	Assault	Undetermined
Spurges	988.2	E865.4	—	E950.9	E962.1	E980.9
Squill (expectorant) NEC	975.5	E858.6	E945.5	E950.4	E962.0	E980.4
rat poison	989.4	E863.7	—	E950.6	E962.1	E980.7
Squirting cucumber (cathartic)	973.1	E858.4	E943.1	E950.4	E962.0	E980.4
SSNRI (selective serotonin and norepinephrine reuptake inhibitors)	969.02	E854.0	E939.0	E950.3	E962.0	E980.3
SSRI (selective serotonin reuptake inhibitors)	969.03	E854.0	E939.0	E950.3	E962.0	E980.3
Stains	989.89	E866.8	—	E950.9	E962.1	E980.9
Stannous - see also Tin fluoride	976.7	E858.7	E946.7	E950.4	E962.0	E980.4
Stanolone	962.1	E858.0	E932.1	E950.4	E962.0	E980.4
Stanozolol	962.1	E858.0	E932.1	E950.4	E962.0	E980.4
Staphisagria or stavesacre (pediculicide)	976.0	E858.7	E946.0	E950.4	E962.0	E980.4
Stelazine	969.1	E853.0	E939.1	E950.3	E962.0	E980.3
Stemetil	969.1	E853.0	E939.1	E950.3	E962.0	E980.3
Sterculia (cathartic) (gum)	973.3	E858.4	E943.3	E950.4	E962.0	E980.4
Sternutator gas	987.8	E869.8	—	E952.8	E962.2	E982.8
Steroids NEC	962.0	E858.0	E932.0	E950.4	E962.0	E980.4
ENT agent	976.6	E858.7	E946.6	E950.4	E962.0	E980.4
ophthalmic preparation	976.5	E858.7	E946.5	E950.4	E962.0	E980.4
topical NEC	976.0	E858.7	E946.0	E950.4	E962.0	E980.4
Stibine	985.8	E866.4	—	E950.9	E962.1	E980.9
Stibophen	961.2	E857	E931.2	E950.4	E962.0	E980.4
Stilbamide, stilbamidine	961.5	E857	E931.5	E950.4	E962.0	E980.4
Stilbestrol	962.2	E858.0	E932.2	E950.4	E962.0	E980.4
Stimulants (central nervous system)	970.9	E854.3	E940.9	E950.4	E962.0	E980.4
analeptics	970.0	E854.3	E940.0	E950.4	E962.0	E980.4
opiate antagonist	970.1	E854.3	E940.1	E950.4	E962.0	E980.4
psychotherapeutic NEC	969.09	E854.0	E939.0	E950.3	E962.0	E980.3
specified NEC	970.89	E854.3	E940.8	E950.4	E962.0	E980.4
Storage batteries (acid) (cells)	983.1	E864.1	—	E950.7	E962.1	E980.6
Stovaine	968.9	E855.2	E938.9	E950.4	E962.0	E980.4
infiltration (subcutaneous)	968.5	E855.2	E938.5	E950.4	E962.0	E980.4
nerve block (peripheral) (plexus)	968.6	E855.2	E938.6	E950.4	E962.0	E980.4
spinal	968.7	E855.2	E938.7	E950.4	E962.0	E980.4
topical (surface)	968.5	E855.2	E938.5	E950.4	E962.0	E980.4
Stovarsal	961.1	E857	E931.1	E950.4	E962.0	E980.4
Stove gas - see Gas, utility	—	—	—	—	—	—
Stoxil	976.5	E858.7	E946.5	E950.4	E962.0	E980.4
STP	969.6	E854.1	E939.6	E950.3	E962.0	E980.3
Stramonium (medicinal) NEC	971.1	E855.4	E941.1	E950.4	E962.0	E980.4
natural state	988.2	E865.4	—	E950.9	E962.1	E980.9

TABLE OF DRUGS AND CHEMICALS / Streptodornase

Substance	Poisoning	External Cause (E Code)				
		Accident	Therapeutic Use	Suicide Attempt	Assault	Undetermined
Streptodornase	964.4	E858.2	E934.4	E950.4	E962.0	E980.4
Streptoduocin	960.6	E856	E930.6	E950.4	E962.0	E980.4
Streptokinase	964.4	E858.2	E934.4	E950.4	E962.0	E980.4
Streptomycin	960.6	E856	E930.6	E950.4	E962.0	E980.4
Streptozocin	960.7	E856	E930.7	E950.4	E962.0	E980.4
Stripper (paint) (solvent)	982.8	E862.9	—	E950.9	E962.1	E980.9
Strobane	989.2	E863.0	—	E950.6	E962.1	E980.7
Strophanthin	972.1	E858.3	E942.1	E950.4	E962.0	E980.4
Strophanthus hispidus or kombe	988.2	E865.4	—	E950.9	E962.1	E980.9
Strychnine (rodenticide) (salts)	989.1	E863.7	—	E950.6	E962.1	E980.7
medicinal NEC	970.89	E854.3	E940.8	E950.4	E962.0	E980.4
Strychnos (ignatii) - see Strychnine	—	—	—	—	—	—
Styramate	968.0	E855.1	E938.0	E950.4	E962.0	E980.4
Styrene	983.0	E864.0	—	E950.7	E962.1	E980.6
Succinimide (anticonvulsant)	966.2	E855.0	E936.2	E950.4	E962.0	E980.4
mercuric - see Mercury	—	—	—	—	—	—
Succinylcholine	975.2	E858.6	E945.2	E950.4	E962.0	E980.4
Succinylsulfathiazole	961.0	E857	E931.0	E950.4	E962.0	E980.4
Sucrose	974.5	E858.5	E944.5	E950.4	E962.0	E980.4
Sulfacetamide	961.0	E857	E931.0	E950.4	E962.0	E980.4
ophthalmic preparation	976.5	E858.7	E946.5	E950.4	E962.0	E980.4
Sulfachlorpyridazine	961.0	E857	E931.0	E950.4	E962.0	E980.4
Sulfacytine	961.0	E857	E931.0	E950.4	E962.0	E980.4
Sulfadiazine	961.0	E857	E931.0	E950.4	E962.0	E980.4
silver (topical)	976.0	E858.7	E946.0	E950.4	E962.0	E980.4
Sulfadimethoxine	961.0	E857	E931.0	E950.4	E962.0	E980.4
Sulfadimidine	961.0	E857	E931.0	E950.4	E962.0	E980.4
Sulfaethidole	961.0	E857	E931.0	E950.4	E962.0	E980.4
Sulfafurazole	961.0	E857	E931.0	E950.4	E962.0	E980.4
Sulfaguanidine	961.0	E857	E931.0	E950.4	E962.0	E980.4
Sulfamerazine	961.0	E857	E931.0	E950.4	E962.0	E980.4
Sulfameter	961.0	E857	E931.0	E950.4	E962.0	E980.4
Sulfamethizole	961.0	E857	E931.0	E950.4	E962.0	E980.4
Sulfamethoxazole	961.0	E857	E931.0	E950.4	E962.0	E980.4
Sulfamethoxydiazine	961.0	E857	E931.0	E950.4	E962.0	E980.4
Sulfamethoxypyridazine	961.0	E857	E931.0	E950.4	E962.0	E980.4
Sulfamethylthiazole	961.0	E857	E931.0	E950.4	E962.0	E980.4
Sulfamylon	976.0	E858.7	E946.0	E950.4	E962.0	E980.4
Sulfan blue (diagnostic dye)	977.8	E858.8	E947.8	E950.4	E962.0	E980.4
Sulfanilamide	961.0	E857	E931.0	E950.4	E962.0	E980.4

◀ New   ◀‖ Revised   ~~deleted~~ Deleted   ● Use Additional Digit(s)

TABLE OF DRUGS AND CHEMICALS / Sutilains

Substance	Poisoning	Accident	Therapeutic Use	Suicide Attempt	Assault	Undetermined
			External Cause (E Code)			
Sulfanilylguanidine	961.0	E857	E931.0	E950.4	E962.0	E980.4
Sulfaphenazole	961.0	E857	E931.0	E950.4	E962.0	E980.4
Sulfaphenylthiazole	961.0	E857	E931.0	E950.4	E962.0	E980.4
Sulfaproxyline	961.0	E857	E931.0	E950.4	E962.0	E980.4
Sulfapyridine	961.0	E857	E931.0	E950.4	E962.0	E980.4
Sulfapyrimidine	961.0	E857	E931.0	E950.4	E962.0	E980.4
Sulfarsphenamine	961.1	E857	E931.1	E950.4	E962.0	E980.4
Sulfasalazine	961.0	E857	E931.0	E950.4	E962.0	E980.4
Sulfasomizole	961.0	E857	E931.0	E950.4	E962.0	E980.4
Sulfasuxidine	961.0	E857	E931.0	E950.4	E962.0	E980.4
Sulfinpyrazone	974.7	E858.5	E944.7	E950.4	E962.0	E980.4
Sulfisoxazole	961.0	E857	E931.0	E950.4	E962.0	E980.4
ophthalmic preparation	976.5	E858.7	E946.5	E950.4	E962.0	E980.4
Sulfomyxin	960.8	E856	E930.8	E950.4	E962.0	E980.4
Sulfonal	967.8	E852.8	E937.8	E950.2	E962.0	E980.2
Sulfonamides (mixtures)	961.0	E857	E931.0	E950.4	E962.0	E980.4
Sulfones	961.8	E857	E931.8	E950.4	E962.0	E980.4
Sulfonethylmethane	967.8	E852.8	E937.8	E950.2	E962.0	E980.2
Sulfonmethane	967.8	E852.8	E937.8	E950.2	E962.0	E980.2
Sulfonphthal, sulfonphthol	977.8	E858.8	E947.8	E950.4	E962.0	E980.4
Sulfonylurea derivatives, oral	962.3	E858.0	E932.3	E950.4	E962.0	E980.4
Sulfoxone	961.8	E857	E931.8	E950.4	E962.0	E980.4
Sulfur, sulfureted, sulfuric, sulfurous, sulfuryl (compounds) NEC	989.89	E866.8	—	E950.9	E962.1	E980.9
acid	983.1	E864.1		E950.7	E962.1	E980.6
dioxide	987.3	E869.1	—	E952.8	E962.2	E982.8
ether - see Ether(s)	—	—	—	—	—	—
hydrogen	987.8	E869.8	—	E952.8	E962.2	E982.8
medicinal (keratolytic) (ointment) NEC	976.4	E858.7	E946.4	E950.4	E962.0	E980.4
pesticide (vapor)	989.4	E863.4	—	E950.6	E962.1	E980.7
vapor NEC	987.8	E869.8	—	E952.8	E962.2	E982.8
Sulkowitch's reagent	977.8	E858.8	E947.8	E950.4	E962.0	E980.4
Sulph - see also Sulf-	—	—	—	—	—	—
Sulphadione	961.8	E857	E931.8	E950.4	E962.0	E980.4
Sulthiame, sultiame	966.3	E855.0	E936.3	E950.4	E962.0	E980.4
Superinone	975.5	E858.6	E945.5	E950.4	E962.0	E980.4
Suramin	961.5	E857	E931.5	E950.4	E962.0	E980.4
Surfacaine	968.5	E855.2	E938.5	E950.4	E962.0	E980.4
Surital	968.3	E855.1	E938.3	E950.4	E962.0	E980.4
Sutilains	976.8	E858.7	E946.8	E950.4	E962.0	E980.4

TABLE OF DRUGS AND CHEMICALS / Suxamethonium

Substance	Poisoning	External Cause (E Code)				
		Accident	Therapeutic Use	Suicide Attempt	Assault	Undetermined
Suxamethonium (bromide) (chloride) (iodide)	975.2	E858.6	E945.2	E950.4	E962.0	E980.4
Suxethonium (bromide)	975.2	E858.6	E945.2	E950.4	E962.0	E980.4
Sweet oil (birch)	976.3	E858.7	E946.3	E950.4	E962.0	E980.4
Sym-dichloroethyl ether	982.3	E862.4	—	E950.9	E962.1	E980.9
Sympatholytics	971.3	E855.6	E941.3	E950.4	E962.0	E980.4
Sympathomimetics	971.2	E855.5	E941.2	E950.4	E962.0	E980.4
Synagis	979.6	E858.8	E949.6	E950.4	E962.0	E980.4
Synalar	976.0	E858.7	E946.0	E950.4	E962.0	E980.4
Synthroid	962.7	E858.0	E932.7	E950.4	E962.0	E980.4
Syntocinon	975.0	E858.6	E945.0	E950.4	E962.0	E950.4
Syrosingopine	972.6	E858.3	E942.6	E950.4	E962.0	E980.4
Systemic agents (primarily)	963.9	E858.1	E933.9	E950.4	E962.0	E980.4
specified NEC	963.8	E858.1	E933.8	E950.4	E962.0	E980.4
Tablets (*see also* specified substance)	977.9	E858.9	E947.9	E950.5	E962.0	E980.5
Tace	962.2	E858.0	E932.2	E950.4	E962.0	E980.4
Tacrine	971.0	E855.3	E941.0	E950.4	E962.0	E980.4
Talbutal	967.0	E851	E937.0	E950.1	E962.0	E980.1
Talc	976.3	E858.7	E946.3	E950.4	E962.0	E980.4
Talcum	976.3	E858.7	E946.3	E950.4	E962.0	E980.4
Tamsulosin	971.3	E855.6	E941.3	E950.4	E962.0	E980.4
Tandearil, tanderil	965.5	E850.5	E935.5	E950.0	E962.0	E980.0
Tannic acid	983.1	E864.1	—	E950.7	E962.1	E980.6
medicinal (astringent)	976.2	E858.7	E946.2	E950.4	E962.0	E980.4
Tannin - *see* Tannic acid	—	—	—	—	—	—
Tansy	988.2	E865.4	—	E950.9	E962.1	E980.9
TAO	960.3	E856	E930.3	E950.4	E962.0	E980.4
Tapazole	962.8	E858.0	E932.8	E950.4	E962.0	E980.4
Tar NEC	983.0	E864.0	—	E950.7	E962.1	E980.6
camphor - *see* Naphthalene	—	—	—	—	—	—
fumes	987.8	E869.8	—	E952.8	E962.2	E982.8
Taractan	969.3	E853.8	E939.3	E950.3	E962.0	E980.3
Tarantula (venomous)	989.5	E905.1	—	E950.9	E962.1	E980.9
Tartar emetic (anti-infective)	961.2	E857	E931.2	E950.4	E962.0	E980.4
Tartaric acid	983.1	E864.1	—	E950.7	E962.1	E980.6
Tartrated antimony (anti-infective)	961.2	E857	E931.2	E950.4	E962.0	E980.4
TCA - *see* Trichloroacetic acid	—	—	—	—	—	—
TDI	983.0	E864.0	—	E950.7	E962.1	E980.6
vapor	987.8	E869.8	—	E952.8	E962.2	E982.8
Tear gas	987.5	E869.3	—	E952.8	E962.2	E982.8

TABLE OF DRUGS AND CHEMICALS / Tetraethylthiuram disulfide

		External Cause (E Code)				
Substance	Poisoning	Accident	Therapeutic Use	Suicide Attempt	Assault	Undetermined
Teclothiazide	974.3	E858.5	E944.3	E950.4	E962.0	E980.4
Tegretol	966.3	E855.0	E936.3	E950.4	E962.0	E980.4
Telepaque	977.8	E858.8	E947.8	E950.4	E962.0	E980.4
Tellurium	985.8	E866.4	—	E950.9	E962.1	E980.9
fumes	985.8	E866.4	—	E950.9	E962.1	E980.9
TEM	963.1	E858.1	E933.1	E950.4	E962.0	E980.4
Temazepam - see Benzodiazepines	—	—	—	—	—	—
TEPA	963.1	E858.1	E933.1	E950.4	E962.0	E980.4
TEPP	989.3	E863.1	—	E950.6	E962.1	E980.7
Terbutaline	971.2	E855.5	E941.2	E950.4	E962.0	E980.4
Teroxalene	961.6	E857	E931.6	E950.4	E962.0	E980.4
Terpin hydrate	975.5	E858.6	E945.5	E950.4	E962.0	E980.4
Terramycin	960.4	E856	E930.4	E950.4	E962.0	E980.4
Tessalon	975.4	E858.6	E945.4	E950.4	E962.0	E980.4
Testosterone	962.1	E858.0	E932.1	E950.4	E962.0	E980.4
Tetanus (vaccine)	978.4	E858.8	E948.4	E950.4	E962.0	E980.4
antitoxin	979.9	E858.8	E949.9	E950.4	E962.0	E980.4
immune globulin (human)	964.6	E858.2	E934.6	E950.4	E962.0	E980.4
toxoid	978.4	E858.8	E948.4	E950.4	E962.0	E980.4
with diphtheria toxoid	978.9	E858.8	E948.9	E950.4	E962.0	E980.4
with pertussis	978.6	E858.8	E948.6	E950.4	E962.0	E980.4
Tetrabenazine	969.5	E853.8	E939.5	E950.3	E962.0	E980.3
Tetracaine (infiltration) (topical)	968.5	E855.2	E938.5	E950.4	E962.0	E980.4
nerve block (peripheral) (plexus)	968.6	E855.2	E938.6	E950.4	E962.0	E980.4
spinal	968.7	E855.2	E938.7	E950.4	E962.0	E980.4
Tetrachlorethylene - see Tetrachloroethylene	—	—	—	—	—	—
Tetrachlormethiazide	974.3	E858.5	E944.3	E950.4	E962.0	E980.4
Tetrachloroethane (liquid) (vapor)	982.3	E862.4	—	E950.9	E962.1	E980.9
paint or varnish	982.3	E861.6	—	E950.9	E962.1	E980.9
Tetrachloroethylene (liquid) (vapor)	982.3	E862.4	—	E950.9	E962.1	E980.9
medicinal	961.6	E857	E931.6	E950.4	E962.0	E980.4
Tetrachloromethane - see Carbon, tetrachloride	—	—	—	—	—	—
Tetracycline	960.4	E856	E930.4	E950.4	E962.0	E980.4
ophthalmic preparation	976.5	E858.7	E946.5	E950.4	E962.0	E980.4
topical NEC	976.0	E858.7	E946.0	E950.4	E962.0	E980.4
Tetraethylammonium chloride	972.3	E858.3	E942.3	E950.4	E962.0	E980.4
Tetraethyl lead (antiknock compound)	984.1	E862.1	—	E950.9	E962.1	E980.9
Tetraethyl pyrophosphate	989.3	E863.1	—	E950.6	E962.1	E980.7
Tetraethylthiuram disulfide	977.3	E858.8	E947.3	E950.4	E962.0	E980.4

◄ New   ◄ Revised   deleted Deleted   ● Use Additional Digit(s)

TABLE OF DRUGS AND CHEMICALS / Tetrahydroaminoacridine

Substance	Poisoning	External Cause (E Code)				
		Accident	Therapeutic Use	Suicide Attempt	Assault	Undetermined
Tetrahydroaminoacridine	971.0	E855.3	E941.0	E950.4	E962.0	E980.4
Tetrahydrocannabinol	969.6	E854.1	E939.6	E950.3	E962.0	E980.3
Tetrahydronaphthalene	982.0	E862.4	—	E950.9	E962.1	E980.9
Tetrahydrozoline	971.2	E855.5	E941.2	E950.4	E962.0	E980.4
Tetralin	982.0	E862.4	—	E950.9	E962.1	E980.9
Tetramethylthiuram (disulfide) NEC	989.4	E863.6	—	E950.6	E962.1	E980.7
medicinal	976.2	E858.7	E946.2	E950.4	E962.0	E980.4
Tetronal	967.8	E852.8	E937.8	E950.2	E962.0	E980.2
Tetryl	983.0	E864.0	—	E950.7	E962.1	E980.6
Thalidomide	967.8	E852.8	E937.8	E950.2	E962.0	E980.2
Thallium (compounds) (dust) NEC	985.8	E866.4	—	E950.9	E962.1	E980.9
pesticide (rodenticide)	985.8	E863.7	—	E950.6	E962.1	E980.7
THC	969.6	E854.1	E939.6	E950.3	E962.0	E980.3
Thebacon	965.09	E850.2	E935.2	E950.0	E962.0	E980.0
Thebaine	965.09	E850.2	E935.2	E950.0	E962.0	E980.0
Theobromine (calcium salicylate)	974.1	E858.5	E944.1	E950.4	E962.0	E980.4
Theophylline (diuretic)	974.1	E858.5	E944.1	E950.4	E962.0	E980.4
ethylenediamine	975.7	E858.6	E945.7	E950.4	E962.0	E980.4
Thiabendazole	961.6	E857	E931.6	E950.4	E962.0	E980.4
Thialbarbital, thialbarbitone	968.3	E855.1	E938.3	E950.4	E962.0	E980.4
Thiamine	963.5	E858.1	E933.5	E950.4	E962.0	E980.4
Thiamylal (sodium)	968.3	E855.1	E938.3	E950.4	E962.0	E980.4
Thiazesim	969.09	E854.0	E939.0	E950.3	E962.0	E980.3
Thiazides (diuretics)	974.3	E858.5	E944.3	E950.4	E962.0	E980.4
Thiethylperazine	963.0	E858.1	E933.0	E950.4	E962.0	E980.4
Thimerosal (topical)	976.0	E858.7	E946.0	E950.4	E962.0	E980.4
ophthalmic preparation	976.5	E858.7	E946.5	E950.4	E962.0	E980.4
Thioacetazone	961.8	E857	E931.8	E950.4	E962.0	E980.4
Thiobarbiturates	968.3	E855.1	E938.3	E950.4	E962.0	E980.4
Thiobismol	961.2	E857	E931.2	E950.4	E962.0	E980.4
Thiocarbamide	962.8	E858.0	E932.8	E950.4	E962.0	E980.4
Thiocarbarsone	961.1	E857	E931.1	E950.4	E962.0	E980.4
Thiocarlide	961.8	E857	E931.8	E950.4	E962.0	E980.4
Thioguanine	963.1	E858.1	E933.1	E950.4	E962.0	E980.4
Thiomercaptomerin	974.0	E858.5	E944.0	E950.4	E962.0	E980.4
Thiomerin	974.0	E858.5	E944.0	E950.4	E962.0	E980.4
Thiopental, thiopentone (sodium)	968.3	E855.1	E938.3	E950.4	E962.0	E980.4
Thiopropazate	969.1	E853.0	E939.1	E950.3	E962.0	E980.3
Thioproperazine	969.1	E853.0	E939.1	E950.3	E962.0	E980.3

TABLE OF DRUGS AND CHEMICALS / Tobacco NEC

Substance	Poisoning	Accident	Therapeutic Use	Suicide Attempt	Assault	Undetermined
Thioridazine	969.1	E853.0	E939.1	E950.3	E962.0	E980.3
Thio-TEPA, thiotepa	963.1	E858.1	E933.1	E950.4	E962.0	E980.4
Thiothixene	969.3	E853.8	E939.3	E950.3	E962.0	E980.3
Thiouracil	962.8	E858.0	E932.8	E950.4	E962.0	E980.4
Thiourea	962.8	E858.0	E932.8	E950.4	E962.0	E980.4
Thiphenamil	971.1	E855.4	E941.1	E950.4	E962.0	E980.4
Thiram NEC	989.4	E863.6	—	E950.6	E962.1	E980.7
medicinal	976.2	E858.7	E946.2	E950.4	E962.0	E980.4
Thonzylamine	963.0	E858.1	E933.0	E950.4	E962.0	E980.4
Thorazine	969.1	E853.0	E939.1	E950.3	E962.0	E980.3
Thornapple	988.2	E865.4	—	E950.9	E962.1	E980.9
Throat preparation (lozenges) NEC	976.6	E858.7	E946.6	E950.4	E962.0	E980.4
Thrombin	964.5	E858.2	E934.5	E950.4	E962.0	E980.4
Thrombolysin	964.4	E858.2	E934.4	E950.4	E962.0	E980.4
Thymol	983.0	E864.0	—	E950.7	E962.1	E980.6
Thymus extract	962.9	E858.0	E932.9	E950.4	E962.0	E980.4
Thyroglobulin	962.7	E858.0	E932.7	E950.4	E962.0	E980.4
Thyroid (derivatives) (extract)	962.7	E858.0	E932.7	E950.4	E962.0	E980.4
Thyrolar	962.7	E858.0	E932.7	E950.4	E962.0	E980.4
Thyrotrophin, thyrotropin	977.8	E858.8	E947.8	E950.4	E962.0	E980.4
Thyroxin(e)	962.7	E858.0	E932.7	E950.4	E962.0	E980.4
Tigan	963.0	E858.1	E933.0	E950.4	E962.0	E980.4
Tigloidine	968.0	E855.1	E938.0	E950.4	E962.0	E980.4
Tin (chloride) (dust) (oxide) NEC	985.8	E866.4	—	E950.9	E962.1	E980.9
anti-infectives	961.2	E857	E931.2	E950.4	E962.0	E980.4
Tinactin	976.0	E858.7	E946.0	E950.4	E962.0	E980.4
Tincture, iodine - see Iodine	—	—	—	—	—	—
Tindal	969.1	E853.0	E939.1	E950.3	E962.0	E980.3
Titanium (compounds) (vapor)	985.8	E866.4	—	E950.9	E962.1	E980.9
ointment	976.3	E858.7	E946.3	E950.4	E962.0	E980.4
Titroid	962.7	E858.0	E932.7	E950.4	E962.0	E980.4
TMTD - see Tetramethylthiuram disulfide	—	—	—	—	—	—
TNT	989.89	E866.8	—	E950.9	E962.1	E980.9
fumes	987.8	E869.8	—	E952.8	E962.2	E982.8
Toadstool	988.1	E865.5	—	E950.9	E962.1	E980.9
Tobacco NEC	989.84	E866.8	—	E950.9	E962.1	E980.9
Indian	988.2	E865.4	—	E950.9	E962.1	E980.9
smoke, second-hand	987.8	E869.4	—	—	—	—

TABLE OF DRUGS AND CHEMICALS / Tocopherol

Substance	Poisoning	External Cause (E Code)				
		Accident	Therapeutic Use	Suicide Attempt	Assault	Undetermined
Tocopherol	963.5	E858.1	E933.5	E950.4	E962.0	E980.4
Tocosamine	975.0	E858.6	E945.0	E950.4	E962.0	E980.4
Tofranil	969.05	E854.0	E939.0	E950.3	E962.0	E980.3
Toilet deodorizer	989.89	E866.8	—	E950.9	E962.1	E980.9
Tolazamide	962.3	E858.0	E932.3	E950.4	E962.0	E980.4
Tolazoline	971.3	E855.6	E941.3	E950.4	E962.0	E980.4
Tolbutamide	962.3	E858.0	E932.3	E950.4	E962.0	E980.4
sodium	977.8	E858.8	E947.8	E950.4	E962.0	E980.4
Tolmetin	965.69	E850.6	E935.6	E950.0	E962.0	E980.0
Tolnaftate	976.0	E858.7	E946.0	E950.4	E962.0	E980.4
Tolpropamine	976.1	E858.7	E946.1	E950.4	E962.0	E980.4
Tolserol	968.0	E855.1	E938.0	E950.4	E962.0	E980.4
Toluene (liquid) (vapor)	982.0	E862.4	—	E950.9	E962.1	E980.9
diisocyanate	983.0	E864.0	—	E950.7	E962.1	E980.6
Toluidine	983.0	E864.0	—	E950.7	E962.1	E980.6
vapor	987.8	E869.8	—	E952.8	E962.2	E982.8
Toluol (liquid) (vapor)	982.0	E862.4	—	E950.9	E962.1	E980.9
Tolylene-2,4-diisocyanate	983.0	E864.0	—	E950.7	E962.1	E980.6
Tonics, cardiac	972.1	E858.3	E942.1	E950.4	E962.0	E980.4
Toxaphene (dust) (spray)	989.2	E863.0	—	E950.6	E962.1	E980.7
Toxoids NEC	978.8	E858.8	E948.8	E950.4	E962.0	E980.4
Tractor fuel NEC	981	E862.1	—	E950.9	E962.1	E980.9
Tragacanth	973.3	E858.4	E943.3	E950.4	E962.0	E980.4
Tramazoline	971.2	E855.5	E941.2	E950.4	E962.0	E980.4
Tranquilizers	969.5	E853.9	E939.5	E950.3	E962.0	E980.3
benzodiazepine-based	969.4	E853.2	E939.4	E950.3	E962.0	E980.3
butyrophenone-based	969.2	E853.1	E939.2	E950.3	E962.0	E980.3
major NEC	969.3	E853.8	E939.3	E950.3	E962.0	E980.3
phenothiazine-based	969.1	E853.0	E939.1	E950.3	E962.0	E980.3
specified NEC	969.5	E853.8	E939.5	E950.3	E962.0	E980.3
Trantoin	961.9	E857	E931.9	E950.4	E962.0	E980.4
Tranxene	969.4	E853.2	E939.4	E950.3	E962.0	E980.3
Tranylcypromine (sulfate)	969.01	E854.0	E939.0	E950.3	E962.0	E980.3
Trasentine	975.1	E858.6	E945.1	E950.4	E962.0	E980.4
Travert	974.5	E858.5	E944.5	E950.4	E962.0	E980.4
Trecator	961.8	E857	E931.8	E950.4	E962.0	E980.4
Tretinoin	976.8	E858.7	E946.8	E950.4	E962.0	E980.4
Triacetin	976.0	E858.7	E946.0	E950.4	E962.0	E980.4

TABLE OF DRUGS AND CHEMICALS / Triflupromazine

| Substance | Poisoning | External Cause (E Code) |||||
		Accident	Therapeutic Use	Suicide Attempt	Assault	Undetermined
Triacetyloleandomycin	960.3	E856	E930.3	E950.4	E962.0	E980.4
Triamcinolone	962.0	E858.0	E932.0	E950.4	E962.0	E980.4
ENT agent	976.6	E858.7	E946.6	E950.4	E962.0	E980.4
ophthalmic preparation	976.5	E858.7	E946.5	E950.4	E962.0	E980.4
topical NEC	976.0	E858.7	E946.0	E950.4	E962.0	E980.4
Triamterene	974.4	E858.5	E944.4	E950.4	E962.0	E980.4
Triaziquone	963.1	E858.1	E933.1	E950.4	E962.0	E980.4
Tribromacetaldehyde	967.3	E852.2	E937.3	E950.2	E962.0	E980.2
Tribromoethanol	968.2	E855.1	E938.2	E950.4	E962.0	E980.4
Tribromomethane	967.3	E852.2	E937.3	E950.2	E962.0	E980.2
Trichlorethane	982.3	E862.4	—	E950.9	E962.1	E980.9
Trichlormethiazide	974.3	E858.5	E944.3	E950.4	E962.0	E980.4
Trichloroacetic acid	983.1	E864.1	—	E950.7	E962.1	E980.6
medicinal (keratolytic)	976.4	E858.7	E946.4	E950.4	E962.0	E980.4
Trichloroethanol	967.1	E852.0	E937.1	E950.2	E962.0	E980.2
Trichloroethylene (liquid) (vapor)	982.3	E862.4	—	E950.9	E962.1	E980.9
anesthetic (gas)	968.2	E855.1	E938.2	E950.4	E962.0	E980.4
Trichloroethyl phosphate	967.1	E852.0	E937.1	E950.2	E962.0	E980.2
Trichlorofluoromethane NEC	987.4	E869.2	—	E952.8	E962.2	E982.8
Trichlorotriethylamine	963.1	E858.1	E933.1	E950.4	E962.0	E980.4
Trichomonacides NEC	961.5	E857	E931.5	E950.4	E962.0	E980.4
Trichomycin	960.1	E856	E930.1	E950.4	E962.0	E980.4
Triclofos	967.1	E852.0	E937.1	E950.2	E962.0	E980.2
Tricresyl phosphate	989.89	E866.8	—	E950.9	E962.1	E980.9
solvent	982.8	E862.4	—	E950.9	E962.1	E980.9
Tricyclamol	966.4	E855.0	E936.4	E950.4	E962.0	E980.4
Tridesilon	976.0	E858.7	E946.0	E950.4	E962.0	E980.4
Tridihexethyl	971.1	E855.4	E941.1	E950.4	E962.0	E980.4
Tridione	966.0	E855.0	E936.0	E950.4	E962.0	E980.4
Triethanolamine NEC	983.2	E864.2	—	E950.7	E962.1	E980.6
detergent	983.2	E861.0	—	E950.7	E962.1	E980.6
trinitrate	972.4	E858.3	E942.4	E950.4	E962.0	E980.4
Triethanomelamine	963.1	E858.1	E933.1	E950.4	E962.0	E980.4
Triethylene melamine	963.1	E858.1	E933.1	E950.4	E962.0	E980.4
Triethylenephosphoramide	963.1	E858.1	E933.1	E950.4	E962.0	E980.4
Triethylenethiophosphoramide	963.1	E858.1	E933.1	E950.4	E962.0	E980.4
Trifluoperazine	969.1	E853.0	E939.1	E950.3	E962.0	E980.3
Trifluperidol	969.2	E853.1	E939.2	E950.3	E962.0	E980.3
Triflupromazine	969.1	E853.0	E939.1	E950.3	E962.0	E980.3

TABLE OF DRUGS AND CHEMICALS / Trihexyphenidyl

Substance	Poisoning	External Cause (E Code)				
		Accident	Therapeutic Use	Suicide Attempt	Assault	Undetermined
Trihexyphenidyl	971.1	E855.4	E941.1	E950.4	E962.0	E980.4
Triiodothyronine	962.7	E858.0	E932.7	E950.4	E962.0	E980.4
Trilene	968.2	E855.1	E938.2	E950.4	E962.0	E980.4
Trimeprazine	963.0	E858.1	E933.0	E950.4	E962.0	E980.4
Trimetazidine	972.4	E858.3	E942.4	E950.4	E962.0	E980.4
Trimethadione	966.0	E855.0	E936.0	E950.4	E962.0	E980.4
Trimethaphan	972.3	E858.3	E942.3	E950.4	E962.0	E980.4
Trimethidinium	972.3	E858.3	E942.3	E950.4	E962.0	E980.4
Trimethobenzamide	963.0	E858.1	E933.0	E950.4	E962.0	E980.4
Trimethylcarbinol	980.8	E860.8	—	E950.9	E962.1	E980.9
Trimethylpsoralen	976.3	E858.7	E946.3	E950.4	E962.0	E980.4
Trimeton	963.0	E858.1	E933.0	E950.4	E962.0	E980.4
Trimipramine	969.05	E854.0	E939.0	E950.3	E962.0	E980.3
Trimustine	963.1	E858.1	E933.1	E950.4	E962.0	E980.4
Trinitrin	972.4	E858.3	E942.4	E950.4	E962.0	E980.4
Trinitrophenol	983.0	E864.0	—	E950.7	E962.1	E980.6
Trinitrotoluene	989.89	E866.8	—	E950.9	E962.1	E980.9
fumes	987.8	E869.8	—	E952.8	E962.2	E982.8
Trional	967.8	E852.8	E937.8	E950.2	E962.0	E980.2
Trioxide of arsenic - *see* Arsenic	—	—	—	—	—	—
Trioxsalen	976.3	E858.7	E946.3	E950.4	E962.0	E980.4
Tripelennamine	963.0	E858.1	E933.0	E950.4	E962.0	E980.4
Triperidol	969.2	E853.1	E939.2	E950.3	E962.0	E980.3
Triprolidine	963.0	E858.1	E933.0	E950.4	E962.0	E980.4
Trisoralen	976.3	E858.7	E946.3	E950.4	E962.0	E980.4
Troleandomycin	960.3	E856	E930.3	E950.4	E962.0	E980.4
Trolnitrate (phosphate)	972.4	E858.3	E942.4	E950.4	E962.0	E980.4
Trometamol	963.3	E858.1	E933.3	E950.4	E962.0	E980.4
Tromethamine	963.3	E858.1	E933.3	E950.4	E962.0	E980.4
Tronothane	968.5	E855.2	E938.5	E950.4	E962.0	E980.4
Tropicamide	971.1	E855.4	E941.1	E950.4	E962.0	E980.4
Troxidone	966.0	E855.0	E936.0	E950.4	E962.0	E980.4
Tryparsamide	961.1	E857	E931.1	E950.4	E962.0	E980.4
Trypsin	963.4	E858.1	E933.4	E950.4	E962.0	E980.4
Tryptizol	969.05	E854.0	E939.0	E950.3	E962.0	E980.3
Tuaminoheptane	971.2	E855.5	E941.2	E950.4	E962.0	E980.4
Tuberculin (old)	977.8	E858.8	E947.8	E950.4	E962.0	E980.4
Tubocurare	975.2	E858.6	E945.2	E950.4	E962.0	E980.4
Tubocurarine	975.2	E858.6	E945.2	E950.4	E962.0	E980.4

◀ New ◀◀◀ Revised ~~deleted~~ Deleted ● Use Additional Digit(s)

TABLE OF DRUGS AND CHEMICALS / Vaccine NEC

Substance	Poisoning	External Cause (E Code)				
		Accident	Therapeutic Use	Suicide Attempt	Assault	Undetermined
Turkish green	969.6	E854.1	E939.6	E950.3	E962.0	E980.3
Turpentine (spirits of) (liquid) (vapor)	982.8	E862.4	—	E950.9	E962.1	E980.9
Tybamate	969.5	E853.8	E939.5	E950.3	E962.0	E980.3
Tyloxapol	975.5	E858.6	E945.5	E950.4	E962.0	E980.4
Tymazoline	971.2	E855.5	E941.2	E950.4	E962.0	E980.4
Typhoid vaccine	978.1	E858.8	E948.1	E950.4	E962.0	E980.4
Typhus vaccine	979.2	E858.8	E949.2	E950.4	E962.0	E980.4
Tyrothricin	976.0	E858.7	E946.0	E950.4	E962.0	E980.4
ENT agent	976.6	E858.7	E946.6	E950.4	E962.0	E980.4
ophthalmic preparation	976.5	E858.7	E946.5	E950.4	E962.0	E980.4
Undecenoic acid	976.0	E858.7	E946.0	E950.4	E962.0	E980.4
Undecylenic acid	976.0	E858.7	E946.0	E950.4	E962.0	E980.4
Unna's boot	976.3	E858.7	E946.3	E950.4	E962.0	E980.4
Uracil mustard	963.1	E858.1	E933.1	E950.4	E962.0	E980.4
Uramustine	963.1	E858.1	E933.1	E950.4	E962.0	E980.4
Urari	975.2	E858.6	E945.2	E950.4	E962.0	E980.4
Urea	974.4	E858.5	E944.4	E950.4	E962.0	E980.4
topical	976.8	E858.7	E946.8	E950.4	E962.0	E980.4
Urethan(e) (antineoplastic)	963.1	E858.1	E933.1	E950.4	E962.0	E980.4
Urginea (maritima) (scilla) - see Squill	—	—	—	—	—	—
Uric acid metabolism agents NEC	974.7	E858.5	E944.7	E950.4	E962.0	E980.4
Urokinase	964.4	E858.2	E934.4	E950.4	E962.0	E980.4
Urokon	977.8	E858.8	E947.8	E950.4	E962.0	E980.4
Urotropin	961.9	E857	E931.9	E950.4	E962.0	E980.4
Urtica	988.2	E865.4	—	E950.9	E962.1	E980.9
Utility gas - see Gas, utility	—	—	—	—	—	—
Vaccine NEC	979.9	E858.8	E949.9	E950.4	E962.0	E980.4
bacterial NEC	978.8	E858.8	E948.8	E950.4	E962.0	E980.4
with	—	—	—	—	—	—
other bacterial component	978.9	E858.8	E948.9	E950.4	E962.0	E980.4
pertussis component	978.6	E858.8	E948.6	E950.4	E962.0	E980.4
viral-rickettsial component	979.7	E858.8	E949.7	E950.4	E962.0	E980.4
mixed NEC	978.9	E858.8	E948.9	E950.4	E962.0	E980.4
BCG	978.0	E858.8	E948.0	E950.4	E962.0	E980.4
cholera	978.2	E858.8	E948.2	E950.4	E962.0	E980.4
diphtheria	978.5	E858.8	E948.5	E950.4	E962.0	E980.4
influenza	979.6	E858.8	E949.6	E950.4	E962.0	E980.4

◀ New   ⬅ Revised   ~~deleted~~ Deleted   ● Use Additional Digit(s)

TABLE OF DRUGS AND CHEMICALS / Vaccine NEC

Substance	Poisoning	External Cause (E Code)				
		Accident	Therapeutic Use	Suicide Attempt	Assault	Undetermined
Vaccine NEC *(Continued)*						
measles	979.4	E858.8	E949.4	E950.4	E962.0	E980.4
meningococcal	978.8	E858.8	E948.8	E950.4	E962.0	E980.4
mumps	979.6	E858.8	E949.6	E950.4	E962.0	E980.4
paratyphoid	978.1	E858.8	E948.1	E950.4	E962.0	E980.4
pertussis (with diphtheria toxoid) (with tetanus toxoid)	978.6	E858.8	E948.6	E950.4	E962.0	E980.4
plague	978.3	E858.8	E948.3	E950.4	E962.0	E980.4
poliomyelitis	979.5	E858.8	E949.5	E950.4	E962.0	E980.4
poliovirus	979.5	E858.8	E949.5	E950.4	E962.0	E980.4
rabies	979.1	E858.8	E949.1	E950.4	E962.0	E980.4
respiratory syncytial virus	979.6	E858.8	E949.6	E950.4	E962.0	E980.4
rickettsial NEC	979.6	E858.8	E949.6	E950.4	E962.0	E980.4
with	—	—	—	—	—	—
bacterial component	979.7	E858.8	E949.7	E950.4	E962.0	E980.4
pertussis component	978.6	E858.8	E948.6	E950.4	E962.0	E980.4
viral component	979.7	E858.8	E949.7	E950.4	E962.0	E980.4
Rocky Mountain spotted fever	979.6	E858.8	E949.6	E950.4	E962.0	E980.4
rotavirus	979.6	E858.8	E949.6	E950.4	E962.0	E980.4
rubella virus	979.4	E858.8	E949.4	E950.4	E962.0	E980.4
sabin oral	979.5	E858.8	E949.5	E950.4	E962.0	E980.4
smallpox	979.0	E858.8	E949.0	E950.4	E962.0	E980.4
tetanus	978.4	E858.8	E948.4	E950.4	E962.0	E980.4
typhoid	978.1	E858.8	E948.1	E950.4	E962.0	E980.4
typhus	979.2	E858.8	E949.2	E950.4	E962.0	E980.4
viral NEC	979.6	E858.8	E949.6	E950.4	E962.0	E980.4
with	—	—	—	—	—	—
bacterial component	979.7	E858.8	E949.7	E950.4	E962.0	E980.4
pertussis component	978.6	E858.8	E948.6	E950.4	E962.0	E980.4
rickettsial component	979.7	E858.8	E949.7	E950.4	E962.0	E980.4
yellow fever	979.3	E858.8	E949.3	E950.4	E962.0	E980.4
Vaccinia immune globulin (human)	964.6	E858.2	E934.6	E950.4	E962.0	E980.4
Vaginal contraceptives	976.8	E858.7	E946.8	E950.4	E962.0	E980.4
Valethamate	971.1	E855.4	E941.1	E950.4	E962.0	E980.4
Valisone	976.0	E858.7	E946.0	E950.4	E962.0	E980.4
Valium	969.4	E853.2	E939.4	E950.3	E962.0	E980.3
Valmid	967.8	E852.8	E937.8	E950.2	E962.0	E980.2
Vanadium	985.8	E866.4	—	E950.9	E962.1	E980.9
Vancomycin	960.8	E856	E930.8	E950.4	E962.0	E980.4

TABLE OF DRUGS AND CHEMICALS / Viagra

Substance	Poisoning	External Cause (E Code)				
		Accident	Therapeutic Use	Suicide Attempt	Assault	Undetermined
Vapor (see also Gas)	987.9	E869.9	—	E952.9	E962.2	E982.9
kiln (carbon monoxide)	986	E868.8	—	E952.1	E962.2	E982.1
lead - see Lead	—	—	—	—	—	—
specified source NEC - (see also specific substance)	987.8	E869.8	—	E952.8	E962.2	E982.8
Varidase	964.4	E858.2	E934.4	E950.4	E962.0	E980.4
Varnish	989.89	E861.6	—	E950.9	E962.1	E980.9
cleaner	982.8	E862.9	—	E950.9	E962.1	E980.9
Vaseline	976.3	E858.7	E946.3	E950.4	E962.0	E980.4
Vasodilan	972.5	E858.3	E942.5	E950.4	E962.0	E980.4
Vasodilators NEC	972.5	E858.3	E942.5	E950.4	E962.0	E980.4
coronary	972.4	E858.3	E942.4	E950.4	E962.0	E980.4
Vasopressin	962.5	E858.0	E932.5	E950.4	E962.0	E980.4
Vasopressor drugs	962.5	E858.0	E932.5	E950.4	E962.0	E980.4
Venom, venomous (bite) (sting)	989.5	E905.9	—	E950.9	E962.1	E980.9
arthropod NEC	989.5	E905.5	—	E950.9	E962.1	E980.9
bee	989.5	E905.3	—	E950.9	E962.1	E980.9
centipede	989.5	E905.4	—	E950.9	E962.1	E980.9
hornet	989.5	E905.3	—	E950.9	E962.1	E980.9
lizard	989.5	E905.0	—	E950.9	E962.1	E980.9
marine animals or plants	989.5	E905.6	—	E950.9	E962.1	E980.9
millipede (tropical)	989.5	E905.4	—	E950.9	E962.1	E980.9
plant NEC	989.5	E905.7	—	E950.9	E962.1	E980.9
marine	989.5	E905.6	—	E950.9	E962.1	E980.9
scorpion	989.5	E905.2	—	E950.9	E962.1	E980.9
snake	989.5	E905.0	—	E950.9	E962.1	E980.9
specified NEC	989.5	E905.8	—	E950.9	E962.1	E980.9
spider	989.5	E905.1	—	E950.9	E962.1	E980.9
wasp	989.5	E905.3	—	E950.9	E962.1	E980.9
Ventolin - see Salbutamol sulfate	—	—	—	—	—	—
Veramon	967.0	E851	E937.0	E950.1	E962.0	E980.1
Veratrum	—	—	—	—	—	—
album	988.2	E865.4	—	E950.9	E962.1	E980.9
alkaloids	972.6	E858.3	E942.6	E950.4	E962.0	E980.4
viride	988.2	E865.4	—	E950.9	E962.1	E980.9
Verdigris (see also Copper)	985.8	E866.4	—	E950.9	E962.1	E980.9
Veronal	967.0	E851	E937.0	E950.1	E962.0	E980.1
Veroxil	961.6	E857	E931.6	E950.4	E962.0	E980.4
Versidyne	965.7	E850.7	E935.7	E950.0	E962.0	E980.0
Viagra	972.5	E858.3	E942.5	E950.4	E962.0	E980.4

◀ New   ◀▦ Revised   deleted Deleted   ● Use Additional Digit(s)

TABLE OF DRUGS AND CHEMICALS / Vienna

Substance	Poisoning	External Cause (E Code) Accident	Therapeutic Use	Suicide Attempt	Assault	Undetermined
Vienna	—	—	—	—	—	—
green	985.1	E866.3	—	E950.8	E962.1	E980.8
insecticide	985.1	E863.4	—	E950.6	E962.1	E980.7
red	989.89	E866.8	—	E950.9	E962.1	E980.9
pharmaceutical dye	977.4	E858.8	E947.4	E950.4	E962.0	E980.4
Vinbarbital, vinbarbitone	967.0	E851	E937.0	E950.1	E962.0	E980.1
Vinblastine	963.1	E858.1	E933.1	E950.4	E962.0	E980.4
Vincristine	963.1	E858.1	E933.1	E950.4	E962.0	E980.4
Vinesthene, vinethene	968.2	E855.1	E938.2	E950.4	E962.0	E980.4
Vinyl	—	—	—	—	—	—
bital	967.0	E851	E937.0	E950.1	E962.0	E980.1
ether	968.2	E855.1	E938.2	E950.4	E962.0	E980.4
Vioform	961.3	E857	E931.3	E950.4	E962.0	E980.4
topical	976.0	E858.7	E946.0	E950.4	E962.0	E980.4
Viomycin	960.6	E856	E930.6	E950.4	E962.0	E980.4
Viosterol	963.5	E858.1	E933.5	E950.4	E962.0	E980.4
Viper (venom)	989.5	E905.0	—	E950.9	E962.1	E980.9
Viprynium (embonate)	961.6	E857	E931.6	E950.4	E962.0	E980.4
Virugon	961.7	E857	E931.7	E950.4	E962.0	E980.4
Visine	976.5	E858.7	E946.5	E950.4	E962.0	E980.4
Vitamins NEC	963.5	E858.1	E933.5	E950.4	E962.0	E980.4
B_{12}	964.1	E858.2	E934.1	E950.4	E962.0	E980.4
hematopoietic	964.1	E858.2	E934.1	E950.4	E962.0	E980.4
K	964.3	E858.2	E934.3	E950.4	E962.0	E980.4
Vleminckx's solution	976.4	E858.7	E946.4	E950.4	E962.0	E980.4
Voltaren - see Diclofenac sodium	—	—	—	—	—	—
Warfarin (potassium) (sodium)	964.2	E858.2	E934.2	E950.4	E962.0	E980.4
rodenticide	989.4	E863.7	—	E950.6	E962.1	E980.7
Wasp (sting)	989.5	E905.3	—	E950.9	E962.1	E980.9
Water	—	—	—	—	—	—
balance agents NEC	974.5	E858.5	E944.5	E950.4	E962.0	E980.4
gas	987.1	E868.1	—	E951.8	E962.2	E981.8
incomplete combustion of - see Carbon, monoxide, fuel, utility	—	—	—	—	—	—
hemlock	988.2	E865.4	—	E950.9	E962.1	E980.9
moccasin (venom)	989.5	E905.0	—	E950.9	E962.1	E980.9
Wax (paraffin) (petroleum)	981	E862.3	—	E950.9	E962.1	E980.9
automobile	989.89	E861.2	—	E950.9	E962.1	E980.9
floor	981	E862.0	—	E950.9	E962.1	E980.9
Weed killers NEC	989.4	E863.5	—	E950.6	E962.1	E980.7

TABLE OF DRUGS AND CHEMICALS / Zerone

Substance	Poisoning	External Cause (E Code) Accident	Therapeutic Use	Suicide Attempt	Assault	Undetermined
Welldorm	967.1	E852.0	E937.1	E950.2	E962.0	E980.2
White	—	—	—	—	—	—
arsenic - *see* Arsenic	—	—	—	—	—	—
hellebore	988.2	E865.4	—	E950.9	E962.1	E980.9
lotion (keratolytic)	976.4	E858.7	E946.4	E950.4	E962.0	E980.4
spirit	981	E862.0	—	E950.9	E962.1	E980.9
Whitewashes	989.89	E861.6	—	E950.9	E962.1	E980.9
Whole blood	964.7	E858.2	E934.7	E950.4	E962.0	E980.4
Wild	—	—	—	—	—	—
black cherry	988.2	E865.4	—	E950.9	E962.1	E980.9
poisonous plants NEC	988.2	E865.4	—	E950.9	E962.1	E980.9
Window cleaning fluid	989.89	E861.3	—	E950.9	E962.1	E980.9
Wintergreen (oil)	976.3	E858.7	E946.3	E950.4	E962.0	E980.4
Witch hazel	976.2	E858.7	E946.2	E950.4	E962.0	E980.4
Wood	—	—	—	—	—	—
alcohol	980.1	E860.2	—	E950.9	E962.1	E980.9
spirit	980.1	E860.2	—	E950.9	E962.1	E980.9
Woorali	975.2	E858.6	E945.2	E950.4	E962.0	E980.4
Wormseed, American	961.6	E857	E931.6	E950.4	E962.0	E980.4
Xanthine diuretics	974.1	E858.5	E944.1	E950.4	E962.0	E980.4
Xanthocillin	960.0	E856	E930.0	E950.4	E962.0	E980.4
Xanthotoxin	976.3	E858.7	E946.3	E950.4	E962.0	E980.4
Xigris	964.2	E858.2	E934.2	E950.4	E962.0	E980.4
Xylene (liquid) (vapor)	982.0	E862.4	—	E950.9	E962.1	E980.9
Xylocaine (infiltration) (topical)	968.5	E855.2	E938.5	E950.4	E962.0	E980.4
nerve block (peripheral) (plexus)	968.6	E855.2	E938.6	E950.4	E962.0	E980.4
spinal	968.7	E855.2	E938.7	E950.4	E962.0	E980.4
Xylol (liquid) (vapor)	982.0	E862.4	—	E950.9	E962.1	E980.9
Xylometazoline	971.2	E855.5	E941.2	E950.4	E962.0	E980.4
Yellow	—	—	—	—	—	—
fever vaccine	979.3	E858.8	E949.3	E950.4	E962.0	E980.4
jasmine	988.2	E865.4	—	E950.9	E962.1	E980.9
Yew	988.2	E865.4	—	E950.9	E962.1	E980.9
Zactane	965.7	E850.7	E935.7	E950.0	E962.0	E980.0
Zaroxolyn	974.3	E858.5	E944.3	E950.4	E962.0	E980.4
Zephiran (topical)	976.0	E858.7	E946.0	E950.4	E962.0	E980.4
ophthalmic preparation	976.5	E858.7	E946.5	E950.4	E962.0	E980.4
Zerone	980.1	E860.2	—	E950.9	E962.1	E980.9

TABLE OF DRUGS AND CHEMICALS / Zinc NEC

		External Cause (E Code)				
Substance	Poisoning	Accident	Therapeutic Use	Suicide Attempt	Assault	Undetermined
Zinc (compounds) (fumes) (salts) (vapor) NEC	985.8	E866.4	—	E950.9	E962.1	E980.9
anti-infectives	976.0	E858.7	E946.0	E950.4	E962.0	E980.4
antivaricose	972.7	E858.3	E942.7	E950.4	E962.0	E980.4
bacitracin	976.0	E858.7	E946.0	E950.4	E962.0	E980.4
chloride	976.2	E858.7	E946.2	E950.4	E962.0	E980.4
gelatin	976.3	E858.7	E946.3	E950.4	E962.0	E980.4
oxide	976.3	E858.7	E946.3	E950.4	E962.0	E980.4
peroxide	976.0	E858.7	E946.0	E950.4	E962.0	E980.4
pesticides	985.8	E863.4	—	E950.6	E962.1	E980.7
phosphide (rodenticide)	985.8	E863.7	—	E950.6	E962.1	E980.7
stearate	976.3	E858.7	E946.3	E950.4	E962.0	E980.4
sulfate (antivaricose)	972.7	E858.3	E942.7	E950.4	E962.0	E980.4
ENT agent	976.6	E858.7	E946.6	E950.4	E962.0	E980.4
ophthalmic solution	976.5	E858.7	E946.5	E950.4	E962.0	E980.4
topical NEC	976.0	E858.7	E946.0	E950.4	E962.0	E980.4
undecylenate	976.0	E858.7	E946.0	E950.4	E962.0	E980.4
Zovant	964.2	E858.2	E934.2	E950.4	E962.0	E980.4
Zoxazolamine	968.0	E855.1	E938.0	E950.4	E962.0	E980.4
Zygadenus (venenosus)	988.2	E865.4	—	E950.9	E962.1	E980.9
Zyprexa	969.3	E853.8	E939.3	E950.3	E962.0	E980.3

SECTION III

INDEX TO EXTERNAL CAUSES OF INJURY (E CODE)

This section contains the index to the codes which classify environmental events, circumstances, and other conditions as the cause of injury and other adverse effects. Where a code from the section Supplementary Classification of External Causes of Injury and Poisoning (E800–E998) is applicable, it is intended that the E code shall be used in addition to a code from the main body of the classification, Chapters 1 to 17.

The alphabetic index to the E codes is organized by main terms which describe the accident, circumstance, event, or specific agent which caused the injury or other adverse effect.

Note: Transport accidents (E800–E848) include accidents involving:

>aircraft and spacecraft (E840–E845)
>watercraft (E830–E838)
>motor vehicle (E810–E825)
>railway (E800–E807)
>other road vehicles (E826–E829)

For definitions and examples related to transport accidents - *see* Supplementary Classification of External Causes of Injury and Poisoning (E800–E999).

The fourth-digit subdivisions for use with categories E800–E848 to identify the injured person are found at the end of this section.

For identifying the place in which an accident or poisoning occurred (circumstances classifiable to categories E850–E869 and E880–E928) - *see* the listing in this section under "Accident, occurring."

See the Table of Drugs and Chemicals (Section 2 of this volume) for identifying the specific agent involved in drug overdose or a wrong substance given or taken in error, and for intoxication or poisoning by a drug or other chemical substance.

The specific adverse effect, reaction, or localized toxic effect to a correct drug or substance properly administered in therapeutic or prophylactic dosage should be classified according to the nature of the adverse effect (e.g., allergy, dermatitis, tachycardia) listed in Section I of this volume.

INDEX TO EXTERNAL CAUSES OF INJURY / Abandonment

A

Abandonment
  causing exposure to weather conditions - *see* Exposure
  child, with intent to injure or kill E968.4
  helpless person, infant, newborn E904.0
    with intent to injure or kill E968.4

Abortion, criminal, injury to child E968.8

Abuse (alleged) (suspected)
  adult
    by
      child E967.4
      ex-partner E967.3
      ex-spouse E967.3
      father E967.0
      grandchild E967.7
      grandparent E967.6
      mother E967.2
      non-related caregiver E967.8
      other relative E967.7
      other specified person E967.1
      partner E967.3
      sibling E967.5
      spouse E967.3
      stepfather E967.0
      stepmother E967.2
      unspecified person E967.9
  child
    by
      boyfriend of parent or guardian E967.0
      child E967.4
      father E967.0
      female partner of parent or guardian E967.2
      girlfriend of parent or guardian E967.2
      grandchild E967.7
      grandparent E967.6
      male partner of parent or guardian E967.0
      mother E967.2
      non-related caregiver E967.8
      other relative E967.7
      other specified person(s) E967.1
      sibling E967.5
      stepfather E967.0
      stepmother E967.2
      unspecified person E967.9

Accident (to) E928.9
  aircraft (in transit) (powered) E841●
    at landing, take-off E840●
    due to, caused by cataclysm - *see* categories E908, E909
    late effect of E929.1
    unpowered (*see also* Collision, aircraft, unpowered) E842●
    while alighting, boarding E843●
  amphibious vehicle
    on
      land - *see* Accident, motor vehicle
      water - *see* Accident, watercraft
  animal, ridden NEC E828●
  animal-drawn vehicle NEC E827●
  balloon (*see also* Collision, aircraft, unpowered) E842●
  caused by, due to
    abrasive wheel (metalworking) E919.3
    animal NEC E906.9
      being ridden (in sport or transport) E828●
    avalanche NEC E909.2
    band saw E919.4
    bench saw E919.4
    bore, earth-drilling or mining (land) (seabed) E919.1
    bulldozer E919.7
    cataclysmic
      earth surface movement or eruption E909.9
      storm E908.9

Accident (*Continued*)
  caused by, due to (*Continued*)
    chain
      hoist E919.2
        agricultural operations E919.0
        mining operations E919.1
      saw E920.1
    circular saw E919.4
    cold (excessive) (*see also* Cold, exposure to) E901.9
    combine E919.0
      conflagration - *see* Conflagration
    corrosive liquid, substance NEC E924.1
    cotton gin E919.8
    crane E919.2
      agricultural operations E919.0
      mining operations E919.1
    cutting or piercing instrument (*see also* Cut) E920.9
    dairy equipment E919.8
    derrick E919.2
      agricultural operations E919.0
      mining operations E919.1
    drill E920.1
      earth (land) (seabed) E919.1
      hand (powered) E920.1
        not powered E920.4
      metalworking E919.3
      woodworking E919.4
    earth(-)
      drilling machine E919.1
      moving machine E919.7
      scraping machine E919.7
    electric
      current (*see also* Electric shock) E925.9
      motor - *see also* Accident, machine, by type of machine
        current (of) - *see* Electric shock
    elevator (building) (grain) E919.2
      agricultural operations E919.0
      mining operations E919.1
    environmental factors NEC E928.9
    excavating machine E919.7
    explosive material (*see also* Explosion) E923.9
    farm machine E919.0
    fire, flames - *see also* Fire
      conflagration - *see* Conflagration
    firearm missile - *see* Shooting
    forging (metalworking) machine E919.3
    forklift (truck) E919.2
      agricultural operations E919.0
      mining operations E919.1
    gas turbine E919.5
    harvester E919.0
    hay derrick, mower, or rake E919.0
    heat (excessive) (*see also* Heat) E900.9
    hoist (*see also* Accident, caused by, due to, lift) E919.2
      chain - *see* Accident, caused by, due to, chain
      shaft E919.1
    hot
      liquid E924.0
        caustic or corrosive E924.1
      object (not producing fire or flames) E924.8
      substance E924.9
        caustic or corrosive E924.1
        liquid (metal) NEC E924.0
        specified type NEC E924.8
    human bite E928.3
    ignition - *see* Ignition E919.4
    internal combustion engine E919.5
    landslide NEC E909.2
    lathe (metalworking) E919.3
      turnings E920.8
      woodworking E919.4

Accident (*Continued*)
  caused by, due to (*Continued*)
    lift, lifting (appliances) E919.2
      agricultural operations E919.0
      mining operations E919.1
      shaft E919.1
    lightning NEC E907
    machine, machinery - *see also* Accident, machine
      drilling, metal E919.3
      manufacturing, for manufacture of steam
        beverages E919.8
        clothing E919.8
        foodstuffs E919.8
        paper E919.8
        textiles E919.8
      milling, metal E919.3
      moulding E919.4
      power press, metal E919.3
      printing E919.8
      rolling mill, metal E919.3
      sawing, metal E919.3
      specified type NEC E919.8
      spinning E919.8
      weaving E919.8
    natural factor NEC E928.9
    overhead plane E919.4
    plane E920.4
      overhead E919.4
    powered
      hand tool NEC E920.1
      saw E919.4
      hand E920.1
    printing machine E919.8
    pulley (block) E919.2
      agricultural operations E919.0
      mining operations E919.1
      transmission E919.6
    radial saw E919.4
    radiation - *see* Radiation
    reaper E919.0
    road scraper E919.7
      when in transport under its own power - *see* categories E810–E825
    roller, coaster E919.8
    sander E919.4
    saw E920.4
      band E919.4
      bench E919.4
      chain E920.1
      circular E919.4
      hand E920.4
        powered E920.1
      powered, except hand E919.4
      radial E919.4
    sawing machine, metal E919.3
    shaft
      hoist E919.1
      lift E919.1
      transmission E919.6
    shears E920.4
      hand E920.4
        powered E920.1
      mechanical E919.3
    shovel E920.4
      steam E919.7
    spinning machine E919.8
    steam - *see also* Burning, steam
      engine E919.5
      shovel E919.7
    thresher E919.0
    thunderbolt NEC E907
    tractor E919.0
      when in transport under its own power - *see* categories E810–E825
    transmission belt, cable, chain, gear, pinion, pulley, shaft E919.6
    turbine (gas) (water driven) E919.5
    under-cutter E919.1
    weaving machine E919.8

INDEX TO EXTERNAL CAUSES OF INJURY / Accident

Accident (Continued)
  caused by, due to (Continued)
    winch E919.2
      agricultural operations E919.0
      mining operations E919.1
    diving E883.0
      with insufficient air supply E913.2
    glider (hang) (see also Collision, aircraft, unpowered) E842 •
    hovercraft
      on
        land - see Accident, motor vehicle
        water - see Accident, watercraft
    ice yacht (see also Accident, vehicle NEC) E848
    in
      medical, surgical procedure
        as, or due to misadventure - see Misadventure
        causing an abnormal reaction or later complication without mention of misadventure - see Reaction, abnormal
    kite carrying a person (see also Collision, involving aircraft, unpowered) E842 •
    land yacht (see also Accident, vehicle NEC) E848
    late effect of - see Late effect
    launching pad E845 •
    machine, machinery (see also Accident, caused by, due to, by specific type of machine) E919.9
      agricultural including animal-powered premises E919.0
      earth-drilling E919.1
      earth moving or scraping E919.7
      excavating E919.7
      involving transport under own power on highway or transport vehicle - see categories E810-E825, E840-E845
      lifting (appliances) E919.2
      metalworking E919.3
      mining E919.1
      prime movers, except electric motors E919.5
        electric motors - see Accident, machine, by specific type of machine
      recreational E919.8
      specified type NEC E919.8
      transmission E919.6
      watercraft (deck) (engine room) (galley) (laundry) (loading) E836 •
      woodworking or forming E919.4
    motor vehicle (on public highway) (traffic) E819 •
      due to cataclysm - see categories E908, E909
      involving
        collision (see also Collision, motor vehicle) E812 •
        nontraffic, not on public highway - see categories E820–E825
        not involving collision - see categories E816–E819
    nonmotor vehicle NEC E829 •
      nonroad - see Accident, vehicle NEC
      road, except pedal cycle, animal-drawn vehicle, or animal being ridden E829 •
    nonroad vehicle NEC - see Accident, vehicle NEC
    not elsewhere classifiable involving
      cable car (not on rails) E847
        on rails E829 •
      coal car in mine E846
      hand truck - see Accident, vehicle NEC
      logging car E846
      sled(ge), meaning snow or ice vehicle E848
      tram, mine or quarry E846

Accident (Continued)
  not elsewhere classifiable involving (Continued)
    truck
      mine or quarry E846
      self-propelled, industrial E846
      station baggage E846
    tub, mine or quarry E846
    vehicle NEC E848
      snow and ice E848
      used only on industrial premises E846
    wheelbarrow E848
  occurring (at) (in)
    apartment E849.0
    baseball field, diamond E849.4
    construction site, any E849.3
    dock E849.8
      yard E849.3
    dormitory E849.7
    factory (building) (premises) E849.3
    farm E849.1
      buildings E849.1
      house E849.0
    football field E849.4
    forest E849.8
    garage (place of work) E849.3
      private (home) E849.0
    gravel pit E849.2
    gymnasium E849.4
    highway E849.5
    home (private) (residential) E849.0
      institutional E849.7
    hospital E849.7
    hotel E849.6
    house (private) (residential) E849.0
      movie E849.6
      public E849.6
    institution, residential E849.7
    jail E849.7
    mine E849.2
    motel E849.6
    movie house E849.6
    office (building) E849.6
    orphanage E849.7
    park (public) E849.4
      mobile home E849.8
      trailer E849.8
    parking lot or place E849.8
    place
      industrial NEC E849.3
      parking E849.8
      public E849.8
        specified place NEC E849.5
      recreational NEC E849.4
      sport NEC E849.4
    playground (park) (school) E849.4
    prison E849.6
    public building NEC E849.6
    quarry E849.2
    railway
      line NEC E849.8
      yard E849.3
    residence
      home (private) E849.0
    resort (beach) (lake) (mountain) (seashore) (vacation) E849.4
    restaurant E849.6
    sand pit E849.2
    school (building) (private) (public) (state) E849.6
      reform E849.7
      riding E849.4
    seashore E849.8
      resort E849.4
    shop (place of work) E849.3
      commercial E849.6
    skating rink E849.4
    sports palace E849.4
    stadium E849.4
    store E849.6
    street E849.5

Accident (Continued)
  occurring (Continued)
    swimming pool (public) E849.4
      private home or garden E849.0
    tennis court E849.4 public
    theatre, theater E849.6
    trailer court E849.8
    tunnel E849.8
      under construction E849.2
    warehouse E849.3
    yard
      dock E849.3
      industrial E849.3
      private (home) E849.0
      railway E849.3
  off-road type motor vehicle (not on public highway) NEC E821 •
    on public highway - see categories E810–E819
  pedal cycle E826 •
  railway E807 •
    due to cataclysm - see categories E908, E909
    involving
      burning by engine, locomotive, train (see also Explosion, railway engine) E803 •
      collision (see also Collision, railway) E800 •
      derailment (see also Derailment, railway) E802 •
      explosion (see also Explosion, railway engine) E803 •
      fall (see also Fall, from, railway rolling stock) E804 •
      fire (see also Explosion, railway engine) E803 •
      hitting by, being struck by
        object falling in, on, from, rolling stock, train, vehicle E806 •
        rolling stock, train, vehicle E805 •
      overturning, railway rolling stock, train, vehicle (see also Derailment, railway) E802 •
      running off rails, railway (see also Derailment, railway) E802 •
      specified circumstances NEC E806 •
      train or vehicle hit by
        avalanche E909.2
        falling object (earth, rock, tree) E806 •
          due to cataclysm - see categories E908, E909
        landslide E909.2
  roller skate E885.1
  scooter (nonmotorized) E885.0
  skateboard E885.2
  ski(ing) E885.3
    jump E884.9
    lift or tow (with chair or gondola) E847
  snow vehicle, motor driven (not on public highway) E820 •
    on public highway - see categories E810–E819
  snowboard E885.4
  spacecraft E845 •
  specified cause NEC E928.8
  street car E829 •
  traffic NEC E819 •
  vehicle NEC (with pedestrian) E848
    battery powered
      airport passenger vehicle E846
      truck (baggage) (mail) E846
    powered commercial or industrial (with other vehicle or object within commercial or industrial premises) E846

◀ New ⬅ Revised ~~deleted~~ Deleted Use Additional Digit(s) ▨ Omit code

615

INDEX TO EXTERNAL CAUSES OF INJURY / Accident

Accident (Continued)
- watercraft E838●
  - with
    - drowning or submersion resulting from
      - accident other than to watercraft E832●
      - accident to watercraft E830●
    - injury, except drowning or submersion, resulting from
      - accident other than to watercraft - see categories E833–E838
      - accident to watercraft E831●
  - due to, caused by cataclysm - see categories E908, E909
  - machinery E836●

Acid throwing E961

Acosta syndrome E902.0

Activity (involving) E030
- aerobic and step exercise (class) E009.2
- alpine skiing E003.2
- animal care NEC E019.9
- arts and handcrafts NEC E012.9
- athletics NEC E008.9
  - played
    - as a team or group NEC E007.9
    - individually NEC E006.9
- baking E015.2
- ballet E005.0
- barbells E010.2
- BASE (Building, Antenna, Span, Earth) jumping E004.2
- baseball E007.3
- basketball E007.6
- bathing (personal) E013.0
- beach volleyball E007.7
- bike riding E006.4
- boogie boarding E002.7
- bowling E006.3
- boxing E008.0
- brass instrument playing E018.3
- building and construction E016.2
- bungee jumping E004.3
- calisthenics E009.1
- canoeing (in calm and turbulent water) E002.5
- capture the flag E007.8
- cardiorespiratory exercise NEC E009.9
- caregiving (providing) NEC E014.9
  - bathing E014.0
  - lifting E014.1
- cellular
  - communication device E011.1
  - telephone E011.1
- challenge course E009.4
- cheerleading E005.4
- circuit training E009.3
- cleaning
  - floor E013.4
- climbing NEC E004.9
  - mountain E004.0
  - rock E004.0
  - wall climbing E004.0
- combatives E008.4
- computer
  - keyboarding E011.0
  - technology NEC E011.9
- confidence course E009.4
- construction (building) E016.2
- cooking and baking E015.2
- cooking and grilling NEC E015.9
- cool down exercises E009.1
- cricket E007.9
- crocheting E012.0
- cross country skiing E003.3
- dancing (all types) E005.0
- digging
  - dirt E016.0
- dirt digging E016.0
- dishwashing E015.0

Activity (Continued)
- diving (platform) (springboard) E002.1
  - underwater E002.4
- dodge ball E007.8
- downhill skiing E003.2
- drum playing E018.1
- dumbbells E010.2
- electronic
  - devices NEC E011.9
    - hand held interactive E011.1
  - game playing (using) (with)
    - interactive device E011.1
    - keyboard or other stationary device E011.0
- elliptical machine E009.0
- exercise(s)
  - machines ((primarily) for)
    - cardiorespiratory conditioning E009.0
    - muscle strengthening E010.0
  - muscle strengthening (non-machine) NEC E010.9
- external motion NEC E017.9
  - roller coaster E017.0
- field hockey E007.4
- figure skating (pairs) (singles) E003.0
- flag football E007.1
- floor mopping and cleaning E013.4
- food preparation and clean up E015.0
- football (American) NOS E007.0
  - flag E007.1
  - tackle E007.0
  - touch E007.1
- four square E007.8
- free weights E010.2
- frisbee (ultimate) E008.3
- furniture
  - building E012.2
  - finishing E012.2
  - repair E012.2
- game playing (electronic)
  - using
    - interactive device E011.1
    - keyboard or other stationary device E011.0
- gardening E016.1
- golf E006.2
- grass drills E009.5
- grilling and smoking food E015.1
- grooming and shearing an animal E019.2
- guerilla drills E009.5
- gymnastics (rhythmic) E005.2
- handball E008.2
- handcrafts NEC E012.9
- hand held interactive electronic device E011.1
- hang gliding E004.4
- hiking (on level or elevated terrain) E001.0
- hockey (ice) E003.1
  - field E007.4
- horseback riding E006.1
- household maintenance NEC E013.9
- ice NEC E003.9
  - dancing E003.0
  - hockey E003.1
  - skating E003.0
- inline roller skating E006.0
- ironing E013.3
- judo E008.4
- jumping (off) NEC E004.9
  - BASE (Building, Antenna, Span, Earth) E004.2
  - bungee E004.3
  - jacks E009.1
  - rope E006.5
- jumping jacks E009.1
- jumping rope E006.5
- karate E008.4
- kayaking (in calm and turbulent water) E002.5
- keyboarding (computer) E011.0
- kickball E007.8

Activity (Continued)
- knitting E012.0
- lacrosse E007.4
- land maintenance NEC E016.9
- landscaping E016.1
- laundry E013.1
- machines (exercise) primarily for cardiorespiratory conditioning E009.0
- maintenance
  - building E016.9
  - household NEC E013.9
  - land E016.9
  - property E016.9
- marching (on level or elevated terrain) E001.0
- martial arts E008.4
- microwave oven E015.2
- mopping (floor) E013.4
- mountain climbing E004.0
- milking an animal E019.1
- muscle strengthening
  - exercises (non-machine) NEC E010.9
  - machines E010.0
- musical keyboard (electronic) playing E018.0
- nordic skiing E003.3
- obstacle course E009.4
- oven (microwave) E015.2
- packing up and unpacking in moving to a new residence E013.5
- parasailing E002.9
- percussion instrument playing NEC E018.1
- personal
  - bathing and showering E013.0
  - hygiene NEC E013.8
  - showering E013.0
- physical
  - games generally associated with school recess, summer camp and children 007.8
  - training NEC E009.9
- piano playing E018.0
- pilates E010.3
- platform diving E002.1
- playing musical instrument
  - brass instrument E018.3
  - drum E018.1
  - musical keyboard (electronic) E018.0
  - percussion instrument NEC E018.1
  - piano E018.0
  - string instrument E018.2
  - wind instrument E018.3
- property maintenance NEC E016.9
- pruning (garden and lawn) E016.1
- pull-ups E010.1
- push-ups E010.1
- racquetball E008.2
- rafting (in calm and turbulent water) E002.5
- raking (leaves) E016.0
- rappelling E004.1
- refereeing a sports activity E029.0
- residential relocation E013.5
- rhythmic
  - gymnastics E005.2
  - movement NEC E005.9
- riding
  - horseback E006.1
  - roller coaster E017.0
- rock climbing E004.0
- roller coaster riding E017.0
- roller skating (inline) E006.0
- rough housing and horseplay E029.2
- rowing (in calm and turbulent water) E002.5
- rugby E007.2
- running E001.1
- SCUBA diving E002.4
- sewing E012.1
- shoveling E016.0
  - dirt E016.0
  - snow E016.0
- showering (personal) E013.0
- sit-ups E010.1

Activity (Continued)
  skateboarding E006.0
  skating (ice) E003.0
    roller E006.0
  skiing (alpine) (downhill) E003.2
    cross country E003.3
    nordic E003.3
  sledding (snow) E003.2
  smoking and grilling food E015.1
  snorkeling E002.4
  snow NEC E003.9
    boarding E003.2
    shoveling E016.0
    sledding E003.2
    tubing E003.2
  soccer E007.5
  softball E007.3
  specified NEC E029.9
  spectator at an event E029.1
  sports NEC E008.9
  sports played as a team or group NEC E007.9
  sports played individually NEC E006.9
  springboard diving E002.1
  squash E008.2
  stationary bike E009.0
  step (stepping) exercise (class) E009.2
  stepper machine E009.0
  stove E015.2
  string instrument playing E018.2
  surfing E002.7
  swimming E002.0
  tackle football E007.0
  tap dancing E005.0
  tennis E008.2
  tobogganing E003.2
  touch football E007.1
  track and field events (non-running) E006.6
    running E001.1
  trampoline E005.3
  treadmill E009.0
  trimming shrubs E016.1
  tubing (in calm and turbulent water) E002.5
    snow E003.2
  ultimate frisbee E008.3
  underwater diving E002.4
  unpacking in moving to a new residence E013.5
  use of stove, oven and microwave oven E015.2
  vacuuming E013.2
  volleyball (beach) (court) E007.7
  wake boarding E002.6
  walking an animal E019.0
  walking (on level or elevated terrain) E001.0
    an animal E019.0
  wall climbing E004.0
  warm up and cool down exercises E009.1
  water NEC E002.9
    aerobics E002.3
    craft NEC E002.9
    exercise E002.3
    polo E002.2
    skiing E002.6
    sliding E002.8
    survival training and testing E002.9
  weeding (garden and lawn) E016.1
  wind instrument playing E018.3
  windsurfing E002.7
  wrestling E008.1
  yoga E005.1
Activity status E000.9
  child assisting in compensated work of other family member E000.8
  civilian
    done for
      financial or other compensation E000.0
      pay or income E000.0
  family member assisting in compensated work of other family member E000.8
  for income E000.0
  hobby or leisure E000.8

Activity status (Continued)
  off duty military E000.8
  military E000.1
    off duty E000.8
  recreation E000.8
  specified NEC E000.8
  sport not for income E000.8
  student E000.8
  volunteer E000.2
Aeroneurosis E902.1
Aero-otitis media - see Effects of, air pressure
Aerosinusitis - see Effects of, air pressure
After-effect, late - see Late effect
Air
  blast
    in
      terrorism E979.2
      war operations E993.9
  embolism (traumatic) NEC E928.9
    in
      infusion or transfusion E874.1
      perfusion E874.2
  sickness E903
Alpine sickness E902.0
Altitude sickness - see Effects of, air pressure
Anaphylactic shock, anaphylaxis (see also Table of Drugs and Chemicals) E947.9
  due to bite or sting (venomous) - see Bite, venomous
Andes disease E902.0
Apoplexy
  heat - see Heat
Arachnidism E905.1
Arson E968.0
Asphyxia, asphyxiation
  by
    chemical
      in
        terrorism E979.7
        war operations E997.2
    explosion - see Explosion E965.8
    food (bone) (regurgitated food) (seed) E911
    foreign object, except food E912
    fumes
      in
        terrorism (chemical weapons) E979.7
        war operations E997.2
    gas - see also Table of Drugs and Chemicals
      in
        terrorism E979.7
        war operations E997.2
      legal
        execution E978
        intervention (tear) E972
      tear E972
    mechanical means (see also Suffocation) E913.9
  from
    conflagration - see Conflagration
    fire - see also Fire E899
      in
        terrorism E979.3
        war operations E990.9
    ignition - see Ignition
Aspiration
  foreign body - see Foreign body, aspiration
  mucus, not of newborn (with asphyxia, obstruction respiratory passage, suffocation) E912
  phlegm (with asphyxia, obstruction respiratory passage, suffocation) E912
  vomitus (with asphyxia, obstruction respiratory passage, suffocation) (see also Foreign body, aspiration, food) E911
Assassination (attempt) (see also Assault) E968.9

Assault (homicidal) (by) (in) E968.9
  acid E961
    swallowed E962.1
  air gun E968.6
  BB gun E968.6
  bite NEC E968.8
    of human being E968.7
  bomb ((placed in) car or house) E965.8
    antipersonnel E965.5
    letter E965.7
    petrol E965.6
  brawl (hand) (fists) (foot) E960.0
  burning, burns (by fire) E968.0
    acid E961
      swallowed E962.1
    caustic, corrosive substance E961
      swallowed E962.1
    chemical from swallowing caustic, corrosive substance NEC E962.1
    hot liquid E968.3
    scalding E968.3
    vitriol E961
      swallowed E962.1
  caustic, corrosive substance E961
    swallowed E962.1
  cut, any part of body E966
  dagger E966
  drowning E964
  explosives E965.9
    bomb (see also Assault, bomb) E965.8
    dynamite E965.8
  fight (hand) (fists) (foot) E960.0
    with weapon E968.9
      blunt or thrown E968.2
      cutting or piercing E966
      firearm - see Shooting, homicide
  fire E968.0
  firearm(s) - see Shooting, homicide
  garrotting E963
  gunshot (wound) - see Shooting, homicide
  hanging E963
  injury NEC E968.9
  knife E966
  late effect of E969
  ligature E963
  poisoning E962.9
    drugs or medicinals E962.0
    gas(es) or vapors, except drugs and medicinals E962.2
    solid or liquid substances, except drugs and medicinals E962.1
  puncture, any part of body E966
  pushing
    before moving object, train, vehicle E968.5
    from high place E968.1
  rape E960.1
  scalding E968.3
  shooting - see Shooting, homicide
  sodomy E960.1
  stab, any part of body E966
  strangulation E963
  submersion E964
  suffocation E963
  transport vehicle E968.5
  violence NEC E968.9
  vitriol E961
    swallowed E962.1
  weapon E968.9
    blunt or thrown E968.2
    cutting or piercing E966
    firearm - see Shooting, homicide
  wound E968.9
    cutting E966
    gunshot - see Shooting, homicide
    knife E966
    piercing E966
    puncture E966
    stab E966
Attack by animal NEC E906.9

INDEX TO EXTERNAL CAUSES OF INJURY / Avalanche

Avalanche E909.2
- falling on or hitting
  - motor vehicle (in motion) (on public highway) E909.2
  - railway train E909.2

Aviators' disease E902.1

B

Barotitis, barodontalgia, berosinusitis, barotrauma (otitic) (sinus) - *see* Effects of, air pressure

Battered
- baby or child (syndrome) - *see* Abuse, child; category E967
- person other than baby or child - *see* Assault

Bayonet wound (*see also* Cut, by bayonet) E920.3
- in
  - legal intervention E974
  - terrorism E979.8
  - war operations E995.2

Bean in nose E912

Bed set on fire NEC E898.0

Beheading (by guillotine)
- homicide E966
- legal execution E978

Bending, injury
- due to
  - repetitive movement E927.3
  - sudden strenuous movement E927.0

Bends E902.0

Bite
- animal NEC E906.5
  - other specified (except arthropod) E906.3
  - venomous NEC E905.9
- arthropod (nonvenomous) NEC E906.4
  - venomous - *see* Sting
- black widow spider E905.1
- cat E906.3
- centipede E905.4
- cobra E905.0
- copperhead snake E905.0
- coral snake E905.0
- dog E906.0
- fer de lance E905.0
- gila monster E905.0
- human being
  - accidental E928.3
  - assault E968.7
- insect (nonvenomous) E906.4
  - venomous - *see* Sting
- krait E905.0
- late effect of - *see* Late effect
- lizard E906.2
  - venomous E905.0
- mamba E905.0
- marine animal
  - nonvenomous E906.3
    - snake E906.2
  - venomous E905.6
    - snake E905.0
- millipede E906.4
  - venomous E905.4
- moray eel E906.3
- rat E906.1
- rattlesnake E905.0
- rodent, except rat E906.3
- serpent - *see* Bite, snake
- shark E906.3
- snake (venomous) E905.0
  - nonvenomous E906.2
  - sea E905.0
- spider E905.1
  - nonvenomous E906.4
- tarantula (venomous) E905.1
- venomous NEC E905.9
  - by specific animal - *see* category E905
- viper E905.0
- water moccasin E905.0

Blast (air)
- in
  - terrorism E979.2
    - from nuclear explosion E979.5
    - underwater E979.0
  - war operations E993.9
    - from nuclear explosion - *see* War operations, injury due to, nuclear weapons
    - underwater E992.9

Blizzard E908.3

Blow E928.9
- by law-enforcing agent, police (on duty) E975
- with blunt object (baton) (nightstick) (stave) (truncheon) E973

Blowing up (*see also* Explosion) E923.9

Brawl (hand) (fists) (foot) E960.0

Breakage (accidental)
- cable of cable car not on rails E847
- ladder (causing fall) E881.0
- part (any) of
  - animal-drawn vehicle E827●
  - ladder (causing fall) E881.0
  - motor vehicle
    - in motion (on public highway) E818●
    - not on public highway E825●
  - nonmotor road vehicle, except animal-drawn vehicle or pedal cycle E829●
  - off-road type motor vehicle (not on public highway) NEC E821●
  - on public highway E818●
  - pedal cycle E826●
- scaffolding (causing fall) E881.1
- snow vehicle, motor-driven (not on public highway) E820●
  - on public highway E818●
- vehicle NEC - *see* Accident, vehicle

Broken
- glass
  - fall on E888.0
  - injury by E920.8
- power line (causing electric shock) E925.1

Bumping against, into (accidentally)
- object (moving) E917.9
  - caused by crowd E917.1
    - with subsequent fall E917.6
  - furniture E917.3
    - with subsequent fall E917.7
  - in
    - running water E917.2
    - sports E917.0
      - with subsequent fall E917.5
  - stationary E917.4
    - with subsequent fall E917.8
- person(s) E917.9
  - with fall E886.9
    - in sports E886.0
  - as, or caused by, a crowd E917.1
    - with subsequent fall E917.6
  - in sports E917.0
    - with fall E886.0

Burning, burns (accidental) (by) (from) (on) E899
- acid (any kind) E924.1
  - swallowed - *see* Table of Drugs and Chemicals
- airgun E928.7
- bedclothes (*see also* Fire, specified NEC) E898.0
- blowlamp (*see also* Fire, specified NEC) E898.1
- blowtorch (*see also* Fire, specified NEC) E898.1
- boat, ship, watercraft - *see* categories E830, E831, E837
- bonfire (controlled) E897
  - uncontrolled E892
- candle (*see also* Fire, specified NEC) E898.1

Burning, burns (*Continued*)
- caustic liquid, substance E924.1
  - swallowed - *see* Table of Drugs and Chemicals
- chemical E924.1
  - from swallowing caustic, corrosive substance - *see* Table of Drugs and Chemicals
  - in
    - terrorism E979.7
    - war operations E997.2
- cigar(s) or cigarette(s) (*see also* Fire, specified NEC) E898.1
- clothes, clothing, nightdress - *see* Ignition, clothes
  - with conflagration - *see* Conflagration
- conflagration - *see* Conflagration
- corrosive liquid, substance E924.1
  - swallowed - *see* Table of Drugs and Chemicals
- electric current (*see also* Electric shock) E925.9
- fire, flames (*see also* Fire) E899
- firearm E928.7
- flare, Verey pistol E922.8
- heat
  - from appliance (electrical) E924.8
  - in local application, or packing during medical or surgical procedure E873.5
- homicide (attempt) (*see also* Assault, burning) E968.0
- hot
  - liquid E924.0
    - caustic or corrosive E924.1
  - object (not producing fire or flames) E924.8
  - substance E924.9
    - caustic or corrosive E924.1
    - liquid (metal) NEC E924.0
    - specified type NEC E924.8
  - tap water E924.2
- ignition - *see also* Ignition
  - clothes, clothing, nightdress - *see also* Ignition, clothes
    - with conflagration - *see* Conflagration
  - highly inflammable material (benzine) (fat) (gasoline) (kerosine) (paraffin) (petrol) E894
- inflicted by other person
  - stated as
    - homicidal, intentional (*see also* Assault, burning) E968.0
    - undetermined whether accidental or intentional (*see also* Burn, stated as undetermined whether accidental or intentional) E988.1
- internal, from swallowed caustic, corrosive liquid, substance - *see* Table of Drugs and Chemicals
- in
  - terrorism E979.3
    - from nuclear explosion E979.5
    - petrol bomb E979.3
  - war operations (from fire-producing device or conventional weapon) E990.9
    - from nuclear explosion (*see also* War operations, injury due to, nuclear weapons) E996.2
    - incendiary bomb E990.0
    - petrol bomb E990.0
- lamp (*see also* Fire, specified NEC) E898.1
- late effect of NEC E929.4
- lighter (cigar) (cigarette) (*see also* Fire, specified NEC) E898.1
- lightning E907
- liquid (boiling) (hot) (molten) E924.0
  - caustic, corrosive (external) E924.1
    - swallowed - *see* Table of Drugs and Chemicals

INDEX TO EXTERNAL CAUSES OF INJURY / Collision

Burning, burns (Continued)
   local application of externally applied substance in medical or surgical care E873.5
   machinery - see Accident, machine
   matches (see also Fire, specified NEC) E898.1
   medicament, externally applied E873.5
   metal, molten E924.0
   object (hot) E924.8
      producing fire or flames - see Fire
   oven (electric) (gas) E924.8
   pipe (smoking) (see also Fire, specified NEC) E898.1
   radiation - see Radiation
   railway engine, locomotive, train (see also Explosion, railway engine) E803●
   self-inflicted (unspecified whether accidental or intentional) E988.1
      caustic or corrosive substance NEC E988.7
      stated as intentional, purposeful E958.1
         caustic or corrosive substance NEC E958.7
      stated as undetermined whether accidental or intentional E988.1
      caustic or corrosive substance NEC E988.7
   steam E924.0
      pipe E924.8
   substance (hot) E924.9
      boiling or molten E924.0
      caustic, corrosive (external) E924.1
         swallowed - see Table of Drugs and Chemicals
   suicidal (attempt) NEC E958.1
      caustic substance E958.7
      late effect of E959
   tanning bed E926.2
   therapeutic misadventure
      overdose of radiation E873.2
   torch, welding (see also Fire, specified NEC) E898.1
   trash fire (see also Burning, bonfire) E897
   vapor E924.0
   vitriol E924.1
   x-rays E926.3
      in medical, surgical procedure - see Misadventure, failure, in dosage, radiation operations
Butted by animal E906.8

C

Cachexia, lead or saturnine E866.0
   from pesticide NEC (see also Table of Drugs and Chemicals) E863.4
Caisson disease E902.2
Capital punishment (any means) E978
Car sickness E903
Casualty (not due to war) NEC E928.9
   terrorism E979.8
   war (see also War operations) E995.9
Cat
   bite E906.3
   scratch E906.8
Cataclysmic (any injury)
   earth surface movement or eruption E909.9
      specified type NEC E909.8
   storm or flood resulting from storm E908.9
      specified type NEC E909.8
Catching fire - see Ignition
Caught
   between
      objects (moving) (stationary and moving) E918
         and machinery - see Accident, machine
   by cable car, not on rails E847
   in
      machinery (moving parts of) - see Accident, machine
      object E918

Cave-in (causing asphyxia, suffocation (by pressure)) (see also Suffocation, due to, cave-in) E913.3
   with injury other than asphyxia or suffocation E916
      with asphyxia or suffocation (see also Suffocation, due to, cave-in) E913.3
   struck or crushed by E916
      with asphyxia or suffocation (see also Suffocation, due to, cave-in) E913.3
Change(s) in air pressure - see also Effects of, air pressure
   sudden, in aircraft (ascent) (descent) (causing aeroneurosis or aviators' disease) E902.1
Chilblains E901.0
   due to manmade conditions E901.1
Choking (on) (any object except food or vomitus) E912
   apple E911
   bone E911
   food, any type (regurgitated) E911
   mucus or phlegm E912
   seed E911
Civil insurrection - see War operations
Cloudburst E908.8
Cold, exposure to (accidental) (excessive) (extreme) (place) E901.9
   causing chilblains or immersion foot E901.0
   due to
      manmade conditions E901.1
      specified cause NEC E901.8
      weather (conditions) E901.0
   late effect of NEC E929.5
   self-inflicted (undetermined whether accidental or intentional) E988.3
      suicidal E958.3
   suicide E958.3
Colic, lead, painters', or saturnine - see category E866
Collapse
   building E916
      burning (uncontrolled fire) E891.8
         in terrorism E979.3
         private E890.8
   dam E909.3
   due to heat - see Heat
   machinery - see Accident, machine or vehicle
   man-made structure E909.3
   postoperative NEC E878.9
   structure
      burning (uncontrolled fire) NEC E891.8
         in terrorism E979.3
Collision (accidental)

> Note: In the case of collisions between different types of vehicles, persons and objects, priority in classification is in the following order:
>
>   Aircraft
>   Watercraft
>   Motor vehicle
>   Railway vehicle
>   Pedal cycle
>   Animal-drawn vehicle
>   Animal being ridden
>   Streetcar or other nonmotor road vehicle
>   Other vehicle
>   Pedestrian or person using pedestrian conveyance
>   Object (except where falling from or set in motion by vehicle, etc. listed above)
>
> In the listing below, the combinations are listed only under the vehicle, etc., having priority. For definitions, see Supplementary Classification of External Causes of Injury and Poisoning (E800–E999).

Collision (Continued)
   aircraft (with object or vehicle) (fixed) (movable) (moving) E841●
      with
         person (while landing, taking off) (without accident to aircraft) E844●
         powered (in transit) (with unpowered aircraft) E841●
            while landing, taking off E840●
         unpowered E842●
            while landing, taking off E840●
   animal being ridden (in sport or transport) E828●
      and
         animal (being ridden) (herded) (unattended) E828●
         nonmotor road vehicle, except pedal cycle or animal-drawn vehicle E828●
         object (fallen) (fixed) (movable) (moving) not falling from or set in motion by vehicle of higher priority E828●
         pedestrian (conveyance or vehicle) E828●
   animal-drawn vehicle E827●
      and
         animal (being ridden) (herded) (unattended) E827●
         nonmotor road vehicle, except pedal cycle E827●
         object (fallen) (fixed) (movable) (moving) not falling from or set in motion by vehicle of higher priority E827●
         pedestrian (conveyance or vehicle) E827●
         streetcar E827●
   motor vehicle (on public highway) (traffic accident) E812●
      after leaving, running off, public highway (without antecedent collision) (without re-entry) E816●
         with antecedent collision on public highway - see categories E810–E815
         with re-entrance collision with another motor vehicle E811●
      and
         abutment (bridge) (overpass) E815●
         animal (herded) (unattended) E815●
            carrying person, property E813●
         animal-drawn vehicle E813●
         another motor vehicle (abandoned) (disabled) (parked) (stalled) (stopped) E812●
            with, involving re-entrance (on same roadway) (across median strip) E811●
         any object, person, or vehicle off the public highway resulting from a noncollision motor vehicle nontraffic accident E816●
         avalanche, fallen or not moving E815●
            falling E909.2
         boundary fence E815●
         culvert E815●
         fallen
            stone E815●
            tree E815●
         guard post or guard rail E815●
         inter-highway divider E815●
         landslide, fallen or not moving E815●
            moving E909.2
         machinery (road) E815●
         nonmotor road vehicle NEC E813●

◀ New   Revised   ~~deleted~~ Deleted   ● Use Additional Digit(s)   Omit code

INDEX TO EXTERNAL CAUSES OF INJURY / Collision

Collision (*Continued*)
  motor vehicle (*Continued*)
    and (*Continued*)
      object (any object, person, or vehicle
        off the public highway resulting
        from a noncollision motor
        vehicle nontraffic accident)
        E815●
        off, normally not on, public
          highway resulting from a
          noncollision motor vehicle
          traffic accident E816●
      pedal cycle E813●
      pedestrian (conveyance) E814●
      person (using pedestrian conveyance)
        E814●
      post or pole (lamp) (light) (signal)
        (telephone) (utility) E815●
      railway rolling stock, train, vehicle
        E810●
      safety island E815●
      street car E813●
      traffic signal, sign, or marker
        (temporary) E815●
      tree E815●
      tricycle E813●
      wall of cut made for road E815●
    due to cataclysm - *see* categories E908,
      E909
    not on public highway, nontraffic accident
      E822●
    and
      animal (carrying person, property)
        (herded) (unattended) E822●
      animal-drawn vehicle E822●
      another motor vehicle (moving),
        except off-road motor vehicle
        E822●
        stationary E823●
      avalanche, fallen, not moving NEC
        E823●
        moving E909.2
      landslide, fallen, not moving
        E823●
        moving E909.2
      nonmotor vehicle (moving)
        E822●
        stationary E823●
      object (fallen) ((normally) (fixed)
        (movable but not in motion)
        (stationary) E823●
        moving, except when falling
          from, set in motion by,
          aircraft or cataclysm E822●
      pedal cycle (moving) E822●
        stationary E823●
      pedestrian (conveyance) E822●
      person (using pedestrian
        conveyance) E822●
      railway rolling stock, train, vehicle
        (moving) E822●
        stationary E823●
      road vehicle (any) (moving) E822●
        stationary E823●
      tricycle (moving) E822●
        stationary E823●
  off-road type motor vehicle (not on public
    highway) E821●
    and
      animal (being ridden) (-drawn vehicle)
        E821●
      another off-road motor vehicle, except
        snow vehicle E821●
      other motor vehicle, not on public
        highway E821●
      other object or vehicle NEC, fixed or
        movable, not set in motion by
        aircraft, motor vehicle on
        highway, or snow vehicle,
        motor-driven E821●
      pedal cycle E821●

Collision (*Continued*)
  off-road type motor vehicle (*Continued*)
    and (*Continued*)
      pedestrian (conveyance) E821●
      railway train E821●
    on public highway - *see* Collision, motor
      vehicle
  pedal cycle E826●
    and
      animal (carrying person, property)
        (herded) (unherded) E826●
      animal-drawn vehicle E826●
      another pedal cycle E826●
      nonmotor road vehicle E826●
      object (fallen) (fixed) (movable)
        (moving) not falling from or set in
        motion by aircraft, motor vehicle,
        or railway train NEC E826●
      pedestrian (conveyance) E826●
      person (using pedestrian conveyance)
        E826●
      street car E826●
  pedestrian(s) (conveyance) E917.9
    with fall E886.9
      in sports E886.0
    and
      crowd, human stampede E917.1
        with subsequent fall E917.6
      furniture E917.3
        with subsequent fall E917.7
      machinery - *see* Accident, machine
      object (fallen) (moving) not falling
        from or set in motion by any
        vehicle classifiable to E800–E848,
        E917.9
        caused by a crowd E917.1
          with subsequent fall E917.6
        furniture E917.3
          with subsequent fall E917.7
        in
          running water E917.2
            with drowning or submersion -
              see Submersion
          sports E917.0
            with subsequent fall E917.5
        stationary E917.4
          with subsequent fall E917.8
      vehicle, nonmotor, nonroad E848
    in
      running water E917.2
        with drowning or submersion - *see*
          Submersion
      sports E917.0
        with fall E886.0
  person(s) (using pedestrian conveyance) (*see
    also* Collision, pedestrian) E917.9
  railway (rolling stock) (train) (vehicle) (with
    (subsequent) derailment, explosion,
    fall or fire) E800●
    with antecedent derailment E802●
    and
      animal (carrying person) (herded)
        (unattended) E801●
      another railway train or vehicle E800●
      buffers E801●
      fallen tree on railway E801●
      farm machinery, nonmotor (in
        transport) (stationary) E801●
      gates E801●
      nonmotor vehicle E801●
      object (fallen) (fixed) (movable)
        (movable) (moving) not falling
        from, set in motion by, aircraft or
        motor vehicle NEC E801●
      pedal cycle E801●
      pedestrian (conveyance) E805●
      person (using pedestrian conveyance)
        E805●
      platform E801●
      rock on railway E801●
      street car E801●

Collision (*Continued*)
  snow vehicle, motor-driven (not on public
    highway) E820●
    and
      animal (being ridden) (-drawn vehicle)
        E820●
      another off-road motor vehicle E820●
      other motor vehicle, not on public
        highway E820●
      other object or vehicle NEC, fixed or
        movable, not set in motion by
        aircraft or motor vehicle on
        highway E820●
      pedal cycle E820●
      pedestrian (conveyance) E820●
      railway train E820●
    on public highway - *see* Collision, motor
      vehicle
  street car(s) E829●
    and
      animal, herded, not being ridden,
        unattended E829●
      nonmotor road vehicle NEC E829●
      object (fallen) (fixed) (movable)
        (moving) not falling from or set
        in motion by aircraft, animal-
        drawn vehicle, animal being
        ridden, motor vehicle, pedal
        cycle, or railway train E829●
      pedestrian (conveyance) E829●
      person (using pedestrian conveyance)
        E829●
  vehicle
    animal-drawn - *see* Collision, animal-
      drawn vehicle
    motor - *see* Collision, motor vehicle
    nonmotor
      nonroad E848
      and
        another nonmotor, nonroad
          vehicle E848
        object (fallen) (fixed) (movable)
          (moving) not falling from
          or set in motion by aircraft,
          animal-drawn vehicle,
          animal being ridden,
          motor vehicle, nonmotor
          road vehicle, pedal cycle,
          railway train, or streetcar
          E848
      road, except animal being ridden,
        animal-drawn vehicle, or pedal
        cycle E829●
      and
        animal, herded, not being
          ridden, unattended E829●
        another nonmotor road vehicle,
          except animal being ridden,
          animal-drawn vehicle, or
          pedal cycle E829●
        object (fallen) (fixed) (movable)
          (moving) not falling from
          or set in motion by,
          aircraft, animal-drawn
          vehicle, animal being
          ridden, motor vehicle,
          pedal cycle, or railway
          train E829●
        pedestrian (conveyance) E829●
        person (using pedestrian
          conveyance) E829●
        vehicle, nonmotor, nonroad
          E829●
  watercraft E838●
    and
      person swimming or water skiing
        E838●
    causing
      drowning, submersion E830●
      injury except drowning, submersion
        E831●

INDEX TO EXTERNAL CAUSES OF INJURY / Cyclone

Combustion, spontaneous - *see* Ignition
Complication of medical or surgical procedure or treatment
  as an abnormal reaction - *see* Reaction, abnormal
  delayed, without mention of misadventure - *see* Reaction, abnormal
  due to misadventure - *see* Misadventure
Compression
  divers' squeeze E902.2
  trachea by
    food E911
    foreign body, except food E912
Conflagration
  building or structure, except private dwelling (barn) (church) (convalescent or residential home) (factory) (farm outbuilding) (hospital) (hotel) or (institution (educational) (dormitory) (residential)) (school) (shop) (store) (theatre) E891.9
    with or causing (injury due to)
      accident or injury NEC E891.9
        specified circumstance NEC E891.8
      burns, burning E891.3
      carbon monoxide E891.2
      fumes E891.2
        polyvinylchloride (PVC) or similar material E891.1
      smoke E891.2
    causing explosion E891.0
    in terrorism E979.3
  not in building or structure E892
  private dwelling (apartment) (boarding house) (camping place) (caravan) (farmhouse) (home (private)) (house) (lodging house) (private garage) (rooming house) (tenement) E890.9
    with or causing (injury due to) accident or injury NEC E890.9
      specified circumstance NEC E890.8
      burns, burning E890.3
      carbon monoxide E890.2
      fumes E890.2
        polyvinylchloride (PVC) or similar material E890.1
      smoke E890.2
    causing explosion E890.0
Constriction, external
  caused by
    hair E928.4
    other object E928.5
Contact with
  dry ice E901.1
  liquid air, hydrogen, nitrogen E901.1
Cramp(s)
  heat - *see* Heat
  swimmers (*see also* category E910) 910.2
    not in recreation or sport E910.3
Cranking (car) (truck) (bus) (engine) injury by E917.9
Crash
  aircraft (in transit) (powered) E841●
    at landing, take-off E840●
    in
      terrorism E979.1
      war operations E994.9
    on runway NEC E840●
    stated as
      homicidal E968.8
      suicidal E958.6
      undetermined whether accidental or intentional E988.6
    unpowered E842●
  glider E842●
  motor vehicle - *see also* Accident, motor vehicle
    homicidal E968.5
    suicidal E958.5
    undetermined whether accidental or intentional E988.5

Crushed (accidentally) E928.9
  between
    boat(s), ship(s), watercraft (and dock or pier) (without accident to watercraft) E838●
      after accident to, or collision, watercraft E831●
    objects (moving) (stationary and moving) E918
  by
    avalanche NEC E909.2
    boat, ship, watercraft after accident to, collision, watercraft E831●
    cave-in E916
      with asphyxiation or suffocation (*see also* Suffocation, due to, cave-in) E913.3
    crowd, human stampede E917.1
    falling
      aircraft (*see also* Accident, aircraft) E841●
        in
          terrorism E979.1
          war operations E994.8
      earth, material E916
        with asphyxiation or suffocation (*see also* Suffocation, due to, cave-in) E913.3
      object E916
        on ship, watercraft E838●
        while loading, unloading watercraft E838●
    firearm E928.7
    landslide NEC E909.2
    lifeboat after abandoning ship E831●
    machinery - *see* Accident, machine
    railway rolling stock, train, vehicle (part of) E805●
    slide trigger mechanism, scope or other part of gun E928.7
    street car E829●
    vehicle NEC - *see* Accident, vehicle NEC
  in
    machinery - *see* Accident, machine
    object E918
    transport accident - *see* categories E800–E848
  late effect of NEC E929.9
Cut, cutting (any part of body) (accidental) E920.9
  by
    arrow E920.8
    axe E920.4
    bayonet (*see also* Bayonet wound) E920.3
      in war operations E995.2
    blender E920.2
    broken glass E920.8
      following fall E888.0
    can opener E920.4
      powered E920.2
    chisel E920.4
    circular saw E919.4
    cutting or piercing instrument - *see also* category E920
      following fall E888.0
      late effect of E929.8
    dagger E920.3
    dart E920.8
    drill - *see* Accident, caused by drill
    edge of stiff paper E920.8
    electric
      beater E920.2
      fan E920.2
      knife E920.2
      mixer E920.2
    firearm component E928.7
    fork E920.4
    garden fork E920.4
    hand saw or tool (not powered) E920.4
      powered E920.1

Cut, cutting (*Continued*)
  by (*Continued*)
    hedge clipper E920.4
      powered E920.1
    hoe E920.4
    ice pick E920.4
    knife E920.3
      electric E920.2
      in war operations E995.2
    lathe turnings E920.8
    lawn mower E920.4
      powered E920.0
      riding E919.8
    machine - *see* Accident, machine
    meat
      grinder E919.8
      slicer E919.8
    nails E920.8
    needle E920.4
      hypodermic E920.5
    object, edged, pointed, sharp - *see* category E920
      following fall E888.0
    paper cutter E920.4
    piercing instrument - *see also* category E920
      late effect of E929.8
    pitchfork E920.4
    powered
      can opener E920.2
      garden cultivator E920.1
        riding E919.8
      hand saw E920.1
      hand tool NEC E920.1
      hedge clipper E920.1
      household appliance or implement E920.2
      lawn mower (hand) E920.0
        riding E919.8
      rivet gun E920.1
      staple gun E920.1
    rake E920.4
    saw
      circular E919.4
      hand E920.4
    scissors E920.4
    screwdriver E920.4
    sewing machine (electric) (powered) E920.2
      not powered E920.4
    shears E920.4
    shovel E920.4
    slide trigger mechanism, scope or other part of gun E928.7
    spade E920.4
    splinters E920.8
    sword E920.3
      in war operations E995.2
    tin can lid E920.8
    wood slivers E920.8
  homicide (attempt) E966
  inflicted by other person
    stated as
      intentional, homicidal E966
      undetermined whether accidental or intentional E986
  late effect of NEC E929.8
  legal
    execution E978
    intervention E974
  self-inflicted (unspecified whether accidental or intentional) E986
    stated as intentional, purposeful E956
  stated as undetermined whether accidental or intentional E986
  suicidal (attempt) E956
  terrorism E979.8
  war operations E995.2
Cyclone E908.1

INDEX TO EXTERNAL CAUSES OF INJURY / Death due to injury occurring one year or more previous

D

Death due to injury occurring one year or more previous - *see* Late effect
Decapitation (accidental circumstances) NEC E928.9
  homicidal E966
  legal execution (by guillotine) E978
Deprivation - *see also* Privation action E913.3
  homicidal intent E968.4
Derailment (accidental)
  railway (rolling stock) (train) (vehicle) (with subsequent collision) E802●
    with
      collision (antecedent) (*see also* Collision, railway) E800●
      explosion (subsequent) (without antecedent collision) E802●
        antecedent collision E803●
      fall (without collision (antecedent)) E802●
      fire (without collision (antecedent)) E802●
  street car E829●
Descent
  parachute (voluntary) (without accident to aircraft) E844●
    due to accident to aircraft - *see* categories E840–E842
Desertion
  child, with intent to injure or kill E968.4
  helpless person, infant, newborn E904.0
    with intent to injure or kill E968.4
Destitution - *see* Privation
Dirty bomb (*see also* War operations, injury due to, nuclear weapons) E996.9
Disability, late effect or sequela of injury - *see* Late effect
Disease
  Andes E902.0
  aviators' E902.1
  caisson E902.2
  range E902.0
Divers' disease, palsy, paralysis, squeeze E902.0
Dog bite E906.0
Dragged by
  cable car (not on rails) E847
    on rails E829●
  motor vehicle (on highway) E814●
    not on highway, nontraffic accident E825●
  street car E829●
Drinking poison (accidental) - *see* Table of Drugs and Chemicals
Drowning - *see* Submersion
Dust in eye E914

E

Earth falling (on) (with asphyxia or suffocation (by pressure)) (*see also* Suffocation, due to, cave-in) E913.3
  as, or due to, a cataclysm (involving any transport vehicle) - *see* categories E908, E909
  not due to cataclysmic action E913.3
    motor vehicle (in motion) (on public highway) E813●
      not on public highway E825●
    nonmotor road vehicle NEC E829●
    pedal cycle E826●
    railway rolling stock, train, vehicle E806●
    street car E829●
  struck or crushed by E916
    with asphyxiation or suffocation E913.3
    with injury other than asphyxia, suffocation E916
Earthquake (any injury) E909.0

Effect(s) (adverse) of
  air pressure E902.9
    at high altitude E902.9
      in aircraft E902.1
      residence or prolonged visit (causing conditions classifiable to E902.0) E902.0
    due to
      diving E902.2
      specified cause NEC E902.8
    in aircraft E902.1
  cold, excessive (exposure to) (*see also* Cold, exposure to) E901.9
  heat (excessive) (*see also* Heat) E900.9
  hot
    place - *see* Heat
    weather E900.0
  insulation - *see* Heat
  late - *see* Late effect of
  motion E903
  nuclear explosion or weapon
    in
      terrorism E979.5
      war operations (*see also* War operations, injury due to, nuclear weapons) E996.9
  radiation - *see* Radiation
  terrorism, secondary E979.9
  travel E903
Electric shock, electrocution (accidental) (from exposed wire, faulty appliance, high voltage cable, live rail, open socket) (by) (in) E925.9
  appliance or wiring
    domestic E925.0
    factory E925.2
    farm (building) E925.8
      house E925.0
    home E925.0
    industrial (conductor) (control apparatus) (transformer) E925.2
    outdoors E925.8
    public building E925.8
    residential institution E925.8
    school E925.8
    specified place NEC E925.8
  caused by other person
    stated as
      intentional, homicidal E968.8
      undetermined whether accidental or intentional E988.4
  electric power generating plant, distribution station E925.1
  electroshock gun (taser) (stun gun) E925.8
    caused by other person E968.8
      legal intervention E975
      stated as accidental E925.8
      stated as intentional E968.8
    due to legal intervention E975
    stated as intentional self-harm (suicidal (attempt)) E958.4
    stated as undetermined whether accidental or intentional E988.4
    suicide (attempt) E958.4
  homicidal (attempt) E968.8
  legal execution E978
  lightning E907
  machinery E925.9
    domestic E925.0
    factory E925.2
    farm E925.8
    home E925.0
  misadventure in medical or surgical procedure
    in electroshock therapy E873.4
  self-inflicted (undetermined whether accidental or intentional) E988.4
  stated as intentional E958.4
  stated as undetermined whether accidental or intentional E988.4

Electric shock, electrocution (*Continued*)
  suicidal (attempt) E958.4
  transmission line E925.1
Electrocution - *see* Electric shock
Embolism E921.1
  air (traumatic) NEC - *see* Air, embolism
Encephalitis
  lead or saturnine E866.0
    from pesticide NEC E863.4
Entanglement
  in
    bedclothes, causing suffocation E913.0
    wheel of pedal cycle E826●
Entry of foreign body, material, any - *see* Foreign body
Execution, legal (any method) E978
Exertion, excessive physical, from prolonged activity E927.2
Exhaustion
  cold - *see* Cold, exposure to
  due to excessive exertion E927.2
  heat - *see* Heat
Explosion (accidental) (in) (of) (on) E923.9
  acetylene E923.2
  aerosol can E921.8
  aircraft (in transit) (powered) E841●
    at landing, take-off E840●
    in
      terrorism E979.1
      war operations
        from
          enemy fire or explosive(s) (device placed on aircraft) E994.0
          own onboard explosives E994.1
    unpowered E842●
  air tank (compressed) (in machinery) E921.1
  anesthetic gas in operating theatre E923.2
  automobile tire NEC E921.8
    causing transport accident - *see* categories E810-E825
  blasting (cap) (materials) E923.1
  boiler (machinery), not on transport vehicle E921.0
    steamship - *see* Explosion, watercraft
  bomb E923.8
    in
      terrorism E979.2
      war operations E993.8
        after cessation of hostilities E998.1
        atom, hydrogen or nuclear (*see also* War operations, injury due to, nuclear weapons) E996.9
        injury by fragments from E991.9
        antipersonnel bomb E991.3
  butane E923.2
  caused by
    other person
      stated as
        intentional, homicidal - *see* Assault, explosive
        undetermined whether accidental or homicidal E985.5
  coal gas E923.2
  detonator E923.1
  dynamite E923.1
  explosive (material) NEC E923.9
    gas(es) E923.2
    missile E923.8
      in
        terrorism E979.2
        war operations E993.1
          injury by fragments from E991.9
          antipersonnel bomb E991.3
    used in blasting operations E923.1
  fire-damp E923.2
  fireworks E923.0
  gas E923.2
    cylinder (in machinery) E921.1
    pressure tank (in machinery) E921.1

INDEX TO EXTERNAL CAUSES OF INJURY / Fall, falling

Explosion (Continued)
  gasoline (fumes) (tank) not in moving motor vehicle E923.2
  grain store (military) (munitions) E923.8
  grenade E923.8
    in
      terrorism E979.2
      war operations E993.8
        injury by fragments from E991.4
  homicide (attempt) - *see* Assault, explosive
  hot water heater, tank (in machinery) E921.0
  in mine (of explosive gases) NEC E923.2
  late effect of NEC E929.8
  machinery - *see also* Accident, machine
  pressure vessel - *see* Explosion, pressure vessel
  methane E923.2
  missile E923.8
    in
      terrorism E979.2
      war operations E993.1
        injury by fragments from E991.4
  motor vehicle (part of)
    in motion (on public highway) E818 ●
    not on public highway E825 ●
  munitions (dump) (factory) E923.8
    in
      terrorism E979.2
      war operations E993.9
  of mine E923.8
    in
      terrorism
        at sea or in harbor E979.0
        land E979.2
        marine E979.0
      war operations
        after cessation of hostilities E998.0
        at sea or in harbor E992.2
        land E993.8
          after cessation of hostilities E998.0
          injury by fragments from E991.4
        marine E992.2
  own weapons
    in
      terrorism (*see also* Suicide) E979.2
      war operations E993.7
        injury by fragments from E991.9
          antipersonnel bomb E991.3
  pressure
    cooker E921.8
    gas tank (in machinery) E921.1
    vessel (in machinery) E921.9
      on transport vehicle - *see* categories E800-E848
      specified type NEC E921.8
  propane E923.2
  railway engine, locomotive, train (boiler) (with subsequent collision, derailment, fall) E803 ●
    with
      collision (antecedent) (*see also* Collision, railway) E800 ●
      derailment (antecedent) E802 ●
      fire (without antecedent collision or derailment) E803 ●
  secondary fire resulting from - *see* Fire
  self-inflicted (unspecified whether accidental or intentional) E985.5
    stated as intentional, purposeful E955.5
  shell (artillery) E923.8
    in
      terrorism E979.2
      war operations E993.2
        injury by fragments from E991.4
    stated as undetermined whether caused accidentally or purposely inflicted E985.5
  steam or water lines (in machinery) E921.0
  suicide (attempted) E955.5
  terrorism - *see* Terrorism, explosion

Explosion (Continued)
  torpedo E923.8
    in
      terrorism E979.0
      war operations E992.0
  transport accident - *see* categories E800–E848
  war operations - *see* War operations, explosion
  watercraft (boiler) E837 ●
    causing drowning, submersion (after jumping from watercraft) E830 ●
Exposure (weather) (conditions) (rain) (wind) E904.3
  with homicidal intent E968.4
  environmental
    to
      algae bloom E928.6
      blue-green algae bloom E928.6
      brown tide E928.6
      cyanobacteria bloom E928.6
      Florida red tide E928.6
      harmful algae
        and toxins E928.6
        bloom E928.6
      pfiesteria piscicida E928.6
      red tide E928.6
  excessive E904.3
    cold (*see also* Cold, exposure to) E901.9
      self-inflicted - *see* Cold, exposure to, self-inflicted
    heat (*see also* Heat) E900.9
  helpless person, infant, newborn due to abandonment or neglect E904.0
  noise E928.1
  prolonged in deep-freeze unit or refrigerator E901.1
  radiation - *see* Radiation
  resulting from transport accident - *see* categories E800–E848
  smoke from, due to
    fire - *see* Fire
    tobacco, second-hand E869.4
  vibration E928.2
External cause status E000.9
  child assisting in compensated work of other family member E000.8
  civilian
    done for
      financial or other compensation E000.0
      pay or income E000.0
  family member assisting in compensated work of other family member E000.8
  for income E000.0
  hobby or leisure E000.8
    off duty military E000.8
  military E000.1
    off duty E000.8
  recreation E000.8
  specified NEC E000.8
  sport not for income E000.8
  student E000.8
  volunteer E000.2

F

Fall, falling (accidental) E888.9
  building E916
    burning E891.8
      private E890.8
  down
    escalator E880.0
    ladder E881.0
      in boat, ship, watercraft E833 ●
    staircase E880.9
    stairs, steps - *see* Fall, from, stairs
  earth (with asphyxia or suffocation (by pressure)) (*see also* Earth, falling) E913.3

Fall, falling (Continued)
  from, off
    aircraft (at landing, take-off) (in-transit) (while alighting, boarding) E843 ●
      resulting from accident to aircraft - *see* categories E840–E842
    animal (in sport or transport) E828 ●
    animal-drawn vehicle E827 ●
    balcony E882
    bed E884.4
    bicycle E826 ●
    boat, ship, watercraft (into water) E832 ●
      after accident to, collision, fire on E830 ●
        and subsequently struck by (part of) boat E831 ●
        and subsequently struck by (part of) while alighting, boat E838 ●
      burning, crushed, sinking E830 ●
        and subsequently struck by (part of) boat E831 ●
    bridge E882
    building E882
      burning (uncontrolled fire) E891.8
        in terrorism E979.3
      private E890.8
    bunk in boat, ship, watercraft E834 ●
      due to accident to watercraft E831 ●
    cable car (not on rails) E847
      on rails E829 ●
    car - *see* Fall from motor vehicle E884.9
    chair E884.2
    cliff E884.1
    commode E884.6
    curb (sidewalk) E880.1
    elevation aboard ship E834 ●
      due to accident to ship E831 ●
    embankment E884.9
    escalator E880.0
    fire escape E882
    flagpole E882
    furniture NEC E884.5
    gangplank (into water) (*see also* Fall, from, boat) E832 ●
      to deck, dock E834 ●
    hammock on ship E834 ●
      due to accident to watercraft E831 ●
    haystack E884.9
    heelies E885.1
    high place NEC E884.9
      stated as undetermined whether accidental or intentional - *see* Jumping, from, high place
    horse (in sport or transport) E828 ●
    in-line skates E885.1
    ladder E881.0
      in boat, ship, watercraft E833 ●
        due to accident to watercraft E831 ●
    machinery - *see also* Accident, machine
      not in operation E884.9
    motor vehicle (in motion) (on public highway) E818 ●
      not on public highway E825 ●
        stationary, except while alighting, boarding, entering, leaving E884.9
        while alighting, boarding, entering, leaving E824 ●
      stationary, except while alighting, boarding, entering, leaving E884.9
      while alighting, boarding, entering, leaving, except off-road type motor vehicle E817 ●
      off-road type - *see* Fall, from, off-road type motor vehicle
    motorized
      mobility scooter E884.3
      wheelchair E884.3

◀ New ⬅ Revised ~~deleted~~ Deleted ● Use Additional Digit(s) ▨ Omit code

INDEX TO EXTERNAL CAUSES OF INJURY / Fall, falling

Fall, falling (Continued)
  from, off (Continued)
    nonmotor road vehicle (while alighting, boarding) NEC E829●
      stationary, except while alighting, boarding, entering, leaving E884.9
    off road type motor vehicle (not on public highway) NEC E821●
      on public highway E818●
        while alighting, boarding, entering, leaving E817●
    snow vehicle - see Fall from snow vehicle, motor-driven
    one
      deck to another on ship E834●
        due to accident to ship E831●
      level to another NEC E884.9
        boat, ship, or watercraft E834●
          due to accident to watercraft E831●
    pedal cycle E826●
    playground equipment E884.0
    railway rolling stock, train, vehicle (while alighting, boarding) E804●
      with
        collision (see also Collision, railway) E800●
        derailment (see also Derailment, railway) E802●
        explosion (see also Explosion, railway engine) E803●
    rigging (aboard ship) E834●
      due to accident to watercraft E831●
    roller skates E885.1
    scaffolding E881.1
    scooter (nonmotorized) E885.0
      motorized mobility E884.3
    sidewalk (curb) E880.1
      moving E885.9
    skateboard E885.2
    skis E885.3
    snow vehicle, motor-driven (not on public highway) E820●
      on public highway E818●
        while alighting, boarding, entering, leaving E817●
    snowboard E885.4
    stairs, steps E880.9
      boat, ship, watercraft E833●
        due to accident to watercraft E831●
      motor bus, motor vehicle - see Fall, from, motor vehicle, while alighting, boarding
      street car E829●
    stationary vehicle NEC E884.9
    stepladder E881.0
    street car (while boarding, alighting) E829●
      stationary, except while boarding or alighting E884.9
    structure NEC E882
      burning (uncontrolled fire) E891.8
        in terrorism E979.3
    table E884.9
    toilet E884.6
    tower E882
    tree E884.9
    turret E882
    vehicle NEC - see also Accident, vehicle NEC
      stationary E884.9
    viaduct E882
    wall E882
    wheelchair (electric) (motorized) E884.3
    wheelies E885.1
    window E882

Fall, falling (Continued)
  in, on
    aircraft (at landing, take-off) (in-transit) E843●
      resulting from accident to aircraft - see categories E840–E842
    boat, ship, watercraft E835●
      due to accident to watercraft E831●
      one level to another NEC E834●
      on ladder, stairs E833●
    cutting or piercing instrument machine E888.0
    deck (of boat, ship, watercraft) E835●
      due to accident to watercraft E831●
    escalator E880.0
    gangplank E835●
    glass, broken E888.0
    knife E888.0
    ladder E881.0
      in boat, ship, watercraft E833●
        due to accident to watercraft E831●
    object
      edged, pointed or sharp E888.0
      other E888.1
    pitchfork E888.0
    railway rolling stock, train, vehicle (while alighting, boarding) E804●
      with
        collision (see also Collision, railway) E800●
        derailment (see also Derailment, railway) E802●
        explosion (see also Explosion, railway engine) E803●
    scaffolding E881.1
    scissors E888.0
    staircase, stairs, steps (see also Fall, from, stairs) E880.9
    street car E829●
    water transport (see also Fall, in, boat) E835●
  into
    cavity E883.9
    dock E883.9
      from boat, ship, watercraft (see also Fall, from, boat) E832●
    hold (of ship) E834●
      due to accident to watercraft E831●
    hole E883.9
    manhole E883.2
    moving part of machinery - see Accident, machine
    opening in surface NEC E883.9
    pit E883.9
    quarry E883.9
    shaft E883.9
    storm drain E883.2
    tank E883.9
    water (with drowning or submersion) E910.9
    well E883.1
  late effect of NEC E929.3
  object (see also Hit by, object, falling) E916
  other E888.8
  over
    animal E885.9
    cliff E884.1
    embankment E884.9
    small object E885.9
  overboard (see also Fall, from, boat) E832●
  resulting in striking against object E888.1
    sharp E888.0
  rock E916
  same level NEC E888.9
    aircraft (any kind) E843●
      resulting from accident to aircraft - see categories E840–E842
    boat, ship, watercraft E835●
      due to accident to, collision, watercraft E831●

Fall, falling (Continued)
  same level NEC (Continued)
    from
      collision, pushing, shoving, by or with other person(s) E886.9
        as, or caused by, a crowd E917.6
        in sports E886.0
      in-line skates E885.1
      roller skates E885.1
      scooter (nonmotorized) E885.0
      skateboard E885.2
      skis E885.3
      slipping, stumbling, tripping E885.9
      snowboard E885.4
    snowslide E916
      as avalanche E909.2
    stone E916
    through
      hatch (on ship) E834●
        due to accident to watercraft E831●
      roof E882
      window E882
    timber E916
    while alighting from, boarding, entering, leaving
      aircraft (any kind) E843●
      motor bus, motor vehicle - see Fall, from, motor vehicle, while alighting, boarding
      nonmotor road vehicle NEC E829●
      railway train E804●
      street car E829●

Fallen on by
  animal (horse) (not being ridden) E906.8
    being ridden (in sport or transport) E828●

Fell or jumped from high place, so stated - see Jumping, from, high place

Felo-de-se (see also Suicide) E958.9

Fever
  heat - see Heat
  thermic - see Heat

Fight (hand) (fist) (foot) (see also Assault, fight) E960.0

Fire (accidental) (caused by great heat from appliance (electrical), hot object, or hot substance) (secondary, resulting from explosion) E899
  conflagration - see Conflagration E892
  controlled, normal (in brazier, fireplace, furnace, or stove) (charcoal) (coal) (coke) (electric) (gas) (wood)
    bonfire E897
    brazier, not in building or structure E897
    in building or structure, except private dwelling (barn) (church) (convalescent or residential home) (factory) (farm outbuilding) (hospital) (hotel) (institution (educational) (dormitory) (residential) (private garage) (school) (shop) (store) (theatre) E896
    in private dwelling (apartment) (boarding house) (camping place) (caravan) (farmhouse) (home (private) (house) (lodging house) (rooming house) (tenement) E895
    not in building or structure E897
    trash E897
  forest (uncontrolled) E892
  grass (uncontrolled) E892
  hay (uncontrolled) E892
  homicide (attempt) E968.0
    late effect of E969
  in, of, on, starting in E892
    aircraft (in transit) (powered) E841●
      at landing, take-off E840●
      stationary E892
      unpowered (balloon) (glider) E842●
    balloon E842●
    boat, ship, watercraft - see categories E830, E831, E837

INDEX TO EXTERNAL CAUSES OF INJURY / High

Fire *(Continued)*
   in, of, on, starting in *(Continued)*
      building or structure, except private dwelling (barn) (church) (convalescent or residential home) (factory) (farm outbuilding) (hospital) (hotel) (institution) (educational) (dormitory) (residential)) (school) (shop) (store) (theatre) *(see also* Conflagration, building or structure, except private dwelling) E891.9
      forest (uncontrolled) E892
      glider E842●
      grass (uncontrolled) E892
      hay (uncontrolled) E892
      lumber (uncontrolled) E892
      machinery - *see* Accident, machine
      mine (uncontrolled) E892
      motor vehicle (in motion) (on public highway) E818●
         not on public highway E825●
         stationary E892
      prairie (uncontrolled) E892
      private dwelling (apartment) (boarding house) (camping place) (caravan) (farmhouse) (home (private)) (house) (lodging house) (private garage) (rooming house) (tenement) *(see also* Conflagration, private dwelling) E890.9
      railway rolling stock, train, vehicle *(see also* Explosion, railway engine) E803●
         stationary E892
      room NEC E898.1
      street car (in motion) E829●
         stationary E892
      terrorism (by fire-producing device) E979.3
         fittings or furniture (burning building) (uncontrolled fire) E979.3
         from nuclear explosion E979.5
      transport vehicle, stationary NEC E892
      tunnel (uncontrolled) E892
      war operations (by fire-producing device or conventional weapon) E990.9
         from nuclear explosion *(see also* War operations, injury due to, nuclear weapons) E996.2
         incendiary bomb E990.0
         petrol bomb E990.0
   late effect of NEC E929.4
   lumber (uncontrolled) E892
   mine (uncontrolled) E892
   prairie (uncontrolled) E892
   self-inflicted (unspecified whether accidental or intentional) E988.1
      stated as intentional, purposeful E958.1
   specified NEC E898.1
      with
         conflagration - *see* Conflagration
         ignition (of)
            clothing - *see* Ignition, clothes
            highly inflammable material (benzine) (fat) (gasoline) (kerosene) (paraffin) (petrol) E894
   started by other person
      stated as
         with intent to injure or kill E968.0
         undetermined whether or not with intent to injure or kill E988.1
   suicide (attempted) E958.1
      late effect of E959
   tunnel (uncontrolled) E892
Fireball effects from nuclear explosion
   in
      terrorism E979.5
      war operations *(see also* War operations, injury due to, nuclear weapons) E996.2

Fireworks (explosion) E923.0
Flash burns from explosion *(see also* Explosion) E923.9
Flood (any injury) (resulting from storm) E908.2
   caused by collapse of dam or manmade structure E909.3
Forced landing (aircraft) E840●
Foreign body, object or material (entrance into (accidental))
   air passage (causing injury) E915
      with asphyxia, obstruction, suffocation E912
         food or vomitus E911
      nose (with asphyxia, obstruction, suffocation) E912
         causing injury without asphyxia, obstruction, suffocation E915
   alimentary canal (causing injury) (with obstruction) E915
      with asphyxia, obstruction respiratory passage, suffocation E912
         food E911
      mouth E915
         with asphyxia, obstruction, suffocation E912
            food E911
      pharynx E915
         with asphyxia, obstruction, suffocation E912
            food E911
   aspiration (with asphyxia, obstruction respiratory passage, suffocation) E912
      causing injury without asphyxia, obstruction respiratory passage, suffocation E915
      food (regurgitated) (vomited) E911
         causing injury without asphyxia, obstruction respiratory passage, suffocation E915
      mucus (not of newborn) E912
      phlegm E912
   bladder (causing injury or obstruction) E915
   bronchus, bronchi - *see* Foreign body, air passages
   conjunctival sac E914
   digestive system - *see* Foreign body, alimentary canal
   ear (causing injury or obstruction) E915
   esophagus (causing injury or obstruction) *(see also* Foreign body, alimentary canal) E915
   eye (any part) E914
   eyelid E914
   hairball (stomach) (with obstruction) E915
   ingestion - *see* Foreign body, alimentary canal
   inhalation - *see* Foreign body, aspiration
   intestine (causing injury or obstruction) E915
   iris E914
   lacrimal apparatus E914
   larynx - *see* Foreign body, air passage
   late effect of NEC E929.8
   lung - *see* Foreign body, air passage
   mouth - *see* Foreign body, alimentary canal, mouth
   nasal passage - *see* Foreign body, air passage, nose
   nose - *see* Foreign body, air passage, nose
   ocular muscle E914
   operation wound (left in) - *see* Misadventure, foreign object
   orbit E914
   pharynx - *see* Foreign body, alimentary canal, pharynx
   rectum (causing injury or obstruction) E915
   stomach (hairball) (causing injury or obstruction) E915
   tear ducts or glands E914
   trachea - *see* Foreign body, air passage
   urethra (causing injury or obstruction) E915
   vagina (causing injury or obstruction) E915

Found dead, injured
   from exposure (to) - *see* Exposure
   on
      public highway E819●
      railway right of way E807●
Fracture (circumstances unknown or unspecified) E887
   due to specified external means - *see* manner of accident
   late effect of NEC E929.3
   occurring in water transport NEC E835●
Freezing - *see* Cold, exposure to
Frostbite E901.0
   due to manmade conditions E901.1
Frozen - *see* Cold, exposure to

G

Garrotting, homicidal (attempted) E963
Gored E906.8
Gunshot wound *(see also* Shooting) E922.9

H

Hailstones, injury by E904.3
Hairball (stomach) (with obstruction) E915
Hanged himself *(see also* Hanging, self-inflicted) E983.0
Hang gliding E842●
Hanging (accidental) E913.8
   caused by other person
      in accidental circumstances E913.8
      stated as
         intentional, homicidal E963
         undetermined whether accidental or intentional E983.0
   homicide (attempt) E963
   in bed or cradle E913.0
   legal execution E978
   self-inflicted (unspecified whether accidental or intentional) E983.0
      in accidental circumstances E913.8
      stated as intentional, purposeful E953.0
   stated as undetermined whether accidental or intentional E983.0
   suicidal (attempt) E953.0
Heat (apoplexy) (collapse) (cramps) (effects of) (excessive) (exhaustion) (fever) (prostration) (stroke) E900.9
   due to
      manmade conditions (as listed in E900.1, except boat, ship, watercraft) E900.1
      weather (conditions) E900.0
   from
      electric heating apparatus causing burning E924.8
      nuclear explosion
         in
            terrorism E979.5
            war operations *(see also* War operations, injury due to, nuclear weapons) E996.2
   generated in, boiler, engine, evaporator, fire room of boat, ship, watercraft E838●
   inappropriate in local application or packing in medical or surgical procedure E873.5
   late effect of NEC E989
Hemorrhage
   delayed following medical or surgical treatment without mention of misadventure - *see* Reaction, abnormal
   during medical or surgical treatment as misadventure - *see* Misadventure, cut
High
   altitude, effects E902.9
   level of radioactivity, effects - *see* Radiation

INDEX TO EXTERNAL CAUSES OF INJURY / **High**

High (Continued)
  pressure effects - *see also* Effects of, air pressure
    from rapid descent in water (causing caisson or divers' disease, palsy, or paralysis) E902.2
  temperature, effects - *see* Heat
Hit, hitting (accidental) by
  aircraft (propeller) (without accident to aircraft) E844●
    unpowered E842●
  avalanche E909.2
  being thrown against object in or part of
    motor vehicle (in motion) (on public highway) E818●
      not on public highway E825●
    nonmotor road vehicle NEC E829●
    street car E829●
  boat, ship, watercraft
    after fall from watercraft E838●
      damaged, involved in accident E831●
    while swimming, water skiing E838●
  bullet (*see also* Shooting) E922.9
    from air gun E922.4
    in
      terrorism E979.4
      war operations E991.2
        rubber E991.0
  flare, Verey pistol (*see also* Shooting) E922.8
  hailstones E904.3
  landslide E909.2
  law-enforcing agent (on duty) E975
    with blunt object (baton) (night stick) (stave) (truncheon) E973
  machine - *see* Accident, machine
  missile
    firearm (*see also* Shooting) E922.9
    in
      terrorism - *see* Terrorism, missile
      war operations - *see* War operations, missile
  motor vehicle (on public highway) (traffic accident) E814●
    not on public highway, nontraffic accident E822●
  nonmotor road vehicle NEC E829●
  object
    falling E916
      from, in, on
        aircraft E844●
          due to accident to aircraft - *see* categories E840–E842
          unpowered E842●
        boat, ship, watercraft E838●
          due to accident to watercraft E831●
        building E916
          burning E891.8
            in terrorism E979.3
            private E890.8
        cataclysmic
          earth surface movement or eruption E909.9
          storm E908.9
        cave-in E916
          with asphyxiation or suffocation (*see also* Suffocation, due to, cave-in) E913.3
        earthquake E909.0
        motor vehicle (in motion) (on public highway) E818●
          not on public highway E825●
          stationary E916
        nonmotor road vehicle NEC E829●
        pedal cycle E826●
        railway rolling stock, train, vehicle E806●
        street car E829●
        structure, burning NEC E891.8
        vehicle, stationary E916

Hit, hitting (Continued)
  object (Continued)
    moving NEC - *see* Striking against, object
    projected NEC - *see* Striking against, object
    set in motion by
      compressed air or gas, spring, striking, throwing - *see* Striking against, object
      explosion - *see* Explosion
    thrown into, on, or towards
      motor vehicle (in motion) (on public highway) E818●
        not on public highway E825●
      nonmotor road vehicle NEC E829●
      pedal cycle E826●
      street car E829●
  off-road type motor vehicle (not on public highway) E821●
    on public highway E814●
  other person(s) E917.9
    with blunt or thrown object E917.9
      in sports E917.0
        with subsequent fall E917.5
      intentionally, homicidal E968.2
    as, or caused by, a crowd E917.1
      with subsequent fall E917.6
    in sports E917.0
  pedal cycle E826●
  police (on duty) E975
    with blunt object (baton) (nightstick) (stave) (truncheon) E973
  railway, rolling stock, train, vehicle (part of) E805●
  shot - *see* Shooting
  snow vehicle, motor-driven (not on highway) E820●
    on public highway E814●
  street car E829●
  vehicle NEC - *see* Accident, vehicle NEC
Homicide, homicidal (attempt) (justifiable) (*see also* Assault) E968.9
Hot
  liquid, object, substance, accident caused by - *see also* Accident, caused by, hot, by type of substance
    late effect of E929.8
  place, effects - *see* Heat
  weather, effects E900.0
Humidity, causing problem E904.3
Hunger E904.1
  resulting from
    abandonment or neglect E904.0
    transport accident - *see* categories E800–E848
Hurricane (any injury) E908.0
Hypobarism, hypobaropathy - *see* Effects of, air pressure
Hypothermia - *see* Cold, exposure to

I

Ictus
  caloris - *see* Heat
  solaris E900.0
Ignition (accidental)
  anesthetic gas in operating theatre E923.2
  bedclothes
    with
      conflagration - *see* Conflagration
      ignition (of)
        clothing - *see* Ignition, clothes
        highly inflammable material
          obstruction (benzine) (fat) (gasoline) (kerosene) (paraffin) (petrol) E894
  benzine E894

Ignition (Continued)
  clothes, clothing (from controlled fire) (in building) E893.9
    with conflagration - *see* Conflagration
    from
      bonfire E893.2
      highly inflammable material E894
      sources or material as listed in E893.8
      trash fire E893.2
      uncontrolled fire - *see* Conflagration
    in
      private dwelling E893.0
      specified building or structure, except of private dwelling E893.1
    not in building or structure E893.2
  explosive material - *see* Explosion
  fat E894
  gasoline E894
  kerosene E894
  material
    explosive - *see* Explosion
    highly inflammable E894
      with conflagration - *see* Conflagration
      with explosion E923.2
  nightdress - *see* Ignition, clothes
  paraffin E894
  petrol E894
Immersion - *see* Submersion
Implantation of quills of porcupine E906.8
Inanition (from) E904.9
  hunger - *see* Lack of, food
  resulting from homicidal intent E968.4
  thirst - *see* Lack of, water
Inattention after, at birth E904.0
  homicidal, infanticidal intent E968.4
Infanticide (*see also* Assault)
Ingestion
  foreign body (causing injury) (with obstruction) - *see* Foreign body, alimentary canal
  poisonous substance NEC - *see* Table of Drugs and Chemicals
Inhalation
  excessively cold substance, manmade E901.1
  foreign body - *see* Foreign body, aspiration
  liquid air, hydrogen, nitrogen E901.1
  mucus, not of newborn (with asphyxia, obstruction respiratory passage, suffocation) E912
  phlegm (with asphyxia, obstruction respiratory passage, suffocation) E912
  poisonous gas - *see* Table of Drugs and Chemicals
  smoke from, due to
    fire - *see* Fire
    tobacco, second-hand E869.4
  vomitus (with asphyxia, obstruction respiratory passage, suffocation) E911
Injury, injured (accidental(ly)) NEC E928.9
  by, caused by, from
    air rifle (B-B gun) E922.4
    animal (not being ridden) NEC E906.9
      being ridden (in sport or transport) E828●
    assault (*see also* Assault) E968.9
    avalanche E909.2
    bayonet (*see also* Bayonet wound) E920.3
    being thrown against some part of, or object in
      motor vehicle (in motion) (on public highway) E818●
        not on public highway E825●
      nonmotor road vehicle NEC E829●
      off-road motor vehicle NEC E821●
      railway train E806●
      snow vehicle, motor-driven E820●
      street car E829●
    bending
      due to
        repetitive movement E927.3
        sudden strenuous movement E927.0

Injury, injured (Continued)
  by, caused by, from (Continued)
    bite, human E928.3
    broken glass E920.8
    bullet - see Shooting
    cave-in (see also Suffocation, due to, cave-in) E913.3
      earth surface movement or eruption E909.9
      storm E908.9
      without asphyxiation or suffocation E916
    cloudburst E908.8
    component of firearm or air gun E928.7
    cutting or piercing instrument (see also Cut) E920.9
    cyclone E908.1
    earth surface movement or eruption E909.9
    earthquake E909.0
    electric current (see also Electric shock) E925.9
    explosion (see also Explosion) E923.9
      of gun part E928.7
    fire - see Fire
    flare, Verey pistol E922.8
    flood E908.2
    foreign body - see Foreign body
    gun recoil E928.7
    hailstones E904.3
    hurricane E908.0
    landslide E909.2
    law-enforcing agent, police, in course of legal intervention - see Legal intervention
    lightning E907
    live rail or live wire - see Electric shock
    machinery - see also Accident, machine
      aircraft, without accident to aircraft E844●
      boat, ship, watercraft (deck) (engine room) (galley) (laundry) (loading) E836●
    mechanism of firearm or air gun E928.7
    missile
      explosive E923.8
      firearm - see Shooting
      in
        terrorism - see Terrorism, missile
        war operations - see War operations, missile
    moving part of motor vehicle (in motion) (on public highway) E818●
      not on public highway, nontraffic accident E825●
      while alighting, boarding, entering, leaving - see Fall, from, motor vehicle, while alighting, boarding
    nail E920.8
    needle (sewing) E920.4
      hypodermic E920.5
    noise E928.1
    object
      fallen on
        motor vehicle (in motion) (on public highway) E818●
          not on public highway E825●
      falling - see Hit by, object, falling
    paintball gun E922.5
    radiation - see Radiation
    railway rolling stock, train, vehicle (part of) E805●
      door or window E806●
    recoil of firearm E928.7
    rotating propeller, aircraft E844●
    rough landing of off-road type motor vehicle (after leaving ground or rough terrain) E821●
    snow vehicle E820●
    saber (see also Wound, saber) E920.3

Injury, injured (Continued)
  by, caused by, from (Continued)
    shot - see Shooting
    sound waves E928.1
    splinter or sliver, wood E920.8
    straining
      due to
        repetitive movement E927.3
        sudden strenuous movement E927.0
    street car (door) E829●
    suicide (attempt) E958.9
    sword E920.3
    terrorism - see Terrorism
    third rail - see Electric shock
    thunderbolt E907
    tidal wave E909.4
      caused by storm E908.0
    tornado E908.1
    torrential rain E908.2
    twisting
      due to
        repetitive movement E927.3
        sudden strenuous movement E927.0
    vehicle NEC - see Accident, vehicle NEC
    vibration E928.2
    volcanic eruption E909.1
    weapon burst, in war operations E993.9
    weightlessness (in spacecraft, real or simulated) E928.0
    wood splinter or sliver E920.8
  due to
    civil insurrection - see War operations
      occurring after cessation of hostilities E993.9
    terrorism - see Terrorism
    war operations - see War operations
      occurring after cessation of hostilities E993.9
    weapon of mass destruction [WMD] E997.3
  homicidal (see also Assault) E968.9
  in, on
    civil insurrection - see War operations
    fight E960.0
    parachute descent (voluntary) (without accident to aircraft) E844●
      with accident to aircraft - see categories E840-E842
    public highway E819●
    railway right of way E807●
    terrorism - see Terrorism
    war operations - see War operations
  inflicted (by)
    in course of arrest (attempted), suppression of disturbance, maintenance of order, by law enforcing agents - see Legal intervention
    law-enforcing agent (on duty) - see Legal intervention
    other person
      stated as
        accidental E928.9
        homicidal, intentional - see Assault
        undetermined whether accidental or intentional - see Injury, stated as undetermined
    police (on duty) - see Legal intervention
  late effect of E929.9
  purposely (inflicted) by other person(s) - see Assault
  self-inflicted (unspecified whether accidental or intentional) E988.9
    stated as
      accidental E928.9
      intentionally, purposely E958.9
  specified cause NEC E928.8

Injury, injured (Continued)
  stated as
    undetermined whether accidentally or purposely inflicted (by) E988.9
    cut (any part of body) E986
    cutting or piercing instrument (classifiable to E920) E986
    drowning E984
    explosive(s) (missile) E985.5
    falling from high place E987.9
      manmade structure, except residential E987.1
      natural site E987.2
      residential premises E987.0
    hanging E983.0
    knife E986
    late effect of E989
    puncture (any part of body) E986
    shooting - see Shooting, stated as undetermined whether accidental or intentional
    specified means NEC E988.8
    stab (any part of body) E986
    strangulation - see Suffocation, stated as undetermined whether accidental or intentional
    submersion E984
    suffocation - see Suffocation, stated as undetermined whether accidental or intentional
  to child due to criminal abortion E968.8

Insufficient nourishment - see also Lack of, food
  homicidal intent E968.4

Insulation, effects - see Heat

Interruption of respiration by
  food lodged in esophagus E911
  foreign body, except food, in esophagus E912

Intervention, legal - see Legal intervention

Intoxication, drug or poison - see Table of Drugs and Chemicals

Irradiation - see Radiation

J

Jammed (accidentally)
  between objects (moving) (stationary and moving) E918
  in object E918

Jumped or fell from high place, so stated - see Jumping, from, high place, stated as in undetermined circumstances

Jumping
  before train, vehicle or other moving object (unspecified whether accidental or intentional) E988.0
    stated as
      intentional, purposeful E958.0
      suicidal (attempt) E958.0
  from
    aircraft
      by parachute (voluntarily) (without accident to aircraft) E844●
      due to accident to aircraft - see categories E840–E842
    boat, ship, watercraft (into water)
      after accident to, fire on, watercraft E830●
        and subsequently struck by (part of) boat E831●
      burning, crushed, sinking E830●
        and subsequently struck by (part of) boat E831●
      voluntarily, without accident (to boat) with injury other than drowning or submersion E883.0
    building - see also Jumping, from, high place
      burning (uncontrolled fire) E891.8
        in terrorism E979.3
        private E890.8

INDEX TO EXTERNAL CAUSES OF INJURY / **Jumping**

Jumping (Continued)
   from (Continued)
      cable car (not on rails) E847
         on rails E829●
      high place
         in accidental circumstances or in
            sport - see categories E880–E884
         stated as
            with intent to injure self E957.9
               man-made structures NEC
                  E957.1
               natural sites E957.2
               residential premises E957.0
            in undetermined circumstances
               E987.9
               man-made structures NEC
                  E987.1
               natural sites E987.2
               residential premises E987.0
            suicidal (attempt) E957.9
               man-made structures NEC
                  E957.1
               natural sites E957.1
               residential premises E957.0
      motor vehicle (in motion) (on public
         highway) - see Fall, from, motor
         vehicle
      nonmotor road vehicle NEC E829●
      street car E829●
      structure - see also Jumping, from, high
         place
         burning NEC (uncontrolled fire)
            E891.8
         in terrorism E979.3
   into water
      with injury other than drowning or
         submersion E883.0
      drowning or submersion - see
         Submersion
   from, off, watercraft - see Jumping, from,
      boat
Justifiable homicide - see Assault

K

Kicked by
   animal E906.8
   person(s) (accidentally) E917.9
      with intent to injure or kill E960.0
      as, or caused by a crowd E917.1
         with subsequent fall E917.6
      in fight E960.0
      in sports E917.0
         with subsequent fall E917.5
Kicking against
   object (moving) E917.9
      in sports E917.0
         with subsequent fall E917.5
      stationary E917.4
         with subsequent fall E917.8
   person - see Striking against, person
Killed, killing (accidentally) NEC (see also
   Injury) E928.9
   in
      action - see War operations
      brawl, fight (hand) (fists) (foot) E960.0
      by weapon - see also Assault
         cutting, piercing E966
         firearm - see Shooting, homicide
   self
      stated as
         accident E928.9
         suicide - see Suicide
         unspecified whether accidental or suicidal
            E988.9
Knocked down (accidentally) (by) NEC E928.9
   animal (not being ridden) E906.8
      being ridden (in sport or transport) E828●
   blast from explosion (see also Explosion)
      E923.9

Knocked down NEC (Continued)
   crowd, human stampede E917.6
   late effect of - see Late effect
   person (accidentally) E917.9
      in brawl, fight E960.0
      in sports E917.5
   transport vehicle - see vehicle involved under
      Hit by
   while boxing E917.5

L

Laceration NEC E928.9
Lack of
   air (refrigerator or closed place), suffocation
      by E913.2
   care (helpless person) (infant) (newborn)
      E904.0
      homicidal intent E968.4
   food except as result of transport accident
      E904.1
      helpless person, infant, newborn due to
         abandonment or neglect E904.0
   water except as result of transport accident
      E904.2
      helpless person, infant, newborn due to
         abandonment or neglect E904.0
Landslide E909.2
   falling on, hitting
      motor vehicle (any) (in motion) (on or off
         public highway) E909.2
      railway rolling stock, train, vehicle E909.2
Late effect of
   accident NEC (accident classifiable to E928.9)
      E929.9
      specified NEC (accident classifiable to
         E910–E928.8) E929.8
   assault E969
   fall,
      accidental (accident classifiable to
         E880–E888) E929.3
   fire, accident caused by (accident classifiable
      to E890–E899) E929.4
   homicide, attempt (any means) E969
   injury due to terrorism E999.1
   injury undetermined whether accidentally or
      purposely inflicted (injury classifiable
      to E980–E988) E989
   legal intervention (injury classifiable to
      E970–E976) E977
   medical or surgical procedure, test or
      therapy
      as, or resulting in, or from
         abnormal or delayed reaction or
            complication - see Reaction,
            abnormal
         misadventure - see Misadventure
   motor vehicle accident (accident classifiable
      to E810–E825) E929.0
   natural or environmental factor, accident due
      to (accident classifiable to E900–E909)
      E929.5
   poisoning, accidental (accident classifiable to
      E850–E858, E860–E869) E929.2
   suicide, attempt (any means) E959
   transport accident NEC (accident classifiable
      to E800–E807, E826–E838, E840–E848)
      E929.1
   war operations, injury due to (injury
      classifiable to E990–E998) E999.0
Launching pad accident E845●
Legal
   execution, any method E978
   intervention (by) (injury from) E976
      baton E973
      bayonet E974
      blow E975
      blunt object (baton) (nightstick) (stave)
         (truncheon) E973
      cutting or piercing instrument E974

Legal (Continued)
   intervention (Continued)
      dynamite E971
      execution, any method E973
      explosive(s) (shell) E971
      firearm(s) E970
      gas (asphyxiation) (poisoning) (tear) E972
      grenade E971
      late effect of E977
      machine gun E970
      manhandling E975
      mortar bomb E971
      nightstick E973
      revolver E970
      rifle E970
      specified means NEC E975
      stabbing E974
      stave E973
      truncheon E973
Lifting, injury
   due to
      repetitive movement E927.3
      sudden strenuous movement E927.0
Lightning (shock) (stroke) (struck by) E907
Liquid (noncorrosive) in eye E914
   corrosive E924.1
Loss of control
   motor vehicle (on public highway) (without
      antecedent collision) E816●
      with
         antecedent collision on public
            highway - see Collision, motor
            vehicle
         involving any object, person or
            vehicle not on public
            highway E816●
      on public highway - see Collision,
         motor vehicle
      not on public highway, nontraffic
         accident E825●
         with antecedent collision - see
            Collision, motor vehicle,
            not on public highway
   off-road type motor vehicle (not on public
      highway) E821●
      on public highway - see Loss of control,
         motor vehicle
   snow vehicle, motor-driven (not on public
      highway) E820●
      on public highway - see Loss of control,
         motor vehicle
Lost at sea E832●
   with accident to watercraft E830●
   in war operations E995.8
Low
   pressure, effects - see Effects of, air pressure
   temperature, effects - see Cold exposure to
**Lying before train, vehicle or other moving
   object** (unspecified whether accidental or
   intentional) E988.0
   stated as intentional, purposeful, suicidal
      (attempt) E958.0
Lynching (see also Assault) E968.9

M

**Malfunction, atomic power plant in water
   transport** E838●
Mangled (accidentally) NEC E928.9
Manhandling (in brawl, fight) E960.0
   legal intervention E975
Manslaughter (nonaccidental) - see Assault
Marble in nose E912
Mauled by animal E906.8
Medical procedure, complication of
   delayed or as an abnormal reaction without
      mention of misadventure - see
      Reaction, abnormal
   due to or as a result of misadventure - see
      Misadventure

Melting of fittings and furniture in burning
 in terrorism E979.3
Minamata disease E865.2
Misadventure(s) to patient(s) during surgical or medical care E876.9
 contaminated blood, fluid, drug or biological substance (presence of agents and toxins as listed in E875) E875.9
  administered (by) NEC E875.9
   infusion E875.0
   injection E875.1
   specified means NEC E875.2
   transfusion E875.0
   vaccination E875.1
 cut, cutting, puncture, perforation or hemorrhage (accidental) (inadvertent) (inappropriate) (during) E870.9
  aspiration of fluid or tissue (by puncture or catheterization, except heart) E870.5
  biopsy E870.8
   needle (aspirating) E870.5
  blood sampling E870.5
  catheterization E870.5
   heart E870.6
  dialysis (kidney) E870.2
  endoscopic examination E870.4
  enema E870.7
  infusion E870.1
  injection E870.3
  lumbar puncture E870.5
  needle biopsy E870.5
  paracentesis, abdominal E870.5
  perfusion E870.2
  specified procedure NEC E870.8
  surgical operation E870.0
  thoracentesis E870.5
  transfusion E870.1
  vaccination E870.3
 excessive amount of blood or other fluid during transfusion or infusion E873.0
 failure
  in dosage E873.9
   electroshock therapy E873.4
   inappropriate temperature (too hot or too cold) in local application and packing E873.5
   infusion
    excessive amount of fluid E873.0
    incorrect dilution of fluid E873.1
   insulin-shock therapy E873.4
   nonadministration of necessary drug or medicinal E873.6
   overdose - see also Overdose
    radiation, in therapy E873.2
   radiation
    inadvertent exposure of patient (receiving radiation for test or therapy) E873.3
    not receiving radiation for test or therapy - see Radiation
    overdose E873.2
   specified procedure NEC E873.8
   transfusion
    excessive amount of blood E873.0
  mechanical, of instrument or apparatus (during procedure) E874.9
   aspiration of fluid or tissue (by puncture or catheterization, except of heart) E874.4
   biopsy E874.8
    needle (aspirating) E874.4
   blood sampling E874.4
   catheterization E874.4
    heart E874.5
   dialysis (kidney) E874.2
   endoscopic examination E874.3
   enema E874.8
   infusion E874.1
   injection E874.8
   lumbar puncture E874.4

Misadventure(s) to patient(s) during surgical or medical care (Continued)
 failure (Continued)
  mechanical, of instrument or apparatus (Continued)
   needle biopsy E874.4
   paracentesis, abdominal E874.4
   perfusion E874.2
   specified procedure NEC E874.8
   surgical operation E874.0
   thoracentesis E874.4
   transfusion E874.1
   vaccination E874.8
  sterile precautions (during procedure) E872.9
   aspiration of fluid or tissue (by puncture or catheterization, except heart) E872.5
   biopsy E872.8
    needle (aspirating) E872.5
   blood sampling E872.5
   catheterization E872.5
    heart E872.6
   dialysis (kidney) E872.2
   endoscopic examination E872.4
   enema E872.8
   infusion E872.1
   injection E872.3
   lumbar puncture E872.5
   needle biopsy E872.5
   paracentesis, abdominal E872.5
   perfusion E872.2
   removal of catheter or packing E872.8
   specified procedure NEC E872.8
   surgical operation E872.0
   thoracentesis E872.5
   transfusion E872.1
   vaccination E872.3
  suture or ligature during surgical procedure E876.2
  to introduce or to remove tube or instrument E876.4
   foreign object left in body - see Misadventure, foreign object
 foreign object left in body (during procedure) E871.9
  aspiration of fluid or tissue (by puncture or catheterization, except heart) E871.5
  biopsy E871.8
   needle (aspirating) E871.5
  blood sampling E871.5
  catheterization E871.5
   heart E871.6
  dialysis (kidney) E871.2
  endoscopic examination E871.4
  enema E871.8
  infusion E871.1
  injection E871.3
  lumbar puncture E871.5
  needle biopsy E871.5
  paracentesis, abdominal E871.5
  perfusion E871.2
  removal of catheter or packing E871.7
  specified procedure NEC E871.8
  surgical operation E871.0
  thoracentesis E871.5
  transfusion E871.1
  vaccination E871.3
 hemorrhage - see Misadventure, cut
 inadvertent exposure of patient to radiation (being received for test or therapy) E873.3
 inappropriate
  temperature (too hot or too cold) in local application or packing E873.5
 infusion - see also Misadventure, by specific type, infusion
  excessive amount of fluid E873.0
  incorrect dilution of fluid E873.1
  wrong fluid E876.1

Misadventure(s) to patient(s) during surgical or medical care (Continued)
 mismatched blood in transfusion E876.0
 nonadministration of necessary drug or medicinal E873.6
 overdose - see also Overdose
  radiation, in therapy E873.2
 perforation - see Misadventure, cut
 performance of correct operation (procedure) on wrong
  body part E876.7
  side E876.7
  site E876.7
 performance of operation (procedure)
  intended for another patient E876.6
  on patient not scheduled for surgery E876.6
  on wrong patient E876.6
 performance of wrong operation on correct patient E876.5
 puncture - see Misadventure, cut
 specified type NEC E876.8
  failure
   suture or ligature during surgical operation E876.2
   to introduce or to remove tube or instrument E876.4
    foreign object left in body E871.9
   infusion of wrong fluid E876.1
   transfusion of mismatched blood E876.0
   wrong
    fluid in infusion E876.1
    placement of endotracheal tube during anesthetic procedure E876.3
 transfusion - see also Misadventure, by specific type, transfusion
  excessive amount of blood E873.0
  mismatched blood E876.0
 wrong
  device implanted into correct surgical site E876.5
  drug given in error - see Table of Drugs and Chemicals
  fluid in infusion E876.1
  placement of endotracheal tube during anesthetic procedure E876.3
  procedure (operation) performed on the correct patient E876.5
Motion (effects) E903
 sickness E903
Mountain sickness E902.0
Mucus aspiration or inhalation, not of newborn (with asphyxia, obstruction respiratory passage, suffocation) E912
Mudslide of cataclysmic nature E909.2
Murder (attempt) (see also Assault) E968.9

N

Nail, injury by E920.8
Needlestick (sewing needle) E920.4
 hypodermic E920.5
Neglect - see also Privation
 criminal E968.4
 homicidal intent E968.4
Noise (causing injury) (pollution) E928.1
Nuclear weapon (see also War operations, injury due to, nuclear weapons) E996.9

O

Object
 falling
  from, in, on, hitting
   aircraft E844
    due to accident to aircraft - see categories E840–E842

INDEX TO EXTERNAL CAUSES OF INJURY / Object

Object (Continued)
  falling (Continued)
    from, in, on, hitting (Continued)
      machinery - see also Accident, machine
        not in operation E916
      motor vehicle (in motion) (on public
        highway) E818●
        not on public highway E825●
        stationary E916
      nonmotor road vehicle NEC E829●
      pedal cycle E826●
      person E916
      railway rolling stock, train, vehicle
        E806●
      street car E829●
      watercraft E838●
        due to accident to watercraft
          E831●
  set in motion by
    accidental explosion of pressure
      vessel - see category E921
    firearm - see category E922
    machine(ry) - see Accident, machine
    transport vehicle - see categories
      E800–E848
  thrown from, in, on, towards
    aircraft E844●
    cable car (not on rails) E847
      on rails E829●
    motor vehicle (in motion) (on public
      highway) E818●
      not on public highway E825●
    nonmotor road vehicle NEC E829●
    pedal cycle E826●
    street car E829●
    vehicle NEC - see Accident, vehicle NEC
Obstruction
  air passages, larynx, respiratory passages
    by
      external means NEC - see Suffocation
      food, any type (regurgitated)
        (vomited) E911
      material or object, except food E912
      mucus E912
      phlegm E912
      vomitus E911
  digestive tract, except mouth or pharynx
    by
      food, any type E915
      foreign body (any) E915
  esophagus
    food E911
    foreign body, except food E912
    without asphyxia or obstruction of
      respiratory passage E915
  mouth or pharynx
    by
      food, any type E911
      material or object, except food E912
  respiration - see Obstruction, air passages
Oil in eye E914
Overdose
  anesthetic (drug) - see Table of Drugs and
    Chemicals
  drug - see Table of Drugs and Chemicals
Overexertion E927.9
  from
    lifting
      repetitive movement E927.3
      sudden strenuous movement E927.0
    maintaining prolonged positions E927.1
      holding E927.1
      sitting E927.1
      standing E927.1
    prolonged static position E927.1
    pulling
      repetitive movement E927.3
      sudden strenuous movement E927.0
    pushing
      repetitive movement E927.3
      sudden strenuous movement E927.0

Overexertion (Continued)
  from (Continued)
    specified NEC E927.8
    sudden strenuous movement E927.0
Overexposure (accidental) (to)
  cold (see also Cold, exposure to) E901.9
    due to manmade conditions E901.1
  heat (see also Heat) E900.9
  radiation - see Radiation
  radioactivity - see Radiation
  sun, except sunburn E900.0
  weather - see Exposure
  wind - see Exposure
Overheated (see also Heat) E900.9
Overlaid E913.0
Overturning (accidental)
  animal-drawn vehicle E827●
  boat, ship, watercraft
    causing
      drowning, submersion E830●
      injury except drowning, submersion
        E831●
  machinery - see Accident, machine
  motor vehicle (see also Loss of control, motor
    vehicle) E816●
    with antecedent collision on public
      highway - see Collision, motor
      vehicle
    not on public highway, nontraffic accident
      E825●
      with antecedent collision - see
        Collision, motor vehicle, not on
        public highway
  nonmotor road vehicle NEC E829●
  off-road type motor vehicle - see Loss of
    control, off-road type motor vehicle
  pedal cycle E826●
  railway rolling stock, train, vehicle (see also
    Derailment, railway) E802●
  street car E829●
  vehicle NEC - see Accident, vehicle NEC

P

Palsy, divers' E902.2
Parachuting (voluntary) (without accident to
  aircraft) E844●
  due to accident to aircraft - see categories
    E840–E842
Paralysis
  divers' E902.2
  lead or saturnine E866.0
    from pesticide NEC E863.4
Pecked by bird E906.8
Performance of correct operation (procedure)
  on wrong
    body part E876.7
    side E876.7
    site E876.7
Performance of operation (procedure)
  intended for another patient E876.6
  on patient not scheduled for surgery
    E876.6
  on wrong patient E876.6
Performance of wrong operation on correct
  patient E876.5
Phlegm aspiration or inhalation (with
  asphyxia, obstruction respiratory
  passage, suffocation) E912
Piercing (see also Cut) E920.9
  by slide trigger mechanism, scope or other
    part of gun E928.7
Pinched
  between objects (moving) (stationary and
    moving) E918
  by slide trigger mechanism, scope or other
    part of gun E928.7
  in object E918
Pinned under
  machine(ry) - see Accident, machine

Place of occurrence of accident - see Accident
  (to), occurring (at) (in)
Plumbism E866.0
  from insecticide NEC E863.4
Poisoning (accidental) (by) - see also Table of
    Drugs and Chemicals
  carbon monoxide
    generated by
      aircraft in transit E844●
      motor vehicle
        in motion (on public highway)
          E818●
        not on public highway
          E825●
      watercraft (in transit) (not in transit)
        E838●
  caused by injection of poisons or toxins into
    or through skin by plant thorns,
    spines, or other mechanism E905.7
    marine or sea plants E905.6
  fumes or smoke due to
    conflagration - see Conflagration
    explosion or fire - see Fire
    ignition - see Ignition
  gas
    in legal intervention E972
    legal execution, by E978
    on watercraft E838●
    used as anesthetic - see Table of Drugs and
      Chemicals
  in
    terrorism (chemical weapons) E979.7
    war operations E997.2
  late effect of - see Late effect
  legal
    execution E978
    intervention
      by gas E972
Pressure, external, causing asphyxia,
  suffocation (see also Suffocation)
  E913.9
Privation E904.9
  food (see also Lack of, food) E904.1
  helpless person, infant, newborn due to
    abandonment or neglect E904.0
  late effect of NEC E929.5
  resulting from transport accident - see
    categories E800–E848
  water (see also Lack of, water) E904.2
Projected objects, striking against or struck
  by - see Striking against, object
Prolonged stay in
  high altitude (causing conditions as listed in
    E902.0) E902.0
  weightless environment E928.0
Prostration
  heat - see Heat
Pulling, injury
  due to
    repetitive movement E927.3
    sudden strenuous movement E927.0
Puncture, puncturing (see also Cut) E920.9
  by
    plant thorns or spines E920.8
      toxic reaction E905.7
      marine or sea plants E905.6
    sea-urchin spine E905.6
Pushing (injury in) (overexertion) E927.8
  by other person(s) (accidental) E917.9
    as, or caused by, a crowd, human
      stampede E917.1
      with subsequent fall E917.6
    before moving vehicle or object
      stated as
        intentional, homicidal E968.5
        undetermined whether accidental
          or intentional E988.8
    from
      high place
        in accidental circumstances - see
          categories E880–E884

Pushing (Continued)
   by other person(s) (Continued)
      from (Continued)
         high place (Continued)
            stated as
               intentional, homicidal E968.1
               undetermined whether accidental
                  or intentional E987.9
               man-made structure, except
                  residential E987.1
               natural site E987.2
               residential E987.0
         motor vehicle (see also Fall, from, motor
            vehicle) E818●
            stated as
               intentional, homicidal E968.5
               undetermined whether accidental
                  or intentional E988.8
   in sports E917.0
      with fall E886.0
   with fall E886.9
      in sports E886.0
   due to
      repetitive movement E927.3
      sudden strenuous movement E927.0

R

Radiation (exposure to) E926.9
   abnormal reaction to medical test or therapy
      E879.2
   arc lamps E926.2
   atomic power plant (malfunction) NEC
      E926.9
      in water transport E838●
   electromagnetic, ionizing E926.3
   gamma rays E926.3
   in
      terrorism (from or following nuclear
         explosion) (direct) (secondary)
         E979.5
         laser E979.8
      war operations (see also War operations,
         injury due to, nuclear weapons)
         E996.3
         laser(s) E997.0
      water transport E838●
   inadvertent exposure of patient (receiving
      test or therapy) E873.3
   infrared (heaters and lamps) E926.1
      excessive heat E900.1
   ionized, ionizing (particles, artificially
      accelerated) E926.8
      electromagnetic E926.3
   isotopes, radioactive - see Radiation,
      radioactive isotopes
   laser(s) E926.4
      in
         terrorism E979.8
         war operations E997.0
   misadventure in medical care - see
      Misadventure, failure, in dosage,
      radiation
   late effect of NEC E929.8
   excessive heat from - see Heat
   light sources (visible) (ultraviolet) E926.2
   misadventure in medical or surgical
      procedure - see Misadventure, failure,
      in dosage, radiation
   overdose (in medical or surgical pacemaker
      procedure) E873.2
   radar E926.0
   radioactive isotopes E926.5
      atomic power plant malfunction E926.5
      in water transport E838●
      misadventure in medical or surgical
         treatment - see Misadventure,
         failure, in dosage, radiation
   radiobiologicals - see Radiation, radioactive
      isotopes

Radiation (Continued)
   radiofrequency E926.0
   radiopharmaceuticals - see Radiation,
      radioactive isotopes
   radium NEC E926.9
   sun E926.2
      excessive heat from E900.0
   tanning bed E926.2
   welding arc or torch E926.2
      excessive heat from E900.1
   x-rays (hard) (soft) E926.3
      misadventure in medical or surgical
         treatment - see Misadventure,
         failure, in dosage, radiation
Rape E960.1
Reaction, abnormal to or following (medical or
   surgical procedure) E879.9
   amputation (of limbs) E878.5
   anastomosis (arteriovenous) (blood vessel)
      (gastrojejunal) (skin) (tendon) (natural,
      artificial material, tissue) E878.2
      external stoma, creation of E878.3
   aspiration (of fluid) E879.4
      tissue E879.8
   biopsy E879.8
   blood
      sampling E879.7
      transfusion
         procedure E879.8
   bypass - see Reaction, abnormal, anastomosis
   catheterization
      cardiac E879.0
      urinary E879.6
   colostomy E878.3
   cystostomy E878.3
   dialysis (kidney) E879.1
   drugs or biologicals - see Table of Drugs and
      Chemicals
   duodenostomy E878.3
   electroshock therapy E879.3
   formation of external stoma E878.3
   gastrostomy E878.3
   graft - see Reaction, abnormal, anastomosis
   hypothermia E879.8
   implant, implantation (of)
      artificial
         internal device (cardiac pacemaker)
            (electrodes in brain) (heart valve
            prosthesis) (orthopedic) E878.1
         material or tissue (for anastomosis or
            bypass) E878.2
            with creation of external stoma
               E878.3
      natural tissues (for anastomosis or
         bypass) E878.2
         as transplantion - see Reaction,
            abnormal, transplant
         with creation of external stoma E878.3
   infusion
      procedure E879.8
   injection
      procedure E879.8
   insertion of gastric or duodenal sound E879.5
   insulin-shock therapy E879.3
   lumbar puncture E879.4
   perfusion E879.1
   procedures other than surgical operation (see
      also Reaction, abnormal, by specific
      type of procedure) E879.9
      specified procedure NEC E879.8
   radiological procedure or therapy E879.2
   removal of organ (partial) (total) NEC
      E878.6
      with
         anastomosis, bypass or graft E878.2
         formation of external stoma E878.3
         implant of artificial internal device
            E878.1
         transplant(ation)
            partial organ E878.4
            whole organ E878.0

Reaction, abnormal to or following (Continued)
   sampling
      blood E879.7
      fluid NEC E879.4
      tissue E879.8
   shock therapy E879.3
   surgical operation (see also Reaction,
      abnormal, by specified type of
      operation) E878.9
      restorative NEC E878.4
         with
            anastomosis, bypass or graft E878.2
            formation of external stoma E878.3
            implant(ation) - see Reaction,
               abnormal, implant
            transplantation - see Reaction,
               abnormal, transplant
      specified operation NEC E878.8
   thoracentesis E879.4
   transfusion
      procedure E879.8
   transplant, transplantation (heart) (kidney)
      (liver) E878.0
      partial organ E878.4
   ureterostomy E878.3
   vaccination E879.8
Reduction in
   atmospheric pressure - see also Effects of, air
      pressure
      while surfacing from
         deep water diving causing caisson or
            divers' disease, palsy or
            paralysis E902.2
         underground E902.8
Repetitive movements NEC E927.8
Residual (effect) - see Late effect
Rock falling on or hitting (accidentally)
   motor vehicle (in motion) (on public
      highway) E818●
      not on public highway E825●
   nonmotor road vehicle NEC E829●
   pedal cycle E826●
   person E916
   railway rolling stock, train, vehicle
      E806●
Running off, away
   animal (being ridden) (in sport or transport)
      E828●
      not being ridden E906.8
   animal-drawn vehicle E827●
   rails, railway (see also Derailment) E802●
   roadway
      motor vehicle (without antecedent
         collision) E816●
         nontraffic accident E825●
            with antecedent collision - see
               categories Collision, motor
               vehicle, not on public
               highway
         with
            antecedent collision - see Collision
               motor vehicle
            subsequent collision
               involving any object, person or
                  vehicle not on public
                  highway E816●
               on public highway E811●
      nonmotor road vehicle NEC E829●
      pedal cycle E826●
Run over (accidentally) (by)
   animal (not being ridden) E906.8
      being ridden (in sport or transport)
         E828●
   animal-drawn vehicle E827●
   machinery - see Accident, machine
   motor vehicle (on public highway) - see Hit
      by, motor vehicle
   nonmotor road vehicle NEC E829●
   railway train E805●
   street car E829●
   vehicle NEC E848

S

Saturnism E866.0
  from insecticide NEC E863.4
Scald, scalding (accidental) (by) (from) (in) E924.0
  acid - *see* Scald, caustic
  boiling tap water E924.2
  caustic or corrosive liquid, substance E924.1
    swallowed - *see* Table of Drugs and Chemicals
  homicide (attempt) - *see* Assault, burning
  inflicted by other person
    stated as
      intentional or homicidal E968.3
      undetermined whether accidental or intentional E988.2
  late effect of NEC E929.8
  liquid (boiling) (hot) E924.0
  local application of externally applied substance in medical or surgical care E873.5
  molten metal E924.0
  self-inflicted (unspecified whether accidental or intentional) E988.2
    stated as intentional, purposeful E958.2
    stated as undetermined whether accidental or intentional E988.2
  steam E924.0
  tap water (boiling) E924.2
  transport accident - *see* categories E800–E848
  vapor E924.0
Scratch, cat E906.8
Sea
  sickness E903
Self-mutilation - *see* Suicide
Sequelae (of)
  in
    terrorism E999.1
    war operations E999.0
Shock
  anaphylactic (*see also* Table of Drugs and Chemicals) E947.9
  due to
    bite (venomous) - *see* Bite, venomous NEC
    sting - *see* Sting
  electric (*see also* Electric shock) E925.9
  from electric appliance or current (*see also* Electric shock) E925.9
Shooting, shot (accidental(ly)) E922.9
  air gun E922.4
  BB gun E922.4
  hand gun (pistol) (revolver) E922.0
  himself (*see also* Shooting, self-inflicted) E985.4
    hand gun (pistol) (revolver) E985.0
    military firearm, except hand gun E985.3
      hand gun (pistol) (revolver) E985.0
    rifle (hunting) E985.2
      military E985.3
    shotgun (automatic) E985.1
    specified firearm NEC E985.4
    Verey pistol E985.4
  homicide (attempt) E965.4
    air gun E968.6
    BB gun E968.6
    hand gun (pistol) (revolver) E965.0
    military firearm, except hand gun E965.3
      hand gun (pistol) (revolver) E965.0
    paintball gun E965.4
    rifle (hunting) E965.2
      military E965.3
    shotgun (automatic) E965.1
    specified firearm NEC E965.4
    Verey pistol E965.4
  inflicted by other person
    in accidental circumstances E922.9
      hand gun (pistol) (revolver) E922.0
      military firearm, except hand gun E922.3
        hand gun (pistol) (revolver) E922.0

Shooting, shot (*Continued*)
  inflicted by other person (*Continued*)
    in accidental circumstances (*Continued*)
      rifle (hunting) E922.2
        military E922.3
      shotgun (automatic) E922.1
      specified firearm NEC E922.8
      Verey pistol E922.8
    stated as
      intentional, homicidal E965.4
        hand gun (pistol) (revolver) E965.0
        military firearm, except hand gun E965.3
          hand gun (pistol) (revolver) E965.0
        paintball gun E965.4
        rifle (hunting) E965.2
          military E965.3
        shotgun (automatic) E965.1
        specified firearm E965.4
        Verey pistol E965.4
      undetermined whether accidental or intentional E985.4
        air gun E985.6
        BB gun E985.6
        hand gun (pistol) (revolver) E985.0
        military firearm, except hand gun E985.3
          hand gun (pistol) (revolver) E985.0
        paintball gun E985.7
        rifle (hunting) E985.2
        shotgun (automatic) E985.1
        specified firearm NEC E985.4
        Verey pistol E985.4
  in
    terrorism - *see* Terrorism, shooting
    war operations - *see* War operations, shooting
  legal
    execution E978
    intervention E970
  military firearm, except hand gun E922.3
    hand gun (pistol) (revolver) E922.0
  paintball gun E922.5
  rifle (hunting) E922.2
    military E922.3
  self-inflicted (unspecified whether accidental or intentional) E985.4
    air gun E985.6
    BB gun E985.6
    hand gun (pistol) (revolver) E985.0
    military firearm, except hand gun E985.3
      hand gun (pistol) (revolver) E985.0
    paintball gun E985.7
    rifle (hunting) E985.2
      military E985.3
    shotgun (automatic) E985.1
    specified firearm NEC E985.4
    stated as
      accidental E922.9
        hand gun (pistol) (revolver) E922.0
        military firearm, except hand gun E922.3
          hand gun (pistol) (revolver) E922.0
        paintball gun E922.5
        rifle (hunting) E922.2
          military E922.3
        shotgun (automatic) E922.1
        specified firearm NEC E922.8
        Verey pistol E922.8
      intentional, purposeful E955.4
        hand gun (pistol) (revolver) E955.0
        military firearm, except hand gun E955.3
          hand gun (pistol) (revolver) E955.0
        paintball gun E955.7
        rifle (hunting) E955.2
          military E955.3

Shooting, shot (*Continued*)
  self-inflicted (*Continued*)
    stated as (*Continued*)
      intentional, purposeful (*Continued*)
        shotgun (automatic) E955.1
        specified firearm NEC E955.4
        Verey pistol E955.4
    shotgun (automatic) E922.1
    specified firearm NEC E922.8
    stated as undetermined whether accidental or intentional E985.4
      hand gun (pistol) (revolver) E985.0
      military firearm, except hand gun E985.3
        hand gun (pistol) (revolver) E985.0
      paintball gun E985.7
      rifle (hunting) E985.2
        military E985.3
      shotgun (automatic) E985.1
      specified firearm NEC E985.4
      Verey pistol E985.4
    suicidal (attempt) E955.4
      air gun E985.6
      BB gun E985.6
      hand gun (pistol) (revolver) E955.0
      military firearm, except hand gun E955.3
        hand gun (pistol) (revolver) E955.0
      paintball gun E955.7
      rifle (hunting) E955.2
        military E955.3
      shotgun (automatic) E955.1
      specified firearm NEC E955.4
      Verey pistol E955.4
  Verey pistol E922.8
Shoving (accidentally) by other person (*see also* Pushing by other person) E917.9
Sickness
  air E903
  alpine E902.0
  car E903
  motion E903
  mountain E902.0
  sea E903
  travel E903
Sinking (accidental)
  boat, ship, watercraft (causing drowning, submersion) E830 ●
    causing injury except drowning, submersion E831 ●
Siriasis E900.0
Skydiving E844 ●
Slashed wrists (*see also* Cut, self-inflicted) E986
Slipping (accidental)
  on
    deck (of boat, ship, watercraft) (icy) (oily) (wet) E835 ●
    ice E885.9
    ladder of ship E833 ●
      due to accident to watercraft E831 ●
    mud E885.9
    oil E885.9
    snow E885.9
    stairs of ship E833 ●
      due to accident to watercraft E831 ●
    surface
      slippery E885.9
      wet E885.9
Sliver, wood, injury by E920.8
Smothering, smothered (*see also* Suffocation) E913.9
Smouldering building or structure in terrorism E979.3
Sodomy (assault) E960.1
Solid substance in eye (any part) or adnexa E914
Sound waves (causing injury) E928.1
Splinter, injury by E920.8
Stab, stabbing E966
  accidental - *see* Cut

INDEX TO EXTERNAL CAUSES OF INJURY / Suffocation

Starvation E904.1
    helpless person, infant, newborn - *see* Lack of food
    homicidal intent E968.4
    late effect of NEC E929.5
    resulting from accident connected with transport - *see* categories E800–E848
Stepped on
    by
        animal (not being ridden) E906.8
            being ridden (in sport or transport) E828●
        crowd E917.1
        person E917.9
            in sports E917.0
    in sports E917.0
Stepping on
    object (moving) E917.9
        in sports E917.0
            with subsequent fall E917.5
        stationary E917.4
            with subsequent fall E917.8
    person E917.9
        as, or caused by a crowd E917.1
            with subsequent fall E917.6
        in sports E917.0
Sting E905.9
    ant E905.5
    bee E905.3
    caterpillar E905.5
    coral E905.6
    hornet E905.3
    insect NEC E905.5
    jelly fish E905.6
    marine animal or plant E905.6
    nematocysts E905.6
    scorpion E905.2
    sea anemone E905.6
    sea cucumber E905.6
    wasp E905.3
    yellow jacket E905.3
Storm E908.9
    specified type NEC E908.8
Straining, injury
    due to
        repetitive movement E927.3
        sudden strenuous movement E927.0
Strangling - *see* Suffocation
Strangulation - *see* Suffocation
Strenuous movements (in recreational or other activities) NEC E927.8
Striking against
    bottom (when jumping or diving into water) E883.0
    object (moving) E917.9
        caused by crowd E917.1
            with subsequent fall E917.6
        furniture E917.3
            with subsequent fall E917.7
        in
            running water E917.2
                with drowning or submersion - *see* Submersion
            sports E917.0
                with subsequent fall E917.5
        stationary E917.4
            with subsequent fall E917.8
    person(s) E917.9
        with fall E886.9
            in sports E886.0
        as, or caused by, a crowd E917.1
            with subsequent fall E917.6
        in sports E917.0
            with fall E886.0
Stroke
    heat - *see* Heat
    lightning E907

Struck by - *see also* Hit by
    bullet
        in
            terrorism E979.4
            war operations E991.2
                rubber E991.0
    lightning E907
    missile
        in terrorism - *see* Terrorism, missile
    object
        falling
            from, in, on
                building
                      burning (uncontrolled fire)
                          in terrorism E979.3
    thunderbolt E907
Stumbling over animal, carpet, curb, rug or (small) object (with fall) E885.9
    without fall - *see* Striking against, object
Submersion (accidental) E910.8
    boat, ship, watercraft (causing drowning, submersion) E830●
        causing injury except drowning, submersion E831●
    by other person
        in accidental circumstances - *see* category E910
        intentional, homicidal E964
        stated as undetermined whether accidental or intentional E984
    due to
        accident
            machinery - *see* Accident, machine
            to boat, ship, watercraft E830●
            transport - *see* categories E800-E848
        avalanche E909.2
        cataclysmic
            earth surface movement or eruption E909.9
            storm E908.9
        cloudburst E908.8
        cyclone E908.1
        fall
            from
                boat, ship, watercraft (not involved in accident) E832●
                burning, crushed E830●
                involved in accident, collision E830●
            gangplank (into water) E832●
            overboard NEC E832●
        flood E908.2
        hurricane E908.0
        jumping into water E910.8
            from boat, ship, watercraft
                burning, crushed, sinking E830●
                involved in accident, collision E830●
                not involved in accident, for swim E910.2
            in recreational activity (without diving equipment) E910.2
                with or using diving equipment E910.1
            to rescue another person E910.3
    homicide (attempt) E964
    in
        bathtub E910.4
        specified activity, not sport, transport or recreational E910.3
        sport or recreational activity (without diving equipment) E910.2
            with or using diving equipment E910.1
            water skiing E910.0
        swimming pool NEC E910.8
        terrorism E979.8
        war operations E995.4
            intentional E995.3
        water transport E832●
            due to accident to boat, ship, watercraft E830●

Submersion (*Continued*)
    landslide E909.2
        overturning boat, ship, watercraft E909.2
        sinking boat, ship, watercraft E909.2
        submersion boat, ship, watercraft E909.2
        tidal wave E909.4
            caused by storm E908.0
        torrential rain E908.2
    late effect of NEC E929.8
    quenching tank E910.8
    self-inflicted (unspecified whether accidental or intentional) E984
        in accidental circumstances - *see* category E910
        stated as intentional, purposeful E954
    stated as undetermined whether accidental or intentional E984
    suicidal (attempted) E954
    while
        attempting rescue of another person E910.3
        engaged in
            marine salvage E910.3
            underwater construction or repairs E910.3
        fishing, not from boat E910.2
        hunting, not from boat E910.2
        ice skating E910.2
        pearl diving E910.3
        placing fishing nets E910.3
        playing in water E910.2
        scuba diving E910.1
            nonrecreational E910.3
        skin diving E910.1
        snorkel diving E910.2
        spear fishing underwater E910.1
        surfboarding E910.2
        swimming (swimming pool) E910.2
        wading (in water) E910.2
        water skiing E910.0
Sucked
    into
        jet (aircraft) E844●
Suffocation (accidental) (by external means) (by pressure) (mechanical) E913.9
    caused by other person
        in accidental circumstances - *see* category E913
        stated as
            intentional, homicidal E963
            undetermined whether accidental or intentional E983.9
                by, in
                      hanging E983.0
                      plastic bag E983.1
                      specified means NEC E983.8
    due to, by
        avalanche E909.2
        bedclothes E913.0
        bib E913.0
        blanket E913.0
        cave-in E913.3
            caused by cataclysmic earth surface movement or eruption E909.9
        conflagration - *see* Conflagration E983.8
        explosion - *see* Explosion
        falling earth, other substance E913.3
        fire - *see* Fire
        food, any type (ingestion) (inhalation) (regurgitated) (vomited) E911
        foreign body, except food (ingestion) (inhalation) E912
        ignition - *see* Ignition
        landslide E909.2
        machine(ry) - *see* Accident, machine
        material, object except food entering by nose or mouth, ingested, inhaled E912
        mucus (aspiration) (inhalation), not of newborn E912
        phlegm (aspiration) (inhalation) E912

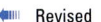

◀ New   ⇚ Revised   ~~deleted~~ Deleted   ● Use Additional Digit(s)   Omit code

633

E CODES

INDEX TO EXTERNAL CAUSES OF INJURY / Suffocation

Suffocation (Continued)
  due to, by (Continued)
    pillow E913.0
    plastic bag - see Suffocation, in, plastic bag
    sheet (plastic) E913.0
    specified means NEC E913.8
    vomitus (aspiration) (inhalation) E911
  homicidal (attempt) E963
    in war operations E995.3
  in
    airtight enclosed place E913.2
    baby carriage E913.0
    bed E913.0
    closed place E913.2
    cot, cradle E913.0
    perambulator E913.0
    plastic bag (in accidental circumstances) E913.1
      homicidal, purposely inflicted by other person E963
      self-inflicted (unspecified whether accidental or intentional) E983.1
        in accidental circumstances E913.1
        intentional, suicidal E953.1
      stated as undetermined whether accidentally or purposely inflicted E983.1
      suicidal, purposely self-inflicted E953.1
    refrigerator E913.2
    war operations E995.3
  self-inflicted - see also Suffocation, stated as undetermined whether accidental or intentional E953.9
    in accidental circumstances - see category E913
    stated as intentional, purposeful - see Suicide, suffocation
  stated as undetermined whether accidental or intentional E983.9
    by, in
      hanging E983.0
      plastic bag E983.1
      specified means NEC E983.8
  suicidal - see Suicide, suffocation

Suicide, suicidal (attempted) (by) E958.9
  burning, burns E958.1
  caustic substance E958.7
    poisoning E950.7
    swallowed E950.7
  cold, extreme E958.3
  cut (any part of body) E956
  cutting or piercing instrument (classifiable to E920) E956
  drowning E954
  electrocution E958.4
  explosive(s) (classifiable to E923) E955.5
  fire E958.1
  firearm (classifiable to E922) - see Shooting, suicidal
  hanging E953.0
  jumping
    before moving object, train, vehicle E958.0
    from high place - see Jumping, from, high place, stated as, suicidal
  knife E956
  late effect of E959
  motor vehicle, crashing of E958.5
  poisoning - see Table of Drugs and Chemicals
  puncture (any part of body) E956
  scald E958.2
  shooting - see Shooting, suicidal
  specified means NEC E958.8
  stab (any part of body) E956
  strangulation - see Suicide, suffocation
  submersion E954
  suffocation E953.9
    by, in
      hanging E953.0
      plastic bag E953.1
      specified means NEC E953.8
  wound NEC E958.9

Sunburn E926.2
Sunstroke E900.0
Supersonic waves (causing injury) E928.1
Surgical procedure, complication of
  delayed or as an abnormal reaction without mention of misadventure, see Reaction, abnormal
  due to or as a result of misadventure - see Misadventure
Swallowed, swallowing
  foreign body - see Foreign body, alimentary canal
  poison - see Table of Drugs and Chemicals
  substance
    caustic - see Table of Drugs and Chemicals
    drugs
    corrosive - see Table of Drugs and Chemicals
    poisonous - see Table of Drugs and Chemicals
Swimmers' cramp (see also category E910) E910.2
  not in recreation or sport E910.3
Syndrome, battered
  baby or child - see Abuse, child
  wife - see Assault

T

Tackle in sport E886.0
Terrorism (by) (in) (injury) E979.8
  air blast E979.2
  aircraft burned, destroyed, exploded, shot down E979.1
    used as a weapon E979.1
  anthrax E979.6
  asphyxia from
    chemical (weapons) E979.7
    fire, conflagration (caused by fire-producing device) E979.3
      from nuclear explosion E979.5
    gas or fumes E979.7
  bayonet E979.8
  biological agents E979.6
  blast (air) (effects) E979.2
    from nuclear explosion E979.5
    underwater E979.0
  bomb (antipersonnel) (mortar) (explosion) (fragments) E979.2
  bullet(s) (from carbine, machine gun, pistol, rifle, shotgun) E979.4
  burn from
    chemical E979.7
    fire, conflagration (caused by fire-producing device) E979.3
      from nuclear explosion E979.5
    gas E979.7
  burning aircraft E979.1
  chemical E979.7
  cholera E979.6
  conflagration E979.3
  crushed by falling aircraft E979.1
  depth-charge E979.0
  destruction of aircraft E979.1
  disability, as sequelae one year or more after injury E999.1
  drowning E979.8
  effect
    of nuclear weapon (direct) (secondary) E979.5
    secondary NEC E979.9
    sequelae E999.1
  explosion (artillery shell) (breech-block) (cannon block) E979.2
    aircraft E979.1
    bomb (antipersonnel) (mortar) E979.2
      nuclear (atom) (hydrogen) E979.5
    depth-charge E979.0
    grenade E979.2
    injury by fragments from E979.2

Terrorism (Continued)
  explosion (Continued)
    land-mine E979.2
    marine weapon E979.0
    mine (land) E979.2
      at sea or in harbor E979.0
      marine E979.0
    missile (explosive) NEC E979.2
    munitions (dump) (factory) E979.2
    nuclear (weapon) E979.5
      other direct and secondary effects of E979.5
    sea-based artillery shell E979.0
    torpedo E979.0
  exposure to ionizing radiation from nuclear explosion E979.5
  falling aircraft E979.1
  fire or fire-producing device E979.3
  firearms E979.4
  fireball effects from nuclear explosion E979.5
  fragments from artillery shell, bomb NEC, grenade, guided missile, land-mine, rocket, shell, shrapnel E979.2
  gas or fumes E979.7
  grenade (explosion) (fragments) E979.2
  guided missile (explosion) (fragments) E979.2
    nuclear E979.5
  heat from nuclear explosion E979.5
  hot substances E979.3
  hydrogen cyanide E979.7
  land-mine (explosion) (fragments) E979.2
  laser(s) E979.8
  late effect of E999.1
  lewisite E979.7
  lung irritant (chemical) (fumes) (gas) E979.7
  marine mine E979.0
  mine E979.2
    at sea E979.0
    in harbor E979.0
    land (explosion) (fragments) E979.2
    marine E979.0
  missile (explosion) (fragments) (guided) E979.2
    marine E979.0
    nuclear weapons E979.5
  mortar bomb (explosion) (fragments) E979.2
  mustard gas E979.7
  nerve gas E979.7
  nuclear weapons E979.5
  pellets (shotgun) E979.4
  petrol bomb E979.3
  phosgene E979.7
  piercing object E979.8
  poisoning (chemical) (fumes) (gas) E979.7
  radiation, ionizing from nuclear explosion E979.5
  rocket (explosion) (fragments) E979.2
  saber, sabre E979.8
  sarin E979.7
  screening smoke E979.7
  sequelae effect (of) E999.1
  shell (aircraft) (artillery) (cannon) (land-based) (explosion) (fragments) E979.2
    sea-based E979.0
  shooting E979.4
    bullet(s) E979.4
    pellet(s) (rifle) (shotgun) E979.4
  shrapnel E979.2
  smallpox E979.7
  stabbing object(s) E979.8
  submersion E979.8
  torpedo E979.0
  underwater blast E979.0
  vesicant (chemical) (fumes) (gas) E979.7
  weapon burst E979.2
Thermic fever E900.9
Thermoplegia E900.9
Thirst - see also Lack of water
  resulting from accident connected with transport - see categories E800–E848

INDEX TO EXTERNAL CAUSES OF INJURY / War operations

Thrown (accidentally)
  against object in or part of vehicle
    by motion of vehicle
      aircraft E844●
      boat, ship, watercraft E838●
      motor vehicle (on public highway) E818●
        not on public highway E825●
        off-road type (not on public highway) E821●
        on public highway E818●
      snow vehicle E820●
        on public highway E818●
      nonmotor road vehicle NEC E829●
      railway rolling stock, train, vehicle E806●
      street car E829●
  from
    animal (being ridden) (in sport or transport) E828●
    high place, homicide (attempt) E968.1
    machinery - see Accident, machine
    vehicle NEC - see Accident, vehicle NEC
  off - see Thrown, from
  overboard (by motion of boat, ship, watercraft) E832●
    by accident to boat, ship, watercraft E830●
Thunderbolt NEC E907
Tidal wave (any injury) E909.4
  caused by storm E908.0
Took
  overdose of drug - see Table of Drugs and Chemicals
  poison - see Table of Drugs and Chemicals
Tornado (any injury) E908.1
Torrential rain (any injury) E908.2
Traffic accident NEC E819●
Trampled by animal E906.8
  being ridden (in sport or transport) E828●
Trapped (accidentally)
  between
    objects (moving) (stationary and moving) E918
  by
    door of
      elevator E918
      motor vehicle (on public highway) (while alighting, boarding) - see Fall, from, motor vehicle, while alighting
      railway train (underground) E806●
      street car E829●
      subway train E806●
  in object E918
Trauma
  cumulative
    from
      repetitive
        impact E927.4
        motion or movements E927.3
    sudden from strenuous movement E927.0
Travel (effects) E903
  sickness E903
Tree
  falling on or hitting E916
    motor vehicle (in motion) (on public highway) E818●
      not on public highway E825●
    nonmotor road vehicle NEC E829●
    pedal cycle E826●
    person E916
    railway rolling stock, train, vehicle E806●
    street car E829●
Trench foot E901.0
Tripping over animal, carpet, curb, rug, or small object (with fall) E885.9
  without fall - see Striking against, object
Tsunami E909.4
Twisting, injury
  due to
    repetitive movement E927.3
    sudden strenuous movement E927.0

V

Violence, nonaccidental (see also Assault) E968.9
Volcanic eruption (any injury) E909.1
Vomitus in air passages (with asphyxia, obstruction or suffocation) E911

W

War operations (during hostilities) (injury) (by) (in) E995.9
  after cessation of hostilities, injury due to E998.9
  air blast E993.9
  aircraft burned, destroyed, exploded, shot down E991.9
  asphyxia from
    chemical E997.2
    fire, conflagration (caused by fire-producing device or conventional weapon) E990.9
      from nuclear explosion (see also War operations, injury due to, nuclear weapons) E996.8
      incendiary bomb E990.0
      petrol bomb E990.0
    fumes E997.2
    gas E997.2
  baton (nightstick) E995.1
  battle wound NEC E995.8
  bayonet E995.2
  biological warfare agents E997.1
  blast (air) (effects) E993.9
    from nuclear explosion - see War operations, injury due to, nuclear weapons
    underwater E992.9
  bomb (mortar) (explosion) E993.2
    after cessation of hostilities E998.1
    fragments, injury by E991.4
      antipersonnel E991.3
  bullet(s) (from carbine, machine gun, pistol, rifle, shotgun) E991.2
    rubber E991.0
  burn from
    chemical E997.2
    fire, conflagration (caused by fire-producing device or conventional weapon) E990.9
      from
        conventional weapon E990.3
        flamethrower E990.1
        incendiary bomb E990.0
        incendiary bullet E990.2
        nuclear explosion E996.2
        petrol bomb E990.0
    gas E997.2
  burning aircraft E994.3
  chemical E997.2
  chlorine E997.2
  conventional warfare, specified form NEC E995.8
  crushing by falling aircraft E994.8
  depth charge E992.1
  destruction of aircraft E994.9
  detonation of own munitions (ammunition) (artillery) (mortars), unintentional E993.6
  disability as sequela one year or more after injury E999.0
  discharge of own munitions launch device (autocannons) (automatic grenade launchers) (missile launchers) (small arms), unintentional E993.7
  drowning E995.4
  effect nuclear weapon (see also War operations, injury due to, nuclear weapons) E996.9

War operations (Continued)
  explosion (breech block) (cannon shell) E993.9
    after cessation of hostilities
      bomb placed in war E998.1
      mine placed in war E998.0
    aircraft E994.1
      due to
        enemy fire or explosives E994.0
        own onboard explosives E994.1
    artillery shell E993.2
    bomb (mortar) E993.2
      aerial E993.0
      atom (see also War operations, injury due to, nuclear weapons) E996.9
      hydrogen (see also War operations, injury due to, nuclear weapons) E996.9
      injury by fragments from E991.4
        antipersonnel E991.3
      nuclear (see also War operations, injury due to, nuclear weapons) E996.9
    depth charge E992.1
    injury by fragments from E991.4
      antipersonnel E991.3
    marine weapon NEC E992.8
    mine
      at sea or in harbor E992.2
      land E993.8
        injury by fragments from E991.4
      marine E992.2
    missile, guided E993.1
    mortar E993.2
    munitions (accidental) (being used in war) (dump) (factory) E993.9
      own E993.7
        ammunition (artillery) (mortars) E993.6
        launch device (autocannons) (automatic grenade launchers) (missile launchers) (small arms) E993.7
    nuclear (weapon) (see also War operations, injury due to, nuclear weapons) E996.9
    own weapons (accidental) E993.7
      injury by fragments from E991.9
        antipersonnel E991.3
    sea-based artillery shell E992.3
    specified NEC E993.8
    torpedo E992.0
  exposure to ionizing radiation from nuclear explosion (see also War operations, injury due to, nuclear weapons) E996.3
  falling aircraft E994.8
  fire or fire-producing device E990.9
    flamethrower E990.1
    incendiary bomb E990.0
    incendiary bullet E990.2
    indirectly caused from conventional weapon E990.3
    petrol bomb E990.0
  fireball effects from nuclear explosion E996.2
  fragments from
    antipersonnel bomb E991.3
    artillery shell E991.4
    bomb NEC E991.4
    grenade E991.4
    guided missile E991.4
    land mine E991.4
    rocket E991.4
    shell E991.4
    shrapnel E991.9
  fumes E997.2
  gas E997.2
  grenade (explosion) E993.8
    fragments, injury by E991.4
  guided missile (explosion) E993.1
    fragments, injury by E991.4
    nuclear (see also War operations, injury due to, nuclear weapons) E996.9

INDEX TO EXTERNAL CAUSES OF INJURY / War operations

War operations (Continued)
   heat from nuclear explosion E996.2
   injury due to
      aerial bomb E993.0
      air blast E993.9
      aircraft shot down E994.0
      artillery shell E993.2
      blast E993.9
         wave E993.9
         wind E993.9
      bomb E993.8
      but occurring after cessation of hostilities E998.9
         explosion of bombs E998.1
         explosion of mines E998.0
         specified NEC E998.8
      conventional warfare E995.9
         specified form NEC E995.8
      depth charge E992.1
      destruction of aircraft E994.9
         due to
            air to air missile E994.0
            collision with other aircraft E994.2
            enemy fire or explosives E994.0
            on board explosion (explosives) E994.1
            on board fire E994.3
            rocket propelled grenade [RPG] E994.0
            small arms fire E994.0
            surface to air missile E994.0
         specified NEC E994.8
      dirty bomb (see also War operations, injury due to, nuclear weapons) E996.9
      drowning E995.4
      explosion (direct pressure) (indirect pressure) (due to) E993.9
         depth charge E992.1
         improvised explosive device [IED]
            person borne E993.3
            roadside E993.5
            specified NEC E993.5
            transport vehicle (air) (land) (water) borne E993.4
            vehicle (air) (land) (water) borne E993.4
         marine mines (in harbor) (at sea) E992.2
         marine weapons E992.9
            specified NEC E992.8
         sea based artillery shell E992.3
         specified NEC E993.8
         torpedo E992.0
         unintentional (of own)
            autocannons E993.7
            automatic grenade launchers E993.7
            launch device discharge E993.7
            munitions detonation (ammunition) (artillery) (mortars) E993.6
            missile launchers E993.7
            small arms E993.7
      fragments (from) E991.9
         artillery E991.8
         artillery shells E991.4
         autocannons E991.8
         automatic grenade launchers [AGL] E991.8
         bombs E991.4
            antipersonnel E991.3
         detonation of unexploded ordnance [UXO] E991.4
         grenade E991.4
         guided missile E991.4
         improvised explosive device [IED]
            person borne E991.5
            roadside E991.7
            specified NEC E991.7
            transport vehicle (air) (land) (water) borne E991.6
            vehicle (air) (land) (water) borne E991.6

War operations (Continued)
   injury due to (Continued)
      fragments (Continued)
         land mine E991.4
         missile launchers E991.8
         mortars E991.8
         munitions (artillery shells) (bombs) (grenades) (rockets) (shells) E991.4
         rockets E991.4
         shells E991.4
         small arms E991.8
         specified NEC E991.9
         weapons (artillery) (autocannons) (mortars) (small arms) E991.8
      grenade E993.8
      guided missile E993.1
      hand to hand combat, unarmed E995.0
      improvised explosive device [IED]
         person borne E993.3
         roadside E993.5
         specified NEC E993.5
         transport vehicle (air) (land) (water) borne E993.4
         vehicle (air) (land) (water) borne E993.4
      inability to surface or obtain air E995.4
      land mine E993.8
      marine mines (in harbor) (at sea) E992.2
      marine weapons E992.9
         specified NEC E992.8
      mortar E993.2
      nuclear weapons E996.9
         beta burns E996.3
         blast debris E996.1
         blast pressure E996.0
         burns due to thermal radiation E996.2
         direct blast effect E996.0
         fallout exposure E996.3
         fireball effect E996.2
         flash burns E996.2
         heat effect E996.2
         indirect blast effect E996.1
         nuclear radiation effects E996.3
         radiation exposure (acute) E996.3
         radiation sickness E996.3
         secondary effects E996.3
         specified effects NEC E996.8
         thermal radiation effect E996.2
      piercing object E995.2
      restriction of airway, intentional E995.3
      sea based artillery shell E992.3
      shrapnel E991.9
      stave E995.1
      strangulation E995.3
      strike by blunt object (baton) (nightstick) (stave) E995.1
      submersion (accidental) (unintentional) E995.4
         intentional E995.3
      suffocation E995.3
         accidental E995.4
      torpedo E992.0
      underwater blast E992.9
      weapon of mass destruction [WMD] E997.3
   knife E995.2
   lacrimator (gas) (chemical) E997.2
   land mine (explosion) E993.8
      after cessation of hostilities E998.0
      fragments, injury by E991.4
   laser(s) E997.0
   late effect of E999.0
   lewisite E997.2
   lung irritant (chemical) (fumes) (gas) E997.2
   marine mine E992.2
   mine
      after cessation of hostilities E998.0
      at sea E992.2
      in harbor E992.2
      land (explosion) E993.8
         fragments, injury by E991.4
      marine E992.2

War operations (Continued)
   missile (guided) (explosion) E993.1
      fragments, injury by E991.4
      marine E992.8
      nuclear (see also War operations, injury due to, nuclear weapons) E996.9
   mortar bomb (explosion) E993.2
      fragments, injury by E991.4
   mustard gas E997.2
   nerve gas E997.2
   phosgene E997.2
   piercing object E995.2
   poisoning (chemical) (fumes) (gas) E997.2
   radiation, ionizing from nuclear explosion (see also War operations, injury due to, nuclear weapons) E996.3
   rocket (explosion) E993.8
      fragments, injury by E991.4
   saber, sabre E995.2
   screening smoke E997.8
   shell (aircraft) (artillery) (cannon) (land based) (explosion) E993.2
      fragments, injury by E991.4
      sea-based E992.3
   shooting E991.2
      after cessation of hostilities E998.8
      bullet(s) E991.2
         rubber E991.0
      pellet(s) (rifle) E991.1
      shrapnel E991.9
   stave E995.2
   strike by blunt object (baton) (nightstick) (stave) E995.1
   submersion E995.4
      intentional E995.3
   sword E995.2
   torpedo E992.0
   unconventional warfare, except by nuclear weapon E997.9
      biological (warfare) E997.1
      gas, fumes, chemicals E997.2
      laser(s) E997.0
      specified type NEC E997.8
   underwater blast E992.9
   vesicant (chemical) (fumes) (gas) E997.2
   weapon burst E993.9

Washed
   away by flood - see Flood
   away by tidal wave - see Tidal wave
   off road by storm (transport vehicle) E908.9
   overboard E832●

Weapon of mass destruction [WMD] E997.3

Weather exposure - see also Exposure
   cold E901.0
   hot E900.0

Weightlessness (causing injury) (effects of) (in spacecraft, real or simulated) E928.0

Wound (accidental) NEC (see also Injury) E928.9
   battle (see also War operations) E995.9
   bayonet E920.3
   in
      legal intervention E974
      war operations E995.2
   gunshot - see Shooting
   incised - see Cut
   saber, sabre E920.3
      in war operations E995.2

Wrong
   body part, performance of correct operation (procedure) on E876.7
   device implanted into correct surgical site E876.5
   patient, performance of operation (procedure) on E876.6
   procedure (operation) performed on correct patient E876.5
   side, performance of correct operation (procedure) on E876.7
   site, performance of correct operation (procedure) on E876.7

PART III

DISEASES: TABULAR LIST VOLUME 1

PART III / Diseases: Tabular List Volume 1 001-003.9

1. INFECTIOUS AND PARASITIC DISEASES (001–139)

Note: Categories for "late effects" of infectious and parasitic diseases are to be found at 137–139.

Includes diseases generally recognized as communicable or transmissible as well as a few diseases of unknown but possibly infectious origin

Excludes *acute respiratory infections (460–466)*
carrier or suspected carrier of infectious organism (V02.0–V02.9)
certain localized infections
influenza (487.0–487.8, 488.01–488.19)

INTESTINAL INFECTIOUS DISEASES (001–009)

Excludes *helminthiases (120.0–129)*
Diseases or infestations caused by parasitic worms

● **001 Cholera**
A serious, often deadly, infectious disease of the small intestine
- 001.0 Due to Vibrio cholerae
- 001.1 Due to Vibrio cholerae el tor
- 001.9 Cholera, unspecified

● **002 Typhoid and paratyphoid fevers**
Caused by Salmonella typhi and Salmonella paratyphi A, B, and C bacteria
- 002.0 Typhoid fever
  Typhoid (fever) (infection) [any site]
- 002.1 Paratyphoid fever A
- 002.2 Paratyphoid fever B
- 002.3 Paratyphoid fever C
- 002.9 Paratyphoid fever, unspecified

Item 1-1 Salmonella is a bacterium that lives in the intestines of fowl and mammals and can spread to humans through improper food preparation and cooking. Salmonellosis is an infection with the bacterium. Symptoms include diarrhea, fever, and abdominal cramps 12 to 72 hours after infection. The illness usually lasts 4 to 7 days, and most persons recover without treatment. The diarrhea may be so severe that the patient needs to be hospitalized. Patients with immunocompromised systems in chronic, ill health are more likely to have the infection invade their bloodstream with life-threatening results. For example, patients with sickle cell disease are more prone to salmonella osteomyelitis than others.

● **003 Other salmonella infections**
Includes infection or food poisoning by Salmonella [any serotype]
- 003.0 Salmonella gastroenteritis
  Salmonellosis
- 003.1 Salmonella septicemia
● 003.2 Localized salmonella infections
  - 003.20 Localized salmonella infection, unspecified
    Specified in the documentation as localized, but unspecified as to type
  - 003.21 Salmonella meningitis
    Specified as localized in the meninges
  - 003.22 Salmonella pneumonia
    Specified as localized in the lungs
  - 003.23 Salmonella arthritis
    Specified as localized in the joints
  - 003.24 Salmonella osteomyelitis
    Specified as localized in bone
  - 003.29 Other
    Specified as localized (because it is still under localized heading) but does not assign into any of the above codes
- 003.8 Other specified salmonella infections
  Any specified salmonella infection which does NOT assign into any of the above codes (not specified as localized)
- 003.9 Salmonella infection, unspecified
  Unspecified in the documentation as to specific type of salmonella

- **004 Shigellosis**
  An infectious disease caused by a group of bacteria (Shigella)
  Includes: bacillary dysentery
  - 004.0 **Shigella dysenteriae**
    Infection by group A Shigella (Schmitz) (Shiga)
  - 004.1 **Shigella flexneri**
    Infection by group B Shigella
  - 004.2 **Shigella boydii**
    Infection by group C Shigella
  - 004.3 **Shigella sonnei**
    Infection by group D Shigella
  - 004.8 **Other specified shigella infections**
  - 004.9 **Shigellosis, unspecified**
- **005 Other food poisoning (bacterial)**
  See Table A, Table of Bacterial Food Poisoning, page 1017
  Excludes: salmonella infections (003.0–003.9)
  toxic effect of:
  food contaminants (989.7)
  noxious foodstuffs (988.0–988.9)
  - 005.0 **Staphylococcal food poisoning**
    Staphylococcal toxemia specified as due to food
  - 005.1 **Botulism food poisoning**
    Botulism NOS
    Food poisoning due to Clostridium botulinum
    Excludes: infant botulism (040.41)
    wound botulism (040.42)
  - 005.2 **Food poisoning due to Clostridium perfringens [C. welchii]**
    Enteritis necroticans
  - 005.3 **Food poisoning due to other Clostridia**
  - 005.4 **Food poisoning due to Vibrio parahaemolyticus**
  - 005.8 **Other bacterial food poisoning**
    Excludes: salmonella food poisoning (003.0–003.9)
    - 005.81 **Food poisoning due to Vibrio vulnificus**
    - 005.89 **Other bacterial food poisoning**
      Food poisoning due to Bacillus cereus
  - 005.9 **Food poisoning, unspecified**
- **006 Amebiasis**
  An intestinal illness caused by the microscopic parasite Entamoeba histolytica
  Includes: infection due to Entamoeba histolytica
  Excludes: amebiasis due to organisms other than Entamoeba histolytica (007.8)
  - 006.0 **Acute amebic dysentery without mention of abscess**
    Acute amebiasis
  - 006.1 **Chronic intestinal amebiasis without mention of abscess**
    Chronic:
    amebiasis
    amebic dysentery
  - 006.2 **Amebic nondysenteric colitis**
  - 006.3 **Amebic liver abscess**
    Hepatic amebiasis
  - 006.4 **Amebic lung abscess**
    Amebic abscess of lung (and liver)
  - 006.5 **Amebic brain abscess**
    Amebic abscess of brain (and liver) (and lung)
  - 006.6 **Amebic skin ulceration**
    Cutaneous amebiasis
  - 006.8 **Amebic infection of other sites**
    Amebic:
    appendicitis
    balanitis
    Ameboma
    Excludes: specific infections by free-living amebae (136.21–136.29)
  - 006.9 **Amebiasis, unspecified**
    Amebiasis NOS
- **007 Other protozoal intestinal diseases**
  Includes: protozoal:
  colitis
  diarrhea
  dysentery
  - 007.0 **Balantidiasis**
    Infection by Balantidium coli
  - 007.1 **Giardiasis**
    Infection by Giardia lamblia
    Lambliasis
  - 007.2 **Coccidiosis**
    Infection by Isospora belli and Isospora hominis
    Isosporiasis
  - 007.3 **Intestinal trichomoniasis**
  - 007.4 **Cryptosporidiosis**
    Coding Clinic: 1997, Q4, P30-31
  - 007.5 **Cyclosporiasis**
  - 007.8 **Other specified protozoal intestinal diseases**
    Amebiasis due to organisms other than Entamoeba histolytica
  - 007.9 **Unspecified protozoal intestinal disease**
    Flagellate diarrhea
    Protozoal dysentery NOS
- **008 Intestinal infections due to other organisms**
  Includes: any condition classifiable to 009.0–009.3 with mention of the responsible organisms
  Excludes: food poisoning by these organisms (005.0–005.9)
  - 008.0 **Escherichia coli [E. coli]**
    Coding Clinic: 1988, Q2, P10
    - 008.00 **E. coli, unspecified**
      E. coli enteritis NOS
    - 008.01 **Enteropathogenic E. coli**
    - 008.02 **Enterotoxigenic E. coli**
    - 008.03 **Enteroinvasive E. coli**
    - 008.04 **Enterohemorrhagic E. coli**
      Coding Clinic: 2011, Q4, P83
    - 008.09 **Other intestinal E. coli infections**
  - 008.1 **Arizona group of paracolon bacilli**
  - 008.2 **Aerobacter aerogenes**
    Enterobacter aerogenes
  - 008.3 **Proteus (mirabilis) (morganii)**
  - 008.4 **Other specified bacteria**
    - 008.41 **Staphylococcus**
      Staphylococcal enterocolitis
    - 008.42 **Pseudomonas**
      Coding Clinic: 1989, Q2, P10
    - 008.43 **Campylobacter**
    - 008.44 **Yersinia enterocolitica**
    - 008.45 **Clostridium difficile**
      Pseudomembranous colitis
    - 008.46 **Other anaerobes**
      Anaerobic enteritis NOS
      Bacteroides (fragilis)
      Gram-negative anaerobes

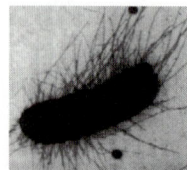

Figure 1-1 Electron micrograph of escherichia coli *(E. coli)* expressing P fimbriae. (From Mandell, Bennett, & Dolin: Principles and Practice of Infectious Diseases, ed 7, Churchill Livingstone, An Imprint of Elsevier, 2009)

Item 1-2 *Escherichia coli [E. coli]* is a gram-negative bacterium found in the intestinal tracts of humans and animals and is usually nonpathogenic. Pathogenic strains can cause diarrhea or pyogenic (pus-producing) infections. Can be a threat to food safety.

008.47 **Other gram-negative bacteria**
Gram-negative enteritis NOS
Excludes: gram-negative anaerobes (008.46)

008.49 **Other**
Coding Clinic: 1989, Q2, P10

● 008.5 **Bacterial enteritis, unspecified**
● 008.6 **Enteritis due to specified virus**

008.61 **Rotavirus**

008.62 **Adenovirus**

008.63 **Norwalk virus**
Norovirus
Norwalk-like agent

008.64 **Other small round viruses [SRV's]**
Small round virus NOS

008.65 **Calicivirus**

008.66 **Astrovirus**

008.67 **Enterovirus NEC**
Coxsackie virus
Echovirus
Excludes: poliovirus (045.0–045.9)

008.69 **Other viral enteritis**
Torovirus
Coding Clinic: 2003, Q1, P10-11

008.8 **Other organism, not elsewhere classified**
Viral:
enteritis NOS
gastroenteritis
Excludes: influenza with involvement of gastrointestinal tract (487.8, 488.09, 488.19)

● 009 **Ill-defined intestinal infections**
Excludes: diarrheal disease or intestinal infection due to specified organism (001.0–008.8)
diarrhea following gastrointestinal surgery (564.4)
intestinal malabsorption (579.0–579.9)
ischemic enteritis (557.0–557.9)
other noninfectious gastroenteritis and colitis (558.1–558.9)
regional enteritis (555.0–555.9)
ulcerative colitis (556)

009.0 **Infectious colitis, enteritis, and gastroenteritis**
Colitis (septic)   Enteritis (septic)
Dysentery: Gastroenteritis (septic)
  NOS
  catarrhal
  hemorrhagic
Coding Clinic: 1988, Q2, P10

009.1 **Colitis, enteritis, and gastroenteritis of presumed infectious origin**
Excludes: colitis NOS (558.9)
enteritis NOS (558.9)
gastroenteritis NOS (558.9)
Coding Clinic: 1999, Q3, P6-7

009.2 **Infectious diarrhea**
Diarrhea:
dysenteric
epidemic
Infectious diarrheal disease NOS

009.3 **Diarrhea of presumed infectious origin**
Excludes: diarrhea NOS (787.91)
Coding Clinic: 1987, Nov-Dec, P7

TUBERCULOSIS (010–018)

Includes: infection by Mycobacterium tuberculosis (human) (bovine)
Excludes: congenital tuberculosis (771.2)
late effects of tuberculosis (137.0–137.4)

The following fifth-digit subclassification is for use with categories 010–018:

0 unspecified
1 bacteriological or histological examination not done
2 bacteriological or histological examination unknown (at present)
3 tubercle bacilli found (in sputum) by microscopy
4 tubercle bacilli not found (in sputum) by microscopy, but found by bacterial culture
5 tubercle bacilli not found by bacteriological examination, but tuberculosis confirmed histologically
6 tubercle bacilli not found by bacteriological or histological examination, but tuberculosis confirmed by other methods [inoculation of animals]

● 010 **Primary tuberculous infection**
Requires fifth digit. See beginning of section 010–018 for codes and definitions.

● 010.0 **Primary tuberculous infection**
[0-6]   Excludes: nonspecific reaction to test for tuberculosis without active tuberculosis (795.51-795.52)
positive PPD (795.51)
positive tuberculin skin test without active tuberculosis (795.51)

● 010.1 **Tuberculous pleurisy in primary progressive**
[0-6] tuberculosis

● 010.8 **Other primary progressive tuberculosis**
[0-6]   Excludes: tuberculous erythema nodosum (017.1)

● 010.9 **Primary tuberculous infection, unspecified**
[0-6]

● 011 **Pulmonary tuberculosis**
Requires fifth digit. See beginning of section 010–018 for codes and definitions.
Use additional code to identify any associated silicosis (502)

● 011.0 **Tuberculosis of lung, infiltrative**
[0-6]

● 011.1 **Tuberculosis of lung, nodular**
[0-6]

● 011.2 **Tuberculosis of lung with cavitation**
[0-6]   Cavitation = pitting
Coding Clinic: 1994, Q4, P36

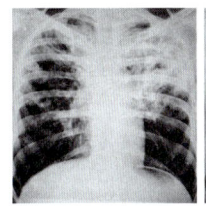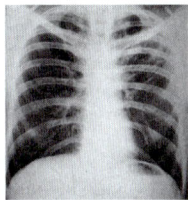

Figure 1–2 Far advanced bilateral pulmonary tuberculosis before and after 8 months of treatment with streptomycin, PAS, and isoniazid. (From Hinshaw HC, Garland LH: Diseases of the Chest, ed 4, Philadelphia, WB Saunders, 1980)

Item 1-3 **Tuberculosis** is a common and deadly infectious disease caused by the *Mycobacterium tuberculosis* organism. The first tuberculosis infection is called the **primary infection** and most commonly attacks the lungs but can affect the central nervous system, lymphatic system, circulatory system, genitourinary system, bones, joints, and even the skin. A **Ghon** lesion is the **initial lesion**. A **secondary lesion** occurs when the tubercle bacilli are carried to other areas.

011.3–016.4 ICD-9-CM

- ● 011.3 Tuberculosis of bronchus
  [0-6]
  Excludes isolated bronchial tuberculosis (012.2)
- ● 011.4 Tuberculous fibrosis of lung
  [0-6]
- ● 011.5 Tuberculous bronchiectasis
  [0-6]
- ● 011.6 Tuberculous pneumonia [any form]
  [0-6]
- ● 011.7 Tuberculous pneumothorax
  [0-6]
- ● 011.8 Other specified pulmonary tuberculosis
  [0-6]
- ●■ 011.9 Pulmonary tuberculosis, unspecified
  [0-6]
  Respiratory tuberculosis NOS
  Tuberculosis of lung NOS
- ● 012 Other respiratory tuberculosis
  Requires fifth digit. See beginning of section 010–018 for codes and definitions.
  Excludes respiratory tuberculosis, unspecified (011.9)
- ● 012.0 Tuberculous pleurisy
  [0-6]
  Tuberculosis of pleura
  Tuberculous empyema
  Tuberculous hydrothorax
  Excludes pleurisy with effusion without mention of cause (511.9)
  tuberculous pleurisy in primary progressive tuberculosis (010.1)
- ● 012.1 Tuberculosis of intrathoracic lymph nodes
  [0-6]
  Tuberculosis of lymph nodes:
  hilar
  mediastinal
  tracheobronchial
  Tuberculous tracheobronchial adenopathy
  Excludes that specified as primary (010.0–010.9)
- ● 012.2 Isolated tracheal or bronchial tuberculosis
  [0-6]
- ● 012.3 Tuberculous laryngitis
  [0-6]
  Tuberculosis of glottis
- ● 012.8 Other specified respiratory tuberculosis
  [0-6]
  Tuberculosis of:
  mediastinum
  nasopharynx
  nose (septum)
  sinus [any nasal]
- ● 013 Tuberculosis of meninges and central nervous system
  Requires fifth digit. See beginning of section 010–018 for codes and definitions.
- ● 013.0 Tuberculous meningitis
  [0-6]
  Tuberculosis of meninges (cerebral) (spinal)
  Tuberculous:
  leptomeningitis
  meningoencephalitis
  Excludes tuberculoma of meninges (013.1)
- ● 013.1 Tuberculoma of meninges
  [0-6]
- ● 013.2 Tuberculoma of brain
  [0-6]
  Tuberculosis of brain (current disease)
- ● 013.3 Tuberculous abscess of brain
  [0-6]
- ● 013.4 Tuberculoma of spinal cord
  [0-6]
- ● 013.5 Tuberculous abscess of spinal cord
  [0-6]

Item 1–4 Although it primarily affects the lungs, the bacteria **Mycobacterium tuberculosis** can travel from the pulmonary circulation to virtually any organ in the body, much as a cancer metastasizes to a secondary site. If the immune system becomes compromised by age or disease, what would otherwise be a self-limiting primary tuberculosis in the lungs will develop in other organs. These are known as extrapulmonary sites.

- ● 013.6 Tuberculous encephalitis or myelitis
  [0-6]
- ● 013.8 Other specified tuberculosis of central nervous system
  [0-6]
- ●■ 013.9 Unspecified tuberculosis of central nervous system
  [0-6]
  Tuberculosis of central nervous system NOS
- ● 014 Tuberculosis of intestines, peritoneum, and mesenteric glands
  Requires fifth digit. See beginning of section 010–018 for codes and definitions.
- ● 014.0 Tuberculous peritonitis
  [0-6]
  Tuberculous ascites
- ● 014.8 Other
  [0-6]
  Tuberculosis (of):
  anus
  intestine (large) (small)
  mesenteric glands
  rectum
  retroperitoneal (lymph nodes)
  Tuberculous enteritis
- ● 015 Tuberculosis of bones and joints
  Requires fifth digit. See beginning of section 010–018 for codes and definitions.
  Use additional code to identify manifestation, as:
  tuberculous:
  arthropathy (711.4)
  necrosis of bone (730.8)
  osteitis (730.8)
  osteomyelitis (730.8)
  synovitis (727.01)
  tenosynovitis (727.01)
- ● 015.0 Vertebral column
  [0-6]
  Pott's disease
  Use additional code to identify manifestation, as:
  curvature of spine [Pott's] (737.4)
  kyphosis (737.4)
  spondylitis (720.81)
- ● 015.1 Hip
  [0-6]
- ● 015.2 Knee
  [0-6]
- ● 015.5 Limb bones
  [0-6]
  Tuberculous dactylitis
- ● 015.6 Mastoid
  [0-6]
  Tuberculous mastoiditis
- ● 015.7 Other specified bone
  [0-6]
- ● 015.8 Other specified joint
  [0-6]
- ●■ 015.9 Tuberculosis of unspecified bones and joints
  [0-6]
- ● 016 Tuberculosis of genitourinary system
  Requires fifth digit. See beginning of section 010–018 for codes and definitions.
- ● 016.0 Kidney
  [0-6]
  Renal tuberculosis
  Use additional code to identify manifestation, as:
  tuberculous:
  nephropathy (583.81)
  pyelitis (590.81)
  pyelonephritis (590.81)
- ● 016.1 Bladder
  [0-6]
- ● 016.2 Ureter
  [0-6]
- ● 016.3 Other urinary organs
  [0-6]
- ● 016.4 Epididymis
  [0-6]

- **016.5 Other male genital organs**
  [0-6]
  Use additional code to identify manifestation, as:
  tuberculosis of:
  prostate (601.4)
  seminal vesicle (608.81)
  testis (608.81)
- **016.6 Tuberculous oophoritis and salpingitis**
  [0-6]
  Oophoritis = inflammation of ovary
  Salpingitis = inflammation of fallopian tube
- **016.7 Other female genital organs**
  [0-6]
  Tuberculous:
  cervicitis
  endometritis
- **016.9 Genitourinary tuberculosis, unspecified**
  [0-6]

- **017 Tuberculosis of other organs**
  Requires fifth digit. See beginning of section 010–018 for codes and definitions.
- **017.0 Skin and subcutaneous cellular tissue**
  [0-6]
  Lupus: Tuberculosis:
  exedens   colliquativa
  vulgaris   cutis
  Scrofuloderma   lichenoides
                  papulonecrotica
                  verrucosa cutis
  Excludes lupus erythematosus (695.4)
  disseminated (710.0)
  lupus NOS (710.0)
  nonspecific reaction to test for tuberculosis
  without active tuberculosis
  (795.51-795.52)
  positive PPD (795.51)
  positive tuberculin skin test without active
  tuberculosis (795.51)
- **017.1 Erythema nodosum with hypersensitivity reaction in tuberculosis**
  [0-6]
  Bazin's disease
  Erythema:
  induratum
  nodosum, tuberculous
  Tuberculosis indurativa
  Excludes erythema nodosum NOS (695.2)
- **017.2 Peripheral lymph nodes**
  [0-6]
  Scrofula
  Scrofulous abscess
  Tuberculous adenitis
  Excludes tuberculosis of lymph nodes:
  bronchial and mediastinal (012.1)
  mesenteric and retroperitoneal (014.8)
  tuberculous tracheobronchial adenopathy (012.1)
- **017.3 Eye**
  [0-6]
  Use additional code to identify manifestation, as:
  tuberculous:
  episcleritis (379.09)
  interstitial keratitis (370.59)
  iridocyclitis, chronic (364.11)
  keratoconjunctivitis (phlyctenular) (370.31)
- **017.4 Ear**
  [0-6]
  Tuberculosis of ear
  Tuberculous otitis media
  Excludes tuberculous mastoiditis (015.6)
- **017.5 Thyroid gland**
  [0-6]
- **017.6 Adrenal glands**
  [0-6]
  Addison's disease, tuberculous
- **017.7 Spleen**
  [0-6]
- **017.8 Esophagus**
  [0-6]

Item 1–5 Miliary tuberculosis can be a life-threatening condition. If a tuberculous lesion enters a blood vessel, immense dissemination of tuberculous organisms can occur if the immune system is weak. High-risk populations—children under 4 years of age, the elderly, or the immunocompromised—are particularly prone to this type of infection. The lesions will have a millet seed-like appearance on chest x-ray. Bronchial washings and biopsy may aid in diagnosis.

- **017.9 Other specified organs**
  [0-6]
  Use additional code to identify manifestation, as:
  tuberculosis of:
  endocardium [any valve] (424.91)
  myocardium (422.0)
  pericardium (420.0)
- **018 Miliary tuberculosis**
  Requires fifth digit. See beginning of section 010–018 for codes and definitions.
  Includes tuberculosis:
  disseminated
  generalized
  miliary, whether of a single specified site,
  multiple sites, or unspecified site
  polyserositis
- **018.0 Acute miliary tuberculosis**
  [0-6]
- **018.8 Other specified miliary tuberculosis**
  [0-6]
- **018.9 Miliary tuberculosis, unspecified**
  [0-6]

ZOONOTIC BACTERIAL DISEASES (020–027)

- **020 Plague**
  Infectious disease caused by Yersinia pestis bacterium, transmitted by rodent flea bite or handling infected animal
  Includes infection by Yersinia [Pasteurella] pestis
  - 020.0 Bubonic
  - 020.1 Cellulocutaneous
  - 020.2 Septicemic
  - 020.3 Primary pneumonic
  - 020.4 Secondary pneumonic
  - 020.5 Pneumonic, unspecified
  - 020.8 Other specified types of plague
    Abortive plague
    Ambulatory plague
    Pestis minor
  - 020.9 Plague, unspecified
- **021 Tularemia**
  Caused by Francisella tularensis bacterium found in rodents, rabbits, and hares; transmitted by contact with infected animal tissues or ticks, biting flies, and mosquitoes
  Includes deerfly fever
  infection by Francisella [Pasteurella] tularensis
  rabbit fever
  - 021.0 Ulceroglandular tularemia
  - 021.1 Enteric tularemia
    Tularemia:
    cryptogenic
    intestinal
    typhoidal
  - 021.2 Pulmonary tularemia
    Bronchopneumonic tularemia
  - 021.3 Oculoglandular tularemia
  - 021.8 Other specified tularemia
    Tularemia:
    generalized or disseminated
    glandular
  - 021.9 Unspecified tularemia

022 Anthrax
An acute infectious disease caused by the spore-forming Bacillus anthracis; it may occur in humans exposed to infected animals or tissue from infected animals

- **022.0 Cutaneous anthrax**
  Malignant pustule
- **022.1 Pulmonary anthrax**
  Respiratory anthrax
  Wool-sorters' disease
- **022.2 Gastrointestinal anthrax**
- **022.3 Anthrax septicemia**
- **022.8 Other specified manifestations of anthrax**
- **022.9 Anthrax, unspecified**

023 Brucellosis
Infectious disease caused by bacterium Brucella. Humans are infected by contact with contaminated animals or animal products. Brucellosis symptoms are similar to flu.

Includes fever:
  Malta
  Mediterranean
  undulant
    Rising and falling

- **023.0 Brucella melitensis**
- **023.1 Brucella abortus**
- **023.2 Brucella suis**
- **023.3 Brucella canis**
- **023.8 Other brucellosis**
  Infection by more than one organism
- **023.9 Brucellosis, unspecified**

024 Glanders
Infection by:
  Actinobacillus mallei
  Malleomyces mallei
  Pseudomonas mallei
  Farcy
  Malleus

025 Melioidosis
Infection by:
  Malleomyces pseudomallei
  Pseudomonas pseudomallei
  Whitmore's bacillus
Pseudoglanders

026 Rat-bite fever
RBF is an infectious disease caused by Streptobacillus moniliformis or Spirillum minus.

- **026.0 Spirillary fever**
  Rat-bite fever due to Spirillum minor [S. minus]
  Sodoku
- **026.1 Streptobacillary fever**
  Epidemic arthritic erythema
  Haverhill fever
  Rat-bite fever due to Streptobacillus moniliformis
- **026.9 Unspecified rat-bite fever**

027 Other zoonotic bacterial diseases
- **027.0 Listeriosis**
  Infection by Listeria monocytogenes
  Septicemia by Listeria monocytogenes
  Use additional code to identify manifestations, as meningitis (320.7)
  Excludes congenital listeriosis (771.2)
- **027.1 Erysipelothrix infection**
  Erysipeloid (of Rosenbach)
  Infection by Erysipelothrix insidiosa [E. rhusiopathiae]
  Septicemia by Erysipelothrix insidiosa [E. rhusiopathiae]
- **027.2 Pasteurellosis**
  Pasteurella pseudotuberculosis infection by Pasteurella multocida [P. septica]
  Mesenteric adenitis by Pasteurella multocida [P. septica]
  Septic infection (cat bite) (dog bite) by Pasteurella multocida [P. septica]
  Excludes infection by:
    Francisella [Pasteurella] tularensis (021.0–021.9)
    Yersinia [Pasteurella] pestis (020.0–020.9)
  Coding Clinic: 2012, Q3, P14
- **027.8 Other specified zoonotic bacterial diseases**
- **027.9 Unspecified zoonotic bacterial disease**

OTHER BACTERIAL DISEASES (030–041)

Excludes bacterial venereal diseases (098.0–099.9)
  bartonellosis (088.0)

030 Leprosy
Also known as Hansen's disease; chronic infectious disease attacking skin, peripheral nerves, and mucous membranes

Includes Hansen's disease
  infection by Mycobacterium leprae

- **030.0 Lepromatous [type L]**
  Lepromatous leprosy (macular) (diffuse) (infiltrated) (nodular) (neuritic)
- **030.1 Tuberculoid [type T]**
  Tuberculoid leprosy (macular) (maculoanesthetic) (major) (minor) (neuritic)
- **030.2 Indeterminate [group I]**
  Indeterminate [uncharacteristic] leprosy (macular) (neuritic)
- **030.3 Borderline [group B]**
  Borderline or dimorphous leprosy (infiltrated) (neuritic)
- **030.8 Other specified leprosy**
- **030.9 Leprosy, unspecified**

031 Diseases due to other mycobacteria
- **031.0 Pulmonary**
  Battey disease
  Infection by Mycobacterium:
    avium
    intracellulare [Battey bacillus]
    kansasii
- **031.1 Cutaneous**
  Buruli ulcer
  Infection by Mycobacterium:
    marinum [M. balnei]
    ulcerans
- **031.2 Disseminated**
  Disseminated mycobacterium avium-intracellulare complex (DMAC)
  Mycobacterium avium-intracellulare complex (MAC) bacteremia
  Coding Clinic: 1997, Q4, P31
- **031.8 Other specified mycobacterial diseases**
- **031.9 Unspecified diseases due to mycobacteria**
  Atypical mycobacterium infection NOS

032 Diphtheria
Highly contagious bacterial disease that results in formation of an adherent membrane in the throat that may lead to suffocation. It may attack the heart and lungs. The exact location is specified in the codes.

Includes infection by Corynebacterium diphtheriae

- **032.0 Faucial diphtheria**
  Membranous angina, diphtheritic
- **032.1 Nasopharyngeal diphtheria**
- **032.2 Anterior nasal diphtheria**
- **032.3 Laryngeal diphtheria**
  Laryngotracheitis, diphtheritic

- **032.8 Other specified diphtheria**
  - 032.81 Conjunctival diphtheria
    - Pseudomembranous diphtheritic conjunctivitis
  - 032.82 Diphtheritic myocarditis
  - 032.83 Diphtheritic peritonitis
  - 032.84 Diphtheritic cystitis
  - 032.85 Cutaneous diphtheria
  - 032.89 Other
- **032.9 Diphtheria, unspecified**
- **033 Whooping cough**

  Pertussis (whooping cough) is a highly contagious disease caused by the bacterium Bordetella pertussis and results in a whooping sound.

  Includes pertussis

  Use additional code to identify any associated pneumonia (484.3)
  - 033.0 Bordetella pertussis [B. pertussis]
  - 033.1 Bordetella parapertussis [B. parapertussis]
  - 033.8 Whooping cough due to other specified organism
    - Bordetella bronchiseptica [B. bronchiseptica]
  - **033.9 Whooping cough, unspecified organism**
- **034 Streptococcal sore throat and scarlet fever**
  - 034.0 Streptococcal sore throat

    Septic:
      angina
      sore throat
    Streptococcal:
      angina
      laryngitis
      pharyngitis
      tonsillitis

    Coding Clinic: 1985, Sept-Oct, P9
  - 034.1 Scarlet fever
    - Scarlatina
    - **Excludes** parascarlatina (057.8)
- 035 Erysipelas
  - **Excludes** postpartum or puerperal erysipelas (670.8)
- **036 Meningococcal infection**

  Most commonly caused by bacteria Streptococcus pneumoniae and Neisseria meningitidis
  - 036.0 Meningococcal meningitis
    - Cerebrospinal fever (meningococcal)
    - Meningitis:
      - cerebrospinal
      - epidemic
  - 036.1 Meningococcal encephalitis
  - 036.2 Meningococcemia
    - Meningococcal septicemia
  - 036.3 Waterhouse-Friderichsen syndrome, meningococcal
    - Meningococcal hemorrhagic adrenalitis
    - Meningococcic adrenal syndrome
    - Waterhouse-Friderichsen syndrome NOS
  - **036.4 Meningococcal carditis**
    - 036.40 Meningococcal carditis, unspecified
    - 036.41 Meningococcal pericarditis
    - 036.42 Meningococcal endocarditis
    - 036.43 Meningococcal myocarditis
  - **036.8 Other specified meningococcal infections**
    - 036.81 Meningococcal optic neuritis
    - 036.82 Meningococcal arthropathy
    - 036.89 Other
  - 036.9 Meningococcal infection, unspecified
    - Meningococcal infection NOS

- 037 Tetanus

  Also indexed as "lockjaw." Do not confuse tetanus with tetany, which is severe muscle twitches, cramps, and spasms (781.7).

  Excludes tetanus:
    complicating:
      abortion (634–638 with .0, 639.0)
      ectopic or molar pregnancy (639.0)
    neonatorum (771.3)
    puerperal (670.8)

- **038 Septicemia**

  Blood poisoning/bacteremia, often associated with serious illness

  Use additional code for systemic inflammatory response syndrome (SIRS) (995.91–995.92).

  Excludes bacteremia (790.7)
    septicemia (sepsis) of newborn (771.81)

  Coding Clinic: 2012, Q3, P12; 2010, Q2, P4; 2004, Q2, P16; 1994, Q2, P13; 1993, Q3, P6; 1988, Q2, P12
  - 038.0 Streptococcal septicemia
    - **Coding Clinic: 1996, Q2, P5**
  - **038.1 Staphylococcal septicemia**
    - 038.10 Staphylococcal septicemia, unspecified
    - 038.11 Methicillin susceptible Staphylococcus aureus septicemia
      - MSSA septicemia
      - Staphylococcus aureus septicemia NOS
      - **Coding Clinic: 2008, Q4, P69-73; 1998, Q4, P41-42**
    - 038.12 Methicillin resistant Staphylococcus aureus septicemia
      - **Coding Clinic: 2011, Q4, P153; Q3, P15; 2008, Q4, P69-73**
    - 038.19 Other staphylococcal septicemia
  - 038.2 Pneumococcal septicemia [Streptococcus pneumoniae septicemia]
    - **Coding Clinic: 1996, Q2, P5; 1991, Q1, P13**
  - 038.3 Septicemia due to anaerobes
    - Septicemia due to bacteroides
    - **Excludes** gas gangrene (040.0)
        that due to anaerobic streptococci (038.0)
  - **038.4 Septicemia due to other gram-negative organisms**
    - 038.40 Gram-negative organism, unspecified
      - Gram-negative septicemia NOS
      - **Coding Clinic: 2007, Q4, P84-86**
    - 038.41 Hemophilus influenzae [H. influenzae]
    - 038.42 Escherichia coli [E. coli]
      - **Coding Clinic: 2003, Q4, P73**
    - 038.43 Pseudomonas
    - 038.44 Serratia
    - 038.49 Other
      - **Coding Clinic: 2012, Q3, P14**
  - 038.8 Other specified septicemias
    - **Excludes** septicemia (due to):
        anthrax (022.3)
        gonococcal (098.89)
        herpetic (054.5)
        meningococcal (036.2)
        septicemic plague (020.2)
  - 038.9 Unspecified septicemia
    - Septicemia NOS
    - **Excludes** bacteremia NOS (790.7)
    - **Coding Clinic: 2012, Q3, P12, 14; 2010, Q2, P4; 2007, Q4, P96-97; 2005, Q2, P18-20; 2004, Q2, P16; 1999, Q3, P9; Q3, P5-6; 1998, Q1, P5; 1996, Q3, P16; Q2, P6; 1995, Q2, P7**

Item 1-6 034.0 is the common **"strep throat"** (sore throat with strep infection). It is grouped in the same three-digit category with scarlet fever. If a patient has both scarlet fever and the strep throat, use both codes. "Streptococcal" must be indicated on the laboratory report to use 034.0; otherwise use 462 for "sore throat" (pharyngitis).

INFECTIOUS AND PARASITIC DISEASES (001–139)

- **039 Actinomycotic infections**
  - Includes: actinomycotic mycetoma
    infection by Actinomycetales, such as species of Actinomyces, Actinomadura, Nocardia, Streptomyces
    maduromycosis (actinomycotic)
    schizomycetoma (actinomycotic)
  - **039.0 Cutaneous**
    Erythrasma
    Trichomycosis axillaris
  - **039.1 Pulmonary**
    Thoracic actinomycosis
  - **039.2 Abdominal**
  - **039.3 Cervicofacial**
  - **039.4 Madura foot**
    - Excludes: madura foot due to mycotic infection (117.4)
  - **039.8 Of other specified sites**
  - **039.9 Of unspecified site**
    Actinomycosis NOS
    Maduromycosis NOS
    Nocardiosis NOS

- **040 Other bacterial diseases**
  - Excludes: bacteremia NOS (790.7)
    bacterial infection NOS (041.9)
  - **040.0 Gas gangrene**
    Gas bacillus infection or gangrene
    Infection by Clostridium:
      histolyticum
      oedematiens
      perfringens [welchii]
      septicum
      sordellii
    Malignant edema
    Myonecrosis, clostridial
    Myositis, clostridial
    Coding Clinic: 1995, Q1, P11
  - **040.1 Rhinoscleroma**
  - **040.2 Whipple's disease**
    Intestinal lipodystrophy
  - **040.3 Necrobacillosis**
    Coding Clinic: 2007, Q4, P84-86
  - **040.4 Other specified botulism**
    Non-foodborne intoxication due to toxins of Clostridium botulinum [C. botulinum]
    - Excludes: botulism NOS (005.1)
      food poisoning due to toxins of Clostridium botulinum (005.1)
    - **040.41 Infant botulism**
      Coding Clinic: 2007, Q4, P60-61
    - **040.42 Wound botulism**
      Non-foodborne botulism NOS
      Use additional code to identify complicated open wound
      Coding Clinic: 2007, Q4, P60-61; 2006, Q2, P7
  - **040.8 Other specified bacterial diseases**
    - **040.81 Tropical pyomyositis**
    - **040.82 Toxic shock syndrome**
      Use additional code to identify the organism
      Coding Clinic: 2002, Q4, P44
    - **040.89 Other**
      Coding Clinic: 1986, Nov-Dec, P7

- **041 Bacterial infection in conditions classified elsewhere and of unspecified site**
  - Note: This category is provided to be used as an additional code to identify the bacterial agent in diseases classified elsewhere. This category will also be used to classify bacterial infections of unspecified nature or site.
  - *Report the disease first, then the bacterium.*
  - Excludes: septicemia (038.0–038.9)
  - Coding Clinic: 2001, Q2, P12; 1984, July-Aug, P19
  - **041.0 Streptococcus**
    Gram-positive bacteria that is the primary cause of strep throat
    - **041.00 Streptococcus, unspecified**
      Specified in documentation as streptococcus, but unspecified as to Group
    - **041.01 Group A**
      Specified as Group A
      Coding Clinic: 2002, Q1, P3-4
    - **041.02 Group B**
      Specified as Group B
    - **041.03 Group C**
      Specified as Group C
    - **041.04 Group D [Enterococcus]**
      Specified as Group D
    - **041.05 Group G**
      Specified as Group G
    - **041.09 Other Streptococcus**
      Streptococcus that is documented but not specified as Group A, B, C, D, or G
  - **041.1 Staphylococcus**
    *"Staph" infections caused by **Staphylococcus aureus** bacteria and range from common skin infections (pimples and boils) to serious infection of surgical wounds, bloodstream infections, and pneumonia*
    Coding Clinic: 1987, Jan-Feb, P14-15
    - **041.10 Staphylococcus, unspecified**
      Coding Clinic: 2006, Q2, P15
    - **041.11 Methicillin susceptible Staphylococcus aureus**
      MSSA
      Staphylococcus aureus NOS
      Coding Clinic: 2008, Q4, P69-73; 2006, Q2, P16-17; 2003, Q4, P104-107; 2001, Q2, P11; 1998, Q4, P42-44, 54.55; 1994, Q3, P6
    - **041.12 Methicillin resistant Staphylococcus aureus**
      Methicillin-resistant staphylococcus aureus (MRSA)
      Coding Clinic: 2009, Q4, P74; 2008, Q4, P69-73
    - **041.19 Other Staphylococcus**
      Coding Clinic: 2008, Q2, P3
  - **041.2 Pneumococcus**
  - **041.3 Klebsiella pneumoniae**
    Coding Clinic: 2008, Q4, P148-149
  - **041.4 Escherichia coli [E. coli]**
    Coding Clinic: 1984, July-Aug, P19
    - **041.41 Shiga toxin-producing Escherichia coli [E. coli] (STEC) O157**
      E. coli O157:H- (nonmotile) with confirmation of Shiga toxin
      E. coli O157 with confirmation of Shiga toxin when H antigen is unknown, or is not H7
      O157:H7 Escherichia coli [E.coli] with or without confirmation of Shiga toxin-production
      Shiga toxin-producing Escherichia coli [E.coli] O157:H7 with or without confirmation of Shiga toxin-production
      STEC O157:H7 with or without confirmation of Shiga toxin-production
      Coding Clinic: 2011, Q4, P83

Item 1-7 Gas gangrene is a necrotizing subcutaneous infection that will cause tissue death. Patients with poor circulation (e.g., diabetes, peripheral nephropathy) will have low oxygen content in their tissues (hypoxia), which allows the Clostridium bacteria to flourish. Gas gangrene often occurs at the site of a surgical wound or trauma. Onset is sudden and dramatic. Treatment can include debridement, amputation, and/or hyperbaric oxygen treatments.

041.42 Other specified Shiga toxin-producing Escherichia coli [E. coli] (STEC)
Non-O157 Shiga toxin-producing Escherichia coli [E.coli]
Non-O157 Shiga toxin-producing Escherichia coli [E.coli] with known O group

041.43 Shiga toxin-producing Escherichia coli [E. coli] (STEC), unspecified
Shiga toxin-producing Escherichia coli [E. coli] with unspecified O group
STEC NOS

041.49 Other and unspecified Escherichia coli [E. coli]
Escherichia coli [E. coli] NOS
Non-Shiga toxin-producing E. coli
Coding Clinic: 2011, Q4, P155

041.5 Hemophilus influenzae [H. influenzae]

041.6 Proteus (mirabilis) (morganii)

041.7 Pseudomonas
Coding Clinic: 1988, Q4, P10

● **041.8** Other specified bacterial infections

041.81 Mycoplasma
Eaton's agent
Pleuropneumonia-like organisms [PPLO]

041.82 Bacteroides fragilis

041.83 Clostridium perfringens

041.84 Other anaerobes
Gram-negative anaerobes
Excludes Helicobacter pylori (041.86)

041.85 Other gram-negative organisms
Aerobacter aerogenes
Gram-negative bacteria NOS
Mima polymorpha
Serratia
Excludes gram-negative anaerobes (041.84)
Coding Clinic: 1994, Q1, P18

041.86 Helicobacter pylori [H. pylori]

041.89 Other specified bacteria
Coding Clinic: 2006, Q2, P7; 2003, Q2, P7-8

041.9 Bacterial infection, unspecified
Coding Clinic: 1991, Q2, P9

OGCR Section I.C.1.a and b

If a patient is admitted for an HIV-related condition, the principal diagnosis should be 042, followed by additional diagnosis codes for all reported HIV-related conditions. If a patient with HIV disease is admitted for an unrelated condition (such as a traumatic injury), the code for the unrelated condition (e.g., the nature of injury code) should be the principal diagnosis. Other diagnoses would be 042 followed by additional diagnosis codes for all reported HIV-related conditions.

HUMAN IMMUNODEFICIENCY VIRUS (HIV) INFECTION (042)

042 Human immunodeficiency virus [HIV] disease
Acquired immune deficiency syndrome
Acquired immunodeficiency syndrome
AIDS
AIDS-like syndrome
AIDS-related complex
ARC
HIV infection, symptomatic
Use additional code(s) to identify all manifestations of HIV
Use additional code to identify HIV-2 infection (079.53)
Excludes asymptomatic HIV infection status (V08)
exposure to HIV virus (V01.79)
nonspecific serologic evidence of HIV (795.71)
Coding Clinic: 2010, Q3, P14; 2007, Q4, P61-64; 2006, Q3, P14-15; 2004, Q2, P11-12; Q1, P5; 2003, Q1, P10-11,15; 1999, Q1, P14; 1997, Q4, P30-31; 1994, Q4, P35-36x2; 1993, Q3, P9; Q1, P20-22; 1990, Q3, P17; 1989, Q1, P9

Item 1-8 AIDS (acquired immune deficiency syndrome) is caused by HIV (human immunodeficiency virus). HIV affects certain white blood cells (T-4 lymphocytes) and destroys the ability of the cells to fight infections, making patients susceptible to a host of infectious diseases (e.g., *Pneumocystis carinii* pneumonia (PCP), Kaposi's sarcoma, and lymphoma). AIDS-related complex (ARC) is an early stage of AIDS in which tests for HIV are positive but the symptoms are mild.

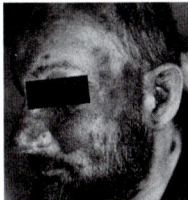

Figure 1-3 Kaposi's sarcoma. There are large confluent hyperpigmented patch-stage lesions with lymphedema. (From Cohen & Powderly: Infectious Diseases, ed 3, Mosby, An Imprint of Elsevier, 2010)

POLIOMYELITIS AND OTHER NON-ARTHROPOD-BORNE VIRAL DISEASES AND PRION DISEASES OF CENTRAL NERVOUS SYSTEM (045-049)

● **045** Acute poliomyelitis
Also called infantile paralysis caused by poliovirus, which enters the body orally and infects the intestinal wall and then enters the bloodstream and central nervous system, causing muscle weakness and paralysis
Excludes late effects of acute poliomyelitis (138)

The following fifth-digit subclassification is for use with category 045:

0 poliovirus, unspecified type
1 poliovirus type I
2 poliovirus type II
3 poliovirus type III

● **045.0** Acute paralytic poliomyelitis specified as bulbar
[0-3] Infantile paralysis (acute) specified as bulbar
Poliomyelitis (acute) (anterior) specified as bulbar
Polioencephalitis (acute) (bulbar)
Polioencephalomyelitis (acute) (anterior) (bulbar)

● **045.1** Acute poliomyelitis with other paralysis
[0-3] Paralysis:
acute atrophic, spinal
infantile, paralytic
Poliomyelitis (acute) with paralysis except bulbar
anterior with paralysis except bulbar
epidemic with paralysis except bulbar

● **045.2** Acute nonparalytic poliomyelitis
[0-3] Poliomyelitis (acute) specified as nonparalytic
anterior specified as nonparalytic
epidemic specified as nonparalytic

● **045.9** Acute poliomyelitis, unspecified
[0-3] Infantile paralysis unspecified whether paralytic or nonparalytic
Poliomyelitis (acute) unspecified whether paralytic or nonparalytic
anterior unspecified whether paralytic or nonparalytic
epidemic unspecified whether paralytic or nonparalytic

INFECTIOUS AND PARASITIC DISEASES (001–139)

- **046 Slow virus infections and prion diseases of central nervous system**
  - **046.0 Kuru**
  - **046.1 Jakob-Creutzfeldt disease** *(JCD)*
    - Use additional code to identify dementia:
      - with behavioral disturbance (294.11)
      - without behavioral disturbance (294.10)
    - **046.11 Variant Creutzfeldt-Jakob disease**
      - vCJD
    - **046.19 Other and unspecified Creutzfeldt-Jakob disease**
      - CJD
      - Familial Creutzfeldt-Jakob disease
      - Iatrogenic Creutzfeldt-Jakob disease
      - Jakob-Creutzfeldt disease, unspecified
      - Sporadic Creutzfeldt-Jakob disease
      - Subacute spongiform encephalopathy
      - **Excludes** *variant Creutzfeldt-Jakob disease (vCJD) (046.11)*
  - **046.2 Subacute sclerosing panencephalitis**
    - Dawson's inclusion body encephalitis
    - Van Bogaert's sclerosing leukoencephalitis
  - **046.3 Progressive multifocal leukoencephalopathy**
    - Multifocal leukoencephalopathy NOS
  - **046.7 Other specified prion diseases of central nervous system**
    - **Excludes** *Creutzfeldt-Jakob disease (046.11-046.19)*
      Jakob-Creutzfeldt disease (046.11-046.19)
      kuru (046.0)
      variant Creutzfeldt-Jakob disease (vCJD) (046.11)
    - **046.71 Gerstmann-Sträussler-Scheinker syndrome**
      - GSS syndrome
    - **046.72 Fatal familial insomnia**
      - FFI
    - **046.79 Other and unspecified prion disease of central nervous system**
  - **046.8 Other specified slow virus infection of central nervous system**
  - **046.9 Unspecified slow virus infection of central nervous system**

- **047 Meningitis due to enterovirus**
  - **Includes** meningitis:
    - abacterial
    - aseptic
    - viral
  - **Excludes** meningitis due to:
    - adenovirus (049.1)
    - arthropod-borne virus (060.0–066.9)
    - leptospira (100.81)
    - virus of:
      - herpes simplex (054.72)
      - herpes zoster (053.0)
      - lymphocytic choriomeningitis (049.0)
      - mumps (072.1)
      - poliomyelitis (045.0–045.9)
    - any other infection specifically classified elsewhere
  - **047.0 Coxsackie virus**
  - **047.1 ECHO virus**
    - Meningo-eruptive syndrome
  - **047.8 Other specified viral meningitis**
  - **047.9 Unspecified viral meningitis**
    - Viral meningitis NOS

- **048 Other enterovirus diseases of central nervous system**
  - Boston exanthem

- **049 Other non-arthropod-borne viral diseases of central nervous system**
  - **Excludes** *late effects of viral encephalitis (139.0)*
  - **049.0 Lymphocytic choriomeningitis**
    - Lymphocytic:
      - meningitis (serous) (benign)
      - meningoencephalitis (serous) (benign)
  - **049.1 Meningitis due to adenovirus**
  - **049.8 Other specified non-arthropod-borne viral diseases of central nervous system**
    - Encephalitis:
      - acute:
        - inclusion body
        - necrotizing
      - epidemic
      - lethargica
      - Rio Bravo
      - von Economo's disease
    - **Excludes** *human herpesvirus 6 encephalitis (058.21)*
      other human herpesvirus encephalitis (058.29)
  - **049.9 Unspecified non-arthropod-borne viral diseases of central nervous system**
    - Viral encephalitis NOS

VIRAL DISEASES GENERALLY ACCOMPANIED BY EXANTHEM (050–059)

Excludes *arthropod-borne viral diseases (060.0–066.9)*
Boston exanthem (048)

- **050 Smallpox**
  - *Caused by variola virus and is a serious, contagious, and sometimes fatal infectious disease*
  - **050.0 Variola major**
    - Hemorrhagic (pustular) smallpox
    - Malignant smallpox
    - Purpura variolosa
  - **050.1 Alastrim**
    - Variola minor
  - **050.2 Modified smallpox**
    - Varioloid
  - **050.9 Smallpox, unspecified**

- **051 Cowpox and paravaccinia**
  - **051.0 Cowpox and vaccinia not from vaccination**
    - Coding Clinic: 2008, Q4, P76-78
    - **051.01 Cowpox**
    - **051.02 Vaccinia not from vaccination**
      - **Excludes** *vaccinia (generalized) (from vaccination) (999.0)*
  - **051.1 Pseudocowpox**
    - Milkers' node
  - **051.2 Contagious pustular dermatitis**
    - Ecthyma contagiosum
    - Orf
  - **051.9 Paravaccinia, unspecified**

- **052 Chickenpox**
  - *Very contagious disease caused by varicella zoster virus; results in itchy outbreak of skin blisters (varicella). The same virus causes shingles (zoster). The Varicella zoster virus is a member of the herpes virus family.*
  - **052.0 Postvaricella encephalitis**
    - Postchickenpox encephalitis
  - **052.1 Varicella (hemorrhagic) pneumonitis**
  - **052.2 Postvaricella myelitis**
    - Postchickenpox myelitis
  - **052.7 With other specified complications**
    - Coding Clinic: 2002, Q1, P3-4
  - **052.8 With unspecified complication**
  - **052.9 Varicella without mention of complication**
    - Chickenpox NOS
    - Varicella NOS

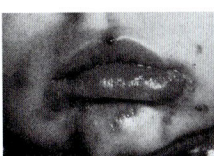

Figure 1-4 Primary herpes simplex in and around the mouth. The infection is usually acquired from siblings or parents and is readily transmitted to other direct contacts. (From Forbes, Jackson: Colour Atlas and Text of Clinical Medicine, International Edition, Mosby, 2002)

Item 1-9 *Herpes* is a viral disease for which there is no cure. There are two types of the herpes simplex virus: **Type I** causes **cold sores** or **fever blisters**, and **Type II** causes **genital herpes**. The virus can be spread from a sore on the lips to the genitals or from the genitals to the lips.

● 053 Herpes zoster
*Also known as **shingles**, caused by same virus as chickenpox. After exposure, the virus lies dormant in nerve tissue and is activated by factors including aging, stress, suppression of the immune system, and certain medication. Begins as a unilateral rash that leads to blisters and sores on skin. Chickenpox NOS is reported with 052.9.*
  Includes shingles
  zona
  053.0 With meningitis
● 053.1 With other nervous system complications
  053.10 With unspecified nervous system complication
  053.11 Geniculate herpes zoster
    Herpetic geniculate ganglionitis
  053.12 Postherpetic trigeminal neuralgia
  053.13 Postherpetic polyneuropathy
  053.14 Herpes zoster myelitis
  053.19 Other
● 053.2 With ophthalmic complications
  053.20 Herpes zoster dermatitis of eyelid
    Herpes zoster ophthalmicus
  053.21 Herpes zoster keratoconjunctivitis
  053.22 Herpes zoster iridocyclitis
  053.29 Other
● 053.7 With other specified complications
  053.71 Otitis externa due to herpes zoster
  053.79 Other
  053.8 With unspecified complication
  053.9 Herpes zoster without mention of complication
    Herpes zoster NOS
● 054 Herpes simplex
  Excludes *congenital herpes simplex (771.2)*
  054.0 Eczema herpeticum
    Kaposi's varicelliform eruption
● 054.1 Genital herpes
  054.10 Genital herpes, unspecified
    Herpes progenitalis
    Coding Clinic: 2010, Q2, P10; 2007, Q4, P61-64; 1985, Jan-Feb, P15-16
  054.11 Herpetic vulvovaginitis
  054.12 Herpetic ulceration of vulva
  054.13 Herpetic infection of penis
  054.19 Other
  054.2 Herpetic gingivostomatitis
  054.3 Herpetic meningoencephalitis
    Herpes encephalitis   Simian B disease
    Excludes *human herpesvirus 6 encephalitis (058.21)*
      other human herpesvirus encephalitis (058.29)
● 054.4 With ophthalmic complications
  054.40 With unspecified ophthalmic complication
  054.41 Herpes simplex dermatitis of eyelid
  054.42 Dendritic keratitis
  054.43 Herpes simplex disciform keratitis
  054.44 Herpes simplex iridocyclitis
  054.49 Other

  054.5 Herpetic septicemia
  054.6 Herpetic whitlow
    Herpetic felon
● 054.7 With other specified complications
  054.71 Visceral herpes simplex
  054.72 Herpes simplex meningitis
  054.73 Herpes simplex otitis externa
  054.74 Herpes simplex myelitis
  054.79 Other
  054.8 With unspecified complication
  054.9 Herpes simplex without mention of complication
● 055 Measles
  Includes morbilli
    rubeola
  The first four combination codes specify condition(s)/complication(s) manifesting after measles.
  055.0 Postmeasles encephalitis
  055.1 Postmeasles pneumonia
  055.2 Postmeasles otitis media

Item 1-10 *Rubeola* (055) and *rubella* (056) are medical terms for two different strains of measles. The MMR (measles, mumps, and rubella) vaccination is an attempt to eradicate these childhood diseases.

● 055.7 With other specified complications
  055.71 Measles keratoconjunctivitis
    Measles keratitis
  055.79 Other
  055.8 With unspecified complication
  055.9 Measles without mention of complication
● 056 Rubella
  Includes German measles
  Excludes *congenital rubella (771.0)*
● 056.0 With neurological complications
  056.00 With unspecified neurological complication
  056.01 Encephalomyelitis due to rubella
    Encephalitis due to rubella
    Meningoencephalitis due to rubella
  056.09 Other
● 056.7 With other specified complications
  056.71 Arthritis due to rubella
  056.79 Other
  056.8 With unspecified complications
  056.9 Rubella without mention of complication
● 057 Other viral exanthemata
  057.0 Erythema infectiosum [fifth disease]
  057.8 Other specified viral exanthemata
    Dukes (-Filatow) disease   Parascarlatina
    Fourth disease   Pseudoscarlatina
    Excludes *exanthema subitum [sixth disease] (058.10–058.12)*
      roseola infantum (058.10–058.12)
  057.9 Viral exanthem, unspecified

058 Other human herpesvirus

Excludes
- congenital herpes (771.2)
- cytomegalovirus (078.5)
- Epstein-Barr virus (075)
- herpes NOS (054.0–054.9)
- herpes simplex (054.0–054.9)
- herpes zoster (053.0–053.9)
- human herpesvirus NOS (054.0–054.9)
- human herpesvirus 1 (054.0–054.9)
- human herpesvirus 2 (054.0–054.9)
- human herpesvirus 3 (052.0–053.9)
- human herpesvirus 4 (075)
- human herpesvirus 5 (078.5)
- varicella (052.0–052.9)
- varicella-zoster virus (052.0–053.9)

058.1 Roseola infantum
Exanthema subitum [sixth disease]

- **058.10 Roseola infantum, unspecified**
  Exanthema subitum [sixth disease], unspecified
- **058.11 Roseola infantum due to human herpesvirus 6**
  Exanthema subitum [sixth disease] due to human herpesvirus 6
- **058.12 Roseola infantum due to human herpesvirus 7**
  Exanthema subitum [sixth disease] due to human herpesvirus 7

058.2 Other human herpesvirus encephalitis
Excludes
- herpes encephalitis NOS (054.3)
- herpes simplex encephalitis (054.3)
- human herpesvirus encephalitis NOS (054.3)
- simian B herpes virus encephalitis (054.3)

Coding Clinic: 2007, Q4, P61-64

- **058.21 Human herpesvirus 6 encephalitis**
- **058.29 Other human herpesvirus encephalitis**
  Human herpesvirus 7 encephalitis

058.8 Other human herpesvirus infections
- **058.81 Human herpesvirus 6 infection**
- **058.82 Human herpesvirus 7 infection**
- **058.89 Other human herpesvirus infection**
  Human herpesvirus 8 infection
  Kaposi's sarcoma-associated herpesvirus infection

Coding Clinic: 2007, Q4, P61-64

059 Other poxvirus infections

Excludes
- contagious pustular dermatitis (051.2)
- cowpox (051.01)
- ecthyma contagiosum (051.2)
- milker's nodule (051.1)
- orf (051.2)
- paravaccinia NOS (051.9)
- pseudocowpox (051.1)
- smallpox (050.0-050.9)
- vaccinia (generalized) (from vaccination) (999.0)
- vaccinia not from vaccination (051.02)

Coding Clinic: 2008, Q4, P76-78

059.0 Other orthopoxvirus infections
- **059.00 Orthopoxvirus infection, unspecified**
- **059.01 Monkeypox**
- **059.09 Other orthopoxvirus infection**

059.1 Other parapoxvirus infections
- **059.10 Parapoxvirus infection, unspecified**
- **059.11 Bovine stomatitis**
- **059.12 Sealpox**
- **059.19 Other parapoxvirus infections**

059.2 Yatapoxvirus infections
- **059.20 Yatapoxvirus infection, unspecified**
- **059.21 Tanapox**
- **059.22 Yaba monkey tumor virus**

059.8 Other poxvirus infections
059.9 Poxvirus infections, unspecified

ARTHROPOD-BORNE VIRAL DISEASES (060–066)

Use additional code to identify any associated meningitis (321.2)

Excludes late effects of viral encephalitis (139.0)

060 Yellow fever

060.0 Sylvatic
Yellow fever:
  jungle
  sylvan

060.1 Urban
060.9 Yellow fever, unspecified

061 Dengue
Breakbone fever

Excludes hemorrhagic fever caused by dengue virus (065.4)

062 Mosquito-borne viral encephalitis
Inflammation of the brain caused most commonly by Herpes Simplex virus. It may be a complication of Lyme disease and is often transmitted by mosquitoes, ticks, or rabid animals.

062.0 Japanese encephalitis
Japanese B encephalitis
062.1 Western equine encephalitis
062.2 Eastern equine encephalitis
Excludes Venezuelan equine encephalitis (066.2)
062.3 St. Louis encephalitis
062.4 Australian encephalitis
Australian arboencephalitis
Australian X disease
Murray Valley encephalitis
062.5 California virus encephalitis
Encephalitis:
  California
  La Crosse
Encephalitis:
  Tahyna fever
062.8 Other specified mosquito-borne viral encephalitis
Encephalitis by Ilheus virus
Excludes West Nile virus (066.40–066.49)
062.9 Mosquito-borne viral encephalitis, unspecified

063 Tick-borne viral encephalitis
Includes diphasic meningoencephalitis

063.0 Russian spring-summer [taiga] encephalitis
063.1 Louping ill
063.2 Central European encephalitis
063.8 Other specified tick-borne viral encephalitis
Langat encephalitis
Powassan encephalitis
063.9 Tick-borne viral encephalitis, unspecified

064 Viral encephalitis transmitted by other and unspecified arthropods
Arthropod-borne viral encephalitis, vector unknown
Negishi virus encephalitis

Excludes viral encephalitis NOS (049.9)

065 Arthropod-borne hemorrhagic fever

065.0 Crimean hemorrhagic fever [CHF Congo virus]
Central Asian hemorrhagic fever
065.1 Omsk hemorrhagic fever
065.2 Kyasanur Forest disease
065.3 Other tick-borne hemorrhagic fever
065.4 Mosquito-borne hemorrhagic fever
Chikungunya hemorrhagic fever
Dengue hemorrhagic fever
Excludes
- Chikungunya fever (066.3)
- dengue (061)
- yellow fever (060.0–060.9)

065.8 Other specified arthropod-borne hemorrhagic fever
Mite-borne hemorrhagic fever
065.9 Arthropod-borne hemorrhagic fever, unspecified
Arbovirus hemorrhagic fever NOS

● 066 Other arthropod-borne viral diseases
  066.0 Phlebotomus fever
        Changuinola fever   Sandfly fever
  066.1 Tick-borne fever
        Nairobi sheep disease
        Tick fever:
            American mountain
            Colorado
            Kemerovo
            Quaranfil
  066.2 Venezuelan equine fever
        Venezuelan equine encephalitis
  066.3 Other mosquito-borne fever
        Fever (viral):   Fever (viral):
            Bunyamwera   Oropouche
            Bwamba   Pixuna
            Chikungunya   Rift valley
            Guama   Ross river
            Mayaro   Wesselsbron
            Mucambo   Zika
            O' Nyong-Nyong
        Excludes dengue (061)
                 yellow fever (060.0–060.9)
● 066.4 West Nile fever
    Also indexed as West Nile virus
    Coding Clinic: 2004, Q4, P50-52; 2002, Q4, P44
    ☐ 066.40 West Nile fever, unspecified
              West Nile fever NOS
              West Nile fever without complications
              West Nile virus NOS
      066.41 West Nile fever with encephalitis
              West Nile encephalitis
              West Nile encephalomyelitis
      066.42 West Nile fever with other neurologic manifestation
              Use additional code to specify the neurologic manifestation
      066.49 West Nile fever with other complications
              Use additional code to specify the other conditions
  066.8 Other specified arthropod-borne viral diseases
        Chandipura fever
        Piry fever
  ☐ 066.9 Arthropod-borne viral disease, unspecified
        Arbovirus infection NOS

OTHER DISEASES DUE TO VIRUSES AND CHLAMYDIAE (070–079)

● 070 Viral hepatitis
    Includes viral hepatitis (acute) (chronic)
    Excludes cytomegalic inclusion virus hepatitis (078.5)

    The following fifth-digit subclassification is for use with categories 070.2 and 070.3:

    0 acute or unspecified, without mention of hepatitis delta
    1 acute or unspecified, with hepatitis delta
    2 chronic, without mention of hepatitis delta
    3 chronic, with hepatitis delta

    Coding Clinic: 2007, Q2, P6-7x3; 2004, Q4, P52-53
    070.0 Viral hepatitis A with hepatic coma
    070.1 Viral hepatitis A without mention of hepatic coma
          Infectious hepatitis
  ● 070.2 Viral hepatitis B with hepatic coma
    [0-3]
  ● 070.3 Viral hepatitis B without mention of hepatic coma
    [0-3] Serum hepatitis
          Coding Clinic: 1993, Q1, P28

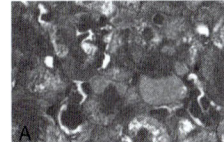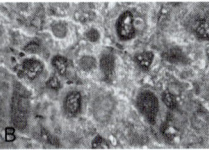

Figure 1–5 Hepatitis B viral infection. **A.** Liver parenchyma showing hepatocytes with diffuse granular cytoplasm, so-called ground glass hepatocytes (H&E). **B.** Immunoperoxidase stains from the same case, showing cytoplasmic inclusions of viral particles. (From Kumar: Robbins and Cotran: Pathologic Basis of Disease, ed 8, Saunders, An Imprint of Elsevier, 2009)

Item 1–11 Hepatitis A (HAV) was formerly called epidemic, infectious, short-incubation, or acute catarrhal jaundice hepatitis. The primary transmission mode is the oral–fecal route. **Hepatitis B (HBV)** was formerly called long-incubation period, serum, or homologous serum hepatitis. Transmission modes are through blood from infected persons and from body fluids of infected mother to neonate. **Hepatitis C (HCV),** caused by the hepatitis C virus, is primarily transfusion associated. **Hepatitis D (HDV),** also called delta hepatitis, is caused by the hepatitis D virus in patients formerly or currently infected with hepatitis B. **Hepatitis E (HEV)** is also called enterically transmitted non-A, non-B hepatitis. The primary transmission mode is the oral–fecal route, usually through contaminated water.

● 070.4 Other specified viral hepatitis with hepatic coma
    070.41 Acute hepatitis C with hepatic coma
    070.42 Hepatitis delta without mention of active hepatitis B disease with hepatic coma
           Hepatitis delta with hepatitis B carrier state
    070.43 Hepatitis E with hepatic coma
    070.44 Chronic hepatitis C with hepatic coma
    070.49 Other specified viral hepatitis with hepatic coma
● 070.5 Other specified viral hepatitis without mention of hepatic coma
    070.51 Acute hepatitis C without mention of hepatic coma
    070.52 Hepatitis delta without mention of active hepatitis B disease or hepatic coma
    070.53 Hepatitis E without mention of hepatic coma
    070.54 Chronic hepatitis C without mention of hepatic coma
           Coding Clinic: 2011, Q1, P23; 2008, Q4, P120; 2007, Q3, P9; 2006, Q2, P13
    070.59 Other specified viral hepatitis without mention of hepatic coma
☐ 070.6 Unspecified viral hepatitis with hepatic coma
    Excludes unspecified viral hepatitis C with hepatic coma (070.71)
● 070.7 Unspecified viral hepatitis C
    ☐ 070.70 Unspecified viral hepatitis C without hepatic coma
              Unspecified viral hepatitis C NOS
    ☐ 070.71 Unspecified viral hepatitis C with hepatic coma
☐ 070.9 Unspecified viral hepatitis without mention of hepatic coma
    Viral hepatitis NOS
    Excludes unspecified viral hepatitis C without hepatic coma (070.70)

071 Rabies
    Viral disease affecting central nervous system and transmitted from infected mammals
    Hydrophobia
    Lyssa

INFECTIOUS AND PARASITIC DISEASES (001–139)

- **072 Mumps**
  An acute, contagious, viral disease that causes painful enlargement of the salivary or parotid glands and is spread by respiratory droplets or direct contact. The following combination codes are specific diseases as an existing complication of mumps.
  - 072.0 Mumps orchitis
  - 072.1 Mumps meningitis
  - 072.2 Mumps encephalitis
    Mumps meningoencephalitis
  - 072.3 Mumps pancreatitis
  - • 072.7 Mumps with other specified complications
    - 072.71 Mumps hepatitis
    - 072.72 Mumps polyneuropathy
    - 072.79 Other
  - ▪ 072.8 Mumps with unspecified complication
  - 072.9 Mumps without mention of complication
    Epidemic parotitis
    Infectious parotitis

- • 073 Ornithosis
  Includes parrot fever
  psittacosis
  - 073.0 With pneumonia
    Lobular pneumonitis due to ornithosis
  - 073.7 With other specified complications
  - ▪ 073.8 With unspecified complication
  - ▪ 073.9 Ornithosis, unspecified

- • 074 Specific diseases due to Coxsackie virus
  Excludes Coxsackie virus:
  infection NOS (079.2)
  meningitis (047.0)
  - 074.0 Herpangina
    Vesicular pharyngitis
  - 074.1 Epidemic pleurodynia
    Bornholm disease   Epidemic:
    Devil's grip   myalgia
                         myositis
  - • 074.2 Coxsackie carditis
    - ▪ 074.20 Coxsackie carditis, unspecified
    - 074.21 Coxsackie pericarditis
    - 074.22 Coxsackie endocarditis
    - 074.23 Coxsackie myocarditis
      Aseptic myocarditis of newborn
  - 074.3 Hand, foot, and mouth disease
    Vesicular stomatitis and exanthem
    Check your documentation—this code is HAND, foot, and mouth disease. Code 078.4 is foot and mouth disease.
  - 074.8 Other specified diseases due to Coxsackie virus
    Acute lymphonodular pharyngitis

- 075 Infectious mononucleosis
  Glandular fever
  Monocytic angina
  Pfeiffer's disease
  Coding Clinic: 2001, Q3, P13-14x2

- • 076 Trachoma
  Excludes *late effect of trachoma (139.1)*
  - 076.0 Initial stage
    Trachoma dubium
  - 076.1 Active stage
    Granular conjunctivitis (trachomatous)
    Trachomatous:
      follicular conjunctivitis
      pannus
  - ▪ 076.9 Trachoma, unspecified
    Trachoma NOS

- • 077 Other diseases of conjunctiva due to viruses and Chlamydiae
  Excludes *ophthalmic complications of viral diseases classified elsewhere*
  - 077.0 Inclusion conjunctivitis
    Paratrachoma
    Swimming pool conjunctivitis
    Excludes *inclusion blennorrhea (neonatal) (771.6)*
  - 077.1 Epidemic keratoconjunctivitis
    Shipyard eye
  - 077.2 Pharyngoconjunctival fever
    Viral pharyngoconjunctivitis
  - 077.3 Other adenoviral conjunctivitis
    Acute adenoviral follicular conjunctivitis
  - 077.4 Epidemic hemorrhagic conjunctivitis
    Apollo:
      conjunctivitis
      disease
    Conjunctivitis due to enterovirus type 70
    Hemorrhagic conjunctivitis (acute) (epidemic)
  - 077.8 Other viral conjunctivitis
    Newcastle conjunctivitis
  - • 077.9 Unspecified diseases of conjunctiva due to viruses and Chlamydiae
    - ▪ 077.98 Due to Chlamydiae
    - ▪ 077.99 Due to viruses
      Viral conjunctivitis NOS

- • 078 Other diseases due to viruses and Chlamydiae
  Excludes *viral infection NOS (079.0–079.9)*
  viremia NOS (790.8)
  - 078.0 Molluscum contagiosum
  - • 078.1 Viral warts
    Viral warts due to human papillomavirus
    Coding Clinic: 1997, Q2, P9
    - ▪ 078.10 Viral warts, unspecified
      Verruca:
        NOS
        Vulgaris
      Warts (infectious)
    - 078.11 Condyloma acuminatum
      Condyloma NOS
      Genital warts NOS
    - 078.12 Plantar wart
      Verruca plantaris
      Coding Clinic: 2008, Q4, P78-79
    - 078.19 Other specified viral warts
      Common wart
      Flat wart
      Verruca plana
  - 078.2 Sweating fever
    Miliary fever
    Sweating disease
  - 078.3 Cat-scratch disease
    Benign lymphoreticulosis (of inoculation)
    Cat-scratch fever
  - 078.4 Foot and mouth disease
    Aphthous fever
    Epizootic:
      aphthae
      stomatitis
    Check your documentation. Code 074.3 is for HAND, foot, and mouth disease.
  - 078.5 Cytomegaloviral disease
    Cytomegalic inclusion disease
    Salivary gland virus disease
    Use additional code to identify manifestation, as:
      cytomegalic inclusion virus:
        hepatitis (573.1)
        pneumonia (484.1)
    Excludes *congenital cytomegalovirus infection (771.1)*
    Coding Clinic: 2011, Q3, P5; 2003, Q1, P11; 1993, Q3, P13; Q2, P11; Q1, P24; 1989, Q1, P9

PART III / Diseases: Tabular List Volume 1   078.6–082.3

078.6 Hemorrhagic nephrosonephritis
Hemorrhagic fever:
epidemic
Korean
Russian with renal syndrome

078.7 Arenaviral hemorrhagic fever
Hemorrhagic fever:
Argentine
Bolivian
Junin virus
Machupo virus

● **078.8 Other specified diseases due to viruses and Chlamydiae**
Excludes: *epidemic diarrhea (009.2)*
lymphogranuloma venereum (099.1)

078.81 Epidemic vertigo

078.82 Epidemic vomiting syndrome
Winter vomiting disease

078.88 Other specified diseases due to Chlamydiae

078.89 Other specified diseases due to viruses
Epidemic cervical myalgia
Marburg disease

● **079 Viral and chlamydial infection in conditions classified elsewhere and of unspecified site**
Note: This category is provided to be used as an additional code to identify the viral agent in diseases classifiable elsewhere. This category will also be used to classify virus infection of unspecified nature or site.

079.0 Adenovirus

079.1 ECHO virus

079.2 Coxsackie virus

079.3 Rhinovirus

079.4 Human papillomavirus
Coding Clinic: 1997, Q2, P9

079.5 Retrovirus
Excludes: *human immunodeficiency virus, type 1 [HIV-1] (042)*
human T-cell lymphotrophic virus, type III [HTLV-III] (042)
lymphadenopathy-associated virus [LAV] (042)

□ **079.50 Retrovirus, unspecified**

079.51 Human T-cell lymphotrophic virus, type I [HTLV-I]

079.52 Human T-cell lymphotrophic virus, type II [HTLV-II]

079.53 Human immunodeficiency virus, type 2 [HIV-2]

079.59 Other specified retrovirus

079.6 Respiratory syncytial virus (RSV)
Coding Clinic: 1996, Q4, P27-28

● **079.8 Other specified viral and chlamydial infections**
Coding Clinic: 1988, Q1, P12; Q1, P12

079.81 Hantavirus

079.82 SARS-associated coronavirus
Coding Clinic: 2003, Q4, P46-48

079.83 Parvovirus B19
Human parvovirus
Parvovirus NOS
Excludes: *erythema infectiosum [fifth disease] (057.0)*
Coding Clinic: 2007, Q4, P64

079.88 Other specified chlamydial infection

079.89 Other specified viral infection
Coding Clinic: 1995, Q1, P7

● **079.9 Unspecified viral and chlamydial infections**
Excludes: *viremia NOS (790.8)*
Coding Clinic: 1988, Q4, P10; 1987, Jan-Feb, P16

□ **079.98 Unspecified chlamydial infection**
Chlamydial infection NOS

□ **079.99 Unspecified viral infection**
Viral infection NOS
Coding Clinic: 1991, Q2, P8

RICKETTSIOSES AND OTHER ARTHROPOD-BORNE DISEASES (080–088)

Excludes: *arthropod-borne viral diseases (060.0–066.9)*

080 Louse-borne [epidemic] typhus
Typhus (fever):
classical
epidemic
Infecting a large number of individuals at the same time
exanthematic NOS
louse-borne

● **081 Other typhus**

081.0 Murine [endemic] typhus
Typhus (fever):
endemic
Restricted to a particular region
flea-borne

081.1 Brill's disease
Brill-Zinsser disease
Recrudescent typhus (fever)

081.2 Scrub typhus
Japanese river fever   Mite-borne typhus
Kedani fever   Tsutsugamushi

□ **081.9 Typhus, unspecified**
Typhus (fever) NOS

● **082 Tick-borne rickettsioses**

082.0 Spotted fevers
Rocky mountain spotted fever
Sao Paulo fever

082.1 Boutonneuse fever
African tick typhus   Marseilles fever
India tick typhus   Mediterranean tick fever
Kenya tick typhus

082.2 North Asian tick fever
Siberian tick typhus

082.3 Queensland tick typhus

Item 1–12 Retrovirus develops by copying its RNA, genetic materials, into the DNA, which then produces new virus particles. It is from the Retroviridae virus family.
Human T-cell lymphotropic virus, Type I (HTLV-I) is also called human T-cell leukemia virus, Type I, and is a retrovirus thought to cause T-cell leukemia/lymphoma.
Human T-cell lymphotropic virus, Type II (HTLV-II), is also called human T-cell leukemia virus, Type II, and is a retrovirus associated with hematologic disorders.
HIV-2 is one of the serotypes of HIV and is usually confined to West Africa, whereas HIV-1 is found worldwide.

Item 1–13 Rickettsioses are diseases spread from ticks, lice, fleas, or mites to humans.
Typhus is spread to humans chiefly by the fleas of rats.
Endemic identifies a disease as being present in low numbers of humans at all times, whereas **epidemic** identifies a disease as being present in high numbers of humans at a specific time. Morbidity (death) is higher in epidemic diseases.
Brill's disease, also known as **Brill-Zinsser disease,** is spread from human to human by body lice and also from the lice of flying squirrels. **Scrub typhus** is spread in the same ways as Brill's disease.
Malaria is spread to humans by mosquitoes.

◀ New   ⇐ Revised   ~~deleted~~ Deleted   Excludes   Includes   Use additional   Code first   Omit code
● Use Additional Digit(s)   □ Unspecified   ● Not first-listed DX   OGCR Official Guidelines   Coding Clinic

- **082.4 Ehrlichiosis**
  - 082.40 Ehrlichiosis, unspecified
  - 082.41 Ehrlichiosis chaffeensis [E. chaffeensis]
  - 082.49 Other ehrlichiosis
- 082.8 Other specified tick-borne rickettsioses
  - Lone star fever
  - *Coding Clinic: 1999, Q4, P19*
- 082.9 Tick-borne rickettsiosis, unspecified
  - Tick-borne typhus NOS

- **083 Other rickettsioses**
  - 083.0 Q fever
  - 083.1 Trench fever
    - Quintan fever
    - Wolhynian fever
  - 083.2 Rickettsialpox
    - Vesicular rickettsiosis
  - 083.8 Other specified rickettsioses
  - 083.9 Rickettsiosis, unspecified

- **084 Malaria**
  Mosquito-borne disease caused by parasite. Left untreated, severe complications and death may result.

  Note: Subcategories 084.0–084.6 exclude the listed conditions with mention of pernicious complications (084.8–084.9).

  Excludes: congenital malaria (771.2)

  - 084.0 Falciparum malaria [malignant tertian]
    - Malaria (fever):
      - by Plasmodium falciparum
      - subtertian
  - 084.1 Vivax malaria [benign tertian]
    - Malaria (fever) by Plasmodium vivax
  - 084.2 Quartan malaria
    - Malaria (fever) by Plasmodium malariae
    - Malariae malaria
  - 084.3 Ovale malaria
    - Malaria (fever) by Plasmodium ovale
  - 084.4 Other malaria
    - Monkey malaria
  - 084.5 Mixed malaria
    - Malaria (fever) by more than one parasite
  - 084.6 Malaria, unspecified
    - Malaria (fever) NOS
  - 084.7 Induced malaria
    - Therapeutically induced malaria
    - Excludes: accidental infection from syringe, blood transfusion, etc. (084.0–084.6, above, according to parasite species)
      - transmission from mother to child during delivery (771.2)
  - 084.8 Blackwater fever
    - Hemoglobinuric:
      - fever (bilious)
      - malaria
    - Malarial hemoglobinuria
  - 084.9 Other pernicious complications of malaria
    - Algid malaria
    - Cerebral malaria
    - Use additional code to identify complication, as:
      - malarial:
        - hepatitis (573.2)
        - nephrosis (581.81)

- **085 Leishmaniasis**
  - 085.0 Visceral [kala-azar]
    - Dumdum fever
    - Infection by Leishmania:
      - donovani
      - infantum
    - Leishmaniasis:
      - dermal, post-kala-azar
      - Mediterranean
      - visceral (Indian)
  - 085.1 Cutaneous, urban
    - Aleppo boil
    - Baghdad boil
    - Delhi boil
    - Infection by Leishmania tropica (minor)
    - Leishmaniasis, cutaneous:
      - dry form
      - late
      - recurrent
      - ulcerating
    - Oriental sore
  - 085.2 Cutaneous, Asian desert
    - Infection by Leishmania tropica major
    - Leishmaniasis, cutaneous:
      - acute necrotizing
      - rural
      - wet form
      - zoonotic form
  - 085.3 Cutaneous, Ethiopian
    - Infection by Leishmania ethiopica
    - Leishmaniasis, cutaneous:
      - diffuse
      - lepromatous
  - 085.4 Cutaneous, American
    - Chiclero ulcer
    - Infection by Leishmania mexicana
    - Leishmaniasis tegumentaria diffusa
  - 085.5 Mucocutaneous (American)
    - Espundia
    - Infection by Leishmania braziliensis
    - Uta
  - 085.9 Leishmaniasis, unspecified

- **086 Trypanosomiasis**
  Human African trypanosomiasis (HAT) is transmitted by fly bites that transmit either Trypanosoma brucei gambiense (causes a chronic infection lasting years) or Trypanosoma brucei rhodesiense (causes acute illness lasting several weeks).

  Use additional code to identify manifestations, as:
  - trypanosomiasis:
    - encephalitis (323.2)
    - meningitis (321.3)

  - 086.0 Chagas' disease with heart involvement
    - American trypanosomiasis with heart involvement
    - Infection by Trypanosoma cruzi with heart involvement
    - Any condition classifiable to 086.2 with heart involvement
  - 086.1 Chagas' disease with other organ involvement
    - American trypanosomiasis with involvement of organ other than heart
    - Infection by Trypanosoma cruzi with involvement of organ other than heart
    - Any condition classifiable to 086.2 with involvement of organ other than heart
  - 086.2 Chagas' disease without mention of organ involvement
    - American trypanosomiasis
    - Infection by Trypanosoma cruzi
  - 086.3 Gambian trypanosomiasis
    - Gambian sleeping sickness
    - Infection by Trypanosoma gambiense
  - 086.4 Rhodesian trypanosomiasis
    - Infection by Trypanosoma rhodesiense
    - Rhodesian sleeping sickness
  - 086.5 African trypanosomiasis, unspecified
    - Sleeping sickness NOS
  - 086.9 Trypanosomiasis, unspecified

PART III / Diseases: Tabular List Volume 1 087-091.9

- **087 Relapsing fever**
  Includes: recurrent fever
  - 087.0 Louse-borne
  - 087.1 Tick-borne
  - 087.9 Relapsing fever, unspecified
- **088 Other arthropod-borne diseases**
  - 088.0 Bartonellosis
    Carrión's disease
    Oroya fever
    Verruga peruana
  - **088.8 Other specified arthropod-borne diseases**
    - 088.81 Lyme disease
      Erythema chronicum migrans
      Coding Clinic: 1990, Q3, P14; 1989, Q2, P10
    - 088.82 Babesiosis
      Babesiasis
    - 088.89 Other
  - 088.9 Arthropod-borne disease, unspecified

SYPHILIS AND OTHER VENEREAL DISEASES (090–099)

Excludes: nonvenereal endemic syphilis (104.0)
urogenital trichomoniasis (131.0)

- **090 Congenital syphilis**
  - 090.0 Early congenital syphilis, symptomatic
    Congenital syphilitic:
      choroiditis
      coryza (chronic)
      hepatomegaly
      mucous patches
      periostitis
      splenomegaly
    Syphilitic (congenital):
      epiphysitis
      osteochondritis
      pemphigus
    Any congenital syphilitic condition specified as early or manifest less than two years after birth
  - 090.1 Early congenital syphilis, latent
    Congenital syphilis without clinical manifestations, with positive serological reaction and negative spinal fluid test, less than two years after birth
  - 090.2 Early congenital syphilis, unspecified
    Congenital syphilis NOS, less than two years after birth
  - 090.3 Syphilitic interstitial keratitis
    Syphilitic keratitis:
      parenchymatous
      punctata profunda
    Excludes: interstitial keratitis NOS (370.50)

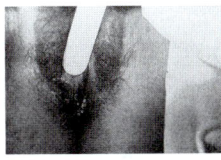

Figure 1-6 Chancre of primary syphilis. (From Mandell, Bennett, & Dolin: Principles and Practice of Infectious Diseases, ed 7, Churchill Livingstone, An Imprint of Elsevier, 2009)

Item 1-14 **Syphilis,** also known as lues, is the most serious of the venereal diseases caused by *Treponema pallidum.* The **primary** stage is characterized by an ulceration known as **chancre**, which usually appears on the genitals but can also develop on the anus, lips, tonsils, breasts, or fingers. Syphilis is easy to cure in its early stages. A single intramuscular injection of penicillin will usually cure a person who has had syphilis for less than a year.
The **secondary** stage is characterized by a rash that can affect any area of the body. **Latent** syphilis is divided into **early,** which is diagnosed within two years of infection, and **late,** which is diagnosed two years or more after infection. Additional doses of penicillin or another antibiotic are needed to treat someone who has had syphilis for longer than a year. For those allergic to penicillin, there are other antibiotic treatments. **Congenital** syphilis is also labeled **early** or **late** based on the time of diagnosis.

- **090.4 Juvenile neurosyphilis**
  Use additional code to identify any associated mental disorder
  - 090.40 Juvenile neurosyphilis, unspecified
    Congenital neurosyphilis
    Dementia paralytica juvenilis
    Juvenile:
      general paresis
      tabes
      taboparesis
  - 090.41 Congenital syphilitic encephalitis
  - 090.42 Congenital syphilitic meningitis
  - 090.49 Other
  - 090.5 Other late congenital syphilis, symptomatic
    Gumma due to congenital syphilis
    Hutchinson's teeth
    Syphilitic saddle nose
    Any congenital syphilitic condition specified as late or manifest two years or more after birth
  - 090.6 Late congenital syphilis, latent
    Congenital syphilis without clinical manifestations, with positive serological reaction and negative spinal fluid test, two years or more after birth
  - 090.7 Late congenital syphilis, unspecified
    Congenital syphilis NOS, two years or more after birth
  - 090.9 Congenital syphilis, unspecified
- **091 Early syphilis, symptomatic**
  Excludes: early cardiovascular syphilis (093.0–093.9)
  early neurosyphilis (094.0–094.9)
  - 091.0 Genital syphilis (primary)
    Genital chancre
  - 091.1 Primary anal syphilis
  - 091.2 Other primary syphilis
    Primary syphilis of:
      breast
      fingers
      lip
      tonsils
  - 091.3 Secondary syphilis of skin or mucous membranes
    Condyloma latum
    Secondary syphilis of:
      anus
      mouth
      pharynx
      skin
      tonsils
      vulva
  - 091.4 Adenopathy due to secondary syphilis
    Syphilitic adenopathy (secondary)
    Syphilitic lymphadenitis (secondary)
  - **091.5 Uveitis due to secondary syphilis**
    - 091.50 Syphilitic uveitis, unspecified
    - 091.51 Syphilitic chorioretinitis (secondary)
    - 091.52 Syphilitic iridocyclitis (secondary)
  - **091.6 Secondary syphilis of viscera and bone**
    - 091.61 Secondary syphilitic periostitis
    - 091.62 Secondary syphilitic hepatitis
      Secondary syphilis of liver
    - 091.69 Other viscera
  - 091.7 Secondary syphilis, relapse
    Secondary syphilis, relapse (treated) (untreated)
  - **091.8 Other forms of secondary syphilis**
    - 091.81 Acute syphilitic meningitis (secondary)
    - 091.82 Syphilitic alopecia
    - 091.89 Other
  - 091.9 Unspecified secondary syphilis

Item 1-15 Notice the placement of 091.4 combination code in with the Infectious and Parasitic Disease codes (syphilis). This uveitis does not appear in the eye code section because it is a manifestation of the underlying disease of syphilis.

- **092 Early syphilis, latent**
  Early syphilis is the disease, latent is the characteristic.
  Includes syphilis (acquired) without clinical manifestations, with positive serological reaction and negative spinal fluid test, less than two years after infection
  - 092.0 Early syphilis, latent, serological relapse after treatment
  - 092.9 Early syphilis, latent, unspecified
- **093 Cardiovascular syphilis**
  - 093.0 Aneurysm of aorta, specified as syphilitic
    Dilatation of aorta, specified as syphilitic
  - 093.1 Syphilitic aortitis
  - **093.2 Syphilitic endocarditis**
    Check documentation for documentation of a specific valve.
    - 093.20 Valve, unspecified
      Syphilitic ostial coronary disease
    - 093.21 Mitral valve
    - 093.22 Aortic valve
      Syphilitic aortic incompetence or stenosis
    - 093.23 Tricuspid valve
    - 093.24 Pulmonary valve
  - **093.8 Other specified cardiovascular syphilis**
    - 093.81 Syphilitic pericarditis
    - 093.82 Syphilitic myocarditis
    - 093.89 Other
  - 093.9 Cardiovascular syphilis, unspecified
- **094 Neurosyphilis**
  Use additional code to identify any associated mental disorder
  - 094.0 Tabes dorsalis
    Locomotor ataxia (progressive)
    Posterior spinal sclerosis (syphilitic)
    Tabetic neurosyphilis
    Use additional code to identify manifestation, as:
      neurogenic arthropathy [Charcot's joint disease] (713.5)
    Coding Clinic: 2012, Q3, P4
  - 094.1 General paresis
    Dementia paralytica
    General paralysis (of the insane) (progressive)
    Paretic neurosyphilis
    Taboparesis
  - 094.2 Syphilitic meningitis
    Meningovascular syphilis
    Excludes acute syphilitic meningitis (secondary) (091.81)
  - 094.3 Asymptomatic neurosyphilis
  - **094.8 Other specified neurosyphilis**
    - 094.81 Syphilitic encephalitis
    - 094.82 Syphilitic Parkinsonism
    - 094.83 Syphilitic disseminated retinochoroiditis
    - 094.84 Syphilitic optic atrophy
    - 094.85 Syphilitic retrobulbar neuritis
    - 094.86 Syphilitic acoustic neuritis
    - 094.87 Syphilitic ruptured cerebral aneurysm
    - 094.89 Other
  - 094.9 Neurosyphilis, unspecified
    Gumma (syphilitic) of central nervous system NOS
    Syphilis (early) (late) of central nervous system NOS
    Syphiloma of central nervous system NOS
- **095 Other forms of late syphilis, with symptoms**
  In the late stages, syphilis can damage organs and body systems.
  Includes gumma (syphilitic)
    Destructive lesions of syphilis
    tertiary, or unspecified stage
  - 095.0 Syphilitic episcleritis
  - 095.1 Syphilis of lung
  - 095.2 Syphilitic peritonitis
  - 095.3 Syphilis of liver
  - 095.4 Syphilis of kidney
  - 095.5 Syphilis of bone
  - 095.6 Syphilis of muscle
    Syphilitic myositis
  - 095.7 Syphilis of synovium, tendon, and bursa
    Syphilitic:
      bursitis
      synovitis
  - 095.8 Other specified forms of late symptomatic syphilis
    Excludes cardiovascular syphilis (093.0–093.9)
      neurosyphilis (094.0–094.9)
  - 095.9 Late symptomatic syphilis, unspecified
- 096 Late syphilis, latent
  Syphilis (acquired) without clinical manifestations, with positive serological reaction and negative spinal fluid test, two years or more after infection
- **097 Other and unspecified syphilis**
  - 097.0 Late syphilis, unspecified
  - 097.1 Latent syphilis, unspecified
    Positive serological reaction for syphilis
  - 097.9 Syphilis, unspecified
    Syphilis (acquired) NOS
    Excludes syphilis NOS causing death under two years of age (090.9)
- **098 Gonococcal infections**
  STD (sexually transmitted disease) caused by Neisseria gonorrhoeae that flourishes in the warm, moist areas of the reproductive tract. Untreated gonorrhea spreads to other parts of the body, causing inflammation of the testes or prostate or pelvic inflammatory disease (PID).
  - 098.0 Acute, of lower genitourinary tract
    Gonococcal:
      Bartholinitis (acute)
      Female only: Bartholin gland
      urethritis (acute)
      vulvovaginitis (acute)
    Gonorrhea (acute):
      NOS
      genitourinary (tract) NOS
  - **098.1 Acute, of upper genitourinary tract**
    - 098.10 Gonococcal infection (acute) of upper genitourinary tract, site unspecified
    - 098.11 Gonococcal cystitis (acute)
      Gonorrhea (acute) of bladder
    - 098.12 Gonococcal prostatitis (acute)
    - 098.13 Gonococcal epididymo-orchitis (acute)
      Gonococcal orchitis (acute)
    - 098.14 Gonococcal seminal vesiculitis (acute)
      Gonorrhea (acute) of seminal vesicle
    - 098.15 Gonococcal cervicitis (acute)
      Gonorrhea (acute) of cervix
    - 098.16 Gonococcal endometritis (acute)
      Gonorrhea (acute) of uterus
    - 098.17 Gonococcal salpingitis, specified as acute
    - 098.19 Other

098.2 Chronic, of lower genitourinary tract
Gonococcal specified as chronic or with duration of two months or more:
Bartholinitis specified as chronic or with duration of two months or more
urethritis specified as chronic or with duration of two months or more
vulvovaginitis specified as chronic or with duration of two months or more
Gonorrhea specified as chronic or with duration of two months or more:
NOS specified as chronic or with duration of two months or more
genitourinary (tract) specified as chronic or with duration of two months or more
Any condition classifiable to 098.0 specified as chronic or with duration of two months or more

098.3 Chronic, of upper genitourinary tract
Any condition classifiable to 098.1 stated as chronic or with a duration of two months or more
- **098.30 Chronic gonococcal infection of upper genitourinary tract, site unspecified**
- **098.31 Gonococcal cystitis, chronic**
  Any condition classifiable to 098.11, specified as chronic
  Gonorrhea of bladder, chronic
- **098.32 Gonococcal prostatitis, chronic**
  Any condition classifiable to 098.12, specified as chronic
- **098.33 Gonococcal epididymo-orchitis, chronic**
  Any condition classifiable to 098.13, specified as chronic
  Chronic gonococcal orchitis
- **098.34 Gonococcal seminal vesiculitis, chronic**
  Any condition classifiable to 098.14, specified as chronic
  Gonorrhea of seminal vesicle, chronic
- **098.35 Gonococcal cervicitis, chronic**
  Any condition classifiable to 098.15, specified as chronic
  Gonorrhea of cervix, chronic
- **098.36 Gonococcal endometritis, chronic**
  Any condition classifiable to 098.16, specified as chronic
- **098.37 Gonococcal salpingitis (chronic)**
- **098.39 Other**

098.4 Gonococcal infection of eye
- **098.40 Gonococcal conjunctivitis (neonatorum)**
  Neonate = newborn
  Gonococcal ophthalmia (neonatorum)
- **098.41 Gonococcal iridocyclitis**
- **098.42 Gonococcal endophthalmia**
- **098.43 Gonococcal keratitis**
- **098.49 Other**

098.5 Gonococcal infection of joint
- **098.50 Gonococcal arthritis**
  Gonococcal infection of joint NOS
- **098.51 Gonococcal synovitis and tenosynovitis**
- **098.52 Gonococcal bursitis**
- **098.53 Gonococcal spondylitis**
- **098.59 Other**
  Gonococcal rheumatism

098.6 Gonococcal infection of pharynx

098.7 Gonococcal infection of anus and rectum
Gonococcal proctitis

098.8 Gonococcal infection of other specified sites
- **098.81 Gonococcal keratosis (blennorrhagica)**
- **098.82 Gonococcal meningitis**
- **098.83 Gonococcal pericarditis**
- **098.84 Gonococcal endocarditis**
- **098.85 Other gonococcal heart disease**
- **098.86 Gonococcal peritonitis**
- **098.89 Other**
  Gonococcemia
  Blood condition

099 Other venereal diseases

099.0 Chancroid
Sexually transmitted infection caused by bacteria (Haemophilus ducreyi)
Bubo (inguinal):
chancroidal
due to Hemophilus ducreyi
Chancre:
Ducrey's simple soft
Ulcus molle (cutis) (skin)

099.1 Lymphogranuloma venereum
Climatic or tropical bubo
(Durand-) Nicolas-Favre disease
Esthiomene
Lymphogranuloma inguinale

099.2 Granuloma inguinale
Donovanosis
Granuloma pudendi (ulcerating)
Granuloma venereum
Pudendal ulcer

099.3 Reiter's disease
Reactive arthritis
Reiter's syndrome
Use additional code for associated:
arthropathy (711.1)
conjunctivitis (372.33)

099.4 Other nongonococcal urethritis [NGU]
- **099.40 Unspecified**
  Nonspecific urethritis
- **099.41 Chlamydia trachomatis**
- **099.49 Other specified organism**

099.5 Other venereal diseases due to Chlamydia trachomatis
Excludes *Chlamydia trachomatis infection of conjunctiva (076.0–076.9, 077.0, 077.9)*
Lymphogranuloma venereum (099.1)
- **099.50 Unspecified site**
- **099.51 Pharynx**
- **099.52 Anus and rectum**
- **099.53 Lower genitourinary sites**
  Excludes *urethra (099.41)*
  Use additional code to specify site of infection, such as:
  bladder (595.4)
  cervix (616.0)
  vagina and vulva (616.11)
- **099.54 Other genitourinary sites**
  Use additional code to specify site of infection, such as:
  pelvic inflammatory disease NOS (614.9)
  testis and epididymis (604.91)
- **099.55 Unspecified genitourinary site**
- **099.56 Peritoneum**
  Perihepatitis
- **099.59 Other specified site**

099.8 Other specified venereal diseases

099.9 Venereal disease, unspecified

OTHER SPIROCHETAL DISEASES (100–104)

- **100 Leptospirosis**
  - **100.0 Leptospirosis icterohemorrhagica**
    - Leptospiral or spirochetal jaundice (hemorrhagic)
    - Weil's disease
  - **100.8 Other specified leptospiral infections**
    - **100.81 Leptospiral meningitis (aseptic)**
    - **100.89 Other**
      - Fever:
        - Fort Bragg
        - pretibial
        - swamp
      - Infection by Leptospira:
        - australis
        - bataviae
        - pyrogenes
  - **100.9 Leptospirosis, unspecified**

- **101 Vincent's angina**
  - Acute necrotizing ulcerative:
    - gingivitis
    - stomatitis
  - Fusospirochetal pharyngitis
  - Spirochetal stomatitis
  - Trench mouth
  - Vincent's:
    - gingivitis
    - infection [any site]

- **102 Yaws**
  - **Includes**   frambesia
                   pian
  - **102.0 Initial lesions**
    - Chancre of yaws
    - Frambesia, initial or primary
    - Initial frambesial ulcer
    - Mother yaw
  - **102.1 Multiple papillomata and wet crab yaws**
    - Butter yaws
    - Frambesioma
    - Pianoma
    - Plantar or palmar papilloma of yaws
  - **102.2 Other early skin lesions**
    - Cutaneous yaws, less than five years after infection
    - Early yaws (cutaneous) (macular) (papular) (maculopapular) (micropapular)
    - Frambeside of early yaws
  - **102.3 Hyperkeratosis**
    - Ghoul hand
    - Hyperkeratosis, palmar or plantar (early) (late) due to yaws
    - Worm-eaten soles
  - **102.4 Gummata and ulcers**
    - Nodular late yaws (ulcerated)
    - Gummatous frambeside
  - **102.5 Gangosa**
    - Rhinopharyngitis mutilans
  - **102.6 Bone and joint lesions**
    - Goundou of yaws (late)
    - Gumma, bone of yaws (late)
    - Gummatous osteitis or periostitis of yaws (late)
    - Hydrarthrosis of yaws (early) (late)
    - Osteitis of yaws (early) (late)
    - Periostitis (hypertrophic) of yaws (early) (late)
  - **102.7 Other manifestations**
    - Juxta-articular nodules of yaws
    - Mucosal yaws
  - **102.8 Latent yaws**
    - Yaws without clinical manifestations, with positive serology
  - **102.9 Yaws, unspecified**

- **103 Pinta**
  - **103.0 Primary lesions**
    - Chancre (primary) of pinta [carate]
    - Papule (primary) of pinta [carate]
    - Pintid of pinta [carate]
  - **103.1 Intermediate lesions**
    - Erythematous plaques of pinta [carate]
    - Hyperchromic lesions of pinta [carate]
    - Hyperkeratosis of pinta [carate]
  - **103.2 Late lesions**
    - Cardiovascular lesions of pinta [carate]
    - Skin lesions of pinta [carate]:
      - achromic of pinta [carate]
      - cicatricial of pinta [carate]
      - dyschromic of pinta [carate]
    - Vitiligo of pinta [carate]
  - **103.3 Mixed lesions**
    - Achromic and hyperchromic skin lesions of pinta [carate]
  - **103.9 Pinta, unspecified**

- **104 Other spirochetal infection**
  - **104.0 Nonvenereal endemic syphilis**
    - Bejel
    - Njovera
  - **104.8 Other specified spirochetal infections**
    - **Excludes**   relapsing fever (087.0–087.9)
                     syphilis (090.0–097.9)
  - **104.9 Spirochetal infection, unspecified**

MYCOSES (110–118)

Use additional code to identify manifestation, as:
- arthropathy (711.6)
- meningitis (321.0–321.1)
- otitis externa (380.15)

Excludes   infection by Actinomycetales, such as species of Actinomyces, Actinomadura, Nocardia, Streptomyces (039.0–039.9)

- **110 Dermatophytosis**

  Also known as tinea or ringworm; condition of scalp, glabrous skin, and/or nails. Caused by fungi (dermatophytes).

  Includes   infection by species of Epidermophyton, Microsporum, and Trichophyton
  tinea, any type except those in 111

  - **110.0 Of scalp and beard**
    - Kerion
    - Sycosis, mycotic
    - Trichophytic tinea [black dot tinea], scalp
  - **110.1 Of nail**
    - Dermatophytic onychia
    - Onychomycosis
    - Tinea unguium
  - **110.2 Of hand**
    - Tinea manuum
  - **110.3 Of groin and perianal area**
    - Dhobie itch
    - Eczema marginatum
    - Tinea cruris
  - **110.4 Of foot**
    - Athlete's foot
    - Tinea pedis
  - **110.5 Of the body**
    - Herpes circinatus
    - Tinea imbricata [Tokelau]
  - **110.6 Deep seated dermatophytosis**
    - Granuloma trichophyticum
    - Majocchi's granuloma
  - **110.8 Of other specified sites**
  - **110.9 Of unspecified site**
    - Favus NOS
    - Microsporic tinea NOS
    - Ringworm NOS

- **111 Dermatomycosis, other and unspecified**
  - **111.0 Pityriasis versicolor**
    - Infection by Malassezia [Pityrosporum] furfur
    - Tinea flava
    - Tinea versicolor
  - **111.1 Tinea nigra**
    - Infection by Cladosporium species
    - Keratomycosis nigricans
    - Microsporosis nigra
    - Pityriasis nigra
    - Tinea palmaris nigra
  - **111.2 Tinea blanca**
    - Infection by Trichosporon (beigelii) cutaneum
    - White piedra
  - **111.3 Black piedra**
    - Infection by Piedraia hortai
  - **111.8 Other specified dermatomycoses**
  - **111.9 Dermatomycosis, unspecified**

- **112 Candidiasis**
  - **Includes** infection by Candida species
    - moniliasis
  - **Excludes** neonatal monilial infection (771.7)
  - **112.0 Of mouth**
    - Thrush (oral)
  - **112.1 Of vulva and vagina**
    - Candidal vulvovaginitis
    - Monilial vulvovaginitis
    - *Coding Clinic: 1994, Q1, P21*
  - **112.2 Of other urogenital sites**
    - Candidal balanitis
    - *Male condition only*
    - *Coding Clinic: 2012, Q3, P12; 2003, Q4, P105-106; 1996, Q4, P33*
  - **112.3 Of skin and nails**
    - Candidal intertrigo
    - Candidal onychia
    - Candidal perionyxis [paronychia]
  - **112.4 Of lung**
    - Candidal pneumonia
    - *Coding Clinic: 1998, Q2, P7*
  - **112.5 Disseminated**
    - Systemic candidiasis
    - *Coding Clinic: 2012, Q3, P12; 1989, Q2, P10*
  - **112.8 Of other specified sites**
    - **112.81 Candidal endocarditis**
    - **112.82 Candidal otitis externa**
      - Otomycosis in moniliasis
    - **112.83 Candidal meningitis**
    - **112.84 Candidal esophagitis**
    - **112.85 Candidal enteritis**
    - **112.89 Other**
      - *Coding Clinic: 1992, Q1, P17; 1991, Q3, P20*
  - **112.9 Of unspecified site**
    - *Coding Clinic: 1996, Q4, P33*

- **114 Coccidioidomycosis**
  - **Includes** infection by Coccidioides (immitis)
    - Posada-Wernicke disease
  - **114.0 Primary coccidioidomycosis (pulmonary)**
    - Acute pulmonary coccidioidomycosis
    - Coccidioidomycotic pneumonitis
    - Desert rheumatism
    - Pulmonary coccidioidomycosis
    - San Joaquin Valley fever
  - **114.1 Primary extrapulmonary coccidioidomycosis**
    - Chancriform syndrome
    - Primary cutaneous coccidioidomycosis
  - **114.2 Coccidioidal meningitis**
  - **114.3 Other forms of progressive coccidioidomycosis**
    - Coccidioidal granuloma
    - Disseminated coccidioidomycosis
  - **114.4 Chronic pulmonary coccidioidomycosis**
  - **114.5 Pulmonary coccidioidomycosis, unspecified**
  - **114.9 Coccidioidomycosis, unspecified**

- **115 Histoplasmosis**
  - The following fifth-digit subclassification is for use with category 115:

0	without mention of manifestation
1	meningitis
2	retinitis
3	pericarditis
4	endocarditis
5	pneumonia
9	other

  - **115.0 Infection by Histoplasma capsulatum**
    - [0-5,9] American histoplasmosis
    - Darling's disease
    - Reticuloendothelial cytomycosis
    - Small form histoplasmosis
  - **115.1 Infection by Histoplasma duboisii**
    - [0-5,9] African histoplasmosis
    - Large form histoplasmosis
  - **115.9 Histoplasmosis, unspecified**
    - [0-5,9] Histoplasmosis NOS

- **116 Blastomycotic infection**
  - *Rare and potentially fatal infections caused by fungus B. dermatitidis inhaled and found in moist soil in temperate climates*
  - **116.0 Blastomycosis**
    - Blastomycotic dermatitis
    - Chicago disease
    - Cutaneous blastomycosis
    - Disseminated blastomycosis
    - Gilchrist's disease
    - Infection by Blastomyces [Ajellomyces] dermatitidis
    - North American blastomycosis
    - Primary pulmonary blastomycosis
  - **116.1 Paracoccidioidomycosis**
    - Brazilian blastomycosis
    - Infection by Paracoccidioides [Blastomyces] brasiliensis
    - Lutz-Splendore-Almeida disease
    - Mucocutaneous-lymphangitic paracoccidioidomycosis
    - Pulmonary paracoccidioidomycosis
    - South American blastomycosis
    - Visceral paracoccidioidomycosis
  - **116.2 Lobomycosis**
    - Infections by Loboa [Blastomyces] loboi
    - Keloidal blastomycosis
    - Lobo's disease

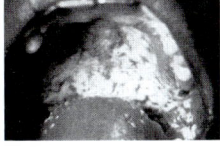

Figure 1-7 Oral candidiasis (thrush). *(Courtesy of Stephen Raffanti, MD, MPH.) (From Mandell, Bennett, & Dolin: Principles and Practice of Infectious Diseases, ed 7, Churchill Livingstone, An Imprint of Elsevier, 2009)*

Item 1-16 Candidiasis, also called oidiomycosis or moniliasis, is a fungal infection. It most often appears on moist cutaneous areas of the body but can also be responsible for a variety of systemic infections such as endocarditis, meningitis, arthritis, and myositis. Antifungal medications cure most yeast infections.

Item 1-17 Bird and bat droppings that fall into the soil give rise to a fungus that can spread airborne spores. When inhaled into the lungs, these spores divide and multiply into lesions. Histoplasmosis capsulatum takes three forms: primary (lodged in the lungs only), chronic (resembles TB), and disseminated (infection has moved to other organs). This is an opportunistic infection in immunosuppressed patients.

● **117 Other mycoses**
    117.0 Rhinosporidiosis
        Infection by Rhinosporidium seeberi
    117.1 Sporotrichosis
        Cutaneous sporotrichosis
        Disseminated sporotrichosis
        Infection by Sporothrix [Sporotrichum] schenckii
        Lymphocutaneous sporotrichosis
        Pulmonary sporotrichosis
        Sporotrichosis of the bones
    117.2 Chromoblastomycosis
        Chromomycosis
        Infection by Cladosporidium carrionii, Fonsecaea compactum, Fonsecaea pedrosoi, Phialophora verrucosa
    117.3 Aspergillosis
        Infection by Aspergillus species, mainly A. fumigatus, A. flavus group, A. terreus group
        Coding Clinic: 1997, Q4, P40
    117.4 Mycotic mycetomas
        Infection by various genera and species of Ascomycetes and Deuteromycetes, such as Acremonium [Cephalosporium] falciforme, Neotestudina rosatii, Madurella grisea, Madurella mycetomii, Pyrenochaeta romeroi, Zopfia [Leptosphaeria] senegalensis
        Madura foot, mycotic
        Maduromycosis, mycotic
        Excludes actinomycotic mycetomas (039.0–039.9)
    117.5 Cryptococcosis
        Busse-Buschke's disease
        European cryptococcosis
        Infection by Cryptococcus neoformans
        Pulmonary cryptococcosis
        Systemic cryptococcosis
        Torula
    117.6 Allescheriosis [Petriellidosis]
        Infections by Allescheria [Petriellidium] boydii [Monosporium apiospermum]
        Excludes mycotic mycetoma (117.4)
    117.7 Zygomycosis [Phycomycosis or Mucormycosis]
        Infection by species of Absidia, Basidiobolus, Conidiobolus, Cunninghamella, Entomophthora, Mucor, Rhizopus, Saksenaea
    117.8 Infection by dematiacious fungi [Phaehyphomycosis]
        Infection by dematiacious fungi, such as Cladosporium trichoides [bantianum], Dreschlera hawaiiensis, Phialophora gougerotii, Phialophora jeanselmi
    117.9 Other and unspecified mycoses
        Coding Clinic: 1995, Q2, P7

  118 Opportunistic mycoses
    Infection of skin, subcutaneous tissues, and/or organs by a wide variety of fungi generally considered to be pathogenic to compromised hosts only (e.g., infection by species of Alternaria, Dreschlera, Fusarium)
    Use additional code to identify manifestation, such as:
        keratitis (370.8)

HELMINTHIASES (120–129)

● **120 Schistosomiasis [bilharziasis]**
    Parasitic disease (worm induced) that leads to chronic illness
    120.0 Schistosoma haematobium
        Vesical schistosomiasis NOS
    120.1 Schistosoma mansoni
        Intestinal schistosomiasis NOS
    120.2 Schistosoma japonicum
        Asiatic schistosomiasis NOS
        Katayama disease or fever
    120.3 Cutaneous
        Cercarial dermatitis
        Infection by cercariae of Schistosoma
        Schistosome dermatitis
        Swimmers' itch
    120.8 Other specified schistosomiasis
        Infection by Schistosoma:
            bovis
            intercalatum
            mattheei
        Infection by Schistosoma spindale
        Schistosomiasis chestermani
    ■ **120.9 Schistosomiasis, unspecified**
        Blood flukes NOS   Hemic distomiasis

● **121 Other trematode infections**
    121.0 Opisthorchiasis
        Infection by:
            cat liver fluke
            Opisthorchis (felineus) (tenuicollis) (viverrini)
    121.1 Clonorchiasis
        Biliary cirrhosis due to clonorchiasis
        Chinese liver fluke disease
        Hepatic distomiasis due to Clonorchis sinensis
        Oriental liver fluke disease
    121.2 Paragonimiasis
        Infection by Paragonimus
        Lung fluke disease (oriental)
        Pulmonary distomiasis
    121.3 Fascioliasis
        Infection by Fasciola:
            gigantica
            hepatica
        Liver flukes NOS
        Sheep liver fluke infection
    121.4 Fasciolopsiasis
        Infection by Fasciolopsis (buski)
        Intestinal distomiasis
    121.5 Metagonimiasis
        Infection by Metagonimus yokogawai
    121.6 Heterophyiasis
        Infection by:
            Heterophyes heterophyes
            Stellantchasmus falcatus
    121.8 Other specified trematode infections
        Infection by:
            Dicrocoelium dendriticum
            Echinostoma ilocanum
            Gastrodiscoides hominis
    ■ **121.9 Trematode infection, unspecified**
        Distomiasis NOS
        Fluke disease NOS

● **122 Echinococcosis**
    Also known as hydatid disease; caused by Echinococcus granulosus, E. multilocularis, and E. vogeli tapeworms; and is contracted from infected food
    Includes echinococciasis
            hydatid disease
            hydatidosis
    122.0 Echinococcus granulosus infection of liver
    122.1 Echinococcus granulosus infection of lung
    122.2 Echinococcus granulosus infection of thyroid
    122.3 Echinococcus granulosus infection, other
    ■ **122.4 Echinococcus granulosus infection, unspecified**
    122.5 Echinococcus multilocularis infection of liver
    122.6 Echinococcus multilocularis infection, other
    ■ **122.7 Echinococcus multilocularis infection, unspecified**
    ■ **122.8 Echinococcosis, unspecified, of liver**
    122.9 Echinococcosis, other and unspecified

- **123 Other cestode infection**
  - **123.0 Taenia solium infection, intestinal form**
    - Pork tapeworm (adult) (infection)
  - **123.1 Cysticercosis**
    - Cysticerciasis
    - Infection by Cysticercus cellulosae [larval form of Taenia solium]
    - Coding Clinic: 1997, Q2, P8
  - **123.2 Taenia saginata infection**
    - Beef tapeworm (infection)
    - Infection by Taeniarhynchus saginatus
  - **123.3 Taeniasis, unspecified**
  - **123.4 Diphyllobothriasis, intestinal**
    - Diphyllobothrium (adult) (latum) (pacificum) infection
    - Fish tapeworm (infection)
  - **123.5 Sparganosis [larval diphyllobothriasis]**
    - Infection by:
      - Diphyllobothrium larvae
      - Sparganum (mansoni) (proliferum)
      - Spirometra larvae
  - **123.6 Hymenolepiasis**
    - Dwarf tapeworm (infection)
    - Hymenolepis (diminuta) (nana) infection
    - Rat tapeworm (infection)
  - **123.8 Other specified cestode infection**
    - Diplogonoporus (grandis) infection
    - Dipylidium (caninum) infection
    - Dog tapeworm (infection)
  - **123.9 Cestode infection, unspecified**
    - Tapeworm (infection) NOS
- **124 Trichinosis**
  - Trichinella spiralis infection
  - Trichinellosis
  - Trichiniasis
- **125 Filarial infection and dracontiasis**
  - **125.0 Bancroftian filariasis**
    - Chyluria due to Wuchereria bancrofti
    - Elephantiasis due to Wuchereria bancrofti
    - Infection due to Wuchereria bancrofti
    - Lymphadenitis due to Wuchereria bancrofti
    - Lymphangitis due to Wuchereria bancrofti
    - Wuchereriasis
  - **125.1 Malayan filariasis**
    - Brugia filariasis due to Brugia [Wuchereria] malayi
    - Chyluria due to Brugia [Wuchereria] malayi
    - Elephantiasis due to Brugia [Wuchereria] malayi
    - Infection due to Brugia [Wuchereria] malayi
    - Lymphadenitis due to Brugia [Wuchereria] malayi
    - Lymphangitis due to Brugia [Wuchereria] malayi
  - **125.2 Loiasis**
    - Eyeworm disease of Africa
    - Loa loa infection
  - **125.3 Onchocerciasis**
    - Onchocerca volvulus infection
    - Onchocercosis
  - **125.4 Dipetalonemiasis**
    - Infection by:
      - Acanthocheilonema perstans
      - Dipetalonema perstans
  - **125.5 Mansonella ozzardi infection**
    - Filariasis ozzardi
  - **125.6 Other specified filariasis**
    - Dirofilaria infection
    - Infection by:
      - Acanthocheilonema streptocerca
      - Dipetalonema streptocerca
  - **125.7 Dracontiasis**
    - Guinea-worm infection
    - Infection by Dracunculus medinensis
  - **125.9 Unspecified filariasis**
- **126 Ancylostomiasis and necatoriasis**
  - Includes: cutaneous larva migrans due to Ancylostoma
    - hookworm (disease) (infection)
    - uncinariasis
  - **126.0 Ancylostoma duodenale**
  - **126.1 Necator americanus**
  - **126.2 Ancylostoma braziliense**
  - **126.3 Ancylostoma ceylanicum**
  - **126.8 Other specified Ancylostoma**
  - **126.9 Ancylostomiasis and necatoriasis, unspecified**
    - Creeping eruption NOS
    - Cutaneous larva migrans NOS
- **127 Other intestinal helminthiases**
  - **127.0 Ascariasis**
    - Ascaridiasis
    - Infection by Ascaris lumbricoides
    - Roundworm infection
  - **127.1 Anisakiasis**
    - Infection by Anisakis larva
  - **127.2 Strongyloidiasis**
    - Infection by Strongyloides stercoralis
    - Excludes: trichostrongyliasis (127.6)
  - **127.3 Trichuriasis**
    - Infection by Trichuris trichiuria
    - Trichocephaliasis
    - Whipworm (disease) (infection)
  - **127.4 Enterobiasis**
    - Infection by Enterobius vermicularis
    - Oxyuriasis
    - Oxyuris vermicularis infection
    - Pinworm (disease) (infection)
    - Threadworm infection
  - **127.5 Capillariasis**
    - Infection by Capillaria philippinensis
    - Excludes: infection by Capillaria hepatica (128.8)
  - **127.6 Trichostrongyliasis**
    - Infection by Trichostrongylus species
  - **127.7 Other specified intestinal helminthiasis**
    - Infection by:
      - Oesophagostomum apiostomum and related species
      - Ternidens diminutus
      - other specified intestinal helminth
    - Physalopteriasis
  - **127.8 Mixed intestinal helminthiasis**
    - Infection by intestinal helminths classified to more than one of the categories 120.0–127.7
    - Mixed helminthiasis NOS
  - **127.9 Intestinal helminthiasis, unspecified**
- **128 Other and unspecified helminthiases**
  - **128.0 Toxocariasis**
    - Larva migrans visceralis
    - Toxocara (canis) (cati) infection
    - Visceral larva migrans syndrome
  - **128.1 Gnathostomiasis**
    - Infection by Gnathostoma spinigerum and related species
  - **128.8 Other specified helminthiasis**
    - Infection by:
      - Angiostrongylus cantonensis
      - Capillaria hepatica
      - other specified helminth
  - **128.9 Helminth infection, unspecified**
    - Helminthiasis NOS
    - Worms NOS
- **129 Intestinal parasitism, unspecified**

Item 1–18 Toxoplasmosis is caused by the protozoa **Toxoplasma gondii**, of which the house cat can be a host. Human infection occurs when contact is made with materials containing the pathogen, such as feces, contaminated soil, or ingestion of infected lamb, goat, or pork. Of the infected, very few have symptoms because a healthy person's immune system keeps the parasite from causing illness. When the immune system is compromised, symptoms may occur. Clinical symptoms include flu-like symptoms, but the disease progresses to include the eyes and the brain in babies.

OTHER INFECTIOUS AND PARASITIC DISEASES (130–136)

- **130 Toxoplasmosis**
  - Includes: infection by toxoplasma gondii
    toxoplasmosis (acquired)
  - Excludes: congenital toxoplasmosis (771.2)
  - **130.0 Meningoencephalitis due to toxoplasmosis**
    Encephalitis due to acquired toxoplasmosis
  - **130.1 Conjunctivitis due to toxoplasmosis**
  - **130.2 Chorioretinitis due to toxoplasmosis**
    Focal retinochoroiditis due to acquired toxoplasmosis
  - **130.3 Myocarditis due to toxoplasmosis**
  - **130.4 Pneumonitis due to toxoplasmosis**
  - **130.5 Hepatitis due to toxoplasmosis**
  - **130.7 Toxoplasmosis of other specified sites**
  - **130.8 Multisystemic disseminated toxoplasmosis**
    Toxoplasmosis of multiple sites
  - **130.9 Toxoplasmosis, unspecified**

- **131 Trichomoniasis**
  A common STD caused by a parasite, Trichomonas vaginalis, affecting both women and men
  - Includes: infection due to Trichomonas (vaginalis)
  - **131.0 Urogenital trichomoniasis**
    - **131.00 Urogenital trichomoniasis, unspecified**
      Fluor (vaginalis) trichomonal or due to Trichomonas (vaginalis)
      Leukorrhea (vaginalis) trichomonal or due to Trichomonas (vaginalis)
    - **131.01 Trichomonal vulvovaginitis**
      Vaginitis, trichomonal or due to Trichomonas (vaginalis)
    - **131.02 Trichomonal urethritis**
    - **131.03 Trichomonal prostatitis**
    - **131.09 Other**
  - **131.8 Other specified sites**
    - Excludes: intestinal (007.3)
  - **131.9 Trichomoniasis, unspecified**

- **132 Pediculosis and phthirus infestation**
  Infestation of lice, Pediculus humanus, specifically capitis infest the head, corporis infest the body-trunk area, and pubis infest the pubic region
  - **132.0 Pediculus capitis [head louse]**
  - **132.1 Pediculus corporis [body louse]**
  - **132.2 Phthirus pubis [pubic louse]**
    Pediculus pubis
  - **132.3 Mixed infestation**
    This is a combination code.
    Infestation classifiable to more than one of the categories 132.0–132.2
  - **132.9 Pediculosis, unspecified**

- **133 Acariasis**
  - **133.0 Scabies**
    Infestation by Sarcoptes scabiei
    Norwegian scabies
    Sarcoptic itch
  - **133.8 Other acariasis**
    Chiggers
    Infestation by:
      Demodex folliculorum
      Trombicula
  - **133.9 Acariasis, unspecified**
    Infestation by mites NOS

- **134 Other infestation**
  - **134.0 Myiasis**
    Infestation by:
      Dermatobia (hominis)
      fly larvae
      Gasterophilus (intestinalis)
      maggots
      Oestrus ovis
  - **134.1 Other arthropod infestation**
    Infestation by:
      chigoe
      Jigger disease
      sand flea
      Scarabiasis
      Tunga penetrans
      Tungiasis
  - **134.2 Hirudiniasis**
    Hirudiniasis (external) (internal)
    Leeches (aquatic) (land)
  - **134.8 Other specified infestations**
  - **134.9 Infestation, unspecified**
    Infestation (skin) NOS
    Skin parasites NOS

- **135 Sarcoidosis**
  Symptom of an inflammation producing tiny lumps of cells (granulomas) in various organs, most commonly the lungs and lymph nodes, that affect organ function
  Besnier-Boeck-Schaumann disease
  Lupoid (miliary) of Boeck
  Lupus pernio (Besnier)
  Lymphogranulomatosis, benign (Schaumann's)
  Sarcoid (any site):
    NOS
    Boeck
    Darier-Roussy
  Uveoparotid fever

- **136 Other and unspecified infectious and parasitic diseases**
  - **136.0 Ainhum**
    Dactylolysis spontanea
  - **136.1 Behçet's syndrome**
  - **136.2 Specific infections by free-living amebae**
    - **136.21 Specific infection due to acanthamoeba**
      Use additional code to identify manifestation, such as:
        keratitis (370.8)
      Coding Clinic: 2008, Q4, P79-81
    - **136.29 Other specific infections by free-living amebae**
      Meningoencephalitis due to Naegleria
      Coding Clinic: 2008, Q4, P79-81
  - **136.3 Pneumocystosis**
    Pneumonia due to Pneumocystis carinii
    Pneumonia due to Pneumocystis jiroveci
    Coding Clinic: 2003, Q1, P15; 1987, Nov-Dec, P5-6
  - **136.4 Psorospermiasis**

136.5 Sarcosporidiosis
Infection by Sarcocystis lindemanni

136.8 Other specified infectious and parasitic diseases
Candiru infestation

136.9 Unspecified infectious and parasitic diseases
Infectious disease NOS
Parasitic disease NOS
Coding Clinic: 1991, Q2, P8

LATE EFFECTS OF INFECTIOUS AND PARASITIC DISEASES (137–139)

137 Late effects of tuberculosis
Note: This category is to be used to indicate conditions classifiable to 010–018 as the cause of late effects, which are themselves classified elsewhere. The "late effects" include those specified as such, as sequelae, or as due to old or inactive tuberculosis, without evidence of active disease.

137.0 Late effects of respiratory or unspecified tuberculosis

137.1 Late effects of central nervous system tuberculosis

137.2 Late effects of genitourinary tuberculosis

137.3 Late effects of tuberculosis of bones and joints

137.4 Late effects of tuberculosis of other specified organs

138 Late effects of acute poliomyelitis
Note: This category is to be used to indicate conditions classifiable to 045 as the cause of late effects, which are themselves classified elsewhere. The "late effects" include conditions specified as such, or as sequelae, or as due to old or inactive poliomyelitis, without evidence of active disease.

139 Late effects of other infectious and parasitic diseases
Note: This category is to be used to indicate conditions classifiable to categories 001–009, 020–041, 046–136 as the cause of late effects, which are themselves classified elsewhere. The "late effects" include conditions specified as such; they also include sequela of diseases classifiable to the above categories if there is evidence that the disease itself is no longer present.

139.0 Late effects of viral encephalitis
Late effects of conditions classifiable to 049.8–049.9, 062–064

139.1 Late effects of trachoma
Late effects of conditions classifiable to 076

139.8 Late effects of other and unspecified infectious and parasitic diseases
Coding Clinic: 2006, Q2, P17-18; 1990, Q3, P14

Item 1-19 Before you assign the late code 137.X, check your documentation. The original problem (tuberculosis, TB) that is causing the current late effect (necrosis) must have been attributable to categories 010–018. A patient who originally had TB of a joint (015.2X) now has a late effect (137.3), which is necrosis of bone (730.8). Because there is no active TB, 015.2X is not coded but serves as an authorization to use the late effect code. Remember to code the manifestation of the late effect, which is the current problem (necrosis).

Item 2-1 Neoplasm: Neo = new, plasm = growth, development, formation. This new growth (mass, tumor) can be malignant or benign, which is confirmed by the pathology report. Do not assign a code to a neoplasm until you review the pathology report. Certain CPT codes will specify benign or malignant lesion, so be certain the diagnosis code supports the procedure code.

2. NEOPLASMS (140–239)

1. Content:
   This chapter contains the following broad groups:
   - 140–195 Malignant neoplasms, stated or presumed to be primary, of specified sites, except of lymphatic and hematopoietic tissue
   - 196–198 Malignant neoplasms, stated or presumed to be secondary, of specified sites
   - 199 Malignant neoplasms, without specification of site
   - 200–208 Malignant neoplasms, stated or presumed to be primary, of lymphatic and hematopoietic tissue
   - 209 Neuroendocrine tumors
   - 210–229 Benign neoplasms
   - 230–234 Carcinoma in situ
   - 235–238 Neoplasms of uncertain behavior [see Note, at beginning of section 235–238]
   - 239 Neoplasms of unspecified nature

2. Functional activity
   All neoplasms are classified in this chapter, whether or not functionally active. An additional code from Chapter 3 may be used to identify such functional activity associated with any neoplasm, e.g.:
   catecholamine-producing malignant pheochromocytoma of adrenal:
   code 194.0, additional code 255.6
   basophil adenoma of pituitary with Cushing's syndrome:
   code 227.3, additional code 255.0

3. Morphology [Histology]
   For those wishing to identify the histological type of neoplasms, a comprehensive coded nomenclature, which comprises the morphology rubrics of the ICD-Oncology, is given after the E-code chapter.

4. Malignant neoplasms overlapping site boundaries
   Categories 140–195 are for the classification of primary malignant neoplasms according to their point of origin. A malignant neoplasm that overlaps two or more subcategories within a three-digit rubric and whose point of origin cannot be determined should be classified to the subcategory .8 "Other." For example, "carcinoma involving tip and ventral surface of tongue" should be assigned to 141.8. On the other hand, "carcinoma of tip of tongue, extending to involve the ventral surface" should be coded to 141.2, as the point of origin, the tip, is known. Three subcategories (149.8, 159.8, 165.8) have been provided for malignant neoplasms that overlap the boundaries of three-digit rubrics within certain systems. Overlapping malignant neoplasms that cannot be classified as indicated above should be assigned to the appropriate subdivision of category 195 (Malignant neoplasm of other and ill-defined sites).

MALIGNANT NEOPLASM OF LIP, ORAL CAVITY, AND PHARYNX (140–149)

Excludes carcinoma in situ (230.0)

● **140 Malignant neoplasm of lip**
Malignant neoplasm is a general term used to describe a cancerous growth or tumor.
Excludes malignant melanoma of skin of lip (172.0)
malignant neoplasm of skin of lip (173.00-173.09)

140.0 Upper lip, vermilion border
Upper lip: Upper lip:
  NOS   lipstick area
  external

140.1 Lower lip, vermilion border
Lower lip: Lower lip:
  NOS   lipstick area
  external

140.3 Upper lip, inner aspect
Upper lip: Upper lip:
  buccal aspect   mucosa
  frenulum   oral aspect

140.4 Lower lip, inner aspect
Lower lip: Lower lip:
  buccal aspect   mucosa
  frenulum   oral aspect

■ **140.5 Lip, unspecified, inner aspect**
Lip, not specified whether upper or lower:
  buccal aspect
  frenulum
  mucosa
  oral aspect

140.6 Commissure of lip
Labial commissure

140.8 Other sites of lip
Malignant neoplasm of contiguous or overlapping sites of lip whose point of origin cannot be determined

■ **140.9 Lip, unspecified, vermilion border**
Lip, not specified as upper or lower:
  NOS
  external
  lipstick area

● **141 Malignant neoplasm of tongue**

141.0 Base of tongue
Dorsal surface of base of tongue
Fixed part of tongue NOS
Coding Clinic: 2006, Q4, P88-91

141.1 Dorsal surface of tongue
Anterior two-thirds of tongue, dorsal surface
Dorsal tongue NOS
Midline of tongue
Excludes dorsal surface of base of tongue (141.0)

141.2 Tip and lateral border of tongue

141.3 Ventral surface of tongue
Anterior two-thirds of tongue, ventral surface
Frenulum linguae

■ **141.4 Anterior two-thirds of tongue, part unspecified**
Mobile part of tongue NOS

Figure 2-1 Anatomical structures of the mouth and lips. **A.** Transitional or vermilion borders. Lips are connected to the gums by frenulum. **B.** Dorsal surface. **C.** Ventral surface.

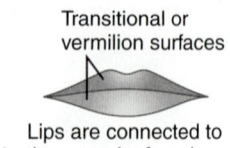
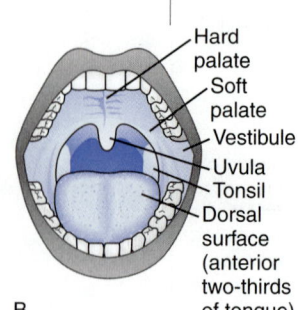
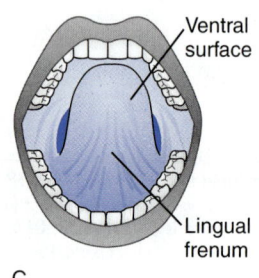

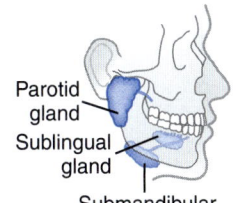

Figure 2-2 Major salivary glands.

- 141.5 **Junctional zone**
  Border of tongue at junction of fixed and mobile parts at insertion of anterior tonsillar pillar
- 141.6 **Lingual tonsil**
- 141.8 **Other sites of tongue**
  Malignant neoplasm of contiguous or overlapping sites of tongue whose point of origin cannot be determined
- 141.9 **Tongue, unspecified**
  Tongue NOS

● 142 **Malignant neoplasm of major salivary glands**
  Includes salivary ducts
  Excludes malignant neoplasm of minor salivary glands:
    NOS (145.9)
    buccal mucosa (145.0)
    soft palate (145.3)
    tongue (141.0–141.9)
    tonsil, palatine (146.0)
- 142.0 **Parotid gland**
- 142.1 **Submandibular gland**
  Submaxillary gland
- 142.2 **Sublingual gland**
- 142.8 **Other major salivary glands**
  Malignant neoplasm of contiguous or overlapping sites of salivary glands and ducts whose point of origin cannot be determined
- 142.9 **Salivary gland, unspecified**
  Salivary gland (major) NOS

● 143 **Malignant neoplasm of gum**
  Includes alveolar (ridge) mucosa
    gingiva (alveolar) (marginal)
    interdental papillae
  Excludes malignant odontogenic neoplasms (170.0–170.1)
- 143.0 **Upper gum**
- 143.1 **Lower gum**
- 143.8 **Other sites of gum**
  Malignant neoplasm of contiguous or overlapping sites of gum whose point of origin cannot be determined
- 143.9 **Gum, unspecified**

● 144 **Malignant neoplasm of floor of mouth**
- 144.0 **Anterior portion**
  Anterior to the premolar-canine junction
- 144.1 **Lateral portion**
- 144.8 **Other sites of floor of mouth**
  Malignant neoplasm of contiguous or overlapping sites of floor of mouth whose point of origin cannot be determined
- 144.9 **Floor of mouth, part unspecified**

● 145 **Malignant neoplasm of other and unspecified parts of mouth**
  Excludes mucosa of lips (140.0–140.9)
- 145.0 **Cheek mucosa**
  Buccal mucosa
  Cheek, inner aspect
- 145.1 **Vestibule of mouth**
  Buccal sulcus (upper) (lower)
  Labial sulcus (upper) (lower)
- 145.2 **Hard palate**
- 145.3 **Soft palate**
  Excludes nasopharyngeal [posterior] [superior] surface of soft palate (147.3)
  Coding Clinic: 1993, 5th Issue, P16
- 145.4 **Uvula**
- 145.5 **Palate, unspecified**
  Junction of hard and soft palate
  Roof of mouth
- 145.6 **Retromolar area**
- 145.8 **Other specified parts of mouth**
  Malignant neoplasm of contiguous or overlapping sites of mouth whose point of origin cannot be determined
- 145.9 **Mouth, unspecified**
  Buccal cavity NOS
  Minor salivary gland, unspecified site
  Oral cavity NOS

● 146 **Malignant neoplasm of oropharynx**
- 146.0 **Tonsil**
  Tonsil: Tonsil:
    NOS   palatine
    faucial
  Excludes lingual tonsil (141.6)
    pharyngeal tonsil (147.1)
  Coding Clinic: 1987, Sept-Oct, P8
- 146.1 **Tonsillar fossa**
- 146.2 **Tonsillar pillars (anterior) (posterior)**
  Faucial pillar
  Glossopalatine fold
  Palatoglossal arch
  Palatopharyngeal arch
- 146.3 **Vallecula**
  Anterior and medial surface of the pharyngoepiglottic fold
- 146.4 **Anterior aspect of epiglottis**
  Epiglottis, free border [margin]
  Glossoepiglottic fold(s)
  Excludes epiglottis:
    NOS (161.1)
    suprahyoid portion (161.1)
- 146.5 **Junctional region**
  Junction of the free margin of the epiglottis, the aryepiglottic fold, and the pharyngoepiglottic fold
- 146.6 **Lateral wall of oropharynx**
- 146.7 **Posterior wall of oropharynx**
- 146.8 **Other specified sites of oropharynx**
  Branchial cleft
  Malignant neoplasm of contiguous or overlapping sites of oropharynx whose point of origin cannot be determined
- 146.9 **Oropharynx, unspecified**
  Coding Clinic: 2002, Q2, P6

● 147 **Malignant neoplasm of nasopharynx**
- 147.0 **Superior wall**
  Roof of nasopharynx
- 147.1 **Posterior wall**
  Adenoid   Pharyngeal tonsil
- 147.2 **Lateral wall**
  Fossa of Rosenmüller   Pharyngeal recess
  Opening of auditory tube
- 147.3 **Anterior wall**
  Floor of nasopharynx
  Nasopharyngeal [posterior] [superior] surface of soft palate
  Posterior margin of nasal septum and choanae
- 147.8 **Other specified sites of nasopharynx**
  Malignant neoplasm of contiguous or overlapping sites of nasopharynx whose point of origin cannot be determined
- 147.9 **Nasopharynx, unspecified**
  Nasopharyngeal wall NOS

148 Malignant neoplasm of hypopharynx
- **148.0** Postcricoid region
  Behind the cricoid cartilage of neck
- **148.1** Pyriform sinus
  Pyriform fossa
- **148.2** Aryepiglottic fold, hypopharyngeal aspect
  Aryepiglottic fold or interarytenoid fold:
  NOS
  marginal zone
  Excludes *aryepiglottic fold or interarytenoid fold, laryngeal aspect (161.1)*
- **148.3** Posterior hypopharyngeal wall
- **148.8** Other specified sites of hypopharynx
  Malignant neoplasm of contiguous or overlapping sites of hypopharynx whose point of origin cannot be determined
- **148.9** Hypopharynx, unspecified
  Hypopharyngeal wall NOS
  Hypopharynx NOS

149 Malignant neoplasm of other and ill-defined sites within the lip, oral cavity, and pharynx
- **149.0** Pharynx, unspecified
- **149.1** Waldeyer's ring
- **149.8** Other
  Malignant neoplasms of lip, oral cavity, and pharynx whose point of origin cannot be assigned to any one of the categories 140–148
  Excludes *"book leaf" neoplasm [ventral surface of tongue and floor of mouth] (145.8)*
- **149.9** Ill-defined

MALIGNANT NEOPLASM OF DIGESTIVE ORGANS AND PERITONEUM (150–159)

Excludes *carcinoma in situ (230.1–230.9)*

150 Malignant neoplasm of esophagus
- **150.0** Cervical esophagus
- **150.1** Thoracic esophagus
- **150.2** Abdominal esophagus
  Excludes *adenocarcinoma (151.0)*
  cardio-esophageal junction (151.0)
- **150.3** Upper third of esophagus
  Proximal third of esophagus
- **150.4** Middle third of esophagus
- **150.5** Lower third of esophagus
  Distal third of esophagus
  Excludes *adenocarcinoma (151.0)*
  cardio-esophageal junction (151.0)
- **150.8** Other specified part
  Malignant neoplasm of contiguous or overlapping sites of esophagus whose point of origin cannot be determined
- **150.9** Esophagus, unspecified

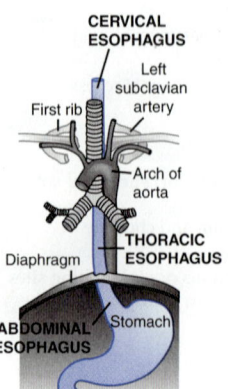

Figure 2-3 The esophagus is the muscular tube that connects the pharynx and the stomach. The 10 inch (25 cm) long esophagus is divided into three parts: **cervical, thoracic,** and **abdominal.**

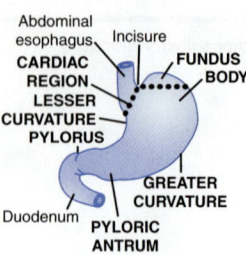

Figure 2-4 Parts of the stomach.

Item 2-2 The esophagus opens into the stomach through the **cardiac orifice,** also called the **cardioesophageal junction.** The **cardia** is adjacent to the cardiac orifice. The stomach widens into the **greater** and **lesser curvatures.** The **pyloric antrum** precedes the **pylorus,** which opens to the duodenum.

151 Malignant neoplasm of stomach
Excludes *benign carcinoid tumor of stomach (209.63)*
malignant carcinoid tumor of stomach (209.23)
- **151.0** Cardia
  Cardiac orifice
  Cardio-esophageal junction
  Excludes *squamous cell carcinoma (150.2, 150.5)*
- **151.1** Pylorus
  Prepylorus
  Pyloric canal
- **151.2** Pyloric antrum
  Antrum of stomach NOS
- **151.3** Fundus of stomach
- **151.4** Body of stomach
- **151.5** Lesser curvature, unspecified
  Lesser curvature, not classifiable to 151.1–151.4
- **151.6** Greater curvature, unspecified
  Greater curvature, not classifiable to 151.0–151.4
- **151.8** Other specified sites of stomach
  Anterior wall, not classifiable to 151.0–151.4
  Posterior wall, not classifiable to 151.0–151.4
  Malignant neoplasm of contiguous or overlapping sites of stomach whose point of origin cannot be determined
- **151.9** Stomach, unspecified
  Carcinoma ventriculi
  Gastric cancer
  Coding Clinic: 2001, Q2, P17-18; 1988, Q2, P11

152 Malignant neoplasm of small intestine, including duodenum
Excludes *benign carcinoid tumor of small intestine and duodenum (209.40-209.43)*
malignant carcinoid tumor of small intestine and duodenum (209.00-209.03)
- **152.0** Duodenum
- **152.1** Jejunum
- **152.2** Ileum
  Excludes *ileocecal valve (153.4)*
- **152.3** Meckel's diverticulum
- **152.8** Other specified sites of small intestine
  Duodenojejunal junction
  Malignant neoplasm of contiguous or overlapping sites of small intestine whose point of origin cannot be determined
- **152.9** Small intestine, unspecified

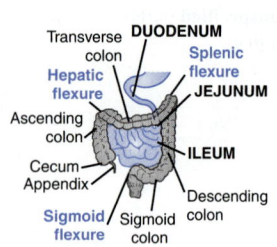

Figure 2-5 Small intestine and colon.

PART III / Diseases: Tabular List Volume 1 — 153-157.4

● **153 Malignant neoplasm of colon**
  [Excludes] benign carcinoid tumor of colon (209.50- 209.56)
  malignant carcinoid tumor of colon (209.10-209.16)

  153.0 Hepatic flexure
   Flexure is a bending in a structure or organ. Note the three flexures illustrated in Figure 2–5. Hepatic = liver, sigmoid = colon, splenic = spleen.

  153.1 Transverse colon

  153.2 Descending colon
   Left colon
   Coding Clinic: 1995, Q1, P4

  153.3 Sigmoid colon
   Sigmoid (flexure)
   [Excludes] rectosigmoid junction (154.0)
   Flexure is a bending in a structure or organ. Note the three flexures illustrated in Figure 2–5. Hepatic = liver, sigmoid = colon, splenic = spleen.

  153.4 Cecum
   Ileocecal valve

  153.5 Appendix

  153.6 Ascending colon
   Right colon

  153.7 Splenic flexure
   Flexure is a bending in a structure or organ. Note the three flexures illustrated in Figure 2–5. Hepatic = liver, sigmoid = colon, splenic = spleen.

  153.8 Other specified sites of large intestine
   Malignant neoplasm of contiguous or overlapping sites of colon whose point of origin cannot be determined
   [Excludes] ileocecal valve (153.4)
   rectosigmoid junction (154.0)

  ■ **153.9 Colon, unspecified**
   Large intestine NOS
   Coding Clinic: 2010, Q2, P12

● **154 Malignant neoplasm of rectum, rectosigmoid junction, and anus**
  [Excludes] benign carcinoid tumor of rectum (209.57)
  malignant carcinoid tumor of rectum (209.17)

  154.0 Rectosigmoid junction
   Colon with rectum   Rectosigmoid (colon)

  154.1 Rectum
   Rectal ampulla

  154.2 Anal canal
   Anal sphincter
   [Excludes] malignant melanoma of skin of anus (172.5)
   malignant neoplasm of skin of anus (173.50-173.59)
   Coding Clinic: 2001, Q1, P8

  ■ **154.3 Anus, unspecified**
   [Excludes] malignant melanoma of:
     anus:
       margin (172.5)
       skin (172.5)
       perianal skin (172.5)
     malignant neoplasm of:
       anus:
         margin (173.50-173.59)
         skin (173.50-173.59)
         perianal skin (173.50-173.59)

  154.8 Other
   Anorectum
   Cloacogenic zone
   Malignant neoplasm of contiguous or overlapping sites of rectum, rectosigmoid junction, and anus whose point of origin cannot be determined

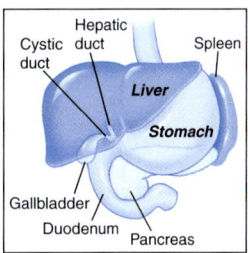

Figure 2-6 Diagram of liver, gallbladder, hepatic duct, pancreas, and spleen. (From Thibodeau and Patton: Anatomy and Physiology, ed 7, Mosby, 2010)

● **155 Malignant neoplasm of liver and intrahepatic bile ducts**

  155.0 Liver, primary
   Carcinoma:
     liver, specified as primary
     hepatocellular
     liver cell
   Hepatoblastoma
   Coding Clinic: 2008, Q4, P82-83

  155.1 Intrahepatic bile ducts
   Canaliculi biliferi   Intrahepatic:
   Interlobular: biliary passages
     bile ducts   canaliculi
     biliary canals   gall duct
   [Excludes] hepatic duct (156.1)

  155.2 Liver, not specified as primary or secondary
   Stated as a liver neoplasm, but not specific as to type

● **156 Malignant neoplasm of gallbladder and extrahepatic bile ducts**
  Extrahepatic = outside the liver

  156.0 Gallbladder

  156.1 Extrahepatic bile ducts
   Biliary duct or passage   Cystic duct
   NOS   Hepatic duct
   Common bile duct   Sphincter of Oddi

  156.2 Ampulla of Vater

  156.8 Other specified sites of gallbladder and extrahepatic bile ducts
   Malignant neoplasm of contiguous or overlapping sites of gallbladder and extrahepatic bile ducts whose point of origin cannot be determined

  ■ **156.9 Biliary tract, part unspecified**
   Malignant neoplasm involving both intrahepatic and extrahepatic bile ducts
   Intra = inside; extra = outside

● **157 Malignant neoplasm of pancreas**
  Check documentation for specific site.

  157.0 Head of pancreas
   Coding Clinic: 2005, Q2, P9-10; 2000, Q4, P39-40

  157.1 Body of pancreas

  157.2 Tail of pancreas

  157.3 Pancreatic duct
   Duct of:
     Santorini
     Wirsung

  157.4 Islets of Langerhans
   Islets of Langerhans, any part of pancreas
   [Use additional] code to identify any functional activity
   Coding Clinic: 2007, Q4, P70-72

Item 2-3 Islets of Langerhans (endocrine producing cells comprising 1% to 2% of the pancreatic mass) make and secrete hormones that regulate the body's production of insulin, glucagon, and stomach acid. Breakdown of the insulin-producing cells can cause diabetes mellitus.
Islet cell tumors can be benign or malignant and include glucagonomas, insulinomas, gastrinomas, and neuroendocrine tumor. The neoplasm table must be consulted for the correct neoplasm code.

◄ New   ◄▥ Revised   ~~deleted~~ Deleted   [Excludes]   [Includes]   [Use additional]   [Code first]   [Omit code]
● Use Additional Digit(s)   ■ Unspecified   ● Not first-listed DX   OGCR Official Guidelines   **Coding Clinic**

157.8 Other specified sites of pancreas
Ectopic pancreatic tissue
Malignant neoplasm of contiguous or overlapping sites of pancreas whose point of origin cannot be determined

157.9 Pancreas, part unspecified
Coding Clinic: 1989, Q4, P11

158 Malignant neoplasm of retroperitoneum and peritoneum

158.0 Retroperitoneum
Periadrenal tissue   Perirenal tissue
Perinephric tissue   Retrocecal tissue

158.8 Specified parts of peritoneum
Cul-de-sac (of Douglas)
Mesentery
Mesocolon
Omentum
Peritoneum:
  parietal
  pelvic
Rectouterine pouch
Malignant neoplasm of contiguous or overlapping sites of retroperitoneum and peritoneum whose point of origin cannot be determined

158.9 Peritoneum, unspecified

159 Malignant neoplasm of other and ill-defined sites within the digestive organs and peritoneum

159.0 Intestinal tract, part unspecified
Intestine NOS

159.1 Spleen, not elsewhere classified
Angiosarcoma of spleen
Fibrosarcoma of spleen
Excludes Hodgkin's disease (201.0–201.9)
  lymphosarcoma (200.1)
  reticulosarcoma (200.0)

159.8 Other sites of digestive system and intra-abdominal organs
Malignant neoplasm of digestive organs and peritoneum whose point of origin cannot be assigned to any one of the categories 150–158
Excludes anus and rectum (154.8)
  cardio-esophageal junction (151.0)
  colon and rectum (154.0)

159.9 Ill-defined
Alimentary canal or tract NOS
Gastrointestinal tract NOS
Excludes abdominal NOS (195.2)
  intra-abdominal NOS (195.2)

MALIGNANT NEOPLASM OF RESPIRATORY AND INTRATHORACIC ORGANS (160–165)

Excludes carcinoma in situ (231.0–231.9)

160 Malignant neoplasm of nasal cavities, middle ear, and accessory sinuses

160.0 Nasal cavities
Cartilage of nose   Septum of nose
Conchae, nasal   Vestibule of nose
Internal nose
Excludes malignant melanoma of skin of nose (172.3)
  malignant neoplasm of skin of nose (173.30–173.39)
  nasal bone (170.0)
  nose NOS (195.0)
  olfactory bulb (192.0)
  posterior margin of septum and choanae (147.3)
  turbinates (170.0)

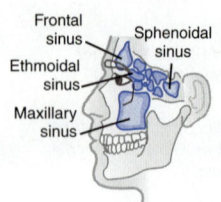

Figure 2-7 Paranasal sinuses. (From Buck CJ: Step-by-Step Medical Coding, ed 2011, Philadelphia, WB Saunders, 2011)

160.1 Auditory tube, middle ear, and mastoid air cells
Antrum tympanicum
Eustachian tube
Tympanic cavity
Excludes bone of ear (meatus) (170.0)
  cartilage of ear (171.0)
  malignant melanoma of:
    auditory canal (external) (172.2)
    ear (external) (skin) (172.2)
  malignant neoplasm of:
    auditory canal (external) (173.20-173.29)
    ear (external) (skin) (173.20-173.29)

160.2 Maxillary sinus
Antrum (Highmore) (maxillary)

160.3 Ethmoidal sinus

160.4 Frontal sinus

160.5 Sphenoidal sinus

160.8 Other
Malignant neoplasm of contiguous or overlapping sites of nasal cavities, middle ear, and accessory sinuses whose point of origin cannot be determined

160.9 Accessory sinus, unspecified

161 Malignant neoplasm of larynx

161.0 Glottis
Intrinsic larynx
Laryngeal commissure (anterior) (posterior)
True vocal cord
True vocal cords (lower vocal folds) produce vocalization when air from lungs passes between them. Check your documentation. Code 161.1 is for malignant neoplasm of false vocal cords.
Vocal cord NOS

161.1 Supraglottis
Aryepiglottic fold or interarytenoid fold, laryngeal aspect
Epiglottis (suprahyoid portion) NOS
Extrinsic larynx
False vocal cords
False vocal cords (upper vocal folds) are not involved in vocalization. Check your documentation. Code 161.0 is for true vocal cords.
Posterior (laryngeal) surface of epiglottis
Ventricular bands
Excludes anterior aspect of epiglottis (146.4)
  aryepiglottic fold or interarytenoid fold:
    NOS (148.2)
    hypopharyngeal aspect (148.2)
    marginal zone (148.2)

161.2 Subglottis

161.3 Laryngeal cartilages
Cartilage: Cartilage:
  arytenoid   cuneiform
  cricoid   thyroid

161.8 Other specified sites of larynx
Malignant neoplasm of contiguous or overlapping sites of larynx whose point of origin cannot be determined
Coding Clinic: 2007, Q3, P8-9

161.9 Larynx, unspecified

- **162 Malignant neoplasm of trachea, bronchus, and lung**
  Excludes benign carcinoid tumor of bronchus (209.61)
  malignant carcinoid tumor of bronchus (209.21)
  Coding Clinic: 2006, Q3, P7-8
  - 162.0 Trachea
    Cartilage of trachea   Mucosa of trachea
  - 162.2 Main bronchus
    Carina   Hilus of lung
  - 162.3 Upper lobe, bronchus or lung
    Coding Clinic: 2004, Q1, P4-5
  - 162.4 Middle lobe, bronchus or lung
  - 162.5 Lower lobe, bronchus or lung
    Coding Clinic: 2010, Q3, P3
  - 162.8 Other parts of bronchus or lung
    Malignant neoplasm of contiguous or overlapping sites of bronchus or lung whose point of origin cannot be determined
    Coding Clinic: 2006, Q3, P7-8
  - 162.9 Bronchus and lung, unspecified
    Coding Clinic: 2010, Q2, P14; 2006, Q3, P14-15; 1997, Q2, P3; 1996, Q4, P47-48; 1993, Q4, P36; 1988, Q2, P10; 1984, May-June, P11, 14

- **163 Malignant neoplasm of pleura**
  Pleura are comprised of serous membrane that lines thoracic cavity (parietal) and covers lungs (visceral).
  - 163.0 Parietal pleura
  - 163.1 Visceral pleura
  - 163.8 Other specified sites of pleura
    Malignant neoplasm of contiguous or overlapping sites of pleura whose point of origin cannot be determined
  - 163.9 Pleura, unspecified

- **164 Malignant neoplasm of thymus, heart, and mediastinum**
  - 164.0 Thymus
    Excludes benign carcinoid tumor of the thymus (209.62)
    malignant carcinoid tumor of the thymus (209.22)
  - 164.1 Heart
    Endocardium   Myocardium
    Epicardium   Pericardium
    Excludes great vessels (171.4)
  - 164.2 Anterior mediastinum
  - 164.3 Posterior mediastinum
  - 164.8 Other
    Malignant neoplasm of contiguous or overlapping sites of thymus, heart, and mediastinum whose point of origin cannot be determined
  - 164.9 Mediastinum, part unspecified

- **165 Malignant neoplasm of other and ill-defined sites within the respiratory system and intrathoracic organs**
  - 165.0 Upper respiratory tract, part unspecified
  - 165.8 Other
    Malignant neoplasm of respiratory and intrathoracic organs whose point of origin cannot be assigned to any one of the categories 160–164
  - 165.9 Ill-defined sites within the respiratory system
    Respiratory tract NOS
    Excludes intrathoracic NOS (195.1)
    thoracic NOS (195.1)

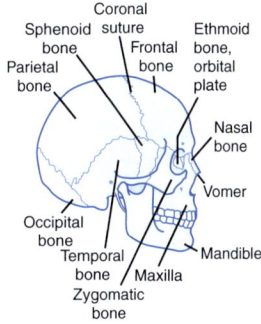

Figure 2–8 Bones of the skull.

MALIGNANT NEOPLASM OF BONE, CONNECTIVE TISSUE, SKIN, AND BREAST (170–176)

Excludes carcinoma in situ:
breast (233.0)
skin (232.0–232.9)

- **170 Malignant neoplasm of bone and articular cartilage**
  Includes cartilage (articular) (joint)
  periosteum
  Excludes bone marrow NOS (202.9)
  cartilage:
  ear (171.0)
  eyelid (171.0)
  larynx (161.3)
  nose (160.0)
  synovia (171.0–171.9)
  - 170.0 Bones of skull and face, except mandible
    Mandible = lower jaw
    Bone: Bone:
    ethmoid   sphenoid
    frontal   temporal
    malar   zygomatic
    nasal   Maxilla (superior)
    occipital   Turbinate
    orbital   Upper jaw bone
    parietal   Vomer
    Excludes carcinoma, any type except intraosseous or odontogenic:
    maxilla, maxillary (sinus) (160.2)
    upper jaw bone (143.0)
    jaw bone (lower) (170.1)
  - 170.1 Mandible
    Inferior maxilla
    Jaw bone NOS
    Lower jaw bone
    Excludes carcinoma, any type except intraosseous or odontogenic:
    jaw bone NOS (143.9)
    lower (143.1)
    upper jaw bone (170.0)
  - 170.2 Vertebral column, excluding sacrum and coccyx
    Spinal column   Vertebra
    Spine
    Excludes sacrum and coccyx (170.6)
  - 170.3 Ribs, sternum, and clavicle
    Costal cartilage   Xiphoid process
    Costovertebral joint
  - 170.4 Scapula and long bones of upper limb
    Acromion   Radius
    Bones NOS of upper limb   Ulna
    Humerus
    Coding Clinic: 1999, Q2, P9

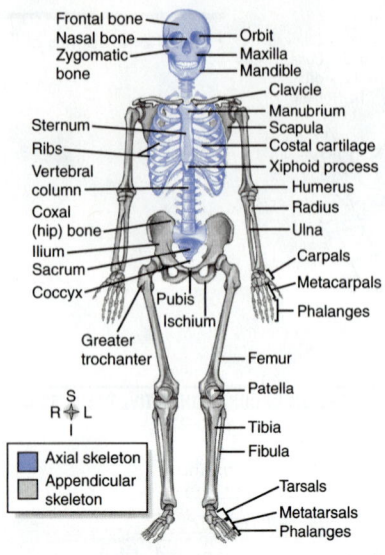

Figure 2-9 Diagram of skeleton of trunk and limbs with bones labeled. (From Thibodeau and Patton: Anatomy and Physiology, ed 7, Mosby, 2010)

170.5 Short bones of upper limb
- Carpal
- Cuneiform, wrist
- Metacarpal
- Navicular, of hand
- Phalanges of hand
- Pisiform
- Scaphoid (of hand)
- Semilunar or lunate
- Trapezium
- Trapezoid
- Unciform

170.6 Pelvic bones, sacrum, and coccyx
- Coccygeal vertebra
- Ilium
- Ischium
- Pubic bone
- Sacral vertebra

170.7 Long bones of lower limb
- Bones NOS of lower limb
- Femur
- Fibula
- Tibia

170.8 Short bones of lower limb
- Astragalus [talus]
- Calcaneus
- Cuboid
- Cuneiform, ankle
- Metatarsal
- Navicular (of ankle)
- Patella
- Phalanges of foot
- Tarsal

170.9 Bone and articular cartilage, site unspecified

● 171 Malignant neoplasm of connective and other soft tissue
- **Includes** blood vessel
  - bursa
  - fascia
  - fat
  - ligament, except uterine
  - muscle
  - peripheral, sympathetic, and parasympathetic nerves and ganglia
  - synovia
  - tendon (sheath)
- **Excludes** cartilage (of):
  - articular (170.0–170.9)
  - larynx (161.3)
  - nose (160.0)
  - connective tissue:
    - breast (174.0–175.9)
    - internal organs—code to malignant neoplasm of the site [e.g., leiomyosarcoma of stomach, 151.9]
    - heart (164.1)
    - uterine ligament (183.4)

171.0 Head, face, and neck
- Cartilage of:
  - ear
  - eyelid

Coding Clinic: 1999, Q2, P6-7

171.2 Upper limb, including shoulder
- Arm
- Finger
- Forearm
- Hand

171.3 Lower limb, including hip
- Foot
- Leg
- Popliteal space
  - *Popliteal space = popliteal cavity, popliteal fossa. Depression in posterior aspect of knee (behind knee).*
- Thigh
- Toe

Coding Clinic: 2012, Q3, P8

171.4 Thorax
- Axilla
- Diaphragm
- Great vessels
- **Excludes** heart (164.1)
  - mediastinum (164.2–164.9)
  - thymus (164.0)

171.5 Abdomen
- Abdominal wall
- Hypochondrium
- **Excludes** peritoneum (158.8)
  - retroperitoneum (158.0)

171.6 Pelvis
- Buttock
- Groin
- Inguinal region
- Perineum
- **Excludes** pelvic peritoneum (158.8)
  - retroperitoneum (158.0)
  - uterine ligament, any (183.3–183.5)

171.7 Trunk, unspecified
- Back NOS
- Flank NOS

171.8 Other specified sites of connective and other soft tissue
- Malignant neoplasm of contiguous or overlapping sites of connective tissue whose point of origin cannot be determined

171.9 Connective and other soft tissue, site unspecified

● 172 Malignant melanoma of skin
- **Includes** melanocarcinoma
  - melanoma in situ of skin
  - melanoma (skin) NOS
- **Excludes** skin of genital organs (184.0–184.9, 187.1–187.9)
  - sites other than skin - code to malignant neoplasm of the site

172.0 Lip
- **Excludes** vermilion border of lip (140.0–140.1, 140.9)

172.1 Eyelid, including canthus

172.2 Ear and external auditory canal
- Auricle (ear)
- Auricular canal, external
- External [acoustic] meatus
- Pinna

172.3 Other and unspecified parts of face
- Cheek (external)
- Chin
- Eyebrow
- Forehead
- Nose, external
- Temple

172.4 Scalp and neck

172.5 Trunk, except scrotum
- Axilla
- Breast
- Buttock
- Groin
- Perianal skin
- Perineum
- Umbilicus
- **Excludes** anal canal (154.2)
  - anus NOS (154.3)
  - scrotum (187.7)

172.6 Upper limb, including shoulder
- Arm
- Finger
- Forearm
- Hand

Item 2-4 Malignant melanoma is a serious form of skin cancer that affects the melanocytes (pigment-forming cells) and is caused by ultraviolet (UV) rays from the sun that damage skin. It is most commonly seen in the 40- to 60-year-olds with fair skin, blue or green eyes, and red or blond hair who sunburn easily. Melanoma can spread very rapidly and is the most deadly form of skin cancer. It is less common than other types of skin cancer. The rate of melanoma is increasing and currently is the leading cause of death from skin disease.

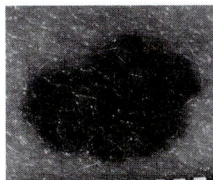

Figure 2-10 Malignant melanoma of skin. (From Goldman: Cecil Textbook of Medicine, ed 22, Saunders, 2004)

- **172.7** Lower limb, including hip
  - Ankle
  - Foot
  - Heel
  - Knee
  - Leg
  - Popliteal area
  - Thigh
  - Toe
- **172.8** Other specified sites of skin
  - Malignant melanoma of contiguous or overlapping sites of skin whose point of origin cannot be determined
- **172.9** Melanoma of skin, site unspecified

- **173** Other and unspecified malignant neoplasm of skin
  - **Includes** malignant neoplasm of:
    - sebaceous glands
    - sudoriferous, sudoriparous glands
    - sweat glands
  - **Excludes** Kaposi's sarcoma (176.0–176.9)
    - malignant melanoma of skin (172.0–172.9)
    - Merkel cell carcinoma of skin (209.31-209.36)
    - skin of genital organs (184.0–184.9, 187.1–187.9)
  - *Coding Clinic: 2000, Q1, P8; 1996, Q2, P12*

- **173.0** Other and unspecified malignant neoplasm of skin of lip
  - **Excludes** vermilion border of lip (140.0–140.1, 140.9)
  - **173.00** Unspecified malignant neoplasm of skin of lip
  - **173.01** Basal cell carcinoma of skin of lip
  - **173.02** Squamous cell carcinoma of skin of lip
  - **173.09** Other specified malignant neoplasm of skin of lip

- **173.1** Other and unspecified malignant neoplasm of eyelid, including canthus
  - **Excludes** cartilage of eyelid (171.0)
  - **173.10** Unspecified malignant neoplasm of eyelid, including canthus
  - **173.11** Basal cell carcinoma of eyelid, including canthus
  - **173.12** Squamous cell carcinoma of eyelid, including canthus
  - **173.19** Other specified malignant neoplasm of eyelid, including canthus

- **173.2** Other and unspecified malignant neoplasm of skin of ear and external auditory canal
  - Auricle (ear)
  - Auricular canal, external
  - External meatus
  - Pinna
  - **Excludes** cartilage of ear (171.0)
  - **173.20** Unspecified malignant neoplasm of skin of ear and external auditory canal
  - **173.21** Basal cell carcinoma of skin of ear and external auditory canal
  - **173.22** Squamous cell carcinoma of skin of ear and external auditory canal
  - **173.29** Other specified malignant neoplasm of skin of ear and external auditory canal

- **173.3** Other and unspecified malignant neoplasm of skin of other and unspecified parts of face
  - Cheek, external
  - Chin
  - Eyebrow
  - Forehead
  - Nose, external
  - Temple
  - *Coding Clinic: 2000, Q1, P3*
  - **173.30** Unspecified malignant neoplasm of skin of other and unspecified parts of face
  - **173.31** Basal cell carcinoma of skin of other and unspecified parts of face
  - **173.32** Squamous cell carcinoma of skin of other and unspecified parts of face
  - **173.39** Other specified malignant neoplasm of skin of other and unspecified parts of face

- **173.4** Other and unspecified malignant neoplasm of scalp and skin of neck
  - **173.40** Unspecified malignant neoplasm of scalp and skin of neck
  - **173.41** Basal cell carcinoma of scalp and skin of neck
  - **173.42** Squamous cell carcinoma of scalp and skin of neck
  - **173.49** Other specified malignant neoplasm of scalp and skin of neck

- **173.5** Other and unspecified malignant neoplasm of skin of trunk, except scrotum
  - Axillary fold
  - Perianal skin
  - Skin of:
    - abdominal wall
    - anus
    - back
    - breast
    - buttock
    - chest wall
    - groin
    - perineum
  - Umbilicus
  - **Excludes** anal canal (154.2)
    - anus NOS (154.3)
    - skin of scrotum (187.7)
  - *Coding Clinic: 2001, Q1, P8*
  - **173.50** Unspecified malignant neoplasm of skin of trunk, except scrotum
  - **173.51** Basal cell carcinoma of skin of trunk, except scrotum
  - **173.52** Squamous cell carcinoma of skin of trunk, except scrotum
  - **173.59** Other specified malignant neoplasm of skin of trunk, except scrotum

- **173.6** Other and unspecified malignant neoplasm of skin of upper limb, including shoulder
  - Arm
  - Finger
  - Forearm
  - Hand
  - **173.60** Unspecified malignant neoplasm of skin of upper limb, including shoulder
  - **173.61** Basal cell carcinoma of skin of upper limb, including shoulder
  - **173.62** Squamous cell carcinoma of skin of upper limb, including shoulder
  - **173.69** Other specified malignant neoplasm of skin of upper limb, including shoulder

- **173.7** Other and unspecified malignant neoplasm of skin of lower limb, including hip
  - Ankle
  - Foot
  - Heel
  - Knee
  - Leg
  - Popliteal area
  - Thigh
  - Toe
  - **173.70** Unspecified malignant neoplasm of skin of lower limb, including hip
  - **173.71** Basal cell carcinoma of skin of lower limb, including hip
  - **173.72** Squamous cell carcinoma of skin of lower limb, including hip
  - **173.79** Other specified malignant neoplasm of skin of lower limb, including hip

173.8–180.9   ICD-9-CM

- **173.8** Other and unspecified malignant neoplasm of other specified sites of skin
  Malignant neoplasm of contiguous or overlapping sites of skin whose point of origin cannot be determined
  - **173.80** Unspecified malignant neoplasm of other specified sites of skin
  - **173.81** Basal cell carcinoma of other specified sites of skin
  - **173.82** Squamous cell carcinoma of other specified sites of skin
  - **173.89** Other specified malignant neoplasm of other specified sites of skin
- **173.9** Other and unspecified malignant neoplasm of skin, site unspecified
  - **173.90** Unspecified malignant neoplasm of skin, site unspecified
    Malignant neoplasm of skin NOS
  - **173.91** Basal cell carcinoma of skin, site unspecified
  - **173.92** Squamous cell carcinoma of skin, site unspecified
  - **173.99** Other specified malignant neoplasm of skin, site unspecified

- **174** Malignant neoplasm of female breast
  This code is for female breast; see 175 for male breast.
  Includes breast (female)
      connective tissue
      soft parts
      Paget's disease of:
        breast
        nipple
  Use additional code to identify estrogen receptor status (V86.0, V86.1)
  Excludes malignant melanoma of skin of breast (172.5)
      malignant neoplasm of skin of breast (173.50-173.59)
  Coding Clinic: 2012, Q1, P11
  - **174.0** Nipple and areola
  - **174.1** Central portion
  - **174.2** Upper-inner quadrant
    Coding Clinic: 1989, Q4, P11
  - **174.3** Lower-inner quadrant
    Coding Clinic: 1989, Q4, P11
  - **174.4** Upper-outer quadrant
    Coding Clinic: 2008, Q4, P152-155; 2004, Q1, P3-4; 1997, Q3, P8; 1984, May-June, P11
  - **174.5** Lower-outer quadrant
  - **174.6** Axillary tail
  - **174.8** Other specified sites of female breast
    Ectopic sites
    Inner breast
    Lower breast
    Malignant neoplasm of contiguous or overlapping sites of breast whose point of origin cannot be determined
    Midline of breast
    Outer breast
    Upper breast
    Coding Clinic: 1985, July-Aug, P11
  - **174.9** Breast (female), unspecified
    Coding Clinic: 2009, Q3, P4; 2005, Q3, P11-12; 1994, Q2, P10x2

Item 2–5 Kaposi's sarcoma is a cancer that causes patches of abnormal tissue to grow under the skin; in the lining of the mouth, nose, and throat; or in other organs, often beginning and spreading to other organs. Patients who have had organ transplants or patients with AIDS are at high risk for this malignancy.

- **175** Malignant neoplasm of male breast
  Use additional code to identify estrogen receptor status (V86.0, V86.1)
  Excludes malignant melanoma of skin of breast (172.5)
      malignant neoplasm of skin of breast (173.50-173.59)
  Coding Clinic: 2012, Q1, P11
  - **175.0** Nipple and areola
  - **175.9** Other and unspecified sites of male breast
    Ectopic breast tissue, male

- **176** Kaposi's sarcoma
  - **176.0** Skin
    Coding Clinic: 2007, Q4, P61-64
  - **176.1** Soft tissue
    Blood vessel   Ligament
    Connective tissue   Lymphatic(s) NEC
    Fascia   Muscle
    Excludes lymph glands and nodes (176.5)
  - **176.2** Palate
  - **176.3** Gastrointestinal sites
  - **176.4** Lung
  - **176.5** Lymph nodes
  - **176.8** Other specified sites
    Oral cavity NEC
  - **176.9** Unspecified
    Viscera NOS

MALIGNANT NEOPLASM OF GENITOURINARY ORGANS (179–189)

Excludes carcinoma in situ (233.1–233.9)

- **179** Malignant neoplasm of uterus, part unspecified
- **180** Malignant neoplasm of cervix uteri
  Includes invasive malignancy [carcinoma]
  Excludes carcinoma in situ (233.1)
  - **180.0** Endocervix
    Inside the cervix
    Cervical canal NOS
    Endocervical canal
    Endocervical gland
  - **180.1** Exocervix
    Outside the cervix
  - **180.8** Other specified sites of cervix
    Cervical stump
    Squamocolumnar junction of cervix
    Malignant neoplasm of contiguous or overlapping sites of cervix uteri whose point of origin cannot be determined
  - **180.9** Cervix uteri, unspecified

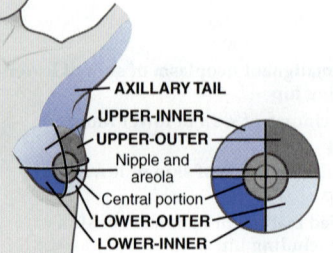

Figure 2–11 Female breast quadrants and axillary tail.

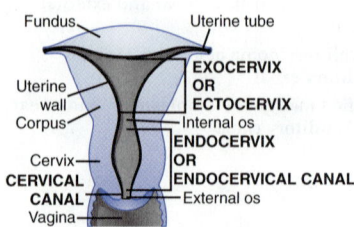

Figure 2–12 Cervix uteri.

181 Malignant neoplasm of placenta
Choriocarcinoma NOS
Chorioepithelioma NOS
Excludes: chorioadenoma (destruens) (236.1)
hydatidiform mole (630)
  malignant (236.1)
invasive mole (236.1)
male choriocarcinoma NOS (186.0–186.9)

● **182 Malignant neoplasm of body of uterus**
Excludes: carcinoma in situ (233.2)

182.0 Corpus uteri, except isthmus
Cornu   Fundus
Endometrium   Myometrium
Coding Clinic: 2009, Q3, P4

182.1 Isthmus
Lower uterine segment

182.8 Other specified sites of body of uterus
Malignant neoplasm of contiguous or overlapping sites of body of uterus whose point of origin cannot be determined
Excludes: uterus NOS (179)

● **183 Malignant neoplasm of ovary and other uterine adnexa**
Excludes: Douglas' cul-de-sac (158.8)

183.0 Ovary
Use additional code to identify any functional activity
Coding Clinic: 2007, Q4, P95-96

183.2 Fallopian tube
Oviduct   Uterine tube

183.3 Broad ligament
Mesovarium   Parovarian region

183.4 Parametrium
Uterine ligament NOS   Uterosacral ligament

183.5 Round ligament

183.8 Other specified sites of uterine adnexa
Tubo-ovarian
Utero-ovarian
Malignant neoplasm of contiguous or overlapping sites of ovary and other uterine adnexa whose point of origin cannot be determined

183.9 Uterine adnexa, unspecified

● **184 Malignant neoplasm of other and unspecified female genital organs**
Excludes: carcinoma in situ (233.30–233.39)

184.0 Vagina
Gartner's duct   Vaginal vault

184.1 Labia majora
Greater vestibular [Bartholin's] gland

184.2 Labia minora

184.3 Clitoris

184.4 Vulva, unspecified
External female genitalia NOS
Pudendum

184.8 Other specified sites of female genital organs
Malignant neoplasm of contiguous or overlapping sites of female genital organs whose point of origin cannot be determined

184.9 Female genital organ, site unspecified
Female genitourinary tract NOS

185 Malignant neoplasm of prostate
Excludes: seminal vesicles (187.8)
Coding Clinic: 2010, Q2, P3; 2003, Q3, P13; 1999, Q3, P5; 1994, Q1, P20; 1992, Q3, P7

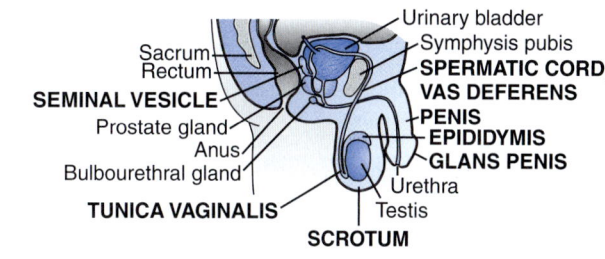

Figure 2-13 Penis and other male genital organs.

● **186 Malignant neoplasm of testis**
Use additional code to identify any functional activity

186.0 Undescended testis
Ectopic testis   Retained testis

186.9 Other and unspecified testis
Testis: Testis:
  NOS   scrotal
  descended

● **187 Malignant neoplasm of penis and other male genital organs**

187.1 Prepuce
Foreskin

187.2 Glans penis

187.3 Body of penis
Corpus cavernosum

187.4 Penis, part unspecified
Skin of penis NOS

187.5 Epididymis

187.6 Spermatic cord
Vas deferens

187.7 Scrotum
Skin of scrotum

187.8 Other specified sites of male genital organs
Seminal vesicle
Tunica vaginalis
Malignant neoplasm of contiguous or overlapping sites of penis and other male genital organs whose point of origin cannot be determined

187.9 Male genital organ, site unspecified
Male genital organ or tract NOS

● **188 Malignant neoplasm of bladder**
Excludes: carcinoma in situ (233.7)

188.0 Trigone of urinary bladder

188.1 Dome of urinary bladder

188.2 Lateral wall of urinary bladder

188.3 Anterior wall of urinary bladder

188.4 Posterior wall of urinary bladder

188.5 Bladder neck
Internal urethral orifice

188.6 Ureteric orifice

188.7 Urachus

188.8 Other specified sites of bladder
Malignant neoplasm of contiguous or overlapping sites of bladder whose point of origin cannot be determined

188.9 Bladder, part unspecified
Bladder wall NOS
Coding Clinic: 2000, Q1, P5

- **189 Malignant neoplasm of kidney and other and unspecified urinary organs**
  - Excludes: benign carcinoid tumor of kidney (209.64)
    malignant carcinoid tumor of kidney (209.24)
  - **189.0 Kidney, except pelvis**
    Kidney NOS   Kidney parenchyma
    Coding Clinic: 2005, Q2, P4-5; 2004, Q2, P4
  - **189.1 Renal pelvis**
    Renal calyces   Ureteropelvic junction
  - **189.2 Ureter**
    Excludes: ureteric orifice of bladder (188.6)
  - **189.3 Urethra**
    Excludes: urethral orifice of bladder (188.5)
  - **189.4 Paraurethral glands**
  - **189.8 Other specified sites of urinary organs**
    Malignant neoplasm of contiguous or overlapping sites of kidney and other urinary organs whose point of origin cannot be determined
  - **189.9 Urinary organ, site unspecified**
    Urinary system NOS
    Excludes: carcinoma in situ (234.0–234.9)

MALIGNANT NEOPLASM OF OTHER AND UNSPECIFIED SITES (190–199)

Excludes: carcinoma in situ (234.0–234.9)

- **190 Malignant neoplasm of eye**
  - Excludes: carcinoma in situ (234.0)
    dark area on retina and choroid (239.81)
    malignant melanoma of eyelid (skin) (172.1)
    cartilage (171.0)
    malignant neoplasm of eyelid (skin) (173.10-173.19)
    optic nerve (192.0)
    orbital bone (170.0)
    retinal freckle (239.81)
  - **190.0 Eyeball, except conjunctiva, cornea, retina, and choroid**
    Note the use of "except" in this code.
    Ciliary body   Sclera
    Crystalline lens Uveal tract
    Iris
  - **190.1 Orbit**
    Connective tissue of orbit
    Extraocular muscle
    Retrobulbar
    Excludes: bone of orbit (170.0)
  - **190.2 Lacrimal gland**
  - **190.3 Conjunctiva**
  - **190.4 Cornea**
  - **190.5 Retina**
  - **190.6 Choroid**
  - **190.7 Lacrimal duct**
    Lacrimal sac   Nasolacrimal duct
  - **190.8 Other specified sites of eye**
    Malignant neoplasm of contiguous or overlapping sites of eye whose point of origin cannot be determined
  - **190.9 Eye, part unspecified**

- **191 Malignant neoplasm of brain**
  - Excludes: cranial nerves (192.0)
    retrobulbar area (190.1)
  - **191.0 Cerebrum, except lobes and ventricles**
    Basal ganglia   Globus pallidus
    Cerebral cortex   Hypothalamus
    Corpus striatum   Thalamus
  - **191.1 Frontal lobe**
    Coding Clinic: 2005, Q4, P117-119; 1993, Q4, P33
  - **191.2 Temporal lobe**
    Hippocampus   Uncus
    Coding Clinic: 2009, Q3, P4; 2006, Q4, P122-123

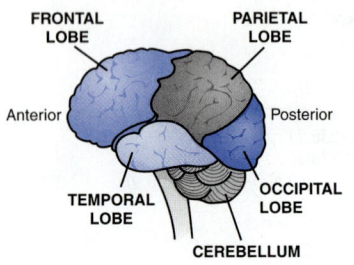

Figure 2-14 The brain.

  - **191.3 Parietal lobe**
  - **191.4 Occipital lobe**
  - **191.5 Ventricles**
    Choroid plexus   Floor of ventricle
  - **191.6 Cerebellum NOS**
    Cerebellopontine angle
  - **191.7 Brain stem**
    Cerebral peduncle Midbrain
    Medulla oblongata Pons
  - **191.8 Other parts of brain**
    Corpus callosum
    Tapetum
    Malignant neoplasm of contiguous or overlapping sites of brain whose point of origin cannot be determined
    Coding Clinic: 2007, Q4, P103-104
  - **191.9 Brain, unspecified**
    Cranial fossa NOS
    Coding Clinic: 2009, Q4, P78; 1994, Q2, P8

- **192 Malignant neoplasm of other and unspecified parts of nervous system**
  - Excludes: peripheral, sympathetic, and parasympathetic nerves and ganglia (171.0–171.9)
  - **192.0 Cranial nerves**
    Olfactory bulb
  - **192.1 Cerebral meninges**
    Dura (mater)   Meninges NOS
    Falx (cerebelli) (cerebri) Tentorium
  - **192.2 Spinal cord**
    Cauda equina
  - **192.3 Spinal meninges**
  - **192.8 Other specified sites of nervous system**
    Malignant neoplasm of contiguous or overlapping sites of other parts of nervous system whose point of origin cannot be determined
  - **192.9 Nervous system, part unspecified**
    Nervous system (central) NOS
    Excludes: meninges NOS (192.1)

- **193 Malignant neoplasm of thyroid gland**
  Thyroglossal duct
  Use additional code to identify any functional activity

- **194 Malignant neoplasm of other endocrine glands and related structures**
  - Excludes: islets of Langerhans (157.4)
    neuroendocrine tumors (209.00–209.69)
    ovary (183.0)
    testis (186.0–186.9)
    thymus (164.0)
  - **194.0 Adrenal gland**
    Adrenal cortex   Suprarenal gland
    Adrenal medulla
  - **194.1 Parathyroid gland**
  - **194.3 Pituitary gland and craniopharyngeal duct**
    Craniobuccal pouch Rathke's pouch
    Hypophysis   Sella turcica
    Coding Clinic: 1985, July-Aug, P9

194.4 Pineal gland
194.5 Carotid body
194.6 Aortic body and other paraganglia
  Coccygeal body   Para-aortic body
  Glomus jugulare
194.8 Other
  Pluriglandular involvement NOS
  Note: If the sites of multiple involvements are known, they should be coded separately.
194.9 Endocrine gland, site unspecified

● **195** Malignant neoplasm of other and ill-defined sites
  Includes malignant neoplasms of contiguous sites, not elsewhere classified, whose point of origin cannot be determined
  Excludes malignant neoplasm:
    lymphatic and hematopoietic tissue (200.0–208.9)
    secondary sites (196.0–198.8)
    unspecified site (199.0–199.1)

  195.0 Head, face, and neck
    Cheek NOS   Nose NOS
    Jaw NOS   Supraclavicular region NOS
    Coding Clinic: 2003, Q4, P107
  195.1 Thorax
    Axilla   Intrathoracic NOS
    Chest (wall) NOS
  195.2 Abdomen
    Intra-abdominal NOS
    Coding Clinic: 1997, Q2, P3
  195.3 Pelvis
    Groin
    Inguinal region NOS
    Presacral region
    Sacrococcygeal region
    Sites overlapping systems within pelvis, as:
      rectovaginal (septum)
      rectovesical (septum)
  195.4 Upper limb
  195.5 Lower limb
  195.8 Other specified sites
    Back NOS   Trunk NOS
    Flank NOS

(See Plate 315 on page NAP-1.)

● **196** Secondary and unspecified malignant neoplasm of lymph nodes
  Excludes any malignant neoplasm of lymph nodes, specified as primary (200.0–202.9)
    Hodgkin's disease (201.0–201.9)
    lymphosarcoma (200.1)
    other forms of lymphoma (202.0–202.9)
    reticulosarcoma (200.0)
    secondary neuroendocrine tumor of (distant) lymph nodes (209.71)
  Coding Clinic: 1992, Q2, P3-4

  196.0 Lymph nodes of head, face, and neck
    Cervical   Scalene
    Cervicofacial   Supraclavicular
    Coding Clinic: 2007, Q3, P8-9
  196.1 Intrathoracic lymph nodes
    Bronchopulmonary   Mediastinal
    Intercostal   Tracheobronchial
    Coding Clinic: 2006, Q3, P7-8
  196.2 Intra-abdominal lymph nodes
    Intestinal   Retroperitoneal
    Mesenteric
    Coding Clinic: 2003, Q4, P111
  196.3 Lymph nodes of axilla and upper limb
    Brachial   Infraclavicular
    Epitrochlear   Pectoral

  196.5 Lymph nodes of inguinal region and lower limb
    Femoral   Popliteal
    Groin   Tibial
  196.6 Intrapelvic lymph nodes
    Hypogastric   Obturator
    Iliac   Parametrial
    Coding Clinic: 2012, Q2, P9
  196.8 Lymph nodes of multiple sites
  196.9 Site unspecified
    Lymph nodes NOS

● **197** Secondary malignant neoplasm of respiratory and digestive systems
  Excludes lymph node metastasis (196.0–196.9)
    secondary neuroendocrine tumor of liver (209.72)
    secondary neuroendocrine tumor of respiratory organs (209.79)

  197.0 Lung
    Bronchus
    Coding Clinic: 2010, Q3, P3; 2006, Q1, P4-5; 1999, Q2, P9
  197.1 Mediastinum
    Coding Clinic: 2006, Q3, P7-8
  197.2 Pleura
    Coding Clinic: 2008, Q1, P16-17; 2007, Q3, P3; 2003, Q4, P110; 1989, Q4, P11
  197.3 Other respiratory organs
    Trachea
  197.4 Small intestine, including duodenum
  197.5 Large intestine and rectum
  197.6 Retroperitoneum and peritoneum
    Coding Clinic: 2011, Q4, P181; 2010, Q3, P3; 2004, Q2, P4; 1989, Q4, P11
  197.7 Liver, specified as secondary
    Coding Clinic: 2010, Q3, P3; 2006, Q1, P4-5; 2005, Q2, P9-10; 1984, May-June, P11
  197.8 Other digestive organs and spleen
    Coding Clinic: 1997, Q2, P3

● **198** Secondary malignant neoplasm of other specified sites
  Excludes lymph node metastasis (196.0–196.9)
    secondary neuroendocrine tumor of other specified sites (209.79)

  198.0 Kidney
  198.1 Other urinary organs
  198.2 Skin
    Skin of breast
  198.3 Brain and spinal cord
    Coding Clinic: 2007, Q3, P4; 1999, Q3, P7-8; 1984, May-June, P14
  198.4 Other parts of nervous system
    Meninges (cerebral) (spinal)
  198.5 Bone and bone marrow
    Coding Clinic: 2007, Q1, P3-8; 2003, Q4, P110; 1999, Q3, P5; 1989, Q4, P12; 1984, May-June, P14
  198.6 Ovary
  198.7 Adrenal gland
    Suprarenal gland
    Coding Clinic: 1988, Q2, P10
● **198.8** Other specified sites
    198.81 Breast
      Excludes skin of breast (198.2)
    198.82 Genital organs
    198.89 Other
      Excludes retroperitoneal lymph nodes (196.2)
      Coding Clinic: 2005, Q2, P4-5; 1997, Q2, P4

● **199 Malignant neoplasm without specification of site**
   Excludes *malignant carcinoid tumor of unknown primary site (209.20)*
   malignant (poorly differentiated) neuroendocrine carcinoma, any site (209.30)
   malignant (poorly differentiated) neuroendocrine tumor, any site (209.30)
   neuroendocrine carcinoma (high grade), any site (209.30)

   ■ **199.0 Disseminated**
      Carcinomatosis unspecified site (primary) (secondary)
      Generalized:
         cancer unspecified site (primary) (secondary)
         malignancy unspecified site (primary) (secondary)
      Multiple cancer unspecified site (primary) (secondary)
      Coding Clinic: 1989, Q4, P10; 1988, Q2, P11

   ■ **199.1 Other**
      Cancer unspecified site (primary) (secondary)
      Carcinoma unspecified site (primary) (secondary)
      Malignancy unspecified site (primary) (secondary)
      Coding Clinic: 2006, Q3, P14-15; Q1, P4-5

   ● **199.2 Malignant neoplasm associated with transplanted organ**
      Code first *complication of transplanted organ (996.80-996.89)*
      Use additional *code for specific malignancy*
      Coding Clinic: 2008, Q4, P82-83

MALIGNANT NEOPLASM OF LYMPHATIC AND HEMATOPOIETIC TISSUE (200–208)

Excludes *autoimmune lymphoproliferative syndrome (279.41)*
secondary neoplasm of:
  bone marrow (198.5)
  spleen (197.8)
secondary and unspecified neoplasm of lymph nodes (196.0–196.9)

The following fifth-digit subclassification is for use with categories 200–202:

```
0  unspecified site, extranodal and solid organ sites
1  lymph nodes of head, face, and neck
2  intrathoracic lymph nodes
3  intra-abdominal lymph nodes
4  lymph nodes of axilla and upper limb
5  lymph nodes of inguinal region and lower limb
6  intrapelvic lymph nodes
7  spleen
8  lymph nodes of multiple sites
```

● **200 Lymphosarcoma and reticulosarcoma and other specified malignant tumors of lymphatic tissue**
   Requires fifth digit. See note before section 200 for codes and definitions.
   Coding Clinic: 2007, Q4, P65-67

   ● **200.0 Reticulosarcoma**
   [0-8]   Lymphoma (malignant):
             histiocytic (diffuse):
                nodular
                pleomorphic cell type
                reticulum cell type
           Reticulum cell sarcoma:
             NOS
             pleomorphic cell type
   Coding Clinic: 2006, Q4, P135-136; 2001, Q3, P12-13

● **200.1 Lymphosarcoma**
   [0-8]   Lymphoblastoma (diffuse)
           Lymphoma (malignant):
             lymphoblastic (diffuse)
             lymphocytic (cell type) (diffuse)
             lymphosarcoma type
           Lymphosarcoma:
             NOS
             diffuse NOS
             lymphoblastic (diffuse)
             lymphocytic (diffuse)
             prolymphocytic
   Excludes *lymphosarcoma:*
             follicular or nodular (202.0)
             mixed cell type (200.8)
           lymphosarcoma cell leukemia (207.8)

● **200.2 Burkitt's tumor or lymphoma**
   [0-8]   Malignant lymphoma, Burkitt's type

● **200.3 Marginal zone lymphoma**
   [0-8]   Extranodal marginal zone B-cell lymphoma
           Mucosa associated lymphoid tissue [MALT]
           Nodal marginal zone B-cell lymphoma
           Splenic marginal zone B-cell lymphoma

● **200.4 Mantle cell lymphoma**
   [0-8]

● **200.5 Primary central nervous system lymphoma**
   [0-8]   Coding Clinic: 2013, Q1, P4

● **200.6 Anaplastic large cell lymphoma**
   [0-8]

● **200.7 Large cell lymphoma**
   [0-8]

● **200.8 Other named variants**
   [0-8]   Lymphoma (malignant):
             lymphoplasmacytoid type
             mixed lymphocytic-histiocytic (diffuse)
           Lymphosarcoma, mixed cell type (diffuse)
           Reticulolymphosarcoma (diffuse)

● **201 Hodgkin's disease**
   Also known as malignant lymphoma/lymphosarcoma and is cancer of the lymphatic system including the lymph nodes and related structures
   Requires fifth digit. See note before section 200 for codes and definitions.

● **201.0 Hodgkin's paragranuloma**
   [0-8]

● **201.1 Hodgkin's granuloma**
   [0-8]

● **201.2 Hodgkin's sarcoma**
   [0-8]

● **201.4 Lymphocytic-histiocytic predominance**
   [0-8]

● **201.5 Nodular sclerosis**
   [0-8]   Hodgkin's disease, nodular sclerosis:
             NOS
             cellular phase

● **201.6 Mixed cellularity**
   [0-8]

● **201.7 Lymphocytic depletion**
   [0-8]   Hodgkin's disease, lymphocytic depletion:
             NOS
             diffuse fibrosis
             reticular type

● ■ **201.9 Hodgkin's disease, unspecified**
   [0-8]   Hodgkin's:
             disease NOS
             lymphoma NOS
           Malignant:
             lymphogranuloma
             lymphogranulomatosis

Item 2-6 Lymphosarcoma, also known as malignant lymphoma, is a cancer of the lymph system exhibiting abnormal cells encompassing an entire lymph node creating a diffuse pattern without any definite organization. Diffuse pattern lymphoma has a more unfavorable survival outlook than those with a follicular or nodular pattern. Reticulosarcoma is the most common aggressive form of non-Hodgkin's lymphoma.

PART III / Diseases: Tabular List Volume 1

- **202 Other malignant neoplasms of lymphoid and histiocytic tissue**
  Requires fifth digit. See note before section 200 for codes and definitions.
  - **202.0 Nodular lymphoma**
    [0-8] Brill-Symmers disease
    Lymphoma:
      follicular (giant) (large cell)
      lymphocytic, nodular
    Lymphosarcoma:
      follicular (giant)
      nodular
    Coding Clinic: 2009, Q3, P5x2
  - **202.1 Mycosis fungoides**
    [0-8] **Excludes** peripheral T-cell lymphoma (202.7)
    Coding Clinic: 1999, Q2, P7-8; 1992, Q2, P4
  - **202.2 Sézary's disease**
    [0-8] Coding Clinic: 1999, Q2, P7-8
  - **202.3 Malignant histiocytosis**
    [0-8] Histiocytic medullary reticulosis
    Malignant:
      reticuloendotheliosis
      reticulosis
  - **202.4 Leukemic reticuloendotheliosis**
    [0-8] Hairy-cell leukemia
  - **202.5 Letterer-Siwe disease**
    [0-8] Acute:
      differentiated progressive histiocytosis
      histiocytosis X (progressive)
      infantile reticuloendotheliosis
      reticulosis of infancy
    Excludes adult pulmonary Langerhans cell histiocytosis (516.5)
      Hand-Schüller-Christian disease (277.89)
      histiocytosis (acute) (chronic) (277.89)
      histiocytosis X (chronic) (277.89)
  - **202.6 Malignant mast cell tumors**
    [0-8] Malignant:
      mastocytoma
      mastocytosis
    Mast cell sarcoma
    Systemic tissue mast cell disease
    Excludes mast cell leukemia (207.8)
  - **202.7 Peripheral T cell lymphoma**
    [0-8]
  - **202.8 Other lymphomas**
    [0-8] Lymphoma (malignant):
      NOS
      diffuse
    Excludes benign lymphoma (229.0)
    Coding Clinic: 2008, Q4, P82-83; Q1, P16-17; 2007, Q3, P3; 2006, Q4, P135-136; Q2, P20-22; 1993, Q4, P33; 1992, Q2, P3-4
  - **202.9 Other and unspecified malignant neoplasms of lymphoid and histiocytic tissue**
    [0-8] Follicular dendritic cell sarcoma
    Interdigitating dendritic cell sarcoma
    Langerhans cell sarcoma
    Malignant neoplasm of bone marrow NOS

- **203 Multiple myeloma and immunoproliferative neoplasms**
  Multiple myeloma is cancer of plasma cell (type of white blood cell) and is incurable but treatable disease. Immunoproliferative neoplasm is term for diseases (mostly cancers) in which immune system cells proliferate.
  The following fifth-digit subclassification is for use with category 203:

0	without mention of having achieved remission failed remission
1	in remission
2	in relapse

  Coding Clinic: 2008, Q4, P83-85
  - **203.0 Multiple myeloma**
    [0-2] Kahler's disease   Myelomatosis
    Excludes solitary myeloma (238.6)
    Coding Clinic: 2012, Q3, P16; 2010, Q2, P6; 2008, Q4, P90-91; 2007, Q2, P9-10; 1999, Q4, P10; 1996, Q1, P16
  - **203.1 Plasma cell leukemia**
    [0-2] Plasmacytic leukemia
  - **203.8 Other immunoproliferative neoplasms**
    [0-2] Coding Clinic: 1990, Q4, P26

- **204 Lymphoid leukemia**
  Includes leukemia: leukemia:
      lymphatic   lymphocytic
      lymphoblastic   lymphogenous
  The following fifth-digit subclassification is for use with category 204:

0	without mention of having achieved remission failed remission
1	in remission
2	in relapse

  Coding Clinic: 2008, Q4, P83-85
  - **204.0 Acute**
    [0-2] **Excludes** acute exacerbation of chronic lymphoid leukemia (204.1)
    Coding Clinic: 2012, Q1, P13-14; 1999, Q3, P4, 6-7; 1993, Q3, P4x2; 1985, May-June, P18-19
  - **204.1 Chronic**
    [0-2]
  - **204.2 Subacute**
    [0-2]
  - **204.8 Other lymphoid leukemia**
    [0-2] Aleukemic leukemia:
      lymphatic
      lymphocytic
      lymphoid
    Coding Clinic: 2009, Q3, P6
  - **204.9 Unspecified lymphoid leukemia**
    [0-2]

NEOPLASMS (140–239)

Item 2-7 Leukemia is a cancer (acute or chronic) of the blood-forming tissues of the bone marrow. Blood cells all start out as stem cells. They mature and become red cells, white cells, or platelets. There are three main types of leukocytes (white cells that fight infection): monocytes, lymphocytes, and granulocytes. **Acute monocytic leukemia** (AML) affects monocytes. **Acute lymphoid leukemia** (ALL) affects lymphocytes, and **acute myeloid leukemia** (AML) affects cells that typically develop into white blood cells (not lymphocytes), though it may develop in other blood cells.

◀ New   ◀▥ Revised   ~~deleted~~ Deleted   Excludes   Includes   Use additional   Code first   Omit code
● Use Additional Digit(s)   ▪ Unspecified   ● Not first-listed DX   OGCR Official Guidelines   Coding Clinic

205 Myeloid leukemia

Includes leukemia: granulocytic, myeloblastic, myelocytic, myelogenous, myelomonocytic, myelosclerotic, myelosis

The following fifth-digit subclassification is for use with category 205:

> 0 without mention of having achieved remission
>   failed remission
> 1 in remission
> 2 in relapse

Coding Clinic: 2008, Q4, P83-85

- **205.0 Acute**
  [0-2] Acute promyelocytic leukemia
  Excludes acute exacerbation of chronic myeloid leukemia (205.1)
  Coding Clinic: 2009, Q4, P78; 2006, Q2, P20-22; 2002, Q1, P11-12; 1993, Q3, P3-4x2

- **205.1 Chronic**
  [0-2] Eosinophilic leukemia
  Neutrophilic leukemia
  Coding Clinic: 2012, Q2, P16-17; 2008, Q4, P140-143; 2000, Q1, P6; 1995, Q2, P12; 1985, July-Aug, P13

- **205.2 Subacute**
  [0-2]

- **205.3 Myeloid sarcoma**
  [0-2] Chloroma
  Granulocytic sarcoma

- **205.8 Other myeloid leukemia**
  [0-2] Aleukemic leukemia:
  granulocytic
  myelogenous
  myeloid
  Aleukemic myelosis

- **205.9 Unspecified myeloid leukemia**
  [0-2] Coding Clinic: 1985, May-June, P18-19

206 Monocytic leukemia

Includes leukemia: histiocytic, monoblastic, monocytoid

The following fifth-digit subclassification is for use with category 206:

> 0 without mention of having achieved remission
>   failed remission
> 1 in remission
> 2 in relapse

Coding Clinic: 2008, Q4, P83-85

- **206.0 Acute**
  [0-2] **Excludes** acute exacerbation of chronic monocytic leukemia (206.1)

- **206.1 Chronic**
  [0-2]

- **206.2 Subacute**
  [0-2]

- **206.8 Other monocytic leukemia**
  [0-2] Aleukemic:
  monocytic leukemia
  monocytoid leukemia

- **206.9 Unspecified monocytic leukemia**
  [0-2]

207 Other specified leukemia

Excludes leukemic reticuloendotheliosis (202.4)
plasma cell leukemia (203.1)

The following fifth-digit subclassification is for use with category 207:

> 0 without mention of having achieved remission
>   failed remission
> 1 in remission
> 2 in relapse

Coding Clinic: 2008, Q4, P83-85

- **207.0 Acute erythremia and erythroleukemia**
  [0-2] Acute erythremic myelosis
  Di Guglielmo's disease
  Erythremic myelosis

- **207.1 Chronic erythremia**
  [0-2] Heilmeyer-Schöner disease

- **207.2 Megakaryocytic leukemia**
  [0-2] Megakaryocytic myelosis
  Thrombocytic leukemia

- **207.8 Other specified leukemia**
  [0-2] Lymphosarcoma cell leukemia

208 Leukemia of unspecified cell type

The following fifth-digit subclassification is for use with category 208:

> 0 without mention of having achieved remission
>   failed remission
> 1 in remission
> 2 in relapse

Coding Clinic: 2008, Q4, P83-85

- **208.0 Acute**
  [0-2] Acute leukemia NOS
  Blast cell leukemia
  Stem cell leukemia
  Excludes acute exacerbation of chronic unspecified leukemia (208.1)
  Coding Clinic: 1987, Mar-April, P12

- **208.1 Chronic**
  [0-2] Chronic leukemia NOS

- **208.2 Subacute**
  [0-2] *Somewhat acute, between acute and chronic*
  Subacute leukemia NOS

- **208.8 Other leukemia of unspecified cell type**
  [0-2] Coding Clinic: 1987, Mar-April, P12

- **208.9 Unspecified leukemia**
  [0-2] Leukemia NOS
  Coding Clinic: 2011, Q4, P148

NEUROENDOCRINE TUMORS (209)

209 Neuroendocrine tumors

Code first any associated multiple endocrine neoplasia syndrome (258.01-258.03)

Use additional code to identify associated endocrine syndrome, such as:
carcinoid syndrome (259.2)

Excludes benign pancreatic islet cell tumors (211.7)
malignant pancreatic islet cell tumors (157.4)

Coding Clinic: 2009, Q4, P78; 2008, Q4, P85-90

- **209.0 Malignant carcinoid tumors of the small intestine**
  - **209.00** Malignant carcinoid tumor of the small intestine, unspecified portion
  - **209.01** Malignant carcinoid tumor of the duodenum
  - **209.02** Malignant carcinoid tumor of the jejunum
  - **209.03** Malignant carcinoid tumor of the ileum

- **209.1** Malignant carcinoid tumors of the appendix, large intestine, and rectum
  - **209.10** Malignant carcinoid tumor of the large intestine, unspecified portion
    Malignant carcinoid tumor of the colon NOS
  - **209.11** Malignant carcinoid tumor of the appendix
  - **209.12** Malignant carcinoid tumor of the cecum
  - **209.13** Malignant carcinoid tumor of the ascending colon
  - **209.14** Malignant carcinoid tumor of the transverse colon
  - **209.15** Malignant carcinoid tumor of the descending colon
  - **209.16** Malignant carcinoid tumor of the sigmoid colon
  - **209.17** Malignant carcinoid tumor of the rectum
- **209.2** Malignant carcinoid tumors of other and unspecified sites
  - **209.20** Malignant carcinoid tumor of unknown primary site
  - **209.21** Malignant carcinoid tumor of the bronchus and lung
  - **209.22** Malignant carcinoid tumor of the thymus
  - **209.23** Malignant carcinoid tumor of the stomach
    Coding Clinic: 2008, Q4, P85-90
  - **209.24** Malignant carcinoid tumor of the kidney
  - **209.25** Malignant carcinoid tumor of the foregut NOS
  - **209.26** Malignant carcinoid tumor of the midgut NOS
  - **209.27** Malignant carcinoid tumor of the hindgut NOS
  - **209.29** Malignant carcinoid tumors of other sites
- **209.3** Malignant poorly differentiated neuroendocrine tumors
  - **209.30** Malignant poorly differentiated neuroendocrine carcinoma, any site
    High grade neuroendocrine carcinoma, any site
    Malignant poorly differentiated neuroendocrine tumor NOS
    Excludes Merkel cell carcinoma (209.31-209.36)
  - **209.31** Merkel cell carcinoma of the face
    Merkel cell carcinoma of the ear
    Merkel cell carcinoma of the eyelid, including canthus
    Merkel cell carcinoma of the lip
  - **209.32** Merkel cell carcinoma of the scalp and neck
  - **209.33** Merkel cell carcinoma of the upper limb
  - **209.34** Merkel cell carcinoma of the lower limb
  - **209.35** Merkel cell carcinoma of the trunk
  - **209.36** Merkel cell carcinoma of other sites
    Merkel cell carcinoma of the buttock
    Merkel cell carcinoma of the genitals
    Merkel cell carcinoma NOS
    Coding Clinic: 2009, Q4, P79
- **209.4** Benign carcinoid tumors of the small intestine
  - **209.40** Benign carcinoid tumor of the small intestine, unspecified portion
  - **209.41** Benign carcinoid tumor of the duodenum
  - **209.42** Benign carcinoid tumor of the jejunum
  - **209.43** Benign carcinoid tumor of the ileum
- **209.5** Benign carcinoid tumors of the appendix, large intestine, and rectum
  - **209.50** Benign carcinoid tumor of the large intestine, unspecified portion
    Benign carcinoid tumor of the colon NOS
  - **209.51** Benign carcinoid tumor of the appendix
  - **209.52** Benign carcinoid tumor of the cecum
  - **209.53** Benign carcinoid tumor of the ascending colon
  - **209.54** Benign carcinoid tumor of the transverse colon
  - **209.55** Benign carcinoid tumor of the descending colon
  - **209.56** Benign carcinoid tumor of the sigmoid colon
  - **209.57** Benign carcinoid tumor of the rectum
- **209.6** Benign carcinoid tumors of other and unspecified sites
  - **209.60** Benign carcinoid tumor of unknown primary site
    Carcinoid tumor NOS
    Neuroendocrine tumor NOS
  - **209.61** Benign carcinoid tumor of the bronchus and lung
    Coding Clinic: 2009, Q4, P79
  - **209.62** Benign carcinoid tumor of the thymus
  - **209.63** Benign carcinoid tumor of the stomach
  - **209.64** Benign carcinoid tumor of the kidney
  - **209.65** Benign carcinoid tumor of the foregut NOS
  - **209.66** Benign carcinoid tumor of the midgut NOS
  - **209.67** Benign carcinoid tumor of the hindgut NOS
  - **209.69** Benign carcinoid tumors of other sites
- **209.7** Secondary neuroendocrine tumors
  Secondary carcinoid tumors
  - **209.70** Secondary neuroendocrine tumor, unspecified site
  - **209.71** Secondary neuroendocrine tumor of distant lymph nodes
    Coding Clinic: 2011, Q4, P181
  - **209.72** Secondary neuroendocrine tumor of liver
  - **209.73** Secondary neuroendocrine tumor of bone
  - **209.74** Secondary neuroendocrine tumor of peritoneum
    Mesentery metastasis of neuroendocrine tumor
    Coding Clinic: 2011, Q4, P181-182; 2009, Q4, P79
  - **209.75** Secondary Merkel cell carcinoma
    Merkel cell carcinoma nodal presentation
    Merkel cell carcinoma visceral metastatic presentation
    Secondary Merkel cell carcinoma, any site
  - **209.79** Secondary neuroendocrine tumor of other sites

BENIGN NEOPLASMS (210–229)

Benign neoplasm: Tumor that does not metastasize to other parts of body and is caused by cell overgrowth, differentiating it from cyst or abscess

- **210** Benign neoplasm of lip, oral cavity, and pharynx
  Excludes cyst (of):
   jaw (526.0–526.2, 526.89)
   oral soft tissue (528.4)
   radicular (522.8)
  - **210.0** Lip
    Frenulum labii
    Lip (inner aspect) (mucosa) (vermilion border)
    Excludes labial commissure (210.4)
     skin of lip (216.0)
  - **210.1** Tongue
    Lingual tonsil
  - **210.2** Major salivary glands
    Gland: Gland:
     parotid   submandibular
     sublingual
    Excludes benign neoplasms of minor salivary glands:
     NOS (210.4)
     buccal mucosa (210.4)
     lips (210.0)
     palate (hard) (soft) (210.4)
     tongue (210.1)
     tonsil, palatine (210.5)
  - **210.3** Floor of mouth
  - **210.4** Other and unspecified parts of mouth
    Gingiva   Oral mucosa
    Gum (upper) (lower) Palate (hard) (soft)
    Labial commissure   Uvula
    Oral cavity NOS
    Excludes benign odontogenic neoplasms of bone (213.0–213.1)
     developmental odontogenic cysts (526.0)
     mucosa of lips (210.0)
     nasopharyngeal [posterior] [superior] surface of soft palate (210.7)

210.5 Tonsil
Tonsil (faucial) (palatine)
Excludes lingual tonsil (210.1)
pharyngeal tonsil (210.7)
tonsillar:
fossa (210.6)
pillars (210.6)

210.6 Other parts of oropharynx
Branchial cleft or vestiges
Epiglottis, anterior aspect
Fauces NOS
Mesopharynx NOS
Tonsillar:
fossa
pillars
Vallecula
Excludes epiglottis:
NOS (212.1)
suprahyoid portion (212.1)

210.7 Nasopharynx
Adenoid tissue
Lymphadenoid tissue
Pharyngeal tonsil
Posterior nasal septum

210.8 Hypopharynx
Arytenoid fold
Laryngopharynx
Postcricoid region
Pyriform fossa

210.9 Pharynx, unspecified
Throat NOS

211 Benign neoplasm of other parts of digestive system
Excludes benign stromal tumors of digestive system (215.5)

211.0 Esophagus

211.1 Stomach
Body of stomach
Cardia of stomach
Fundus of stomach
Cardiac orifice
Pylorus
Excludes benign carcinoid tumors of the stomach (209.63)

211.2 Duodenum, jejunum, and ileum
Small intestine NOS
Excludes ampulla of Vater (211.5)
benign carcinoid tumors of the small intestine (209.40-209.43)
ileocecal valve (211.3)

211.3 Colon
Appendix
Cecum
Ileocecal valve
Large intestine NOS
Excludes benign carcinoid tumors of the large intestine (209.50-209.56)
rectosigmoid junction (211.4)
Coding Clinic: 2005, Q3, P17-18; Q2, P16-17; 2001, Q4, P55-56x2; 1995, Q1, P4; 1992, Q3, P11

211.4 Rectum and anal canal
Anal canal or sphincter
Anus NOS
Rectosigmoid junction
Excludes anus:
margin (216.5)
perianal skin (216.5)
skin (216.5)
benign carcinoid tumors of the rectum (209.57)

211.5 Liver and biliary passages
Ampulla of Vater
Common bile duct
Cystic duct
Gallbladder
Hepatic duct
Sphincter of Oddi

211.6 Pancreas, except islets of Langerhans

211.7 Islets of Langerhans
Islet cell tumor
Use additional code to identify any functional activity

211.8 Retroperitoneum and peritoneum
Mesentery
Mesocolon
Omentum
Retroperitoneal tissue

211.9 Other and unspecified site
Alimentary tract NOS
Digestive system NOS
Gastrointestinal tract NOS
Intestinal tract NOS
Intestine NOS
Spleen, not elsewhere classified

212 Benign neoplasm of respiratory and intrathoracic organs

212.0 Nasal cavities, middle ear, and accessory sinuses
Cartilage of nose
Eustachian tube
Nares
Septum of nose
Sinus:
ethmoidal
frontal
Sinus:
maxillary
sphenoidal
Excludes auditory canal (external) (216.2)
bone of:
ear (213.0)
nose [turbinates] (213.0)
cartilage of ear (215.0)
ear (external) (skin) (216.2)
nose NOS (229.8)
skin (216.3)
olfactory bulb (225.1)
polyp of:
accessory sinus (471.8)
ear (385.30–385.35)
nasal cavity (471.0)
posterior margin of septum and choanae (210.7)
Coding Clinic: 2000, Q3, P10-11

212.1 Larynx
Cartilage:
arytenoid
cricoid
cuneiform
thyroid
Epiglottis (suprahyoid portion) NOS
Glottis
Vocal cords (false) (true)
Excludes epiglottis, anterior aspect (210.6)
polyp of vocal cord or larynx (478.4)

212.2 Trachea

212.3 Bronchus and lung
Carina
Hilus of lung
Excludes benign carcinoid tumors of bronchus and lung (209.61)

212.4 Pleura

212.5 Mediastinum

212.6 Thymus
Excludes benign carcinoid tumors of thymus (209.62)

212.7 Heart
Excludes great vessels (215.4)

212.8 Other specified sites

212.9 Site unspecified
Respiratory organ NOS
Upper respiratory tract NOS
Excludes intrathoracic NOS (229.8)
thoracic NOS (229.8)

● **213 Benign neoplasm of bone and articular cartilage**
  Includes cartilage (articular) (joint)
      periosteum
  Excludes cartilage of:
      ear (215.0)
      eyelid (215.0)
      larynx (212.1)
      nose (212.0)
    exostosis NOS (726.91)
    synovia (215.0–215.9)

  213.0 Bones of skull and face
    Excludes lower jaw bone (213.1)
  213.1 Lower jaw bone
  213.2 Vertebral column, excluding sacrum and coccyx
  213.3 Ribs, sternum, and clavicle
  213.4 Scapula and long bones of upper limb
  213.5 Short bones of upper limb
  213.6 Pelvic bones, sacrum, and coccyx
  213.7 Long bones of lower limb
  213.8 Short bones of lower limb
  213.9 Bone and articular cartilage, site unspecified

● **214 Lipoma**
  Slow growing benign tumors (discrete rubbery masses) of mature fat cells enclosed in a thin fibrous capsule found in subcutaneous tissues of trunk and proximal extremities and in internal organs
  Includes angiolipoma
      fibrolipoma
      hibernoma
      lipoma (fetal) (infiltrating) (intramuscular)
      myelolipoma
      myxolipoma

  214.0 Skin and subcutaneous tissue of face
  214.1 Other skin and subcutaneous tissue
  214.2 Intrathoracic organs
  214.3 Intra-abdominal organs
  214.4 Spermatic cord
  214.8 Other specified sites
    Coding Clinic: 1994, Q3, P7
  214.9 Lipoma, unspecified site

● **215 Other benign neoplasm of connective and other soft tissue**
  Includes blood vessel
      bursa
      fascia
      ligament
      muscle
      peripheral, sympathetic, and parasympathetic nerves and ganglia
      synovia
      tendon (sheath)
  Excludes cartilage:
      articular (213.0–213.9)
      larynx (212.1)
      nose (212.0)
    connective tissue of:
      breast (217)
      internal organ, except lipoma and hemangioma-code to benign neoplasm of the site
    lipoma (214.0–214.9)

  215.0 Head, face, and neck
  215.2 Upper limb, including shoulder
  215.3 Lower limb, including hip
  215.4 Thorax
    Excludes heart (212.7)
      mediastinum (212.5)
      thymus (212.6)
  215.5 Abdomen
    Abdominal wall
    Benign stromal tumors of abdomen
    Hypochondrium
  215.6 Pelvis
    Buttock   Inguinal region
    Groin   Perineum
    Excludes uterine:
      leiomyoma (218.0–218.9)
      ligament, any (221.0)
  215.7 Trunk, unspecified
    Back NOS
    Flank NOS
  215.8 Other specified sites
  215.9 Site unspecified

● **216 Benign neoplasm of skin**
  Includes blue nevus
      dermatofibroma
      hydrocystoma
      pigmented nevus
      syringoadenoma
      syringoma
  Excludes skin of genital organs (221.0–222.9)
  Coding Clinic: 2000, Q1, P21-22

  216.0 Skin of lip
    Excludes vermilion border of lip (210.0)
  216.1 Eyelid, including canthus
    Excludes cartilage of eyelid (215.0)
  216.2 Ear and external auditory canal
    Auricle (ear)
    Auricular canal, external
    External meatus
    Pinna
    Excludes cartilage of ear (215.0)
  216.3 Skin of other and unspecified parts of face
    Cheek, external   Nose, external
    Eyebrow   Temple
  216.4 Scalp and skin of neck
  216.5 Skin of trunk, except scrotum
    Axillary fold
    Perianal skin
    Skin of: Skin of:
      abdominal wall   chest wall
      anus   groin
      back   perineum
      breast
      buttock
    Umbilicus
    Excludes anal canal (211.4)
      anus NOS (211.4)
      skin of scrotum (222.4)
  216.6 Skin of upper limb, including shoulder
  216.7 Skin of lower limb, including hip
  216.8 Other specified sites of skin
  216.9 Skin, site unspecified

  217 Benign neoplasm of breast
    Note no gender difference for this code.
    Breast (male) (female)
      connective tissue
      glandular tissue
      soft parts
    Excludes adenofibrosis (610.2)
      benign cyst of breast (610.0)
      fibrocystic disease (610.1)
      skin of breast (216.5)
    Coding Clinic: 2000, Q1, P4

- **218 Uterine leiomyoma**
  Benign tumors or nodules of the uterine wall
  - **Includes**: fibroid (bleeding) (uterine)
    uterine:
      fibromyoma
      myoma
  - **218.0 Submucous leiomyoma of uterus**
  - **218.1 Intramural leiomyoma of uterus**
    Interstitial leiomyoma of uterus
  - **218.2 Subserous leiomyoma of uterus**
    Subperitoneal leiomyoma of uterus
  - **218.9 Leiomyoma of uterus, unspecified**
    Coding Clinic: 2003, Q1, P4-5; 1995, Q4, P50

- **219 Other benign neoplasm of uterus**
  - **219.0 Cervix uteri**
  - **219.1 Corpus uteri**
    Endometrium   Myometrium
    Fundus
  - **219.8 Other specified parts of uterus**
  - **219.9 Uterus, part unspecified**

- **220 Benign neoplasm of ovary**
  Use additional code to identify any functional activity (256.0–256.1)
  - **Excludes**: cyst:
      corpus albicans (620.2)
      corpus luteum (620.1)
      endometrial (617.1)
      follicular (atretic) (620.0)
      graafian follicle (620.0)
      ovarian NOS (620.2)
      retention (620.2)
    Coding Clinic: 2009, Q4, P79, 82

- **221 Benign neoplasm of other female genital organs**
  - **Includes**: adenomatous polyp
    benign teratoma
  - **Excludes**: cyst:
      epoophoron (752.11)
      fimbrial (752.11)
      Gartner's duct (752.11)
      parovarian (752.11)
  - **221.0 Fallopian tube and uterine ligaments**
    Oviduct
    Parametrium
    Uterine ligament (broad) (round) (uterosacral)
    Uterine tube
  - **221.1 Vagina**
  - **221.2 Vulva**
    Clitoris
    External female genitalia NOS
    Greater vestibular [Bartholin's] gland
    Labia (majora) (minora)
    Pudendum
    - **Excludes**: Bartholin's (duct) (gland) cyst (616.2)
  - **221.8 Other specified sites of female genital organs**
  - **221.9 Female genital organ, site unspecified**
    Female genitourinary tract NOS

- **222 Benign neoplasm of male genital organs**
  - **222.0 Testis**
    Use additional code to identify any functional activity
  - **222.1 Penis**
    Corpus cavernosum
    Glans penis
    Prepuce
  - **222.2 Prostate**
    - **Excludes**: adenomatous hyperplasia of prostate (600.20–600.21)
      prostatic:
        adenoma (600.20–600.21)
        enlargement (600.00–600.01)
        hypertrophy (600.00–600.01)
  - **222.3 Epididymis**
  - **222.4 Scrotum**
    Skin of scrotum
  - **222.8 Other specified sites of male genital organs**
    Seminal vesicle
    Spermatic cord
  - **222.9 Male genital organ, site unspecified**
    Male genitourinary tract NOS

- **223 Benign neoplasm of kidney and other urinary organs**
  - **223.0 Kidney, except pelvis**
    Kidney NOS
    - **Excludes**: benign carcinoid tumors of kidney (209.64)
      renal:
        calyces (223.1)
        pelvis (223.1)
  - **223.1 Renal pelvis**
  - **223.2 Ureter**
    - **Excludes**: ureteric orifice of bladder (223.3)
  - **223.3 Bladder**
  - **223.8 Other specified sites of urinary organs**
    - **223.81 Urethra**
      - **Excludes**: urethral orifice of bladder (223.3)
    - **223.89 Other**
      Paraurethral glands
  - **223.9 Urinary organ, site unspecified**
    Urinary system NOS

- **224 Benign neoplasm of eye**
  - **Excludes**: cartilage of eyelid (215.0)
    eyelid (skin) (216.1)
    optic nerve (225.1)
    orbital bone (213.0)
  - **224.0 Eyeball, except conjunctiva, cornea, retina, and choroid**
    Ciliary body   Sclera
    Iris   Uveal tract
  - **224.1 Orbit**
    - **Excludes**: bone of orbit (213.0)
  - **224.2 Lacrimal gland**
  - **224.3 Conjunctiva**
  - **224.4 Cornea**
  - **224.5 Retina**
    - **Excludes**: hemangioma of retina (228.03)
  - **224.6 Choroid**
  - **224.7 Lacrimal duct**
    Lacrimal sac
    Nasolacrimal duct
  - **224.8 Other specified parts of eye**
  - **224.9 Eye, part unspecified**

Item 2-8 Teratoma: terat = monster, oma = mass, tumor. Alternate terms: dermoid cyst of the ovary, ovarian teratoma. Teratomas are neoplasms and arise from germ cells (ovaries in female and testes in male) and can be benign or malignant. Teratomas have been known to contain hair, nails, and teeth, giving them a bizarre ("monster") appearance.

- **225 Benign neoplasm of brain and other parts of nervous system**
  - Excludes: hemangioma (228.02)
    - neurofibromatosis (237.70–237.79)
    - peripheral, sympathetic, and parasympathetic nerves and ganglia (215.0–215.9)
    - retrobulbar (224.1)
  - 225.0 Brain
  - 225.1 Cranial nerves
    - Coding Clinic: 2004, Q4, P111-113
  - 225.2 Cerebral meninges
    - Meninges NOS
    - Meningioma (cerebral)
  - 225.3 Spinal cord
    - Cauda equina
  - 225.4 Spinal meninges
    - Spinal meningioma
  - 225.8 Other specified sites of nervous system
  - 225.9 Nervous system, part unspecified
    - Nervous system (central) NOS
    - Excludes: meninges NOS (225.2)

- **226 Benign neoplasm of thyroid glands**
  - Use additional code to identify any functional activity

- **227 Benign neoplasm of other endocrine glands and related structures**
  - Use additional code to identify any functional activity
  - Excludes: ovary (220)
    - pancreas (211.6)
    - testis (222.0)
  - 227.0 Adrenal gland
    - Suprarenal gland
  - 227.1 Parathyroid gland
  - 227.3 Pituitary gland and craniopharyngeal duct (pouch)
    - Craniobuccal pouch   Rathke's pouch
    - Hypophysis   Sella turcica
  - 227.4 Pineal gland
    - Pineal body
  - 227.5 Carotid body
  - 227.6 Aortic body and other paraganglia
    - Coccygeal body
    - Glomus jugulare
    - Para-aortic body
    - Coding Clinic: 1984, Nov-Dec, P17
  - 227.8 Other
  - 227.9 Endocrine gland, site unspecified

- **228 Hemangioma and lymphangioma, any site**
  - Includes: angioma (benign) (cavernous) (congenital) NOS
    - cavernous nevus
    - glomus tumor
    - hemangioma (benign) (congenital)
  - Excludes: benign neoplasm of spleen, except hemangioma and lymphangioma (211.9)
    - glomus jugulare (227.6)
    - nevus:
      - NOS (216.0–216.9)
      - blue or pigmented (216.0–216.9)
      - vascular (757.32)

Item 2-9 Hemangiomas are abnormally dense collections of dilated capillaries that occur on the skin or in internal organs. Hemangiomas are both deep and superficial and undergo a rapid growth phase when the size increases rapidly, followed by a rest phase, in which the tumor changes very little, followed by an involutional phase in which the tumor begins to and can disappear altogether. **Lymphangiomas** or cystic hygroma are benign collections of overgrown lymph vessels and, although rare, may occur anywhere but most commonly on the head and neck of children and infants. Visceral organs, lungs, and gastrointestinal tract may also be involved.

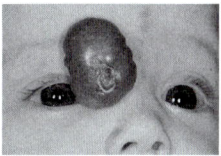

Figure 2-15 Hemangioma of skin and subcutaneous tissue. (From Yanoff: Ophthalmology, ed 3, Mosby, Inc., 2008)

- 228.0 Hemangioma, any site
  - Coding Clinic: 2001, Q1, P18; 1999, Q2, P9
  - 228.00 Of unspecified site
  - 228.01 Of skin and subcutaneous tissue
    - Coding Clinic: 2010, Q3, P16; 1988, Q4, P6
  - 228.02 Of intracranial structures
    - Coding Clinic: 1988, Q4, P6; 1985, Jan-Feb, P15
  - 228.03 Of retina
  - 228.04 Of intra-abdominal structures
    - Peritoneum
    - Retroperitoneal tissue
    - Coding Clinic: 1988, Q4, P6
  - 228.09 Of other sites
    - Systemic angiomatosis
    - Coding Clinic: 1991, Q3, P20
- 228.1 Lymphangioma, any site
  - Congenital lymphangioma
  - Lymphatic nevus

- **229 Benign neoplasm of other and unspecified sites**
  - 229.0 Lymph nodes
    - Excludes: lymphangioma (228.1)
  - 229.8 Other specified sites
    - Intrathoracic NOS
    - Thoracic NOS
  - 229.9 Site unspecified

CARCINOMA IN SITU (230–234)

- Includes: Bowen's disease
  - erythroplasia
  - Queyrat's erythroplasia
- Excludes: leukoplakia - see Alphabetic Index

- **230 Carcinoma in situ of digestive organs**
  - *Cancer involving cells in localized tissues that has not spread to nearby tissues*
  - 230.0 Lip, oral cavity, and pharynx
    - Gingiva   Oropharynx
    - Hypopharynx   Salivary gland or duct
    - Mouth [any part] Tongue
    - Nasopharynx
    - Excludes: aryepiglottic fold or interarytenoid fold, laryngeal aspect (231.0)
      - epiglottis:
        - NOS (231.0)
        - suprahyoid portion (231.0)
      - skin of lip (232.0)
  - 230.1 Esophagus
  - 230.2 Stomach
    - Body of stomach   Cardiac orifice
    - Cardia of stomach   Pylorus
    - Fundus of stomach

230.3 Colon
Appendix Ileocecal valve
Cecum Large intestine NOS
Excludes: rectosigmoid junction (230.4)

230.4 Rectum
Rectosigmoid junction

230.5 Anal canal
Anal sphincter

230.6 Anus, unspecified
Excludes: anus:
margin (232.5)
skin (232.5)
perianal skin (232.5)

230.7 Other and unspecified parts of intestine
Duodenum Jejunum
Ileum Small intestine NOS
Excludes: ampulla of Vater (230.8)

230.8 Liver and biliary system
Ampulla of Vater Gallbladder
Common bile duct Hepatic duct
Cystic duct Sphincter of Oddi

230.9 Other and unspecified digestive organs
Digestive organ NOS
Gastrointestinal tract NOS
Pancreas
Spleen

231 Carcinoma in situ of respiratory system

231.0 Larynx
Cartilage: Epiglottis:
arytenoid NOS
cricoid posterior surface
cuneiform suprahyoid portion
thyroid Vocal cords (false) (true)
Excludes: aryepiglottic fold or interarytenoid fold:
NOS (230.0)
hypopharyngeal aspect (230.0)
marginal zone (230.0)

231.1 Trachea

231.2 Bronchus and lung
Carina
Hilus of lung

231.8 Other specified parts of respiratory system
Accessory sinuses Nasal cavities
Middle ear Pleura
Excludes: ear (external) (skin) (232.2)
nose NOS (234.8)
skin (232.3)

231.9 Respiratory system, part unspecified
Respiratory organ NOS

232 Carcinoma in situ of skin
Includes: pigment cells
Excludes: melanoma in situ of skin (172.0-172.9)

232.0 Skin of lip
Excludes: vermilion border of lip (230.0)

232.1 Eyelid, including canthus

232.2 Ear and external auditory canal

232.3 Skin of other and unspecified parts of face

232.4 Scalp and skin of neck

232.5 Skin of trunk, except scrotum
Anus, margin Skin of:
Axillary fold breast
Perianal skin buttock
Skin of: chest wall
abdominal wall groin
anus perineum
back Umbilicus
Excludes: anal canal (230.5)
anus NOS (230.6)
skin of genital organs (233.30–233.39, 233.5–233.6)

232.6 Skin of upper limb, including shoulder

232.7 Skin of lower limb, including hip

232.8 Other specified sites of skin

232.9 Skin, site unspecified

233 Carcinoma in situ of breast and genitourinary system
This category incorporates specific male and female genitourinary designations (233.0–233.6), while codes 233.7 and 233.9 apply to either male or female organs.

233.0 Breast
Excludes: Paget's disease (174.0–174.9)
skin of breast (232.5)
Coding Clinic: 2012, Q1, P11

233.1 Cervix uteri
Adenocarcinoma in situ of cervix
Cervical intraepithelial glandular neoplasia, grade III
Cervical intraepithelial neoplasia III [CIN III]
Severe dysplasia of cervix
Excludes: cervical intraepithelial neoplasia II [CIN II] (622.12)
cytologic evidence of malignancy without histologic confirmation (795.06)
high grade squamous intraepithelial lesion (HGSIL) (795.04)
moderate dysplasia of cervix (622.12)
Coding Clinic: 1992, Q3, P7-8; 1991, Q1, P11

233.2 Other and unspecified parts of uterus

233.3 Other and unspecified female genital organs
Coding Clinic: 2007, Q4, P67-68

233.30 Unspecified female genital organ

233.31 Vagina
Severe dysplasia of vagina
Vaginal intraepithelial neoplasia [VAIN III]

233.32 Vulva
Severe dysplasia of vulva
Vulvar intraepithelial neoplasia [VIN III]
Coding Clinic: 1995, Q1, P8

233.39 Other female genital organ

233.4 Prostate

233.5 Penis

233.6 Other and unspecified male genital organs

233.7 Bladder
Coding Clinic: 2012, Q2, P10

233.9 Other and unspecified urinary organs

234 Carcinoma in situ of other and unspecified sites

234.0 Eye
Excludes: cartilage of eyelid (234.8)
eyelid (skin) (232.1)
optic nerve (234.8)
orbital bone (234.8)

234.8 Other specified sites
Endocrine gland [any]

234.9 Site unspecified
Carcinoma in situ NOS

NEOPLASMS OF UNCERTAIN BEHAVIOR (235–238)

Note: Categories 235–238 classify by site certain histo-morphologically well-defined neoplasms, the subsequent behavior of which cannot be predicted from the present appearance.

235 Neoplasm of uncertain behavior of digestive and respiratory systems
Excludes stromal tumors of uncertain behavior of digestive system (238.1)

- **235.0 Major salivary glands**
  Gland:
   parotid
   sublingual
   submandibular
  Excludes minor salivary glands (235.1)

- **235.1 Lip, oral cavity, and pharynx**
  Gingiva   Nasopharynx
  Hypopharynx   Oropharynx
  Minor salivary glands   Tongue
  Mouth
  Excludes aryepiglottic fold or interarytenoid fold, laryngeal aspect (235.6)
  epiglottis:
   NOS (235.6)
   suprahyoid portion (235.6)
  skin of lip (238.2)

- **235.2 Stomach, intestines, and rectum**
- **235.3 Liver and biliary passages**
  Ampulla of Vater   Gallbladder
  Bile ducts [any]   Liver
- **235.4 Retroperitoneum and peritoneum**
- **235.5 Other and unspecified digestive organs**
  Anal: Esophagus
   canal   Pancreas
   sphincter   Spleen
  Anus NOS
  Excludes anus:
   margin (238.2)
   skin (238.2)
   perianal skin (238.2)

- **235.6 Larynx**
  Excludes aryepiglottic fold or interarytenoid fold:
   NOS (235.1)
   hypopharyngeal aspect (235.1)
   marginal zone (235.1)

- **235.7 Trachea, bronchus, and lung**
- **235.8 Pleura, thymus, and mediastinum**
- **235.9 Other and unspecified respiratory organs**
  Accessory sinuses   Nasal cavities
  Middle ear   Respiratory organ NOS
  Excludes ear (external) (skin) (238.2)
   nose (238.8)
   skin (238.2)

236 Neoplasm of uncertain behavior of genitourinary organs
- **236.0 Uterus**
- **236.1 Placenta**
  Chorioadenoma (destruens)
  Invasive mole
  Malignant hydatid mole
  Malignant hydatidiform mole
- **236.2 Ovary**
  Use additional code to identify any functional activity
- **236.3 Other and unspecified female genital organs**
- **236.4 Testis**
  Use additional code to identify any functional activity
- **236.5 Prostate**
- **236.6 Other and unspecified male genital organs**
- **236.7 Bladder**
- **236.9 Other and unspecified urinary organs**
  - 236.90 Urinary organ, unspecified
  - 236.91 Kidney and ureter
  - 236.99 Other

237 Neoplasm of uncertain behavior of endocrine glands and nervous system
- **237.0 Pituitary gland and craniopharyngeal duct**
  Use additional code to identify any functional activity
- **237.1 Pineal gland**
- **237.2 Adrenal gland**
  Suprarenal gland
  Use additional code to identify any functional activity
  Pair of glands situated on top of or above each kidney ("suprarenal") responsible for regulating stress response through corticosteroids
- **237.3 Paraganglia**
  Aortic body   Coccygeal body
  Carotid body   Glomus jugulare
  Coding Clinic: 1984, Nov-Dec, P17
- **237.4 Other and unspecified endocrine glands**
  Parathyroid gland   Thyroid gland
- **237.5 Brain and spinal cord**
- **237.6 Meninges**
  Meninges:
   NOS
   cerebral
   spinal
- **237.7 Neurofibromatosis**
  Disorder of nervous system that causes tumors to grow around nerves
  - 237.70 Neurofibromatosis, unspecified
  - 237.71 Neurofibromatosis, type 1 [von Recklinghausen's disease]
  - 237.72 Neurofibromatosis, type 2 [acoustic neurofibromatosis]
  - 237.73 Schwannomatosis
  - 237.79 Other neurofibromatosis
- **237.9 Other and unspecified parts of nervous system**
  Cranial nerves
  Excludes peripheral, sympathetic, and parasympathetic nerves and ganglia (238.1)

238 Neoplasm of uncertain behavior of other and unspecified sites and tissues
- **238.0 Bone and articular cartilage**
  Excludes cartilage:
   ear (238.1)
   eyelid (238.1)
   larynx (235.6)
   nose (235.9)
   synovia (238.1)
  Coding Clinic: 2004, Q4, P128-129
- **238.1 Connective and other soft tissue**
  Peripheral, sympathetic, and parasympathetic nerves and ganglia
  Stromal tumors of digestive system
  Excludes cartilage (of):
   articular (238.0)
   larynx (235.6)
   nose (235.9)
   connective tissue of breast (238.3)
- **238.2 Skin**
  Excludes anus NOS (235.5)
   skin of genital organs (236.3, 236.6)
   vermilion border of lip (235.1)
- **238.3 Breast**
  Excludes skin of breast (238.2)

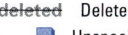

238.4 Polycythemia vera
Primary polycythemia. Secondary polycythemia is 289.0. Check your documentation. Polycythemia is caused by too many red blood cells, which increase thickness of blood (viscosity). This can cause engorgement of the spleen (splenomegaly) with extra RBCs and potential clot formation.

238.5 Histiocytic and mast cells
Mast cell tumor NOS
Mastocytoma NOS

238.6 Plasma cells
Plasmacytoma NOS
Solitary myeloma

● **238.7 Other lymphatic and hematopoietic tissues**
Excludes: *acute myelogenous leukemia (205.0)*
chronic myelomonocytic leukemia (205.1)
myelosclerosis NOS (289.89)
myelosis:
NOS (205.9)
megakaryocytic (207.2)
Coding Clinic: 2006, Q4, P63-66; 2001, Q3, P13-14; 1997, Q1, P5-6

238.71 Essential thrombocythemia
Essential hemorrhagic thrombocythemia
Essential thrombocytosis
Idiopathic (hemorrhagic) thrombocythemia
Primary thrombocytosis
Coding Clinic: 2006, Q4, P64

238.72 Low grade myelodysplastic syndrome lesions
Refractory anemia with excess blasts-1 (RAEB-1)
Refractory anemia (RA)
Refractory anemia with ringed sideroblasts (RARS)
Refractory cytopenia with multilineage dysplasia (RCMD)
Refractory cytopenia with multilineage dysplasia and ringed sideroblasts (RCMD-RS)

238.73 High grade myelodysplastic syndrome lesions
Refractory anemia with excess blasts-2 (RAEB-2)

238.74 Myelodysplastic syndrome with 5q deletion
5q minus syndrome NOS
Excludes: *constitutional 5q deletion (758.39)*
high grade myelodysplastic syndrome with 5q deletion (238.73)

238.75 Myelodysplastic syndrome, unspecified

238.76 Myelofibrosis with myeloid metaplasia
Agnogenic myeloid metaplasia
Idiopathic myelofibrosis (chronic)
Myelosclerosis with myeloid metaplasia
Primary myelofibrosis
Excludes: *myelofibrosis NOS (289.83)*
myelophthisic anemia (284.2)
myelophthisis (284.2)
secondary myelofibrosis (289.83)

● **238.77 Post-transplant lymphoproliferative disorder (PTLD)**
Code first complications of transplant (996.80-996.89)
Coding Clinic: 2008, Q4, P90-91

238.79 Other lymphatic and hematopoietic tissues
Lymphoproliferative disease (chronic) NOS
Megakaryocytic myelosclerosis
Myeloproliferative disease (chronic) NOS
Panmyelosis (acute)

238.8 Other specified sites
Eye
Heart
Excludes: *eyelid (skin) (238.2)*
cartilage (238.1)

238.9 Site unspecified

NEOPLASMS OF UNSPECIFIED NATURE (239)

● **239 Neoplasms of unspecified nature**
Note: Category 239 classifies by site neoplasms of unspecified morphology and behavior. The term "mass," unless otherwise stated, is not to be regarded as a neoplastic growth.
Includes: "growth" NOS
neoplasm NOS
new growth NOS
tumor NOS

239.0 Digestive system
Excludes: *anus:*
margin (239.2)
skin (239.2)
perianal skin (239.2)

239.1 Respiratory system

239.2 Bone, soft tissue, and skin
Excludes: *anal canal (239.0)*
anus NOS (239.0)
bone marrow (202.9)
cartilage:
larynx (239.1)
nose (239.1)
connective tissue of breast (239.3)
skin of genital organs (239.5)
vermilion border of lip (239.0)

239.3 Breast
Excludes: *skin of breast (239.2)*

239.4 Bladder

239.5 Other genitourinary organs

239.6 Brain
Excludes: *cerebral meninges (239.7)*
cranial nerves (239.7)

239.7 Endocrine glands and other parts of nervous system
Excludes: *peripheral, sympathetic, and parasympathetic nerves and ganglia (239.2)*

● **239.8 Other specified sites**
Excludes: *eyelid (skin) (239.2)*
cartilage (239.2)
great vessels (239.2)
optic nerve (239.7)

239.81 Retina and choroid
Dark area on retina
Retinal freckle

239.89 Other specified sites

239.9 Site unspecified

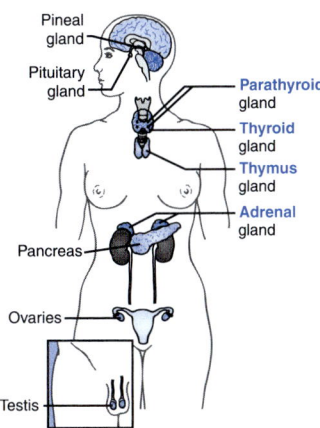

Figure 3-1 The endocrine system. (From Buck CJ: Step-by-Step Medical Coding, ed 2011, Philadelphia, WB Saunders, 2011)

Item 3-1 **Simple** goiter indicates no nodules are present. The most common type of goiter is a **diffuse colloidal**, also called a **nontoxic** or **endemic** goiter. Goiters classifiable to 240.0 or 240.9 are those goiters without mention of nodules.

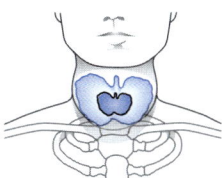

Figure 3-2 Goiter is an enlargement of the thyroid gland.

3. ENDOCRINE, NUTRITIONAL AND METABOLIC DISEASES, AND IMMUNITY DISORDERS (240–279)

Excludes *endocrine and metabolic disturbances specific to the fetus and newborn (775.0–775.9)*

Note: All neoplasms, whether functionally active or not, are classified in Chapter 2. Codes in Chapter 3 (i.e., 242.8, 246.0, 251–253, 255–259) may be used to identify such functional activity associated with any neoplasm, or by ectopic endocrine tissue.

DISORDERS OF THYROID GLAND (240–246)

240 Simple and unspecified goiter
  240.0 Goiter, specified as simple
    Any condition classifiable to 240.9, specified as simple
  240.9 Goiter, unspecified
    Enlargement of thyroid
    Goiter or struma:
      NOS
      diffuse colloid
      endemic
    Goiter or struma:
      hyperplastic
      nontoxic (diffuse)
      parenchymatous
      sporadic
    Excludes *congenital (dyshormonogenic) goiter (246.1)*

241 Nontoxic nodular goiter
  Excludes *adenoma of thyroid (226)*
    cystadenoma of thyroid (226)
  241.0 Nontoxic uninodular goiter
    Thyroid nodule
    Uninodular goiter (nontoxic)
  241.1 Nontoxic multinodular goiter
    Multinodular goiter (nontoxic)
  241.9 Unspecified nontoxic nodular goiter
    Adenomatous goiter
    Nodular goiter (nontoxic) NOS
    Struma nodosa (simplex)

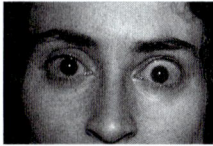

Figure 3-3 Graves' disease. In Graves' disease, exophthalmos often looks more pronounced than it actually is because of the extreme lid retraction that may occur. This patient, for instance, had minimal proptosis of the left eye but marked lid retraction. (Courtesy Dr. HG Scheie. From Yanoff M, Fine BS: Ocular Pathology, ed 6, St. Louis, Mosby, 2008)

Item 3-2 Thyrotoxicosis is a condition caused by excessive amounts of the thyroid hormone thyroxine production or hyperthyroidism. **Graves' disease is associated with hyperthyroidism** (known as **Basedow's disease** in Europe).

242 Thyrotoxicosis with or without goiter
  Excludes *neonatal thyrotoxicosis (775.3)*
  The following fifth-digit subclassification is for use with category 242:

    0 without mention of thyrotoxic crisis or storm
    1 with mention of thyrotoxic crisis or storm

  242.0 Toxic diffuse goiter
    [0-1] Basedow's disease
          Exophthalmic or toxic goiter NOS
          Graves' disease
          Primary thyroid hyperplasia
  242.1 Toxic uninodular goiter
    [0-1] Thyroid nodule, toxic or with hyperthyroidism
          Uninodular goiter, toxic or with hyperthyroidism
  242.2 Toxic multinodular goiter
    [0-1] Secondary thyroid hyperplasia
  242.3 Toxic nodular goiter, unspecified
    [0-1] Adenomatous goiter, toxic or with hyperthyroidism
          Nodular goiter, toxic or with hyperthyroidism
          Struma nodosa, toxic or with hyperthyroidism
          Any condition classifiable to 241.9 specified as toxic or with hyperthyroidism
  242.4 Thyrotoxicosis from ectopic thyroid nodule
    [0-1]
  242.8 Thyrotoxicosis of other specified origin
    [0-1] Overproduction of thyroid-stimulating hormone [TSH]
          Thyrotoxicosis:
            factitia from ingestion of excessive thyroid material
          Use additional E code to identify cause, if drug-induced
  242.9 Thyrotoxicosis without mention of goiter or other
    [0-1] cause
          Hyperthyroidism NOS
          Thyrotoxicosis NOS
          Thyrotoxicosis is also known as thyroid storm.

243 Congenital hypothyroidism
    Congenital thyroid insufficiency
    Cretinism (athyrotic) (endemic)
    Use additional code to identify associated intellectual disabilities
    Excludes *congenital (dyshormonogenic) goiter (246.1)*

244 Acquired hypothyroidism
    Includes athyroidism (acquired)
      hypothyroidism (acquired)
      myxedema (adult) (juvenile)
      thyroid (gland) insufficiency (acquired)
  244.0 Postsurgical hypothyroidism
  244.1 Other postablative hypothyroidism
    Hypothyroidism following therapy, such as irradiation
  244.2 Iodine hypothyroidism
    Hypothyroidism resulting from administration or ingestion of iodide
    Use additional E code to identify drug
    Excludes *hypothyroidism resulting from administration of radioactive iodine (244.1)*

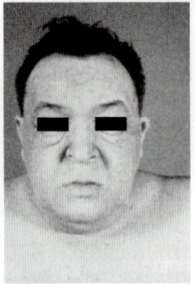

Figure 3-4 Typical appearance of patients with moderately severe primary hypothyroidism or myxedema. (From Larsen: Williams Textbook of Endocrinology, ed 10, Saunders, An Imprint of Elsevier, 2003)

Item 3-3 Hypothyroidism is a condition in which there are insufficient levels of thyroxine.
Cretinism is congenital hypothyroidism, which can result in mental and physical retardation.

244.3 Other iatrogenic hypothyroidism
Hypothyroidism resulting from:
P-aminosalicylic acid [PAS]
Phenylbutazone
Resorcinol
Iatrogenic hypothyroidism NOS
Use additional E code to identify drug

244.8 Other specified acquired hypothyroidism
Secondary hypothyroidism NEC
Coding Clinic: 1985, July-Aug, P9

244.9 Unspecified hypothyroidism
Hypothyroidism, primary or NOS
Myxedema, primary or NOS
Coding Clinic: 1999, Q3, P19-20; 1996, Q4, P29

● **245 Thyroiditis**
Inflammation of thyroid gland, results in inability to convert iodine into thyroid hormone. Common types are autoimmune or chronic lymphatic thyroiditis.

245.0 Acute thyroiditis
Abscess of thyroid
Thyroiditis: Thyroiditis:
nonsuppurative, acute   suppurative
pyogenic
Use additional code to identify organism

245.1 Subacute thyroiditis
Thyroiditis: Thyroiditis:
de Quervain's   granulomatous
giant cell   viral

245.2 Chronic lymphocytic thyroiditis
Hashimoto's disease   Thyroiditis:
Struma lymphomatosa   autoimmune
                        lymphocytic (chronic)

245.3 Chronic fibrous thyroiditis
Struma fibrosa
Thyroiditis: Thyroiditis:
invasive (fibrous)   Riedel's
ligneous

245.4 Iatrogenic thyroiditis
Use additional E to identify cause

245.8 Other and unspecified chronic thyroiditis
Chronic thyroiditis:
NOS
nonspecific

245.9 Thyroiditis, unspecified
Thyroiditis NOS

● **246 Other disorders of thyroid**
246.0 Disorders of thyrocalcitonin secretion
Hypersecretion of calcitonin or thyrocalcitonin

246.1 Dyshormonogenic goiter
Congenital (dyshormonogenic) goiter
Goiter due to enzyme defect in synthesis of thyroid hormone
Goitrous cretinism (sporadic)

246.2 Cyst of thyroid
Excludes *cystadenoma of thyroid (226)*

246.3 Hemorrhage and infarction of thyroid
246.8 Other specified disorders of thyroid
Abnormality of thyroid-binding globulin
Atrophy of thyroid
Hyper-TBG-nemia
Hypo-TBG-nemia
Coding Clinic: 2006, Q2, P5

246.9 Unspecified disorder of thyroid

DISEASES OF OTHER ENDOCRINE GLANDS (249–259)

OGCR Section I.C.3.a.2
If the type of diabetes mellitus is not documented in the medical record the default is type II.

● **249 Secondary diabetes mellitus**
Includes diabetes mellitus (due to) (in) (secondary) (with):
drug-induced or chemical induced
infection
Excludes gestational diabetes (648.8)
hyperglycemia NOS (790.29)
neonatal diabetes mellitus (775.1)
nonclinical diabetes (790.29)
Type I diabetes – see category 250
Type II diabetes – see category 250

The following fifth-digit subclassification is for use with category 249:

0 not stated as uncontrolled
1 uncontrolled

Use additional code to identify any associated insulin use (V58.67)
Coding Clinic: 2008, Q4, P91-95

● **249.0 Secondary diabetes mellitus without mention of complication**
[0-1]
Secondary diabetes mellitus without mention of complication or manifestation classifiable to 249.1-249.9
Secondary diabetes mellitus NOS

● **249.1 Secondary diabetes mellitus with ketoacidosis**
[0-1]
Secondary diabetes mellitus with diabetic acidosis without mention of coma
Secondary diabetes mellitus with diabetic ketosis without mention of coma

● **249.2 Secondary diabetes mellitus with hyperosmolarity**
[0-1]
Secondary diabetes mellitus with hyperosmolar (nonketotic) coma

● **249.3 Secondary diabetes mellitus with other coma**
[0-1]
Secondary diabetes mellitus with diabetic coma (with ketoacidosis)
Secondary diabetes mellitus with diabetic hypoglycemic coma
Secondary diabetes mellitus with insulin coma NOS
Excludes *secondary diabetes mellitus with hyperosmolar coma (249.2)*

● **249.4 Secondary diabetes mellitus with renal manifestations**
[0-1]
Use additional code to identify manifestation, as:
chronic kidney disease (585.1-585.9)
diabetic nephropathy NOS (583.81)
diabetic nephrosis (581.81)
intercapillary glomerulosclerosis (581.81)
Kimmelstiel-Wilson syndrome (581.81)

● **249.5 Secondary diabetes mellitus with ophthalmic manifestations**
[0-1]
Use additional code to identify manifestation, as:
diabetic blindness (369.00-369.9)
diabetic cataract (366.41)
diabetic glaucoma (365.44)
diabetic macular edema (362.07)
diabetic retinal edema (362.07)
diabetic retinopathy (362.01-362.07)

PART III / Diseases: Tabular List Volume 1

● **249.6 Secondary diabetes mellitus with neurological**
[0-1] **manifestations**
Use additional code to identify manifestation, as:
diabetic amyotrophy (353.5)
diabetic gastroparalysis (536.3)
diabetic gastroparesis (536.3)
diabetic mononeuropathy (354.0-355.9)
diabetic neurogenic arthropathy (713.5)
diabetic peripheral autonomic neuropathy (337.1)
diabetic polyneuropathy (357.2)
Coding Clinic: 2008, Q4, P91-95

● **249.7 Secondary diabetes mellitus with peripheral**
[0-1] **circulatory disorders**
Use additional code to identify manifestation, as:
diabetic gangrene (785.4)
diabetic peripheral angiopathy (443.81)

● **249.8 Secondary diabetes mellitus with other specified**
[0-1] **manifestations**
Secondary diabetic hypoglycemia in diabetes mellitus
Secondary hypoglycemic shock in diabetes mellitus
Use additional code to identify manifestation, as:
any associated ulceration (707.10-707.19, 707.8, 707.9)
diabetic bone changes (731.8)

● ■ **249.9 Secondary diabetes mellitus with unspecified**
[0-1] **complication**
OGCR Section I.C.3.a.3

If the documentation in a medical record does not indicate the type of diabetes but does indicate that the patient uses insulin, the appropriate fifth-digit for type II must be used.

An exception to this rule is DKA, which defaults to Type I.

● **250 Diabetes mellitus**
Metabolic disease that results in persistent hyperglycemia. The three primary forms of diabetes mellitus are differentiated by patterns of pancreatic failure—type 1, type 2 and 3.
Excludes gestational diabetes (648.8)
hyperglycemia NOS (790.29)
neonatal diabetes mellitus (775.1)
nonclinical diabetes (790.29)
secondary diabetes (249.0–249.9)

The following fifth-digit subclassification is for use with category 250:

> **0 type II or unspecified type, not stated as uncontrolled**
> Fifth-digit 0 is for use for type II patients, even if the patient requires insulin
> Use additional code, if applicable, for associated long-term (current) insulin use V58.67
> **1 type I [juvenile type], not stated as uncontrolled**
> **2 type II or unspecified type, uncontrolled**
> Fifth-digit 2 is for use for type II patients, even if the patient requires insulin
> Use additional code, if applicable, for associated long-term (current) insulin use V58.67
> **3 type I [juvenile type], uncontrolled**

Coding Clinic: 2006, Q1, P14; 1996, Q3, P5

● **250.0 Diabetes mellitus without mention of complication**
[0-3] Diabetes mellitus without mention of complication or manifestation classifiable to 250.1–250.9
Diabetes (mellitus) NOS
Coding Clinic: 2012, Q2, P19; 2009, Q4, P81-82; 2005, Q2, P21-22; Q1, P15; 2004, Q2, P17; 2003, Q4, P105-106, 108-109, P110; Q2, P6-7, 16; Q1, P5; 2002, Q2, P13; Q1, P7-8; 2001, Q2, P16; 1997, Q4, P33; 1994, Q1, P16-17, 21; 1993, Q4, P42; 5th Issue, P15; 1992, Q2, P15; 1990, Q2, P22; 1985, Nov-Dec, P11; Sept-Oct, P11; Mar-April, P12

● **250.1 Diabetes with ketoacidosis**
[0-3] Diabetic:
acidosis without mention of coma
ketosis without mention of coma
Coding Clinic: 2006, Q2, P19-20; 2003, Q4, P81-82; 1987, Jan-Feb, P15

● **250.2 Diabetes with hyperosmolarity**
[0-3] Hyperosmolar (nonketotic) coma

● **250.3 Diabetes with other coma**
[0-3] Diabetic coma (with ketoacidosis)
Diabetic hypoglycemic coma
Insulin coma NOS
Excludes *diabetes with hyperosmolar coma (250.2)*

● **250.4 Diabetes with renal manifestations**
[0-3] Use additional code to identify manifestation, as:
chronic kidney disease (585.1–585.9) diabetic:
nephropathy NOS (583.81)
nephrosis (581.81)
intercapillary glomerulosclerosis (581.81)
Kimmelstiel-Wilson syndrome (581.81)
Coding Clinic: 2012, Q2, P19; 2003, Q1, P20-21; 1987, Sept-Oct, P9

● **250.5 Diabetes with ophthalmic manifestations**
[0-3] Use additional code to identify manifestation, as:
diabetic:
blindness (369.00–369.9)
cataract (366.41)
glaucoma (365.44)
macular edema (362.07)
retinal edema (362.07)
retinopathy (362.01–362.07)
Coding Clinic: 2005, Q4, P65-67; 1993, Q4, P38; 1985, Sept-Oct, P11

● **250.6 Diabetes with neurological manifestations**
[0-3] Use additional code to identify manifestation, as:
diabetic:
amyotrophy (353.5)
gastroparalysis (536.3)
gastroparesis (536.3)
mononeuropathy (354.0–355.9)
neurogenic arthropathy (713.5)
peripheral autonomic neuropathy (337.1)
polyneuropathy (357.2)
Coding Clinic: 2009, Q4, P81; Q2, P13, 15; 2008, Q3, P5-6; 2004, Q2, P7; 2003, Q4, P105; 1993, Q2, P6; 5th Issue, P15; 1984, Nov-Dec, P9

● **250.7 Diabetes with peripheral circulatory disorders**
[0-3] Use additional code to identify manifestation, as:
diabetic:
gangrene (785.4)
peripheral angiopathy (443.81)
Coding Clinic: 2004, Q1, P14-15; 2002, Q1, P7-8; 1996, Q1, P10; 1994, Q3, P5; Q2, P17; 1990, Q3, P15; 1986, Mar-April, P12

● **250.8 Diabetes with other specified manifestations**
[0-3] Diabetic hypoglycemia NOS
Hypoglycemic shock NOS
Use additional code to identify manifestation, as:
any associated ulceration (707.10-707.19, 707.8, 707.9)
diabetic bone changes (731.8)
Coding Clinic: 1997, Q4, P43; 1994, Q2, P13

● ■ **250.9 Diabetes with unspecified complication**
[0-3] Coding Clinic: 2006, Q1, P14; 1993, Q4, P38; 5th Issue, P15; 5th Issue, P11; 1985, Nov-Dec, P11

● **251 Other disorders of pancreatic internal secretion**
251.0 Hypoglycemic coma
Iatrogenic hyperinsulinism
Non-diabetic insulin coma
Use additional E code to identify cause, if drug-induced
Excludes *hypoglycemic coma in diabetes mellitus (249.3, 250.3)*
Coding Clinic: 1985, Mar-April, P8-9

251.1 Other specified hypoglycemia
Hyperinsulinism:
NOS
ectopic
functional
Hyperplasia of pancreatic islet beta cells NOS
Excludes *hypoglycemia in diabetes mellitus (249.8, 250.8)*
hypoglycemia in infant of diabetic mother (775.0)
hypoglycemic coma (251.0)
neonatal hypoglycemia (775.6)
Use additional E code to identify cause, if drug-induced
Coding Clinic: 2003, Q1, P10

ENDOCRINE, NUTRITIONAL AND METABOLIC DISEASES, AND IMMUNITY DISORDERS (240–279)

ENDOCRINE, NUTRITIONAL AND METABOLIC DISEASES, AND IMMUNITY DISORDERS (240–279)

- **251.2 Hypoglycemia, unspecified**
  Hypoglycemia:
  NOS
  reactive
  spontaneous
  Excludes hypoglycemia:
  with coma (251.0)
  in diabetes mellitus (249.8, 250.8)
  leucine-induced (270.3)
  Coding Clinic: 1985, Mar-April, P8-9

- **251.3 Postsurgical hypoinsulinemia**
  Hypoinsulinemia following complete or partial pancreatectomy
  Postpancreatectomy hyperglycemia
  Use additional code to identify (any associated):
  acquired absence of pancreas (V88.11–V88.12)
  insulin use (V58.67)
  secondary diabetes mellitus (249.00-249.91)
  Excludes transient hyperglycemia post procedure (790.29)
  transient hypoglycemia post procedure (251.2)

- **251.4 Abnormality of secretion of glucagon**
  Hyperplasia of pancreatic islet alpha cells with glucagon excess

- **251.5 Abnormality of secretion of gastrin**
  Hyperplasia of pancreatic alpha cells with gastrin excess
  Zollinger-Ellison syndrome

- **251.8 Other specified disorders of pancreatic internal secretion**
  Coding Clinic: 1998, Q2, P15

- **251.9 Unspecified disorder of pancreatic internal secretion**
  Islet cell hyperplasia NOS

- **252 Disorders of parathyroid gland**
  Excludes hungry bone syndrome (275.5)

  - **252.0 Hyperparathyroidism**
    Excludes ectopic hyperparathyroidism (259.3)
    Coding Clinic: 2004, Q4, P57-59
    - **252.00 Hyperparathyroidism, unspecified**
    - **252.01 Primary hyperparathyroidism**
      Hyperplasia of parathyroid
    - **252.02 Secondary hyperparathyroidism, non-renal**
      Excludes secondary hyperparathyroidism (of renal origin) (588.81)
    - **252.08 Other hyperparathyroidism**
      Tertiary hyperparathyroidism

  - **252.1 Hypoparathyroidism**
    Parathyroiditis (autoimmune)
    Tetany:
    parathyroid
    parathyroprival
    Excludes pseudohypoparathyroidism (275.49)
    pseudopseudohypoparathyroidism (275.49)
    tetany NOS (781.7)
    transitory neonatal hypoparathyroidism (775.4)

  - **252.8 Other specified disorders of parathyroid gland**
    Cyst of parathyroid gland
    Hemorrhage of parathyroid gland

  - **252.9 Unspecified disorder of parathyroid gland**

- **253 Disorders of the pituitary gland and its hypothalamic control**
  Includes the listed conditions whether the disorder is in the pituitary or the hypothalamus
  Excludes Cushing's syndrome (255.0)

  - **253.0 Acromegaly and gigantism**
    Overproduction of growth hormone

  - **253.1 Other and unspecified anterior pituitary hyperfunction**
    Forbes-Albright syndrome
    Excludes overproduction of:
    ACTH (255.3)
    thyroid-stimulating hormone [TSH] (242.8)
    Coding Clinic: 1985, July-Aug, P9

  - **253.2 Panhypopituitarism**
    Cachexia, pituitary
    Necrosis of pituitary (postpartum)
    Pituitary insufficiency NOS
    Sheehan's syndrome
    Simmonds' disease
    Excludes iatrogenic hypopituitarism (253.7)

  - **253.3 Pituitary dwarfism**
    Isolated deficiency of (human) growth hormone [HGH]
    Lorain-Levi dwarfism

  - **253.4 Other anterior pituitary disorders**
    Isolated or partial deficiency of an anterior pituitary hormone, other than growth hormone
    Prolactin deficiency
    Coding Clinic: 1985, July-Aug, P9

  - **253.5 Diabetes insipidus**
    Vasopressin deficiency
    Excludes nephrogenic diabetes insipidus (588.1)

  - **253.6 Other disorders of neurohypophysis**
    Syndrome of inappropriate secretion of antidiuretic hormone [ADH]
    Excludes ectopic antidiuretic hormone secretion (259.3)
    Coding Clinic: 1993, 5th Issue, P8

  - **253.7 Iatrogenic pituitary disorders**
    Hypopituitarism:
    hormone-induced
    hypophysectomy-induced
    postablative
    radiotherapy-induced
    Use additional E code to identify cause

  - **253.8 Other disorders of the pituitary and other syndromes of diencephalohypophyseal origin**
    Abscess of pituitary
    Adiposogenital dystrophy
    Cyst of Rathke's pouch
    Fröhlich's syndrome
    Excludes craniopharyngioma (237.0)

  - **253.9 Unspecified**
    Dyspituitarism

- **254 Diseases of thymus gland**
  Excludes aplasia or dysplasia with immunodeficiency (279.2)
  hypoplasia with immunodeficiency (279.2)
  myasthenia gravis (358.00–358.01)

  - **254.0 Persistent hyperplasia of thymus**
    Hypertrophy of thymus
  - **254.1 Abscess of thymus**
  - **254.8 Other specified diseases of thymus gland**
    Atrophy of thymus
    Cyst of thymus
    Excludes thymoma (212.6)
  - **254.9 Unspecified disease of thymus gland**

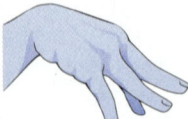

Figure 3–5 Tetany caused by hypoparathyroidism.

Item 3–4 Hyperparathyroidism is an overactive parathyroid gland that secretes excessive parathormone, causing increased levels of circulating calcium. This results in a loss of calcium in the bone (osteoporosis).
Hypoparathyroidism is an underactive parathyroid gland that results in decreased levels of circulating calcium. The primary manifestation is **tetany**, a continuous muscle spasm.

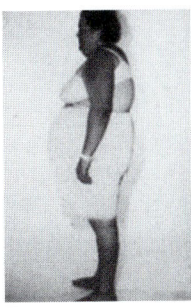

Figure 3-6 Centripetal and generalized obesity and dorsal kyphosis in a 30-year-old woman with Cushing's disease. (From Larsen: Williams Textbook of Endocrinology, ed 10, Saunders, An Imprint of Elsevier, 2003)

● **255 Disorders of adrenal glands**
  Includes: the listed conditions whether the basic disorder is in the adrenals or is pituitary-induced

  255.0 Cushing's syndrome
  Adrenal hyperplasia due to excess ACTH
  Cushing's syndrome:
    NOS
    iatrogenic
    idiopathic
    pituitary-dependent
  Ectopic ACTH syndrome
  Iatrogenic syndrome of excess cortisol
  Overproduction of cortisol
  Use additional E code to identify cause, if drug-induced
  Excludes: congenital adrenal hyperplasia (255.2)

● **255.1 Hyperaldosteronism**
  Coding Clinic: 2003, Q4, P48-50

  ■ **255.10 Hyperaldosteronism, unspecified**
    Aldosteronism NOS
    Primary aldosteronism, unspecified
    Excludes: Conn's syndrome (255.12)

  255.11 Glucocorticoid-remediable aldosteronism
    Familial aldosteronism type I
    Excludes: Conn's syndrome (255.12)

  255.12 Conn's syndrome
  255.13 Bartter's syndrome
  255.14 Other secondary aldosteronism
    Coding Clinic: 2006, Q3, P24

  255.2 Adrenogenital disorders
    Achard-Thiers syndrome
    Adrenogenital syndromes, virilizing or feminizing, whether acquired or associated with congenital adrenal hyperplasia consequent on inborn enzyme defects in hormone synthesis
    Congenital adrenal hyperplasia
    Female adrenal pseudohermaphroditism
    Male:
      macrogenitosomia praecox
      sexual precocity with adrenal hyperplasia
    Virilization (female) (suprarenal)
    Excludes: adrenal hyperplasia due to excess ACTH (255.0)
              isosexual virilization (256.4)

  255.3 Other corticoadrenal overactivity
    Acquired benign adrenal androgenic overactivity
    Overproduction of ACTH

● **255.4 Corticoadrenal insufficiency**
    Excludes: tuberculous Addison's disease (017.6)
    Coding Clinic: 2006, Q3, P24; 1985, July-Aug, P8

  255.41 Glucocorticoid deficiency
    Addisonian crisis
    Addison's disease NOS
    Adrenal atrophy (autoimmune)
    Adrenal calcification
    Adrenal crisis
    Adrenal hemorrhage
    Adrenal infarction
    Adrenal insufficiency NOS
    Combined glucocorticoid and mineralocorticoid deficiency
    Corticoadrenal insufficiency NOS
    Coding Clinic: 2007, Q4, P68-70

  255.42 Mineralocorticoid deficiency
    Hypoaldosteronism
    Excludes: combined glucocorticoid and mineralocorticoid deficiency (255.41)
    Coding Clinic: 2006, Q3, P24

  255.5 Other adrenal hypofunction
    Adrenal medullary insufficiency
    Excludes: Waterhouse-Friderichsen syndrome (meningococcal) (036.3)

  255.6 Medulloadrenal hyperfunction
    Catecholamine secretion by pheochromocytoma

  255.8 Other specified disorders of adrenal glands
    Abnormality of cortisol-binding globulin
    Coding Clinic: 1985, July-Aug, P8

  ■ **255.9 Unspecified disorder of adrenal glands**

● **256 Ovarian dysfunction**
  256.0 Hyperestrogenism
  256.1 Other ovarian hyperfunction
    Hypersecretion of ovarian androgens
    Coding Clinic: 1995, Q3, P15

  256.2 Postablative ovarian failure
    Ovarian failure:
      iatrogenic
      postirradiation
      postsurgical
    Use additional code for states associated with artificial menopause (627.4)
    Excludes: acquired absence of ovary (V45.77)
              asymptomatic age-related (natural) postmenopausal status (V49.81)
    Coding Clinic: 2002, Q2, P12-13

● **256.3 Other ovarian failure**
    Use additional code for states associated with natural menopause (627.2)
    Excludes: asymptomatic age-related (natural) postmenopausal status (V49.81)

  256.31 Premature menopause
  256.39 Other ovarian failure
    Delayed menarche
    Ovarian hypofunction
    Primary ovarian failure NOS

  256.4 Polycystic ovaries
    Isosexual virilization Stein-Leventhal syndrome
  256.8 Other ovarian dysfunction
  ■ **256.9 Unspecified ovarian dysfunction**

● **257 Testicular dysfunction**
  257.0 Testicular hyperfunction
    Hypersecretion of testicular hormones
  257.1 Postablative testicular hypofunction
    Testicular hypofunction:
      iatrogenic
      postirradiation
      postsurgical

Item 3-5 Hyperadrenalism is overactivity of the adrenal cortex, which secretes corticosterioid hormones. Excessive glucocorticoid hormone results in hyperglycemia **(Cushing's syndrome),** and excessive aldosterone results in **Conn's syndrome. Adrenogenital syndrome** is the result of excessive secretion of androgens, male hormones, which stimulates premature sexual development. **Hypoadrenalism, Addison's disease,** is a condition in which the adrenal glands atrophy.

ENDOCRINE, NUTRITIONAL AND METABOLIC DISEASES, AND IMMUNITY DISORDERS (240–279)

257.2 Other testicular hypofunction
Defective biosynthesis of testicular androgen
Eunuchoidism:
  NOS
  hypogonadotropic
Failure:
  Leydig's cell, adult
  seminiferous tubule, adult
Testicular hypogonadism
Excludes: azoospermia (606.0)

257.8 Other testicular dysfunction
Excludes: androgen insensitivity syndrome (259.50–259.52)

257.9 Unspecified testicular dysfunction

● **258 Polyglandular dysfunction and related disorders**

  ● **258.0 Polyglandular activity in multiple endocrine adenomatosis**
  Multiple endocrine neoplasia [MEN] syndromes
  Use additional codes to identify any malignancies and other conditions associated with the syndromes
  Coding Clinic: 2009, Q4, P84x2

  258.01 Multiple endocrine neoplasia [MEN] type I
  Wermer's syndrome
  Coding Clinic: 2008, Q4, P85-90; 2007, Q4, P70-72

  258.02 Multiple endocrine neoplasia [MEN] type IIA
  Sipple's syndrome

  258.03 Multiple endocrine neoplasia [MEN] type IIB

  258.1 Other combinations of endocrine dysfunction
  Lloyd's syndrome
  Schmidt's syndrome

  258.8 Other specified polyglandular dysfunction

  258.9 Polyglandular dysfunction, unspecified

● **259 Other endocrine disorders**

  259.0 Delay in sexual development and puberty, not elsewhere classified
  Delayed puberty

  259.1 Precocious sexual development and puberty, not elsewhere classified
  Sexual precocity:
    NOS
    constitutional
    cryptogenic
    idiopathic

  259.2 Carcinoid syndrome
  Hormone secretion by carcinoid tumors
  Coding Clinic: 2008, Q4, P85-90

  259.3 Ectopic hormone secretion, not elsewhere classified
  Ectopic:
    antidiuretic hormone secretion [ADH]
    hyperparathyroidism
  Excludes: ectopic ACTH syndrome (255.0)

  259.4 Dwarfism, not elsewhere classified
  Dwarfism:
    NOS
    constitutional
  Excludes: dwarfism:
    achondroplastic (756.4)
    intrauterine (759.7)
    nutritional (263.2)
    pituitary (253.3)
    renal (588.0)
    progeria (259.8)

  259.5 Androgen insensitivity syndrome
  Coding Clinic: 2008, Q4, P95-96; 2005, Q4, P53-54

    259.50 Androgen insensitivity, unspecified

    259.51 Androgen insensitivity syndrome
    Complete androgen insensitivity
    de Quervain's syndrome
    Goldberg-Maxwell Syndrome

    259.52 Partial androgen insensitivity
    Partial androgen insensitivity syndrome
    Reifenstein syndrome

  259.8 Other specified endocrine disorders
  Pineal gland dysfunction
  Progeria
  Werner's syndrome

  259.9 Unspecified endocrine disorder
  Disturbance:
    endocrine NOS
    hormone NOS
  Infantilism NOS

NUTRITIONAL DEFICIENCIES (260–269)

Excludes: deficiency anemias (280.0–281.9)

260 Kwashiorkor
Nutritional edema with dyspigmentation of skin and hair
Coding Clinic: 2009, Q3, P6

261 Nutritional marasmus
Nutritional atrophy
Severe calorie deficiency
Severe malnutrition NOS
Coding Clinic: 2013, Q1, P13-14; 2012, Q3, P10; 2007, Q4, P96-97; 2006, Q3, P14-15; Q2, P12

262 Other severe protein-calorie malnutrition
Nutritional edema without mention of dyspigmentation of skin and hair
Coding Clinic: 1985, July-Aug, P12-13

● **263 Other and unspecified protein-calorie malnutrition**

  263.0 Malnutrition of moderate degree
  Coding Clinic: 2012, Q3, P10; 2009, Q3, P6; 1985, July-Aug, P12-13

  263.1 Malnutrition of mild degree
  Coding Clinic: 1985, July-Aug, P12-13

  263.2 Arrested development following protein-calorie malnutrition
  Nutritional dwarfism
  Physical retardation due to malnutrition

  263.8 Other protein-calorie malnutrition

  263.9 Unspecified protein-calorie malnutrition
  Dystrophy due to malnutrition
  Malnutrition (calorie) NOS
  Excludes: nutritional deficiency NOS (269.9)
  Coding Clinic: 2012, Q3, P9; 2006, Q2, P12; 2003, Q4, P109-110; 1984, Nov-Dec, P19

● **264 Vitamin A deficiency**

  264.0 With conjunctival xerosis

  264.1 With conjunctival xerosis and Bitot's spot
  Bitot's spot in the young child

  264.2 With corneal xerosis

  264.3 With corneal ulceration and xerosis

  264.4 With keratomalacia

  264.5 With night blindness

  264.6 With xerophthalmic scars of cornea

  264.7 Other ocular manifestations of vitamin A deficiency
  Xerophthalmia due to vitamin A deficiency

  264.8 Other manifestations of vitamin A deficiency
  Follicular keratosis due to vitamin A deficiency
  Xeroderma due to vitamin A deficiency

  264.9 Unspecified vitamin A deficiency
  Hypovitaminosis A NOS

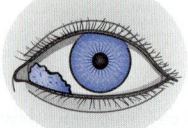

Figure 3–7 Bitot's spot on the conjunctiva.

Item 3–6 **Bitot's spots** are the result of a buildup of keratin debris found on the superficial surface the conjunctiva; oval, triangular, or irregular in shape; and a sign of vitamin A deficiency and associated with night blindness. The disease may progress to **keratomalacia,** which can result in eventual prolapse of the iris and loss of the lens.

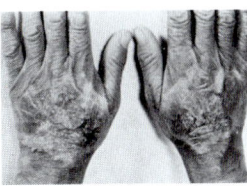

Figure 3-8 The sharply demarcated, characteristic scaling dermatitis of pellagra. (From Kumar: Robbins and Cotran: Pathologic Basis of Disease, ed 8, Saunders, An Imprint of Elsevier, 2009)

Item 3-7 Pellagra is associated with a deficiency of niacin and its precursor, **tryptophan.** Characteristics of the condition include diarrhea, dermatitis on exposed skin surfaces, dementia, and death. It is prevalent in developing countries where nutrition is inadequate. **Beriberi** is associated with thiamine deficiency.

- **265 Thiamine and niacin deficiency states**
  - **265.0 Beriberi**
  - **265.1 Other and unspecified manifestations of thiamine deficiency**
    Other vitamin B_1 deficiency states
  - **265.2 Pellagra**
    Deficiency:
      niacin (-tryptophan)
      nicotinamide
      nicotinic acid
      vitamin PP
    Pellagra (alcoholic)

- **266 Deficiency of B-complex components**
  - **266.0 Ariboflavinosis**
    Riboflavin [vitamin B_2] deficiency
    Coding Clinic: 1986, Sept-Oct, P10
  - **266.1 Vitamin B_6 deficiency**
    Deficiency:
      pyridoxal
      pyridoxamine
      pyridoxine
    Vitamin B_6 deficiency syndrome
    Excludes *vitamin B_6-responsive sideroblastic anemia (285.0)*
  - **266.2 Other B-complex deficiencies**
    Deficiency:
      cyanocobalamin
      folic acid
      vitamin B_{12}
    Excludes *combined system disease with anemia (281.0–281.1)*
    deficiency anemias (281.0–281.9)
    subacute degeneration of spinal cord with anemia (281.0–281.1)
  - **266.9 Unspecified vitamin B deficiency**

- 267 **Ascorbic acid deficiency**
    Deficiency of vitamin C
    Scurvy
    Excludes *scorbutic anemia (281.8)*

- **268 Vitamin D deficiency**
    Excludes *vitamin D-resistant:*
      osteomalacia (275.3)
      rickets (275.3)
  - **268.0 Rickets, active**
    Excludes *celiac rickets (579.0)*
    renal rickets (588.0)
  - **268.1 Rickets, late effect**
    Any condition specified as due to rickets and stated to be a late effect or sequela of rickets
    Code first the nature of late effect
  - **268.2 Osteomalacia, unspecified**
    Softening of bone
  - **268.9 Unspecified vitamin D deficiency**
    Avitaminosis D

- **269 Other nutritional deficiencies**
  - **269.0 Deficiency of vitamin K**
    Excludes *deficiency of coagulation factor due to vitamin K deficiency (286.7)*
    vitamin K deficiency of newborn (776.0)
  - **269.1 Deficiency of other vitamins**
    Deficiency:
      vitamin E
      vitamin P
  - **269.2 Unspecified vitamin deficiency**
    Multiple vitamin deficiency NOS
  - **269.3 Mineral deficiency, not elsewhere classified**
    Deficiency:
      calcium, dietary
      iodine
    Excludes *deficiency:*
      calcium NOS (275.40)
      potassium (276.8)
      sodium (276.1)
  - **269.8 Other nutritional deficiency**
    Excludes *adult failure to thrive (783.7)*
    failure to thrive in childhood (783.41)
    feeding problems (783.3)
    newborn (779.31–779.34)
  - **269.9 Unspecified nutritional deficiency**

OTHER METABOLIC AND IMMUNITY DISORDERS (270–279)

Use additional code to identify any associated intellectual disabilities

- **270 Disorders of amino-acid transport and metabolism**
    Excludes *abnormal findings without manifest disease (790.0–796.9)*
    disorders of purine and pyrimidine metabolism (277.1–277.2)
    gout (274.00–274.9)
  - **270.0 Disturbances of amino-acid transport**
    Cystinosis
    Cystinuria
    Fanconi (-de Toni) (-Debré) syndrome
    Glycinuria (renal)
    Hartnup disease
  - **270.1 Phenylketonuria [PKU]**
    Hyperphenylalaninemia
  - **270.2 Other disturbances of aromatic amino-acid metabolism**
    Albinism
    Alkaptonuria
    Alkaptonuric ochronosis
    Disturbances of metabolism of tyrosine and tryptophan
    Homogentisic acid defects
    Hydroxykynureninuria
    Hypertyrosinemia
    Indicanuria
    Kynureninase defects
    Oasthouse urine disease
    Ochronosis
    Tyrosinosis
    Tyrosinuria
    Waardenburg syndrome
    Excludes *vitamin B_6-deficiency syndrome (266.1)*
    Coding Clinic: 1999, Q3, P20-21
  - **270.3 Disturbances of branched-chain amino-acid metabolism**
    Disturbances of metabolism of leucine, isoleucine, and valine
    Hypervalinemia
    Intermittent branched-chain ketonuria
    Leucine-induced hypoglycemia
    Leucinosis
    Maple syrup urine disease
    Coding Clinic: 2000, Q3, P8

Item 3–8 Any term ending with "emia" will be a blood condition. Any term ending with "uria" will have to do with urine. A term ending with "opathy" is a disease condition. Check for laboratory work.

270.4 Disturbances of sulphur-bearing amino-acid metabolism
Cystathioninemia
Cystathioninuria
Disturbances of metabolism of methionine, homocystine, and cystathionine
Homocystinuria
Hypermethioninemia
Methioninemia
Coding Clinic: 2007, Q2, P9; 2004, Q1, P6

270.5 Disturbances of histidine metabolism
Carnosinemia   Hyperhistidinemia
Histidinemia   Imidazole aminoaciduria

270.6 Disorders of urea cycle metabolism
Argininosuccinic aciduria
Citrullinemia
Disorders of metabolism of ornithine, citrulline, argininosuccinic acid, arginine, and ammonia
Hyperammonemia
Hyperornithinemia

270.7 Other disturbances of straight-chain amino-acid metabolism
Glucoglycinuria
Glycinemia (with methylmalonic acidemia)
Hyperglycinemia
Hyperlysinemia
Pipecolic acidemia
Saccharopinuria
Other disturbances of metabolism of glycine, threonine, serine, glutamine, and lysine
Coding Clinic: 2000, Q3, P8

270.8 Other specified disorders of amino-acid metabolism
Alaninemia   Iminoacidopathy
Ethanolaminuria   Prolinemia
Glycoprolinuria   Prolinuria
Hydroxyprolinemia   Sarcosinemia
Hyperprolinemia

270.9 Unspecified disorder of amino-acid metabolism

● 271 Disorders of carbohydrate transport and metabolism
Excludes abnormality of secretion of glucagon (251.4)
diabetes mellitus (249.0–249.9, 250.0–250.9)
hypoglycemia NOS (251.2)
mucopolysaccharidosis (277.5)

271.0 Glycogenosis
Amylopectinosis
Glucose-6-phosphatase deficiency
Glycogen storage disease
McArdle's disease
Pompe's disease
von Gierke's disease
Coding Clinic: 1998, Q1, P5-6

271.1 Galactosemia
Galactose-1-phosphate uridyl transferase deficiency
Galactosuria

271.2 Hereditary fructose intolerance
Essential benign fructosuria
Fructosemia

271.3 Intestinal disaccharidase deficiencies and disaccharide malabsorption
Intolerance or malabsorption (congenital) (of):
glucose-galactose
lactose
sucrose-isomaltose

271.4 Renal glycosuria
Renal diabetes

271.8 Other specified disorders of carbohydrate transport and metabolism
Essential benign pentosuria   Mannosidosis
Fucosidosis   Oxalosis
Glycolic aciduria   Xylosuria
Hyperoxaluria (primary)   Xylulosuria

271.9 Unspecified disorder of carbohydrate transport and metabolism

● 272 Disorders of lipoid metabolism
Excludes localized cerebral lipidoses (330.1)

272.0 Pure hypercholesterolemia
Familial hypercholesterolemia
Fredrickson Type IIa hyperlipoproteinemia
Hyperbetalipoproteinemia
Hyperlipidemia, Group A
Low-density-lipoid-type [LDL] hyperlipoproteinemia
Coding Clinic: 2005, Q4, P68-69

272.1 Pure hyperglyceridemia
Endogenous hyperglyceridemia
Fredrickson Type IV hyperlipoproteinemia
Hyperlipidemia, Group B
Hyperprebetalipoproteinemia
Hypertriglyceridemia, essential
Very-low-density-lipoid-type [VLDL] hyperlipoproteinemia
Coding Clinic: 1985, Jan-Feb, P15

272.2 Mixed hyperlipidemia
Broad- or floating-betalipoproteinemia
Combined hyperlipidemia
Elevated cholesterol with elevated triglycerides NEC
Fredrickson Type IIb or III hyperlipoproteinemia
Hypercholesterolemia with endogenous hyperglyceridemia
Hyperbetalipoproteinemia with prebetalipoproteinemia
Tubo-eruptive xanthoma
Xanthoma tuberosum

272.3 Hyperchylomicronemia
Bürger-Grütz syndrome
Fredrickson type I or V hyperlipoproteinemia
Hyperlipidemia, Group D
Mixed hyperglyceridemia

272.4 Other and unspecified hyperlipidemia
Alpha-lipoproteinemia
Hyperlipidemia NOS
Hyperlipoproteinemia NOS
Coding Clinic: 2005, Q1, P17

272.5 Lipoprotein deficiencies
Abetalipoproteinemia
Bassen-Kornzweig syndrome
High-density lipoid deficiency
Hypoalphalipoproteinemia
Hypobetalipoproteinemia (familial)

272.6 Lipodystrophy
Barraquer-Simons disease
Progressive lipodystrophy
Use additional E code to identify cause, if iatrogenic
Excludes intestinal lipodystrophy (040.2)

272.7 Lipidoses
Chemically induced lipidosis
Disease:
Anderson's
Fabry's
Gaucher's
I cell [mucolipidosis I]
lipoid storage NOS
Niemann-Pick
pseudo-Hurler's or mucolipidosis III
triglyceride storage, Type I or II
Wolman's or triglyceride storage, Type III
Mucolipidosis II
Primary familial xanthomatosis
Excludes cerebral lipidoses (330.1)
Tay-Sachs disease (330.1)

272.8 Other disorders of lipoid metabolism
Hoffa's disease or liposynovitis prepatellaris
Launois-Bensaude's lipomatosis
Lipoid dermatoarthritis

272.9 Unspecified disorder of lipoid metabolism

● **273 Disorders of plasma protein metabolism**
  Excludes agammaglobulinemia and hypogammaglobulinemia (279.0–279.2)
  coagulation defects (286.0–286.9)
  hereditary hemolytic anemias (282.0–282.9)

  273.0 Polyclonal hypergammaglobulinemia
  Hypergammaglobulinemic purpura:
  benign primary
  Waldenström's

  273.1 Monoclonal paraproteinemia
  Benign monoclonal hypergammaglobulinemia [BMH]
  Monoclonal gammopathy:
  NOS
  associated with lymphoplasmacytic dyscrasias
  benign
  Paraproteinemia:
  benign (familial)
  secondary to malignant or inflammatory disease

  273.2 Other paraproteinemias
  Cryoglobulinemic:
  purpura
  vasculitis
  Mixed cryoglobulinemia
  Coding Clinic: 2008, Q2, P17

  273.3 Macroglobulinemia
  Macroglobulinemia (idiopathic) (primary)
  Waldenström's macroglobulinemia

  273.4 Alpha-1-antitrypsin deficiency
  AAT deficiency
  Coding Clinic: 2004, Q4, P59-60

  273.8 Other disorders of plasma protein metabolism
  Abnormality of transport protein
  Bisalbuminemia
  Coding Clinic: 1998, Q2, P11

  ■**273.9 Unspecified disorder of plasma protein metabolism**
  Coding Clinic: 1998, Q2, P11

● **274 Gout**
  Result of accumulation of uric acid caused by either too much production, or insufficient natural removal of uric acid from body. Results in swollen, red, hot, painful, stiff joints. Also called gouty arthritis.
  Excludes lead gout (984.0–984.9)

  ● **274.0 Gouty arthropathy**
    ■**274.00 Gouty arthropathy, unspecified**
    274.01 Acute gouty arthropathy
    Acute gout   Gout flare
    Gout attack   Podagra
    274.02 Chronic gouty arthropathy without mention of tophus (tophi)
    Chronic gout
    274.03 Chronic gouty arthropathy with tophus (tophi)
    Chronic tophaceous gout
    Gout with tophi NOS
    Coding Clinic: 2009, Q4, P84

  ● **274.1 Gouty nephropathy**
    ■**274.10 Gouty nephropathy, unspecified**
    Coding Clinic: 1985, Nov-Dec, P15
    274.11 Uric acid nephrolithiasis
    274.19 Other

  ● **274.8 Gout with other specified manifestations**
    Tophi = chalky deposit of sodium urate occurring in gout
    274.81 Gouty tophi of ear
    274.82 Gouty tophi of other sites
    Gouty tophi of heart
    Excludes gout with tophi NOS (274.03)
    gouty arthropathy with tophi (274.03)
    274.89 Other
    Use additional code to identify manifestations, as:
    gouty:
    iritis (364.11)
    neuritis (357.4)

  ■**274.9 Gout, unspecified**

● **275 Disorders of mineral metabolism**
  Excludes abnormal findings without manifest disease (790.0–796.9)

  ● **275.0 Disorders of iron metabolism**
    Excludes anemia:
    iron deficiency (280.0–280.9)
    sideroblastic (285.0)
    Coding Clinic: 1997, Q2, P11
    275.01 Hereditary hemochromatosis
    Bronzed diabetes
    Pigmentary cirrhosis (of liver)
    Primary (hereditary) hemochromatosis
    275.02 Hemochromatosis due to repeated red blood cell transfusions
    Iron overload due to repeated red blood cell transfusions
    Transfusion (red blood cell) associated hemochromatosis
    Coding Clinic: 2010, Q4, P78-79
    275.03 Other hemochromatosis
    Hemochromatosis NOS
    275.09 Other disorders of iron metabolism

  275.1 Disorders of copper metabolism
  Hepatolenticular degeneration
  Wilson's disease

  275.2 Disorders of magnesium metabolism
  Hypermagnesemia
  Hypomagnesemia
  Coding Clinic: 2010, Q1, P3-4; 2009, Q3, P6

  275.3 Disorders of phosphorus metabolism
  Familial hypophosphatemia
  Hypophosphatasia
  Vitamin D-resistant:
  osteomalacia
  rickets

  ● **275.4 Disorders of calcium metabolism**
    Excludes hungry bone syndrome (275.5)
    parathyroid disorders (252.00–252.9)
    vitamin D deficiency (268.0–268.9)
    ■**275.40 Unspecified disorder of calcium metabolism**
    275.41 Hypocalcemia
    Coding Clinic: 2007, Q3, P5-6
    275.42 Hypercalcemia
    Coding Clinic: 2012, Q3, P16; 2003, Q4, P110
    275.49 Other disorders of calcium metabolism
    Nephrocalcinosis
    Pseudohypoparathyroidism
    Pseudopseudohypoparathyroidism

  275.5 Hungry bone syndrome
  Coding Clinic: 2008, Q4, P96-97

  275.8 Other specified disorders of mineral metabolism

  ■**275.9 Unspecified disorder of mineral metabolism**

● **276 Disorders of fluid, electrolyte, and acid-base balance**
  Excludes diabetes insipidus (253.5)
  familial periodic paralysis (359.3)

  276.0 Hyperosmolality and/or hypernatremia
  Sodium [Na] excess
  Sodium [Na] overload

  276.1 Hyposmolality and/or hyponatremia
  Sodium [Na] deficiency

  276.2 Acidosis
  Acidosis:
  NOS   metabolic
  lactic   respiratory
  Excludes diabetic acidosis (249.1, 250.1)
  Coding Clinic: 1987, Jan-Feb, P15

  276.3 Alkalosis
  Alkalosis:
  NOS
  metabolic
  respiratory

ENDOCRINE, NUTRITIONAL AND METABOLIC DISEASES, AND IMMUNITY DISORDERS (240–279)

Item 3–9 Circulating fluid volume is regulated by the amount of water and sodium ingested, excreted by the kidneys into the urine, and lost through the gastrointestinal tract, lungs, and skin. To maintain blood volume within a normal range, the kidneys regulate the amount of water and sodium lost into the urine. Too much (**fluid overload**) or too little fluid volume (**volume depletion**) will affect blood pressure. Severe cases of vomiting, diarrhea, bleeding, and burns (fluid loss through exposed burn surface area) can contribute to fluid loss. Internal body environment must maintain a precise balance (homeostasis) between too much fluid and too little fluid. This complex balancing mechanism is critical to good health.

- **276.4 Mixed acid-base balance disorder**
  Hypercapnia with mixed acid-base disorder
- ● **276.5 Volume depletion**
  Excludes hypovolemic shock:
  postoperative (998.09)
  traumatic (958.4)
  Coding Clinic: 2005, Q4, P54-55; Q2, P9-10; 2003, Q1, P5, 20-22; 2002, Q3, P21x2; 1997, Q4, P30-31; 1993, 5th Issue, P1; 1988, Q2, P9-11; 1984, July-Aug, P19-20
  - ■ 276.50 Volume depletion, unspecified
  - 276.51 Dehydration
    Coding Clinic: 2008, Q1, P10-11
  - 276.52 Hypovolemia
    Depletion of volume of plasma
- ● **276.6 Fluid overload**
  Excludes ascites (789.51–789.59)
  localized edema (782.3)
  Coding Clinic: 2007, Q3, P11; 2006, Q4, P136; 1987, Sept-Oct, P9
  - 276.61 Transfusion associated circulatory overload
    Fluid overload due to transfusion (blood) (blood components)
    TACO
    Coding Clinic: 2010, Q4, P80
  - 276.69 Other fluid overload
    Fluid retention
- **276.7 Hyperpotassemia**
  Hyperkalemia
  Potassium [K]:   Potassium [K]:
    excess   overload
    intoxication
  Coding Clinic: 2005, Q1, P9-10; 2001, Q2, P12-13
- **276.8 Hypopotassemia**
  Hypokalemia
  Potassium [K] deficiency
- **276.9 Electrolyte and fluid disorders not elsewhere classified**
  Electrolyte imbalance
  Hyperchloremia
  Hypochloremia
  Excludes electrolyte imbalance:
  associated with hyperemesis gravidarum (643.1)
  complicating labor and delivery (669.0)
  following abortion and ectopic or molar pregnancy (634–638 with .4, 639.4)
  Coding Clinic: 1987, Jan-Feb, P15

● **277 Other and unspecified disorders of metabolism**
- ● **277.0 Cystic fibrosis**
  Fibrocystic disease of the pancreas
  Mucoviscidosis
  Coding Clinic: 2002, Q4, P45-46; 1994, Q3, P7; 1990, Q3, P18
  - 277.00 Without mention of meconium ileus
    Cystic fibrosis NOS
    Coding Clinic: 2003, Q2, P12
  - 277.01 With meconium ileus
    Meconium:
      ileus (of newborn)
      obstruction of intestine in mucoviscidosis
  - 277.02 With pulmonary manifestations
    Cystic fibrosis with pulmonary exacerbation
    Use additional code to identify any infectious organism present, such as:
    pseudomonas (041.7)
    Coding Clinic: 2002, Q4, P46
  - 277.03 With gastrointestinal manifestations
    Excludes with meconium ileus (277.01)
  - 277.09 With other manifestations
- **277.1 Disorders of porphyrin metabolism**
  Hematoporphyria   Porphyrinuria
  Hematoporphyrinuria   Protocoproporphyria
  Hereditary coproporphyria Protoporphyria
  Porphyria   Pyrroloporphyria
- **277.2 Other disorders of purine and pyrimidine metabolism**
  Hypoxanthine-guanine-phosphoribosyltransferase deficiency [HG-PRT deficiency]
  Lesch-Nyhan syndrome
  Xanthinuria
  Excludes gout (274.00–274.9)
  orotic aciduric anemia (281.4)
- ● **277.3 Amyloidosis**
  Disorder resulting from abnormal deposition of particular protein (amyloid) into tissues
  Coding Clinic: 2006, Q4, P66-67; 1997, Q2, P12-13; 1996, Q1, P16; 1985, July-Aug, P9
  - ■ 277.30 Amyloidosis, unspecified
    Amyloidosis NOS
  - 277.31 Familial Mediterranean fever
    Benign paroxysmal peritonitis
    Hereditary amyloid nephropathy
    Periodic familial polyserositis
    Recurrent polyserositis
    Coding Clinic: 2012, Q2, P18-19
  - 277.39 Other amyloidosis
    Hereditary cardiac amyloidosis
    Inherited systemic amyloidosis
    Neuropathic (Portuguese) (Swiss) amyloidosis
    Secondary amyloidosis
    Coding Clinic: 2009, Q1, P17; 2008, Q2, P8-9
- **277.4 Disorders of bilirubin excretion**
  Hyperbilirubinemia: Syndrome:
    congenital   Crigler-Najjar
    constitutional   Dubin-Johnson
                             Gilbert's
                             Rotor's
  Excludes hyperbilirubinemias specific to the perinatal period (774.0–774.7)
- **277.5 Mucopolysaccharidosis**
  Gargoylism
  Hunter's syndrome
  Hurler's syndrome
  Lipochondrodystrophy
  Maroteaux-Lamy syndrome
  Morquio-Brailsford disease
  Osteochondrodystrophy
  Sanfilippo's syndrome
  Scheie's syndrome
- **277.6 Other deficiencies of circulating enzymes**
  Hereditary angioedema
  Coding Clinic: 2010, Q2, P12; 2004, Q4, P59-60
- **277.7 Dysmetabolic syndrome X**
  Use additional code for associated manifestation, such as:
  cardiovascular disease (414.00–414.07)
  obesity (278.00–278.03)
  Coding Clinic: 2001, Q4, P42

● **277.8 Other specified disorders of metabolism**
  Coding Clinic: 2003, Q4, P50-51; 2001, Q2, P18-20
  - **277.81** Primary carnitine deficiency
  - **277.82** Carnitine deficiency due to inborn errors of metabolism
  - **277.83** Iatrogenic carnitine deficiency
    Carnitine deficiency due to:
    Hemodialysis
    Valproic acid therapy
  - **277.84** Other secondary carnitine deficiency
  - **277.85** Disorders of fatty acid oxidation
    Carnitine palmitoyltransferase deficiencies (CPT1, CPT2)
    Glutaric aciduria type II (type IIA, IIB, IIC)
    Long chain 3-hydroxyacyl CoA dehydrogenase deficiency (LCHAD)
    Long chain/very long chain acyl CoA dehydrogenase deficiency (LCAD, VLCAD)
    Medium chain acyl CoA dehydrogenase deficiency (MCAD)
    Short chain acyl CoA dehydrogenase deficiency (SCAD)
    [Excludes] primary carnitine deficiency (277.81)
    Coding Clinic: 2004, Q4, P60-61
  - **277.86** Peroxisomal disorders
    Adrenomyeloneuropathy
    Neonatal adrenoleukodystrophy
    Rhizomelic chondrodysplasia punctata
    X-linked adrenoleukodystrophy
    Zellweger syndrome
    [Excludes] infantile Refsum disease (356.3)
    Coding Clinic: 2004, Q4, P61-62
  - **277.87** Disorders of mitochondrial metabolism
    Kearns-Sayre syndrome
    Mitochondrial Encephalopathy, Lactic Acidosis and Stroke-like episodes (MELAS syndrome)
    Mitochondrial Neurogastrointestinal Encephalopathy syndrome (MNGIE)
    Myoclonus with Epilepsy and with Ragged Red Fibers (MERRF syndrome)
    Neuropathy, Ataxia and Retinitis Pigmentosa (NARP syndrome)
    [Use additional] code for associated conditions
    [Excludes] disorders of pyruvate metabolism (271.8)
    Leber's optic atrophy (377.16)
    Leigh's subacute necrotizing encephalopathy (330.8)
    Reye's syndrome (331.81)
    Coding Clinic: 2004, Q4, P62-63
  - **277.88** Tumor lysis syndrome
    Spontaneous tumor lysis syndrome
    Tumor lysis syndrome following antineoplastic drug therapy
    [Use additional] E code to identify cause, if drug-induced
    Coding Clinic: 2009, Q4, P84
  - **277.89** Other specified disorders of metabolism
    Hand-Schüller-Christian disease
    Histiocytosis (acute) (chronic)
    Histiocytosis X (chronic)
    [Excludes] histiocytosis:
      acute differentiated progressive (202.5)
      adult pulmonary Langerhans cell (516.5)
      X, acute (progressive) (202.5)

■ **277.9 Unspecified disorder of metabolism**
  Enzymopathy NOS
  Coding Clinic: 1987, Sept-Oct, P9

● **278 Overweight, obesity and other hyperalimentation**
  [Excludes] hyperalimentation NOS (783.6)
  poisoning by vitamins NOS (963.5)
  polyphagia (783.6)

● **278.0 Overweight and obesity**
  [Excludes] adiposogenital dystrophy (253.8)
  obesity of endocrine origin NOS (259.9)
  [Use additional] code to identify Body Mass Index (BMI), if known (V85.0–V85.54)
  Coding Clinic: 2005, Q4, P55
  - ■ **278.00** Obesity, unspecified
    Obesity NOS
    Coding Clinic: 2001, Q4, P42; 1999, Q1, P5-6
  - **278.01** Morbid obesity
    Severe obesity
    Coding Clinic: 2010, Q4, P81; 2009, Q2, P11; 2006, Q2, P5-6; 2003, Q3, P3-8
  - **278.02** Overweight
  - **278.03** Obesity hypoventilation syndrome
    Pickwickian syndrome
    Coding Clinic: 2010, Q4, P81

- **278.1** Localized adiposity
  Fat pad
  Coding Clinic: 2006, Q2, P10-11
- **278.2** Hypervitaminosis A
- **278.3** Hypercarotinemia
- **278.4** Hypervitaminosis D
- **278.8** Other hyperalimentation
  Coding Clinic: 2009, Q2, P11

● **279 Disorders involving the immune mechanism**
  [Use additional] code for associated manifestations

● **279.0 Deficiency of humoral immunity**
  - ■ **279.00** Hypogammaglobulinemia, unspecified
    Agammaglobulinemia NOS
  - **279.01** Selective IgA immunodeficiency
  - **279.02** Selective IgM immunodeficiency
  - **279.03** Other selective immunoglobulin deficiencies
    Selective deficiency of IgG
  - **279.04** Congenital hypogammaglobulinemia
    Agammaglobulinemia:
      Bruton's type
      X-linked
  - **279.05** Immunodeficiency with increased IgM
    Immunodeficiency with hyper-IgM:
      autosomal recessive
      X-linked
  - **279.06** Common variable immunodeficiency
    Dysgammaglobulinemia (acquired) (congenital) (primary)
    Hypogammaglobulinemia:
      acquired primary
      congenital non-sex-linked
      sporadic
  - **279.09** Other
    Transient hypogammaglobulinemia of infancy

● **279.1 Deficiency of cell-mediated immunity**
  - ■ **279.10** Immunodeficiency with predominant T-cell defect, unspecified
    Coding Clinic: 1987, Sept-Oct, P10; 1985, Mar-April, P7
  - **279.11** DiGeorge's syndrome
    Pharyngeal pouch syndrome
    Thymic hypoplasia
  - **279.12** Wiskott-Aldrich syndrome
  - **279.13** Nezelof's syndrome
    Cellular immunodeficiency with abnormal immunoglobulin deficiency
  - **279.19** Other
    [Excludes] ataxia-telangiectasia (334.8)
    Coding Clinic: 1985, Mar-April, P7

279.2 Combined immunity deficiency
Agammaglobulinemia:
autosomal recessive
Swiss-type
X-linked recessive
Severe combined immunodeficiency [SCID]
Thymic:
alymphoplasia
aplasia or dysplasia with immunodeficiency
Excludes: *thymic hypoplasia (279.11)*
Coding Clinic: 2011, Q4, P148

279.3 Unspecified immunity deficiency

279.4 Autoimmune disease, not elsewhere classified
Excludes: *transplant failure or rejection (996.80–996.89)*
Coding Clinic: 2008, Q3, P5

279.41 Autoimmune lymphoproliferative syndrome
ALPS

279.49 Autoimmune disease, not elsewhere classified
Autoimmune disease NOS
Coding Clinic: 2012, Q3, P8

279.5 Graft-versus-host disease
Code first underlying cause, such as:
complication of blood transfusion (999.89)
complication of transplanted organ (996.80-996.89)
Use additional code to identify associated manifestations, such as:
desquamative dermatitis (695.89)
diarrhea (787.91)
elevated bilirubin (782.4)
hair loss (704.09)
Coding Clinic: 2008, Q4, P97-100

279.50 *Graft-versus-host disease, unspecified*

279.51 *Acute graft-versus-host disease*
Coding Clinic: 2011, Q4, P148

279.52 *Chronic graft-versus-host disease*

279.53 *Acute on chronic graft-versus-host disease*

279.8 Other specified disorders involving the immune mechanism
Single complement [C_1-C_9] deficiency or dysfunction

279.9 Unspecified disorder of immune mechanism
Coding Clinic: 1996, Q2, P12; 1992, Q3, P13-14

4. DISEASES OF THE BLOOD AND BLOOD-FORMING ORGANS (280–289)

- **280 Iron deficiency anemias**
  Disease characterized by decrease in number of red cells (hemoglobin) in blood, diminishing body's ability to carry adequate amounts of oxygen to cells

  Includes anemia:
  - asiderotic
  - hypochromic-microcytic
  - sideropenic

  Excludes familial microcytic anemia (282.49)

  - **280.0 Secondary to blood loss (chronic)**
    Normocytic anemia due to blood loss
    Excludes acute posthemorrhagic anemia (285.1)
    Coding Clinic: 1993, Q4, P34; 1985, July-Aug, P13

  - **280.1 Secondary to inadequate dietary iron intake**

  - **280.8 Other specified iron deficiency anemias**
    - Paterson-Kelly syndrome
    - Plummer-Vinson syndrome
    - Sideropenic dysphagia

  - **280.9 Iron deficiency anemia, unspecified**
    Anemia:
    - achlorhydric
    - chlorotic
    - idiopathic hypochromic
    - iron [Fe] deficiency NOS

- **281 Other deficiency anemias**

  - **281.0 Pernicious anemia**
    Anemia:
    - Addison's
    - Biermer's
    - congenital pernicious
    Congenital intrinsic factor [Castle's] deficiency
    Excludes combined system disease without mention of anemia (266.2)
    subacute degeneration of spinal cord without mention of anemia (266.2)

  - **281.1 Other vitamin B_{12} deficiency anemia**
    Anemia:
    - vegan's
    - vitamin B_{12} deficiency (dietary)
    - due to selective vitamin B_{12} malabsorption with proteinuria
    Syndrome:
    - Imerslund's
    - Imerslund-Gräsbeck
    Excludes combined system disease without mention of anemia (266.2)
    subacute degeneration of spinal cord without mention of anemia (266.2)

  - **281.2 Folate-deficiency anemia**
    Congenital folate malabsorption
    Folate or folic acid deficiency anemia:
    - NOS
    - dietary
    - drug-induced
    Goat's milk anemia
    Nutritional megaloblastic anemia (of infancy)
    Use additional E code to identify drug

  - **281.3 Other specified megaloblastic anemias, not elsewhere classified**
    Combined B_{12} and folate-deficiency anemia

  - **281.4 Protein-deficiency anemia**
    Amino-acid-deficiency anemia

  - **281.8 Anemia associated with other specified nutritional deficiency**
    Scorbutic anemia

  - **281.9 Unspecified deficiency anemia**
    Anemia:
    - dimorphic
    - macrocytic
    - megaloblastic NOS
    - nutritional NOS
    - simple chronic
    Coding Clinic: 2011, Q1, P16; 1984, Sept-Oct, P16

- **282 Hereditary hemolytic anemias**
  Genetic condition in which bone marrow is unable to compensate for premature destruction of red blood cells

  - **282.0 Hereditary spherocytosis**
    - Acholuric (familial) jaundice
    - Congenital hemolytic anemia (spherocytic)
    - Congenital spherocytosis
    - Minkowski-Chauffard syndrome
    - Spherocytosis (familial)
    Excludes hemolytic anemia of newborn (773.0–773.5)

  - **282.1 Hereditary elliptocytosis**
    - Elliptocytosis (congenital)
    - Ovalocytosis (congenital) (hereditary)

  - **282.2 Anemias due to disorders of glutathione metabolism**
    Anemia:
    - 6-phosphogluconic dehydrogenase deficiency
    - enzyme deficiency, drug-induced
    - erythrocytic glutathione deficiency
    - glucose-6-phosphate dehydrogenase [G-6-PD] deficiency
    - glutathione-reductase deficiency
    - hemolytic nonspherocytic (hereditary), type I
    Disorder of pentose phosphate pathway
    Favism

  - **282.3 Other hemolytic anemias due to enzyme deficiency**
    Anemia:
    - hemolytic nonspherocytic (hereditary), type II
    - hexokinase deficiency
    - pyruvate kinase [PK] deficiency
    - triosephosphate isomerase deficiency

  - **282.4 Thalassemias**
    Hereditary disorders characterized by low production of hemoglobin or excessive destruction of red blood cells
    Excludes sickle-cell:
    disease (282.60–282.69)
    trait (282.5)
    Coding Clinic: 2003, Q4, P51-56

    - **282.40 Thalassemia, unspecified**
      Thalassemia NOS

    - **282.41 Sickle-cell thalassemia without crisis**
      - Microdrepanocytosis
      - Sickle-cell thalassemia NOS
      - Thalassemia Hb-S disease without crisis

    - **282.42 Sickle-cell thalassemia with crisis**
      - Sickle-cell thalassemia with vaso-occlusive pain
      - Thalassemia Hb-S disease with crisis
      Use additional code for type of crisis, such as:
      Acute chest syndrome (517.3)
      Splenic sequestration (289.52)
      Occurs when sickled red blood cells become entrapped in spleen, causing splenomegaly (enlargement) and decreased circulating blood volume

    - **282.43 Alpha thalassemia**
      - Alpha thalassemia major
      - Hemoglobin H Constant Spring
      - Hemoglobin H disease
      - Hydrops fetalis due to alpha thalassemia
      - Severe alpha thalassemia
      - Triple gene defect alpha thalassemia
      Excludes alpha thalassemia trait or minor (282.46)
      hydrops fetalis due to isoimmunization (773.3)
      hydrops fetalis not due to immune hemolysis (778.0)

282.44 Beta thalassemia
   Beta thalassemia major
   Cooley's anemia
   Homozygous beta thalassemia
   Severe beta thalassemia
   Thalassemia intermedia
   Thalassemia major
   Excludes beta thalassemia minor (282.46)
                beta thalassemia trait (282.46)
                delta-beta thalassemia (282.45)
                hemoglobin E beta thalassemia (282.47)
                sickle-cell beta thalassemia (282.41, 282.42)

282.45 Delta-beta thalassemia
   Homozygous delta-beta thalassemia
   Excludes delta-beta thalassemia trait (282.46)

282.46 Thalassemia minor
   Alpha thalassemia minor
   Alpha thalassemia silent carrier
   Alpha thalassemia trait
   Beta thalassemia minor
   Beta thalassemia trait
   Delta-beta thalassemia trait
   Thalassemia trait NOS
   Excludes alpha thalassemia (282.43)
                beta thalassemia (282.44)
                delta-beta thalassemia (282.45)
                hemoglobin E-beta thalassemia (282.47)
                sickle-cell trait (282.5)

282.47 Hemoglobin E-beta thalassemia
   Excludes beta thalassemia (282.44)
                beta thalassemia minor (282.46)
                beta thalassemia trait (282.46)
                delta-beta thalassemia (282.45)
                delta-beta thalassemia trait (282.46)
                hemoglobin E disease (282.7)
                other hemoglobinopathies (282.7)
                sickle-cell beta thalassemia (282.41, 282.42)

282.49 Other thalassemia
   Dominant thalassemia
   Hemoglobin C thalassemia
   Hereditary leptocytosis
   Mediterranean anemia (with other hemoglobinopathy)
   Mixed thalassemia
   Thalassemia with other hemoglobinopathy
   Excludes hemoglobin C disease (282.7)
                hemoglobin E disease (282.7)
                other hemoglobinopathies (282.7)
                sickle-cell anemias (282.60-282.69)
                sickle-cell beta thalassemia (282.41-282.42)

282.5 Sickle-cell trait
   Hb-AS genotype
   Hemoglobin S [Hb-S] trait
   Heterozygous:
      hemoglobin S
      Hb-S
   Excludes that with other hemoglobinopathy (282.60–282.69)
                that with thalassemia (282.41-282.42)
   Coding Clinic: 2012, Q3, P5; 2003, Q4, P51-56

282.6 Sickle-cell disease
   Inherited disease in which red blood cells, normally disc-shaped, become crescent shaped. Small blood clots form, resulting in painful episodes called sickle cell crises.
   Sickle-cell anemia
   Excludes sickle-cell thalassemia (282.41–282.42)
                sickle-cell trait (282.5)

282.60 Sickle-cell disease, unspecified
   Sickle-cell anemia NOS
   Coding Clinic: 1997, Q2, P11

282.61 Hb-SS disease without crisis
   Coding Clinic: 2007, Q2, P9-10

282.62 Hb-SS disease with crisis
   Hb-SS disease with vaso-occlusive pain
   Sickle-cell crisis NOS
   Use additional code for type of crisis, such as:
      Acute chest syndrome (517.3)
      Splenic sequestration (289.52)
   Coding Clinic: 2010, Q4, P78; 2003, Q4, P51-56; 1998, Q2, P8; 1991, Q2, P15

282.63 Sickle-cell/Hb-C disease without crisis
   Hb-S/Hb-C disease without crisis

282.64 Sickle-cell/Hb-C disease with crisis
   Hb-S/Hb-C disease with crisis
   Sickle-cell/Hb-C disease with vaso-occlusive pain
   Use additional code for types of crisis, such as:
      Acute chest syndrome (517.3)
      Splenic sequestration (289.52)

282.68 Other sickle-cell disease without crisis
   Hb-S/Hb-D disease without crisis
   Hb-S/Hb-E disease without crisis
   Sickle-cell/Hb-D disease without crisis
   Sickle-cell/Hb-E disease without crisis

282.69 Other sickle-cell disease with crisis
   Hb-S/Hb-D disease with crisis
   Hb-S/Hb-E disease with crisis
   Other sickle-cell disease with vaso-occlusive pain
   Sickle-cell/Hb-D disease with crisis
   Sickle-cell/Hb-E disease with crisis
   Use additional code for type of crisis, such as:
      Acute chest syndrome (517.3)
      Splenic sequestration (289.52)

282.7 Other hemoglobinopathies
   Abnormal hemoglobin NOS
   Congenital Heinz-body anemia
   Disease:
      hemoglobin C [Hb-C]
      hemoglobin D [Hb-D]
      hemoglobin E [Hb-E]
      hemoglobin Zurich [Hb-Zurich]
   Hemoglobinopathy NOS
   Hereditary persistence of fetal hemoglobin [HPFH]
   Unstable hemoglobin hemolytic disease
   Excludes familial polycythemia (289.6)
                hemoglobin E-beta thalassemia (282.47)
                hemoglobin M [Hb-M] disease (289.7)
                high-oxygen-affinity hemoglobin (289.0)
                other hemoglobinopathies with thalassemia (282.49)

282.8 Other specified hereditary hemolytic anemias
   Stomatocytosis

282.9 Hereditary hemolytic anemia, unspecified
   Hereditary hemolytic anemia NOS

283 Acquired hemolytic anemias
Also known as autoimmune hemolytic or Coombs positive hemolytic anemia. The red blood cells produced are healthy but are destroyed when trapped in the spleen by infection or certain drugs.

- **283.0 Autoimmune hemolytic anemias**
  Autoimmune hemolytic disease (cold type) (warm type)
  Chronic cold hemagglutinin disease
  Cold agglutinin disease or hemoglobinuria
  Hemolytic anemia:
    cold type (secondary) (symptomatic)
    drug-induced
    warm type (secondary) (symptomatic)
  Use additional E code to identify cause, if drug-induced
  Excludes Evans' syndrome (287.32)
  hemolytic disease of newborn (773.0–773.5)
  Coding Clinic: 2008, Q3, P5

- **283.1 Non-autoimmune hemolytic anemias**
  - **283.10 Non-autoimmune hemolytic anemia, unspecified**
  - **283.11 Hemolytic-uremic syndrome**
    Use additional code to identify associated:
      E. coli infection (041.41-041.49)
      Pneumococcal pneumonia (481)
      Shigella dysenteriae (004.0)
  - **283.19 Other non-autoimmune hemolytic anemias**
    Hemolytic anemia:
      mechanical
      microangiopathic
      toxic
    Use additional E code to identify cause

- **283.2 Hemoglobinuria due to hemolysis from external causes**
  Acute intravascular hemolysis
  Hemoglobinuria:
    from exertion
    march
    paroxysmal (cold) (nocturnal)
    due to other hemolysis
  Marchiafava-Micheli syndrome
  Use additional E code to identify cause

- **283.9 Acquired hemolytic anemia, unspecified**
  Acquired hemolytic anemia NOS
  Chronic idiopathic hemolytic anemia

284 Aplastic anemia and other bone marrow failure syndromes
Coding Clinic: 2006, Q4, P67-69

- **284.0 Constitutional aplastic anemia**
  Coding Clinic: 1991, Q1, P14

  - **284.01 Constitutional red blood cell aplasia**
    Aplasia, (pure) red cell:
      congenital
      of infants
      primary
    Blackfan-Diamond syndrome
    Familial hypoplastic anemia
  - **284.09 Other constitutional aplastic anemia**
    Fanconi's anemia
    Pancytopenia with malformations

- **284.1 Pancytopenia**
  Marked deficiency of all the blood elements: Red blood cells (erythrocytes), white blood cells (leukocytes), and platelets (thrombocytes). Check laboratory results.
  Excludes pancytopenia (due to) (with):
    aplastic anemia NOS (284.9)
    bone marrow infiltration (284.2)
    constitutional red blood cell aplasia (284.01)
    hairy cell leukemia (202.4)
    human immunodeficiency virus disease (042)
    leukoerythroblastic anemia (284.2)
    malformations (284.09)
    myelodysplastic syndromes (238.72–238.75)
    myeloproliferative disease (238.79)
    other constitutional aplastic anemia (284.09)
  Coding Clinic: 2011, Q1, P6; 2005, Q3, P11-12

  - **284.11 Antineoplastic chemotherapy induced pancytopenia**
    Excludes aplastic anemia due to antineoplastic chemotherapy (284.89)
    Coding Clinic: 2011, Q4, P92
  - **284.12 Other drug-induced pancytopenia**
    Excludes aplastic anemia due to drugs (284.89)
  - **284.19 Other pancytopenia**

- **284.2 Myelophthisis**
  Leukoerythroblastic anemia
  Myelophthisic anemia
  Code first the underlying disorder, such as:
    malignant neoplasm of breast (174.0–174.9, 175.0–175.9)
    tuberculosis (015.0–015.9)
  Excludes idiopathic myelofibrosis (238.76)
    myelofibrosis NOS (289.83)
    myelofibrosis with myeloid metaplasia (238.76)
    primary myelofibrosis (238.76)
    secondary myelofibrosis (289.83)

- **284.8 Other specified aplastic anemias**
  Coding Clinic: 2007, Q4, P72-73; 2005, Q3, P11-12; 1997, Q1, P5-6; 1991, Q1, P14; 1984, Sept-Oct, P16

  - **284.81 Red cell aplasia (acquired) (adult) (with thymoma)**
    Red cell aplasia NOS
  - **284.89 Other specified aplastic anemias**
    Aplastic anemia (due to):
      chronic systemic disease
      drugs
      infection
      radiation
      toxic (paralytic)
    Use additional E code to identify cause
    Coding Clinic: 2011, Q1, P6; 2009, Q1, P17; 2008, Q2, P6

- **284.9 Aplastic anemia, unspecified**
  Anemia:
    aplastic (idiopathic) NOS
    aregenerative
    hypoplastic NOS
    nonregenerative
  Medullary hypoplasia
  Excludes refractory anemia (238.72)
  Coding Clinic: 2011, Q1, P6

285 Other and unspecified anemias
Coding Clinic: 1990, Q3, P17

285.0 Sideroblastic anemia
Anemia:
  hypochromic with iron loading
  sideroachrestic
  sideroblastic:
    acquired
    congenital
    hereditary
    primary
    secondary (drug-induced) (due to disease)
    sex-linked hypochromic
    vitamin B_6-responsive
Pyridoxine-responsive (hypochromic) anemia
  Excludes refractory sideroblastic anemia (238.72)
  Use additional E code to identify cause, if drug-induced

285.1 Acute posthemorrhagic anemia
Anemia due to acute blood loss
  Excludes anemia due to chronic blood loss (280.0)
    blood loss anemia NOS (280.0)
Coding Clinic: 2011, Q4, P147; 2007, Q1, P19; 2004, Q3, P4; 1993, Q4, P34; 1992, Q2, P15-16

285.2 Anemia of chronic disease
Anemia in (due to) (with) chronic illness

285.21 Anemia in chronic kidney disease
Anemia in end stage renal disease
Erythropoietin-resistant anemia (EPO resistant anemia)
Coding Clinic: 2000, Q4, P39-40

285.22 Anemia in neoplastic disease
  Excludes anemia due to antineoplastic chemotherapy (285.3)
    aplastic anemia due to antineoplastic chemotherapy (284.89)
Coding Clinic: 2009, Q4, P94x2; 2008, Q2, P6; 2000, Q4, P39-40

OGCR   Section I.C.4.a.2
> When assigning code 285.22, Anemia in neoplastic disease, it is also necessary to assign the neoplasm code that is responsible for the anemia. Code 285.22 is for use for anemia that is due to the malignancy, not for anemia due to antineoplastic chemotherapy drugs. Assign the appropriate code for anemia due to antineoplastic chemotherapy.

285.29 Anemia of other chronic disease
Anemia in other chronic illness

285.3 Antineoplastic chemotherapy induced anemia
Anemia due to antineoplastic chemotherapy
  Excludes anemia due to drug NEC – code to type of anemia
    anemia in neoplastic disease (285.22)
    aplastic anemia due to antineoplastic chemotherapy (284.89)
Coding Clinic: 2009, Q4, P94x2

285.8 Other specified anemias
Anemia:
  dyserythropoietic (congenital)
  dyshematopoietic (congenital)
  von Jaksch's
Infantile pseudoleukemia

285.9 Anemia, unspecified
Anemia:
  NOS
  essential
  normocytic, not due to blood loss
  profound
  progressive
  secondary
Oligocythemia
  Excludes anemia (due to):
    blood loss:
      acute (285.1)
      chronic or unspecified (280.0)
    iron deficiency (280.0–280.9)
Coding Clinic: 2011, Q1, P16; 2009, Q1, P17x2; 2007, Q1, P19; 2002, Q1, P14; 1992, Q2, P15-16; 1985, Mar-April, P13

286 Coagulation defects
Can be acquired or genetic and results in inability to control blood clotting. Most common genetic coagulation disorder is hemophilia.
Coding Clinic: 2006, Q2, P17; 1992, Q3, P15

286.0 Congenital factor VIII disorder
Antihemophilic globulin [AHG] deficiency
Factor VIII (functional) deficiency
Hemophilia:
  NOS
  A
  classical
  familial
  hereditary
Subhemophilia
  Excludes factor VIII deficiency with vascular defect (286.4)

286.1 Congenital factor IX disorder
Christmas disease
Deficiency:
  factor IX (functional)
  plasma thromboplastin component [PTC]
Hemophilia B

286.2 Congenital factor XI deficiency
Hemophilia C
Plasma thromboplastin antecedent [PTA] deficiency
Rosenthal's disease

286.3 Congenital deficiency of other clotting factors
Congenital afibrinogenemia
Deficiency:
  AC globulin factor:
    I [fibrinogen]
    II [prothrombin]
    V [labile]
    VII [stable]
    X [Stuart-Prower]
    XII [Hageman]
    XIII [fibrin stabilizing]
  Laki-Lorand factor
  proaccelerin
Disease:
  Owren's
  Stuart-Prower
Dysfibrinogenemia (congenital)
Dysprothrombinemia (constitutional)
Hypoproconvertinemia
Hypoprothrombinemia (hereditary)
Parahemophilia

286.4 von Willebrand's disease
Angiohemophilia (A) (B)
Constitutional thrombopathy
Factor VIII deficiency with vascular defect
Pseudohemophilia type B
Vascular hemophilia
von Willebrand's (-Jürgens') disease
  Excludes factor VIII deficiency:
    NOS (286.0)
    with functional defect (286.0)
    hereditary capillary fragility (287.8)

286.5 Hemorrhagic disorder due to intrinsic circulating anticoagulants, antibodies, or inhibitors
Coding Clinic: 2004, Q3, P7; 1994, Q1, P22; 1993, 5th Issue, P16; 1992, Q3, P15-16; 1990, Q3, P14

286.52 Acquired hemophilia
Autoimmune hemophilia
Autoimmune inhibitors to clotting factors
Secondary hemophilia

286.53 Antiphospholipid antibody with hemorrhagic disorder
Lupus anticoagulant (LAC) with hemorrhagic disorder
Systemic lupus erythematosus [SLE] inhibitor with hemorrhagic disorder

Excludes *antiphospholipid antibody, finding without diagnosis (795.79)*
antiphospholipid antibody syndrome (289.81)
antiphospholipid antibody with hypercoagulable state (289.81)
lupus anticoagulant (LAC) finding without diagnosis (795.79)
lupus anticoagulant (LAC) with hypercoagulable state (289.81)
systemic lupus erythematosus [SLE] inhibitor finding without diagnosis (795.79)
systemic lupus erythematosus [SLE] inhibitor with hypercoagulable state (289.81)

286.59 Other hemorrhagic disorder due to intrinsic circulating anticoagulants, antibodies, or inhibitors
Antithrombinemia
Antithromboplastinemia
Antithromboplastinogenemia
Increase in:
    anti-II (prothrombin)
    anti-VIIIa
    anti-IXa
    anti-Xla

286.6 Defibrination syndrome
Afibrinogenemia, acquired
Consumption coagulopathy
Diffuse or disseminated intravascular coagulation [DIC syndrome]
Fibrinolytic hemorrhage, acquired
Hemorrhagic fibrinogenolysis
Pathologic fibrinolysis
Purpura:
    fibrinolytic
    fulminans

Excludes *that complicating:*
abortion (634–638 with .1, 639.1)
pregnancy or the puerperium (641.3, 666.3)
disseminated intravascular coagulation in newborn (776.2)

286.7 Acquired coagulation factor deficiency
Deficiency of coagulation factor due to:
    liver disease
    vitamin K deficiency
Hypoprothrombinemia, acquired

Excludes *vitamin K deficiency of newborn (776.0)*

Use additional E-code to identify cause, if drug-induced

286.9 Other and unspecified coagulation defects
Defective coagulation NOS
Deficiency, coagulation factor NOS
Delay, coagulation
Disorder:
    coagulation
    hemostasis

Excludes *abnormal coagulation profile (790.92)*
hemorrhagic disease of newborn (776.0)
that complicating:
abortion (634–638 with .1, 639.1)
pregnancy or the puerperium (641.3, 666.3)

Coding Clinic: 1999, Q4, P22-23

287 Purpura and other hemorrhagic conditions
Excludes *hemorrhagic thrombocythemia (238.79)*
purpura fulminans (286.6)

287.0 Allergic purpura
Peliosis rheumatica
Purpura:
    anaphylactoid
    autoimmune
    Henoch's
    nonthrombocytopenic:
        hemorrhagic
        idiopathic
    rheumatica
    Schönlein-Henoch
    vascular
Vasculitis, allergic

Excludes *hemorrhagic purpura (287.39)*
purpura annularis telangiectodes (709.1)

287.1 Qualitative platelet defects
Thrombasthenia (hemorrhagic) (hereditary)
Thrombocytasthenia
Thrombocytopathy (dystrophic)
Thrombopathy (Bernard-Soulier)

Excludes *von Willebrand's disease (286.4)*

287.2 Other nonthrombocytopenic purpuras
Purpura:
    NOS
    senile
    simplex

287.3 Primary thrombocytopenia
Also known as idiopathic thrombocytopenia, may be acquired or congenital and is a common cause of coagulation disorders

Excludes *thrombotic thrombocytopenic purpura (446.6)*
transient thrombocytopenia of newborn (776.1)
Thrombo = clot forming, cyto = cell, penia = deficiency of: deficiency of platelets

287.30 Primary thrombocytopenia unspecified
Megakaryocytic hypoplasia

287.31 Immune thrombocytopenic purpura
Idiopathic thrombocytopenic purpura
Tidal platelet dysgenesis
Coding Clinic: 2005, Q4, P56-57

287.32 Evans' syndrome

287.33 Congenital and hereditary thrombocytopenic purpura
Congenital and hereditary thrombocytopenia
Thrombocytopenia with absent radii (TAR) syndrome

Excludes *Wiskott-Aldrich syndrome (279.12)*

287.39 Other primary thrombocytopenia

● **287.4 Secondary thrombocytopenia**
  Use additional E code to identify cause
  Excludes heparin-induced thrombocytopenia (HIT) (289.84)
  transient thrombocytopenia of newborn (776.1)
  Coding Clinic: 1985, July-Aug, P13; Mar-April, P14

  287.41 Posttransfusion purpura
  Posttransfusion purpura from whole blood (fresh) or blood products
  PTP

  287.49 Other secondary thrombocytopenia
  Thrombocytopenia (due to):
   dilutional
   drugs
   extracorporeal circulation of blood
   massive blood transfusion
   platelet alloimmunization
   secondary NOS

■ **287.5 Thrombocytopenia, unspecified**

287.8 Other specified hemorrhagic conditions
  Capillary fragility (hereditary)
  Vascular pseudohemophilia
  Coding Clinic: 1985, Mar-April, P14

■ **287.9 Unspecified hemorrhagic conditions**
  Hemorrhagic diathesis (familial)

● **288 Diseases of white blood cells**
  Excludes leukemia (204.0–208.9)

● **288.0 Neutropenia**
  Decreased Absolute Neutrophil Count (ANC)
  Use additional code for any associated:
   fever (780.61)
   mucositis (478.11, 528.00–528.09, 538, 616.81)
  Excludes neutropenic splenomegaly (289.53)
   transitory neonatal neutropenia (776.7)
  Coding Clinic: 2005, Q3, P11-12; 1999, Q3, P6-7; 1996, Q3, P16; Q2, P6; 1985, Mar-April, P14

  ■ **288.00 Neutropenia, unspecified**

  288.01 Congenital neutropenia
   Congenital agranulocytosis
   Infantile genetic agranulocytosis
   Kostmann's syndrome

  288.02 Cyclic neutropenia
   Cyclic hematopoiesis
   Periodic neutropenia

  288.03 Drug induced neutropenia
   Use additional E code to identify drug
   Coding Clinic: 2006, Q4, P69-73

  288.04 Neutropenia due to infection

  288.09 Other neutropenia
   Agranulocytosis
   Neutropenia:
    immune
    toxic

288.1 Functional disorders of polymorphonuclear neutrophils
  Chronic (childhood) granulomatous disease
  Congenital dysphagocytosis
  Job's syndrome
  Lipochrome histiocytosis (familial)
  Progressive septic granulomatosis

288.2 Genetic anomalies of leukocytes
  Anomaly (granulation) (granulocyte) or syndrome:
   Alder's (-Reilly)
   Chédiak-Steinbrinck (-Higashi)
   Jordan's
   May-Hegglin
   Pelger-Huet
  Hereditary:
   hypersegmentation
   hyposegmentation
   leukomelanopathy

288.3 Eosinophilia
  Eosinophilia
   allergic
   hereditary
   idiopathic
   secondary
  Eosinophilic leukocytosis
  Excludes Löffler's syndrome (518.3)
   pulmonary eosinophilia (518.3)
  Coding Clinic: 2010, Q3, P16-17; 2000, Q3, P11

288.4 Hemophagocytic syndromes
  Familial hemophagocytic lymphohistiocytosis
  Familial hemophagocytic reticulosis
  Hemophagocytic syndrome, infection-associated
  Histiocytic syndromes
  Macrophage activation syndrome

● **288.5 Decreased white blood cell count**
  Excludes neutropenia (288.01–288.09)

  ■ **288.50 Leukocytopenia, unspecified**
   Decreased leukocytes, unspecified
   Decreased white blood cell count, unspecified
   Leukopenia NOS

  288.51 Lymphocytopenia
   Decreased lymphocytes

  288.59 Other decreased white blood cell count
   Basophilic leukopenia
   Eosinophilic leukopenia
   Monocytopenia
   Plasmacytopenia

● **288.6 Elevated white blood cell count**
  Excludes eosinophilia (288.3)

  ■ **288.60 Leukocytosis, unspecified**
   Elevated leukocytes, unspecified
   Elevated white blood cell count, unspecified

  288.61 Lymphocytosis (symptomatic)
   Elevated lymphocytes

  288.62 Leukemoid reaction
   Basophilic leukemoid reaction
   Lymphocytic leukemoid reaction
   Monocytic leukemoid reaction
   Myelocytic leukemoid reaction
   Neutrophilic leukemoid reaction

  288.63 Monocytosis (symptomatic)
   Excludes infectious mononucleosis (075)

  288.64 Plasmacytosis

  288.65 Basophilia

  288.66 Bandemia
   Bandemia without diagnosis of specific infection
   Excludes confirmed infection – code to infection
    leukemia (204.00–208.9)
   Coding Clinic: 2007, Q4, P73-74

  288.69 Other elevated white blood cell count

288.8 Other specified disease of white blood cells
  Excludes decreased white blood cell counts (288.50–288.59)
   elevated white blood cell counts (288.60–288.69)
   immunity disorders (279.0–279.9)
  Coding Clinic: 1987, Mar-April, P12

■ **288.9 Unspecified disease of white blood cells**

289 Other diseases of blood and blood-forming organs

289.0 Polycythemia, secondary
See 238.4 for primary polycythemia (polycythemia vera).
High-oxygen-affinity hemoglobin
Polycythemia:
  acquired
  benign
  due to:
    fall in plasma volume
    high altitude
  emotional
  erythropoietin
  hypoxemic
  nephrogenous
  relative
  spurious
  stress

Excludes polycythemia:
  neonatal (776.4)
  primary (238.4)
  vera (238.4)

289.1 Chronic lymphadenitis
Chronic:
  adenitis any lymph node, except mesenteric
  lymphadenitis any lymph node, except mesenteric

Excludes acute lymphadenitis (683)
  mesenteric (289.2)
  enlarged glands NOS (785.6)

289.2 Nonspecific mesenteric lymphadenitis
Mesenteric lymphadenitis (acute) (chronic)

289.3 Lymphadenitis, unspecified, except mesenteric
Coding Clinic: 2012, Q2, 18-19; 1992, Q2, P8

289.4 Hypersplenism
"Big spleen" syndrome
Dyssplenism
Hypersplenia

Excludes primary splenic neutropenia (289.53)

289.5 Other diseases of spleen

289.50 Disease of spleen, unspecified

289.51 Chronic congestive splenomegaly

289.52 Splenic sequestration
Code first sickle-cell disease in crisis (282.42, 282.62, 282.64, 282.69)
Coding Clinic: 2003, Q4, P51-56

289.53 Neutropenic splenomegaly

289.59 Other
Lien migrans
Perisplenitis
Splenic:
  abscess
  atrophy
  cyst
Splenic:
  fibrosis
  infarction
  rupture, nontraumatic
Splenitis
Wandering spleen

Excludes bilharzial splenic fibrosis (120.0-120.9)
  hepatolienal fibrosis (571.5)
  splenomegaly NOS (789.2)

289.6 Familial polycythemia
Familial:
  benign polycythemia
  erythrocytosis

289.7 Methemoglobinemia
Congenital NADH [DPNH]-methemoglobin-reductase deficiency
Hemoglobin M [Hb-M] disease
Methemoglobinemia:
  NOS
  acquired (with sulfhemoglobinemia)
  hereditary
  toxic
Stokvis' disease
Sulfhemoglobinemia
Use additional E code to identify cause

289.8 Other specified diseases of blood and blood-forming organs
Coding Clinic: 2003, Q4, P56-57; 2002, Q1, P16-17; 1987, Mar-April, P12

289.81 Primary hypercoagulable state
Activated protein C resistance
Antiphospholipid antibody syndrome
Antithrombin III deficiency
Factor V Leiden mutation
Lupus anticoagulant with hypercoagulable state
Protein C deficiency
Protein S deficiency
Prothrombin gene mutation
Systemic lupus erythematosus [SLE] inhibitor with hypercoagulable state

Excludes anti-phospholipid antibody, finding without diagnosis (795.79)
  anti-phospholipid antibody with hemorrhagic disorder (286.53)
  lupus anticoagulant (LAC) finding without diagnosis (795.79)
  lupus anticoagulant (LAC) with hemorrhagic disorder (286.53)
  secondary activated protein C resistance (289.82)
  secondary antiphospholipid antibody syndrome (289.82)
  secondary lupus anticoagulant with hypercoagulable state (289.82)
  secondary systemic lupus erythematosus [SLE] inhibitor with hypercoagulable state (289.82)
  systemic lupus erythematosus [SLE] inhibitor finding without diagnosis (795.79)
  systemic lupus erythematosus [SLE] inhibitor with hemorrhagic disorder (286.53)

Coding Clinic: 2008, Q3, P16-17

289.82 Secondary hypercoagulable state

Excludes heparin-induced thrombocytopenia (HIT) (289.84)

Coding Clinic: 2008, Q3, P16-17

289.83 Myelofibrosis
Myelofibrosis NOS
Secondary myelofibrosis

Code first the underlying disorder, such as:
  malignant neoplasm of breast (174.0-174.9, 175.0-175.9)

Excludes idiopathic myelofibrosis (238.76)
  leukoerythroblastic anemia (284.2)
  myelofibrosis with myeloid metaplasia (238.76)
  myelophthisic anemia (284.2)
  myelophthisis (284.2)
  primary myelofibrosis (238.76)

Use additional code for associated therapy-related myelodysplastic syndrome, if applicable (238.72, 238.73)

Use additional external cause code if due to anti-neoplastic chemotherapy (E933.1)

289.84 Heparin-induced thrombocytopenia (HIT)
Coding Clinic: 2008, Q4, P100-101

289.89 Other specified diseases of blood and blood-forming organs
Hypergammaglobulinemia
Pseudocholinesterase deficiency

289.9 Unspecified diseases of blood and blood-forming organs
Blood dyscrasia NOS
Erythroid hyperplasia
Coding Clinic: 1985, Mar-April, P14

Item 5-1 Psychosis was a term formerly applied to any mental disorder but is now restricted to disturbances of a great magnitude in which there is a personality disintegration and loss of contact with reality.

5. MENTAL, BEHAVIORAL AND NEURODEVELOPMENTAL DISORDERS (290-319)

PSYCHOSES (290–299)

Excludes intellectual disabilities (317–319)

ORGANIC PSYCHOTIC CONDITIONS (290–294)

Includes psychotic organic brain syndrome

Excludes nonpsychotic syndromes of organic etiology (310.0–310.9)
psychoses classifiable to 295-298 and without impairment of orientation, comprehension, calculation, learning capacity, and judgment, but associated with physical disease, injury, or condition affecting the brain [e.g., following childbirth] (295.0–298.8)

● **290 Dementias**
Progressive decline in cognition along with a short- and long-term memory loss due to brain damage/disease

Code first the associated neurological condition

Excludes dementia due to alcohol (291.0–291.2)
dementia due to drugs (292.82)
dementia not classified as senile, presenile, or arteriosclerotic (294.10–294.11)
psychoses classifiable to 295–298 occurring in the senium without dementia or delirium (295.0–298.8)
senility with mental changes of nonpsychotic severity (310.1)
transient organic psychotic conditions (293.0–293.9)

290.0 Senile dementia, uncomplicated
Senile dementia:
NOS
simple type

Excludes mild memory disturbances, not amounting to dementia, associated with senile brain disease (310.89)
senile dementia with:
delirium or confusion (290.3)
delusional [paranoid] features (290.20)
depressive features (290.21)
Coding Clinic: 1999, Q4, P4-5; 1994, Q1, P21

● **290.1 Presenile dementia**
Brain syndrome with presenile brain disease

Excludes arteriosclerotic dementia (290.40–290.43)
dementia associated with other cerebral conditions (294.10–294.11)

290.10 Presenile dementia, uncomplicated
Presenile dementia:
NOS
simple type
Coding Clinic: 1984, Nov-Dec, P20

290.11 Presenile dementia with delirium
Presenile dementia with acute confusional state
Coding Clinic: 1984, Nov-Dec, P20

290.12 Presenile dementia with delusional features
Presenile dementia, paranoid type
Coding Clinic: 2010, Q3, P16; 1984, Nov-Dec, P20

290.13 Presenile dementia with depressive features
Presenile dementia, depressed type
Coding Clinic: 1984, Nov-Dec, P20

● **290.2 Senile dementia with delusional or depressive features**

Excludes senile dementia:
NOS (290.0)
with delirium and/or confusion (290.3)

290.20 Senile dementia with delusional features
Senile dementia, paranoid type
Senile psychosis NOS

290.21 Senile dementia with depressive features

290.3 Senile dementia with delirium
Senile dementia with acute confusional state

Excludes senile:
dementia NOS (290.0)
psychosis NOS (290.20)
Coding Clinic: 2009, Q3, P6

● **290.4 Vascular dementia**
Multi-infarct dementia or psychosis

Use additional code to identify cerebral atherosclerosis (437.0)

Excludes suspected cases with no clear evidence of arteriosclerosis (290.9)

290.40 Vascular dementia, uncomplicated
Arteriosclerotic dementia:
NOS
simple type

290.41 Vascular dementia with delirium
Arteriosclerotic dementia with acute confusional state

290.42 Vascular dementia with delusions
Arteriosclerotic dementia, paranoid type

290.43 Vascular dementia with depressed mood
Arteriosclerotic dementia, depressed type

290.8 Other specified senile psychotic conditions
Presbyophrenic psychosis
Coding Clinic: 2012, Q2, P9-10

290.9 Unspecified senile psychotic condition

● **291 Alcohol-induced mental disorders**

Excludes alcoholism without psychosis (303.0–303.9)

291.0 Alcohol withdrawal delirium
Alcoholic delirium
Delirium tremens

Excludes alcohol withdrawal (291.81)

291.1 Alcohol-induced persisting amnestic disorder
Alcoholic polyneuritic psychosis
Korsakoff's psychosis, alcoholic
Wernicke-Korsakoff syndrome (alcoholic)

291.2 Alcohol-induced persisting dementia
Alcoholic dementia NOS
Alcoholism associated with dementia NOS
Chronic alcoholic brain syndrome

291.3 Alcohol-induced psychotic disorder with hallucinations
Alcoholic:
hallucinosis (acute)
psychosis with hallucinosis

Excludes alcohol withdrawal with delirium (291.0)
schizophrenia (295.0–295.9) and paranoid states (297.0–297.9) taking the form of chronic hallucinosis with clear consciousness in an alcoholic

291.4 Idiosyncratic alcohol intoxication
Pathologic:
alcohol intoxication
drunkenness

Excludes acute alcohol intoxication (305.0)
in alcoholism (303.0)
simple drunkenness (305.0)

291.5 Alcohol-induced psychotic disorder with delusions
Alcoholic:
paranoia
psychosis, paranoid type

Excludes nonalcoholic paranoid states (297.0–297.9)
schizophrenia, paranoid type (295.3)

● **291.8 Other specified alcohol-induced mental disorders**
Coding Clinic: 1989, Q2, P9

291.81 Alcohol withdrawal
Alcohol:
abstinence syndrome or symptoms
withdrawal syndrome or symptoms
Excludes alcohol withdrawal:
delirium (291.0)
hallucinosis (291.3)
delirium tremens (291.0)
Coding Clinic: 1985, July-Aug, P10

291.82 Alcohol induced sleep disorders
Alcohol induced circadian rhythm sleep disorders
Alcohol induced hypersomnia
Alcohol induced insomnia
Alcohol induced parasomnia

291.89 Other
Alcohol-induced anxiety disorder
Alcohol-induced mood disorder
Alcohol-induced sexual dysfunction

291.9 Unspecified alcohol-induced mental disorders
Alcoholic:
mania NOS
psychosis NOS
Alcoholism (chronic) with psychosis
Alcohol-related disorder NOS

● **292 Drug-induced mental disorders**
Includes organic brain syndrome associated with consumption of drugs
Use additional code for any associated drug dependence (304.0–304.9)
Use additional E code to identify drug
Coding Clinic: 2004, Q3, P8

292.0 Drug withdrawal
Drug:
abstinence syndrome or symptoms
withdrawal syndrome or symptoms
Coding Clinic: 1997, Q1, P12-13

● **292.1 Drug-induced psychotic disorders**

292.11 Drug-induced psychotic disorder with delusions
Paranoid state induced by drugs

292.12 Drug-induced psychotic disorder with hallucinations
Hallucinatory state induced by drugs
Excludes states following LSD or other hallucinogens, lasting only a few days or less ["bad trips"] (305.3)
Coding Clinic: 2004, Q3, P8

292.2 Pathological drug intoxication
Drug reaction resulting in brief psychotic states
NOS
idiosyncratic
pathologic
Excludes expected brief psychotic reactions to hallucinogens ["bad trips"] (305.3)
physiological side-effects of drugs (e.g., dystonias)

● **292.8 Other specified drug-induced mental disorders**

292.81 Drug-induced delirium

292.82 Drug-induced persisting dementia
Coding Clinic: 2004, Q3, P8

292.83 Drug-induced persisting amnestic disorder

292.84 Drug-induced mood disorder
Depressive state induced by drugs

292.85 Drug induced sleep disorders
Drug induced circadian rhythm sleep disorder
Drug induced hypersomnia
Drug induced insomnia
Drug induced parasomnia

292.89 Other
Drug-induced anxiety disorder
Drug-induced organic personality syndrome
Drug-induced sexual dysfunction
Drug intoxication

292.9 Unspecified drug-induced mental disorder
Drug-related disorder NOS
Organic psychosis NOS due to or associated with drugs

● **293 Transient mental disorders due to conditions classified elsewhere**
Includes transient organic mental disorders not associated with alcohol or drugs
Code first the associated physical or neurological condition
Excludes confusional state or delirium superimposed on senile dementia (290.3)
dementia due to:
alcohol (291.0–291.9)
arteriosclerosis (290.40–290.43)
drugs (292.82)
senility (290.0)
Coding Clinic: 2011, Q1, P12

● **293.0 Delirium due to conditions classified elsewhere**
Acute:
confusional state
infective psychosis
organic reaction
posttraumatic organic psychosis
psycho-organic syndrome
Acute psychosis associated with endocrine, metabolic, or cerebrovascular disorder
Epileptic:
confusional state
twilight state
Coding Clinic: 1993, Q3, P11

● **293.1 *Subacute delirium***
Subacute:
confusional state
infective psychosis
organic reaction
posttraumatic organic psychosis
psycho-organic syndrome
psychosis associated with endocrine or metabolic disorder

● **293.8 Other specified transient mental disorders due to conditions classified elsewhere**

● **293.81 *Psychotic disorder with delusions in conditions classified elsewhere***
Transient organic psychotic condition, paranoid type
Coding Clinic: 2011, Q1, P12-13

● **293.82 *Psychotic disorder with hallucinations in conditions classified elsewhere***
Transient organic psychotic condition, hallucinatory type

● **293.83 *Mood disorder in conditions classified elsewhere***
Transient organic psychotic condition, depressive type

● **293.84 *Anxiety disorder in conditions classified elsewhere***
Coding Clinic: 1996, Q4, P29

● **293.89 *Other***
Catatonic disorder in conditions classified elsewhere

● **293.9 Unspecified transient mental disorder in conditions classified elsewhere**
Organic psychosis:
infective NOS
posttraumatic NOS
transient NOS
Psycho-organic syndrome

294 Persistent mental disorders due to conditions classified elsewhere
Includes organic psychotic brain syndromes (chronic), not elsewhere classified

294.0 Amnestic disorder in conditions classified elsewhere
Korsakoff's psychosis or syndrome (nonalcoholic)
Code first underlying condition
Excludes alcoholic:
  amnestic syndrome (291.1)
  Korsakoff's psychosis (291.1)

294.1 Dementia in conditions classified elsewhere
Dementia of the Alzheimer's type
Code first any underlying physical condition as:
  Alzheimer's disease (331.0)
  cerebral lipidoses (330.1)
  dementia with Lewy bodies (331.82)
  dementia with Parkinsonism (331.82)
  epilepsy (345.0–345.9)
  frontal dementia (331.19)
  frontotemporal dementia (331.19)
  general paresis [syphilis] (094.1)
  hepatolenticular degeneration (275.1)
  Huntington's chorea (333.4)
  Jakob-Creutzfeldt disease (046.11–046.19)
  multiple sclerosis (340)
  Parkinson's disease (332.0)
  Pick's disease of the brain (331.11)
  polyarteritis nodosa (446.0)
  syphilis (094.1)
Excludes dementia:
  arteriosclerotic (290.40–290.43)
  presenile (290.10–290.13)
  senile (290.0)
  epileptic psychosis NOS (294.8)
Coding Clinic: 1999, Q1, P14; 1985, Sept-Oct, P12

294.10 Dementia in conditions classified elsewhere without behavioral disturbance
Dementia in conditions classified elsewhere NOS

294.11 Dementia in conditions classified elsewhere with behavioral disturbance
Aggressive behavior
Combative behavior
Violent behavior
Use additional code, where applicable, to identify:
  wandering in conditions classified elsewhere (V40.31)
Coding Clinic: 2000, Q4, P40-41

294.2 Dementia, unspecified
Excludes mild memory disturbances, not amounting to dementia (310.89)

294.20 Dementia, unspecified, without behavioral disturbance
Dementia NOS

294.21 Dementia, unspecified, with behavioral disturbance
Aggressive behavior
Combative behavior
Violent behavior
Use additional code, where applicable, to identify:
  wandering in conditions classified elsewhere (V40.31)
Coding Clinic: 2011, Q4, P96

294.8 Other persistent mental disorders due to conditions classified elsewhere
Amnestic disorder NOS
Epileptic psychosis NOS
Mixed paranoid and affective organic psychotic states
Use additional code for associated epilepsy (345.0–345.9)
Excludes mild memory disturbances, not amounting to dementia (310.89)
Coding Clinic: 2009, Q3, P6x2; 2003, Q3, P14

294.9 Unspecified persistent mental disorders due to conditions classified elsewhere
Cognitive disorder NOS
Organic psychosis (chronic)
Coding Clinic: 2007, Q2, P5

OTHER PSYCHOSES (295–299)

Use additional code to identify any associated physical disease, injury, or condition affecting the brain with psychoses classifiable to 295–298

295 Schizophrenic disorders
Personality disorders characterized by multiple mental and behavioral irregularities
Includes schizophrenia of the types described in 295.0–295.9 occurring in children
Excludes childhood type schizophrenia (299.9)
  infantile autism (299.0)

The following fifth-digit subclassification is for use with category 295:
  0 unspecified
  1 subchronic
  2 chronic
  3 subchronic with acute exacerbation
  4 chronic with acute exacerbation
  5 in remission

295.0 Simple type
[0-5] Schizophrenia simplex
Excludes latent schizophrenia (295.5)

295.1 Disorganized type
[0-5] Hebephrenia
Hebephrenic type schizophrenia

295.2 Catatonic type
[0-5] Catatonic (schizophrenia):   Schizophrenic:
  agitation   catalepsy
  excitation   catatonia
  excited type   flexibilitas cerea
  stupor
  withdrawn type

295.3 Paranoid type
[0-5] Paraphrenic schizophrenia
Excludes involutional paranoid state (297.2)
  paranoia (297.1)
  paraphrenia (297.2)

295.4 Schizophreniform disorder
[0-5] Oneirophrenia
Schizophreniform:
  attack
  psychosis, confusional type
Excludes acute forms of schizophrenia of:
  catatonic type (295.2)
  hebephrenic type (295.1)
  paranoid type (295.3)
  simple type (295.0)
  undifferentiated type (295.8)

295.5 Latent schizophrenia
[0-5] Latent schizophrenic reaction
Schizophrenia: Schizophrenia:
  borderline   prodromal
  incipient   pseudoneurotic
  prepsychotic   pseudopsychopathic
Excludes schizoid personality (301.20–301.22)

295.6 Residual type
[0-5] Chronic undifferentiated schizophrenia
Restzustand (schizophrenic)
Schizophrenic residual state
Coding Clinic: 2006, Q4, P76-78

295.7 Schizoaffective disorder
[0-5] Cyclic schizophrenia
Mixed schizophrenic and affective psychosis
Schizo-affective psychosis
Schizophreniform psychosis, affective type

295.8 Other specified types of schizophrenia
[0-5]
Acute (undifferentiated) schizophrenia
Atypical schizophrenia
Cenesthopathic schizophrenia
Excludes *infantile autism (299.0)*

295.9 Unspecified schizophrenia
[0-5]
Schizophrenia:
  NOS
  mixed NOS
Schizophrenia:
  undifferentiated NOS
  undifferentiated type
Schizophrenic reaction NOS
Schizophreniform psychosis NOS
Coding Clinic: 1995, Q3, P6

296 Episodic mood disorders
Includes episodic affective disorders
Excludes *neurotic depression (300.4)*
reactive depressive psychosis (298.0)
reactive excitation (298.1)
Coding Clinic: 1985, Mar-April, P14

The following fifth-digit subclassification is for use with categories 296.0–296.6:

0 unspecified
1 mild
2 moderate
3 severe, without mention of psychotic behavior
4 severe, specified as with psychotic behavior
5 in partial or unspecified remission
6 in full remission

296.0 Bipolar I disorder, single manic episode
[0-6]
Manic depressive disorder, characterized by moods that swing between periods of exaggerated euphoria, irritability, or both (manic) and episodes of depression
Hypomania (mild) NOS single episode or unspecified
Hypomanic psychosis single episode or unspecified
Mania (monopolar) NOS single episode or unspecified
Manic-depressive psychosis or reaction, single episode or unspecified:
  hypomanic, single episode or unspecified
  manic, single episode or unspecified
Excludes *circular type, if there was a previous attack of depression (296.4)*

296.1 Manic disorder, recurrent episode
[0-6]
Any condition classifiable to 296.0, stated to be recurrent
Excludes *circular type, if there was a previous attack of depression (296.4)*

296.2 Major depressive disorder, single episode
[0-6]
Depressive psychosis, single episode or unspecified
Endogenous depression, single episode or unspecified
Involutional melancholia, single episode or unspecified
Manic-depressive psychosis or reaction, depressed type, single episode or unspecified
Monopolar depression, single episode or unspecified
Psychotic depression, single episode or unspecified
Excludes *circular type, if previous attack was of manic type (296.5)*
depression NOS (311)
reactive depression (neurotic) (300.4)
psychotic (298.0)
Coding Clinic: 2009, Q3, P6x2, 7

296.3 Major depressive disorder, recurrent episode
[0-6]
Any condition classifiable to 296.2, stated to be recurrent
Excludes *circular type, if previous attack was of manic type (296.5)*
depression NOS (311)
reactive depression (neurotic) (300.4)
psychotic (298.0)

296.4 Bipolar I disorder, most recent episode (or current) manic
[0-6]
Bipolar disorder, now manic
Manic-depressive psychosis, circular type but currently manic
Excludes *brief compensatory or rebound mood swings (296.99)*

296.5 Bipolar I disorder, most recent episode (or current) depressed
[0-6]
Bipolar disorder, now depressed
Manic-depressive psychosis, circular type but currently depressed
Excludes *brief compensatory or rebound mood swings (296.99)*
Coding Clinic: 2006, Q1, P10

296.6 Bipolar I disorder, most recent episode (or current) mixed
[0-6]
Manic-depressive psychosis, circular type, mixed

296.7 Bipolar I disorder, most recent episode (or current) unspecified
Atypical bipolar affective disorder NOS
Manic-depressive psychosis, circular type, current condition not specified as either manic or depressive

296.8 Other and unspecified bipolar disorders
296.80 Bipolar disorder, unspecified
Bipolar disorder NOS
Manic-depressive:
  reaction NOS
  syndrome NOS

296.81 Atypical manic disorder

296.82 Atypical depressive disorder

296.89 Other
Bipolar II disorder
Manic-depressive psychosis, mixed type

296.9 Other and unspecified episodic mood disorder
Excludes *psychogenic affective psychoses (298.0–298.8)*

296.90 Unspecified episodic mood disorder
Affective psychosis NOS
Melancholia NOS
Mood disorder NOS
Coding Clinic: 1985, Mar-April, P14

296.99 Other specified episodic mood disorder
Mood swings:
  brief compensatory
  rebound

297 Delusional disorders
Includes paranoid disorders
Excludes *acute paranoid reaction (298.3)*
alcoholic jealousy or paranoid state (291.5)
paranoid schizophrenia (295.3)

297.0 Paranoid state, simple

297.1 Delusional disorder
Chronic paranoid psychosis
Sander's disease
Systematized delusions
Excludes *paranoid personality disorder (301.0)*

297.2 Paraphrenia
Involutional paranoid state
Late paraphrenia
Paraphrenia (involutional)

297.3 Shared psychotic disorder
Folie à deux
Induced psychosis or paranoid disorder

297.8 Other specified paranoid states
Paranoia querulans
Sensitiver Beziehungswahn
Excludes *acute paranoid reaction or state (298.3)*
senile paranoid state (290.20)

297.9 Unspecified paranoid state
Paranoid:
  disorder NOS
  psychosis NOS
  reaction NOS
  state NOS

MENTAL, BEHAVIORAL AND NEURODEVELOPMENTAL DISORDERS (290-319)

- **298 Other nonorganic psychoses**
  - **Includes** psychotic conditions due to or provoked by:
    - emotional stress
    - environmental factors as major part of etiology
  - **298.0 Depressive type psychosis**
    - Psychogenic depressive psychosis
    - Psychotic reactive depression
    - Reactive depressive psychosis
    - **Excludes** manic-depressive psychosis, depressed type (296.2–296.3)
      - neurotic depression (300.4)
      - reactive depression NOS (300.4)
  - **298.1 Excitative type psychosis**
    - Acute hysterical psychosis
    - Psychogenic excitation
    - Reactive excitation
    - **Excludes** manic-depressive psychosis, manic type (296.0–296.1)
  - **298.2 Reactive confusion**
    - Psychogenic confusion
    - Psychogenic twilight state
    - **Excludes** acute confusional state (293.0)
  - **298.3 Acute paranoid reaction**
    - Acute psychogenic paranoid psychosis
    - Bouffée délirante
    - **Excludes** paranoid states (297.0–297.9)
  - **298.4 Psychogenic paranoid psychosis**
    - Protracted reactive paranoid psychosis
  - **298.8 Other and unspecified reactive psychosis**
    - Brief psychotic disorder
    - Brief reactive psychosis NOS
    - Hysterical psychosis
    - Psychogenic psychosis NOS
    - Psychogenic stupor
    - **Excludes** acute hysterical psychosis (298.1)
  - **298.9 Unspecified psychosis**
    - Atypical psychosis
    - Psychosis NOS
    - Psychotic disorder NOS
    - **Coding Clinic: 2006, Q3, P22; 1993, Q3, P11**

- **299 Pervasive developmental disorders**
  - **Excludes** adult type psychoses occurring in childhood, as:
    - affective disorders (296.0–296.9)
    - manic-depressive disorders (296.0–296.9)
    - schizophrenia (295.0–295.9)

  The following fifth-digit subclassification is for use with category 299:

0	current or active state
1	residual state

  - **299.0 Autistic disorder** [0-1]
    - Childhood autism
    - Infantile psychosis
    - Kanner's syndrome
    - **Excludes** disintegrative psychosis (299.1)
      - Heller's syndrome (299.1)
      - schizophrenic syndrome of childhood (299.9)
    - **Coding Clinic: 2012, Q3, P19-20**
  - **299.1 Childhood disintegrative disorder** [0-1]
    - Heller's syndrome
    - **Use additional** code to identify any associated neurological disorder
    - **Excludes** infantile autism (299.0)
      - schizophrenic syndrome of childhood (299.9)
  - **299.8 Other specified pervasive developmental disorders** [0-1]
    - Asperger's disorder
    - Atypical childhood psychosis
    - Borderline psychosis of childhood
    - **Excludes** simple stereotypes without psychotic disturbance (307.3)

- **299.9 Unspecified pervasive developmental disorder** [0-1]
  - Child psychosis NOS
  - Pervasive developmental disorder NOS
  - Schizophrenia, childhood type NOS
  - Schizophrenic syndrome of childhood NOS
  - **Excludes** schizophrenia of adult type occurring in childhood (295.0–295.9)

NEUROTIC DISORDERS, PERSONALITY DISORDERS, AND OTHER NONPSYCHOTIC MENTAL DISORDERS (300–316)

- **300 Anxiety, dissociative and somatoform disorders**
  - **300.0 Anxiety states**
    - **Excludes** anxiety in:
      - acute stress reaction (308.0)
      - transient adjustment reaction (309.24)
      - neurasthenia (300.5)
      - psychophysiological disorders (306.0–306.9)
      - separation anxiety (309.21)
    - **300.00 Anxiety state, unspecified**
      - Anxiety:
        - neurosis
        - reaction
        - state (neurotic)
      - Atypical anxiety disorder
      - **Coding Clinic: 2011, Q3, P6**
    - **300.01 Panic disorder without agoraphobia**
      - Panic:
        - attack
        - state
      - **Excludes** panic disorder with agoraphobia (300.21)
    - **300.02 Generalized anxiety disorder**
    - **300.09 Other**
  - **300.1 Dissociative, conversion and factitious disorders**
    - **Excludes** adjustment reaction (309.0–309.9)
      - anorexia nervosa (307.1)
      - gross stress reaction (308.0–308.9)
      - hysterical personality (301.50–301.59)
      - psychophysiologic disorders (306.0–306.9)
    - **300.10 Hysteria, unspecified**
    - **300.11 Conversion disorder**
      - Astasia-abasia, hysterical
      - Conversion hysteria or reaction
      - Hysterical:
        - blindness
        - deafness
        - paralysis
      - **Coding Clinic: 1985, Nov-Dec, P15**
    - **300.12 Dissociative amnesia**
      - Hysterical amnesia
    - **300.13 Dissociative fugue**
      - Hysterical fugue
    - **300.14 Dissociative identity disorder**
    - **300.15 Dissociative disorder or reaction, unspecified**
    - **300.16 Factitious disorder with predominantly psychological signs and symptoms**
      - Compensation neurosis
      - Ganser's syndrome, hysterical
    - **300.19 Other and unspecified factitious illness**
      - Factitious disorder (with combined psychological and physical signs and symptoms) (with predominantly physical signs and symptoms) NOS
      - **Excludes** multiple operations or hospital addiction syndrome (301.51)

Item 5-2 Anxiety is also known as **generalized disorder** and is evidenced by persistent, excessive, and unrealistic worry about everyday things. **Dissociative disorders** are characterized by a persistent disruption in the integration of memory, consciousness, or identity and a lack of mental connectedness to events. **Somatoform disorders** are characterized by unusual physical symptoms in the absence of any known physical pathology and may lead to unnecessary medical treatments.

PART III / Diseases: Tabular List Volume 1   300.2-301.22

- **300.2 Phobic disorders**
  Irrational fear with avoidance of the feared subject, activity, or situation. Divided into 3 types: specific phobias, social phobias, and agoraphobia.
  Excludes anxiety state not associated with a specific situation or object (300.00–300.09)
  obsessional phobias (300.3)
  - **300.20 Phobia, unspecified**
    Anxiety-hysteria NOS
    Phobia NOS
  - **300.21 Agoraphobia with panic disorder**
    Fear of:
      open spaces with panic attacks
      streets with panic attacks
      travel with panic attacks
    Panic disorder with agoraphobia
    Excludes agoraphobia without panic disorder (300.22)
    panic disorder without agoraphobia (300.01)
  - **300.22 Agoraphobia without mention of panic attacks**
    Any condition classifiable to 300.21 without mention of panic attacks
  - **300.23 Social phobia**
    Fear of:
      eating in public
      public speaking
      washing in public
  - **300.29 Other isolated or specific phobias**
    Acrophobia
    Fear of heights
    Animal phobias
    Claustrophobia
    Fear of closed spaces
    Fear of crowds

- **300.3 Obsessive-compulsive disorders** *(OCD)*
  Anancastic neurosis
  Compulsive neurosis
  Obsessional phobia [any]
  Excludes obsessive-compulsive symptoms occurring in:
    endogenous depression (296.2–296.3)
    organic states (e.g., encephalitis)
    schizophrenia (295.0–295.9)

- **300.4 Dysthymic disorder**
  Anxiety depression
  Depression with anxiety
  Depressive reaction
  Neurotic depressive state
  Reactive depression
  Excludes adjustment reaction with depressive symptoms (309.0–309.1)
    depression NOS (311)
    manic-depressive psychosis, depressed type (296.2–296.3)
    reactive depressive psychosis (298.0)
  Coding Clinic: 2011, Q3, P6

- **300.5 Neurasthenia**
  Fatigue neurosis   Psychogenic:
  Nervous debility   asthenia
                          general fatigue
  Use additional code to identify any associated physical disorder
  Excludes anxiety state (300.00–300.09)
    neurotic depression (300.4)
    psychophysiological disorders (306.0–306.9)
    specific nonpsychotic mental disorders following organic brain damage (310.0–310.9)

- **300.6 Depersonalization disorder**
  Derealization (neurotic)
  Neurotic state with depersonalization episode
  Excludes depersonalization associated with:
    anxiety (300.00–300.09)
    depression (300.4)
    manic-depressive disorder or psychosis (296.0–296.9)
    schizophrenia (295.0–295.9)

- **300.7 Hypochondriasis**
  Hypochondriac
  Body dysmorphic disorder
  Excludes hypochondriasis in:
    hysteria (300.10–300.19)
    manic-depressive psychosis, depressed type (296.2–296.3)
    neurasthenia (300.5)
    obsessional disorder (300.3)
    schizophrenia (295.0–295.9)

- **300.8 Somatoform disorders**
  - **300.81 Somatization disorder**
    Briquet's disorder
    Severe somatoform disorder
  - **300.82 Undifferentiated somatoform disorder**
    Atypical somatoform disorder
    Somatoform disorder NOS
  - **300.89 Other somatoform disorders**
    Occupational neurosis, including writers' cramp
    Psychasthenia
    Psychasthenic neurosis

- **300.9 Unspecified nonpsychotic mental disorder**
  Psychoneurosis NOS

- **301 Personality disorders**
  Long-term patterns of thoughts and behaviors causing serious problems with relationships and work
  Includes character neurosis
  Use additional code to identify any associated neurosis or psychosis, or physical condition
  Excludes nonpsychotic personality disorder associated with organic brain syndromes (310.0–310.9)
  - **301.0 Paranoid personality disorder**
    Fanatic personality
    Paranoid personality (disorder)
    Paranoid traits
    Excludes acute paranoid reaction (298.3)
      alcoholic paranoia (291.5)
      paranoid schizophrenia (295.3)
      paranoid states (297.0–297.9)
  - **301.1 Affective personality disorder**
    Excludes affective psychotic disorders (296.0–296.9)
      neurasthenia (300.5)
      neurotic depression (300.4)
    - **301.10 Affective personality disorder, unspecified**
    - **301.11 Chronic hypomanic personality disorder**
      Chronic hypomanic disorder
      Hypomanic personality
    - **301.12 Chronic depressive personality disorder**
      Chronic depressive disorder
      Depressive character or personality
    - **301.13 Cyclothymic disorder**
      Cycloid personality
      Cyclothymia
      Cyclothymic personality
  - **301.2 Schizoid personality disorder**
    Excludes schizophrenia (295.0–295.9)
    - **301.20 Schizoid personality disorder, unspecified**
    - **301.21 Introverted personality**
    - **301.22 Schizotypal personality disorder**

MENTAL, BEHAVIORAL AND NEURODEVELOPMENTAL DISORDERS (290-319)

301.3 Explosive personality disorder
Aggressive:
    personality
    reaction
Aggressiveness
Emotional instability (excessive)
Pathological emotionality
Quarrelsomeness
> **Excludes** dyssocial personality (301.7)
>   hysterical neurosis (300.10–300.19)

301.4 Obsessive-compulsive personality disorder
Anancastic personality
Obsessional personality
> **Excludes** obsessive-compulsive disorder (300.3)
>   phobic state (300.20–300.29)

● **301.5 Histrionic personality disorder**
> **Excludes** hysterical neurosis (300.10–300.19)

    301.50 Histrionic personality disorder, unspecified
        Hysterical personality NOS

    301.51 Chronic factitious illness with physical symptoms
        Hospital addiction syndrome
        Multiple operations syndrome
        Munchausen syndrome

    301.59 Other histrionic personality disorder
        Personality: Personality:
            emotionally unstable   psychoinfantile
            labile

301.6 Dependent personality disorder
Asthenic personality
Inadequate personality
Passive personality
> **Excludes** neurasthenia (300.5)
>   passive-aggressive personality (301.84)

301.7 Antisocial personality disorder
Amoral personality
Asocial personality
Dyssocial personality
Personality disorder with predominantly sociopathic or asocial manifestation
> **Excludes** disturbance of conduct without specifiable personality disorder (312.0–312.9)
>   explosive personality (301.3)

Coding Clinic: 1984, Sept-Oct, P16

● **301.8 Other personality disorders**
    301.81 Narcissistic personality disorder
    301.82 Avoidant personality disorder
    301.83 Borderline personality disorder
    301.84 Passive-aggressive personality
    301.89 Other
        Personality: Personality:
            eccentric   masochistic
            "haltlose" type   psychoneurotic
            immature
> **Excludes** psychoinfantile personality (301.59)

301.9 Unspecified personality disorder
Pathological personality NOS
Personality disorder NOS
Psychopathic:
    constitutional state
    personality (disorder)

● **302 Sexual and gender identity disorders**
> **Excludes** sexual disorder manifest in:
>   organic brain syndrome (290.0–294.9, 310.0–310.9)
>   psychosis (295.0–298.9)

302.0 Ego-dystonic sexual orientation
Ego-dystonic lesbianism
Sexual orientation conflict disorder
> **Excludes** homosexual pedophilia (302.2)

302.1 Zoophilia
Bestiality

302.2 Pedophilia

302.3 Transvestic fetishism
> **Excludes** trans-sexualism (302.5)

302.4 Exhibitionism

● **302.5 Trans-sexualism**
Sex reassignment surgery status
> **Excludes** transvestism (302.3)

    302.50 With unspecified sexual history
    302.51 With asexual history
    302.52 With homosexual history
    302.53 With heterosexual history

302.6 Gender identity disorder in children
Check age: adolescents and adults separately classified under 302.85
Feminism in boys
Gender identity disorder NOS
> **Excludes** gender identity disorder in adult (302.85)
>   trans-sexualism (302.50–302.53)
>   transvestism (302.3)

● **302.7 Psychosexual dysfunction**
> **Excludes** decreased sexual desire NOS (799.81)
>   impotence of organic origin (607.84)
>   normal transient symptoms from ruptured hymen
>   transient or occasional failures of erection due to fatigue, anxiety, alcohol, or drugs

    302.70 Psychosexual dysfunction, unspecified
        Sexual dysfunction NOS

    302.71 Hypoactive sexual desire disorder
>   **Excludes** decreased sexual desire NOS (799.81)

    302.72 With inhibited sexual excitement
        Female sexual arousal disorder
        Frigidity
        Impotence
        Male erectile disorder

    302.73 Female orgasmic disorder
    302.74 Male orgasmic disorder
    302.75 Premature ejaculation
    302.76 Dyspareunia, psychogenic
    302.79 With other specified psychosexual dysfunctions
        Sexual aversion disorder

● **302.8 Other specified psychosexual disorders**
    302.81 Fetishism
    302.82 Voyeurism
    302.83 Sexual masochism
    302.84 Sexual sadism
    302.85 Gender identity disorder in adolescents or adults
        Use additional code to identify sex reassignment surgery status (302.5)
>   **Excludes** gender identity disorder NOS (302.6)
>   gender identity disorder in children (302.6)

    302.89 Other
        Frotteurism
        Nymphomania
        Satyriasis

302.9 Unspecified psychosexual disorder
Paraphilia NOS
Pathologic sexuality NOS
Sexual deviation NOS
Sexual disorder NOS

303 Alcohol dependence syndrome
Use additional code to identify any associated condition, as:
alcoholic psychoses (291.0–291.9)
drug dependence (304.0–304.9)
physical complications of alcohol, such as:
cerebral degeneration (331.7)
cirrhosis of liver (571.2)
epilepsy (345.0–345.9)
gastritis (535.3)
hepatitis (571.1)
liver damage NOS (571.3)

Excludes drunkenness NOS (305.0)

Coding Clinic: 2010, Q1, P3-4; 1995, Q3, P6

The following fifth-digit subclassification is for use with category 303:

0 unspecified	2 episodic
1 continuous	3 in remission

303.0 Acute alcoholic intoxication
[0-3] Acute drunkenness in alcoholism
Coding Clinic: 1985, July-Aug, P15

303.9 Other and unspecified alcohol dependence
[0-3] Chronic alcoholism
Dipsomania
Coding Clinic: 2012, Q2, P9-10; 2002, Q2, P4; Q1, P3-4; 1989, Q2, P9; 1985, Nov-Dec, P14

304 Drug dependence
For some "dependence" codes there is a corresponding "abuse" code. There is a point at which drug use crosses from "dependence" to "abuse." Check documentation or query provider for patient status.

Excludes nondependent abuse of drugs (305.1–305.9)

Coding Clinic: 2010, Q1, P3

The following fifth-digit subclassification is for use with category 304:

0 unspecified	2 episodic
1 continuous	3 in remission

304.0 Opioid type dependence
[0-3] Heroin
Meperidine
Methadone
Morphine
Opium
Opium alkaloids and their derivatives
Synthetics with morphine-like effects
Coding Clinic: 2011, Q1, P15; 2010, Q2, P13; 2006, Q2, P7; 1988, Q4, P8

304.1 Sedative, hypnotic or anxiolytic dependence
[0-3] Barbiturates
Nonbarbiturate sedatives and tranquilizers with a similar effect:
chlordiazepoxide
diazepam
glutethimide
meprobamate
methaqualone

304.2 Cocaine dependence
[0-3] Coca leaves and derivatives

304.3 Cannabis dependence
[0-3] *Code 305.2 is for abuse of cannabis.*
Hashish
Hemp
Marihuana

304.4 Amphetamine and other psychostimulant dependence
[0-3] Methylphenidate
Phenmetrazine

304.5 Hallucinogen dependence
[0-3] Dimethyltryptamine [DMT]
Lysergic acid diethylamide [LSD] and derivatives
Mescaline
Psilocybin

304.6 Other specified drug dependence
[0-3] Absinthe addiction
Glue sniffing
Inhalant dependence
Phencyclidine dependence

Excludes tobacco dependence (305.1)

304.7 Combinations of opioid type drug with any other
[0-3] Coding Clinic: 1986, Mar-April, P12

304.8 Combinations of drug dependence excluding opioid
[0-3] type drug
Coding Clinic: 1986, Mar-April, P12

304.9 Unspecified drug dependence
[0-3] Drug addiction NOS
Drug dependence NOS
Coding Clinic: 2012, Q2, P16-17; 2003, Q4, P103-104

305 Nondependent abuse of drugs
Note: Includes cases where a person, for whom no other diagnosis is possible, has come under medical care because of the maladaptive effect of a drug on which he is not dependent and that he has taken on his own initiative *(self-medicating)* to the detriment of his health or social functioning.

Excludes alcohol dependence syndrome (303.0–303.9)
drug dependence (304.0–304.9)
drug withdrawal syndrome (292.0)
poisoning by drugs or medicinal substances (960.0–979.9)

Coding Clinic: 2010, Q1, P5

The following fifth-digit subclassification is for use with codes 305.0, 305.2–305.9:

0 unspecified	2 episodic
1 continuous	3 in remission

305.0 Alcohol abuse
[0-3] Drunkenness NOS
Excessive drinking of alcohol NOS
"Hangover" (alcohol)
Inebriety NOS

Excludes acute alcohol intoxication in alcoholism (303.0)
alcoholic psychoses (291.0–291.9)

Coding Clinic: 2009, Q4, P98; Q1, P8; 1996, Q3, P16; 1985, July-Aug, P15

305.1 Tobacco use disorder
Tobacco dependence

Excludes history of tobacco use (V15.82)
smoking complicating pregnancy (649.0)
tobacco use disorder complicating pregnancy (649.0)

Coding Clinic: 2009, Q4, P98; Q1, P8; 1996, Q2, P10; 1984, Nov-Dec, P12

305.2 Cannabis abuse
[0-3] *Code 304.3 is for cannabis dependence.*

305.3 Hallucinogen abuse
[0-3] Acute intoxication from hallucinogens ["bad trips"]
LSD reaction

305.4 Sedative, hypnotic or anxiolytic abuse
[0-3]

305.5 Opioid abuse
[0-3]

305.6 Cocaine abuse
[0-3] Coding Clinic: 1993, Q1, P25; Q1, P25; 1988, Q4, P8

305.7 Amphetamine or related acting sympathomimetic
[0-3] abuse
Coding Clinic: 2003, Q2, P10,11x2

305.8 Antidepressant type abuse
[0-3]

305.9 Other, mixed, or unspecified drug abuse
[0-3] Caffeine intoxication
Inhalant abuse
"Laxative habit"
Misuse of drugs NOS
Nonprescribed use of drugs or patent medicinals
Phencyclidine abuse
Coding Clinic: 1999, Q3, P20; 1994, Q4, P36

- **306 Physiological malfunction arising from mental factors**
    - **Includes:** psychogenic:
        - physical symptoms not involving tissue damage
        - physiological manifestations not involving tissue damage
    - **Excludes:** hysteria (300.11–300.19)
        - physical symptoms secondary to a psychiatric disorder classified elsewhere
        - psychic factors associated with physical conditions involving tissue damage classified elsewhere (316)
        - specific nonpsychotic mental disorders following organic brain damage (310.0–310.9)

    - **306.0 Musculoskeletal**
        - Psychogenic paralysis
        - Psychogenic torticollis
        - **Excludes:** Gilles de la Tourette's syndrome (307.23)
            - paralysis as hysterical or conversion reaction (300.11)
            - tics (307.20–307.22)

    - **306.1 Respiratory**
        - Psychogenic:
            - air hunger
            - cough
            - hiccough
        - Psychogenic:
            - hyperventilation
            - yawning
        - **Excludes:** psychogenic asthma (316 and 493.9)

    - **306.2 Cardiovascular**
        - Cardiac neurosis
        - Cardiovascular neurosis
        - Neurocirculatory asthenia
        - Psychogenic cardiovascular disorder
        - **Excludes:** psychogenic paroxysmal tachycardia (316 and 427.2)
        - *Coding Clinic: 1985, July-Aug, P14*

    - **306.3 Skin**
        - Psychogenic pruritus
        - **Excludes:** psychogenic:
            - alopecia (316 and 704.00)
            - dermatitis (316 and 692.9)
            - eczema (316 and 691.8 or 692.9)
            - urticaria (316 and 708.0–708.9)

    - **306.4 Gastrointestinal**
        - Aerophagy
        - Cyclical vomiting, psychogenic
        - Diarrhea, psychogenic
        - Nervous gastritis
        - Psychogenic dyspepsia
        - **Excludes:** cyclical vomiting NOS (536.2)
            - associated with migraine (346.2)
            - globus hystericus (300.11)
            - mucous colitis (316 and 564.9)
            - psychogenic:
                - cardiospasm (316 and 530.0)
                - duodenal ulcer (316 and 532.0–532.9)
                - gastric ulcer (316 and 531.0–531.9)
                - peptic ulcer NOS (316 and 533.0–533.9)
                - vomiting NOS (307.54)
        - *Coding Clinic: 1989, Q2, P11*

    - **306.5 Genitourinary**
        - **Excludes:** enuresis, psychogenic (307.6)
            - frigidity (302.72)
            - impotence (302.72)
            - psychogenic dyspareunia (302.76)
        - **306.50 Psychogenic genitourinary malfunction, unspecified**
        - **306.51 Psychogenic vaginismus**
            - Functional vaginismus
        - **306.52 Psychogenic dysmenorrhea**
        - **306.53 Psychogenic dysuria**
        - **306.59 Other**

    - **306.6 Endocrine**
    - **306.7 Organs of special sense**
        - **Excludes:** hysterical blindness or deafness (300.11)
            - psychophysical visual disturbances (368.16)
    - **306.8 Other specified psychophysiological malfunction**
        - Bruxism
        - *Sleep-related bruxism, 327.53*
        - Teeth grinding
    - **306.9 Unspecified psychophysiological malfunction**
        - Psychophysiologic disorder NOS
        - Psychosomatic disorder NOS

- **307 Special symptoms or syndromes, not elsewhere classified**
    - **Note:** This category is intended for use if the psychopathology is manifested by a single specific symptom or group of symptoms which is not part of an organic illness or other mental disorder classifiable elsewhere.
    - **Excludes:** those due to mental disorders classified elsewhere
        - those of organic origin

    - **307.0 Adult onset fluency disorder**
        - **Excludes:** childhood onset fluency disorder (315.35)
            - dysphasia (784.59)
            - fluency disorder due to late effect of cerebrovascular accident (438.14)
            - fluency disorder in conditions classified elsewhere (784.52)
            - lisping or lalling (307.9)
            - retarded development of speech (315.31–315.39)

    - **307.1 Anorexia nervosa**
        - **Excludes:** eating disturbance NOS (307.50)
            - feeding problem (783.3)
                - of nonorganic origin (307.59)
            - loss of appetite (783.0)
                - of nonorganic origin (307.59)
        - *Coding Clinic: 2006, Q2, P12; 1989, Q4, P11*

    - **307.2 Tics**
        - **Excludes:** nail-biting or thumb-sucking (307.9)
            - stereotypes occurring in isolation (307.3)
            - tics of organic origin (333.3)
        - **307.20 Tic disorder, unspecified**
            - Tic disorder NOS
        - **307.21 Transient tic disorder**
        - **307.22 Chronic motor or vocal tic disorder**
        - **307.23 Tourette's disorder**
            - Motor-verbal tic disorder

    - **307.3 Stereotypic movement disorder**
        - Body-rocking
        - Head banging
        - Spasmus nutans
        - Stereotypes NOS
        - **Excludes:** tics (307.20–307.23)
            - of organic origin (333.3)

    - **307.4 Specific disorders of sleep of nonorganic origin**
        - **Excludes:** narcolepsy (347.00–347.11)
            - organic hypersomnia (327.10–327.19)
            - organic insomnia (327.00–327.09)
            - those of unspecified cause (780.50–780.59)
        - **307.40 Nonorganic sleep disorder, unspecified**
        - **307.41 Transient disorder of initiating or maintaining sleep**
            - Adjustment insomnia
            - Hyposomnia associated with acute or intermittent emotional reactions or conflicts
            - Insomnia associated with acute or intermittent emotional reactions or conflicts
            - Sleeplessness associated with acute or intermittent emotional reactions or conflicts

307.42 Persistent disorder of initiating or maintaining sleep
  Hyposomnia, insomnia, or sleeplessness associated with:
    anxiety
    conditioned arousal
    depression (major) (minor)
    psychosis
  Idiopathic insomnia
  Paradoxical insomnia
  Primary insomnia
  Psychophysiological insomnia

307.43 Transient disorder of initiating or maintaining wakefulness
  Hypersomnia associated with acute or intermittent emotional reactions or conflicts

307.44 Persistent disorder of initiating or maintaining wakefulness
  Hypersomnia associated with depression (major) (minor)
  Insufficient sleep syndrome
  Primary hypersomnia
  Excludes sleep deprivation (V69.4)

307.45 Circadian rhythm sleep disorder of nonorganic origin

307.46 Sleep arousal disorder
  Night terror disorder
  Night terrors
  Sleep terror disorder
  Sleepwalking
  Somnambulism

307.47 Other dysfunctions of sleep stages or arousal from sleep
  Nightmare disorder
  Nightmares:
    NOS
    REM-sleep type
  Sleep drunkenness

307.48 Repetitive intrusions of sleep
  Repetitive intrusion of sleep with:
    atypical polysomnographic features
    environmental disturbances
    repeated REM-sleep interruptions

307.49 Other
  "Short-sleeper"
  Subjective insomnia complaint

● **307.5** Other and unspecified disorders of eating
  Excludes anorexia:
    nervosa (307.1)
    of unspecified cause (783.0)
    overeating, of unspecified cause (783.6)
    vomiting:
      NOS (787.03)
      cyclical (536.2)
        associated with migraine (346.2)
      psychogenic (306.4)

■ **307.50** Eating disorder, unspecified
  Eating disorder NOS

307.51 Bulimia nervosa
  Overeating of nonorganic origin
  Coding Clinic: 2012, Q3, P9

307.52 Pica
  Perverted appetite of nonorganic origin
  Craving and eating substances such as paint, clay, or dirt to replace a nutritional deficit in the body

307.53 Rumination disorder
  Regurgitation, of nonorganic origin, of food with reswallowing
  Excludes obsessional rumination (300.3)

307.54 Psychogenic vomiting

307.59 Other
  Feeding disorder of infancy or early childhood of nonorganic origin
  Infantile feeding disturbances of nonorganic origin
  Loss of appetite of nonorganic origin

Item 5-3 Enuresis: Bed wetting by children at night. Causes can be either psychological or medical (diabetes, urinary tract infections, or abnormalities).
Encopresis: Overflow incontinence of bowels sometimes resulting from chronic constipation or fecal impaction. Check the documentation for additional diagnoses.

307.6 Enuresis
  Enuresis (primary) (secondary) of nonorganic origin
  Excludes enuresis of unspecified cause (788.3)

307.7 Encopresis
  Encopresis (continuous) (discontinuous) of nonorganic origin
  Excludes encopresis of unspecified cause (787.60-787.63)

● **307.8** Pain disorders related to psychological factors
  ■ **307.80** Psychogenic pain, site unspecified
  307.81 Tension headache
    Excludes headache:
      migraine (346.0–346.9)
      NOS (784.0)
      syndromes (339.00–339.89)
      tension type (339.10–339.12)
    Coding Clinic: 1985, Nov-Dec, P16
  ● **307.89** Other
    Code first to type or site of pain
    Excludes pain disorder exclusively attributed to psychological factors (307.80)
      psychogenic pain (307.80)

307.9 Other and unspecified special symptoms or syndromes, not elsewhere classified
  Communication disorder NOS
  Hair plucking
  Lalling
  Lisping
  Masturbation
  Nail-biting
  Thumb-sucking

● **308** Acute reaction to stress
  Includes catastrophic stress
    combat and operational stress reaction
    combat fatigue
    gross stress reaction (acute)
    transient disorders in response to exceptional physical or mental stress which usually subside within hours or days
  Excludes adjustment reaction or disorder (309.0–309.9)
    chronic stress reaction (309.1–309.9)

308.0 Predominant disturbance of emotions
  Anxiety as acute reaction to exceptional [gross] stress
  Emotional crisis as acute reaction to exceptional [gross] stress
  Panic state as acute reaction to exceptional [gross] stress

308.1 Predominant disturbance of consciousness
  Fugues as acute reaction to exceptional [gross] stress

308.2 Predominant psychomotor disturbance
  Agitation states as acute reaction to exceptional [gross] stress
  Stupor as acute reaction to exceptional [gross] stress

308.3 Other acute reactions to stress
  Acute situational disturbance
  Acute stress disorder
  Excludes prolonged posttraumatic emotional disturbance (309.81)

308.4 Mixed disorders as reaction to stress

■ **308.9** Unspecified acute reaction to stress

● **309 Adjustment reaction**
  Includes adjustment disorders
  reaction (adjustment) to chronic stress
  Excludes acute reaction to major stress (308.0–308.9)
  neurotic disorders (300.0–300.9)

  309.0 Adjustment disorder with depressed mood
  Grief reaction
  Excludes affective psychoses (296.0–296.9)
  neurotic depression (300.4)
  prolonged depressive reaction (309.1)
  psychogenic depressive psychosis (298.0)

  309.1 Prolonged depressive reaction
  Excludes affective psychoses (296.0–296.9)
  brief depressive reaction (309.0)
  neurotic depression (300.4)
  psychogenic depressive psychosis (298.0)

● **309.2 With predominant disturbance of other emotions**
  309.21 Separation anxiety disorder
  309.22 Emancipation disorder of adolescence and early adult life
  309.23 Specific academic or work inhibition
  309.24 Adjustment disorder with anxiety
  309.28 Adjustment disorder with mixed anxiety and depressed mood
  Adjustment reaction with anxiety and depression
  309.29 Other
  Culture shock

  309.3 Adjustment disorder with disturbance of conduct
  Conduct disturbance as adjustment reaction
  Destructiveness as adjustment reaction
  Excludes destructiveness in child (312.9)
  disturbance of conduct NOS (312.9)
  dyssocial behavior without manifest psychiatric disorder (V71.01–V71.02)
  personality disorder with predominantly sociopathic or asocial manifestations (301.7)

  309.4 Adjustment disorder with mixed disturbance of emotions and conduct

● **309.8 Other specified adjustment reactions**
  309.81 Posttraumatic stress disorder
  Chronic posttraumatic stress disorder
  Concentration camp syndrome
  Posttraumatic stress disorder NOS
  Post-Traumatic Stress Disorder (PTSD)
  Excludes acute stress disorder (308.3)
  posttraumatic brain syndrome:
  nonpsychotic (310.2)
  psychotic (293.0–293.9)
  309.82 Adjustment reaction with physical symptoms
  309.83 Adjustment reaction with withdrawal
  Elective mutism as adjustment reaction
  Hospitalism (in children) NOS
  309.89 Other

■ **309.9 Unspecified adjustment reaction**
  Adaptation reaction NOS
  Adjustment reaction NOS

● **310 Specific nonpsychotic mental disorders due to brain damage**
  Excludes neuroses, personality disorders, or other nonpsychotic conditions occurring in a form similar to that seen with functional disorders but in association with a physical condition (300.0–300.9, 301.0–301.9)

  310.0 Frontal lobe syndrome
  Lobotomy syndrome
  Postleucotomy syndrome [state]
  Excludes postcontusion syndrome (310.2)

● **310.1 Personality change due to conditions classified elsewhere**
  Cognitive or personality change of other type, of nonpsychotic severity
  Organic psychosyndrome of nonpsychotic severity
  Presbyophrenia NOS
  Senility with mental changes of nonpsychotic severity
  Excludes mild cognitive impairment (331.83)
  postconcussion syndrome (310.2)
  signs and symptoms involving emotional state (799.21-799.29)
  Coding Clinic: 2005, Q2, P6-7

  310.2 Postconcussion syndrome
  Postcontusion syndrome or encephalopathy
  Posttraumatic brain syndrome, nonpsychotic
  Status postcommotio cerebri
  Excludes any organic psychotic conditions following head injury (293.0–294.0)
  frontal lobe syndrome (310.0)
  postencephalitic syndrome (310.89)
  Use additional code to identify associated post-traumatic headache, if applicable (339.20-339.22)

● **310.8 Other specified nonpsychotic mental disorders following organic brain damage**
  310.81 Pseudobulbar affect
  Involuntary emotional expression disorder
  Code first underlying cause, if known, such as:
  amyotrophic lateral sclerosis (335.20)
  late effect of cerebrovascular accident (438.89)
  late effect of traumatic brain injury (907.0)
  multiple sclerosis (340)
  Coding Clinic: 2011, Q4, P97
  310.89 Other specified nonpsychotic mental disorders following organic brain damage
  Mild memory disturbance
  Other focal (partial) organic psychosyndromes
  Postencephalitic syndrome
  Excludes memory loss of unknown cause (780.93)

■ **310.9 Unspecified nonpsychotic mental disorder following organic brain damage**
  Coding Clinic: 2003, Q4, P103-104

  311 Depressive disorder, not elsewhere classified
  Depressive disorder NOS
  Depressive state NOS
  Depression NOS
  Excludes acute reaction to major stress with depressive symptoms (308.0)
  affective personality disorder (301.10–301.13)
  affective psychoses (296.0–296.9)
  brief depressive reaction (309.0)
  depressive states associated with stressful events (309.0–309.1)
  disturbance of emotions specific to childhood and adolescence, with misery and unhappiness (313.1)
  mixed adjustment reaction with depressive symptoms (309.4)
  neurotic depression (300.4)
  prolonged depressive adjustment reaction (309.1)
  psychogenic depressive psychosis (298.0)
  Coding Clinic: 2011, Q3, P6; 2003, Q4, P75-76

312 Disturbance of conduct, not elsewhere classified

Excludes: adjustment reaction with disturbance of conduct (309.3)
drug dependence (304.0–304.9)
dyssocial behavior without manifest psychiatric disorder (V71.01–V71.02)
personality disorder with predominantly sociopathic or asocial manifestations (301.7)
sexual deviations (302.0–302.9)

The following fifth-digit subclassification is for use with categories 312.0–312.2:

- 0 unspecified
- 1 mild
- 2 moderate
- 3 severe

312.0 Undersocialized conduct disorder, aggressive type
[0-3]
Aggressive outburst
Anger reaction
Unsocialized aggressive disorder

312.1 Undersocialized conduct disorder, unaggressive type
[0-3]
Childhood truancy, unsocialized
Solitary stealing
Tantrums

312.2 Socialized conduct disorder
[0-3]
Childhood truancy, socialized
Group delinquency

Excludes: gang activity without manifest psychiatric disorder (V71.01)

312.3 Disorders of impulse control, not elsewhere classified
- 312.30 Impulse control disorder, unspecified
- 312.31 Pathological gambling
- 312.32 Kleptomania *(stealing)*
- 312.33 Pyromania *(setting fires)*
- 312.34 Intermittent explosive disorder
- 312.35 Isolated explosive disorder
- 312.39 Other
  Trichotillomania
  Pulling or twisting hair until it falls out

312.4 Mixed disturbance of conduct and emotions
Neurotic delinquency

Excludes: compulsive conduct disorder (312.3)

312.8 Other specified disturbances of conduct, not elsewhere classified
- 312.81 Conduct disorder, childhood onset type
- 312.82 Conduct disorder, adolescent onset type
- 312.89 Other conduct disorder
  Conduct disorder of unspecified onset

312.9 Unspecified disturbance of conduct
Delinquency (juvenile)
Disruptive behavior disorder NOS

313 Disturbance of emotions specific to childhood and adolescence

Excludes: adjustment reaction (309.0–309.9)
emotional disorder of neurotic type (300.0–300.9)
masturbation, nail-biting, thumb-sucking, and other isolated symptoms (307.0–307.9)

313.0 Overanxious disorder
Anxiety and fearfulness of childhood and adolescence
Overanxious disorder of childhood and adolescence

Excludes: abnormal separation anxiety (309.21)
anxiety states (300.00–300.09)
hospitalism in children (309.83)
phobic state (300.20–300.29)

313.1 Misery and unhappiness disorder

Excludes: depressive neurosis (300.4)

313.2 Sensitivity, shyness, and social withdrawal disorder

Excludes: infantile autism (299.0)
schizoid personality (301.20–301.22)
schizophrenia (295.0–295.9)

- 313.21 Shyness disorder of childhood
  Sensitivity reaction of childhood or adolescence
- 313.22 Introverted disorder of childhood
  Social withdrawal of childhood or adolescence
  Withdrawal reaction of childhood or adolescence
- 313.23 Selective mutism

  Excludes: elective mutism as adjustment reaction (309.83)

313.3 Relationship problems
Sibling jealousy

Excludes: relationship problems associated with aggression, destruction, or other forms of conduct disturbance (312.0–312.9)

313.8 Other or mixed emotional disturbances of childhood or adolescence
- 313.81 Oppositional defiant disorder
- 313.82 Identity disorder
  Identity problem
- 313.83 Academic underachievement disorder
- 313.89 Other
  Reactive attachment disorder of infancy or early childhood

313.9 Unspecified emotional disturbance of childhood or adolescence
Mental disorder of infancy, childhood or adolescence NOS

314 Hyperkinetic syndrome of childhood

Excludes: hyperkinesis as symptom of underlying disorder-code the underlying disorder

314.0 Attention deficit disorder *(ADD)*
Adult
Child

- 314.00 Without mention of hyperactivity
  Predominantly inattentive type
  Coding Clinic: 2012, Q3, P19; 1997, Q1, P8-9

- 314.01 With hyperactivity
  Attention deficit disorder with hyperactivity = ADHD
  Combined type
  Overactivity NOS
  Predominantly hyperactive/impulsive type
  Simple disturbance of attention with overactivity
  Coding Clinic: 2012, Q3, P19; 1997, Q1, P8-9

314.1 Hyperkinesis with developmental delay
Developmental disorder of hyperkinesis
Use additional code to identify any associated neurological disorder

314.2 Hyperkinetic conduct disorder
Hyperkinetic conduct disorder without developmental delay

Excludes: hyperkinesis with significant delays in specific skills (314.1)

314.8 Other specified manifestations of hyperkinetic syndrome

314.9 Unspecified hyperkinetic syndrome
Hyperkinetic reaction of childhood or adolescence NOS
Hyperkinetic syndrome NOS

- **315 Specific delays in development**
  - **Excludes** *that due to a neurological disorder (320.0–389.9)*
  - **315.0 Specific reading disorder**
    - **315.00** Reading disorder, unspecified
    - 315.01 Alexia
    - 315.02 Developmental dyslexia
    - 315.09 Other
      - Specific spelling difficulty
  - 315.1 Mathematics disorder
    - Dyscalculia
  - 315.2 Other specific learning difficulties
    - Disorder of written expression
    - **Excludes** *specific arithmetical disorder (315.1)*
      specific reading disorder (315.00–315.09)
  - **315.3 Developmental speech or language disorder**
    - 315.31 Expressive language disorder
      - Developmental aphasia
      - Word deafness
      - **Excludes** *acquired aphasia (784.3)*
        elective mutism (309.83, 313.0, 313.23)
    - 315.32 Mixed receptive-expressive language disorder
      - Central auditory processing disorder
      - **Excludes** *acquired auditory processing disorder (388.45)*
      - **Coding Clinic: 2005, Q2, P5-6**
    - 315.34 Speech and language developmental delay due to hearing loss
      - **Coding Clinic: 2007, Q4, P80-81**
    - 315.35 Childhood onset fluency disorder
      - Cluttering NOS
      - Stuttering NOS
      - **Excludes** *adult onset fluency disorder (307.0)*
        fluency disorder due to late effect of cerebrovascular accident (438.14)
        fluency disorder in conditions classified elsewhere (784.52)
    - 315.39 Other
      - Developmental articulation disorder
      - Dyslalia
      - Phonological disorder
      - **Excludes** *lisping and lalling (307.9)*
      - **Coding Clinic: 2007, Q3, P9-10**
  - 315.4 Developmental coordination disorder
    - Clumsiness syndrome
    - Dyspraxia syndrome
    - Specific motor development disorder
  - 315.5 Mixed development disorder
    - **Coding Clinic: 2002, Q2, P11**
  - 315.8 Other specified delays in development
  - **315.9 Unspecified delay in development**
    - Developmental disorder NOS
    - Learning disorder NOS
- 316 Psychic factors associated with diseases classified elsewhere
  - Psychologic factors in physical conditions classified elsewhere
  - Use additional code to identify the associated physical condition, as:
    - psychogenic:
      - asthma (493.9)
      - dermatitis (692.9)
      - duodenal ulcer (532.0–532.9)
      - eczema (691.8, 692.9)
      - gastric ulcer (531.0–531.9)
      - mucous colitis (564.9)
      - paroxysmal tachycardia (427.2)
      - ulcerative colitis (556)
      - urticaria (708.0–708.9)
    - psychosocial dwarfism (259.4)
  - **Excludes** *physical symptoms and physiological malfunctions, not involving tissue damage, of mental origin (306.0–306.9)*

INTELLECTUAL DISABILITIES (317-319)

Use additional code(s) to identify any associated psychiatric or physical condition(s)

- 317 Mild intellectual disabilities
  - High-grade defect
  - IQ 50–70
  - Mild mental subnormality
- **318 Other specified intellectual disabilities**
  - 318.0 Moderate intellectual disabilities
    - IQ 35–49
    - Moderate mental subnormality
  - 318.1 Severe intellectual disabilities
    - IQ 20–34
    - Severe mental subnormality
  - 318.2 Profound intellectual disabilities
    - IQ under 20
    - Profound mental subnormality
- **319 Unspecified intellectual disabilities**
  - Mental deficiency NOS
  - Mental subnormality NOS

(See Plate 164 on page NAP-2.)

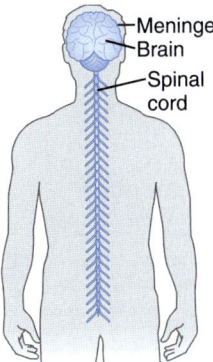

Figure 6-1 The brain and spinal cord make up the central nervous system.

Item 6-1 The two major classifications of the nervous system are the peripheral nervous system and the central nervous system (CNS). The central nervous system is comprised of the brain and the spinal cord. The peripheral nervous system is comprised of the parasympathetic and sympathetic systems. **Encephalitis** is the swelling of the brain. **Meningitis** is swelling of the covering of the brain, the meninges. Types and causes of brain infections are:

Type	Cause
purulent	bacterial
aseptic/abacterial	viral
chronic meningitis	mycobacterial and fungal

6. DISEASES OF THE NERVOUS SYSTEM AND SENSE ORGANS (320–389)

INFLAMMATORY DISEASES OF THE CENTRAL NERVOUS SYSTEM (320–326)

● **320 Bacterial meningitis**
Infection of cerebrospinal fluid surrounding spinal cord and brain
Includes arachnoiditis bacterial
leptomeningitis bacterial
meningitis bacterial
meningoencephalitis bacterial
meningomyelitis bacterial
pachymeningitis bacterial

320.0 Hemophilus meningitis
Meningitis due to Hemophilus influenzae [H. influenzae]

320.1 Pneumococcal meningitis

320.2 Streptococcal meningitis

320.3 Staphylococcal meningitis

● ***320.7 Meningitis in other bacterial diseases classified elsewhere***
Code first underlying disease as:
actinomycosis (039.8)
listeriosis (027.0)
typhoid fever (002.0)
whooping cough (033.0–033.9)
Excludes meningitis (in):
epidemic (036.0)
gonococcal (098.82)
meningococcal (036.0)
salmonellosis (003.21)
syphilis:
NOS (094.2)
congenital (090.42)
meningovascular (094.2)
secondary (091.81)
tuberculosis (013.0)

● **320.8 Meningitis due to other specified bacteria**
320.81 Anaerobic meningitis
Bacteroides (fragilis)
Gram-negative anaerobes

320.82 Meningitis due to gram-negative bacteria, not elsewhere classified
Aerobacter aerogenes
Escherichia coli [E. coli]
Friedlander bacillus
Klebsiella pneumoniae
Proteus morganii
Pseudomonas
Excludes gram-negative anaerobes (320.81)
Coding Clinic: 2011, Q4, P155

320.89 Meningitis due to other specified bacteria
Bacillus pyocyaneus

320.9 Meningitis due to unspecified bacterium
Meningitis: Meningitis:
  bacterial NOS   pyogenic NOS
  purulent NOS   suppurative NOS

● **321 Meningitis due to other organisms**
Includes arachnoiditis due to organisms other than bacteria
leptomeningitis due to organisms other than bacteria
meningitis due to organisms other than bacteria
pachymeningitis due to organisms other than bacteria

● **321.0 Cryptococcal meningitis**
Code first underlying disease (117.5)

● **321.1 Meningitis in other fungal diseases**
Code first underlying disease (110.0–118)
Excludes meningitis in:
candidiasis (112.83)
coccidioidomycosis (114.2)
histoplasmosis (115.01, 115.11, 115.91)

● **321.2 Meningitis due to viruses not elsewhere classified**
Code first underlying disease, as:
meningitis due to arbovirus (060.0–066.9)
Excludes meningitis (due to):
abacterial (047.0–047.9)
adenovirus (049.1)
aseptic NOS (047.9)
Coxsackie (virus) (047.0)
ECHO virus (047.1)
enterovirus (047.0–047.9)
herpes simplex virus (054.72)
herpes zoster virus (053.0)
lymphocytic choriomeningitis virus (049.0)
mumps (072.1)
viral NOS (047.9)
meningo-eruptive syndrome (047.1)
Coding Clinic: 2004, Q4, P50-52

● **321.3 Meningitis due to trypanosomiasis**
Code first underlying disease (086.0–086.9)

● **321.4 Meningitis in sarcoidosis**
Code first underlying disease (135)

● **321.8 Meningitis due to other nonbacterial organisms classified elsewhere**
Code first underlying disease
Excludes leptospiral meningitis (100.81)

● **322 Meningitis of unspecified cause**
    Includes: arachnoiditis with no organism specified as cause
    leptomeningitis with no organism specified as cause
    meningitis with no organism specified as cause
    pachymeningitis with no organism specified as cause

   322.0 Nonpyogenic meningitis
        Meningitis with clear cerebrospinal fluid
   322.1 Eosinophilic meningitis
   322.2 Chronic meningitis
   322.9 Meningitis, unspecified

● **323 Encephalitis, myelitis, and encephalomyelitis**
    Includes: acute disseminated encephalomyelitis
    meningoencephalitis, except bacterial
    meningomyelitis, except bacterial
    myelitis:
        ascending
        transverse
    Excludes: *acute transverse myelitis NOS (341.20)*
    acute transverse myelitis in conditions classified elsewhere (341.21)
    bacterial:
        meningoencephalitis (320.0–320.9)
        meningomyelitis (320.0–320.9)
    idiopathic transverse myelitis (341.22)
    Coding Clinic: 2006, Q4, P58-63

● **323.0 Encephalitis, myelitis, and encephalomyelitis in viral diseases classified elsewhere**
    Code first underlying disease, as:
        cat-scratch disease (078.3)
        human immunodeficiency virus [HIV] disease (042)
        infectious mononucleosis (075)
        ornithosis (073.7)

   ● **323.01 Encephalitis and encephalomyelitis in viral diseases classified elsewhere**
        Excludes: *encephalitis (in):*
            arthropod-borne viral (062.0–064)
            herpes simplex (054.3)
            mumps (072.2)
            other viral diseases of central nervous system (049.8–049.9)
            poliomyelitis (045.0–045.9)
            rubella (056.01)
            slow virus infections of central nervous system (046.0–046.9)
            viral NOS (049.9)
            West Nile (066.41)
        Coding Clinic: 2010, Q3, P14

   ● **323.02 Myelitis in viral diseases classified elsewhere**
        Excludes: *myelitis (in):*
            herpes simplex (054.74)
            herpes zoster (053.14)
            other viral diseases of central nervous system (049.8–049.9)
            poliomyelitis (045.0–045.9)
            rubella (056.01)

● **323.1 Encephalitis, myelitis, and encephalomyelitis in rickettsial diseases classified elsewhere**
    Code first underlying disease (080–083.9)

● **323.2 Encephalitis, myelitis, and encephalomyelitis in protozoal diseases classified elsewhere**
    Code first underlying disease, as:
        malaria (084.0–084.9)
        trypanosomiasis (086.0–086.9)

● **323.4 Other encephalitis, myelitis, and encephalomyelitis due to other infections classified elsewhere**
    Code first underlying disease

   ● **323.41 Other encephalitis and encephalomyelitis due to other infections classified elsewhere**
        Excludes: *encephalitis (in):*
            meningococcal (036.1)
            syphilis:
                NOS (094.81)
                congenital (090.41)
            toxoplasmosis (130.0)
            tuberculosis (013.6)
            meningoencephalitis due to free-living ameba [Naegleria] (136.29)

   ● **323.42 Other myelitis due to other infections classified elsewhere**
        Excludes: *myelitis (in):*
            syphilis (094.89)
            tuberculosis (013.6)

● **323.5 Encephalitis, myelitis, and encephalomyelitis following immunization procedures**
    Use additional E code to identify vaccine

   323.51 Encephalitis and encephalomyelitis following immunization procedures
        Encephalitis postimmunization or postvaccinal
        Encephalomyelitis postimmunization or postvaccinal

   323.52 Myelitis following immunization procedures
        Myelitis postimmunization or postvaccinal

● **323.6 Postinfectious encephalitis, myelitis, and encephalomyelitis**
    Code first underlying disease

   ● **323.61 Infectious acute disseminated encephalomyelitis (ADEM)**
        Acute necrotizing hemorrhagic encephalopathy
        Excludes: *noninfectious acute disseminated encephalomyelitis (323.81)*

   ● **323.62 Other postinfectious encephalitis and encephalomyelitis**
        Excludes: *encephalitis:*
            postchickenpox (052.0)
            postmeasles (055.0)

   ● **323.63 Postinfectious myelitis**

● **323.7 Toxic encephalitis, myelitis, and encephalomyelitis**
    Code first underlying cause, as:
        carbon tetrachloride (982.1)
        hydroxyquinoline derivatives (961.3)
        lead (984.0–984.9)
        mercury (985.0)
        thallium (985.8)

   ● **323.71 Toxic encephalitis and encephalomyelitis**
   ● **323.72 Toxic myelitis**

● **323.8 Other causes of encephalitis, myelitis, and encephalomyelitis**
    Coding Clinic: 1997, Q2, P8-9

   323.81 Other causes of encephalitis and encephalomyelitis
        Noninfectious acute disseminated encephalomyelitis (ADEM)
        Coding Clinic: 2011, Q1, P12; 2010, Q3, P16

   323.82 Other causes of myelitis
        Transverse myelitis NOS

323.9 Unspecified cause of encephalitis, myelitis, and encephalomyelitis
    Coding Clinic: 2010, Q3, P15; 2006, Q1, P8

Item 6-2 Encephalitis is an inflammation of the brain most often caused by a virus but may also be caused by a bacteria and most commonly transmitted by a mosquito. **Myelitis** is an inflammation of the spinal cord that may disrupt CNS function. Untreated myelitis may rapidly lead to permanent damage to the spinal cord. **Encephalomyelitis** is a general term for an inflammation of the brain and spinal cord.

324 Intracranial and intraspinal abscess
Accumulation of pus in either brain or spinal cord

324.0 Intracranial abscess
Abscess (embolic):
- cerebellar
- cerebral

Abscess (embolic) of brain [any part]:
- epidural
- extradural
- otogenic
- subdural

Excludes *tuberculous (013.3)*

324.1 Intraspinal abscess
Abscess (embolic) of spinal cord [any part]:
- epidural
- extradural
- subdural

Excludes *tuberculous (013.5)*

324.9 Of unspecified site
Extradural or subdural abscess NOS

325 Phlebitis and thrombophlebitis of intracranial venous sinuses
Embolism of cavernous, lateral, or other intracranial or unspecified intracranial venous sinus
Endophlebitis of cavernous, lateral, or other intracranial or unspecified intracranial venous sinus
Phlebitis, septic or suppurative of cavernous, lateral, or other intracranial or unspecified intracranial venous sinus
Thrombophlebitis of cavernous, lateral, or other intracranial or unspecified intracranial venous sinus
Thrombosis of cavernous, lateral, or other intracranial or unspecified intracranial venous sinus

Excludes *that specified as:*
complicating pregnancy, childbirth, or the puerperium (671.5)
of nonpyogenic origin (437.6)

326 Late effects of intracranial abscess or pyogenic infection
Note: This category is to be used to indicate conditions whose primary classification is to 320–325 [excluding 320.7, 321.0–321.8, 323.01–323.42, 323.61–323.72] as the cause of late effects, themselves classifiable elsewhere. The "late effects" include conditions specified as such, or as sequelae, which may occur at any time after the resolution of the causal condition.

Use additional code to identify condition, as:
- hydrocephalus (331.4)
- paralysis (342.0–342.9, 344.0–344.9)

ORGANIC SLEEP DISORDERS (327)

327 Organic sleep disorders
Involve difficulties of sleep at all levels, including difficulty falling or staying asleep, falling asleep at inappropriate times, excessive total sleep time, or abnormal behaviors associated with sleep

327.0 Organic disorders of initiating and maintaining sleep [Organic insomnia]
Excludes *insomnia NOS (780.52)*
insomnia not due to a substance or known physiological condition (307.41–307.42)
insomnia with sleep apnea NOS (780.51)

327.00 Organic insomnia, unspecified
327.01 Insomnia due to medical condition classified elsewhere
Code first underlying condition
Excludes *insomnia due to mental disorder (327.02)*

327.02 Insomnia due to mental disorder
Code first mental disorder
Excludes *alcohol induced insomnia (291.82)*
drug induced insomnia (292.85)

327.09 Other organic insomnia

327.1 Organic disorder of excessive somnolence [Organic hypersomnia]
Excludes *hypersomnia NOS (780.54)*
hypersomnia not due to a substance or known physiological condition (307.43–307.44)
hypersomnia with sleep apnea NOS (780.53)

327.10 Organic hypersomnia, unspecified
327.11 Idiopathic hypersomnia with long sleep time
327.12 Idiopathic hypersomnia without long sleep time
327.13 Recurrent hypersomnia
Kleine-Levin syndrome
Menstrual related hypersomnia

327.14 Hypersomnia due to medical condition classified elsewhere
Code first underlying condition
Excludes *hypersomnia due to mental disorder (327.15)*

327.15 Hypersomnia due to mental disorder
Code first mental disorder
Excludes *alcohol induced insomnia (291.82)*
drug induced insomnia (292.85)

327.19 Other organic hypersomnia

327.2 Organic sleep apnea
Characterized by episodes in which breathing stops during sleep, resulting in a lack of prolonged deep sleep and excessive daytime sleepiness

Excludes *Cheyne-Stokes breathing (786.04)*
hypersomnia with sleep apnea NOS (780.53)
insomnia with sleep apnea NOS (780.51)
sleep apnea in newborn (770.81–770.82)
sleep apnea NOS (780.57)

327.20 Organic sleep apnea, unspecified
327.21 Primary central sleep apnea
327.22 High altitude periodic breathing
327.23 Obstructive sleep apnea (adult) (pediatric)
327.24 Idiopathic sleep related nonobstructive alveolar hypoventilation
Sleep related hypoxia

327.25 Congenital central alveolar hypoventilation syndrome

327.26 Sleep related hypoventilation/hypoxemia in conditions classifiable elsewhere
Code first underlying condition

327.27 Central sleep apnea in conditions classified elsewhere
Code first underlying condition

327.29 Other organic sleep apnea

327.3 Circadian rhythm sleep disorder
Involves one of the sleep/wake regulating hormones. The inability to sleep results from a mismatch between the body's internal clock and the external 24-hour schedule.

Organic disorder of sleep wake cycle
Organic disorder of sleep wake schedule

Excludes *alcohol induced circadian rhythm sleep disorder (291.82)*
circadian rhythm sleep disorder of nonorganic origin (307.45)
disruption of 24 hour sleep wake cycle NOS (780.55)
drug induced circadian rhythm sleep disorder (292.85)

327.30 Circadian rhythm sleep disorder, unspecified
327.31 Circadian rhythm sleep disorder, delayed sleep phase type
327.32 Circadian rhythm sleep disorder, advanced sleep phase type
327.33 Circadian rhythm sleep disorder, irregular sleep-wake type
327.34 Circadian rhythm sleep disorder, free-running type

327.35 Circadian rhythm sleep disorder, jet lag type
327.36 Circadian rhythm sleep disorder, shift work type
● **327.37** *Circadian rhythm sleep disorder in conditions classified elsewhere*
   Code first *underlying condition*
327.39 Other circadian rhythm sleep disorder
● **327.4** Organic parasomnia
   Excludes alcohol induced parasomnia (291.82)
             drug induced parasomnia (292.85)
             parasomnia not due to a known physiological condition (307.47)
▪ **327.40** Organic parasomnia, unspecified
327.41 Confusional arousals
327.42 REM sleep behavior disorder
327.43 Recurrent isolated sleep paralysis
● **327.44** *Parasomnia in conditions classified elsewhere*
   Code first *underlying condition*
327.49 Other organic parasomnia
● **327.5** Organic sleep related movement disorders
   Excludes restless legs syndrome (333.94)
             sleep related movement disorder NOS (780.58)
327.51 Periodic limb movement disorder
   Periodic limb movement sleep disorder
327.52 Sleep related leg cramps
327.53 Sleep related bruxism
327.59 Other organic sleep related movement disorders
327.8 Other organic sleep disorders
   Coding Clinic: 2007, Q2, P7-8

HEREDITARY AND DEGENERATIVE DISEASES OF THE CENTRAL NERVOUS SYSTEM (330–337)

   Excludes hepatolenticular degeneration (275.1)
             multiple sclerosis (340)
             other demyelinating diseases of central nervous system (341.0–341.9)

● **330** Cerebral degenerations usually manifest in childhood
   Use additional code to identify associated intellectual disabilities
330.0 Leukodystrophy
   Krabbe's disease
   Leukodystrophy:
      NOS
      globoid cell
      metachromatic
      sudanophilic
   Pelizaeus-Merzbacher disease
   Sulfatide lipidosis
330.1 Cerebral lipidoses
   Amaurotic (familial) idiocy
   Disease:
      Batten
      Jansky-Bielschowsky
      Kufs'
      Spielmeyer-Vogt
      Tay-Sachs
   Gangliosidosis
● **330.2** *Cerebral degeneration in generalized lipidoses*
   Code first *underlying disease, as:*
      Fabry's disease (272.7)
      Gaucher's disease (272.7)
      Niemann-Pick disease (272.7)
      sphingolipidosis (272.7)
● **330.3** *Cerebral degeneration of childhood in other diseases classified elsewhere*
   Code first *underlying disease, as:*
      Hunter's disease (277.5)
      mucopolysaccharidosis (277.5)

330.8 Other specified cerebral degenerations in childhood
   Alpers' disease or gray-matter degeneration
   Infantile necrotizing encephalomyelopathy
   Leigh's disease
   Subacute necrotizing encephalopathy or encephalomyelopathy
   Coding Clinic: 1995, Q1, P9
▪ **330.9** Unspecified cerebral degeneration in childhood
● **331** Other cerebral degenerations
   Use additional code, where applicable, to identify dementia:
      with behavioral disturbance (294.11)
      without behavioral disturbance (294.10)
331.0 Alzheimer's disease
   Coding Clinic: 2000, Q4, P40-41; 1999, Q4, P7; 1994, Q2, P10-11; Q1, P21; 1984, Nov-Dec, P20
● **331.1** Frontotemporal dementia
   331.11 Pick's disease
      Coding Clinic: 2003, Q4, P57-58
   331.19 Other frontotemporal dementia
      Frontal dementia
      Coding Clinic: 2003, Q4, P57-58
331.2 Senile degeneration of brain
   Excludes senility NOS (797)
331.3 Communicating hydrocephalus
   Secondary normal pressure hydrocephalus
   Excludes congenital hydrocephalus (742.3)
             idiopathic normal pressure hydrocephalus (331.5)
             normal pressure hydrocephalus (331.5)
             spina bifida with hydrocephalus (741.0)
   Coding Clinic: 2007, Q4, P74-75; 1985, Sept-Oct, P12
331.4 Obstructive hydrocephalus
   Acquired hydrocephalus NOS
   Excludes congenital hydrocephalus (742.3)
             idiopathic normal pressure hydrocephalus (331.5)
             normal pressure hydrocephalus (331.5)
             spina bifida with hydrocephalus (741.0)
   Coding Clinic: 2007, Q4, P74-75; 2003, Q4, P106-107; 1999, Q1, P9-10
331.5 Idiopathic normal pressure hydrocephalus (INPH)
   Normal pressure hydrocephalus NOS
   Excludes congenital hydrocephalus (742.3)
             secondary normal pressure hydrocephalus (331.3)
             spina bifida with hydrocephalus (741.0)
   Coding Clinic: 2007, Q4, P74-75
331.6 Corticobasal degeneration
● **331.7** *Cerebral degeneration in diseases classified elsewhere*
   Code first *underlying disease, as:*
      alcoholism (303.0–303.9)
      beriberi (265.0)
      cerebrovascular disease (430–438)
      congenital hydrocephalus (741.0, 742.3)
      neoplastic disease (140.0–239.9)
      myxedema (244.0–244.9)
      vitamin B12 deficiency (266.2)
   Excludes cerebral degeneration in:
             Jakob-Creutzfeldt disease (046.11–046.19)
             progressive multifocal leukoencephalopathy (046.3)
             subacute spongiform encephalopathy (046.1)
● **331.8** Other cerebral degeneration
   331.81 Reye's syndrome
   331.82 Dementia with Lewy bodies
      Dementia with Parkinsonism
      Lewy body dementia
      Lewy body disease
      Coding Clinic: 2003, Q4, P57-58

Item 6–3 Leukodystrophy is characterized by degeneration and/or failure of the myelin formation of the central nervous system and sometimes of the peripheral nervous system. The disease is inherited and progressive.

Item 6–4 Pick's disease is the atrophy of the frontal and temporal lobes, causing dementia; **Alzheimer's** is characterized by a more diffuse cerebral atrophy.

331.83 Mild cognitive impairment, so stated
    Excludes altered mental status (780.97)
        cerebral degeneration (331.0–331.9)
        change in mental status (780.9)
        cognitive deficits following (late effects of) cerebral hemorrhage or infarction (438.0)
        cognitive impairment due to intracranial or head injury (850–854, 959.01)
        cognitive impairment due to late effect of intracranial injury (907.0)
        cognitive impairment due to skull fracture (800-801, 803-804)
        dementia (290.0-290.43, 294.20-294.21)
        mild memory disturbance (310.89)
        neurologic neglect syndrome (781.8)
        personality change, nonpsychotic (310.1)
    Coding Clinic: 2006, Q4, P75-76

331.89 Other
    Cerebral ataxia

331.9 Cerebral degeneration, unspecified

332 Parkinson's disease
    Movement disorder (chronic or progressive); cause unknown, and no cure
    Excludes dementia with Parkinsonism (331.82)

332.0 Paralysis agitans
    Parkinsonism or Parkinson's disease:
        NOS
        idiopathic
        primary

332.1 Secondary Parkinsonism
    Neuroleptic-induced Parkinsonism
    Parkinsonism due to drugs
    Use additional E code to identify drug, if drug-induced
    Excludes Parkinsonism (in):
        Huntington's disease (333.4)
        progressive supranuclear palsy (333.0)
        Shy-Drager syndrome (333.0)
        syphilitic (094.82)

333 Other extrapyramidal disease and abnormal movement disorders
    Includes other forms of extrapyramidal, basal ganglia, or striatopallidal disease
    Excludes abnormal movements of head NOS (781.0)
        sleep related movement disorders (327.51–327.59)

333.0 Other degenerative diseases of the basal ganglia
    Atrophy or degeneration:
        olivopontocerebellar [Déjérine-Thomas syndrome]
        pigmentary pallidal [Hallervorden-Spatz disease]
        striatonigral
    Parkinsonian syndrome associated with:
        idiopathic orthostatic hypotension
        symptomatic orthostatic hypotension
    Progressive supranuclear ophthalmoplegia
    Shy-Drager syndrome
    Coding Clinic: 1996, Q2, P8-9

333.1 Essential and other specified forms of tremor
    Benign essential tremor
    Familial tremor
    Medication-induced postural tremor
    Use additional E code to identify drug, if drug-induced
    Excludes tremor NOS (781.0)

333.2 Myoclonus
    Familial essential myoclonus
    Palatal myoclonus
    Excludes progressive myoclonic epilepsy (345.1)
        Unverricht-Lundborg disease (345.1)
    Use additional E code to identify drug, if drug-induced
    Coding Clinic: 1997, Q3, P5; 1987, Mar-April, P12

Item 6–5 **Huntington's chorea** is an inherited degenerative disorder of the central nervous system and is characterized by ceaseless, jerky movements and progressive cognitive and behavioral deterioration.

333.3 Tics of organic origin
    Excludes Gilles de la Tourette's syndrome (307.23)
        habit spasm (307.22)
        tic NOS (307.20)
    Use additional E code to identify drug, if drug-induced

333.4 Huntington's chorea

333.5 Other choreas
    Hemiballism(us)
    Paroxysmal choreo-athetosis
    Excludes Sydenham's or rheumatic chorea (392.0–392.9)
    Use additional E code to identify drug, if drug-induced

333.6 Genetic torsion dystonia
    Dystonia:
        deformans progressiva
        musculorum deformans
    (Schwalbe-) Ziehen-Oppenheim disease
    Coding Clinic: 2006, Q4, P76-78

333.7 Acquired torsion dystonia
    Coding Clinic: 2006, Q4, P76-78

333.71 Athetoid cerebral palsy
    Double athetosis (syndrome)
    Vogt's disease
    Excludes infantile cerebral palsy (343.0–343.9)

333.72 Acute dystonia due to drugs
    Acute dystonic reaction due to drugs
    Neuroleptic-induced acute dystonia
    Use additional E code to identify drug
    Excludes blepharospasm due to drugs (333.85)
        orofacial dyskinesia due to drugs (333.85)
        secondary Parkinsonism (332.1)
        subacute dyskinesia due to drugs (333.85)
        tardive dyskinesia (333.85)

333.79 Other acquired torsion dystonia

333.8 Fragments of torsion dystonia
    Use additional E code to identify drug, if drug-induced

333.81 Blepharospasm
    Excludes blepharospasm due to drugs (333.85)

333.82 Orofacial dyskinesia
    Excludes orofacial dyskinesia due to drugs (333.85)

333.83 Spasmodic torticollis
    Excludes torticollis:
        NOS (723.5)
        hysterical (300.11)
        psychogenic (306.0)

333.84 Organic writers' cramp
    Excludes psychogenic (300.89)

333.85 Subacute dyskinesia due to drugs
    Blepharospasm due to drugs
    Orofacial dyskinesia due to drugs
    Tardive dyskinesia
    Use additional E code to identify drug
    Excludes acute dystonia due to drugs (333.72)
        acute dystonic reaction due to drugs (333.72)
        secondary Parkinsonism (332.1)
    Coding Clinic: 2006, Q4, P76-78

333.89 Other

- **333.9 Other and unspecified extrapyramidal diseases and abnormal movement disorders**
    - **333.90 Unspecified extrapyramidal disease and abnormal movement disorder**
        Medication-induced movement disorders NOS
        Use additional E code to identify drug, if drug-induced
    - 333.91 Stiff-man syndrome
    - 333.92 Neuroleptic malignant syndrome
        Use additional E code to identify drug
        Excludes: neuroleptic induced Parkinsonism (332.1)
    - 333.93 Benign shuddering attacks
    - 333.94 Restless legs syndrome (RLS)
        Coding Clinic: 2006, Q4, P79
    - 333.99 Other
        Neuroleptic-induced acute akathisia
        Use additional E code to identify drug, if drug-induced
        Coding Clinic: 2004, Q2, P12

- **334 Spinocerebellar disease**
    Group of degenerative disorders in which primary symptom is progressive ataxia (jerky, uncoordinated movements)
    Excludes: olivopontocerebellar degeneration (333.0)
    peroneal muscular atrophy (356.1)
    - 334.0 Friedreich's ataxia
    - 334.1 Hereditary spastic paraplegia
    - 334.2 Primary cerebellar degeneration
        Cerebellar ataxia:
            Marie's
            Sanger-Brown
        Dyssynergia cerebellaris myoclonica
        Primary cerebellar degeneration:
            NOS
            hereditary
            sporadic
        Coding Clinic: 1987, Mar-April, P9
    - 334.3 Other cerebellar ataxia
        Cerebellar ataxia NOS
        Use additional E code to identify drug, if drug-induced
    - **334.4 Cerebellar ataxia in diseases classified elsewhere**
        Code first underlying disease, as:
            alcoholism (303.0–303.9)
            myxedema (244.0–244.9)
            neoplastic disease (140.0–239.9)
    - 334.8 Other spinocerebellar diseases
        Ataxia-telangiectasia [Louis-Bar syndrome]
        Corticostriatal-spinal degeneration
    - 334.9 Spinocerebellar disease, unspecified

- **335 Anterior horn cell disease**
    - 335.0 Werdnig-Hoffmann disease
        Infantile spinal muscular atrophy
        Progressive muscular atrophy of infancy
    - **335.1 Spinal muscular atrophy**
        - 335.10 Spinal muscular atrophy, unspecified
        - 335.11 Kugelberg-Welander disease
            Spinal muscular atrophy:
                familial
                juvenile
        - 335.19 Other
            Adult spinal muscular atrophy

- **335.2 Motor neuron disease**
    - 335.20 Amyotrophic lateral sclerosis
        Also listed in the Index as "Lou Gehrig's disease" (ALS)
        Motor neuron disease (bulbar) (mixed type)
        Coding Clinic: 1995, Q4, P81
    - 335.21 Progressive muscular atrophy
        Duchenne-Aran muscular atrophy
        Progressive muscular atrophy (pure)
    - 335.22 Progressive bulbar palsy
    - 335.23 Pseudobulbar palsy
    - 335.24 Primary lateral sclerosis
    - 335.29 Other
    - 335.8 Other anterior horn cell diseases
        Coding Clinic: 2006, Q4, P76-78
    - 335.9 Anterior horn cell disease, unspecified

- **336 Other diseases of spinal cord**
    - 336.0 Syringomyelia and syringobulbia
        Coding Clinic: 1989, Q1, P10
    - 336.1 Vascular myelopathies
        Acute infarction of spinal cord (embolic) (nonembolic)
        Arterial thrombosis of spinal cord
        Edema of spinal cord
        Hematomyelia
        Subacute necrotic myelopathy
    - **336.2 Subacute combined degeneration of spinal cord in diseases classified elsewhere**
        Code first underlying disease, as:
            pernicious anemia (281.0)
            other vitamin B12 deficiency anemia (281.1)
            vitamin B12 deficiency (266.2)
    - **336.3 Myelopathy in other diseases classified elsewhere**
        Code first underlying disease, as:
            myelopathy in neoplastic disease (140.0–239.9)
        Excludes: myelopathy in:
            intervertebral disc disorder (722.70–722.73)
            spondylosis (721.1, 721.41–721.42, 721.91)
        Coding Clinic: 1999, Q3, P5
    - 336.8 Other myelopathy
        Myelopathy:
            drug-induced
            radiation-induced
        Use additional E code to identify cause
    - 336.9 Unspecified disease of spinal cord
        Cord compression NOS
        Myelopathy NOS
        Excludes: myelitis (323.02, 323.1, 323.2, 323.42, 323.52, 323.63, 323.72, 323.82, 323.9)
            spinal (canal) stenosis (723.0, 724.00–724.09)

- **337 Disorders of the autonomic nervous system**
    Includes: disorders of peripheral autonomic, sympathetic, parasympathetic, or vegetative system
    Excludes: familial dysautonomia [Riley-Day syndrome] (742.8)
    - **337.0 Idiopathic peripheral autonomic neuropathy**
        - 337.00 Idiopathic peripheral autonomic neuropathy, unspecified
        - 337.01 Carotid sinus syndrome
            Carotid sinus syncope
            Coding Clinic: 2008, Q4, P101-102
        - 337.09 Other idiopathic peripheral autonomic neuropathy
            Cervical sympathetic dystrophy or paralysis
    - **337.1 Peripheral autonomic neuropathy in disorders classified elsewhere**
        Code first underlying disease, as:
            amyloidosis (277.30–277.39)
            diabetes (249.6, 250.6)
        Coding Clinic: 2009, Q2, P13; 1993, Q2, P6; 1984, Nov-Dec, P9

- **337.2 Reflex sympathetic dystrophy**
  - 337.20 Reflex sympathetic dystrophy, unspecified
    Complex regional pain syndrome type I, unspecified
  - 337.21 Reflex sympathetic dystrophy of the upper limb
    Complex regional pain syndrome type I of the upper limb
  - 337.22 Reflex sympathetic dystrophy of the lower limb
    Complex regional pain syndrome type I of the lower limb
  - 337.29 Reflex sympathetic dystrophy of other specified site
    Complex regional pain syndrome type I of other specified site
  - 337.3 Autonomic dysreflexia
    Use additional code to identify the cause, such as:
    fecal impaction (560.32)
    pressure ulcer (707.00–707.09)
    urinary tract infection (599.0)
    Coding Clinic: 1998, Q4, P37-38
  - 337.9 Unspecified disorder of autonomic nervous system

PAIN (338)

- **338 Pain, not elsewhere classified**
  Use additional code to identify:
  pain associated with psychological factors (307.89)
  Excludes generalized pain (780.96)
  headache syndromes (339.00-339.89)
  localized pain, unspecified type - code to pain by site
  migraines (346.0-346.9)
  pain disorder exclusively attributed to psychological factors (307.80)
  vulvar vestibulitis (625.71)
  vulvodynia (625.70-625.79)
  - 338.0 Central pain syndrome
    Déjérine-Roussy syndrome
    Myelopathic pain syndrome
    Thalamic pain syndrome (hyperesthetic)
- **338.1 Acute pain**
  - 338.11 Acute pain due to trauma
    Coding Clinic: 2007, Q1, P3-8
  - 338.12 Acute post-thoracotomy pain
    Post-thoracotomy pain NOS
  - 338.18 Other acute postoperative pain
    Postoperative pain NOS
    Coding Clinic: 2007, Q2, P13-15; 2003, Q1, P4-5, 8
  - 338.19 Other acute pain
    Excludes neoplasm related acute pain (338.3)
    Coding Clinic: 2007, Q2, P13-15
- **338.2 Chronic pain**
  Excludes causalgia (355.9)
  lower limb (355.71)
  upper limb (354.4)
  chronic pain syndrome (338.4)
  myofascial pain syndrome (729.1)
  neoplasm related chronic pain (338.3)
  reflex sympathetic dystrophy (337.20–337.29)
  Coding Clinic: 2008, Q3, P4
  - 338.21 Chronic pain due to trauma
  - 338.22 Chronic post-thoracotomy pain
  - 338.28 Other chronic postoperative pain
    Coding Clinic: 2007, Q2, P13-15
  - 338.29 Other chronic pain
    Coding Clinic: 2007, Q2, P13-15
  - 338.3 Neoplasm related pain (acute) (chronic)
    Cancer associated pain
    Pain due to malignancy (primary) (secondary)
    Tumor associated pain
    Coding Clinic: 2007, Q2, P13-15
  - 338.4 Chronic pain syndrome
    Chronic pain associated with significant psychosocial dysfunction
    Coding Clinic: 2007, Q2, P13-15

OTHER HEADACHE SYNDROMES (339)

- **339 Other headache syndromes**
  Excludes headache:
  NOS (784.0)
  due to lumbar puncture (349.0)
  migraine (346.0-346.9)
  Coding Clinic: 2008, Q4, P102-109
- **339.0 Cluster headaches and other trigeminal autonomic cephalgias**
  TACS
  - 339.00 Cluster headache syndrome, unspecified
    Ciliary neuralgia
    Cluster headache NOS
    Histamine cephalgia
    Lower half migraine
    Migrainous neuralgia
  - 339.01 Episodic cluster headache
  - 339.02 Chronic cluster headache
  - 339.03 Episodic paroxysmal hemicrania
    Paroxysmal hemicrania NOS
  - 339.04 Chronic paroxysmal hemicrania
  - 339.05 Short lasting unilateral neuralgiform headache with conjunctival injection and tearing
    SUNCT
  - 339.09 Other trigeminal autonomic cephalgias
- **339.1 Tension type headache**
  Excludes tension headache NOS (307.81)
  tension headache related to psychological factors (307.81)
  - 339.10 Tension type headache, unspecified
  - 339.11 Episodic tension type headache
  - 339.12 Chronic tension type headache
- **339.2 Post-traumatic headache**
  - 339.20 Post-traumatic headache, unspecified
    Coding Clinic: 2008, Q4, P102-109
  - 339.21 Acute post-traumatic headache
    Coding Clinic: 2008, Q4, P102-109
  - 339.22 Chronic post-traumatic headache
  - 339.3 Drug induced headache, not elsewhere classified
    Medication overuse headache
    Rebound headache
- **339.4 Complicated headache syndromes**
  - 339.41 Hemicrania continua
  - 339.42 New daily persistent headache
    NDPH
  - 339.43 Primary thunderclap headache
  - 339.44 Other complicated headache syndrome
- **339.8 Other specified headache syndromes**
  - 339.81 Hypnic headache
  - 339.82 Headache associated with sexual activity
    Orgasmic headache
    Preorgasmic headache
  - 339.83 Primary cough headache
  - 339.84 Primary exertional headache
  - 339.85 Primary stabbing headache
  - 339.89 Other specified headache syndromes

Item 6-6 Multiple sclerosis (MS) is a nervous system disease affecting the brain and spinal cord by damaging the myelin sheath surrounding and protecting nerve cells. The damage slows down/blocks messages between the brain and body. Symptoms are: visual disturbances, muscle weakness, coordination and balance issues, numbness, prickling, and thinking and memory problems. The cause is unknown, though it is thought that it may be an autoimmune disease. It affects women more than men, between 20 and 40 years of age. MS can be mild, but it may cause the loss of ability to write, walk, and speak. There is no cure, but medication may slow or control symptoms.

OTHER DISORDERS OF THE CENTRAL NERVOUS SYSTEM (340–349)

340 Multiple sclerosis *(MS)*
Disseminated or multiple sclerosis:
NOS
brain stem
cord
generalized

● **341 Other demyelinating diseases of central nervous system**

341.0 Neuromyelitis optica

341.1 Schilder's disease
Balo's concentric sclerosis
Encephalitis periaxialis:
concentrica [Balo's]
diffusa [Schilder's]

● **341.2 Acute (transverse) myelitis**
Excludes acute (transverse) myelitis (in) (due to):
following immunization procedures (323.52)
infection classified elsewhere (323.42)
postinfectious (323.63)
protozoal diseases classified elsewhere (323.2)
rickettsial diseases classified elsewhere (323.1)
toxic (323.72)
viral diseases classified elsewhere (323.02)
transverse myelitis NOS (323.82)

341.20 Acute (transverse) myelitis NOS

● **341.21 Acute (transverse) myelitis in conditions classified elsewhere**
Code first underlying condition

341.22 Idiopathic transverse myelitis

341.8 Other demyelinating diseases of central nervous system
Central demyelination of corpus callosum
Central pontine myelinosis
Marchiafava (-Bignami) disease
Coding Clinic: 1987, Nov-Dec, P6

■ **341.9 Demyelinating disease of central nervous system, unspecified**

● **342 Hemiplegia and hemiparesis**
Note: This category is to be used when hemiplegia (complete) (incomplete) is reported without further specification, or is stated to be old or long-standing but of unspecified cause. The category is also for use in multiple coding to identify these types of hemiplegia resulting from any cause.
Excludes congenital (343.1)
hemiplegia due to late effect of cerebrovascular accident (438.20–438.22)
infantile NOS (343.4)

The following fifth-digits are for use with codes 342.0–342.9

☐ 0 affecting unspecified side
1 affecting dominant side
2 affecting nondominant side

● **342.0 Flaccid hemiplegia**
[0-2]

● **342.1 Spastic hemiplegia**
[0-2]

● **342.8 Other specified hemiplegia**
[0-2]

● ■ **342.9 Hemiplegia, unspecified**
[0-2] *Coding Clinic: 2006, Q3, P5; 1998, Q4, P87*

Item 6-7 Hemiplegia is complete paralysis of one side of the body—arm, leg, and trunk. **Hemiparesis** is a generalized weakness or incomplete paralysis of one side of the body. If most activities (eating, writing) are performed with the right hand, the right is the dominant side, and the left is the nondominant side. **Quadriplegia,** also called tetraplegia, is the complete paralysis of all four limbs. **Quadriparesis** is the incomplete paralysis of all four limbs. Nerve damage in C1–C4 is associated with lower limb paralysis, and C5–C7 damage is associated with upper limb paralysis. **Diplegia** is the paralysis of the upper limbs. **Monoplegia** is the complete paralysis of one limb. There are separate codes for upper (344.4x) and lower (344.3x) limb. Dominant, nondominant, or unspecified side becomes the fifth digit. Dominant side (right/left) is the side that a person leads with for movement, such as in writing and sports.
Cauda equina syndrome is due to pressure on the roots of the spinal nerves and causes paresthesia (abnormal sensations).

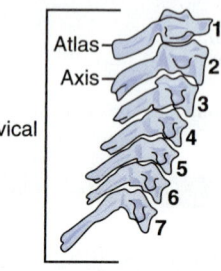

Figure 6–2 Cervical vertebrae.

● **343 Infantile cerebral palsy**
Includes cerebral:
palsy NOS
spastic infantile paralysis
congenital spastic paralysis (cerebral)
Little's disease
paralysis (spastic) due to birth injury:
intracranial
spinal
Excludes athetoid cerebral palsy (333.71)
hereditary cerebral paralysis, such as:
hereditary spastic paraplegia (334.1)
Vogt's disease (333.71)
spastic paralysis specified as noncongenital or noninfantile (344.0–344.9)

343.0 Diplegic
Congenital diplegia
Congenital paraplegia

343.1 Hemiplegic
Congenital hemiplegia
Excludes infantile hemiplegia NOS (343.4)

343.2 Quadriplegic
Tetraplegic

343.3 Monoplegic

343.4 Infantile hemiplegia
Infantile hemiplegia (postnatal) NOS

343.8 Other specified infantile cerebral palsy

■ **343.9 Infantile cerebral palsy, unspecified**
Cerebral palsy NOS
Coding Clinic: 2005, Q4, P89-90

344 Other paralytic syndromes

Note: This category is to be used when the listed conditions are reported without further specification or are stated to be old or long-standing but of unspecified cause. The category is also for use in multiple coding to identify these conditions resulting from any cause.

Includes paralysis (complete) (incomplete), except as classifiable to 342 and 343

Excludes congenital or infantile cerebral palsy (343.0–343.9)
hemiplegia (342.0–342.9)
congenital or infantile (343.1, 343.4)

344.0 Quadriplegia and quadriparesis
- **344.00** Quadriplegia, unspecified
  Coding Clinic: 2003, Q4, P103-104; 1998, Q4, P37-38
- **344.01** C_1-C_4, complete
- **344.02** C_1-C_4, incomplete
- **344.03** C_5-C_7, complete
- **344.04** C_5-C_7, incomplete
- **344.09** Other
  Coding Clinic: 2001, Q1, P12; 1998, Q4, P39-40

344.1 Paraplegia
Paralysis of both lower limbs
Paraplegia (lower)
Coding Clinic: 2003, Q4, P110; 1987, Mar-April, P10-11

344.2 Diplegia of upper limbs
Diplegia (upper)
Paralysis of both upper limbs

344.3 Monoplegia of lower limb
Paralysis of lower limb

Excludes monoplegia of lower limb due to late effect of cerebrovascular accident (438.40–438.42)

- **344.30** Affecting unspecified side
- **344.31** Affecting dominant side
- **344.32** Affecting nondominant side

344.4 Monoplegia of upper limb
Paralysis of upper limb

Excludes monoplegia of upper limb due to late effect of cerebrovascular accident (438.30–438.32)

- **344.40** Affecting unspecified side
- **344.41** Affecting dominant side
- **344.42** Affecting nondominant side

344.5 Unspecified monoplegia

344.6 Cauda equina syndrome
- **344.60** Without mention of neurogenic bladder
- **344.61** With neurogenic bladder
  Acontractile bladder
  Autonomic hyperreflexia of bladder
  Cord bladder
  Detrusor hyperreflexia
  Coding Clinic: 1987, Mar-April, P10-11

344.8 Other specified paralytic syndromes
- **344.81** Locked-in state
- **344.89** Other specified paralytic syndrome
  Coding Clinic: 1999, Q2, P4

344.9 Paralysis, unspecified
Coding Clinic: 1994, Q3, P4

345 Epilepsy and recurrent seizures

The following fifth-digit subclassification is for use with categories 345.0, .1, .4–.9:

> 0 without mention of intractable epilepsy
> 1 with intractable epilepsy
> pharmacoresistant (pharmacologically resistant)
> poorly controlled
> refractory (medically)
> treatment resistant

Excludes hippocampal sclerosis (348.81)
mesial temporal sclerosis (348.81)
temporal sclerosis (348.81)

345.0 Generalized nonconvulsive epilepsy
[0-1]
Absences: Pykno-epilepsy
  atonic   Seizures:
  typical   akinetic
Minor epilepsy   atonic
Petit mal
Coding Clinic: 2004, Q1, P18; 1992, Q2, P8

345.1 Generalized convulsive epilepsy
[0-1]
Epileptic seizures:
  clonic
  myoclonic
  tonic
  tonic-clonic
Grand mal
Major epilepsy
Progressive myoclonic epilepsy
Unverricht-Lundborg disease

Excludes convulsions:
NOS (780.39)
infantile (780.39)
newborn (779.0)
infantile spasms (345.6)
Coding Clinic: 1997, Q3, P5; 1994, Q3, P9

345.2 Petit mal status
Epileptic absence status
Temporary disturbance of brain function caused by abnormal electrical activity

345.3 Grand mal status
Status epilepticus NOS
Grand mal seizure is a generalized tonic-clonic seizure involving the entire body, which involves muscle rigidity, violent muscle contractions, and loss of consciousness.

Excludes epilepsia partialis continua (345.7) status:
psychomotor (345.7)
temporal lobe (345.7)
Coding Clinic: 2005, Q3, P12-13

345.4 Localization-related (focal) (partial) epilepsy and
[0-1] epileptic syndromes with complex partial seizures
Epilepsy:
  limbic system
  partial:
    secondarily generalized
    with impairment of consciousness
    with memory and ideational disturbances
  psychomotor
  psychosensory
  temporal lobe
Epileptic automatism
Coding Clinic: 2009, Q4, P98

345.5-348.2 ICD-9-CM

DISEASES OF THE NERVOUS SYSTEM AND SENSE ORGANS (320–389)

- **345.5** Localization-related (focal) (partial) epilepsy and
- [0-1] epileptic syndromes with simple partial seizures
  Epilepsy:
  Bravais-Jacksonian NOS
  focal (motor) NOS
  Jacksonian NOS
  motor partial
  partial NOS
  without mention of impairment of consciousness
  sensory-induced
  somatomotor
  somatosensory
  visceral
  visual

- **345.6** Infantile spasms
- [0-1] Hypsarrhythmia
  Lightning spasms
  Salaam attacks
  Excludes salaam tic (781.0)
  Coding Clinic: 1984, Nov-Dec, P11

- **345.7** Epilepsia partialis continua
- [0-1] Kojevnikov's epilepsy

- **345.8** Other forms of epilepsy and recurrent seizures
- [0-1] Epilepsy:
  cursive [running]
  gelastic
  Recurrent seizures NOS

- **345.9** Epilepsy, unspecified
- [0-1] Epileptic convulsions, fits, or seizures NOS
  Seizure disorder NOS
  Excludes convulsion (convulsive) disorder (780.39)
  convulsive seizure or fit NOS (780.39)
  recurrent convulsions (780.39)
  Coding Clinic: 2012, Q2, P9-10; 2009, Q2, P10; 2008, Q1, P17; 1993, Q1, P24; 1987, Nov-Dec, P12

- **346** Migraine
  Excludes headache:
  NOS (784.0)
  syndromes (339.00-339.89)
  Coding Clinic: 2008, Q4, P102-109

The following fifth-digit subclassification is for use with category 346:

> 0 without mention of intractable migraine without mention of status migrainosus
>   without mention of refractory migraine without mention of status migrainosus
> 1 with intractable migraine, so stated, without mention of status migrainosus
>   with refractory migraine, so stated, without mention of status migrainosus
> 2 without mention of intractable migraine with status migrainosus
>   without mention of refractory migraine with status migrainosus
> 3 with intractable migraine, so stated, with status migrainosus
>   with refractory migraine, so stated, with status migrainosus

Intractable migraine: Not easily cured or managed; relentless pain from a migraine

- **346.0** Migraine with aura
- [0-3] Basilar migraine
  Classic migraine
  Migraine preceded or accompanied by transient focal neurological phenomena
  Migraine triggered seizures
  Migraine with acute-onset aura
  Migraine with aura without headache (migraine equivalents)
  Migraine with prolonged aura
  Migraine with typical aura
  Retinal migraine
  Excludes persistent migraine aura (346.5, 346.6)

Item 6-8 Migraine headache is described as an intense pulsing or throbbing pain in one area of the head. It can be accompanied by extreme sensitivity to light (photophoic) and sound and is three times more common in women than in men. Symptoms include nausea and vomiting. Research indicates migraine headaches are caused by inherited abnormalities in genes that control the activities of certain cell populations in the brain.

- **346.1** Migraine without aura
- [0-3] Common migraine

- **346.2** Variants of migraine, not elsewhere classified
- [0-3] Abdominal migraine
  Cyclical vomiting associated with migraine
  Ophthalmoplegic migraine
  Periodic headache syndromes in child or adolescent
  Excludes cyclical vomiting NOS (536.2)
  psychogenic cyclical vomiting (306.4)

- **346.3** Hemiplegic migraine
- [0-3] Familial migraine
  Sporadic migraine

- **346.4** Menstrual migraine
- [0-3] Menstrual headache
  Menstrually related migraine
  Premenstrual headache
  Premenstrual migraine
  Pure menstrual migraine

- **346.5** Persistent migraine aura without cerebral
- [0-3] infarction
  Persistent migraine aura NOS

- **346.6** Persistent migraine aura with cerebral
- [0-3] infarction

- **346.7** Chronic migraine without aura
- [0-3] Transformed migraine without aura

- **346.8** Other forms of migraine
- [0-3]

- **346.9** Migraine, unspecified
- [0-3] Coding Clinic: 1985, Nov-Dec, P16

- **347** Cataplexy and narcolepsy
  Cataplexy is a disorder evidenced by seizures. Narcolepsy is difficulty remaining awake during daytime.
  Coding Clinic: 2004, Q4, P74-75

  - **347.0** Narcolepsy
    347.00 Without cataplexy
    Narcolepsy NOS
    347.01 With cataplexy

  - **347.1** Narcolepsy in conditions classified elsewhere
    Code first underlying condition
    - 347.10 Without cataplexy
    - 347.11 With cataplexy

- **348** Other conditions of brain
  348.0 Cerebral cysts
  Arachnoid cyst   Porencephaly, acquired
  Porencephalic cyst   Pseudoporencephaly

  348.1 Anoxic brain damage
  Brain permanently damaged by lack of oxygen perfusion through brain tissues. This is the result of another problem, so use an additional E code to identify the cause.
  Excludes that occurring in:
  abortion (634–638 with .7, 639.8)
  ectopic or molar pregnancy (639.8)
  labor or delivery (668.2, 669.4)
  that of newborn (767.0, 768.0–768.9, 772.1–772.2)
  Use additional E code to identify cause

  348.2 Benign intracranial hypertension
  Pseudotumor cerebri
  Excludes hypertensive encephalopathy (437.2)

- **348.3 Encephalopathy, not elsewhere classified**
  A general term for any degenerative brain disease
  Coding Clinic: 2003, Q4, P58-59; 1997, Q3, P5
  - 348.30 Encephalopathy, unspecified
  - 348.31 Metabolic encephalopathy
    Septic encephalopathy
    Excludes toxic metabolic encephalopathy (349.82)
  - 348.39 Other encephalopathy
    Excludes encephalopathy:
    alcoholic (291.2)
    hepatic (572.2)
    hypertensive (437.2)
    toxic (349.82)
- 348.4 **Compression of brain**
  Compression brain (stem)
  Herniation brain (stem)
  Posterior fossa compression syndrome
  Coding Clinic: 2011, Q3, P11
- 348.5 **Cerebral edema**
  Coding Clinic: 2011, Q4, P100; 2010, Q1, P6; 2009, Q3, P7
- **348.8 Other conditions of brain**
  Coding Clinic: 1992, Q3, P8; 1987, Sept-Oct, P9
  - 348.81 Temporal sclerosis
    Hippocampal sclerosis
    Mesial temporal sclerosis
    Coding Clinic: 2009, Q4, P98
  - 348.82 Brain death
    Coding Clinic: 2011, Q4, P100
  - 348.89 Other conditions of brain
    Cerebral:
    calcification
    fungus
    Excludes brain death (348.82)
- 348.9 **Unspecified condition of brain**
- **349 Other and unspecified disorders of the nervous system**
  - 349.0 **Reaction to spinal or lumbar puncture**
    Headache following lumbar puncture
    Cerebral spinal fluid (CSF) maintains a specific level of pressure inside brain and spinal cord. If this pressure does not return to normal after a puncture, headache will result.
    Coding Clinic: 1999, Q2, P9-10; 1990, Q3, P18
  - 349.1 **Nervous system complications from surgically implanted device**
    Excludes immediate postoperative complications (997.00–997.09)
    mechanical complications of nervous system device (996.2)
  - 349.2 **Disorders of meninges, not elsewhere classified**
    Adhesions, meningeal (cerebral) (spinal)
    Cyst, spinal meninges
    Meningocele, acquired
    Pseudomeningocele, acquired
    Coding Clinic: 2006, Q1, P15-16; 1998, Q2, P18; 1994, Q3, P4; Q1, P22-23
  - 349.3 **Dural tear**
    Coding Clinic: 2008, Q4, P109-110
    - 349.31 Accidental puncture or laceration of dura during a procedure
      Incidental (inadvertent) durotomy
    - 349.39 Other dural tear
  - 349.8 **Other specified disorders of nervous system**
    - 349.81 Cerebrospinal fluid rhinorrhea
      Excludes cerebrospinal fluid otorrhea (388.61)
    - 349.82 Toxic encephalopathy
      Toxic metabolic encephalopathy
      Use additional E code to identify cause
    - 349.89 Other
  - 349.9 **Unspecified disorders of nervous system**
    Disorder of nervous system (central) NOS
    Coding Clinic: 2012, Q3, P4

Item 6-9 The **peripheral nervous system** consists of 31 pairs of spinal nerves, 12 pairs of cranial nerves, and the autonomic nerves, which are divided into the parasympathetic and sympathetic nerves. The cranial nerves are: olfactory (I), optic (II), oculomotor (III), trochlear (IV), trigeminal (V), abducens (VI), facial (VII), vestibulocochlear (VIII), glossopharyngeal (IX), vagus (X), accessory (XI), and hypoglossal (XII).

Item 6-10 Trigeminal neuralgia, tic douloureux, is a pain syndrome diagnosed from the patient's history alone. The condition is characterized by pain and a brief facial spasm or tic. Pain is unilateral and follows the sensory distribution of cranial nerve V, typically radiating to the maxillary (V2) or mandibular (V3) area.

Item 6-11 The most common facial nerve disorder is **Bell's Palsy,** which occurs suddenly and results in facial drooping unilaterally. This disorder is the result of a reaction to a virus that causes the facial nerve in the ear to swell resulting in pressure in the bony canal.

DISORDERS OF THE PERIPHERAL NERVOUS SYSTEM (350–359)

Excludes diseases of:
acoustic [8th] nerve (388.5)
oculomotor [3rd, 4th, 6th] nerves (378.0–378.9)
optic [2nd] nerve (377.0–377.9)
peripheral autonomic nerves (337.0–337.9)
neuralgia NOS or "rheumatic" (729.2)
neuritis NOS or "rheumatic" (729.2)
radiculitis NOS or "rheumatic" (729.2)
peripheral neuritis in pregnancy (646.4)

- **350 Trigeminal nerve disorders**
  Includes disorders of 5th cranial nerve
  - 350.1 Trigeminal neuralgia
    Tic douloureux
    Trifacial neuralgia
    Trigeminal neuralgia NOS
    Excludes postherpetic (053.12)
  - 350.2 Atypical face pain
  - 350.8 Other specified trigeminal nerve disorders
  - 350.9 Trigeminal nerve disorder, unspecified
- **351 Facial nerve disorders**
  Includes disorders of 7th cranial nerve
  Excludes that in newborn (767.5)
  - 351.0 Bell's palsy
    Facial palsy
  - 351.1 Geniculate ganglionitis
    Geniculate ganglionitis NOS
    Excludes herpetic (053.11)
    Coding Clinic: 2002, Q2, P8
  - 351.8 Other facial nerve disorders
    Facial myokymia
    Melkersson's syndrome
    Coding Clinic: 2002, Q3, P12-13
  - 351.9 Facial nerve disorder, unspecified
- **352 Disorders of other cranial nerves**
  - 352.0 Disorders of olfactory [1st] nerve
  - 352.1 Glossopharyngeal neuralgia
    Coding Clinic: 1987, Jan-Feb, P14
  - 352.2 Other disorders of glossopharyngeal [9th] nerve
  - 352.3 Disorders of pneumogastric [10th] nerve
    Disorders of vagal nerve
    Excludes paralysis of vocal cords or larynx (478.30–478.34)
  - 352.4 Disorders of accessory [11th] nerve
  - 352.5 Disorders of hypoglossal [12th] nerve
  - 352.6 Multiple cranial nerve palsies
    Collet-Sicard syndrome
    Polyneuritis cranialis
  - 352.9 Unspecified disorder of cranial nerves

DISEASES OF THE NERVOUS SYSTEM AND SENSE ORGANS (320–389)

- **353 Nerve root and plexus disorders**
  - *Excludes* conditions due to:
    - intervertebral disc disorders (722.0–722.9)
    - spondylosis (720.0–721.9)
    - vertebrogenic disorders (723.0–724.9)
  - **353.0 Brachial plexus lesions**
    - Cervical rib syndrome
    - Costoclavicular syndrome
    - Scalenus anticus syndrome
    - Thoracic outlet syndrome
    - *Excludes* brachial neuritis or radiculitis NOS (723.4)
      - that in newborn (767.6)
    - Coding Clinic: 2006, Q3, P12
  - **353.1 Lumbosacral plexus lesions**
  - **353.2 Cervical root lesions, not elsewhere classified**
  - **353.3 Thoracic root lesions, not elsewhere classified**
  - **353.4 Lumbosacral root lesions, not elsewhere classified**
  - **353.5 Neuralgic amyotrophy**
    - Parsonage-Aldren-Turner syndrome
    - *Phantom limb syndrome: Patients with amputated limbs feel sensations in a limb that no longer exists. There is no separate code for phantom limb pain, and the pain can be part of the syndrome.*
    - *Code first* any associated underlying disease, such as:
      - diabetes mellitus (249.6, 250.6)
  - **353.6 Phantom limb (syndrome)**
  - **353.8 Other nerve root and plexus disorders**
  - **353.9 Unspecified nerve root and plexus disorder**

- **354 Mononeuritis of upper limb and mononeuritis multiplex**
  - **354.0 Carpal tunnel syndrome** (CTS)
    - *Of the wrist*
    - Median nerve entrapment
    - Partial thenar atrophy
  - **354.1 Other lesion of median nerve**
    - Median nerve neuritis
  - **354.2 Lesion of ulnar nerve**
    - Cubital tunnel syndrome
    - Tardy ulnar nerve palsy
  - **354.3 Lesion of radial nerve**
    - Acute radial nerve palsy
    - Coding Clinic: 1987, Nov-Dec, P6
  - **354.4 Causalgia of upper limb**
    - Complex regional pain syndrome type II of the upper limb
    - *Excludes* causalgia:
      - NOS (355.9)
      - lower limb (355.71)
      - complex regional pain syndrome type II of the lower limb (355.71)
  - **354.5 Mononeuritis multiplex**
    - Combinations of single conditions classifiable to 354 or 355
  - **354.8 Other mononeuritis of upper limb**
  - **354.9 Mononeuritis of upper limb, unspecified**

- **355 Mononeuritis of lower limb**
  - Coding Clinic: 1989, Q2, P12
  - **355.0 Lesion of sciatic nerve**
    - *Excludes* sciatica NOS (724.3)
    - Coding Clinic: 1989, Q2, P12
  - **355.1 Meralgia paresthetica**
    - Lateral cutaneous femoral nerve of thigh compression or syndrome
  - **355.2 Other lesion of femoral nerve**
  - **355.3 Lesion of lateral popliteal nerve**
    - Lesion of common peroneal nerve
  - **355.4 Lesion of medial popliteal nerve**
  - **355.5 Tarsal tunnel syndrome**
    - *Of the ankle*
  - **355.6 Lesion of plantar nerve**
    - Morton's metatarsalgia, neuralgia, or neuroma
  - **355.7 Other mononeuritis of lower limb**
    - **355.71 Causalgia of lower limb**
      - *Excludes* causalgia:
        - NOS (355.9)
        - upper limb (354.4)
        - complex regional pain syndrome type II of the upper limb (354.4)
    - **355.79 Other mononeuritis of lower limb**
  - **355.8 Mononeuritis of lower limb, unspecified**
    - Coding Clinic: 2013, Q1, P3
  - **355.9 Mononeuritis of unspecified site**
    - Causalgia NOS
    - Complex regional pain syndrome NOS
    - *Excludes* causalgia:
      - lower limb (355.71)
      - upper limb (354.4)
      - complex regional pain syndrome:
        - lower limb (355.71)
        - upper limb (354.4)

- **356 Hereditary and idiopathic peripheral neuropathy**
  - *Any disease that affects nervous system and of an unknown cause*
  - **356.0 Hereditary peripheral neuropathy**
    - Déjérine-Sottas disease
  - **356.1 Peroneal muscular atrophy**
    - Charcot-Marie-Tooth disease
    - Neuropathic muscular atrophy
  - **356.2 Hereditary sensory neuropathy**
  - **356.3 Refsum's disease**
    - Heredopathia atactica polyneuritiformis
  - **356.4 Idiopathic progressive polyneuropathy**
  - **356.8 Other specified idiopathic peripheral neuropathy**
    - Supranuclear paralysis
  - **356.9 Unspecified**
    - Coding Clinic: 2013, Q1, P3-4

- **357 Inflammatory and toxic neuropathy**
  - **357.0 Acute infective polyneuritis**
    - Guillain-Barre syndrome
    - Postinfectious polyneuritis
    - Coding Clinic: 1998, Q2, P12
  - **357.1 Polyneuropathy in collagen vascular disease**
    - *Code first* underlying disease, as:
      - disseminated lupus erythematosus (710.0)
      - polyarteritis nodosa (446.0)
      - rheumatoid arthritis (714.0)
  - **357.2 Polyneuropathy in diabetes**
    - *Code first* underlying disease (249.6, 250.6)
    - Coding Clinic: 2009, Q4, P98; Q2, P13; 2008, Q3, P5-6; 2003, Q4, P105; 1992, Q2, P15
  - **357.3 Polyneuropathy in malignant disease**
    - *Code first* underlying disease (140.0–208.9)
  - **357.4 Polyneuropathy in other diseases classified elsewhere**
    - *Code first* underlying disease, as:
      - amyloidosis (277.30–277.39)
      - beriberi (265.0)
      - chronic uremia (585.9)
      - deficiency of B vitamins (266.0–266.9)
      - diphtheria (032.0–032.9)
      - hypoglycemia (251.2)
      - pellagra (265.2)
      - porphyria (277.1)
      - sarcoidosis (135)
      - uremia NOS (586)
    - *Excludes* polyneuropathy in:
      - herpes zoster (053.13)
      - mumps (072.72)
    - Coding Clinic: 2008, Q2, P8-9; 1998, Q2, P15
  - **357.5 Alcoholic polyneuropathy**

357.6 Polyneuropathy due to drugs
Use additional E code to identify drug

357.7 Polyneuropathy due to other toxic agents
Use additional E code to identify toxic agent

357.8 Other
Coding Clinic: 2002, Q4, P47-48; 1998, Q2, P12

  357.81 Chronic inflammatory demyelinating polyneuritis

  357.82 Critical illness polyneuropathy
  Acute motor neuropathy
  Coding Clinic: 2003, Q4, P111

  357.89 Other inflammatory and toxic neuropathy
  Coding Clinic: 2013, Q1, P3

357.9 Unspecified

358 Myoneural disorders

358.0 Myasthenia gravis
Acquired and results in fatigable muscle weakness exacerbated by activity and improved with rest. Caused by autoimmune assault against nerve-muscle junction.
Coding Clinic: 2003, Q4, P59-60

  358.00 Myasthenia gravis without (acute) exacerbation

  358.01 Myasthenia gravis with acute exacerbation
  Myasthenia gravis in crisis
  Coding Clinic: 2007, Q4, P108-109; 2004, Q4, P139

358.1 *Myasthenic syndromes in diseases classified elsewhere*
Code first underlying disease, as:
  botulism (005.1, 040.41–040.42)
  hypothyroidism (244.0–244.9)
  malignant neoplasm (140.0–208.9)
  pernicious anemia (281.0)
  thyrotoxicosis (242.0–242.9)

358.2 Toxic myoneural disorders
Use additional E code to identify toxic agent

358.3 Lambert-Eaton syndrome
Eaton-Lambert syndrome

  358.30 Lambert-Eaton syndrome, unspecified
  Lambert-Eaton syndrome NOS
  Coding Clinic: 2011, Q4, P101

  358.31 Lambert-Eaton syndrome in neoplastic disease
  Code first the underlying neoplastic disease

  358.39 Lambert-Eaton syndrome in other diseases classified elsewhere
  Code first the underlying condition

358.8 Other specified myoneural disorders

358.9 Myoneural disorders, unspecified
Coding Clinic: 2002, Q2, P16

359 Muscular dystrophies and other myopathies
Excludes idiopathic polymyositis (710.4)

359.0 Congenital hereditary muscular dystrophy
  Benign congenital myopathy
  Central core disease
  Centronuclear myopathy
  Myotubular myopathy
  Nemaline body disease
Excludes arthrogryposis multiplex congenita (754.89)

359.1 Hereditary progressive muscular dystrophy
  Muscular dystrophy:
    NOS
    distal
    Duchenne
    Erb's
    fascioscapulohumeral
    Gower's
    Landouzy-Déjérine
    limb-girdle
    ocular
    oculopharyngeal

Item 6-12 Muscular dystrophies (MD) are a group of rare inherited muscle diseases. Voluntary muscles become progressively weaker. In the late stages of MD, fat and connective tissue replace muscle fibers. In some types of muscular dystrophy, heart muscles, other involuntary muscles, and other organs are affected. **Myopathies** is a general term for neuromuscular diseases in which the muscle fibers dysfunction for any one of many reasons, resulting in muscular weakness.

359.2 Myotonic disorders
Excludes periodic paralysis (359.3)
Coding Clinic: 2007, Q4, P75-77

  359.21 Myotonic muscular dystrophy
  Dystrophia myotonica
  Myotonia atrophica
  Myotonic dystrophy
  Proximal myotonic myopathy (PROMM)
  Steinert's disease

  359.22 Myotonia congenita
  Acetazolamide responsive myotonia congenita
  Dominant form (Thomsen's disease)
  Myotonia levior
  Recessive form (Becker's disease)

  359.23 Myotonic chondrodystrophy
  Congenital myotonic chondrodystrophy
  Schwartz-Jampel disease

  359.24 Drug-induced myotonia
  Use additional E code to identify drug

  359.29 Other specified myotonic disorder
  Myotonia fluctuans
  Myotonia permanens
  Paramyotonia congenita (of von Eulenburg)

359.3 Periodic paralysis
  Familial periodic paralysis
  Hyperkalemic periodic paralysis
  Hypokalemic familial periodic paralysis
  Hypokalemic periodic paralysis
  Potassium sensitive periodic paralysis
Excludes paramyotonia congenita (of von Eulenburg) (359.29)

359.4 Toxic myopathy
Use additional E code to identify toxic agent

359.5 Myopathy in endocrine diseases classified elsewhere
Code first underlying disease, as:
  Addison's disease (255.41)
  Cushing's syndrome (255.0)
  hypopituitarism (253.2)
  myxedema (244.0–244.9)
  thyrotoxicosis (242.0–242.9)

359.6 Symptomatic inflammatory myopathy in diseases classified elsewhere
Code first underlying disease, as:
  amyloidosis (277.30–277.39)
  disseminated lupus erythematosus (710.0)
  malignant neoplasm (140.0–208.9)
  polyarteritis nodosa (446.0)
  rheumatoid arthritis (714.0)
  sarcoidosis (135)
  scleroderma (710.1)
  Sjögren's disease (710.2)

359.7 Inflammatory and immune myopathies, NEC

  359.71 Inclusion body myositis
  IBM

  359.79 Other inflammatory and immune myopathies, NEC
  Inflammatory myopathy NOS

359.8 Other myopathies
Coding Clinic: 2002, Q4, P47-48; 1990, Q3, P17

  359.81 Critical illness myopathy
  Acute necrotizing myopathy
  Acute quadriplegic myopathy
  Intensive care (ICU) myopathy
  Myopathy of critical illness

  359.89 Other myopathies

359.9 Myopathy, unspecified

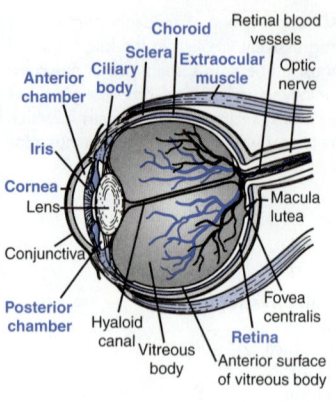

Figure 6-3 Eye and ocular adnexa. (From Buck CJ: Step-by-Step Medical Coding, ed 2011, Philadelphia, WB Saunders, 2011)

DISORDERS OF THE EYE AND ADNEXA (360–379)

Use additional external cause code, if applicable, to identify the cause of the eye condition

- **360 Disorders of the globe**
  - **Includes** disorders affecting multiple structures of eye
  - **360.0 Purulent endophthalmitis**
    - **Excludes** bleb associated endophthalmitis (379.63)
    - 360.00 Purulent endophthalmitis, unspecified
    - 360.01 Acute endophthalmitis
    - 360.02 Panophthalmitis
    - 360.03 Chronic endophthalmitis
    - 360.04 Vitreous abscess
  - **360.1 Other endophthalmitis**
    - **Excludes** bleb associated endophthalmitis (379.63)
    - 360.11 Sympathetic uveitis
    - 360.12 Panuveitis
    - 360.13 Parasitic endophthalmitis NOS
    - 360.14 Ophthalmia nodosa
    - 360.19 Other
      Phacoanaphylactic endophthalmitis
  - **360.2 Degenerative disorders of globe**
    - 360.20 Degenerative disorder of globe, unspecified
    - 360.21 Progressive high (degenerative) myopia
      Malignant myopia
    - 360.23 Siderosis
    - 360.24 Other metallosis
      Chalcosis
    - 360.29 Other
      Excludes xerophthalmia (264.7)
  - **360.3 Hypotony of eye**
    - 360.30 Hypotony, unspecified
    - 360.31 Primary hypotony
    - 360.32 Ocular fistula causing hypotony
    - 360.33 Hypotony associated with other ocular disorders
    - 360.34 Flat anterior chamber
  - **360.4 Degenerated conditions of globe**
    - 360.40 Degenerated globe or eye, unspecified
    - 360.41 Blind hypotensive eye
      Atrophy of globe   Phthisis bulbi
    - 360.42 Blind hypertensive eye
      Absolute glaucoma
    - 360.43 Hemophthalmos, except current injury
      Excludes traumatic (871.0–871.9, 921.0–921.9)
    - 360.44 Leucocoria
  - **360.5 Retained (old) intraocular foreign body, magnetic**
    Use additional code to identify foreign body (V90.11)
    Excludes current penetrating injury with magnetic foreign body (871.5)
    retained (old) foreign body of orbit (376.6)
    - 360.50 Foreign body, magnetic, intraocular, unspecified
    - 360.51 Foreign body, magnetic, in anterior chamber
    - 360.52 Foreign body, magnetic, in iris or ciliary body
    - 360.53 Foreign body, magnetic, in lens
    - 360.54 Foreign body, magnetic, in vitreous
    - 360.55 Foreign body, magnetic, in posterior wall
    - 360.59 Foreign body, magnetic, in other or multiple sites
  - **360.6 Retained (old) intraocular foreign body, nonmagnetic**
    Retained (old) foreign body:
      NOS
      nonmagnetic
    Use additional code to identify foreign body (V90.01-V90.10, V90.12, V90.2-V90.9)
    Excludes current penetrating injury with (nonmagnetic) foreign body (871.6)
    retained (old) foreign body in orbit (376.6)
    - 360.60 Foreign body, intraocular, unspecified
    - 360.61 Foreign body in anterior chamber
    - 360.62 Foreign body in iris or ciliary body
    - 360.63 Foreign body in lens
    - 360.64 Foreign body in vitreous
    - 360.65 Foreign body in posterior wall
    - 360.69 Foreign body in other or multiple sites
  - **360.8 Other disorders of globe**
    - 360.81 Luxation of globe
    - 360.89 Other
  - **360.9 Unspecified disorder of globe**
- **361 Retinal detachments and defects**
  - **361.0 Retinal detachment with retinal defect**
    Rhegmatogenous retinal detachment
    Excludes detachment of retinal pigment epithelium (362.42–362.43)
    retinal detachment (serous) (without defect) (361.2)
    Coding Clinic: 1994, Q1, P17
    - 361.00 Retinal detachment with retinal defect, unspecified
    - 361.01 Recent detachment, partial, with single defect
    - 361.02 Recent detachment, partial, with multiple defects
    - 361.03 Recent detachment, partial, with giant tear
    - 361.04 Recent detachment, partial, with retinal dialysis
      Dialysis (juvenile) of retina (with detachment)
    - 361.05 Recent detachment, total or subtotal
    - 361.06 Old detachment, partial
      Delimited old retinal detachment
    - 361.07 Old detachment, total or subtotal
  - **361.1 Retinoschisis and retinal cysts**
    Excludes juvenile retinoschisis (362.73)
    microcystoid degeneration of retina (362.62)
    parasitic cyst of retina (360.13)
    - 361.10 Retinoschisis, unspecified
    - 361.11 Flat retinoschisis
    - 361.12 Bullous retinoschisis
    - 361.13 Primary retinal cysts
    - 361.14 Secondary retinal cysts
    - 361.19 Other
      Pseudocyst of retina

Item 6-13 Retinal detachments and defects are conditions of the eye in which the retina separates from the underlying tissue. Initial detachment may be localized, requiring rapid treatment (medical emergency) to avoid the entire retina from detaching, which leads to vision loss and blindness.

361.2 Serous retinal detachment
Retinal detachment without retinal defect
Excludes central serous retinopathy (362.41)
retinal pigment epithelium detachment (362.42–362.43)

● **361.3 Retinal defects without detachment**
Excludes chorioretinal scars after surgery for detachment (363.30–363.35)
peripheral retinal degeneration without defect (362.60–362.66)

▫ **361.30 Retinal defect, unspecified**
Retinal break(s) NOS

361.31 Round hole of retina without detachment

361.32 Horseshoe tear of retina without detachment
Operculum of retina without mention of detachment

361.33 Multiple defects of retina without detachment

● **361.8 Other forms of retinal detachment**
361.81 Traction detachment of retina
Traction detachment with vitreoretinal organization

361.89 Other
Coding Clinic: 1999, Q3, P12

▫ **361.9 Unspecified retinal detachment**
Coding Clinic: 1987, Nov-Dec, P10

● **362 Other retinal disorders**
Excludes chorioretinal scars (363.30–363.35)
chorioretinitis (363.0–363.2)

● **362.0 Diabetic retinopathy**
Code first diabetes (249.5, 250.5)
Most common diabetic eye disease and leading cause of blindness in adults. Caused by changes in the blood vessels of retina in which the blood vessels swell and leak fluid into retinal surface.

●**362.01** *Background diabetic retinopathy*
Diabetic retinal microaneurysms
Diabetic retinopathy NOS

●**362.02** *Proliferative diabetic retinopathy*
Coding Clinic: 1996, Q3, P5

●**362.03** *Nonproliferative diabetic retinopathy NOS*

●**362.04** *Mild nonproliferative diabetic retinopathy*

●**362.05** *Moderate nonproliferative diabetic retinopathy*

●**362.06** *Severe nonproliferative diabetic retinopathy*
Coding Clinic: 2005, Q4, P65-67

●**362.07** *Diabetic macular edema*
Diabetic retinal edema
Note: Code 362.07 must be used with a code for diabetic retinopathy (362.01–362.06).

● **362.1 Other background retinopathy and retinal vascular changes**

▫ **362.10 Background retinopathy, unspecified**
Coding Clinic: 2006, Q1, P12

362.11 Hypertensive retinopathy
OGCR Section I.C.7.a.6
Two codes are necessary to identify the condition. First assign the code from subcategory 362.11, Hypertensive retinopathy, then the appropriate code from categories 401–405 to indicate the type of hypertension.

362.12 Exudative retinopathy
Coats' syndrome
Coding Clinic: 1999, Q3, P12

362.13 Changes in vascular appearance
Vascular sheathing of retina
Use additional code for any associated atherosclerosis (440.8)

362.14 Retinal microaneurysms NOS

362.15 Retinal telangiectasia

362.16 Retinal neovascularization NOS
Neovascularization:
choroidal
subretinal

362.17 Other intraretinal microvascular abnormalities
Retinal varices

362.18 Retinal vasculitis
Eales' disease
Retinal:
arteritis
endarteritis
perivasculitis
phlebitis

● **362.2 Other proliferative retinopathy**
▫ **362.20 Retinopathy of prematurity, unspecified**
Retinopathy of prematurity NOS
Coding Clinic: 2008, Q4, P110-111

362.21 Retrolental fibroplasia
Cicatricial retinopathy of prematurity

362.22 Retinopathy of prematurity, stage 0
362.23 Retinopathy of prematurity, stage 1
362.24 Retinopathy of prematurity, stage 2
362.25 Retinopathy of prematurity, stage 3
362.26 Retinopathy of prematurity, stage 4
362.27 Retinopathy of prematurity, stage 5
362.29 Other nondiabetic proliferative retinopathy
Coding Clinic: 1996, Q3, P5

● **362.3 Retinal vascular occlusion**
Blockage in vessel of the retina

▫ **362.30 Retinal vascular occlusion, unspecified**

362.31 Central retinal artery occlusion
362.32 Arterial branch occlusion
362.33 Partial arterial occlusion
Hollenhorst plaque
Retinal microembolism

362.34 Transient arterial occlusion
Amaurosis fugax
Coding Clinic: 2000, Q1, P16

362.35 Central retinal vein occlusion
Coding Clinic: 1993, Q2, P6

362.36 Venous tributary (branch) occlusion

362.37 Venous engorgement
Occlusion:
of retinal vein
incipient of retinal vein
partial of retinal vein

● **362.4 Separation of retinal layers**
Excludes retinal detachment (serous) (361.2)
rhegmatogenous (361.00–361.07)

▫ **362.40 Retinal layer separation, unspecified**
362.41 Central serous retinopathy
362.42 Serous detachment of retinal pigment epithelium
Exudative detachment of retinal pigment epithelium

362.43 Hemorrhagic detachment of retinal pigment epithelium

Item 6-14 Macular degeneration is typically age-related, chronic, and is evidenced by deterioration of the macula (the part of the retina that provides for central field vision), resulting in blurred vision or a blind spot in the center of visual field while not affecting peripheral vision.

- **362.5 Degeneration of macula and posterior pole**
  Excludes: degeneration of optic disc (377.21–377.24)
  hereditary retinal degeneration [dystrophy] (362.70–362.77)

  - 362.50 Macular degeneration (senile), unspecified
  - 362.51 Nonexudative senile macular degeneration
    Senile macular degeneration:
      atrophic
      dry
  - 362.52 Exudative senile macular degeneration
    Kuhnt-Junius degeneration
    Senile macular degeneration:
      disciform
      wet
  - 362.53 Cystoid macular degeneration
    Cystoid macular edema
  - 362.54 Macular cyst, hole, or pseudohole
    Coding Clinic: 2011, Q4, P106
  - 362.55 Toxic maculopathy
    Use additional E code to identify drug, if drug induced
  - 362.56 Macular puckering
    Preretinal fibrosis
  - 362.57 Drusen (degenerative)

- **362.6 Peripheral retinal degenerations**
  Excludes: hereditary retinal degeneration [dystrophy] (362.70–362.77)
  retinal degeneration with retinal defect (361.00–361.07)

  - 362.60 Peripheral retinal degeneration, unspecified
  - 362.61 Paving stone degeneration
  - 362.62 Microcystoid degeneration
    Blessig's cysts
    Iwanoff's cysts
  - 362.63 Lattice degeneration
    Palisade degeneration of retina
  - 362.64 Senile reticular degeneration
  - 362.65 Secondary pigmentary degeneration
    Pseudoretinitis pigmentosa
  - 362.66 Secondary vitreoretinal degenerations

- **362.7 Hereditary retinal dystrophies**
  - 362.70 Hereditary retinal dystrophy, unspecified
  - 362.71 *Retinal dystrophy in systemic or cerebroretinal lipidoses*
    Code first underlying disease, as:
      cerebroretinal lipidoses (330.1)
      systemic lipidoses (272.7)
  - 362.72 *Retinal dystrophy in other systemic disorders and syndromes*
    Code first underlying disease, as:
      Bassen-Kornzweig syndrome (272.5)
      Refsum's disease (356.3)
  - 362.73 Vitreoretinal dystrophies
    Juvenile retinoschisis
  - 362.74 Pigmentary retinal dystrophy
    Retinal dystrophy, albipunctate
    Retinitis pigmentosa
  - 362.75 Other dystrophies primarily involving the sensory retina
    Progressive cone (-rod) dystrophy
    Stargardt's disease
  - 362.76 Dystrophies primarily involving the retinal pigment epithelium
    Fundus flavimaculatus
    Vitelliform dystrophy
  - 362.77 Dystrophies primarily involving Bruch's membrane
    Dystrophy:
      hyaline
      pseudoinflammatory foveal
    Hereditary drusen

- **362.8 Other retinal disorders**
  Excludes: chorioretinal inflammations (363.0–363.2)
  chorioretinal scars (363.30–363.35)

  - 362.81 Retinal hemorrhage
    Hemorrhage:
      preretinal
      retinal (deep) (superficial)
      subretinal
    Coding Clinic: 1996, Q4, P43-44
  - 362.82 Retinal exudates and deposits
  - 362.83 Retinal edema
    Retinal:
      cotton wool spots
      edema (localized) (macular) (peripheral)
  - 362.84 Retinal ischemia
  - 362.85 Retinal nerve fiber bundle defects
  - 362.89 Other retinal disorders

- 362.9 Unspecified retinal disorder

- **363 Chorioretinal inflammations, scars, and other disorders of choroid**

- **363.0 Focal chorioretinitis and focal retinochoroiditis**
  Excludes: focal chorioretinitis or retinochoroiditis in:
    histoplasmosis (115.02, 115.12, 115.92)
    toxoplasmosis (130.2)
    congenital infection (771.2)

  - 363.00 Focal chorioretinitis, unspecified
    Focal:
      choroiditis or chorioretinitis NOS
      retinitis or retinochoroiditis NOS
  - 363.01 Focal choroiditis and chorioretinitis, juxtapapillary
  - 363.03 Focal choroiditis and chorioretinitis of other posterior pole
  - 363.04 Focal choroiditis and chorioretinitis, peripheral
  - 363.05 Focal retinitis and retinochoroiditis, juxtapapillary
    Neuroretinitis
  - 363.06 Focal retinitis and retinochoroiditis, macular or paramacular
  - 363.07 Focal retinitis and retinochoroiditis of other posterior pole
  - 363.08 Focal retinitis and retinochoroiditis, peripheral

- **363.1 Disseminated chorioretinitis and disseminated retinochoroiditis**
  Excludes: disseminated choroiditis or chorioretinitis in:
    secondary syphilis (091.51)
    neurosyphilitic disseminated retinitis or retinochoroiditis (094.83)
    retinal (peri) vasculitis (362.18)

  - 363.10 Disseminated chorioretinitis, unspecified
    Disseminated:
      choroiditis or chorioretinitis NOS
      retinitis or retinochoroiditis NOS
  - 363.11 Disseminated choroiditis and chorioretinitis, posterior pole
  - 363.12 Disseminated choroiditis and chorioretinitis, peripheral
  - 363.13 Disseminated choroiditis and chorioretinitis, generalized
    Code first any underlying disease, as:
      tuberculosis (017.3)

- **363.14** Disseminated retinitis and retinochoroiditis, metastatic
- **363.15** Disseminated retinitis and retinochoroiditis, pigment epitheliopathy
  Acute posterior multifocal placoid pigment epitheliopathy
- **363.2** Other and unspecified forms of chorioretinitis and retinochoroiditis
  Excludes *panophthalmitis (360.02)*
  sympathetic uveitis (360.11)
  uveitis NOS (364.3)
  - **363.20** Chorioretinitis, unspecified
    Choroiditis NOS
    Retinitis NOS
    Uveitis, posterior NOS
  - **363.21** Pars planitis
    Posterior cyclitis
  - **363.22** Harada's disease
- **363.3** Chorioretinal scars
  Scar (postinflammatory) (postsurgical) (posttraumatic):
    choroid
    retina
  - **363.30** Chorioretinal scar, unspecified
  - **363.31** Solar retinopathy
  - **363.32** Other macular scars
  - **363.33** Other scars of posterior pole
  - **363.34** Peripheral scars
  - **363.35** Disseminated scars
- **363.4** Choroidal degenerations
  - **363.40** Choroidal degeneration, unspecified
    Choroidal sclerosis NOS
  - **363.41** Senile atrophy of choroid
  - **363.42** Diffuse secondary atrophy of choroid
  - **363.43** Angioid streaks of choroid
- **363.5** Hereditary choroidal dystrophies
  Hereditary choroidal atrophy:
    partial [choriocapillaris]
    total [all vessels]
  - **363.50** Hereditary choroidal dystrophy or atrophy, unspecified
  - **363.51** Circumpapillary dystrophy of choroid, partial
  - **363.52** Circumpapillary dystrophy of choroid, total
    Helicoid dystrophy of choroid
  - **363.53** Central dystrophy of choroid, partial
    Dystrophy, choroidal:
      central areolar
      circinate
  - **363.54** Central choroidal atrophy, total
    Dystrophy, choroidal:
      central gyrate
      serpiginous
  - **363.55** Choroideremia
  - **363.56** Other diffuse or generalized dystrophy, partial
    Diffuse choroidal sclerosis
  - **363.57** Other diffuse or generalized dystrophy, total
    Generalized gyrate atrophy, choroid
- **363.6** Choroidal hemorrhage and rupture
  - **363.61** Choroidal hemorrhage, unspecified
  - **363.62** Expulsive choroidal hemorrhage
  - **363.63** Choroidal rupture
- **363.7** Choroidal detachment
  - **363.70** Choroidal detachment, unspecified
  - **363.71** Serous choroidal detachment
  - **363.72** Hemorrhagic choroidal detachment
- **363.8** Other disorders of choroid
  Coding Clinic: 2006, Q1, P12
- **363.9** Unspecified disorder of choroid

- **364** Disorders of iris and ciliary body
  - **364.0** Acute and subacute iridocyclitis
    Anterior uveitis, acute, subacute
    Cyclitis, acute, subacute
    Iridocyclitis, acute, subacute
    Iritis, acute, subacute
    Excludes *gonococcal (098.41)*
    herpes simplex (054.44)
    herpes zoster (053.22)
    - **364.00** Acute and subacute iridocyclitis, unspecified
    - **364.01** Primary iridocyclitis
    - **364.02** Recurrent iridocyclitis
    - **364.03** Secondary iridocyclitis, infectious
    - **364.04** Secondary iridocyclitis, noninfectious
      Aqueous:
        cells
        fibrin
        flare
    - **364.05** Hypopyon
  - **364.1** Chronic iridocyclitis
    Excludes *posterior cyclitis (363.21)*
    - **364.10** Chronic iridocyclitis, unspecified
    - **364.11** Chronic iridocyclitis in diseases classified elsewhere
      Code first underlying disease, as:
        sarcoidosis (135)
        tuberculosis (017.3)
      Excludes *syphilitic iridocyclitis (091.52)*
  - **364.2** Certain types of iridocyclitis
    Excludes *posterior cyclitis (363.21)*
    sympathetic uveitis (360.11)
    - **364.21** Fuchs' heterochromic cyclitis
    - **364.22** Glaucomatocyclitic crises
    - **364.23** Lens-induced iridocyclitis
    - **364.24** Vogt-Koyanagi syndrome
  - **364.3** Unspecified iridocyclitis
    Uveitis NOS
  - **364.4** Vascular disorders of iris and ciliary body
    - **364.41** Hyphema
      Hemorrhage of iris or ciliary body
    - **364.42** Rubeosis iridis
      Neovascularization of iris or ciliary body
  - **364.5** Degenerations of iris and ciliary body
    - **364.51** Essential or progressive iris atrophy
    - **364.52** Iridoschisis
    - **364.53** Pigmentary iris degeneration
      Acquired heterochromia of iris
      Pigment dispersion syndrome of iris
      Translucency of iris
    - **364.54** Degeneration of pupillary margin
      Atrophy of sphincter of iris
      Ectropion of pigment epithelium of iris
    - **364.55** Miotic cysts of pupillary margin
    - **364.56** Degenerative changes of chamber angle
    - **364.57** Degenerative changes of ciliary body
    - **364.59** Other iris atrophy
      Iris atrophy (generalized) (sector shaped)
  - **364.6** Cysts of iris, ciliary body, and anterior chamber
    Excludes *miotic pupillary cyst (364.55)*
    parasitic cyst (360.13)
    - **364.60** Idiopathic cysts
    - **364.61** Implantation cysts
      Epithelial down-growth, anterior chamber
      Implantation cysts (surgical) (traumatic)
    - **364.62** Exudative cysts of iris or anterior chamber
    - **364.63** Primary cyst of pars plana
    - **364.64** Exudative cyst of pars plana

- **364.7 Adhesions and disruptions of iris and ciliary body**
  Excludes: flat anterior chamber (360.34)
  - 364.70 Adhesions of iris, unspecified
    Synechiae (iris) NOS
  - 364.71 Posterior synechiae
  - 364.72 Anterior synechiae
  - 364.73 Goniosynechiae
    Peripheral anterior synechiae
  - 364.74 Pupillary membranes
    Iris bombé
    Pupillary:
      occlusion
      seclusion
  - 364.75 Pupillary abnormalities
    Deformed pupil
    Ectopic pupil
    Rupture of sphincter, pupil
  - 364.76 Iridodialysis
    Coding Clinic: 1985, July-Aug, P16
  - 364.77 Recession of chamber angle
- **364.8 Other disorders of iris and ciliary body**
  Coding Clinic: 2007, Q2, P11
  - 364.81 Floppy iris syndrome
    Intraoperative floppy iris syndrome (IFIS)
    Use additional E code to identify cause, such as:
      sympatholytics [antiadrenergics] causing adverse effect in therapeutic use (E941.3)
    Coding Clinic: 2007, Q4, P77-79
  - 364.82 Plateau iris syndrome
    Coding Clinic: 2008, Q4, P112
  - 364.89 Other disorders of iris and ciliary body
    Prolapse of iris NOS
    Excludes: prolapse of iris in recent wound (871.1)
- 364.9 Unspecified disorder of iris and ciliary body

- **365 Glaucoma**
  Intraocular pressure (IOP) is too high. IOP is the result of too much aqueous humor because of excess production or inadequate drainage. Leads to optic nerve damage and vision loss.
  Excludes: blind hypertensive eye [absolute glaucoma] (360.42)
    congenital glaucoma (743.20–743.22)
- **365.0 Borderline glaucoma [glaucoma suspect]**
  - 365.00 Preglaucoma, unspecified
    Coding Clinic: 1990, Q1, P8
  - 365.01 Open angle with borderline findings, low risk
    Open angle, low risk
  - 365.02 Anatomical narrow angle
    Primary angle closure suspect
  - 365.03 Steroid responders
  - 365.04 Ocular hypertension
  - 365.05 Open angle with borderline findings, high risk
    Open angle, high risk
  - 365.06 Primary angle closure without glaucoma damage
- **365.1 Open-angle glaucoma**
  - 365.10 Open-angle glaucoma, unspecified
    Wide-angle glaucoma NOS
    Use additional code to identify glaucoma stage (365.70-365.74)
  - 365.11 Primary open angle glaucoma
    Chronic simple glaucoma
    Use additional code to identify glaucoma stage (365.70-365.74)
  - 365.12 Low tension glaucoma
    Use additional code to identify glaucoma stage (365.70-365.74)
  - 365.13 Pigmentary glaucoma
    Use additional code to identify glaucoma stage (365.70-365.74)
  - 365.14 Glaucoma of childhood
    Infantile or juvenile glaucoma
  - 365.15 Residual stage of open angle glaucoma
- **365.2 Primary angle-closure glaucoma**
  - 365.20 Primary angle-closure glaucoma, unspecified
    Use additional code to identify glaucoma stage (365.70-365.74)
  - 365.21 Intermittent angle-closure glaucoma
    Angle-closure glaucoma:
      interval   subacute
  - 365.22 Acute angle-closure glaucoma
    Acute angle-closure glaucoma attack
    Acute angle-closure glaucoma crisis
  - 365.23 Chronic angle-closure glaucoma
    Chronic primary angle closure glaucoma
    Use additional code to identify glaucoma stage (365.70-365.74)
    Coding Clinic: 1998, Q2, P16
  - 365.24 Residual stage of angle-closure glaucoma
- **365.3 Corticosteroid-induced glaucoma**
  - 365.31 Glaucomatous stage
    Use additional code to identify glaucoma stage (365.70-365.74)
  - 365.32 Residual stage
- **365.4 Glaucoma associated with congenital anomalies, dystrophies, and systemic syndromes**
  - *365.41 Glaucoma associated with chamber angle anomalies*
  - *365.42 Glaucoma associated with anomalies of iris*
  - *365.43 Glaucoma associated with other anterior segment anomalies*
  - *365.44 Glaucoma associated with systemic syndromes*
    Code first associated disease, as:
      neurofibromatosis (237.70-237.79)
      Sturge-Weber (-Dimitri) syndrome (759.6)
- **365.5 Glaucoma associated with disorders of the lens**
  - 365.51 Phacolytic glaucoma
  - 365.52 Pseudoexfoliation glaucoma
    Use additional code to identify glaucoma stage (365.70-365.74)
  - 365.59 Glaucoma associated with other lens disorders
- **365.6 Glaucoma associated with other ocular disorders**
  - 365.60 Glaucoma associated with unspecified ocular disorder
  - 365.61 Glaucoma associated with pupillary block
  - 365.62 Glaucoma associated with ocular inflammations
    Use additional code to identify glaucoma stage (365.70-365.74)
  - 365.63 Glaucoma associated with vascular disorders
    Use additional code to identify glaucoma stage (365.70-365.74)
  - 365.64 Glaucoma associated with tumors or cysts
  - 365.65 Glaucoma associated with ocular trauma
    Use additional code to identify glaucoma stage (365.70-365.74)
- **365.7 Glaucoma stage**
  Code first associated type of glaucoma (365.10-365.13, 365.20, 365.23, 365.31, 365.52, 365.62-365.63, 365.65)
  - *365.70 Glaucoma stage, unspecified*
    Glaucoma stage NOS
  - *365.71 Mild stage glaucoma*
    Early stage glaucoma
  - *365.72 Moderate stage glaucoma*
  - *365.73 Severe stage glaucoma*
    Advanced stage glaucoma
    End-stage glaucoma
  - *365.74 Indeterminate stage glaucoma*

- **365.8 Other specified forms of glaucoma**
  - 365.81 Hypersecretion glaucoma
  - 365.82 Glaucoma with increased episcleral venous pressure
  - 365.83 Aqueous misdirection
    Malignant glaucoma
    Coding Clinic: 2002, Q4, P48
  - 365.89 Other specified glaucoma
    Coding Clinic: 1998, Q2, P16
  - 365.9 Unspecified glaucoma
    Coding Clinic: 2003, Q3, P14; 2001, Q2, P16-17
- **366 Cataract**
  Excludes: congenital cataract (743.30–743.34)
  - **366.0 Infantile, juvenile, and presenile cataract**
    - 366.00 Nonsenile cataract, unspecified
      Coding Clinic: 1987, Mar-April, P9
    - 366.01 Anterior subcapsular polar cataract
    - 366.02 Posterior subcapsular polar cataract
    - 366.03 Cortical, lamellar, or zonular cataract
    - 366.04 Nuclear cataract
    - 366.09 Other and combined forms of nonsenile cataract
  - **366.1 Senile cataract**
    - 366.10 Senile cataract, unspecified
      Coding Clinic: 2003, Q1, P5
    - 366.11 Pseudoexfoliation of lens capsule
    - 366.12 Incipient cataract
      Cataract:
        coronary
        immature NOS
        punctate
      Water clefts
    - 366.13 Anterior subcapsular polar senile cataract
    - 366.14 Posterior subcapsular polar senile cataract
    - 366.15 Cortical senile cataract
    - 366.16 Nuclear sclerosis
      Cataracta brunescens
      Nuclear cataract
      Coding Clinic: 2007, Q4, P77-79; 1985, Sept-Oct, P11
    - 366.17 Total or mature cataract
    - 366.18 Hypermature cataract
      Morgagni cataract
    - 366.19 Other and combined forms of senile cataract
  - **366.2 Traumatic cataract**
    - 366.20 Traumatic cataract, unspecified
    - 366.21 Localized traumatic opacities
      Vossius' ring
    - 366.22 Total traumatic cataract
    - 366.23 Partially resolved traumatic cataract

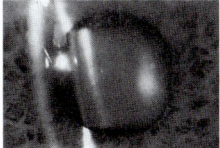

Figure 6–4 Age-related cataract.
Nuclear sclerosis and cortical lens opacities are present. (From Yanoff: Ophthalmology, ed 3, Mosby, Inc., 2008)

Item 6–15 Senile cataracts are linked to the aging process. The most common area for the formation of a cataract is the cortical area of the lens. **Polar cataracts** can be either anterior or posterior. **Anterior polar cataracts** are more common and are small, white, capsular cataracts located on the anterior portion of the lens. **Total cataracts,** also called **complete** or **mature,** cause an opacity of all fibers of the lens. **Hypermature** describes a mature cataract with a swollen, milky cortex that covers the entire lens. **Immature,** also called **incipient,** cataracts have a clear cortex and are only slightly opaque. Treatment for all cataracts is the removal of the lens.

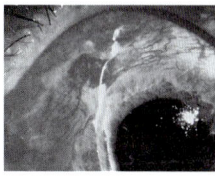

Figure 6–5 Corneal perforation.
Preoperative appearance of a patient who has a small, 1.5 mm corneal perforation at the 10 o'clock limbus. (Courtesy of Dr RK Forster.) (From Yanoff: Ophthalmology, ed 3, Mosby, Inc., 2008)

Item 6–16 Vossius' ring is the result of contusion-type traumatic injury and results in a ring of iris pigment pressed onto the anterior lens capsule.

- **366.3 Cataract secondary to ocular disorders**
  - 366.30 Cataracta complicata, unspecified
  - 366.31 Glaucomatous flecks (subcapsular)
    Code first underlying glaucoma (365.0–365.9)
  - 366.32 Cataract in inflammatory disorders
    Code first underlying condition, as:
      chronic choroiditis (363.0–363.2)
  - 366.33 Cataract with neovascularization
    Code first underlying condition, as:
      chronic iridocyclitis (364.10)
  - 366.34 Cataract in degenerative disorders
    Sunflower cataract
    Code first underlying condition, as:
      chalcosis (360.24)
      degenerative myopia (360.21)
      pigmentary retinal dystrophy (362.74)
- **366.4 Cataract associated with other disorders**
  - 366.41 Diabetic cataract
    Code first diabetes (249.5, 250.5)
    Coding Clinic: 1985, Sept-Oct, P11
  - 366.42 Tetanic cataract
    Code first underlying disease as:
      calcinosis (275.40)
      hypoparathyroidism (252.1)
  - 366.43 Myotonic cataract
    Code first underlying disorder (359.21, 359.23)
  - 366.44 Cataract associated with other syndromes
    Code first underlying condition, as:
      craniofacial dysostosis (756.0)
      galactosemia (271.1)
  - 366.45 Toxic cataract
    Drug-induced cataract
    Use additional E code to identify drug or other toxic substance
    Coding Clinic: 1995, Q4, P51
  - 366.46 Cataract associated with radiation and other physical influences
    Use additional E code to identify cause
- **366.5 After-cataract**
  - 366.50 After-cataract, unspecified
    Secondary cataract NOS
  - 366.51 Soemmering's ring
  - 366.52 Other after-cataract, not obscuring vision
  - 366.53 After-cataract, obscuring vision
  - 366.8 Other cataract
    Calcification of lens
    Coding Clinic: 1994, Q1, P16
  - 366.9 Unspecified cataract
    Coding Clinic: 2009, Q4, P101; 1985, Sept-Oct, P10
- **367 Disorders of refraction and accommodation**
  - 367.0 Hypermetropia
    Far-sightedness
    Hyperopia
  - 367.1 Myopia
    Near-sightedness

Item 6-17 Disorders of refraction: **Hypermetropia**, or far-sightedness, means focus at a distance is adequate but not on close objects. **Myopia** is near-sightedness or short-sightedness and means the focus on nearby objects is clear but distant objects appear blurred. **Astigmatism** is warping of the curvature of the cornea so light rays entering do not meet a single focal point, resulting in a distorted image. **Anisometropia** is unequal refractive power in which one eye may be myopic (near-sighted) and the other hyperopic (far-sighted). **Presbyopia** is the loss of focus on near objects, which occurs with age because the lens loses elasticity.

- **367.2 Astigmatism**
  - 367.20 Astigmatism, unspecified
  - 367.21 Regular astigmatism
  - 367.22 Irregular astigmatism
- **367.3 Anisometropia and aniseikonia**
  - 367.31 Anisometropia
  - 367.32 Aniseikonia
- **367.4 Presbyopia**
- **367.5 Disorders of accommodation**
  - 367.51 Paresis of accommodation
    Cycloplegia
  - 367.52 Total or complete internal ophthalmoplegia
  - 367.53 Spasm of accommodation
- **367.8 Other disorders of refraction and accommodation**
  - 367.81 Transient refractive change
  - 367.89 Other
    Drug-induced disorders of refraction and accommodation
    Toxic disorders of refraction and accommodation
- **367.9 Unspecified disorder of refraction and accommodation**
- **368 Visual disturbances**
  - **Excludes** electrophysiological disturbances (794.11– 794.14)
  - **368.0 Amblyopia ex anopsia**
    - 368.00 Amblyopia, unspecified
    - 368.01 Strabismic amblyopia
      Suppression amblyopia
    - 368.02 Deprivation amblyopia
    - 368.03 Refractive amblyopia
  - **368.1 Subjective visual disturbances**
    - 368.10 Subjective visual disturbance, unspecified
    - 368.11 Sudden visual loss
    - 368.12 Transient visual loss
      Concentric fading
      Scintillating scotoma
    - 368.13 Visual discomfort
      Asthenopia
      Eye strain
      Photophobia
    - 368.14 Visual distortions of shape and size
      Macropsia
      Metamorphopsia
      Micropsia
    - 368.15 Other visual distortions and entoptic phenomena
      Photopsia
      Refractive:
        diplopia
        polyopia
        Visual halos
    - 368.16 Psychophysical visual disturbances
      Prosopagnosia
      Visual:
        agnosia
        disorientation syndrome
        hallucinations
        object agnosia
  - **368.2 Diplopia**
    Double vision
- **368.3 Other disorders of binocular vision**
  - 368.30 Binocular vision disorder, unspecified
  - 368.31 Suppression of binocular vision
  - 368.32 Simultaneous visual perception without fusion
  - 368.33 Fusion with defective stereopsis
  - 368.34 Abnormal retinal correspondence
- **368.4 Visual field defects**
  - 368.40 Visual field defect, unspecified
  - 368.41 Scotoma involving central area
    Scotoma:
      central
      centrocecal
      paracentral
  - 368.42 Scotoma of blind spot area
    Enlarged:
      angioscotoma
      blind spot
    Paracecal scotoma
  - 368.43 Sector or arcuate defects
    Scotoma:
      arcuate
      Bjerrum
      Seidel
  - 368.44 Other localized visual field defect
    Scotoma: Visual field defect:
      NOS   nasal step
      ring   peripheral
  - 368.45 Generalized contraction or constriction
  - 368.46 Homonymous bilateral field defects
    Hemianopsia (altitudinal) (homonymous)
    Quadrant anopia
  - 368.47 Heteronymous bilateral field defects
    Hemianopsia:
      binasal
      bitemporal
- **368.5 Color vision deficiencies**
  Color blindness
  - 368.51 Protan defect
    Protanomaly
    Protanopia
  - 368.52 Deutan defect
    Deuteranomaly
    Deuteranopia
  - 368.53 Tritan defect
    Tritanomaly
    Tritanopia
  - 368.54 Achromatopsia
    Monochromatism (cone) (rod)
  - 368.55 Acquired color vision deficiencies
  - 368.59 Other color vision deficiencies
- **368.6 Night blindness**
  - 368.60 Night blindness, unspecified
  - 368.61 Congenital night blindness
    Hereditary night blindness
    Oguchi's disease
  - 368.62 Acquired night blindness
    Excludes that due to vitamin A deficiency (264.5)
  - 368.63 Abnormal dark adaptation curve
    Abnormal threshold of cones or rods
    Delayed adaptation of cones or rods
  - 368.69 Other night blindness
- **368.8 Other specified visual disturbances**
  Blurred vision NOS
  Coding Clinic: 2002, Q4, P56
- **368.9 Unspecified visual disturbance**
  Coding Clinic: 2006, Q3, P22

369 Blindness and low vision

Excludes correctable impaired vision due to refractive errors (367.0–367.9)

Note: Visual impairment refers to a functional limitation of the eye (e.g., limited visual acuity or visual field). It should be distinguished from visual disability, indicating a limitation of the abilities of the individual (e.g., limited reading skills, vocational skills), and from visual handicap, indicating a limitation of personal and socioeconomic independence (e.g., limited mobility, limited employability).

The levels of impairment defined in the table after 369.9 are based on the recommendations of the WHO Study Group on Prevention of Blindness (Geneva, November 6–10, 1972; WHO Technical Report Series 518), and of the International Council of Ophthalmology (1976).

Note that definitions of blindness vary in different settings.

For international reporting, WHO defines blindness as profound impairment. This definition can be applied to blindness of one eye (369.1, 369.6) and to blindness of the individual (369.0).

For determination of benefits in the U.S.A., the definition of legal blindness as severe impairment is often used. This definition applies to blindness of the individual only.

369.0 Profound impairment, both eyes

- **369.00** Impairment level not further specified
  Blindness:
    NOS according to WHO definition
    both eyes
- **369.01** Better eye: total impairment; lesser eye: total impairment
- **369.02** Better eye: near-total impairment; lesser eye: not further specified
- **369.03** Better eye: near-total impairment; lesser eye: total impairment
- **369.04** Better eye: near-total impairment; lesser eye: near-total impairment
- **369.05** Better eye: profound impairment; lesser eye: not further specified
- **369.06** Better eye: profound impairment; lesser eye: total impairment
- **369.07** Better eye: profound impairment; lesser eye: near-total impairment
- **369.08** Better eye: profound impairment; lesser eye: profound impairment

369.1 Moderate or severe impairment, better eye, profound impairment lesser eye

- **369.10** Impairment level not further specified
  Blindness, one eye, low vision other eye
- **369.11** Better eye: severe impairment; lesser eye: blind, not further specified
- **369.12** Better eye: severe impairment; lesser eye: total impairment
- **369.13** Better eye: severe impairment; lesser eye: near-total impairment
- **369.14** Better eye: severe impairment; lesser eye: profound impairment
- **369.15** Better eye: moderate impairment; lesser eye: blind, not further specified
- **369.16** Better eye: moderate impairment; lesser eye: total impairment
- **369.17** Better eye: moderate impairment; lesser eye: near-total impairment
- **369.18** Better eye: moderate impairment; lesser eye: profound impairment

369.2 Moderate or severe impairment, both eyes

- **369.20** Impairment level not further specified
  Low vision, both eyes NOS
- **369.21** Better eye: severe impairment; lesser eye: not further specified
- **369.22** Better eye: severe impairment; lesser eye: severe impairment
- **369.23** Better eye: moderate impairment; lesser eye: not further specified
- **369.24** Better eye: moderate impairment; lesser eye: severe impairment
- **369.25** Better eye: moderate impairment; lesser eye: moderate impairment

369.3 Unqualified visual loss, both eyes

Excludes blindness NOS:
  legal [U.S.A. definition] (369.4)
  WHO definition (369.00)

369.4 Legal blindness, as defined in U.S.A.
Blindness NOS according to U.S.A. definition

Excludes legal blindness with specification of impairment level (369.01–369.08, 369.11–369.14, 369.21–369.22)

369.6 Profound impairment, one eye
Coding Clinic: 2002, Q3, P20-21

- **369.60** Impairment level not further specified
  Blindness, one eye
- **369.61** One eye: total impairment; other eye: not specified
- **369.62** One eye: total impairment; other eye: near-normal vision
- **369.63** One eye: total impairment; other eye: normal vision
- **369.64** One eye: near-total impairment; other eye: not specified
- **369.65** One eye: near-total impairment; other eye: near-normal vision
- **369.66** One eye: near-total impairment; other eye: normal vision
- **369.67** One eye: profound impairment; other eye: not specified
- **369.68** One eye: profound impairment; other eye: near-normal vision
- **369.69** One eye: profound impairment; other eye: normal vision

369.7 Moderate or severe impairment, one eye

- **369.70** Impairment level not further specified
  Low vision, one eye
- **369.71** One eye: severe impairment; other eye: not specified
- **369.72** One eye: severe impairment; other eye: near-normal vision
- **369.73** One eye: severe impairment; other eye: normal vision
- **369.74** One eye: moderate impairment; other eye: not specified
- **369.75** One eye: moderate impairment; other eye: near-normal vision
- **369.76** One eye: moderate impairment; other eye: normal vision

369.8 Unqualified visual loss, one eye

369.9 Unspecified visual loss

Classification		Levels of Visual Impairment	Additional Descriptors Which May Be Encountered
"Legal"	WHO	Visual Acuity and/or Visual Field Limitation (Whichever Is Worse)	
	(Near-)normal vision	Range of Normal Vision 20/10 20/13 20/16 20/20 20/25 2.0 1.6 1.25 1.0 0.8	
		Near-Normal Vision 20/30 20/40 20/50 20/60 0.7 0.6 0.5 0.4 0.3	
	Low vision	Moderate Visual Impairment 20/70 20/80 20/100 20/125 20/160 0.25 0.20 0.16 0.12	Moderate low vision
Legal Blindness (U.S.A.) both eyes	Blindness (WHO) one or both eyes	Severe Visual Impairment 20/200 20/250 20/320 20/400 0.10 0.08 0.06 0.05 Visual field: 20 degrees or less	Severe low vision, "Legal" blindness
		Profound Visual Impairment 20/500 20/630 20/800 20/1000 0.04 0.03 0.025 0.02 Count fingers at: less than 3 m (10 ft) Visual field: 10 degrees or less	Profound low vision, Moderate blindness
		Near-Total Visual Impairment Visual acuity: less than 0.02 (20/1000) Count fingers: 1 m (3 ft) or less Hand movements: 5 m (15 ft) or less Light projection, light perception Visual field: 5 degrees or less	Severe blindness, Near-total blindness
		Total Visual Impairment No light perception (NLP)	Total blindness

Visual acuity refers to best achievable acuity with correction.
Non-listed Snellen fractions may be classified by converting to the nearest decimal equivalent, e.g., 10/200 = 0.05, 6/30 = 0.20.
CF (count fingers) without designation of distance, may be classified to profound impairment.
HM (hand motion) without designation of distance, may be classified to near-total impairment.
Visual field measurements refer to the largest field diameter for a 1/100 white test object.

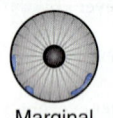 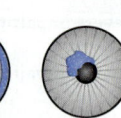 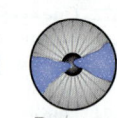 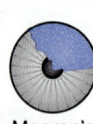

Marginal (catarrhal) ulcer — Ring ulcer — Central corneal ulcer — Rosacea ulcer — Mooren's (rodent) ulcer

Figure 6–6 Corneal ulcers: marginal, ring, central corneal, rosacea, and Mooren's.

Item 6–18 An infected ulcer is usually called a **serpiginous** or **hypopyon** ulcer which is a pus sac in the anterior chamber of the eye.
Marginal ulcers are usually asymptomatic, not primary, and are often superficial and simple. More severe marginal ulcers spread to form a ring ulcer.
Ring ulcers can extend around the entire corneal periphery.
Central corneal ulcers develop when there is an abrasion to the epithelium and an infection develops in the eroded area.
The **pyocyaneal** ulcer is the most serious corneal infection, which, if left untreated, can lead to loss of the eye.

370 Keratitis
- **370.0 Corneal ulcer**
  - Excludes: that due to vitamin A deficiency (264.3)
  - 370.00 Corneal ulcer, unspecified
  - 370.01 Marginal corneal ulcer
  - 370.02 Ring corneal ulcer
  - 370.03 Central corneal ulcer
  - 370.04 Hypopyon ulcer
    - Serpiginous ulcer
  - 370.05 Mycotic corneal ulcer
  - 370.06 Perforated corneal ulcer
  - 370.07 Mooren's ulcer
- **370.2 Superficial keratitis without conjunctivitis**
  - Excludes: dendritic [herpes simplex] keratitis (054.42)
  - 370.20 Superficial keratitis, unspecified
  - 370.21 Punctate keratitis
    - Thygeson's superficial punctate keratitis
  - 370.22 Macular keratitis
    - Keratitis: areolar, nummular, stellate, striate
  - 370.23 Filamentary keratitis
  - 370.24 Photokeratitis
    - Snow blindness
    - Welders' keratitis
    - Coding Clinic: 1996, Q3, P6
- **370.3 Certain types of keratoconjunctivitis**
  - 370.31 Phlyctenular keratoconjunctivitis
    - Phlyctenulosis
    - Use additional code for any associated tuberculosis (017.3)
  - 370.32 Limbal and corneal involvement in vernal conjunctivitis
    - Use additional code for vernal conjunctivitis (372.13)
  - 370.33 Keratoconjunctivitis sicca, not specified as Sjögren's
    - Excludes: Sjögren's syndrome (710.2)
  - 370.34 Exposure keratoconjunctivitis
    - Coding Clinic: 1996, Q3, P6
  - 370.35 Neurotrophic keratoconjunctivitis
- **370.4 Other and unspecified keratoconjunctivitis**
  - 370.40 Keratoconjunctivitis, unspecified
    - Superficial keratitis with conjunctivitis NOS
  - ●370.44 *Keratitis or keratoconjunctivitis in exanthema*
    - Code first underlying condition (050.0–052.9)
    - Excludes: herpes simplex (054.43)
      - herpes zoster (053.21)
      - measles (055.71)
  - 370.49 Other
    - Excludes: epidemic keratoconjunctivitis (077.1)
- **370.5 Interstitial and deep keratitis**
  - 370.50 Interstitial keratitis, unspecified
  - 370.52 Diffuse interstitial keratitis
    - Cogan's syndrome
  - 370.54 Sclerosing keratitis
  - 370.55 Corneal abscess
  - 370.59 Other
    - Excludes: disciform herpes simplex keratitis (054.43)
      - syphilitic keratitis (090.3)
- **370.6 Corneal neovascularization**
  - 370.60 Corneal neovascularization, unspecified
  - 370.61 Localized vascularization of cornea
  - 370.62 Pannus (corneal)
    - Coding Clinic: 2002, Q3, P20-21
  - 370.63 Deep vascularization of cornea
  - 370.64 Ghost vessels (corneal)

- **370.8 Other forms of keratitis**
  Code first underlying condition, such as:
    Acanthamoeba (136.21)
    Fusarium (118)
  Coding Clinic: 2008, Q4, P79-81; 1994, Q3, P5
- **370.9 Unspecified keratitis**

● **371 Corneal opacity and other disorders of cornea**
  ● **371.0 Corneal scars and opacities**
    Excludes that due to vitamin A deficiency (264.6)
    - **371.00 Corneal opacity, unspecified**
      Corneal scar NOS
    - **371.01 Minor opacity of cornea**
      Corneal nebula
    - **371.02 Peripheral opacity of cornea**
      Corneal macula not interfering with central vision
    - **371.03 Central opacity of cornea**
      Corneal:
        leucoma interfering with central vision
        macula interfering with central vision
    - **371.04 Adherent leucoma**
    - ● **371.05 Phthisical cornea**
      Code first underlying tuberculosis (017.3)
  ● **371.1 Corneal pigmentations and deposits**
    - **371.10 Corneal deposit, unspecified**
    - **371.11 Anterior pigmentations**
      Stähli's lines
    - **371.12 Stromal pigmentations**
      Hematocornea
    - **371.13 Posterior pigmentations**
      Krukenberg spindle
    - **371.14 Kayser-Fleischer ring**
    - **371.15 Other deposits associated with metabolic disorders**
    - **371.16 Argentous deposits**
  ● **371.2 Corneal edema**
    - **371.20 Corneal edema, unspecified**
    - **371.21 Idiopathic corneal edema**
    - **371.22 Secondary corneal edema**
    - **371.23 Bullous keratopathy**
    - **371.24 Corneal edema due to wearing of contact lenses**
  ● **371.3 Changes of corneal membranes**
    - **371.30 Corneal membrane change, unspecified**
    - **371.31 Folds and rupture of Bowman's membrane**
    - **371.32 Folds in Descemet's membrane**
    - **371.33 Rupture in Descemet's membrane**
  ● **371.4 Corneal degenerations**
    - **371.40 Corneal degeneration, unspecified**
    - **371.41 Senile corneal changes**
      Arcus senilis   Hassall-Henle bodies
    - **371.42 Recurrent erosion of cornea**
      Excludes Mooren's ulcer (370.07)
    - **371.43 Band-shaped keratopathy**
    - **371.44 Other calcerous degenerations of cornea**
    - **371.45 Keratomalacia NOS**
      Excludes that due to vitamin A deficiency (264.4)
    - **371.46 Nodular degeneration of cornea**
      Salzmann's nodular dystrophy
    - **371.48 Peripheral degenerations of cornea**
      Marginal degeneration of cornea [Terrien's]
    - **371.49 Other**
      Discrete colliquative keratopathy

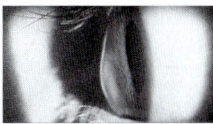

Figure 6–7 Lateral view of the displacement of the cone apex in keratoconus. (From Yanoff: Ophthalmology, ed 3, Mosby, Inc., 2008)

Item 6–19 Keratoconus results in corneal degeneration that begins in childhood, gradually changes the cornea from a round to cone shape, decreasing visual acuity. Treatment includes contact lenses. In severe cases the need for corneal transplant may be the treatment of choice; however, newer technologies may use high frequency radio energy to shrink the edges of the cornea, pulling the central area back to a more normal shape. It can help delay or avoid the need for a corneal transplantation.

  ● **371.5 Hereditary corneal dystrophies**
    - **371.50 Corneal dystrophy, unspecified**
    - **371.51 Juvenile epithelial corneal dystrophy**
    - **371.52 Other anterior corneal dystrophies**
      Corneal dystrophy:
        microscopic cystic
        ring-like
    - **371.53 Granular corneal dystrophy**
    - **371.54 Lattice corneal dystrophy**
    - **371.55 Macular corneal dystrophy**
    - **371.56 Other stromal corneal dystrophies**
      Crystalline corneal dystrophy
    - **371.57 Endothelial corneal dystrophy**
      Combined corneal dystrophy
      Cornea guttata
      Fuchs' endothelial dystrophy
    - **371.58 Other posterior corneal dystrophies**
      Polymorphous corneal dystrophy
  ● **371.6 Keratoconus**
    - **371.60 Keratoconus, unspecified**
    - **371.61 Keratoconus, stable condition**
    - **371.62 Keratoconus, acute hydrops**
  ● **371.7 Other corneal deformities**
    - **371.70 Corneal deformity, unspecified**
    - **371.71 Corneal ectasia**
    - **371.72 Descemetocele**
    - **371.73 Corneal staphyloma**
  ● **371.8 Other corneal disorders**
    - **371.81 Corneal anesthesia and hypoesthesia**
    - **371.82 Corneal disorder due to contact lens**
      Excludes corneal edema due to contact lens (371.24)
    - **371.89 Other**
      Coding Clinic: 1999, Q3, P12
  ● **371.9 Unspecified corneal disorder**

● **372 Disorders of conjunctiva**
  Excludes keratoconjunctivitis (370.3–370.4)
  ● **372.0 Acute conjunctivitis**
    - **372.00 Acute conjunctivitis, unspecified**
    - **372.01 Serous conjunctivitis, except viral**
      Excludes viral conjunctivitis NOS (077.9)
      Coding Clinic: 2008, Q3, P6-7
    - **372.02 Acute follicular conjunctivitis**
      Conjunctival folliculosis NOS
      Excludes conjunctivitis:
        adenoviral (acute follicular) (077.3)
        epidemic hemorrhagic (077.4)
        inclusion (077.0)
        Newcastle (077.8)
      epidemic keratoconjunctivitis (077.1)
      pharyngoconjunctival fever (077.2)

372.03 Other mucopurulent conjunctivitis
Catarrhal conjunctivitis
Excludes blennorrhea neonatorum (gonococcal) (098.40)
neonatal conjunctivitis (771.6)
ophthalmia neonatorum NOS (771.6)

372.04 Pseudomembranous conjunctivitis
Membranous conjunctivitis
Excludes diphtheritic conjunctivitis (032.81)

372.05 Acute atopic conjunctivitis

372.06 Acute chemical conjunctivitis
Acute toxic conjunctivitis
Use additional E code to identify the chemical or toxic agent
Excludes burn of eye and adnexa (940.0–940.9)
chemical corrosion injury of eye (940.2-940.3)

● **372.1 Chronic conjunctivitis**
▪ 372.10 Chronic conjunctivitis, unspecified
372.11 Simple chronic conjunctivitis
372.12 Chronic follicular conjunctivitis
372.13 Vernal conjunctivitis
Coding Clinic: 1996, Q3, P8
372.14 Other chronic allergic conjunctivitis
Coding Clinic: 1996, Q3, P8
● *372.15 Parasitic conjunctivitis*
Code first underlying disease as:
filariasis (125.0–125.9)
mucocutaneous leishmaniasis (085.5)

● **372.2 Blepharoconjunctivitis**
▪ 372.20 Blepharoconjunctivitis, unspecified
372.21 Angular blepharoconjunctivitis
372.22 Contact blepharoconjunctivitis

● **372.3 Other and unspecified conjunctivitis**
▪ 372.30 Conjunctivitis, unspecified
● *372.31 Rosacea conjunctivitis*
Code first underlying rosacea dermatitis (695.3)
● *372.33 Conjunctivitis in mucocutaneous disease*
Code first underlying disease as:
erythema multiforme (695.10–695.19)
Reiter's disease (099.3)
Excludes ocular pemphigoid (694.61)
372.34 Pingueculitis
Excludes pinguecula (372.51)
Coding Clinic: 2008, Q4, P112-113
372.39 Other
Coding Clinic: 2007, Q2, P11

● **372.4 Pterygium**
Excludes pseudopterygium (372.52)
▪ 372.40 Pterygium, unspecified
372.41 Peripheral pterygium, stationary
372.42 Peripheral pterygium, progressive
372.43 Central pterygium
372.44 Double pterygium
372.45 Recurrent pterygium

● **372.5 Conjunctival degenerations and deposits**
▪ 372.50 Conjunctival degeneration, unspecified
372.51 Pinguecula
Excludes pingueculitis (372.34)
372.52 Pseudopterygium
372.53 Conjunctival xerosis
Excludes conjunctival xerosis due to vitamin A deficiency (264.0, 264.1, 264.7)
372.54 Conjunctival concretions
372.55 Conjunctival pigmentations
Conjunctival argyrosis
372.56 Conjunctival deposits

● **372.6 Conjunctival scars**
372.61 Granuloma of conjunctiva
372.62 Localized adhesions and strands of conjunctiva
372.63 Symblepharon
Extensive adhesions of conjunctiva
372.64 Scarring of conjunctiva
Contraction of eye socket (after enucleation)

● **372.7 Conjunctival vascular disorders and cysts**
372.71 Hyperemia of conjunctiva
372.72 Conjunctival hemorrhage
Hyposphagma
Subconjunctival hemorrhage
372.73 Conjunctival edema
Chemosis of conjunctiva
Subconjunctival edema
372.74 Vascular abnormalities of conjunctiva
Aneurysm(ata) of conjunctiva
372.75 Conjunctival cysts

● **372.8 Other disorders of conjunctiva**
372.81 Conjunctivochalasis
Coding Clinic: 2000, Q4, P41
372.89 Other disorders of conjunctiva

▪ **372.9 Unspecified disorder of conjunctiva**

● **373 Inflammation of eyelids**
● **373.0 Blepharitis**
Excludes blepharoconjunctivitis (372.20–372.22)
▪ 373.00 Blepharitis, unspecified
373.01 Ulcerative blepharitis
373.02 Squamous blepharitis

● **373.1 Hordeolum and other deep inflammation of eyelid**
Bacterial infection (staphylococcus) of sebaceous gland of eyelid (stye)
373.11 Hordeolum externum
Hordeolum NOS
Stye
373.12 Hordeolum internum
Infection of meibomian gland
373.13 Abscess of eyelid
Furuncle of eyelid

373.2 Chalazion
Most often caused by accumulation of meibomian gland secretions resulting from blockage of duct
Meibomian (gland) cyst
Excludes infected meibomian gland (373.12)

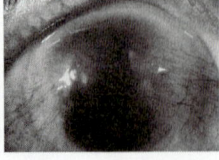

Figure 6–8 Double pterygium. Note both nasal and temporal pterygia in a 57-year-old farmer. (From Yanoff: Ophthalmology, ed 3, Mosby, Inc., 2008)

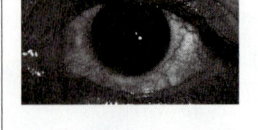

Figure 6–9 Photograph of eyelids with marginal blepharitis. (From Mandell, Bennett, & Dolin: Principles and Practice of Infectious Diseases, ed 7, Churchill Livingstone, An Imprint of Elsevier, 2009)

Item 6–20 **Pterygium** is Greek for batlike. The condition is characterized by a membrane that extends from the limbus to the center of the cornea and resembles a wing.

Item 6–21 **Blepharitis** is a common condition in which the eyelid is swollen and yellow scaling and conjunctivitis develop. Usually the hair on the scalp and brow is involved.

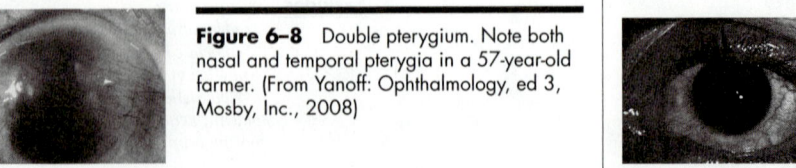

- 373.3 Noninfectious dermatoses of eyelid
  - 373.31 Eczematous dermatitis of eyelid
  - 373.32 Contact and allergic dermatitis of eyelid
  - 373.33 Xeroderma of eyelid
  - 373.34 Discoid lupus erythematosus of eyelid
- 373.4 *Infective dermatitis of eyelid of types resulting in deformity*
  - Code first underlying disease, as:
    - leprosy (030.0–030.9)
    - lupus vulgaris (tuberculous) (017.0)
    - yaws (102.0–102.9)
- 373.5 *Other infective dermatitis of eyelid*
  - Code first underlying disease, as:
    - actinomycosis (039.3)
    - impetigo (684)
    - mycotic dermatitis (110.0–111.9)
    - vaccinia (051.0)
    - postvaccination (999.0)
  - Excludes herpes:
    - simplex (054.41)
    - zoster (053.20)
- 373.6 *Parasitic infestation of eyelid*
  - Code first underlying disease, as:
    - leishmaniasis (085.0–085.9)
    - loiasis (125.2)
    - onchocerciasis (125.3)
    - pediculosis (132.0)
- 373.8 Other inflammations of eyelids
- 373.9 Unspecified inflammation of eyelid
- 374 Other disorders of eyelids
  - 374.0 Entropion and trichiasis of eyelid
    - 374.00 Entropion, unspecified
    - 374.01 Senile entropion
    - 374.02 Mechanical entropion
    - 374.03 Spastic entropion
    - 374.04 Cicatricial entropion
    - 374.05 Trichiasis without entropion
  - 374.1 Ectropion
    - 374.10 Ectropion, unspecified
    - 374.11 Senile ectropion
    - 374.12 Mechanical ectropion
    - 374.13 Spastic ectropion
    - 374.14 Cicatricial ectropion
  - 374.2 Lagophthalmos
    - 374.20 Lagophthalmos, unspecified
    - 374.21 Paralytic lagophthalmos
    - 374.22 Mechanical lagophthalmos
    - 374.23 Cicatricial lagophthalmos
  - 374.3 Ptosis of eyelid
    - *Falling forward, drooping, sagging of eyelid*
    - 374.30 Ptosis of eyelid, unspecified
      - Coding Clinic: 1996, Q2, P11
    - 374.31 Paralytic ptosis
    - 374.32 Myogenic ptosis
    - 374.33 Mechanical ptosis
    - 374.34 Blepharochalasis
      - Pseudoptosis

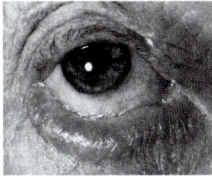

Figure 6–10 Right lower eyelid entropion. Note the inward rotation of the tarsal plate about the horizontal axis and the resultant contact between the mucocutaneous junction and ocular surface. (From Yanoff: Ophthalmology, ed 3, Mosby, Inc., 2008)

Item 6-22 Ptosis of eyelid is drooping of the upper eyelid over the pupil when the eyes are fully opened resulting from nerve or muscle damage, which may require surgical correction.

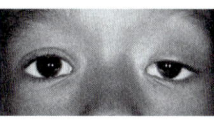

Figure 6–11 Ptosis of eyelid. (From Yanoff: Ophthalmology, ed 3, Mosby, Inc., 2008)

- 374.4 Other disorders affecting eyelid function
  - Excludes blepharoclonus (333.81)
    - blepharospasm (333.81)
    - facial nerve palsy (351.0)
    - third nerve palsy or paralysis (378.51–378.52)
    - tic (psychogenic) (307.20–307.23)
    - organic (333.3)
  - 374.41 Lid retraction or lag
  - 374.43 Abnormal innervation syndrome
    - Jaw-blinking
    - Paradoxical facial movements
  - 374.44 Sensory disorders
  - 374.45 Other sensorimotor disorders
    - Deficient blink reflex
  - 374.46 Blepharophimosis
    - Ankyloblepharon
- 374.5 Degenerative disorders of eyelid and periocular area
  - 374.50 Degenerative disorder of eyelid, unspecified
  - 374.51 Xanthelasma
    - Xanthoma (planum) (tuberosum) of eyelid
    - Code first underlying condition (272.0–272.9)
  - 374.52 Hyperpigmentation of eyelid
    - Chloasma   Dyspigmentation
  - 374.53 Hypopigmentation of eyelid
    - Vitiligo of eyelid
  - 374.54 Hypertrichosis of eyelid
  - 374.55 Hypotrichosis of eyelid
    - Madarosis of eyelid
  - 374.56 Other degenerative disorders of skin affecting eyelid
- 374.8 Other disorders of eyelid
  - 374.81 Hemorrhage of eyelid
    - Excludes black eye (921.0)
  - 374.82 Edema of eyelid
    - Hyperemia of eyelid
    - Coding Clinic: 2008, Q4, P128-131
  - 374.83 Elephantiasis of eyelid
  - 374.84 Cysts of eyelids
    - Sebaceous cyst of eyelid
  - 374.85 Vascular anomalies of eyelid
  - 374.86 Retained foreign body of eyelid
    - Use additional code to identify foreign body (V90.01-V90.9)
  - 374.87 Dermatochalasis
  - 374.89 Other disorders of eyelid
- 374.9 Unspecified disorder of eyelid
- 375 Disorders of lacrimal system
  - 375.0 Dacryoadenitis
    - 375.00 Dacryoadenitis, unspecified
    - 375.01 Acute dacryoadenitis
    - 375.02 Chronic dacryoadenitis
    - 375.03 Chronic enlargement of lacrimal gland
  - 375.1 Other disorders of lacrimal gland
    - 375.11 Dacryops
    - 375.12 Other lacrimal cysts and cystic degeneration
    - 375.13 Primary lacrimal atrophy
    - 375.14 Secondary lacrimal atrophy
    - 375.15 Tear film insufficiency, unspecified
      - Dry eye syndrome
      - Coding Clinic: 1996, Q3, P6
    - 375.16 Dislocation of lacrimal gland

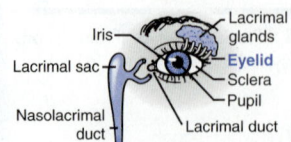

Figure 6-12 Lacrimal apparatus. (From Buck CJ: Step-by-Step Medical Coding. Philadelphia, WB Saunders, 2006, p 302)

- 375.2 Epiphora
  - 375.20 Epiphora, unspecified as to cause
  - 375.21 Epiphora due to excess lacrimation
  - 375.22 Epiphora due to insufficient drainage
- 375.3 Acute and unspecified inflammation of lacrimal passages
  - Excludes: neonatal dacryocystitis (771.6)
  - 375.30 Dacryocystitis, unspecified
  - 375.31 Acute canaliculitis, lacrimal
  - 375.32 Acute dacryocystitis
    - Acute peridacryocystitis
  - 375.33 Phlegmonous dacryocystitis
- 375.4 Chronic inflammation of lacrimal passages
  - 375.41 Chronic canaliculitis
  - 375.42 Chronic dacryocystitis
  - 375.43 Lacrimal mucocele
- 375.5 Stenosis and insufficiency of lacrimal passages
  - 375.51 Eversion of lacrimal punctum
  - 375.52 Stenosis of lacrimal punctum
  - 375.53 Stenosis of lacrimal canaliculi
  - 375.54 Stenosis of lacrimal sac
  - 375.55 Obstruction of nasolacrimal duct, neonatal
    - Excludes: congenital anomaly of nasolacrimal duct (743.65)
  - 375.56 Stenosis of nasolacrimal duct, acquired
  - 375.57 Dacryolith
- 375.6 Other changes of lacrimal passages
  - 375.61 Lacrimal fistula
  - 375.69 Other
- 375.8 Other disorders of lacrimal system
  - 375.81 Granuloma of lacrimal passages
  - 375.89 Other
- 375.9 Unspecified disorder of lacrimal system
- 376 Disorders of the orbit
  - 376.0 Acute inflammation of orbit
    - 376.00 Acute inflammation of orbit, unspecified
    - 376.01 Orbital cellulitis
      - Abscess of orbit
    - 376.02 Orbital periostitis
    - 376.03 Orbital osteomyelitis
    - 376.04 Tenonitis
  - 376.1 Chronic inflammatory disorders of orbit
    - 376.10 Chronic inflammation of orbit, unspecified
    - 376.11 Orbital granuloma
      - Pseudotumor (inflammatory) of orbit
    - 376.12 Orbital myositis
    - ●376.13 Parasitic infestation of orbit
      - *Code first underlying disease, as:*
        - hydatid infestation of orbit (122.3, 122.6, 122.9)
        - myiasis of orbit (134.0)
  - 376.2 Endocrine exophthalmos
    - *Code first underlying thyroid disorder (242.0–242.9)*
    - ●376.21 *Thyrotoxic exophthalmos*
    - ●376.22 *Exophthalmic ophthalmoplegia*
- 376.3 Other exophthalmic conditions
  - 376.30 Exophthalmos, unspecified
  - 376.31 Constant exophthalmos
  - 376.32 Orbital hemorrhage
  - 376.33 Orbital edema or congestion
  - 376.34 Intermittent exophthalmos
  - 376.35 Pulsating exophthalmos
  - 376.36 Lateral displacement of globe
- 376.4 Deformity of orbit
  - 376.40 Deformity of orbit, unspecified
  - 376.41 Hypertelorism of orbit
  - 376.42 Exostosis of orbit
  - 376.43 Local deformities due to bone disease
  - 376.44 Orbital deformities associated with craniofacial deformities
  - 376.45 Atrophy of orbit
  - 376.46 Enlargement of orbit
  - 376.47 Deformity due to trauma or surgery
- 376.5 Enophthalmos
  - 376.50 Enophthalmos, unspecified as to cause
  - 376.51 Enophthalmos due to atrophy of orbital tissue
  - 376.52 Enophthalmos due to trauma or surgery
- 376.6 Retained (old) foreign body following penetrating wound of orbit
  - Retrobulbar foreign body
  - Use additional code to identify foreign body (V90.01-V90.9)
- 376.8 Other orbital disorders
  - 376.81 Orbital cysts
    - Encephalocele of orbit
    - **Coding Clinic: 1999, Q3, P13**
  - 376.82 Myopathy of extraocular muscles
  - 376.89 Other
- 376.9 Unspecified disorder of orbit
- 377 Disorders of optic nerve and visual pathways
  - 377.0 Papilledema
    - 377.00 Papilledema, unspecified
    - 377.01 Papilledema associated with increased intracranial pressure
    - 377.02 Papilledema associated with decreased ocular pressure
    - 377.03 Papilledema associated with retinal disorder
    - 377.04 Foster-Kennedy syndrome
  - 377.1 Optic atrophy
    - 377.10 Optic atrophy, unspecified
    - 377.11 Primary optic atrophy
      - Excludes: neurosyphilitic optic atrophy (094.84)
    - 377.12 Postinflammatory optic atrophy
    - 377.13 Optic atrophy associated with retinal dystrophies
    - 377.14 Glaucomatous atrophy [cupping] of optic disc
    - 377.15 Partial optic atrophy
      - Temporal pallor of optic disc
    - 377.16 Hereditary optic atrophy
      - Optic atrophy:
        - dominant hereditary
        - Leber's

Item 6-23 Papilledema is swelling of the optic disc caused by increased intracranial pressure. It is most often bilateral and occurs quickly (hours) or over weeks of time. It is a common symptom of a brain tumor. The term should not be used to describe optic disc swelling with underlying infectious, infiltrative, or inflammatory etiologies.

- **377.2 Other disorders of optic disc**
  - 377.21 Drusen of optic disc
  - 377.22 Crater-like holes of optic disc
  - 377.23 Coloboma of optic disc
  - 377.24 Pseudopapilledema
- **377.3 Optic neuritis**
  - **Excludes** *meningococcal optic neuritis (036.81)*
  - 377.30 Optic neuritis, unspecified
  - 377.31 Optic papillitis
  - 377.32 Retrobulbar neuritis (acute)
    - **Excludes** *syphilitic retrobulbar neuritis (094.85)*
  - 377.33 Nutritional optic neuropathy
  - 377.34 Toxic optic neuropathy
    - Toxic amblyopia
  - 377.39 Other
    - **Excludes** *ischemic optic neuropathy (377.41)*
- **377.4 Other disorders of optic nerve**
  - 377.41 Ischemic optic neuropathy
  - 377.42 Hemorrhage in optic nerve sheaths
  - 377.43 Optic nerve hypoplasia
    - **Coding Clinic: 2006, Q4, P81-82**
  - 377.49 Other
    - Compression of optic nerve
- **377.5 Disorders of optic chiasm**
  - 377.51 Associated with pituitary neoplasms and disorders
  - 377.52 Associated with other neoplasms
  - 377.53 Associated with vascular disorders
  - 377.54 Associated with inflammatory disorders
- **377.6 Disorders of other visual pathways**
  - 377.61 Associated with neoplasms
  - 377.62 Associated with vascular disorders
  - 377.63 Associated with inflammatory disorders
- **377.7 Disorders of visual cortex**
  - **Excludes** *visual:*
    - *agnosia (368.16)*
    - *hallucinations (368.16)*
    - *halos (368.15)*
  - 377.71 Associated with neoplasms
  - 377.72 Associated with vascular disorders
  - 377.73 Associated with inflammatory disorders
  - 377.75 Cortical blindness
- 377.9 Unspecified disorder of optic nerve and visual pathways
- **378 Strabismus and other disorders of binocular eye movements**
  - **Excludes** *nystagmus and other irregular eye movements (379.50–379.59)*
- **378.0 Esotropia**
  - Convergent concomitant strabismus
  - **Excludes** *intermittent esotropia (378.20–378.22)*
  - 378.00 Esotropia, unspecified
  - 378.01 Monocular esotropia
  - 378.02 Monocular esotropia with A pattern
  - 378.03 Monocular esotropia with V pattern
  - 378.04 Monocular esotropia with other noncomitancies
    - Monocular esotropia with X or Y pattern
  - 378.05 Alternating esotropia
  - 378.06 Alternating esotropia with A pattern
  - 378.07 Alternating esotropia with V pattern
  - 378.08 Alternating esotropia with other noncomitancies
    - Alternating esotropia with X or Y pattern

Item 6-24 Strabismus or esotropia (crossed eyes) is a condition of the extraocular eye muscles, resulting in an inability of the eyes to focus and also affects depth perception.

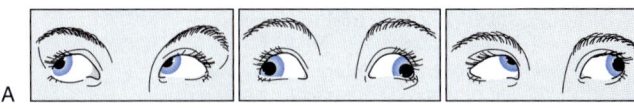
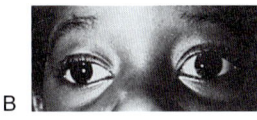

Figure 6-13 **A.** Image of strabismus. **B.** Exotropia. (**A** from Yanoff: Ophthalmology, ed 3, Mosby, Inc., 2008. **B** from Rakel: Textbook of Family Practice, ed 7, Saunders, 2007)

- **378.1 Exotropia**
  - *Misalignment in which one eye deviates outward (away from nose) while other fixates normally*
  - Divergent concomitant strabismus
  - **Excludes** *intermittent exotropia (378.20, 378.23–378.24)*
  - 378.10 Exotropia, unspecified
  - 378.11 Monocular exotropia
  - 378.12 Monocular exotropia with A pattern
  - 378.13 Monocular exotropia with V pattern
  - 378.14 Monocular exotropia with other noncomitancies
    - Monocular exotropia with X or Y pattern
  - 378.15 Alternating exotropia
  - 378.16 Alternating exotropia with A pattern
  - 378.17 Alternating exotropia with V pattern
  - 378.18 Alternating exotropia with other noncomitancies
    - Alternating exotropia with X or Y pattern
- **378.2 Intermittent heterotropia**
  - *Displacement of an organ or part of an organ from normal position*
  - **Excludes** *vertical heterotropia (intermittent) (378.31)*
  - 378.20 Intermittent heterotropia, unspecified
    - Intermittent:
      - esotropia NOS
      - exotropia NOS
  - 378.21 Intermittent esotropia, monocular
  - 378.22 Intermittent esotropia, alternating
  - 378.23 Intermittent exotropia, monocular
  - 378.24 Intermittent exotropia, alternating
- **378.3 Other and unspecified heterotropia**
  - 378.30 Heterotropia, unspecified
  - 378.31 Hypertropia
    - Vertical heterotropia (constant) (intermittent)
  - 378.32 Hypotropia
  - 378.33 Cyclotropia
  - 378.34 Monofixation syndrome
    - Microtropia
  - 378.35 Accommodative component in esotropia
- **378.4 Heterophoria**
  - *Condition in which one or both eyes wander away from position where both eyes are looking*
  - 378.40 Heterophoria, unspecified
  - 378.41 Esophoria
    - *Eye deviates inward (toward nose)*
  - 378.42 Exophoria
    - *Eye deviates outward (toward ear)*
  - 378.43 Vertical heterophoria
  - 378.44 Cyclophoria
  - 378.45 Alternating hyperphoria

- **378.5 Paralytic strabismus**
  - 378.50 Paralytic strabismus, unspecified
  - 378.51 Third or oculomotor nerve palsy, partial
  - 378.52 Third or oculomotor nerve palsy, total
  - 378.53 Fourth or trochlear nerve palsy
    Coding Clinic: 2001, Q2, P21
  - 378.54 Sixth or abducens nerve palsy
  - 378.55 External ophthalmoplegia
    Coding Clinic: 1989, Q2, P12
  - 378.56 Total ophthalmoplegia
- **378.6 Mechanical strabismus**
  - 378.60 Mechanical strabismus, unspecified
  - 378.61 Brown's (tendon) sheath syndrome
  - 378.62 Mechanical strabismus from other musculofascial disorders
  - 378.63 Limited duction associated with other conditions
- **378.7 Other specified strabismus**
  - 378.71 Duane's syndrome
  - 378.72 Progressive external ophthalmoplegia
  - 378.73 Strabismus in other neuromuscular disorders
- **378.8 Other disorders of binocular eye movements**
  Excludes nystagmus (379.50–379.56)
  - 378.81 Palsy of conjugate gaze
  - 378.82 Spasm of conjugate gaze
  - 378.83 Convergence insufficiency or palsy
  - 378.84 Convergence excess or spasm
  - 378.85 Anomalies of divergence
  - 378.86 Internuclear ophthalmoplegia
  - 378.87 Other dissociated deviation of eye movements
    Skew deviation
- **378.9 Unspecified disorder of eye movements**
  Ophthalmoplegia NOS
  Strabismus NOS
  Coding Clinic: 2001, Q2, P21

- **379 Other disorders of eye**
  - **379.0 Scleritis and episcleritis**
    Inflammation of white (sclera and episclera) of eye. Autoimmune disorders are most common cause.
    Excludes syphilitic episcleritis (095.0)
    - 379.00 Scleritis, unspecified
      Episcleritis NOS
    - 379.01 Episcleritis periodica fugax
    - 379.02 Nodular episcleritis
    - 379.03 Anterior scleritis
    - 379.04 Scleromalacia perforans
    - 379.05 Scleritis with corneal involvement
      Scleroperikeratitis
    - 379.06 Brawny scleritis
    - 379.07 Posterior scleritis
      Sclerotenonitis
    - 379.09 Other
      Scleral abscess
  - **379.1 Other disorders of sclera**
    Excludes blue sclera (743.47)
    - 379.11 Scleral ectasia
      Scleral staphyloma NOS
    - 379.12 Staphyloma posticum
    - 379.13 Equatorial staphyloma
    - 379.14 Anterior staphyloma, localized
    - 379.15 Ring staphyloma
    - 379.16 Other degenerative disorders of sclera
    - 379.19 Other
  - **379.2 Disorders of vitreous body**
    - 379.21 Vitreous degeneration
      Vitreous:
        cavitation
        detachment
        liquefaction
    - 379.22 Crystalline deposits in vitreous
      Asteroid hyalitis
      Synchysis scintillans
    - 379.23 Vitreous hemorrhage
      Coding Clinic: 1991, Q3, P15-16
    - 379.24 Other vitreous opacities
      Vitreous floaters
      Small clumps of cells that float in vitreous of the eye, appearing as black specks or dots in field of vision
      Coding Clinic: 1994, Q1, P16
    - 379.25 Vitreous membranes and strands
    - 379.26 Vitreous prolapse
    - 379.27 Vitreomacular adhesion
      Vitreomacular traction
      Excludes traction detachment with vitreoretinal organization (361.81)
      Coding Clinic: 2011, Q4, P106
    - 379.29 Other disorders of vitreous
      Excludes vitreous abscess (360.04)
      Coding Clinic: 1999, Q1, P11
  - **379.3 Aphakia and other disorders of lens**
    Excludes after-cataract (366.50–366.53)
    - 379.31 Aphakia
      Excludes cataract extraction status (V45.61)
    - 379.32 Subluxation of lens
      Coding Clinic: 1994, Q1, P16-17
    - 379.33 Anterior dislocation of lens
    - 379.34 Posterior dislocation of lens
    - 379.39 Other disorders of lens
  - **379.4 Anomalies of pupillary function**
    - 379.40 Abnormal pupillary function, unspecified
    - 379.41 Anisocoria
    - 379.42 Miosis (persistent), not due to miotics
    - 379.43 Mydriasis (persistent), not due to mydriatics
    - 379.45 Argyll Robertson pupil, atypical
      Argyll Robertson phenomenon or pupil, nonsyphilitic
      Excludes Argyll Robertson pupil (syphilitic) (094.89)
    - 379.46 Tonic pupillary reaction
      Adie's pupil or syndrome
    - 379.49 Other
      Hippus
      Pupillary paralysis
  - **379.5 Nystagmus and other irregular eye movements**
    Nystagmus is rapid, involuntary movements of eyes in horizontal or vertical direction.
    - 379.50 Nystagmus, unspecified
      Coding Clinic: 2002, Q4, P68; 2001, Q2, P21
    - 379.51 Congenital nystagmus
    - 379.52 Latent nystagmus
    - 379.53 Visual deprivation nystagmus
    - 379.54 Nystagmus associated with disorders of the vestibular system
    - 379.55 Dissociated nystagmus
    - 379.56 Other forms of nystagmus
    - 379.57 Deficiencies of saccadic eye movements
      Abnormal optokinetic response
    - 379.58 Deficiencies of smooth pursuit movements
    - 379.59 Other irregularities of eye movements
      Opsoclonus

- **379.6 Inflammation (infection) of postprocedural bleb**
  Postprocedural blebitis
  - 379.60 Inflammation (infection) of postprocedural bleb, unspecified
  - 379.61 Inflammation (infection) of postprocedural bleb, stage 1
  - 379.62 Inflammation (infection) of postprocedural bleb, stage 2
    Coding Clinic: 2006, Q4, P82-83
  - 379.63 Inflammation (infection) of postprocedural bleb, stage 3
    Bleb associated endophthalmitis
- 379.8 Other specified disorders of eye and adnexa
- **379.9 Unspecified disorder of eye and adnexa**
  - 379.90 Disorder of eye, unspecified
  - 379.91 Pain in or around eye
  - 379.92 Swelling or mass of eye
  - 379.93 Redness or discharge of eye
  - 379.99 Other ill-defined disorders of eye
    Excludes blurred vision NOS (368.8)

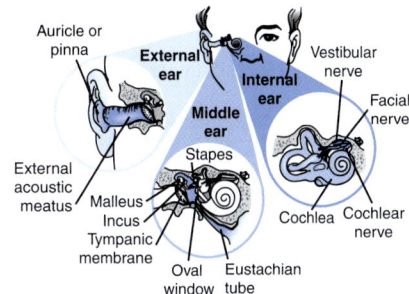

Figure 6-14
Auditory system. (From Buck CJ: Step-by-Step Medical Coding, ed 2010, Philadelphia, WB Saunders, 2010)

DISEASES OF THE EAR AND MASTOID PROCESS (380–389)

Use additional external cause code, if applicable, to identify the cause of the ear condition

- **380 Disorders of external ear**
  - **380.0 Perichondritis and chondritis of pinna**
    Chondritis of auricle
    Perichondritis of auricle
    - 380.00 Perichondritis of pinna, unspecified
    - 380.01 Acute perichondritis of pinna
    - 380.02 Chronic perichondritis of pinna
    - 380.03 Chondritis of pinna
      Coding Clinic: 2004, Q4, P75-76
  - **380.1 Infective otitis externa**
    - 380.10 Infective otitis externa, unspecified
      Otitis externa (acute):
        NOS
        circumscribed
        diffuse
        hemorrhagica
        infective NOS
    - 380.11 Acute infection of pinna
      Excludes furuncular otitis externa (680.0)
    - 380.12 Acute swimmers' ear
      Beach ear   Tank ear
    - ●380.13 *Other acute infections of external ear*
      Code first underlying disease, as:
        erysipelas (035)
        impetigo (684)
        seborrheic dermatitis (690.10–690.18)
      Excludes herpes simplex (054.73)
               herpes zoster (053.71)
    - 380.14 Malignant otitis externa
    - ●380.15 *Chronic mycotic otitis externa*
      Code first underlying disease, as:
        aspergillosis (117.3)
        otomycosis NOS (111.9)
      Excludes candidal otitis externa (112.82)
    - 380.16 Other chronic infective otitis externa
      Chronic infective otitis externa NOS
  - **380.2 Other otitis externa**
    - 380.21 Cholesteatoma of external ear
      Keratosis obturans of external ear (canal)
      Excludes cholesteatoma NOS (385.30–385.35)
               postmastoidectomy (383.32)
    - 380.22 Other acute otitis externa
      Acute otitis externa:
        actinic   eczematoid
        chemical   reactive
        contact
    - 380.23 Other chronic otitis externa
      Chronic otitis externa NOS
  - **380.3 Noninfectious disorders of pinna**
    - 380.30 Disorder of pinna, unspecified
    - 380.31 Hematoma of auricle or pinna
    - 380.32 Acquired deformities of auricle or pinna
      Excludes cauliflower ear (738.7)
      Coding Clinic: 2003, Q3, P12-13
    - 380.39 Other
      Excludes gouty tophi of ear (274.81)
  - 380.4 Impacted cerumen
    Wax in ear
  - **380.5 Acquired stenosis of external ear canal**
    Collapse of external ear canal
    - 380.50 Acquired stenosis of external ear canal, unspecified as to cause
    - 380.51 Secondary to trauma
    - 380.52 Secondary to surgery
    - 380.53 Secondary to inflammation
  - **380.8 Other disorders of external ear**
    - 380.81 Exostosis of external ear canal
    - 380.89 Other
  - 380.9 Unspecified disorder of external ear
- **381 Nonsuppurative otitis media and Eustachian tube disorders**
  Nonsuppurative: not producing pus
  - **381.0 Acute nonsuppurative otitis media**
    Acute tubotympanic catarrh
    Otitis media, acute or subacute:
      catarrhal
      exudative
      transudative
      with effusion
    Excludes otitic barotrauma (993.0)
    - 381.00 Acute nonsuppurative otitis media, unspecified
    - 381.01 Acute serous otitis media
      Acute or subacute secretory otitis media
    - 381.02 Acute mucoid otitis media
      Acute or subacute seromucinous otitis media
      Blue drum syndrome
    - 381.03 Acute sanguinous otitis media
    - 381.04 Acute allergic serous otitis media
    - 381.05 Acute allergic mucoid otitis media
    - 381.06 Acute allergic sanguinous otitis media

- **381.1 Chronic serous otitis media**
  Chronic tubotympanic catarrh
  - 381.10 Chronic serous otitis media, simple or unspecified
  - 381.19 Other
    Serosanguinous chronic otitis media
- **381.2 Chronic mucoid otitis media**
  Glue ear
  Excludes adhesive middle ear disease (385.10–385.19)
  - 381.20 Chronic mucoid otitis media, simple or unspecified
  - 381.29 Other
    Mucosanguinous chronic otitis media
- **381.3 Other and unspecified chronic nonsuppurative otitis media**
  Otitis media, chronic:
    allergic
    exudative
    secretory
    seromucinous
    transudative
    with effusion
- **381.4 Nonsuppurative otitis media, not specified as acute or chronic**
  Otitis media:
    allergic
    catarrhal
    exudative
    mucoid
    secretory
    seromucinous
    serous
    transudative
    with effusion
- **381.5 Eustachian salpingitis**
  - 381.50 Eustachian salpingitis, unspecified
  - 381.51 Acute Eustachian salpingitis
  - 381.52 Chronic Eustachian salpingitis
- **381.6 Obstruction of Eustachian tube**
  Stenosis of Eustachian tube
  Stricture of Eustachian tube
  - 381.60 Obstruction of Eustachian tube, unspecified
  - 381.61 Osseous obstruction of Eustachian tube
    Obstruction of Eustachian tube from cholesteatoma, polyp, or other osseous lesion
  - 381.62 Intrinsic cartilaginous obstruction of Eustachian tube
  - 381.63 Extrinsic cartilaginous obstruction of Eustachian tube
    Compression of Eustachian tube
  - 381.7 Patulous Eustachian tube
- **381.8 Other disorders of Eustachian tube**
  - 381.81 Dysfunction of Eustachian tube
  - 381.89 Other
- 381.9 Unspecified Eustachian tube disorder
- **382 Suppurative and unspecified otitis media**
  - **382.0 Acute suppurative otitis media**
    Suppurative: Discharging pus
    Otitis media, acute:
      necrotizing NOS
      purulent
        pus-filled
    - 382.00 Acute suppurative otitis media without spontaneous rupture of ear drum
    - 382.01 Acute suppurative otitis media with spontaneous rupture of ear drum
    - ● 382.02 *Acute suppurative otitis media in diseases classified elsewhere*
      Code first underlying disease, as:
        influenza (487.8, 488.09, 488.19)
        scarlet fever (034.1)
      Excludes postmeasles otitis (055.2)
- **382.1 Chronic tubotympanic suppurative otitis media**
  Benign chronic suppurative otitis media (with anterior perforation of ear drum)
  Chronic tubotympanic disease (with anterior perforation of ear drum)
- **382.2 Chronic atticoantral suppurative otitis media**
  Chronic atticoantral disease (with posterior or superior marginal perforation of ear drum)
  Persistent mucosal disease (with posterior or superior marginal perforation of ear drum)
- 382.3 Unspecified chronic suppurative otitis media
  Chronic purulent otitis media
  Excludes tuberculous otitis media (017.4)
- 382.4 Unspecified suppurative otitis media
  Purulent otitis media NOS
- 382.9 Unspecified otitis media
  Otitis media:
    NOS
    acute NOS
    chronic NOS
- **383 Mastoiditis and related conditions**
  - **383.0 Acute mastoiditis**
    Abscess of mastoid
    Empyema of mastoid
    - 383.00 Acute mastoiditis without complications
    - 383.01 Subperiosteal abscess of mastoid
    - 383.02 Acute mastoiditis with other complications
      Gradenigo's syndrome
  - 383.1 Chronic mastoiditis
    Caries of mastoid
    Fistula of mastoid
    Excludes tuberculous mastoiditis (015.6)
  - **383.2 Petrositis**
    Coalescing osteitis of petrous bone
    Inflammation of petrous bone
    Osteomyelitis of petrous bone
    - 383.20 Petrositis, unspecified
    - 383.21 Acute petrositis
    - 383.22 Chronic petrositis
  - **383.3 Complications following mastoidectomy**
    - 383.30 Postmastoidectomy complication, unspecified
    - 383.31 Mucosal cyst of postmastoidectomy cavity
    - 383.32 Recurrent cholesteatoma of postmastoidectomy cavity
    - 383.33 Granulations of postmastoidectomy cavity
      Chronic inflammation of postmastoidectomy cavity
  - **383.8 Other disorders of mastoid**
    - 383.81 Postauricular fistula
    - 383.89 Other
  - 383.9 Unspecified mastoiditis
- **384 Other disorders of tympanic membrane**
  - **384.0 Acute myringitis without mention of otitis media**
    - 384.00 Acute myringitis, unspecified
      Acute tympanitis NOS
    - 384.01 Bullous myringitis
      Myringitis bullosa hemorrhagica
    - 384.09 Other
  - 384.1 Chronic myringitis without mention of otitis media
    Chronic tympanitis

Item 6-25 Mastoiditis is an infection of the portion of the temporal bone of the skull that is behind the ear (mastoid process) caused by an untreated otitis media, leading to an infection of the surrounding structures which may include the brain.

- **384.2** Perforation of tympanic membrane
  Perforation of ear drum:
    NOS
    persistent posttraumatic
    postinflammatory
  Excludes *otitis media with perforation of tympanic membrane (382.00–382.9)*
    traumatic perforation [current injury] (872.61)
  - 384.20 Perforation of tympanic membrane, unspecified
  - 384.21 Central perforation of tympanic membrane
  - 384.22 Attic perforation of tympanic membrane
    Pars flaccida
  - 384.23 Other marginal perforation of tympanic membrane
  - 384.24 Multiple perforations of tympanic membrane
  - 384.25 Total perforation of tympanic membrane
- **384.8** Other specified disorders of tympanic membrane
  - 384.81 Atrophic flaccid tympanic membrane
    Healed perforation of ear drum
  - 384.82 Atrophic nonflaccid tympanic membrane
- **384.9** Unspecified disorder of tympanic membrane
- **385** Other disorders of middle ear and mastoid
  Excludes *mastoiditis (383.0–383.9)*
  - **385.0** Tympanosclerosis
    - 385.00 Tympanosclerosis, unspecified as to involvement
    - 385.01 Tympanosclerosis involving tympanic membrane only
    - 385.02 Tympanosclerosis involving tympanic membrane and ear ossicles
    - 385.03 Tympanosclerosis involving tympanic membrane, ear ossicles, and middle ear
    - 385.09 Tympanosclerosis involving other combination of structures
  - **385.1** Adhesive middle ear disease
    Adhesive otitis
    Otitis media: Otitis media:
      chronic adhesive   fibrotic
    Excludes *glue ear (381.20–381.29)*
    - 385.10 Adhesive middle ear disease, unspecified as to involvement
    - 385.11 Adhesions of drum head to incus
    - 385.12 Adhesions of drum head to stapes
    - 385.13 Adhesions of drum head to promontorium
    - 385.19 Other adhesions and combinations
  - **385.2** Other acquired abnormality of ear ossicles
    - 385.21 Impaired mobility of malleus
      Ankylosis of malleus
    - 385.22 Impaired mobility of other ear ossicles
      Ankylosis of ear ossicles, except malleus
    - 385.23 Discontinuity or dislocation of ear ossicles
    - 385.24 Partial loss or necrosis of ear ossicles
  - **385.3** Cholesteatoma of middle ear and mastoid
    Cholesterosis of (middle) ear
    Epidermosis of (middle) ear
    Keratosis of (middle) ear
    Polyp of (middle) ear
    Excludes *cholesteatoma:*
      external ear canal (380.21)
      recurrent of postmastoidectomy cavity (383.32)
    - 385.30 Cholesteatoma, unspecified
    - 385.31 Cholesteatoma of attic
    - 385.32 Cholesteatoma of middle ear
    - 385.33 Cholesteatoma of middle ear and mastoid
      Coding Clinic: 2000, Q3, P10-11
    - 385.35 Diffuse cholesteatosis

- **385.8** Other disorders of middle ear and mastoid
  - 385.82 Cholesterin granuloma
  - 385.83 Retained foreign body of middle ear
    Use additional code to identify foreign body (V90.01-V90.9)
    Coding Clinic: 1987, Nov-Dec, P9
  - 385.89 Other
- **385.9** Unspecified disorder of middle ear and mastoid
- **386** Vertiginous syndromes and other disorders of vestibular system
  Excludes *vertigo NOS (780.4)*
  Coding Clinic: 1985, Mar-April, P12
  - **386.0** Méniére's disease
    Vestibular disorder that produces recurring symptoms including severe and intermittent hearing loss including feeling of ear pressure or pain
    Endolymphatic hydrops
    Lermoyez's syndrome
    Méniére's syndrome or vertigo
    - 386.00 Méniére's disease, unspecified
      Méniére's disease (active)
      Coding Clinic: 1985, Mar-April, P12
    - 386.01 Active Méniére's disease, cochleovestibular
    - 386.02 Active Méniére's disease, cochlear
    - 386.03 Active Méniére's disease, vestibular
    - 386.04 Inactive Méniére's disease
      Méniére's disease in remission
  - **386.1** Other and unspecified peripheral vertigo
    Excludes *epidemic vertigo (078.81)*
    - 386.10 Peripheral vertigo, unspecified
    - 386.11 Benign paroxysmal positional vertigo
      Benign paroxysmal positional nystagmus
    - 386.12 Vestibular neuronitis
      Acute (and recurrent) peripheral vestibulopathy
    - 386.19 Other
      Aural vertigo   Otogenic vertigo
  - 386.2 Vertigo of central origin
    Central positional nystagmus
    Malignant positional vertigo
  - **386.3** Labyrinthitis
    Balance disorder that follows a URI or head injury. The inflammatory process affects the labyrinth that houses vestibular system (senses changes in head position) of inner ear.
    - 386.30 Labyrinthitis, unspecified
    - 386.31 Serous labyrinthitis
      Diffuse labyrinthitis
    - 386.32 Circumscribed labyrinthitis
      Focal labyrinthitis
    - 386.33 Suppurative labyrinthitis
      Purulent labyrinthitis
    - 386.34 Toxic labyrinthitis
    - 386.35 Viral labyrinthitis
  - **386.4** Labyrinthine fistula
    - 386.40 Labyrinthine fistula, unspecified
    - 386.41 Round window fistula
    - 386.42 Oval window fistula
    - 386.43 Semicircular canal fistula
    - 386.48 Labyrinthine fistula of combined sites

- 386.5 **Labyrinthine dysfunction**
  - 386.50 Labyrinthine dysfunction, unspecified
  - 386.51 Hyperactive labyrinth, unilateral
  - 386.52 Hyperactive labyrinth, bilateral
  - 386.53 Hypoactive labyrinth, unilateral
  - 386.54 Hypoactive labyrinth, bilateral
  - 386.55 Loss of labyrinthine reactivity, unilateral
  - 386.56 Loss of labyrinthine reactivity, bilateral
  - 386.58 Other forms and combinations
- 386.8 Other disorders of labyrinth
  Coding Clinic: 2011, Q1, P7
- 386.9 Unspecified vertiginous syndromes and labyrinthine disorders

- **387 Otosclerosis**
  Inherited middle ear spongelike bone growth causing hearing loss because growth prevents vibration from sound waves required for hearing
  Includes otospongiosis
  - 387.0 Otosclerosis involving oval window, nonobliterative
  - 387.1 Otosclerosis involving oval window, obliterative
  - 387.2 Cochlear otosclerosis
    Otosclerosis involving:
      otic capsule
      round window
  - 387.8 Other otosclerosis
  - 387.9 Otosclerosis, unspecified

- **388 Other disorders of ear**
  - 388.0 Degenerative and vascular disorders of ear
    - 388.00 Degenerative and vascular disorders, unspecified
    - 388.01 Presbyacusis
    - 388.02 Transient ischemic deafness
  - 388.1 Noise effects on inner ear
    - 388.10 Noise effects on inner ear, unspecified
    - 388.11 Acoustic trauma (explosive) to ear
      Otitic blast injury
    - 388.12 Noise-induced hearing loss
  - 388.2 Sudden hearing loss, unspecified
  - 388.3 **Tinnitus**
    Perception of sound in absence of external noise and may affect one or both ears and/or head
    - 388.30 Tinnitus, unspecified
    - 388.31 Subjective tinnitus
    - 388.32 Objective tinnitus
  - 388.4 Other abnormal auditory perception
    - 388.40 Abnormal auditory perception, unspecified
    - 388.41 Diplacusis
    - 388.42 Hyperacusis
    - 388.43 Impairment of auditory discrimination
    - 388.44 Recruitment
    - 388.45 Acquired auditory processing disorder
      Auditory processing disorder NOS
      Excludes *central auditory processing disorder (315.32)*
      Coding Clinic: 2007, Q4, P79
  - 388.5 Disorders of acoustic nerve
    Acoustic neuritis
    Degeneration of acoustic or eighth nerve
    Disorder of acoustic or eighth nerve
    Excludes *acoustic neuroma (225.1)*
    syphilitic acoustic neuritis (094.86)
    Coding Clinic: 1987, Mar-April, P8
  - 388.6 Otorrhea
    - 388.60 Otorrhea, unspecified
      Discharging ear NOS
    - 388.61 Cerebrospinal fluid otorrhea
      Excludes *cerebrospinal fluid rhinorrhea (349.81)*
    - 388.69 Other
      Otorrhagia
  - 388.7 Otalgia
    - 388.70 Otalgia, unspecified
      Earache NOS
    - 388.71 Otogenic pain
    - 388.72 Referred pain
      Pain from a diseased area of the body that is not felt directly in that area, but in another part of the body
  - 388.8 Other disorders of ear
  - 388.9 Unspecified disorder of ear

- **389 Hearing loss**
  - 389.0 Conductive hearing loss
    Conductive deafness
    Excludes *mixed conductive and sensorineural hearing loss (389.20–389.22)*
    - 389.00 Conductive hearing loss, unspecified
    - 389.01 Conductive hearing loss, external ear
    - 389.02 Conductive hearing loss, tympanic membrane
    - 389.03 Conductive hearing loss, middle ear
    - 389.04 Conductive hearing loss, inner ear
    - 389.05 Conductive hearing loss, unilateral
    - 389.06 Conductive hearing loss, bilateral
      Coding Clinic: 2007, Q4, P80-81
    - 389.08 Conductive hearing loss of combined types
  - 389.1 Sensorineural hearing loss
    Perceptive hearing loss or deafness
    Excludes *abnormal auditory perception (388.40–388.44)*
    mixed conductive and sensorineural hearing loss (389.20–389.22)
    psychogenic deafness (306.7)
    Coding Clinic: 2007, Q4, P80-81; 2006, Q4, P84
    - 389.10 Sensorineural hearing loss, unspecified
      Coding Clinic: 1993, Q1, P29
    - 389.11 Sensory hearing loss, bilateral
    - 389.12 Neural hearing loss, bilateral
    - 389.13 Neural hearing loss, unilateral
    - 389.14 Central hearing loss
    - 389.15 Sensorineural hearing loss, unilateral
    - 389.16 Sensorineural hearing loss, asymmetrical
    - 389.17 Sensory hearing loss, unilateral
    - 389.18 Sensorineural hearing loss, bilateral
  - 389.2 Mixed conductive and sensorineural hearing loss
    Deafness or hearing loss of type classifiable to 389.00–389.08 with type classifiable to 389.10–389.18
    Coding Clinic: 2007, Q4, P80-81
    - 389.20 Mixed hearing loss, unspecified
    - 389.21 Mixed hearing loss, unilateral
    - 389.22 Mixed hearing loss, bilateral
  - 389.7 Deaf nonspeaking, not elsewhere classifiable
  - 389.8 Other specified forms of hearing loss
  - 389.9 Unspecified hearing loss
    Deafness NOS
    Coding Clinic: 2004, Q1, P15-16

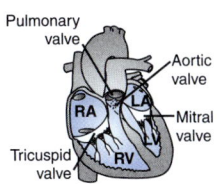

Figure 7-1 Cardiovascular valves.

Item 7-1 **Rheumatic fever** is the inflammation of the valve(s) of the heart, usually the mitral or aortic, which leads to valve damage. Rheumatic heart inflammations are usually **pericarditis** (sac surrounding heart), **endocarditis** (heart cavity), or **myocarditis** (heart muscle).

Item 7-3 **Mitral stenosis** is the narrowing of the mitral valve separating the left atrium from the left ventricle. **Mitral insufficiency** is the improper closure of the mitral valve which may lead to enlargement (hypertrophy) of the left atrium.

Item 7-4 **Aortic stenosis** is the narrowing of the aortic valve located between the left ventricle and the aorta. **Aortic insufficiency** is the improper closure of the aortic valve which may lead to enlargement (hypertrophy) of the left ventricle.

Item 7-5 **Mitral and aortic valve stenosis** is the narrowing of these valves, which leads to enlargement (hypertrophy) of the left atrium and left ventricle respectively, while **mitral and aortic insufficiency** is the improper closure of the mitral and aortic valves resulting in the same outcome as stenosis.

7. DISEASES OF THE CIRCULATORY SYSTEM (390–459)

ACUTE RHEUMATIC FEVER (390–392)

390 Rheumatic fever without mention of heart involvement
  Arthritis, rheumatic, acute or subacute
  Rheumatic fever (active) (acute)
  Rheumatism, articular, acute or subacute
  Excludes that with heart involvement (391.0–391.9)

● **391 Rheumatic fever with heart involvement**
  Excludes chronic heart diseases of rheumatic origin (393–398.99) unless rheumatic fever is also present or there is evidence of recrudescence or activity of the rheumatic process

  391.0 Acute rheumatic pericarditis
    Rheumatic:
      fever (active) (acute) with pericarditis
      pericarditis (acute)
    Any condition classifiable to 390 with pericarditis
    Excludes that not specified as rheumatic (420.0–420.9)

  391.1 Acute rheumatic endocarditis
    Rheumatic:
      endocarditis, acute
      fever (active) (acute) with endocarditis or valvulitis
      valvulitis acute
    Any condition classifiable to 390 with endocarditis or valvulitis

  391.2 Acute rheumatic myocarditis
    Rheumatic fever (active) (acute) with myocarditis
    Any condition classifiable to 390 with myocarditis

  391.8 Other acute rheumatic heart disease
    Rheumatic:
      fever (active) (acute) with other or multiple types of heart involvement
      pancarditis, acute
    Any condition classifiable to 390 with other or multiple types of heart involvement

  391.9 Acute rheumatic heart disease, unspecified
    Rheumatic:
      carditis, acute
      fever (active) (acute) with unspecified type of heart involvement
      heart disease, active or acute
    Any condition classifiable to 390 with unspecified type of heart involvement

● **392 Rheumatic chorea**
  Includes Sydenham's chorea
  Excludes chorea:
    NOS (333.5)
    Huntington's (333.4)

  392.0 With heart involvement
    Rheumatic chorea with heart involvement of any type classifiable to 391

  392.9 Without mention of heart involvement

Item 7-2 **Rheumatic chorea,** also called Sydenham's, juvenile, minor, simple, or St. Vitus' dance, is a major symptom of rheumatic fever and is characterized by ceaseless, involuntary, jerky, purposeless movements.

CHRONIC RHEUMATIC HEART DISEASE (393–398)

393 Chronic rheumatic pericarditis
  Adherent pericardium, rheumatic
  Chronic rheumatic:
    mediastinopericarditis
    myopericarditis
  Excludes pericarditis NOS or not specified as rheumatic (423.0–423.9)

● **394 Diseases of mitral valve**
  Excludes that with aortic valve involvement (396.0–396.9)

  394.0 Mitral stenosis
    Mitral (valve):
      obstruction (rheumatic)
      stenosis NOS

  394.1 Rheumatic mitral insufficiency
    Rheumatic mitral:
      incompetence
      regurgitation
    Excludes that not specified as rheumatic (424.0)
    Coding Clinic: 2005, Q2, P14-15

  394.2 Mitral stenosis with insufficiency
    Mitral stenosis with incompetence or regurgitation
    Coding Clinic: 2007, Q2, P11-12

  394.9 Other and unspecified mitral valve diseases
    Mitral (valve):
      disease (chronic)
      failure

● **395 Diseases of aortic valve**
  Excludes that not specified as rheumatic (424.1)
    that with mitral valve involvement (396.0–396.9)

  395.0 Rheumatic aortic stenosis
    Rheumatic aortic (valve) obstruction
    Coding Clinic: 1988, Q4, P8

  395.1 Rheumatic aortic insufficiency
    Rheumatic aortic:
      incompetence
      regurgitation

  395.2 Rheumatic aortic stenosis with insufficiency
    Rheumatic aortic stenosis with incompetence or regurgitation

  395.9 Other and unspecified rheumatic aortic diseases
    Rheumatic aortic (valve) disease

● **396 Diseases of mitral and aortic valves**
  Includes involvement of both mitral and aortic valves, whether specified as rheumatic or not

  396.0 Mitral valve stenosis and aortic valve stenosis
    Atypical aortic (valve) stenosis
    Mitral and aortic (valve) obstruction (rheumatic)

  396.1 Mitral valve stenosis and aortic valve insufficiency

  396.2 Mitral valve insufficiency and aortic valve stenosis
    Coding Clinic: 2009, Q2, P11; 2000, Q2, P16-17; 1987, Nov-Dec, P8

DISEASES OF THE CIRCULATORY SYSTEM (390–459)

396.3 Mitral valve insufficiency and aortic valve insufficiency
Mitral and aortic (valve):
  incompetence
  regurgitation
Coding Clinic: 2009, Q2, P11; Q1, P8; 1995, Q1, P6

396.8 Multiple involvement of mitral and aortic valves
Stenosis and insufficiency of mitral or aortic valve with stenosis or insufficiency, or both, of the other valve

396.9 Mitral and aortic valve diseases, unspecified

397 Diseases of other endocardial structures
Affects thin serous endothelial tissue that lines inside of heart

397.0 Diseases of tricuspid valve
Tricuspid (valve) (rheumatic):
  disease
  insufficiency
  obstruction
  regurgitation
  stenosis
Coding Clinic: 2006, Q3, P7; 2000, Q2, P16-17

397.1 Rheumatic diseases of pulmonary valve
  Excludes that not specified as rheumatic (424.3)

397.9 Rheumatic diseases of endocardium, valve unspecified
Rheumatic:
  endocarditis (chronic)
  valvulitis (chronic)
  Excludes that not specified as rheumatic (424.90–424.99)

398 Other rheumatic heart disease

398.0 Rheumatic myocarditis
Rheumatic degeneration of myocardium
  Excludes myocarditis not specified as rheumatic (429.0)

398.9 Other and unspecified rheumatic heart diseases

398.90 Rheumatic heart disease, unspecified
Rheumatic:
  carditis
  heart disease NOS
  Excludes carditis not specified as rheumatic (429.89)
  heart disease NOS not specified as rheumatic (429.9)

398.91 Rheumatic heart failure (congestive)
Rheumatic left ventricular failure
Coding Clinic: 2005, Q2, P14-15; 1995, Q1, P6

398.99 Other

HYPERTENSIVE DISEASE (401–405)

Excludes that complicating pregnancy, childbirth, or the puerperium (642.0–642.9)
that involving coronary vessels (410.00–414.9)

401 Essential hypertension
  Includes high blood pressure
  hyperpiesia
  hyperpiesis
  hypertension (arterial) (essential) (primary) (systemic)
  hypertensive vascular:
    degeneration
    disease
  Excludes elevated blood pressure without diagnosis of hypertension (796.2)
  pulmonary hypertension (416.0–416.9)
  that involving vessels of:
    brain (430–438)
    eye (362.11)
Coding Clinic: 1992, Q2, P5

401.0 Malignant
Coding Clinic: 1993, Q4, P37; 5th Issue, P9-10

401.1 Benign

401.9 Unspecified
Coding Clinic: 2012, Q1, P14; 2010, Q4, P124-125, 135; 2009, Q4, P101-102; Q1, P6; 2008, Q2, P16; 2005, Q4, P68-69; Q3, P3-9; 2004, Q4, P77-78; 2003, Q4, P105-106, 108, 111; Q3, P14-15; Q2, P16; 1997, Q4, P35-37; 1989, Q2, P12; 1987, Sept-Oct, P11

Item 7–6 **Hypertension** is caused by high arterial blood pressure in the arteries. **Essential, primary,** or **idiopathic** hypertension occurs without identifiable organic cause.
Secondary hypertension is that which has an organic cause. **Malignant** hypertension is severely elevated blood pressure. **Benign** hypertension is mildly elevated blood pressure.

OGCR Section I.C.7.a.2

Heart conditions (425.8, 429.0-429.3, 429.8, 429.9) are assigned to a code from category 402 when a causal relationship is stated (due to hypertension) or implied (hypertensive). Use an additional code from category 428 to identify the type of heart failure in those patients with heart failure. More than one code from category 428 may be assigned if the patient has systolic or diastolic failure and congestive heart failure. The same heart conditions (425.8, 429.0-429.3, 429.8, 429.9) with hypertension, but without a stated causal relationship, are coded separately. Sequence according to the circumstances of the admission/encounter.

402 Hypertensive heart disease
  Includes hypertensive:
    cardiomegaly
    cardiopathy
    cardiovascular disease
    heart (disease) (failure)
    any condition classifiable to 429.0–429.3, 429.8, 429.9 due to hypertension
  Use additional code to specify type of heart failure (428.0–428.43), if known
Coding Clinic: 1993, Q2, P9; 1987, Nov-Dec, P9

402.0 Malignant

402.00 Without heart failure
Coding Clinic: 2008, Q4, P177-180

402.01 With heart failure

402.1 Benign

402.10 Without heart failure

402.11 With heart failure

402.9 Unspecified
Coding Clinic: 1993, Q2, P9

402.90 Without heart failure

402.91 With heart failure
Coding Clinic: 2002, Q4, P52; 1993, Q1, P19-20; 1989, Q2, P12; 1984, Nov-Dec, P18

OGCR Section I.C.7.a.3

Assign codes from category 403, Hypertensive chronic kidney disease, when conditions classified to category 585 or code 587 are present with hypertension. Unlike hypertension with heart disease, ICD-9-CM presumes a cause-and-effect relationship and classifies chronic kidney disease (CKD) with hypertension as hypertensive chronic kidney disease.

403 Hypertensive chronic kidney disease
  Includes arteriolar nephritis
  arteriosclerosis of:
    kidney
    renal arterioles
  arteriosclerotic nephritis (chronic) (interstitial)
  hypertensive:
    nephropathy
    renal failure
    uremia (chronic)
  nephrosclerosis
  renal sclerosis with hypertension
  any condition classifiable to 585 and 587 with any condition classifiable to 401
  Excludes acute kidney failure (584.5–584.9)
  renal disease stated as not due to hypertension
  renovascular hypertension (405.0–405.9 with fifth-digit 1)
Coding Clinic: 2010, Q3, P13; 2003, Q1, P20-21; 1992, Q2, P5

The following fifth-digit subclassification is for use with category 403:

> 0 with chronic kidney disease stage I through stage IV, or unspecified
> Use additional code to identify the stage of chronic kidney disease (585.1–585.4, 585.9)
> 1 with chronic kidney disease stage V or end stage renal disease
> Use additional code to identify the stage of chronic kidney disease (585.5, 585.6)

- 403.0 **Malignant**
  [0-1]
- 403.1 **Benign**
  [0-1] Coding Clinic: 2010, Q3, P13
- 403.9 **Unspecified**
  [0-1] Coding Clinic: 2010, Q4, P137; 2008, Q1, P7-8, 10-11; 2007, Q2, P3; 2006, Q4, P84-86; 2005, Q4, P68-69; 2004, Q1, P14-15; 2001, Q2, P11; 1987, Sept-Oct, P9, 11; 1985, Nov-Dec, P15

OGCR Section I.C.7.a.4

Assign codes from combination category 404, Hypertensive heart and chronic kidney disease, when both hypertensive kidney disease and hypertensive heart disease are stated in the diagnosis. Assume a relationship between the hypertension and the chronic kidney disease, whether or not the condition is so designated. Assign an additional code from category 428, to identify the type of heart failure. More than one code from category 428 may be assigned if the patient has systolic or diastolic failure and congestive heart failure.

- 404 **Hypertensive heart and chronic kidney disease**
  Includes disease:
  cardiorenal
  cardiovascular renal
  any condition classifiable to 402 with any condition classifiable to 403
  Use additional code to specify type of heart failure (428.0–428.43), if known
  Coding Clinic: 2006, Q4, P84-86; 2005, Q4, P68-69

The following fifth-digit subclassification is for use with category 404:

> 0 without heart failure and with chronic kidney disease stage I through stage IV, or unspecified
> Use additional code to identify the stage of chronic kidney disease (585.1–585.4, 585.9)
> 1 with heart failure and with chronic kidney disease stage I through stage IV, or unspecified
> Use additional code to identify the stage of chronic kidney disease (585.1–585.4, 585.9)
> 2 without heart failure and with chronic kidney disease stage V or end stage renal disease
> Use additional code to identify the stage of chronic kidney disease (585.5, 585.6)
> 3 with heart failure and chronic kidney disease stage V or end stage renal disease
> Use additional code to identify the stage of chronic kidney disease (585.5, 585.6)

- 404.0 **Malignant**
  [0-3]
- 404.1 **Benign**
  [0-3]
- 404.9 **Unspecified**
  [0-3]

- 405 **Secondary hypertension**
  - 405.0 **Malignant**
    - 405.01 Renovascular
    - 405.09 Other
  - 405.1 **Benign**
    - 405.11 Renovascular
    - 405.19 Other
  - 405.9 **Unspecified**
    - 405.91 Renovascular
    - 405.99 Other
    Coding Clinic: 2000, Q3, P4-5; 1987, Sept-Oct, P9, 11

OGCR Section I.C.7.e.1

The ICD-9-CM codes for acute myocardial infarction (AMI) identify the site, such as anterolateral wall or true posterior wall. Subcategories 410.0-410.6 and 410.8 are used for ST elevation myocardial infarction (STEMI). Subcategory 410.7, Subendocardial infarction, is used for non ST elevation myocardial infarction (NSTEMI) and nontransmural MIs.

ISCHEMIC HEART DISEASE (410–414)

Includes that with mention of hypertension
Use additional code to identify presence of hypertension (401.0–405.9)

- 410 **Acute myocardial infarction**
  Includes cardiac infarction
  coronary (artery):
  embolism
  occlusion
  rupture
  thrombosis
  infarction of heart, myocardium, or ventricle
  rupture of heart, myocardium, or ventricle
  ST elevation (STEMI) and non-ST elevation (NSTEMI) myocardial infarction
  any condition classifiable to 414.1–414.9 specified as acute or with a stated duration of 8 weeks or less
  Coding Clinic: 2006, Q2, P9; 1997, Q4, P37; 1994, Q4, P55; 1993, Q4, P39-41; 1992, Q1, P10; 1991, Q3, P18; 1986, Nov-Dec, P12

The following fifth-digit subclassification is for use with category 410:

> 0 episode of care unspecified
> Use when the source document does not contain sufficient information for the assignment of fifth-digit 1 or 2.
> 1 initial episode of care
> Use fifth-digit 1 to designate the first episode of care (regardless of facility site) for a newly diagnosed myocardial infarction. The fifth-digit 1 is assigned regardless of the number of times a patient may be transferred during the initial episode of care.
> 2 subsequent episode of care
> Use fifth-digit 2 to designate an episode of care following the initial episode when the patient is admitted for further observation, evaluation or treatment for a myocardial infarction that has received initial treatment, but is still less than 8 weeks old.

- 410.0 **Of anterolateral wall**
  [0-2] ST elevation myocardial infarction (STEMI) of anterolateral wall
  Coding Clinic: 2009, Q4, P102; 2008, Q4, P69-73; 2001, Q3, P21; 1998, Q3, P15; 1993, 5th Issue, P14, 17-24

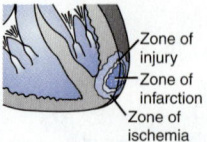

Figure 7-2 Myocardial infarction.

Item 7-7 **Myocardial infarction** is a sudden decrease in the coronary artery blood flow that results in death of the heart muscle. Classifications are based on the affected heart tissue.

- **410.1 Of other anterior wall**
  [0-2]   Infarction:
  anterior (wall) NOS (with contiguous portion of intraventricular septum)
  anteroapical (with contiguous portion of intraventricular septum)
  anteroseptal (with contiguous portion of intraventricular septum)
  ST elevation myocardial infarction (STEMI) of other anterior wall
  Coding Clinic: 2003, Q3, P10-11

- **410.2 Of inferolateral wall**
  [0-2]   ST elevation myocardial infarction (STEMI) of inferolateral wall
  Coding Clinic: 1993, 5th Issue, P17-24

- **410.3 Of inferoposterior wall**
  [0-2]   ST elevation myocardial infarction (STEMI) of inferoposterior wall

- **410.4 Of other inferior wall**
  [0-2]   Infarction:
  diaphragmatic wall NOS (with contiguous portion of intraventricular septum)
  inferior (wall) NOS (with contiguous portion of intraventricular septum)
  ST elevation myocardial infarction (STEMI) of other inferior wall
  Coding Clinic: 2009, Q3, P10; 2006, Q3, P8-9; 2001, Q2, P8-9; 2000, Q1, P7; 1997, Q3, P10; 1993, 5th Issue, P13-14x2

- **410.5 Of other lateral wall**
  [0-2]   Infarction:
  apical-lateral
  basal-lateral
  high lateral
  posterolateral
  ST elevation myocardial infarction (STEMI) of other lateral wall
  Coding Clinic: 2009, Q3, P7

- **410.6 True posterior wall infarction**
  [0-2]   Infarction:
  posterobasal
  strictly posterior
  ST elevation myocardial infarction (STEMI) of true posterior wall

- **410.7 Subendocardial infarction**
  [0-2]   Non-ST elevation myocardial infarction (NSTEMI)
  Nontransmural infarction
  Coding Clinic: 2010, Q2, P9; 2005, Q4, P69-72; Q2, P19-20; 2000, Q1, P7

  OGCR Section I.C.7.e.1

  > The ICD-9-CM codes for acute myocardial infarction (AMI) identify the site, such as anterolateral wall or true posterior wall. Subcategories 410.0–410.6 and 410.8 are used for ST elevation myocardial infarction (STEMI). Subcategory 410.7, Subendocardial infarction, is used for non ST elevation myocardial infarction (NSTEMI) and nontransmural MIs.

- **410.8 Of other specified sites**
  [0-2]   Infarction of:
  atrium
  papillary muscle
  septum alone
  ST elevation myocardial infarction (STEMI) of other specified sites

Item 7-8 "Old" (healed) myocardial infarction: Code 412 cannot be used if the patient is experiencing current ischemic heart disease symptoms. Recent infarctions still under care cannot be coded to 412. This code is only assigned if infarction has some impact on the current episode of care—essentially, it is a history of (H/O) a past, healed MI. (There is no V code for this status/post MI.)

- **410.9 Unspecified site**
  [0-2]   Acute myocardial infarction NOS
  Coronary occlusion NOS
  Myocardial infarction NOS
  Coding Clinic: 2005, Q2, P18-19; 2002, Q3, P5; 1999, Q4, P9; 1993, 5th Issue, P13

  OGCR Section I.C.7.e.2

  > Subcategory 410.9 is the default for the unspecified term acute myocardial infarction. If only STEMI or transmural MI without the site is documented, query the provider as to the site, or assign a code from subcategory 410.9.

- **411 Other acute and subacute forms of ischemic heart disease**
  Coding Clinic: 1994, Q4, P55

  - **411.0 Postmyocardial infarction syndrome**
    Dressler's syndrome

  - **411.1 Intermediate coronary syndrome**
    Impending infarction
    Preinfarction angina
    Preinfarction syndrome
    Unstable angina
    Excludes angina (pectoris) (413.9)
    decubitus (413.0)
    Coding Clinic: 2005, Q4, P103-106; 2004, Q2, P3-4; 2003, Q1, P12-13; 2001, Q3, P15; Q2, P7-9; 1998, Q4, P85-86; 1996, Q2, P10; 1995, Q2, P18-19; 1993, Q4, P39-40; 5th Issue, P17-24; 1991, Q1, P14; 1989, Q4, P10

  - **411.8 Other**

    - **411.81 Acute coronary occlusion without myocardial infarction**
      Acute coronary (artery):
      embolism without or not resulting in myocardial infarction
      obstruction without or not resulting in myocardial infarction
      occlusion without or not resulting in myocardial infarction
      thrombosis without or not resulting in myocardial infarction
      Excludes *obstruction without infarction due to atherosclerosis (414.00–414.07)*
      occlusion without infarction due to atherosclerosis (414.00–414.07)
      Coding Clinic: 2001, Q2, P7-8; 1991, Q3, P18; Q1, P14

    - **411.89 Other**
      Coronary insufficiency (acute)
      Subendocardial ischemia
      Coding Clinic: 2001, Q3, P14; 1992, Q1, P9-10; 1991, Q3, P18

- **412 Old myocardial infarction**
  Healed myocardial infarction
  Past myocardial infarction diagnosed on ECG [EKG] or other special investigation, but currently presenting no symptoms
  Coding Clinic: 2003, Q2, P10; 2001, Q3, P21; Q2, P9; 1998, Q3, P15; 1993, 5th Issue, P17-24

- **413 Angina pectoris**
  Chest pain/discomfort due to lack of oxygen to heart muscle. Principal symptom of myocardial infarction.

  - **413.0 Angina decubitus**
    Nocturnal angina

  - **413.1 Prinzmetal angina**
    Variant angina pectoris
    Coding Clinic: 2006, Q3, P23

413.9 Other and unspecified angina pectoris
Angina:
  NOS
  cardiac
  equivalent
  of effort
Anginal syndrome
Status anginosus
Stenocardia
Syncope anginosa

Excludes: *preinfarction angina (411.1)*

Use additional code(s) for symptoms associated with angina equivalent

Coding Clinic: 2008, Q2, P16; 2003, Q1, P12-13; 2002, Q3, P4-5; 1995, Q2, P18; 1993, 5th Issue, P17-24; 1991, Q3, P16; 1985, Sept-Oct, P9

● **414 Other forms of chronic ischemic heart disease**

Excludes: *arteriosclerotic cardiovascular disease [ASCVD] (429.2)*
  cardiovascular:
    arteriosclerosis or sclerosis (429.2)
    degeneration or disease (429.2)

● **414.0 Coronary atherosclerosis**
Arteriosclerotic heart disease [ASHD]
Atherosclerotic heart disease
Coronary (artery):
  arteriosclerosis
  arteritis or endarteritis
  atheroma
  sclerosis
  stricture

Use additional code, if applicable, to identify chronic total occlusion of coronary artery (414.2)

Excludes: *embolism of graft (996.72)*
  occlusion NOS of graft (996.72)
  thrombus of graft (996.72)

Coding Clinic: 2002, Q3, P3-9; 1994, Q2, P13, 15; Q1, P6-7; 1993, Q1, P20; 5th Issue, P17-24; 5th Issue, P14; 1984, Nov-Dec, P18

■ **414.00 Of unspecified type of vessel, native or graft**
Coding Clinic: 2003, Q2, P16; 2001, Q3, P15; 1997, Q3, P15; 1996, Q4, P31

414.01 Of native coronary artery
Coding Clinic: 2012, Q3, P17; 2009, Q3, P8; 2008, Q3, P10-11; Q2, P16; 2006, Q3, P25; 2005, Q4, P68-69; 2004, Q2, P3-4; 2003, Q4, P105-106, 108-109; Q3, P9.10, 14; 2001, Q3, P15-16; Q2, P8-9; 1997, Q3, P15; 1996, Q2, P10; 1995, Q2, P17-19

414.02 Of autologous biological bypass graft
Coding Clinic: 2010, Q2, P9; 1995, Q2, P18-19

414.03 Of nonautologous biological bypass graft

414.04 Of artery bypass graft
Internal mammary artery

■ **414.05 Of unspecified type of bypass graft**
Bypass graft NOS
Coding Clinic: 1997, Q3, P15; 1996, Q4, P31

414.06 Of native coronary artery of transplanted heart
Coding Clinic: 2003, Q4, P60; 2002, Q4, P53-54; Q4, P53-54

414.07 Of bypass graft (artery) (vein) of transplanted heart
Coding Clinic: 2003, Q4, P60

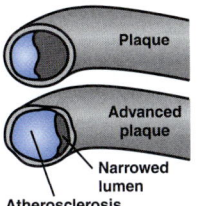

Figure 7-3 Atherosclerosis. (From Buck CJ: Step-by-Step Medical Coding, ed 2008 Philadelphia, WB Saunders, 2008)

● **414.1 Aneurysm and dissection of heart**
414.10 Aneurysm of heart (wall)
Aneurysm (arteriovenous):
  mural
  ventricular

414.11 Aneurysm of coronary vessels
Aneurysm (arteriovenous) of coronary vessels
Coding Clinic: 2010, Q2, P9; 1999, Q1, P17-18

414.12 Dissection of coronary artery
Coding Clinic: 2011, Q1, P3-4; 2002, Q4, P54-55

414.19 Other aneurysm of heart
Arteriovenous fistula, acquired, of heart

● **414.2 Chronic total occlusion of coronary artery**
Complete occlusion of coronary artery
Total occlusion of coronary artery

Code first *coronary atherosclerosis (414.00–414.07)*

Excludes: *acute coronary occlusion with myocardial infarction (410.00–410.92)*
  acute coronary occlusion without myocardial infarction (411.81)

Coding Clinic: 2007, Q4, P82

● **414.3 Coronary atherosclerosis due to lipid rich plaque**
Code first *coronary atherosclerosis (414.00-414.07)*
Coding Clinic: 2008, Q4, P113

● **414.4 Coronary atherosclerosis due to calcified coronary lesion**
Coronary atherosclerosis due to severely calcified coronary lesion

Code first *coronary atherosclerosis (414.00-414.07)*

414.8 Other specified forms of chronic ischemic heart disease
Chronic coronary insufficiency
Ischemia, myocardial (chronic)
Any condition classifiable to 410 specified as chronic, or presenting with symptoms after 8 weeks from date of infarction

Excludes: *coronary insufficiency (acute) (411.89)*

Coding Clinic: 2003, Q2, P10; 2001, Q3, P15-16; 1992, Q1, P10; 1990, Q3, P15; Q2, P19; 1986, Nov-Dec, P12

■ **414.9 Chronic ischemic heart disease, unspecified**
Ischemic heart disease NOS
Coding Clinic: 2001, Q3, P15-16

DISEASES OF PULMONARY CIRCULATION (415–417)

● **415 Acute pulmonary heart disease**
415.0 Acute cor pulmonale

Excludes: *cor pulmonale NOS (416.9)*

● **415.1 Pulmonary embolism and infarction**
Pulmonary (artery) (vein):
  apoplexy
  embolism
  infarction (hemorrhagic)
  thrombosis

Excludes: *chronic pulmonary embolism (416.2)*
  personal history of pulmonary embolism (V12.55)
  that complicating:
    abortion (634–638 with .6, 639.6)
    ectopic or molar pregnancy (639.6)
    pregnancy, childbirth, or the puerperium (673.0–673.8)

415.11 Iatrogenic pulmonary embolism and infarction
Use additional code for associated septic pulmonary embolism, if applicable, 415.12
Coding Clinic: 1990, Q4, P25

Item 7-9 Classification is based on the location of the atherosclerosis. **"Of native coronary artery"** indicates the atherosclerosis is within an original heart artery. **"Of autologous vein bypass graft"** indicates that the atherosclerosis is within a vein graft that was taken from within the patient. **"Of nonautologous biological bypass graft"** indicates the atherosclerosis is within a vessel grafted from other than the patient. **"Of artery bypass graft"** indicates the atherosclerosis is within an artery that was grafted from within the patient.

Item 7-10 Pulmonary heart disease or cor pulmonale is right ventricle hypertrophy or RVH as a result of a respiratory disorder increasing back flow pressure to the right ventricle. Left untreated, cor pulmonale leads to right-heart failure and death.

- **415.12** *Septic pulmonary embolism*
  Septic embolism NOS
  Code first underlying infection, such as:
      septicemia (038.0–038.9)
  Excludes septic arterial embolism (449)
  Coding Clinic: 2007, Q4, P84-86
- **415.13** Saddle embolus of pulmonary artery
- **415.19** Other
  Coding Clinic: 2010, Q3, P11; 1998, Q2, P8

416 Chronic pulmonary heart disease
- **416.0** Primary pulmonary hypertension
  Idiopathic pulmonary arteriosclerosis
  Pulmonary hypertension (essential) (idiopathic) (primary)
  Excludes pulmonary hypertension NOS (416.8)
      secondary pulmonary hypertension (416.8)
  Coding Clinic: 2010, Q2, P11
- **416.1** Kyphoscoliotic heart disease
- **416.2** Chronic pulmonary embolism
  Use additional code, if applicable, for associated long-term (current) use of anticoagulants (V58.61)
  Excludes personal history of pulmonary embolism (V12.55)
- **416.8** Other chronic pulmonary heart diseases
  Pulmonary hypertension NOS
  Pulmonary hypertension, secondary
  Coding Clinic: 2012, Q1, P17; 2011, Q1, P10; 2010, Q3, P13; Q2, P10-11
- **416.9** Chronic pulmonary heart disease, unspecified
  Chronic cardiopulmonary disease
  Cor pulmonale (chronic) NOS

417 Other diseases of pulmonary circulation
- **417.0** Arteriovenous fistula of pulmonary vessels
  Excludes congenital arteriovenous fistula (747.32)
- **417.1** Aneurysm of pulmonary artery
  Excludes congenital aneurysm (747.39)
      congenital arteriovenous aneurysm (747.32)
- **417.8** Other specified diseases of pulmonary circulation
  Pulmonary:
      arteritis
      endarteritis
  Rupture of pulmonary vessel
  Stricture of pulmonary vessel
- **417.9** Unspecified disease of pulmonary circulation

OTHER FORMS OF HEART DISEASE (420–429)

420 Acute pericarditis
Inflammation of the sac surrounding the heart caused by infection. The chest pain is significant on inspiration, and onset is sudden and worst when lying down.
  Includes acute:
      mediastinopericarditis
      myopericarditis
      pericardial effusion
      pleuropericarditis
      pneumopericarditis
  Excludes acute rheumatic pericarditis (391.0)
      postmyocardial infarction syndrome [Dressler's] (411.0)
- **420.0** Acute pericarditis in diseases classified elsewhere
  Code first underlying disease, as:
      actinomycosis (039.8)
      amebiasis (006.8)
      chronic uremia (585.9)
      nocardiosis (039.8)
      tuberculosis (017.9)
      uremia NOS (586)
  Excludes pericarditis (acute) (in):
      Coxsackie (virus) (074.21)
      gonococcal (098.83)
      histoplasmosis (115.0–115.9 with fifth-digit 3)
      meningococcal infection (036.41)
      syphilitic (093.81)
- **420.9** Other and unspecified acute pericarditis
  - **420.90** Acute pericarditis, unspecified
    Pericarditis (acute):
        NOS
        infective NOS
        sicca
    Coding Clinic: 1989, Q2, P12
  - **420.91** Acute idiopathic pericarditis
    Pericarditis, acute:
        benign
        nonspecific
        viral
  - **420.99** Other
    Pericarditis (acute):
        pneumococcal
        purulent
        staphylococcal
        streptococcal
        suppurative
    Pneumopyopericardium
    Pyopericardium
    Excludes pericarditis in diseases classified elsewhere (420.0)

421 Acute and subacute endocarditis
Inflammation/infection of lining of heart, affecting heart valves, usually caused by bacterial infection
- **421.0** Acute and subacute bacterial endocarditis
  Endocarditis (acute) (chronic) (subacute):
      bacterial
      infective NOS
      lenta
      malignant
      purulent
      septic
      ulcerative
      vegetative
  Infective aneurysm
  Subacute bacterial endocarditis [SBE]
  Use additional code, if desired, to identify infectious organism [e.g., Streptococcus 041.0, Staphylococcus 041.1]
  Coding Clinic: 2008, Q4, P69-73; 2006, Q2, P16-17; 1999, Q1, P12; 1991, Q1, P15
- **421.1** Acute and subacute infective endocarditis in diseases classified elsewhere
  Code first underlying disease, as:
      blastomycosis (116.0)
      Q fever (083.0)
      typhoid (fever) (002.0)
  Excludes endocarditis (in):
      Coxsackie (virus) (074.22)
      gonococcal (098.84)
      histoplasmosis (115.0–115.9 with fifth-digit 4)
      meningococcal infection (036.42)
      monilial (112.81)
- **421.9** Acute endocarditis, unspecified
  Endocarditis, acute or subacute
  Myoendocarditis, acute or subacute
  Periendocarditis, acute or subacute
  Excludes acute rheumatic endocarditis (391.1)

422 Acute myocarditis
An inflammation of the heart muscle due to an infection (viral/bacterial)
Excludes *acute rheumatic myocarditis (391.2)*

● 422.0 Acute myocarditis in diseases classified elsewhere
Code first underlying disease, as:
myocarditis (acute):
influenzal (487.8, 488.09, 488.19)
tuberculous (017.9)
Excludes *myocarditis (acute) (due to):*
aseptic, of newborn (074.23)
Coxsackie (virus) (074.23)
diphtheritic (032.82)
meningococcal infection (036.43)
syphilitic (093.82)
toxoplasmosis (130.3)

422.9 Other and unspecified acute myocarditis
422.90 Acute myocarditis, unspecified
Acute or subacute (interstitial) myocarditis

422.91 Idiopathic myocarditis
Myocarditis (acute or subacute):
Fiedler's
giant cell
isolated (diffuse) (granulomatous)
nonspecific granulomatous

422.92 Septic myocarditis
Myocarditis, acute or subacute:
pneumococcal
staphylococcal
Use additional code to identify infectious organism [e.g., Staphylococcus 041.1]
Excludes *myocarditis, acute or subacute:*
in bacterial diseases classified elsewhere (422.0)
streptococcal (391.2)

422.93 Toxic myocarditis
422.99 Other

423 Other diseases of pericardium
Excludes *that specified as rheumatic (393)*

423.0 Hemopericardium
423.1 Adhesive pericarditis
Adherent pericardium
Fibrosis of pericardium
Milk spots
Pericarditis:
adhesive
obliterative
Soldiers' patches

423.2 Constrictive pericarditis
Concato's disease
Pick's disease of heart (and liver)

● 423.3 *Cardiac tamponade*
Code first the underlying cause
Coding Clinic: 2007, Q4, P86-87; 2007, Q2, P11-12

423.8 Other specified diseases of pericardium
Calcification of pericardium
Fistula of pericardium
Coding Clinic: 1989, Q2, P12

423.9 Unspecified disease of pericardium
Coding Clinic: 2007, Q2, P11-12

424 Other diseases of endocardium
Excludes *bacterial endocarditis (421.0–421.9)*
rheumatic endocarditis (391.1, 394.0–397.9)
syphilitic endocarditis (093.20–093.24)

424.0 Mitral valve disorders
Mitral (valve):
incompetence NOS of specified cause, except rheumatic
insufficiency NOS of specified cause, except rheumatic
regurgitation NOS of specified cause, except rheumatic
Excludes *mitral (valve):*
disease (394.9)
failure (394.9)
stenosis (394.0)
the listed conditions:
specified as rheumatic (394.1)
unspecified as to cause but with mention of:
diseases of aortic valve (396.0–396.9)
mitral stenosis or obstruction (394.2)
Coding Clinic: 2006, Q3, P7; 2000, Q2, P16-17; 1998, Q3, P11; 1987, Nov-Dec, P8

424.1 Aortic valve disorders
Aortic (valve):
incompetence NOS of specified cause, except rheumatic
insufficiency NOS of specified cause, except rheumatic
regurgitation NOS of specified cause, except rheumatic
stenosis NOS of specified cause, except rheumatic
Excludes *hypertrophic subaortic stenosis (425.11)*
that specified as rheumatic (395.0–395.9)
that of unspecified cause but with mention of diseases of mitral valve (396.0–396.9)
Coding Clinic: 2011, Q4, P152; 2008, Q4, P177-180; 1988, Q4, P8; 1987, Nov-Dec, P8

424.2 Tricuspid valve disorders, specified as nonrheumatic
Tricuspid valve:
incompetence of specified cause, except rheumatic
insufficiency of specified cause, except rheumatic
regurgitation of specified cause, except rheumatic
stenosis of specified cause, except rheumatic
Excludes *rheumatic or of unspecified cause (397.0)*

424.3 Pulmonary valve disorders
Pulmonic:
incompetence NOS
insufficiency NOS
regurgitation NOS
stenosis NOS
Excludes *that specified as rheumatic (397.1)*

● 424.9 Endocarditis, valve unspecified
424.90 Endocarditis, valve unspecified, unspecified cause
Endocarditis (chronic):
NOS
nonbacterial thrombotic
Valvular:
incompetence of unspecified valve, unspecified cause
insufficiency of unspecified valve, unspecified cause
regurgitation of unspecified valve, unspecified cause
stenosis of unspecified valve, unspecified cause
Valvulitis (chronic)

- **424.91 Endocarditis in diseases classified elsewhere**
  Code first underlying disease, as:
  atypical verrucous endocarditis [Libman-Sacks] (710.0)
  disseminated lupus erythematosus (710.0)
  tuberculosis (017.9)
  Excludes syphilitic (093.20–093.24)

  424.99 Other
  Any condition classifiable to 424.90 with specified cause, except rheumatic
  Excludes endocardial fibroelastosis (425.3)
  that specified as rheumatic (397.9)

- **425 Cardiomyopathy**
  Disease of the heart muscle resulting in abnormally enlarged, weakened, thickened, and/or stiffened muscle causing an inability to pump blood normally and leads to CHF
  Includes myocardiopathy

  425.0 Endomyocardial fibrosis

- **425.1 Hypertrophic cardiomyopathy**
  Excludes ventricular hypertrophy (429.3)

  425.11 Hypertrophic obstructive cardiomyopathy
  Hypertrophic subaortic stenosis (idiopathic)

  425.18 Other hypertrophic cardiomyopathy
  Nonobstructive hypertrophic cardiomyopathy

  425.2 Obscure cardiomyopathy of Africa
  Becker's disease
  Idiopathic mural endomyocardial disease

  425.3 Endocardial fibroelastosis
  Elastomyofibrosis

  425.4 Other primary cardiomyopathies
  Cardiomyopathy:
  NOS
  congestive
  constrictive
  familial
  idiopathic
  obstructive
  restrictive
  Cardiovascular collagenosis
  Coding Clinic: 2009, Q4, P102; 2007, Q1, P20; 2005, Q2, P14-15; 2000, Q1, P22; 1997, Q4, P54-55; 1990, Q2, P19; 1985, Sept-Oct, P15

  425.5 Alcoholic cardiomyopathy
  Coding Clinic: 1985, Sept-Oct, P15; July-Aug, P15

- **425.7 Nutritional and metabolic cardiomyopathy**
  Code first underlying disease, as:
  amyloidosis (277.30–277.39)
  beriberi (265.0)
  cardiac glycogenosis (271.0)
  mucopolysaccharidosis (277.5)
  thyrotoxicosis (242.0–242.9)
  Excludes gouty tophi of heart (274.82)

- **425.8 Cardiomyopathy in other diseases classified elsewhere**
  Code first underlying disease, as:
  Friedreich's ataxia (334.0)
  myotonia atrophica (359.21)
  progressive muscular dystrophy (359.1)
  sarcoidosis (135)
  Excludes cardiomyopathy in Chagas' disease (086.0)
  Coding Clinic: 1993, Q2, P9

  425.9 Secondary cardiomyopathy, unspecified

- **426 Conduction disorders**
  Heart block or atrioventricular block (AV block) caused by conduction problem resulting in arrhythmias/dysrhythmias due to lack of electrical impulses being transmitted normally through heart

  426.0 Atrioventricular block, complete
  Third degree atrioventricular block
  Coding Clinic: 2006, Q2, P14

- **426.1 Atrioventricular block, other and unspecified**

  426.10 Atrioventricular block, unspecified
  Atrioventricular [AV] block (incomplete) (partial)

  426.11 First degree atrioventricular block
  Incomplete atrioventricular block, first degree
  Prolonged P-R interval NOS
  Coding Clinic: 2006, Q2, P14

  426.12 Mobitz (type) II atrioventricular block
  Incomplete atrioventricular block:
  Mobitz (type) II
  second degree, Mobitz (type) II
  Coding Clinic: 2006, Q2, P14

  426.13 Other second degree atrioventricular block
  Incomplete atrioventricular block:
  Mobitz (type) I [Wenckebach's]
  second degree:
  NOS
  Mobitz (type) I
  with 2:1 atrioventricular response [block]
  Wenckebach's phenomenon

  426.2 Left bundle branch hemiblock
  Block:
  left anterior fascicular
  left posterior fascicular

  426.3 Other left bundle branch block
  Left bundle branch block:
  NOS
  anterior fascicular with posterior fascicular
  complete
  main stem

  426.4 Right bundle branch block
  Coding Clinic: 2000, Q3, P3

- **426.5 Bundle branch block, other and unspecified**

  426.50 Bundle branch block, unspecified

  426.51 Right bundle branch block and left posterior fascicular block

  426.52 Right bundle branch block and left anterior fascicular block

  426.53 Other bilateral bundle branch block
  Bifascicular block NOS
  Bilateral bundle branch block NOS
  Right bundle branch with left bundle branch block (incomplete) (main stem)

  426.54 Trifascicular block

  426.6 Other heart block
  Intraventricular block: Sinoatrial block
  NOS   Sinoauricular block
  diffuse
  myofibrillar

  426.7 Anomalous atrioventricular excitation
  Atrioventricular conduction:
  accelerated
  accessory
  pre-excitation
  Ventricular pre-excitation
  Wolff-Parkinson-White syndrome

- **426.8 Other specified conduction disorders**
  - **426.81 Lown-Ganong-Levine syndrome**
    Syndrome of short P-R interval, normal QRS complexes, and supraventricular tachycardias
  - **426.82 Long QT syndrome**
    Coding Clinic: 2005, Q4, P72-73
  - **426.89 Other**
    Dissociation:
      atrioventricular [AV]
      interference
      isorhythmic
    Nonparoxysmal AV nodal tachycardia
- **426.9 Conduction disorder, unspecified**
  Heart block NOS   Stokes-Adams syndrome

- **427 Cardiac dysrhythmias**
  Abnormality in rate, regularity, or sequence of cardiac activation
  Excludes that complicating:
    abortion (634–638 with .7, 639.8)
    ectopic or molar pregnancy (639.8)
    labor or delivery (668.1, 669.4)
  - **427.0 Paroxysmal supraventricular tachycardia**
    Paroxysmal tachycardia:
      atrial [PAT]   junctional
      atrioventricular [AV]   nodal
  - **427.1 Paroxysmal ventricular tachycardia**
    Ventricular tachycardia (paroxysmal)
    Coding Clinic: 2013, Q1, P11; 2008, Q1, P14-15; 2006, Q2, P15-16; 1995, Q3, P9; Q1, P8; 1986, Mar-April, P11-12; 1985, July-Aug, P15
  - **427.2 Paroxysmal tachycardia, unspecified**
    Bouveret-Hoffmann syndrome
    Paroxysmal tachycardia:
      NOS   essential
  - **427.3 Atrial fibrillation and flutter**
    - **427.31 Atrial fibrillation**
      Most common abnormal heart rhythm (arrhythmia) presenting as irregular, rapid beating (tachycardia) of the heart's upper chamber
      Coding Clinic: 2008, Q4, P134-136; 2005, Q3, P3-9; 2004, Q4, P77-78, 121-122; Q3, P7; 2003, Q4, P93-95, 105-106; Q1, P8; 1999, Q2, P17; 1996, Q2, P7x2; 1995, Q3, P8; 1994, Q1, P22; 1985, July-Aug, P15
    - **427.32 Atrial flutter**
      Rapid contractions of the upper heart chamber, but regular, rather than irregular, beats
      Coding Clinic: 2003, Q4, P93-95
  - **427.4 Ventricular fibrillation and flutter**
    - **427.41 Ventricular fibrillation**
      Coding Clinic: 2002, Q3, P5
    - **427.42 Ventricular flutter**
  - **427.5 Cardiac arrest**
    Cardiorespiratory arrest
    Coding Clinic: 2013, Q1, P9-11; 2002, Q3, P5; 2000, Q2, P12; 1995, Q3, P9
  - **427.6 Premature beats**
    - **427.60 Premature beats, unspecified**
      Ectopic beats
      Extrasystoles
      Extrasystolic arrhythmia
      Premature contractions or systoles NOS
    - **427.61 Supraventricular premature beats**
      Atrial premature beats, contractions, or systoles
      Coding Clinic: 1994, Q1, P20
    - **427.69 Other**
      Ventricular premature beats, contractions, or systoles
      Coding Clinic: 1993, Q4, P42-43

- **427.8 Other specified cardiac dysrhythmias**
  - **427.81 Sinoatrial node dysfunction**
    Sinus bradycardia:
      persistent
      severe
    Syndrome:
      sick sinus
      tachycardia-bradycardia
    Excludes sinus bradycardia NOS (427.89)
    Coding Clinic: 2011, Q4, P168
  - **427.89 Other**
    Rhythm disorder:
      coronary sinus
      ectopic
      nodal
    Wandering (atrial) pacemaker
    Excludes carotid sinus syncope (337.0)
      neonatal bradycardia (779.81)
      neonatal tachycardia (779.82)
      reflex bradycardia (337.0)
      tachycardia NOS (785.0)
    Coding Clinic: 2012, Q3, P9; 2000, Q3, P8-9; 1985, July-Aug, P15
- **427.9 Cardiac dysrhythmia, unspecified**
  Arrhythmia (cardiac) NOS
  Coding Clinic: 1989, Q2, P10

- **428 Heart failure**
  Code, if applicable, heart failure due to hypertension first (402.0–402.9, with fifth-digit 1 or 404.0–404.9 with fifth-digit 1 or 3)
  Excludes rheumatic (398.91)
    that complicating:
      abortion (634–638 with .7, 639.8)
      ectopic or molar pregnancy (639.8)
      labor or delivery (668.1, 669.4)
  Coding Clinic: 2005, Q2, P14-15; 2002, Q4, P49-53
  - **428.0 Congestive heart failure, unspecified**
    Congestive heart disease
    Right heart failure (secondary to left heart failure)
    Excludes fluid overload NOS (276.69)
    Coding Clinic: 2012, Q3, P9; 2009, Q4, P106x2; Q1, P6x2; 2008, Q4, P69-73, 177-182; Q3, P12-13x2; 2007, Q3, P11; Q1, P20; 2006, Q3, P7; 2005, Q4, P119-120; Q3, P3-9; Q1, P9; 2004, Q4, P140; Q3, P7; 2003, Q4, P109-110; Q1, P9; 2002, Q4, P52-53; 2001, Q2, P13; 2000, Q4, P47-48; Q2, P16-17; Q1, P22; 1999, Q4, P13-14; Q1, P11; 1998, Q3, P5; 1997, Q4, P54-55; Q3, P10; 1996, Q3, P9; 1991, Q3, P18-20; 1990, Q2, P19; 1989, Q2, P12; 1987, Sept-Oct, P11; 1985, Sept-Oct, P15; Nov-Dec, P14
  - **428.1 Left heart failure**
    Acute edema of lung with heart disease NOS or heart failure
    Acute pulmonary edema with heart disease NOS or heart failure
    Cardiac asthma
    Left ventricular failure
    Coding Clinic: 1990, Q2, P19
  - **428.2 Systolic heart failure**
    Excludes combined systolic and diastolic heart failure (428.40–428.43)
    - **428.20 Unspecified**
    - **428.21 Acute**
      Presenting a short and relatively severe episode

Item 7–11 Congestive heart failure (CHF) is a condition in which the left ventricle of the heart cannot pump enough blood to the body. The blood flow from the heart slows or returns to the heart from the venous system back flow resulting in congestion (fluid accumulation) particularly in the abdomen. Most commonly, fluid collects in the lungs and results in shortness of breath, especially when in a reclining position.

DISEASES OF THE CIRCULATORY SYSTEM (390–459)

- **428.22 Chronic**
  Long-lasting, presenting over time
  Coding Clinic: 2005, Q4, P119-120
- **428.23 Acute on chronic**
  Combination code. What was a chronic condition now has an acute exacerbation (to make more severe). Because two conditions are now present, the combination code reports both.
  Coding Clinic: 2009, Q1, P10; 2003, Q1, P9
- ● **428.3 Diastolic heart failure**
  Excludes combined systolic and diastolic heart failure (428.40–428.43)
  - **428.30 Unspecified**
    Coding Clinic: 2002, Q4, P52
  - **428.31 Acute**
  - **428.32 Chronic**
    Coding Clinic: 2008, Q3, P12-13
  - **428.33 Acute on chronic**
    Coding Clinic: 2009, Q4, P106; 2008, Q3, P12; 2007, Q1, P20
- ● **428.4 Combined systolic and diastolic heart failure**
  - **428.40 Unspecified**
  - **428.41 Acute**
    Coding Clinic: 2004, Q4, P140
  - **428.42 Chronic**
  - **428.43 Acute on chronic**
    Coding Clinic: 2006, Q3, P7; 2002, Q4, P52-53
- **428.9 Heart failure, unspecified**
  Cardiac failure NOS
  Heart failure NOS
  Myocardial failure NOS
  Weak heart
  Coding Clinic: 1989, Q2, P10; 1985, Nov-Dec, P14

● **429 Ill-defined descriptions and complications of heart disease**
- **429.0 Myocarditis, unspecified**
  Myocarditis (with mention of arteriosclerosis):
    NOS (with mention of arteriosclerosis)
    chronic (interstitial) (with mention of arteriosclerosis)
    fibroid (with mention of arteriosclerosis)
    senile (with mention of arteriosclerosis)
  Use additional code to identify presence of arteriosclerosis
  Excludes acute or subacute (422.0–422.9)
    rheumatic (398.0)
    acute (391.2)
    that due to hypertension (402.0–402.9)
- **429.1 Myocardial degeneration**
  Degeneration of heart or myocardium (with mention of arteriosclerosis):
    fatty (with mention of arteriosclerosis)
    mural (with mention of arteriosclerosis)
    muscular (with mention of arteriosclerosis)
  Myocardial (with mention of arteriosclerosis):
    degeneration (with mention of arteriosclerosis)
    disease (with mention of arteriosclerosis)
  Use additional code to identify presence of arteriosclerosis
  Excludes that due to hypertension (402.0–402.9)
- **429.2 Cardiovascular disease, unspecified**
  Arteriosclerotic cardiovascular disease [ASCVD]
  Cardiovascular arteriosclerosis
  Cardiovascular:
    degeneration (with mention of arteriosclerosis)
    disease (with mention of arteriosclerosis)
    sclerosis (with mention of arteriosclerosis)
  Use additional code to identify presence of arteriosclerosis
  Excludes that due to hypertension (402.0–402.9)
  Coding Clinic: 2012, Q3, P17

- **429.3 Cardiomegaly**
  Cardiac:
    dilatation
    hypertrophy
  Ventricular dilatation
  Excludes that due to hypertension (402.0–402.9)
- **429.4 Functional disturbances following cardiac surgery**
  Cardiac insufficiency following cardiac surgery or due to prosthesis
  Heart failure following cardiac surgery or due to prosthesis
  Postcardiotomy syndrome
  Postvalvulotomy syndrome
  Excludes cardiac failure in the immediate postoperative period (997.1)
  Coding Clinic: 2002, Q2, P12-13
- **429.5 Rupture of chordae tendineae**
- **429.6 Rupture of papillary muscle**
- ● **429.7 Certain sequelae of myocardial infarction, not elsewhere classified**
  Use additional code to identify the associated myocardial infarction:
    with onset of 8 weeks or less (410.00–410.92)
    with onset of more than 8 weeks (414.8)
  Excludes congenital defects of heart (745, 746)
    coronary aneurysm (414.11)
    disorders of papillary muscle (429.6, 429.81)
    postmyocardial infarction syndrome (411.0)
    rupture of chordae tendineae (429.5)
  - **429.71 Acquired cardiac septal defect**
    Excludes acute septal infarction (410.00–410.92)
  - **429.79 Other**
    Mural thrombus (atrial) (ventricular) acquired, following myocardial infarction
    Coding Clinic: 1992, Q1, P10
- ● **429.8 Other ill-defined heart diseases**
  - **429.81 Other disorders of papillary muscle**
    Papillary muscle:
      atrophy
      degeneration
      dysfunction
      incompetence
      incoordination
      scarring
  - **429.82 Hyperkinetic heart disease**
  - **429.83 Takotsubo syndrome**
    Broken heart syndrome
    Reversible left ventricular dysfunction following sudden emotional stress
    Stress induced cardiomyopathy
    Transient left ventricular apical ballooning syndrome
    Coding Clinic: 2006, Q4, P87
  - **429.89 Other**
    Carditis
    Excludes that due to hypertension (402.0–402.9)
    Coding Clinic: 2006, Q2, P18-19; 2005, Q3, P14; 1992, Q1, P10
- **429.9 Heart disease, unspecified**
  Heart disease (organic) NOS
  Morbus cordis NOS
  Excludes that due to hypertension (402.0–402.9)
  Coding Clinic: 2009, Q1, P10x2; 1993, Q1, P19-20

CEREBROVASCULAR DISEASE (430–438)

Includes with mention of hypertension (conditions classifiable to 401–405)

Use additional code to identify presence of hypertension

Excludes any condition classifiable to 430–434, 436, 437 occurring during pregnancy, childbirth, or the puerperium, or specified as puerperal (674.0)
iatrogenic cerebrovascular infarction or hemorrhage (997.02)

OGCR Section I.C.7.a.5

First assign codes from 430-438, Cerebrovascular disease, then the appropriate hypertension code from categories 401-405.

430 Subarachnoid hemorrhage
Meningeal hemorrhage
Ruptured:
  berry aneurysm
  (congenital) cerebral aneurysm NOS

Excludes berry aneurysm, nonruptured (437.3)
syphilitic ruptured cerebral aneurysm (094.87)

Coding Clinic: 2000, Q3, P16; 1991, Q3, P15-16

431 Intracerebral hemorrhage
Hemorrhage (of):
  basilar
  bulbar
  cerebellar
  cerebral
  cerebromeningeal
  cortical
  internal capsule
  intrapontine
  pontine
  subcortical
  ventricular
Rupture of blood vessel in brain

Coding Clinic: 2012, Q1, P14; 2010, Q3, P5-6; Q1, P7; 2007, Q3, P4; 1997, Q3, P11

● 432 Other and unspecified intracranial hemorrhage

432.0 Nontraumatic extradural hemorrhage
Nontraumatic epidural hemorrhage

432.1 Subdural hemorrhage
Subdural hematoma, nontraumatic

■ 432.9 Unspecified intracranial hemorrhage
Intracranial hemorrhage NOS

● 433 Occlusion and stenosis of precerebral arteries

The following fifth-digit subclassification is for use with category 433:

  0 without mention of cerebral infarction
  1 with cerebral infarction

Includes embolism of basilar, carotid, and vertebral arteries
narrowing of basilar, carotid, and vertebral arteries
obstruction of basilar, carotid, and vertebral arteries
thrombosis of basilar, carotid, and vertebral arteries

Excludes insufficiency NOS of precerebral arteries (435.0–435.9)

Use additional code, if applicable, to identify status post administration of tPA (rtPA) in a different facility within the last 24 hours prior to admission to current facility (V45.88)

Coding Clinic: 1995, Q2, P16; 1993, Q4, P38-39

● 433.0 Basilar artery
[0-1]

● 433.1 Carotid artery
[0-1] Coding Clinic: 2006, Q1, P17; 2002, Q1, P7-8, 10-11; 2000, Q1, P16; 1995, Q2, P16

● 433.2 Vertebral artery
[0-1]

● 433.3 Multiple and bilateral
[0-1] Coding Clinic: 2006, Q1, P17; 2002, Q1, P10-11

● 433.8 Other specified precerebral artery
[0-1]

● ■ 433.9 Unspecified precerebral artery
[0-1] Precerebral artery NOS

● 434 Occlusion of cerebral arteries

The following fifth-digit subclassification is for use with category 434:

  0 without mention of cerebral infarction
  1 with cerebral infarction

Use additional code, if applicable, to identify status post administration of tPA (rtPA) in a different facility within the last 24 hours prior to admission to current facility (V45.88)

Coding Clinic: 2007, Q3, P12; 1995, Q2, P16; 1993, Q4, P38-39

● 434.0 Cerebral thrombosis
[0-1] Thrombosis of cerebral arteries

● 434.1 Cerebral embolism
[0-1] Coding Clinic: 1997, Q3, P11

● ■ 434.9 Cerebral artery occlusion, unspecified
[0-1] Coding Clinic: 2010, Q3, P5-6; 2008, Q4, P102-109; 2007, Q1, P23-24; 2004, Q4, P77-78; 1998, Q4, P87; 1996, Q2, P5

OGCR Section I.C.7.b

The terms stroke and CVA are often used interchangeably to refer to a cerebral infarction. The terms stroke, CVA, and cerebral infarction NOS are all indexed to the default code 434.91, Cerebral artery occlusion, unspecified, with infarction. Additional code(s) should be assigned for any neurologic deficits associated with the acute CVA, regardless of whether or not the neurologic deficit restores prior to discharge.

● 435 Transient cerebral ischemia

Includes cerebrovascular insufficiency (acute) with transient focal neurological signs and symptoms
insufficiency of basilar, carotid, and vertebral arteries
spasm of cerebral arteries

Excludes acute cerebrovascular insufficiency NOS (437.1)
that due to any condition classifiable to 433 (433.0–433.9)

435.0 Basilar artery syndrome

435.1 Vertebral artery syndrome

435.2 Subclavian steal syndrome

435.3 Vertebrobasilar artery syndrome

435.8 Other specified transient cerebral ischemias

■ 435.9 Unspecified transient cerebral ischemia
Impending cerebrovascular accident
Intermittent cerebral ischemia
Transient ischemic attack [TIA]

Coding Clinic: 1985, Nov-Dec, P12

436 Acute, but ill-defined, cerebrovascular disease
Apoplexy, apoplectic:
NOS
attack
cerebral
seizure
Cerebral seizure
Excludes *any condition classifiable to categories 430–435*
cerebrovascular accident (434.91)
CVA (ischemic) (434.91)
embolic (434.11)
hemorrhagic (430, 431, 432.0–432.9)
thrombotic (434.01)
postoperative cerebrovascular accident (997.02)
stroke (ischemic) (434.91)
embolic (434.11)
hemorrhagic (430, 431, 432.0–432.9)
thrombotic (434.01)
Coding Clinic: 2004, Q4, P77-78; 1999, Q4, P3-4; 1993, Q4, P38-39; Q1, P27

OGCR Section I.C.7.b

The terms stroke and CVA are often used interchangeably to refer to a cerebral vascular infarction. The terms stroke, CVA, and cerebral infarction NOS are all indexed to the default code 434.91, Cerebral artery occlusion, unspecified, with infarction. Additional code(s) should be assigned for any neurologic deficits associated with the acute CVA, regardless of whether or not the neurologic deficit restores prior to discharge.

437 Other and ill-defined cerebrovascular disease
  437.0 Cerebral atherosclerosis
    Atheroma of cerebral arteries
    Cerebral arteriosclerosis
    Coding Clinic: 2010, Q3, P16
  437.1 Other generalized ischemic cerebrovascular disease
    Acute cerebrovascular insufficiency NOS
    Cerebral ischemia (chronic)
    Coding Clinic: 2009, Q1, P10
  437.2 Hypertensive encephalopathy
  437.3 Cerebral aneurysm, nonruptured
    Internal carotid artery, intracranial portion
    Internal carotid artery NOS
    Excludes *congenital cerebral aneurysm, nonruptured (747.81)*
    internal carotid artery, extracranial portion (442.81)
    Coding Clinic: 2009, Q2, P12
  437.4 Cerebral arteritis
    Coding Clinic: 1999, Q4, P21-22
  437.5 Moyamoya disease
  437.6 Nonpyogenic thrombosis of intracranial venous sinus
    Excludes *pyogenic (325)*
  437.7 Transient global amnesia
  437.8 Other
  437.9 Unspecified
    Cerebrovascular disease or lesion NOS
    Coding Clinic: 2009, Q1, P16; 1986, Nov-Dec, P12

OGCR Section I.C.7.d.3

Assign code V12.54, Transient ischemic attack (TIA), and cerebral infarction without residual deficits (and not a code from category 438) as an additional code for history of cerebrovascular disease when no neurologic deficits are present.

438 Late effects of cerebrovascular disease
  Note: This category is to be used to indicate conditions in 430–437 as the cause of late effects. The "late effects" include conditions specified as such, or as sequelae, which may occur at any time after the onset of the causal condition.
  Excludes *personal history of:*
    cerebral infarction without residual deficits (V12.54)
    PRIND (Prolonged reversible ischemic neurologic deficit) (V12.54)
    RIND (Reversible ischemic neurological deficit) (V12.54)
    transient ischemic attack (TIA) (V12.54)
  Coding Clinic: 2006, Q3, P3-4, 6; 1999, Q4, P6-8x2; Q4, P4-5; 1994, Q1, P22-23; 1993, Q1, P27
  438.0 Cognitive deficits
    Coding Clinic: 2007, Q2, P5
  438.1 Speech and language deficits
    438.10 Speech and language deficit, unspecified
    438.11 Aphasia
      Coding Clinic: 2003, Q4, P105-106; 1997, Q4, P35-37
    438.12 Dysphasia
      Coding Clinic: 1999, Q4, P9; Q4, P3-4
    438.13 Dysarthria
    438.14 Fluency disorder
      Stuttering due to late effect of cerebrovascular accident
    438.19 Other speech and language deficits
  438.2 Hemiplegia/hemiparesis
    Coding Clinic: 2005, Q1, P13
    438.20 Hemiplegia affecting unspecified side
      Coding Clinic: 2007, Q4, P92-95; 2003, Q4, P105-106; 1999, Q4, P9; Q4, P3-4
    438.21 Hemiplegia affecting dominant side
    438.22 Hemiplegia affecting nondominant side
      Coding Clinic: 2003, Q4, P105; 2002, Q1, P16
  438.3 Monoplegia of upper limb
    438.30 Monoplegia of upper limb affecting unspecified side
    438.31 Monoplegia of upper limb affecting dominant side
    438.32 Monoplegia of upper limb affecting nondominant side
  438.4 Monoplegia of lower limb
    438.40 Monoplegia of lower limb affecting unspecified side
    438.41 Monoplegia of lower limb affecting dominant side
    438.42 Monoplegia of lower limb affecting nondominant side
  438.5 Other paralytic syndrome
    Use additional code to identify type of paralytic syndrome, such as:
    locked-in state (344.81)
    quadriplegia (344.00–344.09)
    Excludes *late effects of cerebrovascular accident with:*
    hemiplegia/hemiparesis (438.20–438.22)
    monoplegia of lower limb (438.40–438.42)
    monoplegia of upper limb (438.40–438.42)
    438.50 Other paralytic syndrome affecting unspecified side
    438.51 Other paralytic syndrome affecting dominant side
    438.52 Other paralytic syndrome affecting nondominant side
    438.53 Other paralytic syndrome, bilateral
      Coding Clinic: 1998, Q4, P39-40

438.6 Alterations of sensations
  Use additional code to identify the altered sensation
  Coding Clinic: 2002, Q4, P56

438.7 Disturbances of vision
  Use additional code to identify the visual disturbance
  Coding Clinic: 2002, Q4, P56

● **438.8 Other late effects of cerebrovascular disease**
  Coding Clinic: 2005, Q1, P13; 2002, Q4, P56

  438.81 Apraxia

  438.82 Dysphagia
    Use additional code to identify the type of dysphagia, if known (787.20–787.29)
    Coding Clinic: 2007, Q4, P92-95

  438.83 Facial weakness
    Facial droop

  438.84 Ataxia

  438.85 Vertigo
    Coding Clinic: 2002, Q4, P56

  438.89 Other late effects of cerebrovascular disease
    Use additional code to identify the late effect
    Coding Clinic: 2009, Q2, P10; 2005, Q1, P13; 1998, Q4, P39-40

438.9 Unspecified late effects of cerebrovascular disease

DISEASES OF ARTERIES, ARTERIOLES, AND CAPILLARIES (440–449)

● **440 Atherosclerosis**
  Disease in which fatty deposits form on walls of arteries
  Includes: arteriolosclerosis
    arteriosclerosis (obliterans) (senile)
    arteriosclerotic vascular disease
    atheroma
    degeneration:
      arterial
      arteriovascular
      vascular
    endarteritis deformans or obliterans
    senile:
      arteritis
      endarteritis
  Excludes: atheroembolism (445.01–445.89)
    atherosclerosis of bypass graft of the extremities (440.30–440.32)

  440.0 Of aorta
    Coding Clinic: 1993, Q2, P7-8; 1988, Q4, P8

  440.1 Of renal artery
    Excludes: atherosclerosis of renal arterioles (403.00–403.91)

● **440.2 Of native arteries of the extremities**
    Use additional code, if applicable, to identify chronic total occlusion of artery of the extremities (440.4)
    Excludes: atherosclerosis of bypass graft of the extremities (440.30–440.32)
    Coding Clinic: 1994, Q3, P5; 1990, Q3, P15

  440.20 Atherosclerosis of the extremities, unspecified

  440.21 Atherosclerosis of the extremities with intermittent claudication

  440.22 Atherosclerosis of the extremities with rest pain
    Any condition classifiable to 440.21

  440.23 Atherosclerosis of the extremities with ulceration
    Any condition classifiable to 440.21–440.22
    Use additional code for any associated ulceration (707.10-707.19, 707.8, 707.9)

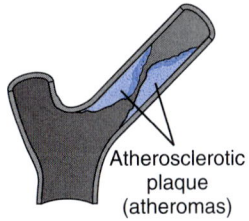

Figure 7-4 Atherosclerotic plaque.

  440.24 Atherosclerosis of the extremities with gangrene
    Any condition classifiable to 440.21, 440.22, and 440.23 with ischemic gangrene 785.4
    Use additional code for any associated ulceration (707.10-707.19, 707.8, 707.9)
    Excludes: gas gangrene 040.0
    Coding Clinic: 2003, Q4, P109-110; Q3, P14x2; 1995, Q1, P11; 1994, Q3, P5

  440.29 Other
    Coding Clinic: 1995, Q1, P11

● **440.3 Of bypass graft of the extremities**
    Excludes: atherosclerosis of native artery of the extremity (440.21–440.24)
    embolism [occlusion NOS] [thrombus] of graft (996.74)

  440.30 Of unspecified graft
  440.31 Of autologous vein bypass graft
  440.32 Of nonautologous vein bypass graft

● **440.4 Chronic total occlusion of artery of the extremities**
    Complete occlusion of artery of the extremities
    Total occlusion of artery of the extremities
    Code first atherosclerosis of arteries of the extremities (440.20–440.29, 440.30–440.32)
    Excludes: acute occlusion of artery of extremity (444.21–444.22)
    Coding Clinic: 2007, Q4, P82-83

  440.8 Of other specified arteries
    Excludes: basilar (433.0)
      carotid (433.1)
      cerebral (437.0)
      coronary (414.00–414.07)
      mesenteric (557.1)
      precerebral (433.0–433.9)
      pulmonary (416.0)
      vertebral (433.2)
    Coding Clinic: 2009, Q3, P9

  440.9 Generalized and unspecified atherosclerosis
    Arteriosclerotic vascular disease NOS
    Excludes: arteriosclerotic cardiovascular disease [ASCVD] (429.2)

● **441 Aortic aneurysm and dissection**
    Excludes: aortic ectasia (447.70-447.73)
      syphilitic aortic aneurysm (093.0)
      traumatic aortic aneurysm (901.0, 902.0)

● **441.0 Dissection of aorta**
    Coding Clinic: 1989, Q4, P10

  441.00 Unspecified site
  441.01 Thoracic
    Coding Clinic: 2009, Q1, P16; 2007, Q4, P86-87
  441.02 Abdominal
  441.03 Thoracoabdominal

  441.1 Thoracic aneurysm, ruptured
    Coding Clinic: 1994, Q2, P15

  441.2 Thoracic aneurysm without mention of rupture
    Coding Clinic: 1992, Q3, P10-11

  441.3 Abdominal aneurysm, ruptured

  441.4 Abdominal aneurysm without mention of rupture
    Coding Clinic: 2000, Q4, P63-64; 1999, Q1, P15-17x2; 1992, Q3, P10-11

441.5 Aortic aneurysm of unspecified site, ruptured
Rupture of aorta NOS

441.6 Thoracoabdominal aneurysm, ruptured

441.7 Thoracoabdominal aneurysm, without mention of rupture
Coding Clinic: 2006, Q2, P16-17

441.9 Aortic aneurysm of unspecified site without mention of rupture
Aneurysm
Dilatation of aorta
Hyaline necrosis of aorta
Coding Clinic: 1992, Q3, P10-11

● **442 Other aneurysm**
Includes aneurysm (ruptured) (cirsoid) (false) (varicose)
aneurysmal varix
Excludes arteriovenous aneurysm or fistula:
acquired (447.0)
congenital (747.60–747.69)
traumatic (900.0–904.9)

442.0 Of artery of upper extremity

442.1 Of renal artery

442.2 Of iliac artery
Coding Clinic: 1999, Q1, P16-17

442.3 Of artery of lower extremity
Aneurysm:
femoral artery
popliteal artery
Coding Clinic: 2008, Q2, P13; 2002, Q3, P24-27; 1999, Q1, P16

● **442.8 Of other specified artery**

442.81 Artery of neck
Aneurysm of carotid artery (common) (external) (internal, extracranial portion)
Excludes internal carotid artery, intracranial portion (437.3)

442.82 Subclavian artery

442.83 Splenic artery

442.84 Other visceral artery
Aneurysm:
celiac artery
gastroduodenal artery
gastroepiploic artery
hepatic artery
pancreaticoduodenal artery
superior mesenteric artery

442.89 Other
Aneurysm: Aneurysm:
mediastinal artery   spinal artery
Excludes cerebral (nonruptured) (437.3)
congenital (747.81)
ruptured (430)
coronary (414.11)
heart (414.10)
pulmonary (417.1)

442.9 Of unspecified site

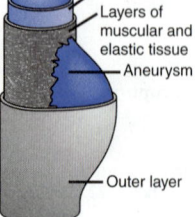

Figure 7-5 An aneurysm is an enclosed swelling on the wall of the vessel.

Item 7-12 Rupture is the tearing of the aneurysm.

● **443 Other peripheral vascular disease**

443.0 Raynaud's syndrome
Resulting from a diminishing oxygen supply to fingers, toes, nose, and ears when exposed to temperature changes or stress with symptoms of pallor, numbness, and feeling cold
Raynaud's:
disease
phenomenon (secondary)
Use additional code to identify gangrene (785.4)

443.1 Thromboangiitis obliterans [Buerger's disease]
Inflammatory occlusive disease resulting in poor circulation to legs, feet, and sometimes hands due to progressive inflammatory narrowing of the small arteries
Presenile gangrene

● **443.2 Other arterial dissection**
Excludes dissection of aorta (441.00–441.03)
dissection of coronary arteries (414.12)
Coding Clinic: 2002, Q4, P54-55

443.21 Dissection of carotid artery

443.22 Dissection of iliac artery

443.23 Dissection of renal artery

443.24 Dissection of vertebral artery

443.29 Dissection of other artery

● **443.8 Other specified peripheral vascular diseases**

●**443.81 Peripheral angiopathy in diseases classified elsewhere**
Code first underlying disease, as:
diabetes mellitus (249.7, 250.7)
Coding Clinic: 2004, Q1, P14-15; 1996, Q1, P10

443.82 Erythromelalgia
Coding Clinic: 2005, Q4, P73-74

443.89 Other
Acrocyanosis
Acroparesthesia:
simple [Schultze's type]
vasomotor [Nothnagel's type]
Erythrocyanosis
Excludes chilblains (991.5)
frostbite (991.0–991.3)
immersion foot (991.4)
Coding Clinic: 2007, Q4, P124

443.9 Peripheral vascular disease, unspecified
Intermittent claudication NOS
Peripheral:
angiopathy NOS
vascular disease NOS
Spasm of artery
Excludes atherosclerosis of the arteries of the extremities (440.20–440.22)
spasm of cerebral artery (435.0–435.9)

● **444 Arterial embolism and thrombosis**
Includes infarction:
embolic
thrombotic
occlusion
Excludes atheroembolism (445.01–445.89)
septic arterial embolism (449)
that complicating:
abortion (634–638 with .6, 639.6)
ectopic or molar pregnancy (639.6)
pregnancy, childbirth, or the puerperium (673.0–673.8)
Coding Clinic: 2003, Q1, P16-18x2; 1992, Q2, P10-11

● **444.0 Of abdominal aorta**
Coding Clinic: 1990, Q4, P27

444.01 Saddle embolus of abdominal aorta
Coding Clinic: 2011, Q4, P109

444.09 Other arterial embolism and thrombosis of abdominal aorta
Aortic bifurcation syndrome
Aortoiliac obstruction
Leriche's syndrome

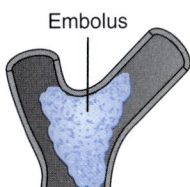

Figure 7-6 An arterial embolus.

Item 7-13 An **embolus** is a mass of undissolved matter present in the blood that is transported by the blood current. A **thrombus** is a blood clot that occludes or shuts off a vessel. When a thrombus is dislodged, it becomes an embolus.

- 444.1 **Of thoracic aorta**
  Embolism or thrombosis of aorta (thoracic)
- 444.2 **Of arteries of the extremities**
  - 444.21 Upper extremity
    Coding Clinic: 1990, Q3, P16
  - 444.22 Lower extremity
    Arterial embolism or thrombosis:
      femoral   popliteal
      peripheral NOS
    Excludes iliofemoral (444.81)
    Coding Clinic: 2007, Q4, P84-86; 2003, Q3, P10
- 444.8 **Of other specified artery**
  - 444.81 Iliac artery
    Coding Clinic: 2003, Q1, P16-17
  - 444.89 Other
    Excludes basilar (433.0)
      carotid (433.1)
      cerebral (434.0–434.9)
      coronary (410.00–410.92)
      mesenteric (557.0)
      ophthalmic (362.30–362.34)
      precerebral (433.0–433.9)
      pulmonary (415.11-415.19)
      renal (593.81)
      retinal (362.30–362.34)
      vertebral (433.2)
- 444.9 **Of unspecified artery**
- 445 **Atheroembolism**
  Includes Atherothrombotic microembolism
    Cholesterol embolism
  Coding Clinic: 2002, Q4, P57-58
- 445.0 **Of extremities**
  - 445.01 Upper extremity
  - 445.02 Lower extremity
- 445.8 **Of other sites**
  - 445.81 Kidney
    Use additional code for any associated acute kidney failure or chronic kidney disease (584, 585)
  - 445.89 Other site
- 446 **Polyarteritis nodosa and allied conditions**
  - 446.0 **Polyarteritis nodosa**
    Disseminated necrotizing periarteritis
    Necrotizing angiitis
    Panarteritis (nodosa)
    Periarteritis (nodosa)
  - 446.1 **Acute febrile mucocutaneous lymph node syndrome [MCLS]**
    Kawasaki disease
  - 446.2 **Hypersensitivity angiitis**
    Excludes antiglomerular basement membrane disease without pulmonary hemorrhage (583.89)
    - 446.20 Hypersensitivity angiitis, unspecified
    - 446.21 Goodpasture's syndrome
      Antiglomerular basement membrane antibody-mediated nephritis with pulmonary hemorrhage
      Use additional code to identify renal disease (583.81)
    - 446.29 Other specified hypersensitivity angiitis
      Coding Clinic: 1995, Q1, P3
  - 446.3 **Lethal midline granuloma**
    Malignant granuloma of face
  - 446.4 **Wegener's granulomatosis**
    Necrotizing respiratory granulomatosis
    Wegener's syndrome
    Coding Clinic: 2000, Q3, P11
  - 446.5 **Giant cell arteritis**
    Cranial arteritis
    Horton's disease
    Temporal arteritis
  - 446.6 **Thrombotic microangiopathy**
    Moschcowitz's syndrome
    Thrombotic thrombocytopenic purpura
  - 446.7 **Takayasu's disease**
    Aortic arch arteritis
    Pulseless disease
- 447 **Other disorders of arteries and arterioles**
  - 447.0 **Arteriovenous fistula, acquired**
    Arteriovenous aneurysm, acquired
    Excludes cerebrovascular (437.3)
      coronary (414.19)
      pulmonary (417.0)
      surgically created arteriovenous shunt or fistula:
        complication (996.1, 996.61–996.62)
        status or presence (V45.11)
      traumatic (900.0–904.9)
  - 447.1 **Stricture of artery**
    Coding Clinic: 1993, Q2, P8; 1987, Jan-Feb, P14
  - 447.2 **Rupture of artery**
    Erosion of artery
    Fistula, except arteriovenous of artery
    Ulcer of artery
    Excludes traumatic rupture of artery (900.0–904.9)
  - 447.3 **Hyperplasia of renal artery**
    Fibromuscular hyperplasia of renal artery
  - 447.4 **Celiac artery compression syndrome**
    Celiac axis syndrome
    Marable's syndrome
  - 447.5 **Necrosis of artery**
  - 447.6 **Arteritis, unspecified**
    Aortitis NOS
    Endarteritis NOS
    Excludes arteritis, endarteritis:
      aortic arch (446.7)
      cerebral (437.4)
      coronary (414.00–414.07)
      deformans (440.0–440.9)
      obliterans (440.0–440.9)
      pulmonary (417.8)
      senile (440.0–440.9)
      polyarteritis NOS (446.0)
      syphilitic aortitis (093.1)
    Coding Clinic: 1999, Q4, P21-22

- **447.7 Aortic ectasia**
  Ectasis aorta
  Excludes aortic aneurysm and dissection (441.00-441.9)
  - 447.70 Aortic ectasia, unspecified site
  - 447.71 Thoracic aortic ectasia
  - 447.72 Abdominal aortic ectasia
  - 447.73 Thoracoabdominal aortic ectasia
- **447.8 Other specified disorders of arteries and arterioles**
  Fibromuscular hyperplasia of arteries, except renal
- **447.9 Unspecified disorders of arteries and arterioles**

- **448 Disease of capillaries**
  - **448.0 Hereditary hemorrhagic telangiectasia**
    Rendu-Osler-Weber disease
  - **448.1 Nevus, non-neoplastic**
    Nevus:
      araneus
      senile
      spider
      stellar
    Excludes neoplastic (216.0–216.9)
      port wine (757.32)
      strawberry (757.32)
  - **448.9 Other and unspecified capillary diseases**
    Capillary:
      hemorrhage
      hyperpermeability
      thrombosis
    Excludes capillary fragility (hereditary) (287.8)

- **449 Septic arterial embolism**
  Code first underlying infection, such as:
    infective endocarditis (421.0)
    lung abscess (513.0)
  Use additional code to identify the site of the embolism (433.0–433.9, 444.01–444.9)
  Excludes septic pulmonary embolism (415.12)
  Coding Clinic: 2007, Q4, P84-86

DISEASES OF VEINS AND LYMPHATICS, AND OTHER DISEASES OF CIRCULATORY SYSTEM (451–459)

- **451 Phlebitis and thrombophlebitis**
  Inflammation of vein with infiltration of walls (phlebitis) and, usually, formation of clot (thrombus) in vein (thrombophlebitis)
  Includes endophlebitis
    inflammation, vein
    periphlebitis
    suppurative phlebitis
  Use additional E code to identify drug if drug-induced
  Excludes that complicating:
    abortion (634–638 with .7, 639.8)
    ectopic or molar pregnancy (639.8)
    pregnancy, childbirth, or the puerperium (671.0–671.9)
    that due to or following:
      implant or catheter device (996.61–996.62)
      infusion, perfusion, or transfusion (999.2)
  Coding Clinic: 2011, Q1, P19; 2004, Q4, P78-80; 1993, Q1, P26; 1992, Q1, P15-16
  - **451.0 Of superficial vessels of lower extremities**
    Saphenous vein (greater) (lesser)
  - **451.1 Of deep vessels of lower extremities**
    Coding Clinic: 1991, Q3, P16
    - 451.11 Femoral vein (deep) (superficial)
    - 451.19 Other
      Femoropopliteal vein
      Popliteal vein
      Tibial vein
  - **451.2 Of lower extremities, unspecified**
    Coding Clinic: 2004, Q4, P78-80
  - **451.8 Of other sites**
    Excludes intracranial venous sinus (325)
      nonpyogenic (437.6)
      portal (vein) (572.1)
    - 451.81 Iliac vein
    - 451.82 Of superficial veins of upper extremities
      Antecubital vein
      Basilic vein
      Cephalic vein
    - 451.83 Of deep veins of upper extremities
      Brachial vein
      Radial vein
      Ulnar vein
    - 451.84 Of upper extremities, unspecified
    - 451.89 Other
      Axillary vein
      Jugular vein
      Subclavian vein
      Thrombophlebitis of breast (Mondor's disease)
  - **451.9 Of unspecified site**

- **452 Portal vein thrombosis**
  Portal (vein) obstruction
  Excludes hepatic vein thrombosis (453.0)
    phlebitis of portal vein (572.1)

- **453 Other venous embolism and thrombosis**
  Excludes that complicating:
    abortion (634–638 with .7, 639.8)
    ectopic or molar pregnancy (639.8)
    pregnancy, childbirth, or the puerperium (671.0–671.9)
  Coding Clinic: 2011, Q1, P19-20; 2004, Q4, P78-80; 1992, Q1, P15-16
  - **453.0 Budd-Chiari syndrome**
    Hepatic vein thrombosis
  - **453.1 Thrombophlebitis migrans**
    "White leg" is the other term used to describe a migrating thrombus.
  - **453.2 Of inferior vena cava**
  - **453.3 Of renal vein**
  - **453.4 Acute venous embolism and thrombosis of deep vessels of lower extremity**
    - 453.40 Acute venous embolism and thrombosis of unspecified deep vessels of lower extremity
      Deep vein thrombosis NOS
      DVT NOS
      Coding Clinic: 2012, Q1, P18
    - 453.41 Acute venous embolism and thrombosis of deep vessels of proximal lower extremity
      Femoral   Thigh
      Iliac   Upper leg NOS
      Popliteal
      Coding Clinic: 2004, Q4, P78-80
    - 453.42 Acute venous embolism and thrombosis of deep vessels of distal lower extremity
      Calf   Peroneal
      Lower leg NOS Tibial
  - **453.5 Chronic venous embolism and thrombosis of deep vessels of lower extremity**
    Use additional code, if applicable, for associated long-term (current) use of anticoagulants (V58.61)
    Excludes personal history of venous thrombosis and embolism (V12.51)
    - 453.50 Chronic venous embolism and thrombosis of unspecified deep vessels of lower extremity
    - 453.51 Chronic venous embolism and thrombosis of deep vessels of proximal lower extremity
      Femoral   Thigh
      Iliac   Upper leg NOS
      Popliteal
    - 453.52 Chronic venous embolism and thrombosis of deep vessels of distal lower extremity
      Calf   Peroneal
      Lower leg NOS Tibial

- **453.6** Venous embolism and thrombosis of superficial vessels of lower extremity
  Saphenous vein (greater) (lesser)
  Use additional code, if applicable, for associated long-term (current) use of anticoagulants (V58.61)

- **453.7** Chronic venous embolism and thrombosis of other specified vessels
  Use additional code, if applicable, for associated long-term (current) use of anticoagulants (V58.61)
  Excludes: personal history of venous thrombosis and embolism (V12.51)

  - **453.71** Chronic venous embolism and thrombosis of superficial veins of upper extremity
    Antecubital vein
    Basilic vein
    Cephalic vein
  - **453.72** Chronic venous embolism and thrombosis of deep veins of upper extremity
    Brachial vein
    Radial vein
    Ulnar vein
  - **453.73** Chronic venous embolism and thrombosis of upper extremity, unspecified
  - **453.74** Chronic venous embolism and thrombosis of axillary veins
  - **453.75** Chronic venous embolism and thrombosis of subclavian veins
  - **453.76** Chronic venous embolism and thrombosis of internal jugular veins
  - **453.77** Chronic venous embolism and thrombosis of other thoracic veins
    Brachiocephalic (innominate)
    Superior vena cava
  - **453.79** Chronic venous embolism and thrombosis of other specified veins

- **453.8** Acute venous embolism and thrombosis of other specified veins
  Excludes: cerebral (434.0–434.9)
  coronary (410.00–410.92)
  intracranial venous sinus (325)
    nonpyogenic (437.6)
  mesenteric (557.0)
  portal (452)
  precerebral (433.0–433.9)
  pulmonary (415.19)
  Coding Clinic: 2004, Q4, P78-80; 1992, Q1, P15-16

  - **453.81** Acute venous embolism and thrombosis of superficial veins of upper extremity
    Antecubital vein
    Basilic vein
    Cephalic vein
  - **453.82** Acute venous embolism and thrombosis of deep veins of upper extremity
    Brachial vein
    Radial vein
    Ulnar vein
  - **453.83** Acute venous embolism and thrombosis of upper extremity, unspecified
  - **453.84** Acute venous embolism and thrombosis of axillary veins
  - **453.85** Acute venous embolism and thrombosis of subclavian veins
  - **453.86** Acute venous embolism and thrombosis of internal jugular veins
  - **453.87** Acute venous embolism and thrombosis of other thoracic veins
    Brachiocephalic (innominate)
    Superior vena cava
  - **453.89** Acute venous embolism and thrombosis of other specified veins

- **453.9** Of unspecified site
  Embolism of vein
  Thrombosis (vein)
  Coding Clinic: 2012, Q1, P18; 2011, Q1, P21

Item 7-14 Varicose/Varicosities (varix = singular, varices = plural): Enlarged, engorged, tortuous, twisted vascular vessels (veins, arteries, lymphatics). As such, the condition can present in various parts of the body, although the most familiar locations are the lower extremities. A common complication of varices is thrombophlebitis. Varicosities of the anus and rectum are called hemorrhoids. There are additional codes for esophageal, sublingual (under the tongue), scrotal, pelvic, vulval, and nasal varices as well.

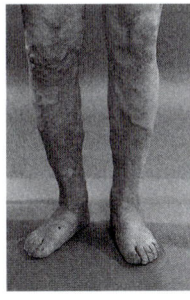

Figure 7-7 Varicose veins of the legs. (From Goldman: Cecil Medicine, ed 23, Saunders, 2008.)

- **454** Varicose veins of lower extremities
  Excludes: that complicating pregnancy, childbirth, or the puerperium (671.0)

  - **454.0** With ulcer
    Varicose ulcer (lower extremity, any part)
    Varicose veins with ulcer of lower extremity [any part] or of unspecified site
    Any condition classifiable to 454.9 with ulcer or specified as ulcerated
    Coding Clinic: 1999, Q4, P18
  - **454.1** With inflammation
    Stasis dermatitis
    Varicose veins with inflammation of lower extremity [any part] or of unspecified site
    Any condition classifiable to 454.9 with inflammation or specified as inflamed
    Coding Clinic: 1991, Q2, P20
  - **454.2** With ulcer and inflammation
    Varicose veins with ulcer and inflammation of lower extremity [any part] or of unspecified site
    Any condition classifiable to 454.9 with ulcer and inflammation
    Coding Clinic: 2004, Q3, P5-6; 1991, Q2, P20
  - **454.8** With other complications
    Edema   Swelling
    Pain
    Coding Clinic: 2002, Q4, P58-60
  - **454.9** Asymptomatic varicose veins
    Phlebectasia of lower extremity [any part] or of unspecified site
    Varicose veins NOS
    Varicose veins of lower extremity [any part] or of unspecified site
    Varix of lower extremity [any part] or of unspecified site

- **455** Hemorrhoids
  Includes: hemorrhoids (anus) (rectum)
    piles
    varicose veins, anus or rectum
  Excludes: that complicating pregnancy, childbirth, or the puerperium (671.8)

  - **455.0** Internal hemorrhoids without mention of complication
    Coding Clinic: 2005, Q3, P17
  - **455.1** Internal thrombosed hemorrhoids
  - **455.2** Internal hemorrhoids with other complication
    Internal hemorrhoids:
      bleeding
      prolapsed
      strangulated
      ulcerated
    Coding Clinic: 2005, Q3, P17; 2003, Q1, P8

455.3 External hemorrhoids without mention of complication
  Coding Clinic: 2007, Q1, P13
455.4 External thrombosed hemorrhoids
455.5 External hemorrhoids with other complication
  External hemorrhoids:
    bleeding
    prolapsed
    strangulated
    ulcerated
  Coding Clinic: 2005, Q3, P17; 2003, Q1, P8
■**455.6** Unspecified hemorrhoids without mention of complication
  Hemorrhoids NOS
■**455.7** Unspecified thrombosed hemorrhoids
  Thrombosed hemorrhoids, unspecified whether internal or external
■**455.8** Unspecified hemorrhoids with other complication
  Hemorrhoids, unspecified whether internal or external:
    bleeding
    prolapsed
    strangulated
    ulcerated
455.9 Residual hemorrhoidal skin tags
  Skin tags, anus or rectum

●**456** Varicose veins of other sites
  456.0 Esophageal varices with bleeding
  456.1 Esophageal varices without mention of bleeding
  ●**456.2** Esophageal varices in diseases classified elsewhere
    Code first underlying disease, as:
      cirrhosis of liver (571.0–571.9)
      portal hypertension (572.3)
    ●**456.20** With bleeding
      Coding Clinic: 1985, Nov-Dec, P14
    ●**456.21** Without mention of bleeding
      Coding Clinic: 2005, Q3, P15-16; 2002, Q2, P4
  456.3 Sublingual varices
  456.4 Scrotal varices
    Varicocele
  456.5 Pelvic varices
    Varices of broad ligament
  456.6 Vulval varices
    Varices of perineum
    Excludes *that complicating pregnancy, childbirth, or the puerperium (671.1)*
  456.8 Varices of other sites
    Varicose veins of nasal septum (with ulcer)
    Excludes *placental varices (656.7)*
      retinal varices (362.17)
      varicose ulcer of unspecified site (454.0)
      varicose veins of unspecified site (454.9)
    Coding Clinic: 2002, Q2, P4

●**457** Noninfectious disorders of lymphatic channels
  457.0 Postmastectomy lymphedema syndrome
    Elephantiasis due to mastectomy
    Obliteration of lymphatic vessel due to mastectomy
    Coding Clinic: 2002, Q2, P12-13
  457.1 Other lymphedema
    Elephantiasis (nonfilarial) NOS
    Lymphangiectasis
    Lymphedema:
      acquired (chronic)
      praecox
      secondary
    Obliteration, lymphatic vessel
    Excludes *elephantiasis (nonfilarial):*
      congenital (757.0)
      eyelid (374.83)
      vulva (624.8)
    Coding Clinic: 2004, Q3, P5-6
  457.2 Lymphangitis
    Lymphangitis:
      NOS
      chronic
      subacute
    Excludes *acute lymphangitis (682.0–682.9)*
  457.8 Other noninfectious disorders of lymphatic channels
    Chylocele (nonfilarial)   Lymph node or vessel:
    Chylous: fistula
      ascites   infarction
      cyst   rupture
    Excludes *chylocele:*
      filarial (125.0–125.9)
      tunica vaginalis (nonfilarial) (608.84)
    Coding Clinic: 2004, Q1, P5; 2003, Q3, P16-17
  ■**457.9** Unspecified noninfectious disorder of lymphatic channels

●**458** Hypotension
  Subnormal arterial blood pressure
  Includes hypopiesis
  Excludes *cardiovascular collapse (785.50)*
    maternal hypotension syndrome (669.2)
    shock (785.50–785.59)
    Shy-Drager syndrome (333.0)
  Coding Clinic: 1994, Q3, P9; 1993, 5th Issue, P6-7
  458.0 Orthostatic hypotension
    Hypotension:
      orthostatic (chronic)
      postural
    Moving from sitting or reclining position to standing position precipitates sudden drop in blood pressure.
    Coding Clinic: 2000, Q3, P8-9
  458.1 Chronic hypotension
    Permanent idiopathic hypotension
  ●**458.2** Iatrogenic hypotension
    Coding Clinic: 2002, Q3, P12; 1993, Q4, P41-42
    458.21 Hypotension of hemodialysis
      Intra-dialytic hypotension
      Coding Clinic: 2003, Q4, P60-61
    458.29 Other iatrogenic hypotension
      Postoperative hypotension
      Coding Clinic: 1993, Q4, P41-42
  458.8 Other specified hypotension
    Coding Clinic: 1997. Q4, P37
  ■**458.9** Hypotension, unspecified
    Hypotension (arterial) NOS

- **459　Other disorders of circulatory system**
  - **459.0　Hemorrhage, unspecified**
    - Rupture of blood vessel NOS
    - Spontaneous hemorrhage NEC
    - **Excludes** *hemorrhage:*
      - *gastrointestinal NOS (578.9)*
      - *in newborn NOS (772.9)*
      - *nontraumatic hematoma of soft tissue (729.92)*
      - *secondary or recurrent following trauma (958.2)*
      - *traumatic rupture of blood vessel (900.0–904.9)*
    - Coding Clinic: 1999, Q4, P18
  - **459.1　Postphlebitic syndrome**
    - Chronic venous hypertension due to deep vein thrombosis
    - **Excludes** *chronic venous hypertension without deep vein thrombosis (459.30–459.39)*
    - Coding Clinic: 2002, Q4, P58-60; 1991, Q2, P20
    - **459.10　Postphlebitic syndrome without complications**
      - Asymptomatic postphlebitic syndrome
      - Postphlebitic syndrome NOS
    - **459.11　Postphlebitic syndrome with ulcer**
    - **459.12　Postphlebitic syndrome with inflammation**
    - **459.13　Postphlebitic syndrome with ulcer and inflammation**
    - **459.19　Postphlebitic syndrome with other complication**
  - **459.2　Compression of vein**
    - Stricture of vein
    - Vena cava syndrome (inferior) (superior)
  - **459.3　Chronic venous hypertension (idiopathic)**
    - Stasis edema
    - **Excludes** *chronic venous hypertension due to deep vein thrombosis (459.10–459.19)*
      - *varicose veins (454.0–454.9)*
    - Coding Clinic: 2002, Q4, P58-60
    - **459.30　Chronic venous hypertension without complications**
      - Asymptomatic chronic venous hypertension
      - Chronic venous hypertension NOS
    - **459.31　Chronic venous hypertension with ulcer**
    - **459.32　Chronic venous hypertension with inflammation**
    - **459.33　Chronic venous hypertension with ulcer and inflammation**
    - **459.39　Chronic venous hypertension with other complication**
  - **459.8　Other specified disorders of circulatory system**
    - **459.81　Venous (peripheral) insufficiency, unspecified**
      - Chronic venous insufficiency NOS
      - Use additional code for any associated ulceration (707.10-707.19, 707.8, 707.9)
      - Coding Clinic: 2004, Q3, P5-6; 1991, Q2, P20
    - **459.89　Other**
      - Collateral circulation (venous), any site
      - Phlebosclerosis
      - Venofibrosis
  - **459.9　Unspecified circulatory system disorder**
    - Coding Clinic: 2013, Q1, P7

8. DISEASES OF THE RESPIRATORY SYSTEM (460–519)

Use additional code to identify infectious organism

ACUTE RESPIRATORY INFECTIONS (460–466)

Excludes pneumonia and influenza (480.0–488.19)

460 Acute nasopharyngitis [common cold]
Coryza (acute)
Nasal catarrh, acute
Nasopharyngitis: Rhinitis:
   NOS   acute
   acute   infective
   infective NOS

Excludes nasopharyngitis, chronic (472.2)
pharyngitis:
    acute or unspecified (462)
    chronic (472.1)
rhinitis:
    allergic (477.0–477.9)
    chronic or unspecified (472.0)
sore throat:
    acute or unspecified (462)
    chronic (472.1)

Coding Clinic: 1988, Q1, P12

●**461 Acute sinusitis**
Code to specific sinus if indicated in documentation.

Includes abscess, acute, of sinus (accessory) (nasal)
empyema, acute, of sinus (accessory) (nasal)
infection, acute, of sinus (accessory) (nasal)
inflammation, acute, of sinus (accessory) (nasal)
suppuration, acute, of sinus (accessory) (nasal)

Excludes chronic or unspecified sinusitis (473.0–473.9)

461.0 Maxillary
       Acute antritis
461.1 Frontal
461.2 Ethmoidal
461.3 Sphenoidal
461.8 Other acute sinusitis
       Acute pansinusitis
■461.9 Acute sinusitis, unspecified
       Acute sinusitis NOS

462 Acute pharyngitis
Acute sore throat NOS
Pharyngitis (acute):
   NOS
   gangrenous
   infective
   phlegmonous
   pneumococcal
   staphylococcal
   suppurative
   ulcerative
Sore throat (viral) NOS
Viral pharyngitis

Excludes abscess:
    peritonsillar [quinsy] (475)
    pharyngeal NOS (478.29)
    retropharyngeal (478.24)
chronic pharyngitis (472.1)
infectious mononucleosis (075)
that specified as (due to):
    Coxsackie (virus) (074.0)
    gonococcus (098.6)
    herpes simplex (054.79)
    influenza (487.1, 488.02, 488.12)
    septic (034.0)
    streptococcal (034.0)

Coding Clinic: 2012, Q2, P18-19; 1985, Sept-Oct, P9

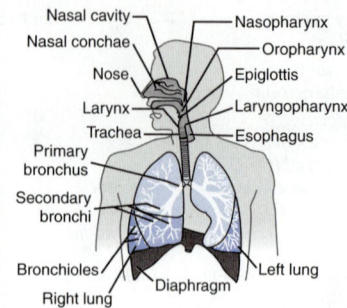

Figure 8-1 Respiratory system. (From Buck CJ: Step-by-Step Medical Coding, ed 2011, Philadelphia, WB Saunders, 2011)

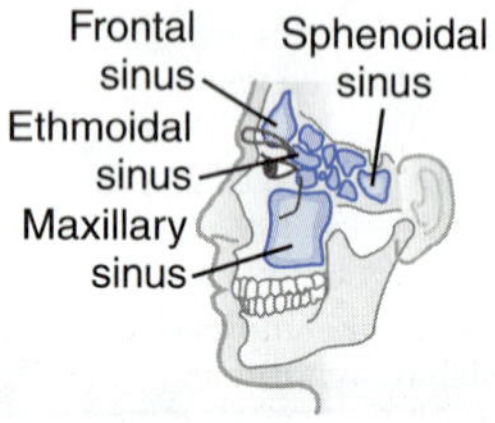

Figure 8-2 Paranasal sinuses. (From Buck CJ: Step-by-Step Medical Coding, ed 2011, Philadelphia, WB Saunders, 2011)

Item 8-1 Pharyngitis is painful inflammation of the pharynx (sore throat). Ninety percent of the infections are caused by a virus with the remaining being bacterial and rarely a fungus (candidiasis). Other irritants such as pollutants, chemicals, or smoke may cause similar symptoms.

463 Acute tonsillitis
Inflammation of pharyngeal tonsils caused by virus/bacteria
Tonsillitis (acute):   Tonsillitis (acute):
   NOS   septic
   follicular   staphylococcal
   gangrenous   suppurative
   infective   ulcerative
   pneumococcal   viral

Excludes chronic tonsillitis (474.0)
hypertrophy of tonsils (474.1)
peritonsillar abscess [quinsy] (475)
sore throat:
    acute or NOS (462)
    septic (034.0)
streptococcal tonsillitis (034.0)

Coding Clinic: 1984, Nov-Dec, P16

●**464 Acute laryngitis and tracheitis**

Excludes that associated with influenza (487.1, 488.02, 488.12)
that due to Streptococcus (034.0)

●**464.0 Acute laryngitis**
Laryngitis (acute):
   NOS
   edematous
   Hemophilus influenzae [H. influenzae]
   pneumococcal
   septic
   suppurative
   ulcerative

Excludes chronic laryngitis (476.0–476.1)
influenzal laryngitis (487.1, 488.02, 488.12)

464.00 Without mention of obstruction
464.01 With obstruction

●**464.1 Acute tracheitis**
Tracheitis (acute):   Tracheitis (acute):
   NOS   viral
   catarrhal

Excludes chronic tracheitis (491.8)

464.10 Without mention of obstruction
464.11 With obstruction

PART III / Diseases: Tabular List Volume 1

Item 8-2 **Laryngitis** is an inflammation of the larynx (voice box) resulting in hoarse voice or the complete loss of the voice. **Tracheitis** is an inflammation of the trachea (often following a URI) commonly caused by *staphylococcus aureus* resulting in inspiratory stridor (crowing sound on inspiration) and a croup-like cough.

- **464.2 Acute laryngotracheitis**
    Laryngotracheitis (acute)
    Tracheitis (acute) with laryngitis (acute)
    Excludes *chronic laryngotracheitis (476.1)*
    - 464.20 Without mention of obstruction
    - 464.21 With obstruction
- **464.3 Acute epiglottitis**
    Viral epiglottitis
    Excludes *epiglottitis, chronic (476.1)*
    - 464.30 Without mention of obstruction
    - 464.31 With obstruction
- 464.4 Croup
    Croup syndrome
- **464.5 Supraglottitis, unspecified**
    - 464.50 Without mention of obstruction
        Coding Clinic: 2001, Q4, P42-43
    - 464.51 With obstruction

- **465 Acute upper respiratory infections of multiple or unspecified sites**
    Excludes *upper respiratory infection due to:*
        influenza (487.1, 488.02, 488.12)
        Streptococcus (034.0)
    - 465.0 Acute laryngopharyngitis
    - 465.8 Other multiple sites
        Multiple URI
        Coding Clinic: 2007, Q4, P84-86
    - 465.9 Unspecified site
        Acute URI NOS
        Upper respiratory infection (acute)
        Coding Clinic: 1990, Q1, P19

- **466 Acute bronchitis and bronchiolitis**
    Includes that with:
        bronchospasm
        obstruction
    - 466.0 Acute bronchitis
        Inflammation/irritation of bronchial tubes lasting 2-3 weeks, which is most commonly caused by a virus
        Bronchitis, acute or   Bronchitis, acute or
            subacute: subacute:
            fibrinous   septic
            membranous   viral
            pneumococcal   with tracheitis
            purulent
        Croupous bronchitis
        Tracheobronchitis, acute
        Excludes *acute bronchitis with chronic obstructive pulmonary disease (491.22)*
        Coding Clinic: 2004, Q4, P81-82,137; Q1, P3; 2002, Q4, P46; 1996, Q4, P27-28; 1993, 5th Issue, P4x2; 1991, Q3, P17-18; 1988, Q1, P12

- **466.1 Acute bronchiolitis**
    Bronchiolitis (acute)
    Capillary pneumonia
    Excludes *respiratory bronchiolitis interstitial lung disease (516.34)*
    Coding Clinic: 1988, Q1, P12
    - 466.11 Acute bronchiolitis due to respiratory syncytial virus (RSV)
        Coding Clinic: 2005, Q1, P10; 1996, Q4, P27-28
    - 466.19 Acute bronchiolitis due to other infectious organisms
        Use additional code to identify organism

OTHER DISEASES OF THE UPPER RESPIRATORY TRACT (470–478)

- 470 **Deviated nasal septum**
    Deflected septum (nasal) (acquired)
    Excludes *congenital (754.0)*
- **471 Nasal polyps**
    Excludes *adenomatous polyps (212.0)*
    - 471.0 Polyp of nasal cavity
        Polyp:
            choanal
            nasopharyngeal
    - 471.1 Polypoid sinus degeneration
        Woakes' syndrome or ethmoiditis
    - 471.8 Other polyp of sinus
        Polyp of sinus:
            accessory
            ethmoidal
            maxillary
            sphenoidal
    - 471.9 Unspecified nasal polyp
        Nasal polyp NOS
- **472 Chronic pharyngitis and nasopharyngitis**
    - 472.0 Chronic rhinitis
        Ozena
        Rhinitis: Rhinitis:
            NOS   obstructive
            atrophic   purulent
            granulomatous   ulcerative
            hypertrophic
        Excludes *allergic rhinitis (477.0–477.9)*
    - 472.1 Chronic pharyngitis
        Chronic sore throat
        Pharyngitis: Pharyngitis:
            atrophic   hypertrophic
            granular (chronic)
    - 472.2 Chronic nasopharyngitis
        Excludes *acute or unspecified nasopharyngitis (460)*

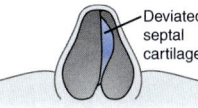
— Deviated septal cartilage

Figure 8-3 Deviated nasal septum.

OGCR Section I.C.8.b.1

Acute bronchitis, 466.0, is due to an infectious organism. When acute bronchitis is documented with COPD, code 491.22, Obstructive chronic bronchitis with acute bronchitis, should be assigned. It is not necessary to also assign code 466.0. If a medical record documents acute bronchitis with COPD with acute exacerbation, only code 491.22 should be assigned. The acute bronchitis included in code 491.22 supersedes the acute exacerbation. If a medical record documents COPD with acute exacerbation without mention of acute bronchitis, only code 491.21 should be assigned.

Item 8-3 A deviated nasal septum is the displacement of the septal cartilage that separates the nares. This displacement causes obstructed air flow through the nasal passages. A child can be born with this displacement (congenital), or the condition may be acquired through trauma, such as a sports injury. Symptoms include nasal block, sinusitis, and related secondary infections. Septoplasty is surgical repair of this condition.

Item 8-4 **Nasal polyps** are an abnormal growth of tissue (tumor) projecting from a mucous membrane and attached to the surface by a narrow elongated stalk (pedunculated). Nasal polyps usually originate in the ethmoid sinus but also may occur in the maxillary sinus. Symptoms are nasal block, sinusitis, anosmia, and secondary infections.

● 473 **Chronic sinusitis**
  Includes: abscess (chronic) of sinus (accessory) (nasal)
  empyema (chronic) of sinus (accessory) (nasal)
  infection (chronic) of sinus (accessory) (nasal)
  suppuration (chronic) of sinus (accessory) (nasal)
  Excludes: acute sinusitis (461.0–461.9)
  473.0 **Maxillary**
    Antritis (chronic)
  473.1 **Frontal**
  473.2 **Ethmoidal**
    Excludes: Woakes' ethmoiditis (471.1)
  473.3 **Sphenoidal**
  473.8 **Other chronic sinusitis**
    Pansinusitis (chronic)
  ■473.9 **Unspecified sinusitis (chronic)**
    Sinusitis (chronic) NOS
● 474 **Chronic disease of tonsils and adenoids**
  ● 474.0 **Chronic tonsillitis and adenoiditis**
    Excludes: acute or unspecified tonsillitis (463)
    474.00 **Chronic tonsillitis**
      Coding Clinic: 1984, Nov-Dec, P16
    474.01 **Chronic adenoiditis**
    474.02 **Chronic tonsillitis and adenoiditis**
  ● 474.1 **Hypertrophy of tonsils and adenoids**
    Enlargement of tonsils or adenoids
    Hyperplasia of tonsils or adenoids
    Hypertrophy of tonsils or adenoids
    Excludes: that with:
      adenoiditis (474.01)
      adenoiditis and tonsillitis (474.02)
      tonsillitis (474.00)
    474.10 **Tonsils with adenoids**
      Coding Clinic: 2005, Q2, P16
    474.11 **Tonsils alone**
      Coding Clinic: 1984, Nov-Dec, P16
    474.12 **Adenoids alone**
  474.2 **Adenoid vegetations**
  474.8 **Other chronic disease of tonsils and adenoids**
    Amygdalolith
    Calculus, tonsil
    Cicatrix of tonsil (and adenoid)
    Tonsillar tag
    Ulcer, tonsil
  ■474.9 **Unspecified chronic disease of tonsils and adenoids**
    Disease (chronic) of tonsils (and adenoids)
  475 **Peritonsillar abscess**
    Abscess of tonsil
    Peritonsillar cellulitis
    Quinsy
    Excludes: tonsillitis:
      acute or NOS (463)
      chronic (474.0)
● 476 **Chronic laryngitis and laryngotracheitis**
  476.0 **Chronic laryngitis**
    Laryngitis: Laryngitis:
      catarrhal   sicca
      hypertrophic
  476.1 **Chronic laryngotracheitis**
    Laryngitis, chronic, with tracheitis (chronic)
    Tracheitis, chronic, with laryngitis
    Excludes: chronic tracheitis (491.8)
      laryngitis and tracheitis, acute or unspecified (464.00–464.51)

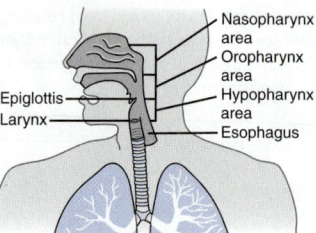

Figure 8-4 The pharynx.

Item 8-5 The **pharynx** is the passage for both food and air between the mouth and the esophagus and is divided into three areas: nasopharynx, oropharynx, and hypopharynx. The hypopharynx branches into the esophagus and the voice box.

● 477 **Allergic rhinitis**
  Includes: allergic rhinitis (nonseasonal) (seasonal)
  hay fever
  spasmodic rhinorrhea
  Excludes: allergic rhinitis with asthma (bronchial) (493.0)
  477.0 **Due to pollen**
    Pollinosis
  477.1 **Due to food**
  477.2 **Due to animal (cat) (dog) hair and dander**
  477.8 **Due to other allergen**
  ■477.9 **Cause unspecified**
    Coding Clinic: 1997, Q2, P9-10
● 478 **Other diseases of upper respiratory tract**
  478.0 **Hypertrophy of nasal turbinates**
  ● 478.1 **Other diseases of nasal cavity and sinuses**
    Excludes: varicose ulcer of nasal septum (456.8)
    Coding Clinic: 1995, Q4, P50; 1990, Q1, P8
    478.11 **Nasal mucositis (ulcerative)**
      Use additional E code to identify adverse effects of therapy, such as:
        antineoplastic and immunosuppressive drugs (E930.7, E933.1)
        radiation therapy (E879.2)
      Coding Clinic: 2006, Q4, P88-91
    478.19 **Other disease of nasal cavity and sinuses**
      Abscess of nose (septum)
      Cyst or mucocele of sinus (nasal)
      Necrosis of nose (septum)
      Rhinolith
      Ulcer of nose (septum)
  ● 478.2 **Other diseases of pharynx, not elsewhere classified**
    ■478.20 **Unspecified disease of pharynx**
    478.21 **Cellulitis of pharynx or nasopharynx**
    478.22 **Parapharyngeal abscess**
    478.24 **Retropharyngeal abscess**
    478.25 **Edema of pharynx or nasopharynx**
    478.26 **Cyst of pharynx or nasopharynx**
    478.29 **Other**
      Abscess of pharynx or nasopharynx
      Excludes: ulcerative pharyngitis (462)
  ● 478.3 **Paralysis of vocal cords or larynx**
    ■478.30 **Paralysis, unspecified**
      Laryngoplegia
      Paralysis of glottis
    478.31 **Unilateral, partial**
    478.32 **Unilateral, complete**
    478.33 **Bilateral, partial**
    478.34 **Bilateral, complete**

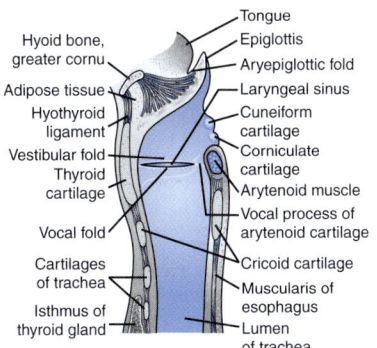

Figure 8-5 Coronal section of the larynx.

Item 8-6 The **larynx** extends from the tongue to the trachea and is divided into an upper and lower portion separated by folds. The framework of the larynx is cartilage composed of the single cricoid, thyroid, and epiglottic cartilages, and the paired arytenoid, cuneiform, and corniculate cartilages.

478.4 **Polyp of vocal cord or larynx**
  Excludes adenomatous polyps (212.1)

478.5 **Other diseases of vocal cords**
  Abscess of vocal cords
  Cellulitis of vocal cords
  Granuloma of vocal cords
  Leukoplakia of vocal cords
  Chorditis (fibrinous) (nodosa) (tuberosa)
  Singers' nodes

478.6 **Edema of larynx**
  Edema (of):
    glottis
    subglottic
    supraglottic

478.7 **Other diseases of larynx, not elsewhere classified**
  478.70 Unspecified disease of larynx
  478.71 Cellulitis and perichondritis of larynx
  478.74 Stenosis of larynx
  478.75 Laryngeal spasm
    Laryngismus (stridulus)
  478.79 Other
    Abscess of larynx
    Necrosis of larynx
    Obstruction of larynx
    Pachyderma of larynx
    Ulcer of larynx
    Excludes ulcerative laryngitis (464.00–464.01)
    Coding Clinic: 1991, Q3, P20

478.8 **Upper respiratory tract hypersensitivity reaction, site unspecified**
  Excludes hypersensitivity reaction of lower respiratory tract, as:
    extrinsic allergic alveolitis (495.0–495.9)
    pneumoconiosis (500–505)

478.9 **Other and unspecified diseases of upper respiratory tract**
  Abscess of trachea
  Cicatrix of trachea

PNEUMONIA AND INFLUENZA (480–488)

Excludes pneumonia:
  allergic or eosinophilic (518.3)
  aspiration:
    NOS (507.0)
    newborn (770.18)
    solids and liquids (507.0–507.8)
  congenital (770.0)
  lipoid (507.1)
  passive (514)
  rheumatic (390)
  ventilator-associated (997.31)

● 480 **Viral pneumonia**
  480.0 Pneumonia due to adenovirus
  480.1 Pneumonia due to respiratory syncytial virus
    Coding Clinic: 2010, Q4, P98; 1996, Q4, P27-28; 1988, Q1, P12
  480.2 Pneumonia due to parainfluenza virus
  480.3 Pneumonia due to SARS-associated coronavirus
    Coding Clinic: 2003, Q4, P46-48
  480.8 Pneumonia due to other virus not elsewhere classified
    Excludes congenital rubella pneumonitis (771.0)
      pneumonia complicating viral diseases classified elsewhere (484.1–484.8)
  480.9 Viral pneumonia, unspecified
    Coding Clinic: 2010, Q4, P135; 1998, Q3, P5

481 **Pneumococcal pneumonia [Streptococcus pneumoniae pneumonia]**
  Lobar pneumonia, organism unspecified
  Coding Clinic: 2009, Q3, P9; 1998, Q2, P7; 1991, Q1, P13; 1988, Q1, P13; 1985, Mar-April, P6

● 482 **Other bacterial pneumonia**
  482.0 Pneumonia due to Klebsiella pneumoniae
  482.1 Pneumonia due to Pseudomonas
  482.2 Pneumonia due to Hemophilus influenzae [H. influenzae]
    Coding Clinic: 2005, Q2, P19-20; 1993, Q4, P39
  ● 482.3 Pneumonia due to Streptococcus
    Excludes Streptococcus pneumoniae pneumonia (481)
    Coding Clinic: 1988, Q1, P13
    482.30 Streptococcus, unspecified
    482.31 Group A
    482.32 Group B
    482.39 Other Streptococcus
  ● 482.4 Pneumonia due to Staphylococcus
    Coding Clinic: 1991, Q3, P16-17
    482.40 Pneumonia due to Staphylococcus, unspecified
    482.41 Methicillin susceptible pneumonia due to Staphylococcus aureus
      MSSA pneumonia
      Pneumonia due to Staphylococcus aureus NOS
      Coding Clinic: 2008, Q4, P69-73
    482.42 Methicillin resistant pneumonia due to Staphylococcus aureus
      Coding Clinic: 2008, Q4, P69-73
    482.49 Other Staphylococcus pneumonia

Item 8-7 Pneumonia is an infection of the lungs, caused by a variety of microorganisms, including viruses, most commonly the *Streptococcus pneumoniae* (pneumococcus) bacteria, fungi, and parasites. Pneumonia occurs when the immune system is weakened, often by a URI or influenza.

DISEASES OF THE RESPIRATORY SYSTEM (460–519)

● **482.8 Pneumonia due to other specified bacteria**
  Excludes *pneumonia complicating infectious disease classified elsewhere (484.1–484.8)*
  Coding Clinic: 1988, Q3, P11

  482.81 Anaerobes
    Bacteroides (melaninogenicus)
    Gram-negative anaerobes

  482.82 Escherichia coli [E. coli]

  482.83 Other gram-negative bacteria
    Gram-negative pneumonia NOS
    Proteus
    Serratia marcescens
    Excludes *gram-negative anaerobes (482.81)*
    Legionnaires' disease (482.84)
    Coding Clinic: 1998, Q2, P5; 1994, Q3, P9; 1993, Q4, P39

  482.84 Legionnaires' disease

  482.89 Other specified bacteria
    Coding Clinic: 1998, Q2, P6; 1997, Q2, P6; 1994, Q1, P17-18

■ **482.9 Bacterial pneumonia unspecified**
  Coding Clinic: 1998, Q2, P4, 6X2; 1997, Q2, P6; 1994, Q1, P17-18

● **483 Pneumonia due to other specified organism**

  483.0 Mycoplasma pneumoniae
    Eaton's agent
    Pleuropneumonia-like organisms [PPLO]
    Coding Clinic: 1987, Nov-Dec, P5-6

  483.1 Chlamydia

  483.8 Other specified organism

● **484 Pneumonia in infectious diseases classified elsewhere**

  ● **484.1 Pneumonia in cytomegalic inclusion disease**
    Code first underlying disease, as: (078.5)

  ● **484.3 Pneumonia in whooping cough**
    Code first underlying disease, as: (033.0–033.9)

  ● **484.5 Pneumonia in anthrax**
    Code first underlying disease (022.1)

  ● **484.6 Pneumonia in aspergillosis**
    Code first underlying disease (117.3)
    Coding Clinic: 1997, Q4, P40

  ● **484.7 Pneumonia in other systemic mycoses**
    Code first underlying disease
    Excludes *pneumonia in:*
      candidiasis (112.4)
      coccidioidomycosis (114.0)
      histoplasmosis (115.0–115.9 with fifth-digit 5)

  ● **484.8 Pneumonia in other infectious diseases classified elsewhere**
    Code first underlying disease, as:
      Q fever (083.0)
      typhoid fever (002.0)
    Excludes *pneumonia in:*
      actinomycosis (039.1)
      measles (055.1)
      nocardiosis (039.1)
      ornithosis (073.0)
      Pneumocystis carinii (136.3)
      salmonellosis (003.22)
      toxoplasmosis (130.4)
      tuberculosis (011.6)
      tularemia (021.2)
      varicella (052.1)

■ **485 Bronchopneumonia, organism unspecified**
  Bronchopneumonia: Pneumonia:
    hemorrhagic   lobular
    terminal   segmental
  Pleurobronchopneumonia
  Excludes *bronchiolitis (acute) (466.11–466.19)*
    chronic (491.8)
    lipoid pneumonia (507.1)

■ **486 Pneumonia, organism unspecified**
  Excludes *hypostatic or passive pneumonia (514)*
    inhalation or aspiration pneumonia due to foreign materials (507.0–507.8)
    pneumonitis due to fumes and vapors (506.0)
  Coding Clinic: 2010, Q4, P137; Q1, P8; 2008, Q4, P140-143; 2006, Q2, P20; 1999, Q4, P6; Q3, P9; 1998, Q3, P7; Q2, P4-5; Q1, P8; 1997, Q3, P9; 1995, Q4, P52; 1994, Q1, P17-18; 1993, Q3, P9; Q1, P21; 1985, Mar-April, P6

● **487 Influenza**
  Influenza caused by unspecified influenza virus
  Excludes *Hemophilus influenzae [H. influenzae]:*
    infection NOS (041.5)
    laryngitis (464.00–464.01)
    meningitis (320.0)
    influenza due to 2009 H1N1 [swine] influenza virus (488.11-488.19)
    influenza due to identified avian influenza virus (488.01-488.09)
    influenza due to identified (novel) 2009 H1N1 influenza virus (488.11-488.19)

  487.0 With pneumonia
    Influenza with pneumonia, any form
    Influenzal:
      bronchopneumonia
      pneumonia
    Use additional code to identify the type of pneumonia (480.0–480.9, 481, 482.0–482.9, 483.0–483.8, 485)
    Coding Clinic: 2010, Q1, P8; 2005, Q2, P18-19

  487.1 With other respiratory manifestations
    Influenza NEC
    Influenza NOS
    Influenzal:
      laryngitis
      pharyngitis
      respiratory infection (upper) (acute)
    Coding Clinic: 2011, Q4, P114; 2005, Q2, P18-19; 1999, Q4, P26; 1987, Jan-Feb, P16

  487.8 With other manifestations
    Encephalopathy due to influenza
    Influenza with involvement of gastrointestinal tract
    Excludes *"intestinal flu" [viral gastroenteritis] (008.8)*

● **488 Influenza due to certain identified influenza viruses**
  Excludes *influenza caused by unspecified or seasonal influenza viruses (487.0-487.8)*
  Coding Clinic: 2007, Q4, P87-88

  ● **488.0 Influenza due to identified avian influenza virus**
    Avian influenza
    Bird flu
    Influenza A/H5N1

    488.01 Influenza due to identified avian influenza virus with pneumonia
      Avian influenzal:
        bronchopneumonia
        pneumonia
      Influenza due to identified avian influenza virus with pneumonia, any form
      Use additional code to identify the type of pneumonia (480.0-480.9, 481, 482.0-482.9, 483.0-483.8, 485)

    488.02 Influenza due to identified avian influenza virus with other respiratory manifestations
      Avian influenzal:
        laryngitis
        pharyngitis
        respiratory infection (acute) (upper)
      Identified avian influenza NOS

    488.09 Influenza due to identified avian influenza virus with other manifestations
      Avian influenza with involvement of gastrointestinal tract
      Encephalopathy due to identified avian influenza
      Excludes *"intestinal flu" [viral gastroenteritis] (008.8)*

- **488.1 Influenza due to identified 2009 H1N1 influenza virus**
  2009 H1N1 swine influenza virus
  (Novel) 2009 influenza H1N1
  Novel H1N1 influenza
  Novel influenza A/H1N1
  > **Excludes** bird influenza virus infection (488.01-488.09)
  > influenza A/H5N1 (488.01-488.09)
  > other human infection with influenza virus of animal origin (488.81-488.89)
  > swine influenza virus infection (488.81-488.89)

  Coding Clinic: 2011, Q4, P114; 2010, Q1, P8

  - **488.11 Influenza due to identified 2009 H1N1 influenza virus with pneumonia**
    Influenza due to identified (novel) 2009 H1N1 with pneumonia, any form
    (Novel) 2009 H1N1 influenzal:
      bronchopneumonia
      pneumonia
    > Use additional code to identify the type of pneumonia (480.0-480.9, 481, 482.0-482.9, 483.0-483.8, 485)

  - **488.12 Influenza due to identified 2009 H1N1 influenza virus with other respiratory manifestations**
    (Novel) 2009 H1N1 influenza NOS
    (Novel) 2009 H1N1 influenzal:
      laryngitis
      pharyngitis
      respiratory infection (acute) (upper)

  - **488.19 Influenza due to identified 2009 H1N1 influenza virus with other manifestations**
    Encephalopathy due to identified (novel) 2009 H1N1 influenza
    (Novel) 2009 H1N1 influenza with involvement of gastrointestinal tract
    > **Excludes** "intestinal flu" [viral gastroenteritis] (008.8)

- **488.8 Influenza due to novel influenza A**
  Infection with influenza viruses occurring in pigs or other animals
  Influenza due to animal origin influenza virus
  Other novel influenza A viruses not previously found in humans
  > **Excludes** bird influenza virus infection (488.01-488.09)
  > influenza A/H5N1 (488.01-488.09)
  > influenza due to identified 2009 H1N1 influenza virus (488.11-488.19)

  - **488.81 Influenza due to identified novel influenza A virus with pneumonia**
    Influenza due to animal origin influenza virus with pneumonia, any form
    Novel influenza A:
      bronchopneumonia
      pneumonia
    > Use additional code to identify the type of pneumonia (480.0-480.9, 481, 482.0-482.9, 483.0-483.8, 485)

  - **488.82 Influenza due to identified novel influenza A virus with other respiratory manifestations**
    Influenza due to animal origin influenza A virus with other respiratory manifestations
    Novel influenza A:
      laryngitis
      pharyngitis
      respiratory infection (acute) (upper)

  - **488.89 Influenza due to identified novel influenza A virus with other manifestations**
    Encephalopathy due to novel influenza A
    Influenza due to animal origin influenza virus with encephalopathy
    Influenza due to animal origin influenza virus with involvement of gastrointestinal tract
    Novel influenza A with involvement of gastrointestinal tract
    > **Excludes** "intestinal flu" [viral gastroenteritis] (008.8)

Item 8-8 **Chronic bronchitis** is usually defined as being present in any patient who has persistent cough with sputum production for at least three months in at least two consecutive years. **Simple chronic bronchitis** is marked by a productive cough but no pathological airflow obstruction. **Chronic obstructive pulmonary disease (COPD)** is a group of conditions—bronchitis, emphysema, asthma, bronchiectasis, allergic alveolitis—marked by dyspnea. **Catarrhal** bronchitis is an acute form of bronchitis marked by profuse mucus and pus production (**mucopurulent** discharge). **Croupous** bronchitis, also known as pseudomembranous, fibrinous, plastic, exudative, or membranous, is marked by a violent cough and dyspnea.

CHRONIC OBSTRUCTIVE PULMONARY DISEASE AND ALLIED CONDITIONS (490–496)

- **490 Bronchitis, not specified as acute or chronic**
  Bronchitis NOS:
    catarrhal
    with tracheitis NOS
  Tracheobronchitis NOS
  > **Excludes** bronchitis:
  > allergic NOS (493.9)
  > asthmatic NOS (493.9)
  > due to fumes and vapors (506.0)

- **491 Chronic bronchitis**
  > **Excludes** chronic obstructive asthma (493.2)

  - **491.0 Simple chronic bronchitis**
    Catarrhal bronchitis, chronic
    Smokers' cough

  - **491.1 Mucopurulent chronic bronchitis**
    Bronchitis (chronic) (recurrent):
      fetid
      mucopurulent
      purulent
    Coding Clinic: 1988, Q2, P11

  - **491.2 Obstructive chronic bronchitis**
    Bronchitis:
      emphysematous
      obstructive (chronic) (diffuse)
    Bronchitis with:
      chronic airway obstruction
      emphysema
    > **Excludes** asthmatic bronchitis (acute) (NOS) 493.9
    > chronic obstructive asthma 493.2

    Coding Clinic: 2004, Q4, P81-82; 2002, Q3, P18, 19x2; 1991, Q2, P21; 1984, Nov-Dec, P17

    - **491.20 Without exacerbation**
      Emphysema with chronic bronchitis
      Coding Clinic: 1997, Q3, P9

    - **491.21 With (acute) exacerbation**
      Acute exacerbation of chronic obstructive pulmonary disease [COPD]
      Decompensated chronic obstructive pulmonary disease [COPD]
      Decompensated chronic obstructive pulmonary disease [COPD] with exacerbation
      > **Excludes** chronic obstructive asthma with acute exacerbation 493.22

      Coding Clinic: 2010, Q1, P9; 2004, Q1, P3; 1996, Q2, P10; 1993, 5th Issue, P5x2

    - **491.22 With acute bronchitis**
      Coding Clinic: 2006, Q3, P20; 2004, Q4, P80-81; Q1, P3

OGCR Section I.C.8.b.1

When acute bronchitis, 466.0, is documented with COPD, code 491.22 should be assigned. It is not necessary to also assign code 466.0. If a medical record documents acute bronchitis with COPD with acute exacerbation, only code 491.22 should be assigned. The acute bronchitis included in code 491.22 supersedes the acute exacerbation. If a medical record documents COPD with acute exacerbation without mention of acute bronchitis, only code 491.21 should be assigned.

491.8 Other chronic bronchitis
Chronic: Chronic:
  tracheitis   tracheobronchitis

491.9 Unspecified chronic bronchitis
Coding Clinic: 1991, Q3, P17-18

● **492 Emphysema**
Coding Clinic: 1991, Q2, P21; 1984, Nov-Dec, P19

492.0 Emphysematous bleb
Giant bullous emphysema
Ruptured emphysematous bleb
Tension pneumatocele
Vanishing lung

492.8 Other emphysema
Emphysema (lung or pulmonary):
  NOS   panacinar
  centriacinar panlobular
  centrilobular unilateral
  obstructive   vesicular
MacLeod's syndrome
Swyer-James syndrome
Unilateral hyperlucent lung
  Excludes emphysema:
    with chronic bronchitis 491.20–491.22)
    compensatory (518.2)
    due to fumes and vapors (506.4)
    interstitial (518.1)
      newborn (770.2)
    mediastinal (518.1)
    surgical (subcutaneous) (998.81)
    traumatic (958.7)
Coding Clinic: 2008, Q4, P174-175; 1993, Q4, P41; 5th Issue, P4

● **493 Asthma**
  Excludes wheezing NOS (786.07)
Coding Clinic: 2003, Q4, P62, 137; 1991, Q1, P13; 1985, July-Aug, P8

The following fifth-digit subclassification is for use with category 493.0–493.2, 493.9:

  0 unspecified
  1 with status asthmaticus
  2 with (acute) exacerbation

● **493.0 Extrinsic asthma**
[0-2] Asthma:
    allergic with stated cause
    atopic
    childhood
    hay
    platinum
  Hay fever with asthma
  Excludes asthma:
    allergic NOS (493.9)
    detergent (507.8)
    miners' (500)
    wood (495.8)
Coding Clinic: 1990, Q2, P20

● **493.1 Intrinsic asthma**
[0-2] Late-onset asthma
Coding Clinic: 1990, Q2, P20

● **493.2 Chronic obstructive asthma**
[0-2] Asthma with chronic obstructive pulmonary disease [COPD]
  Chronic asthmatic bronchitis
  Excludes acute bronchitis (466.0)
    chronic obstructive bronchitis (491.20–491.22)
Coding Clinic: 2009, Q1, P16; 2006, Q3, P20; 2003, Q4, P108; 1993, 5th Issue, P4; 1991, Q2, P21; 1990, Q2, P20

Item 8–9 **Asthma** is a bronchial condition marked by airway obstruction, hyper-responsiveness, and inflammation. **Extrinsic** asthma, also known as allergic asthma, is characterized by the same symptoms that occur with exposure to allergens and is divided into the following types: **atopic, occupational, and allergic bronchopulmonary aspergillosis.** **Intrinsic** asthma occurs in patients who have no history of allergy or sensitivities to allergens and is divided into the following types: **nonreaginic and pharmacologic.** **Status asthmaticus** is the most severe form of asthma attack and can last for days or weeks.

● **493.8 Other forms of asthma**
493.81 Exercise induced bronchospasm
Coding Clinic: 2003, Q4, P62

493.82 Cough variant asthma
Coding Clinic: 2003, Q4, P62

● **493.9 Asthma, unspecified**
[0-2] Asthma (bronchial) (allergic NOS)
  Bronchitis:
    allergic
    asthmatic
Coding Clinic: 2004, Q4, P137; 2003, Q4, P108-109; Q1, P9; 1999, Q4, P25; 1997, Q4, P39-40; Q1, P7; 1996, Q3, P20; 1993, Q4, P32; 1992, Q1, P15; 1990, Q2, P20; 1984, Nov-Dec, P17

● **494 Bronchiectasis**
Bronchiectasis (fusiform) (postinfectious) (recurrent)
Bronchiolectasis
  Excludes congenital (748.61)
    tuberculous bronchiectasis (current disease) (011.5)

494.0 Bronchiectasis without acute exacerbation
494.1 Bronchiectasis with acute exacerbation

● **495 Extrinsic allergic alveolitis**
  Includes allergic alveolitis and pneumonitis due to inhaled organic dust particles of fungal, thermophilic actinomycete, or other origin

495.0 Farmers' lung
495.1 Bagassosis
495.2 Bird-fanciers' lung
  Budgerigar-fanciers' disease or lung
  Pigeon-fanciers' disease or lung
495.3 Suberosis
  Cork-handlers' disease or lung
495.4 Malt workers' lung
  Alveolitis due to Aspergillus clavatus
495.5 Mushroom workers' lung
495.6 Maple bark-strippers' lung
  Alveolitis due to Cryptostroma corticale
495.7 "Ventilation" pneumonitis
  Allergic alveolitis due to fungal, thermophilic actinomycete, and other organisms growing in ventilation [air conditioning] systems
495.8 Other specified allergic alveolitis and pneumonitis
  Cheese-washers' lung
  Coffee workers' lung
  Fish-meal workers' lung
  Furriers' lung
  Grain-handlers' disease or lung
  Pituitary snuff-takers' disease
  Sequoiosis or red-cedar asthma
  Wood asthma
495.9 Unspecified allergic alveolitis and pneumonitis
  Alveolitis, allergic (extrinsic)
  Hypersensitivity pneumonitis

496 Chronic airway obstruction, not elsewhere classified
Chronic:
nonspecific lung disease
obstructive lung disease
obstructive pulmonary disease [COPD] NOS

Note: This code is not to be used with any code from categories 491–493.

Excludes chronic obstructive lung disease [COPD] specified (as) (with):
allergic alveolitis (495.0–495.9)
asthma (493.2)
bronchiectasis (494.0–494.1)
bronchitis (491.20–491.22)
with emphysema (491.20–491.22)
decompensated (491.21)
emphysema (492.0–492.8)

Coding Clinic: 2010, Q1, P9; 2009, Q1, P16; 2006, Q3, P20; 2003, Q4, P109-110; 2000, Q2, P15; 1994, Q1, P19; 1993, Q4, P43; 1992, Q2, P16-17; 1991, Q2, P21; 1988, Q2, P12

OGCR Section I.C.8.a.1
Code 496, Chronic airway obstruction, not elsewhere classified, is a nonspecific code that should only be used when the documentation in a medical record does not specify the type of COPD being treated.

PNEUMOCONIOSES AND OTHER LUNG DISEASES DUE TO EXTERNAL AGENTS (500–508)

500 Coal workers' pneumoconiosis
Anthracosilicosis   Coal workers' lung
Anthracosis   Miners' asthma
Black lung disease

501 Asbestosis

502 Pneumoconiosis due to other silica or silicates
Pneumoconiosis due to talc
Silicotic fibrosis (massive) of lung
Silicosis (simple) (complicated)

503 Pneumoconiosis due to other inorganic dust
Aluminosis (of lung)   Graphite fibrosis (of lung)
Bauxite fibrosis (of lung) Siderosis
Berylliosis   Stannosis

504 Pneumonopathy due to inhalation of other dust
Byssinosis
Cannabinosis
Flax-dressers' disease

Excludes allergic alveolitis (495.0–495.9)
asbestosis (501)
bagassosis (495.1)
farmers' lung (495.0)

505 Pneumoconiosis, unspecified

506 Respiratory conditions due to chemical fumes and vapors
Use additional E code to identify cause
Use additional code to identify associated respiratory conditions, such as:
acute respiratory failure (518.81)

506.0 Bronchitis and pneumonitis due to fumes and vapors
Chemical bronchitis (acute)
Coding Clinic: 2010, Q3, P19; 2008, Q3, P6-7

506.1 Acute pulmonary edema due to fumes and vapors
Chemical pulmonary edema (acute)
Excludes acute pulmonary edema NOS (518.4)
chronic or unspecified pulmonary edema (514)

506.2 Upper respiratory inflammation due to fumes and vapors
Coding Clinic: 2005, Q3, P10

506.3 Other acute and subacute respiratory conditions due to fumes and vapors
Coding Clinic: 2010, Q3, P19

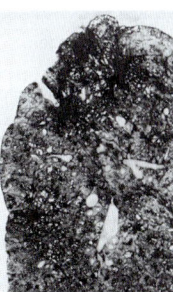

Figure 8–6 Progressive massive fibrosis superimposed on coal workers' pneumoconiosis. The large, blackened scars are located principally in the upper lobe. (From Cotran R, Kumar V, Collins T: Robbins Pathologic Basis of Disease, ed 8, Philadelphia, WB Saunders, 2009. Courtesy of Dr. Warner Laquer, Dr. Jerome Kleinerman, and the National Institute of Occupational Safety and Health, Morgantown, WV)

Item 8–10 Pneumoconiosis refers to a lung condition resulting from exposure to inorganic or organic airborne particles, such as coal dust or moldy hay, as well as chemical fumes and vapors, such as insecticides. In this condition, the lungs retain the airborne particles.

506.4 Chronic respiratory conditions due to fumes and vapors
Emphysema (diffuse) (chronic) due to inhalation of chemical fumes and vapors
Obliterative bronchiolitis (chronic) (subacute) due to inhalation of chemical fumes and vapors
Pulmonary fibrosis (chronic) due to inhalation of chemical fumes and vapors

506.9 Unspecified respiratory conditions due to fumes and vapors
Silo-fillers' disease

507 Pneumonitis due to solids and liquids
Excludes fetal aspiration pneumonitis (770.18)
postprocedural pneumonitis (997.32)
Coding Clinic: 1993, Q2, P9-10

507.0 Due to inhalation of food or vomitus
Aspiration pneumonia (due to):
NOS   milk
food (regurgitated) saliva
gastric secretions   vomitus
Coding Clinic: 2011, Q4, P150; Q1, P16; 2008, Q1, P18-19; Q1, P18-19; 1991, Q3, P16-17; 1989, Q1, P10

507.1 Due to inhalation of oils and essences
Lipoid pneumonia (exogenous)
Excludes endogenous lipoid pneumonia (516.8)
Coding Clinic: 1991, Q3, P16-17

507.8 Due to other solids and liquids
Detergent asthma
Coding Clinic: 1991, Q3, P16-17

508 Respiratory conditions due to other and unspecified external agents
Use additional E code to identify cause
Use additional code to identify associated respiratory conditions, such as:
acute respiratory failure (518.81)

508.0 Acute pulmonary manifestations due to radiation
Radiation pneumonitis

508.1 Chronic and other pulmonary manifestations due to radiation
Fibrosis of lung following radiation

508.2 Respiratory conditions due to smoke inhalation
Smoke inhalation NOS
Excludes smoke inhalation due to chemical fumes and vapors (506.9)

508.8 Respiratory conditions due to other specified external agents

508.9 Respiratory conditions due to unspecified external agent

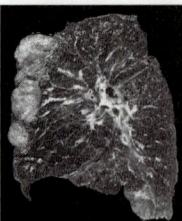

Figure 8–7 Bullous emphysema with large subpleural bullae *(upper left)*. (From Kumar: Robbins and Cotran: Pathologic Basis of Disease, ed 8, Saunders, An Imprint of Elsevier, 2009)

Item 8–11 **Empyema** is a condition in which pus accumulates in a body cavity. Empyema **with fistula** occurs when the pus passes from one cavity to another organ or structure.

OTHER DISEASES OF RESPIRATORY SYSTEM (510–519)

● **510 Empyema**
Use additional code to identify infectious organism (041.0–041.9)
Excludes abscess of lung (513.0)

510.0 With fistula
Fistula:
bronchocutaneous
bronchopleural
hepatopleural
mediastinal
pleural
thoracic
Any condition classifiable to 510.9 with fistula

510.9 Without mention of fistula
Abscess:
pleura
thorax
Empyema (chest) (lung) (pleura)
Fibrinopurulent pleurisy
Pleurisy:
purulent
septic
seropurulent
suppurative
Pyopneumothorax
Pyothorax
Coding Clinic: 2007, Q4, P109-113; 1994, Q3, P6

● **511 Pleurisy**
Occurs when double membrane (pleura) lining chest cavity and lung surface becomes inflamed causing sharp pain on inspiration and expiration
Excludes pleurisy with mention of tuberculosis, current disease (012.0)

511.0 Without mention of effusion or current tuberculosis
Adhesion, lung or pleura
Calcification of pleura
Pleurisy (acute) (sterile):
diaphragmatic
fibrinous
interlobar
Pleurisy:
NOS
pneumococcal
staphylococcal
streptococcal
Thickening of pleura
Coding Clinic: 1994, Q3, P5

511.1 With effusion, with mention of a bacterial cause other than tuberculosis
Pleurisy with effusion (exudative) (serous):
pneumococcal
staphylococcal
streptococcal
other specified nontuberculous bacterial cause

● **511.8 Other specified forms of effusion, except tuberculous**
Excludes traumatic (860.2–860.5, 862.29, 862.39)
Coding Clinic: 2008, Q1, P16-17; 1997, Q1, P10

511.81 Malignant pleural effusion
Code first malignant neoplasm, if known
Coding Clinic: 2008, Q4, P113-114

511.89 Other specified forms of effusion, except tuberculous
Encysted pleurisy
Hemopneumothorax
Hemothorax
Hydropneumothorax
Hydrothorax

■ **511.9 Unspecified pleural effusion**
Pleural effusion NOS
Pleurisy:
exudative
serofibrinous
serous
with effusion NOS
Coding Clinic: 2003, Q2, P7-8; 1991, Q3, P19-20; 1989, Q4, P11; 1988, Q1, P9

● **512 Pneumothorax and air leak**
Collapsed lung

512.0 Spontaneous tension pneumothorax
Tension pneumothorax (most serious type) occurs when air (positive pressure) collects in the pleural space

512.1 Iatrogenic pneumothorax
Postoperative pneumothorax
Coding Clinic: 2011, Q1, P14; 2003, Q3, P19

512.2 Postoperative air leak
Coding Clinic: 2011, Q4, P117

● **512.8 Other pneumothorax and air leak**
Excludes pneumothorax:
congenital (770.2)
traumatic (860.0–860.1, 860.4–860.5)
tuberculous, current disease (011.7)
Coding Clinic: 1993, Q2, P3

512.81 Primary spontaneous pneumothorax

● **512.82 Secondary spontaneous pneumothorax**
Code first underlying condition, such as:
cancer metastatic to lung (197.0)
catamenial pneumothorax due to endometriosis (617.8)
cystic fibrosis (277.02)
eosinophilic pneumonia (518.3)
lymphangioleiomyomatosis (516.4)
Marfan syndrome (759.82)
pneumocystis carinii pneumonia (136.3)
primary lung cancer (162.3-162.9)
spontaneous rupture of the esophagus (530.4)

512.83 Chronic pneumothorax

512.84 Other air leak
Persistent air leak

512.89 Other pneumothorax
Acute pneumothorax
Pneumothorax NOS
Spontaneous pneumothorax NOS

● **513 Abscess of lung and mediastinum**

513.0 Abscess of lung
Abscess (multiple) of lung
Gangrenous or necrotic pneumonia
Pulmonary gangrene or necrosis
Coding Clinic: 2007, Q4, P84-86; 2005, Q2, P14-15; 1998, Q2, P7

513.1 Abscess of mediastinum

514 Pulmonary congestion and hypostasis
Hypostatic:
bronchopneumonia
pneumonia
Passive pneumonia
Pulmonary congestion (chronic) (passive)
Pulmonary edema:
NOS
chronic

> **Excludes** acute pulmonary edema:
> NOS (518.4)
> with mention of heart disease or failure (428.1)
> hypostatic pneumonia due to or specified as a specific type of pneumonia - code to the type of pneumonia (480.0–480.9, 481, 482.0–482.9, 483.0–483.8, 487.0, 488.01, 488.11)

Coding Clinic: 1998, Q2, P6-7

515 Postinflammatory pulmonary fibrosis
Cirrhosis of lung chronic or unspecified
Fibrosis of lung (atrophic) (confluent) (massive) (perialveolar) (peribronchial) chronic or unspecified
Induration of lung chronic or unspecified

516 Other alveolar and parietoalveolar pneumonopathy
  516.0 Pulmonary alveolar proteinosis
  516.1 Idiopathic pulmonary hemosiderosis
  Essential brown induration of lung
  > Code first underlying disease (275.01-275.09)
  > **Excludes** acute idiopathic pulmonary hemorrhage in infants [AIPHI] (786.31)

  516.2 Pulmonary alveolar microlithiasis
  516.3 Idiopathic interstitial pneumonia
    516.30 Idiopathic interstitial pneumonia, not otherwise specified
    Idiopathic fibrosing alveolitis
    516.31 Idiopathic pulmonary fibrosis
    Cryptogenic fibrosing alveolitis
    516.32 Idiopathic non-specific interstitial pneumonitis
    > **Excludes** non-specific interstitial pneumonia NOS, or due to known underlying cause (516.8)

    516.33 Acute interstitial pneumonitis
    Hamman-Rich syndrome
    > **Excludes** pneumocystis pneumonia (136.3)

    516.34 Respiratory bronchiolitis interstitial lung disease
    516.35 Idiopathic lymphoid interstitial pneumonia
    Idiopathic lymphocytic interstitial pneumonitis
    > **Excludes** lymphoid interstitial pneumonia NOS, or due to known underlying cause (516.8)
    > pneumocystis pneumonia (136.3)

    516.36 Cryptogenic organizing pneumonia
    > **Excludes** organizing pneumonia NOS, or due to known underlying cause (516.8)

    516.37 Desquamative interstitial pneumonia
  516.4 Lymphangioleiomyomatosis
  Lymphangiomyomatosis
  516.5 Adult pulmonary Langerhans cell histiocytosis
  Adult PLCH
  516.6 Interstitial lung diseases of childhood
    516.61 Neuroendocrine cell hyperplasia of infancy
    516.62 Pulmonary interstitial glycogenosis
    516.63 Surfactant mutations of the lung
    516.64 Alveolar capillary dysplasia with vein misalignment
    516.69 Other interstitial lung diseases of childhood

  516.8 Other specified alveolar and parietoalveolar pneumonopathies
  Endogenous lipoid pneumonia
  Interstitial pneumonia
  Lymphoid interstitial pneumonia due to known underlying cause
  Lymphoid interstitial pneumonia NOS
  Non-specific interstitial pneumonia due to known underlying cause
  Non-specific interstitial pneumonia NOS
  Organizing pneumonia due to known underlying cause
  Organizing pneumonia NOS
  > Code first, if applicable, underlying cause of pneumonopathy, if known
  > Use additional E code, if applicable, for drug-induced or toxic pneumonopathy
  > **Excludes** cryptogenic organizing pneumonia (516.36)
  > idiopathic lymphoid interstitial pneumonia (516.35)
  > idiopathic non-specific interstitial pneumonitis (516.32)
  > lipoid pneumonia, exogenous or unspecified (507.1)

  Coding Clinic: 2011, Q1, P17; 2010, Q1, P9; 2006, Q2, P20; 1992, Q1, P12

  516.9 Unspecified alveolar and parietoalveolar pneumonopathy

517 Lung involvement in conditions classified elsewhere
> **Excludes** rheumatoid lung (714.81)

  517.1 Rheumatic pneumonia
  > Code first underlying disease (390)

  517.2 Lung involvement in systemic sclerosis
  > Code first underlying disease (710.1)

  517.3 Acute chest syndrome
  > Code first sickle-cell disease in crisis (282.42, 282.62, 282.64, 282.69)

  Coding Clinic: 2003, Q4, P51-56; 1998, Q2, P8

  517.8 Lung involvement in other diseases classified elsewhere
  > Code first underlying disease, as:
  > amyloidosis (277.30–277.39)
  > polymyositis (710.4)
  > sarcoidosis (135)
  > Sjögren's disease (710.2)
  > systemic lupus erythematosus (710.0)
  > **Excludes** syphilis (095.1)

  Coding Clinic: 2003, Q2, P7-8

518 Other diseases of lung
  518.0 Pulmonary collapse
  Atelectasis
  Collapse of lung
  Middle lobe syndrome
  > **Excludes** atelectasis:
  > congenital (partial) (770.5)
  > primary (770.4)
  > tuberculous, current disease (011.8)

  Coding Clinic: 1990, Q4, P25

  518.1 Interstitial emphysema
  Mediastinal emphysema
  > **Excludes** surgical (subcutaneous) emphysema (998.81)
  > that in fetus or newborn (770.2)
  > traumatic emphysema (958.7)

  518.2 Compensatory emphysema
  518.3 Pulmonary eosinophilia
  Eosinophilic asthma
  Löffler's syndrome
  Pneumonia:
  allergic
  eosinophilic
  Tropical eosinophilia
  > **Excludes** pulmonary infiltrate NOS (793.19)

518.4 Acute edema of lung, unspecified
Acute pulmonary edema NOS
Pulmonary edema, postoperative
Excludes pulmonary edema:
  acute, with mention of heart disease or failure (428.1)
  chronic or unspecified (514)
  due to external agents (506.0–508.9)

● 518.5 Pulmonary insufficiency following trauma and surgery
Excludes adult respiratory distress syndrome associated with other conditions (518.82)
pneumonia:
  aspiration (507.0)
  hypostatic (514)
respiratory failure in other conditions (518.81, 518.83–518.84)
Coding Clinic: 2010, Q3, P19; 2004, Q4, P139

518.51 Acute respiratory failure following trauma and surgery
Respiratory failure, not otherwise specified, following trauma and surgery
Excludes acute respiratory failure in other conditions (518.81)

518.52 Other pulmonary insufficiency, not elsewhere classified, following trauma and surgery
Adult respiratory distress syndrome
Pulmonary insufficiency following surgery
Pulmonary insufficiency following trauma
Shock lung related to trauma and surgery
Excludes adult respiratory distress syndrome associated with other conditions (518.82)
  aspiration pneumonia (507.0)
  hypostatic pneumonia (514)
  shock lung, not related to trauma or surgery (518.82)

518.53 Acute and chronic respiratory failure following trauma and surgery
Excludes acute and chronic respiratory failure in other conditions (518.84)

518.6 Allergic bronchopulmonary aspergillosis
Coding Clinic: 1997, Q4, P39-40

518.7 Transfusion related acute lung injury (TRALI)
Coding Clinic: 2006, Q4, P91-92

● 518.8 Other diseases of lung

518.81 Acute respiratory failure
Respiratory failure NOS
Excludes acute and chronic respiratory failure (518.84)
  acute respiratory distress (518.82)
  acute respiratory failure following trauma and surgery (518.51)
  chronic respiratory failure (518.83)
  respiratory arrest (799.1)
  respiratory failure, newborn (770.84)
Coding Clinic: 2012, Q3, P21-22; 2010, Q4, P81; 2009, Q2, P11; 2008, Q1, P18-19; 2007, Q3, P7-8; 2005, Q2, P19-20; Q1, P3-8; 2004, Q4, P139; 2003, Q2, P21-22; Q1, P15; 1993, Q1, P25; 1991, Q3, P14; 1990, Q4, P25; 1987, Nov-Dec, P5-6

518.82 Other pulmonary insufficiency, not elsewhere classified
Acute respiratory distress
Acute respiratory insufficiency
Adult respiratory distress syndrome NEC
Excludes acute interstitial pneumonitis (516.33)
  adult respiratory distress syndrome associated with trauma or surgery (518.52)
  pulmonary insufficiency following trauma or surgery (518.52)
  respiratory distress:
    NOS (786.09)
    newborn (770.89)
    syndrome, newborn (769)
Coding Clinic: 2003, Q4, P105-106; 1995, Q1, P7; 1991, Q2, P21

518.83 Chronic respiratory failure
Coding Clinic: 2003, Q4, P103-104, 111

518.84 Acute and chronic respiratory failure
Acute on chronic respiratory failure
Excludes acute and chronic respiratory failure following trauma or surgery (518.53)

518.89 Other diseases of lung, not elsewhere classified
Broncholithiasis   Lung disease NOS
Calcification of lung   Pulmolithiasis
Coding Clinic: 1988, Q4, P6; 1987, Nov-Dec, P8; 1986, Sept-Oct, P10

● 519 Other diseases of respiratory system

● 519.0 Tracheostomy complications
These complications do not appear in the usual complication range of 996–999.

519.00 Tracheostomy complication, unspecified

519.01 Infection of tracheostomy
Use additional code to identify type of infection, such as:
  abscess or cellulitis of neck (682.1)
  septicemia (038.0–038.9)
Use additional code to identify organism (041.00–041.9)
Coding Clinic: 1998, Q4, P41-42

519.02 Mechanical complication of tracheostomy
Tracheal stenosis due to tracheostomy

519.09 Other tracheostomy complications
Hemorrhage due to tracheostomy
Tracheoesophageal fistula due to tracheostomy

● 519.1 Other diseases of trachea and bronchus, not elsewhere classified
Coding Clinic: 2002, Q3, P18

519.11 Acute bronchospasm
Bronchospasm NOS
Excludes acute bronchitis with bronchospasm (466.0)
  asthma (493.00–493.92)
  exercise induced bronchospasm (493.81)
Coding Clinic: 2006, Q4, P92-93

519.19 Other diseases of trachea and bronchus
Calcification of bronchus or trachea
Stenosis of bronchus or trachea
Ulcer of bronchus or trachea

519.2 Mediastinitis

519.3 Other diseases of mediastinum, not elsewhere classified
Fibrosis of mediastinum
Hernia of mediastinum
Retraction of mediastinum

519.4 Disorders of diaphragm
Diaphragmitis
Paralysis of diaphragm
Relaxation of diaphragm
Excludes congenital defect of diaphragm (756.6)
  diaphragmatic hernia (551–553 with .3)
  congenital (756.6)

519.8 Other diseases of respiratory system, not elsewhere classified
Coding Clinic: 1989, Q4, P12

519.9 Unspecified disease of respiratory system
Respiratory disease (chronic) NOS

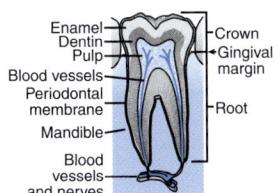

Figure 9-1 Anatomy of a tooth.

Item 9-1 **Anodontia** is the congenital absence of teeth. **Hypodontia** is partial anodontia. **Oligodontia** is the congenital absence of some teeth, whereas **supernumerary** is having more teeth than the normal number. **Mesiodens** are small extra teeth that often appear in pairs, although single small teeth are not uncommon.

9. DISEASES OF THE DIGESTIVE SYSTEM (520–579)

DISEASES OF ORAL CAVITY, SALIVARY GLANDS, AND JAWS (520–529)

- **520 Disorders of tooth development and eruption**

  520.0 Anodontia
  Absence of teeth (complete) (congenital) (partial)
  Hypodontia
  Oligodontia
  Excludes acquired absence of teeth (525.10–525.19)

  520.1 Supernumerary teeth
  Distomolar   Paramolar
  Fourth molar   Supplemental teeth
  Mesiodens
  Excludes supernumerary roots (520.2)

  520.2 Abnormalities of size and form
  Concrescence of teeth   Macrodontia
  Fusion of teeth   Microdontia
  Gemination of teeth   Peg-shaped [conical] teeth
  Dens evaginatus   Supernumerary roots
  Dens in dente   Taurodontism
  Dens invaginatus   Tuberculum paramolare
  Enamel pearls
  Excludes that due to congenital syphilis (090.5)
  tuberculum Carabelli, which is regarded as a normal variation

  520.3 Mottled teeth
  Dental fluorosis
  Mottling of enamel
  Nonfluoride enamel opacities

  520.4 Disturbances of tooth formation
  Aplasia and hypoplasia of cementum
  Dilaceration of tooth
  Enamel hypoplasia (neonatal) (postnatal) (prenatal)
  Horner's teeth
  Hypocalcification of teeth
  Regional odontodysplasia
  Turner's tooth
  Excludes Hutchinson's teeth and mulberry molars in congenital syphilis (090.5)
  mottled teeth (520.3)

  520.5 Hereditary disturbances in tooth structure, not elsewhere classified
  Amelogenesis imperfecta
  Dentinogenesis imperfecta
  Odontogenesis imperfecta
  Dentinal dysplasia
  Shell teeth

  520.6 Disturbances in tooth eruption
  Teeth:
    embedded
    impacted
    natal
    neonatal
    prenatal
    primary [deciduous]:
      persistent
      shedding, premature
  Tooth eruption:
    late
    obstructed
    premature
  Excludes exfoliation of teeth (attributable to disease of surrounding tissues) (525.0–525.19)
  Coding Clinic: 2006, Q1, P18; 2005, Q2, P15-16; 2004, Q1, P17

  520.7 Teething syndrome

  520.8 Other specified disorders of tooth development and eruption
  Color changes during tooth formation
  Pre-eruptive color changes
  Excludes posteruptive color changes (521.7)

  520.9 Unspecified disorder of tooth development and eruption

- **521 Diseases of hard tissues of teeth**

  - **521.0 Dental caries**

    521.00 Dental caries, unspecified

    521.01 Dental caries limited to enamel
    Initial caries
    White spot lesion

    521.02 Dental caries extending into dentin

    521.03 Dental caries extending into pulp

    521.04 Arrested dental caries

    521.05 Odontoclasia
    Infantile melanodontia
    Melanodontoclasia
    Excludes internal and external resorption of teeth (521.40–521.49)

    521.06 Dental caries pit and fissure
    Primary dental caries, pit and fissure origin

    521.07 Dental caries of smooth surface
    Primary dental caries, smooth surface origin

    521.08 Dental caries of root surface
    Primary dental caries, root surface

    521.09 Other dental caries
    Coding Clinic: 2002, Q3, P14

  - **521.1 Excessive attrition (approximal wear) (occlusal wear)**

    521.10 Excessive attrition, unspecified

    521.11 Excessive attrition, limited to enamel

    521.12 Excessive attrition, extending into dentine

    521.13 Excessive attrition, extending into pulp

    521.14 Excessive attrition, localized

    521.15 Excessive attrition, generalized

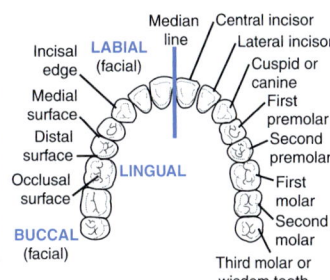

Figure 9-2 The permanent teeth within the dental arch.

Item 9-2 Each dental arch (jaw) normally contains 16 teeth. Tooth decay or **dental caries** is a disease of the enamel, dentin, and cementum of the tooth and can result in a cavity.

DISEASES OF THE DIGESTIVE SYSTEM (520–579)

- **521.2 Abrasion**
  Abrasion of teeth:
    dentifrice
    habitual
    occupational
    ritual
    traditional
  Wedge defect NOS of teeth
  - 521.20 Abrasion, unspecified
  - 521.21 Abrasion, limited to enamel
  - 521.22 Abrasion, extending into dentine
  - 521.23 Abrasion, extending into pulp
  - 521.24 Abrasion, localized
  - 521.25 Abrasion, generalized
- **521.3 Erosion**
  Erosion of teeth:
    NOS
    due to:
      medicine
      persistent vomiting
    idiopathic
    occupational
  - 521.30 Erosion, unspecified
  - 521.31 Erosion, limited to enamel
  - 521.32 Erosion, extending into dentine
  - 521.33 Erosion, extending into pulp
  - 521.34 Erosion, localized
  - 521.35 Erosion, generalized
- **521.4 Pathological resorption**
  - 521.40 Pathological resorption, unspecified
  - 521.41 Pathological resorption, internal
  - 521.42 Pathological resorption, external
  - 521.49 Other pathological resorption
    Internal granuloma of pulp
- 521.5 Hypercementosis
  Cementation hyperplasia
- 521.6 Ankylosis of teeth
- 521.7 Intrinsic posteruptive color changes
  Staining [discoloration] of teeth:
    NOS
    due to:
      drugs
      metals
      pulpal bleeding
  Excludes accretions [deposits] on teeth (523.6)
      extrinsic color changes (523.6)
      pre-eruptive color changes (520.8)
- **521.8 Other specified diseases of hard tissues of teeth**
  - 521.81 Cracked tooth
    Excludes asymptomatic craze lines in enamel - omit code
        broken tooth due to trauma (873.63, 873.73)
        fractured tooth due to trauma (873.63, 873.73)
  - 521.89 Other specified diseases of hard tissues of teeth
    Irradiated enamel
    Sensitive dentin
- 521.9 Unspecified disease of hard tissues of teeth
- **522 Diseases of pulp and periapical tissues**
  - 522.0 Pulpitis
    Pulpal:
      abscess
      polyp
    Pulpitis:
      acute
      chronic (hyperplastic) (ulcerative)
      suppurative
  - 522.1 Necrosis of the pulp
    Pulp gangrene
  - 522.2 Pulp degeneration
    Denticles   Pulp calcifications
    Pulp stones
  - 522.3 Abnormal hard tissue formation in pulp
    Secondary or irregular dentin
  - 522.4 Acute apical periodontitis of pulpal origin
  - 522.5 Periapical abscess without sinus
    Abscess:
      dental
      dentoalveolar
    Excludes periapical abscess with sinus (522.7)
  - 522.6 Chronic apical periodontitis
    Apical or periapical granuloma
    Apical periodontitis NOS
  - 522.7 Periapical abscess with sinus
    Fistula:
      alveolar process
      dental
  - 522.8 Radicular cyst
    Cyst:
      apical (periodontal)
      periapical
      radiculodental
      residual radicular
    Excludes lateral developmental or lateral periodontal cyst (526.0)
  - 522.9 Other and unspecified diseases of pulp and periapical tissues
- **523 Gingival and periodontal diseases**
  - 523.0 Acute gingivitis
    Excludes acute necrotizing ulcerative gingivitis (101)
        herpetic gingivostomatitis (054.2)
    - 523.00 Acute gingivitis, plaque induced
      Acute gingivitis NOS
    - 523.01 Acute gingivitis, non-plaque induced
  - 523.1 Chronic gingivitis
    Gingivitis (chronic):
      desquamative
      hyperplastic
      simple marginal
      ulcerative
    Excludes herpetic gingivostomatitis (054.2)
    - 523.10 Chronic gingivitis, plaque induced
      Chronic gingivitis NOS
      Gingivitis NOS
    - 523.11 Chronic gingivitis, non-plaque induced
  - 523.2 Gingival recession
    Gingival recession (postinfective) (postoperative)
    - 523.20 Gingival recession, unspecified
    - 523.21 Gingival recession, minimal
    - 523.22 Gingival recession, moderate
    - 523.23 Gingival recession, severe
    - 523.24 Gingival recession, localized
    - 523.25 Gingival recession, generalized
  - 523.3 Aggressive and acute periodontitis
    Acute:
      pericementitis
      pericoronitis
    Excludes acute apical periodontitis (522.4)
        periapical abscess (522.5, 522.7)
    - 523.30 Aggressive periodontitis, unspecified
    - 523.31 Aggressive periodontitis, localized
      Periodontal abscess
    - 523.32 Aggressive periodontitis, generalized
    - 523.33 Acute periodontitis

Item 9–3 Acute gingivitis, also known as orilitis or ulitis, is the short-term, severe inflammation of the gums (gingiva) caused by bacteria. **Chronic gingivitis** is persistent inflammation of the gums. When the gingivitis moves into the periodontium it is called periodontitis, also known as paradentitis.

- **523.4 Chronic periodontitis**
  Chronic pericoronitis
  Pericementitis (chronic)
  Periodontitis:
    NOS
    complex
    simplex
  Excludes: chronic apical periodontitis (522.6)
  - 523.40 Chronic periodontitis, unspecified
  - 523.41 Chronic periodontitis, localized
  - 523.42 Chronic periodontitis, generalized
- 523.5 Periodontosis
- 523.6 Accretions on teeth
  Dental calculus:
    subgingival
    supragingival
  Deposits on teeth:
    betel
    materia alba
    soft
    tartar
    tobacco
  Extrinsic discoloration of teeth
  Excludes: intrinsic discoloration of teeth (521.7)
- 523.8 Other specified periodontal diseases
  Giant cell:
    epulis
    peripheral granuloma
  Gingival:
    cysts
    enlargement NOS
    fibromatosis
  Gingival polyp
  Periodontal lesions due to traumatic occlusion
  Peripheral giant cell granuloma
  Excludes: leukoplakia of gingiva (528.6)
- 523.9 Unspecified gingival and periodontal disease
  Coding Clinic: 2002, Q3, P14
- **524 Dentofacial anomalies, including malocclusion**
  - **524.0 Major anomalies of jaw size**
    Excludes: hemifacial atrophy or hypertrophy (754.0)
      unilateral condylar hyperplasia or hypoplasia of mandible
    - 524.00 Unspecified anomaly
    - 524.01 Maxillary hyperplasia
    - 524.02 Mandibular hyperplasia
    - 524.03 Maxillary hypoplasia
    - 524.04 Mandibular hypoplasia
      Coding Clinic: 2012, Q2, P17
    - 524.05 Macrogenia
    - 524.06 Microgenia
    - 524.07 Excessive tuberosity of jaw
      Entire maxillary tuberosity
    - 524.09 Other specified anomaly
  - **524.1 Anomalies of relationship of jaw to cranial base**
    - 524.10 Unspecified anomaly
      Prognathism   Retrognathism
    - 524.11 Maxillary asymmetry
    - 524.12 Other jaw asymmetry
    - 524.19 Other specified anomaly
  - **524.2 Anomalies of dental arch relationship**
    Anomaly of dental arch
    Excludes: hemifacial atrophy or hypertrophy (754.0)
      soft tissue impingement (524.81–524.82)
      unilateral condylar hyperplasia or hypoplasia of mandible (526.89)
    - 524.20 Unspecified anomaly of dental arch relationship
    - 524.21 Malocclusion, Angle's class I
      Neutro-occlusion

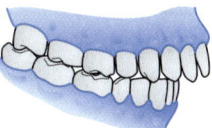

Figure 9-3 Dentofacial malocclusion.

Item 9-4 Hyperplasia is a condition of overdevelopment, whereas **hypoplasia** is a condition of underdevelopment. **Macrogenia** is overdevelopment of the chin, whereas microgenia is underdevelopment of the chin.

- 524.22 Malocclusion, Angle's class II
  Disto-occlusion Division I
  Disto-occlusion Division II
- 524.23 Malocclusion, Angle's class III
  Mesio-occlusion
- 524.24 Open anterior occlusal relationship
  Anterior open bite
- 524.25 Open posterior occlusal relationship
  Posterior open bite
- 524.26 Excessive horizontal overlap
  Excessive horizontal overjet
- 524.27 Reverse articulation
  Anterior articulation
  Crossbite
  Posterior articulation
- 524.28 Anomalies of interarch distance
  Excessive interarch distance
  Inadequate interarch distance
- 524.29 Other anomalies of dental arch relationship
  Other anomalies of dental arch
- **524.3 Anomalies of tooth position of fully erupted teeth**
  Excludes: impacted or embedded teeth with abnormal position of such teeth or adjacent teeth (520.6)
  Coding Clinic: 2004, Q1, P17
  - 524.30 Unspecified anomaly of tooth position
    Diastema of teeth NOS
    Displacement of teeth NOS
    Transposition of teeth NOS
  - 524.31 Crowding of teeth
  - 524.32 Excessive spacing of teeth
  - 524.33 Horizontal displacement of teeth
    Tipped teeth
    Tipping of teeth
  - 524.34 Vertical displacement of teeth
    Extruded tooth
    Infraeruption of teeth
    Intruded tooth
    Supraeruption of teeth
  - 524.35 Rotation of tooth/teeth
  - 524.36 Insufficient interocclusal distance of teeth (ridge)
    Lack of adequate intermaxillary vertical dimension
  - 524.37 Excessive interocclusal distance of teeth
    Excessive intermaxillary vertical dimension
    Loss of occlusal vertical dimension
  - 524.39 Other anomalies of tooth position
- 524.4 Malocclusion, unspecified
- **524.5 Dentofacial functional abnormalities**
  - 524.50 Dentofacial functional abnormality, unspecified
  - 524.51 Abnormal jaw closure
  - 524.52 Limited mandibular range of motion
  - 524.53 Deviation in opening and closing of the mandible
  - 524.54 Insufficient anterior guidance
    Insufficient anterior occlusal guidance
  - 524.55 Centric occlusion maximum intercuspation discrepancy
    Centric occlusion of teeth discrepancy

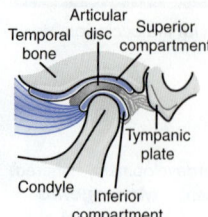

Figure 9-4 Temporomandibular joint.

Item 9-5 Dysfunction of the temporomandibular joint is termed **temporomandibular joint (TMJ) syndrome** and is characterized by pain and tenderness/spasm of the muscles of mastication, joint noise, and in the later stages, limited mandibular movement.

- 524.56 Non-working side interference
  Balancing side interference
- 524.57 Lack of posterior occlusal support
- 524.59 Other dentofacial functional abnormalities
  Abnormal swallowing
  Mouth breathing
  Sleep postures
  Tongue, lip, or finger habits

● **524.6 Temporomandibular joint disorders**
  Excludes current temporomandibular joint:
    dislocation (830.0–830.1)
    strain (848.1)

- 524.60 Temporomandibular joint disorders, unspecified
  Temporomandibular joint-pain-dysfunction syndrome [TMJ]
- 524.61 Adhesions and ankylosis (bony or fibrous)
- 524.62 Arthralgia of temporomandibular joint
- 524.63 Articular disc disorder (reducing or nonreducing)
- 524.64 Temporomandibular joint sounds on opening and/or closing the jaw
- 524.69 Other specified temporomandibular joint disorders

● **524.7 Dental alveolar anomalies**
- 524.70 Unspecified alveolar anomaly
- 524.71 Alveolar maxillary hyperplasia
- 524.72 Alveolar mandibular hyperplasia
- 524.73 Alveolar maxillary hypoplasia
- 524.74 Alveolar mandibular hypoplasia
- 524.75 Vertical displacement of alveolus and teeth
  Extrusion of alveolus and teeth
- 524.76 Occlusal plane deviation
- 524.79 Other specified alveolar anomaly

● **524.8 Other specified dentofacial anomalies**
- 524.81 Anterior soft tissue impingement
- 524.82 Posterior soft tissue impingement
- 524.89 Other specified dentofacial anomalies

- 524.9 Unspecified dentofacial anomalies

● **525 Other diseases and conditions of the teeth and supporting structures**
  525.0 Exfoliation of teeth due to systemic causes
● 525.1 Loss of teeth due to trauma, extraction, or periodontal disease
    Code first class of edentulism (525.40–525.44, 525.50–525.54)
  ●525.10 Acquired absence of teeth, unspecified
    Tooth extraction status, NOS
  ●525.11 Loss of teeth due to trauma
    Check for E code assignment.
  ●525.12 Loss of teeth due to periodontal disease
  ●525.13 Loss of teeth due to caries
  ●525.19 Other loss of teeth

● 525.2 Atrophy of edentulous alveolar ridge
  525.20 Unspecified atrophy of edentulous alveolar ridge
    Atrophy of the mandible NOS
    Atrophy of the maxilla NOS
  525.21 Minimal atrophy of the mandible
  525.22 Moderate atrophy of the mandible
  525.23 Severe atrophy of the mandible
  525.24 Minimal atrophy of the maxilla
  525.25 Moderate atrophy of the maxilla
  525.26 Severe atrophy of the maxilla
  525.3 Retained dental root
● 525.4 Complete edentulism
    Use additional code to identify cause of edentulism (525.10–525.19)
  525.40 Complete edentulism, unspecified
    Edentulism NOS
  525.41 Complete edentulism, class I
  525.42 Complete edentulism, class II
  525.43 Complete edentulism, class III
  525.44 Complete edentulism, class IV
● 525.5 Partial edentulism
    Use additional code to identify cause of edentulism (525.10–525.19)
  525.50 Partial edentulism, unspecified
  525.51 Partial edentulism, class I
  525.52 Partial edentulism, class II
  525.53 Partial edentulism, class III
  525.54 Partial edentulism, class IV
● 525.6 Unsatisfactory restoration of tooth
    Defective bridge, crown, fillings
    Defective dental restoration
    Excludes dental restoration status (V45.84)
      unsatisfactory endodontic treatment (526.61–526.69)
  525.60 Unspecified unsatisfactory restoration of tooth
    Unspecified defective dental restoration
  525.61 Open restoration margins
    Dental restoration failure of marginal integrity
    Open margin on tooth restoration
  525.62 Unrepairable overhanging of dental restorative materials
    Overhanging of tooth restoration
  525.63 Fractured dental restorative material without loss of material
    Excludes cracked tooth (521.81)
      fractured tooth (873.63, 873.73)
  525.64 Fractured dental restorative material with loss of material
    Excludes cracked tooth (521.81)
      fractured tooth (873.63, 873.73)
  525.65 Contour of existing restoration of tooth biologically incompatible with oral health
    Dental restoration failure of periodontal anatomical integrity
    Unacceptable contours of existing restoration
    Unacceptable morphology of existing restoration
  525.66 Allergy to existing dental restorative material
    Use additional code to identify the specific type of allergy
  525.67 Poor aesthetics of existing restoration
    Dental restoration aesthetically inadequate or displeasing
  525.69 Other unsatisfactory restoration of existing tooth

- **525.7 Endosseous dental implant failure**
  - **525.71 Osseointegration failure of dental implant**
    - Failure of dental implant due to infection
    - Failure of dental implant due to unintentional loading
    - Failure of dental implant osseointegration due to premature loading
    - Failure of dental implant to osseointegrate prior to intentional prosthetic loading
    - Hemorrhagic complications of dental implant placement
    - Iatrogenic osseointegration failure of dental implant
    - Osseointegration failure of dental implant due to complications of systemic disease
    - Osseointegration failure of dental implant due to poor bone quality
    - Pre-integration failure of dental implant NOS
    - Pre-osseointegration failure of dental implant
  - **525.72 Post-osseointegration biological failure of dental implant**
    - Failure of dental implant due to lack of attached gingiva
    - Failure of dental implant due to occlusal trauma (caused by poor prosthetic design)
    - Failure of dental implant due to parafunctional habits
    - Failure of dental implant due to periodontal infection (peri-implantitis)
    - Failure of dental implant due to poor oral hygiene
    - Failure of dental implant to osseointegrate following intentional prosthetic loading
    - Iatrogenic post-osseointegration failure of dental implant
    - Post-osseointegration failure of dental implant due to complications of systemic disease
  - **525.73 Post-osseointegration mechanical failure of dental implant**
    - Failure of dental prosthesis causing loss of dental implant
    - Fracture of dental implant
    - Mechanical failure of dental implant NOS
    - **Excludes** *cracked tooth (521.81)*
      fractured dental restorative material with loss of material (525.64)
      fractured dental restorative material without loss of material (525.63)
      fractured tooth (873.63, 873.73)
  - **525.79 Other endosseous dental implant failure**
    - Dental implant failure NOS
- **525.8 Other specified disorders of the teeth and supporting structures**
  - Enlargement of alveolar ridge NOS
  - Irregular alveolar process
- **525.9 Unspecified disorder of the teeth and supporting structures**

- **526 Diseases of the jaws**
  - **526.0 Developmental odontogenic cysts**
    - Cyst:
      - dentigerous
      - eruption
      - follicular
      - lateral developmental
      - lateral periodontal
      - primordial
    - Keratocyst
    - **Excludes** *radicular cyst (522.8)*
  - **526.1 Fissural cysts of jaw**
    - Cyst:
      - globulomaxillary
      - incisor canal
      - median anterior maxillary
      - median palatal
      - nasopalatine
      - palatine of papilla
    - **Excludes** *cysts of oral soft tissues (528.4)*
  - **526.2 Other cysts of jaws**
    - Cyst of jaw:
      - NOS
      - aneurysmal
      - hemorrhagic
      - traumatic
  - **526.3 Central giant cell (reparative) granuloma**
    - **Excludes** *peripheral giant cell granuloma (523.8)*
  - **526.4 Inflammatory conditions**
    - Abscess of jaw (acute) (chronic) (suppurative)
    - Osteitis of jaw (acute) (chronic) (suppurative)
    - Osteomyelitis (neonatal) of jaw (acute) (chronic) (suppurative)
    - Periostitis of jaw (acute) (chronic) (suppurative)
    - Sequestrum of jaw bone
    - **Excludes** *alveolar osteitis (526.5)*
      osteonecrosis of jaw (733.45)
  - **526.5 Alveolitis of jaw**
    - Alveolar osteitis
    - Dry socket
  - **526.6 Periradicular pathology associated with previous endodontic treatment**
    - **526.61 Perforation of root canal space**
    - **526.62 Endodontic overfill**
    - **526.63 Endodontic underfill**
    - **526.69 Other periradicular pathology associated with previous endodontic treatment**
  - **526.8 Other specified diseases of the jaws**
    - **526.81 Exostosis of jaw**
      - Torus mandibularis
      - Torus palatinus
    - **526.89 Other**
      - Cherubism
      - Fibrous dysplasia of jaw(s)
      - Latent bone cyst of jaw(s)
      - Osteoradionecrosis of jaw(s)
      - Unilateral condylar hyperplasia or hypoplasia of mandible
  - **526.9 Unspecified disease of the jaws**

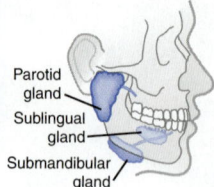

Figure 9–5 Major salivary glands.

Item 9-6 Atrophy is wasting away of a tissue or organ, whereas **hypertrophy** is overdevelopment or enlargement of a tissue or organ. **Sialoadenitis** is salivary gland inflammation. **Parotitis** is the inflammation of the parotid gland. In the epidemic form, parotitis is also known as mumps. **Sialolithiasis** is the formation of calculus within a salivary gland. **Mucocele** is a polyp composed of mucus.

Item 9-7 Stomatitis is the inflammation of the oral mucosa. **Cancrum oris,** also known as **noma** or **gangrenous stomatitis,** begins as an ulcer of the gingiva and results in a progressive gangrenous process. Mucositis is the inflammation of the mucous membranes lining the digestive tract from the mouth to the anus. It is a common side effect of chemotherapy and of radiotherapy that involves any part of the digestive tract.

● **527 Diseases of the salivary glands**
    527.0 Atrophy
    527.1 Hypertrophy
    527.2 Sialoadenitis
        Parotitis: Sialoangitis
           NOS   Sialodochitis
           allergic
           toxic
        Excludes epidemic or infectious parotitis (072.0–072.9)
                           uveoparotid fever (135)
    527.3 Abscess
    527.4 Fistula
        Excludes congenital fistula of salivary gland (750.24)
    527.5 Sialolithiasis
        Calculus of salivary gland or duct
        Stone of salivary gland or duct
        Sialodocholithiasis
    527.6 Mucocele
        Mucous:
            extravasation cyst of salivary gland
            retention cyst of salivary gland
        Ranula
    527.7 Disturbance of salivary secretion
        Hyposecretion   Sialorrhea
        Ptyalism   Xerostomia
    527.8 Other specified diseases of the salivary glands
        Benign lymphoepithelial lesion of salivary gland
        Sialectasia
        Sialosis
        Stenosis of salivary duct
        Stricture of salivary duct
    527.9 Unspecified disease of the salivary glands

● **528 Diseases of the oral soft tissues, excluding lesions specific for gingiva and tongue**
  ● **528.0 Stomatitis and mucositis (ulcerative)**
      Excludes Stevens-Johnson syndrome (695.13)
              stomatitis:
                  acute necrotizing ulcerative (101)
                  aphthous (528.2)
                  cellulitis and abscess of mouth (528.3)
                  diphtheritic stomatitis (032.0)
                  epizootic stomatitis (078.4)
                  gangrenous (528.1)
                  gingivitis (523.0–523.1)
                  herpetic (054.2)
                  oral thrush (112.0)
                  Vincent's (101)
      Coding Clinic: 1999, Q2, P9
    ■ **528.00 Stomatitis and mucositis, unspecified**
        Mucositis NOS
        Ulcerative mucositis NOS
        Ulcerative stomatitis NOS
        Vesicular stomatitis NOS

    528.01 **Mucositis (ulcerative) due to antineoplastic therapy**
        Use additional E code to identify adverse effects of therapy, such as:
            antineoplastic and immunosuppressive drugs (E930.7, E933.1)
            radiation therapy (E879.2)
      Coding Clinic: 2006, Q4, P88-91
    528.02 **Mucositis (ulcerative) due to other drugs**
        Use additional E code to identify drug
    528.09 **Other stomatitis and mucositis (ulcerative)**
  528.1 **Cancrum oris**
      Gangrenous stomatitis
      Noma
  528.2 **Oral aphthae**
      Aphthous stomatitis
      Canker sore
      Periadenitis mucosa necrotica recurrens
      Recurrent aphthous ulcer
      Stomatitis herpetiformis
      Excludes herpetic stomatitis (054.2)
    Coding Clinic: 2012, Q2, P18-19
  528.3 **Cellulitis and abscess**
      Cellulitis of mouth (floor)
      Ludwig's angina
      Oral fistula
      Excludes abscess of tongue (529.0)
                  cellulitis or abscess of lip (528.5)
                  fistula (of):
                      dental (522.7)
                      lip (528.5)
                  gingivitis (523.00–523.11)
  528.4 **Cysts**
      Dermoid cyst of mouth
      Epidermoid cyst of mouth
      Epstein's pearl of mouth
      Lymphoepithelial cyst of mouth
      Nasoalveolar cyst of mouth
      Nasolabial cyst of mouth
      Excludes cyst:
                gingiva (523.8)
                tongue (529.8)
  528.5 **Diseases of lips**
      Abscess of lip(s)   Cheilitis:
      Cellulitis of lip(s)   NOS
      Fistula of lip(s)   angular
      Hypertrophy of lip(s) Cheilodynia
                          Cheilosis
      Excludes actinic cheilitis (692.79)
                  congenital fistula of lip (750.25)
                  leukoplakia of lips (528.6)
    Coding Clinic: 1986, Sept-Oct, P10
  528.6 **Leukoplakia of oral mucosa, including tongue**
      Considered precancerous and evidenced by thickened white patches of epithelium on mucous membranes
      Leukokeratosis of oral mucosa
      Leukoplakia of:
          gingiva
          lips
          tongue
      Excludes carcinoma in situ (230.0, 232.0)
                  leukokeratosis nicotina palati (528.79)

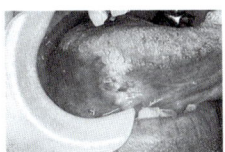

Figure 9-6 Oral leukoplakia and associated squamous carcinoma. (From Feldman: Sleisenger & Fordtran's Gastrointestinal and Liver Disease, ed 8, Saunders, An Imprint of Elsevier, 2006)

- **528.7 Other disturbances of oral epithelium, including tongue**
    - **Excludes** carcinoma in situ (230.0, 232.0)
        leukokeratosis NOS (702.8)
    - 528.71 **Minimal keratinized residual ridge mucosa**
        Minimal keratinization of alveolar ridge mucosa
    - 528.72 **Excessive keratinized residual ridge mucosa**
        Excessive keratinization of alveolar ridge mucosa
    - 528.79 **Other disturbances of oral epithelium, including tongue**
        Erythroplakia of mouth or tongue
        Focal epithelial hyperplasia of mouth or tongue
        Leukoedema of mouth or tongue
        Leukokeratosis nicotina palati
        Other oral epithelium disturbances
- 528.8 **Oral submucosal fibrosis, including of tongue**
- 528.9 **Other and unspecified diseases of the oral soft tissues**
    Cheek and lip biting
    Denture sore mouth
    Denture stomatitis
    Melanoplakia
    Papillary hyperplasia of palate
    Eosinophilic granuloma of oral mucosa
    Irritative hyperplasia of oral mucosa
    Pyogenic granuloma of oral mucosa
    Ulcer (traumatic) of oral mucosa

- **529 Diseases and other conditions of the tongue**
    - 529.0 **Glossitis**
        Abscess of tongue
        Ulceration (traumatic) of tongue
        - **Excludes** glossitis:
            benign migratory (529.1)
            Hunter's (529.4)
            median rhomboid (529.2)
            Moeller's (529.4)
    - 529.1 **Geographic tongue**
        Benign migratory glossitis
        Glossitis areata exfoliativa
    - 529.2 **Median rhomboid glossitis**
    - 529.3 **Hypertrophy of tongue papillae**
        Black hairy tongue
        Coated tongue
        Hypertrophy of foliate papillae
        Lingua villosa nigra
    - 529.4 **Atrophy of tongue papillae**
        Bald tongue   Glossodynia exfoliativa
        Glazed tongue   Smooth atrophic tongue
        Glossitis:
            Hunter's
            Moeller's
    - 529.5 **Plicated tongue**
        Fissured tongue   Scrotal tongue
        Furrowed tongue
        - **Excludes** fissure of tongue, congenital (750.13)
    - 529.6 **Glossodynia**
        Glossopyrosis   Painful tongue
        - **Excludes** glossodynia exfoliativa (529.4)

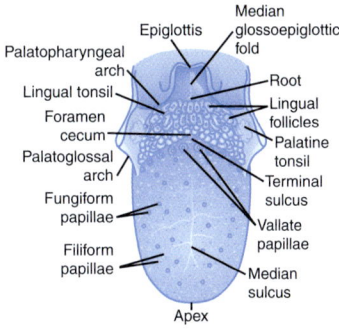

Figure 9-7 Structure of the tongue.

- 529.8 **Other specified conditions of the tongue**
    Atrophy (of) tongue
    Crenated (of) tongue
    Enlargement (of) tongue
    Hypertrophy (of) tongue
    Glossocele
    Glossoptosis
    - **Excludes** erythroplasia of tongue (528.79)
        leukoplakia of tongue (528.6)
        macroglossia (congenital) (750.15)
        microglossia (congenital) (750.16)
        oral submucosal fibrosis (528.8)
- 529.9 **Unspecified condition of the tongue**

DISEASES OF ESOPHAGUS, STOMACH, AND DUODENUM (530–539)

- **530 Diseases of esophagus**
    - **Excludes** esophageal varices (456.0–456.2)
    - 530.0 **Achalasia and cardiospasm**
        Achalasia (of cardia)
        Aperistalsis of esophagus
        Megaesophagus
        - **Excludes** congenital cardiospasm (750.7)
    - **530.1 Esophagitis**
        Esophagitis: Esophagitis:
            chemical   postoperative
            peptic   regurgitant
        Use additional E code to identify cause, if induced by chemical
        - **Excludes** tuberculous esophagitis (017.8)
        Coding Clinic: 1985, Sept-Oct, P9
        - 530.10 **Esophagitis, unspecified**
            Esophagitis NOS
            Coding Clinic: 2005, Q3, P17-18
        - 530.11 **Reflux esophagitis**
            Coding Clinic: 1995, Q4, P82
        - 530.12 **Acute esophagitis**
        - 530.13 **Eosinophilic esophagitis**
            Coding Clinic: 2008, Q4, P115-116
        - 530.19 **Other esophagitis**
            Abscess of esophagus
            Coding Clinic: 2001, Q3, P15
    - **530.2 Ulcer of esophagus**
        Ulcer of esophagus
            fungal
            peptic
        Ulcer of esophagus due to ingestion of:
            aspirin
            chemicals
            medicines
        Use additional E code to identify cause, if induced by chemical or drug
        - 530.20 **Ulcer of esophagus without bleeding**
            Ulcer of esophagus NOS
        - 530.21 **Ulcer of esophagus with bleeding**
            - **Excludes** bleeding esophageal varices (456.0, 456.20)

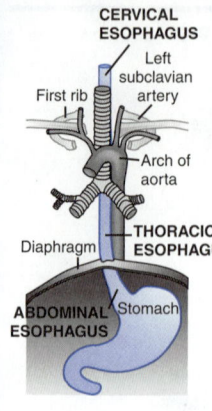

Figure 9–8 The esophagus is the muscular tube that connects the pharynx and the stomach. The 10 inch (25 cm) long esophagus is divided into three parts: **cervical, thoracic,** and **abdominal.**

Figure 9–10 Parts of the stomach.

Item 9–11 Esophageal reflux is the return flow of the contents of the stomach to the esophagus and is referred to as GERD and/or "heartburn." **Gastroesophageal reflux** is the return flow of the contents of the stomach and duodenum to the esophagus. **Esophageal leukoplakia** are white areas on the mucous membrane of the esophagus for which no specific cause can be identified.

Item 9–8 Achalasia is a condition in which the smooth muscle fibers of the esophagus do not relax. Most frequently, this condition occurs at the esophagogastric sphincter. **Cardiospasm,** also known as **megaesophagus,** is achalasia of the thoracic esophagus.

Item 9–9 Dyskinesia is difficulty in moving, and **diverticulum** is a sac or pouch.

- 530.7 Gastroesophageal laceration-hemorrhage syndrome
  Mallory-Weiss syndrome
- ● 530.8 Other specified disorders of esophagus
  - 530.81 Esophageal reflux
    Gastroesophageal reflux
    Excludes reflux esophagitis (530.11)
    Coding Clinic: 2010, Q4, P98; 2001, Q2, P4; 1995, Q1, P7
  - 530.82 Esophageal hemorrhage
    Excludes hemorrhage due to esophageal varices (456.0–456.2)
    Coding Clinic: 2005, Q1, P17-18
  - 530.83 Esophageal leukoplakia
  - 530.84 Tracheoesophageal fistula
    Excludes congenital tracheoesophageal fistula (750.3)
  - 530.85 Barrett's esophagus
    Coding Clinic: 2003, Q4, P63
  - 530.86 Infection of esophagostomy
    Use additional code to specify infection
    Coding Clinic: 2004, Q4, P83
  - 530.87 Mechanical complication of esophagostomy
    Malfunction of esophagostomy
    Coding Clinic: 2004, Q4, P83
  - 530.89 Other
    Excludes Paterson-Kelly syndrome (280.8)
- 530.9 Unspecified disorder of esophagus

- 530.3 Stricture and stenosis of esophagus
  Compression of esophagus
  Obstruction of esophagus
  Excludes congenital stricture of esophagus (750.3)
  Coding Clinic: 2012, Q1, P15-16; 2001, Q2, P4; 1997, Q2, P3; 1988, Q1, P13
- 530.4 Perforation of esophagus
  Rupture of esophagus
  Excludes traumatic perforation of esophagus (862.22, 862.32, 874.4–874.5)
- 530.5 Dyskinesia of esophagus
  Corkscrew esophagus
  Curling esophagus
  Esophagospasm
  Spasm of esophagus
  Excludes cardiospasm (530.0)
  Coding Clinic: 1988, Q1, P13; 1984, Nov-Dec, P19
- 530.6 Diverticulum of esophagus, acquired
  Diverticulum, acquired:
    epiphrenic
    pharyngoesophageal
    pulsion
    subdiaphragmatic
    traction
    Zenker's (hypopharyngeal)
  Esophageal pouch, acquired
  Esophagocele, acquired
  Excludes congenital diverticulum of esophagus (750.4)
  Coding Clinic: 1985, Mar-April, P15

- ● 531 Gastric ulcer
  Includes ulcer (peptic):
    prepyloric
    pylorus
    stomach
  Use additional E code to identify drug, if drug-induced
  Excludes peptic ulcer NOS (533.0–533.9)
  Coding Clinic: 1990, Q4, P27

  The following fifth-digit subclassification is for use with category 531:

0	without mention of obstruction
1	with obstruction

- ● 531.0 Acute with hemorrhage
  [0-1] Coding Clinic: 1984, Nov-Dec, P15
- ● 531.1 Acute with perforation
  [0-1]
- ● 531.2 Acute with hemorrhage and perforation
  [0-1]
- ● 531.3 Acute without mention of hemorrhage or perforation
  [0-1]
- ● 531.4 Chronic or unspecified with hemorrhage
  [0-1]
- ● 531.5 Chronic or unspecified with perforation
  [0-1] Coding Clinic: 2011, Q1, P11-12

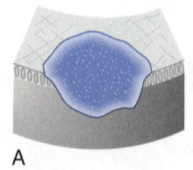
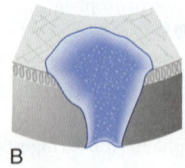
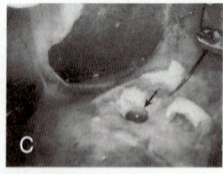

Figure 9–9 A. Ulcer. **B.** Perforated ulcer. **C.** Laparoscopic view of a perforated duodenal ulcer (arrow) with fibrinous exudate on the adjacent peritoneum. (**C** from Feldman: Sleisenger & Fordtran's Gastrointestinal and Liver Disease, ed 8, Saunders, An Imprint of Elsevier, 2006.)

Item 9–10 Gastric ulcers are lesions of the stomach that result in the death of the tissue and a defect of the surface. **Perforated ulcers** are those in which the lesion penetrates the gastric wall, leaving a hole. **Peptic ulcers** are lesions of the stomach or the duodenum.
Peptic refers to the gastric juice, pepsin.

- **531.6** Chronic or unspecified with hemorrhage and perforation
  [0-1]
- **531.7** Chronic without mention of hemorrhage or perforation
  [0-1]
- **531.9** Unspecified as acute or chronic, without mention of hemorrhage or perforation
  [0-1]

- **532** Duodenal ulcer
  - **Includes** erosion (acute) of duodenum
    ulcer (peptic):
      duodenum
      postpyloric
  - Use additional E code to identify drug, if drug-induced
  - **Excludes** peptic ulcer NOS (533.0–533.9)
  - Coding Clinic: 1990, Q4, P27

  The following fifth-digit subclassification is for use with category 532:

0	without mention of obstruction
1	with obstruction

- **532.0** Acute with hemorrhage
  [0-1]
- **532.1** Acute with perforation
  [0-1]
- **532.2** Acute with hemorrhage and perforation
  [0-1]
- **532.3** Acute without mention of hemorrhage or perforation
  [0-1]
- **532.4** Chronic or unspecified with hemorrhage
  [0-1]
- **532.5** Chronic or unspecified with perforation
  [0-1]
- **532.6** Chronic or unspecified with hemorrhage and perforation
  [0-1]
- **532.7** Chronic without mention of hemorrhage or perforation
  [0-1]
- **532.9** Unspecified as acute or chronic, without mention of hemorrhage or perforation
  [0-1]

- **533** Peptic ulcer, site unspecified
  - **Includes** gastroduodenal ulcer NOS
    peptic ulcer NOS
    stress ulcer NOS
  - Use additional E code to identify drug, if drug-induced
  - **Excludes** peptic ulcer:
      duodenal (532.0–532.9)
      gastric (531.0–531.9)
  - Coding Clinic: 1990, Q4, P27

  The following fifth-digit subclassification is for use with category 533:

0	without mention of obstruction
1	with obstruction

- **533.0** Acute with hemorrhage
  [0-1]
- **533.1** Acute with perforation
  [0-1]
- **533.2** Acute with hemorrhage and perforation
  [0-1]
- **533.3** Acute without mention of hemorrhage and perforation
  [0-1]
- **533.4** Chronic or unspecified with hemorrhage
  [0-1]
- **533.5** Chronic or unspecified with perforation
  [0-1]
- **533.6** Chronic or unspecified with hemorrhage and perforation
  [0-1]
- **533.7** Chronic without mention of hemorrhage or perforation
  [0-1]
  - Coding Clinic: 1989, Q2, P16
- **533.9** Unspecified as acute or chronic, without mention of hemorrhage or perforation
  [0-1]

- **534** Gastrojejunal ulcer
  - **Includes** ulcer (peptic) or erosion:
      anastomotic
      gastrocolic
      gastrointestinal
      gastrojejunal
      jejunal
      marginal
      stomal
  - **Excludes** primary ulcer of small intestine (569.82)
  - Coding Clinic: 1990, Q4, P27

  The following fifth-digit subclassification is for use with category 534:

0	without mention of obstruction
1	with obstruction

- **534.0** Acute with hemorrhage
  [0-1]
- **534.1** Acute with perforation
  [0-1]
- **534.2** Acute with hemorrhage and perforation
  [0-1]
- **534.3** Acute without mention of hemorrhage or perforation
  [0-1]
- **534.4** Chronic or unspecified with hemorrhage
  [0-1]
- **534.5** Chronic or unspecified with perforation
  [0-1]
- **534.6** Chronic or unspecified with hemorrhage and perforation
  [0-1]
- **534.7** Chronic without mention of hemorrhage or perforation
  [0-1]
- **534.9** Unspecified as acute or chronic, without mention of hemorrhage or perforation
  [0-1]

- **535** Gastritis and duodenitis
  - Coding Clinic: 2007, Q2, P13; 2005, Q3, P17-18

  The following fifth-digit subclassification is for use with category 535:

0	without mention of hemorrhage
1	with hemorrhage

- **535.0** Acute gastritis
  [0-1]
  - Coding Clinic: 1992, Q2, P8-9; 1986, Nov-Dec, P9
- **535.1** Atrophic gastritis
  [0-1] Gastritis:
    atrophic-hyperplastic   chronic (atrophic)
  - Coding Clinic: 1994, Q1, P18
- **535.2** Gastric mucosal hypertrophy
  [0-1] Hypertrophic gastritis
- **535.3** Alcoholic gastritis
  [0-1]
- **535.4** Other specified gastritis
  [0-1] Gastritis:
    allergic
    bile induced
    irritant
    superficial
    toxic
  - **Excludes** eosinophilic gastritis (535.7)
  - Coding Clinic: 1990, Q4, P27
- **535.5** Unspecified gastritis and gastroduodenitis
  [0-1] Coding Clinic: 2005, Q3, P17-18; 1999, Q4, P25-26; 1992, Q3, P15
- **535.6** Duodenitis
  [0-1] Coding Clinic: 2005, Q3, P17-18
- **535.7** Eosinophilic gastritis
  [0-1] Coding Clinic: 2008, Q4, P115-116

Item 9–12 Gastritis is a severe inflammation of the stomach. **Atrophic gastritis** is a chronic inflammation of the stomach that results in destruction of the cells of the mucosa of the stomach. Duodenitis is an inflammation of the duodenum, the first section of the small intestine.

> **Item 9–13** **Achlorhydria,** also known as gastric anacidity, is the absence of gastric acid. **Gastroparesis** is paralysis of the stomach.

- **536 Disorders of function of stomach**
  > Excludes: functional disorders of stomach specified as psychogenic (306.4)

  536.0 Achlorhydria

  536.1 Acute dilatation of stomach
  Acute distention of stomach

  536.2 Persistent vomiting
  Cyclical vomiting
  Habit vomiting
  Persistent vomiting [not of pregnancy]
  Uncontrollable vomiting
  > Excludes: bilious emesis (vomiting) (787.04)
  > excessive vomiting in pregnancy (643.0–643.9)
  > vomiting NOS (787.03)
  > cyclical, associated with migraine (346.2)
  > vomiting of fecal matter (569.87)

  536.3 Gastroparesis
  Gastroparalysis
  Code first underlying disease, if known, such as:
  diabetes mellitus (249.6, 250.6)
  Coding Clinic: 2004, Q2, P7-8x2; 2001, Q2, P4

  536.4 Gastrostomy complications
  - **536.40** Gastrostomy complication, unspecified
  - **536.41** Infection of gastrostomy
    Use additional code to identify type of infection, such as:
    abscess or cellulitis of abdomen (682.2)
    septicemia (038.0–038.9)
    Use additional code to identify organism (041.00–041.9)
    Coding Clinic: 1998, Q4, P42-44
  - **536.42** Mechanical complication of gastrostomy
  - **536.49** Other gastrostomy complications
    Coding Clinic: 1998, Q4, P42-44

  536.8 Dyspepsia and other specified disorders of function of stomach
  Achylia gastrica
  Hourglass contraction of stomach
  Hyperacidity
  Hyperchlorhydria
  Hypochlorhydria
  Indigestion
  Tachygastria
  > Excludes: achlorhydria (536.0)
  > heartburn (787.1)
  Coding Clinic: 1993, Q2, P6; 1989, Q2, P16; 1984, Nov-Dec, P9

  536.9 Unspecified functional disorder of stomach
  Functional gastrointestinal:
  disorder
  disturbance
  irritation
  Coding Clinic: 2007, Q1, P19

- **537 Other disorders of stomach and duodenum**

  537.0 Acquired hypertrophic pyloric stenosis
  Constriction of pylorus, acquired or adult
  Obstruction of pylorus, acquired or adult
  Stricture of pylorus, acquired or adult
  > Excludes: congenital or infantile pyloric stenosis (750.5)
  Coding Clinic: 2001, Q2, P17-18; 1985, Jan-Feb, P14-15

  537.1 Gastric diverticulum
  > Excludes: congenital diverticulum of stomach (750.7)

  537.2 Chronic duodenal ileus

  537.3 Other obstruction of duodenum
  Cicatrix of duodenum
  Cicatrix = scar
  Stenosis of duodenum
  Stenosis = narrowing
  Stricture of duodenum
  Stricture = narrowing
  Volvulus of duodenum
  Volvulus = twisting/knotting
  > Excludes: congenital obstruction of duodenum (751.1)

  537.4 Fistula of stomach or duodenum
  Gastrocolic fistula
  Gastrojejunocolic fistula
  Coding Clinic: 2012, Q1, P10-11

  537.5 Gastroptosis

  537.6 Hourglass stricture or stenosis of stomach
  Cascade stomach
  > Excludes: congenital hourglass stomach (750.7)
  > hourglass contraction of stomach (536.8)

  537.8 Other specified disorders of stomach and duodenum
  - **537.81** Pylorospasm
    > Excludes: congenital pylorospasm (750.5)
  - **537.82** Angiodysplasia of stomach and duodenum without mention of hemorrhage
    Coding Clinic: 2007, Q2, P9; 1996, Q3, P10
  - **537.83** Angiodysplasia of stomach and duodenum with hemorrhage
    Coding Clinic: 2007, Q2, P9
  - **537.84** Dieulafoy lesion (hemorrhagic) of stomach and duodenum
    Coding Clinic: 2002, Q4, P60-61
  - **537.89** Other
    Gastric or duodenal:
    prolapse
    rupture
    Intestinal metaplasia of gastric mucosa
    Passive congestion of stomach
    > Excludes: diverticula of duodenum (562.00–562.01)
    > gastrointestinal hemorrhage (578.0–578.9)
    Coding Clinic: 2011, Q1, P11; 2005, Q3, P15-16

  537.9 Unspecified disorder of stomach and duodenum

- **538 Gastrointestinal mucositis (ulcerative)**
  Use additional E code to identify adverse effects of therapy, such as:
  antineoplastic and immunosuppressive drugs (E930.7, E933.1)
  radiation therapy (E879.2)
  > Excludes: mucositis (ulcerative) of mouth and oral soft tissue (528.00–528.09)

- **539 Complications of bariatric procedures**
  - **539.0 Complications of gastric band procedure**
    - **539.01** Infection due to gastric band procedure
      Use additional code to specify type of infection, such as:
      abscess or cellulitis of abdomen (682.2)
      septicemia (038.0-038.9)
      Use additional code to identify organism (041.00-041.9)
      Coding Clinic: 2011, Q4, P127
    - **539.09** Other complications of gastric band procedure
      Use additional code(s) to further specify complication
  - **539.8 Complications of other bariatric procedure**
    > Excludes: complications of gastric band surgery (539.01-539.09)
    - **539.81** Infection due to other bariatric procedure
      Use additional code to specify type of infection, such as:
      abscess or cellulitis of abdomen (682.2)
      septicemia (038.0-038.9)
      Use additional code to identify organism (041.00-041.9)
    - **539.89** Other complications of other bariatric procedure
      Use additional code(s) to further specify complication

PART III / Diseases: Tabular List Volume 1

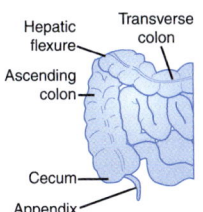

Figure 9-11 Acute appendicitis is the inflammation of the appendix, usually associated with obstruction. Most often this is a disease of adolescents and young adults.

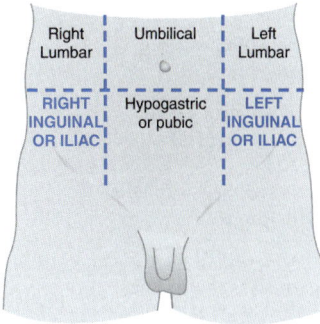

Figure 9-12 Inguinal hernias are those that are located in the inguinal or iliac areas of the abdomen.

APPENDICITIS (540–543)

540 Acute appendicitis

  540.0 With generalized peritonitis
    Appendicitis (acute) with: perforation, peritonitis (generalized), rupture:
      fulminating
      gangrenous
      obstructive
    Cecitis (acute) with: perforation, peritonitis (generalized), rupture
    Rupture of appendix
      Excludes *acute appendicitis with peritoneal abscess (540.1)*
    Coding Clinic: 1984, Nov-Dec, P19

  540.1 With peritoneal abscess
    Abscess of appendix
      With generalized peritonitis
    Coding Clinic: 1984, Nov-Dec, P19

  540.9 Without mention of peritonitis
    Acute:
      appendicitis without mention of perforation, peritonitis, or rupture:
        fulminating
        gangrenous
        inflamed
        obstructive
      cecitis without mention of perforation, peritonitis, or rupture
    Coding Clinic: 2001, Q1, P15-16; 1997, Q4, P52

541 Appendicitis, unqualified
  Coding Clinic: 1990, Q2, P26

542 Other appendicitis
  Appendicitis:
    chronic
    recurrent
    relapsing
    subacute
    Excludes *hyperplasia (lymphoid) of appendix (543.0)*
  Coding Clinic: 2001, Q1, P15-16

543 Other diseases of appendix
  543.0 Hyperplasia of appendix (lymphoid)
  543.9 Other and unspecified diseases of appendix
    Appendicular or appendiceal:
      colic
      concretion
      fistula
    Diverticulum of appendix
    Fecalith of appendix
    Intussusception of appendix
    Mucocele of appendix
    Stercolith of appendix

Item 9-14 Hernias of the groin are the most common type, accounting for 80 percent of all hernias. There are two major types of inguinal hernias: indirect (oblique) affecting men only and direct. **Indirect inguinal hernias** result when the intestines emerge through the abdominal wall in an indirect fashion through the inguinal canal. **Direct inguinal hernias** penetrate through the abdominal wall in a direct fashion. **Femoral hernias** occur at the femoral ring where the femoral vessels enter the thigh and is most common in women. An abdominal wall hernia is also called a ventral or epigastric hernia and occurs in both sexes. Classification is based on location of the hernia and whether there is obstruction or gangrene.

HERNIA OF ABDOMINAL CAVITY (550–553)

Includes hernia:
    acquired
    congenital, except diaphragmatic or hiatal

550 Inguinal hernia
  Includes bubonocele
    inguinal hernia (direct) (double) (indirect) (oblique) (sliding)
    scrotal hernia

The following fifth-digit subclassification is for use with category 550:

> 0 unilateral or unspecified (not specified as recurrent)
>   Unilateral NOS
> 1 unilateral or unspecified, recurrent
> 2 bilateral (not specified as recurrent)
>   Bilateral NOS
> 3 bilateral, recurrent

  550.0 Inguinal hernia, with gangrene
  [0-3]   Inguinal hernia with gangrene (and obstruction)
  550.1 Inguinal hernia, with obstruction, without mention
  [0-3]   **of gangrene**
      Inguinal hernia with mention of incarceration, irreducibility, or strangulation
  550.9 Inguinal hernia, without mention of obstruction or
  [0-3]   **gangrene**
      Inguinal hernia NOS
    Coding Clinic: 2003, Q3, P10-11; 2003, Q1, P4; 1985, Nov-Dec, P12; 1984, May-June, P11

551 Other hernia of abdominal cavity, with gangrene
  Includes that with gangrene (and obstruction)
  551.0 Femoral hernia with gangrene
    551.00 Unilateral or unspecified (not specified as recurrent)
      Femoral hernia NOS with gangrene
    551.01 Unilateral or unspecified, recurrent
    551.02 Bilateral (not specified as recurrent)
    551.03 Bilateral, recurrent
  551.1 Umbilical hernia with gangrene
    Parumbilical hernia specified as gangrenous

DISEASES OF THE DIGESTIVE SYSTEM (520–579)

- **551.2 Ventral hernia with gangrene**
  - ■551.20 Ventral, unspecified, with gangrene
  - 551.21 Incisional, with gangrene
    Hernia:
    postoperative specified as gangrenous
    recurrent, ventral specified as gangrenous
  - 551.29 Other
    Epigastric hernia specified as gangrenous
- 551.3 **Diaphragmatic hernia with gangrene**
  Hernia:
  hiatal (esophageal) (sliding) specified as gangrenous
  paraesophageal specified as gangrenous
  Thoracic stomach specified as gangrenous
  Excludes congenital diaphragmatic hernia (756.6)
- 551.8 **Hernia of other specified sites, with gangrene**
  Any condition classifiable to 553.8 if specified as gangrenous
- ■551.9 **Hernia of unspecified site, with gangrene**
  Any condition classifiable to 553.9 if specified as gangrenous

- **552 Other hernia of abdominal cavity, with obstruction, but without mention of gangrene**
  Excludes that with mention of gangrene (551.0–551.9)
  - **552.0 Femoral hernia with obstruction**
    Femoral hernia specified as incarcerated, irreducible, strangulated, or causing obstruction
    - 552.00 Unilateral or unspecified (not specified as recurrent)
    - 552.01 Unilateral or unspecified, recurrent
    - 552.02 Bilateral (not specified as recurrent)
    - 552.03 Bilateral, recurrent
  - 552.1 **Umbilical hernia with obstruction**
    Parumbilical hernia specified as incarcerated, irreducible, strangulated, or causing obstruction
  - **552.2 Ventral hernia with obstruction**
    Ventral hernia specified as incarcerated, irreducible, strangulated, or causing obstruction
    - ■552.20 Ventral, unspecified, with obstruction
    - 552.21 Incisional, with obstruction
      Hernia:
      postoperative specified as incarcerated, irreducible, strangulated, or causing obstruction
      recurrent, ventral specified as incarcerated, irreducible, strangulated, or causing obstruction
      Coding Clinic: 2012, Q1, P8-9; 2003, Q3, P11
    - 552.29 Other
      Epigastric hernia specified as incarcerated, irreducible, strangulated, or causing obstruction
  - 552.3 **Diaphragmatic hernia with obstruction**
    Hernia:
    hiatal (esophageal) (sliding) specified as incarcerated, irreducible, strangulated, or causing obstruction
    paraesophageal specified as incarcerated, irreducible, strangulated, or causing obstruction
    Thoracic stomach specified as incarcerated, irreducible, strangulated, or causing obstruction
    Excludes congenital diaphragmatic hernia (756.6)
  - 552.8 **Hernia of other specified sites, with obstruction**
    Any condition classifiable to 553.8 if specified as incarcerated, irreducible, strangulated, or causing obstruction
    Coding Clinic: 2004, Q1, P10-11
  - ■552.9 **Hernia of unspecified site, with obstruction**
    Any condition classifiable to 553.9 if specified as incarcerated, irreducible, strangulated, or causing obstruction

- **553 Other hernia of abdominal cavity without mention of obstruction or gangrene**
  Excludes the listed conditions with mention of:
  gangrene (and obstruction) (551.0–551.9)
  obstruction (552.0–552.9)
  - **553.0 Femoral hernia**
    - 553.00 Unilateral or unspecified (not specified as recurrent)
      Femoral hernia NOS
    - 553.01 Unilateral or unspecified, recurrent
    - 553.02 Bilateral (not specified as recurrent)
    - 553.03 Bilateral, recurrent
  - 553.1 **Umbilical hernia**
    Parumbilical hernia
  - 553.2 **Ventral hernia**
    - ■553.20 Ventral, unspecified
      Coding Clinic: 2006, Q2, P10-11; 2003, Q3, P6-7; 1996, Q3, P15
    - 553.21 Incisional
      Hernia:
      postoperative
      recurrent, ventral
      Coding Clinic: 2003, Q3, P6
    - 553.29 Other
      Hernia:
      epigastric
      spigelian
  - 553.3 **Diaphragmatic hernia**
    Hernia:
    hiatal (esophageal) (sliding)
    paraesophageal
    Thoracic stomach
    Excludes congenital:
    diaphragmatic hernia (756.6)
    hiatal hernia (750.6)
    esophagocele (530.6)
    Coding Clinic: 2001, Q2, P6; 2000, Q1, P6
  - 553.8 **Hernia of other specified sites**
    Hernia:
    ischiatic
    ischiorectal
    lumbar
    obturator
    pudendal
    retroperitoneal
    sciatic
    Other abdominal hernia of specified site
    Excludes vaginal enterocele (618.6)
  - ■553.9 **Hernia of unspecified site**
    Enterocele
    Epiplocele
    Hernia:
    NOS
    interstitial
    intestinal
    intra-abdominal
    Rupture (nontraumatic)
    Sarcoepiplocele

Item 9-15 Ventral, epigastric, or incisional hernia occurs on the abdominal surface caused by musculature weakness or a tear at a previous surgical site and is evidenced by a bulge that changes in size, becoming larger with exertion. An **incarcerated** hernia is one in which the intestines become trapped in the hernia. A **strangulated** hernia is one in which the blood supply to the intestines is lost. Hiatal hernia occurs when a loop of the stomach protrudes upward through the small opening in the diaphragm through which the esophagus passes, leaving the abdominal cavity and entering the chest. It occurs in both sexes.

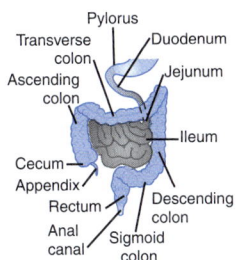

Figure 9-13 Small and large intestines.

Item 9-16 Crohn's disease, also known as **regional enteritis,** is a chronic inflammatory disease of the intestines. Classification is based on location in the small (duodenum, ileum, jejunum) or large (cecum, colon, rectum, anal canal) intestine.

Item 9-17 Ulcerative colitis attacks the colonic mucosa and forms abscesses. The disease involves the intestines. Classification is based on the location:
   Enterocolitis: large and small intestine
   Ileocolitis: ileum and colon
   Proctitis: rectum
   Proctosigmoiditis: sigmoid colon and rectum

NONINFECTIOUS ENTERITIS AND COLITIS (555–558)

- **555 Regional enteritis**
  - Includes: Crohn's disease
    Granulomatous enteritis
  - Excludes: ulcerative colitis (556)
  - **555.0 Small intestine**
    Ileitis:
       regional
       segmental
       terminal
    Regional enteritis or Crohn's disease of:
       duodenum
       ileum
       jejunum
  - **555.1 Large intestine**
    Colitis:
       granulomatous
       regional
       transmural
    Regional enteritis or Crohn's disease of:
       colon
       large bowel
       rectum
    Coding Clinic: 1999, Q3, P8
  - **555.2 Small intestine with large intestine**
    Regional ileocolitis
    Coding Clinic: 2003, Q1, P18
  - **555.9 Unspecified site**
    Crohn's disease NOS
    Regional enteritis NOS
    Coding Clinic: 2009, Q1, P20; 2005, Q2, P11-12; 1999, Q3, P8-9; 1997, Q4, P37; Q2, P3; 1996, Q1, P13; 1988, Q2, P9-10

- **556 Ulcerative colitis**
  - **556.0** Ulcerative (chronic) enterocolitis
  - **556.1** Ulcerative (chronic) ileocolitis
  - **556.2** Ulcerative (chronic) proctitis
  - **556.3** Ulcerative (chronic) proctosigmoiditis
  - **556.4** Pseudopolyposis of colon
  - **556.5** Left-sided ulcerative (chronic) colitis
  - **556.6** Universal ulcerative (chronic) colitis
       Pancolitis
  - **556.8** Other ulcerative colitis
  - **556.9** Ulcerative colitis, unspecified
       Ulcerative enteritis NOS
       Coding Clinic: 2003, Q1, P10-11

- **557 Vascular insufficiency of intestine**
  - Excludes: necrotizing enterocolitis of the newborn (777.50–777.53)
  - **557.0 Acute vascular insufficiency of intestine**
    Acute:
       hemorrhagic enterocolitis
       ischemic colitis, enteritis, or enterocolitis
       massive necrosis of intestine
    Bowel infarction
    Embolism of mesenteric artery
    Fulminant enterocolitis
    Hemorrhagic necrosis of intestine
    Infarction of appendices epiploicae
    Intestinal gangrene
    Intestinal infarction (acute) (agnogenic) (hemorrhagic) (nonocclusive)
    Mesenteric infarction (embolic) (thrombotic)
    Necrosis of intestine
    Terminal hemorrhagic enteropathy
    Thrombosis of mesenteric artery
    Coding Clinic: 2011, Q3, P12; 2008, Q2, P15-16
  - **557.1 Chronic vascular insufficiency of intestine**
    Angina, abdominal
    Chronic ischemic colitis, enteritis, or enterocolitis
    Ischemic stricture of intestine
    Mesenteric:
       angina
       artery syndrome (superior)
       vascular insufficiency
    Coding Clinic: 1996, Q3, P9-10; 1986, Nov-Dec, P11; 1985, Sept-Oct, P9
  - **557.9 Unspecified vascular insufficiency of intestine**
    Alimentary pain due to vascular insufficiency
    Ischemic colitis, enteritis, or enterocolitis NOS

- **558 Other and unspecified noninfectious gastroenteritis and colitis**
  - Excludes: infectious:
       colitis, enteritis, or gastroenteritis (009.0–009.1)
       diarrhea (009.2–009.3)
  - **558.1 Gastroenteritis and colitis due to radiation**
    Radiation enterocolitis
  - **558.2 Toxic gastroenteritis and colitis**
    Use additional E code to identify cause
    Coding Clinic: 2008, Q2, P10-11
  - **558.3 Allergic gastroenteritis and colitis**
    Use additional code to identify type of food allergy (V15.01–V15.05)
    Coding Clinic: 2008, Q4, P115-116; 2003, Q1, P12
- **558.4 Eosinophilic gastroenteritis and colitis**
  - **558.41 Eosinophilic gastroenteritis**
    Eosinophilic enteritis
    Coding Clinic: 2008, Q4, P115-116
  - **558.42 Eosinophilic colitis**
    Coding Clinic: 2008, Q4, P115-116
  - **558.9 Other and unspecified noninfectious gastroenteritis and colitis**
    Colitis, NOS, dietetic, or noninfectious
    Enteritis, NOS, dietetic, or noninfectious
    Gastroenteritis, NOS, dietetic, or noninfectious
    Ileitis, NOS, dietetic or noninfectious
    Jejunitis, NOS, dietetic, or noninfectious
    Sigmoiditis, NOS, dietetic, or noninfectious
    Coding Clinic: 2011, Q3, P12; 2008, Q2, P10-11; Q1, P10-12; 1999, Q3, P4-7; 1987, Nov-Dec, P7-8; 1984, July-Aug, P19-20

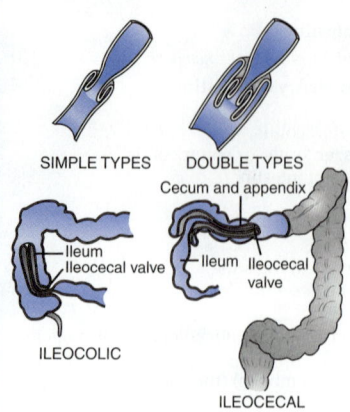

Figure 9-14 Types of intussusception.

Item 9-18 Intussusception is the prolapse (telescoping) of a part of the intestine into another adjacent part of the intestine. Intussusception may be enteric (ileoileal, jejunoileal, jejunojejunal), colic (colocolic), or intracolic (ileocecal, ileocolic).

Item 9-19 Volvulus is the twisting of a segment of the intestine, resulting in obstruction. Paralytic ileus is paralysis of the intestine. It need not be a complete paralysis, but it must prohibit the passage of food through the intestine and lead to intestinal blockage. It is a common aftermath of some types of surgery.

OTHER DISEASES OF INTESTINES AND PERITONEUM (560–569)

● **560 Intestinal obstruction without mention of hernia**
　Excludes duodenum (537.2–537.3)
　　　　　inguinal hernia with obstruction (550.1)
　　　　　intestinal obstruction complicating hernia (552.0–552.9)
　　　　　mesenteric:
　　　　　　embolism (557.0)
　　　　　　infarction (557.0)
　　　　　　thrombosis (557.0)
　　　　　neonatal intestinal obstruction (277.01, 777.1–777.2, 777.4)

　560.0 Intussusception
　　Intussusception (colon) (intestine) (rectum)
　　Invagination of intestine or colon
　　Excludes intussusception of appendix (543.9)
　　Coding Clinic: 1998, Q4, P82-83

　560.1 Paralytic ileus
　　Adynamic ileus
　　Ileus (of intestine) (of bowel) (of colon)
　　Paralysis of intestine or colon
　　Excludes gallstone ileus (560.31)
　　Coding Clinic: 2012, Q1, P6-7; 1987, Jan-Feb, P13-14

　560.2 Volvulus
　　Knotting of intestine, bowel, or colon
　　Strangulation of intestine, bowel, or colon
　　Torsion of intestine, bowel, or colon
　　Twist of intestine, bowel, or colon

● **560.3 Impaction of intestine**
　■ **560.30 Impaction of intestine, unspecified**
　　Impaction of colon
　560.31 Gallstone ileus
　　Obstruction of intestine by gallstone
　560.32 Fecal impaction
　　Excludes constipation (564.00-564.09)
　　　　　incomplete defecation (787.61)
　560.39 Other
　　Concretion of intestine
　　Enterolith
　　Coding Clinic: 1998, Q4, P37-38

● **560.8 Other specified intestinal obstruction**
　560.81 Intestinal or peritoneal adhesions with obstruction (postoperative) (postinfection)
　　Excludes adhesions without obstruction (568.0)
　　Coding Clinic: 2010, Q1, P10-11; 1995, Q3, P6; 1987, Nov-Dec, P9
　560.89 Other
　　Acute pseudo-obstruction of intestine
　　Mural thickening causing obstruction
　　Excludes ischemic stricture of intestine (557.1)
　　Coding Clinic: 1997, Q2, P3

■ **560.9 Unspecified intestinal obstruction**
　Enterostenosis
　Obstruction of intestine or colon
　Occlusion of intestine or colon
　Stenosis of intestine or colon
　Stricture of intestine or colon
　Excludes congenital stricture or stenosis of intestine (751.1–751.2)

● **562 Diverticula of intestine**
　Use additional code to identify any associated:
　　peritonitis (567.0–567.9)
　Excludes congenital diverticulum of colon (751.5)
　　　　　diverticulum of appendix (543.9)
　　　　　Meckel's diverticulum (751.0)

● **562.0 Small intestine**
　562.00 Diverticulosis of small intestine (without mention of hemorrhage)
　　Diverticulosis:
　　　duodenum without mention of diverticulitis
　　　ileum without mention of diverticulitis
　　　jejunum without mention of diverticulitis
　562.01 Diverticulitis of small intestine (without mention of hemorrhage)
　　Diverticulitis (with diverticulosis):
　　　duodenum
　　　ileum
　　　jejunum
　　　small intestine
　562.02 Diverticulosis of small intestine with hemorrhage
　562.03 Diverticulitis of small intestine with hemorrhage

● **562.1 Colon**
　562.10 Diverticulosis of colon (without mention of hemorrhage)
　　Diverticulosis without mention of diverticulitis:
　　　NOS
　　　intestine (large) without mention of diverticulitis
　　Diverticular disease (colon) without mention of diverticulitis
　　Coding Clinic: 2005, Q3, P17-18; 2002, Q3, P14-15
　562.11 Diverticulitis of colon without mention of hemorrhage
　　Diverticulitis (with diverticulosis):
　　　NOS
　　　colon
　　　intestine (large)
　　Coding Clinic: 1996, Q1, P13-14
　562.12 Diverticulosis of colon with hemorrhage
　562.13 Diverticulitis of colon with hemorrhage

Item 9-20 Diverticula of the intestines are acquired herniations of the mucosa. Diverticulum (singular): Pocket or pouch that bulges outward through a weak spot (herniation) in the colon. Diverticula (plural). **Diverticulosis** is the condition of having diverticula. **Diverticulitis** is inflammation of these pouches or herniations. Classification is based on location (small intestine or colon) and whether it occurs with or without hemorrhage.

- **564 Functional digestive disorders, not elsewhere classified**
  - Excludes: functional disorders of stomach (536.0–536.9)
    those specified as psychogenic (306.4)
  - **564.0 Constipation**
    - Excludes: fecal impaction (560.32)
      incomplete defecation (787.61)
      psychogenic constipation (306.4)
    - 564.00 Constipation, unspecified
    - 564.01 Slow transit constipation
    - 564.02 Outlet dysfunction constipation
    - 564.09 Other constipation
  - 564.1 Irritable bowel syndrome
    - Irritable colon
    - Spastic colon
  - 564.2 Postgastric surgery syndromes
    - Dumping syndrome
    - Jejunal syndrome
    - Postgastrectomy syndrome
    - Postvagotomy syndrome
    - Excludes: malnutrition following gastrointestinal surgery (579.3)
      postgastrojejunostomy ulcer (534.0–534.9)
    - Coding Clinic: 1995, Q1, P11
  - 564.3 Vomiting following gastrointestinal surgery
    - Vomiting (bilious) following gastrointestinal surgery
  - 564.4 Other postoperative functional disorders
    - Diarrhea following gastrointestinal surgery
    - Excludes: colostomy and enterostomy complications (569.60–569.69)
  - 564.5 Functional diarrhea
    - Excludes: diarrhea:
      NOS (787.91)
      psychogenic (306.4)
    - Coding Clinic: 1988, Q2, P9-10
  - 564.6 Anal spasm
    - Proctalgia fugax
  - 564.7 Megacolon, other than Hirschsprung's
    - Dilatation of colon
    - Excludes: megacolon:
      congenital [Hirschsprung's] (751.3)
      toxic (556)
  - **564.8 Other specified functional disorders of intestine**
    - Excludes: malabsorption (579.0–579.9)
    - 564.81 Neurogenic bowel
      - Coding Clinic: 2001, Q1, P12
    - 564.89 Other functional disorders of intestine
      - Atony of colon
      - Coding Clinic: 2012, Q3, P22
  - 564.9 Unspecified functional disorder of intestine

- **565 Anal fissure and fistula**
  - 565.0 Anal fissure
    - Excludes: anal sphincter tear (healed) (non-traumatic) (old) (569.43)
      traumatic (863.89, 863.99)
  - 565.1 Anal fistula
    - Fistula:
      anorectal
      rectal
      rectum to skin
    - Excludes: fistula of rectum to internal organs - see Alphabetic Index
      ischiorectal fistula (566)
      rectovaginal fistula (619.1)
    - Coding Clinic: 2007, Q1, P13

- **566 Abscess of anal and rectal regions**
  - Abscess:
    ischiorectal
    perianal
    perirectal
  - Cellulitis:
    anal
    perirectal
    rectal
  - Ischiorectal fistula
  - Coding Clinic: 1999, Q3, P8-9

- **567 Peritonitis and retroperitoneal infections**
  - Excludes: peritonitis:
    benign paroxysmal (277.31)
    pelvic, female (614.5, 614.7)
    periodic familial (277.31)
    puerperal (670.8)
    with or following:
      abortion (634–638 with .0, 639.0)
      appendicitis (540.0–540.1)
      ectopic or molar pregnancy (639.0)
  - **567.0 Peritonitis in infectious diseases classified elsewhere**
    - Code first underlying disease
    - Excludes: peritonitis:
      gonococcal (098.86)
      syphilitic (095.2)
      tuberculous (014.0)
  - 567.1 Pneumococcal peritonitis
  - **567.2 Other suppurative peritonitis**
    - Coding Clinic: 2005, Q4, P74-77; 1998, Q2, P19-20; 1996, Q1, P13-14; 1987, Jan-Feb, P14-15
    - 567.21 Peritonitis (acute) generalized
      - Pelvic peritonitis, male
    - 567.22 Peritoneal abscess
      - Abscess (of):
        abdominopelvic
        mesenteric
        omentum
        peritoneum
      - Abscess (of):
        retrocecal
        subdiaphragmatic
        subhepatic
        subphrenic
    - 567.23 Spontaneous bacterial peritonitis
      - Excludes: bacterial peritonitis NOS (567.29)
    - 567.29 Other suppurative peritonitis
      - Subphrenic peritonitis
      - Coding Clinic: 2010, Q2, P4; 2001, Q2, P11-12; 1999, Q3, P9; 1995, Q3, P5
  - **567.3 Retroperitoneal infections**
    - 567.31 Psoas muscle abscess
    - 567.38 Other retroperitoneal abscess
      - Coding Clinic: 2005, Q4, P74-77; 1998, Q2, P19-20
    - 567.39 Other retroperitoneal infections
  - **567.8 Other specified peritonitis**
    - 567.81 Choleperitonitis
      - Peritonitis due to bile
    - 567.82 Sclerosing mesenteritis
      - Fat necrosis of peritoneum
      - (Idiopathic) sclerosing mesenteric fibrosis
      - Mesenteric lipodystrophy
      - Mesenteric panniculitis
      - Retractile mesenteritis
      - Coding Clinic: 2005, Q4, P74-77
    - 567.89 Other specified peritonitis
      - Chronic proliferative peritonitis
      - Mesenteric saponification
      - Peritonitis due to urine
  - 567.9 Unspecified peritonitis
    - Peritonitis:
      NOS
    - Peritonitis:
      of unspecified cause
    - Coding Clinic: 2004, Q1, P10-11

Item 9–21 A **fissure** is a groove in the surface, whereas a **fistula** is an abnormal passage. An abscess is an accumulation of pus in a tissue cavity resulting from a bacterial or parasitic infection.

Item 9–22 **Peritonitis** is an inflammation of the lining (peritoneum) of the abdominal cavity and surface of the intestines. **Retroperitoneal infections** occur between the posterior parietal peritoneum and posterior abdominal wall where the kidneys, adrenal glands, ureters, duodenum, ascending colon, descending colon, pancreas, and the large vessels and nerves are located. Both are caused by bacteria, parasites, injury, bleeding, or diseases such as systemic lupus erythematosus.

DISEASES OF THE DIGESTIVE SYSTEM (520–579)

- **568 Other disorders of peritoneum**
  - **568.0 Peritoneal adhesions (postoperative) (postinfection)**
    Adhesions (of):
    abdominal (wall)
    diaphragm
    intestine
    male pelvis
    Adhesions (of):
    mesenteric
    omentum
    stomach
    Adhesive bands
    - Excludes adhesions:
      pelvic, female (614.6)
      with obstruction:
      duodenum (537.3)
      intestine (560.81)
    - Coding Clinic: 2012, Q1, P8-9; 2003, Q3, P7&11; 1995, Q3, P7; 1985, Sept-Oct, P11
  - **568.8 Other specified disorders of peritoneum**
    - **568.81** Hemoperitoneum (nontraumatic)
    - **568.82** Peritoneal effusion (chronic)
      - Excludes ascites NOS (789.51–789.59)
    - **568.89** Other
      Peritoneal:
      cyst
      Peritoneal:
      granuloma
  - **568.9 Unspecified disorder of peritoneum**

- **569 Other disorders of intestine**
  - **569.0 Anal and rectal polyp**
    Anal and rectal polyp NOS
    - Excludes adenomatous anal and rectal polyp (211.4)
  - **569.1 Rectal prolapse**
    Procidentia:
    anus (sphincter)
    rectum (sphincter)
    Proctoptosis
    Prolapse:
    anal canal
    rectal mucosa
    - Excludes prolapsed hemorrhoids (455.2, 455.5)
  - **569.2 Stenosis of rectum and anus**
    Stricture of anus (sphincter)
  - **569.3 Hemorrhage of rectum and anus**
    - Excludes gastrointestinal bleeding NOS (578.9)
      melena (578.1)
    - Coding Clinic: 2005, Q3, P17
  - **569.4 Other specified disorders of rectum and anus**
    - **569.41** Ulcer of anus and rectum
      Solitary ulcer of anus (sphincter) or rectum (sphincter)
      Stercoral ulcer of anus (sphincter) or rectum (sphincter)
    - **569.42** Anal or rectal pain
      - Coding Clinic: 2003, Q1, P8; 1996, Q1, P13
    - **569.43** Anal sphincter tear (healed) (old)
      Tear of anus, nontraumatic
      Use additional code for any associated fecal incontinence (787.60-787.63)
      - Excludes anal fissure (565.0)
        anal sphincter tear (healed) (old) complicating delivery (654.8)
    - **569.44** Dysplasia of anus
      Anal intraepithelial neoplasia I and II (AIN I and II) (histologically confirmed)
      Dysplasia of anus NOS
      Mild and moderate dysplasia of anus (histologically confirmed)
      - Excludes abnormal results from anal cytologic examination without histologic confirmation (796.70-796.79)
        anal intraepithelial neoplasia III (230.5, 230.6)
        carcinoma in situ of anus (230.5, 230.6)
        HGSIL of anus (796.74)
        severe dysplasia of anus (230.5, 230.6)
      - Coding Clinic: 2008, Q4, P117-119
  - **569.49** Other
    Granuloma of rectum (sphincter)
    Rupture of rectum (sphincter)
    Hypertrophy of anal papillae
    Proctitis NOS
    Use additional code for any associated fecal incontinence (787.60-787.63)
    - Excludes fistula of rectum to:
      internal organs - see Alphabetic Index
      skin (565.1)
      hemorrhoids (455.0–455.9)
  - **569.5 Abscess of intestine**
    - Excludes appendiceal abscess (540.1)
    - Coding Clinic: 1996, Q1, P13-14
  - **569.6 Colostomy and enterostomy complications**
    - **569.60** Colostomy and enterostomy complication, unspecified
    - **569.61** Infection of colostomy and enterostomy
      Use additional code to specify type of infection, such as:
      abscess or cellulitis of abdomen (682.2)
      septicemia (038.0–038.9)
      Use additional code to identify organism (041.00–041.9)
    - **569.62** Mechanical complication of colostomy and enterostomy
      Malfunction of colostomy and enterostomy
      - Coding Clinic: 2005, Q2, P11-12; 2003, Q1, P10
    - **569.69** Other complication
      Fistula
      Hernia
      Prolapse
  - **569.7 Complications of intestinal pouch**
    - **569.71** Pouchitis
      Inflammation of internal ileoanal pouch
      - Coding Clinic: 2009, Q4, P106
    - **569.79** Other complications of intestinal pouch
  - **569.8 Other specified disorders of intestine**
    - **569.81** Fistula of intestine, excluding rectum and anus
      Fistula:
      abdominal wall
      enterocolic
      enteroenteric
      ileorectal
      - Excludes fistula of intestine to internal organs - see Alphabetic Index
        persistent postoperative fistula (998.6)
      - Coding Clinic: 1999, Q3, P8
    - **569.82** Ulceration of intestine
      Primary ulcer of intestine
      Ulceration of colon
      - Excludes that with perforation (569.83)
    - **569.83** Perforation of intestine
      - Coding Clinic: 2012, Q2, P5-6
    - **569.84** Angiodysplasia of intestine (without mention of hemorrhage)
      - Coding Clinic: 1996, Q3, P9-10
    - **569.85** Angiodysplasia of intestine with hemorrhage
      - Coding Clinic: 1996, Q3, P9-10
    - **569.86** Dieulafoy lesion (hemorrhagic) of intestine
      - Coding Clinic: 2002, Q4, P60-61
    - **569.87** Vomiting of fecal matter
    - **569.89** Other
      Enteroptosis
      Granuloma of intestine
      Prolapse of intestine
      Pericolitis
      Perisigmoiditis
      Visceroptosis
      - Excludes gangrene of intestine, mesentery, or omentum (557.0)
        hemorrhage of intestine NOS (578.9)
        obstruction of intestine (560.0–560.9)
  - **569.9 Unspecified disorder of intestine**

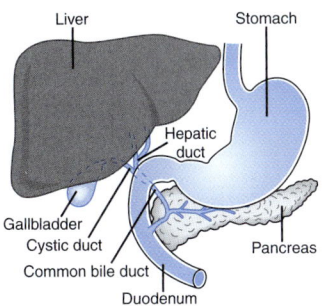

Figure 9–15 Liver and bile ducts.

Item 9–23 **Cirrhosis** is the progressive fibrosis of the liver resulting in loss of liver function. The main causes of cirrhosis of the liver are alcohol abuse, chronic hepatitis (inflammation of the liver), biliary disease, and excessive amounts of iron. **Alcoholic cirrhosis of the liver** is also called portal, Laënnec's, or fatty nutritional cirrhosis.

OTHER DISEASES OF DIGESTIVE SYSTEM (570–579)

570 Acute and subacute necrosis of liver
  Acute hepatic failure
  Acute or subacute hepatitis, not specified as infective
  Necrosis of liver (acute) (diffuse) (massive) (subacute)
  Parenchymatous degeneration of liver
  Yellow atrophy (liver) (acute) (subacute)
  Excludes icterus gravis of newborn (773.0–773.2)
    serum hepatitis (070.2–070.3)
    that with:
      abortion (634–638 with .7, 639.8)
      ectopic or molar pregnancy (639.8)
      pregnancy, childbirth, or the puerperium (646.7)
      viral hepatitis (070.0–070.9)
  Coding Clinic: 2005, Q2, P9-10; 2000, Q1, P22

● **571 Chronic liver disease and cirrhosis**
  571.0 Alcoholic fatty liver
  571.1 Acute alcoholic hepatitis
    Acute alcoholic liver disease
    Coding Clinic: 2002, Q2, P4
  571.2 Alcoholic cirrhosis of liver
    Florid cirrhosis
    Laennec's cirrhosis (alcoholic)
    Coding Clinic: 2011, Q1, P23; 2007, Q3, P9; Q2, P6-7x2; 2002, Q2, P4; Q1, P3; 1985, Nov-Dec, P14
  ☐ **571.3 Alcoholic liver damage, unspecified**
  ● **571.4 Chronic hepatitis**
    Excludes viral hepatitis (acute) (chronic) (070.0–070.9)
    ☐ **571.40 Chronic hepatitis, unspecified**
    571.41 Chronic persistent hepatitis
    571.42 Autoimmune hepatitis
      Coding Clinic: 2008, Q4, P120
    571.49 Other
      Chronic hepatitis:
        active
        aggressive
      Recurrent hepatitis
      Coding Clinic: 1999, Q3, P19
  571.5 Cirrhosis of liver without mention of alcohol
    Cirrhosis of liver: Cirrhosis of liver:
      NOS   micronodular
      cryptogenic   posthepatitic
      macronodular   postnecrotic
    Healed yellow atrophy (liver)
    Portal cirrhosis
    Code first, if applicable, viral hepatitis (acute) (chronic) (070.0-070.9)
    Coding Clinic: 2011, Q1, P23; 2007, Q3, P9

  571.6 Biliary cirrhosis
    Chronic nonsuppurative destructive cholangitis
    Cirrhosis:
      cholangitic
      cholestatic
  571.8 Other chronic nonalcoholic liver disease
    Chronic yellow atrophy (liver)
    Fatty liver, without mention of alcohol
    Coding Clinic: 1996, Q2, P12
  ☐ **571.9 Unspecified chronic liver disease without mention of alcohol**

● **572 Liver abscess and sequelae of chronic liver disease**
  572.0 Abscess of liver
    Excludes amebic liver abscess (006.3)
  572.1 Portal pyemia
    Phlebitis of portal vein
    Portal thrombophlebitis
    Pylephlebitis
    Pylethrombophlebitis
  572.2 Hepatic encephalopathy
    Hepatic coma
    Hepatocerebral intoxication
    Portal-systemic encephalopathy
    Excludes hepatic coma associated with viral hepatitis - see category 070
    Coding Clinic: 2007, Q2, P6; 2005, Q2, P9-10; 2002, Q1, P3; 1995, Q3, P14
  572.3 Portal hypertension
    Use additional code for any associated complications, such as:
      portal hypertensive gastropathy (537.89)
    Coding Clinic: 2005, Q3, P15-16
  572.4 Hepatorenal syndrome
    Excludes that following delivery (674.8)
    Coding Clinic: 1992, Q3, P15
  572.8 Other sequelae of chronic liver disease
    Excludes hepatopulmonary syndrome (573.5)

● **573 Other disorders of liver**
  Excludes amyloid or lardaceous degeneration of liver (277.39)
    congenital cystic disease of liver (751.62)
    glycogen infiltration of liver (271.0)
    hepatomegaly NOS (789.1)
    portal vein obstruction (452)
  573.0 Chronic passive congestion of liver
  ● **573.1 Hepatitis in viral diseases classified elsewhere**
    Code first underlying disease, as:
      Coxsackie virus disease (074.8)
      cytomegalic inclusion virus disease (078.5)
      infectious mononucleosis (075)
    Excludes hepatitis (in):
      mumps (072.71)
      viral (070.0–070.9)
      yellow fever (060.0–060.9)
  ● **573.2 Hepatitis in other infectious diseases classified elsewhere**
    Code first underlying disease, as:
      malaria (084.9)
    Excludes hepatitis in:
      late syphilis (095.3)
      secondary syphilis (091.62)
      toxoplasmosis (130.5)
  ☐ **573.3 Hepatitis, unspecified**
    Toxic (noninfectious) hepatitis
    Use additional E code to identify cause
    Coding Clinic: 1998, Q3, P4; 1990, Q4, P26
  573.4 Hepatic infarction
  ● **573.5 Hepatopulmonary syndrome**
    Code first underlying liver disease, such as:
      alcoholic cirrhosis of liver (571.2)
      cirrhosis of liver without mention of alcohol (571.5)
  573.8 Other specified disorders of liver
    Hepatoptosis
  ☐ **573.9 Unspecified disorder of liver**

574 Cholelithiasis
Presence or formation of gallstones

Excludes retained cholelithiasis following cholecystectomy (997.41)

Coding Clinic: 1990, Q1, P19

The following fifth-digit subclassification is for use with category 574:

- 0 without mention of obstruction
- 1 with obstruction

Check documentation for acute/chronic gallbladder/common bile duct either with or without obstruction.

574.0 Calculus of gallbladder with acute cholecystitis
[0-1]
- Biliary calculus with acute cholecystitis
- Calculus of cystic duct with acute cholecystitis
- Cholelithiasis with acute cholecystitis
- Any condition classifiable to 574.2 with acute cholecystitis

Coding Clinic: 1996, Q4, P32; 1984, Nov-Dec, P18

574.1 Calculus of gallbladder with other cholecystitis
[0-1]
- Biliary calculus with cholecystitis
- Calculus of cystic duct with cholecystitis
- Cholelithiasis with cholecystitis
- Cholecystitis with cholelithiasis NOS
- Any condition classifiable to 574.2 with cholecystitis (chronic)

Coding Clinic: 2003, Q1, P5; 1999, Q3, P9; 1996, Q4, P69; Q2, P13-15; Q1, P7

574.2 Calculus of gallbladder without mention of cholecystitis
[0-1]
- Biliary:
  - calculus NOS
  - colic NOS
- Calculus of cystic duct
- Cholelithiasis NOS
- Colic (recurrent) of gallbladder
- Gallstone (impacted)

Coding Clinic: 1995, Q4, P51-52; 1988, Q1, P14

574.3 Calculus of bile duct with acute cholecystitis
[0-1]
- Calculus of bile duct [any] with acute cholecystitis
- Choledocholithiasis with acute cholecystitis
- Any condition classifiable to 574.5 with acute cholecystitis

574.4 Calculus of bile duct with other cholecystitis
[0-1]
- Calculus of bile duct [any] with cholecystitis (chronic)
- Choledocholithiasis with cholecystitis (chronic)
- Any condition classifiable to 574.5 with cholecystitis (chronic)

Coding Clinic: 1996, Q1, P7

574.5 Calculus of bile duct without mention of cholecystitis
[0-1]
- Calculus of:
  - bile duct [any]
  - common duct
  - hepatic duct
- Choledocholithiasis
- Hepatic:
  - colic (recurrent)
  - lithiasis

Coding Clinic: 1996, Q2, P13-15; 1994, Q3, P11

574.6 Calculus of gallbladder and bile duct with acute cholecystitis
[0-1]
Any condition classifiable to 574.0 and 574.3

574.7 Calculus of gallbladder and bile duct with other cholecystitis
[0-1]
Any condition classifiable to 574.1 and 574.4

574.8 Calculus of gallbladder and bile duct with acute and chronic cholecystitis
[0-1]
Any condition classifiable to 574.6 and 574.7

Coding Clinic: 1996, Q4, P32

574.9 Calculus of gallbladder and bile duct without cholecystitis
[0-1]
Any condition classifiable to 574.2 and 574.5

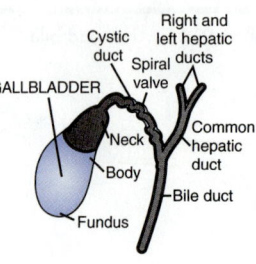

Figure 9-16 Gallbladder and bile ducts.

575 Other disorders of gallbladder
Cholecystitis is chronic or acute inflammation of gallbladder.

575.0 Acute cholecystitis
- Abscess of gallbladder without mention of calculus
- Angiocholecystitis without mention of calculus
- Cholecystitis without mention of calculus:
  - emphysematous (acute)
  - gangrenous
  - suppurative
- Empyema of gallbladder without mention of calculus
- Gangrene of gallbladder without mention of calculus

Excludes that with:
- acute and chronic cholecystitis (575.12)
- choledocholithiasis (574.3)
- choledocholithiasis and cholelithiasis (574.6)
- cholelithiasis (574.0)

Coding Clinic: 1991, Q3, P17-18

575.1 Other cholecystitis
- Cholecystitis without mention of calculus:
  - NOS without mention of calculus
  - chronic without mention of calculus

Excludes that with:
- choledocholithiasis (574.4)
- choledocholithiasis and cholelithiasis (574.8)
- cholelithiasis (574.1)

Coding Clinic: 1991, Q3, P17-18

575.10 Cholecystitis, unspecified
Cholecystitis NOS

575.11 Chronic cholecystitis

575.12 Acute and chronic cholecystitis
Coding Clinic: 1997, Q4, P52; 1996, Q4, P32

575.2 Obstruction of gallbladder
- Occlusion of cystic duct or gallbladder without mention of calculus
- Stenosis of cystic duct or gallbladder without mention of calculus
- Stricture of cystic duct or gallbladder without mention of calculus

575.3 Hydrops of gallbladder
Mucocele of gallbladder

575.4 Perforation of gallbladder
Rupture of cystic duct or gallbladder

575.5 Fistula of gallbladder
- Fistula: cholecystoduodenal
- Fistula: cholecystoenteric

575.6 Cholesterolosis of gallbladder
Strawberry gallbladder

575.8 Other specified disorders of gallbladder
- Adhesions (of) cystic duct gallbladder
- Atrophy (of) cystic duct gallbladder
- Cyst (of) cystic duct gallbladder
- Hypertrophy (of) cystic duct gallbladder
- Nonfunctioning (of) cystic duct gallbladder
- Ulcer (of) cystic duct gallbladder
- Biliary dyskinesia

Excludes Hartmann's pouch of intestine (V44.3)
nonvisualization of gallbladder (793.3)

Coding Clinic: 1989, Q2, P13

575.9 Unspecified disorder of gallbladder

● **576 Other disorders of biliary tract**
  > Excludes: that involving the:
  > cystic duct (575.0–575.9)
  > gallbladder (575.0–575.9)

  576.0 Postcholecystectomy syndrome
  Coding Clinic: 1988, Q1, P10

  576.1 Cholangitis
  Cholangitis: Cholangitis:
    NOS   recurrent
    acute   sclerosing
    ascending   secondary
    chronic   stenosing
    primary   suppurative
  Coding Clinic: 1999, Q2, P13-14; 1995, Q2, P7

  576.2 Obstruction of bile duct
  Occlusion of bile duct, except cystic duct, without mention of calculus
  Stenosis of bile duct, except cystic duct, without mention of calculus
  Stricture of bile duct, except cystic duct, without mention of calculus
  > Excludes: congenital (751.61)
  > that with calculus (574.3–574.5 with fifth-digit 1)
  Coding Clinic: 2003, Q3, P17-18; 2001, Q1, P8-9; 1999, Q2, P13-14

  576.3 Perforation of bile duct
  Rupture of bile duct, except cystic duct

  576.4 Fistula of bile duct
  Choledochoduodenal fistula

  576.5 Spasm of sphincter of Oddi

  576.8 Other specified disorders of biliary tract
  Adhesions of bile duct [any]
  Atrophy of bile duct [any]
  Cyst of bile duct [any]
  Hypertrophy of bile duct [any]
  Stasis of bile duct [any]
  Ulcer of bile duct [any]
  > Excludes: congenital choledochal cyst (751.69)
  Coding Clinic: 2003, Q3, P17-18; 1999, Q2, P14

  576.9 Unspecified disorder of biliary tract

● **577 Diseases of pancreas**
  Pancreatitis is inflammatory process that may be acute or chronic.

  577.0 Acute pancreatitis
  Abscess of pancreas   Pancreatitis:
  Necrosis of pancreas: NOS
    acute   acute (recurrent)
    infective   apoplectic
                               hemorrhagic
                               subacute
                               suppurative
  > Excludes: mumps pancreatitis (072.3)
  Coding Clinic: 1999, Q3, P9; 1998, Q2, P19-20; 1996, Q2, P13-15; 1989, Q2, P9

  577.1 Chronic pancreatitis
  Chronic pancreatitis: Pancreatitis:
    NOS   painless
    infectious   recurrent
    interstitial   relapsing
  Coding Clinic: 2001, Q1, P8-9; 1996, Q2, P13-15; 1994, Q3, P11

  577.2 Cyst and pseudocyst of pancreas

  577.8 Other specified diseases of pancreas
  Atrophy of pancreas   Pancreatic:
  Calculus of pancreas   infantilism
  Cirrhosis of pancreas   necrosis:
  Fibrosis of pancreas   NOS
                               aseptic
                               fat
                             Pancreatolithiasis
  > Excludes: fibrocystic disease of pancreas (277.00–277.09)
  > islet cell tumor of pancreas (211.7)
  > pancreatic steatorrhea (579.4)
  Coding Clinic: 2001, Q1, P8-9

  577.9 Unspecified disease of pancreas

● **578 Gastrointestinal hemorrhage**
  > Excludes: that with mention of:
  > angiodysplasia of stomach and duodenum (537.83)
  > angiodysplasia of intestine (569.85)
  > diverticulitis, intestine:
  > large (562.13)
  > small (562.03)
  > diverticulosis, intestine:
  > large (562.12)
  > small (562.02)
  > gastritis and duodenitis (535.0–535.6)
  > ulcer:
  > duodenal, gastric, gastrojejunal, or peptic (531.00–534.91)
  Coding Clinic: 2007, Q2, P13; 1992, Q2, P9-10; Q2, P8-9

  578.0 Hematemesis
  Vomiting of blood
  Coding Clinic: 2002, Q2, P4

  578.1 Blood in stool
  Melena
  > Excludes: melena of the newborn (772.4, 777.3)
  > occult blood (792.1)
  Coding Clinic: 2006, Q2, P17; 1992, Q2, P8-9

  578.9 Hemorrhage of gastrointestinal tract, unspecified
  Gastric hemorrhage   Intestinal hemorrhage
  Coding Clinic: 2008, Q2, P15-16; 2006, Q4, P91-92; 2005, Q3, P17-18; 1986, Nov-Dec, P9; 1985, Sept-Oct, P9

● **579 Intestinal malabsorption**

  579.0 Celiac disease
  Celiac: Gee (-Herter) disease
    crisis   Gluten enteropathy
    infantilism   Idiopathic steatorrhea
    rickets   Nontropical sprue

  579.1 Tropical sprue
  Sprue:
    NOS
    tropical
  Tropical steatorrhea

  579.2 Blind loop syndrome
  Postoperative blind loop syndrome

  579.3 Other and unspecified postsurgical nonabsorption
  Hypoglycemia following gastrointestinal surgery
  Malnutrition following gastrointestinal surgery
  Coding Clinic: 2003, Q4, P104-105

  579.4 Pancreatic steatorrhea

  579.8 Other specified intestinal malabsorption
  Enteropathy:
    exudative
    protein-losing
  Steatorrhea (chronic)
  Coding Clinic: 2003, Q1, P12

  579.9 Unspecified intestinal malabsorption
  Malabsorption syndrome NOS
  Coding Clinic: 2004, Q4, P57-59

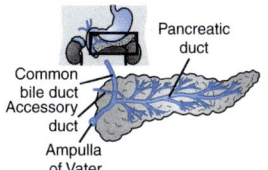

Figure 9–17 Pancreatic ductal system.

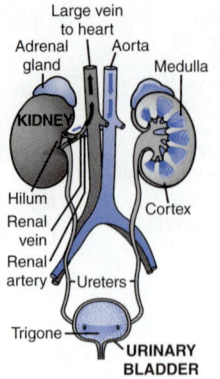

Figure 10-1 Kidneys within the urinary system.

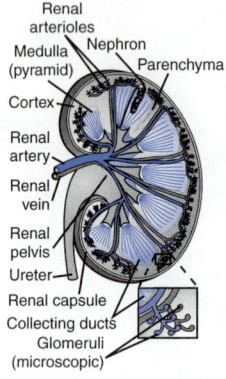

Figure 10-2 Kidney cross section.

Item 10-1 **Glomerulonephritis** is nephritis accompanied by inflammation of the glomeruli of the kidney, resulting in the degeneration of the glomeruli and the nephrons.
Acute glomerulonephritis primarily affects children and young adults and is usually a result of a streptococcal infection.
Proliferative glomerulonephritis is the acute form of the disease resulting from a streptococcal infection.
Rapidly progressive glomerulonephritis, also known as **crescentic** or **malignant glomerulonephritis**, is the acute form of the disease, which leads quickly to rapid and progressive decline in renal function.

Item 10-2 Nephrotic syndrome (NS) is marked by massive proteinuria (protein in the urine) and water retention. Patients with NS are particularly vulnerable to staphylococcal and pneumococcal infections. NS with lesion of proliferative glomerulonephritis results from a streptococcal infection. NS with lesion of membranous glomerulonephritis results in thickening of the capillary walls. NS with lesion of minimal change glomerulonephritis is usually a benign disorder that occurs mostly in children and requires electron microscopy (biopsy) to verify changes in the glomeruli.

10. DISEASES OF THE GENITOURINARY SYSTEM (580–629)

NEPHRITIS, NEPHROTIC SYNDROME, AND NEPHROSIS (580–589)

Excludes hypertensive chronic kidney disease (403.00–403.91, 404.00–404.93)

- **580 Acute glomerulonephritis**
  Includes acute nephritis
  - **580.0 With lesion of proliferative glomerulonephritis**
    Acute (diffuse) proliferative glomerulonephritis
    Acute poststreptococcal glomerulonephritis
  - **580.4 With lesion of rapidly progressive glomerulonephritis**
    Acute nephritis with lesion of necrotizing glomerulitis
  - ● **580.8 With other specified pathological lesion in kidney**
    - ● **580.81 Acute glomerulonephritis in diseases classified elsewhere**
      Code first underlying disease, as:
      infectious hepatitis (070.0–070.9)
      mumps (072.79)
      subacute bacterial endocarditis (421.0)
      typhoid fever (002.0)
    - **580.89 Other**
      Glomerulonephritis, acute, with lesion of:
      exudative nephritis
      interstitial (diffuse) (focal) nephritis
  - **580.9 Acute glomerulonephritis with unspecified pathological lesion in kidney**
    Glomerulonephritis: specified as acute
    NOS specified as acute
    hemorrhagic specified as acute
    Nephritis specified as acute
    Nephropathy specified as acute

- ● **581 Nephrotic syndrome**
  - **581.0 With lesion of proliferative glomerulonephritis**
  - **581.1 With lesion of membranous glomerulonephritis**
    Epimembranous nephritis
    Idiopathic membranous glomerular disease
    Nephrotic syndrome with lesion of:
      focal glomerulosclerosis
      sclerosing membranous glomerulonephritis
      segmental hyalinosis
  - **581.2 With lesion of membranoproliferative glomerulonephritis**
    Nephrotic syndrome with lesion (of):
      endothelial glomerulonephritis
      hypocomplementemic glomerulonephritis persistent glomerulonephritis
      lobular glomerulonephritis
      mesangiocapillary glomerulonephritis
      mixed membranous and proliferative glomerulonephritis
  - **581.3 With lesion of minimal change glomerulonephritis**
    Foot process disease
    Lipoid nephrosis
    Minimal change:
      glomerular disease
      glomerulitis
      nephrotic syndrome
    Coding Clinic: 2007, Q1, P23
  - ● **581.8 With other specified pathological lesion in kidney**
    - ● **581.81 Nephrotic syndrome in diseases classified elsewhere**
      Code first underlying disease, as:
      amyloidosis (277.30–277.39)
      diabetes mellitus (249.4, 250.4)
      malaria (084.9)
      polyarteritis (446.0)
      systemic lupus erythematosus (710.0)
      Excludes nephrosis in epidemic hemorrhagic fever (078.6)
    - **581.89 Other**
      Glomerulonephritis with edema and lesion of:
      exudative nephritis
      interstitial (diffuse) (focal) nephritis
  - **581.9 Nephrotic syndrome with unspecified pathological lesion in kidney**
    Glomerulonephritis with edema NOS
    Nephritis:
      nephrotic NOS
      with edema NOS
    Nephrosis NOS
    Renal disease with edema NOS

Item 10-3 **Chronic glomerulonephritis** (GN) persists over a period of years, with remissions and exacerbation.
Chronic GN with lesion of proliferative glomerulonephritis results from a streptococcal infection.
Chronic GN with lesion of membranous glomerulonephritis, also known as membranous nephropathy, is characterized by deposits along the epithelial side of the basement membrane.
Chronic GN with lesion of membranoproliferative glomerulonephritis (MPGN) is a group of disorders characterized by alterations in the basement membranes of the kidney and the glomerular cells.
Chronic GN with lesion of rapidly progressive glomerulonephritis is characterized by necrosis, endothelial proliferation, and mesangial proliferation. The condition is marked by rapid and progressive decline in renal function.

Item 10-4 **Nephritis** (inflammation) or **nephropathy** (disease) **with lesion of proliferative glomerulonephritis** results from a streptococcal infection.
Nephritis (inflammation) or **nephropathy** (disease) **with lesion of membranous glomerulonephritis** is characterized by deposits along the epithelial side of the basement membrane.
Nephritis (inflammation) or **nephropathy** (disease) **with lesion of membranoproliferative glomerulonephritis** is characterized by alterations in the basement membranes of the kidney and the glomerular cells.
Nephritis (inflammation) or **nephropathy** (disease) **with lesion of rapidly progressive glomerulonephritis** is characterized by rapid and progressive decline in renal function.
Nephritis (inflammation) or **nephropathy** (disease) **with lesion of renal cortical necrosis** is characterized by death of the cortical tissues.
Nephritis (inflammation) or **nephropathy** (disease) **with lesion of renal medullary necrosis** is characterized by death of the tissues that collect urine.

● **582 Chronic glomerulonephritis**
  Includes chronic nephritis
  582.0 With lesion of proliferative glomerulonephritis
    Chronic (diffuse) proliferative glomerulonephritis
  582.1 With lesion of membranous glomerulonephritis
    Chronic glomerulonephritis:
      membranous
      sclerosing
    Focal glomerulosclerosis
    Segmental hyalinosis
    Coding Clinic: 1984, Sept-Oct, P16
  582.2 With lesion of membranoproliferative glomerulonephritis
    Chronic glomerulonephritis:
      endothelial
      hypocomplementemic persistent
      lobular
      membranoproliferative
      mesangiocapillary
      mixed membranous and proliferative
  582.4 With lesion of rapidly progressive glomerulonephritis
    Chronic nephritis with lesion of necrotizing glomerulitis
  ● **582.8 With other specified pathological lesion in kidney**
    ● **582.81 Chronic glomerulonephritis in diseases classified elsewhere**
      Code first underlying disease, as:
        amyloidosis (277.30–277.39)
        systemic lupus erythematosus (710.0)
      582.89 Other
        Chronic glomerulonephritis with lesion of:
          exudative nephritis
          interstitial (diffuse) (focal) nephritis
  ■ **582.9 Chronic glomerulonephritis with unspecified pathological lesion in kidney**
    Glomerulonephritis: specified as chronic
      NOS specified as chronic
      hemorrhagic specified as chronic
    Nephritis specified as chronic
    Nephropathy specified as chronic
    Coding Clinic: 2001, Q2, P12

● **583 Nephritis and nephropathy, not specified as acute or chronic**
  Includes "renal disease" so stated, not specified as acute or chronic but with stated pathology or cause
  583.0 With lesion of proliferative glomerulonephritis
    Proliferative:
      glomerulonephritis (diffuse) NOS
      nephritis NOS
      nephropathy NOS
  583.1 With lesion of membranous glomerulonephritis
    Membranous:
      glomerulonephritis NOS
      nephritis NOS
    Membranous nephropathy NOS
  583.2 With lesion of membranoproliferative glomerulonephritis
    Membranoproliferative:
      glomerulonephritis NOS
      nephritis NOS
      nephropathy NOS
    Nephritis NOS, with lesion of:
      hypocomplementemic persistent glomerulonephritis
      lobular glomerulonephritis
      mesangiocapillary glomerulonephritis
      mixed membranous and proliferative glomerulonephritis
  583.4 With lesion of rapidly progressive glomerulonephritis
    Necrotizing or rapidly progressive:
      glomerulitis NOS
      glomerulonephritis NOS
      nephritis NOS
      nephropathy NOS
    Nephritis, unspecified, with lesion of necrotizing glomerulitis
  583.6 With lesion of renal cortical necrosis
    Nephritis NOS with (renal) cortical necrosis
    Nephropathy NOS with (renal) cortical necrosis
    Renal cortical necrosis NOS
  583.7 With lesion of renal medullary necrosis
    Nephritis NOS with (renal) medullary [papillary] necrosis
    Nephropathy NOS with (renal) medullary [papillary] necrosis
  ● **583.8 With other specified pathological lesion in kidney**
    ● **583.81 Nephritis and nephropathy, not specified as acute or chronic, in diseases classified elsewhere**
      Code first underlying disease, as:
        amyloidosis (277.30–277.39)
        diabetes mellitus (249.4, 250.4)
        gonococcal infection (098.19)
        Goodpasture's syndrome (446.21)
        systemic lupus erythematosus (710.0)
        tuberculosis (016.0)
      Excludes gouty nephropathy (274.10)
        syphilitic nephritis (095.4)
      Coding Clinic: 2012, Q2, P19; 2003, Q2, P7
    583.89 Other
      Glomerulitis with lesion of:
        exudative nephritis
        interstitial nephritis
      Glomerulonephritis with lesion of:
        exudative nephritis
        interstitial nephritis
      Nephritis with lesion of:
        exudative nephritis
        interstitial nephritis
      Nephropathy with lesion of:
        exudative nephritis
        interstitial nephritis
      Renal disease with lesion of:
        exudative nephritis
        interstitial nephritis

■ 583.9 **With unspecified pathological lesion in kidney**
Glomerulitis NOS
Glomerulonephritis NOS
Nephritis NOS
Nephropathy NOS
Excludes *nephropathy complicating pregnancy, labor, or the puerperium (642.0–642.9, 646.2)*
renal disease NOS with no stated cause (593.9)
Coding Clinic: 1994, Q4, P35

● 584 **Acute kidney failure**
Includes Acute renal failure
Excludes *following labor and delivery (669.3)*
posttraumatic (958.5)
that complicating:
abortion (634–638 with .3, 639.3)
ectopic or molar pregnancy (639.3)
Coding Clinic: 2011, Q3, P17; 1992, Q2, P5x2

584.5 **Acute kidney failure with lesion of tubular necrosis**
Lower nephron nephrosis
Renal failure with (acute) tubular necrosis
Tubular necrosis:
 NOS
 acute

584.6 **Acute kidney failure with lesion of renal cortical necrosis**

584.7 **Acute kidney failure with lesion of renal medullary [papillary] necrosis**
Necrotizing renal papillitis

584.8 **Acute kidney failure with other specified pathological lesion in kidney**
Coding Clinic: 2011, Q3, P16-17

■ 584.9 **Acute kidney failure, unspecified**
Acute kidney injury (nontraumatic)
Excludes *traumatic kidney injury (866.00-866.13)*
Coding Clinic: 2011, Q3, P16-17; 2009, Q4, P106; 2008, Q4, P192-193; 2007, Q4, P96-97; 2005, Q2, P18-19; 2003, Q2, P7; 2003, Q1, P22; 2002, Q3, P21x2, 28x2; 2001, Q2, P14x2; 2000, Q3, P9; 2000, Q1, P22; 1996, Q3, P9; 1993, Q4, P34

OGCR Section I.C.10.a.1

> The ICD-9-CM classifies CKD based on severity. The severity of CKD is designated by stages I-V. Stage II, code 585.2, equates to mild CKD; stage III, code 585.3, equates to moderate CKD; and stage IV, code 585.4, equates to severe CKD. Code 585.6, End stage renal disease (ESRD), is assigned when the provider has documented end-stage-renal disease (ESRD). If both a stage of CKD and ESRD are documented, assign code 585.6 only.

● 585 **Chronic kidney disease (CKD)**
Includes Chronic uremia
Code first hypertensive chronic kidney disease, if applicable, (403.00–403.91, 404.00–404.93)
Use additional code to identify:
kidney transplant status, if applicable (V42.0)
manifestation as:
 uremic:
  neuropathy (357.4)
  pericarditis (420.0)

585.1 **Chronic kidney disease, Stage I**
585.2 **Chronic kidney disease, Stage II (mild)**
585.3 **Chronic kidney disease, Stage III (moderate)**
Coding Clinic: 2005, Q4, P68-69
585.4 **Chronic kidney disease, Stage IV (severe)**
585.5 **Chronic kidney disease, Stage V**
Excludes *chronic kidney disease, stage V requiring chronic dialysis (585.6)*
Coding Clinic: 2010, Q4, P137

Item 10–5 Decreased blood flow is the usual cause of **acute renal failure** that offers a good prognosis for recovery. **Chronic renal failure** is usually the result of long-standing kidney disease and is a very serious condition that generally results in death.

585.6 **End stage renal disease**
Chronic kidney disease, stage V requiring chronic dialysis
Coding Clinic: 2011, Q3, P15; 2010, Q3, P13; 2008, Q4, P193; Q1, P7-8; 2007, Q4, P84-86; Q3, P5-6; Q3, P11; 2006, Q4, P136; 2004, Q1, P5

■ 585.9 **Chronic kidney disease, unspecified**
Chronic renal disease
Chronic renal failure NOS
Chronic renal insufficiency
Coding Clinic: 2008, Q1, P7-8, 19; 2007, Q2, P3; 2006, Q4, P84-86; 2003, Q4, P60-61,111-112; 2001, Q2, P11-13x2; Q1, P3; 2000, Q4, P39-40; 1998, Q4, P54-55; Q3, P6-7; Q2, P20-21; 1996, Q3, P9; 1995, Q2, P10; 1987, Sept-Oct, P10; 1985, Nov-Dec, P15

■ 586 **Renal failure, unspecified**
Includes Uremia NOS
Excludes *following labor and delivery (669.3)*
posttraumatic renal failure (958.5)
that complicating:
abortion (634–638 with .3, 639.3)
ectopic or molar pregnancy (639.3)
uremia:
extrarenal (788.9)
prerenal (788.9)
Coding Clinic: 1998, Q3, P6; 1984, Sept-Oct, P16

■ 587 **Renal sclerosis, unspecified**
Includes Atrophy of kidney
Contracted kidney
Renal:
 cirrhosis
 fibrosis
Coding Clinic: 2010, Q4, P137

● 588 **Disorders resulting from impaired renal function**
588.0 **Renal osteodystrophy**
Azotemic osteodystrophy
Phosphate-losing tubular disorders
Renal:
 dwarfism
 infantilism
 rickets

588.1 **Nephrogenic diabetes insipidus**
Excludes *diabetes insipidus NOS (253.5)*

● 588.8 **Other specified disorders resulting from impaired renal function**
Excludes *secondary hypertension (405.0–405.9)*
Coding Clinic: 2004, Q4, P57-59

588.81 **Secondary hyperparathyroidism (of renal origin)**
Secondary hyperparathyroidism NOS

588.89 **Other specified disorders resulting from impaired renal function**
Hypokalemic nephropathy

■ 588.9 **Unspecified disorder resulting from impaired renal function**

● 589 **Small kidney of unknown cause**
589.0 **Unilateral small kidney**
589.1 **Bilateral small kidneys**
■ 589.9 **Small kidney, unspecified**

OTHER DISEASES OF URINARY SYSTEM (590–599)

590 Infections of kidney
Use additional code to identify organism, such as Escherichia coli [E. coli] (041.41-041.49)

590.0 Chronic pyelonephritis
Chronic pyelitis
Chronic pyonephrosis
Code, if applicable, any causal condition first

590.00 Without lesion of renal medullary necrosis
590.01 With lesion of renal medullary necrosis

590.1 Acute pyelonephritis
Acute pyelitis
Acute pyonephrosis

590.10 Without lesion of renal medullary necrosis
590.11 With lesion of renal medullary necrosis

590.2 Renal and perinephric abscess
Abscess:
kidney
nephritic
perirenal
Carbuncle of kidney

590.3 Pyeloureteritis cystica
Infection of renal pelvis and ureter
Ureteritis cystica
Cystica is an infection of the urinary bladder.

590.8 Other pyelonephritis or pyonephrosis, not specified as acute or chronic

590.80 Pyelonephritis, unspecified
Pyelitis NOS
Pyelonephritis NOS
Coding Clinic: 1997, Q4, P40

590.81 Pyelitis or pyelonephritis in diseases classified elsewhere
Code first underlying disease, as:
tuberculosis (016.0)

590.9 Infection of kidney, unspecified
Excludes urinary tract infection NOS (599.0)

591 Hydronephrosis
Hydrocalycosis
Hydronephrosis
Hydroureteronephrosis
Excludes congenital hydronephrosis (753.29)
hydroureter (593.5)
Coding Clinic: 2012, Q3, P12; 1998, Q2, P9

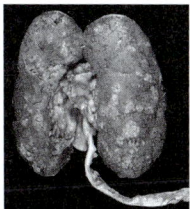

Figure 10–3 Acute pyelonephritis. Cortical surface exhibits grayish white areas of inflammation and abscess formation. (From Kumar: Robbins and Cotran: Pathologic Basis of Disease, ed 8, Saunders, An Imprint of Elsevier, 2009)

Item 10-6 Pyelonephritis is an infection of the kidneys and ureters and may be chronic or acute in one or both kidneys.

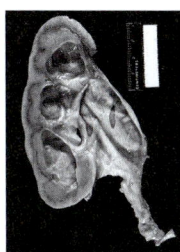

Figure 10–4 Hydronephrosis of the kidney, with marked dilatation of pelvis and calyces and thinning of renal parenchyma. (From Kumar: Robbins and Cotran: Pathologic Basis of Disease, ed 8, Saunders, An Imprint of Elsevier, 2009)

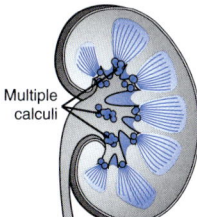

Figure 10–5 Multiple urinary calculi.

592 Calculus of kidney and ureter
Excludes nephrocalcinosis (275.49)

592.0 Calculus of kidney
Nephrolithiasis NOS
Renal calculus or stone
Staghorn calculus
Stone in kidney
Excludes uric acid nephrolithiasis (274.11)
Coding Clinic: 2012, Q3, P12; 2000, Q1, P4; 1993, Q2, P3

592.1 Calculus of ureter
Ureteric stone
Ureterolithiasis
Coding Clinic: 1998, Q2, P9; 1991, Q1, P11

592.9 Urinary calculus, unspecified
Coding Clinic: 1997, Q4, P40

593 Other disorders of kidney and ureter

593.0 Nephroptosis
Floating kidney   Mobile kidney

593.1 Hypertrophy of kidney

593.2 Cyst of kidney, acquired
Cyst (multiple) (solitary) of kidney, not congenital
Peripelvic (lymphatic) cyst
Excludes calyceal or pyelogenic cyst of kidney (591)
congenital cyst of kidney (753.1)
polycystic (disease of) kidney (753.1)

593.3 Stricture or kinking of ureter
Angulation of ureter (postoperative)
Constriction of ureter (postoperative)
Stricture of pelviureteric junction
Coding Clinic: 1994, Q3, P8

593.4 Other ureteric obstruction
Idiopathic retroperitoneal fibrosis
Occlusion NOS of ureter
Excludes that due to calculus (592.1)
Coding Clinic: 2010, Q1, P10; 1997, Q2, P4

593.5 Hydroureter
Excludes congenital hydroureter (753.22)
hydroureteronephrosis (591)

593.6 Postural proteinuria
Benign postural proteinuria
Orthostatic proteinuria
Excludes proteinuria NOS (791.0)

593.7 Vesicoureteral reflux
Occurs when urine flows from bladder back into ureters

593.70 Unspecified or without reflux nephropathy
593.71 With reflux nephropathy, unilateral
593.72 With reflux nephropathy, bilateral
593.73 With reflux nephropathy NOS

DISEASES OF THE GENITOURINARY SYSTEM (580–629)

● **593.8 Other specified disorders of kidney and ureter**
- **593.81 Vascular disorders of kidney**
  - Renal (artery):
    - embolism
    - hemorrhage
    - thrombosis
  - Renal infarction
- **593.82 Ureteral fistula**
  - Intestinoureteral fistula
  - Excludes: fistula between ureter and female genital tract (619.0)
- **593.89 Other**
  - Adhesions, kidney or ureter
  - Periureteritis
  - Polyp of ureter
  - Pyelectasia
  - Ureterocele
  - Excludes: tuberculosis of ureter (016.2)
    - ureteritis cystica (590.3)
  - Coding Clinic: 1984, Nov-Dec, P17

■ **593.9 Unspecified disorder of kidney and ureter**
- Acute renal disease
- Acute renal insufficiency
- Renal disease NOS
- Salt-losing nephritis or syndrome
- Excludes: chronic renal insufficiency (585.9)
  - cystic kidney disease (753.1)
  - nephropathy, so stated (583.0–583.9)
  - renal disease:
    - arising in pregnancy or the puerperium (642.1–642.2, 642.4–642.7, 646.2)
    - not specified as acute or chronic, but with stated pathology or cause (583.0–583.9)
- Coding Clinic: 2005, Q4, P79-80; 1998, Q2, P9

● **594 Calculus of lower urinary tract**
- **594.0 Calculus in diverticulum of bladder**
- **594.1 Other calculus in bladder**
  - Urinary bladder stone
  - Excludes: staghorn calculus (592.0)
- **594.2 Calculus in urethra**
- **594.8 Other lower urinary tract calculus**
  - Coding Clinic: 1985, Jan-Feb, P16
- ■ **594.9 Calculus of lower urinary tract, unspecified**
  - Excludes: calculus of urinary tract NOS (592.9)

● **595 Cystitis**
A general term used to describe an infection of the bladder and irritations in the lower urinary tract
- Excludes: prostatocystitis (601.3)
- Use additional code to identify organism, such as Escherichia coli [E. coli] (041.41-041.49)
- **595.0 Acute cystitis**
  - Excludes: trigonitis (595.3)
  - Coding Clinic: 1999, Q2, P15-16; 1984, Nov-Dec, P15
- **595.1 Chronic interstitial cystitis**
  Describes an ongoing infection of the kidney glomeruli and tubules
  - Hunner's ulcer
  - Panmural fibrosis of bladder
  - Submucous cystitis
- **595.2 Other chronic cystitis**
  - Chronic cystitis NOS
  - Subacute cystitis
  - Excludes: trigonitis (595.3)
- **595.3 Trigonitis**
  Inflammation of triangular area of bladder (where ureters and urethra come together)
  - Follicular cystitis
  - Trigonitis (acute) (chronic)
  - Urethrotrigonitis

● **595.4 Cystitis in diseases classified elsewhere**
- Code first underlying disease, as:
  - actinomycosis (039.8)
  - amebiasis (006.8)
  - bilharziasis (120.0–120.9)
  - Echinococcus infestation (122.3, 122.6)
- Excludes: cystitis:
  - diphtheritic (032.84)
  - gonococcal (098.11, 098.31)
  - monilial (112.2)
  - trichomonal (131.09)
  - tuberculous (016.1)

● **595.8 Other specified types of cystitis**
- **595.81 Cystitis cystica**
- **595.82 Irradiation cystitis**
  - Use additional E code to identify cause
- **595.89 Other**
  - Abscess of bladder
  - Cystitis:
    - bullous
    - emphysematous
    - glandularis

■ **595.9 Cystitis, unspecified**

● **596 Other disorders of bladder**
- Use additional code to identify urinary incontinence (625.6, 788.30–788.39)
- **596.0 Bladder neck obstruction**
  - Contracture (acquired) of bladder neck or vesicourethral orifice
  - Obstruction (acquired) of bladder neck or vesicourethral orifice
  - Stenosis (acquired) of bladder neck or vesicourethral orifice
  - Excludes: congenital (753.6)
  - Coding Clinic: 2002, Q3, P28; 2001, Q2, P14; 1994, Q3, P12
- **596.1 Intestinovesical fistula**
  Passage between bladder and the intestine
  - Fistula:
    - enterovesical
    - vesicocolic
  - Fistula:
    - vesicoenteric
    - vesicorectal
- **596.2 Vesical fistula, not elsewhere classified**
  - Fistula:
    - bladder NOS
    - urethrovesical
  - Fistula:
    - vesicocutaneous
    - vesicoperineal
  - Excludes: fistula between bladder and female genital tract (619.0)
- **596.3 Diverticulum of bladder**
  Formation of a sac from a herniation of the wall of the bladder
  - Diverticulitis of bladder
  - Diverticulum (acquired) (false) of bladder
  - Excludes: that with calculus in diverticulum of bladder (594.0)
- **596.4 Atony of bladder**
  Diminished tone of bladder muscle
  - High compliance bladder
  - Hypotonicity of bladder
  - Inertia of bladder
  - Excludes: neurogenic bladder (596.54)
- ● **596.5 Other functional disorders of bladder**
  - Excludes: cauda equina syndrome with neurogenic bladder (344.61)
  - **596.51 Hypertonicity of bladder**
    - Hyperactivity
    - Overactive bladder
  - **596.52 Low bladder compliance**
  - **596.53 Paralysis of bladder**
  - **596.54 Neurogenic bladder NOS**
    - Coding Clinic: 2001, Q1, P12
  - **596.55 Detrusor sphincter dyssynergia**
  - **596.59 Other functional disorder of bladder**
    - Detrusor instability
    - Coding Clinic: 1995, Q4, P72-73
- **596.6 Rupture of bladder, nontraumatic**

596.7 Hemorrhage into bladder wall
Hyperemia of bladder
Excludes acute hemorrhagic cystitis (595.0)

● **596.8 Other specified disorders of bladder**
Excludes cystocele, female (618.01–618.02, 618.09, 618.2–618.4)
hernia or prolapse of bladder, female (618.01–618.02, 618.09, 618.2–618.4)

596.81 Infection of cystostomy
Use additional code to specify type of infection, such as:
abscess or cellulitis of abdomen (682.2)
septicemia (038.0-038.9)
Use additional code to identify organism (041.00-041.9)
Coding Clinic: 2011, Q4, P129

596.82 Mechanical complication of cystostomy
Malfunction of cystostomy

596.83 Other complication of cystostomy
Fistula   Prolapse
Hernia

596.89 Other specified disorders of bladder
Bladder hemorrhage
Bladder hypertrophy
Calcified bladder
Contracted bladder
Coding Clinic: 2013, Q1, P6

596.9 Unspecified disorder of bladder

● **597 Urethritis, not sexually transmitted, and urethral syndrome**
Inflammation of urethra caused by bacteria or virus
Excludes nonspecific urethritis, so stated (099.4)

597.0 Urethral abscess
Abscess of: Abscess:
bulbourethral gland   periurethral
Cowper's gland   urethral (gland)
Littré's gland   Periurethral cellulitis
Excludes urethral caruncle (599.3)

● **597.8 Other urethritis**
597.80 Urethritis, unspecified
597.81 Urethral syndrome NOS
597.89 Other
Adenitis, Skene's glands
Cowperitis
Meatitis, urethral
Ulcer, urethra (meatus)
Verumontanitis
Excludes trichomonal (131.02)

● **598 Urethral stricture**
Narrowing of lumen of urethra caused by scarring from an infection or injury, which results in functional obstruction
Includes pinhole meatus
stricture of urinary meatus
Use additional code to identify urinary incontinence (625.6, 788.30–788.39)
Excludes congenital stricture of urethra and urinary meatus (753.6)

● **598.0 Urethral stricture due to infection**
598.00 Due to unspecified infection
● **598.01 Due to infective diseases classified elsewhere**
Code first underlying disease, as:
gonococcal infection (098.2)
schistosomiasis (120.0–120.9)
syphilis (095.8)

598.1 Traumatic urethral stricture
Stricture of urethra:
late effect of injury
postobstetric
Excludes postoperative following surgery on genitourinary tract (598.2)

598.2 Postoperative urethral stricture
Postcatheterization stricture of urethra
Coding Clinic: 1997, Q3, P6

598.8 Other specified causes of urethral stricture
Coding Clinic: 1984, Nov-Dec, P9

598.9 Urethral stricture, unspecified

● **599 Other disorders of urethra and urinary tract**
599.0 Urinary tract infection, site not specified
Excludes Candidiasis of urinary tract (112.2)
urinary tract infection of newborn (771.82)
Use additional code to identify organism, such as Escherichia coli [E. coli] (041.41-041.49)
Coding Clinic: 2012, Q2, P20-21; Q1, P11-12; 2011, Q4, P129; 2010, Q1, P11; 2009, Q3, P10x2; 2005, Q3, P12-13; 2004, Q2, P13; 1999, Q4, P6; Q2, P15-16; 1998, Q1, P5; 1996, Q4, P33; 1995, Q2, P7; 1994, Q1, P21; 1992, Q1, P13; 1988, Q4, P10; 1984, Nov-Dec, P15; July-Aug, P19

599.1 Urethral fistula
Fistula:
urethroperineal
urethrorectal
Urinary fistula NOS
Excludes fistula:
urethroscrotal (608.89)
urethrovaginal (619.0)
urethrovesicovaginal (619.0)
Coding Clinic: 1997, Q3, P6

599.2 Urethral diverticulum
599.3 Urethral caruncle
Polyp of urethra
599.4 Urethral false passage
599.5 Prolapsed urethral mucosa
Prolapse of urethra
Urethrocele
Excludes urethrocele, female (618.03, 618.09, 618.2–618.4)

● **599.6 Urinary obstruction**
Use additional code to identify urinary incontinence (625.6, 788.30–788.39)
Excludes obstructive nephropathy NOS (593.89)
Coding Clinic: 2005, Q4, P80-81

599.60 Urinary obstruction, unspecified
Obstructive uropathy NOS
Urinary (tract) obstruction NOS

599.69 Urinary obstruction, not elsewhere classified
Code, if applicable, any causal condition first, such as:
hyperplasia of prostate (600.0–600.9 with fifth-digit 1)

● **599.7 Hematuria**
Hematuria (benign) (essential)
Excludes hemoglobinuria (791.2)
Coding Clinic: 2008, Q4, P121; 2000, Q1, P5; 1995, Q3, P8; 1993, Q1, P26; 5th Issue, P16; 1985, Nov-Dec, P15

599.70 Hematuria, unspecified
599.71 Gross hematuria
Coding Clinic: 2010, Q2, P3
599.72 Microscopic hematuria

● **599.8 Other specified disorders of urethra and urinary tract**
Use additional code to identify urinary incontinence (625.6, 788.30–788.39)
Excludes symptoms and other conditions classifiable to 788.0–788.2, 788.4–788.9, 791.0–791.9

599.81 Urethral hypermobility
599.82 Intrinsic (urethral) sphincter deficiency [ISD]
599.83 Urethral instability
599.84 Other specified disorders of urethra
Rupture of urethra (nontraumatic)
Urethral:
cyst
granuloma
Coding Clinic: 2009, Q1, P20

599.89 Other specified disorders of urinary tract

599.9 Unspecified disorder of urethra and urinary tract

(See Plates 366B and 387 on pages NAP-3 and NAP-5.)

DISEASES OF MALE GENITAL ORGANS (600–608)

● **600 Hyperplasia of prostate**
Benign prostatic hyperplasia (BPH) and is an enlargement of prostate gland usually occurring with age and causing obstructed urine flow
Includes Enlarged prostate
Coding Clinic: 2005, Q3, P20; 2003, Q4, P63-64; 2002, Q3, P28; 1994, Q3, P12-13; 1992, Q3, P7; 1986, Sept-Oct, P12; Nov-Dec, P10; 1984, Nov-Dec, P9

● **600.0 Hypertrophy (benign) of prostate**
Benign prostatic hypertrophy
Enlargement of prostate
Smooth enlarged prostate
Soft enlarged prostate
Coding Clinic: 2003, Q1, P6; 2001, Q2, P14

600.00 Hypertrophy (benign) of prostate without urinary obstruction and other lower urinary tract symptoms (LUTS)
Hypertrophy (benign) of prostate NOS

600.01 Hypertrophy (benign) of prostate with urinary obstruction and other lower urinary tract symptoms (LUTS)
Hypertrophy (benign) of prostate with urinary retention
Use additional code to identify symptoms:
incomplete bladder emptying (788.21)
nocturia (788.43)
straining on urination (788.65)
urinary frequency (788.41)
urinary hesitancy (788.64)
urinary incontinence (788.30–788.39)
urinary obstruction (599.69)
urinary retention (788.20)
urinary urgency (788.63)
weak urinary stream (788.62)
Coding Clinic: 2006, Q4, P93-95

● **600.1 Nodular prostate**
Hard, firm prostate
Multinodular prostate
Excludes malignant neoplasm of prostate (185)

600.10 Nodular prostate without urinary obstruction
Nodular prostate NOS

600.11 Nodular prostate with urinary obstruction
Nodular prostate with urinary retention

● **600.2 Benign localized hyperplasia of prostate**
Adenofibromatous hypertrophy of prostate
Adenoma of prostate
Fibroadenoma of prostate
Fibroma of prostate
Myoma of prostate
Polyp of prostate
Excludes benign neoplasms of prostate (222.2)
hypertrophy of prostate (600.00–600.01)
malignant neoplasm of prostate (185)

600.20 Benign localized hyperplasia of prostate without urinary obstruction and other lower urinary tract symptoms (LUTS)
Benign localized hyperplasia of prostate NOS

600.21 Benign localized hyperplasia of prostate with urinary obstruction and other lower urinary tract symptoms (LUTS)
Benign localized hyperplasia of prostate with urinary retention
Use additional code to identify symptoms:
incomplete bladder emptying (788.21)
nocturia (788.43)
straining on urination (788.65)
urinary frequency (788.41)
urinary hesitancy (788.64)
urinary incontinence (788.30–788.39)
urinary obstruction (599.69)
urinary retention (788.20)
urinary urgency (788.63)
weak urinary stream (788.62)

600.3 Cyst of prostate

● **600.9 Hyperplasia of prostate, unspecified**
Median bar
Prostatic obstruction NOS

600.90 Hyperplasia of prostate, unspecified, without urinary obstruction and other lower urinary tract symptoms (LUTS)
Hyperplasia of prostate NOS

600.91 Hyperplasia of prostate, unspecified, with urinary obstruction and other lower urinary tract symptoms (LUTS)
Hyperplasia of prostate, unspecified, with urinary retention
Use additional code to identify symptoms:
incomplete bladder emptying (788.21)
nocturia (788.43)
straining on urination (788.65)
urinary frequency (788.41)
urinary hesitancy (788.64)
urinary incontinence (788.30–788.39)
urinary obstruction (599.69)
urinary retention (788.20)
urinary urgency (788.63)
weak urinary stream (788.62)

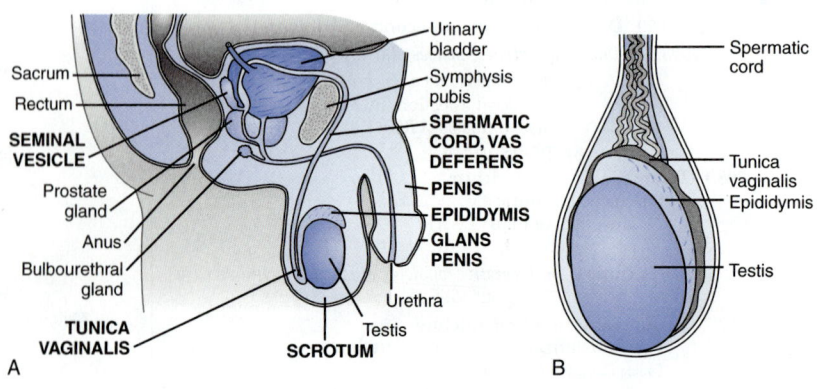

Figure 10–6 **A.** Male genital system. **B.** Testis.

- **601 Inflammatory diseases of prostate**
    Use additional code to identify organism, such as:
        Staphylococcus (041.1), or Streptococcus (041.0)
    - 601.0 Acute prostatitis
    - 601.1 Chronic prostatitis
    - 601.2 Abscess of prostate
    - 601.3 Prostatocystitis
    - ●601.4 Prostatitis in diseases classified elsewhere
        Code first underlying disease, as:
            actinomycosis (039.8)   syphilis (095.8)
            blastomycosis (116.0)   tuberculosis (016.5)
        Excludes prostatitis:
                    gonococcal (098.12, 098.32)
                    monilial (112.2)
                    trichomonal (131.03)
    - 601.8 Other specified inflammatory diseases of prostate
        Prostatitis:
            cavitary
            diverticular
            granulomatous
    - 601.9 Prostatitis, unspecified
        Prostatitis NOS

- **602 Other disorders of prostate**
    - 602.0 Calculus of prostate
        Prostatic stone
    - 602.1 Congestion or hemorrhage of prostate
    - 602.2 Atrophy of prostate
    - 602.3 Dysplasia of prostate
        Prostatic intraepithelial neoplasia I (PIN I)
        Prostatic intraepithelial neoplasia II (PIN II)
        Excludes prostatic intraepithelial neoplasia III (PIN III) (233.4)
    - 602.8 Other specified disorders of prostate
        Fistula of prostate   Stricture of prostate
        Infarction of prostate   Periprostatic adhesions
    - 602.9 Unspecified disorder of prostate

- **603 Hydrocele**
    Includes hydrocele of spermatic cord, testis, or tunica vaginalis
    Excludes congenital (778.6)
    - 603.0 Encysted hydrocele
    - 603.1 Infected hydrocele
        Use additional code to identify organism
    - 603.8 Other specified types of hydrocele
    - 603.9 Hydrocele, unspecified

- **604 Orchitis and epididymitis**
    An inflammation of one or both testes as a result of mumps or other infection, trauma, or metastasis. **Epididymitis** *is an inflammation of the epididymis (the tubular structure that connects testicle with vas deferens).*
    Use additional code to identify organism, such as:
        Escherichia coli [E. coli] (041.41-041.49)
        Staphylococcus (041.10-041.19)
        Streptococcus (041.00-041.09)
    - 604.0 Orchitis, epididymitis, and epididymo-orchitis, with abscess
        Abscess of epididymis or testis
    - ●604.9 Other orchitis, epididymitis, and epididymo-orchitis, without mention of abscess
        - 604.90 Orchitis and epididymitis, unspecified
        - ●604.91 Orchitis and epididymitis in diseases classified elsewhere
            Code first underlying disease, as:
                diphtheria (032.89)
                filariasis (125.0–125.9)
                syphilis (095.8)
            Excludes orchitis:
                        gonococcal (098.13, 098.33)
                        mumps (072.0)
                        tuberculous (016.5)
                        tuberculous epididymitis (016.4)
        - 604.99 Other

- **605 Redundant prepuce and phimosis**
    Adherent prepuce   Phimosis (congenital)
    Paraphimosis   Tight foreskin
    Coding Clinic: 2008, Q3, P9

- **606 Infertility, male**
    Coding Clinic: 1996, Q2, P9
    - 606.0 Azoospermia
        Absolute infertility
        Infertility due to:
            germinal (cell) aplasia
            spermatogenic arrest (complete)
    - 606.1 Oligospermia
        Infertility due to:
            germinal cell desquamation
            hypospermatogenesis
            incomplete spermatogenic arrest
    - 606.8 Infertility due to extratesticular causes
        Infertility due to:
            drug therapy
            infection
            obstruction of efferent ducts
            radiation
            systemic disease
    - 606.9 Male infertility, unspecified

- **607 Disorders of penis**
    Excludes phimosis (605)
    - 607.0 Leukoplakia of penis
        Kraurosis of penis
        Excludes carcinoma in situ of penis (233.5)
                    erythroplasia of Queyrat (233.5)
    - 607.1 Balanoposthitis
        Balanitis
        Use additional code to identify organism

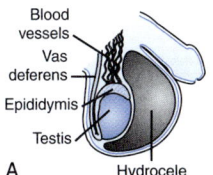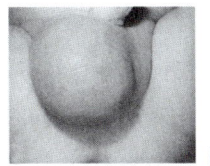

Figure 10–7 A. Hydrocele. **B.** Newborn with large right hydrocele. (**B** from Behrman: Nelson Textbook of Pediatrics, ed 18, Saunders, An Imprint of Elsevier, 2007)

Item 10–7 Hydrocele is a sac of fluid accumulating in the testes membrane.

Item 10-8 Male infertility is the inability of the female sex partner to conceive after one year of unprotected intercourse. **Azoospermia** is no sperm ejaculated and **oligospermia** is few sperm ejaculated—both resulting in infertility. Extratesticular causes such as injury, infections, radiation, and chemotherapy may also cause male infertility.

607.2 Other inflammatory disorders of penis
Abscess of corpus cavernosum or penis
Boil of corpus cavernosum or penis
Carbuncle of corpus cavernosum or penis
Cellulitis of corpus cavernosum or penis
Cavernitis (penis)
Use additional code to identify organism
Excludes herpetic infection (054.13)

607.3 Priapism
Painful erection

●**607.8** Other specified disorders of penis
607.81 Balanitis xerotica obliterans
Induratio penis plastica
607.82 Vascular disorders of penis
Embolism of corpus cavernosum or penis
Hematoma (nontraumatic) of corpus cavernosum or penis
Hemorrhage of corpus cavernosum or penis
Thrombosis of corpus cavernosum or penis
607.83 Edema of penis
607.84 Impotence of organic origin
Excludes nonorganic (302.72)
Coding Clinic: 1985, July-Aug, P9
607.85 Peyronie's disease
Coding Clinic: 2003, Q4, P64-65
607.89 Other
Atrophy of corpus cavernosum or penis
Fibrosis of corpus cavernosum or penis
Hypertrophy of corpus cavernosum or penis
Ulcer (chronic) of corpus cavernosum or penis

607.9 Unspecified disorder of penis

●**608** Other disorders of male genital organs
608.0 Seminal vesiculitis
Abscess of seminal vesicle
Cellulitis of seminal vesicle
Vesiculitis (seminal)
Use additional code to identify organism
Excludes gonococcal infection (098.14, 098.34)
608.1 Spermatocele
●**608.2** Torsion of testis
Coding Clinic: 2006, Q4, P95-96
608.20 Torsion of testis, unspecified
608.21 Extravaginal torsion of spermatic cord
608.22 Intravaginal torsion of spermatic cord
Torsion of spermatic cord NOS
608.23 Torsion of appendix testis
608.24 Torsion of appendix epididymis

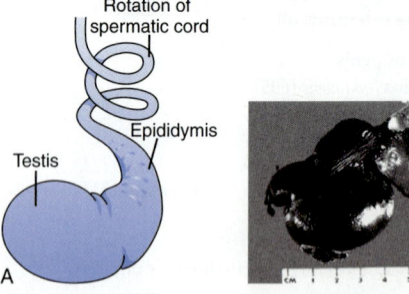

Figure 10–8 A. Torsion of testis. **B.** Torsion of the testis. (**B** from Kumar: Robbins and Cotran: Pathologic Basis of Disease, ed 8, Saunders, An Imprint of Elsevier, 2009)

Item 10–9 Seminal vesiculitis is an inflammation of the seminal vesicle. Spermatocele is a benign cystic accumulation of sperm arising from the head of the epididymis. Torsion of the testis is a medical emergency occurring most commonly in boys 7 to 12 years of age and results from a congenital abnormality of the covering of the testis allowing the testis to twist within its sac and cutting off the blood supply to the testis.

608.3 Atrophy of testis
608.4 Other inflammatory disorders of male genital organs
Abscess of scrotum, spermatic cord, testis [except abscess], tunica vaginalis, or vas deferens
Boil of scrotum, spermatic cord, testis [except abscess], tunica vaginalis, or vas deferens
Carbuncle of scrotum, spermatic cord, testis [except abscess], tunica vaginalis, or vas deferens
Cellulitis of scrotum, spermatic cord, testis [except abscess], tunica vaginalis, or vas deferens
Vasitis
Use additional code to identify organism
Excludes abscess of testis (604.0)

●**608.8** Other specified disorders of male genital organs
●**608.81** Disorders of male genital organs in diseases classified elsewhere
Code first underlying disease, as:
filariasis (125.0–125.9)
tuberculosis (016.5)
608.82 Hematospermia
608.83 Vascular disorders
Hematoma (nontraumatic) of seminal vesicle, spermatic cord, testis, scrotum, tunica vaginalis, or vas deferens
Hemorrhage of seminal vesicle, spermatic cord, testis, scrotum, tunica vaginalis, or vas deferens
Thrombosis of seminal vesicle, spermatic cord, testis, scrotum, tunica vaginalis, or vas deferens
Hematocele NOS, male
Coding Clinic: 2003, Q4, P110
608.84 Chylocele of tunica vaginalis
608.85 Stricture
Stricture of:
spermatic cord
tunica vaginalis
Stricture of:
vas deferens
608.86 Edema
608.87 Retrograde ejaculation
608.89 Other
Atrophy of seminal vesicle, spermatic cord, testis, scrotum tunica vaginalis, or vas deferens
Fibrosis of seminal vesicle, spermatic cord, testis, scrotum tunica vaginalis, or vas deferens
Hypertrophy of seminal vesicle, spermatic cord, testis, scrotum tunica vaginalis, or vas deferens
Ulcer of seminal vesicle, spermatic cord, testis, scrotum tunica vaginalis, or vas deferens
Excludes atrophy of testis (608.3)

608.9 Unspecified disorder of male genital organs

DISORDERS OF BREAST (610–612)

●**610** Benign mammary dysplasias
Benign lumpiness of the breast
610.0 Solitary cyst of breast
Cyst (solitary) of breast
610.1 Diffuse cystic mastopathy
Chronic cystic mastitis
Cystic breast
Fibrocystic disease of breast
Coding Clinic: 2006, Q2, P10
610.2 Fibroadenosis of breast
Fibroadenosis of breast:
NOS
chronic
cystic
Fibroadenosis of breast:
diffuse
periodic
segmental
610.3 Fibrosclerosis of breast

610.4 Mammary duct ectasia
Comedomastitis
Duct ectasia
Mastitis:
  periductal
  plasma cell

610.8 Other specified benign mammary dysplasias
Mazoplasia
Sebaceous cyst of breast
Coding Clinic: 2009, Q2, P9

610.9 Benign mammary dysplasia, unspecified

611 Other disorders of breast
Excludes: that associated with lactation or the puerperium (675.0–676.9)

611.0 Inflammatory disease of breast
Abscess (acute) (chronic) (nonpuerperal) of:
  areola
  breast
Mammillary fistula
Mastitis (acute) (subacute) (nonpuerperal):
  NOS
  infective
  retromammary
  submammary
Excludes: carbuncle of breast (680.2)
  chronic cystic mastitis (610.1)
  neonatal infective mastitis (771.5)
  thrombophlebitis of breast [Mondor's disease] (451.89)

611.1 Hypertrophy of breast
Gynecomastia
Hypertrophy of breast:
  NOS
  massive pubertal
Excludes: breast engorgement in newborn (778.7)
  disproportion of reconstructed breast (612.1)

611.2 Fissure of nipple

611.3 Fat necrosis of breast
Fat necrosis (segmental) of breast
Code first breast necrosis due to breast graft (996.79)

611.4 Atrophy of breast

611.5 Galactocele

611.6 Galactorrhea not associated with childbirth
Excessive or spontaneous flow of milk
Coding Clinic: 1985, July-Aug, P9

611.7 Signs and symptoms in breast
  611.71 Mastodynia
    Pain in breast
  611.72 Lump or mass in breast
    Coding Clinic: 2009, Q4, P108; 2003, Q2, P3-5
  611.79 Other
    Induration of breast
    Inversion of nipple
    Nipple discharge
    Retraction of nipple

611.8 Other specified disorders of breast
Coding Clinic: 2008, Q4, P121-122
  611.81 Ptosis of breast
    Excludes: ptosis of native breast in relation to reconstructed breast (612.1)
  611.82 Hypoplasia of breast
    Micromastia
    Excludes: congenital absence of breast (757.6)
      hypoplasia of native breast in relation to reconstructed breast (612.1)
  611.83 Capsular contracture of breast implant
  611.89 Other specified disorders of breast
    Hematoma (nontraumatic) of breast
    Infarction of breast
    Occlusion of breast duct
    Subinvolution of breast (postlactational) (postpartum)

611.9 Unspecified breast disorder

612 Deformity and disproportion of reconstructed breast
Coding Clinic: 2008, Q4, P123
  612.0 Deformity of reconstructed breast
    Contour irregularity in reconstructed breast
    Excess tissue in reconstructed breast
    Misshapen reconstructed breast
  612.1 Disproportion of reconstructed breast
    Breast asymmetry between native breast and reconstructed breast
    Disproportion between native breast and reconstructed breast

(See Plate 366A on page NAP-3.)

INFLAMMATORY DISEASE OF FEMALE PELVIC ORGANS (614–616)

Use additional code to identify organism, such as Staphylococcus (041.1), or Streptococcus (041.0)
Excludes: that associated with pregnancy, abortion, childbirth, or the puerperium (630–676.9)

614 Inflammatory disease of ovary, fallopian tube, pelvic cellular tissue, and peritoneum
Excludes: endometritis (615.0–615.9)
  major infection following delivery (670.0-670.8)
  that complicating:
    abortion (634–638 with .0, 639.0)
    ectopic or molar pregnancy (639.0)
    pregnancy or labor (646.6)

  614.0 Acute salpingitis and oophoritis
    Any condition classifiable to 614.2, specified as acute or subacute
  614.1 Chronic salpingitis and oophoritis
    Hydrosalpinx
    Salpingitis:
      follicularis
      isthmica nodosa
    Any condition classifiable to 614.2, specified as chronic

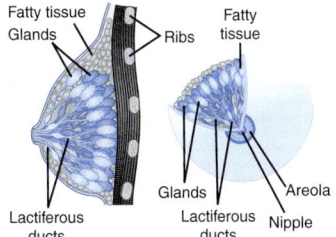

Figure 10–9 Breast.

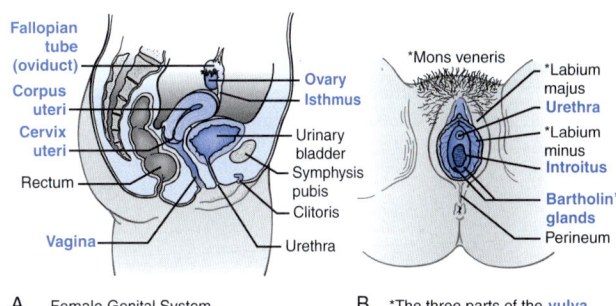

Figure 10–10 **A.** Female genital system. **B.** External female genital system. (From Buck CJ: Step-by-Step Medical Coding, ed 2011, Philadelphia, WB Saunders, 2011)

Item 10-10 **Salpingitis** is an infection of one or both fallopian tubes. **Oophoritis** is an infection of one or both ovaries.

614.2 Salpingitis and oophoritis not specified as acute, subacute, or chronic
Abscess (of):
fallopian tube
ovary
tubo-ovarian
Oophoritis
Perioophoritis
Perisalpingitis
Pyosalpinx
Salpingitis
Salpingo-oophoritis
Tubo-ovarian inflammatory disease
Excludes gonococcal infection (chronic) (098.37)
acute (098.17)
tuberculous (016.6)

614.3 Acute parametritis and pelvic cellulitis
Acute inflammatory pelvic disease
Any condition classifiable to 614.4, specified as acute

614.4 Chronic or unspecified parametritis and pelvic cellulitis
Abscess (of):
broad ligament chronic or NOS
parametrium chronic or NOS
pelvis, female chronic or NOS
pouch of Douglas chronic or NOS
Chronic inflammatory pelvic disease
Pelvic cellulitis, female
Excludes tuberculous (016.7)

614.5 Acute or unspecified pelvic peritonitis, female

614.6 Pelvic peritoneal adhesions, female (postoperative) (postinfection)
Adhesions:
peritubal
tubo-ovarian
Use additional code to identify any associated infertility (628.2)
Coding Clinic: 2003, Q3, P6-7; Q1, P4-5; 1995, Q3, P7

614.7 Other chronic pelvic peritonitis, female
Excludes tuberculous (016.7)

614.8 Other specified inflammatory disease of female pelvic organs and tissues

614.9 Unspecified inflammatory disease of female pelvic organs and tissues
Pelvic infection or inflammation, female NOS
Pelvic inflammatory disease [PID]

615 Inflammatory diseases of uterus, except cervix
Excludes following delivery (670.0-670.8)
hyperplastic endometritis (621.30-621.35)
that complicating:
abortion (634–638 with .0, 639.0)
ectopic or molar pregnancy (639.0)
pregnancy or labor (646.6)

615.0 Acute
Any condition classifiable to 615.9, specified as acute or subacute

615.1 Chronic
Any condition classifiable to 615.9, specified as chronic

615.9 Unspecified inflammatory disease of uterus
Endometritis   Perimetritis
Endomyometritis   Pyometra
Metritis   Uterine abscess
Myometritis

616 Inflammatory disease of cervix, vagina, and vulva
Excludes that complicating:
abortion (634–638 with .0, 639.0)
ectopic or molar pregnancy (639.0)
pregnancy, childbirth, or the puerperium (646.6)

616.0 Cervicitis and endocervicitis
Cervicitis with or without mention of erosion or ectropion
Endocervicitis with or without mention of erosion or ectropion
Nabothian (gland) cyst or follicle
Excludes erosion or ectropion without mention of cervicitis (622.0)

616.1 Vaginitis and vulvovaginitis
Excludes vulvar vestibulitis (625.71)

616.10 Vaginitis and vulvovaginitis, unspecified
Vaginitis:
NOS
postirradiation
Vulvitis NOS
Vulvovaginitis NOS
Use additional code to identify organism, such as:
Escherichia coli [E. coli] (041.41-041.49)
Staphylococcus (041.10-041.19)
Streptococcus (041.00-041.09)
Excludes noninfective leukorrhea (623.5)
postmenopausal or senile vaginitis (627.3)

616.11 Vaginitis and vulvovaginitis in diseases classified elsewhere
Code first underlying disease, as:
pinworm vaginitis (127.4)
Excludes herpetic vulvovaginitis (054.11)
monilial vulvovaginitis (112.1)
trichomonal vaginitis or vulvovaginitis (131.01)

616.2 Cyst of Bartholin's gland
Cysts filled with liquid or semisolid material
Bartholin's duct cyst

616.3 Abscess of Bartholin's gland
Localized collection of pus
Vulvovaginal gland abscess

616.4 Other abscess of vulva
Abscess of vulva
Carbuncle of vulva
Furuncle of vulva

616.5 Ulceration of vulva

616.50 Ulceration of vulva, unspecified
Ulcer NOS of vulva

616.51 Ulceration of vulva in diseases classified elsewhere
Code first underlying disease, as:
Behçet's syndrome (136.1)
tuberculosis (016.7)
Excludes vulvar ulcer (in):
gonococcal (098.0)
herpes simplex (054.12)
syphilitic (091.0)

- **616.8 Other specified inflammatory diseases of cervix, vagina, and vulva**
    Excludes: noninflammatory disorders of:
      cervix (622.0–622.9)
      vagina (623.0–623.9)
      vulva (624.0–624.9)
  - 616.81 Mucositis (ulcerative) of cervix, vagina, and vulva
      Use additional E code to identify adverse effects of therapy, such as:
        antineoplastic and immunosuppressive drugs (E930.7, E933.1)
        radiation therapy (E879.2)
  - 616.89 Other inflammatory disease of cervix, vagina and vulva
      Caruncle, vagina or labium
      Ulcer, vagina
- **616.9 Unspecified inflammatory disease of cervix, vagina, and vulva**

OTHER DISORDERS OF FEMALE GENITAL TRACT (617–629)

- **617 Endometriosis**
  Coding Clinic: 1995, Q1, P7
  - 617.0 Endometriosis of uterus
      Adenomyosis
      Endometriosis:
        cervix
        internal
        myometrium
      Excludes: stromal endometriosis (236.0)
      Coding Clinic: 1992, Q3, P7-8
  - 617.1 Endometriosis of ovary
      Chocolate cyst of ovary
      Endometrial cystoma of ovary
  - 617.2 Endometriosis of fallopian tube
  - 617.3 Endometriosis of pelvic peritoneum
      Endometriosis:
        broad ligament
        cul-de-sac (Douglas')
        parametrium
        round ligament
  - 617.4 Endometriosis of rectovaginal septum and vagina
  - 617.5 Endometriosis of intestine
      Endometriosis:
        appendix
        colon
        rectum
  - 617.6 Endometriosis in scar of skin
  - 617.8 Endometriosis of other specified sites
      Endometriosis:
        bladder
        lung
        umbilicus
        vulva
- **617.9 Endometriosis, site unspecified**

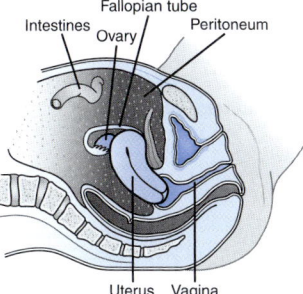

Figure 10–11 Sites of potential endometrial implants.

Item 10–11 Endometriosis is a condition for which no clear cause has been identified. Endometrial tissue is expelled from the uterus into the abdominal cavity and can implant onto a variety of organs. Classification is based on the site of implant of the endometrial tissue.

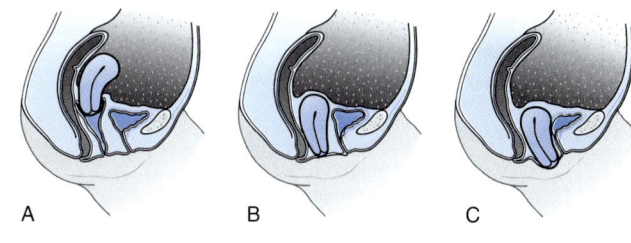

Figure 10–12 Three stages of uterine prolapse. **A.** Uterus is prolapsed. **B.** Vagina and uterus are prolapsed (incomplete uterovaginal prolapse). **C.** Vagina and uterus are completely prolapsed and are exposed through the external genitalia (complete uterovaginal prolapse).

- **618 Genital prolapse**
    Use additional code to identify urinary incontinence (625.6, 788.31, 788.33–788.39)
    Excludes: that complicating pregnancy, labor, or delivery (654.4)
  - **618.0 Prolapse of vaginal walls without mention of uterine prolapse**
      Excludes: that with uterine prolapse (618.2–618.4)
        enterocele (618.6)
        vaginal vault prolapse following hysterectomy (618.5)
      Coding Clinic: 2004, Q4, P83-85
    - 618.00 Unspecified prolapse of vaginal walls
        Vaginal prolapse NOS
    - 618.01 Cystocele, midline
        Cystocele NOS
    - 618.02 Cystocele, lateral
        Paravaginal
    - 618.03 Urethrocele
    - 618.04 Rectocele
        Proctocele
        Use additional code for any associated fecal incontinence (787.60-787.63)
    - 618.05 Perineocele
    - 618.09 Other prolapse of vaginal walls without mention of uterine prolapse
        Cystourethrocele
  - 618.1 Uterine prolapse without mention of vaginal wall prolapse
      Descensus uteri
      Uterine prolapse:
        NOS
        complete
        first degree
        second degree
        third degree
      Excludes: that with mention of cystocele, urethrocele, or rectocele (618.2–618.4)
  - 618.2 Uterovaginal prolapse, incomplete
  - 618.3 Uterovaginal prolapse, complete
  - 618.4 Uterovaginal prolapse, unspecified
  - 618.5 Prolapse of vaginal vault after hysterectomy
  - 618.6 Vaginal enterocele, congenital or acquired
      Pelvic enterocele, congenital or acquired
  - 618.7 Old laceration of muscles of pelvic floor
  - **618.8 Other specified genital prolapse**
    - 618.81 Incompetence or weakening of pubocervical tissue
    - 618.82 Incompetence or weakening of rectovaginal tissue
    - 618.83 Pelvic muscle wasting
        Disuse atrophy of pelvic muscles and anal sphincter
    - 618.84 Cervical stump prolapse
    - 618.89 Other specified genital prolapse
  - 618.9 Unspecified genital prolapse

- **619 Fistula involving female genital tract**
  - **Excludes:** *vesicorectal and intestinovesical fistula (596.1)*
  - **619.0 Urinary-genital tract fistula, female**
    - Fistula:
      - cervicovesical
      - ureterovaginal
      - urethrovaginal
      - urethrovesicovaginal
      - uteroureteric
      - uterovesical
      - vesicocervicovaginal
      - vesicovaginal
  - **619.1 Digestive-genital tract fistula, female**
    - Fistula:
      - intestinouterine
      - intestinovaginal
      - rectovaginal
    - Fistula:
      - rectovulval
      - sigmoidovaginal
      - uterorectal
  - **619.2 Genital tract-skin fistula, female**
    - Fistula:
      - uterus to abdominal wall
      - vaginoperineal
  - **619.8 Other specified fistulas involving female genital tract**
    - Fistula:
      - cervix
      - cul-de-sac (Douglas')
      - uterus
      - vagina
  - **619.9 Unspecified fistula involving female genital tract**

- **620 Noninflammatory disorders of ovary, fallopian tube, and broad ligament**
  - **Excludes:** *hydrosalpinx (614.1)*
  - **620.0 Follicular cyst of ovary**
    - Cyst of graafian follicle
  - **620.1 Corpus luteum cyst or hematoma**
    - Corpus luteum hemorrhage or rupture
    - Lutein cyst
  - **620.2 Other and unspecified ovarian cyst**
    - Cyst of ovary:
      - NOS
      - corpus albicans
      - retention NOS
      - serous
      - theca-lutein
    - Simple cystoma of ovary
    - **Excludes:** *cystadenoma (benign) (serous) (220)*
      - *developmental cysts (752.0)*
      - *neoplastic cysts (220)*
      - *polycystic ovaries (256.4)*
      - *Stein-Leventhal syndrome (256.4)*
  - **620.3 Acquired atrophy of ovary and fallopian tube**
    - Senile involution of ovary
  - **620.4 Prolapse or hernia of ovary and fallopian tube**
    - Displacement of ovary and fallopian tube
    - Salpingocele
  - **620.5 Torsion of ovary, ovarian pedicle, or fallopian tube**
    - Torsion:
      - accessory tube
      - hydatid of Morgagni
  - **620.6 Broad ligament laceration syndrome**
    - Masters-Allen syndrome
  - **620.7 Hematoma of broad ligament**
    - Hematocele, broad ligament
  - **620.8 Other noninflammatory disorders of ovary, fallopian tube, and broad ligament**
    - Cyst of broad ligament or fallopian tube
    - Polyp of broad ligament or fallopian tube
    - Infarction of ovary or fallopian tube
    - Rupture of ovary or fallopian tube
    - Hematosalpinx of ovary or fallopian tube
    - **Excludes:** *hematosalpinx in ectopic pregnancy (639.2)*
      - *peritubal adhesions (614.6)*
      - *torsion of ovary, ovarian pedicle, or fallopian tube (620.5)*
  - **620.9 Unspecified noninflammatory disorder of ovary, fallopian tube, and broad ligament**

- **621 Disorders of uterus, not elsewhere classified**
  - **621.0 Polyp of corpus uteri**
    - Polyp:
      - endometrium
      - uterus NOS
    - **Excludes:** *cervical polyp NOS (622.7)*
  - **621.1 Chronic subinvolution of uterus**
    - **Excludes:** *puerperal (674.8)*
  - **621.2 Hypertrophy of uterus**
    - Bulky or enlarged uterus
    - **Excludes:** *puerperal (674.8)*
  - **621.3 Endometrial hyperplasia**
    - Coding Clinic: 2004, Q4, P85-86
    - **621.30 Endometrial hyperplasia, unspecified**
      - Endometrial hyperplasia NOS
      - Hyperplasia (adenomatous) (cystic) (glandular) of endometrium
      - Hyperplastic endometritis
    - **621.31 Simple endometrial hyperplasia without atypia**
      - **Excludes:** *benign endometrial hyperplasia (621.34)*
    - **621.32 Complex endometrial hyperplasia without atypia**
      - **Excludes:** *benign endometrial hyperplasia (621.34)*
    - **621.33 Endometrial hyperplasia with atypia**
      - **Excludes:** *endometrial intraepithelial neoplasia [EIN] (621.35)*
    - **621.34 Benign endometrial hyperplasia**
    - **621.35 Endometrial intraepithelial neoplasia [EIN]**
      - **Excludes:** *malignant neoplasm of endometrium with endometrium intraepithelial neoplasia [EIN] (182.0)*
  - **621.4 Hematometra**
    - Hemometra
    - **Excludes:** *that in congenital anomaly (752.2–752.39)*
  - **621.5 Intrauterine synechiae**
    - Adhesions of uterus
    - Band(s) of uterus
  - **621.6 Malposition of uterus**
    - Anteversion of uterus
    - Retroflexion of uterus
    - Retroversion of uterus
    - **Excludes:** *malposition complicating pregnancy, labor, or delivery (654.3–654.4)*
      - *prolapse of uterus (618.1–618.4)*
  - **621.7 Chronic inversion of uterus**
    - **Excludes:** *current obstetrical trauma (665.2)*
      - *prolapse of uterus (618.1–618.4)*
  - **621.8 Other specified disorders of uterus, not elsewhere classified**
    - Atrophy, acquired of uterus
    - Cyst of uterus
    - Fibrosis NOS of uterus
    - Old laceration (postpartum) of uterus
    - Ulcer of uterus
    - **Excludes:** *bilharzial fibrosis (120.0–120.9)*
      - *endometriosis (617.0)*
      - *fistulas (619.0–619.8)*
      - *inflammatory diseases (615.0–615.9)*
  - **621.9 Unspecified disorder of uterus**

- **622 Noninflammatory disorders of cervix**
  - **Excludes:** abnormality of cervix complicating pregnancy, labor, or delivery (654.5–654.6)
    - fistula (619.0–619.8)
  - **622.0 Erosion and ectropion of cervix**
    - Eversion of cervix
    - Ulcer of cervix
    - **Excludes:** that in chronic cervicitis (616.0)
  - **622.1 Dysplasia of cervix (uteri)**
    - **Excludes:** abnormal results from cervical cytologic examination without histologic confirmation (795.00–795.09)
      - carcinoma in situ of cervix (233.1)
      - cervical intraepithelial neoplasia III [CIN III] (233.1)
      - HGSIL of cervix (795.04)
    - Coding Clinic: 2004, Q4, P86-88; 1991, Q1, P11
    - **622.10 Dysplasia of cervix, unspecified**
      - Anaplasia of cervix
      - Cervical atypism
      - Cervical dysplasia NOS
    - **622.11 Mild dysplasia of cervix**
      - Cervical intraepithelial neoplasia I [CIN I]
    - **622.12 Moderate dysplasia of cervix**
      - Cervical intraepithelial neoplasia II [CIN II]
      - **Excludes:** carcinoma in situ of cervix (233.1)
        - cervical intraepithelial neoplasia III [CIN III] (233.1)
        - severe dysplasia (233.1)
  - **622.2 Leukoplakia of cervix (uteri)**
    - **Excludes:** carcinoma in situ of cervix (233.1)
  - **622.3 Old laceration of cervix**
    - Adhesions of cervix
    - Band(s) of cervix
    - Cicatrix (postpartum) of cervix
    - **Excludes:** current obstetrical trauma (665.3)
  - **622.4 Stricture and stenosis of cervix**
    - Atresia (acquired) of cervix
    - Contracture of cervix
    - Occlusion of cervix
    - Pinpoint os uteri
    - **Excludes:** congenital (752.49)
      - that complicating labor (654.6)
  - **622.5 Incompetence of cervix**
    - **Excludes:** complicating pregnancy (654.5)
      - that affecting fetus or newborn (761.0)
  - **622.6 Hypertrophic elongation of cervix**
  - **622.7 Mucous polyp of cervix**
    - Polyp NOS of cervix
    - **Excludes:** adenomatous polyp of cervix (219.0)
  - **622.8 Other specified noninflammatory disorders of cervix**
    - Atrophy (senile) of cervix
    - Cyst of cervix
    - Fibrosis of cervix
    - Hemorrhage of cervix
    - **Excludes:** endometriosis (617.0)
      - fistula (619.0–619.8)
      - inflammatory diseases (616.0)
  - **622.9 Unspecified noninflammatory disorder of cervix**

- **623 Noninflammatory disorders of vagina**
  - **Excludes:** abnormality of vagina complicating pregnancy, labor, or delivery (654.7)
    - congenital absence of vagina (752.49)
    - congenital diaphragm or bands (752.49)
    - fistulas involving vagina (619.0–619.8)
  - **623.0 Dysplasia of vagina**
    - Mild and moderate dysplasia of vagina
    - Vaginal intraepithelial neoplasia I and II [VAIN I and II]
    - **Excludes:** abnormal results from vaginal cytological examination without histologic confirmation (795.10-795.19)
      - carcinoma in situ of vagina (233.31)
      - HGSIL of vagina (795.14)
      - severe dysplasia of vagina (233.31)
      - vaginal intraepithelial neoplasia III [VAIN III] (233.31)
  - **623.1 Leukoplakia of vagina**
  - **623.2 Stricture or atresia of vagina**
    - Adhesions (postoperative) (postradiation) of vagina
    - Occlusion of vagina
    - Stenosis, vagina
    - Use additional E code to identify any external cause
    - **Excludes:** congenital atresia or stricture (752.49)
  - **623.3 Tight hymenal ring**
    - Rigid hymen acquired or congenital
    - Tight hymenal ring acquired or congenital
    - Tight introitus acquired or congenital
    - **Excludes:** imperforate hymen (752.42)
  - **623.4 Old vaginal laceration**
    - **Excludes:** old laceration involving muscles of pelvic floor (618.7)
  - **623.5 Leukorrhea, not specified as infective**
    - Leukorrhea NOS of vagina
    - Vaginal discharge NOS
    - **Excludes:** trichomonal (131.00)
  - **623.6 Vaginal hematoma**
    - **Excludes:** current obstetrical trauma (665.7)
  - **623.7 Polyp of vagina**
  - **623.8 Other specified noninflammatory disorders of vagina**
    - Cyst of vagina
    - Hemorrhage of vagina
  - **623.9 Unspecified noninflammatory disorder of vagina**

- **624 Noninflammatory disorders of vulva and perineum**
  - **Excludes:** abnormality of vulva and perineum complicating pregnancy, labor, or delivery (654.8)
    - condyloma acuminatum (078.11)
    - fistulas involving:
      - perineum - see Alphabetic Index
      - vulva (619.0–619.8)
    - vulval varices (456.6)
    - vulvar involvement in skin conditions (690–709.9)
  - **624.0 Dystrophy of vulva**
    - **Excludes:** carcinoma in situ of vulva (233.32)
      - severe dysplasia of vulva (233.32)
      - vulvar intraepithelial neoplasia III [VIN III] (233.32)
    - **624.01 Vulvar intraepithelial neoplasia I [VIN I]**
      - Mild dysplasia of vulva
    - **624.02 Vulvar intraepithelial neoplasia II [VIN II]**
      - Moderate dysplasia of vulva
      - Coding Clinic: 2007, Q4, P90-91
    - **624.09 Other dystrophy of vulva**
      - Kraurosis of vulva
      - Leukoplakia of vulva

624.1 Atrophy of vulva
624.2 Hypertrophy of clitoris
　　Excludes *that in endocrine disorders (255.2, 256.1)*
624.3 Hypertrophy of labia
　　Hypertrophy of vulva NOS
624.4 Old laceration or scarring of vulva
624.5 Hematoma of vulva
　　Excludes *that complicating delivery (664.5)*
624.6 Polyp of labia and vulva
624.8 Other specified noninflammatory disorders of vulva and perineum
　　Cyst of vulva
　　Edema of vulva
　　Stricture of vulva
　　Coding Clinic: 2003, Q1, P13-14; 1995, Q1, P8
624.9 Unspecified noninflammatory disorder of vulva and perineum

● **625** Pain and other symptoms associated with female genital organs
625.0 Dyspareunia
　　Painful intercourse/coitus
　　Excludes *psychogenic dyspareunia (302.76)*
625.1 Vaginismus
　　Colpospasm
　　Vulvismus
　　Excludes *psychogenic vaginismus (306.51)*
625.2 Mittelschmerz
　　Intermenstrual pain
　　Ovulation pain
625.3 Dysmenorrhea
　　Painful menstruation
　　Excludes *psychogenic dysmenorrhea (306.52)*
　　Coding Clinic: 1994, Q2, P12
625.4 Premenstrual tension syndromes
　　Menstrual molimen
　　Premenstrual dysphoric disorder
　　Premenstrual syndrome
　　Premenstrual tension NOS
　　Excludes *menstrual migraine (346.4)*
　　Coding Clinic: 2003, Q4, P116
625.5 Pelvic congestion syndrome
　　Congestion-fibrosis syndrome
　　Taylor's syndrome
625.6 Stress incontinence, female
　　Excludes *mixed incontinence (788.33)*
　　　　　　　stress incontinence, male (788.32)
● **625.7** Vulvodynia
　　Coding Clinic: 2008, Q4, P124
　　625.70 Vulvodynia, unspecified
　　　　Vulvodynia NOS
　　625.71 Vulvar vestibulitis
　　625.79 Other vulvodynia
625.8 Other specified symptoms associated with female genital organs
　　Coding Clinic: 1985, Nov-Dec, P16
625.9 Unspecified symptom associated with female genital organs
　　Coding Clinic: 2006, Q4, P109-110; 1994, Q2, P12; 1985, Nov-Dec, P16

● **626** Disorders of menstruation and other abnormal bleeding from female genital tract
　　Excludes *menopausal and premenopausal bleeding (627.0)*
　　　　　　pain and other symptoms associated with menstrual cycle (625.2–625.4)
　　　　　　postmenopausal bleeding (627.1)
　　　　　　precocious puberty (259.1)
626.0 Absence of menstruation
　　Amenorrhea (primary) (secondary)
　　Coding Clinic: 1985, July-Aug, P9
626.1 Scanty or infrequent menstruation
　　Hypomenorrhea
　　Oligomenorrhea
626.2 Excessive or frequent menstruation
　　Heavy periods　　　　Menorrhagia
　　Menometrorrhagia　　Polymenorrhea
　　Excludes *premenopausal (627.0)*
　　　　　　that in puberty (626.3)
　　Coding Clinic: 2011, Q4, P147; 2006, Q4, P97-98; 2004, Q4, P88-90; 1994, Q2, P12
626.3 Puberty bleeding
　　Excessive bleeding associated with onset of menstrual periods
　　Pubertal menorrhagia
626.4 Irregular menstrual cycle
　　Irregular:　　　　　　Irregular:
　　　bleeding NOS　　　　periods
　　　menstruation
626.5 Ovulation bleeding
　　Regular intermenstrual bleeding
626.6 Metrorrhagia
　　Bleeding unrelated to menstrual cycle
　　Irregular intermenstrual bleeding
626.7 Postcoital bleeding
626.8 Other
　　Dysfunctional or functional uterine hemorrhage NOS
　　Menstruation:　　　　Menstruation:
　　　retained　　　　　　suppression of
626.9 Unspecified

● **627** Menopausal and postmenopausal disorders
　　Excludes *asymptomatic age-related (natural) postmenopausal status (V49.81)*
627.0 Premenopausal menorrhagia
　　Excessive bleeding associated with onset of menopause
　　Menorrhagia:　　　　Menorrhagia:
　　　climacteric　　　　　preclimacteric
　　　menopausal
627.1 Postmenopausal bleeding
627.2 Symptomatic menopausal or female climacteric states
　　Symptoms, such as flushing, sleeplessness, headache, lack of concentration, associated with the menopause
627.3 Postmenopausal atrophic vaginitis
　　Senile (atrophic) vaginitis
627.4 Symptomatic states associated with artificial menopause
　　Postartificial menopause syndromes
　　Any condition classifiable to 627.1, 627.2, or 627.3 which follows induced menopause
627.8 Other specified menopausal and postmenopausal disorders
　　Excludes *premature menopause NOS (256.31)*
627.9 Unspecified menopausal and postmenopausal disorder

- **628 Infertility, female**
  - **Includes** primary and secondary sterility
  - Coding Clinic: 1996, Q2, P9; 1995, Q1, P7
  - **628.0 Associated with anovulation**
    - Anovulatory cycle
    - Use additional code for any associated Stein-Leventhal syndrome (256.4)
  - **628.1 Of pituitary-hypothalamic origin**
    - *Code first underlying disease, as:*
      - adiposogenital dystrophy (253.8)
      - anterior pituitary disorder (253.0–253.4)
  - **628.2 Of tubal origin**
    - Infertility associated with congenital anomaly of tube
    - Tubal:
      - block
      - occlusion
    - Tubal:
      - stenosis
    - Use additional code for any associated peritubal adhesions (614.6)
  - **628.3 Of uterine origin**
    - Infertility associated with congenital anomaly of uterus
    - Nonimplantation
    - Use additional code for any associated tuberculous endometritis (016.7)
  - **628.4 Of cervical or vaginal origin**
    - Infertility associated with:
      - anomaly or cervical mucus
      - congenital structural anomaly
      - dysmucorrhea
  - **628.8 Of other specified origin**
  - **628.9 Of unspecified origin**
- **629 Other disorders of female genital organs**
  - **629.0 Hematocele, female, not elsewhere classified**
    - **Excludes** *hematocele or hematoma:*
      - *broad ligament (620.7)*
      - *fallopian tube (620.8)*
      - *that associated with ectopic pregnancy (633.00–633.91)*
      - *uterus (621.4)*
      - *vagina (623.6)*
      - *vulva (624.5)*
  - **629.1 Hydrocele, canal of Nuck**
    - Cyst of canal of Nuck (acquired)
    - **Excludes** *congenital (752.41)*
  - **629.2 Female genital multilation status**
    - Female circumcision status
    - Female genital cutting
    - **629.20 Female genital mutilation status, unspecified**
      - Female genital cutting status, unspecified
      - Female genital mutilation status NOS
    - **629.21 Female genital mutilation Type I status**
      - Clitorectomy status
      - Female genital cutting Type I status
    - **629.22 Female genital mutilation Type II status**
      - Clitorectomy with excision of labia minora status
      - Female genital cutting Type II status
      - Coding Clinic: 2004, Q4, P88-90
    - **629.23 Female genital mutilation Type III status**
      - Female genital cutting Type III status
      - Infibulation status
    - **629.29 Other female genital mutilation status**
      - Female genital cutting Type IV status
      - Female genital mutilation Type IV status
      - Other female genital cutting status
  - **629.3 Complication of implanted vaginal mesh and other prosthetic materials**
    - **629.31 Erosion of implanted vaginal mesh and other prosthetic materials to surrounding organ or tissue**
      - Erosion of implanted vaginal mesh and other prosthetic materials into pelvic floor muscles
    - **629.32 Exposure of implanted vaginal mesh and other prosthetic materials into vagina**
      - Exposure of vaginal mesh and other prosthetic materials through vaginal wall
  - **629.8 Other specified disorders of female genital organs**
    - **629.81 Recurrent pregnancy loss without current pregnancy**
      - **Excludes** *recurrent pregnancy loss with current pregnancy (646.3)*
      - Coding Clinic: 2006, Q4, P98
    - **629.89 Other specified disorders of female genital organs**
  - **629.9 Unspecified disorder of female genital organs**

(See Plate 375 on page NAP-4.)

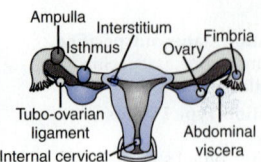

Figure 11-1 Implantation sites of ectopic pregnancy.

Item 11-1 Ectopic pregnancy most often occurs in the fallopian tube. Pregnancy outside the uterus may end in a life-threatening rupture.

Item 11-2 A hydatidiform mole is a benign tumor of the placenta. The tumor secretes a hormone, chorionic gonadotropic hormone (CGH), that indicates a positive pregnancy test.

OGCR Section I.C.11.a.1 and 2

Obstetric cases require codes from chapter 11, codes in the range 630-679, Complications of Pregnancy, Childbirth, and the Puerperium. Chapter 11 codes have sequencing priority over codes from other chapters. Additional codes from other chapters may be used in conjunction with chapter 11 codes to further specify conditions. Should the provider document that the pregnancy is incidental to the encounter, then code V22.2 should be used in place of any chapter 11 codes. It is the provider's responsibility to state that the condition being treated is not affecting the pregnancy.

11. COMPLICATIONS OF PREGNANCY, CHILDBIRTH, AND THE PUERPERIUM (630–679)

ECTOPIC AND MOLAR PREGNANCY (630–633)

Use additional code from category 639 to identify any complications

630 Hydatidiform mole
  Trophoblastic disease NOS
  Vesicular mole
  Excludes chorioadenoma (destruens) (236.1)
    chorionepithelioma (181)
    malignant hydatidiform mole (236.1)

● **631 Other abnormal product of conception**
  631.0 Inappropriate change in quantitative human chorionic gonadotropin (hCG) in early pregnancy
    Biochemical pregnancy
    Chemical pregnancy
    Inappropriate level of quantitative human chorionic gonadotropin (hCG) for gestational age in early pregnancy
    Excludes blighted ovum (631.8)
      molar pregnancy (631.8)
  631.8 Other abnormal products of conception
    Blighted ovum

632 Missed abortion
  Early fetal death before completion of 22 weeks' gestation with retention of dead fetus
  Retained products of conception, not following spontaneous or induced abortion or delivery
  Excludes failed induced abortion (638.0–638.9)
    fetal death (intrauterine) (late) (656.4)
    missed delivery (656.4)
    that with hydatidiform mole (630)
    that with other abnormal products of conception (631.8)
  Coding Clinic: 2001, Q1, P5

● **633 Ectopic pregnancy**
  Includes ruptured ectopic pregnancy
  Coding Clinic: 2002, Q4, P61-62
  ● **633.0 Abdominal pregnancy**
    Intraperitoneal pregnancy
    633.00 Abdominal pregnancy without intrauterine pregnancy
    633.01 Abdominal pregnancy with intrauterine pregnancy
  ● **633.1 Tubal pregnancy**
    Fallopian pregnancy
    Rupture of (fallopian) tube due to pregnancy
    Tubal abortion
    633.10 Tubal pregnancy without intrauterine pregnancy
    633.11 Tubal pregnancy with intrauterine pregnancy
  ● **633.2 Ovarian pregnancy**
    633.20 Ovarian pregnancy without intrauterine pregnancy
    633.21 Ovarian pregnancy with intrauterine pregnancy
  ● **633.8 Other ectopic pregnancy**
    Pregnancy:
      cervical
      combined
      cornual
      intraligamentous
      mesometric
      mural
    633.80 Other ectopic pregnancy without intrauterine pregnancy
    633.81 Other ectopic pregnancy with intrauterine pregnancy
  ● **633.9 Unspecified ectopic pregnancy**
    ■ **633.90 Unspecified ectopic pregnancy without intrauterine pregnancy**
    ■ **633.91 Unspecified ectopic pregnancy with intrauterine pregnancy**

OTHER PREGNANCY WITH ABORTIVE OUTCOME (634–639)

The following fourth digit subdivisions are for use with categories 634-638:

0 Complicated by genital tract and pelvic infection
  Endometritis
  Salpingo-oophoritis
  Sepsis NOS
  Septicemia NOS
  Any condition classifiable to 639.0, with condition classifiable to 634–638
  Excludes urinary tract infection (634–638 with .7)
1 Complicated by delayed or excessive hemorrhage
  Afibrinogenemia
  Defibrination syndrome
  Intravascular hemolysis
  Any condition classifiable to 639.1, with condition classifiable to 634–638
2 Complicated by damage to pelvic organs and tissues
  Laceration, perforation, or tear of:
    bladder
    uterus
  Any condition classifiable to 639.2, with condition classifiable to 634–638
3 Complicated by renal failure
  Oliguria
  Uremia
  Any condition classifiable to 639.3, with condition classifiable to 634–638
4 Complicated by metabolic disorder
  Electrolyte imbalance with conditions classifiable to 634–638

    5 **Complicated by shock**
        Circulatory collapse
        Shock (postoperative) (septic)
        Any condition classifiable to 639.5, with condition classifiable to 634–638
    6 **Complicated by embolism**
        Embolism:
            NOS
            amniotic fluid
            pulmonary
        Any condition classifiable to 639.6, with condition classifiable to 634–638
    7 **With other specified complications**
        Cardiac arrest or failure
        Urinary tract infection
        Any condition classifiable to 639.8, with condition classifiable to 634–638
    8 **With unspecified complications**
    9 **Without mention of complication**

OGCR Section I.C.11.k.1

Fifth-digits are required for abortion categories 634-637. Fifth digit assignment is based on the status of the patient at the beginning (or start) of the encounter. Fifth-digit 1, incomplete, indicates that all of the products of conception have not been expelled from the uterus. Fifth-digit 2, complete, indicates that all products of conception have been expelled from the uterus.

OGCR Section I.C.11.k.5

Subsequent admissions for retained products of conception following a spontaneous or legally induced abortion are assigned the appropriate code from category 634, Spontaneous abortion, or 635 Legally induced abortion, with a fifth digit of "1" (incomplete). This advice is appropriate even when the patient was discharged previously with a discharge diagnosis of complete abortion.

● 634 **Spontaneous abortion**
    Requires fifth digit to identify stage:

    0 unspecified
    1 incomplete
    2 complete

    Includes miscarriage
             spontaneous abortion

● 634.0 **Complicated by genital tract and pelvic**
    [0-2] infection
● 634.1 **Complicated by delayed or excessive hemorrhage**
    [0-2] Coding Clinic: 2003, Q1, P6
● 634.2 **Complicated by damage to pelvic organs or**
    [0-2] tissues
● 634.3 **Complicated by renal failure**
    [0-2]
● 634.4 **Complicated by metabolic disorder**
    [0-2]
● 634.5 **Complicated by shock**
    [0-2]
● 634.6 **Complicated by embolism**
    [0-2]
● 634.7 **With other specified complications**
    [0-2]
● ■ 634.8 **With unspecified complication**
    [0-2]
● 634.9 **Without mention of complication**
    [0-2]

● 635 **Legally induced abortion**
    Requires fifth digit to identify stage:

    0 unspecified
    1 incomplete
    2 complete

    Includes abortion or termination of pregnancy:
             elective
             legal
             therapeutic
    Excludes menstrual extraction or regulation (V25.3)

● 635.0 **Complicated by genital tract and pelvic**
    [0-2] infection
● 635.1 **Complicated by delayed or excessive hemorrhage**
    [0-2]
● 635.2 **Complicated by damage to pelvic organs or**
    [0-2] tissues
● 635.3 **Complicated by renal failure**
    [0-2]
● 635.4 **Complicated by metabolic disorder**
    [0-2]
● 635.5 **Complicated by shock**
    [0-2]
● 635.6 **Complicated by embolism**
    [0-2]
● 635.7 **With other specified complications**
    [0-2]
● ■ 635.8 **With unspecified complication**
    [0-2]
● 635.9 **Without mention of complication**
    [0-2] Coding Clinic: 2010, Q2, P7; 1994, Q2, P14

● 636 **Illegally induced abortion**
    Requires fifth digit to identify stage:

    0 unspecified
    1 incomplete
    2 complete

    Includes abortion:
             criminal
             illegal
             self-induced

● 636.0 **Complicated by genital tract and pelvic**
    [0-2] infection
● 636.1 **Complicated by delayed or excessive hemorrhage**
    [0-2]
● 636.2 **Complicated by damage to pelvic organs or**
    [0-2] tissues
● 636.3 **Complicated by renal failure**
    [0-2]
● 636.4 **Complicated by metabolic disorder**
    [0-2]
● 636.5 **Complicated by shock**
    [0-2]
● 636.6 **Complicated by embolism**
    [0-2]
● 636.7 **With other specified complications**
    [0-2]
● ■ 636.8 **With unspecified complication**
    [0-2]
● 636.9 **Without mention of complication**
    [0-2]

● **637 Unspecified abortion**
Requires following fifth digit to identify stage:
Coding Clinic: 1994, Q2, P14

  ▫ 0 unspecified
  1 incomplete
  2 complete

  Includes abortion NOS
  retained products of conception following abortion, not classifiable elsewhere

  ● 637.0 Complicated by genital tract and pelvic infection
  [0-2]
  ● 637.1 Complicated by delayed or excessive hemorrhage
  [0-2]
  ● 637.2 Complicated by damage to pelvic organs or tissues
  [0-2]
  ● 637.3 Complicated by renal failure
  [0-2]
  ● 637.4 Complicated by metabolic disorder
  [0-2]
  ● 637.5 Complicated by shock
  [0-2]
  ● 637.6 Complicated by embolism
  [0-2]
  ● 637.7 With other specified complications
  [0-2]
  ● ▫ 637.8 With unspecified complication
  [0-2]
  ● 637.9 Without mention of complication
  [0-2]

● **638 Failed attempted abortion**
  Includes failure of attempted induction of (legal) abortion
  Excludes incomplete abortion (634.0–637.9)
  638.0 Complicated by genital tract and pelvic infection
  638.1 Complicated by delayed or excessive hemorrhage
  638.2 Complicated by damage to pelvic organs or tissues
  638.3 Complicated by renal failure
  638.4 Complicated by metabolic disorder
  638.5 Complicated by shock
  638.6 Complicated by embolism
  638.7 With other specified complications
  ▫ 638.8 With unspecified complication
  638.9 Without mention of complication

OGCR Section I.C.11.k.3

Code 639 is to be used for all complications following abortion. Code 639 cannot be assigned with codes from categories 634-638.

● **639 Complications following abortion and ectopic and molar pregnancies**
  Note: This category is provided for use when it is required to classify separately the complications classifiable to the fourth digit level in categories 634–638; for example:
  a) when the complication itself was responsible for an episode of medical care, the abortion, ectopic or molar pregnancy itself having been dealt with at a previous episode
  b) when these conditions are immediate complications of ectopic or molar pregnancies classifiable to 630–633 where they cannot be identified at fourth digit level.

  639.0 Genital tract and pelvic infection
  Endometritis following conditions classifiable to 630–638
  Parametritis following conditions classifiable to 630–638
  Pelvic peritonitis following conditions classifiable to 630–638
  Salpingitis following conditions classifiable to 630–638
  Salpingo-oophoritis following conditions classifiable to 630–638
  Sepsis NOS following conditions classifiable to 630–638
  Septicemia NOS following conditions classifiable to 630–638
  Excludes urinary tract infection (639.8)

  639.1 Delayed or excessive hemorrhage
  Afibrinogenemia following conditions classifiable to 630–638
  Defibrination syndrome following conditions classifiable to 630–638
  Intravascular hemolysis following conditions classifiable to 630–638

  639.2 Damage to pelvic organs and tissues
  Laceration, perforation, or tear of:
  bladder following conditions classifiable to 630–638
  bowel following conditions classifiable to 630–638
  broad ligament following conditions classifiable to 630–638
  cervix following conditions classifiable to 630–638
  periurethral tissue following conditions classifiable to 630–638
  uterus following conditions classifiable to 630–638
  vagina following conditions classifiable to 630–638

  639.3 Kidney failure
  Oliguria following conditions classifiable to 630–638
  Renal (kidney):
  failure (acute) following conditions classifiable to 630–638
  shutdown following conditions classifiable to 630–638
  tubular necrosis following conditions classifiable to 630–638
  Uremia following conditions classifiable to 630–638

  639.4 Metabolic disorders
  Electrolyte imbalance following conditions classifiable to 630–638

  639.5 Shock
  Circulatory collapse following conditions classifiable to 630–638
  Shock (postoperative) (septic) following conditions classifiable to 630–638

  639.6 Embolism
  Embolism:
  NOS following conditions classifiable to 630–638
  air following conditions classifiable to 630–638
  amniotic fluid following conditions classifiable to 630–638
  blood-clot following conditions classifiable to 630–638
  fat following conditions classifiable to 630–638
  pulmonary following conditions classifiable to 630–638
  pyemic following conditions classifiable to 630–638
  septic following conditions classifiable to 630–638
  soap following conditions classifiable to 630–638

  639.8 Other specified complications following abortion or ectopic and molar pregnancy
  Acute yellow atrophy or necrosis of liver following conditions classifiable to 630–638
  Cardiac arrest or failure following conditions classifiable to 630–638
  Cerebral anoxia following conditions classifiable to 630–638
  Urinary tract infection following conditions classifiable to 630–638

  ▫ 639.9 Unspecified complication following abortion or ectopic and molar pregnancy
  Complication(s) not further specified following conditions classifiable to 630–638

OGCR Section I.C.11.k.2
A code from categories 640-649 and 651-659 may be used as additional codes with an abortion code to indicate the complication leading to the abortion. Fifth digit 3 is assigned with codes from these categories when used with an abortion code because the other fifth digits will not apply. Codes from the 660-669 series are not to be used for complications of abortion.

Item 11-3 Placenta previa is a condition in which the opening of the cervix is obstructed by the displaced placenta. The three types, marginal, partial, and total, are varying degrees of placenta displacement. Placenta abruption is the premature breaking away of the placenta from the site of the uterine implant before the delivery of the fetus.

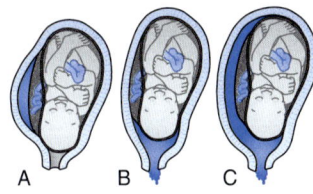

Figure 11-2 Abruptio placentae is classified according to the grade of separation of the placenta from the uterine wall. **A.** Mild separation in which hemorrhage is internal. **B.** Moderate separation in which there is external hemorrhage. **C.** Severe separation in which there is external hemorrhage and extreme separation.

COMPLICATIONS MAINLY RELATED TO PREGNANCY (640–649)

Includes the listed conditions even if they arose or were present during labor, delivery, or the puerperium

The following fifth-digit subclassification is for use with categories 640–649 to denote the current episode of care:

> 0 unspecified as to episode of care or not applicable
> 1 delivered, with or without mention of antepartum condition
>   Antepartum condition with delivery
>   Delivery NOS (with mention of antepartum complication during current episode of care)
>   Intrapartum obstetric condition (with mention of antepartum complication during current episode of care)
>   Pregnancy, delivered (with mention of antepartum complication during current episode of care)
> 2 delivered, with mention of postpartum complication
>   Delivery with mention of puerperal complication during current episode of care
> 3 antepartum condition or complication
>   Antepartum obstetric condition, not delivered during the current episode of care
> 4 postpartum condition or complication
>   Postpartum or puerperal obstetric condition or complication following delivery that occurred:
>   during previous episode of care
>   outside hospital, with subsequent admission for observation or care

● **640 Hemorrhage in early pregnancy**
Requires fifth digit; valid digits are in [brackets] under each code. See beginning of section 640–649 for definitions.
Includes hemorrhage before completion of 22 weeks' gestation

● **640.0 Threatened abortion**
[0,1,3]

● **640.8 Other specified hemorrhage in early pregnancy**
[0,1,3]

● **640.9 Unspecified hemorrhage in early pregnancy**
[0,1,3]

● **641 Antepartum hemorrhage, abruptio placentae, and placenta previa**
Requires fifth digit; valid digits are in [brackets] under each code. See beginning of section 640–649 for definitions.

● **641.0 Placenta previa without hemorrhage**
[0,1,3]   Low implantation of placenta without hemorrhage
Placenta previa noted:
   during pregnancy without hemorrhage
   before labor (and delivered by cesarean delivery) without hemorrhage

● **641.1 Hemorrhage from placenta previa**
[0,1,3]   Low-lying placenta NOS or with hemorrhage (intrapartum)
Placenta previa:
   incomplete NOS or with hemorrhage (intrapartum)
   marginal NOS or with hemorrhage (intrapartum)
   partial NOS or with hemorrhage (intrapartum)
   total NOS or with hemorrhage (intrapartum)
Excludes hemorrhage from vasa previa (663.5)

● **641.2 Premature separation of placenta**
[0,1,3]   Ablatio placentae
Abruptio placentae
Accidental antepartum hemorrhage
Couvelaire uterus
Detachment of placenta (premature)
Premature separation of normally implanted placenta

● **641.3 Antepartum hemorrhage associated with coagulation defects**
[0,1,3]
Antepartum or intrapartum hemorrhage associated with:
   afibrinogenemia
   hyperfibrinolysis
   hypofibrinogenemia
Excludes coagulation defects not associated with antepartum hemorrhage (649.3)

● **641.8 Other antepartum hemorrhage**
[0,1,3]   Antepartum or intrapartum hemorrhage associated with:
   trauma
   uterine leiomyoma

● **641.9 Unspecified antepartum hemorrhage**
[0,1,3]   Hemorrhage:
   antepartum NOS
   intrapartum NOS
   of pregnancy NOS

● **642 Hypertension complicating pregnancy, childbirth, and the puerperium**
Requires fifth digit; valid digits are in [brackets] under each code. See beginning of section 640–649 for definitions.

● **642.0 Benign essential hypertension complicating pregnancy, childbirth, and the puerperium**
[0-4]
Hypertension:
   benign essential specified as complicating, or as a reason for obstetric care during pregnancy, childbirth, or the puerperium
   chronic NOS specified as complicating, or as a reason for obstetric care during pregnancy, childbirth, or the puerperium
   essential specified as complicating, or as a reason for obstetric care during pregnancy, childbirth, or the puerperium
   pre-existing NOS specified as complicating, or as a reason for obstetric care during pregnancy, childbirth, or the puerperium

● **642.1 Hypertension secondary to renal disease, complicating pregnancy, childbirth, and the puerperium**
[0-4]
Hypertension secondary to renal disease, specified as complicating, or as a reason for obstetric care during pregnancy, childbirth, or the puerperium

COMPLICATIONS OF PREGNANCY, CHILDBIRTH, AND THE PUERPERIUM (630–679)

● **642.2** **Other pre-existing hypertension complicating**
[0-4] **pregnancy, childbirth, and the puerperium**
Hypertensive:
chronic kidney disease specified as complicating, or as a reason for obstetric care during pregnancy, childbirth, or the puerperium
heart and chronic kidney disease specified as complicating, or as a reason for obstetric care during pregnancy, childbirth, or the puerperium
heart disease specified as complicating, or as a reason for obstetric care during pregnancy, childbirth, or the puerperium
Malignant hypertension specified as complicating, or as a reason for obstetric care during pregnancy, childbirth, or the puerperium

● **642.3** **Transient hypertension of pregnancy**
[0-4] Gestational hypertension
Transient hypertension, so described, in pregnancy, childbirth, or the puerperium

OGCR Section I.C.7.a.8
Assign code 796.2, Elevated blood pressure reading without diagnosis of hypertension, unless patient has an established diagnosis of hypertension. Assign code 642.3x for transient hypertension of pregnancy.

● **642.4** **Mild or unspecified pre-eclampsia**
[0-4] Hypertension in pregnancy, childbirth, or the puerperium, not specified as pre-existing, with either albuminuria or edema, or both; mild or unspecified
Pre-eclampsia:
  NOS
  mild
Toxemia (pre-eclamptic):
  NOS
  mild

Excludes albuminuria in pregnancy, without mention of hypertension (646.2)
edema in pregnancy, without mention of hypertension (646.1)
Coding Clinic: 2009, Q4, P108

● **642.5** **Severe pre-eclampsia**
[0-4] Hypertension in pregnancy, childbirth, or the puerperium, not specified as pre-existing, with either albuminuria or edema, or both; specified as severe
Pre-eclampsia, severe
Toxemia (pre-eclamptic), severe

● **642.6** **Eclampsia**
[0-4] Toxemia:
eclamptic
with convulsions

● **642.7** **Pre-eclampsia or eclampsia superimposed on pre-**
[0-4] **existing hypertension**
Conditions classifiable to 642.4–642.6, with conditions classifiable to 642.0–642.2

● **642.9** **Unspecified hypertension complicating pregnancy,**
[0-4] **childbirth, or the puerperium**
Hypertension NOS, without mention of albuminuria or edema, complicating pregnancy, childbirth, or the puerperium
Coding Clinic: 2009, Q1, P18

● **643** **Excessive vomiting in pregnancy**
Requires fifth digit; valid digits are in [brackets] under each code. See beginning of section 640–649 for definitions.
Includes hyperemesis arising during pregnancy
vomiting:
  persistent arising during pregnancy
  vicious arising during pregnancy
hyperemesis gravidarum

● **643.0** **Mild hyperemesis gravidarum**
[0,1,3] Hyperemesis gravidarum, mild or unspecified, starting before the end of the 22nd week of gestation

● **643.1** **Hyperemesis gravidarum with metabolic**
[0,1,3] **disturbance**
Hyperemesis gravidarum, starting before the end of the 22nd week of gestation, with metabolic disturbance, such as:
  carbohydrate depletion
  dehydration
  electrolyte imbalance

● **643.2** **Late vomiting of pregnancy**
[0,1,3] Excessive vomiting starting after 22 completed weeks of gestation

● **643.8** **Other vomiting complicating pregnancy**
[0,1,3] Vomiting due to organic disease or other cause, specified as complicating pregnancy, or as a reason for obstetric care during pregnancy
Use additional code to specify cause

● **643.9** **Unspecified vomiting of pregnancy**
[0,1,3] Vomiting as a reason for care during pregnancy, length of gestation unspecified

● **644** **Early or threatened labor**
Requires fifth digit; valid digits are in [brackets] under each code. See beginning of section 640–649 for definitions.

● **644.0** **Threatened premature labor**
[0,3] Premature labor after 22 weeks, but before 37 completed weeks of gestation without delivery
Excludes that occurring before 22 completed weeks of gestation (640.0)

● **644.1** **Other threatened labor**
[0,3] False labor:
  NOS without delivery
  after 37 completed weeks of gestation without delivery
Threatened labor NOS without delivery

● **644.2** **Early onset of delivery**
[0-1] Onset (spontaneous) of delivery before 37 completed weeks of gestation
Premature labor with onset of delivery before 37 completed weeks of gestation
Coding Clinic: 2011, Q3, P3; 1991, Q2, P16

OGCR Section I.C.11.k.4
When an attempted termination of pregnancy results in a liveborn fetus assign code 644.21, Early onset of delivery, with an appropriate code from category V27, Outcome of Delivery. The procedure code for the attempted termination of pregnancy should also be assigned.

● **645** **Late pregnancy**
Requires fifth digit; valid digits are in [brackets] under each code. See beginning of section 640–649 for definitions.
Coding Clinic: 2000, Q1, P17-18

● **645.1** **Post term pregnancy**
[0,1,3] Pregnancy over 40 completed weeks to 42 completed weeks gestation

● **645.2** **Prolonged pregnancy**
[0,1,3] Pregnancy which has advanced beyond 42 completed weeks of gestation

● **646 Other complications of pregnancy, not elsewhere classified**
Use additional code(s) to further specify complication
Requires fifth digit; valid digits are in [brackets] under each code. See beginning of section 640–649 for definitions.

● **646.0 Papyraceous fetus**
[0,1,3]

● **646.1 Edema or excessive weight gain in pregnancy,**
[0-4] **without mention of hypertension**
Gestational edema
Maternal obesity syndrome
Excludes that with mention of hypertension (642.0–642.9)

● ■ **646.2 Unspecified renal disease in pregnancy, without**
[0-4] **mention of hypertension**
Albuminuria in pregnancy or the puerperium, without mention of hypertension
Nephropathy NOS in pregnancy or the puerperium, without mention of hypertension
Renal disease NOS in pregnancy or the puerperium, without mention of hypertension
Uremia in pregnancy or the puerperium, without mention of hypertension
Gestational proteinuria in pregnancy or the puerperium, without mention of hypertension
Excludes that with mention of hypertension (642.0–642.9)

● **646.3 Recurrent pregnancy loss**
[0,1,3]   **Excludes** with current abortion (634.0–634.9)
without current pregnancy (629.81)

● **646.4 Peripheral neuritis in pregnancy**
[0-4]

● **646.5 Asymptomatic bacteriuria in pregnancy**
[0-4]

● **646.6 Infections of genitourinary tract in**
[0-4] **pregnancy**
Conditions classifiable to 590, 595, 597, 599.0, 616 complicating pregnancy, childbirth, or the puerperium
Conditions classifiable to 614.0–614.5, 614.7–614.9, 615 complicating pregnancy or labor
Excludes major puerperal infection (670.0-670.8)
Coding Clinic: 2004, Q4, P88-90

OGCR Section I.C.2.g.
During pregnancy, childbirth or the puerperium, a patient admitted (or presenting for a health care encounter) because of an HIV-related illness should receive a principal diagnosis code of 647.6X, Other specified infectious and parasitic diseases in the mother classifiable elsewhere, but complicating the pregnancy, childbirth or the puerperium, followed by 042 and the code(s) for the HIV-related illness(es). Codes from Chapter 15 always take sequencing priority. Patients with asymptomatic HIV infection status admitted (or presenting for a health care encounter) during pregnancy, childbirth, or the puerperium should receive codes of 647.6X and V08.

● **646.7 Liver and biliary tract disorders in**
[0,1,3] **pregnancy**
Acute yellow atrophy of liver (obstetric) (true) of pregnancy
Icterus gravis of pregnancy
Necrosis of liver of pregnancy
Excludes hepatorenal syndrome following delivery (674.8)
viral hepatitis (647.6)

● **646.8 Other specified complications of pregnancy**
[0-4]   Fatigue during pregnancy
Herpes gestationis
Insufficient weight gain of pregnancy
Coding Clinic: 1998, Q3, P16; 1985, Jan-Feb, P15-16

● ■ **646.9 Unspecified complication of pregnancy**
[0,1,3]

● **647 Infectious and parasitic conditions in the mother classifiable elsewhere, but complicating pregnancy, childbirth, or the puerperium**
Use additional code(s) to further specify complication
Requires fifth digit; valid digits are in [brackets] under each code. See beginning of section 640–649 for definitions.
Includes the listed conditions when complicating the pregnant state, aggravated by the pregnancy, or when a main reason for obstetric care
Excludes those conditions in the mother known or suspected to have affected the fetus (655.0–655.9)

● **647.0 Syphilis**
[0-4]   Conditions classifiable to 090–097

● **647.1 Gonorrhea**
[0-4]   Conditions classifiable to 098

● **647.2 Other venereal diseases**
[0-4]   Conditions classifiable to 099

● **647.3 Tuberculosis**
[0-4]   Conditions classifiable to 010–018

● **647.4 Malaria**
[0-4]   Conditions classifiable to 084

● **647.5 Rubella**
[0-4]   Conditions classifiable to 056

● **647.6 Other viral diseases**
[0-4]   Conditions classifiable to 042, 050-055, 057-079, 795.05, 795.15, 796.75
Coding Clinic: 2010, Q2, P10; 1985, Jan-Feb, P15-16

● **647.8 Other specified infectious and parasitic**
[0-4] **diseases**

● ■ **647.9 Unspecified infection or infestation**
[0-4]

● **648 Other current conditions in the mother classifiable elsewhere, but complicating pregnancy, childbirth, or the puerperium**
Use additional code(s) to identify the condition
Requires fifth digit; valid digits are in [brackets] under each code. See beginning of section 640–649 for definitions.
Includes the listed conditions when complicating the pregnant state, aggravated by the pregnancy, or when a main reason for obstetric care
Excludes those conditions in the mother known or suspected to have affected the fetus (655.0–655.9)

● **648.0 Diabetes mellitus**
[0-4]   Conditions classifiable to 249, 250
Excludes gestational diabetes (648.8)

● **648.1 Thyroid dysfunction**
[0-4]   Conditions classifiable to 240–246

● **648.2 Anemia**
[0-4]   Conditions classifiable to 280–285
Coding Clinic: 2002, Q1, P14

● **648.3 Drug dependence**
[0-4]   Conditions classifiable to 304
Coding Clinic: 1998, Q2, P13-14; 1988, Q4, P8

● **648.4 Mental disorders**
[0-4]   Conditions classifiable to 290–303, 305.0, 305.2–305.9, 306–316, 317–319
Coding Clinic: 1998, Q2, P13-14

● **648.5 Congenital cardiovascular disorders**
[0-4]   Conditions classifiable to 745–747

● **648.6 Other cardiovascular diseases**
[0-4]   Conditions classifiable to 390–398, 410–429
Excludes cerebrovascular disorders in the puerperium (674.0)
peripartum cardiomyopathy (674.5)
venous complications (671.0–671.9)
Coding Clinic: 2012, Q3, P10; 1998, Q3, P11

648.7–651.3   ICD-9-CM

- **648.7** Bone and joint disorders of back, pelvis, and lower limbs
  [0-4]
  Conditions classifiable to 720–724, and those classifiable to 711–719 or 725–738, specified as affecting the lower limbs

- **648.8** Abnormal glucose tolerance
  [0-4]
  Conditions classifiable to 790.21–790.29
  Gestational diabetes
  Use additional code, if applicable, for associated long-term (current) insulin use V58.67
  Coding Clinic: 2004, Q4, P53-56

- **648.9** Other current conditions classifiable elsewhere
  [0-4]
  Conditions classifiable to 440–459, 795.01–795.04, 795.06, 795.10–795.14, 795.16, 796.70–796.74, 796.76
  Nutritional deficiencies [conditions classifiable to 260–269]
  Coding Clinic: 2009, Q1, P17; 2006, Q3, P14; 2004, Q4, P88-90; 2002, Q1, P14-15; 1984, Nov-Dec, P18

- **649** Other conditions or status of the mother complicating pregnancy, childbirth, or the puerperium
  Requires fifth digit; valid digits are in [brackets] under each code. See beginning of section 640-649 for definitions.

- **649.0** Tobacco use disorder complicating pregnancy, childbirth, or the puerperium
  [0-4]
  Smoking complicating pregnancy, childbirth, or the puerperium

- **649.1** Obesity complicating pregnancy, childbirth, or the puerperium
  [0-4]
  Use additional code to identify the obesity (278.00-278.03)

- **649.2** Bariatric surgery status complicating pregnancy, childbirth, or the puerperium
  [0-4]
  Gastric banding status complicating pregnancy, childbirth, or the puerperium
  Gastric bypass status for obesity complicating pregnancy, childbirth, or the puerperium
  Obesity surgery status complicating pregnancy, childbirth, or the puerperium

- **649.3** Coagulation defects complicating pregnancy, childbirth, or the puerperium
  [0-4]
  Conditions classifiable to 286, 287, 289
  Use additional code to identify the specific coagulation defect (286.0–286.9, 287.0-287.9, 289.0-289.9)
  Excludes: coagulation defects causing antepartum hemorrhage (641.3)

- **649.4** Epilepsy complicating pregnancy, childbirth, or the puerperium
  [0-4]
  Conditions classifiable to 345
  Use additional code to identify the specific type of epilepsy (345.00–345.91)
  Excludes: eclampsia (642.6)

- **649.5** Spotting complicating pregnancy
  [0,1,3]
  Excludes: antepartum hemorrhage (641.0–641.9)
  hemorrhage in early pregnancy (640.0–640.9)

OGCR Section I.C.11.h.1
Code 650 is for use in cases when a woman is admitted for a full-term normal delivery and delivers a single, healthy infant without any complications antepartum, during the delivery, or postpartum during the delivery episode. Code 650 is always a principal diagnosis. It is not to be used if any other code from chapter 11 is needed to describe a current complication of the antenatal, delivery, or perinatal period. Additional codes from other chapters may be used with code 650 if they are not related to or are in any way complicating the pregnancy.

OGCR Section I.C.11.h.2
Code 650 may be used if the patient had a complication at some point during her pregnancy, but the complication is not present at the time of the admission for delivery.

OGCR Section I.C.11.h.3
V27.0, Single liveborn, is the only outcome of delivery code appropriate for use with 650.

OGCR Section I.C.11.i.1
The postpartum period begins immediately after delivery and continues for six weeks following delivery. The peripartum period is defined as the last month of pregnancy to five months postpartum.

- **649.6** Uterine size date discrepancy
  [0-4]
  Excludes: suspected problem with fetal growth not found (V89.04)

- **649.7** Cervical shortening
  [0,1,3]
  Excludes: suspected cervical shortening not found (V89.05)
  Coding Clinic: 2008, Q4, P124-125

- **649.8** Onset (spontaneous) of labor after 37 completed weeks of gestation but before 39 completed weeks gestation, with delivery by (planned) cesarean section
  [1-2]
  Delivery by (planned) cesarean section occurring after 37 completed weeks of gestation but before 39 completed weeks gestation due to (spontaneous) onset of labor
  Use additional code to specify reason for planned cesarean section such as:
  cephalopelvic disproportion (normally formed fetus) (653.4)
  previous cesarean delivery (654.2)
  Coding Clinic: 2011, Q4, P133

NORMAL DELIVERY, AND OTHER INDICATIONS FOR CARE IN PREGNANCY, LABOR, AND DELIVERY (650–659)

The following fifth-digit subclassification is for use with categories 651–659 to denote the current episode of care:

0 unspecified as to episode of care or not applicable
1 delivered, with or without mention of antepartum condition
2 delivered, with mention of postpartum complication
3 antepartum condition or complication
4 postpartum condition or complication

- **650** Normal delivery
  Delivery requiring minimal or no assistance, with or without episiotomy, without fetal manipulation [e.g., rotation version] or instrumentation [forceps] of a spontaneous, cephalic, vaginal, full-term, single, live-born infant. This code is for use as a single diagnosis code and is not to be used with any other code in the range 630–676.
  Use additional code to indicate outcome of delivery (V27.0)
  Excludes: breech delivery (assisted) (spontaneous) NOS (652.2)
  delivery by vacuum extractor, forceps, cesarean section, or breech extraction, without specified complication (669.5–669.7)
  Coding Clinic: 2002, Q2, P10; 2001, Q3, P12; 2000, Q3, P5

- **651** Multiple gestation
  Requires fifth digit; valid digits are in [brackets] under each code. See beginning of section 650–659 for definitions.
  Use additional code to specify placenta status (V91.00-V91.99)
  Excludes: fetal conjoined twins (678.1)

- **651.0** Twin pregnancy
  [0,1,3]
  Excludes: fetal conjoined twins (678.1)
  Coding Clinic: 2006, Q3, P16-18; 1992, Q3, P10

- **651.1** Triplet pregnancy
  [0,1,3]

- **651.2** Quadruplet pregnancy
  [0,1,3]

- **651.3** Twin pregnancy with fetal loss and retention of one fetus
  [0,1,3]

OGCR Section I.C.11.k.2
A code from categories 640-649 and 651-659 may be used as additional codes with an abortion code to indicate the complication leading to the abortion. Fifth digit 3 is assigned with codes from these categories when used with an abortion code because the other fifth digits will not apply. Codes from the 660-669 series are not to be used for complications of abortion.

- **651.4** Triplet pregnancy with fetal loss and retention of one or more fetus(es)
  [0,1,3]
- **651.5** Quadruplet pregnancy with fetal loss and retention of one or more fetus(es)
  [0,1,3]
- **651.6** Other multiple pregnancy with fetal loss and retention of one or more fetus(es)
  [0,1,3]
- **651.7** Multiple gestation following (elective) fetal reduction
  [0,1,3]
  Fetal reduction of multiple fetuses reduced to single fetus
  Coding Clinic: 2006, Q3, P16-18; 2005, Q4, P81
- **651.8** Other specified multiple gestation
  [0,1,3]
- **651.9** Unspecified multiple gestation
  [0,1,3]

- **652** Malposition and malpresentation of fetus
  Requires fifth digit; valid digits are in [brackets] under each code. See beginning of section 650–659 for definitions.
  Code first any associated obstructed labor (660.0)
  Coding Clinic: 1995, Q3, P10
- **652.0** Unstable lie
  [0,1,3]
- **652.1** Breech or other malpresentation successfully converted to cephalic presentation
  [0,1,3]
  Cephalic version NOS
- **652.2** Breech presentation without mention of version
  [0,1,3]
  Breech delivery (assisted) (spontaneous) NOS
  Buttocks presentation
  Complete breech
  Frank breech
  Excludes footling presentation (652.8)
  incomplete breech (652.8)
- **652.3** Transverse or oblique presentation
  [0,1,3]
  Oblique lie
  Transverse lie
  Excludes transverse arrest of fetal head (660.3)
- **652.4** Face or brow presentation
  [0,1,3]
  Mentum presentation
- **652.5** High head at term
  [0,1,3]
  Failure of head to enter pelvic brim

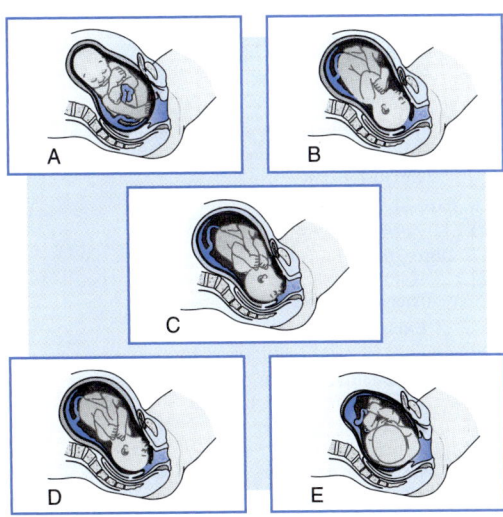

Figure 11-3 Five types of malposition and malpresentation of the fetus: **A.** Breech. **B.** Vertex. **C.** Face. **D.** Brow. **E.** Shoulder.

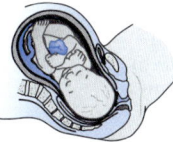

Figure 11-4 Hydrocephalic fetus causing disproportion.

- **652.6** Multiple gestation with malpresentation of one fetus or more
  [0,1,3]
- **652.7** Prolapsed arm
  [0,1,3]
- **652.8** Other specified malposition or malpresentation
  [0,1,3] Compound presentation
- **652.9** Unspecified malposition or malpresentation
  [0,1,3]

- **653** Disproportion
  Requires fifth digit; valid digits are in [brackets] under each code. See beginning of section 650–659 for definitions.
  Code first any associated obstructed labor (660.1)
  Coding Clinic: 1995, Q3, P10
- **653.0** Major abnormality of bony pelvis, not further specified
  [0,1,3]
  Pelvic deformity NOS
- **653.1** Generally contracted pelvis
  [0,1,3] Contracted pelvis NOS
- **653.2** Inlet contraction of pelvis
  [0,1,3] Inlet contraction (pelvis)
- **653.3** Outlet contraction of pelvis
  [0,1,3] Outlet contraction (pelvis)
- **653.4** Fetopelvic disproportion
  [0,1,3] Cephalopelvic disproportion NOS
  Disproportion of mixed maternal and fetal origin, with normally formed fetus
- **653.5** Unusually large fetus causing disproportion
  [0,1,3] Disproportion of fetal origin with normally formed fetus
  Fetal disproportion NOS
  Excludes that when the reason for medical care was concern for the fetus (656.6)
- **653.6** Hydrocephalic fetus causing disproportion
  [0,1,3] **Excludes** that when the reason for medical care was concern for the fetus (655.0)
- **653.7** Other fetal abnormality causing disproportion
  [0,1,3] Fetal: Fetal:
           ascites   sacral teratoma
           hydrops   tumor
           myelomeningocele
  Excludes conjoined twins causing disporportion (678.1)
- **653.8** Disproportion of other origin
  [0,1,3] **Excludes** shoulder (girdle) dystocia (660.4)
- **653.9** Unspecified disproportion
  [0,1,3]

- **654** Abnormality of organs and soft tissues of pelvis
  Requires fifth digit; valid digits are in [brackets] under each code. See beginning of section 650–659 for definitions.
  Includes the listed conditions during pregnancy, childbirth, or the puerperium
  Code first any associated obstructed labor (660.2)
  Excludes trauma to perineum and vulva complicating current delivery (664.0–664.9)
  Coding Clinic: 1995, Q3, P10
- **654.0** Congenital abnormalities of uterus
  [0-4] Double uterus
  Uterus bicornis
- **654.1** Tumors of body of uterus
  [0-4] Uterine fibroids
  Coding Clinic: 1994, Q2, P14
- **654.2** Previous cesarean delivery
  [0,1,3] Uterine scar from previous cesarean delivery
  Coding Clinic: 2011, Q4, P133

654.3 Retroverted and incarcerated gravid uterus
[0-4]

654.4 Other abnormalities in shape or position of gravid uterus and of neighboring structures
[0-4]
- Cystocele
- Pelvic floor repair
- Pendulous abdomen
- Prolapse of gravid uterus
- Rectocele
- Rigid pelvic floor

654.5 Cervical incompetence
[0-4]
Presence of Shirodkar suture with or without mention of cervical incompetence

654.6 Other congenital or acquired abnormality of cervix
[0-4]
- Cicatricial cervix
- Polyp of cervix
- Previous surgery to cervix
- Rigid cervix (uteri)
- Stenosis or stricture of cervix
- Tumor of cervix

654.7 Congenital or acquired abnormality of vagina
[0-4]
- Previous surgery to vagina
- Septate vagina
- Stenosis of vagina (acquired) (congenital)
- Stricture of vagina
- Tumor of vagina

654.8 Congenital or acquired abnormality of vulva
[0-4]
- Anal sphincter tear (healed) (old) complicating delivery
- Fibrosis of perineum
- Persistent hymen
- Previous surgery to perineum or vulva
- Rigid perineum
- Tumor of vulva

Excludes anal sphincter tear (healed) (old) not associated with delivery (569.43)
varicose veins of vulva (671.1)

Coding Clinic: 2003, Q1, P14

654.9 Other and unspecified
[0-4]
Uterine scar NEC

OGCR Section I.C.11.c.2

In cases when in utero surgery is performed on the fetus, a diagnosis code from category 655, Known or suspected fetal abnormalities affecting management of the mother, should be assigned identifying the fetal condition. Procedure code 75.36, Correction of fetal defect, should be assigned on the hospital inpatient record. No code from Chapter 15, the perinatal codes, should be used on the mother's record to identify fetal conditions. Surgery performed in utero on a fetus is still to be coded as an obstetric encounter.

655 Known or suspected fetal abnormality affecting management of mother

Requires fifth digit; valid digits are in [brackets] under each code. See beginning of section 650–659 for definitions.

Includes the listed conditions in the fetus as a reason for observation or obstetrical care of the mother, or for termination of pregnancy

655.0 Central nervous system malformation in fetus
[0,1,3]
Fetal or suspected fetal:
- anencephaly
- hydrocephalus
- spina bifida (with myelomeningocele)

655.1 Chromosomal abnormality in fetus
[0,1,3]

655.2 Hereditary disease in family possibly affecting fetus
[0,1,3]

655.3 Suspected damage to fetus from viral disease in the mother
[0,1,3]
Suspected damage to fetus from maternal rubella

655.4 Suspected damage to fetus from other disease in the mother
[0,1,3]
Suspected damage to fetus from maternal:
- alcohol addiction
- listeriosis
- toxoplasmosis

655.5 Suspected damage to fetus from drugs
[0,1,3]

655.6 Suspected damage to fetus from radiation
[0,1,3]

655.7 Decreased fetal movements
[0,1,3]
Coding Clinic: 1997, Q4, P41

655.8 Other known or suspected fetal abnormality, not elsewhere classified
[0,1,3]
Suspected damage to fetus from:
- environmental toxins
- intrauterine contraceptive device

Coding Clinic: 2006, Q3, P16-18x2

655.9 Unspecified
[0,1,3]
Coding Clinic: 2010, Q2, P7

656 Other known or suspected fetal and placental problems affecting management of mother

Requires fifth digit; valid digits are in [brackets] under each code. See beginning of section 650–659 for definitions.

Excludes fetal hematologic conditions (678.0)
suspected placental problems not found (V89.02)

656.0 Fetal-maternal hemorrhage
[0,1,3]
Leakage (microscopic) of fetal blood into maternal circulation

656.1 Rhesus isoimmunization
[0,1,3]
- Anti-D [Rh] antibodies
- Rh incompatibility

656.2 Isoimmunization from other and unspecified blood-group incompatibility
[0,1,3]
ABO isoimmunization
Coding Clinic: 2006, Q4, P135

656.3 Fetal distress
[0,1,3]
Fetal metabolic acidemia

Excludes abnormal fetal acid-base balance (656.8)
abnormality in fetal heart rate or rhythm (659.7)
fetal bradycardia (659.7)
fetal tachycardia (659.7)
meconium in liquor (656.8)

Coding Clinic: 2010, Q2, P7

656.4 Intrauterine death
[0,1,3]
Fetal death:
- NOS
- after completion of 22 weeks' gestation
- late

Missed delivery

Excludes missed abortion (632)

Coding Clinic: 2010, Q2, P7

656.5 Poor fetal growth
[0,1,3]
- "Light-for-dates"
- "Placental insufficiency"
- "Small-for-dates"

656.6 Excessive fetal growth
[0,1,3]
"Large-for-dates"

656.7 Other placental conditions
[0,1,3]
- Abnormal placenta
- Placental infarct

Excludes placental polyp (674.4)
placentitis (658.4)

656.8 Other specified fetal and placental problems
[0,1,3]
- Abnormal acid-base balance
- Intrauterine acidosis
- Lithopedian
- Meconium in liquor
- Subchorionic hematoma

656.9 Unspecified fetal and placental problem
[0,1,3]

● **657 Polyhydramnios**
[0,1,3] Hydramnios
Requires fifth digit; valid digits are in [brackets] under each code. See beginning of section 650–659 for definitions.
Use 0 as fourth digit for category 657
Excludes *suspected polyhydramnios not found (V89.01)*
Coding Clinic: 2006, Q3, P16-18

● **658 Other problems associated with amniotic cavity and membranes**
Requires fifth digit; valid digits are in [brackets] under each code. See beginning of section 650–659 for definitions.
Excludes *amniotic fluid embolism (673.1)*
suspected problems with amniotic cavity and membranes not found (V89.01)

● **658.0 Oligohydramnios**
[0,1,3] Oligohydramnios without mention of rupture of membranes
Coding Clinic: 2006, Q3, P16-18

● **658.1 Premature rupture of membranes**
[0,1,3] Rupture of amniotic sac less than 24 hours prior to the onset of labor
Coding Clinic: 2001, Q1, P5; 1998, Q4, P76-77

● **658.2 Delayed delivery after spontaneous or unspecified**
[0,1,3] rupture of membranes
Prolonged rupture of membranes NOS
Rupture of amniotic sac 24 hours or more prior to the onset of labor

● **658.3 Delayed delivery after artificial rupture of**
[0,1,3] membranes

● **658.4 Infection of amniotic cavity**
[0,1,3] Amnionitis   Membranitis
        Chorioamnionitis   Placentitis

● **658.8 Other**
[0,1,3] Amnion nodosum
Amniotic cyst

● **658.9 Unspecified**
[0,1,3]

● **659 Other indications for care or intervention related to labor and delivery, not elsewhere classified**
Requires fifth digit; valid digits are in [brackets] under each code. See beginning of section 650–659 for definitions.

● **659.0 Failed mechanical induction**
[0,1,3] Failure of induction of labor by surgical or other instrumental methods

● **659.1 Failed medical or unspecified induction**
[0,1,3] Failed induction NOS
Failure of induction of labor by medical methods, such as oxytocic drugs

● **659.2 Maternal pyrexia during labor, unspecified**
[0,1,3]

● **659.3 Generalized infection during labor**
[0,1,3] Septicemia during labor

● **659.4 Grand multiparity**
[0,1,3] **Excludes** *supervision only, in pregnancy (V23.3)*
without current pregnancy (V61.5)

● **659.5 Elderly primigravida**
[0,1,3] First pregnancy in a woman who will be 35 years of age or older at expected date of delivery
Excludes *supervision only, in pregnancy (V23.81)*
Coding Clinic: 2001, Q3, P12

● **659.6 Elderly multigravida**
[0,1,3] Second or more pregnancy in a woman who will be 35 years of age or older at expected date of delivery
Excludes *elderly primigravida (659.5)*
supervision only, in pregnancy (V23.82)
Coding Clinic: 2013, Q1, P19; 2001, Q3, P12

● **659.7 Abnormality in fetal heart rate or rhythm**
[0,1,3] Depressed fetal heart tones
Fetal:
   bradycardia
   tachycardia
Fetal heart rate decelerations
Non-reassuring fetal heart rate or rhythm
Coding Clinic: 1998, Q4, P47-48

● **659.8 Other specified indications for care or intervention**
[0,1,3] related to labor and delivery
Pregnancy in a female less than 16 years of age at expected date of delivery
Very young maternal age
Coding Clinic: 2001, Q3, P12

● **659.9 Unspecified indication for care or intervention**
[0,1,3] related to labor and delivery

OGCR Section I.C.11.k.2
Codes from the 660-669 series are not to be used for complications of abortion.

COMPLICATIONS OCCURRING MAINLY IN THE COURSE OF LABOR AND DELIVERY (660–669)

The following fifth-digit subclassification is for use with categories 660–669 to denote the current episode of care:

0 unspecified as to episode of care or not applicable
1 delivered, with or without mention of antepartum condition
2 delivered, with mention of postpartum complication
3 antepartum condition or complication
4 postpartum condition or complication

● **660 Obstructed labor**
Requires fifth digit; valid digits are in [brackets] under each code. See beginning of section 660–669 for definitions.
Coding Clinic: 1995, Q3, P10

● **660.0 Obstruction caused by malposition of fetus at onset**
[0,1,3] of labor
Any condition classifiable to 652, causing obstruction during labor
Use additional code from 652.0–652.9 to identify condition
Coding Clinic: 1995, Q3, P10

● **660.1 Obstruction by bony pelvis**
[0,1,3] Any condition classifiable to 653, causing obstruction during labor
Use additional code from 653.0–653.9 to identify condition
Coding Clinic: 1995, Q3, P10

● **660.2 Obstruction by abnormal pelvic soft tissues**
[0,1,3] Prolapse of anterior lip of cervix
Any condition classifiable to 654, causing obstruction during labor
Use additional code from 654.0–654.9 to identify condition
Coding Clinic: 1995, Q3, P10

● **660.3 Deep transverse arrest and persistent occipito-**
[0,1,3] posterior position

● **660.4 Shoulder (girdle) dystocia**
[0,1,3] Impacted shoulders

● **660.5 Locked twins**
[0,1,3]

● **660.6 Failed trial of labor, unspecified**
[0,1,3] Failed trial of labor, without mention of condition or suspected condition

● **660.7 Failed forceps or vacuum extractor, unspecified**
[0,1,3] Application of ventouse or forceps, without mention of condition

● **660.8 Other causes of obstructed labor**
[0,1,3] Use additional code to identify condition

● **660.9 Unspecified obstructed labor**
[0,1,3] Dystocia:
   NOS
   fetal NOS
   maternal NOS

- **661 Abnormality of forces of labor**
  Requires fifth digit; valid digits are in [brackets] under each code. See beginning of section 660–669 for definitions.
  - **661.0 Primary uterine inertia**
    [0,1,3]
    - Failure of cervical dilation
    - Hypotonic uterine dysfunction, primary
    - Prolonged latent phase of labor
    - *Coding Clinic: 1985, July-Aug, P11*
  - **661.1 Secondary uterine inertia**
    [0,1,3]
    - Arrested active phase of labor
    - Hypotonic uterine dysfunction, secondary
    - *Coding Clinic: 1985, July-Aug, P11*
  - **661.2 Other and unspecified uterine inertia**
    [0,1,3]
    - Atony of uterus without hemorrhage
    - Desultory labor
    - Irregular labor
    - Poor contractions
    - Slow slope active phase of labor
    - **Excludes** atony of uterus with hemorrhage (666.1)
      postpartum atony of uterus without hemorrhage (669.8)
    - *Coding Clinic: 1985, July-Aug, P11*
  - **661.3 Precipitate labor**
    [0,1,3]
  - **661.4 Hypertonic, incoordinate, or prolonged uterine contractions**
    [0,1,3]
    - Cervical spasm
    - Contraction ring (dystocia)
    - Dyscoordinate labor
    - Hourglass contraction of uterus
    - Hypertonic uterine dysfunction
    - Incoordinate uterine action
    - Retraction ring (Bandl's) (pathological)
    - Tetanic contractions
    - Uterine dystocia NOS
    - Uterine spasm
  - **661.9 Unspecified abnormality of labor**
    [0,1,3]

- **662 Long labor**
  Requires fifth digit; valid digits are in [brackets] under each code. See beginning of section 660–669 for definitions.
  - **662.0 Prolonged first stage**
    [0,1,3]
  - **662.1 Prolonged labor, unspecified**
    [0,1,3]
  - **662.2 Prolonged second stage**
    [0,1,3]
  - **662.3 Delayed delivery of second twin, triplet, etc.**
    [0,1,3]

- **663 Umbilical cord complications**
  Requires fifth digit; valid digits are in [brackets] under each code. See beginning of section 660–669 for definitions.
  - **663.0 Prolapse of cord**
    [0,1,3]
    - Presentation of cord
  - **663.1 Cord around neck, with compression**
    [0,1,3]
    - Cord tightly around neck
  - **663.2 Other and unspecified cord entanglement, with compression**
    [0,1,3]
    - Entanglement of cords of twins in mono-amniotic sac
    - Knot in cord (with compression)
  - **663.3 Other and unspecified cord entanglement, without mention of compression**
    [0,1,3]
    - *Coding Clinic: 2003, Q2, P9*
  - **663.4 Short cord**
    [0,1,3]
  - **663.5 Vasa previa**
    [0,1,3]
  - **663.6 Vascular lesions of cord**
    [0,1,3]
    - Bruising of cord
    - Hematoma of cord
    - Thrombosis of vessels of cord
  - **663.8 Other umbilical cord complications**
    [0,1,3]
    - Velamentous insertion of umbilical cord
  - **663.9 Unspecified umbilical cord complication**
    [0,1,3]

- **664 Trauma to perineum and vulva during delivery**
  Requires fifth digit; valid digits are in [brackets] under each code. See beginning of section 660–669 for definitions.
  Includes damage from instruments
  that from extension of episiotomy
  Coding Clinic: 2008, Q4, P192; 1992, Q1, P10-11
  - **664.0 First-degree perineal laceration**
    [0,1,4]
    - Perineal laceration, rupture, or tear involving:
      - fourchette
      - hymen
      - labia vulva
      - skin
      - vagina
    - *Coding Clinic: 1984, Nov-Dec, P10*
  - **664.1 Second-degree perineal laceration**
    [0,1,4]
    - Perineal laceration, rupture, or tear (following episiotomy) involving:
      - pelvic floor
      - perineal muscles
      - vaginal muscles
    - **Excludes** that involving anal sphincter (664.2)
    - *Coding Clinic: 2008, Q4, P192; 1984, Nov-Dec, P10*
  - **664.2 Third-degree perineal laceration**
    [0,1,4]
    - Perineal laceration, rupture, or tear (following episiotomy) involving:
      - anal sphincter
      - rectovaginal septum
      - sphincter NOS
    - **Excludes** anal sphincter tear during delivery not associated with third-degree perineal laceration (664.6)
      that with anal or rectal mucosal laceration (664.3)
    - *Coding Clinic: 1984, Nov-Dec, P10*
  - **664.3 Fourth-degree perineal laceration**
    [0,1,4]
    - Perineal laceration, rupture, or tear as classifiable to 664.2 and involving also:
      - anal mucosa
      - rectal mucosa
    - *Coding Clinic: 1984, Nov-Dec, P10*
  - **664.4 Unspecified perineal laceration**
    [0,1,4]
    - Central laceration
  - **664.5 Vulval and perineal hematoma**
    [0,1,4]
    - *Coding Clinic: 1984, Nov-Dec, P10*
  - **664.6 Anal sphincter tear complicating delivery, not associated with third-degree perineal laceration**
    [0,1,4]
    - **Excludes** third-degree perineal laceration (664.2)
    - *Coding Clinic: 2007, Q4, P88-90*
  - **664.8 Other specified trauma to perineum and vulva**
    [0,1,4]
    - Periurethral trauma
    - *Coding Clinic: 2007, Q4, P125*
  - **664.9 Unspecified trauma to perineum and vulva**
    [0,1,4]

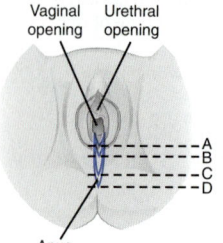

Figure 11–5 Perineal lacerations:
A. First-degree is laceration of superficial tissues.
B. Second-degree is limited to the pelvic floor and may involve the perineal or vaginal muscles.
C. Third-degree involves the anal sphincter.
D. Fourth-degree involves anal or rectal mucosa.

665 Other obstetrical trauma

Requires fifth digit; valid digits are in [brackets] under each code. See beginning of section 660–669 for definitions.

Includes damage from instruments

- **665.0 Rupture of uterus before onset of labor**
  [0,1,3]

- **665.1 Rupture of uterus during labor**
  [0,1] Rupture of uterus NOS

- **665.2 Inversion of uterus**
  [0,2,4]

- **665.3 Laceration of cervix**
  [0,1,4] *Coding Clinic: 1984, Nov-Dec, P10*

- **665.4 High vaginal laceration**
  [0,1,4] Laceration of vaginal wall or sulcus without mention of perineal laceration
  Coding Clinic: 1984, Nov-Dec, P10

- **665.5 Other injury to pelvic organs**
  [0,1,4] Injury to:
  bladder
  urethra
  Excludes periurethral trauma (664.8)
  Coding Clinic: 1984, Nov-Dec, P10, 12

- **665.6 Damage to pelvic joints and ligaments**
  [0,1,4] Avulsion of inner symphyseal cartilage
  Damage to coccyx
  Separation of symphysis (pubis)

- **665.7 Pelvic hematoma**
  [0-2,4] Hematoma of vagina
  Coding Clinic: 1984, Nov-Dec, P10

- **665.8 Other specified obstetrical trauma**
  [0-4]

- **665.9 Unspecified obstetrical trauma**
  [0-4]

666 Postpartum hemorrhage

Requires fifth digit; valid digits are in [brackets] under each code. See beginning of section 660–669 for definitions.

- **666.0 Third-stage hemorrhage**
  [0,2,4] Hemorrhage associated with retained, trapped, or adherent placenta
  Retained placenta NOS
  Coding Clinic: 1988, Q1, P14

- **666.1 Other immediate postpartum hemorrhage**
  [0,2,4] Atony of uterus with hemorrhage
  Hemorrhage within the first 24 hours following delivery of placenta
  Postpartum atony of uterus with hemorrhage
  Postpartum hemorrhage (atonic) NOS
  Excludes atony of uterus without hemorrhage (661.2)
  postpartum atony of uterus without hemorrhage (669.8)
  Coding Clinic: 1988, Q1, P14

- **666.2 Delayed and secondary postpartum hemorrhage**
  [0,2,4] Hemorrhage:
  after the first 24 hours following delivery
  associated with retained portions of placenta or membranes
  Postpartum hemorrhage specified as delayed or secondary
  Retained products of conception NOS, following delivery
  Coding Clinic: 1988, Q1, P14

- **666.3 Postpartum coagulation defects**
  [0,2,4] Postpartum:
  afibrinogenemia
  fibrinolysis

667 Retained placenta without hemorrhage

Requires fifth digit; valid digits are in [brackets] under each code. See beginning of section 660–669 for definitions.

- **667.0 Retained placenta without hemorrhage**
  [0,2,4] Placenta accreta without hemorrhage
  Retained placenta:
  NOS without hemorrhage
  total without hemorrhage
  Coding Clinic: 1988, Q1, P14

- **667.1 Retained portions of placenta or membranes, without hemorrhage**
  [0,2,4] Retained products of conception following delivery, without hemorrhage
  Coding Clinic: 1988, Q1, P14

668 Complications of the administration of anesthetic or other sedation in labor and delivery

Use additional code(s) to further specify complication

Requires fifth digit; valid digits are in [brackets] under each code. See beginning of section 660–669 for definitions.

Includes complications arising from the administration of a general or local anesthetic, analgesic, or other sedation in labor and delivery

Excludes reaction to spinal or lumbar puncture (349.0)
spinal headache (349.0)

- **668.0 Pulmonary complications**
  [0-4] Inhalation [aspiration] of stomach contents or secretions following anesthesia or other sedation in labor or delivery
  Mendelson's syndrome following anesthesia or other sedation in labor or delivery
  Pressure collapse of lung following anesthesia or other sedation in labor or delivery

- **668.1 Cardiac complications**
  [0-4] Cardiac arrest or failure following anesthesia or other sedation in labor and delivery

- **668.2 Central nervous system complications**
  [0-4] Cerebral anoxia following anesthesia or other sedation in labor and delivery

- **668.8 Other complications of anesthesia or other sedation in labor and delivery**
  [0-4] *Coding Clinic: 1999, Q2, P9-10*

- **668.9 Unspecified complication of anesthesia and other sedation**
  [0-4]

669 Other complications of labor and delivery, not elsewhere classified

Requires fifth digit; valid digits are in [brackets] under each code. See beginning of section 660–669 for definitions.

- **669.0 Maternal distress**
  [0-4] Metabolic disturbance in labor and delivery

- **669.1 Shock during or following labor and delivery**
  [0-4] Obstetric shock

- **669.2 Maternal hypotension syndrome**
  [0-4]

- **669.3 Acute kidney failure following labor and delivery**
  [0,2,4]

- **669.4 Other complications of obstetrical surgery and procedures**
  [0-4] Cardiac:
  arrest following cesarean or other obstetrical surgery or procedure, including delivery NOS
  failure following cesarean or other obstetrical surgery or procedure, including delivery NOS
  Cerebral anoxia following cesarean or other obstetrical surgery or procedure, including delivery NOS
  Excludes complications of obstetrical surgical wounds (674.1–674.3)

- **669.5 Forceps or vacuum extractor delivery without mention of indication**
  [0,1]
  Delivery by ventouse, without mention of indication
- **669.6 Breech extraction, without mention of indication**
  [0,1]
  Excludes breech delivery NOS (652.2)
- **669.7 Cesarean delivery, without mention of indication**
  [0,1]
  Coding Clinic: 2001, Q1, P11-12
- **669.8 Other complications of labor and delivery**
  [0-4]
  Coding Clinic: 2006, Q4, P135
- **669.9 Unspecified complication of labor and delivery**
  [0-4]

COMPLICATIONS OF THE PUERPERIUM (670–677)

Note: Categories 671 and 673–676 include the listed conditions even if they occur during pregnancy or childbirth.

The following fifth-digit subclassification is for use with categories 670–676 to denote the current episode of care:

```
0  unspecified as to episode of care or not applicable
1  delivered, with or without mention of antepartum condition
2  delivered, with mention of postpartum complication
3  antepartum condition or complication
4  postpartum condition or complication
```

- **670 Major puerperal infection**
  Requires fifth digit; valid digits are in [brackets] under each code. See beginning of section 670–676 for definitions.
  Excludes infection following abortion (639.0)
  minor genital tract infection following delivery (646.6)
  puerperal fever NOS (672)
  puerperal pyrexia NOS (672)
  puerperal pyrexia of unknown origin (672)
  urinary tract infection following delivery (646.6)
  Coding Clinic: 2007, Q3, P10
- **670.0 Major puerpal infection, unspecified**
  [0,2,4]
- **670.1 Puerpal endometritis**
  [0,2,4]
- **670.2 Puerpal sepsis**
  [0,2,4]
  Puerpal pyemia
  Use additional code to identify severe sepsis (995.92) and any associated acute organ dysfunction, if applicable
  Coding Clinic: 2009, Q4, P108
- **670.3 Puerpal septic thrombophlebitis**
  [0,2,4]
- **670.8 Other major puerpal infection**
  [0,2,4]
  Puerpal:
  pelvic cellulitis
  peritonitis
  salpingitis
- **671 Venous complications in pregnancy and the puerperium**
  Excludes personal history of venous complications prior to pregnancy, such as:
  thrombophlebitis (V12.52)
  thrombosis and embolism (V12.51)
  Requires fifth digit; valid digits are in [brackets] under each code. See beginning of section 670–676 for definitions.
- **671.0 Varicose veins of legs**
  [0-4]
  Varicose veins NOS
- **671.1 Varicose veins of vulva and perineum**
  [0-4]
- **671.2 Superficial thrombophlebitis**
  [0-4]
  Phlebitis NOS
  Thrombophlebitis (superficial)
  Thrombosis NOS
  Use additional code to identify the superficial thrombophlebitis (453.6, 453.71, 453.81)
- **671.3 Deep phlebothrombosis, antepartum**
  [0,1,3]
  Use additional code to identify the deep vein thrombosis (453.40-453.42, 453.50-453.52, 453.72-453.79, 453.82-453.89)
  Use additional code for long-term (current) use of anticoagulants if applicable (V58.61)
  Deep-vein thrombosis, antepartum
- **671.4 Deep phlebothrombosis, postpartum**
  [0,2,4]
  Deep-vein thrombosis, postpartum
  Pelvic thrombophlebitis, postpartum
  Phlegmasia alba dolens (puerperal)
  Use additional code to identify the deep vein thrombosis (453.40-453.42, 453.50-453.52, 453.72-453.79, 453.82-453.89)
  Use additional code for long-term (current) use of anticoagulants if applicable (V58.61)
- **671.5 Other phlebitis and thrombosis**
  [0-4]
  Cerebral venous thrombosis
  Thrombosis of intracranial venous sinus
- **671.8 Other venous complications**
  [0-4]
  Hemorrhoids
- **671.9 Unspecified venous complication**
  [0-4]
- **672 Pyrexia of unknown origin during the puerperium**
  [0,2,4]
  Postpartum fever NOS
  Puerperal fever NOS
  Puerperal pyrexia NOS
  Requires fifth digit; valid digits are in [brackets] under each code. See beginning of section 670–676 for definitions.
  Use 0 as fourth digit for category 672
- **673 Obstetrical pulmonary embolism**
  Requires fifth digit; valid digits are in [brackets] under each code. See beginning of section 670–676 for definitions.
  Includes pulmonary emboli in pregnancy, childbirth, or the puerperium, or specified as puerperal
  Excludes embolism following abortion (639.6)
- **673.0 Obstetrical air embolism**
  [0-4]
- **673.1 Amniotic fluid embolism**
  [0-4]
- **673.2 Obstetrical blood-clot embolism**
  [0-4]
  Puerperal pulmonary embolism NOS
- **673.3 Obstetrical pyemic and septic embolism**
  [0-4]
- **673.8 Other pulmonary embolism**
  [0-4]
  Fat embolism
- **674 Other and unspecified complications of the puerperium, not elsewhere classified**
  Requires fifth digit; valid digits are in [brackets] under each code. See beginning of section 670–676 for definitions.
- **674.0 Cerebrovascular disorders in the puerperium**
  [0-4]
  Any condition classifiable to 430–434, 436–437 occurring during pregnancy, childbirth, or the puerperium, or specified as puerperal
  Excludes intracranial venous sinus thrombosis (671.5)
- **674.1 Disruption of cesarean wound**
  [0,2,4]
  Dehiscence or disruption of uterine wound
  Excludes uterine rupture before onset of labor (665.0)
  uterine rupture during labor (665.1)
- **674.2 Disruption of perineal wound**
  [0,2,4]
  Breakdown of perineum
  Disruption of wound of:
  episiotomy
  perineal laceration
  Secondary perineal tear
  Coding Clinic: 1997, Q1, P9-10

- **674.3 Other complications of obstetrical surgical wounds**
  [0,2,4]
  Hematoma of cesarean section or perineal wound
  Hemorrhage of cesarean section or perineal wound
  Infection of cesarean section or perineal wound
  > **Excludes** *damage from instruments in delivery (664.0–665.9)*
  Coding Clinic: 2009, Q4, P108

- **674.4 Placental polyp**
  [0,2,4]

- **674.5 Peripartum cardiomyopathy**
  [0-4] Postpartum cardiomyopathy
  Coding Clinic: 2012, Q3, P10; 2003, Q4, P65

- **674.8 Other**
  [0,2,4]
  Hepatorenal syndrome, following delivery
  Postpartum:
    subinvolution of uterus
    uterine hypertrophy
  Coding Clinic: 1998, Q3, P16

- **674.9 Unspecified**
  [0,2,4] Sudden death of unknown cause during the puerperium

- **675 Infections of the breast and nipple associated with childbirth**
  Requires fifth digit; valid digits are in [brackets] under each code. See beginning of section 670–676 for definitions.
  > **Includes** the listed conditions during pregnancy, childbirth, or the puerperium

- **675.0 Infections of nipple**
  [0-4] Abscess of nipple

- **675.1 Abscess of breast**
  [0-4]
  Abscess: Mastitis:
    mammary   purulent
    subareolar   retromammary
    submammary   submammary

- **675.2 Nonpurulent mastitis**
  [0-4]
  Lymphangitis of breast
  Mastitis:
    NOS
    interstitial
    parenchymatous

- **675.8 Other specified infections of the breast and nipple**
  [0-4]

- **675.9 Unspecified infection of the breast and nipple**
  [0-4]

- **676 Other disorders of the breast associated with childbirth and disorders of lactation**
  Requires fifth digit; valid digits are in [brackets] under each code. See beginning of section 670–676 for definitions.
  > **Includes** the listed conditions during pregnancy, the puerperium, or lactation

- **676.0 Retracted nipple**
  [0-4]

- **676.1 Cracked nipple**
  [0-4] Fissure of nipple

- **676.2 Engorgement of breasts**
  [0-4]

- **676.3 Other and unspecified disorder of breast**
  [0-4]

- **676.4 Failure of lactation**
  [0-4] Agalactia

- **676.5 Suppressed lactation**
  [0-4]

- **676.6 Galactorrhea**
  [0-4]
  > **Excludes** *galactorrhea not associated with childbirth (611.6)*
  Coding Clinic: 1985, July-Aug, P9

- **676.8 Other disorders of lactation**
  [0-4] Galactocele
  Coding Clinic: 2012, Q3, P7

- **676.9 Unspecified disorder of lactation**
  [0-4]

- **677 Late effect of complication of pregnancy, childbirth, and the puerperium**
  Note: This category is to be used to indicate conditions in 632-648.9 and 651–676.9 as the cause of the late effect, themselves classifiable elsewhere. The "late effects" include conditions specified as such, or as sequelae, which may occur at any time after the puerperium.
  Code first any sequelae
  Coding Clinic: 1997, Q1, P9-10

  OGCR Section I.C.11.j.1-3
  1) **Code 677** Code 677, Late effect of complication of pregnancy, childbirth, and the puerperium is for use in those cases when an initial complication of a pregnancy develops a sequelae requiring care or treatment at a future date.
  2) **After the initial postpartum period** This code may be used at any time after the initial postpartum period.
  3) **Sequencing of Code 677** This code, like all late effect codes, is to be sequenced following the code describing the sequelae of the complication.

OTHER MATERNAL AND FETAL COMPLICATIONS (678-679)

The following fifth-digit subclassification is for use with categories 678-679 to denote the current episode of care:

0	unspecified as to episode of care or not applicable
1	delivered, with or without mention of antepartum condition
2	delivered, with mention of postpartum complication
3	antepartum condition or complication
4	postpartum condition or complication

- **678 Other fetal conditions**
  Requires fifth digit; valid digits are in [brackets] under each code. See beginning of section 678-679 for definitions.
  Coding Clinic: 2008, Q4, P125-127

- **678.0 Fetal hematologic conditions**
  [0,1,3]
  Fetal anemia
  Fetal thrombocytopenia
  Fetal twin to twin transfusion
  > **Excludes** *fetal and neonatal hemorrhage (772.0-772.9)*
  > *fetal hematologic disorders affecting newborn (776.0-776.9)*
  > *fetal-maternal hemorrhage (656.00-656.03)*
  > *isoimmunization incompatibility (656.10-656.13, 656.20-656.23)*

- **678.1 Fetal conjoined twins**
  [0,1,3]

- **679 Complications of in utero procedures**
  Requires fifth digit; valid digits are in [brackets] under each code. See beginning of section 678-679 for definitions.
  Coding Clinic: 2008, Q4, P127-128

- **679.0 Maternal complications from in utero procedure**
  [0-4]
  > **Excludes** *maternal history of in utero procedure during previous pregnancy (V23.86)*

- **679.1 Fetal complications from in utero procedure**
  [0-4] Fetal complications from amniocentesis
  > **Excludes** *newborn affected by in utero procedure (760.61-760.64)*

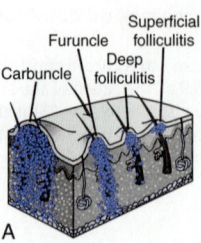
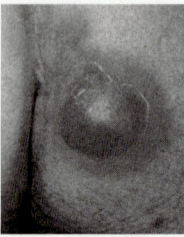

Figure 12-1 Furuncle, also known as a boil, is a staphylococcal infection. The organism enters the body through a hair follicle and so furuncles usually appear in hairy areas of the body. A cluster of furuncles is known as a carbuncle and involves infection into the deep subcutaneous fascia. These usually appear on the back and neck. (**B** from Habif: Clinical Dermatology, ed 5, Mosby, 2009)

12. DISEASES OF THE SKIN AND SUBCUTANEOUS TISSUE (680–709)

INFECTIONS OF SKIN AND SUBCUTANEOUS TISSUE (680–686)

Excludes certain infections of skin classified under "Infectious and Parasitic Diseases," such as:
- erysipelas (035)
- erysipeloid of Rosenbach (027.1)
- herpes:
  - simplex (054.0–054.9)
  - zoster (053.0–053.9)
- molluscum contagiosum (078.0)
- viral warts (078.10-078.19)

● **680 Carbuncle and furuncle**
  Includes boil
  furunculosis

  680.0 Face
   Ear [any part]   Nose (septum)
   Face [any part, except eye]   Temple (region)
   Excludes eyelid (373.13)
           lacrimal apparatus (375.31)
           orbit (376.01)

  680.1 Neck

  680.2 Trunk
   Abdominal wall
   Back [any part, except buttocks]
   Breast
   Chest wall
   Flank
   Groin
   Pectoral region
   Perineum
   Umbilicus
   Excludes buttocks (680.5)
           external genital organs:
             female (616.4)
             male (607.2, 608.4)

  680.3 Upper arm and forearm
   Arm [any part, except hand]
   Axilla
   Shoulder

  680.4 Hand
   Finger [any]   Wrist
   Thumb

  680.5 Buttock
   Anus   Gluteal region

  680.6 Leg, except foot
   Ankle   Knee
   Hip   Thigh

  680.7 Foot
   Heel
   Toe

  680.8 Other specified sites
   Head [any part, except face]
   Scalp
   Excludes external genital organs:
           female (616.4)
           male (607.2, 608.4)

  680.9 Unspecified site
   Boil NOS   Furuncle NOS
   Carbuncle NOS

● **681 Cellulitis and abscess of finger and toe**
  Includes that with lymphangitis
  Use additional code to identify organism, such as:
  Staphylococcus (041.1)

  ● **681.0 Finger**
    681.00 Cellulitis and abscess, unspecified
    681.01 Felon
     Pulp abscess   Whitlow
     Excludes herpetic whitlow (054.6)
    681.02 Onychia and paronychia of finger
     Panaritium of finger
     Perionychia of finger

  ● **681.1 Toe**
    681.10 Cellulitis and abscess, unspecified
     Coding Clinic: 2005, Q1, P14
    681.11 Onychia and paronychia of toe
     Panaritium of toe
     Perionychia of toe

  681.9 Cellulitis and abscess of unspecified digit
   Infection of nail NOS

● **682 Other cellulitis and abscess**
  Includes abscess (acute) (with lymphangitis) except of finger or toe
  cellulitis (diffuse) (with lymphangitis) except of finger or toe
  lymphangitis, acute (with lymphangitis) except of finger or toe
  Use additional code to identify organism, such as:
  Staphylococcus (041.1)
  Excludes lymphangitis (chronic) (subacute) (457.2)

  682.0 Face
   This code reports forehead but not head (682.8).
   Cheek, external   Nose, external
   Chin   Submandibular
   Forehead   Temple (region)
   Excludes ear [any part] (380.10–380.16)
           eyelid (373.13)
           lacrimal apparatus (375.31)
           lip (528.5)
           mouth (528.3)
           nose (internal) (478.1)
           orbit (376.01)

  682.1 Neck

  682.2 Trunk
   Abdominal wall
   Back [any part, except buttock]
   Buttocks see 682.5
   Chest wall
   Flank
   Groin
   Pectoral region
   Perineum
   Umbilicus, except newborn
   Excludes anal and rectal regions (566)
           breast:
             NOS (611.0)
             puerperal (675.1)
           external genital organs:
             female (616.3–616.4)
             male (604.0, 607.2, 608.4)
           umbilicus, newborn (771.4)
   Coding Clinic: 1993, Q1, P26

Item 12-1 Cellulitis is an acute spreading bacterial infection below the surface of the skin characterized by redness (erythema), warmth, swelling, pain, fever, chills, and enlarged lymph nodes ("swollen glands"). **Abscess** is a localized collection of pus in tissues or organs and is a sign of infection resulting in swelling and inflammation. **Onychia** is an inflammation of the tissue surrounding the nail with pus accumulation and loss of the nail, resulting from microscopic pathogens entering through small wounds. **Paronychia** is a nail disease also known as felon or whitlow and is a bacterial or fungal infection.

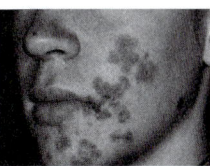

Figure 12-2 Impetigo. A thick, honey-yellow adherent crust covers the entire eroded surface. (From Habif: Clinical Dermatology, ed 4, Mosby, Inc., 2004)

- **682.3 Upper arm and forearm**
  Arm [any part, except hand]
  Axilla
  Shoulder
  `Excludes` hand (682.4)
  Coding Clinic: 2003, Q2, P7-8; 1998, Q4, P42-44

- **682.4 Hand, except fingers and thumb**
  Wrist
  `Excludes` finger and thumb (681.00–681.02)

- **682.5 Buttock**
  Gluteal region
  `Excludes` anal and rectal regions (566)

- **682.6 Leg, except foot**
  Ankle   Knee
  Hip   Thigh
  Coding Clinic: 2012, Q3, P14; 2009, Q1, P18x2; 2004, Q3, P5-6; 2003, Q4, P108; 1995, Q1, P3

- **682.7 Foot, except toes**
  Heel
  `Excludes` toe (681.10–681.11)

- **682.8 Other specified sites**
  Head [except face]
  Scalp
  `Excludes` face (682.0)

- **682.9 Unspecified site**
  Abscess NOS
  Cellulitis NOS
  Lymphangitis, acute NOS
  `Excludes` lymphangitis NOS (457.2)

683 Acute lymphadenitis
  Short term inflammation of lymph nodes which can be regionalized to involve a given area of lymph system or systemic involvement
  Abscess (acute) lymph gland or node, except mesenteric
  Adenitis, acute lymph gland or node, except mesenteric
  Lymphadenitis, acute lymph gland or node, except mesenteric
  `Use additional` code to identify organism such as
  Staphylococcus (041.1)
  `Excludes` enlarged glands NOS (785.6)
  lymphadenitis:
    chronic or subacute, except mesenteric (289.1)
    mesenteric (acute) (chronic) (subacute) (289.2)
    unspecified (289.3)

684 Impetigo
  Contagious skin infection caused by streptococcus or staphylococcus aureus that produces blisters or sores on the face and hands
  Impetiginization of other dermatoses
  Impetigo (contagiosa) [any site] [any organism]:
    bullous neonatorum
    circinate
    simplex
  Pemphigus neonatorum
  `Excludes` impetigo herpetiformis (694.3)

- **685 Pilonidal cyst**
  `Includes` fistula, coccygeal or pilonidal
  sinus, coccygeal or pilonidal

  - **685.0 With abscess**
  - **685.1 Without mention of abscess**
    Coding Clinic: 2011, Q3, P9

Item 12-2 Pilonidal cyst, also called a coccygeal cyst, is the result of a disorder called pilonidal disease. The cyst usually contains hair and pus.

- **686 Other local infections of skin and subcutaneous tissue**
  `Use additional` code to identify any infectious organism (041.0–041.8)

  - **686.0 Pyoderma**
    Dermatitis:
      purulent
      septic
      suppurative
    - **686.00 Pyoderma, unspecified**
    - **686.01 Pyoderma gangrenosum**
      Coding Clinic: 1997, Q4, P42
    - **686.09 Other pyoderma**

  - **686.1 Pyogenic granuloma**
    Granuloma:
      septic
      suppurative
      telangiectaticum
    `Excludes` pyogenic granuloma of oral mucosa (528.9)

  - **686.8 Other specified local infections of skin and subcutaneous tissue**
    Bacterid (pustular)   Ecthyma
    Dermatitis vegetans   Perlèche
    `Excludes` dermatitis infectiosa eczematoides (690.8)
    panniculitis (729.30–729.39)

  - **686.9 Unspecified local infection of skin and subcutaneous tissue**
    Fistula of skin NOS
    Skin infection NOS
    `Excludes` fistula to skin from internal organs—see Alphabetic Index

---

OTHER INFLAMMATORY CONDITIONS OF SKIN AND SUBCUTANEOUS TISSUE (690–698)

`Excludes` panniculitis (729.30–729.39)

- **690 Erythematosquamous dermatosis**
  `Excludes` eczematous dermatitis of eyelid (373.31)
  parakeratosis variegata (696.2)
  psoriasis (696.0–696.1)
  seborrheic keratosis (702.11–702.19)

  - **690.1 Seborrheic dermatitis**
    - **690.10 Seborrheic dermatitis, unspecified**
      Seborrheic dermatitis NOS
    - **690.11 Seborrhea capitis**
      Cradle cap
    - **690.12 Seborrheic infantile dermatitis**
    - **690.18 Other seborrheic dermatitis**
  - **690.8 Other erythematosquamous dermatosis**

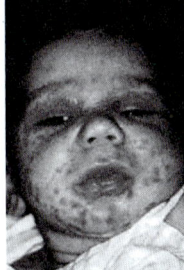

Figure 12-3 Seborrheic dermatitis. (From Cohen BA: Atlas of Pediatric Dermatology. St. Louis, Mosby, 1993)

Item 12-3 Seborrheic dermatitis is characterized by greasy, scaly, red patches and is associated with oily skin and scalp.

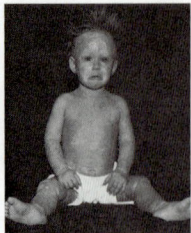

Figure 12-4 Atopic dermatitis. (From Moschella SL, Hurley HJ: Dermatology, ed 3, Philadelphia, WB Saunders, 1993)

Item 12-4 Atopic dermatitis, also known as atopic eczema, infantile eczema, disseminated neurodermatitis, flexural eczema, and *prurigo diathesique* (Besnier), is characterized by intense itching and is often hereditary.

- **691 Atopic dermatitis and related conditions**
  - **691.0 Diaper or napkin rash**
    - Ammonia dermatitis
    - Diaper or napkin:
      - dermatitis
      - erythema
      - rash
    - Psoriasiform napkin eruption
  - **691.8 Other atopic dermatitis and related conditions**
    - Atopic dermatitis
    - Besnier's prurigo
    - Eczema:
      - atopic
      - flexural
      - intrinsic (allergic)
    - Neurodermatitis:
      - atopic
      - diffuse (of Brocq)

- **692 Contact dermatitis and other eczema**
  - **Includes** dermatitis:
    - NOS
    - contact
    - occupational
    - venenata
    - eczema (acute) (chronic):
      - NOS
      - allergic
      - erythematous
      - occupational
  - **Excludes** allergy NOS (995.3)
    - contact dermatitis of eyelids (373.32)
    - dermatitis due to substances taken internally (693.0–693.9)
    - eczema of external ear (380.22)
    - perioral dermatitis (695.3)
    - urticarial reactions (708.0–708.9, 995.1)
  - **692.0 Due to detergents**
  - **692.1 Due to oils and greases**
  - **692.2 Due to solvents**
    - Dermatitis due to solvents of:
      - chlorocompound group
      - cyclohexane group
      - ester group
      - glycol group
      - hydrocarbon group
      - ketone group
  - **692.3 Due to drugs and medicines in contact with skin**
    - Dermatitis (allergic) (contact) due to:
      - arnica
      - fungicides
      - iodine
      - keratolytics
      - mercurials
      - neomycin
      - pediculocides
      - phenols
      - scabicides
      - any drug applied to skin
    - Dermatitis medicamentosa due to drug applied to skin
    - Use additional E code to identify drug
    - **Excludes** allergy NOS due to drugs (995.27)
      - dermatitis due to ingested drugs (693.0)
      - dermatitis medicamentosa NOS (693.0)
  - **692.4 Due to other chemical products**
    - Dermatitis due to:
      - acids
      - adhesive plaster
      - alkalis
      - caustics
      - dichromate
      - insecticide
      - nylon
      - plastic
      - rubber
    - *Coding Clinic: 2008, Q3, P6-7; 1989, Q2, P16*
  - **692.5 Due to food in contact with skin**
    - Dermatitis, contact, due to:
      - cereals
      - fish
      - flour
      - fruit
      - meat
      - milk
    - **Excludes** dermatitis due to:
      - dyes (692.89)
      - ingested foods (693.1)
      - preservatives (692.89)
  - **692.6 Due to plants [except food]**
    - Dermatitis due to:
      - lacquer tree [Rhus verniciflua]
      - poison:
        - ivy [Rhus toxicodendron]
        - oak [Rhus diversiloba]
        - sumac [Rhus venenata]
        - vine [Rhus radicans]
      - primrose [Primula]
      - ragweed [Senecio jacobae]
      - other plants in contact with the skin
    - **Excludes** allergy NOS due to pollen (477.0)
      - nettle rash (708.8)
  - **692.7 Due to solar radiation**
    - **Excludes** sunburn due to other ultraviolet radiation exposure (692.82)
    - **692.70 Unspecified dermatitis due to sun**
    - **692.71 Sunburn**
      - First degree sunburn
      - *See codes 692.76 and 692.77 for second and third degrees.*
      - Sunburn NOS
    - **692.72 Acute dermatitis due to solar radiation**
      - Berloque dermatitis
      - Photoallergic response
      - Phototoxic response
      - Polymorphous light eruption
      - Acute solar skin damage NOS
      - **Excludes** sunburn (692.71, 692.76–692.77)
      - Use additional E code to identify drug, if drug induced
    - **692.73 Actinic reticuloid and actinic granuloma**
    - **692.74 Other chronic dermatitis due to solar radiation**
      - Chronic solar skin damage NOS
      - Solar elastosis
      - **Excludes** actinic [solar] keratosis (702.0)

692.75 Disseminated superficial actinic porokeratosis (DSAP)
692.76 Sunburn of second degree
692.77 Sunburn of third degree
692.79 Other dermatitis due to solar radiation
  Hydroa aestivale
  Photodermatitis (due to sun)
  Photosensitiveness (due to sun)
  Solar skin damage NOS

● **692.8 Due to other specified agents**
  692.81 Dermatitis due to cosmetics
  692.82 Dermatitis due to other radiation
    Infrared rays
    Light, except from sun
    Radiation NOS
    Tanning bed
    Ultraviolet rays, except from sun
    X-rays
    Excludes *that due to solar radiation (692.70–692.79)*
    Coding Clinic: 2000, Q3, P5
  692.83 Dermatitis due to metals
    Jewelry
  692.84 Due to animal (cat) (dog) dander
    Due to animal (cat) (dog) hair
    Coding Clinic: 2004, Q4, P90-91
  692.89 Other
    Dermatitis due to:
      cold weather
      dyes
      hot weather
      preservatives
    Excludes *allergy (NOS) (rhinitis) due to animal hair or dander (477.2)*
    allergy to dust (477.8)
    sunburn (692.71, 692.76–692.77)

■ **692.9 Unspecified cause**
  Dermatitis:
    NOS
    contact NOS
    venenata NOS
  Eczema NOS

● **693 Dermatitis due to substances taken internally**
  Excludes *adverse effect NOS of drugs and medicines (995.20)*
  allergy NOS (995.3)
  contact dermatitis (692.0–692.9)
  urticarial reactions (708.0–708.9, 995.1)
  693.0 Due to drugs and medicines
    Dermatitis medicamentosa NOS
    Use additional E code to identify drug
    Excludes *that due to drugs in contact with skin (692.3)*
    Coding Clinic: 2007, Q2, P9-10
  693.1 Due to food
  693.8 Due to other specified substances taken internally
  ■ **693.9** Due to unspecified substance taken internally
    Excludes *dermatitis NOS (692.9)*

● **694 Bullous dermatoses**
  694.0 Dermatitis herpetiformis
    Dermatosis herpetiformis
    Duhring's disease
    Hydroa herpetiformis
    Excludes *herpes gestationis (646.8)*
    dermatitis herpetiformis:
      juvenile (694.2)
      senile (694.5)
  694.1 Subcorneal pustular dermatosis
    Sneddon-Wilkinson disease or syndrome
  694.2 Juvenile dermatitis herpetiformis
    Juvenile pemphigoid
  694.3 Impetigo herpetiformis

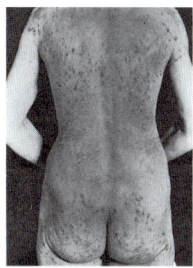

Figure 12-5 Dermatitis herpetiformis. (From Arnold HL, Odom RB, James WD: Andrews' Diseases of the Skin, Clinical Dermatology, ed 8, Philadelphia, WB Saunders, 1990)

Item 12-5 Dermatitis herpetiformis, also known as Duhring's disease, is a systemic disease characterized by small blisters (3 to 5 mm) and occasionally large bullae (+5 mm).

  694.4 Pemphigus
    Pemphigus:
      NOS
      erythematosus
      foliaceus
      malignant
      vegetans
      vulgaris
    Excludes *pemphigus neonatorum (684)*
  694.5 Pemphigoid
    Benign pemphigus NOS
    Bullous pemphigoid
    Herpes circinatus bullosus
    Senile dermatitis herpetiformis
  ● **694.6** Benign mucous membrane pemphigoid
    Cicatricial pemphigoid
    Mucosynechial atrophic bullous dermatitis
    694.60 Without mention of ocular involvement
    694.61 With ocular involvement
      Ocular pemphigus
  694.8 Other specified bullous dermatoses
    Excludes *herpes gestationis (646.8)*
  ■ **694.9** Unspecified bullous dermatoses

● **695 Erythematous conditions**
  695.0 Toxic erythema
    Erythema venenatum
  ● **695.1** Erythema multiforme
    Use additional code to identify associated manifestations, such as:
      arthropathy associated with dermatological disorders (713.3)
      conjunctival edema (372.73)
      conjunctivitis (372.04, 372.33)
      corneal scars and opacities (371.00-371.05)
      corneal ulcer (370.00-370.07)
      edema of eyelid (374.82)
      inflammation of eyelid (373.8)
      keratoconjunctivitis sicca (370.33)
      mechanical lagophthalmos (374.22)
      mucositis (478.11, 528.00, 538, 616.81)
      stomatitis (528.00)
      symblepharon (372.63)
    Use additional E-code to identify drug, if drug-induced
    Use additional code to identify percentage of skin exfoliation (695.50–695.59)
    Excludes *(staphylococcal) scalded skin syndrome (695.81)*
    Coding Clinic: 2008, Q4, P128-131
    ■ **695.10** Erythema multiforme, unspecified
      Erythema iris
      Herpes iris
    695.11 Erythema multiforme minor
    695.12 Erythema multiforme major
    695.13 Stevens-Johnson syndrome

695.14 Stevens-Johnson syndrome-toxic epidermal necrolysis overlap syndrome
SJS-TEN overlap syndrome
Coding Clinic: 2008, Q4, P128-131

695.15 Toxic epidermal necrolysis
Lyell's syndrome

695.19 Other erythema multiforme

695.2 Erythema nodosum
Excludes tuberculous erythema nodosum (017.1)

695.3 Rosacea
Acne:
 erythematosa
 rosacea
Perioral dermatitis
Rhinophyma

695.4 Lupus erythematosus
See 710.0 for designated as systemic lupus erythematosus (SLE).
Lupus:
 erythematodes (discoid)
 erythematosus (discoid), not disseminated
Excludes lupus (vulgaris) NOS (017.0)
systemic [disseminated] lupus erythematosus (710.0)

695.5 Exfoliation due to erythematous conditions according to extent of body surface involved
Code first erythematous condition causing exfoliation, such as:
 Ritter's disease (695.81)
 (Staphylococcal) scalded skin syndrome (695.81)
 Stevens-Johnson syndrome (695.13)
 Stevens-Johnson syndrome-toxic epidermal necrolysis overlap syndrome (695.14)
 toxic epidermal necrolysis (695.15)

- **695.50** *Exfoliation due to erythematous condition involving less than 10 percent of body surface*
Exfoliation due to erythematous condition NOS
- **695.51** *Exfoliation due to erythematous condition involving 10-19 percent of body surface*
- **695.52** *Exfoliation due to erythematous condition involving 20-29 percent of body surface*
- **695.53** *Exfoliation due to erythematous condition involving 30-39 percent of body surface*
Coding Clinic: 2008, Q4, P128-131
- **695.54** *Exfoliation due to erythematous condition involving 40-49 percent of body surface*
- **695.55** *Exfoliation due to erythematous condition involving 50-59 percent of body surface*
- **695.56** *Exfoliation due to erythematous condition involving 60-69 percent of body surface*
- **695.57** *Exfoliation due to erythematous condition involving 70-79 percent of body surface*
- **695.58** *Exfoliation due to erythematous condition involving 80-89 percent of body surface*
- **695.59** *Exfoliation due to erythematous condition involving 90 percent or more of body surface*

695.8 Other specified erythematous conditions
 695.81 Ritter's disease
  Dermatitis exfoliativa neonatorum
  (Staphylococcal) Scalded skin syndrome
  Use additional code to identify percentage of skin exfoliation (695.50-695.59)
 695.89 Other
  Erythema intertrigo
  Intertrigo
  Pityriasis rubra (Hebra)
  Excludes mycotic intertrigo (111.0–111.9)
  Coding Clinic: 1986, Sept-Oct, P10

695.9 Unspecified erythematous condition
Erythema NOS
Erythroderma (secondary)

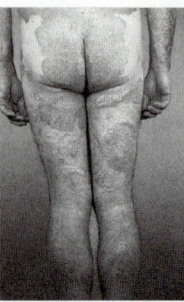

Figure 12-6 Erythematous plaques with silvery scales in a patient with psoriasis. (From Goldman: Cecil Textbook of Medicine, ed 22, Saunders, 2004)

Item 12-6 Psoriasis is a chronic, recurrent inflammatory skin disease characterized by small patches covered with thick silvery scales. **Parapsoriasis** is a treatment-resistant erythroderma. **Pityriasis rosea** is characterized by a herald patch that is a single large lesion and that usually appears on the trunk and is followed by scattered, smaller lesions.

696 Psoriasis and similar disorders
 696.0 Psoriatic arthropathy
 696.1 Other psoriasis
  Acrodermatitis continua
  Dermatitis repens
  Psoriasis:
   NOS
   any type, except arthropathic
  Excludes psoriatic arthropathy (696.0)
  Coding Clinic: 1996, Q2, P12
 696.2 Parapsoriasis
  Parakeratosis variegata
  Parapsoriasis lichenoides chronica
  Pityriasis lichenoides et varioliformis
 696.3 Pityriasis rosea
  Pityriasis circinata (et maculata)
 696.4 Pityriasis rubra pilaris
  Devergie's disease
  Lichen ruber acuminatus
  Excludes pityriasis rubra (Hebra) (695.89)
 696.5 Other and unspecified pityriasis
  Pityriasis:
   NOS
   alba
   streptogenes
  Excludes pityriasis:
   simplex (690.18)
   versicolor (111.0)
 696.8 Other

697 Lichen
 Excludes lichen:
  obtusus corneus (698.3)
  pilaris (congenital) (757.39)
  ruber acuminatus (696.4)
  sclerosus et atrophicus (701.0)
  scrofulosus (017.0)
  simplex chronicus (698.3)
  spinulosus (congenital) (757.39)
  urticatus (698.2)
 697.0 Lichen planus
  Lichen:
   planopilaris
   ruber planus
 697.1 Lichen nitidus
  Pinkus' disease
 697.8 Other lichen, not elsewhere classified
  Lichen:
   ruber moniliforme
   striata
 697.9 Lichen, unspecified

- **698 Pruritus and related conditions**
  Excludes: pruritus specified as psychogenic (306.3)
  - **698.0 Pruritus ani**
    Perianal itch
  - **698.1 Pruritus of genital organs**
  - **698.2 Prurigo**
    Lichen urticatus
    Prurigo:
       NOS
       Hebra's
    Prurigo:
       mitis
       simplex
    Urticaria papulosa (Hebra)
    Excludes: prurigo nodularis (698.3)
  - **698.3 Lichenification and lichen simplex chronicus**
    Hyde's disease
    Neurodermatitis (circumscripta) (local)
    Prurigo nodularis
    Excludes: neurodermatitis, diffuse (of Brocq) (691.8)
  - **698.4 Dermatitis factitia [artefacta]**
    Dermatitis ficta
    Neurotic excoriation
    Use additional code to identify any associated mental disorder
  - **698.8 Other specified pruritic conditions**
    Pruritus:
       hiemalis
       senilis
       Winter itch
  - **698.9 Unspecified pruritic disorder**
    Itch NOS
    Pruritus NOS

OTHER DISEASES OF SKIN AND SUBCUTANEOUS TISSUE (700–709)

Excludes: conditions confined to eyelids (373.0–374.9)
congenital conditions of skin, hair, and nails (757.0–757.9)

- **700 Corns and callosities**
  Callus
  Clavus
- **701 Other hypertrophic and atrophic conditions of skin**
  Excludes: dermatomyositis (710.3)
  hereditary edema of legs (757.0)
  scleroderma (generalized) (710.1)
  - **701.0 Circumscribed scleroderma**
    Addison's keloid
    Dermatosclerosis, localized
    Lichen sclerosus et atrophicus
    Morphea
    Scleroderma, circumscribed or localized
  - **701.1 Keratoderma, acquired**
    Acquired:
       ichthyosis
       keratoderma palmaris et plantaris
    Elastosis perforans serpiginosa
    Hyperkeratosis:
       NOS
       follicularis in cutem penetrans
       palmoplantaris climacterica
    Keratoderma:
       climactericum
       tylodes, progressive
    Keratosis (blennorrhagica)
    Excludes: Darier's disease [keratosis follicularis] (congenital) (757.39)
    keratosis:
       arsenical (692.4)
       gonococcal (098.81)
  - **701.2 Acquired acanthosis nigricans**
    Keratosis nigricans

Item 12-7 Scleroderma means hard skin. It is a group of diseases that causes abnormal growth of connective tissues that support the skin and organs. There are two types: localized scleroderma affecting the skin and systemic scleroderma affecting blood vessels and internal organs and the skin. **Keratoderma** is characterized by firm horny papules that have a cobblestone appearance. **Keratoderma climactericum,** also known as endocrine keratoderma, is hyperkeratosis located on the palms and soles.

  - **701.3 Striae atrophicae**
    Atrophic spots of skin
    Atrophoderma maculatum
    Atrophy blanche (of Milian)
    Degenerative colloid atrophy
    Senile degenerative atrophy
    Striae distensae
  - **701.4 Keloid scar**
    Cheloid
    Hypertrophic scar
    Keloid
    Coding Clinic: 1995, Q3, P14
  - **701.5 Other abnormal granulation tissue**
    Excessive granulation
  - **701.8 Other specified hypertrophic and atrophic conditions of skin**
    Acrodermatitis atrophicans chronica
    Atrophia cutis senilis
    Atrophoderma neuriticum
    Confluent and reticulate papillomatosis
    Cutis laxa senilis
    Elastosis senilis
    Folliculitis ulerythematosa reticulata
    Gougerot-Carteaud syndrome or disease
    Coding Clinic: 2008, Q1, P7-8
  - **701.9 Unspecified hypertrophic and atrophic conditions of skin**
    Atrophoderma
- **702 Other dermatoses**
  Excludes: carcinoma in situ (232.0–232.9)
  - **702.0 Actinic keratosis**
  - **702.1 Seborrheic keratosis**
    - **702.11 Inflamed seborrheic keratosis**
    - **702.19 Other seborrheic keratosis**
      Seborrheic keratosis NOS
  - **702.8 Other specified dermatoses**
- **703 Diseases of nail**
  Excludes: congenital anomalies (757.5)
  onychia and paronychia (681.02, 681.11)
  - **703.0 Ingrowing nail**
    Ingrowing nail with infection
    Unguis incarnatus
    Excludes: infection, nail NOS (681.9)
  - **703.8 Other specified diseases of nail**
    Dystrophia unguium
    Hypertrophy of nail
    Koilonychia
    Leukonychia (punctata) (striata)
    Onychauxis
    Onychogryposis
    Onycholysis
  - **703.9 Unspecified disease of nail**

Item 12-8 **Alopecia** is lack of hair and takes many forms. The most common is male pattern alopecia, also known as **androgenetic alopecia**. **Telogen effluvium** is early and excessive loss of hair resulting from a trauma to the hair follicle (fever, drugs, surgery, etc.).

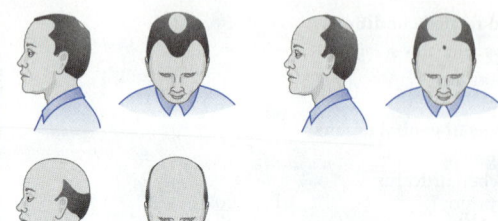

Figure 12-7 Male pattern alopecia.

- **704 Diseases of hair and hair follicles**
  Excludes: congenital anomalies (757.4)
  - **704.0 Alopecia**
    Excludes: madarosis (374.55)
    syphilitic alopecia (091.82)
    - **704.00 Alopecia, unspecified**
      Baldness   Loss of hair
    - **704.01 Alopecia areata**
      Ophiasis
    - **704.02 Telogen effluvium**
    - **704.09 Other**
      Folliculitis decalvans
      Hypotrichosis:
        NOS
        postinfectional NOS
      Pseudopelade
  - **704.1 Hirsutism**
    Excessive growth of hair
    Hypertrichosis:
      NOS
      lanuginosa, acquired
    Polytrichia
    Excludes: hypertrichosis of eyelid (374.54)
  - **704.2 Abnormalities of the hair**
    Atrophic hair   Trichiasis:
    Clastothrix   NOS
    Fragilitas crinium   cicatrical
                             Trichorrhexis (nodosa)
    Excludes: trichiasis of eyelid (374.05)
    Coding Clinic: 2004, Q4, P91-92
  - **704.3 Variations in hair color**
    Canities (premature)
    Grayness, hair (premature)
    Heterochromia of hair
    Poliosis:
      NOS
      circumscripta, acquired
  - **704.4 Pilar and trichilemmal cysts**
    - **704.41 Pilar cyst**
    - **704.42 Trichilemmal cyst**
      Trichilemmal proliferating cyst
      Coding Clinic: 2011, Q4, P135
  - **704.8 Other specified diseases of hair and hair follicles**
    Folliculitis:
      NOS
      abscedens et suffodiens
      pustular
    Perifolliculitis:
      NOS
      capitis abscedens et suffodiens
      scalp
    Sycosis:
      NOS
      barbae [not parasitic]
      lupoid
      vulgaris
    Coding Clinic: 2011, Q1, P8
  - **704.9 Unspecified disease of hair and hair follicles**

- **705 Disorders of sweat glands**
  - **705.0 Anhidrosis**
    Hypohidrosis   Oligohidrosis
  - **705.1 Prickly heat**
    Heat rash   Sudamina
    Miliaria rubra (tropicalis)
  - **705.2 Focal hyperhidrosis**
    Excludes: generalized (secondary) hyperhidrosis (780.8)
    - **705.21 Primary focal hyperhidrosis**
      Focal hyperhidrosis NOS
      Hyperhidrosis NOS
      Hyperhidrosis of:
        axilla   palms
        face   soles
    - **705.22 Secondary focal hyperhidrosis**
      Frey's syndrome
  - **705.8 Other specified disorders of sweat glands**
    - **705.81 Dyshidrosis**
      Cheiropompholyx
      Pompholyx
    - **705.82 Fox-Fordyce disease**
    - **705.83 Hidradenitis**
      Hidradenitis suppurativa
    - **705.89 Other**
      Bromhidrosis   Granulosis rubra nasi
      Chromhidrosis   Urhidrosis
      Excludes: hidrocystoma (216.0-216.9)
      generalized hyperhidrosis (780.8)
  - **705.9 Unspecified disorder of sweat glands**
    Disorder of sweat glands NOS

- **706 Diseases of sebaceous glands**
  - **706.0 Acne varioliformis**
    Acne:
      frontalis
      necrotica
  - **706.1 Other acne**
    Acne:
      NOS
      conglobata
      cystic
      pustular
      vulgaris
    Blackhead
    Comedo
    Excludes: acne rosacea (695.3)
  - **706.2 Sebaceous cyst**
    Atheroma, skin
    Keratin cyst
    Wen
    Excludes: pilar cyst (704.41)
    trichilemmal (proliferating) cyst (704.42)

PART III / Diseases: Tabular List Volume 1   706.3-708.4

706.3 Seborrhea
> Excludes seborrhea:
> capitis (690.11)
> sicca (690.18)
> seborrheic
> dermatitis (690.10)
> keratosis (702.11–702.19)

706.8 Other specified diseases of sebaceous glands
Asteatosis (cutis)
Xerosis cutis

706.9 Unspecified disease of sebaceous glands

707 Chronic ulcer of skin
> Includes non-infected sinus of skin
> non-healing ulcer
> Excludes varicose ulcer (454.0, 454.2)

707.0 Pressure ulcer
Bed sore
Decubitus ulcer
Plaster ulcer
Use additional code to identify pressure ulcer stage (707.20–707.25)
Coding Clinic: 2004, Q4, P92-93; Q1, P14-15; 2003, Q4, P110; 1999, Q4, P20; 1996, Q1, P15; 1990, Q3, P15; 1987, Nov-Dec, P9

707.00 Unspecified site
Coding Clinic: 2012, Q2, P3

707.01 Elbow

707.02 Upper back
Shoulder blades

707.03 Lower back
Coccyx
Sacrum
Coding Clinic: 2008, Q3, P17; 2005, Q1, P16

707.04 Hip

707.05 Buttock
Coding Clinic: 2012, Q2, P3

707.06 Ankle

707.07 Heel
Coding Clinic: 2009, Q4, P108; 2005, Q1, P16

707.09 Other site
Head
Coding Clinic: 2008, Q3, P17

707.1 Ulcer of lower limbs, except pressure ulcer
Ulcer, chronic, of lower limb:
neurogenic of lower limb
trophic of lower limb
Code if applicable, any causal condition first:
atherosclerosis of the extremities with ulceration (440.23)
chronic venous hypertension with ulcer (459.31)
chronic venous hypertension with ulcer and inflammation (459.33)
diabetes mellitus (249.80–249.81, 250.80–250.83)
postphlebitic syndrome with ulcer (459.11)
postphlebitic syndrome with ulcer and inflammation (459.13)
Coding Clinic: 2004, Q1, P14-15; 1999, Q4, P15; 1996, Q1, P10

707.10 Ulcer of lower limb, unspecified
Coding Clinic: 2004, Q3, P5-6

707.11 Ulcer of thigh

707.12 Ulcer of calf

707.13 Ulcer of ankle

707.14 Ulcer of heel and midfoot
Plantar surface of midfoot

707.15 Ulcer of other part of foot
Toes

707.19 Ulcer of other part of lower limb

707.2 Pressure ulcer stages
Code first site of pressure ulcer (707.00-707.09)
Coding Clinic: 2008, Q4, P132-134

707.20 Pressure ulcer, unspecified stage
Healing pressure ulcer NOS
Healing pressure ulcer, unspecified stage

707.21 Pressure ulcer stage I
Healing pressure ulcer, stage I
Pressure pre-ulcer skin changes limited to persistent focal erythema

707.22 Pressure ulcer stage II
Healing pressure ulcer, stage II
Pressure ulcer with abrasion, blister, partial thickness skin loss involving epidermis and/or dermis

707.23 Pressure ulcer stage III
Healing pressure ulcer, stage III
Pressure ulcer with full thickness skin loss involving damage or necrosis of subcutaneous tissue
Coding Clinic: 2009, Q4, P113

707.24 Pressure ulcer stage IV
Healing pressure ulcer, stage IV
Pressure ulcer with necrosis of soft tissues through to underlying muscle, tendon, or bone
Coding Clinic: 2010, Q2, P18

707.25 Pressure ulcer, unstageable

707.8 Chronic ulcer of other specified sites
Ulcer, chronic, of other specified sites:
neurogenic of other specified sites
trophic of other specified sites

707.9 Chronic ulcer of unspecified site
Chronic ulcer NOS   Tropical ulcer NOS
Trophic ulcer NOS   Ulcer of skin NOS

708 Urticaria
> Excludes edema:
> angioneurotic (995.1)
> Quincke's (995.1)
> hereditary angioedema (277.6)
> urticaria:
> giant (995.1)
> papulosa (Hebra) (698.2)
> pigmentosa (juvenile) (congenital) (757.33)

708.0 Allergic urticaria
Coding Clinic: 1984, May-June, P11

708.1 Idiopathic urticaria

708.2 Urticaria due to cold and heat
Thermal urticaria

708.3 Dermatographic urticaria
Dermatographia
Factitial urticaria

708.4 Vibratory urticaria

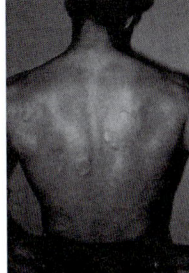

Figure 12–8 Urticaria (hives). *(Courtesy of David Effron, MD.)* (From Marx: Rosen's Emergency Medicine: Concepts and Clinical Practice, ed 6, Mosby, Inc., 2006)

Item 12-9 Urticaria is a vascular reaction in which wheals surrounded by a red halo appear and cause severe itching. The causes of urticaria or hives are extensive and varied (e.g., food, heat, cold, drugs, stress, infections). Dyschromia is any disorder of the pigmentation of the skin or hair.

708.5 Cholinergic urticaria
Coding Clinic: 1995, Q4, P50

708.8 Other specified urticaria
Nettle rash
Urticaria:
  chronic
  recurrent periodic

708.9 Urticaria, unspecified
Hives NOS

709 Other disorders of skin and subcutaneous tissue

709.0 Dyschromia
Excludes: albinism (270.2)
  pigmented nevus (216.0–216.9)
  that of eyelid (374.52–374.53)

709.00 Dyschromia, unspecified
709.01 Vitiligo
709.09 Other

709.1 Vascular disorders of skin
Angioma serpiginosum
Purpura (primary) annularis telangiectodes

709.2 Scar conditions and fibrosis of skin
Adherent scar (skin)
Cicatrix
Disfigurement (due to scar)
Fibrosis, skin NOS
Scar NOS
Excludes: keloid scar (701.4)
Coding Clinic: 1984, Nov-Dec, P19

709.3 Degenerative skin disorders
Calcinosis:
  circumscripta
  cutis
Colloid milium
Degeneration, skin
Deposits, skin
Senile dermatosis NOS
Subcutaneous calcification

709.4 Foreign body granuloma of skin and subcutaneous tissue
Use additional code to identify foreign body (V90.01-V90.9)
Excludes: residual foreign body without granuloma of skin and subcutaneous tissue (729.6)
  that of muscle (728.82)

709.8 Other specified disorders of skin
Epithelial hyperplasia
Menstrual dermatosis
Vesicular eruption
Coding Clinic: 1987, Nov-Dec, P6

709.9 Unspecified disorder of skin and subcutaneous tissue
Dermatosis NOS

13. DISEASES OF THE MUSCULOSKELETAL SYSTEM AND CONNECTIVE TISSUE (710–739)

Use additional external cause code, if applicable, to identify the cause of the musculoskeletal condition

The following fifth-digit subclassification is for use with categories 711–712, 715–716, 718–719, and 730:

- 0 site unspecified
- 1 shoulder region
  - Acromioclavicular joint(s)
  - Clavicle
  - Glenohumeral joint(s)
  - Scapula
  - Sternoclavicular joint(s)
- 2 upper arm
  - Elbow joint
  - Humerus
- 3 forearm
  - Radius
  - Ulna
  - Wrist joint
- 4 hand
  - Carpus
  - Metacarpus
  - Phalanges [fingers]
- 5 pelvic region and thigh
  - Buttock
  - Femur
  - Hip (joint)
- 6 lower leg
  - Fibula
  - Knee joint
  - Patella
  - Tibia
- 7 ankle and foot
  - Ankle joint
  - Digits [toes]
  - Metatarsus
  - Phalanges, foot
  - Tarsus
  - Other joints in foot
- 8 other specified sites
  - Head
  - Neck
  - Ribs
  - Skull
  - Trunk
  - Vertebral column
- 9 multiple sites

ARTHROPATHIES AND RELATED DISORDERS (710–719)

Excludes disorders of spine (720.0–724.9)

710 Diffuse diseases of connective tissue
Includes all collagen diseases whose effects are not mainly confined to a single system

Excludes those affecting mainly the cardiovascular system, i.e., polyarteritis nodosa and allied conditions (446.0–446.7)

710.0 Systemic lupus erythematosus
Autoimmune inflammatory connective tissue disease of unknown cause that occurs most often in women. See 695.4 for nonsystemic.

Disseminated lupus erythematosus
Libman-Sacks disease

Use additional code to identify manifestation, as:
- endocarditis (424.91)
- nephritis (583.81)
  - chronic (582.81)
  - nephrotic syndrome (581.81)

Excludes lupus erythematosus (discoid) NOS (695.4)

Coding Clinic: 2003, Q2, P7x2; 1997, Q2, P8-9; 1987, Sept-Oct, P8

710.1 Systemic sclerosis
Acrosclerosis
CRST syndrome
Progressive systemic sclerosis
Scleroderma

Use additional code to identify manifestation, as:
- lung involvement (517.2)
- myopathy (359.6)

Excludes circumscribed scleroderma (701.0)

710.2 Sicca syndrome
Keratoconjunctivitis sicca
Sjögren's disease

710.3 Dermatomyositis
Poikilodermatomyositis
Polymyositis with skin involvement

710.4 Polymyositis
710.5 Eosinophilia myalgia syndrome
Toxic oil syndrome

Use additional E code to identify drug, if drug induced

710.8 Other specified diffuse diseases of connective tissue
Multifocal fibrosclerosis (idiopathic) NEC
Systemic fibrosclerosing syndrome
Coding Clinic: 1987, Mar-April, P12

710.9 Unspecified diffuse connective tissue disease
Collagen disease NOS

711 Arthropathy associated with infections
Abnormality of a joint

Includes
- arthritis associated with conditions classifiable below
- arthropathy associated with conditions classifiable below
- polyarthritis associated with conditions classifiable below
- polyarthropathy associated with conditions classifiable below

Excludes rheumatic fever (390)

Coding Clinic: 1992, Q1, P16-17

The following fifth-digit subclassification is for use with category 711; valid digits are in [brackets] under each code. See list at beginning of chapter for definitions:

- 0 site unspecified
- 1 shoulder region
- 2 upper arm
- 3 forearm
- 4 hand
- 5 pelvic region and thigh
- 6 lower leg
- 7 ankle and foot
- 8 other specified sites
- 9 multiple sites

711.0 Pyogenic arthritis
[0-9] Arthritis or polyarthritis (due to):
- coliform [Escherichia coli]
- Hemophilus influenzae [H. influenzae]
- pneumococcal
- Pseudomonas
- staphylococcal
- streptococcal

Pyarthrosis

Use additional code to identify infectious organism (041.0–041.8)

Coding Clinic: 1992, Q1, P16-17; 1991, Q1, P15

711.1 Arthropathy associated with Reiter's disease and
[0-9] nonspecific urethritis

Code first underlying disease, as:
- nonspecific urethritis (099.4)
- Reiter's disease (099.3)

711.2 Arthropathy in Behçet's syndrome
[0-9] Code first underlying disease (136.1)

711.3 Postdysenteric arthropathy
[0-9] Code first underlying disease, as:
- dysentery (009.0)
- enteritis, infectious (008.0–009.3)
- paratyphoid fever (002.1–002.9)
- typhoid fever (002.0)

Excludes salmonella arthritis (003.23)

711.4 Arthropathy associated with other bacterial
[0-9] diseases

Code first underlying disease, as:
- diseases classifiable to 010–040, 090–099, except as in 711.1, 711.3, and 713.5
- leprosy (030.0–030.9)
- tuberculosis (015.0–015.9)

Excludes gonococcal arthritis (098.50)
meningococcal arthritis (036.82)

DISEASES OF THE MUSCULOSKELETAL SYSTEM AND CONNECTIVE TISSUE (710–739)

- ● ● **711.5** Arthropathy associated with other viral diseases
  [0-9]
  Code first underlying disease, as:
  diseases classifiable to 045–049, 050–079, 480, 487
  O'nyong-nyong (066.3)
  Excludes *that due to rubella (056.71)*

- ● ● **711.6** Arthropathy associated with mycoses
  [0-9]
  Code first underlying disease (110.0–118)

- ● ● **711.7** Arthropathy associated with helminthiasis
  [0-9]
  Code first underlying disease, as:
  filariasis (125.0–125.9)

- ● ● **711.8** Arthropathy associated with other infectious and
  [0-9] parasitic diseases
  Code first underlying disease, as:
  diseases classifiable to 080–088, 100–104, 130–136
  Excludes *arthropathy associated with sarcoidosis (713.7)*
  Coding Clinic: 1990, Q3, P14

- ● □ **711.9** Unspecified infective arthritis
  [0-9]
  Infective arthritis or polyarthritis (acute) (chronic)
  (subacute) NOS

- ● **712** Crystal arthropathies
  Includes crystal-induced arthritis and synovitis
  Excludes *gouty arthropathy (274.00–274.03)*

  The following fifth-digit subclassification is for use with category 712; valid digits are in [brackets] under each code. See list at beginning of chapter for definitions:

□ 0 site unspecified	5 pelvic region and thigh
1 shoulder region	6 lower leg
2 upper arm	7 ankle and foot
3 forearm	8 other specified sites
4 hand	9 multiple sites

- ● ● **712.1** Chondrocalcinosis due to dicalcium phosphate
  [0-9] crystals
  Chondrocalcinosis due to dicalcium phosphate crystals
  (with other crystals)
  Code first underlying disease (275.49)

- ● ● **712.2** Chondrocalcinosis due to pyrophosphate crystals
  [0-9]
  Code first underlying disease (275.49)

- ● ● □ **712.3** Chondrocalcinosis, unspecified
  [0-9]
  Code first underlying disease (275.49)

- ● **712.8** Other specified crystal arthropathies
  [0-9]

- ● □ **712.9** Unspecified crystal arthropathy
  [0-9]

- ● **713** Arthropathy associated with other disorders classified elsewhere
  Includes arthritis associated with conditions classifiable
  below
  arthropathy associated with conditions classifiable
  below
  polyarthritis associated with conditions classifiable
  below
  polyarthropathy associated with conditions
  classifiable below

- ● **713.0** Arthropathy associated with other endocrine and metabolic
  disorders
  Code first underlying disease, as:
  acromegaly (253.0)
  hemochromatosis (275.01–275.09)
  hyperparathyroidism (252.00–252.08)
  hypogammaglobulinemia (279.00–279.09)
  hypothyroidism (243–244.9)
  lipoid metabolism disorder (272.0–272.9)
  ochronosis (270.2)
  Excludes *arthropathy associated with:*
  amyloidosis (713.7)
  crystal deposition disorders, except gout
  (712.1–712.9)
  diabetic neuropathy (713.5)
  gout (274.00-274.03)

- ● **713.1** Arthropathy associated with gastrointestinal conditions
  other than infections
  Code first underlying disease, as:
  regional enteritis (555.0–555.9)
  ulcerative colitis (556)

- ● **713.2** Arthropathy associated with hematological disorders
  Code first underlying disease, as:
  hemoglobinopathy (282.4–282.7)
  hemophilia (286.0–286.2)
  leukemia (204.0–208.9)
  malignant reticulosis (202.3)
  multiple myelomatosis (203.0)
  Excludes *arthropathy associated with Henoch-Schönlein*
  purpura (713.6)

- ● **713.3** Arthropathy associated with dermatological disorders
  Code first underlying disease, as:
  erythema multiforme (695.10–695.19)
  erythema nodosum (695.2)
  Excludes *psoriatic arthropathy (696.0)*

- ● **713.4** Arthropathy associated with respiratory disorders
  Code first underlying disease, as:
  diseases classifiable to 490–519
  Excludes *arthropathy associated with respiratory infections*
  (711.0, 711.4–711.8)

- ● **713.5** Arthropathy associated with neurological disorders
  Charcot's arthropathy associated with diseases
  classifiable elsewhere
  Neuropathic arthritis associated with diseases classifiable
  elsewhere
  Code first underlying disease, as:
  neuropathic joint disease [Charcot's joints]:
  NOS (094.0)
  diabetic (249.6, 250.6)
  syringomyelic (336.0)
  tabetic [syphilitic] (094.0)
  Coding Clinic: 2012, Q3, P4

- ● **713.6** Arthropathy associated with hypersensitivity reaction
  Code first underlying disease, as:
  Henoch-Schönlein purpura (287.0)
  serum sickness (999.51-999.59)
  Excludes *allergic arthritis NOS (716.2)*

- ● **713.7** Other general diseases with articular involvement
  Code first underlying disease, as:
  amyloidosis (277.30–277.39)
  familial Mediterranean fever (277.31)
  sarcoidosis (135)
  Coding Clinic: 1997, Q2, P12-13

- ● **713.8** Arthropathy associated with other conditions classifiable
  elsewhere
  Code first underlying disease, as:
  conditions classifiable elsewhere except as in
  711.1–711.8, 712, and 713.0–713.7

- ● **714** Rheumatoid arthritis and other inflammatory polyarthropathies
  Excludes *rheumatic fever (390)*
  rheumatoid arthritis of spine NOS (720.0)

  714.0 Rheumatoid arthritis
  Arthritis or polyarthritis:
  atrophic
  rheumatic (chronic)
  Use additional code to identify manifestation, as:
  myopathy (359.6)
  polyneuropathy (357.1)
  Excludes *juvenile rheumatoid arthritis NOS (714.30)*
  Coding Clinic: 2006, Q2, P20; 1995, Q4, P51

  714.1 Felty's syndrome
  Rheumatoid arthritis with splenoadenomegaly and
  leukopenia

  714.2 Other rheumatoid arthritis with visceral or systemic
  involvement
  Rheumatoid carditis

Item 13-1 **Rheumatoid arthritis** (RA) is a chronic systemic inflammatory disease of undetermined etiology involving primarily the synovial membranes and articular structures of multiple joints. The disease is often progressive and results in pain, stiffness, and swelling of joints. In late stages, deformity, ankylosis, and other **inflammatory polyarthropathies** develop.

- **714.3 Juvenile chronic polyarthritis**
  - **714.30 Polyarticular juvenile rheumatoid arthritis, chronic or unspecified**
    - Juvenile rheumatoid arthritis NOS
    - Still's disease
  - **714.31 Polyarticular juvenile rheumatoid arthritis, acute**
  - **714.32 Pauciarticular juvenile rheumatoid arthritis**
  - **714.33 Monoarticular juvenile rheumatoid arthritis**
- **714.4 Chronic postrheumatic arthropathy**
  - Chronic rheumatoid nodular fibrositis
  - Jaccoud's syndrome
- **714.8 Other specified inflammatory polyarthropathies**
  - **714.81 Rheumatoid lung**
    - Caplan's syndrome
    - Diffuse interstitial rheumatoid disease of lung
    - Fibrosing alveolitis, rheumatoid
  - **714.89 Other**
- **714.9 Unspecified inflammatory polyarthropathy**
  - Inflammatory polyarthropathy or polyarthritis NOS
  - **Excludes** polyarthropathy NOS (716.5)

- **715 Osteoarthrosis and allied disorders**
  Degenerative joint disease with breaking down the cartilage causing pain, swelling, and reduced motion in the joints, affecting any joint
  - **Note:** Localized, in the subcategories below, includes bilateral involvement of the same site.
  - **Includes** arthritis or polyarthritis:
    - degenerative
    - hypertrophic
    - degenerative joint disease
    - osteoarthritis
  - **Excludes** Marie-Strümpell spondylitis (720.0)
    osteoarthrosis [osteoarthritis] of spine (721.0–721.9)

The following fifth-digit subclassification is for use with category 715; valid digits are in [brackets] under each code. See list at beginning of chapter for definitions:

0	site unspecified	5	pelvic region and thigh
1	shoulder region	6	lower leg
2	upper arm	7	ankle and foot
3	forearm	8	other specified sites
4	hand	9	multiple sites

- **715.0 Osteoarthrosis, generalized**
  [0,4,9] Degenerative joint disease, involving multiple joints
  Primary generalized hypertrophic osteoarthrosis
  Coding Clinic: 1995, Q2, P5
- **715.1 Osteoarthrosis, localized, primary**
  [0-8] Localized osteoarthropathy, idiopathic
- **715.2 Osteoarthrosis, localized, secondary**
  [0-8] Coxae malum senilis
- **715.3 Osteoarthrosis, localized, not specified whether primary or secondary**
  [0-8] Otto's pelvis
  Coding Clinic: 2004, Q2, P15; 2003, Q2, P18; 1995, Q2, P5
- **715.8 Osteoarthrosis involving, or with mention of more than one site, but not specified as generalized**
  [0,9] Coding Clinic: 1995, Q2, P5
- **715.9 Osteoarthrosis, unspecified whether generalized or localized**
  [0-8] Coding Clinic: 2003, Q2, P18; 1997, Q2, P12-13; 1996, Q1, P16; 1995, Q2, P5

- **716 Other and unspecified arthropathies**
  - **Excludes** cricoarytenoid arthropathy (478.79)

The following fifth-digit subclassification is for use with category 716; valid digits are in [brackets] under each code. See list at beginning of chapter for definitions:

0	site unspecified	5	pelvic region and thigh
1	shoulder region	6	lower leg
2	upper arm	7	ankle and foot
3	forearm	8	other specified sites
4	hand	9	multiple sites

- **716.0 Kaschin-Beck disease**
  [0-9] Endemic polyarthritis
- **716.1 Traumatic arthropathy**
  [0-9] Coding Clinic: 2009, Q2, P11; 2002, Q1, P9-10
- **716.2 Allergic arthritis**
  [0-9] **Excludes** arthritis associated with Henoch-Schönlein purpura or serum sickness (713.6)
- **716.3 Climacteric arthritis**
  [0-9] Menopausal arthritis
- **716.4 Transient arthropathy**
  [0-9] **Excludes** palindromic rheumatism (719.3)
- **716.5 Unspecified polyarthropathy or polyarthritis**
  [0-9]
- **716.6 Unspecified monoarthritis**
  [0-8] Coxitis
- **716.8 Other specified arthropathy**
  [0-9]
- **716.9 Arthropathy, unspecified**
  [0-9] Arthritis (acute) (chronic) (subacute)
  Arthropathy (acute) (chronic) (subacute)
  Articular rheumatism (chronic)
  Inflammation of joint NOS

- **717 Internal derangement of knee**
  - **Includes** degeneration of articular cartilage or meniscus of knee
    rupture, old of articular cartilage or meniscus of knee
    tear, old of articular cartilage or meniscus of knee
  - **Excludes** acute derangement of knee (836.0–836.6)
    ankylosis (718.5)
    contracture (718.4)
    current injury (836.0–836.6)
    deformity (736.4–736.6)
    recurrent dislocation (718.3)
  - **717.0 Old bucket handle tear of medial meniscus**
    Old bucket handle tear of unspecified cartilage
  - **717.1 Derangement of anterior horn of medial meniscus**
  - **717.2 Derangement of posterior horn of medial meniscus**
  - **717.3 Other and unspecified derangement of medial meniscus**
    Degeneration of internal semilunar cartilage
  - **717.4 Derangement of lateral meniscus**
    - **717.40 Derangement of lateral meniscus, unspecified**
    - **717.41 Bucket handle tear of lateral meniscus**
    - **717.42 Derangement of anterior horn of lateral meniscus**
    - **717.43 Derangement of posterior horn of lateral meniscus**
    - **717.49 Other**
  - **717.5 Derangement of meniscus, not elsewhere classified**
    Congenital discoid meniscus
    Cyst of semilunar cartilage
    Derangement of semilunar cartilage NOS
  - **717.6 Loose body in knee**
    Joint mice, knee
    Rice bodies, knee (joint)
  - **717.7 Chondromalacia of patella**
    Chondromalacia patellae
    Degeneration [softening] of articular cartilage of patella
    Coding Clinic: 1985, July-Aug, P14; 1984, Nov-Dec, P9

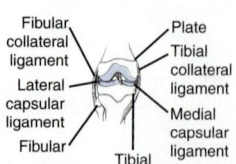

Figure 13-1 Collateral and cruciate ligament of knee. (From DeLee: DeLee and Drez's Orthopaedic Sports Medicine, ed 3, Saunders, 2009)

- **717.8** Other internal derangement of knee
  - 717.81 Old disruption of lateral collateral ligament
  - 717.82 Old disruption of medial collateral ligament
  - 717.83 Old disruption of anterior cruciate ligament
  - 717.84 Old disruption of posterior cruciate ligament
  - 717.85 Old disruption of other ligaments of knee
    - Capsular ligament of knee
  - 717.89 Other
    - Old disruption of ligaments of knee NOS
- **717.9** Unspecified internal derangement of knee
  - Derangement NOS of knee
- **718** Other derangement of joint
  - **Excludes** current injury (830.0–848.9)
    - jaw (524.60–524.69)

The following fifth-digit subclassification is for use with category 718; valid digits are in [brackets] under each code. See list at beginning of chapter for definitions:

0	site unspecified	5	pelvic region and thigh
1	shoulder region	6	lower leg
2	upper arm	7	ankle and foot
3	forearm	8	other specified sites
4	hand	9	multiple sites

- **718.0** Articular cartilage disorder [0-5,7-9]
  - Meniscus:
    - disorder
    - rupture, old
    - tear, old
  - Old rupture of ligament(s) of joint NOS
  - **Excludes** articular cartilage disorder:
    - in ochronosis (270.2)
    - knee (717.0–717.9)
    - chondrocalcinosis (275.49)
    - metastatic calcification (275.40)
- **718.1** Loose body in joint [0-5,7-9]
  - Joint mice
  - **Excludes** knee (717.6)
  - Coding Clinic: 2001, Q2, P14-15
- **718.2** Pathological dislocation [0-9]
  - Dislocation or displacement of joint, not recurrent and not current
- **718.3** Recurrent dislocation of joint [0-9]
  - Coding Clinic: 1987, Nov-Dec, P7
- **718.4** Contracture of joint [0-9]
  - Coding Clinic: 1998, Q4, P39-40
- **718.5** Ankylosis of joint [0-9]
  - Ankylosis of joint (fibrous) (osseous)
  - **Excludes** spine (724.9)
    - stiffness of joint without mention of ankylosis (719.5)
  - Coding Clinic: 1995, Q1, P10
- **718.6** Unspecified intrapelvic protrusion of acetabulum [5]
  - Protrusio acetabuli, unspecified
- **718.7** Developmental dislocation of joint [0-9]
  - **Excludes** congenital dislocation of joint (754.0–755.8)
    - traumatic dislocation of joint (830–839)
- **718.8** Other joint derangement, not elsewhere classified [0-9]
  - Flail joint (paralytic)
  - Instability of joint
  - **Excludes** deformities classifiable to 736 (736.0–736.9)
  - Coding Clinic: 2000, Q2, P14-15
- **718.9** Unspecified derangement of joint [0-5,7-9]
  - **Excludes** knee (717.9)

- **719** Other and unspecified disorders of joint
  - **Excludes** jaw (524.60–524.69)

The following fifth-digit subclassification is for use with codes 719.0–719.6, 719.8–719.9; valid digits are in [brackets] under each code. See list at beginning of chapter for definitions:

0	site unspecified	5	pelvic region and thigh
1	shoulder region	6	lower leg
2	upper arm	7	ankle and foot
3	forearm	8	other specified sites
4	hand	9	multiple sites

- **719.0** Effusion of joint [0-9]
  - Hydrarthrosis
  - Swelling of joint, with or without pain
  - **Excludes** intermittent hydrarthrosis (719.3)
- **719.1** Hemarthrosis [0-9]
  - **Excludes** current injury (840.0–848.9)
- **719.2** Villonodular synovitis [0-9]
- **719.3** Palindromic rheumatism [0-9]
  - Hench-Rosenberg syndrome
  - Intermittent hydrarthrosis
- **719.4** Pain in joint [0-9]
  - Arthralgia
  - Coding Clinic: 2001, Q1, P3-4
- **719.5** Stiffness of joint, not elsewhere classified [0-9]
- **719.6** Other symptoms referable to joint [0-9]
  - Joint crepitus
  - Snapping hip
  - Coding Clinic: 2007, Q2, P7; 1984, Sept-Oct, P15-16
- **719.7** Difficulty in walking
  - **Excludes** abnormality of gait (781.2)
  - Coding Clinic: 2004, Q2, P15
- **719.8** Other specified disorders of joint [0-9]
  - Calcification of joint
  - Fistula of joint
  - **Excludes** temporomandibular joint-pain-dysfunction syndrome [Costen's syndrome] (524.60)
- **719.9** Unspecified disorder of joint [0-9]

DORSOPATHIES (720–724)

Excludes curvature of spine (737.0–737.9)
osteochondrosis of spine (juvenile) (732.0) adult (732.8)

- **720** Ankylosing spondylitis and other inflammatory spondylopathies
  - 720.0 Ankylosing spondylitis
    - Rheumatoid arthritis of spine NOS
    - Spondylitis:
      - Marie-Strümpell
      - rheumatoid
  - 720.1 Spinal enthesopathy
    - Disorder of peripheral ligamentous or muscular attachments of spine
    - Romanus lesion
  - 720.2 Sacroiliitis, not elsewhere classified
    - Inflammation of sacroiliac joint NOS
  - 720.8 Other inflammatory spondylopathies
    - 720.81 Inflammatory spondylopathies in diseases classified elsewhere
      - *Code first* underlying disease, as:
        - tuberculosis (015.0)
    - 720.89 Other
  - 720.9 Unspecified inflammatory spondylopathy
    - Spondylitis NOS

Item 13-2 **Ankylosis** or arthrokleisis is a consolidation of a joint due to disease, injury, or surgical procedure. Spondylosis is the degeneration of the vertebral processes and formation of osteophytes and commonly occurs with age. **Spondylitis** or ankylosing spondylitis is a type of arthritis that affects the spine or backbone causing back pain and stiffness.

PART III / Diseases: Tabular List Volume 1 — 721-723.4

- **721 Spondylosis and allied disorders**
  Coding Clinic: 1989, Q2, P14
  - **721.0 Cervical spondylosis without myelopathy**
    Cervical or cervicodorsal:
    arthritis
    osteoarthritis
    spondylarthritis
  - **721.1 Cervical spondylosis with myelopathy**
    Anterior spinal artery compression syndrome
    Spondylogenic compression of cervical spinal cord
    Vertebral artery compression syndrome
  - **721.2 Thoracic spondylosis without myelopathy**
    Thoracic:
    arthritis
    osteoarthritis
    spondylarthritis
  - **721.3 Lumbosacral spondylosis without myelopathy**
    Lumbar or lumbosacral:
    arthritis
    osteoarthritis
    spondylarthritis
    Coding Clinic: 2002, Q4, P107-108
  - **721.4 Thoracic or lumbar spondylosis with myelopathy**
    - **721.41 Thoracic region**
      Spondylogenic compression of thoracic spinal cord
    - **721.42 Lumbar region**
  - **721.5 Kissing spine**
    Baastrup's syndrome
  - **721.6 Ankylosing vertebral hyperostosis**
  - **721.7 Traumatic spondylopathy**
    Kümmell's disease or spondylitis
  - **721.8 Other allied disorders of spine**
  - **721.9 Spondylosis of unspecified site**
    - **721.90 Without mention of myelopathy**
      Spinal:
      arthritis (deformans) (degenerative) (hypertrophic)
      osteoarthritis NOS
      Spondylarthrosis NOS
    - **721.91 With myelopathy**
      Spondylogenic compression of spinal cord NOS

- **722 Intervertebral disc disorders**
  Coding Clinic: 1989, Q2, P14
  - **722.0 Displacement of cervical intervertebral disc without myelopathy**
    Neuritis (brachial) or radiculitis due to displacement or rupture of cervical intervertebral disc
    Any condition classifiable to 722.2 of the cervical or cervicothoracic intervertebral disc
    Coding Clinic: 1988, Q1, P10
  - **722.1 Displacement of thoracic or lumbar intervertebral disc without myelopathy**
    - **722.10 Lumbar intervertebral disc without myelopathy**
      Lumbago or sciatica due to displacement of intervertebral disc
      Neuritis or radiculitis due to displacement or rupture of lumbar intervertebral disc
      Any condition classifiable to 722.2 of the lumbar or lumbosacral intervertebral disc
      Coding Clinic: 2008, Q4, P183-184; 2007, Q1, P9; 2003, Q3, P12; Q1, P7; 2002, Q4, P107-108; 1994, Q3, P14
    - **722.11 Thoracic intervertebral disc without myelopathy**
      Any condition classifiable to 722.2 of thoracic intervertebral disc
  - **722.2 Displacement of intervertebral disc, site unspecified, without myelopathy**
    Discogenic syndrome NOS
    Herniation of nucleus pulposus NOS
    Intervertebral disc NOS:
    extrusion
    prolapse
    protrusion
    rupture
    Neuritis or radiculitis due to displacement or rupture of intervertebral disc
    Coding Clinic: 1988, Q1, P10
  - **722.3 Schmorl's nodes**
    - **722.30 Unspecified region**
    - **722.31 Thoracic region**
    - **722.32 Lumbar region**
    - **722.39 Other**
  - **722.4 Degeneration of cervical intervertebral disc**
    Degeneration of cervicothoracic intervertebral disc
  - **722.5 Degeneration of thoracic or lumbar intervertebral disc**
    - **722.51 Thoracic or thoracolumbar intervertebral disc**
    - **722.52 Lumbar or lumbosacral intervertebral disc**
      Coding Clinic: 2006, Q2, P18; 2004, Q4, P129-133
  - **722.6 Degeneration of intervertebral disc, site unspecified**
    Degenerative disc disease NOS
    Narrowing of intervertebral disc or space NOS
  - **722.7 Intervertebral disc disorder with myelopathy**
    - **722.70 Unspecified region**
    - **722.71 Cervical region**
    - **722.72 Thoracic region**
    - **722.73 Lumbar region**
  - **722.8 Postlaminectomy syndrome**
    - **722.80 Unspecified region**
    - **722.81 Cervical region**
    - **722.82 Thoracic region**
    - **722.83 Lumbar region**
      Coding Clinic: 1997, Q2, P15x2
  - **722.9 Other and unspecified disc disorder**
    Calcification of intervertebral cartilage or disc
    Discitis
    - **722.90 Unspecified region**
      Coding Clinic: 1984, Nov-Dec, P19
    - **722.91 Cervical region**
    - **722.92 Thoracic region**
    - **722.93 Lumbar region**

- **723 Other disorders of cervical region**
  Excludes conditions due to:
  intervertebral disc disorders (722.0–722.9)
  spondylosis (721.0–721.9)
  Coding Clinic: 1989, Q2, P14
  - **723.0 Spinal stenosis of cervical region**
    Coding Clinic: 2003, Q4, P99-101
  - **723.1 Cervicalgia**
    Pain in neck
  - **723.2 Cervicocranial syndrome**
    Barré-Liéou syndrome
    Posterior cervical sympathetic syndrome
  - **723.3 Cervicobrachial syndrome (diffuse)**
    Coding Clinic: 1985, Nov-Dec, P12
  - **723.4 Brachia neuritis or radiculitis NOS**
    Cervical radiculitis
    Radicular syndrome of upper limbs

■ **723.5 Torticollis, unspecified**
Contracture of neck
Excludes: congenital (754.1)
due to birth injury (767.8)
hysterical (300.11)
ocular torticollis (781.93)
psychogenic (306.0)
spasmodic (333.83)
traumatic, current (847.0)
Coding Clinic: 2001, Q2, P21; 1995, Q1, P7

723.6 Panniculitis specified as affecting neck

723.7 Ossification of posterior longitudinal ligament in cervical region

723.8 Other syndromes affecting cervical region
Cervical syndrome NEC
Klippel's disease
Occipital neuralgia
Coding Clinic: 2000, Q1, P7-8

■ **723.9 Unspecified musculoskeletal disorders and symptoms referable to neck**
Cervical (region) disorder NOS

● **724 Other and unspecified disorders of back**
Excludes: collapsed vertebra (code to cause, e.g., osteoporosis, 733.00–733.09)
conditions due to:
intervertebral disc disorders (722.0–722.9)
spondylosis (721.0–721.9)
Coding Clinic: 1989, Q2, P14

● **724.0 Spinal stenosis, other than cervical**
■ **724.00 Spinal stenosis, unspecified region**
724.01 Thoracic region
724.02 Lumbar region, without neurogenic claudication
Lumbar region NOS
Coding Clinic: 2008, Q4, P109-110; 2007, Q4, P116-120; Q1, P20-21; 1999, Q4, P13-14; 1994, Q3, P14
724.03 Lumbar region, with neurogenic claudication
724.09 Other

724.1 Pain in thoracic spine

724.2 Lumbago
Low back pain   Lumbalgia
Low back syndrome
Coding Clinic: 2007, Q2, P13-15; 1985, Nov-Dec, P12

724.3 Sciatica
Neuralgia or neuritis of sciatic nerve
Excludes: specified lesion of sciatic nerve (355.0)
Coding Clinic: 1989, Q2, P12

■ **724.4 Thoracic or lumbosacral neuritis or radiculitis, unspecified**
Radicular syndrome of lower limbs
Coding Clinic: 1999, Q2, P3-4

■ **724.5 Backache, unspecified**
Vertebrogenic (pain) syndrome NOS

724.6 Disorders of sacrum
Ankylosis, lumbosacral or sacroiliac (joint)
Instability, lumbosacral or sacroiliac (joint)

724.7 Disorders of coccyx
■ **724.70 Unspecified disorder of coccyx**
724.71 Hypermobility of coccyx
724.79 Other
Coccygodynia

724.8 Other symptoms referable to back
Ossification of posterior longitudinal ligament NOS
Panniculitis specified as sacral or affecting back

■ **724.9 Other unspecified back disorders**
Ankylosis of spine NOS
Compression of spinal nerve root NEC
Spinal disorder NOS
Excludes: sacroiliitis (720.2)

Item 13-3 Polymyalgia rheumatica is a syndrome characterized by aching and morning stiffness and is related to aging and hereditary predisposition.

RHEUMATISM, EXCLUDING THE BACK (725–729)

Includes: disorders of muscles and tendons and their attachments, and of other soft tissues

725 Polymyalgia rheumatica

● **726 Peripheral enthesopathies and allied syndromes**
Note: Enthesopathies are disorders of peripheral ligamentous or muscular attachments.
Excludes: spinal enthesopathy (720.1)

726.0 Adhesive capsulitis of shoulder

● **726.1 Rotator cuff syndrome of shoulder and allied disorders**
■ **726.10 Disorders of bursae and tendons in shoulder region, unspecified**
Rotator cuff syndrome NOS
Supraspinatus syndrome NOS
Coding Clinic: 2001, Q2, P12

726.11 Calcifying tendinitis of shoulder
726.12 Bicipital tenosynovitis
726.13 Partial tear of rotator cuff
Excludes: complete rupture of rotator cuff, nontraumatic (727.61)
Coding Clinic: 2011, Q4, P136

726.19 Other specified disorders
Excludes: complete rupture of rotator cuff, nontraumatic (727.61)
Coding Clinic: 2002, Q1, P9-10

726.2 Other affections of shoulder region, not elsewhere classified
Periarthritis of shoulder   Scapulohumeral fibrositis

● **726.3 Enthesopathy of elbow region**
■ **726.30 Enthesopathy of elbow, unspecified**
726.31 Medial epicondylitis
726.32 Lateral epicondylitis
Epicondylitis NOS   Tennis elbow
Golfers' elbow
726.33 Olecranon bursitis
Bursitis of elbow
726.39 Other

726.4 Enthesopathy of wrist and carpus
Bursitis of hand or wrist   Periarthritis of wrist

726.5 Enthesopathy of hip region
Bursitis of hip   Psoas tendinitis
Gluteal tendinitis   Trochanteric tendinitis
Iliac crest spur

● **726.6 Enthesopathy of knee**
■ **726.60 Enthesopathy of knee, unspecified**
Bursitis of knee NOS
726.61 Pes anserinus tendinitis or bursitis
726.62 Tibial collateral ligament bursitis
Pellegrini-Stieda syndrome
726.63 Fibular collateral ligament bursitis
726.64 Patellar tendinitis
726.65 Prepatellar bursitis
Coding Clinic: 2006, Q2, P15
726.69 Other
Bursitis:
infrapatellar
subpatellar

- **726.7 Enthesopathy of ankle and tarsus**
  - **726.70 Enthesopathy of ankle and tarsus, unspecified**
    Metatarsalgia NOS
    Excludes Morton's metatarsalgia (355.6)
  - 726.71 Achilles bursitis or tendinitis
  - 726.72 Tibialis tendinitis
    Tibialis (anterior) (posterior) tendinitis
  - 726.73 Calcaneal spur
  - 726.79 Other
    Peroneal tendinitis
- 726.8 Other peripheral enthesopathies
- **726.9 Unspecified enthesopathy**
  - **726.90 Enthesopathy of unspecified site**
    Capsulitis NOS   Tendinitis NOS
    Periarthritis NOS
  - **726.91 Exostosis of unspecified site**
    Bone spur NOS
    Coding Clinic: 2001, Q2, P13-15

- **727 Other disorders of synovium, tendon, and bursa**
  - **727.0 Synovitis and tenosynovitis**
    - **727.00 Synovitis and tenosynovitis, unspecified**
      Synovitis NOS
      Tenosynovitis NOS
    - **727.01 Synovitis and tenosynovitis in diseases classified elsewhere**
      Code first underlying disease, as:
        tuberculosis (015.0–015.9)
      Excludes crystal-induced (275.49)
        gonococcal (098.51)
        gout (274.00-274.03)
        syphilitic (095.7)
    - 727.02 Giant cell tumor of tendon sheath
    - 727.03 Trigger finger (acquired)
    - 727.04 Radial styloid tenosynovitis
      de Quervain's disease
    - 727.05 Other tenosynovitis of hand and wrist
    - 727.06 Tenosynovitis of foot and ankle
    - 727.09 Other
  - 727.1 Bunion
  - 727.2 Specific bursitides often of occupational origin
    Beat:
      elbow
      hand
      knee
    Chronic crepitant synovitis of wrist
    Miners':
      elbow
      knee
  - 727.3 Other bursitis
    Bursitis NOS
    Excludes bursitis:
      gonococcal (098.52)
      subacromial (726.19)
      subcoracoid (726.19)
      subdeltoid (726.19)
      syphilitic (095.7)
    "frozen shoulder" (726.0)

- **727.4 Ganglion and cyst of synovium, tendon, and bursa**
  - **727.40 Synovial cyst, unspecified**
    Excludes that of popliteal space (727.51)
    Coding Clinic: 1997, Q2, P6
  - 727.41 Ganglion of joint
  - 727.42 Ganglion of tendon sheath
  - **727.43 Ganglion, unspecified**
  - 727.49 Other
    Cyst of bursa
- **727.5 Rupture of synovium**
  - **727.50 Rupture of synovium, unspecified**
  - 727.51 Synovial cyst of popliteal space
    Baker's cyst (knee)
  - 727.59 Other
- **727.6 Rupture of tendon, nontraumatic**
  - **727.60 Nontraumatic rupture of unspecified tendon**
  - 727.61 Complete rupture of rotator cuff
    Excludes partial tear of rotator cuff (726.13)
  - 727.62 Tendons of biceps (long head)
  - 727.63 Extensor tendons of hand and wrist
  - 727.64 Flexor tendons of hand and wrist
  - 727.65 Quadriceps tendon
  - 727.66 Patellar tendon
  - 727.67 Achilles tendon
  - 727.68 Other tendons of foot and ankle
  - 727.69 Other
- **727.8 Other disorders of synovium, tendon, and bursa**
  - 727.81 Contracture of tendon (sheath)
    Short Achilles tendon (acquired)
  - 727.82 Calcium deposits in tendon and bursa
    Calcification of tendon NOS
    Calcific tendinitis NOS
    Excludes peripheral ligamentous or muscular attachments (726.0–726.9)
  - 727.83 Plica syndrome
    Plica knee
  - 727.89 Other
    Abscess of bursa or tendon
    Excludes xanthomatosis localized to tendons (272.7)
    Coding Clinic: 1989, Q2, P15; 1985, July-Aug, P14; 1984, Nov-Dec, P9
  - **727.9 Unspecified disorder of synovium, tendon, and bursa**
- **728 Disorders of muscle, ligament, and fascia**
  Excludes enthesopathies (726.0–726.9)
    muscular dystrophies (359.0–359.1)
    myoneural disorders (358.00–358.9)
    myopathies (359.2–359.9)
    nontraumatic hematoma of muscle (729.92)
    old disruption of ligaments of knee (717.81–717.89)
  - 728.0 Infective myositis
    Myositis:
      purulent
      suppurative
    Excludes myositis:
      epidemic (074.1)
      interstitial (728.81)
      myoneural disorder (358.00–358.9)
      syphilitic (095.6)
      tropical (040.81)
  - **728.1 Muscular calcification and ossification**
    - **728.10 Calcification and ossification, unspecified**
      Massive calcification (paraplegic)
    - 728.11 Progressive myositis ossificans
    - 728.12 Traumatic myositis ossifications
      Myositis ossificans (circumscripta)
    - 728.13 Postoperative heterotopic calcification
    - 728.19 Other
      Polymyositis ossificans

Item 13-4 **Synovitis** is an inflammation of a synovial membrane resulting in pain on motion and is characterized by fluctuating swelling due to effusion in a synovial sac. **Tenosynovitis** is an inflammation of a tendon sheath and occurs most commonly in the wrists, hands, and feet. Bursitis is inflammation of a bursa (fluid filled sac) caused by repetitive use, trauma, infection, or systemic inflammatory disease. Bursae act as protectors and facilitate movement between bones and overlapping muscles (deep bursae) or between bones and tendons/skin (superficial bursae).

728.2 Muscular wasting and disuse atrophy, not elsewhere classified
Amyotrophia NOS
Myofibrosis
Excludes neuralgic amyotrophy (353.5)
pelvic muscle wasting and disuse atrophy (618.83)
progressive muscular atrophy (335.0–335.9)

728.3 Other specific muscle disorders
Arthrogryposis
Immobility syndrome (paraplegic)
Excludes arthrogryposis multiplex congenita (754.89)
stiff-man syndrome (333.91)

728.4 Laxity of ligament

728.5 Hypermobility syndrome

728.6 Contracture of palmar fascia
Dupuytren's contracture

● **728.7 Other fibromatoses**
728.71 Plantar fascial fibromatosis
Contracture of plantar fascia
Plantar fasciitis (traumatic)
728.79 Other
Garrod's or knuckle pads
Nodular fasciitis
Pseudosarcomatous Fibromatosis (proliferative) (subcutaneous)

● **728.8 Other disorders of muscle, ligament, and fascia**
728.81 Interstitial myositis
728.82 Foreign body granuloma of muscle
Talc granuloma of muscle
Use additional code to identify foreign body (V90.01-V90.9)
728.83 Rupture of muscle, nontraumatic
728.84 Diastasis of muscle
Diastasis recti (abdomen)
Excludes diastasis recti complicating pregnancy, labor, and delivery (665.8)
728.85 Spasm of muscle
728.86 Necrotizing fasciitis
Use additional code to identify:
infectious organism (041.00–041.89)
gangrene (785.4), if applicable
728.87 Muscle weakness (generalized)
Excludes generalized weakness (780.79)
Coding Clinic: 2005, Q1, P13
728.88 Rhabdomyolysis
Coding Clinic: 2003, Q4, P66-67; 2001, Q2, P14
728.89 Other
Eosinophilic fasciitis
Use additional E code to identify drug, if drug induced
Coding Clinic: 2006, Q3, P13; 2002, Q3, P28; 2001, Q2, P15

728.9 Unspecified disorder of muscle, ligament, and fascia

● **729 Other disorders of soft tissues**
Excludes acroparesthesia (443.89)
carpal tunnel syndrome (354.0)
disorders of the back (720.0–724.9)
entrapment syndromes (354.0–355.9)
palindromic rheumatism (719.3)
periarthritis (726.0–726.9)
psychogenic rheumatism (306.0)
Coding Clinic: 1984, Nov-Dec, P17

729.0 Rheumatism, unspecified and fibrositis

729.1 Myalgia and myositis, unspecified
Fibromyositis NOS
Coding Clinic: 1984, Nov-Dec, P17

729.2 Neuralgia, neuritis, and radiculitis, unspecified
Excludes brachia radiculitis (723.4)
cervical radiculitis (723.4)
lumbosacral radiculitis (724.4)
mononeuritis (354.0–355.9)
radiculitis due to intervertebral disc involvement (722.0–722.2, 722.7)
sciatica (724.3)

● **729.3 Panniculitis, unspecified**
Inflammation of adipose tissue of heel pad
729.30 Panniculitis, unspecified site
Weber-Christian disease
729.31 Hypertrophy of fat pad, knee
Hypertrophy of infrapatellar fat pad
729.39 Other site
Excludes panniculitis specified as (affecting):
back (724.8)
neck (723.6)
sacral (724.8)

729.4 Fasciitis, unspecified
Excludes necrotizing fasciitis (728.86)
nodular fasciitis (728.79)
Coding Clinic: 1994, Q2, P13

729.5 Pain in limb
Coding Clinic: 2007, Q2, P13-15

729.6 Residual foreign body in soft tissue
Use additional code to identify foreign body (V90.01-V90.9)
Excludes foreign body granuloma:
muscle (728.82)
skin and subcutaneous tissue (709.4)

● **729.7 Nontraumatic compartment syndrome**
Excludes compartment syndrome NOS (958.90)
traumatic compartment syndrome (958.90–958.99)
Code first, if applicable, postprocedural complication (998.89)
729.71 Nontraumatic compartment syndrome of upper extremity
Nontraumatic compartment syndrome of shoulder, arm, forearm, wrist, hand and fingers
Coding Clinic: 2006, Q4, P100-102
729.72 Nontraumatic compartment syndrome of lower extremity
Nontraumatic compartment syndrome of hip, buttock, thigh, leg, foot and toes
729.73 Nontraumatic compartment syndrome of abdomen
729.79 Nontraumatic compartment syndrome of other sites

● **729.8 Other musculoskeletal symptoms referable to limbs**
729.81 Swelling of limb
Coding Clinic: 1988, Q4, P6
729.82 Cramp
729.89 Other
Excludes abnormality of gait (781.2)
tetany (781.7)
transient paralysis of limb (781.4)
Coding Clinic: 1988, Q4, P12

● **729.9 Other and unspecified disorders of soft tissue**
Coding Clinic: 2008, Q4, P134-136
729.90 Disorders of soft tissue, unspecified
729.91 Post-traumatic seroma
Excludes seroma complicating a procedure (998.13)
729.92 Nontraumatic hematoma of soft tissue
Nontraumatic hematoma of muscle
729.99 Other disorders of soft tissue
Polyalgia

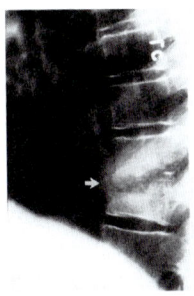

Figure 13-2 Osteomyelitis of the spine. A lateral view of the lower thoracic spine demonstrates destruction of the disk space (arrow) as well as destruction of the adjoining vertebral bodies. (From Mettler: Essentials of Radiology, ed 2, Saunders, An Imprint of Elsevier, 2005)

Item 13-5 Osteomyelitis is an inflammation of the bone. **Acute osteomyelitis** is a rapidly destructive, pus-producing infection capable of causing severe bone destruction. **Chronic osteomyelitis** can remain long after the initial acute episode has passed and may lead to a recurrence of the acute phase. **Brodie's abscess** is an encapsulated focal abscess that must be surgically drained. Periostitis is an inflammation of the periosteum, a dense membrane composed of fibrous connective tissue that closely wraps all bone, except those with articulating surfaces in joints, which are covered by synovial membranes.

OSTEOPATHIES, CHONDROPATHIES, AND ACQUIRED MUSCULOSKELETAL DEFORMITIES (730–739)

- **730 Osteomyelitis, periostitis, and other infections involving bone**
    - Excludes jaw (526.4–526.5)
      petrous bone (383.2)
    - Use additional code to identify organism, such as:
      Staphylococcus (041.1)
    - Coding Clinic: 1997, Q4, P43; 1993, 5th Issue, P3

  The following fifth-digit subclassification is for use with category 730; valid digits are in [brackets] under each code. See list at beginning of chapter for definitions:

0 site unspecified	5 pelvic region and thigh
1 shoulder region	6 lower leg
2 upper arm	7 ankle and foot
3 forearm	8 other specified sites
4 hand	9 multiple sites

  - **730.0 Acute osteomyelitis**
    [0-9] Abscess of any bone except accessory sinus, jaw, or mastoid
    Acute or subacute osteomyelitis, with or without mention of periostitis
    Use additional code to identify major osseous defect, if applicable (731.3)
    Coding Clinic: 2004, Q1, P14-15; 2002, Q1, P3-4

  - **730.1 Chronic osteomyelitis**
    [0-9] Brodie's abscess
    Chronic or old osteomyelitis, with or without mention of periostitis
    Sequestrum
    Sclerosing osteomyelitis of Garré
    Use additional code to identify major osseous defect, if applicable (731.3)
    Excludes aseptic necrosis of bone (733.40–733.49)
    Coding Clinic: 2011, Q3, P15; 2000, Q3, P4

  - **730.2 Unspecified osteomyelitis**
    [0-9] Osteitis or osteomyelitis NOS, with or without mention of periostitis
    Use additional code to identify major osseous defect, if applicable (731.3)

  - **730.3 Periostitis without mention of osteomyelitis**
    [0-9] Abscess of periosteum, without mention of osteomyelitis
    Periostosis, without mention of osteomyelitis
    Excludes that in secondary syphilis (091.61)

  - **730.7 Osteopathy resulting from poliomyelitis**
    [0-9] Code first underlying disease (045.0–045.9)

  - **730.8 Other infections involving bone in disease classified elsewhere**
    [0-9] Code first underlying disease, as:
      tuberculosis (015.0–015.9)
      typhoid fever (002.0)
    Excludes syphilitis of bone NOS (095.5)

  - **730.9 Unspecified infection of bone**
    [0-9]

- **731 Osteitis deformans and osteopathies associated with other disorders classified elsewhere**
  Also known as Paget's Disease; chronic disorder that results in enlarged and deformed bones. The excessive breakdown and formation of bone tissue causes bones to weaken and results in bone pain, arthritis, deformities, and fractures.

  - **731.0 Osteitis deformans without mention of bone tumor**
    Paget's disease of bone
    Coding Clinic: 1994, Q2, P6-7

  - **731.1 Osteitis deformans in diseases classified elsewhere**
    Code first underlying disease, as:
      malignant neoplasm of bone (170.0–170.9)

  - **731.2 Hypertrophic pulmonary osteoarthropathy**
    Bamberger-Marie disease

  - **731.3 Major osseous defects**
    Code first underlying disease, if known, such as:
      aseptic necrosis (733.40–733.49)
      malignant neoplasm of bone (170.0–170.9)
      osteomyelitis (730.00–730.29)
      osteoporosis (733.00–733.09)
      peri-prosthetic osteolysis (996.45)
    Coding Clinic: 2006, Q4, P103-104

  - **731.8 Other bone involvement in diseases classified elsewhere**
    Code first underlying disease, as:
      diabetes mellitus (249.8, 250.8)
    Use additional code to specify bone condition, such as:
      acute osteomyelitis (730.00–730.09)
    Coding Clinic: 2010, Q2, P6; 2004, Q1, P14-15; 1997, Q4, P43

- **732 Osteochondropathies**

  - **732.0 Juvenile osteochondrosis of spine**
    Juvenile osteochondrosis (of):
      marginal or vertebral ephiphysis (of Scheuermann)
      spine NOS
    Vertebral epiphysitis
    Excludes adolescent postural kyphosis (737.0)

  - **732.1 Juvenile osteochondrosis of hip and pelvis**
    Coxa plana
    Ischiopubic synchondrosis (of van Neck)
    Osteochondrosis (juvenile) of:
      acetabulum
      head of femur (of Legg-Calvé-Perthes)
      iliac crest (of Buchanan)
      symphysis pubis (of Pierson)
    Pseudocoxalgia

  - **732.2 Nontraumatic slipped upper femoral epiphysis**
    Slipped upper femoral epiphysis NOS

  - **732.3 Juvenile osteochondrosis of upper extremity**
    Osteochondrosis (juvenile) of:
      capitulum of humerus (of Panner)
      carpal lunate (of Kienbock)
      hand NOS
      head of humerus (of Haas)
      heads of metacarpals (of Mauclaire)
      lower ulna (of Burns)
      radial head (of Brailsford)
      upper extremity NOS

  - **732.4 Juvenile osteochondrosis of lower extremity, excluding foot**
    Osteochondrosis (juvenile) of:
      lower extremity NOS
      primary patellar center (of Köhler)
      proximal tibia (of Blount)
      secondary patellar center (of Sinding-Larsen)
      tibial tubercle (of Osgood-Schlatter)
    Tibia vara

DISEASES OF THE MUSCULOSKELETAL SYSTEM AND CONNECTIVE TISSUE (710–739)

- **732.5 Juvenile osteochondrosis of foot**
  Calcaneal apophysitis
  Epiphysitis, os calcis
  Osteochondrosis (juvenile) of:
    astragalus (of Diaz)
    calcaneum (of Sever)
    foot NOS
    metatarsal:
      second (of Freiberg)
      fifth (of Iselin)
    os tibiale externum (of Haglund)
    tarsal navicular (of Köhler)
- **732.6 Other juvenile osteochondrosis**
  Apophysitis specified as juvenile, of other site, or site NOS
  Epiphysitis specified as juvenile, of other site, or site NOS
  Osteochondritis specified as juvenile, of other site, or site NOS
  Osteochondrosis specified as juvenile, of other site, or site NOS
- **732.7 Osteochondritis dissecans**
- **732.8 Other specified forms of osteochondropathy**
  Adult osteochondrosis of spine
- **732.9 Unspecified osteochondropathy**
  Apophysitis
    NOS
    not specified as adult or juvenile, of unspecified site
  Epiphysitis
    NOS
    not specified as adult or juvenile, of unspecified site
  Osteochondritis
    NOS
    not specified as adult or juvenile, of unspecified site
  Osteochondrosis
    NOS
    not specified as adult or juvenile, of unspecified site

- **733 Other disorders of bone and cartilage**
  Excludes bone spur (726.91)
  cartilage of, or loose body in, joint (717.0–717.9, 718.0–718.9)
  giant cell granuloma of jaw (526.3)
  osteitis fibrosa cystica generalisata (252.01)
  osteomalacia (268.2)
  polyostotic fibrous dysplasia of bone (756.54)
  prognathism, retrognathism (524.1)
  xanthomatosis localized to bone (272.7)

- **733.0 Osteoporosis**
  Condition of excessive skeletal fragility (porous bone) resulting in bone fractures
  Use additional code to identify:
    major osseous defect, if applicable (731.3)
    personal history of pathologic (healed) fracture (V13.51)
  Coding Clinic: 1993, Q4, P25-26
  - **733.00 Osteoporosis, unspecified**
    Wedging of vertebra NOS
    Coding Clinic: 2007, Q4, P91-92; Q1, P22; 2001, Q3, P19; 1998, Q2, P12
  - **733.01 Senile osteoporosis**
    Postmenopausal osteoporosis
    Coding Clinic: 2007, Q1, P3-8
  - **733.02 Idiopathic osteoporosis**
  - **733.03 Disuse osteoporosis**
  - **733.09 Other**
    Drug-induced osteoporosis
    Use additional E code to identify drug
    Coding Clinic: 2003, Q4, P108-109

- **733.1 Pathologic fracture**
  Chronic fracture
  Spontaneous fracture
  Excludes stress fracture (733.93–733.95)
  traumatic fractures (800–829)
  Coding Clinic: 1986, Nov-Dec, P10; 1985, Nov-Dec, P16
  - **733.10 Pathologic fracture, unspecified site**
  - **733.11 Pathologic fracture of humerus**
    Coding Clinic: 2010, Q2, P6
  - **733.12 Pathologic fracture of distal radius and ulna**
    Wrist NOS
  - **733.13 Pathologic fracture of vertebrae**
    Collapse of vertebra NOS
    Coding Clinic: 2008, Q3, P4; 2007, Q1, P3-8,22; 1999, Q3, P5
  - **733.14 Pathologic fracture of neck of femur**
    Femur NOS   Hip NOS
    Coding Clinic: 2001, Q1, P10-11; 1996, Q1, P16; 1993, Q4, P25-26
  - **733.15 Pathologic fracture of other specified part of femur**
    Coding Clinic: 2010, Q2, P6; 1998, Q2, P12; 1994, Q2, P6-7
  - **733.16 Pathologic fracture of tibia and fibula**
    Ankle NOS
  - **733.19 Pathologic fracture of other specified site**

- **733.2 Cyst of bone**
  - **733.20 Cyst of bone (localized), unspecified**
  - **733.21 Solitary bone cyst**
    Unicameral bone cyst
  - **733.22 Aneurysmal bone cyst**
  - **733.29 Other**
    Fibrous dysplasia (monostotic)
    Excludes cyst of jaw (526.0–526.2, 526.89)
    osteitis fibrosa cystica (252.01)
    polyostotic fibrous dysplasia of bone (756.54)

- **733.3 Hyperostosis of skull**
  Hyperostosis interna frontalis
  Leontiasis ossium

- **733.4 Aseptic necrosis of bone**
  Use additional code to identify major osseous defect, if applicable (731.3)
  Excludes osteochondropathies (732.0–732.9)
  Coding Clinic: 2007, Q4, P116-120
  - **733.40 Aseptic necrosis of bone, site unspecified**
  - **733.41 Head of humerus**
  - **733.42 Head and neck of femur**
    Femur NOS
    Excludes Legg-Calvé-Perthes disease (732.1)
  - **733.43 Medial femoral condyle**
  - **733.44 Talus**
  - **733.45 Jaw**
    Use additional E code to identify drug, if drug-induced
    Excludes osteoradionecrosis of jaw (526.89)
    Coding Clinic: 2007, Q4, P91-92
  - **733.49 Other**

- **733.5 Osteitis condensans**
  Piriform sclerosis of ilium

- **733.6 Tietze's disease**
  Costochondral junction syndrome
  Costochondritis

- **733.7 Algoneurodystrophy**
  Disuse atrophy of bone
  Sudeck's atrophy

- **733.8 Malunion and nonunion of fracture**
  - **733.81 Malunion of fracture**
    Fracture ends do not heal together correctly.
  - **733.82 Nonunion of fracture**
    Total failure of fracture healing
    Pseudoarthrosis (bone)
    Coding Clinic: 1994, Q2, P7; 1987, Jan-Feb, P13; 1984, Nov-Dec, P18
- **733.9 Other and unspecified disorders of bone and cartilage**
  Coding Clinic: 2008, Q4, P136-137
  - **733.90 Disorder of bone and cartilage, unspecified**
  - **733.91 Arrest of bone development or growth**
    Epiphyseal arrest
  - **733.92 Chondromalacia**
    Chondromalacia:
      NOS
      localized, except patella
      systemic
      tibial plateau
    Excludes: chondromalacia of patella (717.7)
  - **733.93 Stress fracture of tibia or fibula**
    Stress reaction of tibia or fibula
    Use additional external cause code(s) to identify the cause of the stress fracture
  - **733.94 Stress fracture of the metatarsals**
    Stress reaction of metatarsals
    Use additional external cause code(s) to identify the cause of the stress fracture
    Coding Clinic: 2001, Q4, P48-49
  - **733.95 Stress fracture of other bone**
    Stress reaction of other bone
    Use additional external cause code(s) to identify the cause of the stress fracture
    Excludes: stress fracture of:
      femoral neck (733.96)
      fibula (733.93)
      metatarsals (733.94)
      pelvis (733.98)
      shaft of femur (733.97)
      tibia (733.93)
  - **733.96 Stress fracture of femoral neck**
    Stress reaction of femoral neck
    Use additional external cause code(s) to identify the cause of the stress fracture
  - **733.97 Stress fracture of shaft of femur**
    Stress reaction of shaft of femur
    Use additional external cause code(s) to identify the cause of the stress fracture
  - **733.98 Stress fracture of pelvis**
    Stress reaction of pelvis
    Use additional external cause code(s) to identify the cause of the stress fracture
  - **733.99 Other**
    Diaphysitis
    Hypertrophy of bone
    Relapsing polychondritis
    Coding Clinic: 2011, Q1, P7; 2000, Q3, P4; 1987, Jan-Feb, P14

734 Flat foot
  Pes planus (acquired)
  Talipes planus (acquired)
  Excludes: congenital (754.61)
    rigid flat foot (754.61)
    spastic (everted) flat foot (754.61)

- **735 Acquired deformities of toe**
  Excludes: congenital (754.60–754.69, 755.65–755.66)
  - **735.0 Hallux valgus (acquired)**
  - **735.1 Hallux varus (acquired)**
  - **735.2 Hallux rigidus**
  - **735.3 Hallux malleus**
  - **735.4 Other hammer toe (acquired)**

Item 13–6 Claw toe is caused by a contraction of the flexor tendon producing a flexion deformity characterized by hyperextension of the big toe.

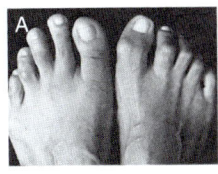
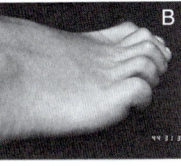
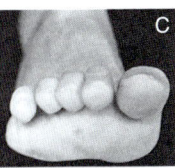

Figure 13–3 A. Claw toes, right foot, secondary to medial and lateral plantar nerve laceration. **B.** Metatarsophalangeal joints of second and third toes could not be flexed to neutral position and none could be flexed past neutral. **C.** Extension posture of claw toes increases plantar pressure on metatarsal heads. (From Canale: Campbell's Operative Orthopaedics, ed 11, Mosby, Inc., 2007)

Figure 13–4 Hallux valgus or bunion.

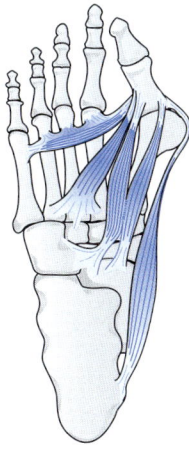

Item 13–7 Hallux valgus, or bunion, is a bursa usually found along the medial aspect of the big toe. It is most often attributed to heredity or poorly fitted shoes.

Item 13–8 Hallux valgus or bunion is a sometimes painful structural deformity caused by an inflammation of the bursal sac at the base of the metatarsophalangeal joint (big toe). **Hallus varus** is a deviation of the great toe to the inner side of the foot or away from the next toe.

  - **735.5 Claw toe (acquired)**
    Coding Clinic: 2007, Q4, P123
  - **735.8 Other acquired deformities of toe**
  - **735.9 Unspecified acquired deformity of toe**

- **736 Other acquired deformities of limbs**
  Excludes: congenital (754.3–755.9)
  - **736.0 Acquired deformities of forearm, excluding fingers**
    - **736.00 Unspecified deformity**
      Deformity of elbow, forearm, hand, or wrist (acquired) NOS
    - **736.01 Cubitus valgus (acquired)**
    - **736.02 Cubitus varus (acquired)**
    - **736.03 Valgus deformity of wrist (acquired)**
    - **736.04 Varus deformity of wrist (acquired)**
    - **736.05 Wrist drop (acquired)**
    - **736.06 Claw hand (acquired)**
    - **736.07 Club hand (acquired)**
    - **736.09 Other**

Item 13–9 Cubitus valgus is a deformity of the elbow resulting in an increased carrying angle in which the arm extends at the side and the palm faces forward, which results in the forearm and hand extended at greater than 15 degrees. **Cubitus varus** is a deformity of the elbow resulting in the arm extended at the side and the palm facing forward so that the forearm and hand are held at less than 5 degrees.

736.1 Mallet finger
● 736.2 Other acquired deformities of finger
 ■ 736.20 Unspecified deformity
  Deformity of finger (acquired) NOS
  736.21 Boutonniere deformity
  736.22 Swan-neck deformity
  736.29 Other
   Excludes trigger finger (727.03)
   Coding Clinic: 2005, Q2, P7; 1989, Q2, P13
● 736.3 Acquired deformities of hip
 Coding Clinic: 2008, Q2, P3-4
 ■ 736.30 Unspecified deformity
  Deformity of hip (acquired) NOS
  736.31 Coxa valga (acquired)
  736.32 Coxa vara (acquired)
  736.39 Other
● 736.4 Genu valgum or varum (acquired)
  736.41 Genu valgum (acquired)
  736.42 Genu varum (acquired)
 736.5 Genu recurvatum (acquired)
 736.6 Other acquired deformities of knee
  Deformity of knee (acquired) NOS
● 736.7 Other acquired deformities of ankle and foot
 Excludes deformities of toe (acquired) (735.0–735.9)
  pes planus (acquired) (734)
 ■ 736.70 Unspecified deformity of ankle and foot, acquired
  736.71 Acquired equinovarus deformity
   Clubfoot, acquired
   Excludes clubfoot not specified as acquired
   (754.5–754.7)
  736.72 Equinus deformity of foot, acquired
  736.73 Cavus deformity of foot
   Excludes that with claw foot (736.74)
  736.74 Claw foot, acquired
  736.75 Cavovarus deformity of foot, acquired
  736.76 Other calcaneus deformity
  736.79 Other
   Acquired:
    pes not elsewhere classified
    talipes not elsewhere classified
● 736.8 Acquired deformities of other parts of limbs
  736.81 Unequal leg length (acquired)
   Coding Clinic: 1995, Q1, P10
  736.89 Other
   Deformity (acquired):
    arm or leg, not elsewhere classified
    shoulder
   Coding Clinic: 2008, Q2, P5-6
■ 736.9 Acquired deformity of limb, site unspecified
 Coding Clinic: 2008, Q2, P3-4

Item 13-11 **Kyphosis** is an abnormal curvature of the spine. **Senile kyphosis** is a result of disc degeneration causing ossification (turning to bone). **Adolescent** or **juvenile kyphosis** is also known as **Scheuermann's disease,** a condition in which the discs of the lower thoracic spine herniate, causing the disc space to narrow and the spine to tilt forward. This condition is attributed to poor posture. Lordosis or swayback is an abnormal curvature of the spine resulting in an inward curve of the lumbar spine just above the buttocks. Scoliosis causes a sideways curve to the spine. The curves are S- or C-shaped, and it is most commonly acquired in late childhood and early teen years, when growth is fast.

● 737 Curvature of spine
 Excludes congenital (754.2)
  737.0 Adolescent postural kyphosis
   Excludes osteochondrosis of spine (juvenile) (732.0)
    adult (732.8)
● 737.1 Kyphosis (acquired)
  737.10 Kyphosis (acquired) (postural)
  737.11 Kyphosis due to radiation
  737.12 Kyphosis, postlaminectomy
  737.19 Other
   Excludes that associated with conditions
    classifiable elsewhere (737.41)
   Coding Clinic: 2007, Q1, P20-21
● 737.2 Lordosis (acquired)
  Abnormal increase in normal curvature of lumbar spine (sway back)
  737.20 Lordosis (acquired) (postural)
  737.21 Lordosis, postlaminectomy
  737.22 Other postsurgical lordosis
  737.29 Other
   Excludes that associated with conditions
    classifiable elsewhere (737.42)
● 737.3 Kyphoscoliosis and scoliosis
  737.30 Scoliosis [and kyphoscoliosis], idiopathic
   Coding Clinic: 2003, Q3, P19x2
  737.31 Resolving infantile idiopathic scoliosis
  737.32 Progressive infantile idiopathic scoliosis
   Coding Clinic: 2002, Q3, P12
  737.33 Scoliosis due to radiation
  737.34 Thoracogenic scoliosis
  737.39 Other
   Excludes that associated with conditions
    classifiable elsewhere (737.43)
    that in kyphoscoliotic heart disease
    (416.1)
   Coding Clinic: 2002, Q2, P16

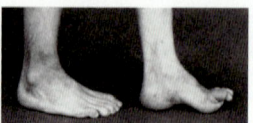

Figure 13-5 Supination and cavus deformity of forefoot. *(Courtesy Jay Cummings, MD.)* (From Canale: Campbell's Operative Orthopaedics, ed 11, Mosby, Inc., 2007)

Item 13-10 **Equinus foot** is a term referring to the hoof of a horse. The deformity is usually congenital or spastic. Talipes equinovarus is referred to as clubfoot. The foot tends to be smaller than normal, with the heel pointing downward and the forefoot turning inward. The heel cord (Achilles tendon) is tight, causing the heel to be drawn up toward the leg.

Item 13-12 **Spondylolisthesis** is a condition caused by the slipping forward of one disc over another.

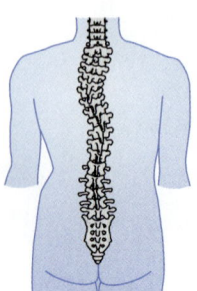

Figure 13-6 Scoliosis is a lateral curvature of the spine.

- **737.4 Curvature of spine associated with other conditions**
  Code first associated condition, as:
  Charcot-Marie-Tooth disease (356.1)
  mucopolysaccharidosis (277.5)
  neurofibromatosis (237.70–237.79)
  osteitis deformans (731.0)
  osteitis fibrosa cystica (252.01)
  osteoporosis (733.00–733.09)
  poliomyelitis (138)
  tuberculosis [Pott's curvature] (015.0)
  - **737.40 Curvature of spine, unspecified**
  - **737.41 Kyphosis**
  - **737.42 Lordosis**
  - **737.43 Scoliosis**
- **737.8 Other curvatures of spine**
- **737.9 Unspecified curvature of spine**
  Curvature of spine (acquired) (idiopathic) NOS
  Hunchback, acquired
  Excludes *deformity of spine NOS (738.5)*

- **738 Other acquired deformity**
  Excludes *congenital (754.0–756.9, 758.0–759.9)*
  dentofacial anomalies (524.0–524.9)
  - **738.0 Acquired deformity of nose**
    Deformity of nose (acquired)
    Overdevelopment of nasal bones
    Excludes *deflected or deviated nasal septum (470)*
  - **738.1 Other acquired deformity of head**
    - **738.10 Unspecified deformity**
    - **738.11 Zygomatic hyperplasia**
    - **738.12 Zygomatic hypoplasia**
    - **738.19 Other specified deformity**
      Coding Clinic: 2006, Q1, P6-7; 2003, Q2, P13
  - **738.2 Acquired deformity of neck**
  - **738.3 Acquired deformity of chest and rib**
    Deformity:
      chest (acquired)
      rib (acquired)
    Pectus:
      carinatum, acquired
      excavatum, acquired
  - **738.4 Acquired spondylolisthesis**
    Degenerative spondylolisthesis
    Spondylolysis, acquired
    Excludes *congenital (756.12)*
    Coding Clinic: 2007, Q4, P116-120
  - **738.5 Other acquired deformity of back or spine**
    Deformity of spine NOS
    Excludes *curvature of spine (737.0–737.9)*
    Coding Clinic: 2007, Q4, P116-120
  - **738.6 Acquired deformity of pelvis**
    Pelvic obliquity
    Excludes *intrapelvic protrusion of acetabulum (718.6)*
    that in relation to labor and delivery (653.0–653.4, 653.8–653.9)
  - **738.7 Cauliflower ear**
  - **738.8 Acquired deformity of other specified site**
    Deformity of clavicle
    Coding Clinic: 2001, Q2, P14-15
  - **738.9 Acquired deformity of unspecified site**

- **739 Nonallopathic lesions, not elsewhere classified**
  Includes segmental dysfunction
  somatic dysfunction
  Coding Clinic: 1995, Q4, P51; 1990, Q1, P18
  - **739.0 Head region**
    Occipitocervical region
  - **739.1 Cervical region**
    Cervicothoracic region
  - **739.2 Thoracic region**
    Thoracolumbar region
  - **739.3 Lumbar region**
    Lumbosacral region
  - **739.4 Sacral region**
    Sacrococcygeal region
    Sacroiliac region
  - **739.5 Pelvic region**
    Hip region
    Pubic region
  - **739.6 Lower extremities**
  - **739.7 Upper extremities**
    Acromioclavicular region
    Sternoclavicular region
  - **739.8 Rib cage**
    Costochondral region
    Costovertebral region
    Sternochondral region
  - **739.9 Abdomen and other**

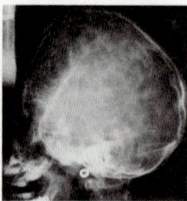

Figure 14–1 Generalized craniosynostosis in a 4-year-old girl without symptoms or signs of increased intracranial pressure. (From Bell WE, McCormick WF: Increased Intracranial Pressure in Children, ed 2, Philadelphia, WB Saunders, 1978)

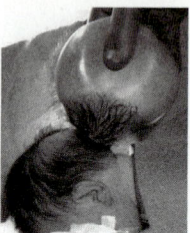

Figure 14–3 An infant with a large occipital encephalocele. The large skin-covered encephalocele is visible. (From Townsend: Sabiston Textbook of Surgery, ed 19, Saunders, An Imprint of Elsevier, 2012)

Item 14–1 Anencephalus is a congenital deformity of the cranial vault. **Craniosynostosis**, also known as craniostenosis and stenocephaly, signifies any form of congenital deformity of the skull that results from the premature closing of the sutures of the skull. **Iniencephaly** is a deformity in which the head and neck are flexed backward to a great extent and the head is very large in comparison to the shortened body.

14. CONGENITAL ANOMALIES (740–759)

- **740 Anencephalus and similar anomalies**
  - **740.0 Anencephalus**
    - Acrania
    - Amyelencephalus
    - Hemianencephaly
    - Hemicephaly
  - **740.1 Craniorachischisis**
  - **740.2 Iniencephaly**

- **741 Spina bifida**
  - **Excludes** spina bifida occulta (756.17)
  - Coding Clinic: 1994, Q3, P7

  The following fifth-digit subclassification is for use with category 741:

0 unspecified region	2 dorsal (thoracic) region
1 cervical region	3 lumbar region

  - **741.0 With hydrocephalus**
    - [0-3] Arnold-Chiari syndrome, type II
    - Any condition classifiable to 741.9 with any condition classifiable to 742.3
    - Chiari malformation, type II
    - Coding Clinic: 1997, Q4, P51; 1987, Sept-Oct, P10
  - **741.9 Without mention of hydrocephalus**
    - [0-3] Hydromeningocele (spinal)
    - Hydromyelocele
    - Meningocele (spinal)
    - Meningomyelocele
    - Myelocele
    - Myelocystocele
    - Rachischisis
    - Spina bifida (aperta)
    - Syringomyelocele
    - Coding Clinic: 1987, Sept-Oct, P10

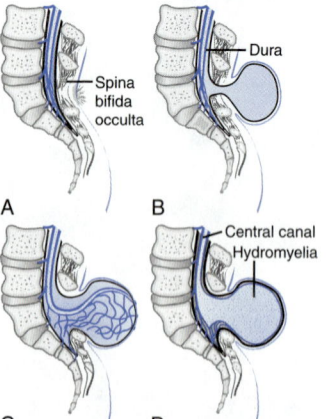

Figure 14–2 A. Spina bifida occulta. **B.** Meningocele. **C.** Myelomeningocele. **D.** Myelocystocele (syringomyelocele) or hydromyelia.

Item 14–2 Spina bifida is a midline spinal defect in which one or more vertebrae fail to fuse, leaving an opening in the vertebral canal. When the defect is not visible, it is called spina bifida occulta, and when it is visible, it is called spina bifida cystica.

- **742 Other congenital anomalies of nervous system**
  - **Excludes** congenital central alveolar hypoventilation syndrome (327.25)
  - **742.0 Encephalocele**
    - *Sac-like protrusions of brain and membranes visible through an opening in various locations in skull*
    - Encephalocystocele
    - Encephalomyelocele
    - Hydroencephalocele
    - Hydromeningocele, cranial
    - Meningocele, cerebral
    - Meningoencephalocele
  - **742.1 Microcephalus**
    - *Describes head size that measures significantly below normal based on standardized charts for age and sex*
    - Hydromicrocephaly
    - Micrencephaly
  - **742.2 Reduction deformities of brain**
    - Absence of part of brain
    - Agenesis of part of brain
    - Agyria
    - Aplasia of part of brain
    - Arhinencephaly
    - Holoprosencephaly
    - Hypoplasia of part of brain
    - Microgyria
    - Coding Clinic: 2003, Q3, P15-16
  - **742.3 Congenital hydrocephalus**
    - *An accumulation of cerebrospinal fluid in ventricles resulting in swelling and enlargement*
    - Aqueduct of Sylvius:
      - anomaly
      - obstruction, congenital
      - stenosis
    - Atresia of foramina of Magendie and Luschka
    - Hydrocephalus in newborn
    - **Excludes** hydrocephalus:
      - acquired (331.3–331.4)
      - due to congenital toxoplasmosis (771.2)
      - with any condition classifiable to 741.9 (741.0)
    - Coding Clinic: 2005, Q4, P82-83
  - **742.4 Other specified anomalies of brain**
    - Congenital cerebral cyst
    - Macroencephaly
    - Macrogyria
    - Megalencephaly
    - Multiple anomalies of brain NOS
    - Porencephaly
    - Ulegyria
    - Coding Clinic: 1999, Q1, P9-10; 1992, Q3, P12
  - **742.5 Other specified anomalies of spinal cord**
    - **742.51 Diastematomyelia**
    - **742.53 Hydromyelia**
      - Hydrorhachis
    - **742.59 Other**
      - Amyelia
      - Atelomyelia
      - Congenital anomaly of spinal meninges
      - Defective development of cauda equina
      - Hypoplasia of spinal cord
      - Myelatelia
      - Myelodysplasia
      - Coding Clinic: 1991, Q2, P14; 1989, Q1, P10

- **742.8** Other specified anomalies of nervous system
    - Agenesis of nerve
    - Displacement of brachial plexus
    - Familial dysautonomia
    - Jaw-winking syndrome
    - Marcus-Gunn syndrome
    - Riley-Day syndrome
    - **Excludes** neurofibromatosis (237.70-237.79)
- **742.9** Unspecified anomaly of brain, spinal cord, and nervous system
    - Anomaly of brain, nervous system, and spinal cord
    - Congenital, of brain, nervous system, and spinal cord:
        - disease of brain, nervous system, and spinal cord
        - lesion of brain, nervous system, and spinal cord
    - Deformity of brain, nervous system, and spinal cord

- **743 Congenital anomalies of eye**
    - **743.0** Anophthalmos
        - *Absence of eye and optic pit*
        - **743.00** Clinical anophthalmos, unspecified
            - Agenesis
            - Congenital absence of eye
            - Anophthalmos NOS
        - **743.03** Cystic eyeball, congenital
        - **743.06** Cryptophthalmos
    - **743.1** Microphthalmos
        - *Partial absence of eye and optic pit*
        - Dysplasia of eye
        - Hypoplasia of eye
        - Rudimentary eye
        - **743.10** Microphthalmos, unspecified
        - **743.11** Simple microphthalmos
        - **743.12** Microphthalmos associated with other anomalies of eye and adnexa
    - **743.2** Buphthalmos
        - *Also known as Sturge-Weber Syndrome and is congenital syndrome characterized by a port-wine nevus covering portions of face and cranium*
        - Glaucoma:
            - congenital
            - newborn
        - Hydrophthalmos
        - **Excludes** glaucoma of childhood (365.14)
            traumatic glaucoma due to birth injury (767.8)
        - **743.20** Buphthalmos, unspecified
        - **743.21** Simple buphthalmos
        - **743.22** Buphthalmos associated with other ocular anomalies
            - Keratoglobus, congenital, associated with buphthalmos
            - Megalocornea associated with buphthalmos
    - **743.3** Congenital cataract and lens anomalies
        - **Excludes** infantile cataract (366.00–366.09)
        - **743.30** Congenital cataract, unspecified
        - **743.31** Capsular and subcapsular cataract
        - **743.32** Cortical and zonular cataract
        - **743.33** Nuclear cataract
        - **743.34** Total and subtotal cataract, congenital
        - **743.35** Congenital aphakia
            - Congenital absence of lens
        - **743.36** Anomalies of lens shape
            - Microphakia   Spherophakia
        - **743.37** Congenital ectopic lens
        - **743.39** Other
    - **743.4** Coloboma and other anomalies of anterior segment
        - **743.41** Anomalies of corneal size and shape
            - Microcornea
            - **Excludes** that associated with buphthalmos (743.22)
        - **743.42** Corneal opacities, interfering with vision, congenital
        - **743.43** Other corneal opacities, congenital
        - **743.44** Specified anomalies of anterior chamber, chamber angle, and related structures
            - Anomaly:
                - Axenfeld's
                - Peters'
                - Rieger's
        - **743.45** Aniridia
            - Coding Clinic: 2010, Q2, P5; 2002, Q3, P20-21
        - **743.46** Other specified anomalies of iris and ciliary body
            - Anisocoria, congenital
            - Atresia of pupil
            - Coloboma of iris
            - Corectopia
        - **743.47** Specified anomalies of sclera
        - **743.48** Multiple and combined anomalies of anterior segment
        - **743.49** Other
    - **743.5** Congenital anomalies of posterior segment
        - **743.51** Vitreous anomalies
            - Congenital vitreous opacity
        - **743.52** Fundus coloboma
        - **743.53** Chorioretinal degeneration, congenital
        - **743.54** Congenital folds and cysts of posterior segment
        - **743.55** Congenital macular changes
        - **743.56** Other retinal changes, congenital
            - Coding Clinic: 1999, Q3, P12
        - **743.57** Specified anomalies of optic disc
            - Coloboma of optic disc (congenital)
        - **743.58** Vascular anomalies
            - Congenital retinal aneurysm
        - **743.59** Other
    - **743.6** Congenital anomalies of eyelids, lacrimal system, and orbit
        - **743.61** Congenital ptosis
        - **743.62** Congenital deformities of eyelids
            - Ablepharon
            - Absence of eyelid
            - Accessory eyelid
            - Congenital:
                - ectropion
                - entropion
            - Coding Clinic: 2000, Q1, P22-23
        - **743.63** Other specified congenital anomalies of eyelid
            - Absence, agenesis, of cilia
        - **743.64** Specified congenital anomalies of lacrimal gland
        - **743.65** Specified congenital anomalies of lacrimal passages
            - Absence, agenesis of:
                - lacrimal apparatus
                - punctum lacrimale
            - Accessory lacrimal canal
        - **743.66** Specified congenital anomalies of orbit
        - **743.69** Other
            - Accessory eye muscles
    - **743.8** Other specified anomalies of eye
        - **Excludes** congenital nystagmus (379.51)
            ocular albinism (270.2)
            optic nerve hypoplasia (377.43)
            retinitis pigmentosa (362.74)
    - **743.9** Unspecified anomaly of eye
        - Congenital:
            - anomaly NOS of eye [any part]
            - deformity NOS of eye [any part]

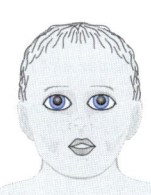

Figure 14–4 Bilateral congenital **hydrophthalmia,** in which the eyes are very large in comparison to the other facial features due to glaucoma.

CONGENITAL ANOMALIES (740–759)

● **744 Congenital anomalies of ear, face, and neck**
  Excludes anomaly of:
  cervical spine (754.2, 756.10–756.19)
  larynx (748.2–748.3)
  nose (748.0–748.1)
  parathyroid gland (759.2)
  thyroid gland (759.2)
  cleft lip (749.10–749.25)

● **744.0 Anomalies of ear causing impairment of hearing**
  Excludes congenital deafness without mention of cause (380.0–389.9)

  744.00 Unspecified anomaly of ear with impairment of hearing

  744.01 Absence of external ear
   Absence of:
   auditory canal (external)
   auricle (ear) (with stenosis or atresia of auditory canal)

  744.02 Other anomalies of external ear with impairment of hearing
   Atresia or stricture of auditory canal (external)

  744.03 Anomaly of middle ear, except ossicles
   Atresia or stricture of osseous meatus (ear)

  744.04 Anomalies of ear ossicles
   Fusion of ear ossicles

  744.05 Anomalies of inner ear
   Congenital anomaly of:
   membranous labyrinth
   organ of Corti

  744.09 Other
   Absence of ear, congenital

  744.1 Accessory auricle
   Accessory tragus   Supernumerary:
   Polyotia   ear
   Preauricular appendage   lobule

● **744.2 Other specified anomalies of ear**
  Excludes that with impairment of hearing (744.00–744.09)

  744.21 Absence of ear lobe, congenital

  744.22 Macrotia
   Enlarged ear

  744.23 Microtia
   Abnormally small ear

  744.24 Specified anomalies of Eustachian tube
   Absence of Eustachian tube

  744.29 Other
   Bat ear
   Darwin's tubercle
   Pointed ear
   Prominence of auricle
   Ridge ear
   Excludes preauricular sinus (744.46)

  744.3 Unspecified anomaly of ear
   Congenital:
   anomaly NOS of ear, NEC
   deformity NOS of ear, NEC

● **744.4 Branchial cleft cyst or fistula; preauricular sinus**

  744.41 Branchial cleft sinus or fistula
   Branchial:
   sinus (external) (internal)
   vestige

  744.42 Branchial cleft cyst

  744.43 Cervical auricle

  744.46 Preauricular sinus or fistula

  744.47 Preauricular cyst

  744.49 Other
   Fistula (of):
   auricle, congenital
   cervicoaural

  744.5 Webbing of neck
   Pterygium colli

● **744.8 Other specified anomalies of face and neck**

  744.81 Macrocheilia
   Hypertrophy of lip, congenital

  744.82 Microcheilia

  744.83 Macrostomia
   Abnormally large mouth

  744.84 Microstomia

  744.89 Other
   Excludes congenital fistula of lip (750.25)
   musculoskeletal anomalies (754.0–754.1, 756.0)

  744.9 Unspecified anomalies of face and neck
   Congenital:
   anomaly NOS of face [any part] or neck [any part]
   deformity NOS of face [any part] or neck [any part]

● **745 Bulbus cordis anomalies and anomalies of cardiac septal closure**

  745.0 Common truncus
   Absent septum between aorta and pulmonary artery
   Communication (abnormal) between aorta and pulmonary artery
   Aortic septal defect
   Common aortopulmonary trunk
   Persistent truncus arteriosus

● **745.1 Transposition of great vessels**

  745.10 Complete transposition of great vessels
   Transposition of great vessels:
   NOS
   classical

  745.11 Double outlet right ventricle
   Dextrotransposition of aorta
   Incomplete transposition of great vessels
   Origin of both great vessels from right ventricle
   Taussig-Bing syndrome or defect

  745.12 Corrected transposition of great vessels

  745.19 Other

  745.2 Tetralogy of Fallot
   Fallot's pentalogy
   Ventricular septal defect with pulmonary stenosis or atresia, dextroposition of aorta, and hypertrophy of right ventricle
   Excludes Fallot's triad (746.09)

  745.3 Common ventricle
   Cor triloculare biatriatum
   Single ventricle

  745.4 Ventricular septal defect
   Eisenmenger's defect or complex
   Gerbode defect
   Interventricular septal defect
   Left ventricular-right atrial communication
   Roger's disease
   Excludes common atrioventricular canal type (745.69)
   single ventricle (745.3)

  745.5 Ostium secundum type atrial septal defect
   Defect: Patent or persistent:
   atrium secundum   foramen ovale
   fossa ovalis   ostium secundum
   Lutembacher's syndrome
   Coding Clinic: 2012, Q2, P3-4; 2009, Q3, P10

● **745.6 Endocardial cushion defects**

  745.60 Endocardial cushion defect, unspecified type

  745.61 Ostium primum defect
   Persistent ostium primum

  745.69 Other
   Absence of atrial septum
   Atrioventricular canal type ventricular septal defect
   Common atrioventricular canal
   Common atrium

745.7 Cor biloculare
Absence of atrial and ventricular septa

745.8 Other

745.9 Unspecified defect of septal closure
Septal defect NOS

● **746 Other congenital anomalies of heart**
Excludes endocardial fibroelastosis (425.3)
Coding Clinic: 2004, Q3, P4-5

● **746.0 Anomalies of pulmonary valve**
Excludes infundibular or subvalvular pulmonic stenosis (746.83)
tetralogy of Fallot (745.2)

746.00 Pulmonary valve anomaly, unspecified

746.01 Atresia, congenital
Congenital absence of pulmonary valve

746.02 Stenosis, congenital
Coding Clinic: 2004, Q1, P16-17

746.09 Other
Congenital insufficiency of pulmonary valve
Fallot's triad or trilogy

746.1 Tricuspid atresia and stenosis, congenital
Absence of tricuspid valve

746.2 Ebstein's anomaly

746.3 Congenital stenosis of aortic valve
Congenital aortic stenosis
Excludes congenital:
subaortic stenosis (746.81)
supravalvular aortic stenosis (747.22)
Coding Clinic: 1988, Q4, P8

746.4 Congenital insufficiency of aortic valve
Bicuspid aortic valve
Congenital aortic insufficiency

746.5 Congenital mitral stenosis
Fused commissure of mitral valve
Parachute deformity of mitral valve
Supernumerary cusps of mitral valve
Coding Clinic: 2007, Q3, P3

746.6 Congenital mitral insufficiency

746.7 Hypoplastic left heart syndrome
Atresia, or marked hypoplasia, of aortic orifice or valve, with hypoplasia of ascending aorta and defective development of left ventricle (with mitral valve atresia)

● **746.8 Other specified anomalies of heart**

746.81 Subaortic stenosis
Coding Clinic: 2007, Q3, P3

746.82 Cor triatriatum

746.83 Infundibular pulmonic stenosis
Subvalvular pulmonic stenosis

746.84 Obstructive anomalies of heart, NEC
Shone's syndrome
Uhl's disease
Use additional code for associated anomalies, such as:
coarctation of aorta (747.10)
congenital mitral stenosis (746.5)
subaortic stenosis (746.81)
Coding Clinic: 2012, Q2, P3-4

746.85 Coronary artery anomaly
Anomalous origin or communication of coronary artery
Arteriovenous malformation of coronary artery
Coronary artery:
absence
arising from aorta or pulmonary trunk
single

746.86 Congenital heart block
Complete or incomplete atrioventricular [AV] block

746.87 Malposition of heart and cardiac apex
Abdominal heart
Dextrocardia
Ectopia cordis
Levocardia (isolated)
Mesocardia
Excludes dextrocardia with complete transposition of viscera (759.3)

746.89 Other
Atresia of cardiac vein
Hypoplasia of cardiac vein
Congenital:
cardiomegaly
diverticulum, left ventricle
pericardial defect
Coding Clinic: 2000, Q3, P3; 1999, Q1, P11; 1995, Q1, P8

746.9 Unspecified anomaly of heart
Congenital:
anomaly of heart NOS
heart disease NOS

● **747 Other congenital anomalies of circulatory system**

747.0 Patent ductus arteriosus (PDA)
Patent ductus Botalli
Persistent ductus arteriosus
Coding Clinic: 2009, Q3, P10-11x2

● **747.1 Coarctation of aorta**

747.10 Coarctation of aorta (preductal) (postductal)
Hypoplasia of aortic arch
Coding Clinic: 2007, Q3, P3; 1999, Q1, P11; 1988, Q4, P8

747.11 Interruption of aortic arch

● **747.2 Other anomalies of aorta**

747.20 Anomaly of aorta, unspecified

747.21 Anomalies of aortic arch
Anomalous origin, right subclavian artery
Dextroposition of aorta
Double aortic arch
Kommerell's diverticulum
Overriding aorta
Persistent:
convolutions, aortic arch
right aortic arch
Vascular ring
Excludes hypoplasia of aortic arch (747.10)
Coding Clinic: 2003, Q1, P15-16

747.22 Atresia and stenosis of aorta
Absence of aorta
Aplasia of aorta
Hypoplasia of aorta
Stricture of aorta
Supra (valvular)-aortic stenosis
Excludes congenital aortic (valvular) stenosis or stricture, so stated (746.3)
hypoplasia of aorta in hypoplastic left heart syndrome (746.7)
Coding Clinic: 1988, Q4, P8

747.29 Other
Aneurysm of sinus of Valsalva
Congenital: Congenital:
aneurysm of aorta   dilation of aorta

- **747.3 Anomalies of pulmonary artery**
  Coding Clinic: 2010, Q3, P9; 2009, Q3, P10x2; 2004, Q1, P16-17; 1994, Q1, P15
  - 747.31 Pulmonary artery coarctation and atresia
    Agenesis of pulmonary artery
    Atresia of pulmonary artery
    Coarctation of pulmonary artery
    Hypoplasia of pulmonary artery
    Stenosis of pulmonary artery
    Coding Clinic: 2012, Q2, P3-4
  - 747.32 Pulmonary arteriovenous malformation
    Pulmonary arteriovenous aneurysm
    Excludes *acquired pulmonary arteriovenous fistula (417.0)*
    Coding Clinic: 2011, Q4, P138
  - 747.39 Other anomalies of pulmonary artery and pulmonary circulation
    Anomaly of pulmonary artery
- **747.4 Anomalies of great veins**
  - 747.40 Anomaly of great veins, unspecified
    Anomaly NOS of: pulmonary veins
    Anomaly NOS of: vena cava
  - 747.41 Total anomalous pulmonary venous connection
    Total anomalous pulmonary venous return [TAPVR]:
      subdiaphragmatic
      supradiaphragmatic
  - 747.42 Partial anomalous pulmonary venous connection
    Partial anomalous pulmonary venous return
  - 747.49 Other anomalies of great veins
    Absence of vena cava (inferior) (superior)
    Congenital stenosis of vena cava (inferior) (superior)
    Persistent:
      left posterior cardinal vein
      left superior vena cava
    Scimitar syndrome
    Transposition of pulmonary veins NOS
- **747.5 Absence or hypoplasia of umbilical artery**
  Single umbilical artery
- **747.6 Other anomalies of peripheral vascular system**
  Absence of artery or vein, NEC
  Anomaly of artery or vein, NEC
  Atresia of artery or vein, NEC
  Arteriovenous aneurysm (peripheral)
  Arteriovenous malformation of the peripheral vascular system
  Congenital:
    aneurysm (peripheral)
    phlebectasia
  Congenital:
    stricture, artery
    varix
  Multiple renal arteries
  Excludes *anomalies of:*
    cerebral vessels (747.81)
    pulmonary artery (747.39)
    congenital retinal aneurysm (743.58)
    hemangioma (228.00–228.09)
    lymphangioma (228.1)
  - 747.60 Anomaly of the peripheral vascular system, unspecified site
  - 747.61 Gastrointestinal vessel anomaly
    Coding Clinic: 1996, Q3, P10
  - 747.62 Renal vessel anomaly
  - 747.63 Upper limb vessel anomaly
  - 747.64 Lower limb vessel anomaly
  - 747.69 Anomalies of other specified sites of peripheral vascular system
    Coding Clinic: 2010, Q3, P9
- **747.8 Other specified anomalies of circulatory system**
  - 747.81 Anomalies of cerebrovascular system
    Arteriovenous malformation of brain
    Cerebral arteriovenous aneurysm, congenital
    Congenital anomalies of cerebral vessels
    Excludes *ruptured cerebral (arteriovenous) aneurysm (430)*
    Coding Clinic: 1985, Jan-Feb, P15
  - 747.82 Spinal vessel anomaly
    Arteriovenous malformation of spinal vessel
    Coding Clinic: 1995, Q3, P5-6
  - 747.83 Persistent fetal circulation
    Persistent pulmonary hypertension
    Primary pulmonary hypertension of newborn
    Coding Clinic: 2002, Q4, P62-63
  - 747.89 Other
    Aneurysm, congenital, specified site not elsewhere classified
    Excludes *congenital aneurysm:*
      coronary (746.85)
      peripheral (747.6)
      pulmonary (747.39)
        arteriovenous (747.32)
      retinal (743.58)
- **747.9 Unspecified anomaly of circulatory system**
- **748 Congenital anomalies of respiratory system**
  Excludes *congenital central alveolar hypoventilation syndrome (327.25)*
  congenital defect of diaphragm (756.6)
  - 748.0 Choanal atresia
    Atresia of nares (anterior) (posterior)
    Congenital stenosis of nares (anterior) (posterior)
  - 748.1 Other anomalies of nose
    Absent nose
    Accessory nose
    Cleft nose
    Deformity of wall of nasal sinus
    Congenital:
      deformity of nose
      notching of tip of nose
      perforation of wall of nasal sinus
    Excludes *congenital deviation of nasal septum (754.0)*
  - 748.2 Web of larynx
    Web of larynx:
      NOS
      glottic
    Web of larynx:
      subglottic
  - 748.3 Other anomalies of larynx, trachea, and bronchus
    Absence or agenesis of:
      bronchus
      larynx
      trachea
    Anomaly (of):
      cricoid cartilage
      epiglottis
    Anomaly (of):
      thyroid cartilage
      tracheal cartilage
    Atresia (of):
      epiglottis
      glottis
    Atresia (of):
      larynx
      trachea
    Cleft thyroid, cartilage, congenital
    Congenital:
      dilation, trachea
      stenosis:
        larynx
        trachea
      tracheocele
    Diverticulum:
      bronchus
      trachea
    Fissure of epiglottis
    Laryngocele
    Posterior cleft of cricoid cartilage (congenital)
    Rudimentary tracheal bronchus
    Stridor, laryngeal, congenital
    Coding Clinic: 1999, Q1, P14

748.4 Congenital cystic lung
Disease, lung:
cystic, congenital
polycystic, congenital
Honeycomb lung, congenital
Excludes *acquired or unspecified cystic lung (518.89)*

748.5 Agenesis, hypoplasia, and dysplasia of lung
Absence of lung (fissures) (lobe)
Aplasia of lung
Hypoplasia of lung (lobe)
Sequestration of lung

● **748.6 Other anomalies of lung**
  748.60 Anomaly of lung, unspecified
  748.61 Congenital bronchiectasis
  748.69 Other
  Accessory lung (lobe)
  Azygos lobe (fissure), lung

748.8 Other specified anomalies of respiratory system
Abnormal communication between pericardial and pleural sacs
Anomaly, pleural folds
Atresia of nasopharynx
Congenital cyst of mediastinum

748.9 Unspecified anomaly of respiratory system
Anomaly of respiratory system NOS

● **749 Cleft palate and cleft lip**
Coding Clinic: 2012, Q2, P17

● **749.0 Cleft palate**
  749.00 Cleft palate, unspecified
  749.01 Unilateral, complete
  749.02 Unilateral, incomplete
  Cleft uvula
  749.03 Bilateral, complete
  749.04 Bilateral, incomplete

● **749.1 Cleft lip**
  Cheiloschisis   Harelip
  Congenital fissure of lip   Labium leporinum
  749.10 Cleft lip, unspecified
  749.11 Unilateral, complete
  749.12 Unilateral, incomplete
  749.13 Bilateral, complete
  749.14 Bilateral, incomplete

● **749.2 Cleft palate with cleft lip**
  Cheilopalatoschisis
  749.20 Cleft palate with cleft lip, unspecified
  749.21 Unilateral, complete
  749.22 Unilateral, incomplete
  749.23 Bilateral, complete
  Coding Clinic: 1996, Q1, P14
  749.24 Bilateral, incomplete
  749.25 Other combinations

● **750 Other congenital anomalies of upper alimentary tract**
Excludes *dentofacial anomalies (524.0–524.9)*

750.0 Tongue tie
Ankyloglossia

● **750.1 Other anomalies of tongue**
  750.10 Anomaly of tongue, unspecified
  750.11 Aglossia
  750.12 Congenital adhesions of tongue
  750.13 Fissure of tongue
  Bifid tongue
  Double tongue
  750.15 Macroglossia
  Congenital hypertrophy of tongue
  750.16 Microglossia
  Hypoplasia of tongue
  750.19 Other

● **750.2 Other specified anomalies of mouth and pharynx**
  750.21 Absence of salivary gland
  750.22 Accessory salivary gland
  750.23 Atresia, salivary gland
  Imperforate salivary duct
  750.24 Congenital fistula of salivary gland
  750.25 Congenital fistula of lip
  Congenital (mucus) lip pits
  750.26 Other specified anomalies of mouth
  Absence of uvula
  750.27 Diverticulum of pharynx
  Pharyngeal pouch
  750.29 Other specified anomalies of pharynx
  Imperforate pharynx

750.3 Tracheoesophageal fistula, esophageal atresia and stenosis
Absent esophagus
Atresia of esophagus
Congenital:
esophageal ring
stenosis of esophagus
stricture of esophagus
Congenital fistula:
esophagobronchial
esophagotracheal
Imperforate esophagus
Webbed esophagus
Coding Clinic: 2012, Q1, P15-16

750.4 Other specified anomalies of esophagus
Dilatation, congenital, of esophagus
Displacement, congenital, of esophagus
Diverticulum of esophagus
Duplication of esophagus
Esophageal pouch
Giant esophagus
Excludes *congenital hiatus hernia (750.6)*

750.5 Congenital hypertrophic pyloric stenosis
Congenital or infantile:
constriction of pylorus
hypertrophy of pylorus
spasm of pylorus
stenosis of pylorus
stricture of pylorus

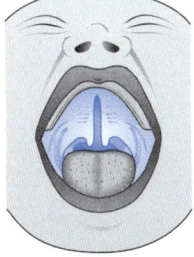

Figure 14–5 Cleft palate.

Item 14-3 A muscle thickening and pyloric stenosis overgrows the pyloric sphincter, resulting in a narrowing of the outlet between the stomach and small intestine. Infants with pyloric stenosis have projectile vomiting, leading to dehydration and electrolyte imbalance.

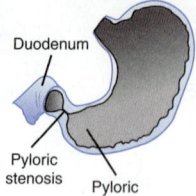

Figure 14-6 Pyloric stenosis.

750.6 **Congenital hiatus hernia**
  Displacement of cardia through esophageal hiatus
  Excludes congenital diaphragmatic hernia (756.6)

750.7 **Other specified anomalies of stomach**
  Congenital:
    cardiospasm
    hourglass stomach
  Displacement of stomach
  Diverticulum of stomach, congenital
  Duplication of stomach
  Megalogastria
  Microgastria
  Transposition of stomach

750.8 **Other specified anomalies of upper alimentary tract**

750.9 **Unspecified anomaly of upper alimentary tract**
  Congenital:
    anomaly NOS of upper alimentary tract [any part, except tongue]
    deformity NOS of upper alimentary tract [any part, except tongue]

● 751 **Other congenital anomalies of digestive system**

751.0 **Meckel's diverticulum**
  Meckel's diverticulum (displaced) (hypertrophic)
  Persistent:
    omphalomesenteric duct
    vitelline duct
  Coding Clinic: 2004, Q1, P10-11

751.1 **Atresia and stenosis of small intestine**
  Atresia of:
    duodenum
    ileum
    intestine NOS
  Congenital:
    absence of small intestine or intestine NOS
    obstruction of small intestine or intestine NOS
    stenosis of small intestine or intestine NOS
    stricture of small intestine or intestine NOS
  Imperforate jejunum

751.2 **Atresia and stenosis of large intestine, rectum, and anal canal**
  Absence:
    anus (congenital)
    appendix, congenital
    large intestine, congenital
    rectum
  Atresia of:
    anus
    colon
    rectum
  Congenital or infantile:
    obstruction of large intestine
    occlusion of anus
    stricture of anus
  Imperforate:
    anus
    rectum
  Stricture of rectum, congenital
  Coding Clinic: 1998, Q2, P16-17

751.3 **Hirschsprung's disease and other congenital functional disorders of colon**
  Absence of ganglion cells in distal colon resulting in functional obstruction
  Aganglionosis
  Congenital dilation of colon
  Congenital megacolon
  Macrocolon

751.4 **Anomalies of intestinal fixation**
  Congenital adhesions:
    omental, anomalous
    peritoneal
  Jackson's membrane
  Malrotation of colon
  Rotation of cecum or colon:
    failure of
    incomplete
    insufficient
  Universal mesentery
  Coding Clinic: 1985, Sept-Oct, P11

751.5 **Other anomalies of intestine**
  Congenital diverticulum, colon
  Dolichocolon
  Duplication of:
    anus
    appendix
    cecum
    intestine
  Ectopic anus
  Megaloappendix
  Megaloduodenum
  Microcolon
  Persistent cloaca
  Transposition of:
    appendix
    colon
    intestine
  Coding Clinic: 2010, Q2, P12; 2002, Q3, P11; 2001, Q3, P8-9

● 751.6 **Anomalies of gallbladder, bile ducts, and liver**
  751.60 **Unspecified anomaly of gallbladder, bile ducts, and liver**

  751.61 **Biliary atresia**
    Congenital:
      absence of bile duct (common) or passage
      hypoplasia of bile duct (common) or passage
      obstruction of bile duct (common) or passage
      stricture of bile duct (common) or passage
    Coding Clinic: 1987, Sept-Oct, P8

  751.62 **Congenital cystic disease of liver**
    Congenital polycystic disease of liver
    Fibrocystic disease of liver

  751.69 **Other anomalies of gallbladder, bile ducts, and liver**
    Absence of:
      gallbladder, congenital
      liver (lobe)
    Accessory:
      hepatic ducts
      liver
    Congenital:
      choledochal cyst
      hepatomegaly
    Duplication of:
      biliary duct
      cystic duct
    Duplication of:
      gallbladder
      liver
    Floating:
      gallbladder
    Floating:
      liver
    Intrahepatic gallbladder
    Coding Clinic: 1987, Sept-Oct, P8

751.7 **Anomalies of pancreas**
  Absence of pancreas
  Accessory pancreas
  Agenesis of pancreas
  Annular pancreas
  Ectopic pancreatic tissue
  Hypoplasia of pancreas
  Pancreatic heterotopia
  Excludes diabetes mellitus (249.0–249.9, (250.0–250.9)
       fibrocystic disease of pancreas (277.00–277.09)
       neonatal diabetes mellitus (775.1)

751.8 Other specified anomalies of digestive system
Absence (complete) (partial) of alimentary tract NOS
Duplication of digestive organs NOS
Malposition, congenital of digestive organs NOS
> **Excludes** congenital diaphragmatic hernia (756.6)
> congenital hiatus hernia (750.6)

751.9 Unspecified anomaly of digestive system
Congenital:
anomaly NOS of digestive system NOS
deformity NOS of digestive system NOS

752 Congenital anomalies of genital organs
> **Excludes** syndromes associated with anomalies in the number and form of chromosomes (758.0–758.9)

752.0 Anomalies of ovaries
Absence, congenital, of ovary
Accessory ovary
Ectopic ovary
Streak of ovary

752.1 Anomalies of fallopian tubes and broad ligaments

752.10 Unspecified anomaly of fallopian tubes and broad ligaments

752.11 Embryonic cyst of fallopian tubes and broad ligaments
Cyst:
epoophoron
fimbrial
parovarian
Coding Clinic: 1985, Sept-Oct, P13

752.19 Other
Absence of fallopian tube or broad ligament
Accessory fallopian tube or broad ligament
Atresia of fallopian tube or broad ligament

752.2 Doubling of uterus
Didelphic uterus
Doubling of uterus [any degree] (associated with doubling of cervix and vagina)

752.3 Other anomalies of uterus
Coding Clinic: 2006, Q3, P18-19

752.31 Agenesis of uterus
Congenital absence of uterus

752.32 Hypoplasia of uterus

752.33 Unicornuate uterus
Unicornate uterus with or without a separate uterine horn
Uterus with only one functioning horn

752.34 Bicornuate uterus
Bicornuate uterus, complete or partial

752.35 Septate uterus
Septate uterus, complete or partial

752.36 Arcuate uterus

752.39 Other anomalies of uterus
Aplasia of uterus NOS
Müllerian anomaly of the uterus, NEC
> **Excludes** anomaly of uterus due to exposure to diethylstilbestrol [DES] in utero (760.76)
> didelphic uterus (752.2)
> doubling of uterus (752.2)

752.4 Anomalies of cervix, vagina, and external female genitalia

752.40 Unspecified anomaly of cervix, vagina, and external female genitalia

752.41 Embryonic cyst of cervix, vagina, and external female genitalia
Cyst of:
canal of Nuck, congenital
Gartner's duct
vagina, embryonal
vulva, congenital

752.42 Imperforate hymen

752.43 Cervical agenesis
Cervical hypoplasia

752.44 Cervical duplication

752.45 Vaginal agenesis
Agenesis of vagina, total or partial

752.46 Transverse vaginal septum

752.47 Longitudinal vaginal septum
Longitudinal vaginal septum with or without obstruction

752.49 Other anomalies of cervix, vagina, and external female genitalia
Absence of clitoris or vulva
Agenesis of clitoris or vulva
Anomalies of cervix, NEC
Anomalies of hymen, NEC
Congenital stenosis or stricture of:
cervical canal
vagina
Müllerian anomalies of the cervix and vagina, NEC
> **Excludes** double vagina associated with total duplication (752.2)
Coding Clinic: 2006, Q3, P18-19

752.5 Undescended and retractile testicle

752.51 Undescended testis
Cryptorchism
Ectopic testis

752.52 Retractile testis

752.6 Hypospadias and epispadias and other penile anomalies

752.61 Hypospadias
Coding Clinic: 2003, Q4, P67-68; 1997, Q3, P6; Q3, P6; 1996, Q4, P34-35

752.62 Epispadias
Anaspadias

752.63 Congenital chordee
Coding Clinic: 1996, Q4, P34-35

752.64 Micropenis

752.65 Hidden penis

752.69 Other penile anomalies

752.7 Indeterminate sex and pseudohermaphroditism
Condition in which internal reproductive organs are opposite external physical characteristics
Gynandrism
Hermaphroditism
Ovotestis
Pseudohermaphroditism (male) (female)
Pure gonadal dysgenesis
> **Excludes** androgen insensitivity (259.50–259.52)
> pseudohermaphroditism:
> female, with adrenocortical disorder (255.2)
> male, with gonadal disorder (257.8)
> with specified chromosomal anomaly (758.0–758.9)
> testicular feminization syndrome (259.50–259.52)

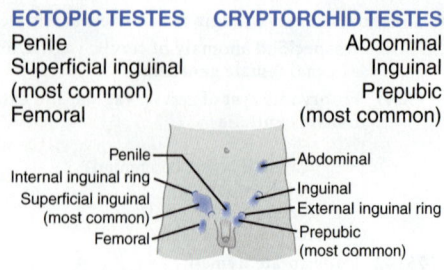

Figure 14-7 Undescended testes and the positions of the testes in various types of cryptorchidism or abnormal paths of descent.

Item 14-4 Testes form in the abdomen of the male and only descend into the scrotum during normal embryonic development. "Ectopic" testes are out of their normal place or "retained" (left behind) in the abdomen. Crypto (hidden) orchism (testicle) is a major risk factor for testicular cancer.

- **752.8** Other specified anomalies of genital organs
  Excludes congenital hydrocele (778.6)
  penile anomalies (752.61–752.69)
  phimosis or paraphimosis (605)
  - **752.81** Scrotal transposition
    Coding Clinic: 2003, Q4, P67-68
  - **752.89** Other specified anomalies of genital organs
    Absence of:
    Check Index for V codes for acquired or congenital.
    prostate
    spermatic cord
    vas deferens
    Anorchism
    Aplasia (congenital) of:
    prostate
    round ligament
    testicle
    Atresia of:
    ejaculatory duct
    vas deferens
    Fusion of testes
    Hypoplasia of testis
    Monorchism
    Polyorchism
- **752.9** Unspecified anomaly of genital organs
  Congenital:
  anomaly NOS of genital organ, NEC
  deformity NOS of genital organ, NEC

- **753** Congenital anomalies of urinary system
  - **753.0** Renal agenesis and dysgenesis
    Atrophy of kidney:
    congenital
    infantile
    Congenital absence of kidney(s)
    Hypoplasia of kidney(s)
  - **753.1** Cystic kidney disease
    Excludes acquired cyst of kidney (593.2)
    - **753.10** Cystic kidney disease, unspecified
    - **753.11** Congenital single renal cyst
    - **753.12** Polycystic kidney, unspecified type
      PKD (polycystic kidney disease)
    - **753.13** Polycystic kidney, autosomal dominant
    - **753.14** Polycystic kidney, autosomal recessive
    - **753.15** Renal dysplasia
    - **753.16** Medullary cystic kidney
      Nephronophthisis
    - **753.17** Medullary sponge kidney
    - **753.19** Other specified cystic kidney disease
      Multicystic kidney
  - **753.2** Obstructive defects of renal pelvis and ureter
    - **753.20** Unspecified obstructive defect of renal pelvis and ureter
    - **753.21** Congenital obstruction of ureteropelvic junction
    - **753.22** Congenital obstruction of ureterovesical junction
      Adynamic ureter
      Congenital hydroureter
    - **753.23** Congenital ureterocele
    - **753.29** Other
  - **753.3** Other specified anomalies of kidney
    Accessory kidney
    Congenital:
    calculus of kidney
    displaced kidney
    Discoid kidney
    Double kidney with double pelvis
    Ectopic kidney
    Fusion of kidneys
    Giant kidney
    Horseshoe kidney
    Hyperplasia of kidney
    Lobulation of kidney
    Malrotation of kidney
    Trifid kidney (pelvis)
    Coding Clinic: 2007, Q1, P23
  - **753.4** Other specified anomalies of ureter
    Absent ureter
    Accessory ureter
    Deviation of ureter
    Displaced ureteric orifice
    Double ureter
    Ectopic ureter
    Implantation, anomalous, of ureter
  - **753.5** Exstrophy of urinary bladder
    Ectopia vesicae
    Extroversion of bladder
  - **753.6** Atresia and stenosis of urethra and bladder neck
    Congenital obstruction:
    bladder neck
    urethra
    Congenital stricture of:
    urethra (valvular)
    urinary meatus
    vesicourethral orifice
    Imperforate urinary meatus
    Impervious urethra
    Urethral valve formation
  - **753.7** Anomalies of urachus
    Cyst (of) urachus
    Fistula (of) urachus
    Patent (of) urachus
    Persistent umbilical sinus
  - **753.8** Other specified anomalies of bladder and urethra
    Absence, congenital of:
    bladder
    urethra
    Accessory:
    bladder
    urethra
    Congenital:
    diverticulum of bladder
    hernia of bladder
    Congenital urethrorectal fistula
    Congenital prolapse of:
    bladder (mucosa)
    urethra
    Double:
    urethra
    urinary meatus
  - **753.9** Unspecified anomaly of urinary system
    Congenital:
    anomaly NOS of urinary system [any part, except urachus]
    deformity NOS of urinary system [any part, except urachus]

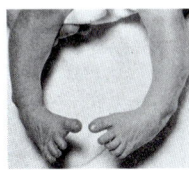

Figure 14–8 Mild to moderate inbowing of the lower leg. (From Jones KL: Smith's Recognizable Patterns of Human Malformation, ed 6, Philadelphia, Saunders, 2005)

● 754 **Certain congenital musculoskeletal deformities**
  Includes nonteratogenic deformities which are considered to be due to intrauterine malposition and pressure

  754.0 **Of skull, face, and jaw**
    Asymmetry of face
    Compression facies
    Depressions in skull
    Deviation of nasal septum, congenital
    Dolichocephaly
    Plagiocephaly
    Potter's facies
    Squashed or bent nose, congenital
    Excludes dentofacial anomalies (524.0–524.9)
    syphilitic saddle nose (090.5)

  754.1 **Of sternocleidomastoid muscle**
    Congenital sternomastoid torticollis
    Congenital wryneck
    Contracture of sternocleidomastoid (muscle)
    Sternomastoid tumor

  754.2 **Of spine**
    Congenital postural:
      lordosis
      scoliosis

● 754.3 **Congenital dislocation of hip**
    754.30 Congenital dislocation of hip, unilateral
      Congenital dislocation of hip NOS
    754.31 Congenital dislocation of hip, bilateral
    754.32 Congenital subluxation of hip, unilateral
      Congenital flexion deformity, hip or thigh
      Predislocation status of hip at birth
      Preluxation of hip, congenital
    754.33 Congenital subluxation of hip, bilateral
    754.35 Congenital dislocation of one hip with subluxation of other hip

● 754.4 **Congenital genu recurvatum and bowing of long bones of leg**
    754.40 Genu recurvatum
      Hyperextension of knee resulting from hypermobility
    754.41 Congenital dislocation of knee (with genu recurvatum)
    754.42 Congenital bowing of femur
    754.43 Congenital bowing of tibia and fibula
    □754.44 Congenital bowing of unspecified long bones of leg

● 754.5 **Varus deformities of feet**
    Foot deformity (pes equino varus) also known as club foot in which there is an inward angulation of distal segment of a bone or joint
    Excludes acquired (736.71, 736.75, 736.79)
    754.50 Talipes varus
      Congenital varus deformity of foot, unspecified
      Pes varus
    754.51 Talipes equinovarus
      Equinovarus (congenital)
    754.52 Metatarsus primus varus
    754.53 Metatarsus varus
    754.59 Other
      Talipes calcaneovarus

● 754.6 **Valgus deformities of feet**
    Inward angulation
    Excludes valgus deformity of foot (acquired) (736.79)
    754.60 Talipes valgus
      Congenital valgus deformity of foot, unspecified
    754.61 Congenital pes planus
      Congenital rocker bottom flat foot
      Flat foot, congenital
      Excludes pes planus (acquired) (734)
    754.62 Talipes calcaneovalgus
    754.69 Other
      Talipes:
        equinovalgus
        planovalgus

● 754.7 **Other deformities of feet**
    Excludes acquired (736.70–736.79)
    □754.70 Talipes, unspecified
      Congenital deformity of foot NOS
    754.71 Talipes cavus
      Cavus foot (congenital)
    754.79 Other
      Asymmetric talipes
      Talipes:
        calcaneus
        equinus

● 754.8 **Other specified nonteratogenic anomalies**
    754.81 Pectus excavatum
      Congenital funnel chest
    754.82 Pectus carinatum
      Congenital pigeon chest [breast]
    754.89 Other
      Club hand (congenital)
      Congenital:
        deformity of chest wall
        dislocation of elbow
      Generalized flexion contractures of lower limb joints, congenital
      Spade-like hand (congenital)

● 755 **Other congenital anomalies of limbs**
    Excludes those deformities classifiable to 754.0–754.8
  ● 755.0 **Polydactyly**
    Also known as hyperdactyly, consists of duplicate fingers or toes
    □755.00 Polydactyly, unspecified digits
      Supernumerary digits
    755.01 Of fingers
      Accessory fingers
    755.02 Of toes
      Accessory toes
  ● 755.1 **Syndactyly**
    Symphalangy
    Webbing of digits
    □755.10 Of multiple and unspecified sites
    755.11 Of fingers without fusion of bone
    755.12 Of fingers with fusion of bone
    755.13 Of toes without fusion of bone
    755.14 Of toes with fusion of bone

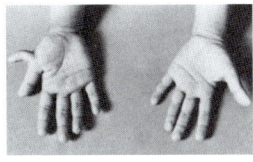

Figure 14–9 Polydactyly, congenital duplicated thumb. (From DeLee: DeLee and Drez's Orthopaedic Sports Medicine, ed 3, Saunders, An Imprint of Elsevier, 2009)

- **755.2 Reduction deformities of upper limb**
  - **755.20 Unspecified reduction deformity of upper limb**
    - Ectromelia NOS of upper limb
      - *Gross hypoplasia or aplasia of one or more long bones of one or more limbs*
    - Hemimelia NOS of upper limb
      - *Absence of one-half of long bone*
    - Shortening of arm, congenital
  - **755.21 Transverse deficiency of upper limb**
    - Amelia of upper limb
    - Congenital absence of:
      - fingers, all (complete or partial)
      - forearm, including hand and fingers
      - upper limb, complete
    - Congenital amputation of upper limb
    - Transverse hemimelia of upper limb
  - **755.22 Longitudinal deficiency of upper limb, NEC**
    - Phocomelia NOS of upper limb
      - *Absence/shortening of long bones primarily as a result of thalidomide*
    - Rudimentary arm
  - **755.23 Longitudinal deficiency, combined, involving humerus, radius, and ulna (complete or incomplete)**
    - Congenital absence of arm and forearm (complete or incomplete) with or without metacarpal deficiency and/or phalangeal deficiency, incomplete
    - Phocomelia, complete, of upper limb
  - **755.24 Longitudinal deficiency, humeral, complete or partial (with or without distal deficiencies, incomplete)**
    - Congenital absence of humerus (with or without absence of some [but not all] distal elements)
    - Proximal phocomelia of upper limb
  - **755.25 Longitudinal deficiency, radioulnar, complete or partial (with or without distal deficiencies, incomplete)**
    - Congenital absence of radius and ulna (with or without absence of some [but not all] distal elements)
    - Distal phocomelia of upper limb
  - **755.26 Longitudinal deficiency, radial, complete or partial (with or without distal deficiencies, incomplete)**
    - Agenesis of radius
    - Congenital absence of radius (with or without absence of some [but not all] distal elements)
  - **755.27 Longitudinal deficiency, ulnar, complete or partial (with or without distal deficiencies, incomplete)**
    - Agenesis of ulna
    - Congenital absence of ulna (with or without absence of some [but not all] distal elements)
  - **755.28 Longitudinal deficiency, carpals or metacarpals, complete or partial (with or without incomplete phalangeal deficiency)**
  - **755.29 Longitudinal deficiency, phalanges, complete or partial**
    - Absence of finger, congenital
    - Aphalangia of upper limb, terminal, complete or partial
    - **Excludes** *terminal deficiency of all five digits (755.21)*
      transverse deficiency of phalanges (755.21)

- **755.3 Reduction deformities of lower limb**
  - **755.30 Unspecified reduction deformity of lower limb**
    - Ectromelia NOS of lower limb
    - Hemimelia NOS of lower limb
    - Shortening of leg, congenital
  - **755.31 Transverse deficiency of lower limb**
    - Amelia of lower limb
    - Congenital absence of:
      - foot
      - leg, including foot and toes
      - lower limb, complete
      - toes, all, complete
    - Transverse hemimelia of lower limb
  - **755.32 Longitudinal deficiency of lower limb, NEC**
    - Phocomelia NOS of lower limb
  - **755.33 Longitudinal deficiency, combined, involving femur, tibia, and fibula (complete or incomplete)**
    - Congenital absence of thigh and (lower) leg (complete or incomplete) with or without metacarpal deficiency and/or phalangeal deficiency, incomplete
    - Phocomelia, complete, of lower limb
  - **755.34 Longitudinal deficiency, femoral, complete or partial (with or without distal deficiencies, incomplete)**
    - Congenital absence of femur (with or without absence of some [but not all] distal elements)
    - Proximal phocomelia of lower limb
  - **755.35 Longitudinal deficiency, tibiofibular, complete or partial (with or without distal deficiencies, incomplete)**
    - Congenital absence of tibia and fibula (with or without absence of some [but not all] distal elements)
    - Distal phocomelia of lower limb
  - **755.36 Longitudinal deficiency, tibia, complete or partial (with or without distal deficiencies, incomplete)**
    - Agenesis of tibia
    - Congenital absence of tibia (with or without absence of some [but not all] distal elements)
  - **755.37 Longitudinal deficiency, fibular, complete or partial (with or without distal deficiencies, incomplete)**
    - Agenesis of fibula
    - Congenital absence of fibula (with or without absence of some [but not all] distal elements)
  - **755.38 Longitudinal deficiency, tarsals or metatarsals, complete or partial (with or without incomplete phalangeal deficiency)**
  - **755.39 Longitudinal deficiency, phalanges, complete or partial**
    - Absence of toe, congenital
    - Aphalangia of lower limb, terminal, complete or partial
    - **Excludes** *terminal deficiency of all five digits (755.31)*
      transverse deficiency of phalanges (755.31)

- **755.4 Reduction deformities, unspecified limb**
  - Absence, congenital (complete or partial) of limb NOS
  - Amelia of unspecified limb
  - Ectromelia of unspecified limb
  - Hemimelia of unspecified limb
  - Phocomelia of unspecified limb

- **755.5 Other anomalies of upper limb, including shoulder girdle**
  - 755.50 Unspecified anomaly of upper limb
  - 755.51 Congenital deformity of clavicle
  - 755.52 Congenital elevation of scapula
    - Sprengel's deformity
  - 755.53 Radioulnar synostosis
  - 755.54 Madelung's deformity
  - 755.55 Acrocephalosyndactyly
    - Apert's syndrome
  - 755.56 Accessory carpal bones
  - 755.57 Macrodactylia (fingers)
  - 755.58 Cleft hand, congenital
    - Lobster-claw hand
  - 755.59 Other
    - Cleidocranial dysostosis
    - Cubitus:
      - valgus, congenital
      - varus, congenital
    - **Excludes** club hand (congenital) (754.89)
      congenital dislocation of elbow (754.89)

- **755.6 Other anomalies of lower limb, including pelvic girdle**
  - 755.60 Unspecified anomaly of lower limb
  - 755.61 Coxa valga, congenital
  - 755.62 Coxa vara, congenital
  - 755.63 Other congenital deformity of hip (joint)
    - Congenital anteversion of femur (neck)
    - **Excludes** congenital dislocation of hip (754.30–754.35)
  - 755.64 Congenital deformity of knee (joint)
    - Congenital:
      - absence of patella
      - genu valgum [knock-knee]
      - genu varum [bowleg]
    - Rudimentary patella
    - Coding Clinic: 1985, July-Aug, P14; 1984, Nov-Dec, P9
  - 755.65 Macrodactylia of toes
  - 755.66 Other anomalies of toes
    - Congenital:
      - hallux valgus
      - hallux varus
      - hammer toe
  - 755.67 Anomalies of foot, NEC
    - Astragaloscaphoid synostosis
    - Calcaneonavicular bar
    - Coalition of calcaneus
    - Talonavicular synostosis
    - Tarsal coalitions
  - 755.69 Other
    - Congenital:
      - angulation of tibia
      - deformity (of):
        - ankle (joint)
        - sacroiliac (joint)
      - fusion of sacroiliac joint

- **755.8 Other specified anomalies of unspecified limb**
- **755.9 Unspecified anomaly of unspecified limb**
  - Congenital:
    - anomaly NOS of unspecified limb
    - deformity NOS of unspecified limb
  - **Excludes** reduction deformity of unspecified limb (755.4)

- **756 Other congenital musculoskeletal anomalies**
  - **Excludes** congenital myotonic chondrodystrophy (359.23)
    those deformities classifiable to 754.0–754.8
  - **756.0 Anomalies of skull and face bones**
    - Absence of skull bones
    - Acrocephaly
    - Congenital deformity of forehead
    - Craniosynostosis
    - Crouzon's disease
    - Hypertelorism
    - Imperfect fusion of skull
    - Oxycephaly
    - Platybasia
    - Premature closure of cranial sutures
    - Tower skull
    - Trigonocephaly
    - **Excludes** acrocephalosyndactyly [Apert's syndrome] (755.55)
      dentofacial anomalies (524.0–524.9)
      skull defects associated with brain anomalies, such as:
        anencephalus (740.0)
        encephalocele (742.0)
        hydrocephalus (742.3)
        microcephalus (742.1)
    - Coding Clinic: 2012, Q2, P17; 1998, Q3, P9-10; 1996, Q3, P15
  - **756.1 Anomalies of spine**
    - 756.10 Anomaly of spine, unspecified
    - 756.11 Spondylolysis, lumbosacral region
      - Prespondylolisthesis (lumbosacral)
    - 756.12 Spondylolisthesis
    - 756.13 Absence of vertebra, congenital
    - 756.14 Hemivertebra
    - 756.15 Fusion of spine [vertebra], congenital
    - 756.16 Klippel-Feil syndrome
    - 756.17 Spina bifida occulta
      - **Excludes** spina bifida (aperta) (741.0–741.9)
    - 756.19 Other
      - Platyspondylia
      - Supernumerary vertebra
  - **756.2 Cervical rib**
    - Supernumerary rib in the cervical region
  - **756.3 Other anomalies of ribs and sternum**
    - Congenital absence of:
      - rib
      - sternum
    - Congenital:
      - fissure of sternum
      - fusion of ribs
    - Sternum bifidum
    - **Excludes** nonteratogenic deformity of chest wall (754.81–754.89)
  - **756.4 Chondrodystrophy**
    - *Skeletal dysplasia (dwarfism) is caused by genetic mutations affecting hyaline cartilage capping long bones and vertebrae*
    - Achondroplasia
    - Chondrodystrophia (fetalis)
    - Dyschondroplasia
    - Enchondromatosis
    - Ollier's disease
    - **Excludes** congenital myotonic chondrodystrophy (359.23)
      lipochondrodystrophy [Hurler's syndrome] (277.5)
      Morquio's disease (277.5)
    - Coding Clinic: 2002, Q2, P16-17; 1987, Sept-Oct, P10

- **756.5 Osteodystrophies**
  Defective bone development; most commonly caused by renal disease or disturbances in calcium and phosphorus metabolism
  - 756.50 Osteodystrophy, unspecified
  - 756.51 Osteogenesis imperfecta
    Fragilitas ossium
    Osteopsathyrosis
  - 756.52 Osteopetrosis
  - 756.53 Osteopoikilosis
  - 756.54 Polyostotic fibrous dysplasia of bone
  - 756.55 Chondroectodermal dysplasia
    Ellis-van Creveld syndrome
  - 756.56 Multiple epiphyseal dysplasia
  - 756.59 Other
    Albright (-McCune)-Sternberg syndrome
- 756.6 Anomalies of diaphragm
  Absence of diaphragm
  Congenital hernia:
    diaphragmatic
    foramen of Morgagni
  Eventration of diaphragm
  Excludes *congenital hiatus hernia (750.6)*
- **756.7 Anomalies of abdominal wall**
  - 756.70 Anomaly of abdominal wall, unspecified
  - 756.71 Prune belly syndrome
    Eagle-Barrett syndrome
    Prolapse of bladder mucosa
  - 756.72 Omphalocele
    Exomphalos
  - 756.73 Gastroschisis
  - 756.79 Other congenital anomalies of abdominal wall
    Excludes *umbilical hernia (551–553 with .1)*
- **756.8 Other specified anomalies of muscle, tendon, fascia, and connective tissue**
  - 756.81 Absence of muscle and tendon
    Absence of muscle (pectoral)
    Coding Clinic: 2010, Q1, P11
  - 756.82 Accessory muscle
  - 756.83 Ehlers-Danlos syndrome
  - 756.89 Other
    Amyotrophia congenita
    Congenital shortening of tendon
    Coding Clinic: 1999, Q3, P16-17
- 756.9 Other and unspecified anomalies of musculoskeletal system
  Congenital:
    anomaly NOS of musculoskeletal system, NEC
    deformity NOS of musculoskeletal system, NEC
- **757 Congenital anomalies of the integument**
  Includes anomalies of skin, subcutaneous tissue, hair, nails, and breast
  Excludes *hemangioma (228.00–228.09)*
  pigmented nevus (216.0–216.9)
  - 757.0 Hereditary edema of legs
    Congenital lymphedema
    Hereditary trophedema
    Milroy's disease
  - 757.1 Ichthyosis congenita
    Congenital ichthyosis
    Harlequin fetus
    Ichthyosiform erythroderma
  - 757.2 Dermatoglyphic anomalies
    Abnormal palmar creases
- **757.3 Other specified anomalies of skin**
  - 757.31 Congenital ectodermal dysplasia
  - 757.32 Vascular hamartomas
    Birthmarks
    Port-wine stain
    Strawberry nevus
    Coding Clinic: 2012, Q2, P7
  - 757.33 Congenital pigmentary anomalies of skin
    Congenital poikiloderma
    Urticaria pigmentosa
    Xeroderma pigmentosum
    Excludes *albinism (270.2)*
    Coding Clinic: 2013, Q1, P14
  - 757.39 Other
    Accessory skin tags, congenital
    Congenital scar
    Epidermolysis bullosa
    Keratoderma (congenital)
    Excludes *pilonidal cyst (685.0–685.1)*
    Coding Clinic: 2013, Q1, P15
  - 757.4 Specified anomalies of hair
    Congenital:
      alopecia
      atrichosis
      beaded hair
      hypertrichosis
      monilethrix
    Persistent lanugo
  - 757.5 Specified anomalies of nails
    Anonychia
    Congenital:
      clubnail
      koilonychia
      leukonychia
      onychauxis
      pachyonychia
  - 757.6 Specified congenital anomalies of breast
    Congenital absent breast or nipple
    Accessory breast or nipple
    Supernumerary breast or nipple
    Excludes *absence of pectoral muscle (756.81)*
    hypoplasia of breast (611.82)
    micromastia (611.82)
  - 757.8 Other specified anomalies of the integument
  - 757.9 Unspecified anomaly of the integument
    Congenital:
      anomaly NOS of integument
      deformity NOS of integument
- **758 Chromosomal anomalies**
  Includes syndromes associated with anomalies in the number and form of chromosomes
  Use additional codes for conditions associated with the chromosomal anomalies
  - 758.0 Down's syndrome
    Mongolism
    Translocation Down's syndrome
    Trisomy:
      21 or 22
      G
  - 758.1 Patau's syndrome
    Trisomy:
      13
      D_1
  - 758.2 Edward's syndrome
    Trisomy:
      18
      E_3

- **758.3 Autosomal deletion syndromes**
  Coding Clinic: 2004, Q4, P93-95; 1995, Q2, P6-7, 11
  - **758.31 Cri-du-chat syndrome**
    Deletion 5p
  - **758.32 Velo-cardio-facial syndrome**
    Deletion 22q11.2
  - **758.33 Other microdeletions**
    Miller-Dieker syndrome
    Smith-Magenis syndrome
  - **758.39 Other autosomal deletions**
- **758.4 Balanced autosomal translocation in normal individual**
- **758.5 Other conditions due to autosomal anomalies**
  Accessory autosomes NEC
- **758.6 Gonadal dysgenesis**
  Ovarian dysgenesis
  Turner's syndrome
  XO syndrome
  > Excludes: pure gonadal dysgenesis (752.7)
- **758.7 Klinefelter's syndrome**
  XXY syndrome
- **758.8 Other conditions due to chromosome anomalies**
  - **758.81 Other conditions due to sex chromosome anomalies**
  - **758.89 Other**
- **758.9 Conditions due to anomaly of unspecified chromosome**

- **759 Other and unspecified congenital anomalies**
  - **759.0 Anomalies of spleen**
    Aberrant spleen   Congenital splenomegaly
    Absent spleen   Ectopic spleen
    Accessory spleen   Lobulation of spleen
  - **759.1 Anomalies of adrenal gland**
    Aberrant adrenal gland
    Absent adrenal gland
    Accessory adrenal gland
    > Excludes: adrenogenital disorders (255.2)
    > congenital disorders of steroid metabolism (255.2)
  - **759.2 Anomalies of other endocrine glands**
    Absent parathyroid gland
    Accessory thyroid gland
    Persistent thyroglossal or thyrolingual duct
    Thyroglossal (duct) cyst
    > Excludes: congenital:
    > goiter (246.1)
    > hypothyroidism (243)
  - **759.3 Situs inversus**
    Situs inversus or transversus:
      abdominalis
      thoracis
    Transposition of viscera:
      abdominal
      thoracic
    > Excludes: dextrocardia without mention of complete transposition (746.87)
  - **759.4 Conjoined twins**
    Craniopagus   Thoracopagus
    Dicephalus   Xiphopagus
    Pygopagus
  - **759.5 Tuberous sclerosis**
    Bourneville's disease
    Epiloia
  - **759.6 Other hamartoses, NEC**
    Syndrome:
      Peutz-Jeghers
      Sturge-Weber (-Dimitri)
      von Hippel-Lindau
    > Excludes: neurofibromatosis (237.70-237.79)
    Coding Clinic: 1992, Q3, P11
  - **759.7 Multiple congenital anomalies, so described**
    Congenital:
      anomaly, multiple NOS
      deformity, multiple NOS
  - **759.8 Other specified anomalies**
    - **759.81 Prader-Willi syndrome**
    - **759.82 Marfan syndrome**
      Coding Clinic: 1993, Q3, P11
    - **759.83 Fragile X syndrome**
    - **759.89 Other**
      Index directs coder to this code for Noonan's syndrome.
      Congenital malformation syndromes affecting multiple systems, NEC
      Laurence-Moon-Biedl syndrome
      Coding Clinic: 2012, Q2, P3-4; 2008, Q3, P3-4; 2006, Q3, P21; 2005, Q2, P17; 2004, Q2, P12; 2001, Q1, P3; 1999, Q3, P17-19x2; 1998, Q3, P8; 1987, Sept-Oct, P9; 1985, Sept-Oct, P11
  - **759.9 Congenital anomaly, unspecified**

OGCR Section I.C.15.a

For coding and reporting purposes the perinatal period is defined as before birth through the 28th day following birth. The following guidelines are provided for reporting purposes. Hospitals may record other diagnoses as needed for internal data use.

1) **Chapter 15 Codes** They are never for use on the maternal record. Codes from Chapter 11, the obstetric chapter, are never permitted on the newborn record. Chapter 15 code may be used throughout the life of the patient if the condition is still present.
2) **Sequencing of perinatal codes** Generally, codes from Chapter 15 should be sequenced as the principal/first-listed diagnosis on the newborn record, with the exception of the appropriate V30 code for the birth episode, followed by codes from any other chapter that provide additional detail. The "use additional code" note at the beginning of the chapter supports this guideline. If the index does not provide a specific code for a perinatal condition, assign code 779.89, Other specified conditions originating in the perinatal period, followed by the code from another chapter that specifies the condition. Codes for signs and symptoms may be assigned when a definitive diagnosis has not been established.
3) **Birth process or community acquired conditions** If a newborn has a condition that may be either due to the birth process or community acquired and the documentation does not indicate which it is, the default is due to the birth process and the code from Chapter 15 should be used. If the condition is community-acquired, a code from Chapter 15 should not be assigned.

15. CERTAIN CONDITIONS ORIGINATING IN THE PERINATAL PERIOD (760–779)

Includes conditions which have their origin in the perinatal period, before birth through the first 28 days after birth, even though death or morbidity occurs later

Use additional code(s) to further specify condition

MATERNAL CAUSES OF PERINATAL MORBIDITY AND MORTALITY (760–763)

● **760 Fetus or newborn affected by maternal conditions which may be unrelated to present pregnancy**

Includes the listed maternal conditions only when specified as a cause of mortality or morbidity of the fetus or newborn

Excludes maternal endocrine and metabolic disorders affecting fetus or newborn (775.0–775.9)

Coding Clinic: 1992, Q2, P12

760.0 Maternal hypertensive disorders
Fetus or newborn affected by maternal conditions classifiable to 642

760.1 Maternal renal and urinary tract diseases
Fetus or newborn affected by maternal conditions classifiable to 580–599

760.2 Maternal infections
Fetus or newborn affected by maternal infectious disease classifiable to 001–136 and 487, but fetus or newborn not manifesting that disease
Excludes congenital infectious diseases (771.0–771.8)
maternal genital tract and other localized infections (760.8)

760.3 Other chronic maternal circulatory and respiratory diseases
Fetus or newborn affected by chronic maternal conditions classifiable to 390–459, 490–519, 745–748

760.4 Maternal nutritional disorders
Fetus or newborn affected by:
maternal disorders classifiable to 260–269
maternal malnutrition NOS
Excludes fetal malnutrition (764.10–764.29)

760.5 Maternal injury
Fetus or newborn affected by maternal conditions classifiable to 800–995

● **760.6 Surgical operation on mother and fetus**
Excludes cesarean section for present delivery (763.4)
damage to placenta from amniocentesis, cesarean section, or surgical induction (762.1)
Coding Clinic: 2008, Q4, P137-138

760.61 Newborn affected by amniocentesis
Excludes fetal complications from amniocentesis (679.1)

760.62 Newborn affected by other in utero procedure
Excludes fetal complications of in utero procedure (679.1)

760.63 Newborn affected by other surgical operations on mother during pregnancy
Excludes newborn affected by previous surgical procedure on mother not associated with pregnancy (760.64)

760.64 Newborn affected by previous surgical procedure on mother not associated with pregnancy

● **760.7 Noxious influences affecting fetus or newborn via placenta or breast milk**
Fetus or newborn affected by noxious substance transmitted via placenta or breast milk
Excludes anesthetic and analgesic drugs administered during labor and delivery (763.5)
drug withdrawal syndrome in newborn (779.5)
Coding Clinic: 1991, Q3, P21

760.70 Unspecified noxious substance
Fetus or newborn affected by:
drug NEC

760.71 Alcohol
Fetal alcohol syndrome

760.72 Narcotics

760.73 Hallucinogenic agents

760.74 Anti-infectives
Antibiotics
Antifungals

760.75 Cocaine
Coding Clinic: 1994, Q3, P6; 1992, Q2, P12

760.76 Diethylstilbestrol [DES]

760.77 Anticonvulsants
Carbamazepine   Phenytoin
Phenobarbital   Valproic acid
Coding Clinic: 2005, Q4, P82-83

760.78 Antimetabolic agents
Methotrexate
Retinoic acid
Statins
Coding Clinic: 2005, Q4, P82-83

760.79 Other
Fetus or newborn affected by:
immune sera transmitted via placenta or breast milk
medicinal agents NEC transmitted via placenta or breast milk
toxic substance NEC transmitted via placenta or breast milk
Coding Clinic: 2010, Q1, P12; 2009, Q3, P12x3

760.8 Other specified maternal conditions affecting fetus or newborn
Maternal genital tract and other localized infection affecting fetus or newborn, but fetus or newborn not manifesting that disease
Excludes maternal urinary tract infection affecting fetus or newborn (760.1)

760.9 Unspecified maternal condition affecting fetus or newborn

- **761 Fetus or newborn affected by maternal complications of pregnancy**
  - *Includes:* the listed maternal conditions only when specified as a cause of mortality or morbidity of the fetus or newborn
  - 761.0 Incompetent cervix
  - 761.1 Premature rupture of membranes
  - 761.2 Oligohydramnios
    - *Scant volume of amniotic fluid*
    - *Excludes:* that due to premature rupture of membranes (761.1)
  - 761.3 Polyhydramnios
    - *Overabundance of amniotic fluid*
    - Hydramnios (acute) (chronic)
  - 761.4 Ectopic pregnancy
    - Pregnancy:
      - abdominal
      - intraperitoneal
      - tubal
  - 761.5 Multiple pregnancy
    - Triplet (pregnancy)
    - Twin (pregnancy)
  - 761.6 Maternal death
  - 761.7 Malpresentation before labor
    - Breech presentation before labor
    - External version before labor
    - Oblique lie before labor
    - Transverse lie before labor
    - Unstable lie before labor
  - 761.8 Other specified maternal complications of pregnancy affecting fetus or newborn
    - Spontaneous abortion, fetus
  - 761.9 Unspecified maternal complication of pregnancy affecting fetus or newborn

- **762 Fetus or newborn affected by complications of placenta, cord, and membranes**
  - *Includes:* the listed maternal conditions only when specified as a cause of mortality or morbidity in the fetus or newborn
  - 762.0 Placenta previa
  - 762.1 Other forms of placental separation and hemorrhage
    - Abruptio placentae
    - Antepartum hemorrhage
    - Damage to placenta from amniocentesis, cesarean section, or surgical induction
    - Maternal blood loss
    - Premature separation of placenta
    - Rupture of marginal sinus
  - 762.2 Other and unspecified morphological and functional abnormalities of placenta
    - Placental:
      - dysfunction
      - infarction
      - insufficiency
  - 762.3 Placental transfusion syndromes
    - Placental and cord abnormality resulting in twin-to-twin or other transplacental transfusion
    - *Use additional* code to indicate resultant condition in newborn:
      - fetal blood loss (772.0)
      - polycythemia neonatorum (776.4)
  - 762.4 Prolapsed cord
    - Cord presentation
  - 762.5 Other compression of umbilical cord
    - Cord around neck   Knot in cord
    - Entanglement of cord   Torsion of cord
    - Coding Clinic: 2003, Q2, P9

- 762.6 Other and unspecified conditions of umbilical cord
  - Short cord
  - Thrombosis of umbilical cord
  - Varices of umbilical cord
  - Velamentous insertion of umbilical cord
  - Vasa previa
  - *Excludes:* infection of umbilical cord (771.4)
    - single umbilical artery (747.5)
- 762.7 Chorioamnionitis
  - Amnionitis
  - Membranitis
  - Placentitis
- 762.8 Other specified abnormalities of chorion and amnion
- 762.9 Unspecified abnormality of chorion and amnion

- **763 Fetus or newborn affected by other complications of labor and delivery**
  - *Includes:* the listed conditions only when specified as a cause of mortality or morbidity in the fetus or newborn
  - *Excludes:* newborn affected by surgical procedures on mother (760.61-760.64)
  - 763.0 Breech delivery and extraction
  - 763.1 Other malpresentation, malposition, and disproportion during labor and delivery
    - Fetus or newborn affected by:
      - abnormality of bony pelvis
      - contracted pelvis
      - persistent occipitoposterior position
      - shoulder presentation
      - transverse lie
      - conditions classifiable to 652, 653, and 660
  - 763.2 Forceps delivery
    - Fetus or newborn affected by forceps extraction
  - 763.3 Delivery by vacuum extractor
  - 763.4 Cesarean delivery
    - *Excludes:* placental separation or hemorrhage from cesarean section (762.1)
  - 763.5 Maternal anesthesia and analgesia
    - Reactions and intoxications from maternal opiates and tranquilizers during labor and delivery
    - *Excludes:* drug withdrawal syndrome in newborn (779.5)
  - 763.6 Precipitate delivery
    - Rapid second stage
  - 763.7 Abnormal uterine contractions
    - Fetus or newborn affected by:
      - contraction ring
      - hypertonic labor
      - hypotonic uterine dysfunction
      - uterine inertia or dysfunction
      - conditions classifiable to 661, except 661.3
  - 763.8 Other specified complications of labor and delivery affecting fetus or newborn
    - 763.81 Abnormality in fetal heart rate or rhythm before the onset of labor
    - 763.82 Abnormality in fetal heart rate or rhythm during labor
      - Coding Clinic: 1998, Q4, P46-47
    - 763.83 Abnormality in fetal heart rate or rhythm, unspecified as to time of onset
    - 763.84 Meconium passage during delivery
      - *Excludes:* meconium aspiration (770.11, 770.12)
        - meconium staining (779.84)
      - Coding Clinic: 2005, Q4, P83-89
    - 763.89 Other specified complications of labor and delivery affecting fetus or newborn
      - Fetus or newborn affected by:
        - abnormality of maternal soft tissues
        - destructive operation on live fetus to facilitate delivery
        - induction of labor (medical)
        - other conditions classifiable to 650–669
        - other procedures used in labor and delivery
  - 763.9 Unspecified complication of labor and delivery affecting fetus or newborn

CERTAIN CONDITIONS ORIGINATING IN THE PERINATAL PERIOD (760–779)

OTHER CONDITIONS ORIGINATING IN THE PERINATAL PERIOD (764–779)

The following fifth-digit subclassification is for use with category 764 and codes 765.0 and 765.1 to denote birthweight:

0	unspecified [weight]	5	1,250–1,499 grams
1	less than 500 grams	6	1,500–1,749 grams
2	500–749 grams	7	1,750–1,999 grams
3	750–999 grams	8	2,000–2,499 grams
4	1,000–1,249 grams	9	2,500 grams and over

- **764 Slow fetal growth and fetal malnutrition**
    Requires fifth digit. See beginning of section 764–779 for codes and definitions.
    Coding Clinic: 2009, Q1, P7; 2004, Q3, P4-5; 1994, Q1, P15; 1989, Q2, P15

    OGCR Section I.C.15.i
    Providers utilize different criteria in determining prematurity. A code for prematurity should not be assigned unless it is documented. The 5th digit assignment for codes from category 764 and subcategories 765.0 and 765.1 should be based on the recorded birth weight and estimated gestational age.

  - **764.0** "Light-for-dates" without mention of fetal
    [0-9]   malnutrition
             Infants underweight for gestational age
             "Small-for-dates"
  - **764.1** "Light-for-dates" with signs of fetal malnutrition
    [0-9]   Infants "light-for-dates" classifiable to 764.0, who in addition show signs of fetal malnutrition, such as dry peeling skin and loss of subcutaneous tissue
  - **764.2** Fetal malnutrition without mention of
    [0-9]   "light-for-dates"
             Infants, not underweight for gestational age, showing signs of fetal malnutrition, such as dry peeling skin and loss of subcutaneous tissue
             Intrauterine malnutrition
  - **764.9** Fetal growth retardation, unspecified
    [0-9]   Intrauterine growth retardation
             Coding Clinic: 1997, Q1, P6

- **765 Disorders relating to short gestation and low birthweight**
    Requires fifth digit. See beginning of section 764–779 for codes and definitions.
    Includes the listed conditions, without further specification, as causes of mortality, morbidity, or additional care, in fetus or newborn
    Coding Clinic: 2002, Q4, P63-64; 1994, Q1, P15; 1991, Q2, P19, 1989, Q2, P15

  - **765.0** Extreme immaturity
    [0-9]   **Note:** Usually implies a birthweight of less than 1,000 grams
             Use additional code for weeks of gestation (765.20–765.29)
             Coding Clinic: 2009, Q1, P12; 2004, Q3, P4-5; 2001, Q4, P50-51

    OGCR Section I.C.15.i
    Providers utilize different criteria in determining prematurity. A code for prematurity should not be assigned unless it is documented. The 5th digit assignment for codes from subcategory 765.0 should be based on the recorded birth weight and estimated gestational age.

  - **765.1** Other preterm infants
    [0-9]   Prematurity NOS
             Prematurity or small size, not classifiable to 765.0 or as "light-for-dates" in 764
             Note: Usually implies birthweight of 1,000–2,499 grams
             Use additional code for weeks of gestation (765.20–765.29)
             Coding Clinic: 2009, Q1, P12; 2008, Q4, P138-140; 2004, Q3, P4-5; 2002, Q4, P64; 1997, Q1, P6; 1994, Q1, P14

    OGCR Section I.C.15.i
    Providers utilize different criteria in determining prematurity. A code for prematurity should not be assigned unless it is documented. The 5th digit assignment for codes from category 764 and subcategories 765.0 and 765.1 should be based on the recorded birth weight and estimated gestational age.

  - **765.2 Weeks of gestation**
    Coding Clinic: 2004, Q3, P4-5

    OGCR Section I.C.15.i
    A code from subcategory 765.2, Weeks of gestation, should be assigned as an additional code with category 764 and codes from 765.0 and 765.1 to specify weeks of gestation as documented by the provider in the record.

    - **765.20** Unspecified weeks of gestation
    - **765.21** Less than 24 completed weeks of gestation
    - **765.22** 24 weeks of gestation
    - **765.23** 25–26 weeks of gestation
      Coding Clinic: 2009, Q1, P6
    - **765.24** 27–28 weeks of gestation
    - **765.25** 29–30 weeks of gestation
    - **765.26** 31–32 weeks of gestation
      Coding Clinic: 2009, Q1, P6; 2008, Q4, P138-140
    - **765.27** 33–34 weeks of gestation
      Coding Clinic: 2010, Q4, P98
    - **765.28** 35–36 weeks of gestation
      Coding Clinic: 2002, Q4, P64
    - **765.29** 37 or more weeks of gestation

- **766 Disorders relating to long gestation and high birthweight**
    Includes the listed conditions, without further specification, as causes of mortality, morbidity, or additional care, in fetus or newborn

  - **766.0** Exceptionally large baby
    Note: Usually implies a birthweight of 4,500 grams or more.
  - **766.1** Other "heavy-for-dates" infants
    Other fetus or infant "heavy-" or "large-for-dates" regardless of period of gestation
  - **766.2** Late infant, not "heavy-for-dates"
    Coding Clinic: 2006, Q2, P12-13; 2003, Q4, P69
    - **766.21** Post-term infant
      Infant with gestation period over 40 completed weeks to 42 completed weeks
      Coding Clinic: 2009, Q1, P6; 2006, Q2, P12-13
    - **766.22** Prolonged gestation of infant
      Infant with gestation period over 42 completed weeks
      Postmaturity NOS
      Coding Clinic: 2009, Q1, P6; 2006, Q2, P12-13

- **767 Birth trauma**
  - **767.0** Subdural and cerebral hemorrhage
    Subdural and cerebral hemorrhage, whether described as due to birth trauma or to intrapartum anoxia or hypoxia
    Subdural hematoma (localized)
    Tentorial tear
    Use additional code to identify cause
    Excludes intraventricular hemorrhage (772.10–772.14) subarachnoid hemorrhage (772.2)
  - **767.1** Injuries to scalp
    Coding Clinic: 2003, Q4, P69-70
    - **767.11** Epicranial subaponeurotic hemorrhage (massive)
      Subgaleal hemorrhage
    - **767.19** Other injuries to scalp
      Caput succedaneum
      Cephalhematoma
      Chignon (from vacuum extraction)
  - **767.2** Fracture of clavicle

767.3 Other injuries to skeleton
Fracture of:
long bones
skull
Excludes congenital dislocation of hip (754.30–754.35)
fracture of spine, congenital (767.4)

767.4 Injury to spine and spinal cord
Dislocation of spine or spinal cord due to birth trauma
Fracture of spine or spinal cord due to birth trauma
Laceration of spine or spinal cord due to birth trauma
Rupture of spine or spinal cord due to birth trauma

767.5 Facial nerve injury
Facial palsy

767.6 Injury to brachial plexus
Palsy or paralysis:
brachial
Erb (-Duchenne)
Klumpke (-Déjérine)

767.7 Other cranial and peripheral nerve injuries
Phrenic nerve paralysis

767.8 Other specified birth trauma
Eye damage
Hematoma of:
liver (subcapsular)
testes
vulva
Rupture of:
liver
spleen
Scalpel wound
Traumatic glaucoma
Excludes hemorrhage classifiable to 772.0–772.9

767.9 Birth trauma, unspecified
Birth injury NOS

● **768 Intrauterine hypoxia and birth asphyxia**
Use only when associated with newborn morbidity classifiable elsewhere
Excludes acidemia NOS of newborn (775.81)
acidosis NOS of newborn (775.81)
cerebral ischemia NOS (779.2)
hypoxia NOS of newborn (770.88)
mixed metabolic and respiratory acidosis of newborn (775.81)
respiratory arrest of newborn (770.87)

768.0 Fetal death from asphyxia or anoxia before onset of labor or at unspecified time

768.1 Fetal death from asphyxia or anoxia during labor

768.2 Fetal distress before onset of labor, in liveborn infant
Fetal metabolic acidemia before onset of labor, in liveborn infant

768.3 Fetal distress first noted during labor and delivery, in liveborn infant
Fetal metabolic acidemia first noted during labor and delivery, in liveborn infant

768.4 Fetal distress, unspecified as to time of onset, in liveborn infant
Fetal metabolic acidemia unspecified as to time of onset, in liveborn infant
Coding Clinic: 1986, Nov-Dec, P10

768.5 Severe birth asphyxia
Birth asphyxia with neurologic involvement
Excludes hypoxic-ischemic encephalopathy (HIE) (768.70-768.73)

768.6 Mild or moderate birth asphyxia
Other specified birth asphyxia (without mention of neurologic involvement)
Excludes hypoxic-ischemic encephalopathy (HIE) (768.70-768.73)

● **768.7 Hypoxic-ischemic encephalopathy (HIE)**
Coding Clinic: 2006, Q4, P104-106

768.70 Hypoxic-ischemic encephalopathy, unspecified

768.71 Mild hypoxic-ischemic encephalopathy

768.72 Moderate hypoxic-ischemic encephalopathy
Coding Clinic: 2009, Q4, P113

768.73 Severe hypoxic-ischemic encephalopathy

768.9 Unspecified birth asphyxia in liveborn infant
Anoxia NOS, in liveborn infant
Asphyxia NOS, in liveborn infant

769 Respiratory distress syndrome
Cardiorespiratory distress syndrome of newborn
Hyaline membrane disease (pulmonary)
Idiopathic respiratory distress syndrome [IRDS or RDS] of newborn
Pulmonary hypoperfusion syndrome
Excludes transient tachypnea of newborn (770.6)
Coding Clinic: 2009, Q3, P12; 1989, Q1, P10

● **770 Other respiratory conditions of fetus and newborn**

770.0 Congenital pneumonia
Infective pneumonia acquired prenatally
Excludes pneumonia from infection acquired after birth (480.0–486)
Coding Clinic: 2005, Q1, P10-11

● **770.1 Fetal and newborn aspiration**
Excludes aspiration of postnatal stomach contents (770.85, 770.86)
meconium passage during delivery (763.84)
meconium staining (779.84)
Coding Clinic: 2005, Q4, P83-89

770.10 Fetal and newborn aspiration, unspecified

770.11 Meconium aspiration without respiratory symptoms
Meconium aspiration NOS

770.12 Meconium aspiration with respiratory symptoms
Meconium aspiration pneumonia
Meconium aspiration pneumonitis
Meconium aspiration syndrome NOS
Use additional code to identify any secondary pulmonary hypertension (416.8), if applicable

770.13 Aspiration of clear amniotic fluid without respiratory symptoms
Aspiration of clear amniotic fluid NOS

770.14 Aspiration of clear amniotic fluid with respiratory symptoms
Aspiration of clear amniotic fluid with pneumonia
Aspiration of clear amniotic fluid with pneumonitis
Use additional code to identify any secondary pulmonary hypertension (416.8), if applicable

770.15 Aspiration of blood without respiratory symptoms
Aspiration of blood NOS

770.16 Aspiration of blood with respiratory symptoms
Aspiration of blood with pneumonia
Aspiration of blood with pneumonitis
Use additional code to identify any secondary pulmonary hypertension (416.8), if applicable

770.17 Other fetal and newborn aspiration without respiratory symptoms

770.18 Other fetal and newborn aspiration with respiratory symptoms
Other aspiration pneumonia
Other aspiration pneumonitis
Use additional code to identify any secondary pulmonary hypertension (416.8), if applicable

770.2 Interstitial emphysema and related conditions
Pneumomediastinum originating in the perinatal period
Pneumopericardium originating in the perinatal period
Pneumothorax originating in the perinatal period

770.3 Pulmonary hemorrhage
Hemorrhage:
alveolar (lung) originating in the perinatal period
intra-alveolar (lung) originating in the perinatal period
massive pulmonary originating in the perinatal period

CERTAIN CONDITIONS ORIGINATING IN THE PERINATAL PERIOD (760–779)

- **770.4 Primary atelectasis**
  Failure of lungs to expand properly at birth
  Pulmonary immaturity NOS
- **770.5 Other and unspecified atelectasis**
  Atelectasis:
     NOS originating in the perinatal period
     partial originating in the perinatal period
     secondary originating in the perinatal period
  Pulmonary collapse originating in the perinatal period
- **770.6 Transitory tachypnea of newborn**
  Idiopathic tachypnea of newborn
  Wet lung syndrome
  Excludes *respiratory distress syndrome (769)*
  Coding Clinic: 2009, Q3, P17x2; 1993, Q3, P7x2; 1989, Q1, P10
- **770.7 Chronic respiratory disease arising in the perinatal period**
  Bronchopulmonary dysplasia
  Interstitial pulmonary fibrosis of prematurity
  Wilson-Mikity syndrome
  Coding Clinic: 2011, Q1, P17; 1991, Q2, P19; 1986, Nov-Dec, P11-12
- **770.8 Other respiratory problems after birth**
  Excludes *mixed metabolic and respiratory acidosis of newborn (775.81)*
  Coding Clinic: 2005, Q4, P83-89; 2002, Q4, P65-66; 1998, Q2, P10; 1996, Q2, P10-11
  - **770.81 Primary apnea of newborn**
    Apneic spells of newborn NOS
    Essential apnea of newborn
    Sleep apnea of newborn
  - **770.82 Other apnea of newborn**
    Obstructive apnea of newborn
    Coding Clinic: 2010, Q4, P98
  - **770.83 Cyanotic attacks of newborn**
  - **770.84 Respiratory failure of newborn**
    Excludes *respiratory distress syndrome (769)*
  - **770.85 Aspiration of postnatal stomach contents without respiratory symptoms**
    Aspiration of postnatal stomach contents NOS
  - **770.86 Aspiration of postnatal stomach contents with respiratory symptoms**
    Aspiration of postnatal stomach contents with pneumonia
    Aspiration of postnatal stomach contents with pneumonitis
    Use additional code to identify any secondary pulmonary hypertension (416.8), if applicable
  - **770.87 Respiratory arrest of newborn**
  - **770.88 Hypoxemia of newborn**
    Hypoxia NOS, in liveborn infant
  - **770.89 Other respiratory problems after birth**
    Coding Clinic: 2009, Q3, P17
- **770.9 Unspecified respiratory condition of fetus and newborn**
- **771 Infections specific to the perinatal period**
  Includes infections acquired before or during birth or via the umbilicus or during the first 28 days after birth
  Excludes *congenital pneumonia (770.0)*
  congenital syphilis (090.0–090.9)
  infant botulism (040.41)
  maternal infectious disease as a cause of mortality or morbidity in fetus or newborn, but fetus or newborn not manifesting the disease (760.2)
  ophthalmia neonatorum due to gonococcus (098.40)
  other infections not specifically classified to this category
  Coding Clinic: 2005, Q1, P10
  - **771.0 Congenital rubella**
    Congenital rubella pneumonitis
  - **771.1 Congenital cytomegalovirus infection**
    Congenital cytomegalic inclusion disease
  - **771.2 Other congenital infections**
    Congenital: Congenital:
      herpes simplex   toxoplasmosis
      listeriosis   tuberculosis
      malaria
  - **771.3 Tetanus neonatorum**
    Tetanus omphalitis
    Excludes *hypocalcemic tetany (775.4)*
  - **771.4 Omphalitis of the newborn**
    Infection: Infection:
      navel cord   umbilical stump
    Excludes *tetanus omphalitis (771.3)*
    Coding Clinic: 2009, Q4, P113
  - **771.5 Neonatal infective mastitis**
    Excludes *noninfective neonatal mastitis (778.7)*
  - **771.6 Neonatal conjunctivitis and dacryocystitis**
    Ophthalmia neonatorum NOS
    Excludes *ophthalmia neonatorum due to gonococcus (098.40)*
  - **771.7 Neonatal Candida infection**
    Neonatal moniliasis
    Thrush in newborn
  - **771.8 Other infections specific to the perinatal period**
    Use additional code to identify organism or specific infection
    - **771.81 Septicemia [sepsis] of newborn**
      Use additional code to identify severe sepsis (995.92) and any associated acute organ dysfunction, if applicable
    - **771.82 Urinary tract infection of newborn**
    - **771.83 Bacteremia of newborn**
    - **771.89 Other infections specific to the perinatal period**
      Intra-amniotic infection of fetus NOS
      Infection of newborn NOS
      Coding Clinic: 2005, Q1, P10
      OGCR Section I.C.15.j
      771.81, Septicemia [sepsis] of newborn, should be assigned with a secondary code from category 041, Bacterial infections in conditions classified elsewhere and of unspecified site, to identify the organism.
- **772 Fetal and neonatal hemorrhage**
  Excludes *fetal hematologic conditions complicating pregnancy (678.0)*
  hematological disorders of fetus and newborn (776.0–776.9)
  - **772.0 Fetal blood loss affecting newborn**
    Fetal blood loss from:
      cut end of co-twin's cord
      placenta
      ruptured cord
      vasa previa
    Fetal exsanguination
    Fetal hemorrhage into:
      co-twin
      mother's circulation
  - **772.1 Intraventricular hemorrhage**
    Intraventricular hemorrhage from any perinatal cause
    Coding Clinic: 1992, Q3, P8; 1988, Q4, P8
    - **772.10 Unspecified grade**
    - **772.11 Grade I**
      Bleeding into germinal matrix
    - **772.12 Grade II**
      Bleeding into ventricle
    - **772.13 Grade III**
      Bleeding with enlargement of ventricle
      Coding Clinic: 2001, Q4, P50-51
    - **772.14 Grade IV**
      Bleeding into cerebral cortex

772.2 Subarachnoid hemorrhage
Subarachnoid hemorrhage from any perinatal cause
Excludes subdural and cerebral hemorrhage (767.0)

772.3 Umbilical hemorrhage after birth
Slipped umbilical ligature

772.4 Gastrointestinal hemorrhage
Excludes swallowed maternal blood (777.3)

772.5 Adrenal hemorrhage

772.6 Cutaneous hemorrhage
Bruising in fetus or newborn
Ecchymoses in fetus or newborn
Petechiae in fetus or newborn
Superficial hematoma in fetus or newborn

772.8 Other specified hemorrhage of fetus or newborn
Excludes hemorrhagic disease of newborn (776.0)
pulmonary hemorrhage (770.3)

772.9 Unspecified hemorrhage of newborn

773 Hemolytic disease of fetus or newborn, due to isoimmunization
Also known as erythroblastosis fetalis as a result of Rh blood factor incompatibilities between mother (Rh negative) and fetus (Rh positive)

773.0 Hemolytic disease due to Rh isoimmunization
Anemia due to RH:
 antibodies
 isoimmunization
 maternal/fetal incompatibility
Erythroblastosis (fetalis) due to RH:
 antibodies
 isoimmunization
 maternal/fetal incompatibility
Hemolytic disease (fetus) (newborn) due to RH:
 antibodies
 isoimmunization
 maternal/fetal incompatibility
Jaundice due to RH:
 antibodies
 isoimmunization
 maternal/fetal incompatibility
Rh hemolytic disease
Rh isoimmunization

773.1 Hemolytic disease due to ABO isoimmunization
ABO hemolytic disease
ABO isoimmunization
Anemia due to ABO:
 antibodies
 isoimmunization
 maternal/fetal incompatibility
Erythroblastosis (fetalis) due to ABO:
 antibodies
 isoimmunization
 maternal/fetal incompatibility
Hemolytic disease (fetus) (newborn) due to ABO:
 antibodies
 isoimmunization
 maternal/fetal incompatibility
Jaundice due to ABO:
 antibodies
 isoimmunization
 maternal/fetal incompatibility
Coding Clinic: 2003, Q2, P14-15; 1992, Q3, P8-9

773.2 Hemolytic disease due to other and unspecified isoimmunization
Erythroblastosis (fetalis) (neonatorum) NOS
Hemolytic disease (fetus) (newborn) NOS
Jaundice or anemia due to other and unspecified blood-group incompatibility
Coding Clinic: 1994, Q1, P13

773.3 Hydrops fetalis due to isoimmunization
Use additional code, if desired, to identify type of isoimmunization (773.0–773.2)

773.4 Kernicterus due to isoimmunization
Use additional code, if desired, to identify type of isoimmunization (773.0–773.2)

773.5 Late anemia due to isoimmunization

774 Other perinatal jaundice

774.0 Perinatal jaundice from hereditary hemolytic anemias
Code first underlying disease (282.0–282.9)

774.1 Perinatal jaundice from other excessive hemolysis
Fetal or neonatal jaundice from:
 bruising
 drugs or toxins transmitted from mother
 infection
 polycythemia
 swallowed maternal blood
Use additional code to identify cause
Excludes jaundice due to isoimmunization (773.0–773.2)

774.2 Neonatal jaundice associated with preterm delivery
Hyperbilirubinemia of prematurity
Jaundice due to delayed conjugation associated with preterm delivery
Coding Clinic: 1994, Q1, P13; 1991, Q3, P21

774.3 Neonatal jaundice due to delayed conjugation from other causes

774.30 Neonatal jaundice due to delayed conjugation, cause unspecified

774.31 Neonatal jaundice due to delayed conjugation in diseases classified elsewhere
Code first underlying diseases, as:
 congenital hypothyroidism (243)
 Crigler-Najjar syndrome (277.4)
 Gilbert's syndrome (277.4)

774.39 Other
Jaundice due to delayed conjugation from causes, such as:
 breast milk inhibitors
 delayed development of conjugating system

774.4 Perinatal jaundice due to hepatocellular damage
Fetal or neonatal hepatitis
Giant cell hepatitis
Inspissated bile syndrome

774.5 Perinatal jaundice from other causes
Code first underlying cause, as:
 congenital obstruction of bile duct (751.61)
 galactosemia (271.1)
 mucoviscidosis (277.00–277.09)

774.6 Unspecified fetal and neonatal jaundice
Icterus neonatorum
Neonatal hyperbilirubinemia (transient)
Physiologic jaundice NOS in newborn
Excludes that in preterm infants (774.2)
Coding Clinic: 1994, Q1, P13

774.7 Kernicterus not due to isoimmunization
Bilirubin encephalopathy
Kernicterus of newborn NOS
Excludes kernicterus due to isoimmunization (773.4)

775 Endocrine and metabolic disturbances specific to the fetus and newborn
Includes transitory endocrine and metabolic disturbances caused by the infant's response to maternal endocrine and metabolic factors, its removal from them, or its adjustment to extrauterine existence

775.0 Syndrome of "infant of a diabetic mother"
Maternal diabetes mellitus affecting fetus or newborn (with hypoglycemia)
Coding Clinic: 2004, Q1, P7-8x3

775.1 Neonatal diabetes mellitus
Diabetes mellitus syndrome in newborn infant

775.2 Neonatal myasthenia gravis

775.3 Neonatal thyrotoxicosis
Neonatal hyperthyroidism (transient)

775.4 Hypocalcemia and hypomagnesemia of newborn
Cow's milk hypocalcemia
Hypocalcemic tetany, neonatal
Neonatal hypoparathyroidism
Phosphate-loading hypocalcemia

775.5 Other transitory neonatal electrolyte disturbances
Dehydration, neonatal
Coding Clinic: 2010, Q1, P12; 2009, Q3, P18; 2008, Q4, P139-140; 2005, Q1, P9-10

775.6 Neonatal hypoglycemia
Excludes infant of mother with diabetes mellitus (775.0)

775.7 Late metabolic acidosis of newborn

775.8 Other neonatal endocrine and metabolic disturbances

775.81 Other acidosis of newborn
Acidemia NOS of newborn
Acidosis of newborn NOS
Mixed metabolic and respiratory acidosis of newborn

775.89 Other neonatal endocrine and metabolic disturbances
Amino-acid metabolic disorders described as transitory

775.9 Unspecified endocrine and metabolic disturbances specific to the fetus and newborn

776 Hematological disorders of newborn
Includes disorders specific to the newborn though possibly originating in utero
Excludes fetal hematologic conditions (678.0)

776.0 Hemorrhagic disease of newborn
Hemorrhagic diathesis of newborn
Vitamin K deficiency of newborn
Excludes fetal or neonatal hemorrhage (772.0–772.9)

776.1 Transient neonatal thrombocytopenia
Lack of sufficient numbers of circulating thrombocytes (platelets)
Neonatal thrombocytopenia due to:
  exchange transfusion
  idiopathic maternal thrombocytopenia
  isoimmunization

776.2 Disseminated intravascular coagulation in newborn

776.3 Other transient neonatal disorders of coagulation
Transient coagulation defect, newborn

776.4 Polycythemia neonatorum
Excess number of thrombocytes (platelets)
Plethora of newborn
Polycythemia due to:
  donor twin transfusion
  maternal-fetal transfusion

776.5 Congenital anemia
Anemia following fetal blood loss
Excludes anemia due to isoimmunization (773.0–773.2, 773.5)
hereditary hemolytic anemias (282.0–282.9)

776.6 Anemia of prematurity

776.7 Transient neonatal neutropenia
Isoimmune neutropenia
Low levels of white blood cells
Maternal transfer neutropenia
Excludes congenital neutropenia (nontransient) (288.01)

776.8 Other specified transient hematological disorders

776.9 Unspecified hematological disorder specific to newborn

777 Perinatal disorders of digestive system
Includes disorders specific to the fetus and newborn
Excludes intestinal obstruction classifiable to 560.0–560.9

777.1 Meconium obstruction
Congenital fecaliths
Stoney feces formations
Delayed passage of meconium
Meconium ileus NOS
Meconium plug syndrome
Excludes meconium ileus in cystic fibrosis (277.01)

777.2 Intestinal obstruction due to inspissated milk
Being thickened, dried, or made less fluid

777.3 Hematemesis and melena due to swallowed maternal blood
Swallowed blood syndrome in newborn
Excludes that not due to swallowed maternal blood (772.4)

777.4 Transitory ileus of newborn
Excludes Hirschsprung's disease (751.3)

777.5 Necrotizing enterocolitis in newborn

777.50 Necrotizing enterocolitis in newborn, unspecified
Necrotizing enterocolitis in newborn, NOS

777.51 Stage I necrotizing enterocolitis in newborn
Necrotizing enterocolitis without pneumatosis, without perforation

777.52 Stage II necrotizing enterocolitis in newborn
Necrotizing enterocolitis with pneumatosis, without perforation

777.53 Stage III necrotizing enterocolitis in newborn
Necrotizing enterocolitis with perforation
Necrotizing enterocolitis with pneumatosis and perforation
Coding Clinic: 2008, Q4, P138-140

777.6 Perinatal intestinal perforation
Meconium peritonitis

777.8 Other specified perinatal disorders of digestive system
Coding Clinic: 2010, Q4, P98

777.9 Unspecified perinatal disorder of digestive system

778 Conditions involving the integument and temperature regulation of fetus and newborn

778.0 Hydrops fetalis not due to isoimmunization
Idiopathic hydrops
Severe, life-threatening problem of edema (swelling) in fetus and newborn
Excludes hydrops fetalis due to isoimmunization (773.3)

778.1 Sclerema neonatorum

778.2 Cold injury syndrome of newborn

778.3 Other hypothermia of newborn

778.4 Other disturbances of temperature regulation of newborn
Dehydration fever in newborn
Environmentally induced pyrexia
Hyperthermia in newborn
Transitory fever of newborn

778.5 Other and unspecified edema of newborn
Edema neonatorum

778.6 Congenital hydrocele
Congenital hydrocele of tunica vaginalis

778.7 Breast engorgement in newborn
Noninfective mastitis of newborn
Excludes infective mastitis of newborn (771.5)

778.8 Other specified conditions involving the integument of fetus and newborn
Urticaria neonatorum
Skin rash
Excludes impetigo neonatorum (684)
pemphigus neonatorum (684)

778.9 Unspecified condition involving the integument and temperature regulation of fetus and newborn

779 Other and ill-defined conditions originating in the perinatal period

779.0 Convulsions in newborn
Fits in newborn
Seizures in newborn
Coding Clinic: 1984, Nov-Dec, P11

779.1 Other and unspecified cerebral irritability in newborn

779.2 Cerebral depression, coma, and other abnormal cerebral signs
Cerebral ischemia NOS of newborn
CNS dysfunction in newborn NOS
Excludes cerebral ischemia due to birth trauma (767.0)
intrauterine cerebral ischemia (768.2–768.9)
intraventricular hemorrhage (772.10–772.14)

- **779.3 Disorder of stomach function and feeding problems in newborn**
  Coding Clinic: 1989, Q2, P15
  - 779.31 **Feeding problems in newborn**
    Slow feeding in newborn
    Excludes *feeding problem in child over 28 days old (783.3)*
    Coding Clinic: 2012, Q3, P7; 2009, Q4, P113
  - 779.32 **Bilious vomiting in newborn**
    Excludes *bilious vomiting in child over 28 days old (787.04)*
  - 779.33 **Other vomiting in newborn**
    Regurgitation of food in newborn
    Excludes *vomiting in child over 28 days old (536.2, 787.01-787.03, 787.04)*
  - 779.34 **Failure to thrive in newborn**
    Excludes *failure to thrive in child over 28 days old (783.41)*
- 779.4 **Drug reactions and intoxications specific to newborn**
  Gray syndrome from chloramphenicol administration in newborn
  Excludes *fetal alcohol syndrome (760.71)
  reactions and intoxications from maternal opiates and tranquilizers (763.5)*
- 779.5 **Drug withdrawal syndrome in newborn**
  Drug withdrawal syndrome in infant of dependent mother
  Excludes *fetal alcohol syndrome (760.71)*
  Coding Clinic: 1994, Q3, P6
- 779.6 **Termination of pregnancy (fetus)**
  Fetal death due to:
  induced abortion
  termination of pregnancy
  Excludes *spontaneous abortion (fetus) (761.8)*
- 779.7 **Periventricular leukomalacia**
  Coding Clinic: 2001, Q4, P50-51

- **779.8 Other specified conditions originating in the perinatal period**
  Coding Clinic: 2006, Q1, P18; 2002, Q4, P67; 1994, Q1, P15
  - 779.81 **Neonatal bradycardia**
    Excludes *abnormality in fetal heart rate or rhythm complicating labor and delivery (763.81-763.83)
    bradycardia due to birth asphyxia (768.5-768.9)*
  - 779.82 **Neonatal tachycardia**
    Excludes *abnormality in fetal heart rate or rhythm complicating labor and delivery (763.81-763.83)*
  - 779.83 **Delayed separation of umbilical cord**
    Coding Clinic: 2003, Q4, P71
  - 779.84 **Meconium staining**
    Excludes *meconium aspiration (770.11, 770.12)
    meconium passage during delivery (763.84)*
    Coding Clinic: 2005, Q4, P83-89x2
  - 779.85 **Cardiac arrest of newborn**
  - 779.89 **Other specified conditions originating in the perinatal period**
    Use additional code to specify condition
    Coding Clinic: 2012, Q3, P5; 2011, Q3, P3-4; 2005, Q2, P15-16; Q1, P9
    OGCR Section I.C.15.a.2
    If the index does not provide a specific code for a perinatal condition, assign code 779.89 followed by the code from another chapter that specifies the condition.
- 779.9 **Unspecified condition originating in the perinatal period**
  Congenital debility NOS
  Stillbirth NEC

16. SYMPTOMS, SIGNS, AND ILL-DEFINED CONDITIONS (780–799)

This section includes symptoms, signs, abnormal results of laboratory or other investigative procedures, and ill-defined conditions regarding which no diagnosis classifiable elsewhere is recorded.

Signs and symptoms that point rather definitely to a given diagnosis are assigned to some category in the preceding part of the classification. In general, categories 780–796 include the more ill-defined conditions and symptoms that point with perhaps equal suspicion to two or more diseases or to two or more systems of the body, and without the necessary study of the case to make a final diagnosis. Practically all categories in this group could be designated as "not otherwise specified," or as "unknown etiology," or as "transient." The Alphabetic Index should be consulted to determine which symptoms and signs are to be allocated here and which to more specific sections of the classification; the residual subcategories numbered .9 are provided for other relevant symptoms which cannot be allocated elsewhere in the classification.

The conditions and signs or symptoms included in categories 780–796 consist of: (a) cases for which no more specific diagnosis can be made even after all facts bearing on the case have been investigated; (b) signs or symptoms existing at the time of initial encounter that proved to be transient and whose causes could not be determined; (c) provisional diagnoses in a patient who failed to return for further investigation or care; (d) cases referred elsewhere for investigation or treatment before the diagnosis was made; (e) cases in which a more precise diagnosis was not available for any other reason; (f) certain symptoms which represent important problems in medical care and which it might be desired to classify in addition to a known cause.

SYMPTOMS (780–789)

- **780 General symptoms**
  - **780.0 Alteration of consciousness**
    - Excludes: alteration of consciousness due to:
      - intracranial injuries (850.0-854.19)
      - skull fractures (800.00-801.99, 803.00-804.99)
      - coma:
        - diabetic (249.2–249.3, 250.2–250.3)
        - hepatic (572.2)
        - originating in the perinatal period (779.2)
    - **780.01 Coma**
      - Coding Clinic: 2012, Q1, P14; 1996, Q3, P16
    - **780.02 Transient alteration of awareness**
    - **780.03 Persistent vegetative state**
    - **780.09 Other**
      - Drowsiness
      - Semicoma
      - Somnolence
      - Stupor
      - Unconsciousness
  - **780.1 Hallucinations**
    - Hallucinations:
      - NOS
      - auditory
      - gustatory
      - olfactory
      - tactile
    - Excludes: those associated with mental disorders, as
      - functional psychoses (295.0–298.9)
      - organic brain syndromes (290.0–294.9, 310.0–310.9)
      - visual hallucinations (368.16)
  - **780.2 Syncope and collapse**
    - Blackout
    - Fainting
    - (Near) (Pre)syncope
    - Vasovagal attack
    - Excludes: carotid sinus syncope (337.0)
      - heat syncope (992.1)
      - neurocirculatory asthenia (306.2)
      - orthostatic hypotension (458.0)
      - shock NOS (785.50)
    - Coding Clinic: 2002, Q1, P6; 2000, Q3, P12; 1995, Q4, P50-51; Q3, P14; 1992, Q3, P16; 1990, Q1, P9; 1985, Nov-Dec, P12
  - **780.3 Convulsions**
    - Excludes: convulsions:
      - epileptic (345.10–345.91)
      - in newborn (779.0)
    - Coding Clinic: 2012, Q2, P9-10; 1984, Nov-Dec, P11
    - **780.31 Febrile convulsions (simple), unspecified**
      - Febrile seizures NOS
      - Coding Clinic: 2005, Q3, P12-13; 1987, Nov-Dec, P11
    - **780.32 Complex febrile convulsions**
      - Febrile seizure:
        - atypical
        - complex
        - complicated
      - Excludes: status epilepticus (345.3)
      - Coding Clinic: 2006, Q4, P106-107
    - **780.33 Post traumatic seizures**
      - Excludes: post traumatic epilepsy (345.00-345.91)
      - Coding Clinic: 2010, Q4, P93
    - **780.39 Other convulsions**
      - Convulsive disorder NOS
      - Fits NOS
      - Recurrent convulsions NOS
      - Seizure NOS
      - Seizures NOS
      - Coding Clinic: 2012, Q2, P9-10; 2008, Q1, P17; 2006, Q3, P22; 2004, Q4, P50-52; 2003, Q1, P7; 1998, Q4, P39-40; 1997, Q2, P8; Q1, P12-13; 1994, Q3, P9; 1993, Q1, P24; 1987, Nov-Dec, P12; 1985, July-Aug, P10; 1984, May-June, P14
  - **780.4 Dizziness and giddiness**
    - Light-headedness
    - Vertigo NOS
    - Excludes: Ménière's disease and other specified vertiginous syndromes (386.0–386.9)
    - Coding Clinic: 2003, Q2, P11; 2000, Q3, P12; 1997, Q2, P9-10; 1991, Q2, P17
  - **780.5 Sleep disturbances**
    - Excludes: circadian rhythm sleep disorders (327.30–327.39)
      - organic hypersomnia (327.10 327.19)
      - organic insomnia (327.00–327.09)
      - organic sleep apnea (327.20–327.29)
      - organic sleep related movement disorders (327.51–327.59)
      - parasomnias (327.40–327.49)
      - that of nonorganic origin (307.40–307.49)
    - **780.50 Sleep disturbance, unspecified**
    - **780.51 Insomnia with sleep apnea, unspecified**
      - Coding Clinic: 1993, Q1, P28-29
    - **780.52 Insomnia, unspecified**
    - **780.53 Hypersomnia with sleep apnea, unspecified**
      - Coding Clinic: 1993, Q1, P28-29
    - **780.54 Hypersomnia, unspecified**
    - **780.55 Disruptions of 24 hour sleep wake cycle, unspecified**
    - **780.56 Dysfunctions associated with sleep stages or arousal from sleep**
    - **780.57 Unspecified sleep apnea**
      - Coding Clinic: 2001, Q1, P6-7; 1997, Q1, P5; 1993, Q1, P28-29
    - **780.58 Sleep related movement disorder, unspecified**
      - Excludes: restless legs syndrome (333.94)
      - Coding Clinic: 2004, Q4, P95-96
    - **780.59 Other**

- **780.6 Fever and other physiologic disturbances of temperature regulation**
  - **Excludes** effects of reduced environmental temperature (991.0-991.9)
  - effects of heat and light (992.0-992.9)
  - fever, chills or hypothermia associated with confirmed infection – code to infection
  - Coding Clinic: 2008, Q4, P140-143; 2005, Q3, P16-17; 2000, Q3, P13; 1991, Q2, P8x2; 1990, Q1, P8; 1985, July-Aug, P13

  - **780.60 Fever, unspecified**
    - Chills with fever
    - Fever NOS
    - Fever of unknown origin (FUO)
    - Hyperpyrexia NOS
    - Pyrexia NOS
    - Pyrexia of unknown origin
    - **Excludes** chills without fever (780.64)
      - neonatal fever (778.4)
      - pyrexia of unknown origin (during):
        - in newborn (778.4)
        - labor (659.2)
        - the puerperium (672)

  - **780.61 Fever presenting with conditions classified elsewhere**
    - Code first underlying condition when associated fever is present, such as with:
      - leukemia (conditions classifiable to 204-208)
      - neutropenia (288.00-288.09)
      - sickle-cell disease (282.60-282.69)
    - Coding Clinic: 2012, Q2, P18-19; 2008, Q4, P140-143

  - **780.62 Postprocedural fever**
    - **Excludes** posttransfusion fever (780.66)
      - postvaccination fever (780.63)

  - **780.63 Postvaccination fever**
    - Postimmunization fever

  - **780.64 Chills (without fever)**
    - Chills NOS
    - **Excludes** chills with fever (780.60)

  - **780.65 Hypothermia not associated with low environmental temperature**
    - **Excludes** hypothermia:
      - associated with low environmental temperature (991.6)
      - due to anesthesia (995.89)
      - of newborn (778.2, 778.3)

  - **780.66 Febrile nonhemolytic transfusion reaction**
    - FNHTR
    - Posttransfusion fever

- **780.7 Malaise and fatigue**
  - **Excludes** debility, unspecified (799.3)
    - fatigue (during):
      - combat (308.0–308.9)
      - heat (992.6)
      - pregnancy (646.8)
    - neurasthenia (300.5)
    - senile asthenia (797)

  - **780.71 Chronic fatigue syndrome**
    - Coding Clinic: 1998, Q4, P48-49

  - **780.72 Functional quadriplegia**
    - Complete immobility due to severe physical disability or frailty
    - **Excludes** hysterical paralysis (300.11)
      - immobility syndrome (728.3)
      - neurologic quadriplegia (344.00-344.09)
      - quadriplegia NOS (344.00)
    - Coding Clinic: 2008, Q4, P143

  - **780.79 Other malaise and fatigue**
    - Asthenia NOS
    - Lethargy
    - Postviral (asthenic) syndrome
    - Tiredness
    - Coding Clinic: 2004, Q4, P77-78; 2000, Q1, P6

- **780.8 Generalized hyperhidrosis**
  - Diaphoresis
  - Excessive sweating
  - Secondary hyperhidrosis
  - **Excludes** focal (localized) (primary) (secondary) hyperhidrosis (705.21–705.22)
    - Frey's syndrome (705.22)

- **780.9 Other general symptoms**
  - **Excludes** hypothermia:
    - NOS (accidental) (991.6)
    - due to anesthesia (995.89)
    - memory disturbance as part of a pattern of mental disorder
    - of newborn (778.2–778.3)
  - Coding Clinic: 2002, Q4, P67-68

  - **780.91 Fussy infant (baby)**

  - **780.92 Excessive crying of infant (baby)**
    - **Excludes** excessive crying of child, adolescent or adult (780.95)
    - Coding Clinic: 2005, Q4, P89-90

  - **780.93 Memory loss**
    - Amnesia (retrograde)
    - Memory loss NOS
    - **Excludes** memory loss due to:
      - intracranial injuries (850.0-854.19)
      - skull fractures (800.00-801.99, 803.00-804.99)
      - mild memory disturbance due to organic brain damage (310.89)
      - transient global amnesia (437.7)
    - Coding Clinic: 2003, Q4, P71

  - **780.94 Early satiety**
    - Coding Clinic: 2003, Q4, P72

  - **780.95 Excessive crying of child, adolescent, or adult**
    - **Excludes** excessive crying of infant (baby) (780.92)
    - Coding Clinic: 2005, Q4, P89-90

  - **780.96 Generalized pain**
    - Pain NOS

  - **780.97 Altered mental status**
    - Change in mental status
    - **Excludes** altered level of consciousness (780.01–780.09)
      - altered mental status due to known condition - code to condition
      - delirium NOS (780.09)
    - Coding Clinic: 2006, Q4, P107-108; 1993, Q3, P11

  - **780.99 Other general symptoms**
    - Coding Clinic: 2003, Q4, P103-104; 1999, Q4, P10; 1985, Nov-Dec, P12

- **781 Symptoms involving nervous and musculoskeletal systems**
  - **Excludes** depression NOS (311)
    - disorders specifically relating to:
      - back (724.0–724.9)
      - hearing (388.0–389.9)
      - joint (718.0–719.9)
      - limb (729.0–729.9)
      - neck (723.0–723.9)
      - vision (368.0–369.9)
    - pain in limb (729.5)

  - **781.0 Abnormal involuntary movements**
    - Abnormal head movements
    - Fasciculation
    - Spasms NOS
    - Tremor NOS
    - **Excludes** abnormal reflex (796.1)
      - chorea NOS (333.5)
      - infantile spasms (345.60–345.61)
      - spastic paralysis (342.1, 343.0–344.9)
      - specified movement disorders classifiable to 333 (333.0–333.9)
      - that of nonorganic origin (307.2–307.3)

  - **781.1 Disturbances of sensation of smell and taste**
    - Anosmia
    - Parosmia
    - Parageusia

781.2 Abnormality of gait
Gait:
  ataxic
  paralytic
  spastic
  staggering
  Excludes ataxia:
    NOS (781.3)
    difficulty in walking (719.7)
    locomotor (progressive) (094.0)
  Coding Clinic: 2011, Q1, P9; 2005, Q2, P6-7; 2004, Q2, P15

781.3 Lack of coordination
Ataxia NOS
Muscular incoordination
  Excludes ataxic gait (781.2)
    cerebellar ataxia (334.0–334.9)
    difficulty in walking (719.7)
    vertigo NOS (780.4)
  Coding Clinic: 2004, Q4, P50-52; 1997, Q3, P12-13

781.4 Transient paralysis of limb
Monoplegia, transient NOS
  Excludes paralysis (342.0–344.9)

781.5 Clubbing of fingers

781.6 Meningismus
Dupre's syndrome   Meningism
Coding Clinic: 2000, Q3, P13

781.7 Tetany
Carpopedal spasm
  Excludes tetanus neonatorum (771.3)
    tetany:
      hysterical (300.11)
      newborn (hypocalcemic) (775.4)
      parathyroid (252.1)
      psychogenic (306.0)

781.8 Neurologic neglect syndrome
Asomatognosia   Left-sided neglect
Hemi-akinesia   Sensory extinction
Hemi-inattention   Sensory neglect
Hemispatial neglect   Visuospatial neglect
  Excludes visuospatial deficit (799.53)

● **781.9 Other symptoms involving nervous and musculoskeletal systems**
  781.91 Loss of height
    Excludes osteoporosis (733.00–733.09)
  781.92 Abnormal posture
  781.93 Ocular torticollis
    Coding Clinic: 2002, Q4, P68; Q4, P68
  781.94 Facial weakness
    Facial droop
    Excludes facial weakness due to late effect of cerebrovascular accident (438.83)
    Coding Clinic: 2003, Q4, P72
  781.99 Other symptoms involving nervous and musculoskeletal systems

● **782 Symptoms involving skin and other integumentary tissue**
  Excludes symptoms relating to breast (611.71–611.79)

782.0 Disturbance of skin sensation
Anesthesia of skin
Burning or prickling sensation
Hyperesthesia
Hypoesthesia
Numbness
Paresthesia
Tingling
Coding Clinic: 2009, Q4, P113

782.1 Rash and other nonspecific skin eruption
Exanthem
  Excludes vesicular eruption (709.8)

782.2 Localized superficial swelling, mass, or lump
Subcutaneous nodules
  Excludes localized adiposity (278.1)

782.3 Edema
Anasarca
Dropsy
Localized edema NOS
  Excludes ascites (789.51–789.59)
    edema of:
      newborn NOS (778.5)
      pregnancy (642.0–642.9, 646.1)
    fluid retention (276.69)
    hydrops fetalis (773.3, 778.0)
    hydrothorax (511.81–511.89)
    nutritional edema (260, 262)
  Coding Clinic: 2000, Q2, P18

■ **782.4 Jaundice, unspecified, not of newborn**
Cholemia NOS
Icterus NOS
  Excludes due to isoimmunization (773.0–773.2, 773.4)
    jaundice in newborn (774.0–774.7)

782.5 Cyanosis
  Excludes newborn (770.83)

● **782.6 Pallor and flushing**
  782.61 Pallor
  782.62 Flushing
    Excessive blushing

782.7 Spontaneous ecchymoses
Petechiae
  Excludes ecchymosis in fetus or newborn (772.6)
    purpura (287.0–287.9)

782.8 Changes in skin texture
Induration of skin
Thickening of skin

782.9 Other symptoms involving skin and integumentary tissues

● **783 Symptoms concerning nutrition, metabolism, and development**

783.0 Anorexia
Loss of appetite
  Excludes anorexia nervosa (307.1)
    loss of appetite of nonorganic origin (307.59)

783.1 Abnormal weight gain
  Excludes excessive weight gain in pregnancy (646.1)
    obesity (278.00)
      morbid (278.01)

● **783.2 Abnormal loss of weight and underweight**
  Use additional code to identify Body Mass Index (BMI), if known (V85.0–V85.54)
  783.21 Loss of weight
  783.22 Underweight

783.3 Feeding difficulties and mismanagement
Feeding problem (elderly) (infant)
  Excludes feeding disturbance or problems:
    in newborn (779.31–779.34)
    of nonorganic origin (307.50–307.59)
  Coding Clinic: 1997, Q3, P12-13; 1994, Q2, P10-11

● **783.4 Lack of expected normal physiological development in childhood**
  Excludes delay in sexual development and puberty (259.0)
    gonadal dysgenesis (758.6)
    pituitary dwarfism (253.3)
    slow fetal growth and fetal malnutrition (764.00–764.99)
    specific delays in mental development (315.0–315.9)
  Coding Clinic: 1997, Q3, P5

■ **783.40 Lack of normal physiological development, unspecified**
Inadequate development
Lack of development

783.41 Failure to thrive
Failure to gain weight
Excludes *failure to thrive in newborn (779.34)*
Coding Clinic: 2003, Q1, P12

783.42 Delayed milestones
Late talker
Late walker

783.43 Short stature
Growth failure
Growth retardation
Lack of growth
Physical retardation
Coding Clinic: 2004, Q2, P3

783.5 Polydipsia
Excessive thirst

783.6 Polyphagia
Excessive eating
Hyperalimentation NOS
Excludes *disorders of eating of nonorganic origin (307.50–307.59)*

783.7 Adult failure to thrive

783.9 Other symptoms concerning nutrition, metabolism, and development
Hypometabolism
Excludes *abnormal basal metabolic rate (794.7)*
dehydration (276.51)
other disorders of fluid, electrolyte, and acid-base balance (276.0–276.9)
Coding Clinic: 2004, Q2, P3

● **784 Symptoms involving head and neck**
Excludes *encephalopathy NOS (348.30)*
specific symptoms involving neck classifiable to 723 (723.0–723.9)

784.0 Headache
Facial pain   Pain in head NOS
Excludes *atypical face pain (350.2)*
migraine (346.0–346.9)
tension headache (307.81)
Coding Clinic: 2006, Q3, P22; Q2, P17-18; 2000, Q3, P13; 1992, Q3, P14; 1990, Q1, P9

784.1 Throat pain
Excludes *dysphagia (787.20–787.29)*
neck pain (723.1)
sore throat (462)
chronic (472.1)

784.2 Swelling, mass, or lump in head and neck
Space-occupying lesion, intracranial NOS
Coding Clinic: 2003, Q1, P8

784.3 Aphasia
Excludes *aphasia due to late effects of cerebrovascular disease (438.11)*
developmental aphasia (315.31)
Coding Clinic: 2010, Q3, P5; 2004, Q4, P77-78; 1998, Q4, P87; 1997, Q3, P12-13

● **784.4 Voice and resonance disorders**
  784.40 Voice and resonance disorder, unspecified
  784.41 Aphonia
Loss of voice
  784.42 Dysphonia
Hoarseness
  784.43 Hypernasality
  784.44 Hyponasality
  784.49 Other voice and resonance disorders
Change in voice

● **784.5 Other speech disturbance**
Excludes *speech disorder due to late effect of cerebrovascular accident (438.10-438.19)*
stuttering (315.35)

  784.51 Dysarthria
Excludes *dysarthria due to late effect of cerebrovascular accident (438.13)*

● **784.52 Fluency disorder in conditions classified elsewhere**
Stuttering in conditions classified elsewhere
Code first underlying disease or condition, such as:
Parkinson's disease (332.0)
Excludes *adult onset fluency disorder (307.0)*
childhood onset fluency disorder (315.35)
fluency disorder due to late effect of cerebrovascular accident (438.14)

  784.59 Other speech disturbance
Dysphasia
Slurred speech
Speech disturbance NOS

● **784.6 Other symbolic dysfunction**
Excludes *developmental learning delays (315.0–315.9)*

  784.60 Symbolic dysfunction, unspecified
  784.61 Alexia and dyslexia
Alexia (with agraphia)
Loss of ability to read
  784.69 Other
Acalculia
Difficulty performing simple mathematical tasks
Agnosia
Loss of ability to recognize objects, persons, sounds, shapes, or smells
Agraphia NOS
Apraxia
Loss of the ability to execute or carry out movements

784.7 Epistaxis
Hemorrhage from nose   Nosebleed
Coding Clinic: 2004, Q3, P7; 1995, Q1, P5

784.8 Hemorrhage from throat
Excludes *hemoptysis (786.30–786.39)*
Spitting blood

● **784.9 Other symptoms involving head and neck**
  784.91 Postnasal drip
  784.92 Jaw pain
Mandibular pain
Maxilla pain
Excludes *temporomandibular joint arthralgia (524.62)*
Coding Clinic: 2010, Q4, P94

  784.99 Other symptoms involving head and neck
Choking sensation
Feeling of foreign body in throat
Halitosis
Bad breath
Mouth breathing
Sneezing
Excludes *foreign body in throat (933.0)*

● **785 Symptoms involving cardiovascular system**
Excludes *heart failure NOS (428.9)*

  785.0 Tachycardia, unspecified
Rapid heart beat
Excludes *neonatal tachycardia (779.82)*
paroxysmal tachycardia (427.0–427.2)
Coding Clinic: 2003, Q2, P11

  785.1 Palpitations
Awareness of heart beat
Excludes *specified dysrhythmias (427.0–427.9)*

785.2 Undiagnosed cardiac murmurs
Heart murmur NOS

785.3 Other abnormal heart sounds
Cardiac dullness, increased or decreased
Friction fremitus, cardiac
Precordial friction

785.4 Gangrene
Gangrene:
  NOS
  spreading cutaneous
Gangrene:
  Gangrenous cellulitis
  Phagedena
Rapidly spreading destructive ulceration of soft tissue
Code first any associated underlying condition
Excludes gangrene of certain sites-see Alphabetic Index
  gangrene with atherosclerosis of the extremities (440.24)
  gas gangrene (040.0)
Coding Clinic: 2004, Q1, P14-15; 1994, Q3, P5; 1990, Q3, P15; 1986, Mar-April, P12

● **785.5 Shock without mention of trauma**
  ■ **785.50 Shock, unspecified**
    Failure of peripheral circulation
    Resulting in significant blood pressure drop
  785.51 Cardiogenic shock
    Coding Clinic: 2008, Q4, P180-182; 2005, Q3, P14
  ● **785.52 Septic shock**
    Endotoxic
    Gram-negative
    Code first underlying infection
    Use additional code, if applicable, to identify systemic inflammatory response syndrome due to infectious process with organ dysfunction (995.92)
    Coding Clinic: 2010, Q2, P4; 2005, Q3, P23; Q2, P18-20x2; 2003, Q4, P73, 79-81
  785.59 Other
    Shock:
      hypovolemic
    Decreased blood volume
    Excludes shock (due to):
      anesthetic (995.4)
      anaphylactic (995.0)
        due to serum (999.41-999.49)
      electric (994.8)
      following abortion (639.5)
      lightning (994.0)
      obstetrical (669.1)
      postoperative (998.00-998.09)
      traumatic (958.4)
    Coding Clinic: 2008, Q4, P97-100

785.6 Enlargement of lymph nodes
Lymphadenopathy
"Swollen glands"
Excludes lymphadenitis (chronic) (289.1–289.3)
  acute (683)

785.9 Other symptoms involving cardiovascular system
Bruit (arterial)   Weak pulse

● **786 Symptoms involving respiratory system and other chest symptoms**
  ● **786.0 Dyspnea and respiratory abnormalities**
    ■ **786.00 Respiratory abnormality, unspecified**
    786.01 Hyperventilation
      Excludes hyperventilation, psychogenic (306.1)
    786.02 Orthopnea
    786.03 Apnea
      Excludes apnea of newborn (770.81, 770.82)
        sleep apnea (780.51, 780.53, 780.57)
      Coding Clinic: 1998, Q2, P10
    786.04 Cheyne-Stokes respiration
      Abnormal pattern of breathing with gradually increasing and decreasing tidal volume with some periods of apnea
    786.05 Shortness of breath
      Coding Clinic: 1999, Q4, P25; Q1, P6
    786.06 Tachypnea
      Excludes transitory tachypnea of newborn (770.6)
      Coding Clinic: 2011, Q1, P17
    786.07 Wheezing
      Excludes asthma (493.00–493.92)
    786.09 Other
      Respiratory:
        distress
        insufficiency
      Excludes respiratory distress:
        following trauma and surgery (518.52)
        newborn (770.89)
        respiratory failure (518.81, 518.83–518.84)
        newborn (770.84)
        syndrome (newborn) (769)
        adult (518.52)
      Coding Clinic: 1990, Q1, P9

  786.1 Stridor
    Excludes congenital laryngeal stridor (748.3)
  786.2 Cough
    Excludes cough:
      psychogenic (306.1)
      smokers' (491.0)
      with hemorrhage (786.39)
    Coding Clinic: 1995, Q4, P50; 1990, Q1, P8
  ● **786.3 Hemoptysis**
    Coding Clinic: 2006, Q2, P17
    ■ **786.30 Hemoptysis, unspecified**
      Pulmonary hemorrhage NOS
    786.31 Acute idiopathic pulmonary hemorrhage in infants [AIPHI]
      Acute idiopathic pulmonary hemorrhage in infant over 28 days old
      Excludes pulmonary hemorrhage of newborn under 28 days old (770.3)
        von Willebrand's disease (286.4)
    786.39 Other hemoptysis
      Cough with hemorrhage
  786.4 Abnormal sputum
    Abnormal:
      amount of sputum
      color of sputum
      odor of sputum
    Excessive sputum
  ● **786.5 Chest pain**
    ■ **786.50 Chest pain, unspecified**
      Coding Clinic: 2007, Q1, P19; 2006, Q2, P7-8; 2003, Q1, P6-7; 2002, Q1, P4-5; 1999, Q4, P25-26; 1993, Q1, P25
    786.51 Precordial pain
      Coding Clinic: 1984, May-June, P11
    786.52 Painful respiration
      Pain:
        anterior chest wall
        pleuritic
        Pleurodynia
      Excludes epidemic pleurodynia (074.1)
      Coding Clinic: 1984, Nov-Dec, P17
    786.59 Other
      Discomfort in chest
      Pressure in chest
      Tightness in chest
      Excludes pain in breast (611.71)
      Coding Clinic: 2007, Q1, P19; 2002, Q1, P6

786.6 Swelling, mass, or lump in chest
  Excludes *lump in breast (611.72)*

786.7 Abnormal chest sounds
  Abnormal percussion, chest
  Friction sounds, chest
  Rales
    Wet rattling, clicking, crackling sounds on auscultation
  Tympany, chest
  Excludes *wheezing (786.07)*

786.8 Hiccough
  Excludes *psychogenic hiccough (306.1)*

786.9 Other symptoms involving respiratory system and chest
  Breath-holding spell

● **787 Symptoms involving digestive system**
  Excludes *constipation (564.0–564.9)*
    pylorospasm (537.81)
    congenital (750.5)

● **787.0 Nausea and vomiting**
  Emesis
  Excludes *hematemesis NOS (578.0)*
    vomiting:
      bilious, following gastrointestinal surgery (564.3)
      cyclical (536.2)
        associated with migraine (346.2)
        psychogenic (306.4)
      excessive, in pregnancy (643.0–643.9)
      fecal matter (569.87)
      habit (536.2)
      of newborn (779.32, 779.33)
      persistent (536.2)
      psychogenic NOS (307.54)

  787.01 Nausea with vomiting
    Concurrent conditions
    Coding Clinic: 2003, Q1, P5

  787.02 Nausea alone
    Separate condition
    Coding Clinic: 2000, Q3, P12; 1997, Q2, P9-10

  787.03 Vomiting alone
    Separate condition
    Coding Clinic: 1985, Mar-April, P11

  787.04 Bilious emesis
    Bilious vomiting
    Excludes *bilious emesis (vomiting) in newborn (779.32)*

787.1 Heartburn
  Pyrosis
  Waterbrash
  Excludes *dyspepsia or indigestion (536.8)*
  Coding Clinic: 2001, Q2, P6

● **787.2 Dysphagia**
  Code first, if applicable, dysphagia due to late effect of cerebrovascular accident (438.82)
  Coding Clinic: 2007, Q3, P8-9; 2003, Q4, P103-104, 109-110; 2001, Q2, P4-6; 1993, 5th Issue, P16; 1986, Nov-Dec, P10

  787.20 Dysphagia, unspecified
    Difficulty in swallowing NOS
  787.21 Dysphagia, oral phase
  787.22 Dysphagia, oropharyngeal phase
    Coding Clinic: 2007, Q4, P92-95
  787.23 Dysphagia, pharyngeal phase
  787.24 Dysphagia, pharyngoesophageal phase
  787.29 Other dysphagia
    Cervical dysphagia
    Neurogenic dysphagia

787.3 Flatulence, eructation, and gas pain
  Abdominal distention (gaseous)
  Bloating
  Tympanites (abdominal) (intestinal)
  Excludes *aerophagy (306.4)*

787.4 Visible peristalsis
  Hyperperistalsis

787.5 Abnormal bowel sounds
  Absent bowel sounds
  Hyperactive bowel sounds

● **787.6 Incontinence of feces**
  Encopresis NOS
  Incontinence of sphincter ani
  Excludes *that of nonorganic origin (307.7)*
  Coding Clinic: 1997, Q1, P9-10

  787.60 Full incontinence of feces
    Fecal incontinence NOS
  787.61 Incomplete defecation
    Excludes *constipation (564.00-564.09)*
      fecal impaction (560.32)
  787.62 Fecal smearing
    Fecal soiling
  787.63 Fecal urgency

787.7 Abnormal feces
  Bulky stools
  Excludes *abnormal stool content (792.1)*
    melena:
      NOS (578.1)
      newborn (772.4, 777.3)

● **787.9 Other symptoms involving digestive system**
  Excludes *gastrointestinal hemorrhage (578.0–578.9)*
    intestinal obstruction (560.0–560.9)
    specific functional digestive disorders:
      esophagus (530.0–530.9)
      stomach and duodenum (536.0–536.9)
      those not elsewhere classified (564.0–564.9)

  787.91 Diarrhea
    Diarrhea NOS
    Coding Clinic: 2010, Q2, P12; 2008, Q4, P97-100
  787.99 Other
    Change in bowel habits
    Tenesmus (rectal)

● **788 Symptoms involving urinary system**
  Excludes *hematuria (599.70–599.72)*
    nonspecific findings on examination of the urine (791.0–791.9)
    small kidney of unknown cause (589.0–589.9)
    uremia NOS (586)
    urinary obstruction (599.60, 599.69)

  788.0 Renal colic
    Colic (recurrent) of:
      kidney
      ureter
    Coding Clinic: 2004, Q3, P8

  788.1 Dysuria
    Painful urination
    Strangury

● **788.2 Retention of urine**
  Code first, if applicable, hyperplasia of prostate (600.0–600.9 with fifth-digit 1)
  Coding Clinic: 2003, Q3, P13; 1994, Q1, P20; 1986, Sept-Oct, P12

  788.20 Retention of urine, unspecified
    Coding Clinic: 2013, Q1, P6; 2006, Q4, P93-95; 2004, Q2, P18; 2003, Q3, P12; Q1, P6; 1996, Q3, P10-11; 1994, Q3, P13
  788.21 Incomplete bladder emptying
  788.29 Other specified retention of urine

788.3 Urinary incontinence
Excludes *functional urinary incontinence (788.91)*
that of nonorganic origin (307.6)
urinary incontinence associated with cognitive impairment (788.91)
Code, if applicable, any causal condition first, such as:
congenital ureterocele (753.23)
genital prolapse (618.00–618.9)
hyperplasia of prostate (600.0–600.9 with fifth-digit 1)
Coding Clinic: 2005, Q3, P20

788.30 Urinary incontinence, unspecified
Enuresis NOS
Coding Clinic: 2009, Q1, P18; 1995, Q4, P72-73

788.31 Urge incontinence
Coding Clinic: 2000, Q1, P19-20

788.32 Stress incontinence, male
Excludes *stress incontinence, female (625.6)*
Coding Clinic: 1995, Q4, P72-73

788.33 Mixed incontinence (female) (male)
Urge and stress

788.34 Incontinence without sensory awareness

788.35 Post-void dribbling

788.36 Nocturnal enuresis

788.37 Continuous leakage

788.38 Overflow incontinence
Coding Clinic: 2004, Q4, P96

788.39 Other urinary incontinence

788.4 Frequency of urination and polyuria
Code first, if applicable, hyperplasia of prostate (600.0–600.9 with fifth-digit 1)

788.41 Urinary frequency
Frequency of micturition

788.42 Polyuria

788.43 Nocturia

788.5 Oliguria and anuria
Deficient secretion of urine
Suppression of urinary secretion
Excludes *that complicating:*
abortion (634–638 with .3, 639.3)
ectopic or molar pregnancy (639.3)
pregnancy, childbirth, or the puerperium (642.0–642.9, 646.2)

788.6 Other abnormality of urination
Code first, if applicable, hyperplasia of prostate (600.0–600.9 with fifth-digit 1)

788.61 Splitting of urinary stream
Intermittent urinary stream

788.62 Slowing of urinary stream
Weak stream

788.63 Urgency of urination
Excludes *urge incontinence (788.31, 788.33)*
Coding Clinic: 2003, Q4, P74

788.64 Urinary hesitancy

788.65 Straining on urination

788.69 Other

788.7 Urethral discharge
Penile discharge
Urethrorrhea

788.8 Extravasation of urine
Leakage, discharge

788.9 Other symptoms involving urinary system
Coding Clinic: 2005, Q1, P12-13

788.91 Functional urinary incontinence
Urinary incontinence due to cognitive impairment, or severe physical disability or immobility
Excludes *urinary incontinence due to physiologic condition (788.30-788.39)*
Coding Clinic: 2008, Q4, P144-145

788.99 Other symptoms involving urinary system
Extrarenal uremia
Vesical:
pain
tenesmus

789 Other symptoms involving abdomen and pelvis
The following fifth-digit subclassification is to be used for codes 789.0, 789.3, 789.4, 789.6

```
0  unspecified site          5  periumbilic
1  right upper quadrant      6  epigastric
2  left upper quadrant       7  generalized
3  right lower quadrant      9  other specified site
4  left lower quadrant          multiple sites
```

Excludes *symptoms referable to genital organs:*
female (625.0–625.9)
male (607.0–608.9)
psychogenic (302.70–302.79)

789.0 Abdominal pain
[0-7,9] Cramps, abdominal
Coding Clinic: 2002, Q1, P5; 1995, Q1, P3; 1990, Q2, P26

789.1 Hepatomegaly
Enlargement of liver

789.2 Splenomegaly
Enlargement of spleen

789.3 Abdominal or pelvic swelling, mass, or lump
[0-7,9] Diffuse or generalized swelling or mass:
abdominal NOS
umbilical
Excludes *abdominal distention (gaseous) (787.3)*
ascites (789.51–789.59)

789.4 Abdominal rigidity
[0-7,9]

789.5 Ascites
Fluid in peritoneal cavity
Coding Clinic: 2008, Q1, P16-18; 2007, Q4, P95-96; 2005, Q2, P8; 1989, Q4, P11

789.51 *Malignant ascites*
Code first malignancy, such as:
malignant neoplasm of ovary (183.0)
secondary malignant neoplasm of retroperitoneum and peritoneum (197.6)
Coding Clinic: 2008, Q1, P16-17

789.59 Other ascites

789.6 Abdominal tenderness
[0-7,9] Rebound tenderness

789.7 Colic
Colic NOS
Infantile colic
Excludes *colic in adult and child over 12 months old (789.0)*
renal colic (788.0)

789.9 Other symptoms involving abdomen and pelvis
Umbilical: Umbilical:
bleeding   discharge

NONSPECIFIC ABNORMAL FINDINGS (790–796)

- **790 Nonspecific findings on examination of blood**
  - **Excludes:** *abnormality of:*
    - *platelets (287.0–287.9)*
    - *thrombocytes (287.0–287.9)*
    - *white blood cells (288.00–288.9)*

- **790.0 Abnormality of red blood cells**
  - **Excludes:** *anemia:*
    - *congenital (776.5)*
    - *newborn, due to isoimmunization (773.0–773.2, 773.5)*
    - *of premature infant (776.6)*
    - *other specified types (280.0–285.9)*
    - *hemoglobin disorders (282.5–282.7)*
    - *polycythemia:*
      - *familial (289.6)*
      - *neonatorum (776.4)*
      - *secondary (289.0)*
      - *vera (238.4)*

  - **790.01 Precipitous drop in hematocrit**
    - Drop in hematocrit
    - Drop in hemoglobin
    - *Decrease in red blood cells*

  - **790.09 Other abnormality of red blood cells**
    - Abnormal red cell morphology NOS
    - Abnormal red cell volume NOS
    - Anisocytosis
      - *Red blood cells of unequal size*
    - Poikilocytosis
      - *Red blood cells of abnormal shape*

- **790.1 Elevated sedimentation rate**

- **790.2 Abnormal glucose**
  - **Excludes:** *diabetes mellitus (249.00–249.91, 250.00–250.93)*
    - *dysmetabolic syndrome X (277.7)*
    - *gestational diabetes (648.8)*
    - *glycosuria (791.5)*
    - *hypoglycemia (251.2)*
    - *that complicating pregnancy, childbirth, or the puerperium (648.8)*
  - Coding Clinic: 2012, Q1, P17; 2011, Q1, P10; 2003, Q4, P74-75

  - **790.21 Impaired fasting glucose**
    - Elevated fasting glucose

  - **790.22 Impaired glucose tolerance test (oral)**
    - Elevated glucose tolerance test

  - **790.29 Other abnormal glucose**
    - Abnormal glucose NOS
    - Abnormal non-fasting glucose
    - Hyperglycemia NOS
    - Pre-diabetes NOS
    - Coding Clinic: 2009, Q3, P18; 2005, Q2, P21-22; 2004, Q4, P53-56

- **790.3 Excessive blood level of alcohol**
  - Elevated blood-alcohol

- **790.4 Nonspecific elevation of levels of transaminase or lactic acid dehydrogenase [LDH]**

- **790.5 Other nonspecific abnormal serum enzyme levels**
  - Abnormal serum level of:
    - acid phosphatase
    - alkaline phosphatase
    - amylase
    - lipase
  - **Excludes:** *deficiency of circulating enzymes (277.6)*

- **790.6 Other abnormal blood chemistry**
  - Abnormal blood levels of:
    - cobalt
    - copper
    - iron
    - lead
    - lithium
    - magnesium
    - mineral
    - zinc
  - **Excludes:** *abnormality of electrolyte or acid-base balance (276.0–276.9)*
    - *hypoglycemia NOS (251.2)*
    - *lead poisoning (984.0–984.9)*
    - *specific finding indicating abnormality of:*
      - *amino-acid transport and metabolism (270.0–270.9)*
      - *carbohydrate transport and metabolism (271.0–271.9)*
      - *lipid metabolism (272.0–272.9)*
    - *uremia NOS (586)*

- **790.7 Bacteremia**
  - **Excludes:** *bacteremia of newborn (771.83)*
    - *septicemia (038)*
  - Use additional code to identify organism (041)
  - Coding Clinic: 2003, Q2, P7-8

- **790.8 Viremia, unspecified**
  - Coding Clinic: 1988, Q4, P10

- **790.9 Other nonspecific findings on examination of blood**
  - **790.91 Abnormal arterial blood gases**
  - **790.92 Abnormal coagulation profile**
    - Abnormal or prolonged:
      - bleeding time
      - coagulation time
      - partial thromboplastin time [PTT]
      - prothrombin time [PT]
    - **Excludes:** *coagulation (hemorrhagic) disorders (286.0–286.9)*
    - Coding Clinic: 1994, Q1, P22
  - **790.93 Elevated prostate specific antigen [PSA]**
  - **790.94 Euthyroid sick syndrome**
  - **790.95 Elevated C-reactive protein (CRP)**
    - Coding Clinic: 2004, Q4, P96-97
  - **790.99 Other**
    - Coding Clinic: 2012, Q3, P18; 2011, Q3, P4

- **791 Nonspecific findings on examination of urine**
  - **Excludes:** *hematuria NOS (599.70–599.72)*
    - *specific findings indicating abnormality of:*
      - *amino-acid transport and metabolism (270.0–270.9)*
      - *carbohydrate transport and metabolism (271.0–271.9)*

  - **791.0 Proteinuria**
    - Albuminuria
    - Bence-Jones proteinuria
    - **Excludes:** *postural proteinuria (593.6)*
      - *that arising during pregnancy or the puerperium (642.0–642.9, 646.2)*
    - Coding Clinic: 2012, Q2, P19

  - **791.1 Chyluria**
    - *White milky urine*
    - **Excludes:** *filarial (125.0–125.9)*

  - **791.2 Hemoglobinuria**
  - **791.3 Myoglobinuria**
  - **791.4 Biliuria**

791.5 Glycosuria
  Excludes renal glycosuria (271.4)
791.6 Acetonuria
  Ketonuria
791.7 Other cells and casts in urine
791.9 Other nonspecific findings on examination of urine
  Crystalluria
  Elevated urine levels of:
    17-ketosteroids
    catecholamines
    indolacetic acid
    vanillylmandelic acid [VMA]
  Melanuria
  Coding Clinic: 2005, Q1, P12

● **792 Nonspecific abnormal findings in other body substances**
  Excludes that in chromosomal analysis (795.2)
  792.0 Cerebrospinal fluid
  792.1 Stool contents
    Abnormal stool color   Occult blood
    Fat in stool   Pus in stool
    Mucus in stool
    Excludes blood in stool [melena] (578.1)
      newborn (772.4, 777.3)
    Coding Clinic: 1992, Q2, P9-10; Q2, P9
  792.2 Semen
    Abnormal spermatozoa
    Excludes azoospermia (606.0)
      oligospermia (606.1)
  792.3 Amniotic fluid
  792.4 Saliva
    Excludes that in chromosomal analysis (795.2)
  792.5 Cloudy (hemodialysis) (peritoneal) dialysis effluent
  792.9 Other nonspecific abnormal findings in body substances
    Peritoneal fluid   Synovial fluid
    Pleural fluid   Vaginal fluids

● **793 Nonspecific (abnormal) findings on radiological and other examination of body structure**
  Includes nonspecific abnormal findings of:
    thermography
    ultrasound examination [echogram]
    x-ray examination
  Excludes abnormal results of function studies and radioisotope scans (794.0–794.9)
  793.0 Skull and head
    Excludes nonspecific abnormal echoencephalogram (794.01)
    Coding Clinic: 2006, Q3, P22
  ● **793.1** Lung field
    793.11 Solitary pulmonary nodule
      Coin lesion lung
      Solitary pulmonary nodule, subsegmental branch of the bronchial tree
    793.19 Other nonspecific abnormal finding of lung field
      Pulmonary infiltrate NOS
      Shadow, lung
      Coding Clinic: 2011, Q4, P139
  793.2 Other intrathoracic organ
    Abnormal:
      echocardiogram
      heart shadow
      ultrasound cardiogram
      Mediastinal shift
    Coding Clinic: 2012, Q1, P17
  793.3 Biliary tract
    Nonvisualization of gallbladder
  793.4 Gastrointestinal tract
  793.5 Genitourinary organs
    Filling defect:
      bladder
      kidney
      ureter
  793.6 Abdominal area, including retroperitoneum
  793.7 Musculoskeletal system
  ● **793.8** Breast
    793.80 Abnormal mammogram, unspecified
    793.81 Mammographic microcalcification
      Excludes mammographic calcification (793.89)
        mammographic calculus (793.89)
    793.82 Inconclusive mammogram
      Dense breasts NOS
      Inconclusive mammogram NEC
      Inconclusive mammography due to dense breasts
      Inconclusive mammography NEC
      Coding Clinic: 2009, Q4, P113
    793.89 Other (abnormal) findings on radiological examination of breast
      Mammographic calcification
      Mammographic calculus
  ● **793.9** Other
    Excludes abnormal finding by radioisotope localization of placenta (794.9)
    793.91 Image test inconclusive due to excess body fat
      Use additional code to identify Body Mass Index (BMI), if known (V85.0–V85.54)
      Coding Clinic: 2006, Q4, P109-110
    793.99 Other nonspecific (abnormal) findings on radiological and other examinations of body structure
      Abnormal:
        placental finding by x-ray or ultrasound method
        radiological findings in skin and subcutaneous tissue

● **794 Nonspecific abnormal results of function studies**
  Includes radioisotope:
    scans
    uptake studies
    scintiphotography
  ● **794.0** Brain and central nervous system
    794.00 Abnormal function study, unspecified
    794.01 Abnormal echoencephalogram
    794.02 Abnormal electroencephalogram [EEG]
    794.09 Other
      Abnormal brain scan
  ● **794.1** Peripheral nervous system and special senses
    794.10 Abnormal response to nerve stimulation, unspecified
    794.11 Abnormal retinal function studies
      Abnormal electroretinogram [ERG]
    794.12 Abnormal electro-oculogram [EOG]
    794.13 Abnormal visually evoked potential
    794.14 Abnormal oculomotor studies
    794.15 Abnormal auditory function studies
      Coding Clinic: 2011, Q3, P3; 2004, Q1, P15-16
    794.16 Abnormal vestibular function studies
    794.17 Abnormal electromyogram [EMG]
      Excludes that of eye (794.14)
    794.19 Other

794.2 Pulmonary
Abnormal lung scan
Reduced:
ventilatory capacity
vital capacity

● **794.3 Cardiovascular**
▪ **794.30** Abnormal function study, unspecified
794.31 Abnormal electrocardiogram [ECG] [EKG]
Excludes long QT syndrome (426.82)
Coding Clinic: 1985, Mar-April, P13

794.39 Other
Abnormal:
ballistocardiogram
phonocardiogram
vectorcardiogram

794.4 Kidney
Abnormal renal function test

794.5 Thyroid
Abnormal thyroid:
scan
uptake

794.6 Other endocrine function study

794.7 Basal metabolism
Abnormal basal metabolic rate [BMR]

794.8 Liver
Abnormal liver scan

794.9 Other
Bladder   Placenta
Pancreas   Spleen

● **795 Other and nonspecific abnormal cytological, histological, immunological, and DNA test findings**
Excludes abnormal cytologic smear of anus and anal HPV (796.70-796.79)
nonspecific abnormalities of red blood cells (790.01–790.09)
Coding Clinic: 2002, Q4, P69-70

● **795.0 Abnormal Papanicolaou smear of cervix and cervical HPV**
Abnormal thin preparation smear of cervix
Abnormal cervical cytology
Excludes abnormal cytologic smear of vagina and vaginal HPV (795.10-795.19)
carcinoma in situ of cervix (233.1)
cervical intraepithelial neoplasia I (CIN I) (622.11)
cervical intraepithelial neoplasia II (CIN II) (622.12)
cervical intraepithelial neoplasia III (CIN III) (233.1)
dysplasia (histologically confirmed) of cervix (uteri) NOS (622.10)
mild cervical dysplasia (histologically confirmed) (622.11)
moderate cervical dysplasia (histologically confirmed) (622.12)
severe cervical dysplasia (histologically confirmed) (233.1)
Coding Clinic: 2008, Q4, P145-148; 2004, Q4, P97-99

795.00 Abnormal glandular Papanicolaou smear of cervix
Atypical endocervical cells NOS
Atypical endometrial cells NOS
Atypical cervical glandular cells NOS

795.01 Papanicolaou smear of cervix with atypical squamous cells of undetermined significance (ASC-US)
Coding Clinic: 2006, Q2, P3,4

795.02 Papanicolaou smear of cervix with atypical squamous cells cannot exclude high grade squamous intraepithelial lesion (ASC-H)

795.03 Papanicolaou smear of cervix with low grade squamous intraepithelial lesion (LGSIL)

795.04 Papanicolaou smear of cervix with high grade squamous intraepithelial lesion (HGSIL)

795.05 Cervical high risk human papillomavirus (HPV) DNA test positive

795.06 Papanicolaou smear of cervix with cytologic evidence of malignancy

795.07 Satisfactory cervical smear but lacking transformation zone

795.08 Unsatisfactory cervical cytology smear
Inadequate cervical cytology sample
Coding Clinic: 2006, Q2, P3,4

795.09 Other abnormal Papanicolaou smear of cervix and cervical HPV
Cervical low risk human papillomavirus (HPV) DNA test positive
Use additional code for associated human papillomavirus (079.4)
Excludes encounter for Papanicolaou cervical smear to confirm findings of recent normal smear following initial abnormal smear (V72.32)

● **795.1 Abnormal Papanicolaou smear of vagina and vaginal HPV**
Abnormal thin preparation smear of vagina NOS
Abnormal vaginal cytology NOS
Use additional code to identify acquired absence of uterus and cervix, if applicable (V88.01-V88.03)
Excludes abnormal cytologic smear of cervix and cervical HPV (795.00-795.09)
carcinoma in situ of vagina (233.31)
carcinoma in situ of vulva (233.32)
dysplasia (histologically confirmed) of vagina NOS (623.0, 233.31)
dysplasia (histologically confirmed) of vulva NOS (624.01, 624.02, 233.32)
mild vaginal dysplasia (histologically confirmed) (623.0)
mild vulvar dysplasia (histologically confirmed) (624.01)
moderate vaginal dysplasia (histologically confirmed) (623.0)
moderate vulvar dysplasia (histologically confirmed) (624.02)
severe vaginal dysplasia (histologically confirmed) (233.31)
severe vulvar dysplasia (histologically confirmed) (233.32)
vaginal intraepithelial neoplasia I (VAIN I) (623.0)
vaginal intraepithelial neoplasia II (VAIN II) (623.0)
vaginal intraepithelial neoplasia III (VAIN III) (233.31)
vulvar intraepithelial neoplasia I (VIN I) (624.01)
vulvar intraepithelial neoplasia II (VIN II) (624.02)
vulvar intraepithelial neoplasia III (VIN III) (233.32)
Coding Clinic: 2008, Q4, P145-148

795.10 Abnormal glandular Papanicolaou smear of vagina
Atypical vaginal glandular cells NOS

795.11 Papanicolaou smear of vagina with atypical squamous cells of undetermined significance (ASC-US)

795.12 Papanicolaou smear of vagina with atypical squamous cells cannot exclude high grade squamous intraepithelial lesion (ASC-H)

795.13 Papanicolaou smear of vagina with low grade squamous intraepithelial lesion (LGSIL)

795.14 Papanicolaou smear of vagina with high grade squamous intraepithelial lesion (HGSIL)

795.15 Vaginal high risk human papillomavirus (HPV) DNA test positive
- Excludes: *condyloma acuminatum (078.11)*
  genital warts (078.11)

795.16 Papanicolaou smear of vagina with cytologic evidence of malignancy
Coding Clinic: 2004, Q2, P11

795.18 Unsatisfactory vaginal cytology smear
Inadequate vaginal cytology sample

795.19 Other abnormal Papanicolaou smear of vagina and vaginal HPV
Vaginal low risk human papillomavirus (HPV) DNA test positive
Use additional code for associated human papillomavirus (079.4)

795.2 Nonspecific abnormal findings on chromosomal analysis
Abnormal karyotype

● **795.3** Nonspecific positive culture findings
Positive culture findings in:
  nose
  sputum
  throat
  wound
- Excludes: *that of:*
  blood (790.7–790.8)
  urine (791.9)

795.31 Nonspecific positive findings for anthrax
Positive findings by nasal swab
Coding Clinic: 2002, Q4, P70

795.39 Other nonspecific positive culture findings
- Excludes: *colonization status (V02.0-V02.9)*

795.4 Other nonspecific abnormal histological findings

● **795.5** Nonspecific reaction to test for tuberculosis

795.51 Nonspecific reaction to tuberculin skin test without active tuberculosis
Abnormal result of Mantoux test
PPD positive
Tuberculin (skin test) positive
Tuberculin (skin test) reactor
- Excludes: *nonspecific reaction to cell mediated immunity measurement of gamma interferon antigen response without active tuberculosis (795.52)*
Coding Clinic: 2011, Q4, P183

795.52 Nonspecific reaction to cell mediated immunity measurement of gamma interferon antigen response without active tuberculosis
Nonspecific reaction to QuantiFERON-TB test (QFT) without active tuberculosis
- Excludes: *nonspecific reaction to tuberculin skin test without active tuberculosis (795.51)*
  positive tuberculin skin test (795.51)

795.6 False positive serological test for syphilis
False positive Wassermann reaction

● **795.7** Other nonspecific immunological findings
- Excludes: *abnormal tumor markers (795.81–795.89)*
  elevated prostate specific antigen [PSA] (790.93)
  elevated tumor associated antigens (795.81–795.89)
  isoimmunization, in pregnancy (656.1–656.2)
  affecting fetus or newborn (773.0–773.2)

795.71 Nonspecific serologic evidence of human immunodeficiency virus [HIV]
Inconclusive human immunodeficiency virus [HIV] test (adult) (infant)
Note: This code is ONLY to be used when a test finding is reported as nonspecific. Asymptomatic positive findings are coded to V08. If any HIV infection symptom or condition is present, see code 042. Negative findings are not coded.
- Excludes: *acquired immunodeficiency syndrome [AIDS] (042)*
  asymptomatic human immunodeficiency virus [HIV] infection status (V08)
  HIV infection, symptomatic (042)
  human immunodeficiency virus [HIV] disease (042)
  positive (status) NOS (V08)

OGCR Section I.C.1.a.2.e
Patients with inconclusive HIV serology, but no definitive diagnosis or manifestations of the illness, may be assigned code 795.71, Inconclusive serologic test for Human Immunodeficiency Virus [HIV].

795.79 Other and unspecified nonspecific immunological findings
Raised antibody titer
Raised level of immunoglobulins
Coding Clinic: 1993, Q2, P6

● **795.8** Abnormal tumor markers
Elevated tumor associated antigens [TAA]
Elevated tumor specific antigens [TSA]
- Excludes: *elevated prostate specific antigen [PSA] (790.93)*
Coding Clinic: 2006, Q4, P111-112; 1993, Q1, P21-22; 1992, Q2, P11

795.81 Elevated carcinoembryonic antigen [CEA]

795.82 Elevated cancer antigen 125 [CA 125]

795.89 Other abnormal tumor markers

● **796** Other nonspecific abnormal findings

796.0 Nonspecific abnormal toxicological findings
Abnormal levels of heavy metals or drugs in blood, urine, or other tissue
Use additional code for retained foreign body, if applicable, (V90.01-V90.9)
- Excludes: *excessive blood level of alcohol (790.3)*
Coding Clinic: 1997, Q1, P16

796.1 Abnormal reflex

796.2 Elevated blood pressure reading without diagnosis of hypertension
Note: This category is to be used to record an episode of elevated blood pressure in a patient in whom no formal diagnosis of hypertension has been made, or as an incidental finding.
Coding Clinic: 2003, Q2, P11; 1993, 5th Issue, P6-7

OGCR Section I.C.7.a.8
Assign code 796.2, Elevated blood pressure reading without diagnosis of hypertension, unless patient has an established diagnosis of hypertension. Assign code 642.3x for transient hypertension of pregnancy.

796.3 Nonspecific low blood pressure reading

796.4 **Other abnormal clinical findings**
Coding Clinic: 1995, Q3, P13

796.5 **Abnormal finding on antenatal screening**

796.6 **Abnormal findings on neonatal screening**
- Excludes: nonspecific serologic evidence of human immunodeficiency virus [HIV] (795.71)

Coding Clinic: 2004, Q4, P99-100

● 796.7 **Abnormal cytologic smear of anus and anal HPV**
- Excludes: abnormal cytologic smear of cervix and cervical HPV (795.00-795.09)
  abnormal cytologic smear of vagina and vaginal HPV (795.10-795.19)
  anal intraepithelial neoplasia I (AIN I) (569.44)
  anal intraepithelial neoplasia II (AIN II) (569.44)
  anal intraepithelial neoplasia III (AIN III) (230.5, 230.6)
  carcinoma in situ of anus (230.5, 230.6)
  dysplasia (histologically confirmed) of anus NOS (569.44)
  mild anal dysplasia (histologically confirmed) (569.44)
  moderate anal dysplasia (histologically confirmed) (569.44)
  severe anal dysplasia (histologically confirmed) (230.5, 230.6)

Coding Clinic: 2008, Q4, P117-119

796.70 **Abnormal glandular Papanicolaou smear of anus**
Atypical anal glandular cells NOS

796.71 **Papanicolaou smear of anus with atypical squamous cells of undetermined significance (ASC-US)**

796.72 **Papanicolaou smear of anus with atypical squamous cells cannot exclude high grade squamous intraepithelial lesion (ASC-H)**

796.73 **Papanicolaou smear of anus with low grade squamous intraepithelial lesion (LGSIL)**

796.74 **Papanicolaou smear of anus with high grade squamous intraepithelial lesion (HGSIL)**

796.75 **Anal high risk human papillomavirus (HPV) DNA test positive**

796.76 **Papanicolaou smear of anus with cytologic evidence of malignancy**

796.77 **Satisfactory anal smear but lacking transformation zone**

796.78 **Unsatisfactory anal cytology smear**
Inadequate anal cytology sample

796.79 **Other abnormal Papanicolaou smear of anus and anal HPV**
Anal low risk human papillomavirus (HPV) DNA test positive
Use additional code for associated human papillomavirus (079.4)

796.9 **Other**

ILL-DEFINED AND UNKNOWN CAUSES OF MORBIDITY AND MORTALITY (797–799)

797 **Senility without mention of psychosis**
Frailty
Old age
Senescence
Senile asthenia
Senile:
  debility
  exhaustion
- Excludes: senile psychoses (290.0–290.9)

● 798 **Sudden death, cause unknown**

798.0 **Sudden infant death syndrome** (SIDS)
Cot death
Crib death
Sudden death of nonspecific cause in infancy

798.1 **Instantaneous death**

798.2 **Death occurring in less than 24 hours from onset of symptoms, not otherwise explained**
Death known not to be violent or instantaneous, for which no cause could be discovered
Died without sign of disease

798.9 **Unattended death**
Death in circumstances where the body of the deceased was found and no cause could be discovered
Found dead

● 799 **Other ill-defined and unknown causes of morbidity and mortality**

● 799.0 **Asphyxia and hypoxemia**
- Excludes: asphyxia and hypoxemia (due to):
  carbon monoxide (986)
  hypercapnia (786.09)
  inhalation of food or foreign body (932–934.9)
  newborn (768.0–768.9)
  traumatic (994.7)

Coding Clinic: 2005, Q4, P90; 1990, Q1, P20

799.01 **Asphyxia**

799.02 **Hypoxemia**
Coding Clinic: 2009, Q3, P18; 2006, Q2, P24,25

799.1 **Respiratory arrest**
Cardiorespiratory failure
- Excludes: cardiac arrest (427.5)
  failure of peripheral circulation (785.50)
  respiratory distress:
    NOS (786.09)
    acute (518.82)
    following trauma or surgery (518.52)
    newborn (770.89)
    syndrome (newborn) (769)
      adult (following trauma or surgery) (518.52)
      other (518.82)
  respiratory failure (518.81, 518.83–518.84)
    newborn (770.84)
  respiratory insufficiency (786.09)
    acute (518.82)

● 799.2 **Signs and symptoms involving emotional state**
- Excludes: anxiety (293.84, 300.00-300.09)
  depression (311)

799.21 **Nervousness**
Nervous
Coding Clinic: 2009, Q4, P120

799.22 **Irritability**
Irritable
Coding Clinic: 2009, Q4, P120

799.23 **Impulsiveness**
Impulsive
- Excludes: impulsive neurosis (300.3)

799.24 **Emotional lability**

799.25 **Demoralization and apathy**
Apathetic

799.29 **Other signs and symptoms involving emotional state**

799.3 **Debility, unspecified**
- Excludes: asthenia (780.79)
  nervous debility (300.5)
  neurasthenia (300.5)
  senile asthenia (797)

Coding Clinic: 1997, Q3, P11-12

799.4 Cachexia
  Wasting disease
  Code first underlying condition, if known
  Coding Clinic: 2013, Q1, P14; 2006, Q3, P14-15x2; 1990, Q3, P17

● **799.5 Signs and symptoms involving cognition**
  Excludes: amnesia (780.93)
  amnestic syndrome (294.0)
  attention deficit disorder (314.00-314.01)
  late effects of cerebrovascular disease (438)
  memory loss (780.93)
  mild cognitive impairment, so stated (331.83)
  specific problems in developmental delay (315.00-315.9)
  transient global amnesia (437.7)
  visuospatial neglect 781.8
  Coding Clinic: 2012, Q3, P19

  799.51 Attention or concentration deficit
    Coding Clinic: 2012, Q3, P20
  799.52 Cognitive communication deficit
    Coding Clinic: 2012, Q3, P19-21
  799.53 Visuospatial deficit
  799.54 Psychomotor deficit
    Coding Clinic: 2010, Q4, P97
  799.55 Frontal lobe and executive function deficit
    Coding Clinic: 2012, Q3, P20
  799.59 Other signs and symptoms involving cognition

● **799.8 Other ill-defined conditions**
  799.81 Decreased libido
    Decreased sexual desire
    Excludes: psychosexual dysfunction with inhibited sexual desire (302.71)
    Coding Clinic: 2003, Q4, P75-76; Q4, P75-76
  799.82 Apparent life threatening event in infant
    ALTE
    Apparent life threatening event in newborn and infant
    Code first confirmed diagnosis, if known
    Use additional code(s) for associated signs and symptoms if no confirmed diagnosis established, or if signs and symptoms are not associated routinely with confirmed diagnosis, or provide additional information for cause of ALTE
    Coding Clinic: 2010, Q4, P98
  799.89 Other ill-defined conditions

799.9 Other unknown and unspecified cause
  Undiagnosed disease, not specified as to site or system involved
  Unknown cause of morbidity or mortality
  Coding Clinic: 1998, Q1, P4; 1990, Q1, P22

PART III / Diseases: Tabular List Volume 1

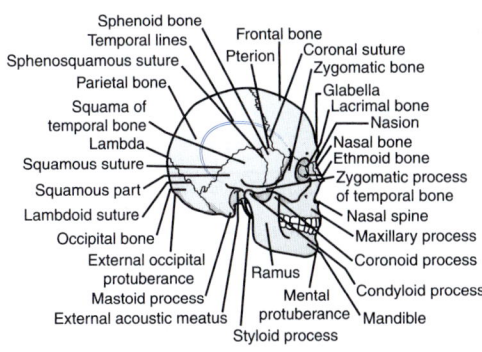

Figure 17-1 Lateral view of skull.

Figure 17-2 Frontal view of skull.

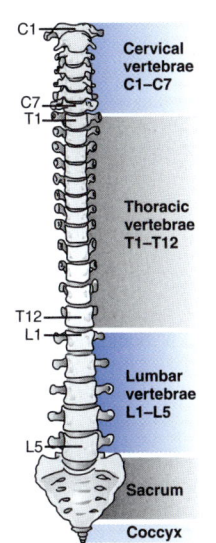

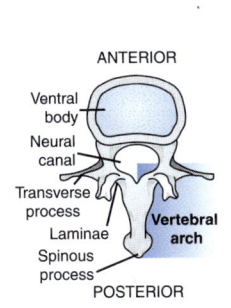

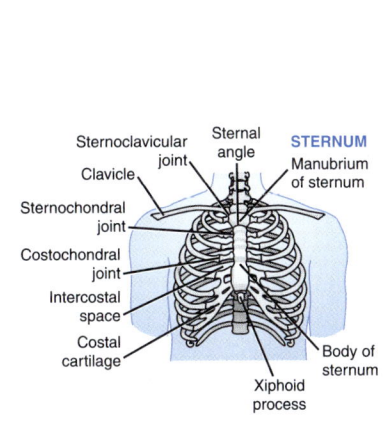

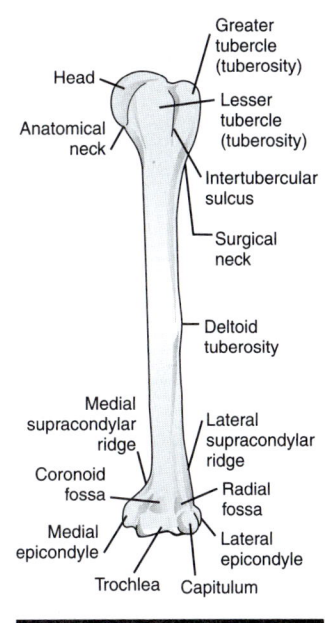

Figure 17-3 Anterior view of vertebral column.

Figure 17-4 Vertebra viewed from above.

Figure 17-5 Anterior view of rib cage.

Figure 17-6 Anterior aspect of left humerus.

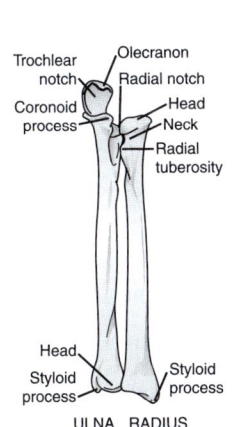

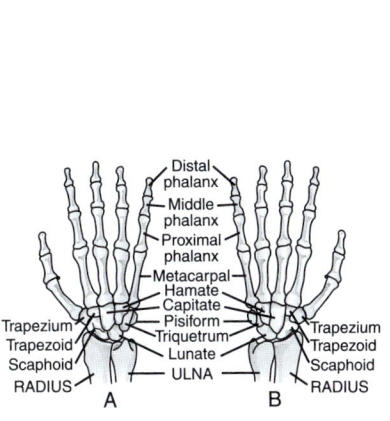

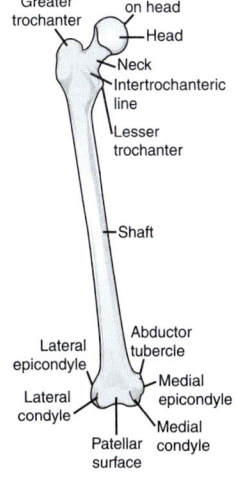

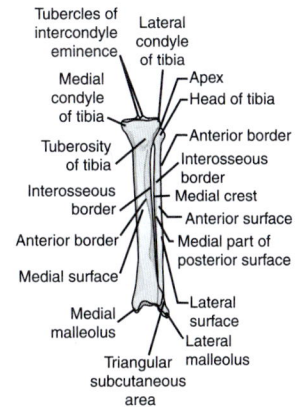

Figure 17-7 Anterior aspect of left radius and ulna.

Figure 17-8 Right hand and wrist: **A.** Dorsal surface. **B.** Palmar surface.

Figure 17-9 Anterior aspect of right femur.

Figure 17-10 Anterior aspect of left tibia and fibula.

◀ New ◀▬ Revised ~~deleted~~ Deleted Excludes   Includes   Use additional   Code first   Omit code
● Use Additional Digit(s)   Unspecified   ● Not first-listed DX   **OGCR** Official Guidelines   **Coding Clinic**

885

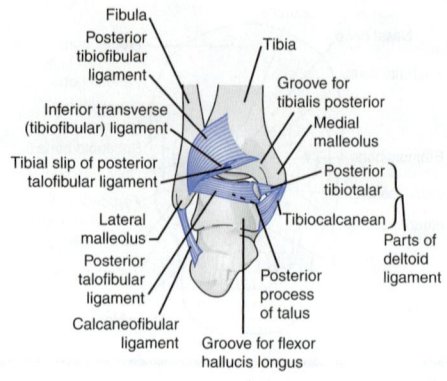

Figure 17-11 Posterior aspect of the left ankle joint.

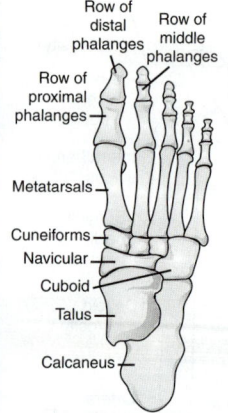

Figure 17-12 Right foot viewed from above.

OGCR Section I.C.17.a

When coding injuries, assign separate codes for each injury unless a combination code is provided, in which case the combination code is assigned. Multiple injury codes are provided in ICD-9-CM, but should not be assigned unless information for a more specific code is not available. These traumatic injury codes are not to be used for normal, healing surgical wounds or to identify complications of surgical wounds.

The code for the most serious injury, as determined by the provider and the focus of treatment, is sequenced first.

1) **Superficial injuries:** Superficial injuries such as abrasions or contusions are not coded when associated with more severe injuries of the same site.

2) **Primary injury with damage to nerves/blood vessels:** When a primary injury results in minor damage to peripheral nerves or blood vessels, the primary injury is sequenced first with additional code(s) from categories 950-957, Injury to nerves and spinal cord, and/or 900-904, Injury to blood vessels. When the primary injury is to the blood vessels or nerves, that injury should be sequenced first.

17. INJURY AND POISONING (800–999)

Use E code(s) to identify the cause and intent of the injury or poisoning (E800–E999).

> **Use additional** code for retained foreign body, if applicable, V90.01-V90.9.

Note:
1. The principle of multiple coding of injuries should be followed wherever possible. Combination categories for multiple injuries are provided for use when there is insufficient detail as to the nature of the individual conditions, or for primary tabulation purposes when it is more convenient to record a single code; otherwise, the component injuries should be coded separately.

Where multiple sites of injury are specified in the titles, the word "with" indicates involvement of both sites, and the word "and" indicates involvement of either or both sites. The word "finger" includes thumb.
2. Categories for "late effect" of injuries are to be found at 905–909.

FRACTURES (800–829)

Excludes malunion (733.81)
nonunion (733.82)
pathologic or spontaneous fracture (733.10–733.19)
stress fracture (733.93–733.95)

The terms "condyle," "coronoid process," "ramus," and "symphysis" indicate the portion of the bone fractured, not the name of the bone involved.

The descriptions "closed" and "open" used in the fourth-digit subdivisions include the following terms:
closed (with or without delayed healing):
  comminuted
  depressed
  elevated
  fissured
  fracture NOS
  greenstick
  impacted
  linear
  simple
  slipped epiphysis
  spiral
open (with or without delayed healing):
  compound
  infected
  missile
  puncture
  with foreign body

Note: A fracture not indicated as closed or open should be classified as closed.

FRACTURE OF SKULL (800–804)

Includes traumatic brain injury due to fracture of skull

The following fifth-digit subclassification is for use with the appropriate codes in categories 800, 801, 803, and 804:

- 0 unspecified state of consciousness
- 1 with no loss of consciousness
- 2 with brief [less than one hour] loss of consciousness
- 3 with moderate [1–24 hours] loss of consciousness
- 4 with prolonged [more than 24 hours] loss of consciousness and return to pre-existing conscious level
- 5 with prolonged [more than 24 hours] loss of consciousness, without return to pre-existing conscious level
  Use fifth-digit 5 to designate when a patient is unconscious and dies before regaining consciousness, regardless of the duration of the loss of consciousness
- 6 with loss of consciousness of unspecified duration
- 9 with concussion, unspecified

● **800 Fracture of vault of skull**
Requires fifth digit. See beginning of section 800–804 for codes and definitions.

Includes frontal bone
parietal bone

● **800.0** Closed without mention of intracranial injury
[0-6,9]

● **800.1** Closed with cerebral laceration and contusion
[0-6,9]

● **800.2** Closed with subarachnoid, subdural, and extradural
[0-6,9] hemorrhage

● **800.3** Closed with other and unspecified intracranial
[0-6,9] hemorrhage

- **800.4** Closed with intracranial injury of other and unspecified nature [0-6,9]
- **800.5** Open without mention of intracranial injury [0-6,9]
- **800.6** Open with cerebral laceration and contusion [0-6,9]
- **800.7** Open with subarachnoid, subdural, and extradural hemorrhage [0-6,9]
- **800.8** Open with other and unspecified intracranial hemorrhage [0-6,9]
- **800.9** Open with intracranial injury of other and unspecified nature [0-6,9]

- **801 Fracture of base of skull**

    Requires fifth digit. See beginning of section 800–804 for codes and definitions.

    Includes fossa:
    anterior
    middle
    posterior
    occiput bone
    orbital roof
    sinus:
    ethmoid
    frontal
    sphenoid bone
    temporal bone

- **801.0** Closed without mention of intracranial injury [0-6,9]
- **801.1** Closed with cerebral laceration and contusion [0-6,9]
    Coding Clinic: 1996, Q4, P36.37
- **801.2** Closed with subarachnoid, subdural, and extradural hemorrhage [0-6,9]
- **801.3** Closed with other and unspecified intracranial hemorrhage [0-6,9]
- **801.4** Closed with intracranial injury of other and unspecified nature [0-6,9]
- **801.5** Open without mention of intracranial injury [0-6,9]
- **801.6** Open with cerebral laceration and contusion [0-6,9]
- **801.7** Open with subarachnoid, subdural, and extradural hemorrhage [0-6,9]
- **801.8** Open with other and unspecified intracranial hemorrhage [0-6,9]
- **801.9** Open with intracranial injury of other and unspecified nature [0-6,9]

- **802 Fracture of face bones**
    - **802.0** Nasal bones, closed
    - **802.1** Nasal bones, open
    - **802.2** Mandible, closed
        Inferior maxilla
        Lower jaw (bone)
        - **802.20** Unspecified site
        - **802.21** Condylar process
        - **802.22** Subcondylar
        - **802.23** Coronoid process
        - **802.24** Ramus, unspecified
        - **802.25** Angle of jaw
        - **802.26** Symphysis of body
        - **802.27** Alveolar border of body
        - **802.28** Body, other and unspecified
        - **802.29** Multiple sites
    - **802.3** Mandible, open
        - **802.30** Unspecified site
        - **802.31** Condylar process
        - **802.32** Subcondylar
        - **802.33** Coronoid process
        - **802.34** Ramus, unspecified
        - **802.35** Angle of jaw
        - **802.36** Symphysis of body
        - **802.37** Alveolar border of body
        - **802.38** Body, other and unspecified
        - **802.39** Multiple sites
    - **802.4** Malar and maxillary bones, closed
        Superior maxilla   Zygoma
        Upper jaw (bone)   Zygomatic arch
    - **802.5** Malar and maxillary bones, open
    - **802.6** Orbital floor (blow-out), closed
    - **802.7** Orbital floor (blow-out), open
    - **802.8** Other facial bones, closed
        Alveolus
        Orbit:
            NOS
            part other than roof or floor
        Palate
        Excludes orbital:
            floor (802.6)
            roof (801.0–801.9)
    - **802.9** Other facial bones, open

- **803 Other and unqualified skull fractures**

    Requires fifth digit. See beginning of section 800–804 for codes and definitions.

    Includes skull NOS
    skull multiple NOS

- **803.0** Closed without mention of intracranial injury [0-6,9]
- **803.1** Closed with cerebral laceration and contusion [0-6,9]
- **803.2** Closed with subarachnoid, subdural, and extradural hemorrhage [0-6,9]
- **803.3** Closed with other and unspecified intracranial hemorrhage [0-6,9]
- **803.4** Closed with intracranial injury of other and unspecified nature [0-6,9]
- **803.5** Open without mention of intracranial injury [0-6,9]
- **803.6** Open with cerebral laceration and contusion [0-6,9]
- **803.7** Open with subarachnoid, subdural, and extradural hemorrhage [0-6,9]
- **803.8** Open with other and unspecified intracranial hemorrhage [0-6,9]
- **803.9** Open with intracranial injury of other and unspecified nature [0-6,9]

- **804 Multiple fractures involving skull or face with other bones**

    Requires fifth digit. See beginning of section 800–804 for codes and definitions.

- **804.0** Closed without mention of intracranial injury [0-6,9]
- **804.1** Closed with cerebral laceration and contusion [0-6,9]
    Coding Clinic: 2006, Q1, P6-7
- **804.2** Closed with subarachnoid, subdural, and extradural hemorrhage [0-6,9]
- **804.3** Closed with other and unspecified intracranial hemorrhage [0-6,9]
- **804.4** Closed with intracranial injury of other and unspecified nature [0-6,9]
- **804.5** Open without mention of intracranial injury [0-6,9]
- **804.6** Open with cerebral laceration and contusion [0-6,9]
- **804.7** Open with subarachnoid, subdural, and extradural hemorrhage [0-6,9]
- **804.8** Open with other and unspecified intracranial hemorrhage [0-6,9]
- **804.9** Open with intracranial injury of other and unspecified nature [0-6,9]

FRACTURE OF NECK AND TRUNK (805–809)

● **805 Fracture of vertebral column without mention of spinal cord injury**

  Includes neural arch
  spine
  spinous process
  transverse process
  vertebra
  Coding Clinic: 1985, Nov-Dec, P16

The following fifth-digit subclassification is for use with codes 805.0–805.1:

> 0 cervical vertebra, unspecified level
> 1 first cervical vertebra
> 2 second cervical vertebra
> 3 third cervical vertebra
> 4 fourth cervical vertebra
> 5 fifth cervical vertebra
> 6 sixth cervical vertebra
> 7 seventh cervical vertebra
> 8 multiple cervical vertebrae

● 805.0 Cervical, closed
  [0-8]   Atlas
          Axis
● 805.1 Cervical, open
  [0-8]
  805.2 Dorsal [thoracic], closed
  805.3 Dorsal [thoracic], open
  805.4 Lumbar, closed
    Coding Clinic: 2007, Q1, P3-8
  805.5 Lumbar, open
  805.6 Sacrum and coccyx, closed
  805.7 Sacrum and coccyx, open
  805.8 Unspecified, closed
  805.9 Unspecified, open

● **806 Fracture of vertebral column with spinal cord injury**
  Includes any condition classifiable to 805 with:
    complete or incomplete transverse lesion (of cord)
    hematomyelia
    injury to:
      cauda equina
      nerve
    paralysis
    paraplegia
    quadriplegia
    spinal concussion

● 806.0 Cervical, closed
  ■ 806.00 C_1-C_4 level with unspecified spinal cord injury
        Cervical region NOS with spinal cord injury NOS
    806.01 C_1-C_4 level with complete lesion of cord
    806.02 C_1-C_4 level with anterior cord syndrome
    806.03 C_1-C_4 level with central cord syndrome
    806.04 C_1-C_4 level with other specified spinal cord injury
        C_1-C_4 level with:
          incomplete spinal cord lesion NOS
          posterior cord syndrome
  ■ 806.05 C_5-C_7 level with unspecified spinal cord injury
    806.06 C_5-C_7 level with complete lesion of cord
    806.07 C_5-C_7 level with anterior cord syndrome
    806.08 C_5-C_7 level with central cord syndrome
    806.09 C_5-C_7 level with other specified spinal cord injury
        C_5-C_7 level with:
          incomplete spinal cord lesion NOS
          posterior cord syndrome

● 806.1 Cervical, open
  ■ 806.10 C_1-C_4 level with unspecified spinal cord injury
    806.11 C_1-C_4 level with complete lesion of cord
    806.12 C_1-C_4 level with anterior cord syndrome
    806.13 C_1-C_4 level with central cord syndrome
    806.14 C_1-C_4 level with other specified spinal cord injury
        C_1-C_4 level with:
          incomplete spinal cord lesion NOS
          posterior cord syndrome
  ■ 806.15 C_5-C_7 level with unspecified spinal cord injury
    806.16 C_5-C_7 level with complete lesion of cord
    806.17 C_5-C_7 level with anterior cord syndrome
    806.18 C_5-C_7 level with central cord syndrome
    806.19 C_5-C_7 level with other specified spinal cord injury
        C_5-C_7 level with:
          incomplete spinal cord lesion NOS
          posterior cord syndrome

● 806.2 Dorsal [thoracic], closed
  ■ 806.20 T_1-T_6 level with unspecified spinal cord injury
        Thoracic region NOS with spinal cord injury NOS
    806.21 T_1-T_6 level with complete lesion of cord
    806.22 T_1-T_6 level with anterior cord syndrome
    806.23 T_1-T_6 level with central cord syndrome
    806.24 T_1-T_6 level with other specified spinal cord injury
        T_1-T_6 level with:
          incomplete spinal cord lesion NOS
          posterior cord syndrome
  ■ 806.25 T_7-T_{12} level with unspecified spinal cord injury
    806.26 T_7-T_{12} level with complete lesion of cord
    806.27 T_7-T_{12} level with anterior cord syndrome
    806.28 T_7-T_{12} level with central cord syndrome
    806.29 T_7-T_{12} level with other specified spinal cord injury
        T_7-T_{12} level with:
          incomplete spinal cord lesion NOS
          posterior cord syndrome

● 806.3 Dorsal [thoracic], open
  ■ 806.30 T_1-T_6 level with unspecified spinal cord injury
    806.31 T_1-T_6 level with complete lesion of cord
    806.32 T_1-T_6 level with anterior cord syndrome
    806.33 T_1-T_6 level with central cord syndrome
    806.34 T_1-T_6 level with other specified spinal cord injury
        T_1-T_6 level with:
          incomplete spinal cord lesion NOS
          posterior cord syndrome
  ■ 806.35 T_7-T_{12} level with unspecified spinal cord injury
    806.36 T_7-T_{12} level with complete lesion of cord
    806.37 T_7-T_{12} level with anterior cord syndrome
    806.38 T_7-T_{12} level with central cord syndrome
    806.39 T_7-T_{12} level with other specified spinal cord injury
        T_7-T_{12} level with:
          incomplete spinal cord lesion NOS
          posterior cord syndrome

  806.4 Lumbar, closed
    Coding Clinic: 1999, Q4, P11-13
  806.5 Lumbar, open
● 806.6 Sacrum and coccyx, closed
  ■ 806.60 With unspecified spinal cord injury
    806.61 With complete cauda equina lesion
    806.62 With other cauda equina injury
    806.69 With other spinal cord injury
● 806.7 Sacrum and coccyx, open
  ■ 806.70 With unspecified spinal cord injury
    806.71 With complete cauda equina lesion
    806.72 With other cauda equina injury
    806.79 With other spinal cord injury
  ■ 806.8 Unspecified, closed
  ■ 806.9 Unspecified, open

PART III / Diseases: Tabular List Volume 1

807 Fracture of rib(s), sternum, larynx, and trachea

The following fifth-digit subclassification is for use with codes 807.0–807.1:

0 rib(s), unspecified	6 six ribs
1 one rib	7 seven ribs
2 two ribs	8 eight or more ribs
3 three ribs	9 multiple ribs, unspecified
4 four ribs	
5 five ribs	

- **807.0 Rib(s), closed**
  [0-9]
  Coding Clinic: 2013, Q1, P15
- **807.1 Rib(s), open**
  [0-9]
- 807.2 Sternum, closed
- 807.3 Sternum, open
- 807.4 Flail chest
  Unstable chest due to sternum and/or rib fracture
- 807.5 Larynx and trachea, closed
  Hyoid bone
  Thyroid cartilage
  Trachea
- 807.6 Larynx and trachea, open

808 Fracture of pelvis

- 808.0 Acetabulum, closed
- 808.1 Acetabulum, open
- 808.2 Pubis, closed
  Coding Clinic: 2008, Q1, P9-10
- 808.3 Pubis, open
- **808.4 Other specified part, closed**
  - 808.41 Ilium
  - 808.42 Ischium
  - 808.43 Multiple closed pelvic fractures with disruption of pelvic circle
    Multiple closed pelvic fractures with disruption of pelvic ring
    Coding Clinic: 2008, Q1, P9-10
  - 808.44 Multiple closed pelvic fractures without disruption of pelvic circle
    Multiple closed pelvic fractures without disruption of pelvic ring
  - 808.49 Other
    Innominate bone
    Pelvic rim
- **808.5 Other specified part, open**
  - 808.51 Ilium
  - 808.52 Ischium
  - 808.53 Multiple open pelvic fractures with disruption of pelvic circle
    Multiple open pelvic fractures with disruption of pelvic ring
  - 808.54 Multiple open pelvic fractures without disruption of pelvic circle
    Multiple open pelvic fractures without disruption of pelvic ring
  - 808.59 Other
- 808.8 Unspecified, closed
- 808.9 Unspecified, open

809 Ill-defined fractures of bones of trunk

Includes bones of trunk with other bones except those of skull and face
multiple bones of trunk

Excludes multiple fractures of:
pelvic bones alone (808.0–808.9)
ribs alone (807.0–807.1, 807.4)
ribs or sternum with limb bones (819.0–819.1, 828.0–828.1)
skull or face with other bones (804.0–804.9)

- 809.0 Fracture of bones of trunk, closed
- 809.1 Fracture of bones of trunk, open

FRACTURE OF UPPER LIMB (810–819)

810 Fracture of clavicle

Includes collar bone
interligamentous part of clavicle

The following fifth-digit subclassification is for use with category 810:

0 unspecified part	2 shaft of clavicle
Clavicle NOS	3 acromial end of clavicle
1 sternal end of clavicle	

- **810.0 Closed**
  [0-3]
- **810.1 Open**
  [0-3]

811 Fracture of scapula

Includes shoulder blade

The following fifth-digit subclassification is for use with category 811:

0 unspecified part	3 glenoid cavity and neck of scapula
1 acromial process	
Acromion (process)	9 other
2 coracoid process	

- **811.0 Closed**
  [0-3,9]
- **811.1 Open**
  [0-3,9]

812 Fracture of humerus

- **812.0 Upper end, closed**
  - 812.00 Upper end, unspecified part
    Proximal end   Shoulder
  - 812.01 Surgical neck
    Neck of humerus NOS
  - 812.02 Anatomical neck
  - 812.03 Greater tuberosity
  - 812.09 Other
    Head   Upper epiphysis
- **812.1 Upper end, open**
  - 812.10 Upper end, unspecified part
  - 812.11 Surgical neck
  - 812.12 Anatomical neck
  - 812.13 Greater tuberosity
  - 812.19 Other
- **812.2 Shaft or unspecified part, closed**
  - 812.20 Unspecified part of humerus
    Humerus NOS   Upper arm NOS
  - 812.21 Shaft of humerus
    Coding Clinic: 2005, Q4, P127-129; 1999, Q3, P14-15
- **812.3 Shaft or unspecified part, open**
  - 812.30 Unspecified part of humerus
  - 812.31 Shaft of humerus

- **812.4 Lower end, closed**
  Distal end of humerus
  Elbow
  - 812.40 Lower end, unspecified part
  - 812.41 Supracondylar fracture of humerus
  - 812.42 Lateral condyle
    External condyle
  - 812.43 Medial condyle
    Internal epicondyle
  - 812.44 Condyle(s), unspecified
    Articular process NOS
    Lower epiphysis
  - 812.49 Other
    Multiple fractures of lower end
    Trochlea
- **812.5 Lower end, open**
  - 812.50 Lower end, unspecified part
  - 812.51 Supracondylar fracture of humerus
  - 812.52 Lateral condyle
  - 812.53 Medial condyle
  - 812.54 Condyle(s), unspecified
  - 812.59 Other

- **813 Fracture of radius and ulna**
  - **813.0 Upper end, closed**
    Proximal end
    - 813.00 Upper end of forearm, unspecified
    - 813.01 Olecranon process of ulna
    - 813.02 Coronoid process of ulna
    - 813.03 Monteggia's fracture
    - 813.04 Other and unspecified fractures of proximal end of ulna (alone)
      Multiple fractures of ulna, upper end
    - 813.05 Head of radius
    - 813.06 Neck of radius
    - 813.07 Other and unspecified fractures of proximal end of radius (alone)
      Multiple fractures of radius, upper end
    - 813.08 Radius with ulna, upper end [any part]
  - **813.1 Upper end, open**
    - 813.10 Upper end of forearm, unspecified
    - 813.11 Olecranon process of ulna
    - 813.12 Coronoid process of ulna
    - 813.13 Monteggia's fracture
    - 813.14 Other and unspecified fractures of proximal end of ulna (alone)
    - 813.15 Head of radius
    - 813.16 Neck of radius
    - 813.17 Other and unspecified fractures of proximal end of radius (alone)
    - 813.18 Radius with ulna, upper end [any part]
  - **813.2 Shaft, closed**
    - 813.20 Shaft, unspecified
    - 813.21 Radius (alone)
    - 813.22 Ulna (alone)
    - 813.23 Radius with ulna
      Coding Clinic: 2009, Q4, P120
  - **813.3 Shaft, open**
    - 813.30 Shaft, unspecified
    - 813.31 Radius (alone)
    - 813.32 Ulna (alone)
    - 813.33 Radius with ulna

- **813.4 Lower end, closed**
  Distal end
  - 813.40 Lower end of forearm, unspecified
  - 813.41 Colles' fracture
    Smith's fracture
  - 813.42 Other fractures of distal end of radius (alone)
    Dupuytren's fracture, radius
    Radius, lower end
  - 813.43 Distal end of ulna (alone)
    Ulna: Ulna:
      head   lower epiphysis
      lower end   styloid process
  - 813.44 Radius with ulna, lower end
    Coding Clinic: 2007, Q1, P3-8
  - 813.45 Torus fracture of radius (alone)
    Excludes *torus fracture of radius and ulna (813.47)*
    Coding Clinic: 2002, Q4, P70-71
  - 813.46 Torus fracture of ulna (alone)
    Excludes *torus fracture of radius and ulna (813.47)*
  - 813.47 Torus fracture of radius and ulna
- **813.5 Lower end, open**
  - 813.50 Lower end of forearm, unspecified
  - 813.51 Colles' fracture
  - 813.52 Other fractures of distal end of radius (alone)
  - 813.53 Distal end of ulna (alone)
  - 813.54 Radius with ulna, lower end
- **813.8 Unspecified part, closed**
  - 813.80 Forearm, unspecified
  - 813.81 Radius (alone)
    Coding Clinic: 1998, Q2, P19
  - 813.82 Ulna (alone)
  - 813.83 Radius with ulna
- **813.9 Unspecified part, open**
  - 813.90 Forearm, unspecified
  - 813.91 Radius (alone)
  - 813.92 Ulna (alone)
  - 813.93 Radius with ulna

- **814 Fracture of carpal bone(s)**
  The following fifth-digit subclassification is for use with category 814:

  ```
  0  carpal bone, unspecified
       Wrist NOS
  1  navicular [scaphoid] of wrist
  2  lunate [semilunar] bone of wrist
  3  triquetral [cuneiform] bone of wrist
  4  pisiform
  5  trapezium bone [larger multangular]
  6  trapezoid bone [smaller multangular]
  7  capitate bone [os magnum]
  8  hamate [unciform] bone
  9  other
  ```

  - **814.0 Closed**
    [0-9]
  - **814.1 Open**
    [0-9]

PART III / Diseases: Tabular List Volume 1

- **815 Fracture of metacarpal bone(s)**
  - **Includes** hand [except finger]
    metacarpus

  The following fifth-digit subclassification is for use with category 815:

  - 0 metacarpal bone(s), site unspecified
  - 1 base of thumb [first] metacarpal
      Bennett's fracture
  - 2 base of other metacarpal bone(s)
  - 3 shaft of metacarpal bone(s)
  - 4 neck of metacarpal bone(s)
  - 9 multiple sites of metacarpus

  - **815.0 Closed**
    [0-4,9] *Coding Clinic: 1994, Q2, P6*
  - **815.1 Open**
    [0-4,9]

- **816 Fracture of one or more phalanges of hand**
  - **Includes** finger(s)
    thumb

  The following fifth-digit subclassification is for use with category 816:

  - 0 phalanx or phalanges, unspecified
  - 1 middle or proximal phalanx or phalanges
  - 2 distal phalanx or phalanges
  - 3 multiple sites

  - **816.0 Closed**
    [0-3]
  - **816.1 Open**
    [0-3] *Coding Clinic: 2003, Q4, P76-78*

- **817 Multiple fractures of hand bones**
  - **Includes** metacarpal bone(s) with phalanx or phalanges of same hand
  - 817.0 Closed
  - 817.1 Open

- **818 Ill-defined fractures of upper limb**
  - **Includes** arm NOS
    multiple bones of same upper limb
  - **Excludes** multiple fractures of:
    metacarpal bone(s) with phalanx or phalanges (817.0–817.1)
    phalanges of hand alone (816.0–816.1)
    radius with ulna (813.0–813.9)
  - 818.0 Closed
  - 818.1 Open

  OGCR Section I.C.17.b.4
  Multiple fracture categories 819 and 828 classify bilateral fractures of both upper limbs (819) and both lower limbs (828), but without any detail at the fourth-digit level other than open and closed type of fractures.

- **819 Multiple fractures involving both upper limbs, and upper limb with rib(s) and sternum**
  - **Includes** arm(s) with rib(s) or sternum
    both arms [any bones]
  - 819.0 Closed
  - 819.1 Open

FRACTURE OF LOWER LIMB (820–829)

- **820 Fracture of neck of femur**
  - **820.0 Transcervical fracture, closed**
    - 820.00 Intracapsular section, unspecified
    - 820.01 Epiphysis (separation) (upper)
        Transepiphyseal
        Fracture and separation across growth plate
    - 820.02 Midcervical section
        Transcervical NOS
        Coding Clinic: 2003, Q3, P12-13
    - 820.03 Base of neck
        Cervicotrochanteric section
    - 820.09 Other
        Head of femur   Subcapital
  - **820.1 Transcervical fracture, open**
    - 820.10 Intracapsular section, unspecified
    - 820.11 Epiphysis (separation) (upper)
    - 820.12 Midcervical section
    - 820.13 Base of neck
    - 820.19 Other
  - **820.2 Pertrochanteric fracture, closed**
    - 820.20 Trochanteric section, unspecified
        Trochanter:
           NOS
           greater
           lesser
    - 820.21 Intertrochanteric section
        Coding Clinic: 1994, Q2, P6; 1984, May-June, P11
    - 820.22 Subtrochanteric section
  - **820.3 Pertrochanteric fracture, open**
    - 820.30 Trochanteric section, unspecified
    - 820.31 Intertrochanteric section
    - 820.32 Subtrochanteric section
  - 820.8 Unspecified part of neck of femur, closed
    Hip NOS   Neck of femur NOS
    Coding Clinic: 1994, Q2, P9; 1985, Nov-Dec, P16
  - 820.9 Unspecified part of neck of femur, open

- **821 Fracture of other and unspecified parts of femur**
  - **821.0 Shaft or unspecified part, closed**
    - 821.00 Unspecified part of femur
        Thigh   Upper leg
        Excludes hip NOS (820.8)
    - 821.01 Shaft
        Coding Clinic: 2007, Q1, P3-8; 1999, Q1, P5
  - **821.1 Shaft or unspecified part, open**
    - 821.10 Unspecified part of femur
    - 821.11 Shaft
  - **821.2 Lower end, closed**
    Distal end
    - 821.20 Lower end, unspecified part
    - 821.21 Condyle, femoral
    - 821.22 Epiphysis, lower (separation)
    - 821.23 Supracondylar fracture of femur
    - 821.29 Other
        Multiple fractures of lower end
  - **821.3 Lower end, open**
    - 821.30 Lower end, unspecified part
    - 821.31 Condyle, femoral
    - 821.32 Epiphysis, lower (separation)
    - 821.33 Supracondylar fracture of femur
    - 821.39 Other

- **822 Fracture of patella**
  - 822.0 Closed
  - 822.1 Open

- **823 Fracture of tibia and fibula**
  - Excludes: Dupuytren's fracture (824.4–824.5)
    - ankle (824.4–824.5)
    - radius (813.42, 813.52)
    - Pott's fracture (824.4–824.5)
    - that involving ankle (824.0–824.9)

  The following fifth-digit subclassification is for use with category 823:

  > 0 tibia alone
  > 1 fibula alone
  > 2 fibula with tibia

  - **823.0 Upper end, closed**
    [0-2]
    - Head
    - Proximal end
    - Tibia:
      - condyles
      - tuberosity
  - **823.1 Upper end, open**
    [0-2]
  - **823.2 Shaft, closed**
    [0-2]
  - **823.3 Shaft, open**
    [0-2]
  - **823.4 Torus fracture**
    [0-2]
    Coding Clinic: 2002, Q4, P70-71
  - **823.8 Unspecified part, closed**
    [0-2]
    - Lower leg NOS
    Coding Clinic: 1997, Q1, P8
  - **823.9 Unspecified part, open**
    [0-2]

- **824 Fracture of ankle**
  - **824.0 Medial malleolus, closed**
    - Tibia involving:
      - ankle
      - malleolus
    Coding Clinic: 2004, Q1, P9
  - **824.1 Medial malleolus, open**
  - **824.2 Lateral malleolus, closed**
    - Fibula involving:
      - ankle
      - malleolus
    Coding Clinic: 2002, Q2, P3
  - **824.3 Lateral malleolus, open**
  - **824.4 Bimalleolar, closed**
    - Dupuytren's fracture, fibula
    - Pott's fracture
    Coding Clinic: 2012, Q2, P11
  - **824.5 Bimalleolar, open**
  - **824.6 Trimalleolar, closed**
    - Lateral and medial malleolus with anterior or posterior lip of tibia
  - **824.7 Trimalleolar, open**
  - **824.8 Unspecified, closed**
    - Ankle NOS
    Coding Clinic: 2000, Q3, P12; 1994, Q2, P7
  - **824.9 Unspecified, open**

- **825 Fracture of one or more tarsal and metatarsal bones**
  - **825.0 Fracture of calcaneus, closed**
    - Heel bone
    - Os calcis
  - **825.1 Fracture of calcaneus, open**
  - **825.2 Fracture of other tarsal and metatarsal bones, closed**
    - **825.20 Unspecified bone(s) of foot [except toes]**
      - Instep
    - **825.21 Astragalus**
      - Talus
    - **825.22 Navicular [scaphoid], foot**
    - **825.23 Cuboid**
    - **825.24 Cuneiform, foot**
    - **825.25 Metatarsal bone(s)**
    - **825.29 Other**
      - Tarsal with metatarsal bone(s) only
      - Excludes: calcaneus (825.0)
      Coding Clinic: 1994, Q2, P5
  - **825.3 Fracture of other tarsal and metatarsal bones, open**
    - **825.30 Unspecified bone(s) of foot [except toes]**
    - **825.31 Astragalus**
    - **825.32 Navicular [scaphoid], foot**
    - **825.33 Cuboid**
    - **825.34 Cuneiform, foot**
    - **825.35 Metatarsal bone(s)**
    - **825.39 Other**

- **826 Fracture of one or more phalanges of foot**
  - Includes: toe(s)
  - **826.0 Closed**
  - **826.1 Open**

- **827 Other, multiple, and ill-defined fractures of lower limb**
  - Includes: leg NOS
    - multiple bones of same lower limb
  - Excludes: multiple fractures of:
    - ankle bones alone (824.4–824.9)
    - phalanges of foot alone (826.0–826.1)
    - tarsal with metatarsal bones (825.29, 825.39)
    - tibia with fibula (823.0–823.9 with fifth-digit 2)
  - **827.0 Closed**
  - **827.1 Open**

- **828 Multiple fractures involving both lower limbs, lower with upper limb, and lower limb(s) with rib(s) and sternum**
  - Includes: arm(s) with leg(s) [any bones]
    - both legs [any bones]
    - leg(s) with rib(s) or sternum

  OGCR Section I.C.17.b.4

  > Multiple fracture categories 819 and 828 classify bilateral fractures of both upper limbs (819) and both lower limbs (828), but without any detail at the fourth-digit level other than open and closed type of fractures.

  - **828.0 Closed**
  - **828.1 Open**

- **829 Fracture of unspecified bones**
  - **829.0 Unspecified bone, closed**
  - **829.1 Unspecified bone, open**

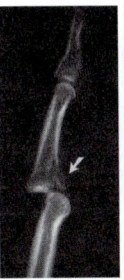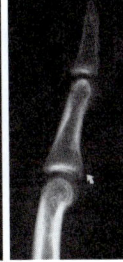

Figure 17–13 Dislocation including displacement and subluxation. (From Grainger & Allison's Diagnostic Radiology: A Textbook of Medical Imaging, ed 4, Churchill Livingstone, 2011)

A   B

DISLOCATION (830–839)

Includes   displacement
subluxation
Out of position

Excludes   congenital dislocation (754.0–755.8)
pathological dislocation (718.2)
recurrent dislocation (718.3)

The descriptions "closed" and "open," used in the fourth-digit subdivisions, include the following terms:

closed:
  complete
  dislocation NOS
  partial
  simple
  uncomplicated
open:
  compound
  infected
  with foreign body

Note: A dislocation not indicated as closed or open should be classified as closed.

● **830 Dislocation of jaw**
  Includes   jaw (cartilage) (meniscus)
  mandible
  maxilla (inferior)
  temporomandibular (joint)
  830.0 Closed dislocation
  830.1 Open dislocation

● **831 Dislocation of shoulder**
  Excludes   sternoclavicular joint (839.61, 839.71)
  sternum (839.61, 839.71)

The following fifth-digit subclassification is for use with category 831:

```
0  shoulder, unspecified
     Humerus NOS
1  anterior dislocation of humerus
2  posterior dislocation of humerus
3  inferior dislocation of humerus
4  acromioclavicular (joint)
     Clavicle
9  other
     Scapula
```

● **831.0 Closed dislocation**
[0-4,9] **Coding Clinic: 1987, Nov-Dec, P7**
● **831.1 Open dislocation**
[0-4,9]

● **832 Dislocation of elbow**
The following fifth-digit subclassification is for use with subcategories 832.0 and 832.1:

```
0  elbow unspecified
1  anterior dislocation of elbow
2  posterior dislocation of elbow
3  medial dislocation of elbow
4  lateral dislocation of elbow
9  other
```

● **832.0 Closed dislocation**
[0-4,9]
● **832.1 Open dislocation**
[0-4,9]
  832.2 Nursemaid's elbow
     Subluxation of radial head

● **833 Dislocation of wrist**
The following fifth-digit subclassification is for use with category 833:

```
0  wrist, unspecified part
     Carpal (bone)
     Radius, distal end
1  radioulnar (joint), distal
2  radiocarpal (joint)
3  midcarpal (joint)
4  carpometacarpal (joint)
5  metacarpal (bone), proximal end
9  other
     Ulna, distal end
```

● **833.0 Closed dislocation**
[0-5,9]
● **833.1 Open dislocation**
[0-5,9]

● **834 Dislocation of finger**
  Includes   finger(s)
  phalanx of hand
  thumb

The following fifth-digit subclassification is for use with category 834:

```
0  finger, unspecified part
1  metacarpophalangeal (joint)
     Metacarpal (bone), distal end
2  interphalangeal (joint), hand
```

● **834.0 Closed dislocation**
[0-2]
● **834.1 Open dislocation**
[0-2]

● **835 Dislocation of hip**
The following fifth-digit subclassification is for use with category 835:

```
0  dislocation of hip, unspecified
1  posterior dislocation
2  obturator dislocation
3  other anterior dislocation
```

● **835.0 Closed dislocation**
[0-3]
● **835.1 Open dislocation**
[0-3]

836 Dislocation of knee

Excludes dislocation of knee:
- old or pathological (718.2)
- recurrent (718.3)
- internal derangement of knee joint (717.0–717.5, 717.8–717.9)
- old tear of cartilage or meniscus of knee (717.0–717.5, 717.8–717.9)

- 836.0 Tear of medial cartilage or meniscus of knee, current
  - Bucket handle tear:
    - NOS current injury
    - medial meniscus current injury
- 836.1 Tear of lateral cartilage or meniscus of knee, current
- 836.2 Other tear of cartilage or meniscus of knee, current
  - Tear of:
    - cartilage (semilunar) current injury, not specified as medial or lateral
    - meniscus current injury, not specified as medial or lateral
- 836.3 Dislocation of patella, closed
- 836.4 Dislocation of patella, open
- 836.5 Other dislocation of knee, closed
  - 836.50 Dislocation of knee, unspecified
  - 836.51 Anterior dislocation of tibia, proximal end
    - Posterior dislocation of femur, distal end, closed
  - 836.52 Posterior dislocation of tibia, proximal end
    - Anterior dislocation of femur, distal end, closed
  - 836.53 Medial dislocation of tibia, proximal end
  - 836.54 Lateral dislocation of tibia, proximal end
  - 836.59 Other
- 836.6 Other dislocation of knee, open
  - 836.60 Dislocation of knee, unspecified
  - 836.61 Anterior dislocation of tibia, proximal end
    - Posterior dislocation of femur, distal end, open
  - 836.62 Posterior dislocation of tibia, proximal end
    - Anterior dislocation of femur, distal end, open
  - 836.63 Medial dislocation of tibia, proximal end
  - 836.64 Lateral dislocation of tibia, proximal end
  - 836.69 Other

837 Dislocation of ankle

Includes
- astragalus
- fibula, distal end
- navicular, foot
- scaphoid, foot
- tibia, distal end

- 837.0 Closed dislocation
- 837.1 Open dislocation

838 Dislocation of foot

The following fifth-digit subclassification is for use with category 838:

- 0 foot, unspecified
- 1 tarsal (bone), joint unspecified
- 2 midtarsal (joint)
- 3 tarsometatarsal (joint)
- 4 metatarsal (bone), joint unspecified
- 5 metatarsophalangeal (joint)
- 6 interphalangeal (joint), foot
- 9 other
  - Phalanx of foot
  - Toe(s)

- 838.0 Closed dislocation [0-6,9]
- 838.1 Open dislocation [0-6,9]

839 Other, multiple, and ill-defined dislocations
Coding Clinic: 1995, Q4, P51

- 839.0 Cervical vertebra, closed
  - Cervical spine
  - Neck
  - 839.00 Cervical vertebra, unspecified
  - 839.01 First cervical vertebra
  - 839.02 Second cervical vertebra
  - 839.03 Third cervical vertebra
  - 839.04 Fourth cervical vertebra
  - 839.05 Fifth cervical vertebra
  - 839.06 Sixth cervical vertebra
  - 839.07 Seventh cervical vertebra
  - 839.08 Multiple cervical vertebrae
- 839.1 Cervical vertebra, open
  - 839.10 Cervical vertebra, unspecified
  - 839.11 First cervical vertebra
  - 839.12 Second cervical vertebra
  - 839.13 Third cervical vertebra
  - 839.14 Fourth cervical vertebra
  - 839.15 Fifth cervical vertebra
  - 839.16 Sixth cervical vertebra
  - 839.17 Seventh cervical vertebra
  - 839.18 Multiple cervical vertebrae
- 839.2 Thoracic and lumbar vertebra, closed
  - 839.20 Lumbar vertebra
  - 839.21 Thoracic vertebra
    - Dorsal [thoracic] vertebra
- 839.3 Thoracic and lumbar vertebra, open
  - 839.30 Lumbar vertebra
  - 839.31 Thoracic vertebra
- 839.4 Other vertebra, closed
  - 839.40 Vertebra, unspecified site
    - Spine NOS
  - 839.41 Coccyx
  - 839.42 Sacrum
    - Sacroiliac (joint)
  - 839.49 Other
- 839.5 Other vertebra, open
  - 839.50 Vertebra, unspecified site
  - 839.51 Coccyx
  - 839.52 Sacrum
  - 839.59 Other
- 839.6 Other location, closed
  - 839.61 Sternum
    - Sternoclavicular joint
  - 839.69 Other
    - Pelvis
- 839.7 Other location, open
  - 839.71 Sternum
  - 839.79 Other
- 839.8 Multiple and ill-defined, closed
  - Arm
  - Back
  - Hand
  - Multiple locations, except fingers or toes alone
  - Other ill-defined locations
  - Unspecified location
- 839.9 Multiple and ill-defined, open

SPRAINS AND STRAINS OF JOINTS AND ADJACENT MUSCLES (840–848)

Includes: avulsion of joint capsule, ligament, muscle, tendon
hemarthrosis of joint capsule, ligament, muscle, tendon
Bleeding into joint space
laceration of joint capsule, ligament, muscle, tendon
rupture of joint capsule, ligament, muscle, tendon
sprain of joint capsule, ligament, muscle, tendon
strain of joint capsule, ligament, muscle, tendon
tear of joint capsule, ligament, muscle, tendon

Excludes: laceration of tendon in open wounds (880–884 and 890–894 with .2)

840 Sprains and strains of shoulder and upper arm
Sprains are an injury to ligaments when one or more is stretched/torn and strains are caused by twisting or pulling a muscle(s) or tendon.

- 840.0 Acromioclavicular (joint) (ligament)
- 840.1 Coracoclavicular (ligament)
- 840.2 Coracohumeral (ligament)
- 840.3 Infraspinatus (muscle) (tendon)
- 840.4 Rotator cuff (capsule)
  - **Excludes:** complete rupture of rotator cuff, nontraumatic (727.61)
- 840.5 Subscapularis (muscle)
- 840.6 Supraspinatus (muscle) (tendon)
- 840.7 Superior glenoid labrum lesion
  - SLAP lesion
  - Coding Clinic: 2012, Q2, P15; 2001, Q4, P52
- 840.8 Other specified sites of shoulder and upper arm
- 840.9 Unspecified site of shoulder and upper arm
  - Arm NOS   Shoulder NOS

841 Sprains and strains of elbow and forearm
- 841.0 Radial collateral ligament
- 841.1 Ulnar collateral ligament
- 841.2 Radiohumeral (joint)
- 841.3 Ulnohumeral (joint)
- 841.8 Other specified sites of elbow and forearm
- 841.9 Unspecified site of elbow and forearm
  - Elbow NOS

842 Sprains and strains of wrist and hand
- 842.0 Wrist
  - 842.00 Unspecified site
  - 842.01 Carpal (joint)
  - 842.02 Radiocarpal (joint) (ligament)
  - 842.09 Other
    - Radioulnar joint, distal
- 842.1 Hand
  - 842.10 Unspecified site
  - 842.11 Carpometacarpal (joint)
  - 842.12 Metacarpophalangeal (joint)
  - 842.13 Interphalangeal (joint)
  - 842.19 Other
    - Midcarpal (joint)

843 Sprains and strains of hip and thigh
- 843.0 Iliofemoral (ligament)
- 843.1 Ischiocapsular (ligament)
- 843.8 Other specified sites of hip and thigh
- 843.9 Unspecified site of hip and thigh
  - Hip NOS   Thigh NOS

844 Sprains and strains of knee and leg
- 844.0 Lateral collateral ligament of knee
- 844.1 Medial collateral ligament of knee
- 844.2 Cruciate ligament of knee
- 844.3 Tibiofibular (joint) (ligament), superior
- 844.8 Other specified sites of knee and leg
- 844.9 Unspecified site of knee and leg
  - Knee NOS   Leg NOS

845 Sprains and strains of ankle and foot
- 845.0 Ankle
  - 845.00 Unspecified site
    - Coding Clinic: 2002, Q2, P3
  - 845.01 Deltoid (ligament), ankle
    - Internal collateral (ligament), ankle
  - 845.02 Calcaneofibular (ligament)
  - 845.03 Tibiofibular (ligament), distal
    - Coding Clinic: 2004, Q1, P9
  - 845.09 Other
    - Achilles tendon
- 845.1 Foot
  - 845.10 Unspecified site
  - 845.11 Tarsometatarsal (joint) (ligament)
  - 845.12 Metatarsophalangeal (joint)
  - 845.13 Interphalangeal (joint), toe
  - 845.19 Other

846 Sprains and strains of sacroiliac region
- 846.0 Lumbosacral (joint) (ligament)
- 846.1 Sacroiliac ligament
- 846.2 Sacrospinatus (ligament)
- 846.3 Sacrotuberous (ligament)
- 846.8 Other specified sites of sacroiliac region
- 846.9 Unspecified site of sacroiliac region

847 Sprains and strains of other and unspecified parts of back
Excludes: lumbosacral (846.0)
- 847.0 Neck
  - Anterior longitudinal (ligament), cervical
  - Atlanto-axial (joints)
  - Atlanto-occipital (joints)
  - Whiplash injury
  - **Excludes:** neck injury NOS (959.09)
    - thyroid region (848.2)
- 847.1 Thoracic
- 847.2 Lumbar
- 847.3 Sacrum
  - Sacrococcygeal (ligament)
- 847.4 Coccyx
- 847.9 Unspecified site of back
  - Back NOS

848 Other and ill-defined sprains and strains
- 848.0 Septal cartilage of nose
- 848.1 Jaw
  - Temporomandibular (joint) (ligament)
- 848.2 Thyroid region
  - Cricoarytenoid (joint) (ligament)
  - Cricothyroid (joint) (ligament)
  - Thyroid cartilage
- 848.3 Ribs
  - Chondrocostal (joint) without mention of injury to sternum
  - Costal cartilage without mention of injury to sternum
- 848.4 Sternum
  - 848.40 Unspecified site
  - 848.41 Sternoclavicular (joint) (ligament)
  - 848.42 Chondrosternal (joint)
  - 848.49 Other
    - Xiphoid cartilage
- 848.5 Pelvis
  - Symphysis pubis
  - **Excludes:** that in childbirth (665.6)
- 848.8 Other specified sites of sprains and strains
- 848.9 Unspecified site of sprain and strain

INTRACRANIAL INJURY, EXCLUDING THOSE WITH SKULL FRACTURE (850–854)

Includes: traumatic brain injury without skull fracture

Excludes: intracranial injury with skull fracture (800–801 and 803–804, except .0 and .5)
open wound of head without intracranial injury (870.0–873.9)
skull fracture alone (800–801 and 803–804 with .0, .5)

Note: The description "with open intracranial wound," used in the fourth-digit subdivisions, includes those specified as open or with mention of infection or foreign body.

The following fifth-digit subclassification is for use with categories 851–854:

- 0 unspecified state of consciousness
- 1 with no loss of consciousness
- 2 with brief [less than one hour] loss of consciousness
- 3 with moderate [1–24 hours] loss of consciousness
- 4 with prolonged [more than 24 hours] loss of consciousness and return to pre-existing conscious level
- 5 with prolonged [more than 24 hours] loss of consciousness without return to pre-existing conscious level
  Use fifth-digit 5 to designate when a patient is unconscious and dies before regaining consciousness, regardless of the duration of the loss of consciousness
- 6 with loss of consciousness of unspecified duration
- 9 with concussion, unspecified

850 Concussion
Includes: commotio cerebri
Excludes: concussion with:
cerebral laceration or contusion (851.0–851.9)
cerebral hemorrhage (852–853)
head injury NOS (959.01)
Coding Clinic: 1993, Q1, P22-23

- **850.0 With no loss of consciousness**
  Concussion with mental confusion or disorientation, without loss of consciousness
  Coding Clinic: 1992, Q2, P5-6
- **850.1 With brief loss of consciousness**
  Loss of consciousness for less than one hour
  Coding Clinic: 2003, Q4, P76; 1999, Q1, P10; 1992, Q2, P5-6
  - 850.11 With loss of consciousness of 30 minutes or less
  - 850.12 With loss of consciousness from 31 to 59 minutes
    Coding Clinic: 2010, Q4, P111
- **850.2 With moderate loss of consciousness**
  Loss of consciousness for 1–24 hours
- **850.3 With prolonged loss of consciousness and return to pre-existing conscious level**
  Loss of consciousness for more than 24 hours with complete recovery
- **850.4 With prolonged loss of consciousness, without return to pre-existing conscious level**
- **850.5 With loss of consciousness of unspecified duration**
- **850.9 Concussion, unspecified**

851 Cerebral laceration and contusion
Cerebral lacerations are tears in brain tissue. Cerebral contusions are bruises on brain.
Requires fifth digit. See beginning of section 850–854 for codes and definitions.
Coding Clinic: 1993, Q1, P22-23

- **851.0** [0-6,9] **Cortex (cerebral) contusion without mention of open intracranial wound**
  Coding Clinic: 2010, Q4, P93
- **851.1** [0-6,9] **Cortex (cerebral) contusion with open intracranial wound**
- **851.2** [0-6,9] **Cortex (cerebral) laceration without mention of open intracranial wound**
- **851.3** [0-6,9] **Cortex (cerebral) laceration with open intracranial wound**
- **851.4** [0-6,9] **Cerebellar or brain stem contusion without mention of open intracranial wound**
- **851.5** [0-6,9] **Cerebellar or brain stem contusion with open intracranial wound**
- **851.6** [0-6,9] **Cerebellar or brain stem laceration without mention of open intracranial wound**
- **851.7** [0-6,9] **Cerebellar or brain stem laceration with open intracranial wound**
- **851.8** [0-6,9] **Other and unspecified cerebral laceration and contusion, without mention of open intracranial wound**
  Brain (membrane) NOS
  Coding Clinic: 1996, Q4, P36.37
- **851.9** [0-6,9] **Other and unspecified cerebral laceration and contusion, with open intracranial wound**

852 Subarachnoid, subdural, and extradural hemorrhage, following injury
Requires fifth digit. See beginning of section 850–854 for codes and definitions.
Excludes: cerebral contusion or laceration (with hemorrhage) (851.0–851.9)

- **852.0** [0-6,9] **Subarachnoid hemorrhage following injury without mention of open intracranial wound**
  Middle meningeal hemorrhage following injury
  Coding Clinic: 2010, Q2, P17; 1991, Q3, P15-16
- **852.1** [0-6,9] **Subarachnoid hemorrhage following injury with open intracranial wound**
  Coding Clinic: 1991, Q3, P15-16
- **852.2** [0-6,9] **Subdural hemorrhage following injury without mention of open intracranial wound**
  Coding Clinic: 2011, Q4, P100; 2007, Q4, P105-107; 1996, Q4, P43-44
- **852.3** [0-6,9] **Subdural hemorrhage following injury with open intracranial wound**
- **852.4** [0-6,9] **Extradural hemorrhage following injury without mention of open intracranial wound**
  Epidural hematoma following injury
- **852.5** [0-6,9] **Extradural hemorrhage following injury with open intracranial wound**

853 Other and unspecified intracranial hemorrhage following injury
Requires fifth digit. See beginning of section 850–854 for codes and definitions.

- **853.0** [0-6,9] **Without mention of open intracranial wound**
  Cerebral compression due to injury
  Intracranial hematoma following injury
  Traumatic cerebral hemorrhage
  Coding Clinic: 1990, Q3, P14
- **853.1** [0-6,9] **With open intracranial wound**

854 Intracranial injury of other and unspecified nature
Requires fifth digit. See beginning of section 850-854 for codes and definitions.
Includes: injury:
brain NOS
cavernous sinus
intracranial
traumatic brain NOS
Excludes: any condition classifiable to 850–853
head injury NOS (959.01)
Coding Clinic: 1999, Q1, P10; 1992, Q2, P5-6

- **854.0** [0-6,9] **Without mention of open intracranial wound**
  Coding Clinic: 2009, Q4, P120; 2005, Q2, P6-7
- **854.1** [0-6,9] **With open intracranial wound**

Item 17-1 **Pneumothorax** is a collection of gas (positive air pressure) in the pleural space resulting in the lung collapsing. A tension pneumothorax is life-threatening and is a result of air in the pleural space causing a displacement in the mediastinal structures and cardiopulmonary function compromise. A traumatic pneumothorax results from blunt or penetrating injury that disrupts the parietal/visceral pleura. **Hemothorax** is blood or bloody fluid in the pleural cavity as a result of traumatic blood vessel rupture or inflammation of the lungs from pneumonia.

INTERNAL INJURY OF THORAX, ABDOMEN, AND PELVIS (860–869)

Includes
blast injuries of internal organs
blunt trauma of internal organs
bruise of internal organs
concussion injuries (except cerebral) of internal organs
crushing of internal organs
hematoma of internal organs
laceration of internal organs
puncture of internal organs
tear of internal organs
traumatic rupture of internal organs

Excludes
concussion NOS (850.0–850.9)
flail chest (807.4)
foreign body entering through orifice (930.0–939.9)
injury to blood vessels (901.0–902.9)

Note: The description "with open wound," used in the fourth-digit subdivisions, includes those with mention of infection or foreign body.

● 860 Traumatic pneumothorax and hemothorax
  860.0 Pneumothorax without mention of open wound into thorax
    Coding Clinic: 1993, Q2, P4-5
  860.1 Pneumothorax with open wound into thorax
    Coding Clinic: 1995, Q3, P17; 1993, Q2, P4-5
  860.2 Hemothorax without mention of open wound into thorax
  860.3 Hemothorax with open wound into thorax
    Coding Clinic: 1995, Q3, P17
  860.4 Pneumohemothorax without mention of open wound into thorax
  860.5 Pneumohemothorax with open wound into thorax
    Coding Clinic: 1995, Q3, P17

● 861 Injury to heart and lung
  Excludes injury to blood vessels of thorax (901.0–901.9)
  Coding Clinic: 1992, Q1, P9-10
  ● 861.0 Heart, without mention of open wound into thorax
    861.00 Unspecified injury
    861.01 Contusion
      Cardiac contusion
      Myocardial contusion
    861.02 Laceration without penetration of heart chambers
    861.03 Laceration with penetration of heart chambers
  ● 861.1 Heart, with open wound into thorax
    861.10 Unspecified injury
    861.11 Contusion
    861.12 Laceration without penetration of heart chambers
    861.13 Laceration with penetration of heart chambers
  ● 861.2 Lung, without mention of open wound into thorax
    861.20 Unspecified injury
    861.21 Contusion
    861.22 Laceration
  ● 861.3 Lung, with open wound into thorax
    861.30 Unspecified injury
    861.31 Contusion
    861.32 Laceration

● 862 Injury to other and unspecified intrathoracic organs
  Excludes injury to blood vessels of thorax (901.0–901.9)
  862.0 Diaphragm, without mention of open wound into cavity
  862.1 Diaphragm, with open wound into cavity
  ● 862.2 Other specified intrathoracic organs, without mention of open wound into cavity
    862.21 Bronchus
    862.22 Esophagus
    862.29 Other
      Pleura
      Thymus gland
  ● 862.3 Other specified intrathoracic organs, with open wound into cavity
    862.31 Bronchus
    862.32 Esophagus
    862.39 Other
  862.8 Multiple and unspecified intrathoracic organs, without mention of open wound into cavity
    Crushed chest
    Multiple intrathoracic organs
  862.9 Multiple and unspecified intrathoracic organs, with open wound into cavity

● 863 Injury to gastrointestinal tract
  Trauma to any structure from the stomach to the anus
  Excludes anal sphincter laceration during delivery (664.2)
    bile duct (868.0–868.1 with fifth-digit 2)
    gallbladder (868.0–868.1 with fifth-digit 2)
  863.0 Stomach, without mention of open wound into cavity
  863.1 Stomach, with open wound into cavity
  ● 863.2 Small intestine, without mention of open wound into cavity
    863.20 Small intestine, unspecified site
    863.21 Duodenum
    863.29 Other
  ● 863.3 Small intestine, with open wound into cavity
    863.30 Small intestine, unspecified site
    863.31 Duodenum
    863.39 Other
  ● 863.4 Colon or rectum, without mention of open wound into cavity
    863.40 Colon, unspecified site
    863.41 Ascending [right] colon
    863.42 Transverse colon
    863.43 Descending [left] colon
    863.44 Sigmoid colon
    863.45 Rectum
    863.46 Multiple sites in colon and rectum
    863.49 Other
  ● 863.5 Colon or rectum, with open wound into cavity
    863.50 Colon, unspecified site
    863.51 Ascending [right] colon
    863.52 Transverse colon
    863.53 Descending [left] colon
    863.54 Sigmoid colon
    863.55 Rectum
    863.56 Multiple sites in colon and rectum
    863.59 Other
  ● 863.8 Other and unspecified gastrointestinal sites, without mention of open wound into cavity
    863.80 Gastrointestinal tract, unspecified site
    863.81 Pancreas, head
    863.82 Pancreas, body
    863.83 Pancreas, tail
    863.84 Pancreas, multiple and unspecified sites
    863.85 Appendix
    863.89 Other
      Intestine NOS

- **863.9** Other and unspecified gastrointestinal sites, with open wound into cavity
  - 863.90 Gastrointestinal tract, unspecified site
  - 863.91 Pancreas, head
  - 863.92 Pancreas, body
  - 863.93 Pancreas, tail
  - 863.94 Pancreas, multiple and unspecified sites
  - 863.95 Appendix
  - 863.99 Other

- **864 Injury to liver**

  The following fifth-digit subclassification is for use with category 864:

  - 0 unspecified injury
  - 1 hematoma and contusion
  - 2 laceration, minor
    Laceration involving capsule only, or without significant involvement of hepatic parenchyma [i.e., less than 1 cm deep]
  - 3 laceration, moderate
    Laceration involving parenchyma but without major disruption of parenchyma [i.e., less than 10 cm long and less than 3 cm deep]
  - 4 laceration, major
    Laceration with significant disruption of hepatic parenchyma [i.e., 10 cm long and 3 cm deep]
    Multiple moderate lacerations, with or without hematoma
    Stellate lacerations of liver
  - 5 laceration, unspecified
  - 9 other

  - **864.0** Without mention of open wound into cavity [0-5,9]
  - **864.1** With open wound into cavity [0-5,9]

- **865 Injury to spleen**

  The following fifth-digit subclassification is for use with category 865:

  - 0 unspecified injury
  - 1 hematoma without rupture of capsule
  - 2 capsular tears, without major disruption of parenchyma
  - 3 laceration extending into parenchyma
  - 4 massive parenchymal disruption
  - 9 other

  - **865.0** Without mention of open wound into cavity [0-4,9]
  - **865.1** With open wound into cavity [0-4,9]

- **866 Injury to kidney**

  The following fifth-digit subclassification is for use with category 866:

  - 0 unspecified injury
  - 1 hematoma without rupture of capsule
  - 2 laceration
  - 3 complete disruption of kidney parenchyma

  Excludes *acute kidney injury (nontraumatic) (584.9)*

  - **866.0** Without mention of open wound into cavity [0-3]
    Coding Clinic: 2008, Q4, P192-193
  - **866.1** With open wound into cavity [0-3]

- **867 Injury to pelvic organs**

  Excludes *injury during delivery (664.0–665.9)*

  - **867.0** Bladder and urethra, without mention of open wound into cavity
    Coding Clinic: 2009, Q1, P8; 1985, Nov-Dec, P15; 1984, Nov-Dec, P15
  - **867.1** Bladder and urethra, with open wound into cavity
    Coding Clinic: 1984, Nov-Dec, P12
  - **867.2** Ureter, without mention of open wound into cavity
  - **867.3** Ureter, with open wound into cavity
  - **867.4** Uterus, without mention of open wound into cavity
  - **867.5** Uterus, with open wound into cavity
  - **867.6** Other specified pelvic organs, without mention of open wound into cavity
    - Fallopian tube
    - Ovary
    - Prostate
    - Seminal vesicle
    - Vas deferens
  - **867.7** Other specified pelvic organs, with open wound into cavity
  - **867.8** Unspecified pelvic organ, without mention of open wound into cavity
  - **867.9** Unspecified pelvic organ, with open wound into cavity

- **868 Injury to other intra-abdominal organs**

  The following fifth-digit subclassification is for use with category 868:

  - 0 unspecified intra-abdominal organ
  - 1 adrenal gland
  - 2 bile duct and gallbladder
  - 3 peritoneum
  - 4 retroperitoneum
  - 9 other and multiple intra-abdominal organs

  - **868.0** Without mention of open wound into cavity [0-4,9]
  - **868.1** With open wound into cavity [0-4,9]

- **869 Internal injury to unspecified or ill-defined organs**

  Includes internal injury NOS
  multiple internal injury NOS

  - **869.0** Without mention of open wound into cavity
  - **869.1** With open wound into cavity

OPEN WOUNDS (870–897)

Includes
- animal bite
- avulsion
- cut
- laceration
- puncture wound
- traumatic amputation

Excludes
- *burn (940.0–949.5)*
- *crushing (925–929.9)*
- *puncture of internal organs (860.0–869.1)*
- *superficial injury (910.0–919.9)*
- *that incidental to:*
  - *dislocation (830.0–839.9)*
  - *fracture (800.0–829.1)*
  - *internal injury (860.0–869.1)*
  - *intracranial injury (851.0–854.1)*

Note: The description "complicated" used in the fourth-digit subdivisions includes those with mention of delayed healing, delayed treatment, foreign body, or infection.

OPEN WOUND OF HEAD, NECK, AND TRUNK (870–879)

- **870 Open wound of ocular adnexa**
  - **870.0** Laceration of skin of eyelid and periocular area
  - **870.1** Laceration of eyelid, full-thickness, not involving lacrimal passages
  - **870.2** Laceration of eyelid involving lacrimal passages
  - **870.3** Penetrating wound of orbit, without mention of foreign body
  - **870.4** Penetrating wound of orbit with foreign body
    Excludes *retained (old) foreign body in orbit (376.6)*
  - **870.8** Other specified open wounds of ocular adnexa
  - **870.9** Unspecified open wound of ocular adnexa

- **871 Open wound of eyeball**
  - Excludes: 2nd cranial nerve [optic] injury (950.0–950.9)
    3rd cranial nerve [oculomotor] injury (951.0)
  - 871.0 Ocular laceration without prolapse of intraocular tissue
    Coding Clinic: 1996, Q3, P7
  - 871.1 Ocular laceration with prolapse or exposure of intraocular tissue
  - 871.2 Rupture of eye with partial loss of intraocular tissue
  - 871.3 Avulsion of eye
    Traumatic enucleation
  - 871.4 Unspecified laceration of eye
  - 871.5 Penetration of eyeball with magnetic foreign body
    Excludes: retained (old) magnetic foreign body in globe (360.50–360.59)
  - 871.6 Penetration of eyeball with (nonmagnetic) foreign body
    Excludes: retained (old) (nonmagnetic) foreign body in globe (360.60–360.69)
  - 871.7 Unspecified ocular penetration
  - 871.9 Unspecified open wound of eyeball
- **872 Open wound of ear**
  - 872.0 External ear, without mention of complication
    - 872.00 External ear, unspecified site
    - 872.01 Auricle, ear
      Pinna
    - 872.02 Auditory canal
  - 872.1 External ear, complicated
    - 872.10 External ear, unspecified site
    - 872.11 Auricle, ear
    - 872.12 Auditory canal
  - 872.6 Other specified parts of ear, without mention of complication
    - 872.61 Ear drum
      Drumhead Tympanic membrane
    - 872.62 Ossicles
    - 872.63 Eustachian tube
    - 872.64 Cochlea
    - 872.69 Other and multiple sites
  - 872.7 Other specified parts of ear, complicated
    - 872.71 Ear drum
    - 872.72 Ossicles
    - 872.73 Eustachian tube
    - 872.74 Cochlea
    - 872.79 Other and multiple sites
  - 872.8 Ear, part unspecified, without mention of complication
    Ear NOS
  - 872.9 Ear, part unspecified, complicated
- **873 Other open wound of head**
  - 873.0 Scalp, without mention of complication
  - 873.1 Scalp, complicated
  - 873.2 Nose, without mention of complication
    - 873.20 Nose, unspecified site
    - 873.21 Nasal septum
    - 873.22 Nasal cavity
    - 873.23 Nasal sinus
    - 873.29 Multiple sites
  - 873.3 Nose, complicated
    - 873.30 Nose, unspecified site
    - 873.31 Nasal septum
    - 873.32 Nasal cavity
    - 873.33 Nasal sinus
    - 873.39 Multiple sites
  - 873.4 Face, without mention of complication
    - 873.40 Face, unspecified site
    - 873.41 Cheek
    - 873.42 Forehead
      Eyebrow
      Coding Clinic: 1996, Q4, P43-44
    - 873.43 Lip
    - 873.44 Jaw
    - 873.49 Other and multiple sites
  - 873.5 Face, complicated
    - 873.50 Face, unspecified site
    - 873.51 Cheek
    - 873.52 Forehead
    - 873.53 Lip
    - 873.54 Jaw
    - 873.59 Other and multiple sites
  - 873.6 Internal structures of mouth, without mention of complication
    - 873.60 Mouth, unspecified site
    - 873.61 Buccal mucosa
    - 873.62 Gum (alveolar process)
    - 873.63 Tooth (broken) (fractured) (due to trauma)
      Excludes: cracked tooth (521.81)
      Coding Clinic: 2004, Q1, P17
    - 873.64 Tongue and floor of mouth
    - 873.65 Palate
    - 873.69 Other and multiple sites
  - 873.7 Internal structures of mouth, complicated
    - 873.70 Mouth, unspecified site
    - 873.71 Buccal mucosa
    - 873.72 Gum (alveolar process)
    - 873.73 Tooth (broken) (fractured) (due to trauma)
      Excludes: cracked tooth (521.81)
      Coding Clinic: 2004, Q1, P17
    - 873.74 Tongue and floor of mouth
    - 873.75 Palate
    - 873.79 Other and multiple sites
  - 873.8 Other and unspecified open wound of head without mention of complication
    Head NOS
  - 873.9 Other and unspecified open wound of head, complicated
- **874 Open wound of neck**
  - 874.0 Larynx and trachea, without mention of complication
    - 874.00 Larynx with trachea
    - 874.01 Larynx
    - 874.02 Trachea
  - 874.1 Larynx and trachea, complicated
    - 874.10 Larynx with trachea
    - 874.11 Larynx
    - 874.12 Trachea
  - 874.2 Thyroid gland, without mention of complication
  - 874.3 Thyroid gland, complicated
  - 874.4 Pharynx, without mention of complication
    Cervical esophagus
  - 874.5 Pharynx, complicated
  - 874.8 Other and unspecified parts, without mention of complication
    Nape of neck Throat NOS
    Supraclavicular region
  - 874.9 Other and unspecified parts, complicated

875-887.2 ICD-9-CM

- **875 Open wound of chest (wall)**
  Excludes *open wound into thoracic cavity (860.0–862.9)*
  traumatic pneumothorax and hemothorax (860.1, 860.3, 860.5)
  Coding Clinic: 1995, Q3, P17
  - 875.0 Without mention of complication
  - 875.1 Complicated
- **876 Open wound of back**
  Includes loin
  lumbar region
  Excludes *open wound into thoracic cavity (860.0–862.9)*
  traumatic pneumothorax and hemothorax (860.1, 860.3, 860.5)
  Coding Clinic: 1995, Q3, P17
  - 876.0 Without mention of complication
    Coding Clinic: 1993, Q2, P4-5
  - 876.1 Complicated
- **877 Open wound of buttock**
  Includes sacroiliac region
  - 877.0 Without mention of complication
  - 877.1 Complicated
- **878 Open wound of genital organs (external), including traumatic amputation**
  Excludes *injury during delivery (664.0–665.9)*
  internal genital organs (867.0–867.9)
  - 878.0 Penis, without mention of complication
  - 878.1 Penis, complicated
  - 878.2 Scrotum and testes, without mention of complication
  - 878.3 Scrotum and testes, complicated
  - 878.4 Vulva, without mention of complication
    Labium (majus) (minus)
  - 878.5 Vulva, complicated
  - 878.6 Vagina, without mention of complication
  - 878.7 Vagina, complicated
  - 878.8 Other and unspecified parts, without mention of complication
  - 878.9 Other and unspecified parts, complicated
- **879 Open wound of other and unspecified sites, except limbs**
  - 879.0 Breast, without mention of complication
  - 879.1 Breast, complicated
  - 879.2 Abdominal wall, anterior, without mention of complication
    Abdominal wall NOS   Pubic region
    Epigastric region   Umbilical region
    Hypogastric region
  - 879.3 Abdominal wall, anterior, complicated
  - 879.4 Abdominal wall, lateral, without mention of complication
    Flank   Iliac (region)
    Groin Inguinal region
    Hypochondrium
  - 879.5 Abdominal wall, lateral, complicated
  - 879.6 Other and unspecified parts of trunk, without mention of complication
    Pelvic region   Trunk NOS
    Perineum
  - 879.7 Other and unspecified parts of trunk, complicated
  - 879.8 Open wound(s) (multiple) of unspecified site(s) without mention of complication
    Multiple open wounds NOS
    Open wound NOS
  - 879.9 Open wound(s) (multiple) of unspecified site(s), complicated

OPEN WOUND OF UPPER LIMB (880–887)

- **880 Open wound of shoulder and upper arm**
  The following fifth-digit subclassification is for use with category 880:

0	shoulder region
1	scapular region
2	axillary region
3	upper arm
9	multiple sites

  - 880.0 Without mention of complication
    [0-3,9]
  - 880.1 Complicated
    [0-3,9]   Coding Clinic: 2006, Q2, P7
  - 880.2 With tendon involvement
    [0-3,9]
- **881 Open wound of elbow, forearm, and wrist**
  The following fifth-digit subclassification is for use with category 881:

0	forearm
1	elbow
2	wrist

  - 881.0 Without mention of complication
    [0-2]
  - 881.1 Complicated
    [0-2]
  - 881.2 With tendon involvement
    [0-2]
- **882 Open wound of hand except finger(s) alone**
  - 882.0 Without mention of complication
  - 882.1 Complicated
    Coding Clinic: 2008, Q4, P149-152
  - 882.2 With tendon involvement
- **883 Open wound of finger(s)**
  Includes fingernail
  thumb (nail)
  - 883.0 Without mention of complication
    Avulsion of fingernail reported with this code
  - 883.1 Complicated
  - 883.2 With tendon involvement
- **884 Multiple and unspecified open wound of upper limb**
  Includes arm NOS
  multiple sites of one upper limb
  upper limb NOS
  - 884.0 Without mention of complication
  - 884.1 Complicated
  - 884.2 With tendon involvement
- **885 Traumatic amputation of thumb (complete) (partial)**
  Includes thumb(s) (with finger(s) of either hand)
  - 885.0 Without mention of complication
    Coding Clinic: 2003, Q1, P7
  - 885.1 Complicated
- **886 Traumatic amputation of other finger(s) (complete) (partial)**
  Includes finger(s) of one or both hands, without mention of thumb(s)
  - 886.0 Without mention of complication
  - 886.1 Complicated
- **887 Traumatic amputation of arm and hand (complete) (partial)**
  - 887.0 Unilateral, below elbow, without mention of complication
  - 887.1 Unilateral, below elbow, complicated
  - 887.2 Unilateral, at or above elbow, without mention of complication

- **887.3** Unilateral, at or above elbow, complicated
- **887.4** Unilateral, level not specified, without mention of complication
- **887.5** Unilateral, level not specified, complicated
- **887.6** Bilateral [any level], without mention of complication
  One hand and other arm
- **887.7** Bilateral [any level], complicated

OPEN WOUND OF LOWER LIMB (890–897)

- **890** Open wound of hip and thigh
  - **890.0** Without mention of complication
  - **890.1** Complicated
  - **890.2** With tendon involvement

- **891** Open wound of knee, leg [except thigh], and ankle
  - **Includes:** leg NOS
    multiple sites of leg, except thigh
  - **Excludes:** that of thigh (890.0–890.2)
    with multiple sites of lower limb (894.0–894.2)
  - **891.0** Without mention of complication
  - **891.1** Complicated
  - **891.2** With tendon involvement

- **892** Open wound of foot except toe(s) alone
  - **Includes:** heel
  - **892.0** Without mention of complication
  - **892.1** Complicated
    Coding Clinic: 1985, Sept-Oct, P10
  - **892.2** With tendon involvement

- **893** Open wound of toe(s)
  - **Includes:** toenail
  - **893.0** Without mention of complication
  - **893.1** Complicated
    Coding Clinic: 2008, Q4, P69-73
  - **893.2** With tendon involvement

- **894** Multiple and unspecified open wound of lower limb
  - **Includes:** lower limb NOS
    multiple sites of one lower limb, with thigh
  - **894.0** Without mention of complication
  - **894.1** Complicated
  - **894.2** With tendon involvement

- **895** Traumatic amputation of toe(s) (complete) (partial)
  - **Includes:** toe(s) of one or both feet
  - **895.0** Without mention of complication
  - **895.1** Complicated

- **896** Traumatic amputation of foot (complete) (partial)
  - **896.0** Unilateral, without mention of complication
  - **896.1** Unilateral, complicated
  - **896.2** Bilateral, without mention of complication
    - **Excludes:** one foot and other leg (897.6–897.7)
  - **896.3** Bilateral, complicated

- **897** Traumatic amputation of leg(s) (complete) (partial)
  - **897.0** Unilateral, below knee, without mention of complication
  - **897.1** Unilateral, below knee, complicated
  - **897.2** Unilateral, at or above knee, without mention of complication
  - **897.3** Unilateral, at or above knee, complicated
  - **897.4** Unilateral, level not specified, without mention of complication
  - **897.5** Unilateral, level not specified, complicated
  - **897.6** Bilateral [any level], without mention of complication
    One foot and other leg
  - **897.7** Bilateral [any level], complicated

INJURY TO BLOOD VESSELS (900–904)

Includes: arterial hematoma of blood vessel, secondary to other injuries, e.g., fracture or open wound
avulsion of blood vessel, secondary to other injuries, e.g., fracture or open wound
cut of blood vessel, secondary to other injuries, e.g., fracture or open wound
laceration of blood vessel, secondary to other injuries, e.g., fracture or open wound
rupture of blood vessel, secondary to other injuries, e.g., fracture or open wound
traumatic aneurysm or fistula (arteriovenous) of blood vessel, secondary to other injuries, e.g., fracture or open wound

Excludes: accidental puncture or laceration during medical procedure (998.2)
intracranial hemorrhage following injury (851.0–854.1)

- **900** Injury to blood vessels of head and neck
  - **900.0** Carotid artery
    - **900.00** Carotid artery, unspecified
    - **900.01** Common carotid artery
    - **900.02** External carotid artery
    - **900.03** Internal carotid artery
  - **900.1** Internal jugular vein
  - **900.8** Other specified blood vessels of head and neck
    - **900.81** External jugular vein
      Jugular vein NOS
    - **900.82** Multiple blood vessels of head and neck
    - **900.89** Other
  - **900.9** Unspecified blood vessel of head and neck

- **901** Injury to blood vessels of thorax
  - **Excludes:** traumatic hemothorax (860.2–860.5)
  - **901.0** Thoracic aorta
  - **901.1** Innominate and subclavian arteries
  - **901.2** Superior vena cava
  - **901.3** Innominate and subclavian veins
  - **901.4** Pulmonary blood vessels
    - **901.40** Pulmonary vessel(s), unspecified
    - **901.41** Pulmonary artery
    - **901.42** Pulmonary vein
  - **901.8** Other specified blood vessels of thorax
    - **901.81** Intercostal artery or vein
    - **901.82** Internal mammary artery or vein
    - **901.83** Multiple blood vessels of thorax
    - **901.89** Other
      Azygos vein
      Hemiazygos vein
  - **901.9** Unspecified blood vessel of thorax

- **902** Injury to blood vessels of abdomen and pelvis
  - **902.0** Abdominal aorta
  - **902.1** Inferior vena cava
    - **902.10** Inferior vena cava, unspecified
    - **902.11** Hepatic veins
    - **902.19** Other
  - **902.2** Celiac and mesenteric arteries
    - **902.20** Celiac and mesenteric arteries, unspecified
    - **902.21** Gastric artery
    - **902.22** Hepatic artery
    - **902.23** Splenic artery
    - **902.24** Other specified branches of celiac axis
    - **902.25** Superior mesenteric artery (trunk)
    - **902.26** Primary branches of superior mesenteric artery
      Ileo-colic artery
    - **902.27** Inferior mesenteric artery
    - **902.29** Other

- 902.3 Portal and splenic veins
  - 902.31 Superior mesenteric vein and primary subdivisions
    - Ileo-colic vein
  - 902.32 Inferior mesenteric vein
  - 902.33 Portal vein
  - 902.34 Splenic vein
  - 902.39 Other
    - Cystic vein
    - Gastric vein
- 902.4 Renal blood vessels
  - 902.40 Renal vessel(s), unspecified
  - 902.41 Renal artery
  - 902.42 Renal vein
  - 902.49 Other
    - Suprarenal arteries
- 902.5 Iliac blood vessels
  - 902.50 Iliac vessel(s), unspecified
  - 902.51 Hypogastric artery
  - 902.52 Hypogastric vein
  - 902.53 Iliac artery
  - 902.54 Iliac vein
  - 902.55 Uterine artery
  - 902.56 Uterine vein
  - 902.59 Other
- 902.8 Other specified blood vessels of abdomen and pelvis
  - 902.81 Ovarian artery
  - 902.82 Ovarian vein
  - 902.87 Multiple blood vessels of abdomen and pelvis
  - 902.89 Other
- 902.9 Unspecified blood vessel of abdomen and pelvis

- 903 Injury to blood vessels of upper extremity
  - 903.0 Axillary blood vessels
    - 903.00 Axillary vessel(s), unspecified
    - 903.01 Axillary artery
    - 903.02 Axillary vein
  - 903.1 Brachial blood vessels
  - 903.2 Radial blood vessels
  - 903.3 Ulnar blood vessels
  - 903.4 Palmar artery
  - 903.5 Digital blood vessels
  - 903.8 Other specified blood vessels of upper extremity
    - Multiple blood vessels of upper extremity
  - 903.9 Unspecified blood vessel of upper extremity

- 904 Injury to blood vessels of lower extremity and unspecified sites
  - 904.0 Common femoral artery
    - Femoral artery above profunda origin
    - *Profunda = deep and posterior*
  - 904.1 Superficial femoral artery
  - 904.2 Femoral veins
  - 904.3 Saphenous veins
    - Saphenous vein (greater) (lesser)
  - 904.4 Popliteal blood vessels
    - 904.40 Popliteal vessel(s), unspecified
    - 904.41 Popliteal artery
    - 904.42 Popliteal vein
  - 904.5 Tibial blood vessels
    - 904.50 Tibial vessel(s), unspecified
    - 904.51 Anterior tibial artery
    - 904.52 Anterior tibial vein
    - 904.53 Posterior tibial artery
    - 904.54 Posterior tibial vein
  - 904.6 Deep plantar blood vessels
  - 904.7 Other specified blood vessels of lower extremity
    - Multiple blood vessels of lower extremity
  - 904.8 Unspecified blood vessel of lower extremity
  - 904.9 Unspecified site
    - Injury to blood vessel NOS

LATE EFFECTS OF INJURIES, POISONINGS, TOXIC EFFECTS, AND OTHER EXTERNAL CAUSES (905–909)

Note: These categories are to be used to indicate conditions classifiable to 800–999 as the cause of late effects, which are themselves classified elsewhere. The "late effects" include those specified as such, or as sequelae, which may occur at any time after the acute injury.

- 905 Late effects of musculoskeletal and connective tissue injuries
  - 905.0 Late effect of fracture of skull and face bones
    - Late effect of injury classifiable to 800–804
    - Coding Clinic: 1997, Q3, P12-13
  - 905.1 Late effect of fracture of spine and trunk without mention of spinal cord lesion
    - Late effects of injury classifiable to 805, 807–809
    - Coding Clinic: 2007, Q1, P20-21
  - 905.2 Late effect of fracture of upper extremities
    - Late effect of injury classifiable to 810–819
  - 905.3 Late effect of fracture of neck of femur
    - Late effect of injury classifiable to 820
  - 905.4 Late effect of fracture of lower extremities
    - Late effect of injury classifiable to 821–827
    - Coding Clinic: 1995, Q1, P10; 1994, Q2, P7
  - 905.5 Late effect of fracture of multiple and unspecified bones
    - Late effect of injury classifiable to 828–829
  - 905.6 Late effect of dislocation
    - Late effect of injury classifiable to 830–839
  - 905.7 Late effect of sprain and strain without mention of tendon injury
    - Late effect of injury classifiable to 840–848, except tendon injury
  - 905.8 Late effect of tendon injury
    - Late effect of tendon injury due to:
      - open wound [injury classifiable to 880–884 with .2, 890–894 with .2]
      - sprain and strain [injury classifiable to 840–848]
    - Coding Clinic: 1989, Q2, P15; Q2, P13
  - 905.9 Late effect of traumatic amputation
    - Late effect of injury classifiable to 885–887, 895–897
    - Excludes: late amputation stump complication (997.60–997.69)

- 906 Late effects of injuries to skin and subcutaneous tissues
  - 906.0 Late effect of open wound of head, neck, and trunk
    - Late effect of injury classifiable to 870–879
  - 906.1 Late effect of open wound of extremities without mention of tendon injury
    - Late effect of injury classifiable to 880–884, 890–894 except .2
    - Coding Clinic: 1993, 5th Issue, P3
  - 906.2 Late effect of superficial injury
    - Late effect of injury classifiable to 910–919
  - 906.3 Late effect of contusion
    - Late effect of injury classifiable to 920–924
  - 906.4 Late effect of crushing
    - Late effect of injury classifiable to 925–929
  - 906.5 Late effect of burn of eye, face, head, and neck
    - Late effect of injury classifiable to 940–941
    - Coding Clinic: 2004, Q4, P75-76
  - 906.6 Late effect of burn of wrist and hand
    - Late effect of injury classifiable to 944
  - 906.7 Late effect of burn of other extremities
    - Late effect of injury classifiable to 943 or 945

906.8 Late effect of burns of other specified sites
Late effect of injury classifiable to 942, 946–947

906.9 Late effect of burn of unspecified site
Late effect of injury classifiable to 948–949

OGCR Section I.C.17.c.7
Encounters for the treatment of the late effects of burns (i.e., scars or joint contractures) should be coded to the residual condition (sequelae) followed by the appropriate late effect code (906.5–906.9). A late effect E code may also be used, if desired.

907 Late effects of injuries to the nervous system

907.0 Late effect of intracranial injury without mention of skull fracture
Late effect of injury classifiable to 850–854
Coding Clinic: 2012, Q3, P20; 2011, Q4, P97; 2010, Q4, P97; 2009, Q4, P120; 2008, Q4, P102-109; 2003, Q4, P103-104; 1987, Nov-Dec, P12

907.1 Late effect of injury to cranial nerve
Late effect of injury classifiable to 950–951

907.2 Late effect of spinal cord injury
Late effect of injury classifiable to 806, 952
Coding Clinic: 2003, Q4, P103-104; 1998, Q4, P37-38; 1994, Q3, P4

907.3 Late effect of injury to nerve root(s), spinal plexus(es), and other nerves of trunk
Late effect of injury classifiable to 953–954
Coding Clinic: 2007, Q2, P13-15

907.4 Late effect of injury to peripheral nerve of shoulder girdle and upper limb
Late effect of injury classifiable to 955

907.5 Late effect of injury to peripheral nerve of pelvic girdle and lower limb
Late effect of injury classifiable to 956

907.9 Late effect of injury to other and unspecified nerve
Late effect of injury classifiable to 957

908 Late effects of other and unspecified injuries

908.0 Late effect of internal injury to chest
Late effect of injury classifiable to 860–862

908.1 Late effect of internal injury to intra-abdominal organs
Late effect of injury classifiable to 863–866, 868

908.2 Late effect of internal injury to other internal organs
Late effect of injury classifiable to 867 or 869

908.3 Late effect of injury to blood vessel of head, neck, and extremities
Late effect of injury classifiable to 900, 903–904

908.4 Late effect of injury to blood vessel of thorax, abdomen, and pelvis
Late effect of injury classifiable to 901–902

908.5 Late effect of foreign body in orifice
Late effect of injury classifiable to 930–939

908.6 Late effect of certain complications of trauma
Late effect of complications classifiable to 958

908.9 Late effect of unspecified injury
Late effect of injury classifiable to 959
Coding Clinic: 2000, Q3, P4

909 Late effects of other and unspecified external causes

909.0 Late effect of poisoning due to drug, medicinal or biological substance
Late effect of conditions classifiable to 960–979
Excludes Late effect of adverse effect of drug, medicinal or biological substance (909.5)
Coding Clinic: 2003, Q4, P103-104; 1984, Sept-Oct, P16

909.1 Late effect of toxic effects of nonmedical substances
Late effect of conditions classifiable to 980–989

909.2 Late effect of radiation
Late effect of conditions classifiable to 990
Coding Clinic: 1984, Nov-Dec, P19

909.3 Late effect of complications of surgical and medical care
Late effect of conditions classifiable to 996–999
Coding Clinic: 1993, Q1, P29

909.4 Late effect of certain other external causes
Late effect of conditions classifiable to 991–994

909.5 Late effect of adverse effect of drug, medicinal or biological substance
Excludes late effect of poisoning due to drug, medicinal or biological substances (909.0)

909.9 Late effect of other and unspecified external causes

SUPERFICIAL INJURY (910–919)

Excludes burn (blisters) (940.0–949.5)
contusion (920–924.9)
foreign body:
  granuloma (728.82)
  inadvertently left in operative wound (998.4)
  residual, in soft tissue (729.6)
  insect bite, venomous (989.5)
  open wound with incidental foreign body (870.0–897.7)

910 Superficial injury of face, neck, and scalp except eye
Includes cheek   lip
ear   nose
gum   throat
Excludes eye and adnexa (918.0–918.9)

910.0 Abrasion or friction burn without mention of infection
910.1 Abrasion or friction burn, infected
910.2 Blister without mention of infection
910.3 Blister, infected
910.4 Insect bite, nonvenomous, without mention of infection
910.5 Insect bite, nonvenomous, infected
910.6 Superficial foreign body (splinter) without major open wound and without mention of infection
910.7 Superficial foreign body (splinter) without major open wound, infected
910.8 Other and unspecified superficial injury of face, neck, and scalp without mention of infection
910.9 Other and unspecified superficial injury of face, neck, and scalp, infected

911 Superficial injury of trunk
Includes abdominal wall   interscapular region
anus   labium (majus) (minus)
back   penis
breast   perineum
buttock   scrotum
chest wall   testis
flank   vagina
groin   vulva
Excludes hip (916.0–916.9)
scapular region (912.0–912.9)

911.0 Abrasion or friction burn without mention of infection
Coding Clinic: 2001, Q3, P10
911.1 Abrasion or friction burn, infected
911.2 Blister without mention of infection
911.3 Blister, infected
911.4 Insect bite, nonvenomous, without mention of infection
911.5 Insect bite, nonvenomous, infected
911.6 Superficial foreign body (splinter) without major open wound and without mention of infection
911.7 Superficial foreign body (splinter) without major open wound, infected
911.8 Other and unspecified superficial injury of trunk without mention of infection
911.9 Other and unspecified superficial injury of trunk, infected

● 912 **Superficial injury of shoulder and upper arm**
  Includes axilla
            scapular region
  912.0 Abrasion or friction burn without mention of infection
  912.1 Abrasion or friction burn, infected
  912.2 Blister without mention of infection
  912.3 Blister, infected
  912.4 Insect bite, nonvenomous, without mention of infection
  912.5 Insect bite, nonvenomous, infected
  912.6 Superficial foreign body (splinter) without major open wound and without mention of infection
  912.7 Superficial foreign body (splinter) without major open wound, infected
  912.8 Other and unspecified superficial injury of shoulder and upper arm without mention of infection
  912.9 Other and unspecified superficial injury of shoulder and upper arm, infected

● 913 **Superficial injury of elbow, forearm, and wrist**
  913.0 Abrasion or friction burn without mention of infection
  913.1 Abrasion or friction burn, infected
  913.2 Blister without mention of infection
  913.3 Blister, infected
  913.4 Insect bite, nonvenomous, without mention of infection
  913.5 Insect bite, nonvenomous, infected
  913.6 Superficial foreign body (splinter) without major open wound and without mention of infection
  913.7 Superficial foreign body (splinter) without major open wound, infected
  913.8 Other and unspecified superficial injury of elbow, forearm, and wrist without mention of infection
  913.9 Other and unspecified superficial injury of elbow, forearm, and wrist, infected

● 914 **Superficial injury of hand(s) except finger(s) alone**
  914.0 Abrasion or friction burn without mention of infection
  914.1 Abrasion or friction burn, infected
  914.2 Blister without mention of infection
  914.3 Blister, infected
  914.4 Insect bite, nonvenomous, without mention of infection
  914.5 Insect bite, nonvenomous, infected
  914.6 Superficial foreign body (splinter) without major open wound and without mention of infection
  914.7 Superficial foreign body (splinter) without major open wound, infected
  914.8 Other and unspecified superficial injury of hand without mention of infection
  914.9 Other and unspecified superficial injury of hand, infected

● 915 **Superficial injury of finger(s)**
  Includes fingernail
            thumb (nail)
  915.0 Abrasion or friction burn without mention of infection
  915.1 Abrasion or friction burn, infected
  915.2 Blister without mention of infection
  915.3 Blister, infected
  915.4 Insect bite, nonvenomous, without mention of infection
  915.5 Insect bite, nonvenomous, infected
  915.6 Superficial foreign body (splinter) without major open wound and without mention of infection
  915.7 Superficial foreign body (splinter) without major open wound, infected
  915.8 Other and unspecified superficial injury of fingers without mention of infection
    Coding Clinic: 2001, Q3, P10
  915.9 Other and unspecified superficial injury of fingers, infected

● 916 **Superficial injury of hip, thigh, leg, and ankle**
  916.0 Abrasion or friction burn without mention of infection
    Coding Clinic: 2000, Q4, P61
  916.1 Abrasion or friction burn, infected
  916.2 Blister without mention of infection
  916.3 Blister, infected
  916.4 Insect bite, nonvenomous, without mention of infection
  916.5 Insect bite, nonvenomous, infected
  916.6 Superficial foreign body (splinter) without major open wound and without mention of infection
  916.7 Superficial foreign body (splinter) without major open wound, infected
  916.8 Other and unspecified superficial injury of hip, thigh, leg, and ankle without mention of infection
  916.9 Other and unspecified superficial injury of hip, thigh, leg, and ankle, infected

● 917 **Superficial injury of foot and toe(s)**
  Includes heel
            toenail
  917.0 Abrasion or friction burn without mention of infection
  917.1 Abrasion or friction burn, infected
  917.2 Blister without mention of infection
  917.3 Blister, infected
  917.4 Insect bite, nonvenomous, without mention of infection
  917.5 Insect bite, nonvenomous, infected
  917.6 Superficial foreign body (splinter) without major open wound and without mention of infection
  917.7 Superficial foreign body (splinter) without major open wound, infected
  917.8 Other and unspecified superficial injury of foot and toes without mention of infection
    Coding Clinic: 2003, Q1, P13
  917.9 Other and unspecified superficial injury of foot and toes, infected
    Coding Clinic: 2003, Q1, P13

● 918 **Superficial injury of eye and adnexa**
  Excludes burn (940.0–940.9)
            foreign body on external eye (930.0–930.9)
  918.0 Eyelids and periocular area
        Abrasion
        Insect bite
        Superficial foreign body (splinter)
  918.1 Cornea
        Corneal abrasion
        Superficial laceration
    Excludes corneal injury due to contact lens (371.82)
  918.2 Conjunctiva
  918.9 Other and unspecified superficial injuries of eye
        Eye (ball) NOS

● 919 **Superficial injury of other, multiple, and unspecified sites**
  Excludes multiple sites classifiable to the same three-digit category (910.0–918.9)
  919.0 Abrasion or friction burn without mention of infection
  919.1 Abrasion or friction burn, infected
  919.2 Blister without mention of infection
  919.3 Blister, infected
  919.4 Insect bite, nonvenomous, without mention of infection
  919.5 Insect bite, nonvenomous, infected
  919.6 Superficial foreign body (splinter) without major open wound and without mention of infection
  919.7 Superficial foreign body (splinter) without major open wound, infected
  919.8 Other and unspecified superficial injury without mention of infection
  919.9 Other and unspecified superficial injury, infected

CONTUSION WITH INTACT SKIN SURFACE (920–924)

Includes bruise without fracture or open wound
hematoma without fracture or open wound

Excludes concussion (850.0–850.9)
hemarthrosis (840.0–848.9)
internal organs (860.0–869.1)
that incidental to:
    crushing injury (925–929.9)
    dislocation (830.0–839.9)
    fracture (800.0–829.1)
    internal injury (860.0–869.1)
    intracranial injury (850.0–854.1)
    nerve injury (950.0–957.9)
    open wound (870.0–897.7)

920 Contusion of face, scalp, and neck except eye(s)
Cheek   Mandibular joint area
Ear (auricle)   Nose
Gum   Throat
Lip

921 Contusion of eye and adnexa
921.0 Black eye, NOS
921.1 Contusion of eyelids and periocular area
921.2 Contusion of orbital tissues
921.3 Contusion of eyeball
Coding Clinic: 1985, July-Aug, P16
921.9 Unspecified contusion of eye
Injury of eye NOS

922 Contusion of trunk
922.0 Breast
922.1 Chest wall
922.2 Abdominal wall
Flank
Groin
922.3 Back
    922.31 Back
        Excludes interscapular region (922.33)
        Coding Clinic: 1999, Q3, P14-15
    922.32 Buttock
    922.33 Interscapular region
        Excludes scapular region (923.01)
922.4 Genital organs
Labium (majus) (minus)   Testis
Penis   Vagina
Perineum   Vulva
Scrotum
922.8 Multiple sites of trunk
922.9 Unspecified part
Trunk NOS

923 Contusion of upper limb
923.0 Shoulder and upper arm
    923.00 Shoulder region
    923.01 Scapular region
    923.02 Axillary region
    923.03 Upper arm
    923.09 Multiple sites
923.1 Elbow and forearm
    923.10 Forearm
    923.11 Elbow
923.2 Wrist and hand(s), except finger(s) alone
    923.20 Hand(s)
    923.21 Wrist
923.3 Finger
Fingernail   Thumb (nail)
923.8 Multiple sites of upper limb
923.9 Unspecified part of upper limb
Arm NOS

924 Contusion of lower limb and of other and unspecified sites
924.0 Hip and thigh
    924.00 Thigh
        Coding Clinic: 2009, Q1, P10x2
    924.01 Hip
924.1 Knee and lower leg
    924.10 Lower leg
    924.11 Knee
924.2 Ankle and foot, excluding toe(s)
    924.20 Foot
        Heel
    924.21 Ankle
924.3 Toe
Toenail
924.4 Multiple sites of lower limb
924.5 Unspecified part of lower limb
Leg NOS
924.8 Multiple sites, not elsewhere classified
Coding Clinic: 2003, Q1, P7
924.9 Unspecified site

CRUSHING INJURY (925–929)

Use additional code to identify any associated injuries, such as:
    fractures (800–829)
    internal injuries (860.0–869.1)
    intracranial injury (850.0–854.1)

925 Crushing injury of face, scalp, and neck
Cheek   Pharynx
Ear   Throat
Larynx
Coding Clinic: 2003, Q4, P76-78
925.1 Crushing injury of face and scalp
Cheek   Ear
925.2 Crushing injury of neck
Larynx   Pharynx
Throat

926 Crushing injury of trunk
Coding Clinic: 2003, Q4, P76-78
926.0 External genitalia
Labium (majus) (minus)
Penis
Scrotum
Testis
Vulva
926.1 Other specified sites
    926.11 Back
    926.12 Buttock
    926.19 Other
        Breast
926.8 Multiple sites of trunk
926.9 Unspecified site
Trunk NOS

927 Crushing injury of upper limb
927.0 Shoulder and upper arm
    927.00 Shoulder region
    927.01 Scapular region
    927.02 Axillary region
    927.03 Upper arm
    927.09 Multiple sites
927.1 Elbow and forearm
    927.10 Forearm
    927.11 Elbow
927.2 Wrist and hand(s), except finger(s) alone
    927.20 Hand(s)
    927.21 Wrist

927.3 Finger(s)
Coding Clinic: 2003, Q4, P76-78
927.8 Multiple sites of upper limb
927.9 Unspecified site
Arm NOS

● 928 Crushing injury of lower limb
Coding Clinic: 2003, Q4, P76-78
● 928.0 Hip and thigh
928.00 Thigh
928.01 Hip
● 928.1 Knee and lower leg
928.10 Lower leg
928.11 Knee
● 928.2 Ankle and foot, excluding toe(s) alone
928.20 Foot
Heel
928.21 Ankle
928.3 Toe(s)
928.8 Multiple sites of lower limb
928.9 Unspecified site
Leg NOS

● 929 Crushing injury of multiple and unspecified sites
Coding Clinic: 2003, Q4, P76-78
929.0 Multiple sites, not elsewhere classified
929.9 Unspecified site

EFFECTS OF FOREIGN BODY ENTERING THROUGH ORIFICE (930–939)

Excludes *foreign body:*
granuloma (728.82)
inadvertently left in operative wound (998.4, 998.7)
in open wound (800–839, 851–897)
residual, in soft tissues (729.6)
superficial without major open wound (910–919 with .6 or .7)

● 930 Foreign body on external eye
Excludes *foreign body in penetrating wound of:*
eyeball (871.5–871.6)
retained (old) (360.5–360.6)
ocular adnexa (870.4)
retained (old) (376.6)
930.0 Corneal foreign body
930.1 Foreign body in conjunctival sac
930.2 Foreign body in lacrimal punctum
930.8 Other and combined sites
930.9 Unspecified site
External eye NOS

931 Foreign body in ear
Auditory canal
Auricle

932 Foreign body in nose
Nasal sinus
Nostril

● 933 Foreign body in pharynx and larynx
933.0 Pharynx
Nasopharynx
Throat NOS
933.1 Larynx
Asphyxia due to foreign body
Choking due to:
food (regurgitated)
phlegm

● 934 Foreign body in trachea, bronchus, and lung
934.0 Trachea
934.1 Main bronchus
934.8 Other specified parts
Bronchioles
Lung
934.9 Respiratory tree, unspecified
Inhalation of liquid or vomitus, lower respiratory tract NOS

● 935 Foreign body in mouth, esophagus, and stomach
935.0 Mouth
935.1 Esophagus
Coding Clinic: 1988, Q1, P13
935.2 Stomach
Coding Clinic: 1985, Jan-Feb, P14-15

936 Foreign body in intestine and colon

937 Foreign body in anus and rectum
Rectosigmoid (junction)

938 Foreign body in digestive system, unspecified
Alimentary tract NOS
Swallowed foreign body

● 939 Foreign body in genitourinary tract
939.0 Bladder and urethra
939.1 Uterus, any part
Excludes *intrauterine contraceptive device: complications from (996.32, 996.65) presence of (V45.51)*
939.2 Vulva and vagina
939.3 Penis
939.9 Unspecified site

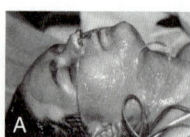
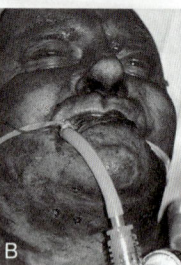

Figure 17–14 **A.** Second-degree burn. **B.** Third-degree burn. (From Cummings: Otolaryngology: Head & Neck Surgery, ed 4, Mosby, 2005)

OGCR Section I.C.17.c
Current burns (940-948) are classified by depth, extent and by agent (E code). Burns are classified by depth as first degree (erythema), second degree (blistering), and third degree (full-thickness involvement).

OGCR Section I.C.17.c.1
Sequence first the code that reflects the highest degree of burn when more than one burn is present.

OGCR Section I.C.17.c.2
Classify burns of the same local site (three-digit category level, 940-947) but of different degrees to the subcategory identifying the highest degree recorded in the diagnosis.

BURNS (940–949)

Includes burns from:
- electrical heating appliance
- electricity
- flame
- hot object
- lightning
- radiation
- chemical burns (external) (internal)
- scalds

Excludes friction burns (910–919 with .0, .1)
sunburn (692.71, 692.76–692.77)

- **940 Burn confined to eye and adnexa**
  - 940.0 Chemical burn of eyelids and periocular area
  - 940.1 Other burns of eyelids and periocular area
  - 940.2 Alkaline chemical burn of cornea and conjunctival sac
  - 940.3 Acid chemical burn of cornea and conjunctival sac
  - 940.4 Other burn of cornea and conjunctival sac
  - 940.5 Burn with resulting rupture and destruction of eyeball
  - 940.9 Unspecified burn of eye and adnexa

- **941 Burn of face, head, and neck**

  Excludes mouth (947.0)

  The following fifth-digit subclassification is for use with category 941:

0	face and head, unspecified site
1	ear [any part]
2	eye (with other parts of face, head, and neck)
3	lip(s)
4	chin
5	nose (septum)
6	scalp [any part]
	Temple (region)
7	forehead and cheek
8	neck
9	multiple sites [except with eye] of face, head, and neck

  - 941.0 Unspecified degree
    [0-9]
  - 941.1 Erythema [first degree]
    [0-9] *Coding Clinic: 2010, Q3, P19; 2005, Q3, P10-11*
  - 941.2 Blisters, epidermal loss [second degree]
    [0-9]
  - 941.3 Full-thickness skin loss [third degree NOS]
    [0-9]
  - 941.4 Deep necrosis of underlying tissues [deep third
    [0-9] degree] without mention of loss of a body part
  - 941.5 Deep necrosis of underlying tissues [deep third
    [0-9] degree] with loss of a body part

- **942 Burn of trunk**

  Excludes scapular region (943.0–943.5 with fifth-digit 6)

  The following fifth-digit subclassification is for use with category 942:

0	trunk, unspecified site	
1	breast	
2	chest wall, excluding breast and nipple	
3	abdominal wall	
	Flank	
	Groin	
4	back [any part]	
	Buttock	
	Interscapular region	
5	genitalia	
	Labium (majus) (minus)	Scrotum
	Penis	Testis
	Perineum	Vulva
9	other and multiple sites of trunk	

  - 942.0 Unspecified degree
    [0-5,9]
  - 942.1 Erythema [first degree]
    [0-5,9]
  - 942.2 Blisters, epidermal loss [second degree]
    [0-5,9] *Coding Clinic: 1984, Nov-Dec, P13*
  - 942.3 Full-thickness skin loss [third degree NOS]
    [0-5,9]
  - 942.4 Deep necrosis of underlying tissues [deep third
    [0-5,9] degree] without mention of loss of a body part
  - 942.5 Deep necrosis of underlying tissues [deep third
    [0-5,9] degree] with loss of a body part

- **943 Burn of upper limb, except wrist and hand**

  The following fifth-digit subclassification is for use with category 943:

0	upper limb, unspecified site
1	forearm
2	elbow
3	upper arm
4	axilla
5	shoulder
6	scapular region
9	multiple sites of upper limb, except wrist and hand

  - 943.0 Unspecified degree
    [0-6,9] *Coding Clinic: 2010, Q3, P19*
  - 943.1 Erythema [first degree]
    [0-6,9]
  - 943.2 Blisters, epidermal loss [second degree]
    [0-6,9]
  - 943.3 Full-thickness skin loss [third degree NOS]
    [0-6,9]
  - 943.4 Deep necrosis of underlying tissues [deep third
    [0-6,9] degree] without mention of loss of a body part
  - 943.5 Deep necrosis of underlying tissues [deep third
    [0-6,9] degree] with loss of a body part

- **944 Burn of wrist(s) and hand(s)**

  The following fifth-digit subclassification is for use with category 944:

0	hand, unspecified site
1	single digit [finger (nail)] other than thumb
2	thumb (nail)
3	two or more digits, not including thumb
4	two or more digits including thumb
5	palm
6	back of hand
7	wrist
8	multiple sites of wrist(s) and hand(s)

  - 944.0 Unspecified degree
    [0-8]
  - 944.1 Erythema [first degree]
    [0-8]
  - 944.2 Blisters, epidermal loss [second degree]
    [0-8]
  - 944.3 Full-thickness skin loss [third degree NOS]
    [0-8]
  - 944.4 Deep necrosis of underlying tissues [deep third
    [0-8] degree] without mention of loss of a body part
  - 944.5 Deep necrosis of underlying tissues [deep third
    [0-8] degree] with loss of a body part

● 945 **Burn of lower limb(s)**
The following fifth-digit subclassification is for use with category 945:

> 0 lower limb [leg], unspecified site
> 1 toe(s) (nail)
> 2 foot
> 3 ankle
> 4 lower leg
> 5 knee
> 6 thigh [any part]
> 9 multiple sites of lower limb(s)

● ■ **945.0 Unspecified degree**
[0-6,9]
● **945.1 Erythema [first degree]**
[0-6,9]
● **945.2 Blisters, epidermal loss [second degree]**
[0-6,9]
● **945.3 Full-thickness skin loss [third degree NOS]**
[0-6,9]
● **945.4 Deep necrosis of underlying tissues [deep third**
[0-6,9] **degree] without mention of loss of a body part**
● **945.5 Deep necrosis of underlying tissues [deep third**
[0-6,9] **degree] with loss of a body part**

OGCR Section I.C.17.c.5

When coding burns, assign separate codes for each burn site. Category 946 should only be used if the location of the burns are not documented.

● 946 **Burns of multiple specified sites**
Documented as multiple sites but not specified as to location
Includes burns of sites classifiable to more than one three-digit category in 940–945
Excludes multiple burns NOS (949.0–949.5)

■ **946.0 Unspecified degree**
946.1 Erythema [first degree]
946.2 Blisters, epidermal loss [second degree]
946.3 Full-thickness skin loss [third degree NOS]
946.4 Deep necrosis of underlying tissues [deep third degree] without mention of loss of a body part
946.5 Deep necrosis of underlying tissues [deep third degree] with loss of a body part

● 947 **Burn of internal organs**
Includes burns from chemical agents (ingested)
947.0 Mouth and pharynx
Gum
Tongue
947.1 Larynx, trachea, and lung
947.2 Esophagus
947.3 Gastrointestinal tract
Colon
Rectum
Small intestine
Stomach
Coding Clinic: 2012, Q2, P8
947.4 Vagina and uterus
947.8 Other specified sites
■ **947.9 Unspecified site**

OGCR Section I.C.17.c.6

Fourth-digit identifies percentage of **total body surface** involved in a burn (all degrees). **Fifth-digit** identifies the percentage of body surface involved in **third-degree burn.** Fifth-digit zero (0) assigned when less than 10 percent or when no body surface is involved in a third-degree burn.

Category 948 is based on the classic "rule of nines" in estimating body surface involved: head and neck are assigned nine percent, each arm nine percent, each leg 18 percent, the anterior trunk 18 percent, posterior trunk 18 percent, and genitalia one percent. Providers may change these percentage assignments where necessary to accommodate infants and children who have proportionately larger heads than adults and patients who have large buttocks, thighs, or abdomen that involve burns.

● 948 **Burns classified according to extent of body surface involved**
Excludes sunburn (692.71, 692.76–692.77)
Note: This category is to be used when the site of the burn is unspecified, or with categories 940–947 when the site is specified.
Coding Clinic: 1984, Nov-Dec, P13

The following fifth-digit subclassification is for use with category 948 to indicate the percent of body surface with third degree burn; valid digits are in [brackets] under each code:

> 0 less than 10 percent or unspecified
> 1 10–19%
> 2 20–29%
> 3 30–39%
> 4 40–49%
> 5 50–59%
> 6 60–69%
> 7 70–79%
> 8 80–89%
> 9 90% or more of body surface

● **948.0 Burn [any degree] involving less than 10 percent of**
[0] **body surface**
● **948.1 10–19 percent of body surface**
[0-1] Coding Clinic: 1984, Nov-Dec, P13
● **948.2 20–29 percent of body surface**
[0-2] Coding Clinic: 1984, Nov-Dec, P13
● **948.3 30–39 percent of body surface**
[0-3]
● **948.4 40–49 percent of body surface**
[0-4]
● **948.5 50–59 percent of body surface**
[0-5]
● **948.6 60–69 percent of body surface**
[0-6]
● **948.7 70–79 percent of body surface**
[0-7]
● **948.8 80–89 percent of body surface**
[0-8]
● **948.9 90 percent or more of body surface**
[0-9]

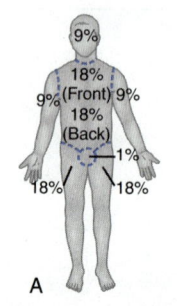
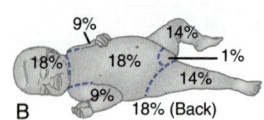

Figure 17-15 Rule of nines: percentages of total body area. (From Marx: Rosen's Emergency Medicine: Concepts and Clinical Practice, ed 6, Mosby, 2006)

OGCR Section I.C.17.c.5
When coding burns, assign separate codes for each burn site. Category 946 Burns of Multiple specified sites, should only be used if the location of the burns are not documented. Category 949, Burn, unspecified, is extremely vague and should rarely be used.

- **949 Burn, unspecified**
  - Includes: burn NOS
    - multiple burns NOS
  - Excludes: burn of unspecified site but with statement of the extent of body surface involved (948.0–948.9)
  - 949.0 Unspecified degree
  - 949.1 Erythema [first degree]
  - 949.2 Blisters, epidermal loss [second degree]
  - 949.3 Full-thickness skin loss [third degree NOS]
  - 949.4 Deep necrosis of underlying tissues [deep third degree] without mention of loss of a body part
  - 949.5 Deep necrosis of underlying tissues [deep third degree] with loss of a body part
    - Includes: division of nerve
      - lesion in continuity (with open wound)
      - traumatic neuroma (with open wound)
      - traumatic transient paralysis (with open wound)
    - Excludes: accidental puncture or laceration during medical procedure (998.2)

INJURY TO NERVES AND SPINAL CORD (950–957)

- **950 Injury to optic nerve and pathways**
  - 950.0 Optic nerve injury
    - Second cranial nerve
  - 950.1 Injury to optic chiasm
  - 950.2 Injury to optic pathways
  - 950.3 Injury to visual cortex
  - 950.9 Unspecified
    - Traumatic blindness NOS

- **951 Injury to other cranial nerve(s)**
  - 951.0 Injury to oculomotor nerve
    - Third cranial nerve
  - 951.1 Injury to trochlear nerve
    - Fourth cranial nerve
  - 951.2 Injury to trigeminal nerve
    - Fifth cranial nerve
  - 951.3 Injury to abducens nerve
    - Sixth cranial nerve
  - 951.4 Injury to facial nerve
    - Seventh cranial nerve
  - 951.5 Injury to acoustic nerve
    - Auditory nerve
    - Eighth cranial nerve
    - Traumatic deafness NOS
  - 951.6 Injury to accessory nerve
    - Eleventh cranial nerve
  - 951.7 Injury to hypoglossal nerve
    - Twelfth cranial nerve
  - 951.8 Injury to other specified cranial nerves
    - Glossopharyngeal [9th cranial] nerve
    - Olfactory [1st cranial] nerve
    - Pneumogastric [10th cranial] nerve
    - Traumatic anosmia NOS
    - Vagus [10th cranial] nerve
  - 951.9 Injury to unspecified cranial nerve

- **952 Spinal cord injury without evidence of spinal bone injury**
  - **952.0 Cervical**
    - 952.00 C_1-C_4 level with unspecified spinal cord injury
      - Spinal cord injury, cervical region NOS
    - 952.01 C_1-C_4 level with complete lesion of spinal cord
    - 952.02 C_1-C_4 level with anterior cord syndrome
    - 952.03 C_1-C_4 level with central cord syndrome
    - 952.04 C_1-C_4 level with other specified spinal cord injury
      - Incomplete spinal cord lesion at C_1-C_4 level:
        - NOS
        - with posterior cord syndrome
    - 952.05 C_5-C_7 level with unspecified spinal cord injury
    - 952.06 C_5-C_7 level with complete lesion of spinal cord
    - 952.07 C_5-C_7 level with anterior cord syndrome
    - 952.08 C_5-C_7 level with central cord syndrome
    - 952.09 C_5-C_7 level with other specified spinal cord injury
      - Incomplete spinal cord lesion at C_5-C_7 level:
        - NOS
        - with posterior cord syndrome
  - **952.1 Dorsal [thoracic]**
    - 952.10 T_1-T_6 level with unspecified spinal cord injury
      - Spinal cord injury, thoracic region NOS
    - 952.11 T_1-T_6 level with complete lesion of spinal cord
    - 952.12 T_1-T_6 level with anterior cord syndrome
    - 952.13 T_1-T_6 level with central cord syndrome
    - 952.14 T_1-T_6 level with other specified spinal cord injury
      - Incomplete spinal cord lesion at T_1-T_6 level:
        - NOS
        - with posterior cord syndrome
    - 952.15 T_7-T_{12} level with unspecified spinal cord injury
    - 952.16 T_7-T_{12} level with complete lesion of spinal cord
    - 952.17 T_7-T_{12} level with anterior cord syndrome
    - 952.18 T_7-T_{12} level with central cord syndrome
    - 952.19 T_7-T_{12} level with other specified spinal cord injury
      - Incomplete spinal cord lesion at T_7-T_{12} level:
        - NOS
        - with posterior cord syndrome
  - 952.2 Lumbar
  - 952.3 Sacral
  - 952.4 Cauda equina
  - 952.8 Multiple sites of spinal cord
  - 952.9 Unspecified site of spinal cord

- **953 Injury to nerve roots and spinal plexus**
  - 953.0 Cervical root
  - 953.1 Dorsal root
  - 953.2 Lumbar root
  - 953.3 Sacral root
  - 953.4 Brachial plexus
  - 953.5 Lumbosacral plexus
  - 953.8 Multiple sites
  - 953.9 Unspecified site

- **954 Injury to other nerve(s) of trunk, excluding shoulder and pelvic girdles**
  - 954.0 Cervical sympathetic
  - 954.1 Other sympathetic
    - Celiac ganglion or plexus   Splanchnic nerve(s)
    - Inferior mesenteric plexus   Stellate ganglion
  - 954.8 Other specified nerve(s) of trunk
  - 954.9 Unspecified nerve of trunk

- **955 Injury to peripheral nerve(s) of shoulder girdle and upper limb**
  - 955.0 Axillary nerve
  - 955.1 Median nerve
  - 955.2 Ulnar nerve
  - 955.3 Radial nerve
  - 955.4 Musculocutaneous nerve
  - 955.5 Cutaneous sensory nerve, upper limb
  - 955.6 Digital nerve
  - 955.7 Other specified nerve(s) of shoulder girdle and upper limb
  - 955.8 Multiple nerves of shoulder girdle and upper limb
  - 955.9 Unspecified nerve of shoulder girdle and upper limb

- **956 Injury to peripheral nerve(s) of pelvic girdle and lower limb**
  - 956.0 Sciatic nerve
  - 956.1 Femoral nerve
  - 956.2 Posterior tibial nerve
  - 956.3 Peroneal nerve
  - 956.4 Cutaneous sensory nerve, lower limb
  - 956.5 Other specified nerve(s) of pelvic girdle and lower limb
  - 956.8 Multiple nerves of pelvic girdle and lower limb
  - 956.9 Unspecified nerve of pelvic girdle and lower limb

- **957 Injury to other and unspecified nerves**
  - 957.0 Superficial nerves of head and neck
  - 957.1 Other specified nerve(s)
  - 957.8 Multiple nerves in several parts
    - Multiple nerve injury NOS
  - 957.9 Unspecified site
    - Nerve injury NOS

CERTAIN TRAUMATIC COMPLICATIONS AND UNSPECIFIED INJURIES (958–959)

- **958 Certain early complications of trauma**
  - **Excludes** adult respiratory distress syndrome (518.52)
    - flail chest (807.4)
    - post-traumatic seroma (729.91)
    - shock lung related to trauma and surgery (518.52)
    - that occurring during or following medical procedures (996.0–999.9)
  - 958.0 Air embolism
    - Pneumathemia
    - **Excludes** that complicating:
      - abortion (634–638 with .6, 639.6)
      - ectopic or molar pregnancy (639.6)
      - pregnancy, childbirth, or the puerperium (673.0)
  - 958.1 Fat embolism
    - **Excludes** that complicating:
      - abortion (634–638 with .6, 639.6)
      - pregnancy, childbirth, or the puerperium (673.8)
  - 958.2 Secondary and recurrent hemorrhage
  - 958.3 Posttraumatic wound infection, not elsewhere classified
    - **Excludes** infected open wounds - code to complicated open wound of site
    - Coding Clinic: 1993, 5th Issue, P3; 1985, Sept-Oct, P10; 1984, Nov-Dec, P20
    - **OGCR** Section I.C.17.c.4
    - Assign code 958.3, Posttraumatic wound infection, not elsewhere classified, as an additional code for any documented infected burn site.
  - 958.4 Traumatic shock
    - Shock (immediate) (delayed) following injury
    - **Excludes** shock:
      - anaphylactic (995.0)
      - due to serum (999.41-999.49)
      - anesthetic (995.4)
      - electric (994.8)
      - following abortion (639.5)
      - lightning (994.0)
      - nontraumatic NOS (785.50)
      - obstetric (669.1)
      - postoperative (998.00-998.09)
  - 958.5 Traumatic anuria
    - Crush syndrome
    - Renal failure following crushing
    - **Excludes** that due to a medical procedure (997.5)
  - 958.6 Volkmann's ischemic contracture
    - Posttraumatic muscle contracture
  - 958.7 Traumatic subcutaneous emphysema
    - **Excludes** subcutaneous emphysema resulting from a procedure (998.81)
  - 958.8 Other early complications of trauma
    - Coding Clinic: 1992, Q2, P13
  - 958.9 Traumatic compartment syndrome
    - **Excludes** nontraumatic compartment syndrome (729.71–729.79)
    - 958.90 Compartment syndrome, unspecified
    - 958.91 Traumatic compartment syndrome of upper extremity
      - Traumatic compartment syndrome of shoulder, arm, forearm, wrist, hand, and fingers
    - 958.92 Traumatic compartment syndrome of lower extremity
      - Traumatic compartment syndrome of hip, buttock, thigh, leg, foot, and toes
    - 958.93 Traumatic compartment syndrome of abdomen
      - Coding Clinic: 2006, Q4, P100-102
    - 958.99 Traumatic compartment syndrome of other sites

- **959 Injury, other and unspecified**
  - **Includes** injury NOS
  - **Excludes** injury NOS of:
    - blood vessels (900.0–904.9)
    - eye (921.0–921.9)
    - internal organs (860.0–869.1)
    - intracranial sites (854.0–854.1)
    - nerves (950.0–951.9, 953.0–957.9)
    - spinal cord (952.0–952.9)
  - Coding Clinic: 1984, Nov-Dec, P9
  - 959.0 Head, face, and neck
    - 959.01 Head injury, unspecified
      - **Excludes** concussion (850.0–850.9)
        - with head injury NOS (850.0–850.9)
        - head injury NOS with loss of consciousness (850.1–850.5)
        - specified head injuries (850.0–854.1)
      - Coding Clinic: 2008, Q4, P102-109; 1999, Q1, P10
    - 959.09 Injury of face and neck
  - 959.1 Trunk
    - **Excludes** scapular region (959.2)
    - 959.11 Other injury of chest wall
    - 959.12 Other injury of abdomen
    - 959.13 Fracture of corpus cavernosum penis
    - 959.14 Other injury of external genitals
    - 959.19 Other injury of other sites of trunk
      - Injury of trunk NOS
  - 959.2 Shoulder and upper arm
    - Axilla
    - Scapular region
  - 959.3 Elbow, forearm, and wrist
    - Coding Clinic: 1997, Q1, P8
  - 959.4 Hand, except finger
  - 959.5 Finger
    - Fingernail
    - Thumb (nail)
  - 959.6 Hip and thigh
    - Upper leg
  - 959.7 Knee, leg, ankle, and foot
  - 959.8 Other specified sites, including multiple
    - **Excludes** multiple sites classifiable to the same four-digit category (959.0–959.7)
  - 959.9 Unspecified site
    - Coding Clinic: 1984, Nov-Dec, P9

OGCR Section I.C.17.e.2

Poisoning. Errors made in drug prescription or in the administration of the drug by provider, nurse, patient, or other person, use the appropriate poisoning code from the 960-979 series. If an overdose of a drug was **intentionally** taken or administered and resulted in drug toxicity, it would be coded as a poisoning (960-979 series). If a **nonprescribed** drug or medicinal agent was taken in combination with a correctly prescribed and properly administered drug, any drug toxicity or other reaction resulting from the interaction of the two drugs would be classified as a poisoning.

When a reaction results from the interaction of a drug(s) and alcohol, this would be classified as poisoning.

Sequencing of poisoning: When coding a poisoning or reaction to the improper use of a medication (e.g., wrong dose, wrong substance, wrong route of administration) the poisoning code is sequenced first, followed by a code for the manifestation. If there is also a diagnosis of drug abuse or dependence to the substance, the abuse or dependence is coded as an additional code.

See Section I.C.3.a.6.b. if poisoning is the result of insulin pump malfunctions and Section I.C.19 for general use of E-codes.

POISONING BY DRUGS, MEDICINAL AND BIOLOGICAL SUBSTANCES (960–979)

Includes overdose of these substances
wrong substance given or taken in error

Excludes adverse effects ["hypersensitivity," "reaction," etc.] of correct substance properly administered. Such cases are to be classified according to the nature of the adverse effect, such as:
adverse effect NOS (995.20)
allergic lymphadenitis (289.3)
aspirin gastritis (535.4)
blood disorders (280.0–289.9)
dermatitis:
  contact (692.0–692.9)
  due to ingestion (693.0–693.9)
nephropathy (583.9)
[The drug giving rise to the adverse effect may be identified by use of categories E930–E949.]
drug dependence (304.0–304.9)
drug reaction and poisoning affecting the newborn (760.0–779.9)
nondependent abuse of drugs (305.0–305.9)
pathological drug intoxication (292.2)

Use additional code to specify the effects of the poisoning

960 Poisoning by antibiotics
Excludes antibiotics:
ear, nose, and throat (976.6)
eye (976.5)
local (976.0)

960.0 Penicillins
Ampicillin   Cloxacillin
Carbenicillin   Penicillin G

960.1 Antifungal antibiotics
Amphotericin B   Nystatin
Griseofulvin   Trichomycin
Excludes preparations intended for topical use (976.0–976.9)

960.2 Chloramphenicol group
Chloramphenicol   Thiamphenicol

960.3 Erythromycin and other macrolides
Oleandomycin   Spiramycin

960.4 Tetracycline group
Doxycycline   Oxytetracycline
Minocycline

960.5 Cephalosporin group
Cephalexin   Cephaloridine
Cephaloglycin   Cephalothin

960.6 Antimycobacterial antibiotics
Cycloserine   Rifampin
Kanamycin   Streptomycin

960.7 Antineoplastic antibiotics
Actinomycin such as:
Bleomycin   Dactinomycin
Cactinomycin   Daunorubicin
                   Mitomycin

960.8 Other specified antibiotics

960.9 Unspecified antibiotic

961 Poisoning by other anti-infectives
Excludes anti-infectives:
ear, nose, and throat (976.6)
eye (976.5)
local (976.0)

961.0 Sulfonamides
Sulfadiazine
Sulfafurazole
Sulfamethoxazole

961.1 Arsenical anti-infectives

961.2 Heavy metal anti-infectives
Compounds of: Compounds of:
  antimony   lead
  bismuth   mercury
Excludes mercurial diuretics (974.0)

961.3 Quinoline and hydroxyquinoline derivatives
Chiniofon
Diiodohydroxyquin
Excludes antimalarial drugs (961.4)

961.4 Antimalarials and drugs acting on other blood protozoa
Chloroquine
Cycloguanil
Primaquine
Proguanil [chloroguanide]
Pyrimethamine
Quinine

961.5 Other antiprotozoal drugs
Emetine

961.6 Anthelmintics
Hexylresorcinol   Thiabendazole
Piperazine

961.7 Antiviral drugs
Methisazone
Excludes amantadine (966.4)
cytarabine (963.1)
idoxuridine (976.5)

961.8 Other antimycobacterial drugs
Ethambutol
Ethionamide
Isoniazid
Para-aminosalicylic acid derivatives
Sulfones

961.9 Other and unspecified anti-infectives
Flucytosine
Nitrofuran derivatives

962 Poisoning by hormones and synthetic substitutes
Excludes oxytocic hormones (975.0)

962.0 Adrenal cortical steroids
Cortisone derivatives
Desoxycorticosterone derivatives
Fluorinated corticosteroids

962.1 Androgens and anabolic congeners
Methandriol   Oxymetholone
Nandrolone   Testosterone

962.2 Ovarian hormones and synthetic substitutes
Contraceptives, oral
Estrogens
Estrogens and progestogens, combined
Progestogens

962.3 Insulins and antidiabetic agents
Acetohexamide
Biguanide derivatives, oral
Chlorpropamide
Glucagon
Insulin
Phenformin
Sulfonylurea derivatives, oral
Tolbutamide

962.4 Anterior pituitary hormones
Corticotropin
Gonadotropin
Somatotropin [growth hormone]

962.5 Posterior pituitary hormones
Vasopressin
Excludes oxytocic hormones (975.0)

962.6 Parathyroid and parathyroid derivatives

962.7 Thyroid and thyroid derivatives
Dextrothyroxin
Levothyroxine sodium
Liothyronine
Thyroglobulin

962.8 Antithyroid agents
Iodides
Thiouracil
Thiourea

962.9 Other and unspecified hormones and synthetic substitutes

963 Poisoning by primarily systemic agents

963.0 Antiallergic and antiemetic drugs
Antihistamines
Chlorpheniramine
Diphenhydramine
Diphenylpyraline
Thonzylamine
Tripelennamine
Excludes phenothiazine-based tranquilizers (969.1)

963.1 Antineoplastic and immunosuppressive drugs
Azathioprine
Busulfan
Chlorambucil
Cyclophosphamide
Cytarabine
Fluorouracil
Mercaptopurine
thio-TEPA
Excludes antineoplastic antibiotics (960.7)

963.2 Acidifying agents

963.3 Alkalizing agents

963.4 Enzymes, not elsewhere classified
Penicillinase

963.5 Vitamins, not elsewhere classified
Vitamin A
Vitamin D
Excludes nicotinic acid (972.2)
vitamin K (964.3)

963.8 Other specified systemic agents
Heavy metal antagonists

963.9 Unspecified systemic agent

964 Poisoning by agents primarily affecting blood constituents

964.0 Iron and its compounds
Ferric salts
Ferrous sulfate and other ferrous salts

964.1 Liver preparations and other antianemic agents
Folic acid

964.2 Anticoagulants
Coumarin
Heparin
Phenindione
Warfarin sodium
Coding Clinic: 1994, Q1, P22

964.3 Vitamin K [phytonadione]

964.4 Fibrinolysis-affecting drugs
Aminocaproic acid
Streptodornase
Streptokinase
Urokinase

964.5 Anticoagulant antagonists and other coagulants
Hexadimethrine
Protamine sulfate

964.6 Gamma globulin

964.7 Natural blood and blood products
Blood plasma
Human fibrinogen
Packed red cells
Whole blood
Excludes transfusion reactions (999.41-999.8)

964.8 Other specified agents affecting blood constituents
Macromolecular blood substitutes
Plasma expanders

964.9 Unspecified agents affecting blood constituents

965 Poisoning by analgesics, antipyretics, and antirheumatics
Use additional code to identify:
drug dependence (304.0–304.9)
nondependent abuse (305.0–305.9)

965.0 Opiates and related narcotics

965.00 Opium (alkaloids), unspecified
Coding Clinic: 2007, Q3, P7-8

965.01 Heroin
Diacetylmorphine

965.02 Methadone

965.09 Other
Codeine [methylmorphine]
Meperidine [pethidine]
Morphine
Coding Clinic: 2007, Q3, P7-8

965.1 Salicylates
Acetylsalicylic acid [aspirin]
Salicylic acid salts
Coding Clinic: 1984, Nov-Dec, P15

965.4 Aromatic analgesics, not elsewhere classified
Acetanilid
Paracetamol [acetaminophen]
Phenacetin [acetophenetidin]

965.5 Pyrazole derivatives
Aminophenazone [aminopyrine]
Phenylbutazone

965.6 Antirheumatics [antiphlogistics]
Excludes salicylates (965.1)
steroids (962.0–962.9)

965.61 Propionic acid derivatives
Fenoprofen
Flurbiprofen
Ibuprofen
Ketoprofen
Naproxen
Oxaprozin
Coding Clinic: 1998, Q4, P42-44

965.69 Other antirheumatics
Gold salts
Indomethacin

965.7 Other non-narcotic analgesics
Pyrabital

965.8 Other specified analgesics and antipyretics
Pentazocine

965.9 Unspecified analgesic and antipyretic

966 Poisoning by anticonvulsants and anti-Parkinsonism drugs

966.0 Oxazolidine derivatives
Paramethadione
Trimethadione

966.1 Hydantoin derivatives
Phenytoin

966.2 Succinimides
Ethosuximide
Phensuximide

966.3 Other and unspecified anticonvulsants
Primidone
Excludes barbiturates (967.0)
sulfonamides (961.0)

966.4 Anti-Parkinsonism drugs
Amantadine
Ethopropazine [profenamine]
Levodopa [L-dopa]

● **967 Poisoning by sedatives and hypnotics**
  Use additional code to identify:
    drug dependence (304.0–304.9)
    nondependent abuse (305.0–305.9)

  967.0 Barbiturates
    Amobarbital [amylobarbitone]
    Barbital [barbitone]
    Butabarbital [butabarbitone]
    Pentobarbital [pentobarbitone]
    Phenobarbital [phenobarbitone]
    Secobarbital [quinalbarbitone]
    Excludes: thiobarbiturate anesthetics (968.3)

  967.1 Chloral hydrate group
  967.2 Paraldehyde
  967.3 Bromine compounds
    Bromide
    Carbromal (derivatives)
  967.4 Methaqualone compounds
  967.5 Glutethimide group
  967.6 Mixed sedatives, not elsewhere classified
  967.8 Other sedatives and hypnotics
  ■ **967.9 Unspecified sedative or hypnotic**
    Sleeping: Sleeping:
      drug NOS   tablet NOS
      pill NOS

● **968 Poisoning by other central nervous system depressants and anesthetics**
  Use additional code to identify:
    drug dependence (304.0–304.9)
    nondependent abuse (305.0–305.9)

  968.0 Central nervous system muscle-tone depressants
    Chlorphenesin (carbamate)
    Mephenesin
    Methocarbamol
  968.1 Halothane
  968.2 Other gaseous anesthetics
    Ether
    Halogenated hydrocarbon derivatives, except halothane
    Nitrous oxide
  968.3 Intravenous anesthetics
    Ketamine
    Methohexital [methohexitone]
    Thiobarbiturates, such as thiopental sodium
  968.4 Other and unspecified general anesthetics
  968.5 Surface (topical) and infiltration anesthetics
    Cocaine (topical)   Procaine
    Lidocaine [lignocaine] Tetracaine
    Excludes: poisoning by cocaine used as a central nervous system stimulant (970.81)
    Coding Clinic: 1993, Q1, P25
  968.6 Peripheral nerve- and plexus-blocking anesthetics
  968.7 Spinal anesthetics
  968.9 Other and unspecified local anesthetics

● **969 Poisoning by psychotropic agents**
  Use additional code to identify:
    drug dependence (304.0–304.9)
    nondependent abuse (305.0–305.9)

  ● **969.0 Antidepressants**
    Coding Clinic: 2007, Q3, P7-8; 1991, Q3, P14
    ■ **969.00 Antidepressant, unspecified**
    969.01 Monoamine oxidase inhibitors
      MAOI
    969.02 Selective serotonin and norepinephrine reuptake inhibitors
      SSNRI antidepressants
    969.03 Selective serotonin reuptake inhibitors
      SSRI antidepressants
    969.04 Tetracyclic antidepressants
    969.05 Tricyclic antidepressants
      Coding Clinic: 2009, Q4, P129
    969.09 Other antidepressants
  969.1 Phenothiazine-based tranquilizers
    Chlorpromazine   Prochlorperazine
    Fluphenazine   Promazine
  969.2 Butyrophenone-based tranquilizers
    Haloperidol   Trifluperidol
    Spiperone
  969.3 Other antipsychotics, neuroleptics, and major tranquilizers
  969.4 Benzodiazepine-based tranquilizers
    Chlordiazepoxide Lorazepam
    Diazepam   Medazepam
    Flurazepam   Nitrazepam
    Coding Clinic: 2009, Q4, P129; 1991, Q3, P14
  969.5 Other tranquilizers
    Hydroxyzine
    Meprobamate
  969.6 Psychodysleptics [hallucinogens]
    Cannabis (derivatives)
    Lysergide [LSD]
    Marihuana (derivatives)
      Marijuana
    Mescaline
    Psilocin
    Psilocybin
  ● **969.7 Psychostimulants**
    Excludes: central appetite depressants (977.0)
    Coding Clinic: 2003, Q2, P11
    ■ **969.70 Psychostimulant, unspecified**
    969.71 Caffeine
    969.72 Amphetamines
      Methamphetamines
    969.73 Methylphenidate
    969.79 Other psychostimulants
  969.8 Other specified psychotropic agents
  ■ **969.9 Unspecified psychotropic agent**

● **970 Poisoning by central nervous system stimulants**
  970.0 Analeptics
    Lobeline
    Nikethamide
  970.1 Opiate antagonists
    Levallorphan
    Nalorphine
    Naloxone
  ● **970.8 Other specified central nervous system stimulants**
    970.81 Cocaine
      Crack
    970.89 Other central nervous system stimulants
  ■ **970.9 Unspecified central nervous system stimulant**

● **971 Poisoning by drugs primarily affecting the autonomic nervous system**
  971.0 Parasympathomimetics [cholinergics]
    Acetylcholine
    Anticholinesterase:
      organophosphorus
      reversible
    Pilocarpine
  971.1 Parasympatholytics [anticholinergics and antimuscarinics] and spasmolytics
    Atropine
    Homatropine
    Hyoscine [scopolamine]
    Quaternary ammonium derivatives
    Excludes: papaverine (972.5)

971.2 Sympathomimetics [adrenergics]
Epinephrine [adrenalin]
Levarterenol [noradrenalin]

971.3 Sympatholytics [antiadrenergics]
Phenoxybenzamine
Tolazoline hydrochloride

■971.9 Unspecified drug primarily affecting autonomic nervous system

●972 Poisoning by agents primarily affecting the cardiovascular system

972.0 Cardiac rhythm regulators
Practolol
Procainamide
Propranolol
Quinidine
Excludes lidocaine (968.5)

972.1 Cardiotonic glycosides and drugs of similar action
Digitalis glycosides
Digoxin
Strophanthins

972.2 Antilipemic and antiarteriosclerotic drugs
Clofibrate
Nicotinic acid derivatives

972.3 Ganglion-blocking agents
Pentamethonium bromide

972.4 Coronary vasodilators
Dipyridamole
Nitrates [nitroglycerin]
Nitrites

972.5 Other vasodilators
Cyclandelate
Diazoxide
Papaverine
Excludes nicotinic acid (972.2)

972.6 Other antihypertensive agents
Clonidine
Guanethidine
Rauwolfia alkaloids
Reserpine

972.7 Antivaricose drugs, including sclerosing agents
Sodium morrhuate
Zinc salts

972.8 Capillary-active drugs
Adrenochrome derivatives
Metaraminol

972.9 Other and unspecified agents primarily affecting the cardiovascular system

●973 Poisoning by agents primarily affecting the gastrointestinal system

973.0 Antacids and antigastric secretion drugs
Aluminum hydroxide
Magnesium trisilicate
Coding Clinic: 2003, Q1, P19

973.1 Irritant cathartics
Bisacodyl
Castor oil
Phenolphthalein

973.2 Emollient cathartics
Dioctyl sulfosuccinates

973.3 Other cathartics, including intestinal atonia drugs
Magnesium sulfate

973.4 Digestants
Pancreatin
Papain
Pepsin

973.5 Antidiarrheal drugs
Kaolin
Pectin
Excludes anti-infectives (960.0–961.9)

973.6 Emetics

973.8 Other specified agents primarily affecting the gastrointestinal system

■973.9 Unspecified agent primarily affecting the gastrointestinal system

●974 Poisoning by water, mineral, and uric acid metabolism drugs

974.0 Mercurial diuretics
Chlormerodrin
Mercaptomerin
Mersalyl

974.1 Purine derivative diuretics
Theobromine
Theophylline
Excludes aminophylline [theophylline ethylenediamine] (975.7)
caffeine (969.71)

974.2 Carbonic acid anhydrase inhibitors
Acetazolamide

974.3 Saluretics
Benzothiadiazides
Chlorothiazide group

974.4 Other diuretics
Ethacrynic acid
Furosemide

974.5 Electrolytic, caloric, and water-balance agents

974.6 Other mineral salts, not elsewhere classified

974.7 Uric acid metabolism drugs
Allopurinol
Colchicine
Probenecid

●975 Poisoning by agents primarily acting on the smooth and skeletal muscles and respiratory system

975.0 Oxytocic agents
Ergot alkaloids
Oxytocin
Prostaglandins

975.1 Smooth muscle relaxants
Adiphenine
Metaproterenol [orciprenaline]
Excludes papaverine (972.5)

975.2 Skeletal muscle relaxants

975.3 Other and unspecified drugs acting on muscles

975.4 Antitussives
Dextromethorphan
Pipazethate

975.5 Expectorants
Acetylcysteine
Guaifenesin
Terpin hydrate

975.6 Anti-common cold drugs

975.7 Antiasthmatics
Aminophylline [theophylline ethylenediamine]

975.8 Other and unspecified respiratory drugs

●976 Poisoning by agents primarily affecting skin and mucous membrane, ophthalmological, otorhinolaryngological, and dental drugs

976.0 Local anti-infectives and anti-inflammatory drugs

976.1 Antipruritics

976.2 Local astringents and local detergents

976.3 Emollients, demulcents, and protectants

976.4 Keratolytics, keratoplastics, other hair treatment drugs and preparations

976.5 Eye anti-infectives and other eye drugs
Idoxuridine

976.6 Anti-infectives and other drugs and preparations for ear, nose, and throat

976.7 Dental drugs topically applied
Excludes anti-infectives (976.0)
local anesthetics (968.5)

976.8 Other agents primarily affecting skin and mucous membrane
Spermicides [vaginal contraceptives]

■976.9 Unspecified agent primarily affecting skin and mucous membrane

- **977 Poisoning by other and unspecified drugs and medicinal substances**
  - 977.0 Dietetics
    - Central appetite depressants
  - 977.1 Lipotropic drugs
  - 977.2 Antidotes and chelating agents, not elsewhere classified
  - 977.3 Alcohol deterrents
  - 977.4 Pharmaceutical excipients
    - Pharmaceutical adjuncts
  - 977.8 Other specified drugs and medicinal substances
    - Contrast media used for diagnostic x-ray procedures
    - Diagnostic agents and kits
  - 977.9 Unspecified drug or medicinal substance
    - Coding Clinic: 1986, Mar-April, P12

- **978 Poisoning by bacterial vaccines**
  - 978.0 BCG
  - 978.1 Typhoid and paratyphoid
  - 978.2 Cholera
  - 978.3 Plague
  - 978.4 Tetanus
  - 978.5 Diphtheria
  - 978.6 Pertussis vaccine, including combinations with a pertussis component
  - 978.8 Other and unspecified bacterial vaccines
  - 978.9 Mixed bacterial vaccines, except combinations with a pertussis component

- **979 Poisoning by other vaccines and biological substances**
  - Excludes gamma globulin (964.6)
  - 979.0 Smallpox vaccine
  - 979.1 Rabies vaccine
  - 979.2 Typhus vaccine
  - 979.3 Yellow fever vaccine
  - 979.4 Measles vaccine
  - 979.5 Poliomyelitis vaccine
  - 979.6 Other and unspecified viral and rickettsial vaccines
    - Mumps vaccine
  - 979.7 Mixed viral-rickettsial and bacterial vaccines, except combinations with a pertussis component
    - Excludes combinations with a pertussis component (978.6)
  - 979.9 Other and unspecified vaccines and biological substances

TOXIC EFFECTS OF SUBSTANCES CHIEFLY NONMEDICINAL AS TO SOURCE (980–989)

Excludes burns from chemical agents (ingested) (947.0–947.9)
localized toxic effects indexed elsewhere (001.0–799.9)
respiratory conditions due to external agents (506.0–508.9)
respiratory conditions due to smoke inhalation NOS (508.2)

Use additional code to identify:
  personal history of retained foreign body fully removed (V15.53)
  retained foreign body status, if applicable (V90.01-V90.9)
Use additional code to specify the nature of the toxic effect

- **980 Toxic effect of alcohol**
  - 980.0 Ethyl alcohol
    - Denatured alcohol
    - Ethanol
    - Grain alcohol
    - Use additional code to identify any associated:
      - acute alcohol intoxication (305.0)
      - in alcoholism (303.0)
      - drunkenness (simple) (305.0)
      - pathological (291.4)
    - Coding Clinic: 2009, Q4, P129; 1996, Q3, P16; 1991, Q3, P14

OGCR Section I.C.17.e.3
When a harmful substance is ingested or comes in contact with a person, this is classified as a toxic effect. The toxic effect codes are in categories 980-989. A toxic effect code should be sequenced first, followed by the code(s) that identify the result of the toxic effect. An external cause code from categories E860-E869 for accidental exposure, codes E950.6 or E950.7 for intentional self-harm, category E962 for assault, or categories E980-E982, for undetermined, should also be assigned to indicate intent.

  - 980.1 Methyl alcohol
    - Methanol
    - Wood alcohol
  - 980.2 Isopropyl alcohol
    - Dimethyl carbinol
    - Isopropanol
    - Rubbing alcohol
  - 980.3 Fusel oil
    - Alcohol:
      - amyl
      - butyl
      - propyl
  - 980.8 Other specified alcohols
  - 980.9 Unspecified alcohol

- 981 **Toxic effect of petroleum products**
  - Benzine
  - Gasoline
  - Kerosene
  - Paraffin wax
  - Petroleum:
    - ether
    - naphtha
    - spirit

- **982 Toxic effect of solvents other than petroleum based**
  - 982.0 Benzene and homologues
  - 982.1 Carbon tetrachloride
  - 982.2 Carbon disulfide
    - Carbon bisulfide
  - 982.3 Other chlorinated hydrocarbon solvents
    - Tetrachloroethylene
    - Trichloroethylene
    - Excludes chlorinated hydrocarbon preparations other than solvents (989.2)
    - Coding Clinic: 2008, Q3, P6, 7x2
  - 982.4 Nitroglycol
  - 982.8 Other nonpetroleum-based solvents
    - Acetone

- **983 Toxic effect of corrosive aromatics, acids, and caustic alkalis**
  - 983.0 Corrosive aromatics
    - Carbolic acid or phenol
    - Cresol
  - 983.1 Acids
    - Acid:
      - hydrochloric
      - nitric
      - sulfuric
  - 983.2 Caustic alkalis
    - Lye
    - Potassium hydroxide
    - Sodium hydroxide
  - 983.9 Caustic, unspecified

- **984 Toxic effect of lead and its compounds (including fumes)**
  - Includes that from all sources except medicinal substances
  - 984.0 Inorganic lead compounds
    - Lead dioxide
    - Lead salts
  - 984.1 Organic lead compounds
    - Lead acetate
    - Tetraethyl lead
  - 984.8 Other lead compounds
  - 984.9 Unspecified lead compound

985-992.4 ICD-9-CM

- **985 Toxic effect of other metals**
  - **Includes** that from all sources except medicinal substances
  - 985.0 Mercury and its compounds
    - Minamata disease
  - 985.1 Arsenic and its compounds
  - 985.2 Manganese and its compounds
  - 985.3 Beryllium and its compounds
  - 985.4 Antimony and its compounds
  - 985.5 Cadmium and its compounds
  - 985.6 Chromium
  - 985.8 Other specified metals
    - Brass fumes
    - Copper salts
    - Iron compounds
    - Nickel compounds
  - 985.9 Unspecified metal

- 986 Toxic effect of carbon monoxide

- **987 Toxic effect of other gases, fumes, or vapors**
  - 987.0 Liquefied petroleum gases
    - Butane
    - Propane
  - 987.1 Other hydrocarbon gas
  - 987.2 Nitrogen oxides
    - Nitrogen dioxide
    - Nitrous fumes
  - 987.3 Sulfur dioxide
  - 987.4 Freon
    - Dichloromonofluoromethane
  - 987.5 Lacrimogenic gas
    - Bromobenzyl cyanide
    - Chloroacetophenone
    - Ethyliodoacetate
  - 987.6 Chlorine gas
  - 987.7 Hydrocyanic acid gas
  - 987.8 Other specified gases, fumes, or vapors
    - Phosgene
    - Polyester fumes
  - 987.9 Unspecified gas, fume, or vapor
    - **Coding Clinic: 2005, Q3, P10-11**

- **988 Toxic effect of noxious substances eaten as food**
  - **Excludes** allergic reaction to food, such as:
    - gastroenteritis (558.3)
    - rash (692.5, 693.1)
    - food poisoning (bacterial) (005.0–005.9)
    - toxic effects of food contaminants, such as:
      - aflatoxin and other mycotoxin (989.7)
      - mercury (985.0)
  - 988.0 Fish and shellfish
  - 988.1 Mushrooms
  - 988.2 Berries and other plants
  - 988.8 Other specified noxious substances eaten as food
  - 988.9 Unspecified noxious substance eaten as food

- **989 Toxic effect of other substances, chiefly nonmedicinal as to source**
  - 989.0 Hydrocyanic acid and cyanides
    - Potassium cyanide
    - Sodium cyanide
    - **Excludes** gas and fumes (987.7)
  - 989.1 Strychnine and salts
  - 989.2 Chlorinated hydrocarbons
    - Aldrin
    - Chlordane
    - DDT
    - Dieldrin
    - **Excludes** chlorinated hydrocarbon solvents (982.0–982.3)
  - 989.3 Organophosphate and carbamate
    - Carbaryl
    - Dichlorvos
    - Malathion
    - Parathion
    - Phorate
    - Phosdrin
  - 989.4 Other pesticides, not elsewhere classified
    - Mixtures of insecticides
  - 989.5 Venom
    - Bites of venomous snakes, lizards, and spiders
    - Tick paralysis
  - 989.6 Soaps and detergents
  - 989.7 Aflatoxin and other mycotoxin [food contaminants]

- **989.8 Other substances, chiefly nonmedicinal as to source**
  - 989.81 Asbestos
    - **Excludes** asbestosis (501)
      - exposure to asbestos (V15.84)
  - 989.82 Latex
  - 989.83 Silicone
    - **Excludes** silicone used in medical devices, implants and grafts (996.00–996.79)
  - 989.84 Tobacco
  - 989.89 Other
- 989.9 Unspecified substance, chiefly nonmedicinal as to source

OTHER AND UNSPECIFIED EFFECTS OF EXTERNAL CAUSES (990–995)

- **990 Effects of radiation, unspecified**
  - Complication of:
    - phototherapy
    - radiation therapy
  - Radiation sickness
  - **Excludes** specified adverse effects of radiation. Such conditions are to be classified according to the nature of the adverse effect, as:
    - burns (940.0–949.5)
    - dermatitis (692.7–692.8)
    - leukemia (204.0–208.9)
    - pneumonia (508.0)
    - sunburn (692.71, 692.76–692.77)
  - [The type of radiation giving rise to the adverse effect may be identified by use of the E codes.]

- **991 Effects of reduced temperature**
  - 991.0 Frostbite of face
  - 991.1 Frostbite of hand
  - 991.2 Frostbite of foot
  - 991.3 Frostbite of other and unspecified sites
  - 991.4 Immersion foot
    - Trench foot
  - 991.5 Chilblains
    - Erythema pernio
    - Perniosis
  - 991.6 Hypothermia
    - Hypothermia (accidental)
    - **Excludes** hypothermia following anesthesia (995.89)
      - hypothermia not associated with low environmental temperature (780.65)
  - 991.8 Other specified effects of reduced temperature
  - 991.9 Unspecified effect of reduced temperature
    - Effects of freezing or excessive cold NOS

- **992 Effects of heat and light**
  - **Excludes** burns (940.0–949.5)
    - diseases of sweat glands due to heat (705.0–705.9)
    - malignant hyperpyrexia following anesthesia (995.86)
    - sunburn (692.71, 692.76–692.77)
  - 992.0 Heat stroke and sunstroke
    - Heat apoplexy
    - Heat pyrexia
    - Ictus solaris
    - Siriasis
    - Thermoplegia
    - Use additional code(s) to identify any associated complication of heat stroke, such as:
      - alterations of consciousness (780.01-780.09)
      - systemic inflammatory response syndrome (995.93-995.94)
  - 992.1 Heat syncope
    - Heat collapse
  - 992.2 Heat cramps
  - 992.3 Heat exhaustion, anhydrotic
    - Heat prostration due to water depletion
    - **Excludes** that associated with salt depletion (992.4)
  - 992.4 Heat exhaustion due to salt depletion
    - Heat prostration due to salt (and water) depletion

992.5 Heat exhaustion, unspecified
Heat prostration NOS

992.6 Heat fatigue, transient

992.7 Heat edema

992.8 Other specified heat effects

992.9 Unspecified

993 Effects of air pressure

993.0 Barotrauma, otitic
Aero-otitis media
Effects of high altitude on ears

993.1 Barotrauma, sinus
Aerosinusitis
Effects of high altitude on sinuses

993.2 Other and unspecified effects of high altitude
Alpine sickness
Andes disease
Anoxia due to high altitude
Hypobaropathy
Mountain sickness

993.3 Caisson disease
Bends
Compressed-air disease
Decompression sickness
Divers' palsy or paralysis

993.4 Effects of air pressure caused by explosion

993.8 Other specified effects of air pressure

993.9 Unspecified effect of air pressure

994 Effects of other external causes
Excludes *certain adverse effects not elsewhere classified (995.0–995.8)*

994.0 Effects of lightning
Shock from lightning
Struck by lightning NOS
Excludes *burns (940.0–949.5)*

994.1 Drowning and nonfatal submersion
Bathing cramp
Immersion

994.2 Effects of hunger
Deprivation of food
Starvation

994.3 Effects of thirst
Deprivation of water

994.4 Exhaustion due to exposure

994.5 Exhaustion due to excessive exertion
Exhaustion due to overexertion

994.6 Motion sickness
Air sickness
Seasickness
Travel sickness

994.7 Asphyxiation and strangulation
Suffocation (by):
bedclothes
cave-in
constriction
mechanical
plastic bag
pressure
strangulation
Excludes *asphyxia from:*
carbon monoxide (986)
inhalation of food or foreign body (932–934.9)
other gases, fumes, and vapors (987.0–987.9)

994.8 Electrocution and nonfatal effects of electric current
Shock from electric current
Shock from electroshock gun (taser)
Excludes *electric burns (940.0–949.5)*

994.9 Other effects of external causes
Effects of:
abnormal gravitational [G] forces or states
weightlessness

995 Certain adverse effects not elsewhere classified
Excludes *complications of surgical and medical care (996.0–999.9)*
Coding Clinic: 2008, Q1, P12-13

995.0 Other anaphylactic reaction
Allergic shock NOS or due to adverse effect of correct medicinal substance properly administered
Anaphylactic reaction NOS or due to adverse effect of correct medicinal substance properly administered
Anaphylactic shock NOS or due to adverse effect of correct medicinal substance properly administered
Anaphylactoid reaction NOS
Anaphylaxis NOS or due to adverse effect of correct medicinal substance properly administered
Excludes *anaphylactic reaction to serum (999.41-999.49)*
anaphylactic shock or reaction due to adverse food reaction (995.60-995.69)

Use additional E code to identify external cause, such as: adverse effects of correct medicinal substance properly administered [E930–E949]

995.1 Angioneurotic edema
Allergic angioedema
Giant urticaria
Excludes *urticaria:*
due to serum (999.51-999.59)
other specified (698.2, 708.0–708.9, 757.33)

995.2 Other and unspecified adverse effect of drug, medicinal and biological substance
Excludes *pathological drug intoxication (292.2)*
Coding Clinic: 2010, Q2, P4; 2006, Q4, P112-113; 1997, Q2, P12; 1995, Q3, P13; 1992, Q3, P16-17

995.20 Unspecified adverse effect of unspecified drug, medicinal and biological substance
Unspecified adverse effect of unspecified medicinal substance properly administered

995.21 Arthus phenomenon
Arthus reaction
Hypersensitivity reaction resulting from immune complex reactions

995.22 Unspecified adverse effect of anesthesia

995.23 Unspecified adverse effect of insulin

995.24 Failed moderate sedation during procedure
Failed conscious sedation during procedure

995.27 Other drug allergy
Allergic reaction NEC (due) to correct medical substance properly administered
Drug allergy NOS
Drug hypersensitivity NOS
Hypersensitivity (due) to correct medical substance properly administered

995.29 Unspecified adverse effect of other drug, medicinal and biological substance
Unspecified adverse effect of medicinal substance NEC properly administered

995.3 Allergy, unspecified
Allergic reaction NOS   Idiosyncrasy NOS
Hypersensitivity NOS
Excludes *allergic reaction NOS to correct medicinal substance properly administered (995.27)*
allergy to existing dental restorative materials (525.66)
specific types of allergic reaction, such as:
allergic diarrhea (558.3)
dermatitis (691.0–693.9)
hayfever (477.0–477.9)

995.4 Shock due to anesthesia
Shock due to anesthesia in which the correct substance was properly administered
> **Excludes** complications of anesthesia in labor or delivery (668.0–668.9)
> overdose or wrong substance given (968.0–969.9)
> postoperative shock NOS (998.00)
> specified adverse effects of anesthesia classified elsewhere, such as:
> anoxic brain damage (348.1)
> hepatitis (070.0–070.9), etc.
> unspecified adverse effect of anesthesia (995.22)

● 995.5 Child maltreatment syndrome
Use additional code(s), if applicable, to identify any associated injuries
Use additional E code to identify:
nature of abuse (E960–E968)
perpetrator (E967.0–E967.9)
Coding Clinic: 1998, Q1, P11; 1984, Sept-Oct, P16; 1984, Nov-Dec, P9

995.50 Child abuse, unspecified
Coding Clinic: 2012, Q2, P12-13

995.51 Child emotional/psychological abuse
Coding Clinic: 2012, Q2, P12-13

995.52 Child neglect (nutritional)
Use additional code to identify intent of neglect (E904.0, E968.4)
Coding Clinic: 2012, Q2, P12-13

995.53 Child sexual abuse
Coding Clinic: 2012, Q2, P12-13

995.54 Child physical abuse
Battered baby or child syndrome
> **Excludes** Shaken infant syndrome (995.55)
Coding Clinic: 2012, Q2, P12-13; 1999, Q3, P14-15

995.55 Shaken infant syndrome
Use additional code(s) to identify any associated injuries
Coding Clinic: 2012, Q2, P12-13; 1996, Q4, P43-44

995.59 Other child abuse and neglect
Multiple forms of abuse
Use additional code to identify intent of neglect (E904.0, E968.4)
Coding Clinic: 2012, Q2, P12-13

● 995.6 Anaphylactic reaction due to food
Anaphylactic reaction due to adverse food reaction
Anaphylactic shock or reaction due to nonpoisonous foods
Anaphylactoid reaction due to food

995.60 Anaphylactic reaction due to unspecified food

995.61 Anaphylactic reaction due to peanuts

995.62 Anaphylactic reaction due to crustaceans

995.63 Anaphylactic reaction due to fruits and vegetables

995.64 Anaphylactic reaction due to tree nuts and seeds
Coding Clinic: 2008, Q1, P12-13

995.65 Anaphylactic reaction due to fish

995.66 Anaphylactic reaction due to food additives

995.67 Anaphylactic reaction due to milk products

995.68 Anaphylactic reaction due to eggs

995.69 Anaphylactic reaction due to other specified food

995.7 Other adverse food reactions, not elsewhere classified
Use additional code to identify the type of reaction, such as:
hives (708.0)
wheezing (786.07)
> **Excludes** anaphylactic reaction or shock due to adverse food reaction (995.60-995.69)
> asthma (493.0, 493.9)
> dermatitis due to food (693.1)
> in contact with the skin (692.5)
> gastroenteritis and colitis due to food (558.3)
> rhinitis due to food (477.1)

● 995.8 Other specified adverse effects, not elsewhere classified

995.80 Adult maltreatment, unspecified
Abused person NOS
Use additional code to identify:
any associated injury
nature of abuse (E960–E968)
perpetrator (E967.0–E967.9)
Coding Clinic: 2012, Q2, P12-13

995.81 Adult physical abuse
Battered:
person syndrome NEC
man
spouse
woman
Use additional code to identify:
any associated injury
nature of abuse (E960–E968)
perpetrator (E967.0–E967.9)
Coding Clinic: 2012, Q2, P12-13; 1996, Q4, P43-44; 1984, Sept-Oct, P16

995.82 Adult emotional/psychological abuse
Use additional E code to identify perpetrator (E967.0–E967.9)
Coding Clinic: 2012, Q2, P12-13

995.83 Adult sexual abuse
Use additional code to identify:
any associated injury
perpetrator (E967.0–E967.9)
Coding Clinic: 2012, Q2, P12-13

995.84 Adult neglect (nutritional)
Use additional code to identify:
intent of neglect (E904.0–E968.4)
perpetrator (E967.0–E967.9)
Coding Clinic: 2012, Q2, P12-13

995.85 Other adult abuse and neglect
Multiple forms of abuse and neglect
Use additional code to identify:
any associated injury
intent of neglect (E904.0, E968.4)
nature of abuse (E960–E968)
perpetrator (E967.0–E967.9)
Coding Clinic: 2012, Q2, P12-13

995.86 Malignant hyperthermia
Malignant hyperpyrexia due to anesthesia
Extremely high body temperature—greater than 106° F or 41.1° C
Coding Clinic: 2012, Q2, P12-13

995.89 Other
Hypothermia due to anesthesia
Coding Clinic: 2004, Q2, P18; 2003, Q3, P12

● 995.9 Systemic inflammatory response syndrome (SIRS)
Coding Clinic: 2010, Q1, P12; 2006, Q4, P113-116; 2005, Q3, P23; 2004, Q2, P16; 2002, Q4, P71-73

995.90 Systemic inflammatory response syndrome, unspecified SIRS NOS

● 995.91 Sepsis
Systemic inflammatory response syndrome due to infectious process without acute organ dysfunction
Code first underlying infection
> **Excludes** sepsis with acute organ dysfunction (995.92)
> sepsis with multiple organ dysfunction (995.92)
> severe sepsis (995.92)
Coding Clinic: 2012, Q3, P12, 14; 2011, Q3, P15; 2008, Q4, P69-73; 2007, Q4, P84-86; 2004, Q2, P16

PART III / Diseases: Tabular List Volume 1   995.92–996.09

OGCR Section I.C.1.b.2.12

Only one code from subcategory 995.9 should be assigned. Therefore, when a non-infectious condition leads to an infection resulting in sepsis or severe sepsis, assign either code 995.91 or 995.92. Do not additionally assign code 995.93, Systemic inflammatory response syndrome due to noninfectious process without acute organ dysfunctiion, or 995.94, Systemic inflammatory response syndrome with acute organ dysfunction.

● **995.92 Severe sepsis**
   Sepsis with acute organ dysfunction
   Sepsis with multiple organ dysfunction (MOD)
   Systemic inflammatory response syndrome due to infectious process with acute organ dysfunction

   Code first underlying infection

   Use additional code to specify acute organ dysfunction, such as:
      acute kidney failure (584.5–584.9)
      acute respiratory failure (518.81)
      critical illness myopathy (359.81)
      critical illness polyneuropathy (357.82)
      disseminated intravascular coagulopathy (DIC) syndrome (286.6)
      encephalopathy (348.31)
      hepatic failure (570)
      septic shock (785.52)

   Coding Clinic: 2012, Q3, P12; 2011, Q4, P153; Q3, P15; 2010, Q2, P4; 2009, Q4, P129; 2007, Q4, P96-97; 2005, Q2, P18-20x2; 2004, Q2, P16; 2003, Q4, P73, 79-81

● **995.93 Systemic inflammatory response syndrome due to noninfectious process without acute organ dysfunction**

   Code first underlying conditions, such as:
      acute pancreatitis (577.0)
      trauma

   Excludes: systemic inflammatory response syndrome due to noninfectious process with acute organ dysfunction (995.94)

   Coding Clinic: 2011, Q1, P22; 2010, Q1, P12

● **995.94 Systemic inflammatory response syndrome due to non-infectious process with acute organ dysfunction**

   Code first underlying conditions, such as:
      acute pancreatitis (577.0)
      heat stroke (992.0)
      trauma

   Use additional code to specify acute organ dysfunction, such as:
      acute kidney failure (584.5–584.9)
      acute respiratory failure (518.81)
      critical illness myopathy (359.81)
      critical illness polyneuropathy (357.82)
      disseminated intravascular coagulopathy (DIC) syndrome (286.6)
      encephalopathy (348.31)
      hepatic failure (570)

   Excludes: severe sepsis (995.92)

   Coding Clinic: 2010, Q1, P12; 2005, Q2, P19-20

OGCR Section I.C.19.a.7

An external cause code is not appropriate with a code from subcategory 995.9, unless the patient also has another condition for which an E code would be appropriate (such as an injury, poisoning, or adverse effect of drugs).

COMPLICATIONS OF SURGICAL AND MEDICAL CARE, NOT ELSEWHERE CLASSIFIED (996–999)

Excludes: adverse effects of medicinal agents (001.0–799.9, 995.0–995.8)
   burns from local applications and irradiation (940.0–949.5)
   complications of:
      conditions for which the procedure was performed
      surgical procedures during abortion, labor, and delivery (630–676.9)
      poisoning and toxic effects of drugs and chemicals (960.0–989.9)
      postoperative conditions in which no complications are present, such as:
         artificial opening status (V44.0–V44.9)
         closure of external stoma (V55.0–V55.9)
         fitting of prosthetic device (V52.0–V52.9)
      specified complications classified elsewhere:
         anesthetic shock (995.4)
         electrolyte imbalance (276.0–276.9)
         postlaminectomy syndrome (722.80–722.83)
         postmastectomy lymphedema syndrome (457.0)
         postoperative psychosis (293.0–293.9)
      any other condition classified elsewhere in the Alphabetic Index when described as due to a procedure

● **996 Complications peculiar to certain specified procedures**

   Includes: complications, not elsewhere classified, in the use of artificial substitutes [e.g., Dacron, metal, Silastic, Teflon] or natural sources [e.g., bone] involving:
      anastomosis (internal)
      graft (bypass) (patch)
      implant
      internal device:
         catheter
         electronic
         fixation
         prosthetic
         reimplant
         transplant

   Excludes: accidental puncture or laceration during procedure (998.2)
      capsular contracture of breast implant (611.83)
      complications of internal anastomosis of:
         gastrointestinal tract (997.49)
         urinary tract (997.5)
      endosseous dental implant failures (525.71–525.79)
      intraoperative floppy iris syndrome (IFIS) (364.81)
      mechanical complication of respirator (V46.14)
      other specified complications classified elsewhere, such as:
         hemolytic anemia (283.1)
         functional cardiac disturbances (429.4)
         serum hepatitis (070.2–070.3)

● **996.0 Mechanical complication of cardiac device, implant, and graft**
   Breakdown (mechanical)   Obstruction, mechanical
   Displacement   Perforation
   Leakage   Protrusion

   Coding Clinic: 2007, Q3, P7-8

   996.00 Unspecified device, implant, and graft

   996.01 Due to cardiac pacemaker (electrode)
      Coding Clinic: 2006, Q2, P15-16; 1999, Q2, P11-12

   996.02 Due to heart valve prosthesis
      Coding Clinic: 1999, Q2, P4

   996.03 Due to coronary bypass graft
      Excludes: atherosclerosis of graft (414.02, 414.03)
         embolism [occlusion NOS] [thrombus] of graft (996.72)
      Coding Clinic: 1993, Q4, P40-41

   996.04 Due to automatic implantable cardiac defibrillator
      Coding Clinic: 2005, Q2, P3

   996.09 Other
      Coding Clinic: 2013, Q1, P5; 1993, Q2, P9**

INJURY AND POISONING (800–999)

996.1 **Mechanical complication of other vascular device, implant, and graft**
Mechanical complications involving:
aortic (bifurcation) graft (replacement)
arteriovenous:
dialysis catheter
fistula surgically created
shunt surgically created
balloon (counterpulsation) device, intra-aortic
carotid artery bypass graft
femoral-popliteal bypass graft
umbrella device, vena cava

Excludes atherosclerosis of biological graft (440.30–440.32)
embolism [occlusion NOS] [thrombus] of (biological) (synthetic) graft (996.74)
peritoneal dialysis catheter (996.56)

Coding Clinic: 2012, Q1, P18; 2011, Q1, P6; 2006, Q1, P10-11; 2005, Q2, P8; 2002, Q1, P13; 1995, Q1, P3

996.2 **Mechanical complication of nervous system device, implant, and graft**
Mechanical complications involving:
dorsal column stimulator
electrodes implanted in brain [brain "pacemaker"]
peripheral nerve graft
ventricular (communicating) shunt

Coding Clinic: 1987, Sept-Oct, P10

996.3 **Mechanical complication of genitourinary device, implant, and graft**

996.30 Unspecified device, implant, and graft
996.31 Due to urethral [indwelling] catheter
996.32 Due to intrauterine contraceptive device
996.39 Other
Prosthetic reconstruction of vas deferens
Repair (graft) of ureter without mention of resection

Excludes complications due to:
external stoma of urinary tract (596.81-596.83)
internal anastomosis of urinary tract (997.5)

996.4 **Mechanical complication of internal orthopedic device, implant, and graft**
Mechanical complications involving:
external (fixation) device utilizing internal screw(s), pin(s) or other methods of fixation
grafts of bone, cartilage, muscle, or tendon
internal (fixation) device such as nail, plate, rod, etc.
Use additional code to identify prosthetic joint with mechanical complication (V43.60–V43.69)

Excludes complications of external orthopedic device, such as:
pressure ulcer due to cast (707.00–707.09)

Coding Clinic: 2005, Q4, P91-93, 110-112; 1999, Q2, P10-11; 1998, Q2, P19; 1996, Q2, P11; 1985, Nov-Dec, P11; 1984, Nov-Dec, P18

996.40 Unspecified mechanical complication of internal orthopedic device, implant, and graft
996.41 Mechanical loosening of prosthetic joint
Aseptic loosening
Coding Clinic: 2005, Q4, P91-93
996.42 Dislocation of prosthetic joint
Instability of prosthetic joint
Subluxation of prosthetic joint
996.43 Broken prosthetic joint implant
Breakage (fracture) of prosthetic joint
996.44 Peri-prosthetic fracture around prosthetic joint
Coding Clinic: 2005, Q4, P91-93
996.45 Peri-prosthetic osteolysis
Use additional code to identify major osseous defect, if applicable (731.3)
Coding Clinic: 2006, Q4, P103-104
996.46 Articular bearing surface wear of prosthetic joint
996.47 Other mechanical complication of prosthetic joint implant
Mechanical complication of prosthetic joint NOS
Prosthetic joint implant failure NOS
996.49 Other mechanical complication of other internal orthopedic device, implant, and graft
Breakage of internal fixation device in bone
Dislocation of internal fixation device in bone

Excludes mechanical complication of prosthetic joint implant (996.41–996.46)

Coding Clinic: 2010, Q1, P13

996.5 **Mechanical complication of other specified prosthetic device, implant, and graft**
Mechanical complications involving:
prosthetic implant in:
bile duct
breast
chin
orbit of eye
nonabsorbable surgical material NOS
other graft, implant, and internal device, not elsewhere classified

996.51 Due to corneal graft
Coding Clinic: 2010, Q2, P5
996.52 Due to graft of other tissue, not elsewhere classified
Skin graft failure or rejection

Excludes failure of artificial skin graft (996.55)
failure of decellularized allodermis (996.55)
sloughing of temporary skin allografts or xenografts (pigskin)- omit code

Coding Clinic: 2012, Q3, P6-7; 1996, Q1, P10; 1990, Q3, P15

996.53 Due to ocular lens prosthesis
Excludes contact lenses—code to condition
Coding Clinic: 2000, Q1, P9-10
996.54 Due to breast prosthesis
Breast capsule (prosthesis)
Mammary implant
Coding Clinic: 1998, Q2, P14; 1992, Q3, P4-5
996.55 Due to artificial skin graft and decellularized allodermis
Dislodgement   Non-adherence
Displacement   Poor incorporation
Failure   Shearing
Coding Clinic: 2012, Q3, P6; 1998, Q4, P52-53
996.56 Due to peritoneal dialysis catheter
Excludes mechanical complication of arteriovenous dialysis catheter (996.1)
Coding Clinic: 1998, Q4, P54
996.57 Due to insulin pump
Coding Clinic: 2003, Q4, P81-82

OGCR Section I.C.3.a.6.a

An underdose of insulin due to an insulin pump failure should be assigned 996.57, Mechanical complication due to insulin pump, as the principal or first listed code, followed by the appropriate diabetes mellitus code based on documentation.

OGCR Section I.C.3.a.6.b

The principal or first listed code for an encounter due to an insulin pump malfunction resulting in an overdose of insulin, should also be 996.57, Mechanical complication due to insulin pump, followed by 962.3, Poisoning by insulins and antidiabetic agents, and the appropriate diabetes mellitus code based on documentation.

996.59 Due to other implant and internal device, not elsewhere classified
Nonabsorbable surgical material NOS
Prosthetic implant in:
bile duct
chin
orbit of eye
Coding Clinic: 2011, Q1, P11; 1999, Q2, P13-14; 1997, Q3, P7; 1994, Q3, P7x2

● **996.6 Infection and inflammatory reaction due to internal prosthetic device, implant, and graft**
Infection (causing obstruction) due to (presence of) any device, implant, and graft classifiable to 996.0–996.5
Inflammation due to (presence of) any device, implant, and graft classifiable to 996.0–996.5
Use additional code to identify specified infections
Coding Clinic: 2008, Q2, P9-10; 1987, Jan-Feb, P14-15

■ **996.60 Due to unspecified device, implant and graft**

996.61 Due to cardiac device, implant and graft
Cardiac pacemaker or defibrillator:
electrode(s), lead(s)
pulse generator
subcutaneous pocket
Coronary artery bypass graft
Heart valve prosthesis

996.62 Due to vascular device, implant and graft
Arterial graft
Arteriovenous fistula or shunt
Infusion pump
Vascular catheter (arterial) (dialysis) (peripheral venous)
Excludes infection due to:
central venous catheter (999.31-999.32)
Hickman catheter (999.31-999.32)
peripherally inserted central catheter (PICC) (999.31-999.32)
portacath (port-a-cath) (999.31-999.32)
triple lumen catheter (999.31-999.32)
umbilical venous catheter (999.31-999.32)
Coding Clinic: 2010, Q2, P8; 2007, Q4, P84-86; 2004, Q2, P16; Q1, P5; 2003, Q4, P111-112; Q2, P7-8; 1994, Q2, P13

996.63 Due to nervous system device, implant and graft
Electrodes implanted in brain
Peripheral nerve graft
Spinal canal catheter
Ventricular (communicating) shunt (catheter)

996.64 Due to indwelling urinary catheter
Use additional code to identify specified infections, such as:
cystitis (595.0–595.9)
sepsis (038.0–038.9)
Excludes complications due to:
external stoma of urinary tract (596.81-596.83)
Coding Clinic: 2012, Q2, P20-21; Q1, P11-12; 2009, Q3, P18-19; 1993, Q3, P6

996.65 Due to other genitourinary device, implant and graft
Intrauterine contraceptive device
Coding Clinic: 2000, Q1, P15-16

996.66 Due to internal joint prosthesis
Use additional code to identify infected prosthetic joint (V43.60–V43.69)
Coding Clinic: 2008, Q2, P3-5x3; 2007, Q2, P8-9; 2005, Q4, P110-112; 1991, Q2, P18

996.67 Due to other internal orthopedic device, implant and graft
Bone growth stimulator (electrode)
Internal fixation device (pin) (rod) (screw)

996.68 Due to peritoneal dialysis catheter
Exit-site infection or inflammation
Coding Clinic: 2001, Q2, P11; 1998, Q4, P55

996.69 Due to other internal prosthetic device, implant, and graft
Breast prosthesis
Ocular lens prosthesis
Prosthetic orbital implant
Coding Clinic: 2011, Q1, P11; 2008, Q2, P9-11; 2003, Q4, P108; 1998, Q4, P52-53

● **996.7 Other complications of internal (biological) (synthetic) prosthetic device, implant, and graft**
Complication NOS due to (presence of) any device, implant, and graft classifiable to 996.0–996.5
occlusion NOS
Embolism due to (presence of) any device, implant, and graft classifiable to 996.0–996.5
Fibrosis due to (presence of) any device, implant, and graft classifiable to 996.0–996.5
Hemorrhage due to (presence of) any device, implant, and graft classifiable to 996.0–996.5
Pain due to (presence of) any device, implant, and graft classifiable to 996.0–996.5
Stenosis due to (presence of) any device, implant, and graft classifiable to 996.0–996.5
Thrombus due to (presence of) any device, implant, and graft classifiable to 996.0–996.5
Use additional code to identify complication, such as:
pain due to presence of device, implant or graft (338.18–338.19, 338.28–338.29)
venous embolism and thrombosis (453.2-453.9)
Excludes disruption (dehiscence) of internal suture material (998.31)
transplant rejection (996.80-996.89)
Coding Clinic: 2012, Q2, P5; Q1, P18; 2010, Q2, P9; 2007, Q2, P13-15; 2004, Q2, P7-8; 1989, Q1, P9&10; 1984, Nov-Dec, P18

■ **996.70 Due to unspecified device, implant, and graft**

996.71 Due to heart valve prosthesis
Coding Clinic: 2008, Q2, P9-10

996.72 Due to other cardiac device, implant, and graft
Cardiac pacemaker or defibrillator:
electrode(s), lead(s)
subcutaneous pocket
Coronary artery bypass (graft)
Excludes occlusion due to atherosclerosis (414.00–414.07)
Coding Clinic: 2010, Q2, P9; 2008, Q3, P10-11; 2006, Q3, P8-9, 25; 2001, Q3, P20

996.73 Due to renal dialysis device, implant, and graft
Coding Clinic: 1991, Q2, P18

996.74 Due to vascular device, implant, and graft
Excludes occlusion of biological graft due to atherosclerosis (440.30–440.32)
Coding Clinic: 2012, Q1, P18; 2003, Q1, P16-18x2; 2000, Q1, P10

996.75 Due to nervous system device, implant, and graft

996.76 Due to genitourinary device, implant, and graft
Excludes complications of implanted vaginal mesh (629.31-629.32)
Coding Clinic: 2009, Q1, P13; 2000, Q1, P15-16

996.77 Due to internal joint prosthesis
Use additional code to identify prosthetic joint (V43.60–V43.69)

OGCR Section I.C.17.f.2.a

Transplant complications other than kidney: Codes under subcategory 996.8, Complications of transplanted organ, are for use for both complications and rejection of transplanted organs. A transplant complication code is only assigned if the complication affects the function of the transplanted organ. Two codes are required to fully describe a transplant complication, the appropriate code from subcategory 996.8 and a secondary code that identifies the complication.

Pre-existing conditions or conditions that develop after the transplant are not coded as complications unless they affect the function of the transplanted organs.

See I.C.18.d.3 for transplant organ removal status
See I.C.2.i for malignant neoplasm associated with transplanted organ.

996.78 Due to other internal orthopedic device, implant, and graft
Coding Clinic: 2003, Q2, P14

996.79 Due to other internal prosthetic device, implant, and graft
Coding Clinic: 2004, Q2, P7; 2001, Q1, P8-9; 1995, Q3, P14; 1992, Q3, P4-5

● **996.8 Complications of transplanted organ**
Transplant failure or rejection
Use additional code to identify nature of complication, such as:
  cytomegalovirus [CMV] infection (078.5)
  graft-versus-host disease (279.50–279.53)
  malignancy associated with organ transplant (199.2)
  post-transplant lymphoproliferative disorder (PTLD) (238.77)
Coding Clinic: 2003, Q1, P11; 2002, Q4, P53-54; 2001, Q3, P12-13; 1993, Q2, P11; Q1, P24

996.80 Transplanted organ, unspecified

996.81 Kidney
Coding Clinic: 2012, Q2, P6-7; 2010, Q1, P15; 2008, Q4, P82-83; 2003, Q3, P16-17; 1998, Q3, P6x2&7; 1994, Q3, P8; Q2, P9; 1993, Q4, P32-33; Q1, P24-25

996.82 Liver
Coding Clinic: 2008, Q4, P82-83, 97-100; 2003, Q3, P16x2&17; 1998, Q3, P4

996.83 Heart
Coding Clinic: 2003, Q3, P16; 2002, Q4, P53-54; 2001, Q3, P13-14x2; 1998, Q3, P5; 1993, Q3, P13

996.84 Lung
Coding Clinic: 2003, Q2, P12; 1998, Q3, P5

996.85 Bone marrow
Coding Clinic: 2012, Q1, P13-14; 2011, Q1, P9; 2008, Q4, P90-91

996.86 Pancreas

996.87 Intestine
Coding Clinic: 2000, Q4, P47-48

996.88 Stem cell
Complications from stem cells from:
  peripheral blood
  umbilical cord
Coding Clinic: 2011, Q4, P148

996.89 Other specified transplanted organ
Coding Clinic: 2011, Q1, P9; 1994, Q3, P5

● **996.9 Complications of reattached extremity or body part**

996.90 Unspecified extremity
996.91 Forearm
996.92 Hand
996.93 Finger(s)
996.94 Upper extremity, other and unspecified
996.95 Foot and toe(s)
996.96 Lower extremity, other and unspecified
996.99 Other specified body part

● **997 Complications affecting specified body systems, not elsewhere classified**
Use additional code to identify complication
Excludes the listed conditions when specified as:
  causing shock (998.00-998.09)
  complications of:
    anesthesia:
      adverse effect (001.0–799.9, 995.0–995.8)
      in labor or delivery (668.0–668.9)
      poisoning (968.0–969.9)
    implanted device or graft (996.0–996.9)
    obstetrical procedures (669.0–669.4)
    reattached extremity (996.90–996.96)
    transplanted organ (996.80–996.89)
Coding Clinic: 2011, Q4, P150; Q1, P16; 1995, Q2, P7; 1993, Q2, P9-10; 1992, Q1, P13

● **997.0 Nervous system complications**

997.00 Nervous system complication, unspecified

997.01 Central nervous system complication
Anoxic brain damage
Cerebral hypoxia
Excludes Cerebrovascular hemorrhage or infarction (997.02)
Coding Clinic: 2007, Q1, P22-23; 2006, Q1, P15-16

997.02 Iatrogenic cerebrovascular infarction or hemorrhage
Postoperative stroke
Coding Clinic: 2010, Q3, P5; 2006, Q3, P6; 2004, Q2, P8-9

OGCR Section I.C.7.c

A cerebrovascular hemorrhage or infarction that occurs as a result of medical intervention is coded to 997.02. Documentation should clearly specify cause-and-effect relationship between the medical intervention and the cerebrovascular accident in order to assign this code. A secondary code from the code range 430-432 or from a code from subcategories 433 or 434 with a fifth digit of "1" should also be used to identify the type of hemorrhage or infarct.

997.09 Other nervous system complications

997.1 Cardiac complications
Cardiac:
  arrest during or resulting from a procedure
  insufficiency during or resulting from a procedure
Cardiorespiratory failure during or resulting from a procedure
Heart failure during or resulting from a procedure
Excludes the listed conditions as long-term effects of cardiac surgery or due to the presence of cardiac prosthetic device (429.4)
Coding Clinic: 2013, Q1, P11; 2011, Q1, P3-4; 2008, Q4, P177-180; 2000, Q2, P12; 1994, Q3, P9; Q1, P20; 1993, Q4, P37, 39-43; 5th Issue, P6-7

997.2 Peripheral vascular complications
Phlebitis or thrombophlebitis during or resulting from a procedure
Excludes the listed conditions due to:
  implant or catheter device (996.62)
  infusion, perfusion, or transfusion (999.2)
  complications affecting blood vessels (997.71–997.79)
Coding Clinic: 2003, Q1, P6-7; 2002, Q3, P24-27; 1993, Q1, P26

- **997.3 Respiratory complications**
  - Excludes: iatrogenic [postoperative] pneumothorax (512.1)
    - iatrogenic pulmonary embolism (415.11)
    - specified complications classified elsewhere, such as:
      - adult respiratory distress syndrome (518.52)
      - pulmonary edema, postoperative (518.4)
      - respiratory insufficiency, acute, postoperative (518.52)
      - shock lung
        - related to trauma and surgery (518.52)
      - tracheostomy complications (519.00–519.09)
      - transfusion related acute lung injury (TRALI) (518.7)
  - Coding Clinic: 1997, Q1, P10; 1993, Q4, P43; Q2, P9-10; Q2, P3-4; 1990, Q4, P25x2; 1989, Q1, P10
  - **997.31 Ventilator associated pneumonia**
    - Ventilator associated pneumonitis
    - Use additional code to identify organism
    - Coding Clinic: 2008, Q4, P148-149; 2006, Q2, P25
  - **997.32 Postprocedural aspiration pneumonia**
    - Chemical pneumonitis resulting from a procedure
    - Mendelson's syndrome resulting from a procedure
    - Excludes: aspiration pneumonia during labor and delivery (668.0)
    - Coding Clinic: 2011, Q4, P150
  - **997.39 Other respiratory complications**
    - Coding Clinic: 2011, Q1, P16
- **997.4 Digestive system complications**
  - Complications of:
    - intestinal (internal) anastomosis and bypass, not elsewhere classified, except that involving urinary tract
  - Hepatic failure specified as due to a procedure
  - Hepatorenal syndrome specified as due to a procedure
    - *Acute renal failure occurring along with cirrhosis or fulminant liver failure associated with portal hypertension*
  - Intestinal obstruction NOS specified as due to a procedure
  - Excludes: complications of gastric band procedure (539.01-539.09)
    - complications of other bariatric procedure (539.81-539.89)
    - specified gastrointestinal complications classified elsewhere, such as:
      - blind loop syndrome (579.2)
      - colostomy or enterostomy complications (569.60–569.69)
      - complications of intestinal pouch (569.71–569.79)
      - gastrojejunal ulcer (534.0–534.9)
      - gastrostomy complications (536.40–536.49)
      - infection of esophagostomy (530.86)
      - infection of external stoma (569.61)
      - mechanical complication of esophagostomy (530.87)
      - pelvic peritoneal adhesions, female (614.6)
      - peritoneal adhesions (568.0)
      - peritoneal adhesions with obstruction (560.81)
      - postcholecystectomy syndrome (576.0)
      - postgastric surgery syndromes (564.2)
      - pouchitis (569.71)
      - vomiting following gastrointestinal surgery (564.3)
  - Coding Clinic: 2009, Q4, P129; 2003, Q1, P18; 2001, Q2, P4-6x2; 1999, Q3, P4-5; Q2, P14; 1997, Q3, P7; Q1, P11; 1995, Q3, P7, 16; Q2, P7; 1993, Q1, P26; 1992, Q3, P15; 1989, Q2, P15; 1988, Q1, P14; 1987, Nov-Dec, P9; 1985, Sept-Oct, P11; Mar-April, P11
  - **997.41 Retained cholelithiasis following cholecystectomy**
  - **997.49 Other digestive system complications**
    - Coding Clinic: 2012, Q1, P6-7
- **997.5 Urinary complications**
  - Complications of:
    - internal anastomosis and bypass of urinary tract, including that involving intestinal tract
  - Oliguria or anuria specified as due to procedure
  - Renal (kidney):
    - failure (acute) specified as due to procedure
    - insufficiency (acute) specified as due to procedure
  - Tubular necrosis (acute) specified as due to procedure
  - Excludes: complications of cystostomy (596.81-596.83)
    - complications of external stoma of urinary tract (596.81-596.83)
    - specified complications classified elsewhere, such as:
      - postoperative stricture of:
        - ureter (593.3)
        - urethra (598.2)
  - Coding Clinic: 2012, Q1, P11-12; 2003, Q3, P13; 1996, Q3, P10-11,15; 1995, Q4, P72-73; 1994, Q1, P20; 1992, Q1, P13; 1989, Q2, P16
- **997.6 Amputation stump complication**
  - Excludes: admission for treatment for a current traumatic amputation - code to complicated traumatic amputation
    - phantom limb (syndrome) (353.6)
  - Coding Clinic: 1996, Q4, P45-46
  - **997.60 Unspecified complication**
  - **997.61 Neuroma of amputation stump**
  - **997.62 Infection (chronic)**
    - Use additional code to identify the organism
    - Coding Clinic: 2005, Q1, P14-15; 2003, Q3, P14; 1996, Q4, P45-46
  - **997.69 Other**
    - Coding Clinic: 2005, Q1, P15
- **997.7 Vascular complications of other vessels**
  - Excludes: peripheral vascular complications (997.2)
  - **997.71 Vascular complications of mesenteric artery**
    - Coding Clinic: 2001, Q4, P53
  - **997.72 Vascular complications of renal artery**
  - **997.79 Vascular complications of other vessels**
- **997.9 Complications affecting other specified body systems, not elsewhere classified**
  - Excludes: specified complications classified elsewhere, such as:
    - broad ligament laceration syndrome (620.6)
    - postartificial menopause syndrome (627.4)
    - postoperative stricture of vagina (623.2)
  - Coding Clinic: 1994, Q1, P16; 1993, Q4, P41-42
  - **997.91 Hypertension**
    - Excludes: Essential hypertension (401.0–401.9)
  - **997.99 Other**
    - Vitreous touch syndrome
    - Coding Clinic: 1994, Q2, P12; Q1, P17; Q1, P16-17
- **998 Other complications of procedures, NEC**
  - Excludes: fluid overload due to transfusion (blood) (276.61)
    - TACO (276.61)
    - transfusion associated circulatory overload (276.61)
  - **998.0 Postoperative shock**
    - Shock during or resulting from a surgical procedure
    - Excludes: shock:
      - anaphylactic due to serum (999.41-999.49)
      - anesthetic (995.4)
      - electric (994.8)
      - following abortion (639.5)
      - obstetric (669.1)
      - traumatic (958.4)
    - **998.00 Postoperative shock, unspecified**
      - Collapse, not otherwise specified, during or resulting from a surgical procedure
      - Failure of peripheral circulation, postoperative
    - **998.01 Postoperative shock, cardiogenic**
      - Coding Clinic: 2011, Q4, P152

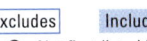

- **998.02** *Postoperative shock, septic*
  Postoperative endotoxic shock
  Postoperative gram-negative shock
  Code first underlying infection
  Use additional code, to identify severe sepsis (995.92) and any associated acute organ dysfunction, if applicable
  Coding Clinic: 2011, Q4, P153

  998.09 Postoperative shock, other
  Postoperative hypovolemic shock

- **998.1 Hemorrhage or hematoma or seroma complicating a procedure**
  Excludes hemorrhage, hematoma or seroma:
      complicating cesarean section or puerperal perineal wound (674.3)
      due to implanted device or graft (996.70–996.79)
  Coding Clinic: 2003, Q3, P13; 1993, Q1, P26; 1992, Q2, P15-16; 1987, Sept-Oct, P8

  998.11 Hemorrhage complicating a procedure
  Coding Clinic: 2003, Q3, P13; Q1, P4; 1997, Q4, P52; Q1, P10; 1994, Q1, P19-20

  998.12 Hematoma complicating a procedure
  Coding Clinic: 2006, Q3, P12; 2003, Q1, P6-7; 2002, Q3, P24-25; 1994, Q1, P20

  998.13 Seroma complicating a procedure
  Pocket of clear serous fluid that sometimes develops in the body after surgery
  Coding Clinic: 1996, Q4, P46

  998.2 Accidental puncture or laceration during a procedure
  Accidental perforation by catheter or other instrument during a procedure on:
      blood vessel
      nerve
      organ
  Excludes iatrogenic [postoperative] pneumothorax (512.1)
      puncture or laceration caused by implanted device intentionally left in operation wound (996.0–996.5)
      specified complications classified elsewhere, such as:
          broad ligament laceration syndrome (620.6)
          dural tear (349.31)
          incidental durotomy (349.31)
          trauma from instruments during delivery (664.0–665.9)
  Coding Clinic: 2012, Q2, P5-6, 8; 2011, Q1, P3-4; 2010, Q1, P15; 2007, Q2, P11-12; 2006, Q1, P15; 2002, Q3, P24-27; 1994, Q3, P6; 1994, Q1, P17; 1990, Q3, P17-18; 1984, Nov-Dec, P12

- **998.3 Disruption of wound**
  Dehiscence of operation wound
  Splitting open
  Disruption of any suture materials or other closure method
  Rupture of operation wound
  Excludes disruption of:
      amputation of stump (997.69)
      cesarean wound (674.1)
      perineal wound, puerperal (674.2)
  Coding Clinic: 2008, Q4, P149-152; 2002, Q4, P73; 1993, Q1, P19

  ▪ 998.30 Disruption of wound, unspecified
  Disruption of wound NOS

  998.31 Disruption of internal operation surgical wound
  Disruption or dehiscence of closure of:
      fascia, superficial or muscular
      internal organ
      muscle or muscle flap
      ribs or rib cage
      skull or craniotomy
      sternum or sternotomy
      tendon or ligament
  Deep disruption or dehiscence of operation wound NOS
  Excludes complications of internal anastomosis of:
      gastrointestinal tract (997.49)
      urinary tract (997.5)
  Coding Clinic: 2010, Q4, P131

  998.32 Disruption of external operation (surgical) wound
  Disruption or dehiscence of closure of:
      cornea
      mucosa
      skin
      subcutaneous tissue
  Full-thickness skin disruption or dehiscence
  Superficial disruption or dehiscence of operation wound
  Coding Clinic: 2006, Q1, P8; 2005, Q1, P11; 2003, Q4, P104-107

  998.33 Disruption of traumatic injury wound repair
  Disruption or dehiscence of closure of traumatic laceration (external) (internal)

  998.4 Foreign body accidentally left during a procedure
  Adhesions due to foreign body accidentally left in operative wound or body cavity during a procedure
  Obstruction due to foreign body accidentally left in operative wound or body cavity during a procedure
  Perforation due to foreign body accidentally left in operative wound or body cavity during a procedure
  Excludes obstruction or perforation caused by implanted device intentionally left in body (996.0–996.5)
  Coding Clinic: 2012, Q1, P12-13; 2011, Q1, P5-6; 2009, Q1, P13; 1989, Q1, P9

- **998.5 Postoperative infection**
  Excludes bleb associated endophthalmitis (379.63)
      infection due to:
          implanted device (996.60–996.69)
          infusion, perfusion, or transfusion (999.31–999.39)
      postoperative obstetrical wound infection (674.3)
  Coding Clinic: 1996, Q4, P45-46; 1995, Q2, P7; 1994, Q3, P6; 1987, Jan-Feb, P13-14

  998.51 Infected postoperative seroma
  Use additional code to identify organism
  Coding Clinic: 1996, Q4, P46

  998.59 Other postoperative infection
  Abscess: postoperative
      intra-abdominal postoperative
      stitch postoperative
      subphrenic postoperative
      wound postoperative
  Septicemia postoperative
  Use additional code to identify infection
  Coding Clinic: 2011, Q4, P153; 2006, Q2, P23-24; 2004, Q4, P75-76; 2003, Q4, P104-107; 1995, Q3, P5; Q2, P7, 11; 1993, Q1, P19

  OGCR Section I.C.1.b.10.b
  > Sepsis due to postprocedural infection: In cases of postprocedural sepsis, the complication code, such as code 998.59, Other postoperative infection, or 674.3x, Other complications of obstetrical surgical wounds should be coded first followed by the appropriate sepsis codes (systemic infection code and either code 995.91 or 995.92). An additional code(s) for any acute organ dysfunction should also be assigned for cases of severe sepsis.

  998.6 Persistent postoperative fistula
  Coding Clinic: 1987, Jan-Feb, P14

  998.7 Acute reaction to foreign substance accidentally left during a procedure
  Peritonitis:
      aseptic
      chemical

- **998.8 Other specified complications of procedures, not elsewhere classified**
  Coding Clinic: 1993, 5th Issue, P8, 15; 1989, Q1, P9; 1987, Jan-Feb, P13
  - 998.81 Emphysema (subcutaneous) (surgical) resulting from a procedure
  - 998.82 Cataract fragments in eye following cataract surgery
  - 998.83 Non-healing surgical wound
    Coding Clinic: 1996, Q4, P47
  - 998.89 Other specified complications
    Coding Clinic: 2009, Q2, P11; 2006, Q3, P9-10; 2005, Q3, P16-17; 1999, Q3, P13; 1998, Q2, P16

- **998.9 Unspecified complication of procedure, not elsewhere classified**
  Postoperative complication NOS
  Excludes complication NOS of obstetrical surgery or procedure (669.4)
  Coding Clinic: 1993, Q4, P41-42

- **999 Complications of medical care, not elsewhere classified**
  Includes complications, not elsewhere classified, of:
  dialysis (hemodialysis) (peritoneal) (renal)
  extracorporeal circulation
  hyperalimentation therapy
  immunization
  infusion
  inhalation therapy
  injection
  inoculation
  perfusion
  transfusion
  vaccination
  ventilation therapy

  Use additional code, where applicable, to identify specific complication

  Excludes specified complications classified elsewhere such as:
  complications of implanted device (996.0–996.9)
  contact dermatitis due to drugs (692.3)
  dementia dialysis (294.8)
    transient (293.9)
  dialysis disequilibrium syndrome (276.0–276.9)
  poisoning and toxic effects of drugs and chemicals (960.0–989.9)
  postvaccinal encephalitis (323.51)
  water and electrolyte imbalance (276.0–276.9)

  - 999.0 Generalized vaccinia
    Excludes vaccinia not from vaccine (051.02)

  - 999.1 Air embolism
    Air embolism to any site following infusion, perfusion, or transfusion
    Excludes embolism specified as:
      complicating:
        abortion (634–638 with .6, 639.6)
        ectopic or molar pregnancy (639.6)
        pregnancy, childbirth, or the puerperium (673.0)
      due to implanted device (996.7)
      traumatic (958.0)

  - 999.2 Other vascular complications
    Phlebitis following infusion, perfusion, or transfusion
    Thromboembolism following infusion, perfusion, or transfusion
    Thrombophlebitis following infusion, perfusion, or transfusion
    Excludes extravasation of vesicant drugs (999.81, 999.82)
      the listed conditions when specified as:
        due to implanted device (996.61–996.62, 996.72–996.74)
        postoperative NOS (997.2, 997.71–997.79)
    Coding Clinic: 1997, Q2, P5

- **999.3 Other infection**
  Infection following infusion, injection, transfusion, or vaccination
  Sepsis following infusion, injection, transfusion, or vaccination
  Septicemia following infusion, injection, transfusion, or vaccination
  Use additional code to identify the specified infection, such as:
  septicemia (038.0–038.9)
  Excludes the listed conditions when specified as:
    due to implanted device (996.60–996.69)
    postoperative NOS (998.51–998.59)
  Coding Clinic: 2001, Q2, P11-12; 1987, Jan-Feb, P14-15

  - 999.31 Other and unspecified infection due to central venous catheter
    Central line-associated infection
    Infection due to:
      central venous catheter NOS
      Hickman catheter
      peripherally inserted central catheter (PICC)
      triple lumen catheter
      umbilical venous catheter
    Excludes infection due to:
      arterial catheter (996.62)
      catheter NOS (996.69)
      peripheral venous catheter (996.62)
      urinary catheter (996.64)
    Coding Clinic: 2012, Q2, P16-17; 2010, Q2, P8; 2008, Q4, P69-73, 192-193; 2007, Q4, P96-97

  - 999.32 Bloodstream infection due to central venous catheter
    Bloodstream infection due to:
      Hickman catheter
      peripherally inserted central catheter (PICC)
      portacath (port-a-cath)
      triple lumen catheter
      umbilical venous catheter
    Catheter-related bloodstream infection (CRBSI) NOS
    Central line-associated bloodstream infection (CLABSI)

  - 999.33 Local infection due to central venous catheter
    Exit or insertion site infection
    Local infection due to:
      Hickman catheter
      peripherally inserted central catheter (PICC)
      portacath (port-a-cath)
      triple lumen catheter
      umbilical venous catheter
    Port or reservoir infection
    Tunnel infection

  - 999.34 Acute infection following transfusion, infusion, or injection of blood and blood products
    Coding Clinic: 2011, Q4, P155

  - 999.39 Infection following other infusion, injection, transfusion, or vaccination

- **999.4 Anaphylactic reaction due to serum**
    Allergic shock
    Anaphylactic shock due to serum
    Anaphylactoid reaction due to serum
    Anaphylaxis
    Excludes ABO incompatibility reaction due to transfusion
        of blood or blood products (999.60-999.69)
        reaction:
            allergic NOS (995.0)
            anaphylactic:
                due to drugs and chemicals (995.0)
                NOS (995.0)
            other serum (999.51-999.59)
        shock:
            allergic NOS (995.0)
            anaphylactic:
                due to drugs and chemicals (995.0)
                NOS (995.0)

    999.41 **Anaphylactic reaction due to administration of blood and blood products**
        Coding Clinic: 2011, Q4, P147

    999.42 **Anaphylactic reaction due to vaccination**

    999.49 **Anaphylactic reaction due to other serum**

- **999.5 Other serum reaction**
    Intoxication by serum   Serum sickness
    Protein sickness   Urticaria due to serum
    Serum rash
    Excludes serum hepatitis (070.2–070.3)

    999.51 **Other serum reaction due to administration of blood and blood products**

    999.52 **Other serum reaction due to vaccination**

    999.59 **Other serum reaction**

- **999.6 ABO incompatibility reaction due to transfusion of blood or blood products**
    Excludes minor blood group antigens reactions (Duffy)
        (E) (K(ell)) (Kidd) (Lewis) (M) (N) (P) (S)
        (999.75-999.79)

    999.60 **ABO incompatibility reaction, unspecified**
        ABO incompatible blood transfusion NOS
        Reaction to ABO incompatibility from
            transfusion NOS

    999.61 **ABO incompatibility with hemolytic transfusion reaction not specified as acute or delayed**
        ABO incompatibility with hemolytic transfusion
            reaction at unspecified time after
            transfusion
        Hemolytic transfusion reaction (HTR) due to
            ABO incompatibility

    999.62 **ABO incompatibility with acute hemolytic transfusion reaction**
        ABO incompatibility with hemolytic transfusion
            reaction less than 24 hours after transfusion
        Acute hemolytic transfusion reaction (AHTR)
            due to ABO incompatibility

    999.63 **ABO incompatibility with delayed hemolytic transfusion reaction**
        ABO incompatibility with hemolytic transfusion
            reaction 24 hours or more after transfusion
        Delayed hemolytic transfusion reaction (DHTR)
            due to ABO incompatibility

    999.69 **Other ABO incompatibility reaction**
        Delayed serologic transfusion reaction (DSTR)
            from ABO incompatibility
        Other ABO incompatible blood transfusion
        Other reaction to ABO incompatibility from
            transfusion

- **999.7 Rh and other non-ABO incompatibility reaction due to transfusion of blood or blood products**

    999.70 **Rh incompatibility reaction, unspecified**
        Reaction due to Rh factor in transfusion NOS
        Rh incompatible blood transfusion NOS
        Unspecified reaction due to incompatibility
            related to Rh antigens (C) (c) (D) (E) (e)
        Unspecified reaction to Rh incompatibility

    999.71 **Rh incompatibility with hemolytic transfusion reaction not specified as acute or delayed**
        Hemolytic transfusion reaction (HTR) due to Rh
            incompatibility
        HTR due to incompatibility related to Rh
            antigens (C) (c) (D) (E) (e), not specified as
            acute or delayed
        Rh incompatibility with hemolytic transfusion
            reaction at unspecified time after
            transfusion

    999.72 **Rh incompatibility with acute hemolytic transfusion reaction**
        Acute hemolytic transfusion reaction (AHTR)
            due to Rh incompatibility
        AHTR due to incompatibility related to Rh
            antigens (C) (c) (D) (E) (e)
        Rh incompatibility with hemolytic transfusion
            reaction less than 24 hours after transfusion

    999.73 **Rh incompatibility with delayed hemolytic transfusion reaction**
        Delayed hemolytic transfusion reaction (DHTR)
            due to Rh incompatibility
        DHTR due to incompatibility related to Rh
            antigens (C) (c) (D) (E) (e)
        Rh incompatibility with hemolytic transfusion
            reaction 24 hours or more after transfusion

    999.74 **Other Rh incompatibility reaction**
        Delayed serologic transfusion reaction (DSTR)
            from Rh incompatibility
        Other reaction due to incompatibility related to
            Rh antigens (C) (c) (D) (E) (e)
        Other reaction to Rh incompatible blood
            transfusion

    999.75 **Non-ABO incompatibility reaction, unspecified**
        Non-ABO incompatible blood transfusion NOS
        Reaction to non-ABO antigen incompatibility
            from transfusion NOS
        Unspecified reaction due to incompatibility
            related to minor antigens (Duffy) (Kell)
            (Kidd) (Lewis) (M) (N) (P) (S)

    999.76 **Non-ABO incompatibility with hemolytic transfusion reaction not specified as acute or delayed**
        Hemolytic transfusion reaction (HTR) due to
            non-ABO incompatibility
        HTR from incompatibility related to minor
            antigens (Duffy) (Kell) (Kidd) (Lewis) (M)
            (N) (P) (S)
        Non-ABO incompatibility with hemolytic
            transfusion reaction at unspecified time
            after transfusion

    999.77 **Non-ABO incompatibility with acute hemolytic transfusion reaction**
        Acute hemolytic transfusion reaction (AHTR)
            due to non-ABO incompatibility
        AHTR from incompatibility related to minor
            antigens (Duffy) (Kell) (Kidd) (Lewis) (M)
            (N) (P) (S)
        Non-ABO incompatibility with hemolytic
            transfusion reaction less than 24 hours after
            transfusion

999.78 Non-ABO incompatibility with delayed hemolytic transfusion reaction
Delayed hemolytic transfusion reaction (DHTR) due to non-ABO incompatibility
DHTR from incompatibility related to minor antigens (Duffy) (Kell) (Kidd) (Lewis) (M) (N) (P) (S)
Non-ABO incompatibility with hemolytic transfusion reaction 24 hours or more after transfusion

999.79 Other non-ABO incompatibility reaction
Delayed serologic transfusion reaction (DSTR) from non-ABO incompatibility
Other non-ABO incompatible blood transfusion
Other reaction due to incompatibility related to minor antigens (Duffy) (Kell) (Kidd) (Lewis) (M) (N) (P) (S)
Other reaction to non-ABO incompatibility from transfusion

● **999.8 Other and unspecified infusion and transfusion reaction**
Excludes: *ABO incompatibility reactions (999.60-999.69)*
febrile nonhemolytic transfusion reaction (FNHTR) (780.66)
hemochromatosis due to repeated red blood cell transfusions (275.02)
non-ABO incompatibility reactions (999.70-999.79)
postoperative shock (998.00-998.09)
posttransfusion purpura (287.41)
Rh incompatibility reactions (999.70-999.74)
transfusion associated circulatory overload (TACO) (276.61)
transfusion related acute lung injury (TRALI) (518.7)
Coding Clinic: 2008, Q4, P152-155; 2000, Q3, P9

999.80 Transfusion reaction, unspecified
Incompatible blood transfusion NOS
Reaction to blood group incompatibility in infusion or transfusion NOS

999.81 Extravasation of vesicant chemotherapy
Infiltration of vesicant chemotherapy
Coding Clinic: 2008, Q4, P152-155

999.82 Extravasation of other vesicant agent
Infiltration of other vesicant agent

999.83 Hemolytic transfusion reaction, incompatibility unspecified
Hemolytic transfusion reaction (HTR) with antigen incompatibility unspecified, not specified as acute or delayed
HTR with incompatibility unspecified at unspecified time after transfusion

999.84 Acute hemolytic transfusion reaction, incompatibility unspecified
Acute hemolytic transfusion reaction (AHTR) with antigen incompatibility unspecified
AHTR, incompatibility unspecified

999.85 Delayed hemolytic transfusion reaction, incompatibility unspecified
Delayed hemolytic transfusion reaction (DHTR) with antigen incompatibility unspecified
DHTR, incompatibility unspecified

999.88 Other infusion reaction

999.89 Other transfusion reaction
Delayed serologic transfusion reaction (DSTR), incompatibility unspecified
Use additional code to identify graft-versus-host reaction (279.5)

999.9 Other and unspecified complications of medical care, not elsewhere classified
Complications, not elsewhere classified, of:
electroshock therapy   ultrasound therapy
inhalation therapy   ventilation therapy
Unspecified misadventure of medical care
Excludes: *unspecified complication of:*
phototherapy (990)
radiation therapy (990)
ventilator associated pneumonia (997.31)
Coding Clinic: 2006, Q2, P25; 2003, Q1, P19; 1997, Q2, P5; 1994, Q3, P9

SUPPLEMENTARY CLASSIFICATION OF FACTORS INFLUENCING HEALTH STATUS AND CONTACT WITH HEALTH SERVICES (V01–V91)

This classification is provided to deal with occasions when circumstances other than a disease or injury classifiable to categories 001–999 (the main part of ICD) are recorded as "diagnoses" or "problems." This can arise mainly in three ways:

a) When a person who is not currently sick encounters the health services for some specific purpose, such as to act as a donor of an organ or tissue, to receive prophylactic vaccination, or to discuss a problem which is in itself not a disease or injury. This will be a fairly rare occurrence among hospital inpatients, but will be relatively more common among hospital outpatients and patients of family practitioners, health clinics, etc.

b) When a person with a known disease or injury, whether it is current or resolving, encounters the health care system for a specific treatment of that disease or injury (e.g., dialysis for renal disease; chemotherapy for malignancy; cast change).

c) When some circumstance or problem is present which influences the person's health status but is not in itself a current illness or injury. Such factors may be elicited during population surveys, when the person may or may not be currently sick, or be recorded as an additional factor to be borne in mind when the person is receiving care for some current illness or injury classifiable to categories 001–999.

In the latter circumstances the V code should be used only as a supplementary code and should not be the one selected for use in primary, single cause tabulations. Examples of these circumstances are a personal history of certain diseases, or a person with an artificial heart valve in situ.

PERSONS WITH POTENTIAL HEALTH HAZARDS RELATED TO COMMUNICABLE DISEASES (V01–V06)

Excludes family history of infectious and parasitic diseases (V18.8)
personal history of infectious and parasitic diseases (V12.0)

● **V01 Contact with or exposure to communicable diseases**
Coding Clinic: 2001, Q1, P10

V01.0 Cholera
Conditions classifiable to 001

V01.1 Tuberculosis
Conditions classifiable to 010–018

V01.2 Poliomyelitis
Conditions classifiable to 045

OGCR Section I.C.18.b
V codes use in any healthcare setting V codes are for use in any healthcare setting. V codes may be used as either a first listed (principal diagnosis code in the inpatient setting) or secondary code, depending on the circumstances of the encounter. Certain V codes may only be used as first listed, others only as secondary codes. See Section I.C.18.e, V Codes That May Only be Principal/First-Listed Diagnosis.

OGCR Section I.C.18.d.1
Category V01 indicates contact with or exposure to communicable diseases. These codes are for patients who do not show any sign or symptom of a disease but have been exposed to it by close personal contact with an infected individual or are in an area where a disease is epidemic. These codes may be used as a first listed code to explain an encounter for testing, or, more commonly, as a secondary code to identify a potential risk.

V01.3 Smallpox
Conditions classifiable to 050

V01.4 Rubella
Conditions classifiable to 056

V01.5 Rabies
Conditions classifiable to 071

V01.6 Venereal diseases
Conditions classifiable to 090–099
Coding Clinic: 2007, Q4, P124-125x2

● **V01.7 Other viral diseases**
Conditions classifiable to 042–078, and V08, except as above

V01.71 Varicella
V01.79 Other viral diseases
Coding Clinic: 1992, Q2, P11

● **V01.8 Other communicable diseases**
Conditions classifiable to 001–136, except as above

V01.81 Anthrax
V01.82 Exposure to SARS-associated coronavirus
Coding Clinic: 2003, Q4, P46-48
V01.83 Escherichia coli (E. coli)
V01.84 Meningococcus
V01.89 Other communicable diseases

V01.9 Unspecified communicable disease

● **V02 Carrier or suspected carrier of infectious diseases**
Includes Colonization status

V02.0 Cholera
V02.1 Typhoid
V02.2 Amebiasis
V02.3 Other gastrointestinal pathogens
V02.4 Diphtheria
● **V02.5 Other specified bacterial diseases**
V02.51 Group B streptococcus
Coding Clinic: 2006, Q3, P14; 2002, Q1, P14-15; 1998, Q4, P56; 1994, Q3, P4
V02.52 Other streptococcus
V02.53 Methicillin susceptible Staphylococcus aureus
MSSA colonization
Coding Clinic: 2008, Q4, P69-73
V02.54 Methicillin resistant Staphylococcus aureus
MRSA colonization
Coding Clinic: 2008, Q4, P69-73
V02.59 Other specified bacterial diseases
Meningococcal
Staphylococcal

● **V02.6 Viral hepatitis**
V02.60 Viral hepatitis carrier, unspecified
V02.61 Hepatitis B carrier
V02.62 Hepatitis C carrier
V02.69 Other viral hepatitis carrier

V02.7 Gonorrhea
V02.8 Other venereal diseases
V02.9 Other specified infectious organism
Coding Clinic: 1994, Q4, P36; 1993, Q1, P22

OGCR Section I.C.18.d.2
Categories V03-V06 are for encounters for inoculations and vaccinations. They indicate that a patient is being seen to receive a prophylactic inoculation against a disease. The injection itself must be represented by the appropriate procedure code. A code from V03-V06 may be used as a secondary code if the inoculation is given as a routine part of preventive health care, such as a well-baby visit.

● **V03 Need for prophylactic vaccination and inoculation against bacterial diseases**
Excludes vaccination not carried out (V64.00–V64.09)
vaccines against combinations of diseases (V06.0–V06.9)

V03.0 Cholera alone
V03.1 Typhoid-paratyphoid alone [TAB]
V03.2 Tuberculosis [BCG]
V03.3 Plague
V03.4 Tularemia
V03.5 Diphtheria alone
V03.6 Pertussis alone
V03.7 Tetanus toxoid alone

- **V03.8** Other specified vaccinations against single bacterial diseases
  - V03.81 Hemophilus influenza, type B [Hib]
  - V03.82 Streptococcus pneumoniae [pneumococcus]
  - V03.89 Other specified vaccination
    Coding Clinic: 2000, Q2, P9
- V03.9 Unspecified single bacterial disease

- **V04** Need for prophylactic vaccination and inoculation against certain diseases
  - Excludes: vaccines against combinations of diseases (V06.0–V06.9)
  - V04.0 Poliomyelitis
  - V04.1 Smallpox
  - V04.2 Measles alone
  - V04.3 Rubella alone
  - V04.4 Yellow fever
  - V04.5 Rabies
  - V04.6 Mumps alone
  - V04.7 Common cold
  - **V04.8** Other viral diseases
    - V04.81 Influenza
    - V04.82 Respiratory syncytial virus (RSV)
      Coding Clinic: 2009, Q1, P5; 2001, Q1, P4
    - V04.89 Other viral diseases
      Coding Clinic: 2007, Q2, P11

- **V05** Need for prophylactic vaccination and inoculation against single diseases
  - Excludes: vaccines against combinations of diseases (V06.0–V06.9)
  - V05.0 Arthropod-borne viral encephalitis
  - V05.1 Other arthropod-borne viral diseases
  - V05.2 Leishmaniasis
  - V05.3 Viral hepatitis
  - V05.4 Varicella
    Chicken pox
  - V05.8 Other specified disease
    Coding Clinic: 2001, Q1, P4; 1991, Q3, P20-21
  - V05.9 Unspecified single disease

- **V06** Need for prophylactic vaccination and inoculation against combinations of diseases
  - Note: Use additional single vaccination codes from categories V03–V05 to identify any vaccinations not included in a combination code.
  - Coding Clinic: 2012, Q1, P11
  - V06.0 Cholera with typhoid-paratyphoid [cholera TAB]
  - V06.1 Diphtheria-tetanus-pertussis, combined [DTP] [DTaP]
    Coding Clinic: 1998, Q3, P13-14
  - V06.2 Diphtheria-tetanus-pertussis with typhoid-paratyphoid [DTP TAB]
  - V06.3 Diphtheria-tetanus-pertussis with poliomyelitis [DTP+polio]
  - V06.4 Measles-mumps-rubella [MMR]
  - V06.5 Tetanus-diphtheria [Td] [DT]
  - V06.6 Streptococcus pneumoniae [pneumococcus] and influenza
  - V06.8 Other combinations
    Excludes: multiple single vaccination codes (V03.0–V05.9)
    Coding Clinic: 2012, Q1, P11; 1994, Q1, P19
  - V06.9 Unspecified combined vaccine

PERSONS WITH NEED FOR ISOLATION, OTHER POTENTIAL HEALTH HAZARDS AND PROPHYLACTIC MEASURES (V07–V09)

- **V07** Need for isolation and other prophylactic or treatment measures
  - Excludes: long-term (current) (prophylactic) use of certain specific drugs (V58.61–V58.69)
    prophylactic organ removal (V50.41–V50.49)
  - V07.0 Isolation
    Admission to protect the individual from his surroundings or for isolation of individual after contact with infectious diseases
  - V07.1 Desensitization to allergens
  - V07.2 Prophylactic immunotherapy
    Administration of:
      antivenin
      immune sera [gamma globulin]
      RhoGAM
      tetanus antitoxin
  - **V07.3** Other prophylactic chemotherapy
    - V07.31 Prophylactic fluoride administration
    - V07.39 Other prophylactic chemotherapy
      Excludes: maintenance chemotherapy following disease (V58.11)
  - V07.4 Hormone replacement therapy (postmenopausal)
  - **V07.5** Use of agents affecting estrogen receptors and estrogen levels
    Code first, if applicable:
      malignant neoplasm of breast (174.0-174.9, 175.0-175.9)
      malignant neoplasm of prostate (185)
    Use additional code, if applicable, to identify:
      estrogen receptor positive status (V86.0)
      family history of breast cancer (V16.3)
      genetic susceptibility to cancer (V84.01-V84.09)
      personal history of breast cancer (V10.3)
      personal history of prostate cancer (V10.46)
      postmenopausal status (V49.81)
    Excludes: hormone replacement therapy (postmenopausal) (V07.4)
    - V07.51 Use of selective estrogen receptor modulators (SERMs)
      Use of:
        raloxifene (Evista)
        tamoxifen (Nolvadex)
        toremifene (Fareston)
    - V07.52 Use of aromatase inhibitors
      Use of:
        anastrozole (Arimidex)
        exemestane (Aromasin)
        letrozole (Femara)
    - V07.59 Use of other agents affecting estrogen receptors and estrogen levels
      Use of:
        estrogen receptor downregulators
        fulvestrant (Faslodex)
        gonadotropin-releasing hormone (GnRH) agonist
        goserelin acetate (Zoladex)
        leuprolide acetate (leuprorelin) (Lupron)
        megestrol acetate (Megace)
  - V07.8 Other specified prophylactic or treatment measure
    Coding Clinic: 2013, Q1, P9; 2010, Q2, P6, 14; 1992, Q1, P11
  - V07.9 Unspecified prophylactic or treatment measure

> **OGCR** Section I.C.1.d
> V08, Asymptomatic human immunodeficiency virus [HIV] infection, is to be applied when the patient without any documentation of symptoms is listed as being "HIV positive," "known HIV," "HIV test positive," or similar terminology. Do not use this code if the term "AIDS" is used or if the patient is treated for any HIV-related illness or is described as having any condition(s) resulting from HIV positive status; use 042 in these cases.

V08 Asymptomatic human immunodeficiency virus [HIV] infection status
   HIV positive NOS
   Note: This code is ONLY to be used when NO HIV infection symptoms or conditions are present. If any HIV infection symptoms or conditions are present, see code 042.
   Excludes AIDS (042)
      human immunodeficiency virus [HIV] disease (042)
      exposure to HIV (V01.79)
      nonspecific serologic evidence of HIV (795.71)
      symptomatic human immunodeficiency virus [HIV] infection (042)
   Coding Clinic: 2004, Q2, P11; 1999, Q2, P8

● **V09 Infection with drug-resistant microorganisms**
   Note: This category is intended for use as an additional code for infectious conditions classified elsewhere to indicate the presence of drug-resistance of the infectious organism.
   Coding Clinic: 2008, Q4, P69-73

   V09.0 Infection with microorganisms resistant to penicillins
      Coding Clinic: 2006, Q2, P16-17; 2003, Q4, P104-107; 1994, Q3, P4
   V09.1 Infection with microorganisms resistant to cephalosporins and other B-lactam antibiotics
   V09.2 Infection with microorganisms resistant to macrolides
   V09.3 Infection with microorganisms resistant to tetracyclines
   V09.4 Infection with microorganisms resistant to aminoglycosides
● **V09.5 Infection with microorganisms resistant to quinolones and fluoroquinolones**
      V09.50 Without mention of resistance to multiple quinolones and fluoroquinoles
      V09.51 With resistance to multiple quinolones and fluoroquinoles
   V09.6 Infection with microorganisms resistant to sulfonamides
● **V09.7 Infection with microorganisms resistant to other specified antimycobacterial agents**
      Excludes Amikacin (V09.4)
         Kanamycin (V09.4)
         Streptomycin [SM] (V09.4)
      V09.70 Without mention of resistance to multiple antimycobacterial agents
      V09.71 With resistance to multiple antimycobacterial agents
● **V09.8 Infection with microorganisms resistant to other specified drugs**
      Vancomycin (glycopeptide) intermediate staphylococcus aureus (VISA/GISA)
      Vancomycin (glycopeptide) resistant enterococcus (VRE)
      Vancomycin (glycopeptide) resistant staphylococcus aureus (VRSA/GRSA)
      V09.80 Without mention of resistance to multiple drugs
      V09.81 With resistance to multiple drugs
● ■**V09.9 Infection with drug-resistant microorganisms, unspecified**
      Drug resistance NOS
      V09.90 Without mention of multiple drug resistance
      V09.91 With multiple drug resistance
         Multiple drug resistance NOS

> **OGCR** Section I.C.2.d
> When a primary malignancy has been previously excised or eradicated from its site and there is no further treatment directed to that site and there is no evidence of any existing primary malignancy, a code from category V10 should be used to indicate the former site of the malignancy. Any mention of extension, invasion, or metastasis to another site is coded as a secondary malignant neoplasm to that site. The secondary site may be the principal or first-listed with the V10 code used as a secondary code.

> **OGCR** Section I.C.18.d.4
> Personal history codes explain a patient's past medical condition that no longer exists and is not receiving any treatment, but that has the potential for recurrence, and therefore may require continued monitoring. The exceptions to this general rule are category V14, Personal history of allergy to medicinal agents, and subcategory V15.0, Allergy, other than to medicinal agents. A person who has had an allergic episode to a substance or food in the past should always be considered allergic to the substance.

PERSONS WITH POTENTIAL HEALTH HAZARDS RELATED TO PERSONAL AND FAMILY HISTORY (V10–V19)

   Excludes obstetric patients where the possibility that the fetus might be affected is the reason for observation or management during pregnancy (655.0–655.9)

● **V10 Personal history of malignant neoplasm**
   Coding Clinic: 1994, Q2, P8
   ● **V10.0 Gastrointestinal tract**
      History of conditions classifiable to 140–159
      Excludes personal history of malignant carcinoid tumor (V10.91)
         personal history of malignant neuroendocrine tumor (V10.91)
      ■**V10.00** Gastrointestinal tract, unspecified
      V10.01 Tongue
      V10.02 Other and unspecified oral cavity and pharynx
      V10.03 Esophagus
      V10.04 Stomach
      V10.05 Large intestine
         Coding Clinic: 1999, Q3, P7-8; 1995, Q1, P3-4
      V10.06 Rectum, rectosigmoid junction, and anus
      V10.07 Liver
      V10.09 Other
         Coding Clinic: 2003, Q4, P111
   ● **V10.1 Trachea, bronchus, and lung**
      History of conditions classifiable to 162
      Excludes personal history of malignant carcinoid tumor (V10.91)
         personal history of malignant neuroendocrine tumor (V10.91)
      V10.11 Bronchus and lung
         Coding Clinic: 2013, Q1, P8
      V10.12 Trachea
   ● **V10.2 Other respiratory and intrathoracic organs**
      History of conditions classifiable to 160, 161, 163–165
      ■**V10.20** Respiratory organ, unspecified
      V10.21 Larynx
         Coding Clinic: 2003, Q4, P108,110
      V10.22 Nasal cavities, middle ear, and accessory sinuses
      V10.29 Other
   V10.3 Breast
      History of conditions classifiable to 174 and 175
      Coding Clinic: 2012, Q1, P11; 2007, Q3, P4; Q1, P3-8; 2003, Q2, P3-5; 2001, Q4, P66; 1997, Q4, P50; 1995, Q4, P53; 1990, Q1, P21

PART III / Diseases: Tabular List Volume 1

- **V10.4 Genital organs**
  History of conditions classifiable to 179–187
  - V10.40 Female genital organ, unspecified
  - V10.41 Cervix uteri
    Coding Clinic: 2007, Q4, P99-101
  - V10.42 Other parts of uterus
  - V10.43 Ovary
  - V10.44 Other female genital organs
  - V10.45 Male genital organ, unspecified
  - V10.46 Prostate
    Coding Clinic: 2009, Q1, P5; 1994, Q2, P12; 1984, May-June, P10
  - V10.47 Testis
  - V10.48 Epididymis
  - V10.49 Other male genital organs
- **V10.5 Urinary organs**
  History of conditions classifiable to 188 and 189
  Excludes personal history of malignant carcinoid tumor (V10.91)
  personal history of malignant neuroendocrine tumor (V10.91)
  Coding Clinic: 1995, Q2, P8
  - V10.50 Urinary organ, unspecified
  - V10.51 Bladder
    Coding Clinic: 1995, Q2, P8; 1985, July-Aug, P16
  - V10.52 Kidney
    Excludes renal pelvis (V10.53)
    Coding Clinic: 2004, Q2, P4
  - V10.53 Renal pelvis
  - V10.59 Other
- **V10.6 Leukemia**
  Conditions classifiable to 204–208
  Excludes leukemia in remission (204–208)
  Coding Clinic: 1992, Q2, P13; 1985, May-June, P8-9
  - V10.60 Leukemia, unspecified
  - V10.61 Lymphoid leukemia
  - V10.62 Myeloid leukemia
  - V10.63 Monocytic leukemia
  - V10.69 Other
- **V10.7 Other lymphatic and hematopoietic neoplasms**
  Conditions classifiable to 200–203
  Excludes listed conditions in 200–203 in remission
  Coding Clinic: 1985, May-June, P8-9
  - V10.71 Lymphosarcoma and reticulosarcoma
  - V10.72 Hodgkin's disease
  - V10.79 Other
- **V10.8 Personal history of malignant neoplasm of other sites**
  History of conditions classifiable to 170–173, 190–195
  Excludes personal history of malignant carcinoid tumor (V10.91)
  personal history of malignant neuroendocrine tumor (V10.91)
  - V10.81 Bone
    Coding Clinic: 2003, Q2, P13
  - V10.82 Malignant melanoma of skin
  - V10.83 Other malignant neoplasm of skin
  - V10.84 Eye
  - V10.85 Brain
    Coding Clinic: 2001, Q1, P6-7
  - V10.86 Other parts of nervous system
    Excludes peripheral, sympathetic, and parasympathetic nerves (V10.89)
  - V10.87 Thyroid
  - V10.88 Other endocrine glands and related structures
  - V10.89 Other
- **V10.9 Other and unspecified personal history of malignant neoplasm**
  - V10.90 Personal history of unspecified malignant neoplasm
    Personal history of malignant neoplasm NOS
    Excludes personal history of malignant carcinoid tumor (V10.91)
    personal history of malignant neuroendocrine tumor (V10.91)
    personal history of Merkel cell carcinoma (V10.91)
  - V10.91 Personal history of malignant neuroendocrine tumor
    Personal history of malignant carcinoid tumor NOS
    Personal history of malignant neuroendocrine tumor NOS
    Personal history of Merkel cell carcinoma NOS
    Code first any continuing functional activity, such as:
    carcinoid syndrome (259.2)
- **V11 Personal history of mental disorder**
  - V11.0 Schizophrenia
    Excludes that in remission (295.0–295.9 with fifth-digit 5)
    Coding Clinic: 1995, Q3, P6
  - V11.1 Affective disorders
    Personal history of manic-depressive psychosis
    Excludes that in remission (296.0–296.6 with fifth-digit 5, 6)
  - V11.2 Neurosis
  - V11.3 Alcoholism
  - V11.4 Combat and operational stress reaction
  - V11.8 Other mental disorders
  - V11.9 Unspecified mental disorder
- **V12 Personal history of certain other diseases**
  Coding Clinic: 2005, Q4, P94-100; 1992, Q3, P11
  - **V12.0 Infectious and parasitic diseases**
    Excludes personal history of infectious diseases specific to a body system
    - V12.00 Unspecified infectious and parasitic disease
    - V12.01 Tuberculosis
    - V12.02 Poliomyelitis
    - V12.03 Malaria
    - V12.04 Methicillin resistant Staphylococcus aureus
      MRSA
      Coding Clinic: 2008, Q4, P69-73
    - V12.09 Other
  - V12.1 Nutritional deficiency
  - V12.2 Personal history endocrine, metabolic, and immunity disorders
    Excludes history of allergy (V14.0–V14.9, V15.01–V15.09)
    Coding Clinic: 2007, Q3, P5-6
    - V12.21 Gestational diabetes
    - V12.29 Other endocrine, metabolic, and immunity disorders
  - V12.3 Diseases of blood and blood-forming organs
  - **V12.4 Disorders of nervous system and sense organs**
    - V12.40 Unspecified disorder of nervous system and sense organs
    - V12.41 Benign neoplasm of the brain
    - V12.42 Infections of the central nervous system
      Encephalitis   Meningitis
    - V12.49 Other disorders of nervous system and sense organs
      Coding Clinic: 1998, Q4, P59-60

- **V12.5 Diseases of circulatory system**
  Excludes: history of anaphylactic shock (V13.81)
  old myocardial infarction (412)
  postmyocardial infarction syndrome (411.0)
  - V12.50 Unspecified circulatory disease
  - V12.51 Venous thrombosis and embolism
    Excludes: pulmonary embolism (V12.55)
    Coding Clinic: 2011, Q1, P20; 2006, Q3, P12; 2003, Q4, P108; 2002, Q1, P15-16
  - V12.52 Thrombophlebitis
  - V12.53 Sudden cardiac arrest
    Sudden cardiac death successfully resuscitated
    Coding Clinic: 2007, Q4, P99-101
  - V12.54 Transient ischemic attack (TIA), and cerebral infarction without residual deficits
    Prolonged reversible ischemic neurological deficit (PRIND)
    Reversible ischemic neurologic deficit (RIND)
    Stroke NOS without residual deficits
    Excludes: history of traumatic brain injury (V15.52)
    late effects of cerebrovascular disease (438.0–438.9)
    Coding Clinic: 2007, Q4, P99-101; 2007, Q2, P3
    OGCR Section I.C.7.d.3
    Assign code V12.54, Transient ischemic attack (TIA), and cerebral infarction without residual deficits (and not a code from category 438) as an additional code for history of cerebrovascular disease when no neurologic deficits are present.
  - V12.55 Pulmonary embolism
  - V12.59 Other
    Coding Clinic: 2007, Q2, P3; 1997, Q4, P35-37
- **V12.6 Diseases of respiratory system**
  Excludes: tuberculosis (V12.01)
  - V12.60 Unspecified disease of respiratory system
  - V12.61 Pneumonia (recurrent)
  - V12.69 Other diseases of respiratory system
- **V12.7 Diseases of digestive system**
  Coding Clinic: 1995, Q1, P3; 1992, Q3, P11; 1989, Q2, P16
  - V12.70 Unspecified digestive disease
  - V12.71 Peptic ulcer disease
  - V12.72 Colonic polyps
    Coding Clinic: 2002, Q3, P14-15
  - V12.79 Other

- **V13 Personal history of other diseases**
  - **V13.0 Disorders of urinary system**
    - V13.00 Unspecified urinary disorder
    - V13.01 Urinary calculi
    - V13.02 Urinary (tract) infection
    - V13.03 Nephrotic syndrome
    - V13.09 Other
      Coding Clinic: 1996, Q2, P7x2
  - V13.1 Trophoblastic disease
    Excludes: supervision during a current pregnancy (V23.1)
  - V13.2 Other genital system and obstetric disorders
    Excludes: supervision during a current pregnancy of a woman with poor obstetric history (V23.0–V23.9)
    recurrent pregnancy loss (646.3)
    without current pregnancy (629.81)
    - V13.21 Personal history of pre-term labor
      Excludes: current pregnancy with history of pre-term labor (V23.41)
    - V13.22 Personal history of cervical dysplasia
      Personal history of conditions classifiable to 622.10–622.12
      Excludes: personal history of malignant neoplasm of cervix uteri (V10.41)
      Coding Clinic: 2007, Q4, P99-101
    - V13.23 Personal history of vaginal dysplasia
      Personal history of conditions classifiable to 623.0
      Excludes: personal history of malignant neoplasm of vagina (V10.44)
    - V13.24 Personal history of vulvar dysplasia
      Personal history of conditions classifiable to 624.01-624.02
      Excludes: personal history of malignant neoplasm of vulva (V10.44)
    - V13.29 Other genital system and obstetric disorders
  - V13.3 Diseases of skin and subcutaneous tissue
  - V13.4 Arthritis
  - **V13.5 Other musculoskeletal disorders**
    - V13.51 Pathologic fracture
      Healed pathologic fracture
      Excludes: personal history of traumatic fracture (V15.51)
    - V13.52 Stress fracture
      Healed stress fracture
      Excludes: personal history of traumatic fracture (V15.51)
    - V13.59 Other musculoskeletal disorders
  - **V13.6 Congenital (corrected) malformations**
    - V13.61 Personal history of (corrected) hypospadias
    - V13.62 Personal history of other (corrected) congenital malformations of genitourinary system
    - V13.63 Personal history of (corrected) congenital malformations of nervous system
    - V13.64 Personal history of (corrected) congenital malformations of eye, ear, face and neck
      Corrected cleft lip and palate
    - V13.65 Personal history of (corrected) congenital malformations of heart and circulatory system
      Coding Clinic: 2010, Q4, P137
    - V13.66 Personal history of (corrected) congenital malformations of respiratory system
    - V13.67 Personal history of (corrected) congenital malformations of digestive system
    - V13.68 Personal history of (corrected) congenital malformations of integument, limbs, and musculoskeletal systems
    - V13.69 Personal history of other (corrected) congenital malformations
      Coding Clinic: 2004, Q1, P16-17
  - V13.7 Perinatal problems
    Excludes: low birth weight status (V21.30–V21.35)
  - **V13.8 Other specified diseases**
    Coding Clinic: 2012, Q1, P11
    - V13.81 Anaphylaxis
    - V13.89 Other specified diseases
  - V13.9 Unspecified disease

- **V14 Personal history of allergy to medicinal agents**
  - V14.0 Penicillin
  - V14.1 Other antibiotic agent
  - V14.2 Sulfonamides
  - V14.3 Other anti-infective agent
  - V14.4 Anesthetic agent
  - V14.5 Narcotic agent
  - V14.6 Analgesic agent
  - V14.7 Serum or vaccine
  - V14.8 Other specified medicinal agents
  - V14.9 Unspecified medicinal agent

- **V15 Other personal history presenting hazards to health**
  - Excludes: personal history of drug therapy (V87.41–V87.49)
  - **V15.0 Allergy, other than to medicinal agents**
    - Excludes: allergy to food substance used as base for medicinal agent (V14.0–V14.9)
    - V15.01 Allergy to peanuts
    - V15.02 Allergy to milk products
      - Excludes: lactose intolerance (271.3)
      - Coding Clinic: 2003, Q1, P12
    - V15.03 Allergy to eggs
    - V15.04 Allergy to seafood
      - Seafood (octopus) (squid) ink
      - Shellfish
    - V15.05 Allergy to other foods
      - Food additives
      - Nuts other than peanuts
    - V15.06 Allergy to insects and arachnids
      - Bugs
      - Insect bites and stings
      - Spiders
    - V15.07 Allergy to latex
      - Latex sensitivity
    - V15.08 Allergy to radiographic dye
      - Contrast media used for diagnostic x-ray procedures
    - V15.09 Other allergy, other than to medicinal agents
  - V15.1 Surgery to heart and great vessels
    - Excludes: replacement by transplant or other means (V42.1–V42.2, V43.2–V43.4)
    - Coding Clinic: 2004, Q1, P16-17
  - **V15.2 Surgery to other organs**
    - Excludes: replacement by transplant or other means (V42.0–V43.8)
    - V15.21 Personal history of undergoing in utero procedure during pregnancy
    - V15.22 Personal history of undergoing in utero procedure while a fetus
    - V15.29 Surgery to other organs
  - V15.3 Irradiation
    - Previous exposure to therapeutic or other ionizing radiation
  - **V15.4 Psychological trauma**
    - Excludes: history of condition classifiable to 290–316 (V11.0–V11.9)
    - V15.41 History of physical abuse
      - Rape
      - Coding Clinic: 1999, Q3, P15
    - V15.42 History of emotional abuse
      - Neglect
      - Coding Clinic: 1999, Q3, P15
    - V15.49 Other
      - Coding Clinic: 1999, Q3, P15
  - **V15.5 Injury**
    - V15.51 Traumatic fracture
      - Healed traumatic fracture
      - Excludes: personal history of pathologic and stress fracture (V13.51, V13.52)
    - V15.52 History of traumatic brain injury
      - Excludes: personal history of cerebrovascular accident (cerebral infarction) without residual deficits (V12.54)
    - V15.53 Personal history of retained foreign body fully removed
    - V15.59 Other injury
  - V15.6 Poisoning
  - V15.7 Contraception
    - Excludes: current contraceptive management (V25.0–V25.4)
      presence of intrauterine contraceptive device as incidental finding (V45.5)
  - **V15.8 Other specified personal history presenting hazards to health**
    - Excludes: contact with and (suspected) exposure to:
      - aromatic compounds and dyes (V87.11-V87.19)
      - arsenic and other metals (V87.01-V87.09)
      - molds (V87.31)
    - V15.80 History of failed moderate sedation
      - History of failed conscious sedation
    - V15.81 Noncompliance with medical treatment
      - Excludes: noncompliance with renal dialysis (V45.12)
      - Coding Clinic: 2012, Q2, P16-17; 2007, Q3, P11; 2006, Q4, P136; 2003, Q2, P7-8; 2001, Q2, P13; 1999, Q2, P17; Q1, P13-14; 1997, Q2, P11; 1996, Q3, P9
    - V15.82 History of tobacco use
      - Excludes: tobacco dependence (305.1)
      - Coding Clinic: 2009, Q1, P15
    - V15.83 Underimmunization status
      - Delinquent immunization status
      - Lapsed immunization schedule status
    - V15.84 Contact with and (suspected) exposure to asbestos
    - V15.85 Contact with and (suspected) exposure to potentially hazardous body fluids
    - V15.86 Contact with and (suspected) exposure to lead
    - V15.87 History of extracorporeal membrane oxygenation [ECMO]
    - V15.88 History of fall
      - At risk for falling
      - Coding Clinic: 2005, Q4, P94-100
    - V15.89 Other
      - Excludes: contact with and (suspected) exposure to other potentially hazardous chemicals (V87.2)
        contact with and (suspected) exposure to other potentially hazardous substances (V87.39)
      - Coding Clinic: 2008, Q3, P6-7; 2007, Q3, P6; 1990, Q1, P21
  - V15.9 Unspecified personal history presenting hazards to health

V16-V20.2 ICD-9-CM

OGCR Section I.C.18.d.3
Family history codes are for use when a patient has a family member(s) who has had a particular disease that causes the patient to be at higher risk of also contracting the disease.

- **V16 Family history of malignant neoplasm**
  Coding Clinic: 1985, Nov-Dec, P13
  - V16.0 Gastrointestinal tract
    Family history of condition classifiable to 140–159
    Coding Clinic: 1999, Q1, P4
  - V16.1 Trachea, bronchus, and lung
    Family history of condition classifiable to 162
  - V16.2 Other respiratory and intrathoracic organs
    Family history of condition classifiable to 160–161, 163–165
  - V16.3 Breast
    Family history of condition classifiable to 174
    Coding Clinic: 2004, Q4, P106-107; 2003, Q2, P3-5; 2000, Q2, P8-9; 1995, Q4, P61; 1992, Q1, P11; 1990, Q1, P21
  - V16.4 Genital organs
    Family history of condition classifiable to 179–187
    - V16.40 Genital organ, unspecified
    - V16.41 Ovary
      Coding Clinic: 2009, Q3, P21
    - V16.42 Prostate
    - V16.43 Testis
    - V16.49 Other
      Coding Clinic: 2006, Q2, P3,4
  - V16.5 Urinary organs
    Family history of condition classifiable to 188–189
    - V16.51 Kidney
    - V16.52 Bladder
    - V16.59 Other
  - V16.6 Leukemia
    Family history of condition classifiable to 204–208
  - V16.7 Other lymphatic and hematopoietic neoplasms
    Family history of condition classifiable to 200–203
  - V16.8 Other specified malignant neoplasm
    Family history of other condition classifiable to 140–199
  - V16.9 Unspecified malignant neoplasm

- **V17 Family history of certain chronic disabling diseases**
  Coding Clinic: 1985, Nov-Dec, P13
  - V17.0 Psychiatric condition
    Excludes family history of intellectual disabilities (V18.4)
  - V17.1 Stroke (cerebrovascular)
  - V17.2 Other neurological diseases
    Epilepsy   Huntington's chorea
  - V17.3 Ischemic heart disease
  - V17.4 Other cardiovascular diseases
    Coding Clinic: 2004, Q1, P6-7
    - V17.41 Family history of sudden cardiac death (SCD)
      Excludes family history of ischemic heart disease (V17.3)
      family history of myocardial infarction (V17.3)
    - V17.49 Family history of other cardiovascular diseases
      Family history of cardiovascular disease NOS
  - V17.5 Asthma
  - V17.6 Other chronic respiratory conditions
  - V17.7 Arthritis
  - V17.8 Other musculoskeletal diseases
    - V17.81 Osteoporosis
    - V17.89 Other musculoskeletal diseases

- **V18 Family history of certain other specific conditions**
  Coding Clinic: 1985, Nov-Dec, P13
  - V18.0 Diabetes mellitus
    Coding Clinic: 2005, Q2, P21; 2004, Q1, P8
  - V18.1 Other endocrine and metabolic diseases
    - V18.11 Multiple endocrine neoplasia [MEN] syndrome
    - V18.19 Other endocrine and metabolic diseases
  - V18.2 Anemia
  - V18.3 Other blood disorders
  - V18.4 Intellectual disabilities
  - V18.5 Digestive disorders
    - V18.51 Colonic polyps
      Excludes family history of malignant neoplasm of gastrointestinal tract (V16.0)
    - V18.59 Other digestive disorders
  - V18.6 Kidney diseases
    - V18.61 Polycystic kidney
    - V18.69 Other kidney diseases
  - V18.7 Other genitourinary diseases
  - V18.8 Infectious and parasitic diseases
  - V18.9 Genetic disease carrier

- **V19 Family history of other conditions**
  Coding Clinic: 1985, Nov-Dec, P13
  - V19.0 Blindness or visual loss
  - V19.1 Other eye disorders
    - V19.11 Glaucoma
    - V19.19 Other specified eye disorder
  - V19.2 Deafness or hearing loss
  - V19.3 Other ear disorders
  - V19.4 Skin conditions
  - V19.5 Congenital anomalies
  - V19.6 Allergic disorders
  - V19.7 Consanguinity
  - V19.8 Other condition

PERSONS ENCOUNTERING HEALTH SERVICES IN CIRCUMSTANCES RELATED TO REPRODUCTION AND DEVELOPMENT (V20–V29)

- **V20 Health supervision of infant or child**
  - V20.0 Foundling
  - V20.1 Other healthy infant or child receiving care
    Medical or nursing care supervision of healthy infant in cases of:
      maternal illness, physical or psychiatric
      socioeconomic adverse condition at home
      too many children at home preventing or interfering with normal care
    Coding Clinic: 2000, Q1, P25; 1993, Q4, P36; 1989, Q3, P14
  - V20.2 Routine infant or child health check
    Developmental testing of infant or child
    Health check for child over 28 days old
    Immunizations appropriate for age
    Routine vision and hearing testing
    Excludes health check for child under 29 days old (V20.31-V20.32)
    newborn health supervision (V20.31-V20.32)
    special screening for developmental handicaps (V79.3)
    Use additional code(s) to identify:
    Special screening examination(s) performed (V73.0–V82.9)
    Coding Clinic: 2009, Q1, P15; 2004, Q1, P15-16x2

- **V20.3** Newborn health supervision
  Health check for child under 29 days old
  Excludes health check for child over 28 days old (V20.2)
  - **V20.31** Health supervision for newborn under 8 days old
    Health check for newborn under 8 days old
  - **V20.32** Health supervision for newborn 8 to 28 days old
    Health check for newborn 8 to 28 days old
    Newborn weight check
    Coding Clinic: 2009, Q4, P151

- **V21** Constitutional states in development
  - **V21.0** Period of rapid growth in childhood
  - **V21.1** Puberty
  - **V21.2** Other adolescence
  - **V21.3** Low birth weight status
    Excludes history of perinatal problems (V13.7)
    - **V21.30** Low birth weight status, unspecified
    - **V21.31** Low birth weight status, less than 500 grams
    - **V21.32** Low birth weight status, 500–999 grams
    - **V21.33** Low birth weight status, 1000–1499 grams
    - **V21.34** Low birth weight status, 1500–1999 grams
    - **V21.35** Low birth weight status, 2000–2500 grams
  - **V21.8** Other specified constitutional states in development
  - **V21.9** Unspecified constitutional state in development

- **V22** Normal pregnancy
  Excludes pregnancy examination or test, pregnancy unconfirmed (V72.40)
  Coding Clinic: 2012, Q1, P10; 2007, Q4, P124-125

  OGCR Section I.C.11.b.1
  For routine outpatient prenatal visits when no complications are present codes V22.0, Supervision of normal first pregnancy, and V22.1, Supervision of other normal pregnancy, should be used as the first-listed diagnoses. These codes should not be used in conjunction with chapter 11 codes.

  - **V22.0** Supervision of normal first pregnancy
    Coding Clinic: 1999, Q3, P16; 1990, Q1, P10; 1984, Nov-Dec, P18
  - **V22.1** Supervision of other normal pregnancy
    Coding Clinic: 1999, Q3, P16; 1990, Q1, P10
  - **V22.2** Pregnant state, incidental
    Pregnant state NOS
    Coding Clinic: 1998, Q2, P13-14; 1994, Q2, P14

  OGCR Section I.C.11.b.2
  For routine prenatal outpatient visits for patients with high-risk pregnancies, a code from category V23, Supervision of high-risk pregnancy, should be used as the first-listed diagnosis. Secondary chapter 11 codes may be used in conjunction with these codes if appropriate.

- **V23** Supervision of high-risk pregnancy
  Coding Clinic: 2012, Q1, P10; 1990, Q1, P10
  - **V23.0** Pregnancy with history of infertility
  - **V23.1** Pregnancy with history of trophoblastic disease
    Pregnancy with history of:
      hydatidiform mole
      vesicular mole
    Excludes that without current pregnancy (V13.1)
  - **V23.2** Pregnancy with history of abortion
    Pregnancy with history of conditions classifiable to 634–638
    Excludes recurrent pregnancy loss:
      care during pregnancy (646.3)
      that without current pregnancy (629.81)
  - **V23.3** Grand multiparity
    Excludes care in relation to labor and delivery (659.4)
    that without current pregnancy (V61.5)
  - **V23.4** Pregnancy with other poor obstetric history
    Pregnancy with history of other conditions classifiable to 630–676
    - **V23.41** Pregnancy with history of pre-term labor
    - **V23.42** Pregnancy with history of ectopic pregnancy
    - **V23.49** Pregnancy with other poor obstetric history
  - **V23.5** Pregnancy with other poor reproductive history
    Pregnancy with history of stillbirth or neonatal death
  - **V23.7** Insufficient prenatal care
    History of little or no prenatal care
  - **V23.8** Other high-risk pregnancy
    Coding Clinic: 1998, Q4, P50-51
    - **V23.81** Elderly primigravida
      First pregnancy in a woman who will be 35 years of age or older at expected date of delivery
      Excludes elderly primigravida complicating pregnancy (659.5)
      Coding Clinic: 1998, Q4, P58
    - **V23.82** Elderly multigravida
      Second or more pregnancy in a woman who will be 35 years of age or older at expected date of delivery
      Excludes elderly multigravida complicating pregnancy (659.6)
      Coding Clinic: 2013, Q1, P19; 2011, Q4, P133
    - **V23.83** Young primigravida
      First pregnancy in a female less than 16 years old at expected date of delivery
      Excludes young primigravida complicating pregnancy (659.8)
    - **V23.84** Young multigravida
      Second or more pregnancy in a female less than 16 years old at expected date of delivery
      Excludes young multigravida complicating pregnancy (659.8)
    - **V23.85** Pregnancy resulting from assisted reproductive technology
      Pregnancy resulting from in vitro fertilization
    - **V23.86** Pregnancy with history of in utero procedure during previous pregnancy
      Excludes management of pregnancy affected by in utero procedure during current pregnancy (679.0–679.1)
    - **V23.87** Pregnancy with inconclusive fetal viability
      Encounter to determine fetal viability of pregnancy
    - **V23.89** Other high-risk pregnancy
      Coding Clinic: 2006, Q3, P14
  - **V23.9** Unspecified high-risk pregnancy

OGCR Section I.C.18.d.8
The follow-up codes (V24, V67 and V89), are used to explain continuing surveillance following completed treatment of a disease, condition, or injury. They imply that the condition has been fully treated and no longer exists. They should not be confused with aftercare codes that explain current treatment for a healing condition or its sequelae. Follow-up codes may be used in conjunction with history codes to provide the full picture of the healed condition and its treatment. The follow-up code is sequenced first, followed by the history code. A follow-up code may be used to explain repeated visits. Should a condition be found to have recurred on the follow-up visit, then the diagnosis code should be used in place of the follow-up code.

● **V24 Postpartum care and examination**
   V24.0 Immediately after delivery
      Care and observation in uncomplicated cases
      Coding Clinic: 2006, Q3, P11

   OGCR Section I.C.10.i.5
   When the mother delivers outside the hospital prior to admission and is admitted for routine postpartum care and no complications are noted, code V24.0, Postpartum care and examination immediately after delivery, should be assigned as the principal diagnosis.

   V24.1 Lactating mother
      Supervision of lactation
      Coding Clinic: 2012, Q3, P7
   V24.2 Routine postpartum follow-up

● **V25 Encounter for contraceptive management**
  ● **V25.0 General counseling and advice**
    V25.01 Prescription of oral contraceptives
    V25.02 Initiation of other contraceptive measures
      Fitting of diaphragm
      Prescription of foams, creams, or other agents
      Coding Clinic: 1997, Q3, P7
    V25.03 Encounter for emergency contraceptive counseling and prescription
      Encounter for postcoital contraceptive counseling and prescription
    V25.04 Counseling and instruction in natural family planning to avoid pregnancy
      Coding Clinic: 2007, Q4, P99-101
    V25.09 Other
      Family planning advice
  ● **V25.1 Encounter for insertion or removal of intrauterine contraceptive device**
    Excludes encounter for routine checking of intrauterine contraceptive device (V25.42)
    V25.11 Encounter for insertion of intrauterine contraceptive device
    V25.12 Encounter for removal of intrauterine contraceptive device
    V25.13 Encounter for removal and reinsertion of intrauterine contraceptive device
      Encounter for replacement of intrauterine contraceptive device
   V25.2 Sterilization
      Admission for interruption of fallopian tubes or vas deferens
   V25.3 Menstrual extraction
      Menstrual regulation
  ● **V25.4 Surveillance of previously prescribed contraceptive methods**
      Checking, reinsertion, or removal of contraceptive device
      Repeat prescription for contraceptive method
      Routine examination in connection with contraceptive maintenance
    V25.40 Contraceptive surveillance, unspecified
    V25.41 Contraceptive pill
    V25.42 Intrauterine contraceptive device
      Checking of intrauterine device
      Excludes insertion or removal of intrauterine contraceptive device (V25.11-V25.13)
      presence of intrauterine contraceptive device as incidental finding (V45.5)
    V25.43 Implantable subdermal contraceptive
    V25.49 Other contraceptive method
      Coding Clinic: 1997, Q3, P7
   V25.5 Insertion of implantable subdermal contraceptive
   V25.8 Other specified contraceptive management
      Postvasectomy sperm count
    Excludes sperm count following sterilization reversal (V26.22)
      sperm count for fertility testing (V26.21)
    Coding Clinic: 1996, Q3, P9
  ■ **V25.9 Unspecified contraceptive management**

● **V26 Procreative management**
   V26.0 Tuboplasty or vasoplasty after previous sterilization
      Coding Clinic: 1995, Q2, P10
   V26.1 Artificial insemination
  ● **V26.2 Investigation and testing**
    Excludes postvasectomy sperm count (V25.8)
    Coding Clinic: 1996, Q2, P9; 1985, Nov-Dec, P15
    V26.21 Fertility testing
      Fallopian insufflation
      Sperm count for fertility testing
      Excludes genetic counseling and testing (V26.31–V26.39)
    V26.22 Aftercare following sterilization reversal
      Fallopian insufflation following sterilization reversal
      Sperm count following sterilization reversal
    V26.29 Other investigation and testing

   OGCR Section I.C.18.d.3
   If the purpose of the encounter is genetic counseling associated with procreative management, a code from subcategory V26.3 should be assigned as the first-listed code, followed by a code from category V84, Genetic susceptibility to disease. Additional codes should be assigned for any applicable family or personal history.

  ● **V26.3 Genetic counseling and testing**
    Excludes fertility testing (V26.21)
      nonprocreative genetic screening (V82.71, V82.79)
    Coding Clinic: 2006, Q4, P117; 2005, Q4, P94-100
    V26.31 Testing of female genetic disease carrier status
    V26.32 Other genetic testing of female
      Use additional code to identify recurrent pregnancy loss (629.81, 646.3)
    V26.33 Genetic counseling
    V26.34 Testing of male for genetic disease carrier status
    V26.35 Encounter for testing of male partner of female with recurrent pregnancy loss
    V26.39 Other genetic testing of male
  ● **V26.4 General counseling and advice**
    V26.41 Procreative counseling and advice using natural family planning
      Coding Clinic: 2007, Q4, P99-101
    V26.42 Encounter for fertility preservation counseling
      Encounter for fertility preservation counseling prior to cancer therapy
      Encounter for fertility preservation counseling prior to surgical removal of gonads
    V26.49 Other procreative management counseling and advice

- **V26.5** Sterilization status
  - **V26.51** Tubal ligation status
    - [Excludes] *infertility not due to previous tubal ligation (628.0–628.9)*
  - **V26.52** Vasectomy status
- **V26.8** Other specified procreative management
  - **V26.81** Encounter for assisted reproductive fertility procedure cycle
    - Patient undergoing in vitro fertilization cycle
    - [Use additional] code to identify the type of infertility
    - [Excludes] *pre-cycle diagnosis and testing - code to reason for encounter*
    - Coding Clinic: 2007, Q4, P99-101
  - **V26.82** Encounter for fertility preservation procedure
    - Encounter for fertility preservation counseling prior to cancer therapy
    - Encounter for fertility preservation procedure prior to surgical removal of gonads
  - **V26.89** Other specified procreative management
- **V26.9** Unspecified procreative management

OGCR Section I.C.11.h.3
V27.0, Single liveborn, is the only outcome of delivery code appropriate for use with 650.

OGCR Section I.C.11.k.4
When an attempted termination of pregnancy results in a liveborn fetus assign code 644.21 with an appropriate code from category V27, Outcome of Delivery. The procedure code for the attempted termination of pregnancy should also be assigned.

OGCR Section I.C.11.b.5
An outcome of delivery code, V27.0-V27.9, should be included on every maternal record when a delivery has occurred. These codes are not to be used on subsequent records or on the newborn record.

- **V27** Outcome of delivery
  - **Note:** This category is intended for the coding of the outcome of delivery on the mother's record.
  - Coding Clinic: 1991, Q2, P16
  - **V27.0** Single liveborn
    - Coding Clinic: 2011, Q4, P133; 2008, Q4, P192; 2005, Q4, P81; 2003, Q2, P9; 2002, Q2, P10; 2000, Q3, P5; 1998, Q4, P76-77
  - **V27.1** Single stillborn
    - Coding Clinic: 2001, Q1, P11-12
  - **V27.2** Twins, both liveborn
    - Coding Clinic: 1992, Q3, P10
  - **V27.3** Twins, one liveborn and one stillborn
  - **V27.4** Twins, both stillborn
  - **V27.5** Other multiple birth, all liveborn
  - **V27.6** Other multiple birth, some liveborn
  - **V27.7** Other multiple birth, all stillborn
  - **V27.9** Unspecified outcome of delivery
    - Routine prenatal care (V22.0–V23.9)
- **V28** Encounter for antenatal screening of mother
  - [Excludes] *abnormal findings on screening - code to findings*
    - *suspected fetal conditions affecting management of pregnancy (655.00–655.93, 656.00–656.93, 657.00–657.03, 658.00–658.93)*
    - *suspected fetal conditions not found (V89.01-V89.09)*

OGCR Section I.C.18.d.5
See V28, Antenatal screening; V73-V82 to report special screening examinations.

  - **V28.0** Screening for chromosomal anomalies by amniocentesis
  - **V28.1** Screening for raised alpha-fetoprotein levels in amniotic fluid
  - **V28.2** Other screening based on amniocentesis
  - **V28.3** Encounter for routine screening for malformation using ultrasonics
    - Encounter for routine fetal ultrasound NOS
    - [Excludes] *encounter for fetal anatomic survey (V28.81) genetic counseling and testing (V26.31–V26.39)*
  - **V28.4** Screening for fetal growth retardation using ultrasonics
  - **V28.5** Screening for isoimmunization
  - **V28.6** Screening for Streptococcus B
  - **V28.8** Other specified antenatal screening
    - Coding Clinic: 1999, Q3, P16
    - **V28.81** Encounter for fetal anatomic survey
    - **V28.82** Encounter for screening for risk of pre-term labor
    - **V28.89** Other specified antenatal screening
      - Chorionic villus sampling
      - Genomic screening
      - Nuchal translucency testing
      - Proteomic screening
  - **V28.9** Unspecified antenatal screening
- **V29** Observation and evaluation of newborns for suspected condition not found
  - **Note:** This category is to be used for newborns, within the neonatal period (the first 28 days of life), who are suspected of having an abnormal condition resulting from exposure from the mother or the birth process, but without signs or symptoms, and which, after examination and observation, is found not to exist.
  - [Excludes] *suspected fetal conditions not found (V89.01–V89.09)*
  - Coding Clinic: 2000, Q1, P25-26
  - **V29.0** Observation for suspected infectious condition
    - Coding Clinic: 2001, Q1, P10
  - **V29.1** Observation for suspected neurological condition

OGCR Section I.C.15.d.1
Assign a code from category V29, Observation and evaluation of newborns and infants for suspected conditions not found, to identify those instances when a healthy newborn is evaluated for a suspected condition that is determined after study not to be present. Do not use a code from category V29 when the patient has identified signs or symptoms of a suspected problem; in such cases, code the sign or symptom. A code from category V29 may also be assigned as a principal code for readmissions or encounters when the V30 code no longer applies. Codes from category V29 are for use only for healthy newborns and infants for which no condition after study is found to be present.

OGCR Section I.C.15.d.2
A V29 code is to be used as a secondary code after the V30.

OGCR Section I.C.18.d.6
There are three observation V code categories. They are for use in very limited circumstances when a person is being observed for a suspected condition that is ruled out. The observation codes are not for use if an injury or illness or any signs or symptoms related to the suspected condition are present. In such cases the diagnosis/symptom code is used with the corresponding E code to identify any external cause. The observation codes are to be used as principal diagnosis only. The only exception to this is when the principal diagnosis is required to be a code from the V30, Live born infant, category. Then the V29 observation code is sequenced after the V30 code. Additional codes may be used in addition to the observation code but only if they are unrelated to the suspected condition being observed.

  - **V29.2** Observation for suspected respiratory condition
  - **V29.3** Observation for suspected genetic or metabolic condition
    - Coding Clinic: 2005, Q2, P21; 2004, Q1, P8; 1998, Q4, P59
  - **V29.8** Observation for other specified suspected condition
    - Coding Clinic: 2003, Q2, P15-16
  - **V29.9** Observation for unspecified suspected condition
    - Coding Clinic: 2002, Q1, P6-7

OGCR Section I.C.15.b
When coding the birth of an infant, assign a code from categories V30-V39, according to the type of birth. A code from this series is assigned as a principal diagnosis, and assigned only once to a newborn at the time of birth.

OGCR Section I.C.15.c
If the newborn is transferred to another institution, the V30 series is not used at the receiving hospital.

LIVEBORN INFANTS ACCORDING TO TYPE OF BIRTH (V30–V39)

Note: These categories are intended for the coding of liveborn infants who are consuming health care [e.g., crib or bassinet occupancy].

The following fourth-digit subdivisions are for use with categories V30–V39:

0 Born in hospital
1 Born before admission to hospital
2 Born outside hospital and not hospitalized

The following two fifths-digits are for use with the fourth-digit .0, Born in hospital:

0 delivered without mention of cesarean delivery
1 delivered by cesarean delivery

- **V30 Single liveborn**
  Coding Clinic: 2012, Q3, P5; Q2, P17; 2009, Q4, P151x2; 2006, Q3, P10-11; 2005, Q4, P83-89; Q2, P21; 2004, Q1, P8, 16; 2003, Q4, P67-68; Q2, P9; 2001, Q4, P50-51; 2000, Q1, P25-26; 1998, Q4, P46-47, 59; 1994, Q3, P4; 1993, Q4, P36

- **V31 Twin, mate liveborn**
  Coding Clinic: 1992, Q3, P10

- **V32 Twin, mate stillborn**

- **V33 Twin, unspecified**

- **V34 Other multiple, mates all liveborn**

- **V35 Other multiple, mates all stillborn**

- **V36 Other multiple, mates live- and stillborn**

- **V37 Other multiple, unspecified**

- **V39 Unspecified**

PERSONS WITH A CONDITION INFLUENCING THEIR HEALTH STATUS (V40–V49)

Note: These categories are intended for use when these conditions are recorded as "diagnoses" or "problems."

- **V40 Mental and behavioral problems**
  V40.0 Problems with learning
  V40.1 Problems with communication [including speech]
  V40.2 Other mental problems
  - **V40.3 Other behavioral problems**
    - **V40.31 Wandering in diseases classified elsewhere**
      Code first underlying disorder such as:
      Alzheimer's disease (331.0)
      autism or pervasive developmental disorder (299.0-299.9)
      dementia, unspecified, with behavioral disturbance (294.21)
      intellectual disabilities (317-319)
    V40.39 Other specified behavioral problem
  V40.9 Unspecified mental or behavioral problem

- **V41 Problems with special senses and other special functions**
  V41.0 Problems with sight
  V41.1 Other eye problems
  V41.2 Problems with hearing
  V41.3 Other ear problems
  V41.4 Problems with voice production
  V41.5 Problems with smell and taste
  V41.6 Problems with swallowing and mastication
  V41.7 Problems with sexual function
    Excludes marital problems (V61.10)
    psychosexual disorders (302.0–302.9)
  V41.8 Other problems with special functions
  V41.9 Unspecified problem with special functions

- **V42 Organ or tissue replaced by transplant**
  Includes homologous or heterologous (animal) (human) transplant organ status
  Coding Clinic: 1998, Q3, P5

  OGCR Section I.C.17.f.2.a
  Transplant complications other than kidney: Codes under subcategory 996.8, Complications of transplanted organ, are for use for both complications and rejection of transplanted organs. A transplant complication code is only assigned if the complication affects the function of the transplanted organ. Two codes are required to fully describe a transplant complication, the appropriate code from subcategory 996.8 and a secondary code that identifies the complication.
  Pre-existing conditions or conditions that develop after the transplant are not coded as complications unless they affect the function of the transplanted organs.
  See I.C.18.d.3) for transplant organ removal status.
  See I.C.2.i for malignant neoplasm associated with transplanted organ.

  V42.0 Kidney
    Coding Clinic: 2008, Q1, P10-13; 2003, Q1, P10-11; 2001, Q3, P12-13; 1994, Q2, P9x2

    OGCR Section I.C.17.f.2.b
    Patients who have undergone kidney transplant may still have some form of chronic kidney disease (CKD) because the kidney transplant may not fully restore kidney function. Code 996.81 should be assigned for documented complications of a kidney transplant, such as transplant failure or rejection or other transplant complication. Code 996.81 should not be assigned for post kidney transplant patients who have chronic kidney (CKD) unless a transplant complication such as transplant failure or rejection is documented. If the documentation is unclear as to whether the patient has a complication of the transplant, query the provider. For patients with CKD following a kidney transplant, but who do not have a complication such as failure or rejection, *see section I.C.10.a.2, Chronic kidney disease and kidney transplant status.*

  V42.1 Heart
    Coding Clinic: 2011, Q3, P5; 2003, Q3, P16; 2001, Q3, P13-14x2; 1994, Q2, P13
  V42.2 Heart valve
  V42.3 Skin
  V42.4 Bone
  V42.5 Cornea
  V42.6 Lung
  V42.7 Liver
    Coding Clinic: 2011, Q3, P6
  - **V42.8 Other specified organ or tissue**
    V42.81 Bone marrow
      Coding Clinic: 2012, Q1, P13-14
    V42.82 Peripheral stem cells
    V42.83 Pancreas
      Coding Clinic: 2003, Q1, P10-11; 2001, Q2, P16
    V42.84 Intestines
      Coding Clinic: 2000, Q4, P47-48
    V42.89 Other
  V42.9 Unspecified organ or tissue

- **V43 Organ or tissue replaced by other means**
  - **Includes** organ or tissue assisted by other means
    replacement of organ by:
    artificial device
    mechanical device
    prosthesis
  - **Excludes** cardiac pacemaker in situ (V45.01)
    fitting and adjustment of prosthetic device (V52.0–V52.9)
    renal dialysis status (V45.11)
  - V43.0 Eye globe
  - V43.1 Lens
    Pseudophakos
  - **V43.2 Heart**
    - V43.21 Heart assist device
    - V43.22 Fully implantable artificial heart
  - V43.3 Heart valve
    Coding Clinic: 2006, Q3, P7; 2002, Q3, P13-15
  - V43.4 Blood vessel
  - V43.5 Bladder
  - **V43.6 Joint**
    Coding Clinic: 1991, Q1, P15
    - V43.60 Unspecified joint
    - V43.61 Shoulder
    - V43.62 Elbow
    - V43.63 Wrist
    - V43.64 Hip
      Coding Clinic: 2009, Q1, P15; 2008, Q2, P3-5; 2006, Q3, P4-5; 2005, Q4, P83-89, 110-112; 2004, Q2, P15
    - V43.65 Knee
      Coding Clinic: 2006, Q3, P5
    - V43.66 Ankle
    - V43.69 Other
  - V43.7 Limb
  - **V43.8 Other organ or tissue**
    - V43.81 Larynx
    - V43.82 Breast
    - V43.83 Artificial skin
    - V43.89 Other
- **V44 Artificial opening status**
  - **Excludes** artificial openings requiring attention or management (V55.0–V55.9)
  - V44.0 Tracheostomy
    Coding Clinic: 2003, Q4, P103-104, 107, 111; 2001, Q1, P6-7
  - V44.1 Gastrostomy
    Coding Clinic: 2003, Q4, P103-104, 107-108, 110; 2001, Q1, P12; 1998, Q4, P42-44; 1997, Q3, P12-13; 1993, Q1, P26
  - V44.2 Ileostomy
    Coding Clinic: 1988, Q2, P9-10
  - V44.3 Colostomy
    Coding Clinic: 2003, Q4, P110
  - V44.4 Other artificial opening of gastrointestinal tract
  - **V44.5 Cystostomy**
    - V44.50 Cystostomy, unspecified
    - V44.51 Cutaneous-vesicostomy
    - V44.52 Appendico-vesicostomy
    - V44.59 Other cystostomy
  - V44.6 Other artificial opening of urinary tract
    Nephrostomy
    Ureterostomy
    Urethrostomy
    Coding Clinic: 2012, Q3, P12
  - V44.7 Artificial vagina
  - V44.8 Other artificial opening status
  - V44.9 Unspecified artificial opening status
- **V45 Other postprocedural states**
  - **Excludes** aftercare management (V51–V58.9)
    malfunction or other complication-code to condition
  - **V45.0 Cardiac device in situ**
    - **Excludes** artificial heart (V43.22)
      heart assist device (V43.21)
    - Coding Clinic: 1994, Q2, P10x2; 1993, 5th Issue, P12
    - V45.00 Unspecified cardiac device
    - V45.01 Cardiac pacemaker
      - **Excludes** cardiac defibrillator with synchronous cardiac pacemaker (V45.02)
    - V45.02 Automatic implantable cardiac defibrillator
      With synchronous cardiac pacemaker
    - V45.09 Other specified cardiac device
      Carotid sinus pacemaker in situ
  - **V45.1 Renal dialysis status**
    - **Excludes** admission for dialysis treatment or session (V56.0)
    - Coding Clinic: 2008, Q1, P7-8; 2007, Q4, P84-86; Q3, P11; 2006, Q4, P136; 2004, Q1, P22,23; 2001, Q2, P12-13; 1987, Sept-Oct, P8; Jan-Feb, P15
    - V45.11 Renal dialysis status
      Hemodialysis status
      Patient requiring intermittent renal dialysis
      Peritoneal dialysis status
      Presence of arterial-venous shunt (for dialysis)
      Coding Clinic: 2011, Q3, P15; 2008, Q4, P193; 2004, Q1, P23
    - V45.12 Noncompliance with renal dialysis
      Coding Clinic: 2006, Q4, P136
  - V45.2 Presence of cerebrospinal fluid drainage device
    Cerebral ventricle (communicating) shunt, valve, or device in situ
    - **Excludes** malfunction (996.2)
    - Coding Clinic: 2003, Q4, P106-107
  - V45.3 Intestinal bypass or anastomosis status
    - **Excludes** bariatric surgery status (V45.86)
      gastric bypass status (V45.86)
      obesity surgery status (V45.86)
  - V45.4 Arthrodesis status
    Coding Clinic: 1984, Nov-Dec, P18
  - **V45.5 Presence of contraceptive device**
    - V45.51 Intrauterine contraceptive device
      - **Excludes** checking of device (V25.42)
        complication from device (996.32)
        insertion and removal of device (V25.11-V25.13)
    - V45.52 Subdermal contraceptive implant
      Coding Clinic: 1995, Q3, P14
    - V45.59 Other
  - **V45.6 States following surgery of eye and adnexa**
    - **Excludes** aphakia (379.31)
      artificial:
      eye globe (V43.0)
    - V45.61 Cataract extraction status
      Use additional code for associated artificial lens status (V43.1)
    - V45.69 Other states following surgery of eye and adnexa
      Coding Clinic: 2001, Q2, P16-17

- **V45.7 Acquired absence of organ**
  - **V45.71** Acquired absence of breast and nipple
    - **Excludes** congenital absence of breast and nipple (757.6)
    - Coding Clinic: 2001, Q4, P66; 1997, Q4, P50
  - **V45.72** Acquired absence of intestine (large) (small)
  - **V45.73** Acquired absence of kidney
  - **V45.74** Other parts of urinary tract
    - Bladder
  - **V45.75** Stomach
  - **V45.76** Lung
  - **V45.77** Genital organs
    - **Excludes** acquired absence of cervix and uterus (V88.01–V88.03)
      female genital mutilation status (629.20–629.29)
    - Coding Clinic: 2003, Q1, P13-14x2
  - **V45.78** Eye
  - **V45.79** Other acquired absence of organ
    - **Excludes** acquired absence of pancreas (V88.11-V88.12)
- **V45.8 Other postprocedural status**
  - **V45.81** Aortocoronary bypass status
    - Coding Clinic: 2011, Q4, P153; 2010, Q4, P131; 2003, Q4, P105-106; 2001, Q3, P15; 1997, Q3, P16
  - **V45.82** Percutaneous transluminal coronary angioplasty status
    - Coding Clinic: 1995, Q2, P18
  - **V45.83** Breast implant removal status
  - **V45.84** Dental restoration status
    - Dental crowns status
    - Dental fillings status
  - **V45.85** Insulin pump status
  - **V45.86** Bariatric surgery status
    - Gastric banding status
    - Gastric bypass status for obesity
    - Obesity surgery status
    - **Excludes** bariatric surgery status complicating pregnancy, childbirth or the puerperium (649.2)
      intestinal bypass or anastomosis status (V45.3)
    - Coding Clinic: 2009, Q2, P10
  - **V45.87** Transplanted organ removal status
    - Transplanted organ previously removed due to complication, failure, rejection or infection
    - **Excludes** encounter for removal of transplanted organ – code to complication of transplanted organ (996.80–996.89)
  - **V45.88** Status post administration of tPA (rtPA) in a different facility within the last 24 hours prior to admission to the current facility
    - Code first condition requiring tPA administration, such as:
      acute cerebral infarction (433.0–433.9 with fifth-digit 1, 434.0–434.9 with fifth digit 1)
      acute myocardial infarction (410.00–410.92)
  - **V45.89** Other
    - Presence of neuropacemaker or other electronic device
    - **Excludes** artificial heart valve in situ (V43.3)
      vascular prosthesis in situ (V43.4)
    - Coding Clinic: 1995, Q1, P11

- **V46 Other dependence on machines and devices**
  - **V46.0** Aspirator
  - **V46.1** Respirator [Ventilator]
    - Iron lung
    - Coding Clinic: 2005, Q4, P94-100; 2004, Q4, P100-101
    - **V46.11** Dependence on respirator, status
      - Coding Clinic: 2003, Q4, P104-105; 2001, Q1, P12
    - **V46.12** Encounter for respirator dependence during power failure
    - **V46.13** Encounter for weaning from respirator [ventilator]
    - **V46.14** Mechanical complication of respirator [ventilator]
      - Mechanical failure of respirator [ventilator]
  - **V46.2** Supplemental oxygen
    - Long-term oxygen therapy
  - **V46.3** Wheelchair dependence
    - Wheelchair confinement status
    - Code first cause of dependence, such as:
      muscular dystrophy (359.1)
      obesity (278.00-278.03)
  - **V46.8** Other enabling machines
    - Hyperbaric chamber
    - Possum [Patient-Operated-Selector-Mechanism]
    - **Excludes** cardiac pacemaker (V45.0)
      kidney dialysis machine (V45.11)
  - **V46.9** Unspecified machine dependence
- **V47 Other problems with internal organs**
  - **V47.0** Deficiencies of internal organs
  - **V47.1** Mechanical and motor problems with internal organs
  - **V47.2** Other cardiorespiratory problems
    - Cardiovascular exercise intolerance with pain (with):
      at rest
      less than ordinary activity
      ordinary activity
  - **V47.3** Other digestive problems
  - **V47.4** Other urinary problems
  - **V47.5** Other genital problems
  - **V47.9** Unspecified
- **V48 Problems with head, neck, and trunk**
  - **V48.0** Deficiencies of head
    - **Excludes** deficiencies of ears, eyelids, and nose (V48.8)
  - **V48.1** Deficiencies of neck and trunk
  - **V48.2** Mechanical and motor problems with head
  - **V48.3** Mechanical and motor problems with neck and trunk
  - **V48.4** Sensory problem with head
  - **V48.5** Sensory problem with neck and trunk
  - **V48.6** Disfigurements of head
  - **V48.7** Disfigurements of neck and trunk
  - **V48.8** Other problems with head, neck, and trunk
  - **V48.9** Unspecified problem with head, neck, or trunk
- **V49 Other conditions influencing health status**
  - **V49.0** Deficiencies of limbs
  - **V49.1** Mechanical problems with limbs
  - **V49.2** Motor problems with limbs
  - **V49.3** Sensory problems with limbs
  - **V49.4** Disfigurements of limbs
  - **V49.5** Other problems of limbs

- **V49.6** Upper limb amputation status
  Coding Clinic: 1998, Q4, P42-44
  - V49.60 Unspecified level
  - V49.61 Thumb
  - V49.62 Other finger(s)
    Coding Clinic: 2005, Q2, P7
  - V49.63 Hand
  - V49.64 Wrist
    Disarticulation of wrist
  - V49.65 Below elbow
  - V49.66 Above elbow
    Disarticulation of elbow
  - V49.67 Shoulder
    Disarticulation of shoulder
- **V49.7** Lower limb amputation status
  Coding Clinic: 2006, Q3, P5; 1998, Q4, P42-44
  - V49.70 Unspecified level
  - V49.71 Great toe
  - V49.72 Other toe(s)
  - V49.73 Foot
  - V49.74 Ankle
    Disarticulation of ankle
  - V49.75 Below knee
  - V49.76 Above knee
    Disarticulation of knee
    Coding Clinic: 2005, Q2, P14
  - V49.77 Hip
    Disarticulation of hip
- **V49.8** Other specified conditions influencing health status
  - V49.81 Asymptomatic postmenopausal status (age-related) (natural)
    Excludes menopausal and premenopausal disorders (627.0–627.9)
    postsurgical menopause (256.2)
    premature menopause (256.31)
    symptomatic menopause (627.0–627.9)
    Coding Clinic: 2009, Q4, P151; 2000, Q4, P53-54
  - V49.82 Dental sealant status
  - V49.83 Awaiting organ transplant status
    Coding Clinic: 2004, Q4, P101
  - V49.84 Bed confinement status
    Coding Clinic: 2005, Q4, P94-100
  - V49.85 Dual sensory impairment
    Blindness with deafness
    Combined visual hearing impairment
    Code first:
    hearing impairment (389.00–389.9)
    visual impairment (369.00–369.9)
    Coding Clinic: 2007, Q4, P99-101
  - V49.86 Do not resuscitate status
    Coding Clinic: 2012, Q1, P14
  - V49.87 Physical restraints status
    Excludes restraint due to a procedure – omit code
  - V49.89 Other specified conditions influencing health status
- **V49.9** Unspecified

PERSONS ENCOUNTERING HEALTH SERVICES FOR SPECIFIC PROCEDURES AND AFTERCARE (V50–V59)

Note: Categories V51–V58 are intended for use to indicate a reason for care in patients who may have already been treated for some disease or injury not now present, or who are receiving care to consolidate the treatment, to deal with residual states, or to prevent recurrence.

Excludes follow-up examination for medical surveillance following treatment (V67.0–V67.9)

- **V50** Elective surgery for purposes other than remedying health states
  - V50.0 Hair transplant
  - V50.1 Other plastic surgery for unacceptable cosmetic appearance
    Breast augmentation or reduction
    Face-lift
    Excludes encounter for breast reduction (611.1)
    plastic surgery following healed injury or operation (V51.0–V51.8)
  - V50.2 Routine or ritual circumcision
    Circumcision in the absence of significant medical indication
  - V50.3 Ear piercing
  - V50.4 Prophylactic organ removal
    Excludes organ donations (V59.0–V59.9)
    therapeutic organ removal-code to condition
    Coding Clinic: 2009, Q3, P21
    - V50.41 Breast
      Coding Clinic: 2004, Q4, P106-107
    - V50.42 Ovary
      Coding Clinic: 2009, Q3, P21x2
    - V50.49 Other
      Coding Clinic: 2009, Q3, P21
  - V50.8 Other
  - V50.9 Unspecified
    OGCR Section I.C.18.d.14
    For encounters specifically for prophylactic removal of breasts, ovaries, or another organ due to a genetic susceptibility to cancer or a family history of cancer, the principal or first listed code should be a code from subcategory V50.4, Prophylactic organ removal, followed by the appropriate genetic susceptibility code and the appropriate family history code.
- **V51** Aftercare involving the use of plastic surgery
  Includes plastic surgery following healed injury or operation
  Excludes cosmetic plastic surgery (V50.1)
  plastic surgery as treatment for current condition or injury - code to condition or injury
  repair of scar tissue - code to scar
  - V51.0 Encounter for breast reconstruction following mastectomy
    Excludes deformity and disproportion of reconstructed breast (612.0–612.1)
  - V51.8 Other aftercare involving the use of plastic surgery
- **V52** Fitting and adjustment of prosthetic device and implant
  Includes removal of device
  Excludes malfunction or complication of prosthetic device (996.0–996.7)
  status only, without need for care (V43.0–V43.8)
  - V52.0 Artificial arm (complete) (partial)
  - V52.1 Artificial leg (complete) (partial)
  - V52.2 Artificial eye
  - V52.3 Dental prosthetic device

V52.4–V54.19 ICD-9-CM

V52.4 Breast prosthesis and implant
Elective implant exchange (different material) (different size)
Removal of tissue expander without synchronous insertion of permanent implant
> **Excludes** admission for initial breast implant insertion for breast augmentation (V50.1)
> complications of breast implant (996.54, 996.69, 996.79)
> encounter for breast reconstruction following mastectomy (V51.0)
>
> Coding Clinic: 1995, Q4, P80.81

V52.8 Other specified prosthetic device
Coding Clinic: 2002, Q3, P12; Q2, P16-17

V52.9 Unspecified prosthetic device

V53 Fitting and adjustment of other device
> **Includes** removal of device
> replacement of device
>
> **Excludes** status only, without need for care (V45.0–V45.8)

V53.0 Devices related to nervous system and special senses

- **V53.01** Fitting and adjustment of cerebral ventricle (communicating) shunt
  Coding Clinic: 1997, Q4, P51
- **V53.02** Neuropacemaker (brain) (peripheral nerve) (spinal cord)
- **V53.09** Fitting and adjustment of other devices related to nervous system and special senses
  Auditory substitution device
  Visual substitution device
  Coding Clinic: 1999, Q2, P3-4

V53.1 Spectacles and contact lenses

V53.2 Hearing aid

V53.3 Cardiac device
Reprogramming
Coding Clinic: 1992, Q3, P3

- **V53.31** Cardiac pacemaker
  > **Excludes** automatic implantable cardiac defibrillator with synchronous cardiac pacemaker (V53.32)
  > mechanical complication of cardiac pacemaker (996.01)
  >
  > Coding Clinic: 2010, Q3, P10; 2002, Q1, P3; 1984, Nov-Dec, P18
- **V53.32** Automatic implantable cardiac defibrillator
  With synchronous cardiac pacemaker
  Coding Clinic: 2005, Q3, P3-9
- **V53.39** Other cardiac device
  Coding Clinic: 2010, Q4, P124-125; 2008, Q2, P9-10; 2007, Q1, P20

V53.4 Orthodontic devices

V53.5 Other gastrointestinal appliance and device
> **Excludes** colostomy (V55.3)
> ileostomy (V55.2)
> other artifical opening of digestive tract (V55.4)

- **V53.50** Fitting and adjustment of intestinal appliance and device
- **V53.51** Fitting and adjustment of gastric lap band
- **V53.59** Fitting and adjustment of other gastrointestinal appliance and device

V53.6 Urinary devices
Urinary catheter
> **Excludes** cystostomy (V55.5)
> nephrostomy (V55.6)
> ureterostomy (V55.6)
> urethrostomy (V55.6)

V53.7 Orthopedic devices
Orthopedic:
  brace
  cast
  corset
  shoes
> **Excludes** other orthopedic aftercare (V54)

V53.8 Wheelchair

V53.9 Other and unspecified device
Coding Clinic: 2003, Q2, P6-7

- **V53.90** Unspecified device
- **V53.91** Fitting and adjustment of insulin pump
  Insulin pump titration
- **V53.99** Other device
  Coding Clinic: 2009, Q2, P10

V54 Other orthopedic aftercare
> **Excludes** fitting and adjustment of orthopedic devices (V53.7)
> malfunction of internal orthopedic device (996.40–996.49)
> other complication of nonmechanical nature (996.60–996.79)

V54.0 Aftercare involving internal fixation device
> **Excludes** malfunction of internal orthopedic device (996.40–996.49)
> other complication of nonmechanical nature (996.60–996.79)
> removal of external fixation device (V54.89)

- **V54.01** Encounter for removal of internal fixation device
- **V54.02** Encounter for lengthening/adjustment of growth rod
- **V54.09** Other aftercare involving internal fixation device
  Coding Clinic: 2009, Q1, P15

V54.1 Aftercare for healing traumatic fracture
> **Excludes** aftercare following joint replacement (V54.81)
> aftercare for amputation stump (V54.89)

- **V54.10** Aftercare for healing traumatic fracture of arm, unspecified
- **V54.11** Aftercare for healing traumatic fracture of upper arm
- **V54.12** Aftercare for healing traumatic fracture of lower arm
  Coding Clinic: 2007, Q1, P3-8
- **V54.13** Aftercare for healing traumatic fracture of hip
  Coding Clinic: 2009, Q1, P15; 2007, Q1, P3-8; 2003, Q4, P103-105
- **V54.14** Aftercare for healing traumatic fracture of leg, unspecified
- **V54.15** Aftercare for healing traumatic fracture of upper leg
  > **Excludes** aftercare for healing traumatic fracture of hip (V54.13)
  >
  > Coding Clinic: 2006, Q3, P6
- **V54.16** Aftercare for healing traumatic fracture of lower leg
  Coding Clinic: 2009, Q1, P14
- **V54.17** Aftercare for healing traumatic fracture of vertebrae
- **V54.19** Aftercare for healing traumatic fracture of other bone
  Coding Clinic: 2005, Q1, P13

- **V54.2 Aftercare for healing pathologic fracture**
  Excludes *aftercare following joint replacement (V54.81)*
  - **V54.20** Aftercare for healing pathologic fracture of arm, unspecified
  - V54.21 Aftercare for healing pathologic fracture of upper arm
  - V54.22 Aftercare for healing pathologic fracture of lower arm
  - V54.23 Aftercare for healing pathologic fracture of hip
  - **V54.24** Aftercare for healing pathologic fracture of leg, unspecified
  - V54.25 Aftercare for healing pathologic fracture of upper leg
    Excludes *aftercare for healing pathologic fracture of hip (V54.23)*
  - V54.26 Aftercare for healing pathologic fracture of lower leg
  - V54.27 Aftercare for healing pathologic fracture of vertebrae
    Coding Clinic: 2008, Q3, P4; 2003, Q4, P108-109
  - V54.29 Aftercare for healing pathologic fracture of other bone
- **V54.8 Other orthopedic aftercare**
  Coding Clinic: 2001, Q3, P19; 1999, Q4, P5x2; 1990, Q1, P10, 20
  - V54.81 Aftercare following joint replacement
    Use additional code to identify joint replacement site (V43.60–V43.69)
    Coding Clinic: 2011, Q1, P9; 2009, Q1, P14; 2006, Q3, P4; 2004, Q3, P12; Q2, P15
  - V54.82 Aftercare following explantation of joint prosthesis
    Aftercare following explantation of joint prosthesis, staged procedure
    Encounter for joint prosthesis insertion following prior explantation of joint prosthesis
  - V54.89 Other orthopedic aftercare
    Aftercare for healing fracture NOS
    Coding Clinic: 2007, Q2, P8-9
- **V54.9** Unspecified orthopedic aftercare

- **V55 Attention to artificial openings**
  Includes adjustment or repositioning of catheter
  closure
  passage of sounds or bougies
  reforming
  removal or replacement of catheter
  toilet or cleansing
  Excludes *complications of external stoma (519.00-519.09, 569.60-569.69, 596.81-596.83, 997.49)*
  status only, without need for care (V44.0–V44.9)
  Coding Clinic: 1995, Q3, P13
  - V55.0 Tracheostomy
  - V55.1 Gastrostomy
    Coding Clinic: 1999, Q4, P9; 1997, Q3, P7-8; 1996, Q1, P14; 1995, Q3, P13
  - V55.2 Ileostomy
  - V55.3 Colostomy
    Coding Clinic: 2009, Q1, P14; 2005, Q2, P4-5; 1997, Q3, P9-10
  - V55.4 Other artificial opening of digestive tract
    Coding Clinic: 2005, Q2, P14; 2003, Q1, P10
  - V55.5 Cystostomy
  - V55.6 Other artificial opening of urinary tract
    Nephrostomy
    Ureterostomy
    Urethrostomy
  - V55.7 Artificial vagina
  - V55.8 Other specified artificial opening
  - **V55.9** Unspecified artificial opening

- **V56 Encounter for dialysis and dialysis catheter care**
  Use additional code to identify the associated condition
  Excludes *dialysis preparation-code to condition*
  Coding Clinic: 1993, Q1, P29
  - V56.0 Extracorporeal dialysis
    Dialysis (renal) NOS
    Excludes *dialysis status (V45.11)*
    Coding Clinic: 2005, Q4, P77-79; 2004, Q1, P23; 2000, Q4, P39-40; 1998, Q3, P6; Q2, P20-21; 1993, Q4, P34
  - V56.1 Fitting and adjustment of extracorporeal dialysis catheter
    Removal or replacement of catheter
    Toilet or cleansing
    Use additional code for any concurrent extracorporeal dialysis (V56.0)
    Coding Clinic: 1998, Q2, P20-21
  - V56.2 Fitting and adjustment of peritoneal dialysis catheter
    Use additional code for any concurrent peritoneal dialysis (V56.8)
    Coding Clinic: 1998, Q4, P55
  - **V56.3 Encounter for adequacy testing for dialysis**
    - V56.31 Encounter for adequacy testing for hemodialysis
    - V56.32 Encounter for adequacy testing for peritoneal dialysis
      Peritoneal equilibration test
  - V56.8 Other dialysis
    Peritoneal dialysis
    Coding Clinic: 1998, Q4, P55

- **V57 Care involving use of rehabilitation procedures**
  Use additional code to identify underlying condition
  Coding Clinic: 2002, Q1, P18-19; 1997, Q3, P12
  - V57.0 Breathing exercises
  - V57.1 Other physical therapy
    Therapeutic and remedial exercises, except breathing
    Coding Clinic: 2006, Q3, P4; 2004, Q2, P15; 2002, Q4, P56; 1999, Q4, P5
  - **V57.2 Occupational therapy and vocational rehabilitation**
    - V57.21 Encounter for occupational therapy
      Coding Clinic: 1999, Q4, P7
    - V57.22 Encounter for vocational therapy
  - V57.3 Speech-language therapy
    Coding Clinic: 1997, Q4, P35-37
  - V57.4 Orthoptic training
  - **V57.8 Other specified rehabilitation procedure**
    - V57.81 Orthotic training
      Gait training in the use of artificial limbs
    - V57.89 Other
      Multiple training or therapy
      Coding Clinic: 2007, Q4, P92-95; 2006, Q3, P6; 2003, Q4, P105-106, 108-109; Q2, P16; 2002, Q1, P16; 2001, Q3, P21; 1997, Q3, P11-13
  - **V57.9** Unspecified rehabilitation procedure

OGCR Section I.C.2.e.2
If a patient admission/encounter is solely for the administration of chemotherapy, immunotherapy or radiation therapy assign code V58.0, Encounter for radiation therapy, or V58.11, Encounter for antineoplastic chemotherapy, or V58.12, Encounter for antineoplastic immunotherapy as the first-listed or principal diagnosis. If a patient receives more than one of these therapies during the same admission more than one of these codes may be assigned, in any sequence.
The malignancy for which the therapy is being administered should be assigned as a secondary diagnosis.

- **V58 Encounter for other and unspecified procedures and aftercare**
    - Excludes: convalescence and palliative care (V66.0–V66.9)
    - **V58.0 Radiotherapy**
        Encounter or admission for radiotherapy
        - Excludes: encounter for radioactive implant-code to condition
            radioactive iodine therapy-code to condition
        - Coding Clinic: 2013, Q1, P8; 1994, Q2, P10x2; 1993, Q4, P 36; 1987, Jan-Feb, P13
- **V58.1 Encounter for chemotherapy and immunotherapy for neoplastic conditions**
    Encounter or admission for chemotherapy
    - Excludes: chemotherapy and immunotherapy for nonneoplastic conditions-code to condition
    - Coding Clinic: 2005, Q4, P94-100; 2004, Q1, P13-14; 2003, Q2, P16-17; 2000, Q1, P23; 1993, Q4, P34, 36; Q3, P4x5; 1992, Q2, P16-17; 1991, Q2, P17; 1987, Sept-Oct, P8
    - **V58.11 Encounter for antineoplastic chemotherapy**
        - Coding Clinic: 2012, Q1, P13-14; 2009, Q4, P152x2; 2008, Q4, P82-83, 152-155; 2007, Q4, P103-104; 2006, Q2, P20-22; 2004, Q1, P13-14
    - **V58.12 Encounter for antineoplastic immunotherapy**
        - Coding Clinic: 2004, Q1, P13-14
    - **V58.2 Blood transfusion, without reported diagnosis**
        - Coding Clinic: 1994, Q1, P22
- **V58.3 Attention to dressings and sutures**
    Change or removal of wound packing
    - Excludes: attention to drains (V58.49)
        planned postoperative wound closure (V58.41)
    - Coding Clinic: 2006, Q4, P117-118; 2005, Q2, P14
    - **V58.30 Encounter for change or removal of nonsurgical wound dressing**
        Encounter for change or removal of wound dressing NOS
        - Coding Clinic: 2009, Q4, P152x2
    - **V58.31 Encounter for change or removal of surgical wound dressing**
    - **V58.32 Encounter for removal of sutures**
        Encounter for removal of staples
- **V58.4 Other aftercare following surgery**
    Note: Codes from this subcategory should be used in conjunction with other aftercare codes to fully identify the reason for the aftercare encounter.
    - Excludes: aftercare following sterilization reversal surgery (V26.22)
        attention to artificial openings (V55.0–V55.9)
        orthopedic aftercare (V54.0–V54.9)
    - Coding Clinic: 1999, Q4, P8-9
    - **V58.41 Encounter for planned post-operative wound closure**
        - Excludes: disruption of operative wound (998.31–998.32)
            encounter for dressings and suture aftercare (V58.30–V58.32)
        - Coding Clinic: 1999, Q4, P15
    - **V58.42 Aftercare following surgery for neoplasm**
        Conditions classifiable to 140–239
    - **V58.43 Aftercare following surgery for injury and trauma**
        Conditions classifiable to 800–999
        - Excludes: aftercare for healing traumatic fracture (V54.10–V54.19)
        - Coding Clinic: 2007, Q2, P8-9; 1987, Nov-Dec, P9
    - **V58.44 Aftercare following organ transplant**
        - Use additional code to identify the organ transplanted (V42.0–V42.9)
        - Coding Clinic: 2011, Q3, P5; 2004, Q4, P101
    - **V58.49 Other specified aftercare following surgery**
        Change or removal of drains
        - Coding Clinic: 1996, Q1, P8-9x2
    - **V58.5 Orthodontics**
        - Excludes: fitting and adjustment of orthodontic device (V53.4)

OGCR Section I.C.18.d.3
Codes from this subcategory (V58) indicate a patient's continuous use of a prescribed drug (including such things as aspirin therapy) for the long-term treatment of a condition or for prophylactic use. It is not for use for patients who have addictions to drugs. This subcategory is not for use of medications for detoxification or maintenance programs to prevent withdrawal symptoms in patients with drug dependence (e.g., methadone maintenance for opiate dependence). Assign the appropriate code for the drug dependence instead.
Assign a code from subcategory V58.6 Long-term (current) drug use, if the patient is receiving a medication for an extended period as a prophylactic measure (such as for the prevention of deep vein thrombosis) or as treatment of a chronic condition (such as arthritis) or a disease requiring a lengthy course of treatment (such as cancer). Do not assign a code from subcategory V58.6 for medication being administered for a brief period of time to treat an acute illness or injury (such as a course of antibiotics to treat acute bronchitis).

- **V58.6 Long-term (current) drug use**
    Long-term (current) prophylactic drug use
    - Excludes: drug abuse (305.00–305.93)
        drug abuse and dependence complicating pregnancy (648.3–648.4)
        drug dependence (304.00–304.93)
        hormone replacement therapy (postmenopausal) (V07.4)
        use of agents affecting estrogen receptors and estrogen levels (V07.51–V07.59)
    - Coding Clinic: 2011, Q1, P15; 2010, Q2, P13
    - **V58.61 Long-term (current) use of anticoagulants**
        - Excludes: long-term (current) use of aspirin (V58.66)
        - Coding Clinic: 2008, Q4, P134-136; 2006, Q3, P13; 2004, Q3, P7; 2003, Q4, P108; 2003, Q1, P11-12; 2002, Q3, P13-16; Q1, P16
    - **V58.62 Long-term (current) use of antibiotics**
        - Coding Clinic: 1998, Q4, P59-60
    - **V58.63 Long-term (current) use of antiplatelets/antithrombotics**
        - Excludes: long-term (current) use of aspirin (V58.66)
    - **V58.64 Long-term (current) use of non-steroidal anti-inflammatories (NSAID)**
        - Excludes: long-term (current) use of aspirin (V58.66)
    - **V58.65 Long-term (current) use of steroids**
    - **V58.66 Long-term (current) use of aspirin**
        - Coding Clinic: 2004, Q4, P102-103; 2003, Q1, P11-12

V58.67 Long-term (current) use of insulin
Coding Clinic: 2004, Q4, P53-56

V58.68 Long term (current) use of bisphosphonates

V58.69 Long-term (current) use of other medications
Long term current use of methadone for pain control
Long term current use of opiate analgesic
Other high-risk medications
Excludes *methadone maintenance NOS (304.00)*
methadone use NOS (304.00)
Coding Clinic: 2011, Q1, P15; 2010, Q2, P10, 13; 2009, Q4, P152; Q3, P21; 2004, Q2, P10; Q1, P13-14; 2003, Q1, P11-12; 2000, Q2, P8-9; 1999, Q3, 13-14; 1996, Q3, P20; Q2, P7x2; 1995, Q4, P51, 61

● **V58.7** Aftercare following surgery to specified body systems, not elsewhere classified
Note: Codes from this subcategory should be used in conjunction with other aftercare codes to fully identify the reason for the aftercare encounter.
Excludes *aftercare following organ transplant (V58.44)*
aftercare following surgery for neoplasm (V58.42)
Coding Clinic: 2003, Q4, P104-105

V58.71 Aftercare following surgery of the sense organs, NEC
Conditions classifiable to 360–379, 380–389

V58.72 Aftercare following surgery of the nervous system, NEC
Conditions classifiable to 320–359
Excludes *aftercare following surgery of the sense organs, NEC (V58.71)*

V58.73 Aftercare following surgery of the circulatory system, NEC
Conditions classifiable to 390–459
Coding Clinic: 2009, Q2, P12

V58.74 Aftercare following surgery of the respiratory system, NEC
Conditions classifiable to 460–519

V58.75 Aftercare following surgery of the teeth, oral cavity and digestive system, NEC
Conditions classifiable to 520–579
Coding Clinic: 2005, Q2, P14

V58.76 Aftercare following surgery of the genitourinary system, NEC
Conditions classifiable to 580–629
Excludes *aftercare following sterilization reversal (V26.22)*
Coding Clinic: 2005, Q1, P11,12

V58.77 Aftercare following surgery of the skin and subcutaneous tissue, NEC
Conditions classifiable to 680–709

V58.78 Aftercare following surgery of the musculoskeletal system, NEC
Conditions classifiable to 710–739
Excludes *orthopedic aftercare (V54.01–V54.9)*

● **V58.8** Other specified procedures and aftercare
Coding Clinic: 1994, Q2, P8x2

V58.81 Fitting and adjustment of vascular catheter
Removal or replacement of catheter
Toilet or cleansing
Excludes *complications of renal dialysis (996.73)*
complications of vascular catheter (996.74)
dialysis preparation—code to condition
encounter for dialysis (V56.0–V56.8)
fitting and adjustment of dialysis catheter (V56.1)

V58.82 Fitting and adjustment of non-vascular catheter NEC
Removal or replacement of catheter
Toilet or cleansing
Excludes *fitting and adjustment of peritoneal dialysis catheter (V56.2)*
fitting and adjustment of urinary catheter (V53.6)

V58.83 Encounter for therapeutic drug monitoring
Use additional code for any associated long-term (current) drug use (V58.61–V58.69)
Excludes *blood-drug testing for medicolegal reasons (V70.4)*
Coding Clinic: 2004, Q2, P10-11; Q1, P13-14; 2002, Q3, P13-16

V58.89 Other specified aftercare
Coding Clinic: 2003, Q4, P106-107; 1998, Q4, P59-60

■ **V58.9** Unspecified aftercare
OGCR Section I.C.18.d.9
Category V59 is the donor codes. They are used for living individuals who are donating blood or other body tissue. These codes are only for individuals donating for others, not for self donations. They are not for use to identify cadaveric donations.

● **V59** Donors
Excludes *examination of potential donor (V70.8)*
self-donation of organ or tissue--code to condition
Coding Clinic: 2008, Q2, P8-9; 1995, Q4, P50x2

● **V59.0** Blood
Coding Clinic: 1990, Q1, P9-10
V59.01 Whole blood
V59.02 Stem cells
Coding Clinic: 1995, Q4, P51
V59.09 Other

V59.1 Skin
V59.2 Bone
V59.3 Bone marrow
Coding Clinic: 1985, Jan-Feb, P15
V59.4 Kidney
V59.5 Cornea
V59.6 Liver

● **V59.7** Egg (oocyte) (ovum)
■ **V59.70** Egg (oocyte) (ovum) donor, unspecified
V59.71 Egg (oocyte) (ovum) donor, under age 35, anonymous recipient
Egg donor, under age 35 NOS
V59.72 Egg (oocyte) (ovum) donor, under age 35, designated recipient
V59.73 Egg (oocyte) (ovum) donor, age 35 and over, anonymous recipient
Egg donor, age 35 and over NOS
V59.74 Egg (oocyte) (ovum) donor, age 35 and over, designated recipient

V59.8 Other specified organ or tissue
Coding Clinic: 2002, Q3, P20-21

■ **V59.9** Unspecified organ or tissue

PERSONS ENCOUNTERING HEALTH SERVICES IN OTHER CIRCUMSTANCES (V60–V69)

- **V60 Housing, household, and economic circumstances**
  - **V60.0 Lack of housing**
    - Hobos
    - Social migrants
    - Tramps
    - Transients
    - Vagabonds
  - **V60.1 Inadequate housing**
    - Lack of heating
    - Restriction of space
    - Technical defects in home preventing adequate care
  - **V60.2 Inadequate material resources**
    - Economic problem
    - Poverty NOS
  - **V60.3 Person living alone**
  - **V60.4 No other household member able to render care**
    - Person requiring care (has) (is):
      - family member too handicapped, ill, or otherwise unsuited to render care
      - partner temporarily away from home
      - temporarily away from usual place of abode
    - *Excludes* holiday relief care (V60.5)
  - **V60.5 Holiday relief care**
    - Provision of health care facilities to a person normally cared for at home, to enable relatives to take a vacation
  - **V60.6 Person living in residential institution**
    - Boarding school resident
  - **V60.8 Other specified housing or economic circumstances**
    - **V60.81 Foster care (status)**
    - **V60.89 Other specified housing or economic circumstances**
  - **V60.9 Unspecified housing or economic circumstance**

- **V61 Other family circumstances**
  - *Includes* when these circumstances or fear of them, affecting the person directly involved or others, are mentioned as the reason, justified or not, for seeking or receiving medical advice or care
  - **V61.0 Family disruption**
    - **V61.01 Family disruption due to family member on military deployment**
      - Individual or family affected by other family member being on deployment
      - *Excludes* family disruption due to family member on non-military extended absence from home (V61.08)
    - **V61.02 Family disruption due to return of family member from military deployment**
      - Individual or family affected by other family member having returned from deployment (current or past conflict)
    - **V61.03 Family disruption due to divorce or legal separation**
    - **V61.04 Family disruption due to parent-child estrangement**
      - *Excludes* other family estrangement (V61.09)
    - **V61.05 Family disruption due to child in welfare custody**
    - **V61.06 Family disruption due to child in foster care or in care of non-parental family member**
    - **V61.07 Family disruption due to death of family member**
      - *Excludes* bereavement (V62.82)
    - **V61.08 Family disruption due to other extended absence of family member**
      - *Excludes* family disruption due to family member on military deployment (V61.01)
    - **V61.09 Other family disruption**
      - Family estrangement NOS

  - **V61.1 Counseling for marital and partner problems**
    - *Excludes* problems related to:
      - psychosexual disorders (302.0–302.9)
      - sexual function (V41.7)
    - **V61.10 Counseling for marital and partner problems, unspecified**
      - Marital conflict
      - Marital relationship problem
      - Partner conflict
      - Partner relationship problem
    - **V61.11 Counseling for victim of spousal and partner abuse**
      - *Excludes* encounter for treatment of current injuries due to abuse (995.80–995.85)
    - **V61.12 Counseling for perpetrator of spousal and partner abuse**
  - **V61.2 Parent-child problems**
    - **V61.20 Counseling for parent-child problem, unspecified**
      - Concern about behavior of child
      - Parent-child conflict
      - Parent-child relationship problem
    - **V61.21 Counseling for victim of child abuse**
      - Child battering
      - Child neglect
      - *Excludes* current injuries due to abuse (995.50–995.59)
    - **V61.22 Counseling for perpetrator of parental child abuse**
      - *Excludes* counseling for non-parental abuser (V62.83)
    - **V61.23 Counseling for parent-biological child problem**
      - Concern about behavior of biological child
      - Parent-biological child conflict
      - Parent-biological child relationship problem
    - **V61.24 Counseling for parent-adopted child problem**
      - Concern about behavior of adopted child
      - Parent-adopted child conflict
      - Parent-adopted child relationship problem
    - **V61.25 Counseling for parent (guardian)-foster child problem**
      - Concern about behavior of foster child
      - Parent (guardian)-foster child conflict
      - Parent (guardian)-foster child relationship problem
    - **V61.29 Other parent-child problems**
      - Coding Clinic: 1999, Q3, P16
  - **V61.3 Problems with aged parents or in-laws**
  - **V61.4 Health problems within family**
    - **V61.41 Alcoholism in family**
    - **V61.42 Substance abuse in family**
    - **V61.49 Other**
      - Care of sick or handicapped person in family or household
      - Presence of sick or handicapped person in family or household
  - **V61.5 Multiparity**
  - **V61.6 Illegitimacy or illegitimate pregnancy**
  - **V61.7 Other unwanted pregnancy**
  - **V61.8 Other specified family circumstances**
    - Problems with family members NEC
    - Sibling relationship problem
    - Coding Clinic: 1994, Q1, P21
  - **V61.9 Unspecified family circumstance**

V62 Other psychosocial circumstances

Includes: those circumstances or fear of them, affecting the person directly involved or others, mentioned as the reason, justified or not, for seeking or receiving medical advice or care

Excludes: previous psychological trauma (V15.41–V15.49)

- **V62.0 Unemployment**
  - **Excludes:** circumstances when main problem is economic inadequacy or poverty (V60.2)
- **V62.1 Adverse effects of work environment**
- **V62.2 Other occupational circumstances or maladjustment**
  - **V62.21 Personal current military deployment status**
    - Individual (civilian or military) currently deployed in theater or in support of military war, peacekeeping and humanitarian operations
  - **V62.22 Personal history of return from military deployment**
    - Individual (civilian or military) with past history of military war, peacekeeping and humanitarian deployment (current or past conflict)
  - **V62.29 Other occupational circumstances or maladjustment**
    - Career choice problem
    - Dissatisfaction with employment
    - Occupational problem
- **V62.3 Educational circumstances**
  - Academic problem
  - Dissatisfaction with school environment
  - Educational handicap
- **V62.4 Social maladjustment**
  - Acculturation problem
  - Cultural deprivation
  - Political, religious, or sex discrimination
  - Social:
    - isolation
    - persecution
- **V62.5 Legal circumstances**
  - Imprisonment
  - Legal investigation
  - Litigation
  - Prosecution
- **V62.6 Refusal of treatment for reasons of religion or conscience**
- **V62.8 Other psychological or physical stress, not elsewhere classified**
  - **V62.81 Interpersonal problems, not elsewhere classified**
    - Relational problem NOS
  - **V62.82 Bereavement, uncomplicated**
    - **Excludes:** bereavement as adjustment reaction (309.0)
    - family disruption due to death of family member (V61.07)
  - **V62.83 Counseling for perpetrator of physical/sexual abuse**
    - **Excludes:** counseling for perpetrator of parental child abuse (V61.22)
    - counseling for perpetrator of spousal and partner abuse (V61.12)
  - **V62.84 Suicidal ideation**
    - **Excludes:** suicidal tendencies (300.9)
    - Coding Clinic: 2005, Q4, P94-100
  - **V62.85 Homicidal ideation**
  - **V62.89 Other**
    - Borderline intellectual functioning
    - Life circumstance problems
    - Phase of life problems
    - Religious or spiritual problem
- **V62.9 Unspecified psychosocial circumstance**

V63 Unavailability of other medical facilities for care

- **V63.0 Residence remote from hospital or other health care facility**
- **V63.1 Medical services in home not available**
  - **Excludes:** no other household member able to render care (V60.4)
  - Coding Clinic: 2001, Q4, P67; Q1, P12
- **V63.2 Person awaiting admission to adequate facility elsewhere**
  - Coding Clinic: 1994, Q1, P22-23
- **V63.8 Other specified reasons for unavailability of medical facilities**
  - Person on waiting list undergoing social agency investigation
- **V63.9 Unspecified reason for unavailability of medical facilities**

V64 Persons encountering health services for specific procedures, not carried out

- **V64.0 Vaccination not carried out**
  - **V64.00 Vaccination not carried out, unspecified reason**
  - **V64.01 Vaccination not carried out because of acute illness**
  - **V64.02 Vaccination not carried out because of chronic illness or condition**
  - **V64.03 Vaccination not carried out because of immune compromised state**
  - **V64.04 Vaccination not carried out because of allergy to vaccine or component**
  - **V64.05 Vaccination not carried out because of caregiver refusal**
    - Guardian refusal
    - Parent refusal
    - **Excludes:** vaccination not carried out because of caregiver refusal for religious reasons (V64.07)
    - Coding Clinic: 2007, Q1, P12
  - **V64.06 Vaccination not carried out because of patient refusal**
  - **V64.07 Vaccination not carried out for religious reasons**
  - **V64.08 Vaccination not carried out because patient had disease being vaccinated against**
  - **V64.09 Vaccination not carried out for other reason**
- **V64.1 Surgical or other procedure not carried out because of contraindication**
  - Coding Clinic: 1993, 5th Issue, P9-10; 1985, Mar-April, P13; 1984, May-June, P11
- **V64.2 Surgical or other procedure not carried out because of patient's decision**
  - Coding Clinic: 2001, Q2, P8-9; 1999, Q1, P13-14; 1987, Jan-Feb, P13; 1985, July-Aug, P14
- **V64.3 Procedure not carried out for other reasons**
- **V64.4 Closed surgical procedure converted to open procedure**
  - **V64.41 Laparoscopic surgical procedure converted to open procedure**
    - Coding Clinic: 2011, Q1, P14-15; 1997, Q4, P52
  - **V64.42 Thoracoscopic surgical procedure converted to open procedure**
  - **V64.43 Arthroscopic surgical procedure converted to open procedure**

- **V65 Other persons seeking consultation**
  - **V65.0 Healthy person accompanying sick person**
    Boarder
    Coding Clinic: 1993, Q4, P36
  - **V65.1 Person consulting on behalf of another person**
    Advice or treatment for nonattending third party
    Excludes concern (normal) about sick person in family (V61.41–V61.49)
    - V65.11 Pediatric pre-birth visit for expectant parent(s)
      Pre-adoption visit for adoptive parent(s)
    - V65.19 Other person consulting on behalf of another person
  - V65.2 Person feigning illness
    Malingerer   Peregrinating patient
    Coding Clinic: 1999, Q3, P20
  - V65.3 Dietary surveillance and counseling
    Dietary surveillance and counseling (in):
    NOS
    colitis
    diabetes mellitus
    food allergies or intolerance
    gastritis
    hypercholesterolemia
    hypoglycemia
    obesity
    Use additional code to identify Body Mass Index (BMI), if known (V85.0–V85.54)
  - **V65.4 Other counseling, not elsewhere classified**
    Health:
    advice
    education
    instruction
    Excludes counseling (for):
    contraception (V25.40–V25.49)
    genetic (V26.31–V26.39)
    on behalf of third party (V65.11–V65.19)
    procreative management (V26.41–V26.49)
    - V65.40 Counseling NOS
    - V65.41 Exercise counseling
    - V65.42 Counseling on substance use and abuse
    - V65.43 Counseling on injury prevention
    - V65.44 Human immunodeficiency virus [HIV] counseling
      Coding Clinic: 1994, Q4, P35x3
      OGCR Section I.C.1.h
      When a patient returns to be informed of HIV test results use V65.44 if the results of the test are negative.
    - V65.45 Counseling on other sexually transmitted diseases
    - V65.46 Encounter for insulin pump training
    - V65.49 Other specified counseling
      Coding Clinic: 2000, Q2, P8-9
  - V65.5 Person with feared complaint in whom no diagnosis was made
    Feared condition not demonstrated
    Problem was normal state
    "Worried well"
    Coding Clinic: 1984, July-Aug, P20
  - V65.8 Other reasons for seeking consultation
    Excludes specified symptoms
    Coding Clinic: 1992, Q3, P4
  - V65.9 Unspecified reason for consultation

- **V66 Convalescence and palliative care**
  - V66.0 Following surgery
  - V66.1 Following radiotherapy
  - V66.2 Following chemotherapy
  - V66.3 Following psychotherapy and other treatment for mental disorder
  - V66.4 Following treatment of fracture
  - V66.5 Following other treatment
  - V66.6 Following combined treatment
  - V66.7 Encounter for palliative care
    End-of-life care   Terminal care
    Hospice care
    Code first underlying disease
    Coding Clinic: 2012, Q1, P14; 2010, Q3, P18; 2008, Q3, P13-14; 2005, Q2, P9-10; 2003, Q4, P107; 1996, Q4, P47-48
  - V66.9 Unspecified convalescence
    Coding Clinic: 2012, Q3, P16; 1999, Q4, P8

  OGCR Section I.C.18.d.8
  The follow-up codes are used to explain continuing surveillance following completed treatment of a disease, condition, or injury. They imply that the condition has been fully treated and no longer exists. They should not be confused with aftercare codes that explain current treatment for a healing condition or its sequelae. Follow-up codes may be used in conjunction with history codes to provide the full picture of the healed condition and its treatment. The follow-up code is sequenced first, followed by the history code. A follow-up code may be used to explain repeated visits. Should a condition be found to have recurred on the follow-up visit, then the diagnosis code should be used in place of the follow-up code.

- **V67 Follow-up examination**
  Includes surveillance only following completed treatment
  Excludes surveillance of contraception (V25.40–V25.49)
  Coding Clinic: 2009, Q1, P14; 2003, Q2, P5
  - **V67.0 Following surgery**
    Coding Clinic: 1997, Q4, P50; 1995, Q1, P4; 1992, Q3, P11; 1985, July-Aug, P16
    - V67.00 Following surgery, unspecified
    - V67.01 Follow-up vaginal pap smear
      Vaginal pap smear, status-post hysterectomy for malignant condition
      Use additional code to identify:
      acquired absence of uterus (V88.01–V88.03)
      personal history of malignant neoplasm (V10.40–V10.44)
      Excludes vaginal pap smear status-post hysterectomy for non-malignant condition (V76.47)
    - V67.09 Following other surgery
      Excludes sperm count following sterilization reversal (V26.22)
      sperm count for fertility testing (V26.21)
      Coding Clinic: 2008, Q3, P6; 2003, Q3, P16; 2002, Q3, P14-15; 1995, Q4, P53; Q2, P8; 1993, Q4, P32; 1992, Q3, P11; 1984, May-June, P10
  - V67.1 Following radiotherapy
    Coding Clinic: 1985, July-Aug, P16
  - V67.2 Following chemotherapy
    Cancer chemotherapy follow-up
    Coding Clinic: 1985, July-Aug, P16
  - V67.3 Following psychotherapy and other treatment for mental disorder
  - V67.4 Following treatment of healed fracture
    Excludes current (healing) fracture aftercare (V54.0–V54.9)
    Coding Clinic: 2009, Q1, P14

- **V67.5** Following other treatment
  - **V67.51** Following completed treatment with high-risk medication, not elsewhere classified
    - Excludes long-term (current) drug use (V58.61–V58.69)
    - Coding Clinic: 1999, Q1, P5-6x2; 1990, Q1, P18
  - **V67.59** Other
  - **V67.6** Following combined treatment
  - **V67.9** Unspecified follow-up examination
- **V68** Encounters for administrative purposes
  - **V68.0** Issue of medical certificates
    - Excludes encounter for general medical examination (V70.0–V70.9)
    - **V68.01** Disability examination
      - Use additional code(s) to identify: specific examination(s), screening and testing performed (V72.0–V82.9)
      - Coding Clinic: 2007, Q4, P99-101
    - **V68.09** Other issue of medical certificates
  - **V68.1** Issue of repeat prescriptions
    - Issue of repeat prescription for:
      - appliance
      - glasses
      - medications
    - Excludes repeat prescription for contraceptives (V25.41–V25.49)
  - **V68.2** Request for expert evidence
  - **V68.8** Other specified administrative purpose
    - **V68.81** Referral of patient without examination or treatment
    - **V68.89** Other
  - **V68.9** Unspecified administrative purpose
- **V69** Problems related to lifestyle
  - **V69.0** Lack of physical exercise
  - **V69.1** Inappropriate diet and eating habits
    - Excludes anorexia nervosa (307.1)
      bulimia (783.6)
      malnutrition and other nutritional deficiencies (260–269.9)
      other and unspecified eating disorders (307.50–307.59)
  - **V69.2** High-risk sexual behavior
  - **V69.3** Gambling and betting
    - Excludes pathological gambling (312.31)
  - **V69.4** Lack of adequate sleep
    - Sleep deprivation
    - Excludes insomnia (780.52)
    - Coding Clinic: 2004, Q4, P104
  - **V69.5** Behavioral insomnia of childhood
  - **V69.8** Other problems related to lifestyle
    - Self-damaging behavior
  - **V69.9** Problem related to lifestyle, unspecified

PERSONS WITHOUT REPORTED DIAGNOSIS ENCOUNTERED DURING EXAMINATION AND INVESTIGATION OF INDIVIDUALS AND POPULATIONS (V70–V82)

Note: Nonspecific abnormal findings disclosed at the time of these examinations are classifiable to categories 790–796.

- **V70** General medical examination
  - Use additional code(s) to identify any special screening examination(s) performed (V73.0–V82.9)
  - Coding Clinic: 1993, Q1, P28; 1985, Nov-Dec, P13
  - **V70.0** Routine general medical examination at a health care facility
    - Health checkup
    - Excludes health checkup of infant or child over 28 days old (V20.2)
      health supervision of newborn 8 to 28 days old (V20.32)
      health supervision of newborn under 8 days old (V20.31)
      pre-procedural general physical examination (V72.83)
  - **V70.1** General psychiatric examination, requested by the authority
  - **V70.2** General psychiatric examination, other and unspecified
  - **V70.3** Other medical examination for administrative purposes
    - General medical examination for:
      - admission to old age home
      - adoption
      - camp
      - driving license
      - immigration and naturalization
      - insurance certification
      - marriage
      - prison
      - school admission
      - sports competition
    - Excludes attendance for issue of medical certificates (V68.0)
      pre-employment screening (V70.5)
    - Coding Clinic: 2008, Q3, P6
  - **V70.4** Examination for medicolegal reasons
    - Blood-alcohol tests
    - Blood-drug tests
    - Paternity testing
    - Excludes examination and observation following:
      accidents (V71.3, V71.4)
      assault (V71.6)
      rape (V71.5)
  - **V70.5** Health examination of defined subpopulations
    - Armed forces personnel
    - Inhabitants of institutions
    - Occupational health examinations
    - Pre-employment screening
    - Preschool children
    - Prisoners
    - Prostitutes
    - Refugees
    - School children
    - Students
  - **V70.6** Health examination in population surveys
    - Excludes special screening (V73.0–V82.9)
  - **V70.7** Examination of participant in clinical trial
    - Examination of participant or control in clinical research
    - Coding Clinic: 2006, Q2, P5-6
  - **V70.8** Other specified general medical examinations
    - Examination of potential donor of organ or tissue
  - **V70.9** Unspecified general medical examination

OGCR Section I.C.18.d.6

There are three observation V code categories. They are for use in very limited circumstances when a person is being observed for a suspected condition that is ruled out. The observation codes are not for use if an injury or illness or any signs or symptoms related to the suspected condition are present. In such cases the diagnosis/symptom code is used with the corresponding E code to identify any external cause. The observation codes are to be used as principal diagnosis only. The only exception to this is when the principal diagnosis is required to be a code from the V30, Live born infant, category. Then the V29 observation code is sequenced after the V30 code. Additional codes may be used in addition to the observation code but only if they are unrelated to the suspected condition being observed.

● **V71 Observation and evaluation for suspected conditions not found**

> Note: This category is to be used when persons without a diagnosis are suspected of having an abnormal condition, without signs or symptoms, which requires study, but after examination and observation, is found not to exist. This category is also for use for administrative and legal observation status.

| Excludes | suspected maternal and fetal conditions not found (V89.01–V89.09) |

Coding Clinic: 1990, Q1, P19; 1985, Nov-Dec, P10, 13

● **V71.0 Observation for suspected mental condition**

V71.01 Adult antisocial behavior
Dyssocial behavior or gang activity in adult without manifest psychiatric disorder

V71.02 Childhood or adolescent antisocial behavior
Dyssocial behavior or gang activity in child or adolescent without manifest psychiatric disorder

V71.09 Other suspected mental condition

V71.1 Observation for suspected malignant neoplasm
Coding Clinic: 1990, Q1, P21

V71.2 Observation for suspected tuberculosis

V71.3 Observation following accident at work

V71.4 Observation following other accident
Examination of individual involved in motor vehicle traffic accident
Coding Clinic: 2006, Q1, P9; 2004, Q1, P6-7

V71.5 Observation following alleged rape or seduction
Examination of victim or culprit

V71.6 Observation following other inflicted injury
Examination of victim or culprit

V71.7 Observation for suspected cardiovascular disease
Coding Clinic: 2004, Q1, P6-7; 1993, 5th Issue, P17-24; 1990, Q1, P19; 1987, Sept-Oct, P10

● **V71.8 Observation and evaluation for other specified suspected conditions**

| Excludes | contact with and (suspected) exposure to (potentially) hazardous substances (V15.84–V15.86, V87.0–V87.31) |

Coding Clinic: 1990, Q1, P19

V71.81 Abuse and neglect

| Excludes | adult abuse and neglect (995.80–995.85) child abuse and neglect (995.50–995.59) |

Coding Clinic: 2000, Q4, P54-55

V71.82 Observation and evaluation for suspected exposure to anthrax

V71.83 Observation and evaluation for suspected exposure to other biological agent
Coding Clinic: 2003, Q4, P46-48

V71.89 Other specified suspected conditions
Coding Clinic: 2008, Q3, P6-7; 2003, Q2, P15-16

■ **V71.9 Observation for unspecified suspected condition**
Coding Clinic: 2002, Q1, P6-7

● **V72 Special investigations and examinations**

| Includes | routine examination of specific system |
| Excludes | general medical examination (V70.0–70.4) general screening examination of defined population groups (V70.5, V70.6, V70.7) health supervision of newborn 8 to 28 days old (V20.32) health supervision of newborn under 8 days old (V20.31) routine examination of infant or child over 28 days old (V20.2) |

Use additional code(s) to identify any special screening examination(s) performed (V73.0–V82.9)
Coding Clinic: 2004, Q1, P15-16; 1985, Nov-Dec, P13

V72.0 Examination of eyes and vision

● **V72.1 Examination of ears and hearing**
Coding Clinic: 2004, Q1, P15-16

V72.11 Encounter for hearing examination following failed hearing screening
Coding Clinic: 2011, Q3, P3; 2006, Q4, P118

V72.12 Encounter for hearing conservation and treatment
Coding Clinic: 2007, Q4, P99-101

V72.19 Other examination of ears and hearing

V72.2 Dental examination

● **V72.3 Gynecological examination**

| Excludes | cervical Papanicolaou smear without general gynecological examination (V76.2) routine examination in contraceptive management (V25.40–V25.49) |

Coding Clinic: 2004, Q4, P104-105

V72.31 Routine gynecological examination
General gynecological examination with or without Papanicolaou cervical smear
Pelvic examination (annual) (periodic)
Use additional code to identify:
human papillomavirus (HPV) screening (V73.81)
routine vaginal Papanicolaou smear (V76.47)
Coding Clinic: 2006, Q2, P3,4

V72.32 Encounter for Papanicolaou cervical smear to confirm findings of recent normal smear following initial abnormal smear
Coding Clinic: 2006, Q2, P3-4

● **V72.4 Pregnancy examination or test**
Coding Clinic: 2005, Q4, P94-100; 2004, Q4, P105

V72.40 Pregnancy examination or test, pregnancy unconfirmed
Possible pregnancy, not (yet) confirmed

V72.41 Pregnancy examination or test, negative result

V72.42 Pregnancy examination or test, positive result

V72.5 Radiological examination, not elsewhere classified
Routine chest x-ray

| Excludes | radiologic examinations as part of pre-procedural testing (V72.81-V72.84) |

Coding Clinic: 1990, Q1, P8, 10, 19-21; 1985, Nov-Dec, P13

OGCR Section I.C.18.d.13 (outpatient)

Codes V72.5 and V72.62 may be used if the reason for the patient encounter is for routine laboratory/radiology testing in the absence of any signs, symptoms, or associated diagnosis. If routine testing is performed during the same encounter as a test to evaluate a sign, symptom, or diagnosis, it is appropriate to assign both the V code and the code describing the reason for the non-routine test.

- **V72.6 Laboratory examination**
  Encounters for blood and urine testing
  Coding Clinic: 2006, Q2, P4; 1994, Q4, P35; 1990, Q1, P22; 1985, Nov-Dec, P13

  OGCR Section I.C.18.d.13 (outpatient)
  Codes V72.5 and V72.62 may be used if the reason for the patient encounter is for routine laboratory/radiology testing in the absence of any signs, symptoms, or associated diagnosis. If routine testing is performed during the same encounter as a test to evaluate a sign, symptom, or diagnosis, it is appropriate to assign both the V code and the code describing the reason for the non-routine test.

  - V72.60 Laboratory examination, unspecified
  - V72.61 Antibody response examination
    Immunity status testing
    Excludes: encounter for allergy testing (V72.7)
  - V72.62 Laboratory examination ordered as part of a routine general medical examination
    Blood tests for routine general physical examination
  - V72.63 Pre-procedural laboratory examination
    Blood tests prior to treatment or procedure
    Pre-operative laboratory examination
  - V72.69 Other laboratory examination

- **V72.7 Diagnostic skin and sensitization tests**
  Allergy tests
  Skin tests for hypersensitivity
  Excludes: diagnostic skin tests for bacterial diseases (V74.0–V74.9)
  Coding Clinic: 1985, Nov-Dec, P13

- **V72.8 Other specified examinations**
  Excludes: pre-procedural laboratory examinations (V72.63)
  Coding Clinic: 1995, Q4, P51-52; 1990, Q1, P10; 1985, Nov-Dec, P13

  - V72.81 Preoperative cardiovascular examination
    Pre-procedural cardiovascular examination
    Coding Clinic: 1995, Q4, P51-52
  - V72.82 Preoperative respiratory examination
    Pre-procedural respiratory examination
    Coding Clinic: 1996, Q3, P14
  - V72.83 Other specified preoperative examination
    Examination prior to chemotherapy
    Other pre-procedural examination
    Pre-procedural general physical examination
    Excludes: routine general medical examination (V70.0)
    Coding Clinic: 1996, Q3, P14; 1995, Q4, P52
  - V72.84 Preoperative examination, unspecified
    Pre-procedural examination, unspecified
    Coding Clinic: 1995, Q4, P52
  - V72.85 Other specified examination
    Coding Clinic: 2012, Q1, P10; 2004, Q1, P12-13
  - V72.86 Encounter for blood typing

- V72.9 Unspecified examination

- **V73 Special screening examination for viral and chlamydial diseases**
  - V73.0 Poliomyelitis
  - V73.1 Smallpox
  - V73.2 Measles
  - V73.3 Rubella
  - V73.4 Yellow fever
  - V73.5 Other arthropod-borne viral diseases
    Dengue fever
    Hemorrhagic fever
    Viral encephalitis:
      mosquito-borne
      tick-borne
  - V73.6 Trachoma

- V73.8 Other specified viral and chlamydial diseases
  - V73.81 Human papillomavirus (HPV)
    Coding Clinic: 2007, Q4, P99-101
  - V73.88 Other specified chlamydial diseases
    Coding Clinic: 2007, Q4, P124-125
  - V73.89 Other specified viral diseases

  OGCR Section I.C.1.h.
  If a patient is being seen to determine his/her HIV status, use V73.89, Screening for other specified viral disease. Use V69.8, Other problems related to lifestyle, as a secondary code if an asymptomatic patient is in a known high risk group for HIV. Should a patient with signs or symptoms or illness, or a confirmed HIV related diagnosis be tested for HIV, code the signs and symptoms or the diagnosis. An additional counseling code V65.44 may be used if counseling is provided during the encounter for the test.

- V73.9 Unspecified viral and chlamydial disease
  - V73.98 Unspecified chlamydial disease
  - V73.99 Unspecified viral disease

- **V74 Special screening examination for bacterial and spirochetal diseases**
  Includes: diagnostic skin tests for these diseases
  - V74.0 Cholera
  - V74.1 Pulmonary tuberculosis
  - V74.2 Leprosy [Hansen's disease]
  - V74.3 Diphtheria
  - V74.4 Bacterial conjunctivitis
  - V74.5 Venereal disease
    Screening for bacterial and spirochetal sexually transmitted diseases
    Screening for sexually transmitted diseases NOS
    Excludes: special screening for nonbacterial sexually transmitted diseases (V73.81–V73.89, V75.4, V75.8)
    Coding Clinic: 2007, Q4, P124-125
  - V74.6 Yaws
  - V74.8 Other specified bacterial and spirochetal diseases
    Brucellosis
    Leptospirosis
    Plague
    Tetanus
    Whooping cough
  - V74.9 Unspecified bacterial and spirochetal disease

- **V75 Special screening examination for other infectious diseases**
  - V75.0 Rickettsial diseases
  - V75.1 Malaria
  - V75.2 Leishmaniasis
  - V75.3 Trypanosomiasis
    Chagas' disease
    Sleeping sickness
  - V75.4 Mycotic infections
  - V75.5 Schistosomiasis
  - V75.6 Filariasis
  - V75.7 Intestinal helminthiasis
  - V75.8 Other specified parasitic infections
  - V75.9 Unspecified infectious disease

- **V76 Special screening for malignant neoplasms**
  - V76.0 Respiratory organs
  - V76.1 Breast
    - V76.10 Breast screening, unspecified
    - V76.11 Screening mammogram for high-risk patient
      Coding Clinic: 2003, Q2, P3-5
    - V76.12 Other screening mammogram
      Coding Clinic: 2009, Q4, P153; 2006, Q2, P10; Q2, P3-5
    - V76.19 Other screening breast examination

V76.2 Cervix
        Routine cervical Papanicolaou smear
        Excludes special screening for human papillomavirus (V73.81)
                  that as part of a general gynecological examination (V72.31)
V76.3 Bladder
● V76.4 Other sites
    V76.41 Rectum
    V76.42 Oral cavity
    V76.43 Skin
    V76.44 Prostate
    V76.45 Testis
    V76.46 Ovary
    V76.47 Vagina
        Vaginal pap smear status-post hysterectomy for non-malignant condition
        Use additional code to identify acquired absence of uterus (V88.01–V88.03)
        Excludes vaginal pap smear status-post hysterectomy for malignant condition (V67.01)
    V76.49 Other sites
        Coding Clinic: 1999, Q1, P4
● V76.5 Intestine
    ☐ V76.50 Intestine, unspecified
    V76.51 Colon
        Screening colonoscopy NOS
        Excludes rectum (V76.41)
        Coding Clinic: 2004, Q1, P11-12; 2001, Q4, P55-56x2
    V76.52 Small intestine
● V76.8 Other neoplasm
    V76.81 Nervous system
    V76.89 Other neoplasm
☐ V76.9 Unspecified
● V77 Special screening for endocrine, nutritional, metabolic, and immunity disorders
    V77.0 Thyroid disorders
    V77.1 Diabetes mellitus
    V77.2 Malnutrition
    V77.3 Phenylketonuria [PKU]
    V77.4 Galactosemia
    V77.5 Gout
    V77.6 Cystic fibrosis
        Screening for mucoviscidosis
    V77.7 Other inborn errors of metabolism
    V77.8 Obesity
    ● V77.9 Other and unspecified endocrine, nutritional, metabolic, and immunity disorders
        V77.91 Screening for lipoid disorders
            Screening cholesterol level
            Screening for hypercholesterolemia
            Screening for hyperlipidemia
        V77.99 Other and unspecified endocrine, nutritional, metabolic, and immunity disorders
● V78 Special screening for disorders of blood and blood-forming organs
    V78.0 Iron deficiency anemia
    V78.1 Other and unspecified deficiency anemia
    V78.2 Sickle-cell disease or trait
    V78.3 Other hemoglobinopathies
    V78.8 Other disorders of blood and blood-forming organs
    ☐ V78.9 Unspecified disorder of blood and blood-forming organs

● V79 Special screening for mental disorders and developmental handicaps
    V79.0 Depression
    V79.1 Alcoholism
    V79.2 Intellectual disabilities
    V79.3 Developmental handicaps in early childhood
    V79.8 Other specified mental disorders and developmental handicaps
    ☐ V79.9 Unspecified mental disorder and developmental handicap
● V80 Special screening for neurological, eye, and ear diseases
    ● V80.0 Neurological conditions
        V80.01 Traumatic brain injury
        V80.09 Other neurological conditions
    V80.1 Glaucoma
    V80.2 Other eye conditions
        Screening for:
            cataract
            congenital anomaly of eye
            senile macular lesions
        Excludes general vision examination (V72.0)
    V80.3 Ear diseases
        Excludes general hearing examination (V72.11–V72.19)
● V81 Special screening for cardiovascular, respiratory, and genitourinary diseases
    V81.0 Ischemic heart disease
    V81.1 Hypertension
    V81.2 Other and unspecified cardiovascular conditions
    V81.3 Chronic bronchitis and emphysema
    V81.4 Other and unspecified respiratory conditions
        Excludes screening for:
            lung neoplasm (V76.0)
            pulmonary tuberculosis (V74.1)
    V81.5 Nephropathy
        Screening for asymptomatic bacteriuria
    V81.6 Other and unspecified genitourinary conditions
● V82 Special screening for other conditions
    V82.0 Skin conditions
    V82.1 Rheumatoid arthritis
    V82.2 Other rheumatic disorders
    V82.3 Congenital dislocation of hip
    V82.4 Maternal postnatal screening for chromosomal anomalies
        Excludes antenatal screening by amniocentesis (V28.0)
    V82.5 Chemical poisoning and other contamination
        Screening for:
            heavy metal poisoning
            ingestion of radioactive substance
            poisoning from contaminated water supply
            radiation exposure
    V82.6 Multiphasic screening
    ● V82.7 Genetic screening
        Excludes genetic testing for procreative management (V26.31–V26.39)
        Coding Clinic: 2006, Q4, P118
        V82.71 Screening for genetic disease carrier status
        V82.79 Other genetic screening
    ● V82.8 Other specified conditions
        V82.81 Osteoporosis
            Use additional code to identify:
                hormone replacement therapy (postmenopausal) status (V07.4)
                postmenopausal (natural) status (V49.81)
            Coding Clinic: 2000, Q4, P53-54
        V82.89 Other specified conditions
    ☐ V82.9 Unspecified condition

PART III / Diseases: Tabular List Volume 1

GENETICS (V83–V84)

OGCR Section I.C.18.d.3
Genetic carrier status indicates that a person carries a gene, associated with a particular disease, which may be passed to offspring who may develop that disease. The person does not have the disease and is not at risk of developing the disease.

- **V83 Genetic carrier status**
  - **V83.0 Hemophilia A carrier**
    - V83.01 Asymptomatic hemophilia A carrier
    - V83.02 Symptomatic hemophilia A carrier
  - **V83.8 Other genetic carrier status**
    - V83.81 Cystic fibrosis gene carrier
    - V83.89 Other genetic carrier status

OGCR Section I.C.18.d.3
Genetic susceptibility indicates that a person has a gene that increases the risk of that person developing the disease. Codes from category V84, Genetic susceptibility to disease, should not be used as principal or first-listed codes.

- **V84 Genetic susceptibility to disease**
  - **Includes** Confirmed abnormal gene
  - **Excludes** chromosomal anomalies (758.0-758.9)
  - Use additional code, if applicable, for any associated family history of the disease (V16–V19)
  - **V84.0 Genetic susceptibility to malignant neoplasm**
    - *Code first*, if applicable, any current malignant neoplasms (140.0–195.8, 200.0–208.9, 230.0–234.9)
    - Use additional code, if applicable, for any personal history of malignant neoplasm (V10.0–V10.9)
    - V84.01 Genetic susceptibility to malignant neoplasm of breast
      - Coding Clinic: 2004, Q4, P106-107
    - V84.02 Genetic susceptibility to malignant neoplasm of ovary
    - V84.03 Genetic susceptibility to malignant neoplasm of prostate
    - V84.04 Genetic susceptibility to malignant neoplasm of endometrium
    - V84.09 Genetic susceptibility to other malignant neoplasm
  - **V84.8 Genetic susceptibility to other disease**
    - V84.81 Genetic susceptibility to multiple endocrine neoplasia [MEN]
      - **Excludes** multiple endocrine neoplasia [MEN] syndromes (258.01-258.03)
      - Coding Clinic: 2007, Q4, P99-101
    - V84.89 Genetic susceptibility to other disease

BODY MASS INDEX (V85)

- **V85 Body mass index (BMI)**
  - Kilograms per meters squared
  - Note: BMI adult codes are for use for persons over 20 years old
  - Coding Clinic: 2012, Q2, P13; 2008, Q4, P191; 2005, Q4, P94-100
  - **V85.0 Body Mass Index less than 19, adult**
  - **V85.1 Body Mass Index between 19–24, adult**
  - **V85.2 Body Mass Index between 25–29, adult**
    - V85.21 Body Mass Index 25.0–25.9, adult
    - V85.22 Body Mass Index 26.0–26.9, adult
    - V85.23 Body Mass Index 27.0–27.9, adult
    - V85.24 Body Mass Index 28.0–28.9, adult
    - V85.25 Body Mass Index 29.0–29.9, adult
  - **V85.3 Body Mass Index between 30–39, adult**
    - V85.30 Body Mass Index 30.0–30.9, adult
    - V85.31 Body Mass Index 31.0–31.9, adult
    - V85.32 Body Mass Index 32.0–32.9, adult
    - V85.33 Body Mass Index 33.0–33.9, adult
    - V85.34 Body Mass Index 34.0–34.9, adult
    - V85.35 Body Mass Index 35.0–35.9, adult
    - V85.36 Body Mass Index 36.0–36.9, adult
    - V85.37 Body Mass Index 37.0–37.9, adult
    - V85.38 Body Mass Index 38.0–38.9, adult
    - V85.39 Body Mass Index 39.0–39.9, adult
  - **V85.4 Body Mass Index 40 and over, adult**
    - Coding Clinic: 2010, Q4, P81
    - V85.41 Body Mass Index 40.0–44.9, adult
    - V85.42 Body Mass Index 45.0–49.9, adult
    - V85.43 Body Mass Index 50.0–59.9, adult
    - V85.44 Body Mass Index 60.0–69.9, adult
    - V85.45 Body Mass Index 70 and over, adult
  - **V85.5 Body Mass Index, pediatric**
    - Note: BMI pediatric codes are for use for persons age 2–20 years old. These percentiles are based on the growth charts published by the Centers for Disease Control and Prevention (CDC)
    - V85.51 Body Mass Index, pediatric, less than 5th percentile for age
    - V85.52 Body Mass Index, pediatric, 5th percentile to less than 85th percentile for age
    - V85.53 Body Mass Index, pediatric, 85th percentile to less than 95th percentile for age
    - V85.54 Body Mass Index, pediatric, greater than or equal to 95th percentile for age

ESTROGEN RECEPTOR STATUS (V86)

- **V86 Estrogen receptor status**
  - *Code first* malignant neoplasm of breast (174.0–174.9, 175.0–175.9)
  - **V86.0 Estrogen receptor positive status [ER+]**
  - **V86.1 Estrogen receptor negative status [ER-]**

OTHER SPECIFIED PERSONAL EXPOSURES AND HISTORY PRESENTING HAZARDS TO HEALTH (V87)

- **V87 Other specified personal exposures and history presenting hazards to health**
  - **V87.0 Contact with and (suspected) exposure to hazardous metals**
    - **Excludes** exposure to lead (V15.86)
      toxic effect of metals (984.0-985.9)
    - V87.01 Arsenic
    - V87.02 Contact with and (suspected) exposure to uranium
      - **Excludes** retained depleted uranium fragments (V90.01)
    - V87.09 Other hazardous metals
      - Chromium compounds
      - Nickel dust
  - **V87.1 Contact with and (suspected) exposure to hazardous aromatic compounds**
    - **Excludes** toxic effects of aromatic compounds (982.0, 983.0)
    - V87.11 Aromatic amines
    - V87.12 Benzene
    - V87.19 Other hazardous aromatic compounds
      - Aromatic dyes NOS
      - Polycyclic aromatic hydrocarbons

V87.2 Contact with and (suspected) exposure to other potentially hazardous chemicals
Dyes NOS
Excludes: *exposure to asbestos (V15.84)*
toxic effect of chemicals (980–989)

● **V87.3** Contact with and (suspected) exposure to other potentially hazardous substances
Excludes: *contact with and (suspected) exposure to potentially hazardous body fluids (V15.85)*
personal history of retained foreign body fully removed (V15.53)
toxic effect of substances (980–989)

V87.31 Exposure to mold
V87.32 Contact with and (suspected) exposure to algae bloom
V87.39 Contact with and (suspected) exposure to other potentially hazardous substances

● **V87.4** Personal history of drug therapy
Excludes: *long-term (current) drug use (V58.61-V58.69)*

V87.41 Personal history of antineoplastic chemotherapy
V87.42 Personal history of monoclonal drug therapy
V87.43 Personal history of estrogen therapy
V87.44 Personal history of inhaled steroid therapy
V87.45 Personal history of systemic steroid therapy
Personal history of steroid therapy NOS
V87.46 Personal history of immunosuppression therapy
Excludes: *personal history of steroid therapy (V87.44, V87.45)*
V87.49 Personal history of other drug therapy

ACQUIRED ABSENCE OF OTHER ORGANS AND TISSUE (V88)

● **V88** Acquired absence of other organs and tissue
● **V88.0** Acquired absence of cervix and uterus
V88.01 Acquired absence of both cervix and uterus
Acquired absence of uterus NOS
Status post total hysterectomy
V88.02 Acquired absence of uterus with remaining cervical stump
Status post partial hysterectomy with remaining cervical stump
V88.03 Acquired absence of cervix with remaining uterus

● **V88.1** Acquired absence of pancreas
Use additional code to identify any associated:
insulin use (V58.67)
secondary diabetes mellitus (249.00-249.91)
V88.11 Acquired total absence of pancreas
Acquired absence of pancreas NOS
V88.12 Acquired partial absence of pancreas

● **V88.2** Acquired absence of joint
Acquired absence of joint following prior explantation of joint prosthesis
Joint prosthesis explantation status
V88.21 Acquired absence of hip joint
Acquired absence of hip joint following explantation of joint prosthesis, with or without presence of antibiotic-impregnated cement spacer
V88.22 Acquired absence of knee joint
Acquired absence of knee joint following explantation of joint prosthesis, with or without presence of antibiotic-impregnated cement spacer
V88.29 Acquired absence of other joint
Acquired absence of other joint following explantation of joint prosthesis, with or without presence of antibiotic-impregnated cement spacer

OTHER SUSPECTED CONDITIONS NOT FOUND (V89)

● **V89** Other suspected conditions not found
● **V89.0** Suspected maternal and fetal conditions not found
Excludes: *known or suspected fetal anomalies affecting management of mother, not ruled out (655.00 655.93, 656.00–656.93, 657.00–657.03, 658.00–658.93)*
newborn and perinatal conditions – code to condition

V89.01 Suspected problem with amniotic cavity and membrane not found
Suspected oligohydramnios not found
Suspected polyhydramnios not found
V89.02 Suspected placental problem not found
V89.03 Suspected fetal anomaly not found
V89.04 Suspected problem with fetal growth not found
V89.05 Suspected cervical shortening not found
V89.09 Other suspected maternal and fetal condition not found

RETAINED FOREIGN BODY (V90)

● **V90** Retained foreign body
Embedded fragment (status)
Embedded splinter (status)
Retained foreign body status
Excludes: *artificial joint prosthesis status (V43.60-V43.69)*
foreign body accidentally left during a procedure (998.4)
foreign body entering through orifice (930.0-939.9)
in situ cardiac devices (V45.00-V45.09)
organ or tissue replaced by other means (V43.0-V43.89)
organ or tissue replaced by transplant (V42.0-V42.9)
personal history of retained foreign body removed (V15.53)
superficial foreign body (splinter) (categories 910-917 and 919 with 4th character 6 or 7, 918.0)

● **V90.0** Retained radioactive fragment
V90.01 Retained depleted uranium fragments
V90.09 Other retained radioactive fragments
Other retained depleted isotope fragments
Retained nontherapeutic radioactive fragments

● **V90.1** Retained metal fragments
Excludes: *retained radioactive metal fragments (V90.01-V90.09)*
■ **V90.10** Retained metal fragments, unspecified
Retained metal fragment NOS
V90.11 Retained magnetic metal fragments
V90.12 Retained nonmagnetic metal fragments

V90.2 Retained plastic fragments
Acrylics fragments
Diethylhexylphthalates fragments
Isocyanate fragments

● **V90.3** Retained organic fragments
V90.31 Retained animal quills or spines
V90.32 Retained tooth
V90.33 Retained wood fragments
V90.39 Other retained organic fragments

● **V90.8** Other specified retained foreign body
V90.81 Retained glass fragments
V90.83 Retained stone or crystalline fragments
Retained concrete or cement fragments
V90.89 Other specified retained foreign body

■ **V90.9** Retained foreign body, unspecified material

MULTIPLE GESTATION PLACENTA STATUS (V91)

- **V91 Multiple gestation placenta status**
  Code first multiple gestation (651.0-651.9)
  - **V91.0 Twin gestation placenta status**
    - V91.00 Twin gestation, unspecified number of placenta, unspecified number of amniotic sacs
    - V91.01 Twin gestation, monochorionic/monoamniotic (one placenta, one amniotic sac)
    - V91.02 Twin gestation, monochorionic/diamniotic (one placenta, two amniotic sacs)
    - V91.03 Twin gestation, dichorionic/diamniotic (two placentae, two amniotic sacs)
    - V91.09 Twin gestation, unable to determine number of placenta and number of amniotic sacs
  - **V91.1 Triplet gestation placenta status**
    - V91.10 Triplet gestation, unspecified number of placenta and unspecified number of amniotic sacs
    - V91.11 Triplet gestation, with two or more monochorionic fetuses
    - V91.12 Triplet gestation, with two or more monoamniotic fetuses
    - V91.19 Triplet gestation, unable to determine number of placenta and number of amniotic sacs
- **V91.2 Quadruplet gestation placenta status**
  - V91.20 Quadruplet gestation, unspecified number of placenta and unspecified number of amniotic sacs
  - V91.21 Quadruplet gestation, with two or more monochorionic fetuses
  - V91.22 Quadruplet gestation, with two or more monoamniotic fetuses
  - V91.29 Quadruplet gestation, unable to determine number of placenta and number of amniotic sacs
- **V91.9 Other specified multiple gestation placenta status**
  Placenta status for multiple gestations greater than quadruplets
  - V91.90 Other specified multiple gestation, unspecified number of placenta and unspecified number of amniotic sacs
  - V91.91 Other specified multiple gestation, with two or more monochorionic fetuses
  - V91.92 Other specified multiple gestation, with two or more monoamniotic fetuses
  - V91.99 Other specified multiple gestation, unable to determine number of placenta and number of amniotic sacs

Medicare Code Edit: E-codes are ICD-9-CM codes beginning with the letter E. They describe the circumstance causing an injury, not the nature of the injury, and therefore should not be used as a principal diagnosis.

SUPPLEMENTARY CLASSIFICATION OF EXTERNAL CAUSES OF INJURY AND POISONING (E000-E999)

This section is provided to permit the classification of environmental events, circumstances, and conditions as the cause of injury, poisoning, and other adverse effects. Where a code from this section is applicable, it is intended that it shall be used in addition to a code from one of the main chapters of ICD-9-CM, indicating the nature of the condition. Certain other conditions which may be stated to be due to external causes are classified in Chapters 1 to 16 of ICD-9-CM. For these, the "E" code classification should be used as an additional code for more detailed analysis.

Machinery accidents [other than those connected with transport] are classifiable to category E919, in which the fourth digit allows a broad classification of the type of machinery involved.

Categories for "late effects" of accidents and other external causes are to be found at E929, E959, E969, E977, E989, and E999.

(a) A transport accident (E800–E848) is any accident involving a device designed primarily for, or being used at the time primarily for, conveying persons or goods from one place to another.

> **Includes** accidents involving:
> aircraft and spacecraft (E840–E845)
> watercraft (E830–E838)
> motor vehicle (E810–E825)
> railway (E800–E807)
> other road vehicles (E826–E829)

In classifying accidents which involve more than one kind of transport, the above order of precedence of transport accidents should be used.

Accidents involving agricultural and construction machines, such as tractors, cranes, and bulldozers, are regarded as transport accidents only when these vehicles are under their own power on a highway [otherwise the vehicles are regarded as machinery]. Vehicles which can travel on land or water, such as hovercraft and other amphibious vehicles, are regarded as watercraft when on the water, as motor vehicles when on the highway, and as off-road motor vehicles when on land, but off the highway.

> **Excludes** accidents:
> in sports which involve the use of transport but where the transport vehicle itself was not involved in the accident
> involving vehicles which are part of industrial equipment used entirely on industrial premises
> occurring during transportation but unrelated to the hazards associated with the means of transportation [e.g., injuries received in a fight on board ship; transport vehicle involved in a cataclysm such as an earthquake]
> to persons engaged in the maintenance or repair of transport equipment or vehicle not in motion, unless injured by another vehicle in motion

(b) A railway accident is a transport accident involving a railway train or other railway vehicle operated on rails, whether in motion or not.

> **Excludes** accidents:
> in repair shops
> in roundhouse or on turntable
> on railway premises but not involving a train or other railway vehicle

(c) A railway train or railway vehicle is any device with or without cars coupled to it, designed for traffic on a railway.

> **Includes** interurban:
> electric car (operated chiefly on its own right-of-way, not open to other traffic)
> streetcar (operated chiefly on its own right-of-way, not open to other traffic)
> railway train, any power [diesel] [electric] [steam]
> funicular
> monorail or two-rail
> subterranean or elevated
> other vehicle designed to run on a railway track

> **Excludes** interurban electric cars [streetcars] specified to be operating on a right-of-way that forms part of the public street or highway [definition (n)]

(d) A railway or railroad is a right-of-way designed for traffic on rails, which is used by carriages or wagons transporting passengers or freight, and by other rolling stock, and which is not open to other public vehicular traffic

(e) A motor vehicle accident is a transport accident involving a motor vehicle. It is defined as a motor vehicle traffic accident or as a motor vehicle nontraffic accident according to whether the accident occurs on a public highway or elsewhere.

> **Excludes** injury or damage due to cataclysm
> injury or damage while a motor vehicle, not under its own power, is being loaded on, or unloaded from, another conveyance

(f) A motor vehicle traffic accident is any motor vehicle accident occurring on a public highway [i.e., originating, terminating, or involving a vehicle partially on the highway]. A motor vehicle accident is assumed to have occurred on the highway unless another place is specified, except in the case of accidents involving only off-road motor vehicles which are classified as nontraffic accidents unless the contrary is stated.

(g) A motor vehicle nontraffic accident is any motor vehicle accident which occurs entirely in any place other than a public highway.

(h) A public highway [trafficway] or street is the entire width between property lines [or other boundary lines] of every way or place, of which any part is open to the use of the public for purposes of vehicular traffic as a matter of right or custom. A roadway is that part of the public highway designed, improved, and ordinarily used, for vehicular travel.

> **Includes** approaches (public) to:
> docks
> public building
> station

> **Excludes** driveway (private)
> parking lot
> ramp
> roads in:
> airfield
> farm
> industrial premises
> mine
> private grounds
> quarry

(i) A motor vehicle is any mechanically or electrically powered device, not operated on rails, upon which any person or property may be transported or drawn upon a highway. Any object such as a trailer, coaster, sled, or wagon being towed by a motor vehicle is considered a part of the motor vehicle.

Includes automobile [any type]
bus
construction machinery, farm and industrial machinery, steam roller, tractor, army tank, highway grader, or similar vehicle on wheels or treads, while in transport under own power
fire engine (motorized)
motorcycle
motorized bicycle [moped] or scooter
trolley bus not operating on rails
truck
van

Excludes devices used solely to move persons or materials within the confines of a building and its premises, such as:
building elevator
coal car in mine
electric baggage or mail truck used solely within a railroad station
electric truck used solely within an industrial plant
moving overhead crane

(j) A motorcycle is a two-wheeled motor vehicle having one or two riding saddles and sometimes having a third wheel for the support of a sidecar. The sidecar is considered part of the motorcycle.

Includes motorized:
bicycle [moped]
scooter
tricycle

(k) An off-road motor vehicle is a motor vehicle of special design, to enable it to negotiate rough or soft terrain or snow. Examples of special design are high construction, special wheels and tires, driven by treads, or support on a cushion of air.

Includes all terrain vehicle [ATV]
army tank
hovercraft, on land or swamp
snowmobile

(l) A driver of a motor vehicle is the occupant of the motor vehicle operating it or intending to operate it. A motorcyclist is the driver of a motorcycle. Other authorized occupants of a motor vehicle are passengers.

(m) An other road vehicle is any device, except a motor vehicle, in, on, or by which any person or property may be transported on a highway.

Includes animal carrying a person or goods
animal-drawn vehicle
animal harnessed to conveyance
bicycle [pedal cycle]
streetcar
tricycle (pedal)

Excludes pedestrian conveyance [definition (q)]

(n) A streetcar is a device designed and used primarily for transporting persons within a municipality, running on rails, usually subject to normal traffic control signals, and operated principally on a right-of-way that forms part of the traffic way. A trailer being towed by a streetcar is considered a part of the streetcar.

Includes interurban or intraurban electric or streetcar, when specified to be operating on a street or public highway
tram (car)
trolley (car)

(o) A pedal cycle is any road transport vehicle operated solely by pedals.

Includes bicycle
pedal cycle
tricycle

Excludes motorized bicycle [definition (i)]

(p) A pedal cyclist is any person riding on a pedal cycle or in a sidecar attached to such a vehicle.

(q) A pedestrian conveyance is any human powered device by which a pedestrian may move other than by walking or by which a walking person may move another pedestrian.

Includes baby carriage
coaster wagon
heelies
ice skates
motorized mobility scooter
perambulator
pushcart
pushchair
roller skates
scooter
skateboard
skis
sled
wheelchair (electric)
wheelies

(r) A pedestrian is any person involved in an accident who was not at the time of the accident riding in or on a motor vehicle, railroad train, streetcar, animal-drawn or other vehicle, or on a bicycle or animal.

Includes person:
changing tire of vehicle
in or operating a pedestrian conveyance
making adjustment to motor of vehicle
on foot

(s) A watercraft is any device for transporting passengers or goods on the water.

(t) A small boat is any watercraft propelled by paddle, oars, or small motor, with a passenger capacity of less than ten.

Includes boat NOS
canoe
coble
dinghy
punt
raft
rowboat
rowing shell
scull
skiff
small motorboat

Excludes barge
lifeboat (used after abandoning ship)
raft (anchored) being used as a diving platform
yacht

(u) An aircraft is any device for transporting passengers or goods in the air.

Includes airplane [any type]
balloon
bomber
dirigible
glider (hang)
military aircraft
parachute

(v) A commercial transport aircraft is any device for collective passenger or freight transportation by air, whether run on commercial lines for profit or by government authorities, with the exception of military craft.

EXTERNAL CAUSE STATUS (E000)

Note: A code from category E000 should be used in conjunction with the external cause code(s) assigned to a record to indicate the status of the person at the time the event occurred. A single code from category E000 should be assigned for an encounter.

● **E000 External cause status**

    E000.0 Civilian activity done for income or pay
        Civilian activity done for financial or other compensation
        Excludes: military activity (E000.1)
        Coding Clinic: 2009, Q4, P130

    E000.1 Military activity
        Excludes: activity of off duty military personnel (E000.8)

    E000.2 Volunteer activity
        Excludes: activity of child or other family member assisting in compensated work of other family member (E000.8)
        Coding Clinic: 2010, Q4, P111

    E000.8 Other external cause status
        Activity NEC
        Activity of child or other family member assisting in compensated work of other family member
        Hobby not done for income
        Leisure activity
        Off-duty activity of military personnel
        Recreation or sport not for income or while a student
        Student activity
        Excludes: civilian activity done for income or compensation (E000.0)
        military activity (E000.1)
        Coding Clinic: 2010, Q4, P93; 2009, Q4, P130

    E000.9 Unspecified external cause status

ACTIVITY (E001-E030)

Note: Categories E001 to E030 are provided for use to indicate the activity of the person seeking healthcare for an injury or health condition, such as a heart attack while shoveling snow, which resulted from, or was contributed to, by the activity. These codes are appropriate for use for both acute injuries, such as those from chapter 17, and conditions that are due to the long-term, cumulative effects of an activity, such as those from chapter 13. They are also appropriate for use with external cause codes for cause and intent if identifying the activity provides additional information on the event.

These codes should be used in conjunction with other external cause codes for external cause status (E000) and place of occurrence (E849).

This section contains the following broad activity categories:

E001 Activities involving walking and running
E002 Activities involving water and water craft
E003 Activities involving ice and snow
E004 Activities involving climbing, rappelling, and jumping off
E005 Activities involving dancing and other rhythmic movement
E006 Activities involving other sports and athletics played individually
E007 Activities involving other sports and athletics played as a team or group
E008 Activities involving other specified sports and athletics
E009 Activity involving other cardiorespiratory exercise
E010 Activity involving other muscle strengthening exercises
E011 Activities involving computer technology and electronic devices
E012 Activities involving arts and handcrafts
E013 Activities involving personal hygiene and household maintenance
E014 Activities involving person providing caregiving
E015 Activities involving food preparation, cooking and grilling
E016 Activities involving property and land maintenance, building and construction
E017 Activities involving roller coasters and other types of external motion
E018 Activities involving playing musical instrument
E019 Activities involving animal care
E029 Other activity
E030 Unspecified activity

● **E001 Activities involving walking and running**
    Excludes: walking an animal (E019.0)
        walking or running on a treadmill (E009.0)

    E001.0 Walking, marching and hiking
        Walking, marching and hiking on level or elevated terrain
        Excludes: mountain climbing (E004.0)
        Coding Clinic: 2009, Q4, P141

    E001.1 Running

● **E002 Activities involving water and water craft**
    Excludes: activities involving ice (E003.0-E003.9)
        boating and other watercraft transport accidents (E830-E838)

    E002.0 Swimming
    E002.1 Springboard and platform diving
    E002.2 Water polo
    E002.3 Water aerobics and water exercise
    E002.4 Underwater diving and snorkeling
        SCUBA diving
    E002.5 Rowing, canoeing, kayaking, rafting and tubing
        Canoeing, kayaking, rafting and tubing in calm and turbulent water
    E002.6 Water skiing and wake boarding
    E002.7 Surfing, windsurfing and boogie boarding
    E002.8 Water sliding
    E002.9 Other activity involving water and watercraft
        Activity involving water NOS
        Parasailing
        Water survival training and testing
        Coding Clinic: 2010, Q2, P16

● **E003 Activities involving ice and snow**
    Excludes: shoveling ice and snow (E016.0)

    E003.0 Ice skating
        Figure skating (singles) (pairs)
        Ice dancing
        Excludes: ice hockey (E003.1)
    E003.1 Ice hockey
    E003.2 Snow (alpine) (downhill) skiing, snow boarding, sledding, tobogganing and snow tubing
        Excludes: cross country skiing (E003.3)
    E003.3 Cross country skiing
        Nordic skiing
    E003.9 Other activity involving ice and snow
        Activity involving ice and snow NOS

- **E004 Activities involving climbing, rappelling and jumping off**
  > **Excludes** hiking on level or elevated terrain (E001.0)
  > jumping rope (E006.5)
  > sky diving (E840-E844)
  > trampoline jumping (E005.3)

  E004.0 Mountain climbing, rock climbing and wall climbing
  E004.1 Rappelling
  E004.2 BASE jumping
      Building, Antenna, Span, Earth jumping
  E004.3 Bungee jumping
  E004.4 Hang gliding
  E004.9 Other activity involving climbing, rappelling and jumping off

- **E005 Activities involving dancing and other rhythmic movement**
  > **Excludes** martial arts (E008.4)

  E005.0 Dancing
  E005.1 Yoga
  E005.2 Gymnastics
      Rhythmic gymnastics
  > **Excludes** trampoline (E005.3)

  E005.3 Trampoline
  E005.4 Cheerleading
  E005.9 Other activity involving dancing and other rhythmic movements

- **E006 Activities involving other sports and athletics played individually**
  > **Excludes** dancing (E005.0)
  > gymnastics (E005.2)
  > trampoline (E005.3)
  > yoga (E005.1)

  E006.0 Roller skating (inline) and skateboarding
      Coding Clinic: 2010, Q4, P93
  E006.1 Horseback riding
  E006.2 Golf
  E006.3 Bowling
  E006.4 Bike riding
  > **Excludes** transport accident involving bike riding (E800-E829)

  E006.5 Jumping rope
  E006.6 Non-running track and field events
  > **Excludes** running (any form) (E001.1)

  E006.9 Other activity involving other sports and athletics played individually
  > **Excludes** activities involving climbing, rappelling, and jumping (E004.0-E004.9)
  > activities involving ice and snow (E003.0-E003.9)
  > activities involving walking and running (E001.0-E001.9)
  > activities involving water and watercraft (E002.0-E002.9)

- **E007 Activities involving other sports and athletics played as a team or group**
  > **Excludes** ice hockey (E003.1)
  > water polo (E002.2)

  E007.0 American tackle football
      Football NOS
  E007.1 American flag or touch football
  E007.2 Rugby
  E007.3 Baseball
      Softball
  E007.4 Lacrosse and field hockey
  E007.5 Soccer
  E007.6 Basketball
  E007.7 Volleyball (beach) (court)
  E007.8 Physical games generally associated with school recess, summer camp and children
      Capture the flag
      Dodge ball
      Four square
      Kickball
  E007.9 Other activity involving other sports and athletics played as a team or group
      Cricket

- **E008 Activities involving other specified sports and athletics**
  E008.0 Boxing
  E008.1 Wrestling
  E008.2 Racquet and hand sports
      Handball
      Racquetball
      Squash
      Tennis
  E008.3 Frisbee
      Ultimate frisbee
  E008.4 Martial arts
      Combatives
  E008.9 Other specified sports and athletics activity
  > **Excludes** sports and athletics activities specified in categories E001-E007

- **E009 Activity involving other cardiorespiratory exercise**
  Activity involving physical training

  E009.0 Exercise machines primarily for cardiorespiratory conditioning
      Elliptical and stepper machines
      Stationary bike
      Treadmill
  E009.1 Calisthenics
      Jumping jacks
      Warm up and cool down
  E009.2 Aerobic and step exercise
  E009.3 Circuit training
  E009.4 Obstacle course
      Challenge course
      Confidence course
  E009.5 Grass drills
      Guerilla drills
  E009.9 Other activity involving other cardiorespiratory exercise
  > **Excludes** activities involving cardiorespiratory exercise specified in categories E001-E008

- **E010 Activity involving other muscle strengthening exercises**
  E010.0 Exercise machines primarily for muscle strengthening
  E010.1 Push-ups, pull-ups, sit-ups
  E010.2 Free weights
      Barbells
      Dumbbells
  E010.3 Pilates
  E010.9 Other activity involving other muscle strengthening exercises
  > **Excludes** activities involving muscle strengthening specified in categories E001-E009

- **E011** Activities involving computer technology and electronic devices

  > **Excludes** electronic musical keyboard or instruments (E018.0)

  - E011.0 Computer keyboarding
    Electronic game playing using keyboard or other stationary device
  - E011.1 Hand held interactive electronic device
    Cellular telephone and communication device
    Electronic game playing using interactive device
    > **Excludes** electronic game playing using keyboard or other stationary device (E011.0)
  - E011.9 Other activity involving computer technology and electronic devices

- **E012** Activities involving arts and handcrafts

  > **Excludes** activities involving playing musical instrument (E018.0-E018.3)

  - E012.0 Knitting and crocheting
  - E012.1 Sewing
  - E012.2 Furniture building and finishing
    Furniture repair
  - E012.9 Activity involving other arts and handcrafts

- **E013** Activities involving personal hygiene and household maintenance

  > **Excludes** activities involving cooking and grilling (E015.0-E015.9)
  > activities involving property and land maintenance, building and construction (E016.0-E016.9)
  > activity involving persons providing caregiving (E014.0-E014.9)
  > dishwashing (E015.0)
  > food preparation (E015.0)
  > gardening (E016.1)

  - E013.0 Personal bathing and showering
  - E013.1 Laundry
  - E013.2 Vacuuming
  - E013.3 Ironing
  - E013.4 Floor mopping and cleaning
  - E013.5 Residential relocation
    Packing up and unpacking involved in moving to a new residence
  - E013.8 Other personal hygiene activity
  - E013.9 Other household maintenance

- **E014** Activities involving person providing caregiving
  - E014.0 Caregiving involving bathing
  - E014.1 Caregiving involving lifting
  - E014.9 Other activity involving person providing caregiving

- **E015** Activities involving food preparation, cooking and grilling
  - E015.0 Food preparation and clean up
    Dishwashing
  - E015.1 Grilling and smoking food
  - E015.2 Cooking and baking
    Use of stove, oven and microwave oven
  - E015.9 Other activity involving cooking and grilling

- **E016** Activities involving property and land maintenance, building and construction
  - E016.0 Digging, shoveling and raking
    Dirt digging
    Raking leaves
    Snow shoveling
    Coding Clinic: 2009, Q4, P141
  - E016.1 Gardening and landscaping
    Pruning, trimming shrubs, weeding
  - E016.2 Building and construction
  - E016.9 Other activity involving property and land maintenance, building and construction

- **E017** Activities involving roller coasters and other types of external motion
  - E017.0 Roller coaster riding
  - E017.9 Other activity involving external motion

- **E018** Activities involving playing musical instrument
  Activity involving playing electric musical instrument
  - E018.0 Piano playing
    Musical keyboard (electronic) playing
  - E018.1 Drum and other percussion instrument playing
  - E018.2 String instrument playing
  - E018.3 Wind and brass instrument playing

- **E019** Activities involving animal care
  > **Excludes** horseback riding (E006.1)
  - E019.0 Walking an animal
  - E019.1 Milking an animal
  - E019.2 Grooming and shearing an animal
  - E019.9 Other activity involving animal care

- **E029** Other activity
  Coding Clinic: 2010, Q4, P111
  - E029.0 Refereeing a sports activity
  - E029.1 Spectator at an event
  - E029.2 Rough housing and horseplay
  - E029.9 Other activity

  - E030 Unspecified activity

TRANSPORT ACCIDENTS (E800-E848)

Definitions and examples related to transport accidents

(a) A transport accident (E800-E848) is any accident involving a device designed primarily for, or being used at the time primarily for, conveying persons or goods from one place to another.

RAILWAY ACCIDENTS (E800-E807)

Note: For definitions of railway accident and related terms see definitions (a) to (d).

Excludes *accidents involving railway train and:*
aircraft (E840.0-E845.9)
motor vehicle (E810.0-E825.9)
watercraft (E830.0-E838.9)

The following fourth-digit subdivisions are for use with categories E800-E807 to identify the injured person:

0 Railway employee
Any person who by virtue of his employment in connection with a railway, whether by the railway company or not, is at increased risk of involvement in a railway accident, such as:
catering staff of train
driver
guard
porter
postal staff on train
railway fireman
shunter
sleeping car attendant

1 Passenger on railway
Any authorized person traveling on a train, except a railway employee.
Excludes *intending passenger waiting at station (8)*
unauthorized rider on railway vehicle (8)

2 Pedestrian
See definition (r)

3 Pedal cyclist
See definition (p)

8 Other specified person
Intending passenger or bystander waiting at station
Unauthorized rider on railway vehicle

9 Unspecified person

E800 Railway accident involving collision with rolling stock
Requires fourth digit. See beginning of section E800-E845 for codes and definitions.
Includes collision between railway trains or railway vehicles, any kind
collision NOS on railway
derailment with antecedent collision with rolling stock or NOS

E801 Railway accident involving collision with other object
Requires fourth digit. See beginning of section E800-E845 for codes and definitions.
Includes collision of railway train with:
buffers
fallen tree on railway
gates
platform
rock on railway
streetcar
other nonmotor vehicle
other object
Excludes *collision with:*
aircraft (E840.0-E842.9)
motor vehicle (E810.0-E810.9, E820.0-E822.9)

E802 Railway accident involving derailment without antecedent collision
Requires fourth digit. See beginning of section E800-E845 for codes and definitions.

E803 Railway accident involving explosion, fire, or burning
Requires fourth digit. See beginning of section E800-E845 for codes and definitions.
Excludes *explosion or fire, with antecedent derailment (E802.0-E802.9)*
explosion or fire, with mention of antecedent collision (E800.0-E801.9)

E804 Fall in, on, or from railway train
Requires fourth digit. See beginning of section E800-E845 for codes and definitions.
Includes fall while alighting from or boarding railway train
Excludes *fall related to collision, derailment, or explosion of railway train (E800.0-E803.9)*

E805 Hit by rolling stock
Requires fourth digit. See beginning of section E800-E845 for codes and definitions.
Includes crushed by railway train or part
injured by railway train or part
killed by railway train or part
knocked down by railway train or part
run over by railway train or part
Excludes *pedestrian hit by object set in motion by railway train (E806.0-E806.9)*

E806 Other specified railway accident
Requires fourth digit. See beginning of section E800-E845 for codes and definitions.
Includes hit by object falling in railway train
injured by door or window on railway train
nonmotor road vehicle or pedestrian hit by object set in motion by railway train
railway train hit by falling:
earth NOS
rock
tree
other object
Excludes *railway accident due to cataclysm (E908-E909)*

E807 Railway accident of unspecified nature
Requires fourth digit. See beginning of section E800-E845 for codes and definitions.
Includes found dead on railway right-of-way NOS
injured on railway right-of-way NOS
railway accident NOS

MOTOR VEHICLE TRAFFIC ACCIDENTS (E810-E819)

Note: For definitions of motor vehicle traffic accident, and related terms, see definitions (e) to (k).

Excludes accidents involving motor vehicle and aircraft (E840.0-E845.9)

The following fourth-digit subdivisions are for use with categories E810-E819 to identify the injured person:

> 0 Driver of motor vehicle other than motorcycle
>   See definition (l)
> 1 Passenger in motor vehicle other than motorcycle
>   See definition (l)
> 2 Motorcyclist
>   See definition (l)
> 3 Passenger on motorcycle
>   See definition (l)
> 4 Occupant of streetcar
> 5 Rider of animal; occupant of animal-drawn vehicle
> 6 Pedal cyclist
>   See definition (p)
> 7 Pedestrian
>   See definition (r)
> 8 Other specified person
>   Occupant of vehicle other than above
>   Person in railway train involved in accident
>   Unauthorized rider of motor vehicle
> 9 Unspecified person

● **E810 Motor vehicle traffic accident involving collision with train**
Requires fourth digit. See beginning of section E800-E845 for codes and definitions.
Excludes motor vehicle collision with object set in motion by railway train (E815.0-E815.9)
railway train hit by object set in motion by motor vehicle (E818.0-E818.9)

● **E811 Motor vehicle traffic accident involving re-entrant collision with another motor vehicle**
Requires fourth digit. See beginning of section E800-E845 for codes and definitions.
Includes collision between motor vehicle which accidentally leaves the roadway then re-enters the same roadway, or the opposite roadway on a divided highway, and another motor vehicle
Excludes collision on the same roadway when none of the motor vehicles involved have left and re-entered the roadway (E812.0-E812.9)

● **E812 Other motor vehicle traffic accident involving collision with motor vehicle**
Requires fourth digit. See beginning of section E800-E845 for codes and definitions.
Includes collision with another motor vehicle parked, stopped, stalled, disabled, or abandoned on the highway
motor vehicle collision NOS
Excludes collision with object set in motion by another motor vehicle (E815.0-E815.9)
re-entrant collision with another motor vehicle (E811.0-E811.9)
Coding Clinic: 2011, Q4, P100; 2007, Q4, P105-107; 1996, Q4, P36-37

● **E813 Motor vehicle traffic accident involving collision with other vehicle**
Requires fourth digit. See beginning of section E800-E845 for codes and definitions.
Includes collision between motor vehicle, any kind, and: other road (nonmotor transport) vehicle, such as:
animal carrying a person
animal-drawn vehicle
pedal cycle
streetcar
Excludes collision with:
object set in motion by nonmotor road vehicle (E815.0-E815.9)
pedestrian (E814.0-E814.9)
nonmotor road vehicle hit by object set in motion by motor vehicle (E818.0-E818.9)

● **E814 Motor vehicle traffic accident involving collision with pedestrian**
Requires fourth digit. See beginning of section E800-E845 for codes and definitions.
Includes collision between motor vehicle, any kind, and pedestrian
pedestrian dragged, hit, or run over by motor vehicle, any kind
Excludes pedestrian hit by object set in motion by motor vehicle (E818.0-E818.9)
Coding Clinic: 2010, Q4, P93; 1996, Q4, P36-37

● **E815 Other motor vehicle traffic accident involving collision on the highway**
Requires fourth digit. See beginning of section E800-E845 for codes and definitions.
Includes collision (due to loss of control) (on highway) between motor vehicle, any kind, and:
abutment (bridge) (overpass)
animal (herded) (unattended)
fallen stone, traffic sign, tree, utility pole
guard rail or boundary fence
interhighway divider
landslide (not moving)
object set in motion by railway train or road vehicle (motor) (nonmotor)
object thrown in front of motor vehicle
safety island
temporary traffic sign or marker
wall of cut made for road
other object, fixed, movable, or moving
Excludes collision with:
any object off the highway (resulting from loss of control) (E816.0-E816.9)
any object which normally would have been off the highway and is not stated to have been on it (E816.0-E816.9)
motor vehicle parked, stopped, stalled, disabled, or abandoned on highway (E812.0-E812.9)
moving landslide (E909.2)
motor vehicle hit by object:
set in motion by railway train or road vehicle (motor) (nonmotor) (E818.0-E818.9)
thrown into or on vehicle (E818.0-E818.9)

● **E816 Motor vehicle traffic accident due to loss of control, without collision on the highway**

Requires fourth digit. See beginning of section E800-E845 for codes and definitions.

Includes motor vehicle:
  failing to make curve and:
    colliding with object off the highway
    overturning
    stopping abruptly off the highway
  going out of control (due to)
    blowout and:
      colliding with object off the highway
      overturning
      stopping abruptly off the highway
    burst tire and:
      colliding with object off the highway
      overturning
      stopping abruptly off the highway
    driver falling asleep and:
      colliding with object off the highway
      overturning
      stopping abruptly off the highway
    driver inattention and:
      colliding with object off the highway
      overturning
      stopping abruptly off the highway
    excessive speed and:
      colliding with object off the highway
      overturning
      stopping abruptly off the highway
    failure of mechanical part and:
      colliding with object off the highway
      overturning
      stopping abruptly off the highway

Excludes collision on highway following loss of control (E810.0-E815.9)
loss of control of motor vehicle following collision on the highway (E810.0-E815.9)

● **E817 Noncollision motor vehicle traffic accident while boarding or alighting**

Requires fourth digit. See beginning of section E800-E845 for codes and definitions.

Includes fall down stairs of motor bus while boarding or alighting
fall from car in street while boarding or alighting
injured by moving part of the vehicle while boarding or alighting
trapped by door of motor bus boarding or alighting while boarding or alighting

● **E818 Other noncollision motor vehicle traffic accident**

Requires fourth digit. See beginning of section E800-E845 for codes and definitions.

Includes accidental poisoning from exhaust gas generated by motor vehicle while in motion
breakage of any part of motor vehicle while in motion
explosion of any part of motor vehicle while in motion
fall, jump, or being accidentally pushed from motor vehicle while in motion
fire starting in motor vehicle while in motion
hit by object thrown into or on motor vehicle while in motion
injured by being thrown against some part of, or object in motor vehicle while in motion
injury from moving part of motor vehicle while in motion
object falling in or on motor vehicle while in motion
object thrown on motor vehicle while in motion
collision of railway train or road vehicle except motor vehicle, with object set in motion by motor vehicle
motor vehicle hit by object set in motion by railway train or road vehicle (motor) (nonmotor)
pedestrian, railway train, or road vehicle (motor) (nonmotor) hit by object set in motion by motor vehicle

Excludes collision between motor vehicle and:
  object set in motion by railway train or road vehicle (motor) (nonmotor) (E815.0-E815.9)
  object thrown towards the motor vehicle (E815.0-E815.9)
person overcome by carbon monoxide generated by stationary motor vehicle off the roadway with motor running (E868.2)

● ■ **E819 Motor vehicle traffic accident of unspecified nature**

Requires fourth digit. See beginning of section E800-E845 for codes and definitions.

Includes motor vehicle traffic accident NOS
traffic accident NOS

Coding Clinic: 2009, Q4, P141; 2008, Q4, P96-97; 2006, Q4, P100-102; 2003, Q1, P7; 1999, Q4, P11-12; Q1, P10; 1993, Q2, P4-5

MOTOR VEHICLE NONTRAFFIC ACCIDENTS (E820-E825)

Note: For definitions of motor vehicle nontraffic accident and related terms see definition (a) to (k).

Includes: accidents involving motor vehicles being used in recreational or sporting activities off the highway
collision and noncollision motor vehicle accidents occurring entirely off the highway

Excludes: accidents involving motor vehicle and:
aircraft (E840.0-E845.9)
watercraft (E830.0-E838.9)
accidents, not on the public highway, involving agricultural and construction machinery but not involving another motor vehicle (E919.0, E919.2, E919.7)

The following fourth-digit subdivisions are for use with categories E820-E825 to identify the injured person:

0 **Driver of motor vehicle other than motorcycle**
  See definition (l)
1 **Passenger in motor vehicle other than motorcycle**
  See definition (l)
2 **Motorcyclist**
  See definition (l)
3 **Passenger on motorcycle**
  See definition (l)
4 **Occupant of streetcar**
5 **Rider of animal; occupant of animal-drawn vehicle**
6 **Pedal cyclist**
  See definition (p)
7 **Pedestrian**
  See definition (r)
8 **Other specified person**
  Occupant of vehicle other than above
  Person on railway train involved in accident
  Unauthorized rider of motor vehicle
9 **Unspecified person**

● **E820 Nontraffic accident involving motor-driven snow vehicle**

Requires fourth digit. See beginning of section E800-E845 for codes and definitions.

Includes: breakage of part of motor-driven snow vehicle (not on public highway)
fall from motor-driven snow vehicle (not on public highway)
hit by motor-driven snow vehicle (not on public highway)
overturning of motor-driven snow vehicle (not on public highway)
run over or dragged by motor-driven snow vehicle (not on public highway)
collision of motor-driven snow vehicle with:
  animal (being ridden) (-drawn vehicle)
  another off-road motor vehicle
  other motor vehicle, not on public highway
  railway train
  other object, fixed or movable
injury caused by rough landing of motor-driven snow vehicle (after leaving ground on rough terrain)

Excludes: accident on the public highway involving motor driven snow vehicle (E810.0-E819.9)

● **E821 Nontraffic accident involving other off-road motor vehicle**

Requires fourth digit. See beginning of section E800-E845 for codes and definitions.

Includes: breakage of part of off-road motor vehicle, except snow vehicle (not on public highway)
fall from off-road motor vehicle, except snow vehicle (not on public highway)
hit by off-road motor vehicle, except snow vehicle (not on public highway)
overturning of off-road motor vehicle, except snow vehicle (not on public highway)
run over or dragged by off-road motor vehicle, except snow vehicle (not on public highway)
thrown against some part of or object in off-road motor vehicle, except snow vehicle (not on public highway)
collision with:
  animal (being ridden) (-drawn vehicle)
  another off-road motor vehicle, except snow vehicle
  other motor vehicle, not on public highway
  other object, fixed or movable

Excludes: accident on public highway involving off-road motor vehicle (E810.0-E819.9)
collision between motor driven snow vehicle and other off-road motor vehicle (E820.0-E820.9)
hovercraft accident on water (E830.0-E838.9)

● **E822 Other motor vehicle nontraffic accident involving collision with moving object**

Requires fourth digit. See beginning of section E800-E845 for codes and definitions.

Includes: collision, not on public highway, between motor vehicle, except off-road motor vehicle and:
  animal
  nonmotor vehicle
  other motor vehicle, except off-road motor vehicle
  pedestrian
  railway train
  other moving object

Excludes: collision with:
motor-driven snow vehicle (E820.0-E820.9)
other off-road motor vehicle (E821.0-E821.9)

● **E823 Other motor vehicle nontraffic accident involving collision with stationary object**

Requires fourth digit. See beginning of section E800-E845 for codes and definitions.

Includes: collision, not on public highway, between motor vehicle, except off-road motor vehicle, and any object, fixed or movable, but not in motion

● **E824 Other motor vehicle nontraffic accident while boarding and alighting**

Requires fourth digit. See beginning of section E800-E845 for codes and definitions.

Includes: fall while boarding or alighting from motor vehicle except off-road motor vehicle, not on public highway
injury from moving part of motor vehicle while boarding or alighting from motor vehicle except off-road motor vehicle, not on public highway
trapped by door of motor vehicle while boarding or alighting from motor vehicle except off-road motor vehicle, not on public highway

Coding Clinic: 2010, Q4, P111

● **E825** Other motor vehicle nontraffic accident of other and unspecified nature

Requires fourth digit. See beginning of section E800-E845 for codes and definitions.

Includes accidental poisoning from carbon monoxide generated by motor vehicle while in motion, not on public highway
breakage of any part of motor vehicle while in motion, not on public highway
explosion of any part of motor vehicle while in motion, not on public highway
fall, jump, or being accidentally pushed from motor vehicle while in motion, not on public highway
fire starting in motor vehicle while in motion, not on public highway
hit by object thrown into, towards, or on motor vehicle while in motion, not on public highway
injured by being thrown against some part of, or object in motor vehicle while in motion, not on public highway
injury from moving part of motor vehicle while in motion, not on public highway
object falling in or on motor vehicle while in motion, not on public highway
motor vehicle nontraffic accident NOS

Excludes *fall from or in stationary motor vehicle (E884.9, E885.9)*
overcome by carbon monoxide or exhaust gas generated by stationary motor vehicle off the roadway with motor running (E868.2)
struck by falling object from or in stationary motor vehicle (E916)

OTHER ROAD VEHICLE ACCIDENTS (E826-E829)

Note: Other road vehicle accidents are transport accidents involving road vehicles other than motor vehicles. For definitions of other road vehicle and related terms see definitions (m) to (o).

Includes accidents involving other road vehicles being used in recreational or sporting activities

Excludes *collision of other road vehicle [any] with:*
aircraft (E840.0-E845.9)
motor vehicle (E813.0-E813.9, E820.0-E822.9)
railway train (E801.0-E801.9)

The following fourth-digit subdivisions are for use with categories E826-E829 to identify the injured person:

0 Pedestrian
   See definition (r)
1 Pedal cyclist
   See definition (p)
2 Rider of animal
3 Occupant of animal-drawn vehicle
4 Occupant of streetcar
8 Other specified person
9 Unspecified person

● **E826** Pedal cycle accident
[0-9]
Requires fourth digit. See beginning of section E800-E845 for codes and definitions.

Includes breakage of any part of pedal cycle
collision between pedal cycle and:
   animal (being ridden) (herded) (unattended)
   another pedal cycle
   nonmotor road vehicle, any
   pedestrian
   other object, fixed, movable, or moving, not set in motion by motor vehicle, railway train, or aircraft
entanglement in wheel of pedal cycle
fall from pedal cycle
hit by object falling or thrown on the pedal cycle
pedal cycle accident NOS
pedal cycle overturned

● **E827** Animal-drawn vehicle accident
[0,2-4,8,9]
Requires fourth digit. See beginning of section E800-E845 for codes and definitions.

Includes breakage of any part of vehicle
collision between animal-drawn vehicle and:
   animal (being ridden) (herded) (unattended)
   nonmotor road vehicle, except pedal cycle
   pedestrian, pedestrian conveyance, or pedestrian vehicle
   other object, fixed, movable, or moving, not set in motion by motor vehicle, railway train, or aircraft
fall from animal-drawn vehicle
knocked down by animal-drawn vehicle
overturning of animal-drawn vehicle
run over by animal-drawn vehicle
thrown from animal-drawn vehicle

Excludes *collision of animal-drawn vehicle with pedal cycle (E826.0-E826.9)*

● **E828** Accident involving animal being ridden
[0,2,4,8,9]
Requires fourth digit. See beginning of section E800-E845 for codes and definitions.

Includes collision between animal being ridden and:
   another animal
   nonmotor road vehicle, except pedal cycle, and animal-drawn vehicle
   pedestrian, pedestrian conveyance, or pedestrian vehicle
   other object, fixed, movable, or moving, not set in motion by motor vehicle, railway train, or aircraft
fall from animal being ridden
knocked down by animal being ridden
thrown from animal being ridden
trampled by animal being ridden
ridden animal stumbled and fell

Excludes *collision of animal being ridden with:*
animal-drawn vehicle (E827.0-E827.9)
pedal cycle (E826.0-E826.9)

E829-E831 ICD-9-CM

- **E829 Other road vehicle accidents**
  [0,4,8,9]
  Requires fourth digit. See beginning of section E800-E845 for codes and definitions.

  Includes accident while boarding or alighting from
      streetcar
      nonmotor road vehicle not classifiable to
          E826-E828
    blow from object in
      streetcar
      nonmotor road vehicle not classifiable to
          E826-E828
    breakage of any part of
      streetcar
      nonmotor road vehicle not classifiable to
          E826-E828
    caught in door of
      streetcar
      nonmotor road vehicle not classifiable to
          E826-E828
    derailment of
      streetcar
      nonmotor road vehicle not classifiable to
          E826-E828
    fall in, on, or from
      streetcar
      nonmotor road vehicle not classifiable to
          E826-E828
    fire in
      streetcar
      nonmotor road vehicle not classifiable to
          E826-E828
    collision between streetcar or nonmotor road
      vehicle, except as in E826-E828, and:
      animal (not being ridden)
      another nonmotor road vehicle not
        classifiable to E826-E828
      pedestrian
      other object, fixed, movable, or moving, not
        set in motion by motor vehicle, railway
        train, or aircraft
    nonmotor road vehicle accident NOS
    streetcar accident NOS

  Excludes collision with:
      animal being ridden (E828.0-E828.9)
      animal-drawn vehicle (E827.0-E827.9)
      pedal cycle (E826.0-E826.9)

WATER TRANSPORT ACCIDENTS (E830-E838)

Note: For definitions of water transport accident and related terms see definitions (a), (s), and (t).

Includes watercraft accidents in the course of recreational activities

Excludes *accidents involving both aircraft, including objects set in motion by aircraft, and watercraft (E840.0-E845.9)*

The following fourth-digit subdivisions are for use with categories E830-E838 to identify the injured person:

```
0  Occupant of small boat, unpowered
1  Occupant of small boat, powered
     See definition (t)
     Excludes  water skier (4)
2  Occupant of other watercraft-crew
     Persons:
        engaged in operation of watercraft
        providing passenger services [cabin attendants,
           ship's physician, catering personnel]
        working on ship during voyage in other capacity
           [musician in band, operators of shops and
           beauty parlors]
3  Occupant of other watercraft -- other than crew
     Passenger
     Occupant of lifeboat, other than crew, after
        abandoning ship
4  Water skier
5  Swimmer
6  Dockers, stevedores
     Longshoreman employed on the dock in loading
        and unloading ships
7  Occupant of military watercraft, any type
8  Other specified person
     Immigration and custom officials on board ship
     Person:
        accompanying passenger or member of crew
           visiting boat
     Pilot (guiding ship into port)
9  Unspecified person
```

- **E830 Accident to watercraft causing submersion**
  Requires fourth digit. See beginning of section E800-E845 for codes and definitions.

  Includes submersion and drowning due to:
      boat overturning
      boat submerging
      falling or jumping from burning ship
      falling or jumping from crushed watercraft
      ship sinking
      other accident to watercraft

- **E831 Accident to watercraft causing other injury**
  Requires fourth digit. See beginning of section E800-E845 for codes and definitions.

  Includes any injury, except submersion and drowning, as
      a result of an accident to watercraft
    burned while ship on fire
    crushed between ships in collision
    crushed by lifeboat after abandoning ship
    fall due to collision or other accident to
      watercraft
    hit by falling object due to accident to watercraft
    injured in watercraft accident involving
      collision
    struck by boat or part thereof after fall or jump
      from damaged boat

  Excludes *burns from localized fire or explosion on board ship (E837.0-E837.9)*

- **E832 Other accidental submersion or drowning in water transport accident**

    Requires fourth digit. See beginning of section E800-E845 for codes and definitions.

    Includes submersion or drowning as a result of an accident other than accident to the watercraft, such as:
    fall:
    from gangplank
    from ship
    overboard
    thrown overboard by motion of ship
    washed overboard

    Excludes submersion or drowning of swimmer or diver who voluntarily jumps from boat not involved in an accident (E910.0-E910.9)

- **E833 Fall on stairs or ladders in water transport**

    Requires fourth digit. See beginning of section E800-E845 for codes and definitions.

    Excludes fall due to accident to watercraft (E831.0-E831.9)

- **E834 Other fall from one level to another in water transport**

    Requires fourth digit. See beginning of section E800-E845 for codes and definitions.

    Excludes fall due to accident to watercraft (E831.0-E831.9)

- **E835 Other and unspecified fall in water transport**

    Requires fourth digit. See beginning of section E800-E845 for codes and definitions.

    Excludes fall due to accident to watercraft (E831.0-E831.9)

- **E836 Machinery accident in water transport**

    Requires fourth digit. See beginning of section E800-E845 for codes and definitions.

    Includes injuries in water transport caused by:
    deck machinery
    engine room machinery
    galley machinery
    laundry machinery
    loading machinery

- **E837 Explosion, fire, or burning in watercraft**

    Requires fourth digit. See beginning of section E800-E845 for codes and definitions.

    Includes explosion of boiler on steamship
    localized fire on ship

    Excludes burning ship (due to collision or explosion) resulting in:
    submersion or drowning (E830.0-E830.9)
    other injury (E831.0-E831.9)

- **E838 Other and unspecified water transport accident**

    Requires fourth digit. See beginning of section E800-E845 for codes and definitions.

    Includes accidental poisoning by gases or fumes on ship
    atomic power plant malfunction in watercraft
    crushed between ship and stationary object [wharf]
    crushed between ships without accident to watercraft
    crushed by falling object on ship or while loading or unloading
    hit by boat while water skiing
    struck by boat or part thereof (after fall from boat)
    watercraft accident NOS

AIR AND SPACE TRANSPORT ACCIDENTS (E840-E845)

Note: For definition of aircraft and related terms see definitions (u) and (v).

The following fourth-digit subdivisions are for use with categories E840-E845 to identify the injured person:

> 0 Occupant of spacecraft
> 1 Occupant of military aircraft, any
>   Crew in military aircraft [air force] [army] [national guard] [navy]
>   Passenger (civilian) (military) in military aircraft [air force] [army] [national guard] [navy]
>   Troops in military aircraft [air force] [army] [national guard] [navy]
>   **Excludes** occupants of aircraft operated under jurisdiction of police departments (5) parachutist (7)
> 2 Crew of commercial aircraft (powered) in surface-to-surface transport
> 3 Other occupant of commercial aircraft (powered) in surface-to-surface transport
>   Flight personnel:
>   not part of crew
>   on familiarization flight
>   Passenger on aircraft (powered) NOS
> 4 Occupant of commercial aircraft (powered) in surface-to-air transport
>   Occupant [crew] [passenger] of aircraft (powered) engaged in activities, such as:
>   aerial spraying (crops) (fire retardants)
>   air drops of emergency supplies
>   air drops of parachutists, except from military craft
>   crop dusting
>   lowering of construction material [bridge or telephone pole]
>   sky writing
> 5 Occupant of other powered aircraft
>   Occupant [crew] [passenger] of aircraft [powered] engaged in activities, such as:
>   aerobatic flying
>   aircraft racing
>   rescue operation
>   storm surveillance
>   traffic surveillance
>   Occupant of private plane NOS
> 6 Occupant of unpowered aircraft, except parachutist
>   Occupant of aircraft classifiable to E842
> 7 Parachutist (military) (other)
>   Person making voluntary descent
>   **Excludes** person making descent after accident to aircraft (.1-.6)
> 8 Ground crew, airline employee
>   Persons employed at airfields (civil) (military) or launching pads, not occupants of aircraft
> 9 Other person

- **E840 Accident to powered aircraft at takeoff or landing**

    Requires fourth digit. See beginning of section E800-E845 for codes and definitions.

    Includes collision of aircraft with any object, fixed, movable, or moving while taking off or landing
    crash while taking off or landing
    explosion on aircraft while taking off or landing
    fire on aircraft while taking off or landing
    forced landing

● **E841 Accident to powered aircraft, other and unspecified**
　　Requires fourth digit. See beginning of section E800-E845 for codes and definitions.
　　Includes　aircraft accident NOS
　　　　　　　aircraft crash or wreck NOS
　　　　　　　any accident to powered aircraft while in transit or when not specified whether in transit, taking off, or landing
　　　　　　　collision of aircraft with another aircraft, bird, or any object, while in transit
　　　　　　　explosion on aircraft while in transit
　　　　　　　fire on aircraft while in transit

● **E842 Accident to unpowered aircraft**
[6-9]　Requires fourth digit. See beginning of section E800-E845 for codes and definitions.
　　Includes　any accident, except collision with powered aircraft, to:
　　　　　　　balloon
　　　　　　　glider
　　　　　　　hang glider
　　　　　　　kite carrying a person
　　　　　　　hit by object falling from unpowered aircraft

● **E843 Fall in, on, or from aircraft**
[0-9]　Requires fourth digit. See beginning of section E800-E845 for codes and definitions.
　　Includes　accident in boarding or alighting from aircraft, any kind
　　　　　　　fall in, on, or from aircraft [any kind], while in transit, taking off, or landing, except when as a result of an accident to aircraft

● **E844 Other specified air transport accidents**
[0-9]　Requires fourth digit. See beginning of section E800-E845 for codes and definitions.
　　Includes　hit by aircraft without accident to aircraft
　　　　　　　hit by object falling from aircraft without accident to aircraft
　　　　　　　injury by or from machinery on aircraft without accident to aircraft
　　　　　　　injury by or from rotating propeller without accident to aircraft
　　　　　　　injury by or from voluntary parachute descent without accident to aircraft
　　　　　　　poisoning by carbon monoxide from aircraft while in transit without accident to aircraft
　　　　　　　sucked into jet without accident to aircraft
　　　　　　　any accident involving other transport vehicle (motor) (nonmotor) due to being hit by object set in motion by aircraft (powered)
　　Excludes　air sickness (E903)
　　　　　　　effects of:
　　　　　　　　high altitude (E902.0-E902.1)
　　　　　　　　pressure change (E902.0-E902.1)
　　　　　　　injury in parachute descent due to accident to aircraft (E840.0-E842.9)

● **E845 Accident involving spacecraft**
[0,8,9]　Requires fourth digit. See beginning of section E800-E845 for codes and definitions.
　　Includes　launching pad accident
　　Excludes　effects of weightlessness in spacecraft (E928.0)

VEHICLE ACCIDENTS NOT ELSEWHERE CLASSIFIABLE (E846-E848)

E846 Accidents involving powered vehicles used solely within the buildings and premises of industrial or commercial establishment
　　Accident to, on, or involving:
　　　battery-powered airport passenger vehicle
　　　battery-powered trucks (baggage) (mail)
　　　coal car in mine
　　　logging car
　　　self-propelled truck, industrial
　　　station baggage truck (powered)
　　　tram, truck, or tub (powered) in mine or quarry
　　Breakage of any part of vehicle
　　Collision with:
　　　pedestrian
　　　other vehicle or object within premises
　　Explosion of powered vehicle, industrial or commercial
　　Fall from powered vehicle, industrial or commercial
　　Overturning of powered vehicle, industrial or commercial
　　Struck by powered vehicle, industrial or commercial
　　Excludes　accidental poisoning by exhaust gas from vehicle not elsewhere classifiable (E868.2)
　　　　　　　injury by crane, lift (fork), or elevator (E919.2)

E847 Accidents involving cable cars not running on rails
　　Accident to, on, or involving:
　　　cable car, not on rails
　　　ski chair-lift
　　　ski-lift with gondola
　　　teleferique
　　Breakage of cable
　　　caught or dragged by cable car, not on rails
　　　fall or jump from cable car, not on rails
　　　object thrown from or in cable car not on rails

E848 Accidents involving other vehicles, not elsewhere classifiable
　　Accident to, on, or involving:
　　　ice yacht
　　　land yacht
　　　nonmotor, nonroad vehicle NOS

OGCR　Section I.C.19.b
Use an additional code from category E849 to indicate the Place of Occurrence. The Place of Occurrence describes the place where the event occurred and not the patient's activity at the time of the event. Do not use E849.9 if the place of occurrence is not stated.

PLACE OF OCCURRENCE (E849)

● **E849 Place of Occurrence**
　　Note:　The following category is for use to denote the place where the injury or poisoning occurred.
　　E849.0 Home
　　　　Apartment
　　　　Boarding house
　　　　Farm house
　　　　Home premises
　　　　House (residential)
　　　　Noninstitutional place of residence
　　　　Private:
　　　　　driveway
　　　　　garage
　　　　　garden
　　　　　home
　　　　　walk
　　　　Swimming pool in private house or garden
　　　　Yard of home
　　　　Excludes　home under construction but not yet occupied (E849.3)
　　　　　　　　　institutional place of residence (E849.7)

E849.1 **Farm**
  Buildings
  Land under cultivation
  > Excludes: farm house and home premises of farm (E849.0)

E849.2 **Mine and quarry**
  Gravel pit
  Sand pit
  Tunnel under construction

E849.3 **Industrial place and premises**
  Building under construction
  Dockyard
  Dry dock
  Factory
    building
    premises
  Garage (place of work)
  Industrial yard
  Loading platform (factory) (store)
  Plant, industrial
  Railway yard
  Shop (place of work)
  Warehouse
  Workhouse
  Coding Clinic: 2010, Q4, P111; 2003, Q4, P76-78

E849.4 **Place for recreation and sport**
  Amusement park
  Baseball field
  Basketball court
  Beach resort
  Cricket ground
  Fives court
  Football field
  Golf course
  Gymnasium
  Hockey field
  Holiday camp
  Ice palace
  Lake resort
  Mountain resort
  Playground, including school playground
  Public park
  Racecourse
  Resort NOS
  Riding school
  Rifle range
  Seashore resort
  Skating rink
  Sports palace
  Stadium
  Swimming pool, public
  Tennis court
  Vacation resort
  > Excludes: that in private house or garden (E849.0)

E849.5 **Street and highway**
  Coding Clinic: 2011, Q4, P100; 2010, Q4, P93; 2009, Q4, P144; 1995, Q1, P10

E849.6 **Public building**
  Building (including adjacent grounds) used by the general public or by a particular group of the public, such as:
    airport
    bank
    cafe
    casino
    church
    cinema
    clubhouse
    courthouse
    dance hall
    garage building (for car storage)
    hotel
    market (grocery or other commodity)
    movie house
    music hall
    nightclub
    office
    office building
    opera house
    post office
    public hall
    radio broadcasting station
    restaurant
    school (state) (public) (private)
    shop, commercial
    station (bus) (railway)
    store
    theater
  > Excludes: home garage (E849.0)
  > industrial building or workplace (E849.3)

E849.7 **Residential institution**
  Children's home
  Dormitory
  Hospital
  Jail
  Old people's home
  Orphanage
  Prison
  Reform School

E849.8 **Other specified places**
  Beach NOS
  Canal
  Caravan site NOS
  Derelict house
  Desert
  Dock
  Forest
  Harbor
  Hill
  Lake NOS
  Mountain
  Parking lot
  Parking place
  Pond or pool (natural)
  Prairie
  Public place NOS
  Railway line
  Reservoir
  River
  Sea
  Seashore NOS
  Stream
  Swamp
  Trailer court
  Woods

E849.9 **Unspecified place**

ACCIDENTAL POISONING BY DRUGS, MEDICINAL SUBSTANCES, AND BIOLOGICALS (E850-E858)

> Includes: accidental overdose of drug, wrong drug given or taken in error, and drug taken inadvertently
> accidents in the use of drugs and biologicals in medical and surgical procedures

> Excludes: administration with suicidal or homicidal intent or intent to harm, or in circumstances classifiable to E980-E989 (E950.0-E950.5, E962.0, E980.0-E980.5)
> correct drug properly administered in therapeutic or prophylactic dosage, as the cause of adverse effect (E930.0-E949.9)

Note: See Alphabetic Index for more complete list of specific drugs to be classified under the fourth-digit subdivisions. The American Hospital Formulary numbers can be used to classify new drugs listed by the American Hospital Formulary Service (AHFS). See Appendix C.

E850 **Accidental poisoning by analgesics, antipyretics, and antirheumatics**
Coding Clinic: 2008, Q3, P21

E850.0 **Heroin**
  Diacetylmorphine

E850.1 **Methadone**

E850.2 **Other opiates and related narcotics**
  Codeine [methylmorphine]
  Meperidine [pethidine]
  Morphine
  Opium (alkaloids)

E850.3 **Salicylates**
  Acetylsalicylic acid [aspirin]
  Amino derivatives of salicylic acid
  Salicylic acid salts

- **E850.4** Aromatic analgesics, not elsewhere classified
  - Acetanilid
  - Paracetamol [acetaminophen]
  - Phenacetin [acetophenetidin]
- **E850.5** Pyrazole derivatives
  - Aminophenazone [amidopyrine]
  - Phenylbutazone
- **E850.6** Antirheumatics [antiphlogistics]
  - Gold salts
  - Indomethacin
  - **Excludes**: salicylates (E850.3)
    steroids (E858.0)
- **E850.7** Other non-narcotic analgesics
  - Pyrabital
- **E850.8** Other specified analgesics and antipyretics
  - Pentazocine
- **E850.9** Unspecified analgesic or antipyretic

E851 Accidental poisoning by barbiturates
- Amobarbital [amylobarbitone]
- Barbital [barbitone]
- Butabarbital [butabarbitone]
- Pentobarbital [pentobarbitone]
- Phenobarbital [phenobarbitone]
- Secobarbital [quinalbarbitone]
- **Excludes**: thiobarbiturates (E855.1)

E852 Accidental poisoning by other sedatives and hypnotics
- **E852.0** Chloral hydrate group
- **E852.1** Paraldehyde
- **E852.2** Bromine compounds
  - Bromides
  - Carbromal (derivatives)
- **E852.3** Methaqualone compounds
- **E852.4** Glutethimide group
- **E852.5** Mixed sedatives, not elsewhere classified
- **E852.8** Other specified sedatives and hypnotics
- **E852.9** Unspecified sedative or hypnotic
  - Sleeping:
    - drug NOS
    - pill NOS
    - tablet NOS

E853 Accidental poisoning by tranquilizers
- **E853.0** Phenothiazine-based tranquilizers
  - Chlorpromazine
  - Fluphenazine
  - Prochlorperazine
  - Promazine
- **E853.1** Butyrophenone-based tranquilizers
  - Haloperidol
  - Spiperone
  - Trifluperidol
- **E853.2** Benzodiazepine-based tranquilizers
  - Chlordiazepoxide
  - Diazepam
  - Flurazepam
  - Lorazepam
  - Medazepam
  - Nitrazepam
  - **Coding Clinic: 2009, Q4, P150; 1991, Q3, P14**
- **E853.8** Other specified tranquilizers
  - Hydroxyzine
  - Meprobamate
- **E853.9** Unspecified tranquilizer

E854 Accidental poisoning by other psychotropic agents
- **E854.0** Antidepressants
  - Amitriptyline
  - Imipramine
  - Monoamine oxidase [MAO] inhibitors
  - **Coding Clinic: 2009, Q4, P150; 1991, Q3, P14**
- **E854.1** Psychodysleptics [hallucinogens]
  - Cannabis derivatives
  - Lysergide [LSD]
  - Marihuana (derivatives)
  - Mescaline
  - Psilocin
  - Psilocybin
- **E854.2** Psychostimulants
  - Amphetamine
  - Caffeine
  - **Excludes**: central appetite depressants (E858.8)
  - **Coding Clinic: 2003, Q2, P11**
- **E854.3** Central nervous system stimulants
  - Analeptics
  - Opiate antagonists
- **E854.8** Other psychotropic agents

E855 Accidental poisoning by other drugs acting on central and autonomic nervous system
- **E855.0** Anticonvulsant and anti-Parkinsonism drugs
  - Amantadine
  - Hydantoin derivatives
  - Levodopa [L-dopa]
  - Oxazolidine derivatives [paramethadione] [trimethadione]
  - Succinimides
- **E855.1** Other central nervous system depressants
  - Ether
  - Gaseous anesthetics
  - Halogenated hydrocarbon derivatives
  - Intravenous anesthetics
  - Thiobarbiturates, such as thiopental sodium
- **E855.2** Local anesthetics
  - Cocaine
  - Lidocaine [lignocaine]
  - Procaine
  - Tetracaine
- **E855.3** Parasympathomimetics [cholinergics]
  - Acetylcholine
  - Anticholinesterase:
    - organophosphorus
    - reversible
  - Pilocarpine
- **E855.4** Parasympatholytics [anticholinergics and antimuscarinics] and spasmolytics
  - Atropine
  - Homatropine
  - Hyoscine [scopolamine]
  - Quaternary ammonium derivatives
- **E855.5** Sympathomimetics [adrenergics]
  - Epinephrine [adrenalin]
  - Levarterenol [noradrenalin]
- **E855.6** Sympatholytics [antiadrenergics]
  - Phenoxybenzamine
  - Tolazoline hydrochloride
- **E855.8** Other specified drugs acting on central and autonomic nervous systems
- **E855.9** Unspecified drug acting on central and autonomic nervous systems

E856 Accidental poisoning by antibiotics

E857 Accidental poisoning by other anti-infectives

E858 Accidental poisoning by other drugs
- **Coding Clinic: 2008, Q3, P21**
- **E858.0** Hormones and synthetic substitutes
- **E858.1** Primarily systemic agents
- **E858.2** Agents primarily affecting blood constituents
- **E858.3** Agents primarily affecting cardiovascular system
- **E858.4** Agents primarily affecting gastrointestinal system
- **E858.5** Water, mineral, and uric acid metabolism drugs
- **E858.6** Agents primarily acting on the smooth and skeletal muscles and respiratory system
- **E858.7** Agents primarily affecting skin and mucous membrane, ophthalmological, otorhinolaryngological, and dental drugs
- **E858.8** Other specified drugs
  - Central appetite depressants
- **E858.9** Unspecified drug

ACCIDENTAL POISONING BY OTHER SOLID AND LIQUID SUBSTANCES, GASES, AND VAPORS (E860-E869)

Note: Categories in this section are intended primarily to indicate the external cause of poisoning states classifiable to 980–989. They may also be used to indicate external causes of localized effects classifiable to 001–799.

- **E860 Accidental poisoning by alcohol, not elsewhere classified**
  - **E860.0 Alcoholic beverages**
    Alcohol in preparations intended for consumption
    Coding Clinic: 2009, Q4, P150; 1996, Q3, P161; 1991, Q3, P14
  - **E860.1 Other and unspecified ethyl alcohol and its products**
    Denatured alcohol
    Ethanol NOS
    Grain alcohol NOS
    Methylated spirit
  - **E860.2 Methyl alcohol**
    Methanol
    Wood alcohol
  - **E860.3 Isopropyl alcohol**
    Dimethyl carbinol
    Isopropanol
    Rubbing alcohol substitute
    Secondary propyl alcohol
  - **E860.4 Fusel oil**
    Alcohol:
      amyl
      butyl
      propyl
  - **E860.8 Other specified alcohols**
  - **E860.9 Unspecified alcohol**

- **E861 Accidental poisoning by cleansing and polishing agents, disinfectants, paints, and varnishes**
  - **E861.0 Synthetic detergents and shampoos**
  - **E861.1 Soap products**
  - **E861.2 Polishes**
  - **E861.3 Other cleansing and polishing agents**
    Scouring powders
  - **E861.4 Disinfectants**
    Household and other disinfectants not ordinarily used on the person
    Excludes *carbolic acid or phenol (E864.0)*
  - **E861.5 Lead paints**
  - **E861.6 Other paints and varnishes**
    Lacquers
    Oil colors
    Paints, other than lead
    Whitewashes
  - **E861.9 Unspecified**

- **E862 Accidental poisoning by petroleum products, other solvents and their vapors, not elsewhere classified**
  - **E862.0 Petroleum solvents**
    Petroleum:
      ether
      benzine
      naphtha
  - **E862.1 Petroleum fuels and cleaners**
    Antiknock additives to petroleum fuels
    Gas oils
    Gasoline or petrol
    Kerosene
    Excludes *kerosene insecticides (E863.4)*
  - **E862.2 Lubricating oils**
  - **E862.3 Petroleum solids**
    Paraffin wax
  - **E862.4 Other specified solvents**
    Benzene
    Coding Clinic: 2008, Q3, P6-7
  - **E862.9 Unspecified solvent**

- **E863 Accidental poisoning by agricultural and horticultural chemical and pharmaceutical preparations other than plant foods and fertilizers**
    Excludes *plant foods and fertilizers (E866.5)*
  - **E863.0 Insecticides of organochlorine compounds**
    Benzene hexachloride   Dieldrin
    Chlordane   Endrine
    DDT   Toxaphene
  - **E863.1 Insecticides of organophosphorus compounds**
    Demeton   Parathion
    Diazinon   Phenylsulphthion
    Dichlorvos   Phorate
    Malathion   Phosdrin
    Methyl parathion
  - **E863.2 Carbamates**
    Aldicarb   Propoxur
    Carbaryl
  - **E863.3 Mixtures of insecticides**
  - **E863.4 Other and unspecified insecticides**
    Kerosene insecticides
  - **E863.5 Herbicides**
    2,4-Dichlorophenoxyacetic acid [2, 4-D]
    2,4,5-Trichlorophenoxyacetic acid [2, 4, 5-T]
    Chlorates
    Diquat
    Mixtures of plant foods and fertilizers with herbicides
    Paraquat
  - **E863.6 Fungicides**
    Organic mercurials (used in seed dressing)
    Pentachlorophenols
  - **E863.7 Rodenticides**
    Fluoroacetates   Warfarin
    Squill and derivatives   Zinc phosphide
    Thallium
  - **E863.8 Fumigants**
    Cyanides   Phosphine
    Methyl bromide
  - **E863.9 Other and unspecified**

- **E864 Accidental poisoning by corrosives and caustics, not elsewhere classified**
    Excludes *those as components of disinfectants (E861.4)*
  - **E864.0 Corrosive aromatics**
    Carbolic acid or phenol
  - **E864.1 Acids**
    Acid:
      hydrochloric
      nitric
      sulfuric
  - **E864.2 Caustic alkalis**
    Lye
  - **E864.3 Other specified corrosives and caustics**
  - **E864.4 Unspecified corrosives and caustics**

- **E865 Accidental poisoning from poisonous foodstuffs and poisonous plants**
    Includes any meat, fish, or shellfish
    plants, berries, and fungi eaten as, or in mistake for food, or by a child
    Excludes *anaphylactic shock due to adverse food reaction (995.60–995.69)*
    food poisoning (bacterial) (005.0–005.9)
    poisoning and toxic reactions to venomous plants (E905.6–E905.7)
  - **E865.0 Meat**
  - **E865.1 Shellfish**
  - **E865.2 Other fish**
  - **E865.3 Berries and seeds**
  - **E865.4 Other specified plants**
  - **E865.5 Mushrooms and other fungi**
  - **E865.8 Other specified foods**
  - **E865.9 Unspecified foodstuff or poisonous plant**

● **E866 Accidental poisoning by other and unspecified solid and liquid substances**
Excludes: these substances as a component of:
medicines (E850.0-E858.9)
paints (E861.5-E861.6)
pesticides (E863.0-E863.9)
petroleum fuels (E862.1)

- E866.0 Lead and its compounds and fumes
- E866.1 Mercury and its compounds and fumes
- E866.2 Antimony and its compounds and fumes
- E866.3 Arsenic and its compounds and fumes
- E866.4 Other metals and their compounds and fumes
    Beryllium (compounds)
    Brass fumes
    Cadmium (compounds)
    Copper salts
    Iron (compounds)
    Manganese (compounds)
    Nickel (compounds)
    Thallium (compounds)
- E866.5 Plant foods and fertilizers
    Excludes: mixtures with herbicides (E863.5)
- E866.6 Glues and adhesives
- E866.7 Cosmetics
- E866.8 Other specified solid or liquid substances
    Coding Clinic: 1990, Q4, P25
- ■ E866.9 Unspecified solid or liquid substance

E867 Accidental poisoning by gas distributed by pipeline
Carbon monoxide from incomplete combustion of piped gas
Coal gas NOS
Liquefied petroleum gas distributed through pipes (pure or mixed with air)
Piped gas (natural) (manufactured)

● **E868 Accidental poisoning by other utility gas and other carbon monoxide**

- E868.0 Liquefied petroleum gas distributed in mobile containers
    Butane or carbon monoxide from incomplete combustion of these gases
    Liquefied hydrocarbon gas NOS or carbon monoxide from incomplete combustion of these gases
    Propane or carbon monoxide from incomplete combustion of these gases
- E868.1 Other and unspecified utility gas
    Acetylene or carbon monoxide from incomplete combustion of these gases
    Gas NOS used for lighting, heating, or cooking or carbon monoxide from incomplete combustion of these gases
    Water gas or carbon monoxide from incomplete combustion of these gases
- E868.2 Motor vehicle exhaust gas
    Exhaust gas from:
        farm tractor, not in transit
        gas engine
        motor pump
        motor vehicle, not in transit
        any type of combustion engine not in watercraft
    Excludes: poisoning by carbon monoxide from:
        aircraft while in transit (E844.0-E844.9)
        motor vehicle while in transit (E818.0-E818.9)
        watercraft whether or not in transit (E838.0-E838.9)
- E868.3 Carbon monoxide from incomplete combustion of other domestic fuels
    Carbon monoxide from incomplete combustion of:
        coal in domestic stove or fireplace
        coke in domestic stove or fireplace
        kerosene in domestic stove or fireplace
        wood in domestic stove or fireplace
    Excludes: carbon monoxide from smoke and fumes due to conflagration (E890.0-E893.9)
- E868.8 Carbon monoxide from other sources
    Carbon monoxide from:
        blast furnace gas
        incomplete combustion of fuels in industrial use
        kiln vapor
- ■ E868.9 Unspecified carbon monoxide

● **E869 Accidental poisoning by other gases and vapors**
Excludes: effects of gases used as anesthetics (E855.1, E938.2)
fumes from heavy metals (E866.0-E866.4)
smoke and fumes due to conflagration or explosion (E890.0-E899)

- E869.0 Nitrogen oxides
- E869.1 Sulfur dioxide
- E869.2 Freon
- E869.3 Lacrimogenic gas [tear gas]
    Bromobenzyl cyanide
    Chloroacetophenone
    Ethyliodoacetate
- E869.4 Second-hand tobacco smoke
    Coding Clinic: 1996, Q2, P10
- E869.8 Other specified gases and vapors
    Chlorine
    Hydrocyanic acid gas
- ■ E869.9 Unspecified gases and vapors

MISADVENTURES TO PATIENTS DURING SURGICAL AND MEDICAL CARE (E870-E876)

Excludes: accidental overdose of drug and wrong drug given in error (E850.0-E858.9)
surgical and medical procedures as the cause of abnormal reaction by the patient, without mention of misadventure at the time of procedure (E878.0-E879.9)

OGCR Section I.C.19.h.1
Assign a code in the range of E870-E876 if misadventures are stated by the provider. **When applying the E code guidelines pertaining to sequencing, these E codes are considered causal codes.**

● **E870 Accidental cut, puncture, perforation, or hemorrhage during medical care**

- E870.0 Surgical operation
    Coding Clinic: 2010, Q1, P20-21
- E870.1 Infusion or transfusion
- E870.2 Kidney dialysis or other perfusion
- E870.3 Injection or vaccination
- E870.4 Endoscopic examination
- E870.5 Aspiration of fluid or tissue, puncture, and catheterization
    Abdominal paracentesis
    Aspirating needle biopsy
    Blood sampling
    Lumbar puncture
    Thoracentesis
    Excludes: heart catheterization (E870.6)
- E870.6 Heart catheterization
- E870.7 Administration of enema
- E870.8 Other specified medical care
- ■ E870.9 Unspecified medical care

- **E871** Foreign object left in body during procedure
  - E871.0 Surgical operation
  - E871.1 Infusion or transfusion
  - E871.2 Kidney dialysis or other perfusion
  - E871.3 Injection or vaccination
  - E871.4 Endoscopic examination
  - E871.5 Aspiration of fluid or tissue, puncture, and catheterization
    - Abdominal paracentesis
    - Aspiration needle biopsy
    - Blood sampling
    - Lumbar puncture
    - Thoracentesis
    - **Excludes** *heart catheterization (E871.6)*
  - E871.6 Heart catheterization
  - E871.7 Removal of catheter or packing
  - E871.8 Other specified procedures
  - E871.9 Unspecified procedure

- **E872** Failure of sterile precautions during procedure
  - E872.0 Surgical operation
  - E872.1 Infusion or transfusion
  - E872.2 Kidney dialysis and other perfusion
  - E872.3 Injection or vaccination
  - E872.4 Endoscopic examination
  - E872.5 Aspiration of fluid or tissue, puncture, and catheterization
    - Abdominal paracentesis
    - Aspirating needle biopsy
    - Blood sampling
    - Lumbar puncture
    - Thoracentesis
    - **Excludes** *heart catheterization (E872.6)*
  - E872.6 Heart catheterization
  - E872.8 Other specified procedures
  - E872.9 Unspecified procedure

- **E873** Failure in dosage
  - **Excludes** *accidental overdose of drug, medicinal or biological substance (E850.0-E858.9)*
  - E873.0 Excessive amount of blood or other fluid during transfusion or infusion
  - E873.1 Incorrect dilution of fluid during infusion
  - E873.2 Overdose of radiation in therapy
  - E873.3 Inadvertent exposure of patient to radiation during medical care
  - E873.4 Failure in dosage in electroshock or insulin-shock therapy
  - E873.5 Inappropriate [too hot or too cold] temperature in local application and packing
  - E873.6 Nonadministration of necessary drug or medicinal substance
  - E873.8 Other specified failure in dosage
  - E873.9 Unspecified failure in dosage

- **E874** Mechanical failure of instrument or apparatus during procedure
  - E874.0 Surgical operation
  - E874.1 Infusion and transfusion
    - Air in system
  - E874.2 Kidney dialysis and other perfusion
  - E874.3 Endoscopic examination
  - E874.4 Aspiration of fluid or tissue, puncture, and catheterization
    - Abdominal paracentesis
    - Aspirating needle biopsy
    - Blood sampling
    - Lumbar puncture
    - Thoracentesis
    - **Excludes** *heart catheterization (E874.5)*
  - E874.5 Heart catheterization
    - Coding Clinic: 2013, Q1, P5
  - E874.8 Other specified procedures
  - E874.9 Unspecified procedure

- **E875** Contaminated or infected blood, other fluid, drug, or biological substance
  - **Includes** presence of:
    - bacterial pyrogens
    - endotoxin-producing bacteria
    - serum hepatitis-producing agent
  - E875.0 Contaminated substance transfused or infused
  - E875.1 Contaminated substance injected or used for vaccination
  - E875.2 Contaminated drug or biological substance administered by other means
  - E875.8 Other
  - E875.9 Unspecified

- **E876** Other and unspecified misadventures during medical care
  - E876.0 Mismatched blood in transfusion
  - E876.1 Wrong fluid in infusion
  - E876.2 Failure in suture and ligature during surgical operation
  - E876.3 Endotracheal tube wrongly placed during anesthetic procedure
  - E876.4 Failure to introduce or to remove other tube or instrument
    - **Excludes** *foreign object left in body during procedure (E871.0-E871.9)*
  - E876.5 Performance of wrong operation (procedure) on correct patient
    - Wrong device implanted into correct surgical site
    - **Excludes** *correct operation (procedure) performed on wrong body part (E876.7)*
    - Coding Clinic: 2006, Q3, P9-10
  - E876.6 Performance of operation (procedure) on patient not scheduled for surgery
    - Performance of operation (procedure) intended for another patient
    - Performance of operation (procedure) on wrong patient
  - E876.7 Performance of correct operation (procedure) on wrong side/body part
    - Performance of correct operation (procedure) on wrong side
    - Performance of correct operation (procedure) on wrong site
    - Coding Clinic: 2009, Q4, P150-151
  - E876.8 Other specified misadventures during medical care
    - Performance of inappropriate treatment, NEC
    - Coding Clinic: 2012, Q2, P8; 2009, Q2, P11; 2008, Q4, P152-155
  - E876.9 Unspecified misadventure during medical care

SURGICAL AND MEDICAL PROCEDURES AS THE CAUSE OF ABNORMAL REACTION OF PATIENT OR LATER COMPLICATION, WITHOUT MENTION OF MISADVENTURE AT THE TIME OF PROCEDURE (E878-E879)

Includes: procedures as the cause of abnormal reaction, such as:
- displacement or malfunction of prosthetic device
- hepatorenal failure, postoperative
- malfunction of external stoma
- postoperative intestinal obstruction
- rejection of transplanted organ

Excludes: anesthetic management properly carried out as the cause of adverse effect (E937.0-E938.9)
infusion and transfusion, without mention of misadventure in the technique of procedure (E930.0-E949.9)

OGCR Section I.C.19.h.2
Assign a code in the range of E878-E879 if the provider attributes an abnormal reaction or later complication to a surgical or medical procedure, but does not mention misadventure at the time of the procedure as the cause of the reaction.

- **E878** Surgical operation and other surgical procedures as the cause of abnormal reaction of patient, or of later complication, without mention of misadventure at the time of operation
  - **E878.0** Surgical operation with transplant of whole organ
    - Transplantation of:
      - heart
      - kidney
      - liver
  - **E878.1** Surgical operation with implant of artificial internal device
    - Cardiac pacemaker
    - Electrodes implanted in brain
    - Heart valve prosthesis
    - Internal orthopedic device
  - **E878.2** Surgical operation with anastomosis, bypass, or graft, with natural or artificial tissues used as implant
    - Anastomosis:
      - arteriovenous
      - gastrojejunal
    - Graft of blood vessel, tendon, or skin
    - **Excludes**: external stoma (E878.3)
    - Coding Clinic: 2010, Q2, P9
  - **E878.3** Surgical operation with formation of external stoma
    - Colostomy
    - Cystostomy
    - Duodenostomy
    - Gastrostomy
    - Ureterostomy
  - **E878.4** Other restorative surgery
  - **E878.5** Amputation of limb(s)
  - **E878.6** Removal of other organ (partial) (total)
  - **E878.8** Other specified surgical operations and procedures
  - **E878.9** Unspecified surgical operations and procedures
- **E879** Other procedures, without mention of misadventure at the time of procedure, as the cause of abnormal reaction of patient, or of later complication
  - **E879.0** Cardiac catheterization
  - **E879.1** Kidney dialysis
    - Coding Clinic: 2003, Q4, P60-61; 1994, Q3, P9
  - **E879.2** Radiological procedure and radiotherapy
    - **Excludes**: radio-opaque dyes for diagnostic x-ray procedures (E947.8)
    - Coding Clinic: 2006, Q4, P88-91
  - **E879.3** Shock therapy
    - Electroshock therapy
    - Insulin-shock therapy
  - **E879.4** Aspiration of fluid
    - Lumbar puncture
    - Thoracentesis
  - **E879.5** Insertion of gastric or duodenal sound
  - **E879.6** Urinary catheterization
  - **E879.7** Blood sampling
  - **E879.8** Other specified procedures
    - Blood transfusion
    - Coding Clinic: 2013, Q1, P15; 1993, Q2, P3-4
  - **E879.9** Unspecified procedure

ACCIDENTAL FALLS (E880-E888)

Excludes: falls (in or from):
- burning building (E890.8, E891.8)
- into fire (E890.0-E899)
- into water (with submersion or drowning) (E910.0-E910.9)
- machinery (in operation) (E919.0-E919.9)
- on edged, pointed, or sharp object (E920.0-E920.9)
- transport vehicle (E800.0-E845.9)
- vehicle not elsewhere classifiable (E846-E848)

- **E880** Fall on or from stairs or steps
  - **E880.0** Escalator
  - **E880.1** Fall on or from sidewalk curb
    - **Excludes**: fall from moving sidewalk (E885.9)
  - **E880.9** Other stairs or steps
- **E881** Fall on or from ladders or scaffolding
  - **E881.0** Fall from ladder
    - Coding Clinic: 2007, Q1, P3-8
  - **E881.1** Fall from scaffolding
    - Coding Clinic: 1999, Q4, P13
  - **E882** Fall from or out of building or other structure
    - Fall from:
      - balcony
      - bridge
      - building
      - flagpole
      - tower
      - turret
      - viaduct
      - wall
      - window
    - Fall through roof
    - **Excludes**: collapse of a building or structure (E916)
      fall or jump from burning building (E890.8, E891.8)
- **E883** Fall into hole or other opening in surface
  - **Includes**: fall into:
    - cavity
    - dock
    - hole
    - pit
    - quarry
    - shaft
    - swimming pool
    - tank
    - well
  - **Excludes**: fall into water NOS (E910.9)
    that resulting in drowning or submersion without mention of injury (E910.0-E910.9)
  - **E883.0** Accident from diving or jumping into water [swimming pool]
    - Strike or hit:
      - against bottom when jumping or diving into water
      - wall or board of swimming pool
      - water surface
    - **Excludes**: diving with insufficient air supply (E913.2)
      effects of air pressure from diving (E902.2)
  - **E883.1** Accidental fall into well
  - **E883.2** Accidental fall into storm drain or manhole
  - **E883.9** Fall into other hole or other opening in surface

- **E884 Other fall from one level to another**
  - **E884.0 Fall from playground equipment**
    - Excludes: recreational machinery (E919.8)
    - Coding Clinic: 2007, Q1, P3-8
  - **E884.1 Fall from cliff**
  - **E884.2 Fall from chair**
  - **E884.3 Fall from wheelchair**
    - Fall from motorized mobility scooter
    - Fall from motorized wheelchair
    - Coding Clinic: 2010, Q4, P135
  - **E884.4 Fall from bed**
  - **E884.5 Fall from other furniture**
  - **E884.6 Fall from commode**
    - Toilet
  - **E884.9 Other fall from one level to another**
    - Fall from:
      - embankment
      - haystack
      - stationary vehicle
      - tree

- **E885 Fall on same level from slipping, tripping, or stumbling**
  - **E885.0 Fall from (nonmotorized) scooter**
    - Excludes: fall from motorized mobility scooter (E884.3)
    - Coding Clinic: 2002, Q4, P73
  - **E885.1 Fall from roller skates**
    - Heelies
    - In-line skates
    - Wheelies
  - **E885.2 Fall from skateboard**
    - Coding Clinic: 2000, Q4, P61
  - **E885.3 Fall from skis**
    - Coding Clinic: 2007, Q2, P3-4
  - **E885.4 Fall from snowboard**
  - **E885.9 Fall from other slipping, tripping, or stumbling**
    - Fall on moving sidewalk
    - Coding Clinic: 2009, Q4, P150

- **E886 Fall on same level from collision, pushing, or shoving, by or with other person**
  - Excludes: crushed or pushed by a crowd or human stampede (E917.1, E917.6)
  - **E886.0 In sports**
    - Tackles in sports
    - Excludes: kicked, stepped on, struck by object, in sports (E917.0, E917.5)
    - Coding Clinic: 2007, Q2, P3-4
  - **E886.9 Other and unspecified**
    - Fall from collision of pedestrian (conveyance) with another pedestrian (conveyance)

- **E887 Fracture, cause unspecified**

- **E888 Other and unspecified fall**
  - Accidental fall NOS
  - Fall on same level NOS
  - Coding Clinic: 1993, Q4, P25-26
  - **E888.0 Fall resulting in striking against sharp object**
    - Use additional external cause code to identify object (E920)
  - **E888.1 Fall resulting in striking against other object**
  - **E888.8 Other fall**
  - **E888.9 Unspecified fall**
    - Fall NOS

ACCIDENTS CAUSED BY FIRE AND FLAMES (E890-E899)

Includes:
- asphyxia or poisoning due to conflagration or ignition
- burning by fire
- secondary fires resulting from explosion

Excludes:
- arson (E968.0)
- fire in or on:
  - machinery (in operation) (E919.0-E919.9)
  - transport vehicle other than stationary vehicle (E800.0-E845.9)
  - vehicle not elsewhere classifiable (E846-E848)

- **E890 Conflagration in private dwelling**
  - Includes: conflagration in:
    - apartment
    - boarding house
    - camping place
    - caravan
    - farmhouse
    - house
    - lodging house
    - mobile home
    - private garage
    - rooming house
    - tenement
  - conflagration originating from sources classifiable to E893-E898 in the above buildings
  - **E890.0 Explosion caused by conflagration**
  - **E890.1 Fumes from combustion of polyvinylchloride [PVC] and similar material in conflagration**
  - **E890.2 Other smoke and fumes from conflagration**
    - Carbon monoxide from conflagration in private building
    - Fumes NOS from conflagration in private building
    - Smoke NOS from conflagration in private building
    - Coding Clinic: 2010, Q3, P19; 2005, Q3, P10-11
  - **E890.3 Burning caused by conflagration**
  - **E890.8 Other accident resulting from conflagration**
    - Collapse of burning private building
    - Fall from burning private building
    - Hit by object falling from burning private building
    - Jump from burning private building
  - **E890.9 Unspecified accident resulting from conflagration in private dwelling**

- **E891 Conflagration in other and unspecified building or structure**
  - Conflagration in:
    - barn
    - church
    - convalescent and other residential home
    - dormitory of educational institution
    - factory
    - farm outbuildings
    - hospital
    - hotel
    - school
    - store
    - theater
  - Conflagration originating from sources classifiable to E893-E898, in the above buildings
  - **E891.0 Explosion caused by conflagration**
  - **E891.1 Fumes from combustion of polyvinylchloride [PVC] and similar material in conflagration**
  - **E891.2 Other smoke and fumes from conflagration**
    - Carbon monoxide from conflagration in building or structure
    - Fumes NOS from conflagration in building or structure
    - Smoke NOS from conflagration in building or structure
  - **E891.3 Burning caused by conflagration**
  - **E891.8 Other accident resulting from conflagration**
    - Collapse of burning building or structure
    - Fall from burning building or structure
    - Hit by object falling from burning building or structure
    - Jump from burning building or structure
  - **E891.9 Unspecified accident resulting from conflagration of other and unspecified building or structure**

E892 Conflagration not in building or structure
　　Fire (uncontrolled) (in) (of):
　　　forest
　　　grass
　　　hay
　　　lumber
　　　mine
　　　prairie
　　　transport vehicle [any], except while in transit
　　　tunnel

● **E893 Accident caused by ignition of clothing**
　　Excludes ignition of clothing:
　　　　from highly inflammable material (E894)
　　　　with conflagration (E890.0-E892)

　E893.0 From controlled fire in private dwelling
　　Ignition of clothing from:
　　　normal fire (charcoal) (coal) (electric) (gas)
　　　　(wood) in:
　　　　brazier in private dwelling (as listed in E890)
　　　　fireplace in private dwelling (as listed in E890)
　　　　furnace in private dwelling (as listed in E890)
　　　　stove in private dwelling (as listed in E890)

　E893.1 From controlled fire in other building or structure
　　Ignition of clothing from:
　　　normal fire (charcoal) (coal) (electric) (gas)
　　　　(wood) in:
　　　　brazier in other building or structure (as listed in E891)
　　　　fireplace in other building or structure (as listed in E891)
　　　　furnace in other building or structure (as listed in E891)
　　　　stove in other building or structure (as listed in E891)

　E893.2 From controlled fire not in building or structure
　　Ignition of clothing from:
　　　bonfire (controlled)
　　　brazier fire (controlled), not in building or structure
　　　trash fire (controlled)
　　Excludes conflagration not in building (E892)
　　　　trash fire out of control (E892)

　E893.8 From other specified sources
　　Ignition of clothing from:
　　　blowlamp
　　　blowtorch
　　　burning bedspread
　　　candle
　　　cigar
　　　cigarette
　　　lighter
　　　matches
　　　pipe
　　　welding torch

　■**E893.9 Unspecified source**
　　Ignition of clothing (from controlled fire NOS) (in building NOS) NOS

E894 Ignition of highly inflammable material
　　Ignition of:
　　　benzine (with ignition of clothing)
　　　gasoline (with ignition of clothing)
　　　fat (with ignition of clothing)
　　　kerosene (with ignition of clothing)
　　　paraffin (with ignition of clothing)
　　　petrol (with ignition of clothing)
　　Excludes ignition of highly inflammable material with:
　　　　conflagration (E890.0-E892)
　　　　explosion (E923.0-E923.9)

E895 Accident caused by controlled fire in private dwelling
　　Burning by (flame of) normal fire (charcoal) (coal) (electric) (gas) (wood) in:
　　　brazier in private dwelling (as listed in E890)
　　　fireplace in private dwelling (as listed in E890)
　　　furnace in private dwelling (as listed in E890)
　　　stove in private dwelling (as listed in E890)
　　Excludes burning by hot objects not producing fire or flames (E924.0-E924.9)
　　　　ignition of clothing from these sources (E893.0)
　　　　poisoning by carbon monoxide from incomplete combustion of fuel (E867-E868.9)
　　　　that with conflagration (E890.0-E890.9)

E896 Accident caused by controlled fire in other and unspecified building or structure
　　Burning by (flame of) normal fire (charcoal) (coal) (electric) (gas) (wood) in:
　　　brazier in other building or structure (as listed in E891)
　　　fireplace in other building or structure (as listed in E891)
　　　furnace in other building or structure (as listed in E891)
　　　stove in other building or structure (as listed in E891)
　　Excludes burning by hot objects not producing fire or flames (E924.0-E924.9)
　　　　ignition of clothing from these sources (E893.1)
　　　　poisoning by carbon monoxide from incomplete combustion of fuel (E867-E868.9)
　　　　that with conflagration (E891.0-E891.9)

E897 Accident caused by controlled fire not in building or structure
　　Burns from flame of:
　　　bonfire (controlled)
　　　brazier fire (controlled), not in building or structure
　　　trash fire (controlled)
　　Excludes ignition of clothing from these sources (E893.2)
　　　　trash fire out of control (E892)
　　　　that with conflagration (E892)

● **E898 Accident caused by other specified fire and flames**
　　Excludes conflagration (E890.0-E892)
　　　　that with ignition of:
　　　　　clothing (E893.0-E893.9)
　　　　　highly inflammable material (E894)

　E898.0 Burning bedclothes
　　　Bed set on fire NOS

　E898.1 Other
　　　Burning by:　　　　　　Burning by:
　　　　blowlamp　　　　　　　lamp
　　　　blowtorch　　　　　　 lighter
　　　　candle　　　　　　　　matches
　　　　cigar　　　　　　　　　pipe
　　　　cigarette　　　　　　 welding torch
　　　　fire in room NOS

■**E899 Accident caused by unspecified fire**
　　Burning NOS

ACCIDENTS DUE TO NATURAL AND ENVIRONMENTAL FACTORS (E900-E909)

- **E900 Excessive heat**
    - **E900.0 Due to weather conditions**
        Excessive heat as the external cause of:
        - ictus solaris
        - siriasis
        - sunstroke
    - **E900.1 Of man-made origin**
        Heat (in):
        - boiler room
        - drying room
        - factory
        - furnace room
        - generated in transport vehicle
        - kitchen
    - **E900.9 Of unspecified origin**

- **E901 Excessive cold**
    - **E901.0 Due to weather conditions**
        Excessive cold as the cause of:
        - chilblains NOS
        - immersion foot
    - **E901.1 Of man-made origin**
        Contact with or inhalation of:
        - dry ice
        - liquid air
        - liquid hydrogen
        - liquid nitrogen
        Prolonged exposure in:
        - deep freeze unit
        - refrigerator
    - **E901.8 Other specified origin**
    - **E901.9 Of unspecified origin**

- **E902 High and low air pressure and changes in air pressure**
    - **E902.0 Residence or prolonged visit at high altitude**
        Residence or prolonged visit at high altitude as the cause of:
        - Acosta syndrome
        - Alpine sickness
        - altitude sickness
        - Andes disease
        - anoxia, hypoxia
        - barotitis, barodontalgia, barosinusitis, otitic barotrauma
        - hypobarism, hypobaropathy
        - mountain sickness
        - range disease
    - **E902.1 In aircraft**
        Sudden change in air pressure in aircraft during ascent or descent as the cause of:
        - aeroneurosis
        - aviators' disease
    - **E902.2 Due to diving**
        High air pressure from rapid descent in water as the cause of:
        - caisson disease
        - divers' disease
        - divers' palsy or paralysis
        Reduction in atmospheric pressure while surfacing from deep water diving as the cause of:
        - caisson disease
        - divers' disease
        - divers' palsy or paralysis
    - **E902.8 Due to other specified causes**
        Reduction in atmospheric pressure while surfacing from under ground
    - **E902.9 Unspecified cause**

- E903 Travel and motion

- **E904 Hunger, thirst, exposure, and neglect**
    Excludes any condition resulting from homicidal intent (E968.0-E968.9)
    hunger, thirst, and exposure resulting from accidents connected with transport (E800.0-E848)
    - **E904.0 Abandonment or neglect of infants and helpless persons**
        Desertion of newborn
        Exposure to weather conditions resulting from abandonment or neglect
        Hunger or thirst resulting from abandonment or neglect
        Inattention at or after birth
        Lack of care (helpless person) (infant)
        Excludes criminal [purposeful] neglect (E968.4)
        OGCR Section I.C.19.e.2
        In cases of neglect when the intent is determined to be accidental E code E904.0 should be the first listed E code.
    - **E904.1 Lack of food**
        Lack of food as the cause of:
        - inanition
        - insufficient nourishment
        - starvation
        Excludes hunger resulting from abandonment or neglect (E904.0)
    - **E904.2 Lack of water**
        Lack of water as the cause of:
        - dehydration
        - inanition
        Excludes dehydration due to acute fluid loss (276.51)
    - **E904.3 Exposure (to weather conditions), not elsewhere classifiable**
        - Exposure NOS
        - Humidity
        - Struck by hailstones
        Excludes struck by lightning (E907)
    - **E904.9 Privation, unqualified**
        Destitution

- **E905 Venomous animals and plants as the cause of poisoning and toxic reactions**
    Includes chemical released by animal
    insects
    release of venom through fangs, hairs, spines, tentacles, and other venom apparatus
    Excludes eating of poisonous animals or plants (E865.0-E865.9)
    - **E905.0 Venomous snakes and lizards**
        - Cobra
        - Copperhead snake
        - Coral snake
        - Fer de lance
        - Gila monster
        - Krait
        - Mamba
        - Rattlesnake
        - Sea snake
        - Snake (venomous)
        - Viper
        - Water moccasin
        Excludes bites of snakes and lizards known to be nonvenomous (E906.2)
    - **E905.1 Venomous spiders**
        - Black widow spider
        - Brown spider
        - Tarantula (venomous)
    - **E905.2 Scorpion**

E905.3 Hornets, wasps, and bees
　　　　Yellow jacket
E905.4 Centipede and venomous millipede (tropical)
E905.5 Other venomous arthropods
　　　　Sting of:
　　　　　ant
　　　　　caterpillar
E905.6 Venomous marine animals and plants
　　　　Puncture by sea urchin spine
　　　　Sting of:
　　　　　coral
　　　　　jelly fish
　　　　　nematocysts
　　　　　sea anemone
　　　　　sea cucumber
　　　　　other marine animal or plant
　　　　Excludes bites and other injuries caused by
　　　　　　nonvenomous marine animal
　　　　　　(E906.2-E906.8)
　　　　　　bite of sea snake (venomous) (E905.0)
E905.7 Poisoning and toxic reactions caused by other plants
　　　　Injection of poisons or toxins into or through skin
　　　　　　by plant thorns, spines, or other mechanisms
　　　　Excludes puncture wound NOS by plant thorns or
　　　　　　spines (E920.8)
E905.8 Other specified
E905.9 Unspecified
　　　　Sting NOS
　　　　Venomous bite NOS

● E906 Other injury caused by animals
　　　　Excludes poisoning and toxic reactions caused by venomous
　　　　　　animals and insects (E905.0-E905.9)
　　　　　　road vehicle accident involving animals
　　　　　　(E827.0-E828.9)
　　　　　　tripping or falling over an animal (E885.9)
　　E906.0 Dog bite
　　E906.1 Rat bite
　　E906.2 Bite of nonvenomous snakes and lizards
　　E906.3 Bite of other animal except arthropod
　　　　　Cats
　　　　　Moray eel
　　　　　Rodents, except rats
　　　　　Shark
　　E906.4 Bite of nonvenomous arthropod
　　　　　Insect bite NOS
　　E906.5 Bite by unspecified animal
　　　　　Animal bite NOS
　　E906.8 Other specified injury caused by animal
　　　　　Butted by animal
　　　　　Fallen on by horse or other animal, not being
　　　　　　ridden
　　　　　Gored by animal
　　　　　Implantation of quills of porcupine
　　　　　Pecked by bird
　　　　　Run over by animal, not being ridden
　　　　　Stepped on by animal, not being ridden
　　　　　Excludes injury by animal being ridden
　　　　　　(E828.0-E828.9)
　　E906.9 Unspecified injury caused by animal

E907 Lightning
　　　　Excludes injury from:
　　　　　fall of tree or other object caused by lightning
　　　　　　(E916)
　　　　　fire caused by lightning (E890.0-E892)

● E908 Cataclysmic storms, and floods resulting from storms
　　　　Excludes collapse of dam or man-made structure causing flood
　　　　　　(E909.3)
　　E908.0 Hurricane
　　　　　Storm surge
　　　　　"Tidal wave" caused by storm action
　　　　　Typhoon
　　E908.1 Tornado
　　　　　Cyclone　　　　　Twisters
　　E908.2 Floods
　　　　　Torrential rainfall　　Flash flood
　　　　　Excludes collapse of dam or man-made structure
　　　　　　causing flood (E909.3)
　　E908.3 Blizzard (snow) (ice)
　　E908.4 Dust storm
　　E908.8 Other cataclysmic storms
　　E908.9 Unspecified cataclysmic storms, and floods resulting
　　　　　from storms
　　　　　Storm NOS

● E909 Cataclysmic earth surface movements and eruptions
　　E909.0 Earthquakes
　　E909.1 Volcanic eruptions
　　　　　Burns from lava　　Ash inhalation
　　E909.2 Avalanche, landslide, or mudslide
　　E909.3 Collapse of dam or man-made structure
　　E909.4 Tidal wave caused by earthquake
　　　　　Tidal wave NOS　　Tsunami
　　　　　Excludes tidal wave caused by tropical storm
　　　　　　(E908.0)
　　E909.8 Other cataclysmic earth surface movements and
　　　　　eruptions
　　E909.9 Unspecified cataclysmic earth surface movements
　　　　　and eruptions

ACCIDENTS CAUSED BY SUBMERSION, SUFFOCATION, AND FOREIGN BODIES (E910-E915)

● E910 Accidental drowning and submersion
　　　　Includes immersion
　　　　　　swimmers' cramp
　　　　Excludes diving accident (NOS) (resulting in injury except
　　　　　　drowning) (E883.0)
　　　　　diving with insufficient air supply (E913.2)
　　　　　drowning and submersion due to:
　　　　　　cataclysm (E908-E909)
　　　　　　machinery accident (E919.0-E919.9)
　　　　　　transport accident (E800.0-E845.9)
　　　　　　effect of high and low air pressure (E902.2)
　　　　　injury from striking against objects while in
　　　　　　running water (E917.2)
　　E910.0 While water-skiing
　　　　　Fall from water skis with submersion or drowning
　　　　　Excludes accident to water-skier involving a
　　　　　　watercraft and resulting in
　　　　　　submersion or other injury (E830.4,
　　　　　　E831.4)
　　E910.1 While engaged in other sport or recreational activity
　　　　　with diving equipment
　　　　　Scuba diving NOS
　　　　　Skin diving NOS
　　　　　Underwater spear fishing NOS

E910.2 **While engaged in other sport or recreational activity without diving equipment**
- Fishing or hunting, except from boat or with diving equipment
- Ice skating
- Playing in water
- Surfboarding
- Swimming NOS
- Voluntarily jumping from boat, not involved in accident, for swim NOS
- Wading in water

Excludes jumping into water to rescue another person (E910.3)

E910.3 **While swimming or diving for purposes other than recreation or sport**
- Marine salvage (with diving equipment)
- Pearl diving (with diving equipment)
- Placement of fishing nets (with diving equipment)
- Rescue (attempt) of another person (with diving equipment)
- Underwater construction or repairs (with diving equipment)

E910.4 **In bathtub**

E910.8 **Other accidental drowning or submersion**
- Drowning in:
  - quenching tank
  - swimming pool

E910.9 **Unspecified accidental drowning or submersion**
- Accidental fall into water NOS
- Drowning NOS

E911 **Inhalation and ingestion of food causing obstruction of respiratory tract or suffocation**
- Aspiration and inhalation of food [any] (into respiratory tract) NOS
- Asphyxia by food [including bone, seed in food, regurgitated food]
- Choked on food [including bone, seed in food, regurgitated food]
- Suffocation by food [including bone, seed in food, regurgitated food]
- Compression of trachea by food lodged in esophagus
- Interruption of respiration by food lodged in esophagus
- Obstruction of respiration by food lodged in esophagus
- Obstruction of pharynx by food (bolus)

Excludes injury, except asphyxia and obstruction of respiratory passage, caused by food (E915)
obstruction of esophagus by food without mention of asphyxia or obstruction of respiratory passage (E915)

E912 **Inhalation and ingestion of other object causing obstruction of respiratory tract or suffocation**
- Aspiration and inhalation of foreign body except food (into respiratory tract) NOS
- Compression by foreign body in esophagus
- Foreign object [bean] [marble] in nose
- Interruption of respiration by foreign body in esophagus
- Obstruction of pharynx by foreign body
- Obstruction of respiration by foreign body in esophagus

Excludes injury, except asphyxia and obstruction of respiratory passage, caused by foreign body (E915)
obstruction of esophagus by foreign body without mention of asphyxia or obstruction in respiratory passage (E915)

● E913 **Accidental mechanical suffocation**

Excludes mechanical suffocation from or by:
- accidental inhalation or ingestion of:
  - food (E911)
  - foreign object (E912)
- cataclysm (E908-E909)
- explosion (E921.0-E921.9, E923.0-E923.9)
- machinery accident (E919.0-E919.9)

E913.0 **In bed or cradle**
Excludes suffocation by plastic bag (E913.1)

E913.1 **By plastic bag**

E913.2 **Due to lack of air (in closed place)**
- Accidentally closed up in refrigerator or other airtight enclosed space
- Diving with insufficient air supply

Excludes suffocation by plastic bag (E913.1)

E913.3 **By falling earth or other substance**
- Cave-in NOS

Excludes cave-in caused by cataclysmic earth surface movements and eruptions (E909.8)
struck by cave-in without asphyxiation or suffocation (E916)

E913.8 **Other specified means**
- Accidental hanging, except in bed or cradle

■ E913.9 **Unspecified means**
- Asphyxia, mechanical NOS
- Strangulation NOS
- Suffocation NOS

E914 **Foreign body accidentally entering eye and adnexa**

Excludes corrosive liquid (E924.1)

E915 **Foreign body accidentally entering other orifice**

Excludes aspiration and inhalation of foreign body, any, (into respiratory tract) NOS (E911-E912)

OTHER ACCIDENTS (E916-E928)

E916 **Struck accidentally by falling object**
- Collapse of building, except on fire
- Falling:
  - rock
  - snowslide NOS
  - stone
  - tree
- Object falling from:
  - machine, not in operation
  - stationary vehicle

Code first collapse of building on fire (E890.0-E891.9)
- falling object in:
  - cataclysm (E908-E909)
  - machinery accidents (E919.0-E919.9)
  - transport accidents (E800.0-E845.9)
  - vehicle accidents not elsewhere classifiable (E846-E848)
- object set in motion by:
  - explosion (E921.0-E921.9, E923.0-E923.9)
  - firearm (E922.0-E922.9)
  - projected object (E917.0-E917.9)

● **E917 Striking against or struck accidentally by objects or persons**
  Includes bumping into or against
          object (moving) (projected) (stationary)
          pedestrian conveyance
          person
       colliding with
          object (moving) (projected) (stationary)
          pedestrian conveyance
          person
       kicking against
          object (moving) (projected) (stationary)
          pedestrian conveyance
          person
       stepping on
          object (moving) (projected) (stationary)
          pedestrian conveyance
          person
       struck by
          object (moving) (projected) (stationary)
          pedestrian conveyance
          person
  Excludes fall from:
         collision with another person, except when caused by a crowd (E886.0-E886.9)
         stumbling over object (E885.9)
         fall resulting in striking against object (E888.0-E888.1)
         injury caused by:
            assault (E960.0-E960.1, E967.0-E967.9)
            cutting or piercing instrument (E920.0-E920.9)
            explosion (E921.0-E921.9, E923.0-E923.9)
            firearm (E922.0-E922.9)
            machinery (E919.0-E919.9)
            transport vehicle (E800.0-E845.9)
            vehicle not elsewhere classifiable (E846-E848)

  E917.0 In sports without subsequent fall
      Kicked or stepped on during game (football) (rugby)
      Struck by hit or thrown ball
      Struck by hockey stick or puck
      Coding Clinic: 2007, Q2, P3-4; 2006, Q1, P8; 2004, Q1, P9

  E917.1 Caused by a crowd, by collective fear or panic without subsequent fall
      Crushed by crowd or human stampede
      Pushed by crowd or human stampede
      Stepped on by crowd or human stampede

  E917.2 In running water without subsequent fall
      Excludes drowning or submersion (E910.0-E910.9)
              that in sports (E917.0, E917.5)

  E917.3 Furniture without subsequent fall
      Excludes fall from furniture (E884.2, E884.4–E884.5)

  E917.4 Other stationary object without subsequent fall
      Bath tub
      Fence
      Lamp-post

  E917.5 Object in sports with subsequent fall
      Knocked down while boxing
      Coding Clinic: 2007, Q2, P3-4

  E917.6 Caused by a crowd, by collective fear or panic with subsequent fall

  E917.7 Furniture with subsequent fall
      Excludes fall from furniture (E884.2, E884.4–E884.5)

  E917.8 Other stationary object with subsequent fall
      Bath tub
      Fence
      Lamp-post

  E917.9 Other striking against with or without subsequent fall

E918 Caught accidentally in or between objects
  Caught, crushed, jammed, or pinched in or between moving or stationary objects, such as:
     escalator
     folding object
     hand tools, appliances, or implements
     sliding door and door frame
     under packing crate
     washing machine wringer
  Excludes injury caused by:
          cutting or piercing instrument (E920.0- E920.9)
          machinery (E919.0-E919.9)
          mechanism or component of firearm and air gun (E928.7)
          transport vehicle (E800.0-E845.9)
          vehicle not elsewhere classifiable (E846-E848)
       struck accidentally by:
          falling object (E916)
          object (moving) (projected) (E917.0-E917.9)

● **E919 Accidents caused by machinery**
  Includes burned by machinery (accident)
       caught between machinery and other object
       caught in (moving parts of) machinery (accident)
       collapse of machinery (accident)
       crushed by machinery (accident)
       cut or pierced by machinery (accident)
       drowning or submersion caused by machinery (accident)
       explosion of, on, in machinery (accident)
       fall from or into moving part of machinery (accident)
       fire starting in or on machinery (accident)
       mechanical suffocation caused by machinery (accident)
       object falling from, on, in motion by machinery (accident)
       overturning of machinery (accident)
       pinned under machinery (accident)
       run over by machinery (accident)
       struck by machinery (accident)
       thrown from machinery (accident)
       machinery accident NOS
  Excludes accidents involving machinery, not in operation (E884.9, E916-E918)
       injury caused by:
          electric current in connection with machinery (E925.0-E925.9)
          escalator (E880.0, E918)
          explosion of pressure vessel in connection with machinery (E921.0-E921.9)
          mechanism or component of firearm and air gun (E928.7)
          moving sidewalk (E885.9)
          powered hand tools, appliances, and implements (E916-E918, E920.0-E921.9, E923.0-E926.9)
          transport vehicle accidents involving machinery (E800.0-E848.9)
          poisoning by carbon monoxide generated by machine (E868.8)

E919.0 Agricultural machines
Animal-powered agricultural machine
Combine
Derrick, hay
Farm machinery NOS
Farm tractor
Harvester
Hay mower or rake
Reaper
Thresher
  Excludes: that being towed by another vehicle on the highway (E810.0-E819.9, E827.0-E827.9, E829.0-E829.9)
  that in transport under own power on the highway (E810.0-E819.9)
  that involved in accident classifiable to E820-E829 (E820.0-E829.9)

E919.1 Mining and earth-drilling machinery
Bore or drill (land) (seabed)
Shaft hoist
Shaft lift
Under-cutter
  Excludes: coal car, tram, truck, and tub in mine (E846)

E919.2 Lifting machines and appliances
Chain hoist except in agricultural or mining operations
Crane except in agricultural or mining operations
Derrick except in agricultural or mining operations
Elevator (building) (grain) except in agricultural or mining operations
Forklift truck except in agricultural or mining operations
Lift except in agricultural or mining operations
Pulley block except in agricultural or mining operations
Winch except in agricultural or mining operations
  Excludes: that being towed by another vehicle on the highway (E810.0-E819.9, E827.0-E827.9, E829.0-E829.9)
  that in transport under own power on the highway (E810.0-E819.9)
  that involved in accident classifiable to E820-E829 (E820.0-E829.9)

E919.3 Metalworking machines
Abrasive wheel
Forging machine
Lathe
Mechanical shears
Metal:
  drilling machine
Metal:
  milling machine
  power press
  rolling-mill
  sawing machine
Coding Clinic: 2003, Q4, P76-78

E919.4 Woodworking and forming machines
Band saw
Bench saw
Circular saw
Molding machine
Overhead plane
Powered saw
Radial saw
Sander
  Excludes: hand saw (E920.1)

E919.5 Prime movers, except electrical motors
Gas turbine
Internal combustion engine
Steam engine
Water driven turbine
  Excludes: that being towed by other vehicle on the highway (E810.0-E819.9, E827.0-E827.9, E829.0-E829.9)
  that in transport under own power on the highway (E810.0-E819.9)

E919.6 Transmission machinery
Transmission:
  belt
  cable
  chain
  gear
Transmission:
  pinion
  pulley
  shaft

E919.7 Earth moving, scraping, and other excavating machines
Bulldozer
Road scraper
Steam shovel
  Excludes: that being towed by other vehicle on the highway (E810.0-E819.9)
  that in transport under own power on the highway (E810.0-E819.9)

E919.8 Other specified machinery
Machines for manufacture of:
  clothing
  foodstuffs and beverages
  paper
Printing machine
Recreational machinery
Spinning, weaving, and textile machines

E919.9 Unspecified machinery

E920 Accidents caused by cutting and piercing instruments or objects
  Includes: accidental injury (by) object:
    edged
    pointed
    sharp
  Excludes: injury caused by mechanism or component of firearm and air gun (E928.7)

E920.0 Powered lawn mower

E920.1 Other powered hand tools
Any powered hand tool [compressed air] [electric] [explosive cartridge] [hydraulic power], such as:
  drill
  hand saw
  hedge clipper
  rivet gun
  snow blower
  staple gun
  Excludes: band saw (E919.4)
    bench saw (E919.4)

E920.2 Powered household appliances and implements
Blender
Electric:
  beater or mixer
  can opener
  fan
  knife
  sewing machine
Garbage disposal appliance

E920.3 Knives, swords, and daggers

E920.4 Other hand tools and implements
Axe
Can opener NOS
Chisel
Fork
Hand saw
Hoe
Ice pick
Needle (sewing)
Paper cutter
Pitchfork
Rake
Scissors
Screwdriver
Sewing machine, not powered
Shovel

E920.5 Hypodermic needle
Contaminated needle
Needle stick

E920.8 **Other specified cutting and piercing instruments or objects**
    Arrow
    Broken glass
    Dart
    Edge of stiff paper
    Lathe turnings
    Nail
    Plant thorn
    Splinter
    Tin can lid

    Excludes: animal spines or quills (E906.8)
             flying glass due to explosion (E921.0-E923.9)

    Coding Clinic: 2001, Q3, P10

E920.9 **Unspecified cutting and piercing instrument or object**

● **E921** **Accident caused by explosion of pressure vessel**
    Includes: accidental explosion of pressure vessels, whether or not part of machinery
    Excludes: explosion of pressure vessel on transport vehicle (E800.0-E845.9)

E921.0 **Boilers**
    Coding Clinic: 2005, Q3, P10-11

E921.1 **Gas cylinders**
    Air tank
    Pressure gas tank

E921.8 **Other specified pressure vessels**
    Aerosol can
    Automobile tire
    Pressure cooker

E921.9 **Unspecified pressure vessel**

● **E922** **Accident caused by firearm and air gun missile**
    Excludes: injury caused by mechanism or component of firearm and air gun (E928.7)

E922.0 **Handgun**
    Pistol
    Revolver
    Excludes: Verey pistol (E922.8)

E922.1 **Shotgun (automatic)**

E922.2 **Hunting rifle**

E922.3 **Military firearms**
    Army rifle
    Machine gun

E922.4 **Air gun**
    BB gun
    Pellet gun

E922.5 **Paintball gun**
    Coding Clinic: 2002, Q4, P74

E922.8 **Other specified firearm missile**
    Verey pistol [flare]

E922.9 **Unspecified firearm missile**
    Gunshot wound NOS
    Shot NOS

● **E923** **Accident caused by explosive material**
    Includes: flash burns and other injuries resulting from explosion of explosive material
             ignition of highly explosive material with explosion
    Excludes: explosion:
             in or on machinery (E919.0-E919.9)
             on any transport vehicle, except stationary motor vehicle (E800.0-E848)
             with conflagration (E890.0, E891.0, E892)
             injury caused by mechanism or component of firearm and air gun (E928.7)
             secondary fires resulting from explosion (E890.0-E899)

E923.0 **Fireworks**

E923.1 **Blasting materials**
    Blasting cap
    Detonator
    Dynamite
    Explosive [any] used in blasting operations

E923.2 **Explosive gases**
    Acetylene
    Butane
    Coal gas
    Explosion in mine NOS
    Fire damp
    Gasoline fumes
    Methane
    Propane

E923.8 **Other explosive materials**
    Bomb
    Explosive missile
    Grenade
    Mine
    Shell
    Torpedo
    Explosion in munitions:
        dump
        factory

E923.9 **Unspecified explosive material**
    Explosion NOS

● **E924** **Accident caused by hot substance or object, caustic or corrosive material, and steam**
    Excludes: burning NOS (E899)
             chemical burn resulting from swallowing a corrosive substance (E860.0-E864.4)
             fire caused by these substances and objects (E890.0-E894)
             radiation burns (E926.0-E926.9)
             therapeutic misadventures (E870.0-E876.9)

E924.0 **Hot liquids and vapors, including steam**
    Burning or scalding by:
        boiling water
        hot or boiling liquids not primarily caustic or corrosive
        liquid metal
        other hot vapor
        steam
    Excludes: hot (boiling) tap water (E924.2)

E924.1 **Caustic and corrosive substances**
    Burning by:
        acid [any kind]
        ammonia
        caustic oven cleaner or other substance
        corrosive substance
        lye
        vitriol

E924.2 **Hot (boiling) tap water**

E924.8 **Other**
    Burning by:
        heat from electric heating appliance
        hot object NOS
        light bulb
        steam pipe

E924.9 **Unspecified**

● **E925** **Accident caused by electric current**
    Includes: electric current from exposed wire, faulty appliance, high voltage cable, live rail, or open electric socket as the cause of:
        burn
        cardiac fibrillation
        convulsion
        electric shock
        electrocution
        puncture wound
        respiratory paralysis
    Excludes: burn by heat from electrical appliance (E924.8)
             lightning (E907)

E925.0 **Domestic wiring and appliances**

E925.1 **Electric power generating plants, distribution stations, transmission lines**
    Broken power line

E925.2 **Industrial wiring, appliances, and electrical machinery**
    Conductors
    Control apparatus
    Electrical equipment and machinery
    Transformers

E925.8 Other electric current
  Wiring and appliances in or on:
    farm [not farmhouse]
    outdoors
    public building
    residential institutions
    schools

E925.9 Unspecified electric current
  Burns or other injury from electric current NOS
  Electric shock NOS
  Electrocution NOS

● **E926** Exposure to radiation
  Excludes: *abnormal reaction to or complication of treatment without mention of misadventure (E879.2)*
  atomic power plant malfunction in water transport (E838.0-E838.9)
  misadventure to patient in surgical and medical procedures (E873.2-E873.3)
  use of radiation in war operations (E996-E997.9)

E926.0 Radiofrequency radiation
  Overexposure to:
    microwave radiation from:
      high-powered radio and television transmitters
      industrial radiofrequency induction heaters
      radar installations
    radar radiation from:
      high-powered radio and television transmitters
      industrial radiofrequency induction heaters
      radar installations
    radiofrequency from:
      high-powered radio and television transmitters
      industrial radiofrequency induction heaters
      radar installations
    radiofrequency radiation [any] from:
      high-powered radio and television transmitters
      industrial radiofrequency induction heaters
      radar installations

E926.1 Infra-red heaters and lamps
  Exposure to infra-red radiation from heaters and lamps as the cause of:
    blistering   charring
    burning   inflammatory change
  Excludes: *physical contact with heater or lamp (E924.8)*

E926.2 Visible and ultraviolet light sources
  Arc lamps
  Black light sources
  Electrical welding arc
  Oxygas welding torch
  Sun rays
  Tanning bed
  Excludes: *excessive heat from these sources (E900.1-E900.9)*
  Coding Clinic: 1996, Q3, P6

E926.3 X-rays and other electromagnetic ionizing radiation
  Gamma rays
  X-rays (hard) (soft)

E926.4 Lasers

E926.5 Radioactive isotopes
  Radiobiologicals
  Radiopharmaceuticals

E926.8 Other specified radiation
  Artificially accelerated beams of ionized particles generated by:
    betatrons
    synchrotrons

■ **E926.9** Unspecified radiation
  Radiation NOS

● **E927** Overexertion and strenuous and repetitive movements or loads
  Use additional code to identify activity (E001-E030)
  Coding Clinic: 2009, Q3, P18; 2008, Q3, P21

E927.0 Overexertion from sudden strenuous movement
  Sudden trauma from strenuous movement

E927.1 Overexertion from prolonged static position
  Overexertion from maintaining prolonged positions, such as:
    holding
    sitting
    standing

E927.2 Excessive physical exertion from prolonged activity

E927.3 Cumulative trauma from repetitive motion
  Cumulative trauma from repetitive movements
  Coding Clinic: 2009, Q3, P20

E927.4 Cumulative trauma from repetitive impact
  Coding Clinic: 2009, Q3, P20x3, 21

E927.8 Other overexertion and strenuous and repetitive movements or loads

■ **E927.9** Unspecified overexertion and strenuous and repetitive movements or loads

● **E928** Other and unspecified environmental and accidental causes

E928.0 Prolonged stay in weightless environment
  Weightlessness in spacecraft (simulator)

E928.1 Exposure to noise
  Noise (pollution)
  Sound waves
  Supersonic waves

E928.2 Vibration

E928.3 Human bite

E928.4 External constriction caused by hair

E928.5 External constriction caused by other object

E928.6 Environmental exposure to harmful algae and toxins
  Algae bloom NOS
  Blue-green algae bloom
  Brown tide
  Cyanobacteria bloom
  Florida red tide
  Harmful algae bloom
  Pfiesteria piscicida
  Red tide
  Coding Clinic: 2007, Q4, P101-102

E928.7 Mechanism or component of firearm and air gun
  Injury due to:
    explosion of gun parts
    recoil
  Pierced, cut, crushed, or pinched by slide trigger mechanism, scope or other gun part
  Powder burn from firearm or air gun
  Excludes: *accident caused by firearm and air gun missile (E922.0-E922.9)*

E928.8 Other

■ **E928.9** Unspecified accident
  Accident NOS stated as accidentally inflicted
  Blow NOS stated as accidentally inflicted
  Casualty (not due to war) stated as accidentally inflicted
  Decapitation stated as accidentally inflicted
  Injury [any part of body, or unspecified] stated as accidentally inflicted, but not otherwise specified
  Killed stated as accidentally inflicted, but not otherwise specified
  Knocked down stated as accidentally inflicted, but not otherwise specified
  Mangled stated as accidentally inflicted, but not otherwise specified
  Wound stated as accidentally inflicted, but not otherwise specified
  Excludes: *fracture, cause unspecified (E887)*
  injuries undetermined whether accidentally or purposely inflicted (E980.0-E989)
  Coding Clinic: 1996, Q3, P7; 1985, Nov-Dec, P15; 1984, Nov-Dec, P15

LATE EFFECTS OF ACCIDENTAL INJURY (E929)

Note: This category is to be used to indicate accidental injury as the cause of death or disability from late effects, which are themselves classifiable elsewhere. The "late effects" include conditions reported as such or as sequelae, which may occur at any time after the acute accidental injury.

● **E929 Late effects of accidental injury**
  Excludes late effects of:
    surgical and medical procedures (E870.0-E879.9)
    therapeutic use of drugs and medicines (E930.0-E949.9)

  E929.0 Late effects of motor vehicle accident
    Late effects of accidents classifiable to E810-E825
    Coding Clinic: 2008, Q4, P102-109; 1997, Q3, P12-13; 1995, Q1, P10; 1994, Q3, P4

  E929.1 Late effects of other transport accident
    Late effects of accidents classifiable to E800-E807, E826-E838, E840-E848

  E929.2 Late effects of accidental poisoning
    Late effects of accidents classifiable to E850-E858, E860-E869

  E929.3 Late effects of accidental fall
    Late effects of accidents classifiable to E880-E888

  E929.4 Late effects of accident caused by fire
    Late effects of accidents classifiable to E890-E899

  E929.5 Late effects of accident due to natural and environmental factors
    Late effects of accidents classifiable to E900-E909

  E929.8 Late effects of other accidents
    Late effects of accidents classifiable to E910-E928.8

  ■ **E929.9 Late effects of unspecified accident**
    Late effects of accidents classifiable to E928.9

OGCR Section I.C.17.e.1

Adverse Effect: When the drug was correctly prescribed and properly administered, code the reaction plus the appropriate code from the E930-E949 series. Codes from the E930-E949 series must be used to identify the causative substance for an adverse effect of drug, medicinal and biological substances, correctly prescribed and properly administered. The effect, such as tachycardia, delirium, gastrointestinal hemorrhaging, vomiting, hypokalemia, hepatitis, renal failure, or respiratory failure, is coded and followed by the appropriate code from the E930-E949 series.

DRUGS, MEDICINAL AND BIOLOGICAL SUBSTANCES CAUSING ADVERSE EFFECTS IN THERAPEUTIC USE (E930-E949)

  Includes correct drug properly administered in therapeutic or prophylactic dosage, as the cause of any adverse effect including allergic or hypersensitivity reactions

  Excludes accidental overdose of drug and wrong drug given or taken in error (E850.0-E858.9)
    accidents in the technique of administration of drug or biological substance such as accidental puncture during injection, or contamination of drug (E870.0-E876.9)
    administration with suicidal or homicidal intent or intent to harm, or in circumstances classifiable to E950.0-E950.5, E962.0, E980.0-E980.5

  See Alphabetic Index for more complete list of specific drugs to be classified under the fourth-digit subdivisions. The American Hospital Formulary numbers can be used to classify new drugs listed by the American Hospital Formulary Service (AHFS). See appendix C.

● **E930 Antibiotics**
  Excludes that used as eye, ear, nose, and throat [ENT], and local anti-infectives (E946.0-E946.9)
  Coding Clinic: 2008, Q3, P21

  E930.0 Penicillins
    Natural
    Synthetic
    Semisynthetic, such as:
      ampicillin
      cloxacillin
      nafcillin
      oxacillin
    Coding Clinic: 2008, Q4, P128-131

  E930.1 Antifungal antibiotics
    Amphotericin B
    Griseofulvin
    Hachimycin [trichomycin]
    Nystatin

  E930.2 Chloramphenicol group
    Chloramphenicol
    Thiamphenicol

  E930.3 Erythromycin and other macrolides
    Oleandomycin
    Spiramycin

  E930.4 Tetracycline group
    Doxycycline
    Minocycline
    Oxytetracycline
    Coding Clinic: 1988, Q2, P9-10

  E930.5 Cephalosporin group
    Cephalexin
    Cephaloglycin
    Cephaloridine
    Cephalothin

  E930.6 Antimycobacterial antibiotics
    Cycloserine
    Kanamycin
    Rifampin
    Streptomycin

  E930.7 Antineoplastic antibiotics
    Actinomycins, such as:
      bleomycin
      cactinomycin
      dactinomycin
      daunorubicin
      mitomycin
    Excludes other antineoplastic drugs (E933.1)
    Coding Clinic: 2007, Q2, P9-10

  E930.8 Other specified antibiotics
    Coding Clinic: 1993, Q1, P29

  ■ **E930.9 Unspecified antibiotic**

● **E931 Other anti-infectives**
  Excludes ENT, and local anti-infectives (E946.0-E946.9)

  E931.0 Sulfonamides
    Sulfadiazine
    Sulfafurazole
    Sulfamethoxazole

  E931.1 Arsenical anti-infectives

  E931.2 Heavy metal anti-infectives
    Compounds of:
      antimony
      bismuth
      lead
      mercury
    Excludes mercurial diuretics (E944.0)

E931.3 Quinoline and hydroxyquinoline derivatives
Chiniofon
Diiodohydroxyquin
Excludes antimalarial drugs (E931.4)

E931.4 Antimalarials and drugs acting on other blood protozoa
Chloroquine phosphate
Cycloguanil
Primaquine
Proguanil [chloroguanide]
Pyrimethamine
Quinine (sulphate)

E931.5 Other antiprotozoal drugs
Emetine

E931.6 Anthelmintics
Hexylresorcinol
Male fern oleoresin
Piperazine
Thiabendazole

E931.7 Antiviral drugs
Methisazone
Excludes amantadine (E936.4)
cytarabine (E933.1)
idoxuridine (E946.5)

E931.8 Other antimycobacterial drugs
Ethambutol
Ethionamide
Isoniazid
Para-aminosalicylic acid derivatives
Sulfones

E931.9 Other and unspecified anti-infectives
Flucytosine
Nitrofuran derivatives

● **E932 Hormones and synthetic substitutes**

E932.0 Adrenal cortical steroids
Cortisone derivatives
Desoxycorticosterone derivatives
Fluorinated corticosteroids
Coding Clinic: 2008, Q4, P91-95; 2003, Q4, P108-109; 2000, Q3, P4-5

E932.1 Androgens and anabolic congeners
Nandrolone phenpropionate
Oxymetholone
Testosterone and preparations
Coding Clinic: 1985, July-Aug, P8

E932.2 Ovarian hormones and synthetic substitutes
Contraceptives, oral
Estrogens
Estrogens and progestogens combined
Progestogens

E932.3 Insulins and antidiabetic agents
Acetohexamide
Biguanide derivatives, oral
Chlorpropamide
Glucagon
Insulin
Phenformin
Sulfonylurea derivatives, oral
Tolbutamide
Excludes adverse effect of insulin administered for shock therapy (E879.3)

E932.4 Anterior pituitary hormones
Corticotropin
Gonadotropin
Somatotropin [growth hormone]
Coding Clinic: 1995, Q3, P15

E932.5 Posterior pituitary hormones
Vasopressin
Excludes oxytocic agents (E945.0)

E932.6 Parathyroid and parathyroid derivatives

E932.7 Thyroid and thyroid derivatives
Dextrothyroxine
Levothyroxine sodium
Liothyronine
Thyroglobulin

E932.8 Antithyroid agents
Iodides
Thiouracil
Thiourea

E932.9 Other and unspecified hormones and synthetic substitutes

● **E933 Primarily systemic agents**

E933.0 Antiallergic and antiemetic drugs
Antihistamines
Chlorpheniramine
Diphenhydramine
Diphenylpyraline
Thonzylamine
Tripelennamine
Excludes phenothiazine-based tranquilizers (E939.1)
Coding Clinic: 1997, Q2, P9-10

E933.1 Antineoplastic and immunosuppressive drugs
Azathioprine
Busulfan
Chlorambucil
Cyclophosphamide
Cytarabine
Fluorouracil
Mechlorethamine hydrochloride
Mercaptopurine
Triethylenethiophosphoramide [thio-TEPA]
Excludes antineoplastic antibiotics (E930.7)
Coding Clinic: 2011, Q4, P92; 2010, Q2, P12; 2009, Q4, P151; 2008, Q2, P6, 10-11; 2006, Q4, P69-73; Q2, P20; 2005, Q3, P11-12; 1999, Q3, P6-7; Q2, P9; 1996, Q2, P12; 1985, Mar-April, P14

E933.2 Acidifying agents

E933.3 Alkalizing agents

E933.4 Enzymes, not elsewhere classified
Penicillinase

E933.5 Vitamins, not elsewhere classified
Vitamin A
Vitamin D
Excludes nicotinic acid (E942.2)
vitamin K (E934.3)

E933.6 Oral bisphosphonates
Coding Clinic: 2007, Q4, P91-92, 102

E933.7 Intravenous bisphosphonates
Coding Clinic: 2007, Q4, P102

E933.8 Other systemic agents, not elsewhere classified
Heavy metal antagonists

■ **E933.9 Unspecified systemic agent**

● **E934 Agents primarily affecting blood constituents**
Coding Clinic: 1993, 5th Issue, P16

E934.0 Iron and its compounds
Ferric salts
Ferrous sulphate and other ferrous salts

E934.1 Liver preparations and other antianemic agents
Folic acid

E934.2 Anticoagulants
Coumarin
Heparin
Phenindione
Prothrombin synthesis inhibitor
Warfarin sodium
Coding Clinic: 2008, Q4, P134-136; 2006, Q3, P12-13; Q2, P17; 2004, Q3, P7; 1994, Q1, P22; 1990, Q3, P14

E934.3 Vitamin K [phytonadione]

E934.4	Fibrinolysis-affecting drugs Aminocaproic acid Streptodornase Streptokinase Urokinase *Coding Clinic: 2010, Q3, P5*	E937	Sedatives and hypnotics
E934.5	Anticoagulant antagonists and other coagulants Hexadimethrine bromide Protamine sulfate	E937.0	Barbiturates Amobarbital [amylobarbitone] Barbital [barbitone] Butabarbital [butabarbitone] Pentobarbital [pentobarbitone] Phenobarbital [phenobarbitone] Secobarbital [quinalbarbitone] **Excludes** thiobarbiturates (E938.3)

E934.4 Fibrinolysis-affecting drugs
Aminocaproic acid
Streptodornase
Streptokinase
Urokinase
Coding Clinic: 2010, Q3, P5

E934.5 Anticoagulant antagonists and other coagulants
Hexadimethrine bromide
Protamine sulfate

E934.6 Gamma globulin

E934.7 Natural blood and blood products
Blood plasma
Human fibrinogen
Packed red cells
Whole blood
Coding Clinic: 2011, Q4, P147; 2010, Q4, P79; 2006, Q4, P91-92; 2000, Q3, P9; 1997, Q2, P11

E934.8 Other agents affecting blood constituents
Macromolecular blood substitutes

▪E934.9 Unspecified agent affecting blood constituents

●E935 Analgesics, antipyretics, and antirheumatics

E935.0 Heroin
Diacetylmorphine

E935.1 Methadone

E935.2 Other opiates and related narcotics
Codeine [methylmorphine]
Morphine
Opium (alkaloids)
Meperidine [pethidine]

E935.3 Salicylates
Acetylsalicylic acid [aspirin]
Amino derivatives of salicylic acid
Salicylic acid salts
Coding Clinic: 1984, Nov-Dec, P15

E935.4 Aromatic analgesics, not elsewhere classified
Acetanilid
Paracetamol [acetaminophen]
Phenacetin [acetophenetidin]

E935.5 Pyrazole derivatives
Aminophenazone [aminopyrine]
Phenylbutazone
Coding Clinic: 1990, Q4, P26

E935.6 Antirheumatics [antiphlogistics]
Gold salts
Indomethacin
Excludes salicylates (E935.3)
steroids (E932.0)

E935.7 Other non-narcotic analgesics
Pyrabital

E935.8 Other specified analgesics and antipyretics
Pentazocine
Coding Clinic: 1992, Q3, P16-17

▪E935.9 Unspecified analgesic and antipyretic

●E936 Anticonvulsants and anti-Parkinsonism drugs

E936.0 Oxazolidine derivatives
Paramethadione
Trimethadione

E936.1 Hydantoin derivatives
Phenytoin

E936.2 Succinimides
Ethosuximide
Phensuximide

E936.3 Other and unspecified anticonvulsants
Beclamide
Primidone

E936.4 Anti-Parkinsonism drugs
Amantadine
Ethopropazine [profenamine]
Levodopa [L-dopa]

●E937 Sedatives and hypnotics

E937.0 Barbiturates
Amobarbital [amylobarbitone]
Barbital [barbitone]
Butabarbital [butabarbitone]
Pentobarbital [pentobarbitone]
Phenobarbital [phenobarbitone]
Secobarbital [quinalbarbitone]
Excludes thiobarbiturates (E938.3)

E937.1 Chloral hydrate group

E937.2 Paraldehyde

E937.3 Bromine compounds
Bromide
Carbromal (derivatives)

E937.4 Methaqualone compounds

E937.5 Glutethimide group

E937.6 Mixed sedatives, not elsewhere classified

E937.8 Other sedatives and hypnotics

▪E937.9 Unspecified
Sleeping:
   drug NOS
   pill NOS
   tablet NOS

●E938 Other central nervous system depressants and anesthetics

E938.0 Central nervous system muscle-tone depressants
Chlorphenesin (carbamate)
Mephenesin
Methocarbamol

E938.1 Halothane

E938.2 Other gaseous anesthetics
Ether
Halogenated hydrocarbon derivatives, except halothane
Nitrous oxide

E938.3 Intravenous anesthetics
Ketamine
Methohexital [methohexitone]
Thiobarbiturates, such as thiopental sodium

E938.4 Other and unspecified general anesthetics

E938.5 Surface and infiltration anesthetics
Cocaine
Lidocaine [lignocaine]
Procaine
Tetracaine

E938.6 Peripheral nerve- and plexus-blocking anesthetics

E938.7 Spinal anesthetics
Coding Clinic: 2004, Q2, P18; 2003, Q3, P12; 1987, Jan-Feb, P13-14

E938.9 Other and unspecified local anesthetics

●E939 Psychotropic agents

E939.0 Antidepressants
Amitriptyline
Imipramine
Monoamine oxidase [MAO] inhibitors
Coding Clinic: 2003, Q4, P75-76; 1992, Q3, P16

E939.1 Phenothiazine-based tranquilizers
Chlorpromazine   Prochlorperazine
Fluphenazine   Promazine
Phenothiazine

E939.2 Butyrophenone-based tranquilizers
Haloperidol
Spiperone
Trifluperidol

E939.3 Other antipsychotics, neuroleptics, and major tranquilizers
Coding Clinic: 2010, Q1, P20-21; 2006, Q4, P76-78

E939.4 Benzodiazepine-based tranquilizers
Chlordiazepoxide   Lorazepam
Diazepam   Medazepam
Flurazepam   Nitrazepam

E939.5 **Other tranquilizers**
  Hydroxyzine
  Meprobamate

E939.6 **Psychodysleptics [hallucinogens]**
  Cannabis (derivatives)
  Lysergide [LSD]
  Marihuana (derivatives)
  Mescaline
  Psilocin
  Psilocybin

E939.7 **Psychostimulants**
  Amphetamine
  Caffeine
  Excludes central appetite depressants (E947.0)

E939.8 **Other psychotropic agents**

E939.9 **Unspecified psychotropic agent**

● E940 **Central nervous system stimulants**

E940.0 **Analeptics**
  Lobeline
  Nikethamide

E940.1 **Opiate antagonists**
  Levallorphan
  Nalorphine
  Naloxone

E940.8 **Other specified central nervous system stimulants**

E940.9 **Unspecified central nervous system stimulant**

● E941 **Drugs primarily affecting the autonomic nervous system**

E941.0 **Parasympathomimetics [cholinergics]**
  Acetylcholine
  Anticholinesterase:
    organophosphorus
    reversible
  Pilocarpine

E941.1 **Parasympatholytics [anticholinergics and antimuscarinics] and spasmolytics**
  Atropine
  Homatropine
  Hyoscine [scopolamine]
  Quaternary ammonium derivatives
  Excludes papaverine (E942.5)

E941.2 **Sympathomimetics [adrenergics]**
  Epinephrine [adrenalin]
  Levarterenol [noradrenalin]
  Coding Clinic: 2002, Q3, P12

E941.3 **Sympatholytics [antiadrenergics]**
  Phenoxybenzamine
  Tolazoline hydrochloride
  Coding Clinic: 2007, Q4, P77-79

E941.9 **Unspecified drug primarily affecting the autonomic nervous system**

● E942 **Agents primarily affecting the cardiovascular system**

E942.0 **Cardiac rhythm regulators**
  Practolol
  Procainamide
  Propranolol
  Quinidine
  Coding Clinic: 1986, Mar-April, P11-12

E942.1 **Cardiotonic glycosides and drugs of similar action**
  Digitalis glycosides
  Digoxin
  Strophanthins

E942.2 **Antilipemic and antiarteriosclerotic drugs**
  Cholestyramine
  Clofibrate
  Nicotinic acid derivatives
  Sitosterols
  Excludes dextrothyroxine (E932.7)

E942.3 **Ganglion-blocking agents**
  Pentamethonium bromide

E942.4 **Coronary vasodilators**
  Dipyridamole
  Nitrates [nitroglycerin]
  Nitrites
  Prenylamine

E942.5 **Other vasodilators**
  Cyclandelate
  Diazoxide
  Hydralazine
  Papaverine

E942.6 **Other antihypertensive agents**
  Clonidine
  Guanethidine
  Rauwolfia alkaloids
  Reserpine

E942.7 **Antivaricose drugs, including sclerosing agents**
  Monoethanolamine
  Zinc salts

E942.8 **Capillary-active drugs**
  Adrenochrome derivatives
  Bioflavonoids
  Metaraminol

E942.9 **Other and unspecified agents primarily affecting the cardiovascular system**

● E943 **Agents primarily affecting gastrointestinal system**

E943.0 **Antacids and antigastric secretion drugs**
  Aluminum hydroxide
  Magnesium trisilicate

E943.1 **Irritant cathartics**
  Bisacodyl
  Castor oil
  Phenolphthalein

E943.2 **Emollient cathartics**
  Sodium dioctyl sulfosuccinate

E943.3 **Other cathartics, including intestinal atonia drugs**
  Magnesium sulfate

E943.4 **Digestants**
  Pancreatin
  Papain
  Pepsin

E943.5 **Antidiarrheal drugs**
  Bismuth subcarbonate
  Kaolin
  Pectin
  Excludes anti-infectives (E930.0-E931.9)

E943.6 **Emetics**

E943.8 **Other specified agents primarily affecting the gastrointestinal system**

E943.9 **Unspecified agent primarily affecting the gastrointestinal system**

● E944 **Water, mineral, and uric acid metabolism drugs**

E944.0 **Mercurial diuretics**
  Chlormerodrin
  Mercaptomerin
  Mercurophylline
  Mersalyl

E944.1 **Purine derivative diuretics**
  Theobromine
  Theophylline
  Excludes aminophylline [theophylline ethylenediamine] (E945.7)

E944.2 **Carbonic acid anhydrase inhibitors**
  Acetazolamide

E944.3 **Saluretics**
  Benzothiadiazides
  Chlorothiazide group

E944.4 **Other diuretics**
  Ethacrynic acid
  Furosemide

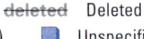

E944.5 Electrolytic, caloric, and water-balance agents
E944.6 Other mineral salts, not elsewhere classified
E944.7 Uric acid metabolism drugs
- Cinchophen and congeners
- Colchicine
- Phenoquin
- Probenecid

- E945 **Agents primarily acting on the smooth and skeletal muscles and respiratory system**
  - E945.0 Oxytocic agents
    - Ergot alkaloids
    - Prostaglandins
  - E945.1 Smooth muscle relaxants
    - Adiphenine
    - Metaproterenol [orciprenaline]
    - Excludes: papaverine (E942.5)
  - E945.2 Skeletal muscle relaxants
    - Alcuronium chloride
    - Suxamethonium chloride
  - E945.3 Other and unspecified drugs acting on muscles
  - E945.4 Antitussives
    - Dextromethorphan
    - Pipazethate hydrochloride
  - E945.5 Expectorants
    - Acetylcysteine
    - Cocillana
    - Guaifenesin [glyceryl guaiacolate]
    - Ipecacuanha
    - Terpin hydrate
  - E945.6 Anti-common cold drugs
  - E945.7 Antiasthmatics
    - Aminophylline [theophylline ethylenediamine]
  - E945.8 Other and unspecified respiratory drugs

- E946 **Agents primarily affecting skin and mucous membrane, ophthalmological, otorhinolaryngological, and dental drugs**
  - E946.0 Local anti-infectives and anti-inflammatory drugs
  - E946.1 Antipruritics
  - E946.2 Local astringents and local detergents
  - E946.3 Emollients, demulcents, and protectants
  - E946.4 Keratolytics, keratoplastics, other hair treatment drugs and preparations
  - E946.5 Eye anti-infectives and other eye drugs
    - Idoxuridine
  - E946.6 Anti-infectives and other drugs and preparations for ear, nose, and throat
  - E946.7 Dental drugs topically applied
  - E946.8 Other agents primarily affecting skin and mucous membrane
    - Spermicides
  - E946.9 Unspecified agent primarily affecting skin and mucous membrane

- E947 **Other and unspecified drugs and medicinal substances**
  - E947.0 Dietetics
  - E947.1 Lipotropic drugs
  - E947.2 Antidotes and chelating agents, not elsewhere classified
  - E947.3 Alcohol deterrents
  - E947.4 Pharmaceutical excipients
  - E947.8 Other drugs and medicinal substances
    - Contrast media used for diagnostic x-ray procedures
    - Diagnostic agents and kits
  - E947.9 Unspecified drug or medicinal substance

- E948 Bacterial vaccines
  - E948.0 BCG vaccine
  - E948.1 Typhoid and paratyphoid
  - E948.2 Cholera
  - E948.3 Plague
  - E948.4 Tetanus
  - E948.5 Diphtheria
  - E948.6 Pertussis vaccine, including combinations with a pertussis component
  - E948.8 Other and unspecified bacterial vaccines
  - E948.9 Mixed bacterial vaccines, except combinations with a pertussis component

- E949 Other vaccines and biological substances
  - Excludes: gamma globulin (E934.6)
  - Coding Clinic: 2008, Q3, P21
  - E949.0 Smallpox vaccine
  - E949.1 Rabies vaccine
  - E949.2 Typhus vaccine
  - E949.3 Yellow fever vaccine
  - E949.4 Measles vaccine
  - E949.5 Poliomyelitis vaccine
  - E949.6 Other and unspecified viral and rickettsial vaccines
    - Mumps vaccine
  - E949.7 Mixed viral-rickettsial and bacterial vaccines, except combinations with a pertussis component
    - Excludes: combinations with a pertussis component (E948.6)
  - E949.9 Other and unspecified vaccines and biological substances

SUICIDE AND SELF-INFLICTED INJURY (E950-E959)

Includes: injuries in suicide and attempted suicide
self-inflicted injuries specified as intentional

- E950 Suicide and self-inflicted poisoning by solid or liquid substances
  - E950.0 Analgesics, antipyretics, and antirheumatics
    - Coding Clinic: 1998, Q4, P50-51
  - E950.1 Barbiturates
  - E950.2 Other sedatives and hypnotics
  - E950.3 Tranquilizers and other psychotropic agents
  - E950.4 Other specified drugs and medicinal substances
  - E950.5 Unspecified drug or medicinal substance
  - E950.6 Agricultural and horticultural chemical and pharmaceutical preparations other than plant foods and fertilizers
  - E950.7 Corrosive and caustic substances
    - Suicide and self-inflicted poisoning by substances classifiable to E864
  - E950.8 Arsenic and its compounds
  - E950.9 Other and unspecified solid and liquid substances

- E951 Suicide and self-inflicted poisoning by gases in domestic use
  - E951.0 Gas distributed by pipeline
  - E951.1 Liquefied petroleum gas distributed in mobile containers
  - E951.8 Other utility gas

- E952 Suicide and self-inflicted poisoning by other gases and vapors
  - E952.0 Motor vehicle exhaust gas
  - E952.1 Other carbon monoxide
  - E952.8 Other specified gases and vapors
  - E952.9 Unspecified gases and vapors

- **E953** Suicide and self-inflicted injury by hanging, strangulation, and suffocation
  - E953.0 Hanging
  - E953.1 Suffocation by plastic bag
  - E953.8 Other specified means
  - E953.9 Unspecified means

- E954 Suicide and self-inflicted injury by submersion [drowning]

- **E955** Suicide and self-inflicted injury by firearms, air guns and explosives
  - E955.0 Handgun
  - E955.1 Shotgun
  - E955.2 Hunting rifle
  - E955.3 Military firearms
  - E955.4 Other and unspecified firearm
    Gunshot NOS
    Shot NOS
  - E955.5 Explosives
  - E955.6 Air gun
    BB gun
    Pellet gun
  - E955.7 Paintball gun
  - E955.9 Unspecified

- E956 Suicide and self-inflicted injury by cutting and piercing instrument

- **E957** Suicide and self-inflicted injuries by jumping from high place
  - E957.0 Residential premises
  - E957.1 Other man-made structures
  - E957.2 Natural sites
  - E957.9 Unspecified

- **E958** Suicide and self-inflicted injury by other and unspecified means
  - E958.0 Jumping or lying before moving object
  - E958.1 Burns, fire
  - E958.2 Scald
  - E958.3 Extremes of cold
  - E958.4 Electrocution
  - E958.5 Crashing of motor vehicle
  - E958.6 Crashing of aircraft
  - E958.7 Caustic substances, except poisoning
    Excludes *poisoning by caustic substance (E950.7)*
  - E958.8 Other specified means
  - E958.9 Unspecified means

- E959 Late effects of self-inflicted injury
  - Note: This category is to be used to indicate circumstances classifiable to E950-E958 as the cause of death or disability from late effects, which are themselves classifiable elsewhere. The "late effects" include conditions reported as such or as sequelae which may occur at any time after the attempted suicide or self-inflicted injury.

OGCR Section I.C.19.d.1

When the cause of an injury or neglect is intentional child or adult abuse, the first listed E code should be assigned from categories E960-E968, Homicide and injury purposely inflicted by other persons, (except category E967). An E code from category E967, Child and adult battering and other maltreatment, should be added as an additional code to identify the perpetrator, if known.

HOMICIDE AND INJURY PURPOSELY INFLICTED BY OTHER PERSONS (E960-E969)

Includes injuries inflicted by another person with intent to injure or kill, by any means

Excludes *injuries due to:*
legal intervention (E970-E978)
operations of war (E990-E999)
terrorism (E979)

- **E960** Fight, brawl, rape
  - E960.0 Unarmed fight or brawl
    Beatings NOS
    Brawl or fight with hands, fists, feet
    Injured or killed in fight NOS
    Excludes *homicidal:*
    injury by weapons (E965.0-E966, E969)
    strangulation (E963)
    submersion (E964)
  - E960.1 Rape
    Coding Clinic: 1999, Q3, P15

- E961 Assault by corrosive or caustic substance, except poisoning
  Injury or death purposely caused by corrosive or caustic substance, such as:
  acid [any]
  corrosive substance
  vitriol
  Excludes *burns from hot liquid (E968.3)*
  chemical burns from swallowing a corrosive substance (E962.0-E962.9)

- **E962** Assault by poisoning
  - E962.0 Drugs and medicinal substances
    Homicidal poisoning by any drug or medicinal substance
  - E962.1 Other solid and liquid substances
  - E962.2 Other gases and vapors
  - E962.9 Unspecified poisoning

- E963 Assault by hanging and strangulation
  Homicidal (attempt):
  garrotting or ligature
  hanging
  strangulation
  suffocation

- E964 Assault by submersion [drowning]

- **E965** Assault by firearms and explosives
  - E965.0 Handgun
    Pistol
    Revolver
  - E965.1 Shotgun
  - E965.2 Hunting rifle
  - E965.3 Military firearms
  - E965.4 Other and unspecified firearm
  - E965.5 Antipersonnel bomb
  - E965.6 Gasoline bomb
  - E965.7 Letter bomb
  - E965.8 Other specified explosive
    Bomb NOS (placed in):
    car
    house
    Dynamite
  - E965.9 Unspecified explosive

E966 Assault by cutting and piercing instrument
Assassination (attempt), homicide (attempt) by any instrument classifiable under E920
Homicidal:
  cut any part of body
  puncture any part of body
  stab any part of body
Stabbed any part of body
Coding Clinic: 1993, Q2, P4-5

● **E967 Perpetrator of child and adult abuse**
  Note: Selection of the correct perpetrator code is based on the relationship between the perpetrator and the victim.

  E967.0 By father, stepfather, or boyfriend
    Male partner of child's parent or guardian

  E967.1 By other specified person
    Coding Clinic: 1999, Q3, P14-15

  E967.2 By mother, stepmother, or girlfriend
    Female partner of child's parent or guardian
    Coding Clinic: 1996, Q4, P43-44

  E967.3 By spouse or partner
    Abuse of spouse or partner by ex-spouse or ex-partner
    Coding Clinic: 1996, Q4, P43-44

  E967.4 By child
  E967.5 By sibling
  E967.6 By grandparent
  E967.7 By other relative
  E967.8 By non-related caregiver
  E967.9 By unspecified person

● **E968 Assault by other and unspecified means**

  E968.0 Fire
    Arson
    Homicidal burns NOS
    Excludes: burns from hot liquid (E968.3)

  E968.1 Pushing from a high place

  E968.2 Striking by blunt or thrown object
    Coding Clinic: 1996, Q4, P43-44

  E968.3 Hot liquid
    Homicidal burns by scalding

  E968.4 Criminal neglect
    Abandonment of child, infant, or other helpless person with intent to injure or kill

  E968.5 Transport vehicle
    Being struck by other vehicle or run down with intent to injure
    Pushed in front of, thrown from, or dragged by moving vehicle with intent to injure

  E968.6 Air gun
    BB gun
    Pellet gun

  E968.7 Human bite

  E968.8 Other specified means
    Coding Clinic: 1999, Q3, P14-15x2

  E968.9 Unspecified means
    Assassination (attempt) NOS
    Homicidal (attempt):
      injury NOS
      wound NOS
    Manslaughter (nonaccidental)
    Murder (attempt) NOS
    Violence, non-accidental

E969 Late effects of injury purposely inflicted by other person
  Note: This category is to be used to indicate circumstances classifiable to E960-E968 as the cause of death or disability from late effects, which are themselves classifiable elsewhere. The "late effects" include conditions reported as such, or as sequelae which may occur at any time after the injury purposely inflicted by another person.

LEGAL INTERVENTION (E970-E978)

Includes: injuries inflicted by the police or other law-enforcing agents, including military on duty, in the course of arresting or attempting to arrest lawbreakers, suppressing disturbances, maintaining order, and other legal action
legal execution

Excludes: injuries caused by civil insurrections (E990.0-E999)

E970 Injury due to legal intervention by firearms
  Gunshot wound
  Injury by:
    machine gun
    revolver
    rifle pellet or rubber bullet
    shot NOS

E971 Injury due to legal intervention by explosives
  Injury by:
    dynamite
    explosive shell
    grenade
    motor bomb

E972 Injury due to legal intervention by gas
  Asphyxiation by gas
  Injury by tear gas
  Poisoning by gas

E973 Injury due to legal intervention by blunt object
  Hit, struck by:
    baton (nightstick)
    blunt object
    stave

E974 Injury due to legal intervention by cutting and piercing instrument
  Cut
  Incised wound
  Injured by bayonet
  Stab wound

E975 Injury due to legal intervention by other specified means
  Blow
  Manhandling

E976 Injury due to legal intervention by unspecified means

E977 Late effects of injuries due to legal intervention
  Note: This category is to be used to indicate circumstances classifiable to E970-E976 as the cause of death or disability from late effects, which are themselves classifiable elsewhere. The "late effects" include conditions reported as such, or as sequelae which may occur at any time after the injury due to legal intervention.

E978 Legal execution
  All executions performed at the behest of the judiciary or ruling authority [whether permanent or temporary] as:
    asphyxiation by gas
    beheading, decapitation (by guillotine)
    capital punishment
    electrocution
    hanging
    poisoning
    shooting
    other specified means

OGCR Section I.C.19.j.1-3

When the cause of an injury is identified by the Federal Government (FBI) as terrorism, the first-listed E-code should be a code from category E979, Terrorism. The definition of terrorism employed by the FBI is found at the inclusion note at E979. The terrorism E-code is the only E-code that should be assigned. Additional E codes from the assault categories should not be assigned.

When the cause of an injury is suspected to be the result of terrorism a code from category E979 should not be assigned. Assign a code in the range of E codes based circumstances on the documentation of intent and mechanism.

Assign code E979.9, Terrorism, secondary effects, for conditions occurring subsequent to the terrorist event. This code should not be assigned for conditions that are due to the initial terrorist act.

TERRORISM (E979)

● **E979 Terrorism**
Injuries resulting from the unlawful use of force or violence against persons or property to intimidate or coerce a Government, the civilian population, or any segment thereof, in furtherance of political or social objective
Coding Clinic: 2002, Q4, P74-77

E979.0 Terrorism involving explosion of marine weapons
Depth-charge
Marine mine
Mine NOS, at sea or in harbour
Sea-based artillery shell
Torpedo
Underwater blast

E979.1 Terrorism involving destruction of aircraft
Aircraft:
burned
exploded
shot down
Aircraft used as a weapon
Crushed by falling aircraft

E979.2 Terrorism involving other explosions and fragments
Antipersonnel bomb (fragments)
Blast NOS
Explosion (of):
artillery shell
breech-block
cannon block
mortar bomb
munitions being used in terrorism
NOS
Fragments from:
artillery shell
bomb
grenade
guided missile
land-mine
rocket
shell
shrapnel
Mine NOS

E979.3 Terrorism involving fires, conflagration and hot substances
Burning building or structure:
collapse of
fall from
hit by falling object in
jump from
Conflagration NOS
Fire (causing):
asphyxia
burns
NOS
other injury
Melting of fittings and furniture in burning
Petrol bomb
Smouldering building or structure

E979.4 Terrorism involving firearms
Bullet:
carbine
machine gun
pistol
rifle
rubber (rifle)
Pellets (shotgun)

E979.5 Terrorism involving nuclear weapons
Blast effects
Exposure to ionizing radiation from nuclear weapon
Fireball effects
Heat from nuclear weapon
Other direct and secondary effects of nuclear weapons

E979.6 Terrorism involving biological weapons
Anthrax
Cholera
Smallpox

E979.7 Terrorism involving chemical weapons
Gases, fumes, chemicals
Hydrogen cyanide
Phosgene
Sarin

E979.8 Terrorism involving other means
Drowning and submersion
Lasers
Piercing or stabbing instruments
Terrorism NOS

E979.9 Terrorism secondary effects
Note: This code is for use to identify conditions occurring subsequent to a terrorist attack not those that are due to the initial terrorist attack
Excludes late effect of terrorist attack (E999.1)

INJURY UNDETERMINED WHETHER ACCIDENTALLY OR PURPOSELY INFLICTED (E980-E989)

Note: Categories E980-E989 are for use when it is unspecified or it cannot be determined whether the injuries are accidental (unintentional), suicide (attempted), or assault.

● **E980 Poisoning by solid or liquid substances, undetermined whether accidentally or purposely inflicted**
E980.0 Analgesics, antipyretics, and antirheumatics
E980.1 Barbiturates
E980.2 Other sedatives and hypnotics
E980.3 Tranquilizers and other psychotropic agents
E980.4 Other specified drugs and medicinal substances
■ E980.5 Unspecified drug or medicinal substance
E980.6 Corrosive and caustic substances
Poisoning, undetermined whether accidental or purposeful, by substances classifiable to E864
E980.7 Agricultural and horticultural chemical and pharmaceutical preparations other than plant foods and fertilizers
E980.8 Arsenic and its compounds
E980.9 Other and unspecified solid and liquid substances

● **E981 Poisoning by gases in domestic use, undetermined whether accidentally or purposely inflicted**
E981.0 Gas distributed by pipeline
E981.1 Liquefied petroleum gas distributed in mobile containers
E981.8 Other utility gas

- **E982** Poisoning by other gases, undetermined whether accidentally or purposely inflicted
  - E982.0 Motor vehicle exhaust gas
  - E982.1 Other carbon monoxide
  - E982.8 Other specified gases and vapors
  - E982.9 Unspecified gases and vapors
- **E983** Hanging, strangulation, or suffocation, undetermined whether accidentally or purposely inflicted
  - E983.0 Hanging
  - E983.1 Suffocation by plastic bag
  - E983.8 Other specified means
  - E983.9 Unspecified means
- E984 Submersion [drowning], undetermined whether accidentally or purposely inflicted
- **E985** Injury by firearms, air guns and explosives, undetermined whether accidentally or purposely inflicted
  - E985.0 Handgun
  - E985.1 Shotgun
  - E985.2 Hunting rifle
  - E985.3 Military firearms
  - E985.4 Other and unspecified firearm
  - E985.5 Explosives
  - E985.6 Air gun
    - BB gun
    - Pellet gun
  - E985.7 Paintball gun
- E986 Injury by cutting and piercing instruments, undetermined whether accidentally or purposely inflicted
- **E987** Falling from high place, undetermined whether accidentally or purposely inflicted
  - E987.0 Residential premises
  - E987.1 Other man-made structures
  - E987.2 Natural sites
  - E987.9 Unspecified site
- **E988** Injury by other and unspecified means, undetermined whether accidentally or purposely inflicted
  - E988.0 Jumping or lying before moving object
  - E988.1 Burns, fire
  - E988.2 Scald
  - E988.3 Extremes of cold
  - E988.4 Electrocution
  - E988.5 Crashing of motor vehicle
  - E988.6 Crashing of aircraft
  - E988.7 Caustic substances, except poisoning
  - E988.8 Other specified means
    - Coding Clinic: 2012, Q2, P16-17
  - E988.9 Unspecified means
- E989 Late effects of injury, undetermined whether accidentally or purposely inflicted
  - Note: This category is to be used to indicate circumstances classifiable to E980-E988 as the cause of death or disability from late effects, which are themselves classifiable elsewhere. The "late effects" include conditions reported as such or as sequelae which may occur at any time after injury, undetermined whether accidentally or purposely inflicted.

INJURY RESULTING FROM OPERATIONS OF WAR (E990-E999)

Includes: injuries to military personnel and civilians caused by war and civil insurrections and occurring during the time of war and insurrection, and peacekeeping missions

Excludes: accidents during training of military personnel, manufacture of war material and transport, unless attributable to enemy action

- **E990** Injury due to war operations by fires and conflagrations
  - **Includes**: asphyxia, burns, or other injury originating from fire caused by a fire-producing device or indirectly by any conventional weapon
  - E990.0 From gasoline bomb
    - Incendiary bomb
  - E990.1 From flamethrower
  - E990.2 From incendiary bullet
  - E990.3 From fire caused indirectly from conventional weapon
    - **Excludes**: fire aboard military aircraft (E994.3)
  - E990.9 From other and unspecified source
- **E991** Injury due to war operations by bullets and fragments
  - **Excludes**: injury due to bullets and fragments due to war operations, but occurring after cessation of hostilities (E998.0)
    injury due to explosion of artillery shells and mortars (E993.2)
    injury due to explosion of improvised explosive device [IED] (E993.3-E993.5)
    injury due to sea-based artillery shell (E992.3)
  - E991.0 Rubber bullets (rifle)
  - E991.1 Pellets (rifle)
  - E991.2 Other bullets
    - Bullet [any, except rubber bullets and pellets]
      - carbine
      - machine gun
      - pistol
      - rifle
      - shotgun
  - E991.3 Antipersonnel bomb (fragments)
  - E991.4 Fragments from munitions
    - Fragments from:
      - artillery shell
      - bombs, except antipersonnel
      - detonation of unexploded ordnance [UXO]
      - grenade
      - guided missile
      - land mine
      - rockets
      - shell
  - E991.5 Fragments from person-borne improvised explosive device [IED]
  - E991.6 Fragments from vehicle-borne improvised explosive device [IED]
    - IED borne by land, air, or water transport vehicle
  - E991.7 Fragments from other improvised explosive device [IED]
    - Roadside IED

E991.8 Fragments from weapons
Fragments from:
artillery
autocannons
automatic grenade launchers
missile launchers
mortars
small arms

E991.9 Other and unspecified fragments
Shrapnel NOS

● **E992 Injury due to war operations by explosion of marine weapons**

E992.0 Torpedo

E992.1 Depth charge

E992.2 Marine mines
Marine mines at sea or in harbor

E992.3 Sea-based artillery shell

E992.8 Other by other marine weapons

E992.9 Unspecified marine weapon
Underwater blast NOS

● **E993 Injury due to war operations by other explosion**
Injuries due to direct or indirect pressure or air blast of an explosion occurring during war operations

Excludes injury due to fragments resulting from an explosion (E991.0-E991.9)
injury due to detonation of unexploded ordnance but occurring after cessation of hostilities (E998.0-E998.9)
injury due to nuclear weapons (E996.0-E996.9)

E993.0 Aerial bomb

E993.1 Guided missile

E993.2 Mortar
Artillery shell

E993.3 Person-borne improvised explosive device [IED]

E993.4 Vehicle-borne improvised explosive device [IED]
IED borne by land, air, or water transport vehicle

E993.5 Other improvised explosive device [IED]
Roadside IED

E993.6 Unintentional detonation of own munitions
Unintentional detonation of own ammunition (artillery) (mortars)

E993.7 Unintentional discharge of own munitions launch device
Unintentional explosion of own:
autocannons
automatic grenade launchers
missile launchers
small arms

E993.8 Other specified explosion
Bomb
Grenade
Land mine

E993.9 Unspecified explosion
Air blast NOS
Blast NOS
Blast wave NOS
Blast wind NOS
Explosion NOS

● **E994 Injury due to war operations by destruction of aircraft**

E994.0 Destruction of aircraft due to enemy fire or explosives
Air to air missile
Explosive device placed on aircraft
Rocket propelled grenade [RPG]
Small arms fire
Surface to air missile

E994.1 Unintentional destruction of aircraft due to own onboard explosives

E994.2 Destruction of aircraft due to collision with other aircraft

E994.3 Destruction of aircraft due to onboard fire

E994.8 Other destruction of aircraft

E994.9 Unspecified destruction of aircraft

● **E995 Injury due to war operations by other and unspecified forms of conventional warfare**

E995.0 Unarmed hand-to-hand combat

Excludes intentional restriction of airway (E995.3)

E995.1 Struck by blunt object
Baton (nightstick)
Stave

E995.2 Piercing object
Bayonet
Knife
Sword

E995.3 Intentional restriction of air and airway
Intentional submersion
Strangulation
Suffocation

E995.4 Unintentional drowning due to inability to surface or obtain air
Submersion

E995.8 Other forms of conventional warfare

E995.9 Unspecified form of conventional warfare

● **E996 Injury due to war operations by nuclear weapons**
Dirty bomb NOS

Excludes late effects of injury due to nuclear weapons (E999.1, E999.0)

E996.0 Direct blast effect of nuclear weapon
Injury to bodily organs due to blast pressure

E996.1 Indirect blast effect of nuclear weapon
Injury due to being thrown by blast
Injury due to being struck or crushed by blast debris

E996.2 Thermal radiation effect of nuclear weapon
Burns due to thermal radiation
Fireball effects
Flash burns
Heat effects

E996.3 Nuclear radiation effects
Acute radiation exposure
Beta burns
Fallout exposure
Radiation sickness
Secondary effects of nuclear weapons

E996.8 Other effects of nuclear weapons

E996.9 Unspecified effect of nuclear weapon

- **E997 Injury due to war operations by other forms of unconventional warfare**
  - E997.0 Lasers
  - E997.1 Biological warfare
  - E997.2 Gases, fumes, and chemicals
  - ▫ E997.3 Weapon of mass destruction [WMD], unspecified
  - E997.8 Other specified forms of unconventional warfare
  - ▫ E997.9 Unspecified form of unconventional warfare
- **E998 Injury due to war operations but occurring after cessation of hostilities**

  Injuries due to operations of war but occurring after cessation of hostilities by any means classifiable under E990-E997

  Injuries by explosion of bombs or mines placed in the course of operations of war, if the explosion occurred after cessation of hostilities
  - E998.0 Explosion of mines
  - E998.1 Explosion of bombs
  - E998.8 Injury due to other war operations but occurring after cessation of hostilities
  - ▫ E998.9 Injury due to unspecified war operations but occurring after cessation of hostilities

- **E999 Late effect of injury due to war operations and terrorism**

  Note: This category is to be used to indicate circumstances classifiable to E979, E990-E998 as the cause of death or disability from late effects, which are themselves classifiable elsewhere. The "late effects" include conditions reported as such or as sequelae which may occur at any time after injury resulting from operations of war or terrorism.
  - E999.0 Late effect of injury due to war operations
    Coding Clinic: 2012, Q3, P21; 1998, Q1, P4; 1996, Q2, P12
  - E999.1 Late effect of injury due to terrorism

APPENDIX A

MORPHOLOGY OF NEOPLASMS

The World Health Organization has published an adaptation of the International Classification of Diseases for Oncology (ICD-O). It contains a coded nomenclature for the morphology of neoplasms, which is reproduced here for those who wish to use it in conjunction with Chapter 2 of the International Classification of Diseases, 9th Revision, Clinical Modification.

The morphology code numbers consist of five digits; the first four identify the histological type of the neoplasm and the fifth indicates its behavior. The one-digit behavior code is as follows:

/0 Benign
/1 Uncertain whether benign or malignant
   Borderline malignancy
/2 Carcinoma in situ
   Intraepithelial
   Noninfiltrating
   Noninvasive
/3 Malignant, primary site
/6 Malignant, metastatic site
   Secondary site
/9 Malignant, uncertain whether primary or metastatic site

In the nomenclature below, the morphology code numbers include the behavior code appropriate to the histological type of neoplasm, but this behavior code should be changed if other reported information makes this necessary. For example, "chordoma (M9370/3)" is assumed to be malignant; the term "benign chordoma" should be coded M9370/0. Similarly, "superficial spreading adenocarcinoma (M8143/3)" described as "noninvasive" should be coded M8143/2 and "melanoma (M8720/3)" described as "secondary" should be coded M8720/6.

The following table shows the correspondence between the morphology code and the different sections of Chapter 2:

Morphology Code Histology/Behavior		ICD-9-CM Chapter 2	
Any	0	210-229	Benign neoplasms
M8000-M8004	1	239	Neoplasms of unspecified nature
M8010+	1	235-238	Neoplasms of uncertain behavior
Any	2	230-234	Carcinoma in situ
Any	3	140-195 200-208	Malignant neoplasms, stated or presumed to be primary
Any	6	196-198	Malignant neoplasms, stated or presumed to be secondary

The ICD-O behavior digit /9 is inapplicable in an ICD context, since all malignant neoplasms are presumed to be primary (/3) or secondary (/6) according to other information on the medical record.

Only the first-listed term of the full ICD-O morphology nomenclature appears against each code number in the list below. The ICD-9-CM Alphabetical Index (Volume 2), however, includes all the ICD-O synonyms as well as a number of other morphological names still likely to be encountered on medical records but omitted from ICD-O as outdated or otherwise undesirable.

A coding difficulty sometimes arises where a morphological diagnosis contains two qualifying adjectives that have different code numbers. An example is "transitional cell epidermoid carcinomas." "Transitional cell carcinoma NOS" is M8120/3 and "epidermoid carcinoma NOS" is M8070/3. In such circumstances, the higher number (M8120/3 in this example) should be used, as it is usually more specific.

CODED NOMENCLATURE FOR MORPHOLOGY OF NEOPLASMS

M800	Neoplasms NOS
M8000/0	Neoplasm, benign
M8000/1	Neoplasm, uncertain whether benign or malignant
M8000/3	Neoplasm, malignant
M8000/6	Neoplasm, metastatic
M8000/9	Neoplasm, malignant, uncertain whether primary or metastatic
M8001/0	Tumor cells, benign
M8001/1	Tumor cells, uncertain whether benign or malignant
M8001/3	Tumor cells, malignant
M8002/3	Malignant tumor, small cell type
M8003/3	Malignant tumor, giant cell type
M8004/3	Malignant tumor, fusiform cell type

M801-M804	Epithelial neoplasms NOS
M8010/0	Epithelial tumor, benign
M8010/2	Carcinoma in situ NOS
M8010/3	Carcinoma NOS
M8010/6	Carcinoma, metastatic NOS
M8010/9	Carcinomatosis
M8011/0	Epithelioma, benign
M8011/3	Epithelioma, malignant
M8012/3	Large cell carcinoma NOS
M8020/3	Carcinoma, undifferentiated type NOS
M8021/3	Carcinoma, anaplastic type NOS
M8022/3	Pleomorphic carcinoma
M8030/3	Giant cell and spindle cell carcinoma
M8031/3	Giant cell carcinoma
M8032/3	Spindle cell carcinoma
M8033/3	Pseudosarcomatous carcinoma
M8034/3	Polygonal cell carcinoma
M8035/3	Spheroidal cell carcinoma
M8040/1	Tumorlet
M8041/3	Small cell carcinoma NOS
M8042/3	Oat cell carcinoma
M8043/3	Small cell carcinoma, fusiform cell type

M805-M808	Papillary and squamous cell neoplasms
M8050/0	Papilloma NOS (except Papilloma of urinary bladder M8120/1)
M8050/2	Papillary carcinoma in situ
M8050/3	Papillary carcinoma NOS
M8051/0	Verrucous papilloma
M8051/3	Verrucous carcinoma NOS
M8052/0	Squamous cell papilloma
M8052/3	Papillary squamous cell carcinoma
M8053/0	Inverted papilloma
M8060/0	Papillomatosis NOS
M8070/2	Squamous cell carcinoma in situ NOS
M8070/3	Squamous cell carcinoma NOS
M8070/6	Squamous cell carcinoma, metastatic NOS
M8071/3	Squamous cell carcinoma, keratinizing type NOS
M8072/3	Squamous cell carcinoma, large cell, nonkeratinizing type
M8073/3	Squamous cell carcinoma, small cell, nonkeratinizing type
M8074/3	Squamous cell carcinoma, spindle cell type
M8075/3	Adenoid squamous cell carcinoma
M8076/2	Squamous cell carcinoma in situ with questionable stromal invasion
M8076/3	Squamous cell carcinoma, microinvasive
M8080/2	Queyrat's erythroplasia
M8081/2	Bowen's disease
M8082/3	Lymphoepithelial carcinoma

M809-M811	Basal cell neoplasms
M8090/1	Basal cell tumor
M8090/3	Basal cell carcinoma NOS
M8091/3	Multicentric basal cell carcinoma
M8092/3	Basal cell carcinoma, morphea type
M8093/3	Basal cell carcinoma, fibroepithelial type
M8094/3	Basosquamous carcinoma
M8095/3	Metatypical carcinoma
M8096/0	Intraepidermal epithelioma of Jadassohn
M8100/0	Trichoepithelioma
M8101/0	Trichofolliculoma
M8102/0	Tricholemmoma
M8110/0	Pilomatrixoma

M812-M813	Transitional cell papillomas and carcinomas
M8120/0	Transitional cell papilloma NOS
M8120/1	Urothelial papilloma
M8120/2	Transitional cell carcinoma in situ
M8120/3	Transitional cell carcinoma NOS
M8121/0	Schneiderian papilloma
M8121/1	Transitional cell papilloma, inverted type
M8121/3	Schneiderian carcinoma
M8122/3	Transitional cell carcinoma, spindle cell type
M8123/3	Basaloid carcinoma
M8124/3	Cloacogenic carcinoma
M8130/3	Papillary transitional cell carcinoma

M814-M838	**Adenomas and adenocarcinomas**
M8140/0	Adenoma NOS
M8140/1	Bronchial adenoma NOS
M8140/2	Adenocarcinoma in situ
M8140/3	Adenocarcinoma NOS
M8140/6	Adenocarcinoma, metastatic NOS
M8141/3	Scirrhous adenocarcinoma
M8142/3	Linitis plastica
M8143/3	Superficial spreading adenocarcinoma
M8144/3	Adenocarcinoma, intestinal type
M8145/3	Carcinoma, diffuse type
M8146/0	Monomorphic adenoma
M8147/0	Basal cell adenoma
M8150/0	Islet cell adenoma
M8150/3	Islet cell carcinoma
M8151/0	Insulinoma NOS
M8151/3	Insulinoma, malignant
M8152/0	Glucagonoma NOS
M8152/3	Glucagonoma, malignant
M8153/1	Gastrinoma NOS
M8153/3	Gastrinoma, malignant
M8154/3	Mixed islet cell and exocrine adenocarcinoma
M8160/0	Bile duct adenoma
M8160/3	Cholangiocarcinoma
M8161/0	Bile duct cystadenoma
M8161/3	Bile duct cystadenocarcinoma
M8170/0	Liver cell adenoma
M8170/3	Hepatocellular carcinoma NOS
M8180/0	Hepatocholangioma, benign
M8180/3	Combined hepatocellular carcinoma and cholangiocarcinoma
M8190/0	Trabecular adenoma
M8190/3	Trabecular adenocarcinoma
M8191/0	Embryonal adenoma
M8200/0	Eccrine dermal cylindroma
M8200/3	Adenoid cystic carcinoma
M8201/3	Cribriform carcinoma
M8210/0	Adenomatous polyp NOS
M8210/3	Adenocarcinoma in adenomatous polyp
M8211/0	Tubular adenoma NOS
M8211/3	Tubular adenocarcinoma
M8220/0	Adenomatous polyposis coli
M8220/3	Adenocarcinoma in adenomatous polyposis coli
M8221/0	Multiple adenomatous polyps
M8230/3	Solid carcinoma NOS
M8231/3	Carcinoma simplex
M8240/1	Carcinoid tumor NOS
M8240/3	Carcinoid tumor, malignant
M8241/1	Carcinoid tumor, argentaffin NOS
M8241/3	Carcinoid tumor, argentaffin, malignant
M8242/1	Carcinoid tumor, nonargentaffin NOS
M8242/3	Carcinoid tumor, nonargentaffin, malignant
M8243/3	Mucocarcinoid tumor, malignant
M8244/3	Composite carcinoma
M8250/1	Pulmonary adenomatosis
M8250/3	Bronchiolo-alveolar adenocarcinoma
M8251/0	Alveolar adenoma
M8251/3	Alveolar adenocarcinoma
M8260/0	Papillary adenoma NOS
M8260/3	Papillary adenocarcinoma NOS
M8261/1	Villous adenoma NOS
M8261/3	Adenocarcinoma in villous adenoma
M8262/3	Villous adenocarcinoma
M8263/0	Tubulovillous adenoma
M8270/0	Chromophobe adenoma
M8270/3	Chromophobe carcinoma
M8280/0	Acidophil adenoma
M8280/3	Acidophil carcinoma
M8281/0	Mixed acidophil-basophil adenoma
M8281/3	Mixed acidophil-basophil carcinoma
M8290/0	Oxyphilic adenoma
M8290/3	Oxyphilic adenocarcinoma
M8300/0	Basophil adenoma
M8300/3	Basophil carcinoma
M8310/0	Clear cell adenoma
M8310/3	Clear cell adenocarcinoma NOS
M8311/1	Hypernephroid tumor
M8312/3	Renal cell carcinoma
M8313/0	Clear cell adenofibroma
M8320/3	Granular cell carcinoma
M8321/0	Chief cell adenoma
M8322/0	Water-clear cell adenoma
M8322/3	Water-clear cell adenocarcinoma
M8323/0	Mixed cell adenoma
M8323/3	Mixed cell adenocarcinoma
M8324/0	Lipoadenoma
M8330/0	Follicular adenoma
M8330/3	Follicular adenocarcinoma NOS
M8331/3	Follicular adenocarcinoma, well differentiated type
M8332/3	Follicular adenocarcinoma, trabecular type
M8333/0	Microfollicular adenoma
M8334/0	Macrofollicular adenoma
M8340/3	Papillary and follicular adenocarcinoma
M8350/3	Nonencapsulated sclerosing carcinoma
M8360/1	Multiple endocrine adenomas
M8361/1	Juxtaglomerular tumor
M8370/0	Adrenal cortical adenoma NOS
M8370/3	Adrenal cortical carcinoma
M8371/0	Adrenal cortical adenoma, compact cell type
M8372/0	Adrenal cortical adenoma, heavily pigmented variant
M8373/0	Adrenal cortical adenoma, clear cell type
M8374/0	Adrenal cortical adenoma, glomerulosa cell type
M8375/0	Adrenal cortical adenoma, mixed cell type
M8380/0	Endometrioid adenoma NOS
M8380/1	Endometrioid adenoma, borderline malignancy
M8380/3	Endometrioid carcinoma
M8381/0	Endometrioid adenofibroma NOS
M8381/1	Endometrioid adenofibroma, borderline malignancy
M8381/3	Endometrioid adenofibroma, malignant
M839-M842	**Adnexal and skin appendage neoplasms**
M8390/0	Skin appendage adenoma
M8390/3	Skin appendage carcinoma
M8400/0	Sweat gland adenoma
M8400/1	Sweat gland tumor NOS
M8400/3	Sweat gland adenocarcinoma
M8401/0	Apocrine adenoma
M8401/3	Apocrine adenocarcinoma
M8402/0	Eccrine acrospiroma
M8403/0	Eccrine spiradenoma
M8404/0	Hidrocystoma
M8405/0	Papillary hydradenoma
M8406/0	Papillary syringadenoma
M8407/0	Syringoma NOS
M8410/0	Sebaceous adenoma
M8410/3	Sebaceous adenocarcinoma
M8420/0	Ceruminous adenoma
M8420/3	Ceruminous adenocarcinoma
M843	**Mucoepidermoid neoplasms**
M8430/1	Mucoepidermoid tumor
M8430/3	Mucoepidermoid carcinoma
M844-M849	**Cystic, mucinous, and serous neoplasms**
M8440/0	Cystadenoma NOS
M8440/3	Cystadenocarcinoma NOS
M8441/0	Serous cystadenoma NOS
M8441/1	Serous cystadenoma, borderline malignancy
M8441/3	Serous cystadenocarcinoma NOS
M8450/0	Papillary cystadenoma NOS
M8450/1	Papillary cystadenoma, borderline malignancy
M8450/3	Papillary cystadenocarcinoma NOS
M8460/0	Papillary serous cystadenoma NOS
M8460/1	Papillary serous cystadenoma, borderline malignancy
M8460/3	Papillary serous cystadenocarcinoma
M8461/0	Serous surface papilloma NOS
M8461/1	Serous surface papilloma, borderline malignancy
M8461/3	Serous surface papillary carcinoma
M8470/0	Mucinous cystadenoma NOS
M8470/1	Mucinous cystadenoma, borderline malignancy
M8470/3	Mucinous cystadenocarcinoma NOS
M8471/0	Papillary mucinous cystadenoma NOS
M8471/1	Papillary mucinous cystadenoma, borderline malignancy
M8471/3	Papillary mucinous cystadenocarcinoma
M8480/0	Mucinous adenoma
M8480/3	Mucinous adenocarcinoma
M8480/6	Pseudomyxoma peritonei
M8481/3	Mucin-producing adenocarcinoma
M8490/3	Signet ring cell carcinoma
M8490/6	Metastatic signet ring cell carcinoma

PART III / Appendix A Morphology of Neoplasms

M850-M854	**Ductal, lobular, and medullary neoplasms**		M8722/3	Balloon cell melanoma
M8500/2	Intraductal carcinoma, noninfiltrating NOS		M8723/0	Halo nevus
M8500/3	Infiltrating duct carcinoma		M8724/0	Fibrous papule of the nose
M8501/2	Comedocarcinoma, noninfiltrating		M8725/0	Neuronevus
M8501/3	Comedocarcinoma NOS		M8726/0	Magnocellular nevus
M8502/3	Juvenile carcinoma of the breast		M8730/0	Nonpigmented nevus
M8503/0	Intraductal papilloma		M8730/3	Amelanotic melanoma
M8503/2	Noninfiltrating intraductal papillary adenocarcinoma		M8740/0	Junctional nevus
M8504/0	Intracystic papillary adenoma		M8740/3	Malignant melanoma in junctional nevus
M8504/2	Noninfiltrating intracystic carcinoma		M8741/2	Precancerous melanosis NOS
M8505/0	Intraductal papillomatosis NOS		M8741/3	Malignant melanoma in precancerous melanosis
M8506/0	Subareolar duct papillomatosis		M8742/2	Hutchinson's melanotic freckle
M8510/3	Medullary carcinoma NOS		M8742/3	Malignant melanoma in Hutchinson's melanotic freckle
M8511/3	Medullary carcinoma with amyloid stroma		M8743/3	Superficial spreading melanoma
M8512/3	Medullary carcinoma with lymphoid stroma		M8750/0	Intradermal nevus
M8520/2	Lobular carcinoma in situ		M8760/0	Compound nevus
M8520/3	Lobular carcinoma NOS		M8761/1	Giant pigmented nevus
M8521/3	Infiltrating ductular carcinoma		M8761/3	Malignant melanoma in giant pigmented nevus
M8530/3	Inflammatory carcinoma		M8770/0	Epithelioid and spindle cell nevus
M8540/3	Paget's disease, mammary		M8771/3	Epithelioid cell melanoma
M8541/3	Paget's disease and infiltrating duct carcinoma of breast		M8772/3	Spindle cell melanoma NOS
M8542/3	Paget's disease, extramammary (except Paget's disease of bone)		M8773/3	Spindle cell melanoma, type A
			M8774/3	Spindle cell melanoma, type B
M855	**Acinar cell neoplasms**		M8775/3	Mixed epithelioid and spindle cell melanoma
M8550/0	Acinar cell adenoma		M8780/0	Blue nevus NOS
M8550/1	Acinar cell tumor		M8780/3	Blue nevus, malignant
M8550/3	Acinar cell carcinoma		M8790/0	Cellular blue nevus
M856-M858	**Complex epithelial neoplasms**		**M880**	**Soft tissue tumors and sarcomas NOS**
M8560/3	Adenosquamous carcinoma		M8800/0	Soft tissue tumor, benign
M8561/0	Adenolymphoma		M8800/3	Sarcoma NOS
M8570/3	Adenocarcinoma with squamous metaplasia		M8800/9	Sarcomatosis NOS
M8571/3	Adenocarcinoma with cartilaginous and osseous metaplasia		M8801/3	Spindle cell sarcoma
M8572/3	Adenocarcinoma with spindle cell metaplasia		M8802/3	Giant cell sarcoma (except of bone M9250/3)
M8573/3	Adenocarcinoma with apocrine metaplasia		M8803/3	Small cell sarcoma
M8580/0	Thymoma, benign		M8804/3	Epithelioid cell sarcoma
M8580/3	Thymoma, malignant		**M881-M883**	**Fibromatous neoplasms**
M859-M867	**Specialized gonadal neoplasms**		M8810/0	Fibroma NOS
M8590/1	Sex cord-stromal tumor		M8810/3	Fibrosarcoma NOS
M8600/0	Thecoma NOS		M8811/0	Fibromyxoma
M8600/3	Theca cell carcinoma		M8811/3	Fibromyxosarcoma
M8610/0	Luteoma NOS		M8812/0	Periosteal fibroma
M8620/1	Granulosa cell tumor NOS		M8812/3	Periosteal fibrosarcoma
M8620/3	Granulosa cell tumor, malignant		M8813/0	Fascial fibroma
M8621/1	Granulosa cell-theca cell tumor		M8813/3	Fascial fibrosarcoma
M8630/0	Androblastoma, benign		M8814/3	Infantile fibrosarcoma
M8630/1	Androblastoma NOS		M8820/0	Elastofibroma
M8630/3	Androblastoma, malignant		M8821/1	Aggressive fibromatosis
M8631/0	Sertoli-Leydig cell tumor		M8822/1	Abdominal fibromatosis
M8632/1	Gynandroblastoma		M8823/1	Desmoplastic fibroma
M8640/0	Tubular androblastoma NOS		M8830/0	Fibrous histiocytoma NOS
M8640/3	Sertoli cell carcinoma		M8830/1	Atypical fibrous histiocytoma
M8641/0	Tubular androblastoma with lipid storage		M8830/3	Fibrous histiocytoma, malignant
M8650/0	Leydig cell tumor, benign		M8831/0	Fibroxanthoma NOS
M8650/1	Leydig cell tumor NOS		M8831/1	Atypical fibroxanthoma
M8650/3	Leydig cell tumor, malignant		M8831/3	Fibroxanthoma, malignant
M8660/0	Hilar cell tumor		M8832/0	Dermatofibroma NOS
M8670/0	Lipid cell tumor of ovary		M8832/1	Dermatofibroma protuberans
M8671/0	Adrenal rest tumor		M8832/3	Dermatofibrosarcoma NOS
M868-M871	**Paragangliomas and glomus tumors**		**M884**	**Myxomatous neoplasms**
M8680/1	Paraganglioma NOS		M8840/0	Myxoma NOS
M8680/3	Paraganglioma, malignant		M8840/3	Myxosarcoma
M8681/1	Sympathetic paraganglioma		**M885-M888**	**Lipomatous neoplasms**
M8682/1	Parasympathetic paraganglioma		M8850/0	Lipoma NOS
M8690/1	Glomus jugulare tumor		M8850/3	Liposarcoma NOS
M8691/1	Aortic body tumor		M8851/0	Fibrolipoma
M8692/1	Carotid body tumor		M8851/3	Liposarcoma, well differentiated type
M8693/1	Extra-adrenal paraganglioma NOS		M8852/0	Fibromyxolipoma
M8693/3	Extra-adrenal paraganglioma, malignant		M8852/3	Myxoid liposarcoma
M8700/0	Pheochromocytoma NOS		M8853/3	Round cell liposarcoma
M8700/3	Pheochromocytoma, malignant		M8854/3	Pleomorphic liposarcoma
M8710/3	Glomangiosarcoma		M8855/3	Mixed type liposarcoma
M8711/0	Glomus tumor		M8856/0	Intramuscular lipoma
M8712/0	Glomangioma		M8857/0	Spindle cell lipoma
M872-M879	**Nevi and melanomas**		M8860/0	Angiomyolipoma
M8720/0	Pigmented nevus NOS		M8860/3	Angiomyoliposarcoma
M8720/3	Malignant melanoma NOS		M8861/0	Angiolipoma NOS
M8721/3	Nodular melanoma		M8861/1	Angiolipoma, infiltrating
M8722/0	Balloon cell nevus			

M8870/0	Myelolipoma
M8880/0	Hibernoma
M8881/0	Lipoblastomatosis
M889-M892	**Myomatous neoplasms**
M8890/0	Leiomyoma NOS
M8890/1	Intravascular leiomyomatosis
M8890/3	Leiomyosarcoma NOS
M8891/1	Epithelioid leiomyoma
M8891/3	Epithelioid leiomyosarcoma
M8892/1	Cellular leiomyoma
M8893/0	Bizarre leiomyoma
M8894/0	Angiomyoma
M8894/3	Angiomyosarcoma
M8895/0	Myoma
M8895/3	Myosarcoma
M8900/0	Rhabdomyoma NOS
M8900/3	Rhabdomyosarcoma NOS
M8901/3	Pleomorphic rhabdomyosarcoma
M8902/3	Mixed type rhabdomyosarcoma
M8903/0	Fetal rhabdomyoma
M8904/0	Adult rhabdomyoma
M8910/3	Embryonal rhabdomyosarcoma
M8920/3	Alveolar rhabdomyosarcoma
M893-M899	**Complex mixed and stromal neoplasms**
M8930/3	Endometrial stromal sarcoma
M8931/1	Endolymphatic stromal myosis
M8932/0	Adenomyoma
M8940/0	Pleomorphic adenoma
M8940/3	Mixed tumor, malignant NOS
M8950/3	Mullerian mixed tumor
M8951/3	Mesodermal mixed tumor
M8960/1	Mesoblastic nephroma
M8960/3	Nephroblastoma NOS
M8961/3	Epithelial nephroblastoma
M8962/3	Mesenchymal nephroblastoma
M8970/3	Hepatoblastoma
M8980/3	Carcinosarcoma NOS
M8981/3	Carcinosarcoma, embryonal type
M8982/0	Myoepithelioma
M8990/0	Mesenchymoma, benign
M8990/1	Mesenchymoma NOS
M8990/3	Mesenchymoma, malignant
M8991/3	Embryonal sarcoma
M900-M903	**Fibroepithelial neoplasms**
M9000/0	Brenner tumor NOS
M9000/1	Brenner tumor, borderline malignancy
M9000/3	Brenner tumor, malignant
M9010/0	Fibroadenoma NOS
M9011/0	Intracanalicular fibroadenoma NOS
M9012/0	Pericanalicular fibroadenoma
M9013/0	Adenofibroma NOS
M9014/0	Serous adenofibroma
M9015/0	Mucinous adenofibroma
M9020/0	Cellular intracanalicular fibroadenoma
M9020/1	Cystosarcoma phyllodes NOS
M9020/3	Cystosarcoma phyllodes, malignant
M9030/0	Juvenile fibroadenoma
M904	**Synovial neoplasms**
M9040/0	Synovioma, benign
M9040/3	Synovial sarcoma NOS
M9041/3	Synovial sarcoma, spindle cell type
M9042/3	Synovial sarcoma, epithelioid cell type
M9043/3	Synovial sarcoma, biphasic type
M9044/3	Clear cell sarcoma of tendons and aponeuroses
M905	**Mesothelial neoplasms**
M9050/0	Mesothelioma, benign
M9050/3	Mesothelioma, malignant
M9051/0	Fibrous mesothelioma, benign
M9051/3	Fibrous mesothelioma, malignant
M9052/0	Epithelioid mesothelioma, benign
M9052/3	Epithelioid mesothelioma, malignant
M9053/0	Mesothelioma, biphasic type, benign
M9053/3	Mesothelioma, biphasic type, malignant
M9054/0	Adenomatoid tumor NOS
M906-M909	**Germ cell neoplasms**
M9060/3	Dysgerminoma
M9061/3	Seminoma NOS
M9062/3	Seminoma, anaplastic type
M9063/3	Spermatocytic seminoma
M9064/3	Germinoma
M9070/3	Embryonal carcinoma NOS
M9071/3	Endodermal sinus tumor
M9072/3	Polyembryoma
M9073/1	Gonadoblastoma
M9080/0	Teratoma, benign
M9080/1	Teratoma NOS
M9080/3	Teratoma, malignant NOS
M9081/3	Teratocarcinoma
M9082/3	Malignant teratoma, undifferentiated type
M9083/3	Malignant teratoma, intermediate type
M9084/0	Dermoid cyst
M9084/3	Dermoid cyst with malignant transformation
M9090/0	Struma ovarii NOS
M9090/3	Struma ovarii, malignant
M9091/1	Strumal carcinoid
M910	**Trophoblastic neoplasms**
M9100/0	Hydatidiform mole NOS
M9100/1	Invasive hydatidiform mole
M9100/3	Choriocarcinoma
M9101/3	Choriocarcinoma combined with teratoma
M9102/3	Malignant teratoma, trophoblastic
M911	**Mesonephromas**
M9110/0	Mesonephroma, benign
M9110/1	Mesonephric tumor
M9110/3	Mesonephroma, malignant
M9111/1	Endosalpingioma
M912-M916	**Blood vessel tumors**
M9120/0	Hemangioma NOS
M9120/3	Hemangiosarcoma
M9121/0	Cavernous hemangioma
M9122/0	Venous hemangioma
M9123/0	Racemose hemangioma
M9124/3	Kupffer cell sarcoma
M9130/0	Hemangioendothelioma, benign
M9130/1	Hemangioendothelioma NOS
M9130/3	Hemangioendothelioma, malignant
M9131/0	Capillary hemangioma
M9132/0	Intramuscular hemangioma
M9140/3	Kaposi's sarcoma
M9141/0	Angiokeratoma
M9142/0	Verrucous keratotic hemangioma
M9150/0	Hemangiopericytoma, benign
M9150/1	Hemangiopericytoma NOS
M9150/3	Hemangiopericytoma, malignant
M9160/0	Angiofibroma NOS
M9161/1	Hemangioblastoma
M917	**Lymphatic vessel tumors**
M9170/0	Lymphangioma NOS
M9170/3	Lymphangiosarcoma
M9171/0	Capillary lymphangioma
M9172/0	Cavernous lymphangioma
M9173/0	Cystic lymphangioma
M9174/0	Lymphangiomyoma
M9174/1	Lymphangiomyomatosis
M9175/0	Hemolymphangioma
M918-M920	**Osteomas and osteosarcomas**
M9180/0	Osteoma NOS
M9180/3	Osteosarcoma NOS
M9181/3	Chondroblastic osteosarcoma
M9182/3	Fibroblastic osteosarcoma
M9183/3	Telangiectatic osteosarcoma
M9184/3	Osteosarcoma in Paget's disease of bone
M9190/3	Juxtacortical osteosarcoma
M9191/0	Osteoid osteoma NOS
M9200/0	Osteoblastoma
M921-M924	**Chondromatous neoplasms**
M9210/0	Osteochondroma
M9210/1	Osteochondromatosis NOS
M9220/0	Chondroma NOS

PART III / Appendix A Morphology of Neoplasms

M9220/1	Chondromatosis NOS
M9220/3	Chondrosarcoma NOS
M9221/0	Juxtacortical chondroma
M9221/3	Juxtacortical chondrosarcoma
M9230/0	Chondroblastoma NOS
M9230/3	Chondroblastoma, malignant
M9240/3	Mesenchymal chondrosarcoma
M9241/0	Chondromyxoid fibroma
M925	**Giant cell tumors**
M9250/1	Giant cell tumor of bone NOS
M9250/3	Giant cell tumor of bone, malignant
M9251/1	Giant cell tumor of soft parts NOS
M9251/3	Malignant giant cell tumor of soft parts
M926	**Miscellaneous bone tumors**
M9260/3	Ewing's sarcoma
M9261/3	Adamantinoma of long bones
M9262/0	Ossifying fibroma
M927-M934	**Odontogenic tumors**
M9270/0	Odontogenic tumor, benign
M9270/1	Odontogenic tumor NOS
M9270/3	Odontogenic tumor, malignant
M9271/0	Dentinoma
M9272/0	Cementoma NOS
M9273/0	Cementoblastoma, benign
M9274/0	Cementifying fibroma
M9275/0	Gigantiform cementoma
M9280/0	Odontoma NOS
M9281/0	Compound odontoma
M9282/0	Complex odontoma
M9290/0	Ameloblastic fibro-odontoma
M9290/3	Ameloblastic odontosarcoma
M9300/0	Adenomatoid odontogenic tumor
M9301/0	Calcifying odontogenic cyst
M9310/0	Ameloblastoma NOS
M9310/3	Ameloblastoma, malignant
M9311/0	Odontoameloblastoma
M9312/0	Squamous odontogenic tumor
M9320/0	Odontogenic myxoma
M9321/0	Odontogenic fibroma NOS
M9330/0	Ameloblastic fibroma
M9330/3	Ameloblastic fibrosarcoma
M9340/0	Calcifying epithelial odontogenic tumor
M935-M937	**Miscellaneous tumors**
M9350/1	Craniopharyngioma
M9360/1	Pinealoma
M9361/1	Pineocytoma
M9362/3	Pineoblastoma
M9363/0	Melanotic neuroectodermal tumor
M9370/3	Chordoma
M938-M948	**Gliomas**
M9380/3	Glioma, malignant
M9381/3	Gliomatosis cerebri
M9382/3	Mixed glioma
M9383/1	Subependymal glioma
M9384/1	Subependymal giant cell astrocytoma
M9390/0	Choroid plexus papilloma NOS
M9390/3	Choroid plexus papilloma, malignant
M9391/3	Ependymoma NOS
M9392/3	Ependymoma, anaplastic type
M9393/1	Papillary ependymoma
M9394/1	Myxopapillary ependymoma
M9400/3	Astrocytoma NOS
M9401/3	Astrocytoma, anaplastic type
M9410/3	Protoplasmic astrocytoma
M9411/3	Gemistocytic astrocytoma
M9420/3	Fibrillary astrocytoma
M9421/3	Pilocytic astrocytoma
M9422/3	Spongioblastoma NOS
M9423/3	Spongioblastoma polare
M9430/3	Astroblastoma
M9440/3	Glioblastoma NOS
M9441/3	Giant cell glioblastoma
M9442/3	Glioblastoma with sarcomatous component
M9443/3	Primitive polar spongioblastoma
M9450/3	Oligodendroglioma NOS
M9451/3	Oligodendroglioma, anaplastic type
M9460/3	Oligodendroblastoma
M9470/3	Medulloblastoma NOS
M9471/3	Desmoplastic medulloblastoma
M9472/3	Medullomyoblastoma
M9480/3	Cerebellar sarcoma NOS
M9481/3	Monstrocellular sarcoma
M949-M952	**Neuroepitheliomatous neoplasms**
M9490/0	Ganglioneuroma
M9490/3	Ganglioneuroblastoma
M9491/0	Ganglioneuromatosis
M9500/3	Neuroblastoma NOS
M9501/3	Medulloepithelioma NOS
M9502/3	Teratoid medulloepithelioma
M9503/3	Neuroepithelioma NOS
M9504/3	Spongioneuroblastoma
M9505/1	Ganglioglioma
M9506/0	Neurocytoma
M9507/0	Pacinian tumor
M9510/3	Retinoblastoma NOS
M9511/3	Retinoblastoma, differentiated type
M9512/3	Retinoblastoma, undifferentiated type
M9520/3	Olfactory neurogenic tumor
M9521/3	Esthesioneurocytoma
M9522/3	Esthesioneuroblastoma
M9523/3	Esthesioneuroepithelioma
M953	**Meningiomas**
M9530/0	Meningioma NOS
M9530/1	Meningiomatosis NOS
M9530/3	Meningioma, malignant
M9531/0	Meningotheliomatous meningioma
M9532/0	Fibrous meningioma
M9533/0	Psammomatous meningioma
M9534/0	Angiomatous meningioma
M9535/0	Hemangioblastic meningioma
M9536/0	Hemangiopericytic meningioma
M9537/0	Transitional meningioma
M9538/1	Papillary meningioma
M9539/3	Meningeal sarcomatosis
M954-M957	**Nerve sheath tumor**
M9540/0	Neurofibroma NOS
M9540/1	Neurofibromatosis NOS
M9540/3	Neurofibrosarcoma
M9541/0	Melanotic neurofibroma
M9550/0	Plexiform neurofibroma
M9560/0	Neurilemmoma NOS
M9560/1	Neurinomatosis
M9560/3	Neurilemmoma, malignant
M9570/0	Neuroma NOS
M958	**Granular cell tumors and alveolar soft part sarcoma**
M9580/0	Granular cell tumor NOS
M9580/3	Granular cell tumor, malignant
M9581/3	Alveolar soft part sarcoma
M959-M963	**Lymphomas, NOS or diffuse**
M9590/0	Lymphomatous tumor, benign
M9590/3	Malignant lymphoma NOS
M9591/3	Malignant lymphoma, non Hodgkin's type
M9600/3	Malignant lymphoma, undifferentiated cell type NOS
M9601/3	Malignant lymphoma, stem cell type
M9602/3	Malignant lymphoma, convoluted cell type NOS
M9610/3	Lymphosarcoma NOS
M9611/3	Malignant lymphoma, lymphoplasmacytoid type
M9612/3	Malignant lymphoma, immunoblastic type
M9613/3	Malignant lymphoma, mixed lymphocytic-histiocytic NOS
M9614/3	Malignant lymphoma, centroblastic-centrocytic, diffuse
M9615/3	Malignant lymphoma, follicular center cell NOS
M9620/3	Malignant lymphoma, lymphocytic, well differentiated NOS
M9621/3	Malignant lymphoma, lymphocytic, intermediate differentiation NOS
M9622/3	Malignant lymphoma, centrocytic
M9623/3	Malignant lymphoma, follicular center cell, cleaved NOS
M9630/3	Malignant lymphoma, lymphocytic, poorly differentiated NOS
M9631/3	Prolymphocytic lymphosarcoma
M9632/3	Malignant lymphoma, centroblastic type NOS
M9633/3	Malignant lymphoma, follicular center cell, noncleaved NOS

M964	**Reticulosarcomas**		**M981**	**Compound leukemias**
M9640/3	Reticulosarcoma NOS		M9810/3	Compound leukemia
M9641/3	Reticulosarcoma, pleomorphic cell type		**M982**	**Lymphoid leukemias**
M9642/3	Reticulosarcoma, nodular		M9820/3	Lymphoid leukemia NOS
M965-M966	**Hodgkin's disease**		M9821/3	Acute lymphoid leukemia
M9650/3	Hodgkin's disease NOS		M9822/3	Subacute lymphoid leukemia
M9651/3	Hodgkin's disease, lymphocytic predominance		M9823/3	Chronic lymphoid leukemia
M9652/3	Hodgkin's disease, mixed cellularity		M9824/3	Aleukemic lymphoid leukemia
M9653/3	Hodgkin's disease, lymphocytic depletion NOS		M9825/3	Prolymphocytic leukemia
M9654/3	Hodgkin's disease, lymphocytic depletion, diffuse fibrosis		**M983**	**Plasma cell leukemias**
M9655/3	Hodgkin's disease, lymphocytic depletion, reticular type		M9830/3	Plasma cell leukemia
M9656/3	Hodgkin's disease, nodular sclerosis NOS		**M984**	**Erythroleukemias**
M9657/3	Hodgkin's disease, nodular sclerosis, cellular phase		M9840/3	Erythroleukemia
M9660/3	Hodgkin's paragranuloma		M9841/3	Acute erythremia
M9661/3	Hodgkin's granuloma		M9842/3	Chronic erythremia
M9662/3	Hodgkin's sarcoma		**M985**	**Lymphosarcoma cell leukemias**
M969	**Lymphomas, nodular or follicular**		M9850/3	Lymphosarcoma cell leukemia
M9690/3	Malignant lymphoma, nodular NOS		**M986**	**Myeloid leukemias**
M9691/3	Malignant lymphoma, mixed lymphocytic-histiocytic, nodular		M9860/3	Myeloid leukemia NOS
M9692/3	Malignant lymphoma, centroblastic-centrocytic, follicular		M9861/3	Acute myeloid leukemia
M9693/3	Malignant lymphoma, lymphocytic, well differentiated, nodular		M9862/3	Subacute myeloid leukemia
M9694/3	Malignant lymphoma, lymphocytic, intermediate differentiation, nodular		M9863/3	Chronic myeloid leukemia
			M9864/3	Aleukemic myeloid leukemia
M9695/3	Malignant lymphoma, follicular center cell, cleaved, follicular		M9865/3	Neutrophilic leukemia
M9696/3	Malignant lymphoma, lymphocytic, poorly differentiated, nodular		M9866/3	Acute promyelocytic leukemia
			M987	**Basophilic leukemias**
M9697/3	Malignant lymphoma, centroblastic type, follicular		M9870/3	Basophilic leukemia
M9698/3	Malignant lymphoma, follicular center cell, noncleaved, follicular		**M988**	**Eosinophilic leukemias**
			M9880/3	Eosinophilic leukemia
M970	**Mycosis fungoides**		**M989**	**Monocytic leukemias**
M9700/3	Mycosis fungoides		M9890/3	Monocytic leukemia NOS
M9701/3	Sezary's disease		M9891/3	Acute monocytic leukemia
M971-M972	**Miscellaneous reticuloendothelial neoplasms**		M9892/3	Subacute monocytic leukemia
M9710/3	Microglioma		M9893/3	Chronic monocytic leukemia
M9720/3	Malignant histiocytosis		M9894/3	Aleukemic monocytic leukemia
M9721/3	Histiocytic medullary reticulosis		**M990-M994**	**Miscellaneous leukemias**
M9722/3	Letterer-Siwe's disease		M9900/3	Mast cell leukemia
M973	**Plasma cell tumors**		M9910/3	Megakaryocytic leukemia
M9730/3	Plasma cell myeloma		M9920/3	Megakaryocytic myelosis
M9731/0	Plasma cell tumor, benign		M9930/3	Myeloid sarcoma
M9731/1	Plasmacytoma NOS		M9940/3	Hairy cell leukemia
M9731/3	Plasma cell tumor, malignant		**M995-M997**	**Miscellaneous myeloproliferative and lymphoproliferative disorders**
M974	**Mast cell tumors**			
M9740/1	Mastocytoma NOS		M9950/1	Polycythemia vera
M9740/3	Mast cell sarcoma		M9951/1	Acute panmyelosis
M9741/3	Malignant mastocytosis		M9960/1	Chronic myeloproliferative disease
M975	**Burkitt's tumor**		M9961/1	Myelosclerosis with myeloid metaplasia
M9750/3	Burkitt's tumor		M9962/1	Idiopathic thrombocythemia
M980-M994	**Leukemias**		M9970/1	Chronic lymphoproliferative disease
M980	**Leukemias NOS**			
M9800/3	Leukemia NOS			
M9801/3	Acute leukemia NOS			
M9802/3	Subacute leukemia NOS			
M9803/3	Chronic leukemia NOS			
M9804/3	Aleukemic leukemia NOS			

APPENDIX B
GLOSSARY OF MENTAL DISORDERS

Deleted as of October 1, 2004

APPENDIX C

CLASSIFICATION OF DRUGS BY AMERICAN HOSPITAL FORMULARY SERVICES LIST NUMBER AND THEIR ICD-9-CM EQUIVALENTS

The coding of adverse effects of drugs is keyed to the continually revised Hospital Formulary of the American Hospital Formulary Service (AHFS) published under the direction of the American Society of Hospital Pharmacists.

The following section gives the ICD-9-CM diagnosis code for each AHFS list.

AHFS List		ICD-9-CM Diagnosis Code
4:00	**ANTIHISTAMINE DRUGS**	**963.0**
8:00	**ANTI-INFECTIVE AGENTS**	
8:04	Amebicides	961.5
	hydroxyquinoline derivatives	961.3
	arsenical anti-infectives	961.1
8:08	Anthelmintics	961.6
	quinoline derivatives	961.3
8:12.04	Antifungal Antibiotics	960.1
	nonantibiotics	961.9
8:12.06	Cephalosporins	960.5
8:12.08	Chloramphenicol	960.2
8:12.12	The Erythromycins	960.3
8:12.16	The Penicillins	960.0
8:12.20	The Streptomycins	960.6
8:12.24	The Tetracyclines	960.4
8:12.28	Other Antibiotics	960.8
	antimycobacterial antibiotics	960.6
	macrolides	960.3
8:16	Antituberculars	961.8
	antibiotics	960.6
8:18	Antivirals	961.7
8:20	Plasmodicides (antimalarials)	961.4
8:24	Sulfonamides	961.0
8:26	The Sulfones	961.8
8:28	Treponemicides	961.2
8:32	Trichomonacides	961.5
	hydroxyquinoline derivatives	961.3
	nitrofuran derivatives	961.9
8:36	Urinary Germicides	961.9
	quinoline derivatives	961.3
8:40	Other Anti-Infectives	961.9
10:00	**ANTINEOPLASTIC AGENTS**	**963.1**
	antibiotics	960.7
	progestogens	962.2
12:00	**AUTONOMIC DRUGS**	
12:04	Parasympathomimetic (Cholinergic) Agents	971.0
12:08	Parasympatholytic (Cholinergic Blocking) Agents	971.1
12:12	Sympathomimetic (Adrenergic) Agents	971.2
12:16	Sympatholytic (Adrenergic Blocking) Agents	971.3
12:20	Skeletal Muscle Relaxants	975.2
	central nervous system muscle-tone depressants	968.0
16:00	**BLOOD DERIVATIVES**	**964.7**
20:00	**BLOOD FORMATION AND COAGULATION**	
20:04	Antianemia Drugs	964.1
20:04.04	Iron Preparations	964.0
20:04.08	Liver and Stomach Preparations	964.1
20:12.04	Anticoagulants	964.2
20:12.08	Antiheparin agents	964.5
20:12.12	Coagulants	964.5
20:12.16	Hemostatics	964.5
	capillary-active drugs	972.8
	fibrinolysis-affecting agents	964.4
	natural products	964.7
24:00	**CARDIOVASCULAR DRUGS**	
24:04	Cardiac Drugs	972.9
	cardiotonic agents	972.1
	rhythm regulators	972.0
24:06	Antilipemic Agents	972.2
	thyroid derivatives	962.7
24:08	Hypotensive Agents	972.6
	adrenergic blocking agents	971.3
	ganglion-blocking agents	972.3
	vasodilators	972.5
24:12	Vasodilating Agents	972.5
	coronary	972.4
	nicotinic acid derivatives	972.2
24:16	Sclerosing Agents	972.7
28:00	**CENTRAL NERVOUS SYSTEM DRUGS**	
28:04	General Anesthetics	968.4
	gaseous anesthetics	968.2
	halothane	968.1
	intravenous anesthetics	968.3
28:08	Analgesics and Antipyretics	965.9
	antirheumatics	965.6
	aromatic analgesics	965.4
	non-narcotics NEC	965.7
	opium alkaloids	965.00
	heroin	965.01
	methadone	965.02
	specified type NEC	965.09
	pyrazole derivatives	965.5
	salicylates	965.1
	specified type NEC	965.8
28:10	Narcotic Antagonists	970.1
28:12	Anticonvulsants	966.3
	barbiturates	967.0
	benzodiazepine-based tranquilizers	969.4
	bromides	967.3
	hydantoin derivatives	966.1
	oxazolidine derivative	966.0
	succinimides	966.2
28:16.04	Antidepressants	969.0
28:16.08	Tranquilizers	969.5
	benzodiazepine-based	969.4
	butyrophenone-based	969.2
	major NEC	969.3
	phenothiazine-based	969.1
28:16.12	Other Psychotherapeutic Agents	969.8
28:20	Respiratory and Cerebral Stimulants	970.9
	analeptics	970.0
	anorexigenic agents	977.0
	psychostimulants	969.7
	specified type NEC	970.8
28:24	Sedatives and Hypnotics	967.9
	barbiturates	967.0
	benzodiazepine-based tranquilizers	969.4
	chloral hydrate group	967.1
	glutethimide group	967.5
	intravenous anesthetics	968.3
	methaqualone	967.4
	paraldehyde	967.2
	phenothiazine-based tranquilizers	969.1
	specified type NEC	967.8
	thiobarbiturates	968.3
	tranquilizer NEC	969.5
36:00	**DIAGNOSTIC AGENTS**	**977.8**
40:00	**ELECTROLYTE, CALORIC, AND WATER BALANCE AGENTS NEC**	**974.5**
40:04	Acidifying Agents	963.2
40:08	Alkalinizing Agents	963.3
40:10	Ammonia Detoxicants	974.5
40:12	Replacement Solutions NEC	974.5
	plasma volume expanders	964.8
40:16	Sodium-Removing Resins	974.5
40:18	Potassium-Removing Resins	974.5
40:20	Caloric Agents	974.5
40:24	Salt and Sugar Substitutes	974.5

PART III / Appendix C Classification of Drugs by American Hospital Formulary Services

40:28	Diuretics NEC	974.4		68:28	Pituitary	
	carbonic acid anhydrase inhibitors	974.2			anterior	962.4
	mercurials	974.0			posterior	962.5
	purine derivatives	974.1		68:32	Progestogens	962.2
	saluretics	974.3		68:34	Other Corpus Luteum Hormones	962.2
40:36	Irrigating Solutions	974.5		68:36	Thyroid and Antithyroid	
40:40	Uricosuric Agents	974.7			antithyroid	962.8
44:00	**ENZYMES NEC**	**963.4**			thyroid	962.7
	fibrinolysis-affecting agents	964.4		**72:00**	**LOCAL ANESTHETICS NEC**	**968.9**
	gastric agents	973.4			topical (surface) agents	968.5
48:00	**EXPECTORANTS AND COUGH PREPARATIONS**				infiltrating agents (intradermal) (subcutaneous) (submucosal)	968.5
	antihistamine agents	963.0			nerve blocking agents (peripheral) (plexus) (regional)	968.6
	antitussives	975.4				
	codeine derivatives	965.09			spinal	968.7
	expectorants	975.5		**76:00**	**OXYTOCICS**	**975.0**
	narcotic agents NEC	965.09		**78:00**	**RADIOACTIVE AGENTS**	**990**
52:00	**EYE, EAR, NOSE, AND THROAT PREPARATIONS**			**80:00**	**SERUMS, TOXOIDS, AND VACCINES**	
52:04	Anti-Infectives			80:04	Serums	979.9
	ENT	976.6			immune globulin (gamma) (human)	964.6
	ophthalmic	976.5		80:08	Toxoids NEC	978.8
52:04.04	Antibiotics				diphtheria	978.5
	ENT	976.6			and tetanus	978.9
	ophthalmic	976.5			with pertussis component	978.6
52:04.06	Antivirals				tetanus	978.4
	ENT	976.6			and diphtheria	978.9
	ophthalmic	976.5			with pertussis component	978.6
52:04.08	Sulfonamides			80:12	Vaccines NEC	979.9
	ENT	976.6			bacterial NEC	978.8
	ophthalmic	976.5			with	
52:04.12	Miscellaneous Anti-Infectives				other bacterial component	978.9
	ENT	976.6			pertussis component	978.6
	ophthalmic	976.5			viral and rickettsial component	979.7
52:08	Anti-Inflammatory Agents				rickettsial NEC	979.6
	ENT	976.6			with	
	ophthalmic	976.5			bacterial component	979.7
52:10	Carbonic Anhydrase Inhibitors	974.2			pertussis component	978.6
52:12	Contact Lens Solutions	976.5			viral component	979.7
52:16	Local Anesthetics	968.5			viral NEC	979.6
52:20	Miotics	971.0			with	
52:24	Mydriatics				bacterial component	979.7
	adrenergics	971.2			pertussis component	978.6
	anticholinergics	971.1			rickettsial component	979.7
	antimuscarinics	971.1		**84:00**	**SKIN AND MUCOUS MEMBRANE PREPARATIONS**	
	parasympatholytics	971.1				
	spasmolytics	971.1		84:04	Anti-Infectives	976.0
	sympathomimetics	971.2		84:04.04	Antibiotics	976.0
52:28	Mouth Washes and Gargles	976.6		84:04.08	Fungicides	976.0
52:32	Vasoconstrictors	971.2		84:04.12	Scabicides and Pediculicides	976.0
52:36	Unclassified Agents			84:04.16	Miscellaneous Local Anti-Infectives	976.0
	ENT	976.6		84:06	Anti-Inflammatory Agents	976.0
	ophthalmic	976.5		84:08	Antipruritics and Local Anesthetics	
56:00	**GASTROINTESTINAL DRUGS**				antipruritics	976.1
56:04	Antacids and Absorbents	973.0			local anesthetics	968.5
56:08	Anti-Diarrhea Agents	973.5		84:12	Astringents	976.2
56:10	Antiflatulents	973.8		84:16	Cell Stimulants and Proliferants	976.8
56:12	Cathartics NEC	973.3		84:20	Detergents	976.2
	emollients	973.2		84:24	Emollients, Demulcents, and Protectants	976.3
	irritants	973.1		84:28	Keratolytic Agents	976.4
56:16	Digestants	973.4		84:32	Keratoplastic Agents	976.4
56:20	Emetics and Antiemetics			84:36	Miscellaneous Agents	976.8
	antiemetics	963.0		**86:00**	**SPASMOLYTIC AGENTS**	**975.1**
	emetics	973.6			antiasthmatics	975.7
56:24	Lipotropic Agents	977.1			papaverine	972.5
60:00	**GOLD COMPOUNDS**	**965.6**			theophylline	974.1
64:00	**HEAVY METAL ANTAGONISTS**	**963.8**		**88:00**	**VITAMINS**	
68:00	**HORMONES AND SYNTHETIC SUBSTITUTES**			88:04	Vitamin A	963.5
				88:08	Vitamin B Complex	963.5
68:04	Adrenals	962.0			hematopoietic vitamin	964.1
68:08	Androgens	962.1			nicotinic acid derivatives	972.2
68:12	Contraceptives	962.2		88:12	Vitamin C	963.5
68:16	Estrogens	962.2		88:16	Vitamin D	963.5
68:18	Gonadotropins	962.4		88:20	Vitamin E	963.5
68:20	Insulins and Antidiabetic Agents	962.3		88:24	Vitamin K Activity	964.3
68:20.08	Insulins	962.3		88:28	Multivitamin Preparations	963.5
68:24	Parathyroid	962.6		**92:00**	**UNCLASSIFIED THERAPEUTIC AGENTS**	**977.8**

APPENDIX D

CLASSIFICATION OF INDUSTRIAL ACCIDENTS ACCORDING TO AGENCY

Annex B to the Resolution concerning Statistics of Employment Injuries adopted by the Tenth International Conference of Labor Statisticians on 12 October 1962

1 MACHINES

11 **Prime-Movers, except Electrical Motors**
    111 *Steam engines*
    112 *Internal combustion engines*
    119 *Others*

12 **Transmission Machinery**
    121 *Transmission shafts*
    122 *Transmission belts, cables, pulleys, pinions, chains, gears*
    129 *Others*

13 **Metalworking Machines**
    131 *Power presses*
    132 *Lathes*
    133 *Milling machines*
    134 *Abrasive wheels*
    135 *Mechanical shears*
    136 *Forging machines*
    137 *Rolling-mills*
    139 *Others*

14 **Wood and Assimilated Machines**
    141 *Circular saws*
    142 *Other saws*
    143 *Molding machines*
    144 *Overhand planes*
    149 *Others*

15 **Agricultural Machines**
    151 *Reapers (including combine reapers)*
    152 *Threshers*
    159 *Others*

16 **Mining Machinery**
    161 *Under-cutters*
    169 *Others*

19 **Other Machines Not Elsewhere Classified**
    191 *Earth-moving machines, excavating and scraping machines, except means of transport*
    192 *Spinning, weaving and other textile machines*
    193 *Machines for the manufacture of foodstuffs and beverages*
    194 *Machines for the manufacture of paper*
    195 *Printing machines*
    199 *Others*

2 MEANS OF TRANSPORT AND LIFTING EQUIPMENT

21 **Lifting Machines and Appliances**
    211 *Cranes*
    212 *Lifts and elevators*
    213 *Winches*
    214 *Pulley blocks*
    219 *Others*

22 **Means of Rail Transport**
    221 *Inter-urban railways*
    222 *Rail transport in mines, tunnels, quarries, industrial establishments, docks, etc.*
    229 *Others*

23 **Other Wheeled Means of Transport, Excluding Rail Transport**
    231 *Tractors*
    232 *Lorries*
    233 *Trucks*
    234 *Motor vehicles, not elsewhere classified*
    235 *Animal-drawn vehicles*
    236 *Hand-drawn vehicles*
    239 *Others*

24 **Means of Air Transport**

25 **Means of Water Transport**
    251 *Motorized means of water transport*
    252 *Non-motorized means of water transport*

26 **Other Means of Transport**
    261 *Cable-cars*
    262 *Mechanical conveyors, except cable-cars*
    269 *Others*

3 OTHER EQUIPMENT

31 **Pressure Vessels**
    311 *Boilers*
    312 *Pressurized containers*
    313 *Pressurized piping and accessories*
    314 *Gas cylinders*
    315 *Caissons, diving equipment*
    319 *Others*

32 **Furnaces, Ovens, Kilns**
    321 *Blast furnaces*
    322 *Refining furnaces*
    323 *Other furnaces*
    324 *Kilns*
    325 *Ovens*

33 **Refrigerating Plants**

34 **Electrical Installations, Including Electric Motors, but Excluding Electric Hand Tools**
    341 *Rotating machines*
    342 *Conductors*
    343 *Transformers*
    344 *Control apparatus*
    349 *Others*

35 **Electric Hand Tools**

36 **Tools, Implements, and Appliances, Except Electric Hand Tools**
    361 *Power-driven hand tools, except electric hand tools*
    362 *Hand tools, not power-driven*
    369 *Others*

37 **Ladders, Mobile Ramps**

38 **Scaffolding**

39 **Other Equipment, Not Elsewhere Classified**

4 MATERIALS, SUBSTANCES, AND RADIATIONS

41 **Explosives**

42 **Dusts, Gases, Liquids and Chemicals, Excluding Explosives**
    421 *Dusts*
    422 *Gases, vapors, fumes*
    423 *Liquids, not elsewhere classified*
    424 *Chemicals, not elsewhere classified*

43 **Flying Fragments**

44 **Radiations**
    441 *Ionizing radiations*
    449 *Others*

49 **Other Materials and Substances Not Elsewhere Classified**

5 WORKING ENVIRONMENT

51 **Outdoor**
    511 *Weather*
    512 *Traffic and working surfaces*
    513 *Water*
    519 *Others*

PART III / Appendix D Classification of Industrial Accidents According to Agency

52	**Indoor**
	521 *Floors*
	522 *Confined quarters*
	523 *Stairs*
	524 *Other traffic and working surfaces*
	525 *Floor openings and wall openings*
	526 *Environmental factors (lighting, ventilation, temperature, noise, etc.)*
	529 *Others*
53	**Underground**
	531 *Roofs and faces of mine roads and tunnels, etc.*
	532 *Floors of mine roads and tunnels, etc.*
	533 *Working-faces of mines, tunnels, etc.*
	534 *Mine shafts*
	535 *Fire*
	536 *Water*
	539 *Others*

6 OTHER AGENCIES, NOT ELSEWHERE CLASSIFIED

61	**Animals**
	611 *Live animals*
	612 *Animals products*
69	**Other Agencies, Not Elsewhere Classified**

7 AGENCIES NOT CLASSIFIED FOR LACK OF SUFFICIENT DATA

APPENDIX E

LIST OF THREE-DIGIT CATEGORIES

1. INFECTIOUS AND PARASITIC DISEASES

Intestinal infectious diseases (001–009)
- 001 Cholera
- 002 Typhoid and paratyphoid fevers
- 003 Other salmonella infections
- 004 Shigellosis
- 005 Other food poisoning (bacterial)
- 006 Amebiasis
- 007 Other protozoal intestinal diseases
- 008 Intestinal infections due to other organisms
- 009 Ill-defined intestinal infections

Tuberculosis (010–018)
- 010 Primary tuberculous infection
- 011 Pulmonary tuberculosis
- 012 Other respiratory tuberculosis
- 013 Tuberculosis of meninges and central nervous system
- 014 Tuberculosis of intestines, peritoneum, and mesenteric glands
- 015 Tuberculosis of bones and joints
- 016 Tuberculosis of genitourinary system
- 017 Tuberculosis of other organs
- 018 Miliary tuberculosis

Zoonotic bacterial diseases (020–027)
- 020 Plague
- 021 Tularemia
- 022 Anthrax
- 023 Brucellosis
- 024 Glanders
- 025 Melioidosis
- 026 Rat-bite fever
- 027 Other zoonotic bacterial diseases

Other bacterial diseases (030–041)
- 030 Leprosy
- 031 Diseases due to other mycobacteria
- 032 Diphtheria
- 033 Whooping cough
- 034 Streptococcal sore throat and scarlet fever
- 035 Erysipelas
- 036 Meningococcal infection
- 037 Tetanus
- 038 Septicemia
- 039 Actinomycotic infections
- 040 Other bacterial diseases
- 041 Bacterial infection in conditions classified elsewhere and of unspecified site

Human immunodeficiency virus (042)
- 042 Human immunodeficiency virus [HIV] disease

Poliomyelitis and other non-arthropod-borne viral diseases of central nervous system (045–049)
- 045 Acute poliomyelitis
- 046 Slow virus infection of central nervous system
- 047 Meningitis due to enterovirus
- 048 Other enterovirus diseases of central nervous system
- 049 Other non-arthropod-borne viral diseases of central nervous system

Viral diseases accompanied by exanthem (050–059)
- 050 Smallpox
- 051 Cowpox and paravaccinia
- 052 Chickenpox
- 053 Herpes zoster
- 054 Herpes simplex
- 055 Measles
- 056 Rubella
- 057 Other viral exanthemata
- 058 Other human herpesvirus
- 059 Other poxvirus infections

Arthropod-borne viral diseases (060–066)
- 060 Yellow fever
- 061 Dengue
- 062 Mosquito-borne viral encephalitis
- 063 Tick-borne viral encephalitis
- 064 Viral encephalitis transmitted by other and unspecified arthropods
- 065 Arthropod-borne hemorrhagic fever
- 066 Other arthropod-borne viral diseases

Other diseases due to viruses and Chlamydiae (070–079)
- 070 Viral hepatitis
- 071 Rabies
- 072 Mumps
- 073 Ornithosis
- 074 Specific diseases due to Coxsackie virus
- 075 Infectious mononucleosis
- 076 Trachoma
- 077 Other diseases of conjunctiva due to viruses and Chlamydiae
- 078 Other diseases due to viruses and Chlamydiae
- 079 Viral infection in conditions classified elsewhere and of unspecified site

Rickettsioses and other arthropod-borne diseases (080–088)
- 080 Louse-borne [epidemic] typhus
- 081 Other typhus
- 082 Tick-borne rickettsioses
- 083 Other rickettsioses
- 084 Malaria
- 085 Leishmaniasis
- 086 Trypanosomiasis
- 087 Relapsing fever
- 088 Other arthropod-borne diseases

Syphilis and other venereal diseases (090–099)
- 090 Congenital syphilis
- 091 Early syphilis, symptomatic
- 092 Early syphilis, latent
- 093 Cardiovascular syphilis
- 094 Neurosyphilis
- 095 Other forms of late syphilis, with symptoms
- 096 Late syphilis, latent
- 097 Other and unspecified syphilis
- 098 Gonococcal infections
- 099 Other venereal diseases

Other spirochetal diseases (100–104)
- 100 Leptospirosis
- 101 Vincent's angina
- 102 Yaws
- 103 Pinta
- 104 Other spirochetal infection

Mycoses (110–118)
- 110 Dermatophytosis
- 111 Dermatomycosis, other and unspecified
- 112 Candidiasis
- 114 Coccidioidomycosis
- 115 Histoplasmosis
- 116 Blastomycotic infection
- 117 Other mycoses
- 118 Opportunistic mycoses

Helminthiases (120–129)
- 120 Schistosomiasis [bilharziasis]
- 121 Other trematode infections
- 122 Echinococcosis
- 123 Other cestode infection
- 124 Trichinosis
- 125 Filarial infection and dracontiasis
- 126 Ancylostomiasis and necatoriasis
- 127 Other intestinal helminthiases
- 128 Other and unspecified helminthiases
- 129 Intestinal parasitism, unspecified

Other infectious and parasitic diseases (130–136)
- 130 Toxoplasmosis
- 131 Trichomoniasis
- 132 Pediculosis and phthirus infestation
- 133 Acariasis
- 134 Other infestation
- 135 Sarcoidosis
- 136 Other and unspecified infectious and parasitic diseases

Late effects of infectious and parasitic diseases (137–139)
- 137 Late effects of tuberculosis
- 138 Late effects of acute poliomyelitis
- 139 Late effects of other infectious and parasitic diseases

PART III / Appendix E List of Three-Digit Categories

2. NEOPLASMS

Malignant neoplasm of lip, oral cavity, and pharynx (140–149)
140 Malignant neoplasm of lip
141 Malignant neoplasm of tongue
142 Malignant neoplasm of major salivary glands
143 Malignant neoplasm of gum
144 Malignant neoplasm of floor of mouth
145 Malignant neoplasm of other and unspecified parts of mouth
146 Malignant neoplasm of oropharynx
147 Malignant neoplasm of nasopharynx
148 Malignant neoplasm of hypopharynx
149 Malignant neoplasm of other and ill-defined sites within the lip, oral cavity, and pharynx

Malignant neoplasm of digestive organs and peritoneum (150–159)
150 Malignant neoplasm of esophagus
151 Malignant neoplasm of stomach
152 Malignant neoplasm of small intestine, including duodenum
153 Malignant neoplasm of colon
154 Malignant neoplasm of rectum, rectosigmoid junction, and anus
155 Malignant neoplasm of liver and intrahepatic bile ducts
156 Malignant neoplasm of gallbladder and extrahepatic bile ducts
157 Malignant neoplasm of pancreas
158 Malignant neoplasm of retroperitoneum and peritoneum
159 Malignant neoplasm of other and ill-defined sites within the digestive organs and peritoneum

Malignant neoplasm of respiratory and intrathoracic organs (160–165)
160 Malignant neoplasm of nasal cavities, middle ear, and accessory sinuses
161 Malignant neoplasm of larynx
162 Malignant neoplasm of trachea, bronchus, and lung
163 Malignant neoplasm of pleura
164 Malignant neoplasm of thymus, heart, and mediastinum
165 Malignant neoplasm of other and ill-defined sites within the respiratory system and intrathoracic organs

Malignant neoplasm of bone, connective tissue, skin, and breast (170–176)
170 Malignant neoplasm of bone and articular cartilage
171 Malignant neoplasm of connective and other soft tissue
172 Malignant melanoma of skin
173 Other malignant neoplasm of skin
174 Malignant neoplasm of female breast
175 Malignant neoplasm of male breast

Kaposi's sarcoma (176)
176 Kaposi's sarcoma

Malignant neoplasm of genitourinary organs (179–189)
179 Malignant neoplasm of uterus, part unspecified
180 Malignant neoplasm of cervix uteri
181 Malignant neoplasm of placenta
182 Malignant neoplasm of body of uterus
183 Malignant neoplasm of ovary and other uterine adnexa
184 Malignant neoplasm of other and unspecified female genital organs
185 Malignant neoplasm of prostate
186 Malignant neoplasm of testis
187 Malignant neoplasm of penis and other male genital organs
188 Malignant neoplasm of bladder
189 Malignant neoplasm of kidney and other and unspecified urinary organs

Malignant neoplasm of other and unspecified sites (190–199)
190 Malignant neoplasm of eye
191 Malignant neoplasm of brain
192 Malignant neoplasm of other and unspecified parts of nervous system
193 Malignant neoplasm of thyroid gland
194 Malignant neoplasm of other endocrine glands and related structures
195 Malignant neoplasm of other and ill-defined sites
196 Secondary and unspecified malignant neoplasm of lymph nodes
197 Secondary malignant neoplasm of respiratory and digestive systems
198 Secondary malignant neoplasm of other specified sites
199 Malignant neoplasm without specification of site

Malignant neoplasm of lymphatic and hematopoietic tissue (200–208)
200 Lymphosarcoma and reticulosarcoma
201 Hodgkin's disease
202 Other malignant neoplasm of lymphoid and histiocytic tissue
203 Multiple myeloma and immunoproliferative neoplasms
204 Lymphoid leukemia
205 Myeloid leukemia
206 Monocytic leukemia
207 Other specified leukemia
208 Leukemia of unspecified cell type

Neuroendocrine tumors (209)
209 Neuroendocrine tumors

Benign neoplasms (210–229)
210 Benign neoplasm of lip, oral cavity, and pharynx
211 Benign neoplasm of other parts of digestive system
212 Benign neoplasm of respiratory and intrathoracic organs
213 Benign neoplasm of bone and articular cartilage
214 Lipoma
215 Other benign neoplasm of connective and other soft tissue
216 Benign neoplasm of skin
217 Benign neoplasm of breast
218 Uterine leiomyoma
219 Other benign neoplasm of uterus
220 Benign neoplasm of ovary
221 Benign neoplasm of other female genital organs
222 Benign neoplasm of male genital organs
223 Benign neoplasm of kidney and other urinary organs
224 Benign neoplasm of eye
225 Benign neoplasm of brain and other parts of nervous system
226 Benign neoplasm of thyroid gland
227 Benign neoplasm of other endocrine glands and related structures
228 Hemangioma and lymphangioma, any site
229 Benign neoplasm of other and unspecified sites

Carcinoma in situ (230–234)
230 Carcinoma in situ of digestive organs
231 Carcinoma in situ of respiratory system
232 Carcinoma in situ of skin
233 Carcinoma in situ of breast and genitourinary system
234 Carcinoma in situ of other and unspecified sites

Neoplasms of uncertain behavior (235–238)
235 Neoplasm of uncertain behavior of digestive and respiratory systems
236 Neoplasm of uncertain behavior of genitourinary organs
237 Neoplasm of uncertain behavior of endocrine glands and nervous system
238 Neoplasm of uncertain behavior of other and unspecified sites and tissues

Neoplasms of unspecified nature (239)
239 Neoplasm of unspecified nature

3. ENDOCRINE, NUTRITIONAL AND METABOLIC DISEASES, AND IMMUNITY DISORDERS

Disorders of thyroid gland (240–246)
240 Simple and unspecified goiter
241 Nontoxic nodular goiter
242 Thyrotoxicosis with or without goiter
243 Congenital hypothyroidism
244 Acquired hypothyroidism
245 Thyroiditis
246 Other disorders of thyroid

Diseases of other endocrine glands (249–259)
249 Secondary diabetes mellitus
250 Diabetes mellitus
251 Other disorders of pancreatic internal secretion
252 Disorders of parathyroid gland
253 Disorders of the pituitary gland and its hypothalamic control
254 Diseases of thymus gland
255 Disorders of adrenal glands
256 Ovarian dysfunction
257 Testicular dysfunction
258 Polyglandular dysfunction and related disorders
259 Other endocrine disorders

ICD-9-CM

Nutritional deficiencies (260–269)
260 Kwashiorkor
261 Nutritional marasmus
262 Other severe protein-calorie malnutrition
263 Other and unspecified protein-calorie malnutrition
264 Vitamin A deficiency
265 Thiamine and niacin deficiency states
266 Deficiency of B-complex components
267 Ascorbic acid deficiency
268 Vitamin D deficiency
269 Other nutritional deficiencies

Other metabolic disorders and immunity disorders (270–279)
270 Disorders of amino-acid transport and metabolism
271 Disorders of carbohydrate transport and metabolism
272 Disorders of lipoid metabolism
273 Disorders of plasma protein metabolism
274 Gout
275 Disorders of mineral metabolism
276 Disorders of fluid, electrolyte, and acid-base balance
277 Other and unspecified disorders of metabolism
278 Obesity and other hyperalimentation
279 Disorders involving the immune mechanism

4. DISEASES OF BLOOD AND BLOOD-FORMING ORGANS

Diseases of the blood and blood-forming organs (280–289)
280 Iron deficiency anemias
281 Other deficiency anemias
282 Hereditary hemolytic anemias
283 Acquired hemolytic anemias
284 Aplastic anemia
285 Other and unspecified anemias
286 Coagulation defects
287 Purpura and other hemorrhagic conditions
288 Diseases of white blood cells
289 Other diseases of blood and blood-forming organs

5. MENTAL DISORDERS

Organic psychotic conditions (290–294)
290 Senile and presenile organic psychotic conditions
291 Alcoholic psychoses
292 Drug psychoses
293 Transient organic psychotic conditions
294 Other organic psychotic conditions (chronic)

Other psychoses (295–299)
295 Schizophrenic psychoses
296 Affective psychoses
297 Paranoid states
298 Other nonorganic psychoses
299 Psychoses with origin specific to childhood

Neurotic disorders, personality disorders, and other nonpsychotic mental disorders (300–316)
300 Neurotic disorders
301 Personality disorders
302 Sexual deviations and disorders
303 Alcohol dependence syndrome
304 Drug dependence
305 Nondependent abuse of drugs
306 Physiological malfunction arising from mental factors
307 Special symptoms or syndromes, not elsewhere classified
308 Acute reaction to stress
309 Adjustment reaction
310 Specific nonpsychotic mental disorders following organic brain damage
311 Depressive disorder, not elsewhere classified
312 Disturbance of conduct, not elsewhere classified
313 Disturbance of emotions specific to childhood and adolescence
314 Hyperkinetic syndrome of childhood
315 Specific delays in development
316 Psychic factors associated with diseases classified elsewhere

Mental retardation (317–319)
317 Mild mental retardation
318 Other specified mental retardation
319 Unspecified mental retardation

6. DISEASES OF THE NERVOUS SYSTEM AND SENSE ORGANS

Inflammatory diseases of the central nervous system (320–326)
320 Bacterial meningitis
321 Meningitis due to other organisms
322 Meningitis of unspecified cause
323 Encephalitis, myelitis, and encephalomyelitis
324 Intracranial and intraspinal abscess
325 Phlebitis and thrombophlebitis of intracranial venous sinuses
326 Late effects of intracranial abscess or pyogenic infection
327 Organic sleep disorders

Hereditary and degenerative diseases of the central nervous system (330–337)
330 Cerebral degenerations usually manifest in childhood
331 Other cerebral degenerations
332 Parkinson's disease
333 Other extrapyramidal disease and abnormal movement disorders
334 Spinocerebellar disease
335 Anterior horn cell disease
336 Other diseases of spinal cord
337 Disorders of the autonomic nervous system

Pain (338)
338 Pain, not elsewhere classified

Other headache syndromes (339)
339 Other headache syndromes

Other disorders of the central nervous system (340–349)
340 Multiple sclerosis
341 Other demyelinating diseases of central nervous system
342 Hemiplegia and hemiparesis
343 Infantile cerebral palsy
344 Other paralytic syndromes
345 Epilepsy
346 Migraine
347 Cataplexy and narcolepsy
348 Other conditions of brain
349 Other and unspecified disorders of the nervous system

Disorders of the peripheral nervous system (350–359)
350 Trigeminal nerve disorders
351 Facial nerve disorders
352 Disorders of other cranial nerves
353 Nerve root and plexus disorders
354 Mononeuritis of upper limb and mononeuritis multiplex
355 Mononeuritis of lower limb
356 Hereditary and idiopathic peripheral neuropathy
357 Inflammatory and toxic neuropathy
358 Myoneural disorders
359 Muscular dystrophies and other myopathies

Disorders of the eye and adnexa (360–379)
360 Disorders of the globe
361 Retinal detachments and defects
362 Other retinal disorders
363 Chorioretinal inflammations and scars and other disorders of choroid
364 Disorders of iris and ciliary body
365 Glaucoma
366 Cataract
367 Disorders of refraction and accommodation
368 Visual disturbances
369 Blindness and low vision
370 Keratitis
371 Corneal opacity and other disorders of cornea
372 Disorders of conjunctiva
373 Inflammation of eyelids
374 Other disorders of eyelids
375 Disorders of lacrimal system
376 Disorders of the orbit
377 Disorders of optic nerve and visual pathways
378 Strabismus and other disorders of binocular eye movements
379 Other disorders of eye

Diseases of the ear and mastoid process (380–389)
380 Disorders of external ear
381 Nonsuppurative otitis media and Eustachian tube disorders

382	Suppurative and unspecified otitis media
383	Mastoiditis and related conditions
384	Other disorders of tympanic membrane
385	Other disorders of middle ear and mastoid
386	Vertiginous syndromes and other disorders of vestibular system
387	Otosclerosis
388	Other disorders of ear
389	Hearing loss

7. DISEASES OF THE CIRCULATORY SYSTEM

Acute rheumatic fever (390–392)

390	Rheumatic fever without mention of heart involvement
391	Rheumatic fever with heart involvement
392	Rheumatic chorea

Chronic rheumatic heart disease (393–398)

393	Chronic rheumatic pericarditis
394	Diseases of mitral valve
395	Diseases of aortic valve
396	Diseases of mitral and aortic valves
397	Diseases of other endocardial structures
398	Other rheumatic heart disease

Hypertensive disease (401–405)

401	Essential hypertension
402	Hypertensive heart disease
403	Hypertensive renal disease
404	Hypertensive heart and renal disease
405	Secondary hypertension

Ischemic heart disease (410–414)

410	Acute myocardial infarction
411	Other acute and subacute form of ischemic heart disease
412	Old myocardial infarction
413	Angina pectoris
414	Other forms of chronic ischemic heart disease

Diseases of pulmonary circulation (415–417)

415	Acute pulmonary heart disease
416	Chronic pulmonary heart disease
417	Other diseases of pulmonary circulation

Other forms of heart disease (420–429)

420	Acute pericarditis
421	Acute and subacute endocarditis
422	Acute myocarditis
423	Other diseases of pericardium
424	Other diseases of endocardium
425	Cardiomyopathy
426	Conduction disorders
427	Cardiac dysrhythmias
428	Heart failure
429	Ill-defined descriptions and complications of heart disease

Cerebrovascular disease (430–438)

430	Subarachnoid hemorrhage
431	Intracerebral hemorrhage
432	Other and unspecified intracranial hemorrhage
433	Occlusion and stenosis of precerebral arteries
434	Occlusion of cerebral arteries
435	Transcient cerebral ischemia
436	Acute but ill-defined cerebrovascular disease
437	Other and ill-defined cerebrovascular disease
438	Late effects of cerebrovascular disease

Diseases of arteries, arterioles, and capillaries (440–448)

440	Atherosclerosis
441	Aortic aneurysm and dissection
442	Other aneurysm
443	Other peripheral vascular disease
444	Arterial embolism and thrombosis
445	Atheroembolism
446	Polyarteritis nodosa and allied conditions
447	Other disorders of arteries and arterioles
448	Diseases of capillaries

Diseases of veins and lymphatics, and other diseases of circulatory system (451–459)

451	Phlebitis and thrombophlebitis
452	Portal vein thrombosis
453	Other venous embolism and thrombosis
454	Varicose veins of lower extremities
455	Hemorrhoids
456	Varicose veins of other sites
457	Noninfective disorders of lymphatic channels
458	Hypotension
459	Other disorders of circulatory system

8. DISEASES OF THE RESPIRATORY SYSTEM

Acute respiratory infections (460–466)

460	Acute nasopharyngitis [common cold]
461	Acute sinusitis
462	Acute pharyngitis
463	Acute tonsillitis
464	Acute laryngitis and tracheitis
465	Acute upper respiratory infections of multiple or unspecified sites
466	Acute bronchitis and bronchiolitis

Other diseases of upper respiratory tract (470–478)

470	Deviated nasal septum
471	Nasal polyps
472	Chronic pharyngitis and nasopharyngitis
473	Chronic sinusitis
474	Chronic disease of tonsils and adenoids
475	Peritonsillar abscess
476	Chronic laryngitis and laryngotracheitis
477	Allergic rhinitis
478	Other diseases of upper respiratory tract

Pneumonia and influenza (480–488)

480	Viral pneumonia
481	Pneumococcal pneumonia [*Streptococcus pneumoniae* pneumonia]
482	Other bacterial pneumonia
483	Pneumonia due to other specified organism
484	Pneumonia in infectious diseases classified elsewhere
485	Bronchopneumonia, organism unspecified
486	Pneumonia, organism unspecified
487	Influenza
488	Influenza due to identified avian influenza virus

Chronic obstructive pulmonary disease and allied conditions (490–496)

490	Bronchitis, not specified as acute or chronic
491	Chronic bronchitis
492	Emphysema
493	Asthma
494	Bronchiectasis
495	Extrinsic allergic alveolitis
496	Chronic airways obstruction, not elsewhere classified

Pneumoconioses and other lung diseases due to external agents (500–508)

500	Coalworkers' pneumoconiosis
501	Asbestosis
502	Pneumoconiosis due to other silica or silicates
503	Pneumoconiosis due to other inorganic dust
504	Pneumopathy due to inhalation of other dust
505	Pneumoconiosis, unspecified
506	Respiratory conditions due to chemical fumes and vapors
507	Pneumonitis due to solids and liquids
508	Respiratory conditions due to other and unspecified external agents

Other diseases of respiratory system (510–519)

510	Empyema
511	Pleurisy
512	Pneumothorax
513	Abscess of lung and mediastinum
514	Pulmonary congestion and hypostasis
515	Postinflammatory pulmonary fibrosis
516	Other alveolar and parietoalveolar pneumopathy
517	Lung involvement in conditions classified elsewhere
518	Other diseases of lung
519	Other diseases of respiratory system

9. DISEASES OF THE DIGESTIVE SYSTEM

Diseases of oral cavity, salivary glands, and jaws (520–529)
520 Disorders of tooth development and eruption
521 Diseases of hard tissues of teeth
522 Diseases of pulp and periapical tissues
523 Gingival and periodontal diseases
524 Dentofacial anomalies, including malocclusion
525 Other diseases and conditions of the teeth and supporting structures
526 Diseases of the jaws
527 Diseases of the salivary glands
528 Diseases of the oral soft tissues, excluding lesions specific for gingiva and tongue
529 Diseases and other conditions of the tongue

Diseases of esophagus, stomach, and duodenum (530–538)
530 Diseases of esophagus
531 Gastric ulcer
532 Duodenal ulcer
533 Peptic ulcer, site unspecified
534 Gastrojejunal ulcer
535 Gastritis and duodenitis
536 Disorders of function of stomach
537 Other disorders of stomach and duodenum
538 Gastrointestinal mucositis (ulcerative)

Appendicitis (540–543)
540 Acute appendicitis
541 Appendicitis, unqualified
542 Other appendicitis
543 Other diseases of appendix

Hernia of abdominal cavity (550–553)
550 Inguinal hernia
551 Other hernia of abdominal cavity, with gangrene
552 Other hernia of abdominal cavity, with obstruction, but without mention of gangrene
553 Other hernia of abdominal cavity without mention of obstruction or gangrene

Noninfective enteritis and colitis (555–558)
555 Regional enteritis
556 Ulcerative colitis
557 Vascular insufficiency of intestine
558 Other noninfective gastroenteritis and colitis

Other diseases of intestines and peritoneum (560–569)
560 Intestinal obstruction without mention of hernia
562 Diverticula of intestine
564 Functional digestive disorders, not elsewhere classified
565 Anal fissure and fistula
566 Abscess of anal and rectal regions
567 Peritonitis
568 Other disorders of peritoneum
569 Other disorders of intestine

Other diseases of digestive system (570–579)
570 Acute and subacute necrosis of liver
571 Chronic liver disease and cirrhosis
572 Liver abscess and sequelae of chronic liver disease
573 Other disorders of liver
574 Cholelithiasis
575 Other disorders of gallbladder
576 Other disorders of biliary tract
577 Diseases of pancreas
578 Gastrointestinal hemorrhage
579 Intestinal malabsorption

10. DISEASES OF THE GENITOURINARY SYSTEM

Nephritis, nephrotic syndrome, and nephrosis (580–589)
580 Acute glomerulonephritis
581 Nephrotic syndrome
582 Chronic glomerulonephritis
583 Nephritis and nephropathy, not specified as acute or chronic
584 Acute renal failure
585 Chronic renal failure
586 Renal failure, unspecified
587 Renal sclerosis, unspecified
588 Disorders resulting from impaired renal function
589 Small kidney of unknown cause

Other diseases of urinary system (590–599)
590 Infections of kidney
591 Hydronephrosis
592 Calculus of kidney and ureter
593 Other disorders of kidney and ureter
594 Calculus of lower urinary tract
595 Cystitis
596 Other disorders of bladder
597 Urethritis, not sexually transmitted, and urethral syndrome
598 Urethral stricture
599 Other disorders of urethra and urinary tract

Diseases of male genital organs (600–608)
600 Hyperplasia of prostate
601 Inflammatory diseases of prostate
602 Other disorders of prostate
603 Hydrocele
604 Orchitis and epididymitis
605 Redundant prepuce and phimosis
606 Infertility, male
607 Disorders of penis
608 Other disorders of male genital organs

Disorders of breast (610–611)
610 Benign mammary dysplasias
611 Other disorders of breast
612 Deformity and disproportion of reconstructed breast

Inflammatory disease of female pelvic organs (614–616)
614 Inflammatory disease of ovary, fallopian tube, pelvic cellular tissue, and peritoneum
615 Inflammatory diseases of uterus, except cervix
616 Inflammatory disease of cervix, vagina, and vulva

Other disorders of female genital tract (617–629)
617 Endometriosis
618 Genital prolapse
619 Fistula involving female genital tract
620 Noninflammatory disorders of ovary, fallopian tube, and broad ligament
621 Disorders of uterus, not elsewhere classified
622 Noninflammatory disorders of cervix
623 Noninflammatory disorders of vagina
624 Noninflammatory disorders of vulva and perineum
625 Pain and other symptoms associated with female genital organs
626 Disorders of menstruation and other abnormal bleeding from female genital tract
627 Menopausal and postmenopausal disorders
628 Infertility, female
629 Other disorders of female genital organs

11. COMPLICATIONS OF PREGNANCY, CHILDBIRTH, AND THE PUERPERIUM

Ectopic and molar pregnancy and other pregnancy with abortive outcome (630–639)
630 Hydatidiform mole
631 Other abnormal product of conception
632 Missed abortion
633 Ectopic pregnancy
634 Spontaneous abortion
635 Legally induced abortion
636 Illegally induced abortion
637 Unspecified abortion
638 Failed attempted abortion
639 Complications following abortion and ectopic and molar pregnancies

Complications mainly related to pregnancy (640–649)
640 Hemorrhage in early pregnancy
641 Antepartum hemorrhage, abruptio placentae, and placenta previa
642 Hypertension complicating pregnancy, childbirth, and the puerperium
643 Excessive vomiting in pregnancy
644 Early or threatened labor
645 Prolonged pregnancy
646 Other complications of pregnancy, not elsewhere classified
647 Infective and parasitic conditions in the mother classifiable elsewhere but complicating pregnancy, childbirth, and the puerperium

648 Other current conditions in the mother classifiable elsewhere but complicating pregnancy, childbirth, and the puerperium
649 Other conditions or status of the mother complicating pregnancy, childbirth, or the puerperium

Normal delivery, and other indications for care in pregnancy, labor, and delivery (650–659)
650 Normal delivery
651 Multiple gestation
652 Malposition and malpresentation of fetus
653 Disproportion
654 Abnormality of organs and soft tissues of pelvis
655 Known or suspected fetal abnormality affecting management of mother
656 Other fetal and placental problems affecting management of mother
657 Polyhydramnios
658 Other problems associated with amniotic cavity and membranes
659 Other indications for care or intervention related to labor and delivery and not elsewhere classified

Complications occurring mainly in the course of labor and delivery (660–669)
660 Obstructed labor
661 Abnormality of forces of labor
662 Long labor
663 Umbilical cord complications
664 Trauma to perineum and vulva during delivery
665 Other obstetrical trauma
666 Postpartum hemorrhage
667 Retained placenta or membranes, without hemorrhage
668 Complications of the administration of anesthetic or other sedation in labor and delivery
669 Other complications of labor and delivery, not elsewhere classified

Complications of the puerperium (670–677)
670 Major puerperal infection
671 Venous complications in pregnancy and the puerperium
672 Pyrexia of unknown origin during the puerperium
673 Obstetrical pulmonary embolism
674 Other and unspecified complications of the puerperium, not elsewhere classified
675 Infections of the breast and nipple associated with childbirth
676 Other disorders of the breast associated with childbirth, and disorders of lactation
677 Late effect of complication of pregnancy, childbirth, and the puerperium

Other Maternal and Fetal Complications (678-679)
678 Other fetal conditions
679 Complications of in utero procedures

12. DISEASES OF THE SKIN AND SUBCUTANEOUS TISSUE

Infections of skin and subcutaneous tissue (680–686)
680 Carbuncle and furuncle
681 Cellulitis and abscess of finger and toe
682 Other cellulitis and abscess
683 Acute lymphadenitis
684 Impetigo
685 Pilonidal cyst
686 Other local infections of skin and subcutaneous tissue

Other inflammatory conditions of skin and subcutaneous tissue (690–698)
690 Erythematosquamous dermatosis
691 Atopic dermatitis and related conditions
692 Contact dermatitis and other eczema
693 Dermatitis due to substances taken internally
694 Bullous dermatoses
695 Erythematous conditions
696 Psoriasis and similar disorders
697 Lichen
698 Pruritus and related conditions

Other diseases of skin and subcutaneous tissue (700–709)
700 Corns and callosities
701 Other hypertrophic and atrophic conditions of skin
702 Other dermatoses
703 Diseases of nail
704 Diseases of hair and hair follicles
705 Disorders of sweat glands
706 Diseases of sebaceous glands
707 Chronic ulcer of skin
708 Urticaria
709 Other disorders of skin and subcutaneous tissue

13. DISEASES OF THE MUSCULOSKELETAL SYSTEM AND CONNECTIVE TISSUE

Arthropathies and related disorders (710–719)
710 Diffuse diseases of connective tissue
711 Arthropathy associated with infections
712 Crystal arthropathies
713 Arthropathy associated with other disorders classified elsewhere
714 Rheumatoid arthritis and other inflammatory polyarthropathies
715 Osteoarthrosis and allied disorders
716 Other and unspecified arthropathies
717 Internal derangement of knee
718 Other derangement of joint
719 Other and unspecified disorder of joint

Dorsopathies (720–724)
720 Ankylosing spondylitis and other inflammatory spondylopathies
721 Spondylosis and allied disorders
722 Intervertebral disc disorders
723 Other disorders of cervical region
724 Other and unspecified disorders of back

Rheumatism, excluding the back (725–729)
725 Polymyalgia rheumatica
726 Peripheral enthesopathies and allied syndromes
727 Other disorders of synovium, tendon, and bursa
728 Disorders of muscle, ligament, and fascia
729 Other disorders of soft tissues

Osteopathies, chondropathies, and acquired musculoskeletal deformities (730–739)
730 Osteomyelitis, periostitis, and other infections involving bone
731 Osteitis deformans and osteopathies associated with other disorders classified elsewhere
732 Osteochondropathies
733 Other disorders of bone and cartilage
734 Flat foot
735 Acquired deformities of toe
736 Other acquired deformities of limbs
737 Curvature of spine
738 Other acquired deformity
739 Nonallopathic lesions, not elsewhere classified

14. CONGENITAL ANOMALIES

Congenital anomalies (740–759)
740 Anencephalus and similar anomalies
741 Spina bifida
742 Other congenital anomalies of nervous system
743 Congenital anomalies of eye
744 Congenital anomalies of ear, face, and neck
745 Bulbus cordis anomalies and anomalies of cardiac septal closure
746 Other congenital anomalies of heart
747 Other congenital anomalies of circulatory system
748 Congenital anomalies of respiratory system
749 Cleft palate and cleft lip
750 Other congenital anomalies of upper alimentary tract
751 Other congenital anomalies of digestive system
752 Congenital anomalies of genital organs
753 Congenital anomalies of urinary system
754 Certain congenital musculoskeletal deformities
755 Other congenital anomalies of limbs
756 Other congenital musculoskeletal anomalies
757 Congenital anomalies of the integument
758 Chromosomal anomalies
759 Other and unspecified congenital anomalies

15. CERTAIN CONDITIONS ORIGINATING IN THE PERINATAL PERIOD

Maternal causes of perinatal morbidity and mortality (760–763)
- 760 Fetus or newborn affected by maternal conditions which may be unrelated to present pregnancy
- 761 Fetus or newborn affected by maternal complications of pregnancy
- 762 Fetus or newborn affected by complications of placenta, cord, and membranes
- 763 Fetus or newborn affected by other complications of labor and delivery

Other conditions originating in the perinatal period (764–779)
- 764 Slow fetal growth and fetal malnutrition
- 765 Disorders relating to short gestation and unspecified low birthweight
- 766 Disorders relating to long gestation and high birthweight
- 767 Birth trauma
- 768 Intrauterine hypoxia and birth asphyxia
- 769 Respiratory distress syndrome
- 770 Other respiratory conditions of fetus and newborn
- 771 Infections specific to the perinatal period
- 772 Fetal and neonatal hemorrhage
- 773 Hemolytic disease of fetus or newborn, due to isoimmunization
- 774 Other perinatal jaundice
- 775 Endocrine and metabolic disturbances specific to the fetus and newborn
- 776 Hematological disorders of fetus and newborn
- 777 Perinatal disorders of digestive system
- 778 Conditions involving the integument and temperature regulation of fetus and newborn
- 779 Other and ill-defined conditions originating in the perinatal period

16. SYMPTOMS, SIGNS, AND ILL-DEFINED CONDITIONS

Symptoms (780–789)
- 780 General symptoms
- 781 Symptoms involving nervous and musculoskeletal systems
- 782 Symptoms involving skin and other integumentary tissue
- 783 Symptoms concerning nutrition, metabolism, and development
- 784 Symptoms involving head and neck
- 785 Symptoms involving cardiovascular system
- 786 Symptoms involving respiratory system and other chest symptoms
- 787 Symptoms involving digestive system
- 788 Symptoms involving urinary system
- 789 Other symptoms involving abdomen and pelvis

Nonspecific abnormal findings (790–796)
- 790 Nonspecific findings on examination of blood
- 791 Nonspecific findings on examination of urine
- 792 Nonspecific abnormal findings in other body substances
- 793 Nonspecific abnormal findings on radiological and other examination of body structure
- 794 Nonspecific abnormal results of function studies
- 795 Nonspecific abnormal histological and immunological findings
- 796 Other nonspecific abnormal findings

Ill-defined and unknown causes of morbidity and mortality (797–799)
- 797 Senility without mention of psychosis
- 798 Sudden death, cause unknown
- 799 Other ill-defined and unknown causes of morbidity and mortality

17. INJURY AND POISONING

Fracture of skull (800–804)
- 800 Fracture of vault of skull
- 801 Fracture of base of skull
- 802 Fracture of face bones
- 803 Other and unqualified skull fractures
- 804 Multiple fractures involving skull or face with other bones

Fracture of spine and trunk (805–809)
- 805 Fracture of vertebral column without mention of spinal cord lesion
- 806 Fracture of vertebral column with spinal cord lesion
- 807 Fracture of rib(s), sternum, larynx, and trachea
- 808 Fracture of pelvis
- 809 Ill-defined fractures of bones of trunk

Fracture of upper limb (810–819)
- 810 Fracture of clavicle
- 811 Fracture of scapula
- 812 Fracture of humerus
- 813 Fracture of radius and ulna
- 814 Fracture of carpal bone(s)
- 815 Fracture of metacarpal bone(s)
- 816 Fracture of one or more phalanges of hand
- 817 Multiple fractures of hand bones
- 818 Ill-defined fractures of upper limb
- 819 Multiple fractures involving both upper limbs, and upper limb with rib(s) and sternum

Fracture of lower limb (820–829)
- 820 Fracture of neck of femur
- 821 Fracture of other and unspecified parts of femur
- 822 Fracture of patella
- 823 Fracture of tibia and fibula
- 824 Fracture of ankle
- 825 Fracture of one or more tarsal and metatarsal bones
- 826 Fracture of one or more phalanges of foot
- 827 Other, multiple, and ill-defined fractures of lower limb
- 828 Multiple fractures involving both lower limbs, lower with upper limb, and lower limb(s) with rib(s) and sternum
- 829 Fracture of unspecified bones

Dislocation (830–839)
- 830 Dislocation of jaw
- 831 Dislocation of shoulder
- 832 Dislocation of elbow
- 833 Dislocation of wrist
- 834 Dislocation of finger
- 835 Dislocation of hip
- 836 Dislocation of knee
- 837 Dislocation of ankle
- 838 Dislocation of foot
- 839 Other, multiple, and ill-defined dislocations

Sprains and strains of joints and adjacent muscles (840–848)
- 840 Sprains and strains of shoulder and upper arm
- 841 Sprains and strains of elbow and forearm
- 842 Sprains and strains of wrist and hand
- 843 Sprains and strains of hip and thigh
- 844 Sprains and strains of knee and leg
- 845 Sprains and strains of ankle and foot
- 846 Sprains and strains of sacroiliac region
- 847 Sprains and strains of other and unspecified parts of back
- 848 Other and ill-defined sprains and strains

Intracranial injury, excluding those with skull fracture (850–854)
- 850 Concussion
- 851 Cerebral laceration and contusion
- 852 Subarachnoid, subdural, and extradural hemorrhage, following injury
- 853 Other and unspecified intracranial hemorrhage following injury
- 854 Intracranial injury of other and unspecified nature

Internal injury of chest, abdomen, and pelvis (860–869)
- 860 Traumatic pneumothorax and hemothorax
- 861 Injury to heart and lung
- 862 Injury to other and unspecified intrathoracic organs
- 863 Injury to gastrointestinal tract
- 864 Injury to liver
- 865 Injury to spleen
- 866 Injury to kidney
- 867 Injury to pelvic organs
- 868 Injury to other intra-abdominal organs
- 869 Internal injury to unspecified or ill-defined organs

Open wound of head, neck, and trunk (870–879)
- 870 Open wound of ocular adnexa
- 871 Open wound of eyeball
- 872 Open wound of ear
- 873 Other open wound of head
- 874 Open wound of neck
- 875 Open wound of chest (wall)
- 876 Open wound of back
- 877 Open wound of buttock
- 878 Open wound of genital organs (external), including traumatic amputation
- 879 Open wound of other and unspecified sites, except limbs

PART III / Appendix E List of Three-Digit Categories

Open wound of upper limb (880–887)
880 Open wound of shoulder and upper arm
881 Open wound of elbow, forearm, and wrist
882 Open wound of hand except finger(s) alone
883 Open wound of finger(s)
884 Multiple and unspecified open wound of upper limb
885 Traumatic amputation of thumb (complete) (partial)
886 Traumatic amputation of other finger(s) (complete) (partial)
887 Traumatic amputation of arm and hand (complete) (partial)

Open wound of lower limb (890–897)
890 Open wound of hip and thigh
891 Open wound of knee, leg [except thigh], and ankle
892 Open wound of foot except toe(s) alone
893 Open wound of toe(s)
894 Multiple and unspecified open wound of lower limb
895 Traumatic amputation of toe(s) (complete) (partial)
896 Traumatic amputation of foot (complete) (partial)
897 Traumatic amputation of leg(s) (complete) (partial)

Injury to blood vessels (900–904)
900 Injury to blood vessels of head and neck
901 Injury to blood vessels of thorax
902 Injury to blood vessels of abdomen and pelvis
903 Injury to blood vessels of upper extremity
904 Injury to blood vessels of lower extremity and unspecified sites

Late effects of injuries, poisonings, toxic effects, and other external causes (905–909)
905 Late effects of musculoskeletal and connective tissue injuries
906 Late effects of injuries to skin and subcutaneous tissues
907 Late effects of injuries to the nervous system
908 Late effects of other and unspecified injuries
909 Late effects of other and unspecified external causes

Superficial injury (910–919)
910 Superficial injury of face, neck, and scalp except eye
911 Superficial injury of trunk
912 Superficial injury of shoulder and upper arm
913 Superficial injury of elbow, forearm, and wrist
914 Superficial injury of hand(s) except finger(s) alone
915 Superficial injury of finger(s)
916 Superficial injury of hip, thigh, leg, and ankle
917 Superficial injury of foot and toe(s)
918 Superficial injury of eye and adnexa
919 Superficial injury of other, multiple, and unspecified sites

Contusion with intact skin surface (920–924)
920 Contusion of face, scalp, and neck except eye(s)
921 Contusion of eye and adnexa
922 Contusion of trunk
923 Contusion of upper limb
924 Contusion of lower limb and of other and unspecified sites

Crushing injury (925–929)
925 Crushing injury of face, scalp, and neck
926 Crushing injury of trunk
927 Crushing injury of upper limb
928 Crushing injury of lower limb
929 Crushing injury of multiple and unspecified sites

Effects of foreign body entering through orifice (930–939)
930 Foreign body on external eye
931 Foreign body in ear
932 Foreign body in nose
933 Foreign body in pharynx and larynx
934 Foreign body in trachea, bronchus, and lung
935 Foreign body in mouth, esophagus, and stomach
936 Foreign body in intestine and colon
937 Foreign body in anus and rectum
938 Foreign body in digestive system, unspecified
939 Foreign body in genitourinary tract

Burns (940–949)
940 Burn confined to eye and adnexa
941 Burn of face, head, and neck
942 Burn of trunk
943 Burn of upper limb, except wrist and hand
944 Burn of wrist(s) and hand(s)
945 Burn of lower limb(s)
946 Burns of multiple specified sites
947 Burn of internal organs
948 Burns classified according to extent of body surface involved
949 Burn, unspecified

Injury to nerves and spinal cord (950–957)
950 Injury to optic nerve and pathways
951 Injury to other cranial nerve(s)
952 Spinal cord injury without evidence of spinal bone injury
953 Injury to nerve roots and spinal plexus
954 Injury to other nerve(s) of trunk excluding shoulder and pelvic girdles
955 Injury to peripheral nerve(s) of shoulder girdle and upper limb
956 Injury to peripheral nerve(s) of pelvic girdle and lower limb
957 Injury to other and unspecified nerves

Certain traumatic complications and unspecified injuries (958–959)
958 Certain early complications of trauma
959 Injury, other and unspecified

Poisoning by drugs, medicinals and biological substances (960–979)
960 Poisoning by antibiotics
961 Poisoning by other anti-infectives
962 Poisoning by hormones and synthetic substitutes
963 Poisoning by primarily systemic agents
964 Poisoning by agents primarily affecting blood constituents
965 Poisoning by analgesics, antipyretics, and antirheumatics
966 Poisoning by anticonvulsants and anti-Parkinsonism drugs
967 Poisoning by sedatives and hypnotics
968 Poisoning by other central nervous system depressants and anesthetics
969 Poisoning by psychotropic agents
970 Poisoning by central nervous system stimulants
971 Poisoning by drugs primarily affecting the autonomic nervous system
972 Poisoning by agents primarily affecting the cardiovascular system
973 Poisoning by agents primarily affecting the gastrointestinal system
974 Poisoning by water, mineral, and uric acid metabolism drugs
975 Poisoning by agents primarily acting on the smooth and skeletal muscles and respiratory system
976 Poisoning by agents primarily affecting skin and mucous membrane, ophthalmological, otorhinolaryngological, and dental drugs
977 Poisoning by other and unspecified drugs and medicinals
978 Poisoning by bacterial vaccines
979 Poisoning by other vaccines and biological substances

Toxic effects of substances chiefly nonmedicinal as to source (980–989)
980 Toxic effect of alcohol
981 Toxic effect of petroleum products
982 Toxic effect of solvents other than petroleum-based
983 Toxic effect of corrosive aromatics, acids, and caustic alkalis
984 Toxic effect of lead and its compounds (including fumes)
985 Toxic effect of other metals
986 Toxic effect of carbon monoxide
987 Toxic effect of other gases, fumes, or vapors
988 Toxic effect of noxious substances eaten as food
989 Toxic effect of other substances, chiefly nonmedicinal as to source

Other and unspecified effects of external causes (990–995)
990 Effects of radiation, unspecified
991 Effects of reduced temperature
992 Effects of heat and light
993 Effects of air pressure
994 Effects of other external causes
995 Certain adverse effects, not elsewhere classified

Complications of surgical and medical care, not elsewhere classified (996–999)
996 Complications peculiar to certain specified procedures
997 Complications affecting specified body systems, not elsewhere classified
998 Other complications of procedures, not elsewhere classified
999 Complications of medical care, not elsewhere classified

ICD-9-CM

SUPPLEMENTARY CLASSIFICATION OF FACTORS INFLUENCING HEALTH STATUS AND CONTACT WITH HEALTH SERVICES (V01–V86)

Persons with potential health hazards related to communicable diseases (V01–V09)
- V01 Contact with or exposure to communicable diseases
- V02 Carrier or suspected carrier of infectious diseases
- V03 Need for prophylactic vaccination and inoculation against bacterial diseases
- V04 Need for prophylactic vaccination and inoculation against certain viral diseases
- V05 Need for other prophylactic vaccination and inoculation against single diseases
- V06 Need for prophylactic vaccination and inoculation against combinations of diseases
- V07 Need for isolation and other prophylactic measures
- V08 Asymptomatic human immunodeficiency virus [HIV] infection status
- V09 Infection with drug-resistant microorganisms

Persons with potential health hazards related to personal and family history (V10–V19)
- V10 Personal history of malignant neoplasm
- V11 Personal history of mental disorder
- V12 Personal history of certain other diseases
- V13 Personal history of other diseases
- V14 Personal history of allergy to medicinal agents
- V15 Other personal history presenting hazards to health
- V16 Family history of malignant neoplasm
- V17 Family history of certain chronic disabling diseases
- V18 Family history of certain other specific conditions
- V19 Family history of other conditions

Persons encountering health services in circumstances related to reproduction and development (V20–V29)
- V20 Health supervision of infant or child
- V21 Constitutional states in development
- V22 Normal pregnancy
- V23 Supervision of high-risk pregnancy
- V24 Postpartum care and examination
- V25 Encounter for contraceptive management
- V26 Procreative management
- V27 Outcome of delivery
- V28 Antenatal screening
- V29 Observation and evaluation of newborns and infants for suspected condition not found

Liveborn infants according to type of birth (V30–V39)
- V30 Single liveborn
- V31 Twin, mate liveborn
- V32 Twin, mate stillborn
- V33 Twin, unspecified
- V34 Other multiple, mates all liveborn
- V35 Other multiple, mates all stillborn
- V36 Other multiple, mates live- and stillborn
- V37 Other multiple, unspecified
- V39 Unspecified

Persons with a condition influencing their health status (V40–V49)
- V40 Mental and behavioral problems
- V41 Problems with special senses and other special functions
- V42 Organ or tissue replaced by transplant
- V43 Organ or tissue replaced by other means
- V44 Artificial opening status
- V45 Other postsurgical states
- V46 Other dependence on machines
- V47 Other problems with internal organs
- V48 Problems with head, neck, and trunk
- V49 Problems with limbs and other problems

Persons encountering health services for specific procedures and aftercare (V50–V59)
- V50 Elective surgery for purposes other than remedying health states
- V51 Aftercare involving the use of plastic surgery
- V52 Fitting and adjustment of prosthetic device
- V53 Fitting and adjustment of other device
- V54 Other orthopedic aftercare
- V55 Attention to artificial openings
- V56 Encounter for dialysis and dialysis catheter care
- V57 Care involving use of rehabilitation procedures
- V58 Other and unspecified aftercare
- V59 Donors

Persons encountering health services in other circumstances (V60–V69)
- V60 Housing, household, and economic circumstances
- V61 Other family circumstances
- V62 Other psychosocial circumstances
- V63 Unavailability of other medical facilities for care
- V64 Persons encountering health services for specific procedures, not carried out
- V65 Other persons seeking consultation without complaint or sickness
- V66 Convalescence and palliative care
- V67 Follow-up examination
- V68 Encounters for administrative purposes
- V69 Problems related to lifestyle

Persons without reported diagnosis encountered during examination and investigation of individuals and populations (V70–V82)
- V70 General medical examination
- V71 Observation and evaluation for suspected conditions
- V72 Special investigations and examinations
- V73 Special screening examination for viral and chlamydial diseases
- V74 Special screening examination for bacterial and spirochetal diseases
- V75 Special screening examination for other infectious diseases
- V76 Special screening for malignant neoplasms
- V77 Special screening for endocrine, nutritional, metabolic, and immunity disorders
- V78 Special screening for disorders of blood and blood-forming organs
- V79 Special screening for mental disorders and developmental handicaps
- V80 Special screening for neurological, eye, and ear diseases
- V81 Special screening for cardiovascular, respiratory, and genitourinary diseases
- V82 Special screening for other conditions

Genetics (V83–V84)
- V83 Genetic carrier status
- V84 Genetic susceptibility to malignant neoplasm

Body Mass Index (V85)
- V85 Body mass index

Estrogen Receptor Status (V86)
- V86 Estrogen receptor status

Other specified personal exposures and history presenting hazards to health (V87)
- V87 Other specified personal exposures and history presenting hazards to health

Acquired absence of other organs and tissue (V88)
- V88 Acquired absence of other organs and tissue

Other suspected conditions not found (V89)
- V89 Other suspected conditions not found

SUPPLEMENTARY CLASSIFICATION OF EXTERNAL CAUSES OF INJURY AND POISONING (E800–E899)

Railway accidents (E800–E807)
- E800 Railway accident involving collision with rolling stock
- E801 Railway accident involving collision with other object
- E802 Railway accident involving derailment without antecedent collision
- E803 Railway accident involving explosion, fire, or burning
- E804 Fall in, on, or from railway train
- E805 Hit by rolling stock
- E806 Other specified railway accident
- E807 Railway accident of unspecified nature

Motor vehicle traffic accidents (E810–E819)
- E810 Motor vehicle traffic accident involving collision with train
- E811 Motor vehicle traffic accident involving re-entrant collision with another motor vehicle
- E812 Other motor vehicle traffic accident involving collision with another motor vehicle
- E813 Motor vehicle traffic accident involving collision with other vehicle
- E814 Motor vehicle traffic accident involving collision with pedestrian

E815 Other motor vehicle traffic accident involving collision on the highway
E816 Motor vehicle traffic accident due to loss of control, without collision on the highway
E817 Noncollision motor vehicle traffic accident while boarding or alighting
E818 Other noncollision motor vehicle traffic accident
E819 Motor vehicle traffic accident of unspecified nature

Motor vehicle nontraffic accidents (E820–E825)
E820 Nontraffic accident involving motor-driven snow vehicle
E821 Nontraffic accident involving other off-road motor vehicle
E822 Other motor vehicle nontraffic accident involving collision with moving object
E823 Other motor vehicle nontraffic accident involving collision with stationary object
E824 Other motor vehicle nontraffic accident while boarding and alighting
E825 Other motor vehicle nontraffic accident of other and unspecified nature

Other road vehicle accidents (E826–E829)
E826 Pedal cycle accident
E827 Animal-drawn vehicle accident
E828 Accident involving animal being ridden
E829 Other road vehicle accidents

Water transport accidents (E830–E838)
E830 Accident to watercraft causing submersion
E831 Accident to watercraft causing other injury
E832 Other accidental submersion or drowning in water transport accident
E833 Fall on stairs or ladders in water transport
E834 Other fall from one level to another in water transport
E835 Other and unspecified fall in water transport
E836 Machinery accident in water transport
E837 Explosion, fire, or burning in watercraft
E838 Other and unspecified water transport accident

Air and space transport accidents (E840–E845)
E840 Accident to powered aircraft at takeoff or landing
E841 Accident to powered aircraft, other and unspecified
E842 Accident to unpowered aircraft
E843 Fall in, on, or from aircraft
E844 Other specified air transport accidents
E845 Accident involving spacecraft

Vehicle accidents, not elsewhere classifiable (E846–E849)
E846 Accidents involving powered vehicles used solely within the buildings and premises of an industrial or commercial establishment
E847 Accidents involving cable cars not running on rails
E848 Accidents involving other vehicles, not elsewhere classifiable
E849 Place of occurrence

Accidental poisoning by drugs, medicinal substances, and biologicals (E850–E858)
E850 Accidental poisoning by analgesics, antipyretics, and antirheumatics
E851 Accidental poisoning by barbiturates
E852 Accidental poisoning by other sedatives and hypnotics
E853 Accidental poisoning by tranquilizers
E854 Accidental poisoning by other psychotropic agents
E855 Accidental poisoning by other drugs acting on central and autonomic nervous systems
E856 Accidental poisoning by antibiotics
E857 Accidental poisoning by anti-infectives
E858 Accidental poisoning by other drugs

Accidental poisoning by other solid and liquid substances, gases, and vapors (E860–E869)
E860 Accidental poisoning by alcohol, not elsewhere classified
E861 Accidental poisoning by cleansing and polishing agents, disinfectants, paints, and varnishes
E862 Accidental poisoning by petroleum products, other solvents and their vapors, not elsewhere classified
E863 Accidental poisoning by agricultural and horticultural chemical and pharmaceutical preparations other than plant foods and fertilizers
E864 Accidental poisoning by corrosives and caustics, not elsewhere classified
E865 Accidental poisoning from poisonous foodstuffs and poisonous plants
E866 Accidental poisoning by other and unspecified solid and liquid substances
E867 Accidental poisoning by gas distributed by pipeline
E868 Accidental poisoning by other utility gas and other carbon monoxide
E869 Accidental poisoning by other gases and vapors

Misadventures to patients during surgical and medical care (E870–E876)
E870 Accidental cut, puncture, perforation, or hemorrhage during medical care
E871 Foreign object left in body during procedure
E872 Failure of sterile precautions during procedure
E873 Failure in dosage
E874 Mechanical failure of instrument or apparatus during procedure
E875 Contaminated or infected blood, other fluid, drug, or biological substance
E876 Other and unspecified misadventures during medical care

Surgical and medical procedures as the cause of abnormal reaction of patient or later complication, without mention of misadventure at the time of procedure (E878–E879)
E878 Surgical operation and other surgical procedures as the cause of abnormal reaction of patient, or of later complication, without mention of misadventure at the time of operation
E879 Other procedures, without mention of misadventure at the time of procedure, as the cause of abnormal reaction of patient, or of later complication

Accidental falls (E880–E888)
E880 Fall on or from stairs or steps
E881 Fall on or from ladders or scaffolding
E882 Fall from or out of building or other structure
E883 Fall into hole or other opening in surface
E884 Other fall from one level to another
E885 Fall on same level from slipping, tripping, or stumbling
E886 Fall on same level from collision, pushing, or shoving, by or with other person
E887 Fracture, cause unspecified
E888 Other and unspecified fall

Accidents caused by fire and flames (E890–E899)
E890 Conflagration in private dwelling
E891 Conflagration in other and unspecified building or structure
E892 Conflagration not in building or structure
E893 Accident caused by ignition of clothing
E894 Ignition of highly inflammable material
E895 Accident caused by controlled fire in private dwelling
E896 Accident caused by controlled fire in other and unspecified building or structure
E897 Accident caused by controlled fire not in building or structure
E898 Accident caused by other specified fire and flames
E899 Accident caused by unspecified fire

Accidents due to natural and environmental factors (E900–E909)
E900 Excessive heat
E901 Excessive cold
E902 High and low air pressure and changes in air pressure
E903 Travel and motion
E904 Hunger, thirst, exposure, and neglect
E905 Venomous animals and plants as the cause of poisoning and toxic reactions
E906 Other injury caused by animals
E907 Lightning
E908 Cataclysmic storms, and floods resulting from storms
E909 Cataclysmic earth surface movements and eruptions

Accidents caused by submersion, suffocation, and foreign bodies (E910–E915)
E910 Accidental drowning and submersion
E911 Inhalation and ingestion of food causing obstruction of respiratory tract or suffocation
E912 Inhalation and ingestion of other object causing obstruction of respiratory tract or suffocation
E913 Accidental mechanical suffocation
E914 Foreign body accidentally entering eye and adnexa
E915 Foreign body accidentally entering other orifice

Other accidents (E916–E928)
- E916 Struck accidentally by falling object
- E917 Striking against or struck accidentally by objects or persons
- E918 Caught accidentally in or between objects
- E919 Accidents caused by machinery
- E920 Accidents caused by cutting and piercing instruments or objects
- E921 Accident caused by explosion of pressure vessel
- E922 Accident caused by firearm missile
- E923 Accident caused by explosive material
- E924 Accident caused by hot substance or object, caustic or corrosive material, and steam
- E925 Accident caused by electric current
- E926 Exposure to radiation
- E927 Overexertion and strenuous movements
- E928 Other and unspecified environmental and accidental causes

Late effects of accidental injury (E929)
- E929 Late effects of accidental injury

Drugs, medicinal and biological substances causing adverse effects in therapeutic use (E930–E949)
- E930 Antibiotics
- E931 Other anti-infectives
- E932 Hormones and synthetic substitutes
- E933 Primarily systemic agents
- E934 Agents primarily affecting blood constituents
- E935 Analgesics, antipyretics, and antirheumatics
- E936 Anticonvulsants and anti-Parkinsonism drugs
- E937 Sedatives and hypnotics
- E938 Other central nervous system depressants and anesthetics
- E939 Psychotropic agents
- E940 Central nervous system stimulants
- E941 Drugs primarily affecting the autonomic nervous system
- E942 Agents primarily affecting the cardiovascular system
- E943 Agents primarily affecting gastrointestinal system
- E944 Water, mineral, and uric acid metabolism drugs
- E945 Agents primarily acting on the smooth and skeletal muscles and respiratory system
- E946 Agents primarily affecting skin and mucous membrane, ophthalmological, otorhinolaryngological, and dental drugs
- E947 Other and unspecified drugs and medicinal substances
- E948 Bacterial vaccines
- E949 Other vaccines and biological substances

Suicide and self-inflicted injury (E950–E959)
- E950 Suicide and self-inflicted poisoning by solid or liquid substances
- E951 Suicide and self-inflicted poisoning by gases in domestic use
- E952 Suicide and self-inflicted poisoning by other gases and vapors
- E953 Suicide and self-inflicted injury by hanging, strangulation, and suffocation
- E954 Suicide and self-inflicted injury by submersion [drowning]
- E955 Suicide and self-inflicted injury by firearms and explosives
- E956 Suicide and self-inflicted injury by cutting and piercing instruments
- E957 Suicide and self-inflicted injuries by jumping from high place
- E958 Suicide and self-inflicted injury by other and unspecified means
- E959 Late effects of self-inflicted injury

Homicide and injury purposely inflicted by other persons (E960–E969)
- E960 Fight, brawl, and rape
- E961 Assault by corrosive or caustic substance, except poisoning
- E962 Assault by poisoning
- E963 Assault by hanging and strangulation
- E964 Assault by submersion [drowning]
- E965 Assault by firearms and explosives
- E966 Assault by cutting and piercing instrument
- E967 Child and adult battering and other maltreatment
- E968 Assault by other and unspecified means
- E969 Late effects of injury purposely inflicted by other person

Legal intervention (E970–E978)
- E970 Injury due to legal intervention by firearms
- E971 Injury due to legal intervention by explosives
- E972 Injury due to legal intervention by gas
- E973 Injury due to legal intervention by blunt object
- E974 Injury due to legal intervention by cutting and piercing instruments
- E975 Injury due to legal intervention by other specified means
- E976 Injury due to legal intervention by unspecified means
- E977 Late effects of injuries due to legal intervention
- E978 Legal execution
- E979 Terrorism

Injury undetermined whether accidentally or purposely inflicted (E980–E989)
- E980 Poisoning by solid or liquid substances, undetermined whether accidentally or purposely inflicted
- E981 Poisoning by gases in domestic use, undetermined whether accidentally or purposely inflicted
- E982 Poisoning by other gases, undetermined whether accidentally or purposely inflicted
- E983 Hanging, strangulation, or suffocation, undetermined whether accidentally or purposely inflicted
- E984 Submersion [drowning], undetermined whether accidentally or purposely inflicted
- E985 Injury by firearms and explosives, undetermined whether accidentally or purposely inflicted
- E986 Injury by cutting and piercing instruments, undetermined whether accidentally or purposely inflicted
- E987 Falling from high place, undetermined whether accidentally or purposely inflicted
- E988 Injury by other and unspecified means, undetermined whether accidentally or purposely inflicted
- E989 Late effects of injury, undetermined whether accidentally or purposely inflicted

Injury resulting from operations of war (E990–E999)
- E990 Injury due to war operations by fires and conflagrations
- E991 Injury due to war operations by bullets and fragments
- E992 Injury due to war operations by explosion of marine weapons
- E993 Injury due to war operations by other explosion
- E994 Injury due to war operations by destruction of aircraft
- E995 Injury due to war operations by other and unspecified forms of conventional warfare
- E996 Injury due to war operations by nuclear weapons
- E997 Injury due to war operations by other forms of unconventional warfare
- E998 Injury due to war operations but occurring after cessation of hostilities
- E999 Late effects of injury due to war operations

TABLE A

TABLE OF BACTERIAL FOOD POISONING

Bacteria Responsible	Description	Habitat	Types of Foods	Symptoms	Cause	Temperature Sensitivity
Staphylococcus aureus	Produces a heat-stable toxin.	Nose and throat of 30 to 50 percent of healthy population; also skin and superficial wounds.	Meat and seafood salads, sandwich spreads, and high salt foods.	Nausea, vomiting, and diarrhea within 4 to 6 hours. No fever.	Poor personal hygiene and subsequent temperature abuse.	No growth below 40° F. Bacteria are destroyed by normal cooking, but toxin is heat-stable.
Clostridium perfringens	Produces a spore and prefers low oxygen atmosphere. Live cells must be ingested.	Dust, soil, and gastrointestinal tracts of animals and man.	Meat and poultry dishes, sauces and gravies.	Cramps and diarrhea within 12 to 24 hours. No vomiting or fever.	Improper temperature control of hot foods and recontamination.	No growth below 40° F. Bacteria are killed by normal cooking, but a heat-stable spore can survive.
Clostridium botulinum	Produces a spore and requires a low oxygen atmosphere. Produces a heat-sensitive toxin.	Soils, plants, marine sediments, and fish.	Home-canned foods.	Blurred vision, respiratory distress, and possible DEATH.	Improper methods of home-processing foods.	Type E and Type B can grow at 38° F. Bacteria destroyed by cooking and the toxin is destroyed by boiling for 5 to 10 minutes. Heat-resistant spore can survive.
Vibrio parahaemolyticus	Requires salt for growth.	Fish and shellfish.	Raw and cooked seafood.	Diarrhea, cramps, vomiting, headache, and fever within 12 to 24 hours.	Recontamination of cooked foods or eating raw seafood.	No growth below 40° F. Bacteria killed by normal cooking.

Trust Elsevier.
We've got you covered.

When it comes to preparing for ICD-10,

we've got you covered.

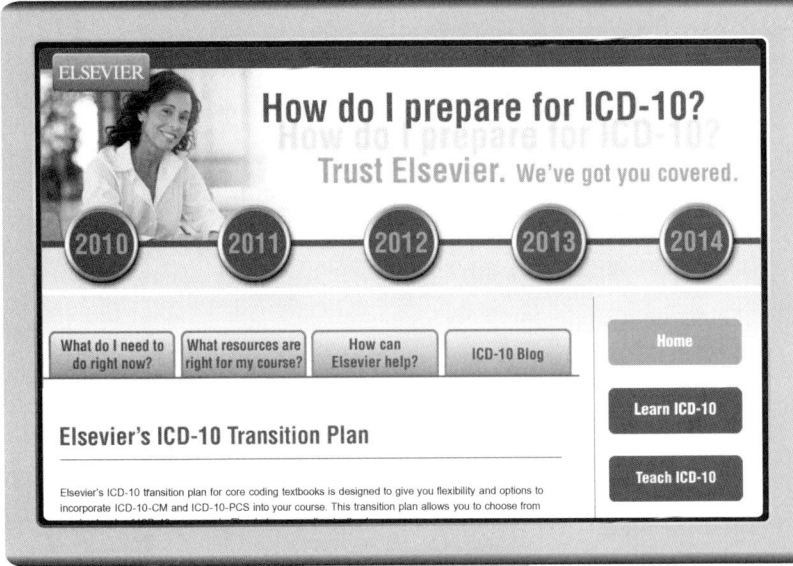

- Learn how to transition from ICD-9-CM to ICD-10-CM/PCS.

- Develop your plan to teach ICD-10-CM/PCS to students.

- Articles, updates, and webinars provide guidance for integrating ICD-10 into your program.

Count on the leader in coding education for everything you need to train your staff, teach your students, and transition your program.

Learn more at www.icd10educators.com!

Stay up to date!
Access the latest ICD-9-CM and HCPCS code updates throughout the year

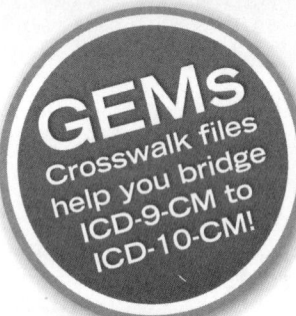

- Access the mid-year code updates as soon as they are published by the government.
- Sign up now for email alerts that let you know when new codes are posted.

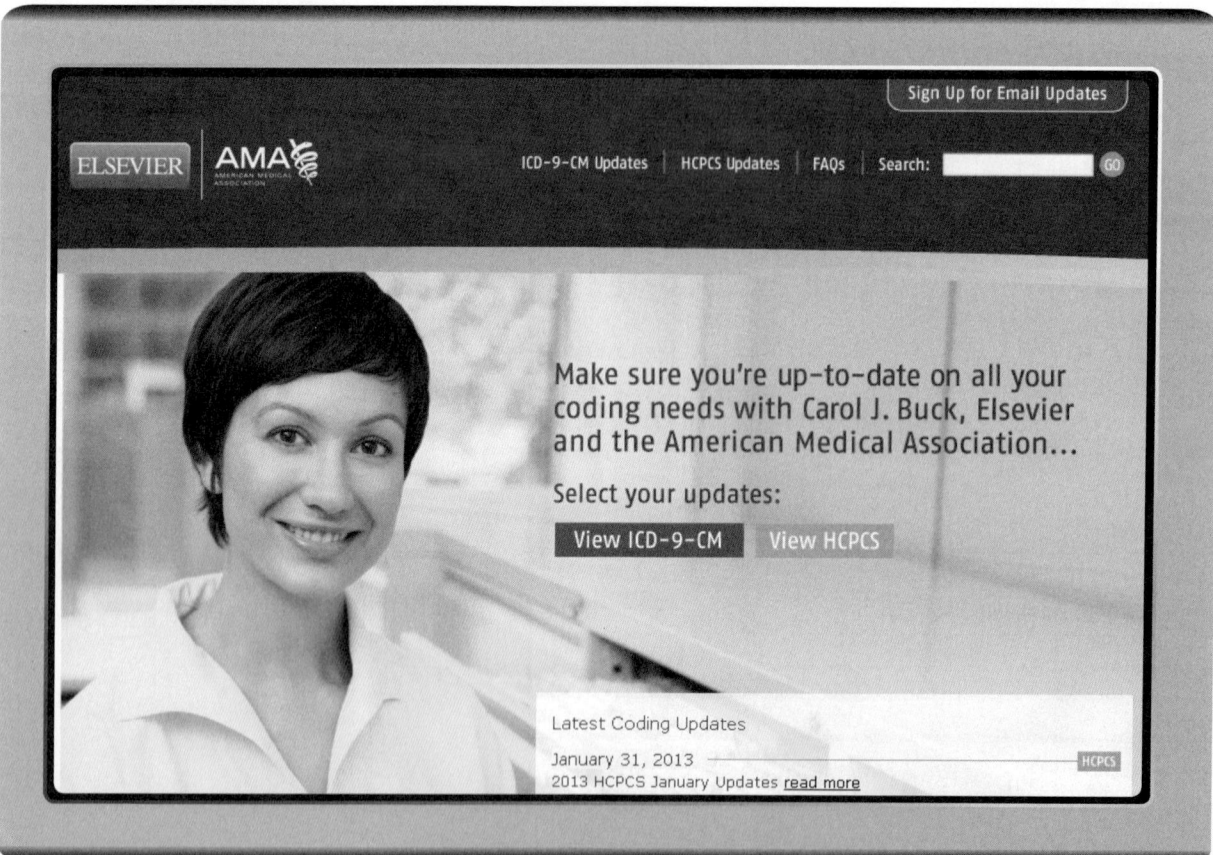

Trust Carol J. Buck, the AMA, and Elsevier to give you quick access to the most up-to-date codes!

www.codingupdates.com

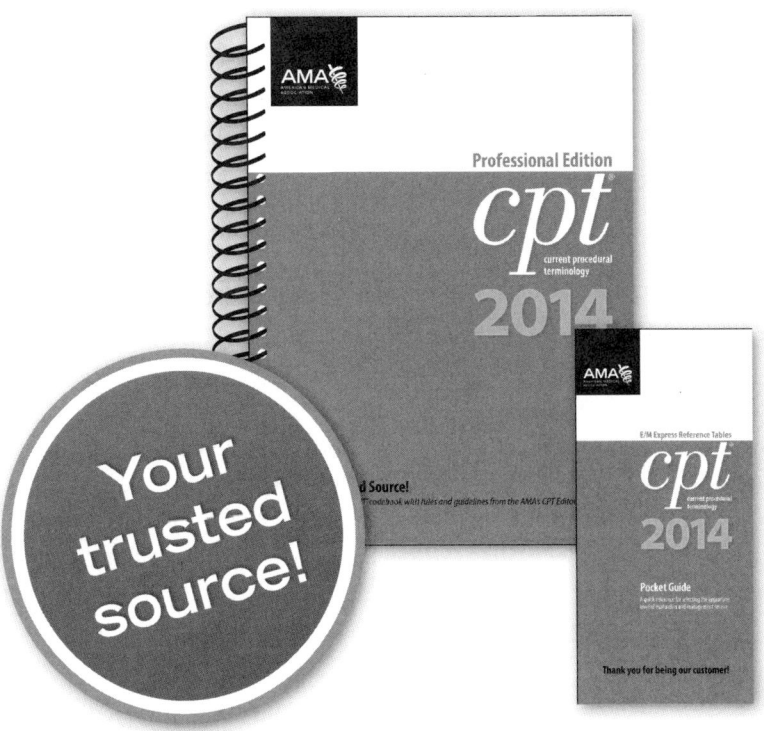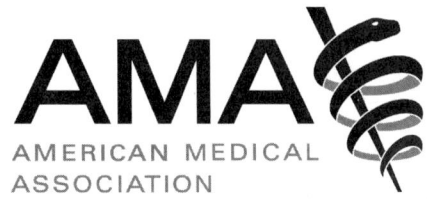

Learn to implement and code for ICD-10
with help from the American Medical Association

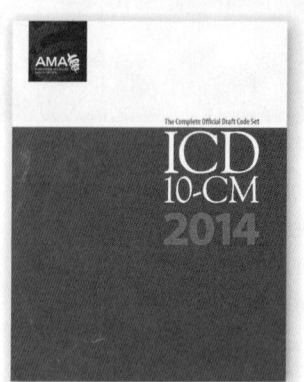

ICD-10-CM 2014: The Complete Official Draft Code Set presents the most comprehensive government draft of the entire ICD-10-CM code set with color-coding, symbols, illustrations, and coding guidelines.
Available September 2013

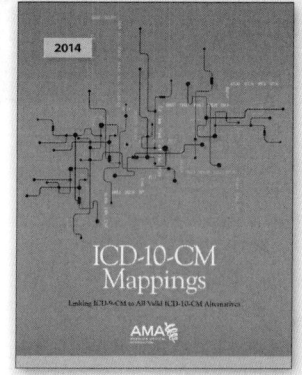

ICD-10-CM Mappings 2014 links ICD-9-CM codes to all valid ICD-10-CM alternatives and allows you to know what code choices are available so you can make the most appropriate selection.
Available October 2013

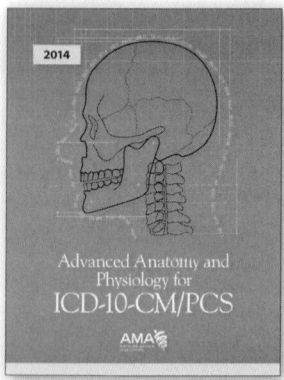

Advanced Anatomy and Physiology for ICD-10-CM/PCS guides you through all of the body systems as they relate to both ICD-10 code sets and offers chapter quizzes to help you test your understanding of the material.
Available October 2013

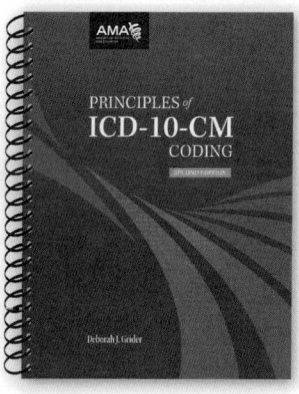

Principles of ICD-10-CM Coding, Second Edition teaches the self-learner, classroom student, and advanced coder how to make the correct diagnosis coding decision when using ICD-10-CM.
Available Now

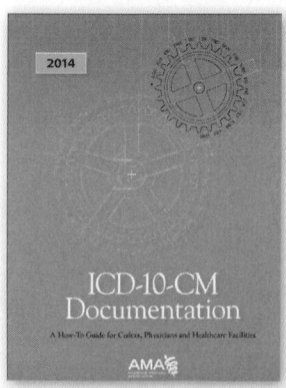

ICD-10-CM Documentation: A How-To Guide for Coder, Physicians and Health Care Facilities identifies detailed documentation requirements and elements and provides tools for effective documentation analysis.
Available October 2013

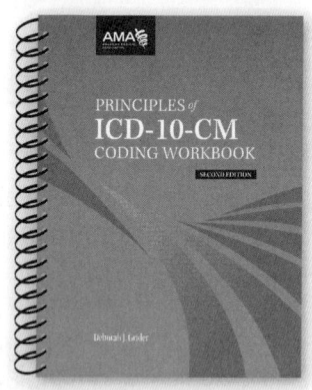

Principles of ICD-10-CM Coding Workbook, Second Edition delivers practical experience to all levels of coders by offering real-life chart notes, case studies, and exercises.
Available Now

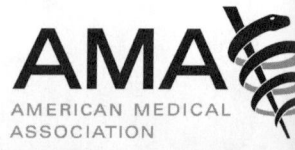

View full product descriptions OR order online at *amastore.com*; OR call (800) 621-8335.

Interactive ICD-10-CM workshops are hosted by the AMA in Chicago and throughout the country. Visit Training & Events at *amastore.com* to learn more and register.

Develop a more productive and prosperous medical practice
with proven resources from the American Medical Association

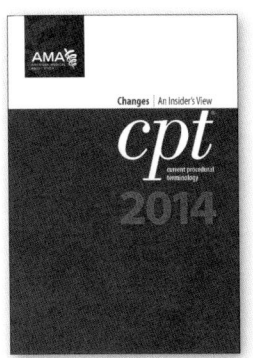

**CPT® Changes 2014:
An Insider's View**
An indispensable guide for CPT® codebook users, this title provides rationales for every new, revised, and deleted CPT code and guideline in the 2014 code set.
Available November 2013

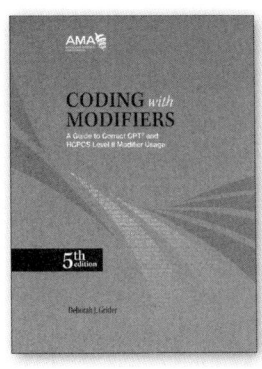

**Coding With Modifiers,
Fifth Edition**
Provides guidance on how and when to use modifiers in order to avoid costly payment delays and denials.
Available December 2013

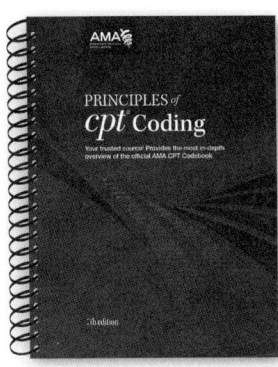

**Principles of CPT® Coding,
Seventh Edition**
Designed to supplement the CPT® codebook, this textbook provides an in-depth review of the CPT guidelines and serves as a guide for proper application of the CPT codes.
Available Now

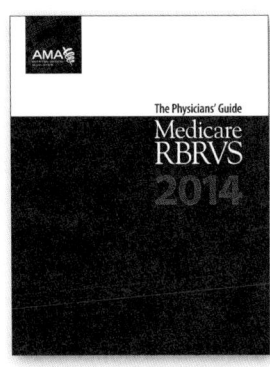

**Medicare RBRVS:
The Physicians' Guide 2014**
The 23rd edition of this authoritative text provides information on new 2014 payment rules and how they may affect your practice.
Available March 2014

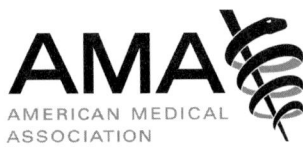

For more information on these popular resources or to view our recent digital catalog, visit *ama-assn.org/go/online-catalog*.

Order online or call (800) 621-8335 today!

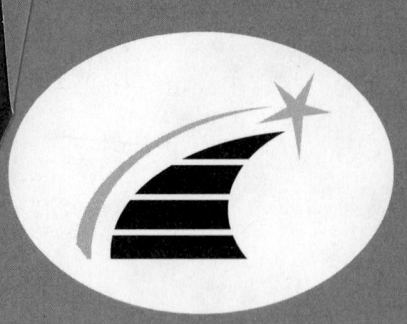

Trust Carol J. Buck and Elsevier for the resources you need at each step of your coding career!

2014

Track your progress toward complete coding success!

Step 1: Learn

- ☐ Step-by-Step Medical Coding, 2014 Edition • ISBN: 978-1-4557-4635-4
- ☐ Workbook for Step-by-Step Medical Coding, 2014 Edition • ISBN: 978-1-4557-4630-9
- ☐ Medical Coding Online for Step-by-Step Medical Coding, 2014 Edition • ISBN: 978-1-4557-4631-6

Step 2: Practice

- ☐ The Next Step: Advanced Medical Coding and Auditing, 2014 Edition • ISBN: 978-1-4557-5897-5
- ☐ E/M Auditing Step, Third Edition • ISBN: 978-1-4557-5199-0
- ☐ **Capstone** Online Internship for Medical Coding, 2014 Edition • ISBN: 978-0-323-23937-0

Step 3: Certify

- ☐ Physician Coding Exam Review 2014: The Certification Step with ICD-9-CM • ISBN: 978-1-4557-2287-7
- ☐ Facility Coding Exam Review 2014: The Certification Step with ICD-10-CM/PCS • ISBN: 978-1-4557-4574-6

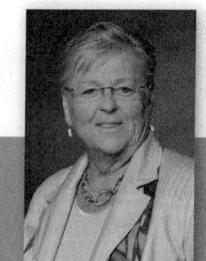

Author and Educator
Carol J. Buck,
MS, CPC,
CPC-H, CCS-P

Step 4: Professional Resources

- ☐ 2014 ICD-9-CM for Physicians, Volumes 1 & 2, Professional Edition • ISBN: 978-0-323-18676-6
- ☐ 2014 ICD-9-CM for Hospitals, Volumes 1, 2, & 3, Professional Edition • ISBN: 978-0-323-18674-2
- ☐ 2014 ICD-9-CM for Physicians, Volumes 1 & 2, Standard Edition • ISBN: 978-0-323-18677-3
- ☐ 2014 ICD-9-CM for Hospitals, Volumes 1, 2, & 3, Standard Edition • ISBN: 978-0-323-18675-9
- ☐ 2014 HCPCS Level II Professional Edition • ISBN: 978-1-4557-7504-0
- ☐ 2014 HCPCS Level II Standard Edition • ISBN: 978-1-4557-7505-7
- ☐ 2014 ICD-10-CM Draft Manual • ISBN: 978-1-4557-2290-7
- ☐ 2014 ICD-10-PCS Draft Manual • ISBN: 978-1-4557-2289-1
- ☐ ICD-10-CM Online Training Modules (by Buck) • ISBN: 978-0-323-22145-0
- ☐ ICD-10-PCS Online Training Modules (by Lovaasen) • ISBN: 978-0-323-22811-4

Order today!

- Order securely at **www.us.elsevierhealth.com**.
- Call toll-free **1-800-545-2522**.
- Visit your **local bookstore**.

ELSEVIER